THE LUNG
Scientific Foundations
Volume 2

THE LUNG
Scientific Foundations
Volume 2

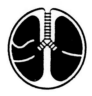

EDITORS-IN-CHIEF

Ronald G. Crystal, M.D.
Chief, Pulmonary Branch
National Heart, Lung and Blood Institute
National Institutes of Health
Bethesda, Maryland

John B. West, M.D., Ph.D.,
D.Sc., F.R.C.P., F.R.A.C.P.
Professor of Medicine and Physiology
Department of Medicine
University of California San Diego
La Jolla, California

ASSOCIATE EDITORS

Peter J. Barnes, M.A., D.M.,
D.Sc., F.R.C.P.
Professor and Chairman
Department of Thoracic Medicine
National Heart and Lung Institute
Brompton Hospital
London, England

Neil S. Cherniack, M.D.
Professor of Medicine and Physiology
School of Medicine
Case Western Reserve University
Cleveland, Ohio

Ewald R. Weibel, M.D., D.Sc.
Professor of Anatomy
University of Berne
Berne, Switzerland

RAVEN PRESS ☙ NEW YORK

Raven Press, Ltd., 1185 Avenue of the Americas, New York, New York 10036

Made in the United States of America

Library of Congress Cataloging-in-Publication Data

The Lung : scientific foundations / editors-in-chief, Ronald G.
   Crystal, John B. West ; associate editors, Peter J. Barnes, Neil S.
Cherniack, Ewald R. Weibel.
      p. cm.
   Includes bibliographical references.
   Includes index.
   ISBN 0-88167-629-2
   1. Lungs—Physiology.   2. Lungs—Pathophysiology.   I. Crystal,
Ronald G.   II. West, John B. (John Burnard)
   [DNLM: 1. Lung.   WF 600 L96357]
   QP121.L87   1991
   612.2—dc20
   DNLM/DLC
   for Library of Congress   90-9015
                                                                 CIP

The material contained in this volume was submitted as previously unpublished material, except in the instances in which credit has been given to the source from which some of the illustrative material was derived.

Great care has been taken to maintain the accuracy of the information contained in the volume. However, neither Raven Press nor the editors can be held responsible for errors or for any consequences arising from the use of the information contained herein.

Materials appearing in this book prepared by individuals as part of their official duties as U.S. Government employees are not covered by the above-mentioned copyright.

9 8 7 6 5 4 3 2 1

To my family
Janet and Zachary

RGC

To my wife Penelope

JBW

To my family
Olivia, Adam, Toby, and Julian

PJB

To my family
Evan, Andy, Emily, and Sandy

NSC

To my wife Verena

ERW

Preface

Everyone interested in respiratory sciences is aware of the great burgeoning of information over the past 5 to 10 years. This explosion of activity is exemplified by an exponential increase in the number of scientific articles, monographs, and textbooks in the area and by the emergence of two new journals on pulmonary biology. Much of this new information relates to great advances in cellular biology of the lung, which, in turn, reflect the spectacular innovations in molecular and cell biology that have characterized the life sciences over the past 10 years. In addition to these advances in cell biology, major progress is being made in biochemistry, morphology, pathology, pharmacology, and physiology of the lung. Everywhere, knowledge is increasing at an unprecedented rate.

Because nobody can hope to keep abreast of all the expanding areas, textbooks and handbooks that distill the information and make it available for the nonspecialist in each area become increasingly valuable. There are several excellent textbooks of respiratory diseases, and there are outstanding handbooks in some areas, notably the handbooks of respiratory physiology published by the American Physiological Society. However, there is no compendium that covers the whole field of the scientific foundations of the lung in health and disease and that includes cell biology, biochemistry, morphology, physiology, pharmacology, and general pathological processes. About 2 years ago, Raven Press perceptively identified the need for such a book, and these two volumes are the result. They take their place alongside similar textbooks of broad scope by the same publisher in a number of fields of biomedical science, including cardiology, renal disease, gastrointestinal disease, and liver disease.

This two-volume set is divided into eight sections: a general introduction; general biologic processes; major components of the lung; integrated morphology; integrated physiology and pathophysiology; development and aging; injury, defense, and repair; and special environments and interventions. It surveys the whole territory of respiratory science. It is written to be used by a broad group of basic researchers and clinicians, and we expect that it will be valuable to investigators at all levels who are interested in the pulmonary field. It is also intended as a reference text for all libraries that include books on the lung and the sciences basic to the understanding of the lung.

A common criticism of texts such as this is that they are out of date by the time they are published. Great pains were taken by the editors and publisher to ensure the timeliness of these chapters. While a large compendium like this cannot compete with a journal for publication promptness, this book is not far behind. We thank the very large number of contributors, and we hope that the value of the book to the pulmonary science community will fully justify their efforts.

Ronald G. Crystal
John B. West
Peter J. Barnes
Neil S. Cherniack
Ewald R. Weibel

Acknowledgments

It is a pleasure to acknowledge the enterprise, efficiency, enthusiasm, and general helpfulness of the people at Raven Press, especially the President, Dr. Alan M. Edelson, the Medical Editor, John Molyneux, the Production Editor, Wanda Woloszyn, the Copy Editor, Robert Golden, and the Proofreader, Lee Stump.

Contents

Volume Two

Subject Index follows page 2224

Contributors

Stuart L. Abramson, MD, PhD
Bacterial Diseases Section
Laboratory of Clinical Investigation
National Institute of Allergy and
*   Infectious Diseases*
National Institutes of Health
Bethesda, Maryland 20892
Present address:
Texas Childrens' Hospital
Allergy and Immunology Section
Houston, Texas 77030

Ian Y. R. Adamson, PhD
Department of Pathology
Faculty of Medicine
University of Manitoba
Winnepeg, Manitoba R3E OW3, Canada

W. Keith Adkins, BS
Department of Physiology
University of South Alabama College of
*   Medicine*
Mobile, Alabama 36688

C. R. Adolphson, MS
Departments of Immunology and
*   Medicine*
Mayo Medical School
Mayo Clinic and Foundation
Rochester, Minnesota 55905

Björn A. Afzelius, MD
Department of Ultrastructure Research
The Wenner–Gren Institute
University of Stockholm
S-106 91 Stockholm, Sweden

R. B. Armstrong, PhD
Department of Physical Education
University of Georgia
Athens, Georgia 30602

Tak Yee Aw, PhD
Department of Biochemistry and Winship
*   Cancer Center*
Emory University
Atlanta, Georgia 30322

Hans Bachofen, MD
Department of Medicine
University of Berne
Inselspital
CH-3010 Berne 9, Switzerland

Marianne Bachofen, MD
Department of Medicine
University of Berne
Inselspital
CH-3010 Berne 9, Switzerland

M. Safwan Badr, MD
The John Rankin Laboratory of
*   Pulmonary Medicine*
William S. Middleton Memorial Veterans
*   Hospital*
Madison, Wisconsin 53705
and
Departments of Preventive Medicine and
*   Medicine*
University of Wisconsin—Madison
Madison, Wisconsin 53705

Scott A. Barman, PhD
Department of Physiology
University of South Albama College of
*   Medicine*
Mobile, Alabama 36688

Joseph W. Barnard, PhD
Department of Physiology
University of South Alabama College of
*   Medicine*
Mobile, Alabama 36688

Peter J. Barnes, DM, DSc, FRCP
Department of Thoracic Medicine
National Heart and Lung Institute
London SW3 6LY, England

Francoise Basset, MD
INSERM U82
Faculté Xavier Bichart
75017 Paris, France

Christian Bauer, MD
Department of Physiology
University of Zurich
CH-8057 Zurich, Switzerland

Douglas A. Bayliss, PhD
Department of Physiology
University of North Carolina
Chapel Hill, North Carolina 27599

Joe D. Beckmann, PhD
Pulmonary and Critical Care Medicine
* Section*
University of Nebraska Medical Center
Omaha, Nebraska 68105

I. Berezin, PhD
Department of Biomedical Sciences
McMaster University Health Science
* Centre*
Hamilton, Ontario L8N 3Z5, Canada

Richard A. Berg, PhD
Department of Biochemistry
University of Medicine and Dentistry of
* New Jersey—Robert Wood Johnson*
* Medical School*
Piscataway, New Jersey 08854

J. F. Bernaudin, MD, PhD
INSERM U139
Clinique de pathologie respiratoire et de
* l'environnement et Département*
* d'Histologie*
Hôpital Henri Mondor et Faculté de
* Médecine*
Université Paris-Val-de-Marne
94010 Créteil, France

Robert S. Bienkowski, PhD
Pediatric Research Center
Long Island Jewish Medical Center
New Hyde Park, New York 11042
and
Departments of Pediatrics and Physiology
* and Biophysics*
Albert Einstein College of Medicine
Bronx, New York 10461

J. Bignon, MD
INSERM U139
Clinique de pathologie respiratoire et de
* l'environnement et Département*
* d'Histologie*
Hôpital Henri Mondor et Faculté de
* Médecine*
Université Paris-Val-de-Marne
94010 Créteil, France

Peter B. Bitterman, MD
Pulmonary Division
Department of Medicine
University of Minnesota
Minneapolis, Minnesota 55455

Richard D. Bland, MD
Department of Pediatrics
Children's Research Center
University of Utah School of Medicine
Salt Lake City, Utah 84132

S. R. Bloom, MD, FRCP
Department of Histochemistry
Royal Postgraduate Medical School
London W12 ONN, England

Mark L. Brantly, MD
Pulmonary Branch
National Heart, Lung and Blood Institute
National Institutes of Health
Bethesda, Maryland 20892

Jerome Brody, MD
Pulmonary Center and Department of
* Medicine*
Boston University School of Medicine
Boston, Massachusetts 02118

Roy G. Brower, MD
Division of Pulmonary and Critical Care
* Medicine*
The Johns Hopkins University School of
* Medicine*
Baltimore, Maryland 21205

Alan R. Buckpitt, PhD
Departments of Anatomy and Veterinary
* Pharmacology and Toxicology*
and
California Primate Research Center
University of California
School of Veterinary Medicine
Davis, California 95616

Peter H. Burri, MD
Institute of Anatomy
University of Berne
CH-3000 Berne 9, Switzerland

E. J. M. Campbell, MD, FRCP(C)
Department of Medicine
McMaster University Medical Center
Hamilton, Ontario L8N 3Z5, Canada

Don M. Carlson, PhD
Department of Biochemistry and
*   Biophysics*
University of California—Davis
Davis, California 95616

Cristina Casals, PhD
Department of Biochemistry and
*   Molecular Biology*
Faculty of Chemistry
Complutense University
28040 Madrid, Spain

Sidney Cassin, PhD
Department of Physiology
University of Florida College of Medicine
Gainesville, Florida 32610

Paolo Cerretelli, MD
Département de Physiologie
Centre Médical Universitaire
1211 Geneva, Switzerland

Neil S. Cherniack, MD
Department of Medicine
Case Western Reserve University School
*   of Medicine*
Cleveland, Ohio 44106

Daniel F. Church, PhD
Biodynamics Institute
Louisiana State University
Baton Rouge, Louisiana 70803

Andrew Churg, MD
Department of Pathology and University
*   Hospital*
University of British Columbia
Vancouver, B.C. V6T 2B5, Canada

James M. Clark, MD, PhD
Departments of Environmental Medicine
*   and Pharmacology*
Institute for Environmental Medicine
University of Pennsylvania Medical
*   Center*
Philadelphia, Pennsylvania 19104

Stewart W. Clarke, MD, FRCP
Department of Thoracic Medicine
The Royal Free Hospital and School of
*   Medicine*
Hampstead, London NW3 2QG, England

Charles B. Cochrane, MD
Division of Vascular Biology and
*   Inflammation*
Department of Immunology Research
Scripps Clinic
La Jolla, California 92037

Hazel M. Coleridge, MB, ChB
Cardiovascular Research Institute and
*   Department of Physiology*
University of California—San Francisco
San Francisco, California 94143

John C. G. Coleridge, MB, ChB
Cardiovascular Research Institute and
*   Department of Physiology*
University of California—San Francisco
San Francisco, California 94143

Harvey R. Colten, MD
Edward Mallinckrodt Department of
*   Pediatrics*
Washington University School of
*   Medicine*
St. Louis, Missouri 63110

J. D. Cooper, MD
Department of Thoracic Surgery
Washington University School of
*   Medicine*
St. Louis, Missouri 63110

Edward D. Crandall, PhD, MD
Department of Medicine
Will Rogers Institute Pulmonary Research
*   Program*
Cornell University Medical College
New York, New York 10021
and
University of Southern California
Los Angeles, California 90033

James D. Crapo, MD
Division of Allergy, Critical Care, and
*   Respiratory Medicine*
Duke University Medical Center
Durham, North Carolina 27710

A. B. H. Crawford, MD
Department of Thoracic Medicine
Westmead Hospital
Sydney, New South Wales 2145, Australia

Christian Crone, MD, PhD
Institute of Medical Physiology
University of Copenhagen
The Panum Institute
DK-2200 Copenhagen N, Denmark

Carroll E. Cross, MD
Departments of Internal Medicine and
 Human Physiology
School of Medicine
University of California—Davis
Davis, California 95616
Present address:
Pulmonary–Critical Care Medicine
University of California—Davis
Sacramento, California 95817

Edmond C. Crouch, MD, PhD
Department of Pathology
Jewish Hospital of St. Louis
Washington University Medical Center
St. Louis, Missouri 63110

Ronald G. Crystal, MD
Pulmonary Branch
National Heart, Lung and Blood Institute
National Institutes of Health
Bethesda, Maryland 20892

Maria F. Czyzyk-Krzeska, MD, PhD
Department of Physiology
University of North Carolina
Chapel Hill, North Carolina 27599

E. E. Daniel, PhD
Department of Biomedical Sciences
McMaster University Health Science
 Centre
Hamilton, Ontario L8N 3Z5, Canada

V. P. Daniel, MEd
Department of Biomedical Sciences
McMaster University Health Science
 Centre
Hamilton, Ontario L8N 3Z5, Canada

David R. Dantzker, MD
Division of Pulmonary and Critical Care
 Medicine
Department of Internal Medicine
University of Texas Health Science
 Center
Houston, Texas 77030
Present address:
Department of Medicine
Long Island Jewish Medical Center
New Hyde Park, New York 11042

Carlos C. Daughaday, MD
Department of Medicine
Washington University School of
 Medicine
St. Louis, Missouri 63110
and
Respiratory Care Center
John Cochran Veterans Administration
 Medical Center
St. Louis, Missouri 63125

W. Bruce Davis, MD
Division of Pulmonary and Critical Care
Department of Internal Medicine
The Ohio State University
Columbus, Ohio 43210

Jay B. Dean, PhD
Department of Physiology
University of North Carolina
Chapel Hill, North Carolina 27599

Mark E. Deffebach, MD
Division of Pulmonary and Critical Care
 Medicine
Department of Medicine
University of Washington School of
 Medicine
Seattle, Washington 98195

Daphne deMello, MD
Department of Pathology
St. Louis University School of Medicine
and
Department of Pathology
Cardinal Glennon Children's Hospital
St. Louis, Missouri 63104

William C. Dement, MD, PhD
Sleep Disorders Center
Stanford University School of Medicine
Stanford, California 94305

Colby W. Dempesy, PhD
Department of Neurosurgery
Tulane Medical School
New Orleans, Louisiana 70112

Jerome A. Dempsey, PhD
The John Rankin Laboratory of
 Pulmonary Medicine
William S. Middleton Memorial Veterans
 Hospital
Madison, Wisconsin 53705
and
Departments of Preventive Medicine and
 Medicine
University of Wisconsin—Madison
Madison, Wisconsin 53705

Patricia A. Detmers, PhD
Laboratory of Cellular Physiology and
*   Immunology*
The Rockefeller University
New York, New York 10021

André De Troyer, MD, PhD
Department of Medicine and Physiology
Brussels School of Medicine
1070 Brussels, Belgium
and
Respiratory Research Unit
Erasme University Hospital
1070 Brussels, Belgium

Bruce Dinger, PhD
Department of Physiology
University of Utah School of Medicine
Salt Lake City, Utah 84108

Pietro Enrico di Prampero, MD
Istituto di Biologia
Università di Udine
33100 Udine, Italy.

Jeffrey M. Drazen, MD
Department of Medicine
Beth Israel, Children's, Brigham and
*   Women's Hospital and Harvard*
*   Medical School*
Boston, Massachusetts 02215

Roland M. du Bois, MA, MD, FRCP
Interstitial Disease Unit
National Heart and Lung Institute
London SW3 6LR, England

Brian R. Duling, PhD
Department of Physiology
University of Virginia School of Medicine
Charlottesville, Virginia 22908

W. Y. Durand-Arczynska, PhD
Department of Physiology
University of Fribourg
CH-1700 Fribourg, Switzerland

Norman H. Edelman, MD
Division of Pulmonary and Critical Care
*   Medicine*
Department of Medicine
University of Medicine and Dentistry of
*   New Jersey—Robert Wood Johnson*
*   Medical School*
New Brunswick, New Jersey 08903

Richard M. Effros, MD
Division of Pulmonary and Critical Care
*   Medicine*
Medical College of Wisconsin
Milwaukee, Wisconsin 53226

Thomas M. Egan, MD
Department of Thoracic Surgery
Washington University Medical School
St. Louis, Missouri 63110
Present address:
Department of Surgery
University of North Carolina
School of Medicine
Chapel Hill, North Carolina 27599

L. A. Engel, MD
Department of Thoracic Medicine
Westmead Hospital
Sydney, New South Wales 2145, Australia

Jeffery T. Erickson, MD
Department of Physiology
University of North Carolina
Chapel Hill, North Carolina 27599

Barry L. Fanburg, MD
Pulmonary Division
New England Medical Center
Tufts University
Boston, Massachusetts 02111

Victor J. Ferrans, MD, PhD
Pathology Branch
National Heart, Lung and Blood Institute
National Institutes of Health
Bethesda, Maryland 20892

Salvatore J. Fidone, PhD
Department of Physiology
University of Utah School of Medicine
Salt Lake City, Utah 84108

Alan Fine, MD
Pulmonary Section
Boston D.V.A. Medical Center
Boston, Massachusetts 02130

Aron B. Fisher, MD
Institute for Environmental Medicine
University of Pennsylvania
Philadelphia, Pennsylvania 19104

J. Fleury, MD
INSERM U139
Clinique de pathologie respiratoire et de
*   l'environnement et Département*
*   d'Histologie*
Hôpital Henri Mondor et Faculté de
*   Médecine*
Université Paris-Val-de-Marne
94010 Créteil, France

James B. Forrest, MD, PhD, FRCP
Department of Anaesthesia
McMaster University
Hamilton, Ontario L8N 3Z5, Canada

Hubert V. Forster, PhD
Department of Physiology
Medical College of Wisconsin
Milwaukee, Wisconsin 53226
and
Department of Physiology
Veterans Administration Medical Center
Milwaukee, Wisconsin 53226

Philip J. Fracica, MD
Division of Allergy, Critical Care, and
*   Respiratory Medicine*
Duke University Medical Center
Durham, North Carolina 27710

Yuh Fukuda, MD
Department of Pathology
Nippon Medical School
Bunkyo-Ku, Tokyo 113, Japan

R. W. Fuller, MD, MRCP
Department of Clinical Pharmacology
Royal Postgraduate Medical School
London W12 ONN, England

Y. C. Fung, PhD
Department of Applied Mechanics and
*   Engineering Sciences*
University of California—San Diego
La Jolla, California 92093

James E. Gadek, MD
Pulmonary and Critical Care Division
Department of Medicine
Ohio State University
Columbus, Ohio 43210

John I. Gallin, MD
Division of Intramural Research
National Institute of Allergy and
*   Infectious Diseases*
National Institutes of Health
Bethesda, Maryland 20892

Eve A. Gallman, PhD
Department of Physiology
University of North Carolina
Chapel Hill, North Carolina 27599

S. C. Gandevia, MD, PhD
Department of Clinical Neurophysiology
Institute of Neurological Sciences
The Prince Henry Hospital
and
Department of Respiratory Medicine
The Prince of Wales Hospital
and
Department of Respiratory Medicine
University of New South Wales
School of Medicine
Sydney, New South Wales 2036, Australia

Thomas E. J. Gayeski, MD, PhD.
Departments of Physiology and
*   Anesthesiology*
University of Rochester
Rochester, New York 14642

M. Ge, MD
Department of Physiology and Cell
*   Biology*
The Albany Medical College
Albany, New York 12208
and
Wadsworth Center for Laboratories and
*   Research*
New York State Department of Health
Albany, New York 12201

G. J. Gleich, MD
Departments of Immunology and
*   Medicine*
Mayo Medical School
Mayo Clinic and Foundation
Rochester, Minnesota 55905

D. J. Godden, MD
University of British Columbia Pulmonary
*   Research Laboratory*
St. Paul's Hospital
Vancouver, British Columbia V6Z 1Y6,
*   Canada*

Jon Goerke, MD
Cardiovascular Research Institute and
*   Department of Physiology*
School of Medicine
University of California—San Francisco
San Francisco, California 94143

Ronald H. Goldstein, MD
Pulmonary Section
Boston D.V.A. Medical Center
Boston, Massachusetts 02130

Angela Gomez-Niño, MD, PhD
Department of Physiology
University of Utah School of Medicine
Salt Lake City, Utah 84108

Constancio Gonzalez, MD, PhD
Department of Physiology
University of Utah School of Medicine
Salt Lake City, Utah 84108
Present address:
Department of Biochemistry and
* Physiology*
University of Valladolid
Valladolid, Spain

A. E. Grassino, MD
Meakins–Christie Laboratories,
McGill University and
Notre Dame Hospital
University of Montreal
Montreal, Quebec, Canada

Karlfried Groebe, DrMed
Department of Physiology
University of Mainz
6500 Mainz, West Germany

Christian Guilleminault, MD
Sleep Disorders Center
Stanford University School of Medicine
Stanford, California 94305

Guillermo Gutierrez, MD, PhD
Pulmonary and Critical Care Division
University of Texas Health Science
* Center at Houston*
Houston, Texas 77030

P. E. Habb, MD
Department of Physiology
University of Fribourg
CH-1700 Fribourg, Switzerland

Jesse Hall, MD
Section of Pulmonary and Critical Care
* Medicine*
University of Chicago
Chicago, Illinois 60637

Barry Halliwell, PhD, DSc
Department of Biochemistry
King's College
University of London
London WC2R 2LS, England

Dale E. Hammerschmidt, MD
Division of Hematology
Department of Medicine
University of Minnesota Hospital
Minneapolis, Minnesota 55455

M. D. Hammond, MD
Division of Pulmonary, Critical Care and
* Occupational Medicine*
Department of Medicine
University of South Florida College of
* Medicine and James A. Haley Veterans*
* Administration Hospital*
Tampa, Florida 33612

Allan J. Hance, MD
INSERM U82
Faculté Bichat
75018 Paris, France

Richard Harding, PhD
Department of Physiology
Monash University
Melbourne 3168, Australia

Keith R. Harmon, MD
Pulmonary Division
Department of Medicine
University of Minnesota
Minneapolis, Minnesota 55455

John H. Hartwig, PhD
Hematology Unit
Massachusetts General Hospital
Boston, Massachusetts 02114
and
Department of Medicine and Department
* of Anatomy and Cellular Biology*
Harvard Medical School
Boston, Massachusetts 02115

Vincent E. Hascall, PhD
Bone Research Branch
National Institute of Dental Research
National Institutes of Health
Bethesda, Maryland 20892

Paul M. Hassoun, MD
Pulmonary Division
New England Medical Center
Tufts University
Boston, Massachusetts 02111

Samuel Hawgood, MD
Department of Pediatrics
Cardiovascular Research Institute
University of California—San Francisco
San Francisco, California 94143

Göran Hedenstierna, MD
Department of Clinical Physiology
Uppsala University Hospital
S-751 85 Uppsala, Sweden

John E. Heffner, MD
Division of Pulmonary and Critical Care
  Medicine
Medical University of South Carolina
Charleston, South Carolina 29425
Present address:
Medical Intensive Care Unit
Department of Medicine
St. Joseph's Hospital and Medical Center
Phoenix, Arizona 85013

Craig A. Henke, MD
Pulmonary Division
Department of Medicine
University of Minnesota
Minneapolis, Minnesota 55455

Kathe G. Henke, PhD
The John Rankin Laboratory of
  Pulmonary Medicine
William S. Middleton Memorial Veterans
  Hospital
Madison, Wisconsin 53705
and
Departments of Preventive Medicine and
  Medicine
University of Wisconsin—Madison
Madison, Wisconsin 53705
Present address:
Department of Thoracic Medicine
University of Sydney
Sydney, New South Wales 2006, Australia

Peter M. Henson, PhD
Department of Pediatrics
National Jewish Center for Immunology
  and Respiratory Disease
Denver, Colorado 80206

Michael P. Hlastala, PhD
Division of Pulmonary and Critical Care
  Medicine
University of Washington School of
  Medicine
Seattle, Washington 98195

W. Alan Hodson, MD
Pediatric Department
Division of Neonatal and Respiratory
  Diseases
University of Washington School of
  Medicine
Seattle, Washington 98195

James C. Hogg, MD, PhD
University of British Columbia
Pulmonary Research Laboratory
St. Paul's Hospital
Vancouver, British Columbia V6Z 1Y6,
  Canada

Stephen T. Holgate, MD, FRCP
Immunopharmacology Group
Clinical Pharmacology and Medicine 1
Southampton General Hospital
Southampton SO9 4XY Hampshire,
  England

Kenneth J. Holroyd, MD
Pulmonary Branch
National Heart, Lung and Blood Institute
National Institutes of Health
Bethesda, Maryland 20892

Carl R. Honig, MD
Departments of Physiology and
  Anesthesiology
University of Rochester
Rochester, New York 14642

L. Hoofd, PhD
Department of Physiology
University of Nijmegen
NL-6500 HB Nijmegen, The Netherlands

H. Hoppeler, MD
Institute of Anatomy
University of Berne
CH-3000 Berne 9, Switzerland

Thomas F. Hornbein, MD
Department of Anesthesiology and
  Department of Physiology and
  Biophysics
University of Washington
Seattle, Washington 98195

Keith Horsfield, DSc, PhD, MD
King Edward VII Hospital
Midhurst, West Sussex GU29 0BL,
  England

Richard C. Hubbard, MD
Pulmonary Branch
National Heart, Lung and Blood Institute
National Institutes of Health
Bethesda, Maryland 20892

David W. Hudgel, MD
Department of Medicine
Case Western Reserve University School
  of Medicine
Cleveland, Ohio 44106
and
Division of Pulmonary and Critical Care
  Medicine
MetroHealth Medical Center
Cleveland, Ohio 44109
and
Sleep Laboratory
MetroHealth Medical Center
Cleveland, Ohio 44109

Thomas F. Huff, PhD
Department of Microbiology and
  Immunology
Medical College of Virginia
Virginia Commonwealth University
Richmond, Virginia 23298

J. M. B. Hughes, DM, FRCP
Department of Medicine
Royal Postgraduate Medical School
Hammersmith Hospital
London W12 ONN, England

Ernst B. Hunziker, MD
Institute for Biomechanics
University of Berne
CH-3010 Berne 9, Switzerland

Robert E. Hyatt, MD
1912 Lake Ridge Drive
Vandalia, Illinois 62471

Dallas M. Hyde, PhD
Departments of Anatomy and Veterinary
  Pharmacology and Toxicology
and
California Primate Research Center
University of California School of
  Veterinary Medicine
Davis, California 95616

Albert L. Hyman, MD
Department of Surgery
Tulane Medical School
New Orleans, Louisiana 70112

Harry S. Jacob, MD
Division of Hematology
Department of Medicine
University of Minnesota Hospital
Minneapolis, Minnesota 55455

M. C. Jaurand, PhD
INSERM U139
Clinique de pathologie respiratoire et de
  l'environnement et Département
  d'Histologie
Hôpital Henri Mondor et Faculté de
  Médecine
Université Paris-Val-de-Marne
94010 Créteil, France

Kent J. Johnson, MD
Department of Pathology
University of Michigan Medical School
Ann Arbor, Michigan 48109

Dean P. Jones, PhD
Department of Biochemistry and Winship
  Cancer Center
Emory University
Atlanta, Georgia 30322

Norman L. Jones, MD
Department of Medicine
McMaster University
Hamilton, Ontario L8N 3Z5, Canada

David Jordan, D Phil
Department of Physiology
Royal Free Hospital School of Medicine
University of London
London NW3 2PF, England

Alain F. Junod, MD
Division de Pneumologie
Universitaire de Geneve
Hôpital Cantonal
1211 Geneva 4, Switzerland

Sandra E. Juul, MD
Department of Pediatrics
University of Washington
Seattle, Washington 98195

Michael A. Kaliner, MD
Allergic Diseases Section
National Institute of Allergy and
  Infectious Disease
National Institutes of Health
Bethesda, Maryland 20892

H. Benfer Kaltreider, MD
Respiratory Care Section
VA Medical Center—San Francisco
San Francisco, California 94121
and
Department of Medicine
University of California—San Francisco
San Francisco, California 94143

Roger D. Kamm, PhD
Department of Mechanical Engineering
Massachusetts Institute of Technology
Cambridge, Massachusetts 02139

S. R. Kayar, PhD
Department of Physiology
Robert Wood Johnson Medical School
Piscataway, New Jersey 08854

Homayoun Kazemi, MD
Pulmonary and Critical Care Unit
Department of Medicine
Harvard Medical School
and
Massachusetts General Hospital
Boston, Massachusetts 02114

Michael C. K. Khoo, PhD
Biomedical Engineering Department
University of Southern California
Los Angeles, California 90089

Kieran J. Killian, MD, BCh
Department of Medicine
McMaster University Medical Center
Hamilton, Ontario L8N 3Z5, Canada

Kwang-Jin Kim, PhD
Departments of Medicine and Physiology
Will Rogers Institute Pulmonary Research
 Program
Cornell University Medical College
New York, New York 10021
and
University of Southern California
Los Angeles, California 90033

Robert A. Klocke, MD
Departments of Medicine and Physiology
State University of New York—Buffalo
Buffalo, New York 14214

Ronald J. Knudson, MD
Department of Internal Medicine
Division of Respiratory Sciences
University of Arizona College of Medicine
Tucson, Arizona 85724

Theodor Kolobow, MD
Section on Pulmonary and Cardiac Assist
 Devices
National Heart, Lung and Blood Institute
National Institutes of Health
Bethesda, Maryland 20892

F. Kreuzer, MD
Department of Physiology
University of Nijmegen
NL-6500 HB Nijmegen, The Netherlands

Klaus E. Kuettner, PhD
Department of Biochemistry
Rush-Presbyterian–St. Luke's Medical
 Center
Chicago, Illinois 60612

Hugo Lagercrantz, MD, PhD
Department of Pediatrics and the Nobel
 Institute for Neurophysiology
Karolinska Institute
S-104 01 Stockholm, Sweden

Sukhamay Lahiri, D Phil
Department of Physiology
University of Pennsylvania School of
 Medicine
Philadelphia, Pennsylvania 19104

Stephen J. Lai-Fook, PhD
Biomedical Engineering Center
Wenner-Gren Research Laboratory
University of Kentucky
Lexington, Kentucky 40506

Annika Laitinen, PhD
Department of Electron Microscopy
University of Helsinki
SF-00280 Helsinki, Finland
and
Department of Medical and Physiological
 Chemistry
University of Lund
S-221 00 Lund, Sweden

Lauri A. Laitinen, MD
Department of Pulmonary Medicine
University of Lund
University Hospital of Lund
S-221 85 Lund, Sweden
and
Explorative Clinical Research
AB Draco
S-221 00 Lund, Sweden

Gary L. Larsen, MD
Section of Pediatric Pulmonary and
*   Critical Care Medicine*
Department of Pediatrics
University of Colorado School of
*   Medicine*
and National Jewish Center for
*   Immunology and Respiratory Medicine*
Denver, Colorado 80206

M. Harold Laughlin, PhD
Departments of Veterinary Biomedical
*   Sciences and Medical Physiology*
and Dalton Research Center
University of Missouri
Columbia, Missouri 65211

Lee V. Leak, PhD
Department of Anatomy
College of Medicine
Howard University
Washington, D.C. 20059

Robert M. K. W. Lee, PhD
Department of Anaesthesia
McMaster University
Hamilton, Ontario L8N 3Z5, Canada

Lawrence M. Lichtenstein, MD, PhD
Division of Clinical Immunology
Department of Medicine
The Johns Hopkins University School of
*   Medicine*
Baltimore, Maryland 21239

Howard L. Lippton, MD
Department of Surgery
Tulane Medical School
New Orleans, Louisiana 70112
and
Department of Pulmonary and Critical
*   Care Medicine*
Louisiana State University Medical
*   School*
New Orleans, Louisiana 70112

Lawrence D. Longo, MD
Department of Physiology
Loma Linda University
Loma Linda, California 92350

Robert G. Loudon, MD, BCh
Pulmonary Disease Division
Medical Science Building
University of Cincinnati
College of Medicine
Cincinnati, Ohio 45267

Edgar C. Lucey, PhD
Pulmonary Section
Boston D.V.A. Medical Center
Boston, Massachusetts 02130

Claes Lundgren, MD, PhD
Center for Research in Special
*   Environments*
Department of Physiology
State University of New York—Buffalo
Buffalo, New York 14214

Donald W. MacGlashan, Jr., MD, PhD
Division of Clinical Immunology
Department of Medicine
The Johns Hopkins University School of
*   Medicine*
Baltimore, Maryland 21239

P. T. Macklem, MD, CM
Montreal Chest Hospital Centre and
*   Meakins–Christie Laboratories*
McGill University
Montreal, Quebec, Canada

Harry L. Malech, MD
Bacterial Diseases Section
Laboratory of Clinical Investigation
National Institute of Allergy and
*   Infectious Diseases*
National Institutes of Health
Bethesda, Maryland 20892

A. B. Malik, PhD
Department of Physiology and Cell
*   Biology*
The Albany Medical College
Albany, New York 12208
and
Wadsworth Center for Laboratories and
*   Research*
New York State Department of Health
Albany, New York 12201

Vincent C. Manganiello, MD, PhD
Laboratory of Cellular Metabolism
National Heart, Lung and Blood Institute
National Institutes of Health
Bethesda, Maryland 20892

William A. Marinelli, MD
Pulmonary Division
Department of Medicine
University of Minnesota
Minneapolis, Minnesota 55455

Bryan E. Marshall, MD, FRCP
Center for Research in Anesthesia
University of Pennsylvania School of
Medicine
Philadelphia, Pennsylvania 19104

Carol Marshall, PhD
Center for Research in Anesthesia
University of Pennsylvania School of
Medicine
Philadelphia, Pennsylvania 19104

George R. Martin, PhD
National Institute on Aging
Gerontology Research Center
Baltimore, Maryland 21224

W. J. Martin II, MD
Division of Pulmonary and Critical Care
Medicine
Indiana University School of Medicine
Indianapolis, Indiana 46202

Robert J. Mason, MD
Respiratory Medicine and Pulmonary
Division
University of Colorado
and
Department of Medicine
National Jewish Center for Immunology
and Respiratory Disease
Denver, Colorado 80206

Donald Massaro, MD
Sol Katz Laboratory of Respiratory
Biology
Georgetown University School of
Medicine
Washington, D.C. 20007

Gloria D. Massaro, MD
Sol Katz Laboratory of Respiratory
Biology
Georgetown University School of
Medicine
Washington, D.C. 20007

O. Mathieu-Costello, PhD
Department of Medicine
University of California—San Diego
School of Medicine
La Jolla, California 92093

Joe L. Mauderly, DVM
Inhalation Toxicology Research Institute
Albuquerque, New Mexico 87185

John A. McDonald, MD, PhD
Respiratory and Critical Care Division
Washington University School of
Medicine
St. Louis, Missouri 63110

E. R. McFadden, Jr., MD
Airway Disease Center
University Hospitals of Cleveland
Cleveland, Ohio 44106
and
Department of Medicine
Case Western Reserve University School
of Medicine
Cleveland, Ohio 44106

D. K. McKenzie, PhD
Department of Clinical Neurophysiology
Institute of Neurological Sciences
The Prince Henry Hospital
and
Department of Respiratory Medicine
The Prince of Wales Hospital
and
Department of Respiratory Medicine
University of New South Wales
School of Medicine
Sydney, New South Wales 2036, Australia

Robert P. Mecham, PhD
Departments of Cell Biology and
Medicine
Jewish Hospital at Washington University
Medical School
St. Louis, Missouri 63110

Joseph Milerad, MD, PhD
Department of Pediatrics and the Nobel
Institute for Neurophysiology
Karolinska Institute
S-104 01 Stockholm, Sweden

J. Milic-Emili, PhD
Meakins–Christie Laboratories
McGill University
Montreal, Quebec H2X 2P2, Canada

David E. Millhorn, PhD
Department of Physiology
University of North Carolina
Chapel Hill, North Carolina 27599

Giuseppe Miserocchi, MD
Istituto di Fisiologia Umana
Università degli Studi, Milano
20133 Milano, Italy

Wayne Mitzner, PhD
School of Hygiene and Public Health
Department of Environmental Health
  Sciences
The Johns Hopkins University
Baltimore, Maryland 21205

Masaji Mochizuki, MD
Nishimaruyama Hospital
Geriatric Respiratory Research Center
064 Sapporo/Chuo-Ku, Japan

Jacopo P. Mortola, MD
Department of Physiology
McGill University
Montreal, Quebec H3G 1Y6, Canada

Joel Moss, MD, PhD
Laboratory of Cellular Metabolism
National Heart, Lung and Blood Institute
National Institutes of Health
Bethesda, Maryland 20892

David C. F. Muir, MD
Occupational Health Program
McMaster University
Hamilton, Ontario L8N 3Z5, Canada

Raymond L. H. Murphy, MD
Department of Medicine
Tufts University School of Medicine
Boston, Massachusetts 02130
and
Pulmonary Services
Faulkner and Lemuel Shattuck Hospitals
Boston, Massachusetts 02130

Judith A. Neubauer, PhD
Division of Pulmonary and Critical Care
  Medicine
Department of Medicine
University of Medicine and Dentistry of
  New Jersey—Robert Wood Johnson
  Medical School
New Brunswick, New Jersey 08903

Ana Obeso, MD, PhD
Department of Physiology
University of Utah School of Medicine
Salt Lake City, Utah 84108
Present address:
Department of Biochemistry and
  Physiology
University of Valladolid
Valladolid, Spain

John Orem, PhD
Department of Physiology
Texas Tech University Health Sciences
  Center
Lubbock, Texas 79430

Eric R. Pacht, MD
Division of Pulmonary and Critical Care
Department of Internal Medicine
The Ohio State University
Columbus, Ohio 43210

M. Paiva, MD
Institute of Interdisciplinary Research and
  Respiratory Research Unit
School of Medicine
University of Brussels
B-1070 Brussels, Belgium

George E. Palade, MD
Department of Cell Biology
Yale School of Medicine
New Haven, Connecticut 06510

Lawrence G. Pan, PhD
Department of Physiology
Medical College of Wisconsin
Milwaukee, Wisconsin 53226
and
Department of Physical Therapy
Marquette University
Milwaukee, Wisconsin 53226

P. D. Pare, MD
University of British Columbia Pulmonary
  Research Laboratory
St. Paul's Hospital
Vancouver, British Columbia V6Z 1Y6,
  Canada

Polly E. Parsons, MD
Department of Medicine
National Jewish Center for Immunology
  and Respiratory Disease
Denver, Colorado 80206

Demetri Pavia, PhD, FInstP
Institute of Intramural Research
Medical Division
Boehringer Ingelheim (UK), Ltd.
Bracknell, Berkshire RG12 4YS, England

Timothy J. Pedley, PhD
Department of Applied Mathematical
  Studies
University of Leeds
Leeds LS2 9JT, England

David H. Perlmutter, MD
Edward Mallinckrodt Department of
  Pediatrics
Washington University School of
  Medicine
St. Louis, Missouri 63110

Solbert Permutt, MD
Division of Pulmonary and Critical Care
  Medicine
The Johns Hopkins Center for Asthma
  and Allergy
Hopkins Bayview Research Campus at
  the Francis Scott Key Medical Center
Baltimore, Maryland 21224

Claude A. Piantodosi, MD
Division of Allergy, Critical Care, and
  Respiratory Medicine
Duke University Medical Center
Durham, North Carolina 27710

Johannes Piiper, MD
Institute for Physiology
Ruhr University
Bochum, D-4630
and
Department of Physiology
Max Planck Institute for Experimental
  Medicine
D-3400 Göttingen, Federal Republic of
  Germany

Charles G. Plopper, PhD
Departments of Anatomy and Veterinary
  Pharmacology and Toxicology and
  California Primate Research Center
University of California School of
  Veterinary Medicine
Davis, California 95616

J. M. Polak, DSc, MD, FRCP
Department of Histochemistry
Royal Postgraduate Medical School
London W12 ONN, England

Martin Post, PhD
Research Institute
The Hospital for Sick Children
Toronto, Ontario M5G 1X8, Canada

Ian W. Prosser, MB, BS
Department of Hematology
University of Adelaide
Institute of Medical and Veterinary
  Sciences
Adelaide, South Australia 5000

David Proud, PhD
The Johns Hopkins University School of
  Medicine
Johns Hopkins Asthma and Allergy
  Center
Baltimore, Maryland 21224

William A. Pryor, PhD
Biodynamics Institute
Louisiana State University
Baton Rouge, Louisiana 70803

D. Eugene Rannels, PhD
Departments of Cellular and Molecular
  Physiology and Anesthesia
College of Medicine
The Pennsylvania State University
Hershey, Pennsylvania 17033

Robert Blake Reeves, PhD
Department of Physiology
School of Medicine
State University of New York—Buffalo
Buffalo, New York 14226

Lynne M. Reid, MD
Department of Pathology
Harvard Medical School
Boston, Massachusetts 02115
and
Children's Hospital
Boston, Massachusetts 02115

Stephen I. Rennard, MD
Pulmonary and Critical Care Medicine
  Section
University of Nebraska Medical Center
Omaha, Nebraska 68105

John E. Repine, MD
Department of Medicine
Webb Waring Lung Institute
University of Colorado Health Sciences
  Center
Denver, Colorado 80262

Herbert Y. Reynolds, MD
Department of Medicine
The Milton S. Hershey Medical Center
The Pennsylvania State University
Hershey, Pennsylvania 17033

Donald E. Richardson, MD
Department of Neurosurgery
Tulane Medical School
New Orleans, Louisiana 70112

Luca Richeldi, MD
Institute for Tuberculosis and Pulmonary
    Diseases
University of Modena
Modena 4110, Italy

David J. Riley, MD
Division of Pulmonary and Critical Care
    Medicine
Department of Medicine
University of Medicine and Dentistry of
    New Jersey—Robert Wood Johnson
    Medical School
New Brunswick, New Jersey 08903

Bengt Rippe, MD, PhD
Department of Physiology
University of Göteborg
400 33 Göteborg, Sweden

Richard A. Robbins, MD
Pulmonary and Critical Care Medicine
    Section
University of Nebraska Medical Center
Omaha, Nebraska 68105

Clive Robinson, MB, BS
Immunopharmacology Group
Clinical Pharmacology and Medicine 1
Southampton General Hospital
Southampton S09 4XY Hampshire,
    England

David M. Rodman, MD
Cardiovascular Pulmonary Research
    Laboratory
University of Colorado Health Sciences
    Center
Denver, Colorado 80262

William N. Rom, MD, MPH
Division of Pulmonary and Critical Care
    Center
New York University Medical Center
New York, New York 10016

Jesse Roman, MD
Respiratory and Critical Care Division
Washington University School of
    Medicine
St. Louis, Missouri 63110

Giovanni A. Rossi, MD
1° Divisione di Pneumologia
Ospedale San Martino
16132 Genova, Italy

Luigi Rossi-Bernardi, MD
Via Selice Poggi 14
Milano 20131, Italy

C. Roussos, MD, PhD
Critical Care Department
Evangelismos Hospital
Athens, Greece

Louise A. Russo, PhD
Departments of Cellular and Molecular
    Physiology and Anesthesia
College of Medicine
The Pennsylvania State University
Hershey, Pennsylvania 17033

T. J. Ryan, PhD
Department of Physiology and Cell
    Biology
The Albany Medical College
Albany, New York 12208
and
Wadsworth Center for Laboratories and
    Research
New York State Department of Health
Albany, New York 12201

Kent Sahlin, MD
Department of Clinical Physiology
Karolinska Institute
Huddinge University Hospital
S-141 86 Huddinge, Sweden

B. Saltin, MD
August Krogh Institute
University of Copenhagen
DK-2100 Copenhagen, Denmark

Cesare Saltini, MD
Pulmonary Branch
National Heart, Lung and Blood Institute
National Institutes of Health
Bethesda, Maryland 20892
and
Institute for Tuberculosis and Pulmonary
    Diseases
University of Modena
Modena 4110, Italy

Jonathan M. Samet, MD
Pulmonary Division
Department of Medicine
University of New Mexico School of
    Medicine
Albuquerque, New Mexico 87131

Franca B. Sant'Ambrogio, DrNS, PhD
Department of Physiology and Biophysics
The University of Texas Medical Branch
Galveston, Texas 77550

Giuseppe Sant'Ambrogio, MD
Department of Physiology and Biophysics
The University of Texas Medical Branch
Galveston, Texas 77550

Peter Scheid, MD
Institute for Physiology
Ruhr University
Bochum, D-4630
and
Department of Physiology
Max Planck Institute for Experimental
*   Medicine*
D-3400 Göttingen, Federal Republic of
*   Germany*

Dietrich W. Scheuermann, MD
Institute of Histology and Microscopic
*   Anatomy*
University of Antwerp
B-2020 Antwerp, Belgium

Eveline E. Schneeberger, MD
Department of Pathology
Massachusetts General Hospital
Boston, Massachusetts 02114

Ingrid U. Schraufstätter, MD
Division of Vascular Biology and
*   Inflammation*
Department of Immunology Research
Scripps Clinic
La Jolla, California 92037

Paul T. Schumacker, PhD
Section of Pulmonary and Critical Care
*   Medicine*
The University of Chicago
Chicago, Illinois 60637

Samuel Schürch, PhD
Departments of Medical Physiology and
*   Medicine*
University of Calgary
Calgary, Alberta T2N 4N1, Canada

Lawrence B. Schwartz, MD, PhD
Division of Rheumatology, Allergy, and
*   Immunology*
Department of Medicine
Medical College of Virginia
Virginia Commonwealth University
Richmond, Virginia 23298

Robert M. Senior, MD
Washington University School of
*   Medicine*
St Louis, Missouri 63110
and
Respiratory and Critical Care Division
Jewish Hospital at Washington University
*   Medical Center*
St. Louis, Missouri 63110

J. T. Sharp, MD
Division of Pulmonary, Critical Care and
*   Occupational Medicine*
Department of Medicine
University of South Florida College of
*   Medicine and James A. Haley Veterans*
*   Administration Hospital*
Tampa, Florida 33612

Maya Simionescu, PhD
Institute of Cellular Biology and
*   Pathology*
Department of Biological Structures
Bucharest 79691, Romania

James B. Skatrud, MD
The John Rankin Laboratory of
*   Pulmonary Medicine*
William S. Middleton Memorial Veterans
*   Hospital*
Madison, Wisconsin 53705
and
Departments of Preventive Medicine and
*   Medicine*
University of Wisconsin—Madison
Madison, Wisconsin 53705

Michael A. Sleigh, PhD
Department of Biology
University of Southampton
Bassett Crescent East
Southampton SO9 3TU, England

Arthur S. Slutsky, MD
Department of Medicine
Mount Sinai Hospital
Toronto, Ontario M5G 1X5, Canada

Barry T. Smith, MD, FRCP(C)
Research Institute
The Hospital for Sick Children
Toronto, Ontario M5G 1X8, Canada

Robert M. Smith, MD
Department of Medicine
Division of Pulmonary and Critical Care
*   Medicine*
University of California—San Diego
La Jolla, California 92093

Gordon L. Snider, MD
Pulmonary Section
Boston D.V.A. Medical Center
Boston, Massachusetts 02130

Roger G. Spragg, MD
Department of Medicine
Division of Pulmonary and Critical Care
Medicine
University of California—San Diego
La Jolla, California 92093

D. R. Springall, PhD
Department of Histochemistry
Royal Postgraduate Medical School
London W12 ONN, England

Phillip J. Stone, PhD
Department of Biochemistry
Boston University School of Medicine
Boston, Massachusetts 02118

Kingman P. Strohl, MD
Department of Medicine
Case Western Reserve University School
of Medicine
Cleveland, Ohio 44106
and
Division of Pulmonary and Critical Care
Medicine
University Hospitals of Cleveland
Cleveland, Ohio 44106

Robert C. Strunk, MD
Edward Mallinckrodt Department of
Pediatrics
Washington University School of
Medicine
St. Louis, Missouri 63110

Caroline L. Szymeczek, MS
Department of Physiology
University of North Carolina
Chapel Hill, North Carolina 27599

Aubrey E. Taylor, PhD
Department of Physiology
University of South Alabama College of
Medicine
Mobile, Alabama 36688

C. Richard Taylor, PhD
Museum of Comparative Zoology
Harvard University
Cambridge, Massachusetts 02138

William M. Thurlbeck, MB, FRCP
Department of Pathology
Faculty of Medicine
University of British Columbia
Vancouver, British Columbia V6T 1W5,
Canada

Mary L. Tod, PhD
Division of Pulmonary and Critical Care
Medicine
Department of Medicine
University of Maryland School of
Medicine
Baltimore, Maryland 21201

Leif Tokics, MD
Department of Anesthesia
Huddinge University Hospital
S-14186 Huddinge, Sweden

Z. Turek, MD, PhD
Department of Physiology
University of Nijmegen
NL-6500 HB Nijmegen, The Netherlands

Lambert M. G. van Golde, PhD
Laboratory of Veterinary Biochemistry
University of Utrecht
3508 TD Utrect, The Netherlands

Erik van Lunteren, MD
Departments of Medicine and
Neurosciences
Case Western Reserve University School
of Medicine
Cleveland, Ohio 44106

Martha Vaughan, MD
Laboratory of Cellular Metabolism
National Heart, Lung and Blood Institute
National Institutes of Health
Bethesda, Maryland 20892

Gregory M. Vercellotti, MD
Division of Hematology
Department of Medicine
University of Minnesota Hospital
Minneapolis, Minnesota 55455

Norbert F. Voelkel, MD
Cardiovascular Pulmonary Research
Laboratory
University of Colorado Health Sciences
Center
Denver, Colorado 80262

Curt von Euler, MD, PhD
Nobel Institute for Neurophysiology
Karolinska Institute
S-104 01 Stockholm, Sweden

Peter D. Wagner, MD
Department of Medicine
University of California—San Diego
La Jolla, California 92093-0623

David W. Walker, PhD
Department of Physiology
Monash University
Melbourne, Victoria 3168, Australia

M. Wang, MD
Department of Biomedical Sciences
McMaster University Health Science
*   Centre*
Hamilton, Ontario L8N 3Z5, Canada

Peter A. Ward, PhD
Department of Pathology
University of Michigan Medical School
Ann Arbor, Michigan 48109

Jeffrey S. Warren, M.D
Department of Pathology
University of Michigan Medical School
Ann Arbor, Michigan 48109

Karlman Wasserman, MD, PhD
Division of Respiratory and Critical Care
*   Physiology and Medicine*
Harbor–UCLA Medical Center
Torrance, California 90509

Ewald R. Weibel, MD, DSc
Department of Anatomy
University of Berne
CH-3000 Berne 9, Switzerland

Michael J. Welsh, PhD
Howard Hughes Medical Institute
and
Departments of Internal Medicine and
*   Physiology and Biophysics*
University of Iowa College of Medicine
Iowa City, Iowa 52242

John B. West, MD, PhD, DSc, FRCP,
**   FRACP**
Department of Medicine
University of California—San Diego
La Jolla, California 92093

Mark D. Wewers, MD
Pulmonary and Critical Care Division
Department of Medicine
Ohio State University
Columbus, Ohio 43210

Brian J. Whipp, PhD, DSc
Department of Physiology
University of California—Los Angeles
School of Medicine
Los Angeles, California 90024

Martha V. White, MD
Allergic Diseases Section
National Institute of Allergy and
*   Infectious Diseases*
National Institutes of Health
Bethesda, Maryland 20892

Jeffrey A. Whitsett, MD
Division of Pulmonary Biology
Children's Hospital Research Foundation
Children's Hospital Medical Center
Cincinnati, Ohio 45267
and
Division of Neonatology
Department of Pediatrics
University of Cincinnati College of
*   Medicine*
Cincinnati, Ohio 45267

J. H. Widdicombe, MD
Cardiovascular Research Institute
University of California—San Francisco
San Francisco, California 94143

John Widdicombe, MD, PhD
Department of Physiology
St. George's Hospital Medical School
London SW17 ORE, England

Thomas N. Wight, PhD
Department of Pathology
University of Washington
Seattle, Washington 98195

Mary C. Williams, PhD
Cardiovascular Research Institute and
*   Department of Anatomy*
School of Medicine
University of California—San Francisco
San Francisco, California 94143

Theodore A. Wilson, PhD
Department of Aerospace Engineering
*   and Mechanics*
University of Minnesota
Minneapolis, Minnesota 55455

Robert M. Winslow, MD
Blood Research Department
Letterman Army Institute of Research
Presidio of San Francisco
San Francisco, California 94129

Lawrence D. H. Wood, MD, PhD
Section of Pulmonary and Critical Care
* Medicine*
University of Chicago
Chicago, Illinois 60637

G. Scott Worthen, MD
Department of Medicine
National Jewish Center for Immunology
* and Respiratory Disease*
Denver, Colorado 80206

Samuel D. Wright, PhD
Laboratory of Cellular Physiology and
* Immunology*
The Rockefeller University
New York, New York 10021

Reen Wu, PhD
California Primate Research Center
University of California—Davis
Davis, California 95616

Donovan B. Yeates, PhD
Section of Environmental and
* Occupational Medicine*
Department of Medicine
Goldberg Research Center
University of Illinois at Chicago
Chicago, Illinois 60680

Katsuaki Yoshizaki, PhD
Department of Physiology
University of Utah School of Medicine
Salt Lake City, Utah 84108
Present address:
Department of Physiology
University of Akita School of Medicine
Akita City, Japan

Warren M. Zapol, MD
Department of Anesthesia
Massachusetts General Hospital
Boston, Massachusetts 02114

THE LUNG: Scientific Foundations
edited by R.G. Crystal, J.B. West et al.
Raven Press, Ltd., New York © 1991.

CHAPTER 5.3.1

Ventilation

Michael P. Hlastala

In order to transfer gases in the lung in an efficient manner, blood and outside air must be brought into close proximity in the lung. Ventilation is the movement of fresh air from the outside to the alveoli for gas exchange, along with the subsequent movement of alveolar air back to the outside.

GAS PRESSURE

Atmospheric or barometric pressure (P_B) is the total pressure exerted by the kinetic energy of all the molecules in the atmospheric mixture. P_B decreases with increasing altitude, but at sea level, atmospheric pressure will raise a column of mercury in an evacuated tube to a height of 760 mm (this is equivalent to 29.92 inches).

In previous chapters, pressure in the chest or lungs was expressed relative to atmospheric pressure ($P_{atm} = 0$). This is termed "gauge pressure" and is also used when measuring blood pressure. However, for gas pressure in atmosphere, alveoli, and blood, absolute pressure terms are expressed in mmHg or torr (1 torr = 1 mmHg under standard gravitational conditions). In absolute pressure terms, a pleural pressure of -13 cmH$_2$O or -10 mmHg (gauge) is equal to 750 mmHg (absolute).

Atmospheric air is a mixture consisting of oxygen (20.95%), nitrogen (78.09%), argon (0.93%), and carbon dioxide (0.03%), with water vapor varying from 0% to 2% and diluting the other gases accordingly. For practical purposes we usually assume oxygen 21% and nitrogen 79% and ignore carbon dioxide and argon. Water vapor varies with the degree of humidification.

M. P. Hlastala: Division of Pulmonary and Critical Care Medicine, University of Washington School of Medicine, Seattle, Washington 98195.

PARTIAL PRESSURE

In a mixture of gases, the pressure exerted by the kinetic energy of each separate gas is referred to as its "partial pressure." If the mixture were enclosed in a sealed container, it would develop a pressure on the walls of the container by virtue of the collisions between the gas molecules and the container walls. The pressure developed by all the molecules of the mixture as they bounce off the container walls is the "total pressure" developed by the gas. The "partial pressure" of any component gas is the pressure developed by the molecules of that component acting alone. Since the random motion causing collisions is the same motion that allows diffusion to take place, the partial pressure of a gas is a measure of its tendency to diffuse through either gas or fluid media.

The total pressure of a mixture of gases is equal to the sum of the partial pressure of each gas in the mixture (Dalton's law). In the gas phase, partial pressure is proportional to concentration. The partial pressure of a gas is found by multiplying the fraction of the gas by the total pressure. P_{O_2} in air is expressed as

$$P_{O_2} = F_{O_2} \times P_B = 0.21 \times 760 \text{ mmHg}$$

$$= 160 \text{ mmHg} \quad [1]$$

The sum of the partial pressures in the lung equals total pressure:

$$P_{CO_2} + P_{O_2} + P_{N_2} + P_{H_2O} = P_B \quad [2]$$

WATER VAPOR

Water vapor behaves differently from the other respiratory gases. When a gas mixture is in contact with liquid and is saturated with the vapor of that liquid, the partial pressure of water vapor depends on temperature.

Atmospheric gas is cooler than body temperature and, though containing some water, is rarely 100% saturated. Inspired gas entering the respiratory system is warmed to body temperature and humidified to full saturation with water vapor. At 37°C, water vapor has a partial pressure of 47 mmHg (water vapor pressure at saturation = 17.5 mmHg at 20°C, 47.0 mmHg at 37°C, and 760 mmHg at 100°C). This pressure does not vary with changes in barometric pressure or changes in the other components in the gas mixture. If P_B is 760 mmHg, and P_{H_2O} is 47 mmHg, the difference, 713 mmHg, is the total partial pressure of the remaining inspired gases. Of this total, 21% is oxygen and 79% is nitrogen. The relative humidity is the actual water vapor partial pressure expressed as a fraction of the saturated vapor pressure at the same temperature. For example, at 20°C, a P_{H_2O} of 8.0 mmHg corresponds to a 46% (8.0/17.5) relative humidity.

After humidification, $P_{I_{O_2}}$ can be calculated as

$$P_{I_{O_2}} = F_{I_{O_2}} \times (P_B - P_{H_2O})$$

$$= 0.21 \times 713 = 150 \text{ mmHg} \qquad [3]$$

$$P_{I_{N_2}} = 0.79 \times 713 = 563 \text{ mmHg}$$

INSPIRED AIR WARMING AND HUMIDIFICATION

The volume occupied by an amount of gas is directly proportional to its absolute temperature (in degrees Kelvin), is inversely proportional to its total pressure, and is affected by the amount of water vapor present. Exhaled gas collected in a spirometer or bag is saturated at ambient temperature and pressure (ATPS). Lung and ventilatory volumes are conventionally converted to body temperature and pressure, saturated (BTPS) conditions, an expansion of about 9–10%. Gas transfer quantities ($\dot{V}_{O_2}$, $\dot{V}_{CO_2}$, and diffusing capacity) are conventionally expressed at standard temperature (273 K), pressure (760 torr), dry (STPD) conditions. Corrections can be made using the following relationship:

$$\frac{V_1 \times (P_1 - P_{1_{H_2O}})}{T_1} = \frac{V_2 \times (P_2 - P_{2_{H_2O}})}{T_2} \qquad [4]$$

TOTAL VENTILATION

The total ventilation or minute volume can be determined by collecting exhaled gas for a measured time ($\dot{V}_E$ = volume exhaled per minute). The volume of gas exhaled during one normal respiratory cycle is the tidal volume ($\dot{V}_T$). The total ventilation is equal to the tidal volume multiplied by the breathing frequency:

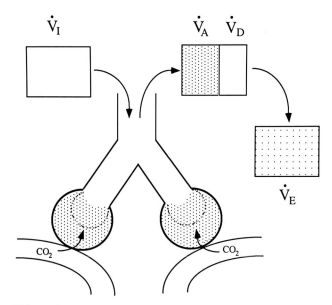

FIG. 1. Schematic of ventilation in the lung. Inspired ventilation is divided between the dead space and the alveolar space, where it picks up CO_2. On exhalation, ventilation from the dead space ($\dot{V}_D$) and from the alveolar space ($\dot{V}_A$) mix to form the total ventilation ($\dot{V}_E$).

$$\dot{V}_E = \dot{V}_T \times f \qquad [5]$$

Alveolar Ventilation

Gas exchange occurs in the alveolar acinus when fresh air comes in close proximity to capillary blood. However, not all the air inspired reaches the alveoli to participate in gas exchange (Fig. 1). The inspired air must first pass through the conducting airways: the nose, mouth, pharynx, larynx, trachea, bronchi, and bronchioles. These airways "conduct" air from the atmosphere to the alveoli. Because they contain no alveoli, they do not participate in gas exchange. However, airways do participate in the warming and humidification of inspired air. At the end of inspiration, the volume of air remaining in the conducting airways is called the "anatomic dead space" ("dead" because it does not participate in gas exchange). The effect of the conducting airways on ventilation and gas exchange can be considered in two ways. After inspiration, humidified and warmed atmospheric air remains in these airways and leaves as the first gas out on the subsequent exhalation. After expiration, alveolar gas (with CO_2 added and O_2 partially removed) fills the anatomic dead space and reenters the alveoli with the next breath. Thus a tidal breath may inspire 600 ml of air and will cause a 600 ml expansion of the alveolar volume followed by the expiration of 600 ml, but the volume of fresh air delivered to the alveoli and the volume of alveolar air exhaled to the atmosphere

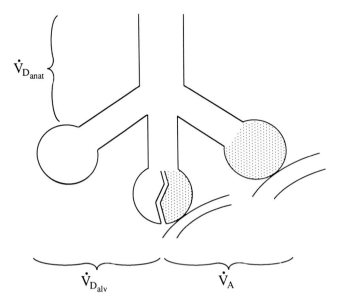

FIG. 2. Schematic of dead-space ventilation. Physiologic dead space is composed of anatomic dead space and alveolar dead space.

will each be less than 600 ml by the volume of the anatomic dead space.

In addition to the conducting airways, any alveoli that are ventilated with air but not perfused with blood do not participate in gas exchange. The volume of ventilation going to these alveoli also acts as dead-space ventilation and is called "alveolar dead space." Ventilation to areas of lung which have reduced perfusion behaves as if one portion were going to alveoli with normal perfusion and another portion were going to alveoli with no perfusion. The latter portion is also part of the alveolar dead space. These dead-space components are shown schematically in Fig. 2. The sum of anatomic and alveolar dead space makes up the physiologic dead space.

$$V_{D_{physiol}} = V_{D_{anat}} + V_{D_{alv}} \qquad [6]$$

In this chapter the symbols V_D and $\dot{V}_D$ without further qualifiers will always mean the physiologic dead space and its ventilation. The physiologic dead space (V_D) or wasted ventilation ($\dot{V}_D$) is usually expressed as a fraction of the tidal volume (V_D/V_T) or of the total ventilation ($\dot{V}_D/\dot{V}_E$).

The physiologic dead space may be increased with lung disease, primarily because of an increase in the alveolar component. The volume of air that does participate in gas exchange because it is in contact with perfused alveoli is the alveolar ventilation ($\dot{V}_A = \dot{V}_E - \dot{V}_{D_{physiol}}$). The volume per minute of alveolar ventilation is critical, because it determines the amount of air presented to alveoli into which CO_2 can be added and from which O_2 can be removed.

ALVEOLAR GAS COMPOSITION

Carbon Dioxide Exchange

The body's CO_2 production is eliminated only by ventilation. $\dot{V}CO_2$ equals the volume of CO_2 exhaled per minute ($\dot{V}_ECO_2$) minus the volume of CO_2 inhaled (negligible). Because all the CO_2 in the expired gas must have come from alveolar ventilation, we have

$$\dot{V}CO_2 = \dot{V}_A \times F_ACO_2 \qquad [7]$$

where F_ACO_2 is the concentration of CO_2 in the alveolar space. Rearranging, we obtain

$$F_ACO_2 = \frac{\dot{V}CO_2}{\dot{V}_A} \qquad [8]$$

and because

$$F_ACO_2 \times (P_B - 47) = P_ACO_2 \qquad [9]$$

we obtain

$$P_ACO_2 = \frac{\dot{V}CO_2}{\dot{V}_A} (P_B - 47) \qquad [10]$$

Equation 10 is the alveolar ventilation equation. Alveolar PCO_2 is directly related to the production of CO_2 and is inversely related to alveolar ventilation ($\dot{V}_A$). The body maintains a normal arterial and alveolar PCO_2 of 40 mmHg by adjusting ventilation appropriately for the $\dot{V}CO_2$ determined by metabolic production. When using Eq. 10, both $\dot{V}_A$ and $\dot{V}CO_2$ must be expressed in the same units (i.e., either BTPS or STPD).

"Hyperventilation" is defined as ventilation in excess of metabolic needs. It follows from the alveolar ventilation equation that a P_aCO_2 less than normal indicates alveolar hyperventilation. Conversely, a P_aCO_2 greater than normal indicates alveolar hypoventilation. Alveolar ventilation can be altered by changes in either total ventilation or wasted ventilation ($\dot{V}_A = \dot{V}_E - \dot{V}_D$). Any depression in central nervous system function can change $\dot{V}_E$; for example, many drugs such as analgesics and sedatives can reduce $\dot{V}_E$. Any increase in $\dot{V}_D$ will reduce $\dot{V}_A$ unless $\dot{V}_E$ increases accordingly. Many disease processes increase physiologic dead space, which is a contributing cause of respiratory failure when the patient can no longer increase total ventilation.

Alveolar PCO_2 reflects a balance between (a) the CO_2 delivery to the alveoli ($\dot{V}CO_2$) and (b) the CO_2 elimination from the lungs by ventilation ($\dot{V}_ECO_2$). In a steady state, production and excretion must be the same. Under resting conditions, $\dot{V}CO_2$ is relatively constant at approximately 200 ml/min for a normal-sized individual. With transient hyperventilation, CO_2 will be exhaled at a greater rate than our CO_2 production;

P_ACO_2 (and arterial PCO_2) will fall. As P_ACO_2 falls, the CO_2 exhaled per minute will decrease until it is again equal to CO_2 production and a new steady state is established. With hypoventilation, the rate of CO_2 exhalation initially falls, and then P_ACO_2 (and arterial PCO_2) rises until a new steady state is reached where excretion again equals production with less ventilation, but each liter of gas leaving the alveoli carries more CO_2. This mechanism allows patients with severe lung disease and high work of breathing to excrete their CO_2 production at less energy cost.

Energy necessary for life processes is produced by oxidation of carbohydrates, protein, and fats, producing mainly CO_2 and H_2O as breakdown products. The respiratory quotient (RQ) is the ratio of metabolic CO_2 production to the oxygen consumption ($\dot{V}CO_2/\dot{V}O_2$) of the tissues. When metabolizing carbohydrate, the RQ equals 1.0:

$$C_6H_{12}O_6 + 6O_2 \rightarrow 6CO_2 + 6H_2O \qquad [11]$$

$$RQ = \frac{\dot{V}CO_2}{\dot{V}O_2} = \frac{6}{6} = 1 \qquad [12]$$

When metabolizing fat, RQ = 0.7 and the RQ of protein has an average value of 0.8. Thus the RQ for the entire body varies with the percentages of carbohydrate, fat, and protein being oxidized at any given time. The respiratory exchange ratio (R) relates the volume of CO_2 eliminated to the lungs and the net volume of O_2 taken up from the lungs. In a steady state or over a long period of time, R must equal RQ, but R may vary transiently with factors other than metabolism. If an individual suddenly increases ventilation, R rises because CO_2 is being "blown off" from blood and tissue stores (but little O_2 can be added).

Oxygen Exchange

The level of alveolar O_2 also reflects a balance of two processes: (i) O_2 delivery to the alveoli by ventilation and (ii) O_2 removal from the alveoli by capillary blood. Oxygen delivery to alveoli is determined by the ventilation ($\dot{V}_A$) and the fraction of inspired O_2 (F_IO_2). But oxygen is also carried away in exhaled air. The air leaving alveoli has the alveolar oxygen concentration (F_AO_2). Thus the net O_2 delivery is given by $\dot{V}_A \times (F_IO_2 - F_AO_2)$. Oxygen removal is governed by tissue O_2 consumption. It varies with disease and activity, but under resting conditions it is approximately 250 ml/min for an average-sized person. In a steady state the alveolar O_2 level is not changing, so these processes of delivery and removal are equal. This relationship can be written as a conservation-of-mass equation stating that the oxygen consumed ($\dot{V}O_2$) equals that removed from the alveolar ventilation (none is removed from dead-space ventilation); thus

$$\dot{V}O_2 = \dot{V}_A(F_IO_2 - F_AO_2) \qquad [13]$$

Rearranging, we obtain

$$F_IO_2 - F_AO_2 = \frac{\dot{V}O_2}{\dot{V}_A} \qquad [14]$$

Converting to partial pressure and multiplying both sides by $P_B - 47$, we obtain

$$P_IO_2 - P_AO_2 = \frac{\dot{V}O_2}{\dot{V}_A}(P_B - 47) \qquad [15]$$

This is analogous to the alveolar ventilation equation (Eq. 10), for CO_2. Equation 15 shows that alveolar PO_2 is determined only by P_IO_2, $\dot{V}_A$, and $\dot{V}O_2$. If P_IO_2 and $\dot{V}O_2$ are constant and $\dot{V}_A$ goes up (hyperventilation), then P_AO_2 must go up, and if $\dot{V}_A$ goes down (hypoventilation), then P_AO_2 must go down.

Since $\dot{V}CO_2$ is the metabolic product of the O_2 consumption, the quantities $\dot{V}CO_2$ and $\dot{V}O_2$ are linked to one another. If they are identical ($R = 1$), then Eqs. 10 and 15 are identical on the right and show that the fall in PO_2 from inspired to alveolar air is exactly the same as the rise in PCO_2 from 0 to the alveolar level:

$$P_IO_2 - P_AO_2 = P_ACO_2 \qquad [16]$$

To understand arterial blood gas values in patients, it will be useful to estimate the P_AO_2. From the discussion above we can see that if $\dot{V}CO_2 = \dot{V}O_2$, then (rearranging the previous equation)

$$P_AO_2 = P_IO_2 - P_ACO_2 \qquad [17]$$

Since the arterial P_aCO_2 that we measure is very close to the P_ACO_2, we can rewrite Eq. 17:

$$P_AO_2 = P_IO_2 - P_aCO_2 \qquad [18]$$

$\dot{V}CO_2$ and $\dot{V}O_2$ are not necessarily identical but are closely linked, and their ratio ($\dot{V}CO_2/\dot{V}O_2$) is the respiratory quotient (RQ) or respiratory exchange ratio (R).

The approximate relationship described in Eq. 18 implicitly assumes that $R = 1$, $\dot{V}CO_2 = \dot{V}O_2$, and $\dot{V}_E = \dot{V}_I$. Under normal conditions, $R < 1$, $\dot{V}CO_2 < \dot{V}O_2$, and $\dot{V}_E > \dot{V}_I$. A more complete form of this alveolar gas equation that accounts for the change in gas volume is

$$P_AO_2 = P_IO_2 - P_aCO_2\left(F_IO_2 + \frac{1 - F_IO_2}{R}\right) \qquad [19]$$

When breathing 100% oxygen ($F_IO_2 = 1$), P_aCO_2 and P_AO_2 always equal P_IO_2, for any R.

For typical normal values ($R = 0.8$; $F_IO_2 = 0.21$; $P_IO_2 = 150$ mmHg; $P_aCO_2 = 40$ mmHg), P_AO_2 turns out to be about 100 mmHg:

$$P_AO_2 = 150 - 40\left(0.21 + \frac{1 - 0.21}{0.8}\right)$$

$$= 102 \text{ mmHg} \qquad [20]$$

This equation is often misinterpreted as indicating that alveolar O_2 is displaced by CO_2. This is incorrect, because the removal of O_2 and addition of CO_2 proceed as independent processes in the lung. But since the normal RQ in the tissues is approximately equal to 1, the loss of O_2 from the inspired air to the blood is approximately equal to the gain in CO_2.

Nitrogen Exchange

When $R \neq 1$, $\dot{V}_{CO_2} \neq \dot{V}_{O_2}$. Under such circumstances, the total amount of gas in the alveolus changes. Because the exchange of N_2 is so small, the total number of N_2 molecules in the alveolus remains unchanged. If the alveolar gas volume decreases (when $R < 1$), the relative fraction of N_2 increases and P_{N_2} increases. On the other hand, when $R > 1$, the opposite will occur and P_{N_2} decreases. Under normal circumstances, if $R = 0.8$, the alveolar P_{N_2} (and alveolar end-capillary blood P_{N_2}) is greater than inspired P_{N_2} (humidified) by about 10 mmHg. This difference occurs even though there is only minimal net nitrogen exchange.

Alveolar P_{O_2} and P_{CO_2} are both changing during the respiratory cycle because ventilation is periodic while $\dot{V}_{O_2}$ and $\dot{V}_{CO_2}$ are relatively constant. During inspiration, fresh air is delivered to the alveolus, causing P_{CO_2} to decrease and P_{O_2} to increase. During expiration, continuing gas exchange causes P_{CO_2} to increase and P_{O_2} to decrease. Even though the alveolar gas equations predict constant values for P_{CO_2} and P_{O_2}, the values actually fluctuate about the mean values by 3 mmHg and 5 mmHg for P_{CO_2} and P_{O_2}, respectively.

DEAD-SPACE VENTILATION

Anatomic Dead Space

The volume of the anatomic dead space in a normal adult male is 150–180 ml. (A commonly used approximation is that the V_D in milliliters equals lean body weight in pounds.) In a young normal individual the volume of the physiologic dead space is only slightly greater than this or about 25–35% of an average tidal volume (referred to as the V_D/V_T ratio). The anatomic dead space is not fixed; instead, it increases at higher lung volumes because the intrapulmonary airways increase in size along with the surrounding lung tissue. Breathing with an increased tidal volume is associated with only a modest decrease in V_D/V_T ratio. With exercise, tidal volume may increase to 2.5–3.0 liters and V_D/V_T normally falls to 10–15%. A contributing factor is the increase in pulmonary blood flow, which tends to eliminate any poorly perfused alveolar dead space. At the other extreme, it would seem that as tidal volume became small, approaching the anatomic dead

space, alveolar ventilation should fall to zero and gas exchange would be impossible. However, it has been demonstrated that gas exchange can be maintained even with tidal volumes equal to or smaller than the measured anatomic dead space if ventilation occurs at a sufficiently high frequency. Some fresh gas reaches alveoli because of interaction of physical mixing induced by high breathing frequencies (see Chapter 8.2.3).

Physiologic Dead Space

The ventilation wasted by ventilating dead space includes that going to anatomic dead space plus that to unperfused alveoli and a portion of that to poorly perfused alveoli. These poorly perfused (or excessively ventilated) areas can be considered as if they were made up of some perfect alveoli (normal gas exchange) and some unperfused alveoli. Thus the total physiologic dead space is not an anatomically identifiable volume but is, instead, an "as if" volume that we obtain by calculation. It reflects the inefficiency of ventilation as it affects CO_2 exchange.

The total expired volume of air per minute is considered to come from two sources: (i) ideal alveoli with $P_{A_{CO_2}} = P_{a_{CO_2}}$ and (ii) unperfused areas (conducting airways or alveolar dead space) with $P_{I_{CO_2}} = $ inspired $P_{CO_2} = 0$. The total expired volume of CO_2 comes entirely from the effective (non-dead-space) alveolar ventilation ($\dot{V}_E - \dot{V}_D$):

$$\dot{V}_{CO_2} = \dot{V}_E \times F_{E_{CO_2}}$$

$$= (\dot{V}_E - \dot{V}_D) \times F_{A_{CO_2}} + \dot{V}_D \times 0 \quad [21]$$

Algebraic manipulation yields

$$\dot{V}_D \times F_{A_{CO_2}} = \dot{V}_E \times F_{A_{CO_2}} - \dot{V}_E \times F_{E_{CO_2}} \quad [22]$$

$$\frac{V_D}{V_T} = \frac{F_{A_{CO_2}} - F_{E_{CO_2}}}{F_{A_{CO_2}}} \quad [23]$$

Multiplying top and bottom by $P_B - 47$ converts fraction to partial pressure:

$$\frac{V_D}{V_T} = \frac{P_{A_{CO_2}} - P_{E_{CO_2}}}{P_{A_{CO_2}}} \quad [24]$$

$P_{A_{CO_2}}$ cannot be measured easily, but since ideal alveoli with $P_{A_{CO_2}} = P_{a_{CO_2}}$ are assumed, the measured arterial blood gas value can be used. $P_{E_{CO_2}}$ is obtained from a collection of expired gas:

$$\frac{V_D}{V_T} = \frac{P_{a_{CO_2}} - P_{E_{CO_2}}}{P_{a_{CO_2}}} \quad [25]$$

By convention, V_D/V_T is referred to as the "wasted fraction" of each tidal breath. Multiplying this fraction by the tidal volume or minute ventilation gives the volume of physiologic dead space or wasted ventilation. Dead space thus has the effect of diluting the CO_2 content of expired air below the alveolar level. Since the body needs to expire a certain volume of CO_2 per minute, the effect of a low $P_{E}CO_2$ is to require more total ventilation to maintain homeostasis.

In carrying out a measurement of physiologic dead space, it must be remembered that the volume of air in mouthpiece, connections, and valve (mechanical dead space) will also contribute CO_2-free air to the expired collection.

SUGGESTED READING

Bohr C. Über die Lungenathmung. *Skand Arch Physiol* 1891;2:236–268.

Coffey RL, Albert RK, Robertson HT. Mechanisms of physiological dead space response to PEEP after acute oleic acid lung injury. *J Appl Physiol* 1973;224:838–847.

Enghoff H. Volumen inefficax. Bemerkungen zur Frage des schädlichen Raumes. *Upsala Laekarefoeren Foerh* 1938;44:191–218.

Fowler WS. Lung function studies. II. The respiratory dead space. *Am J Physiol* 1948;154:405–416.

Hlastala MP. A model of fluctuating alveolar gas exchange during the respiratory cycle. *Respir Physiol* 1972;15:224–232.

Riley RL, Lilienthal JL Jr, Proemmel D, Franke RE. On the determination of the physiologically effective pressure of oxygen and carbon dioxide in alveolar air. *Am J Physiol* 1946;147:191–198.

Severinghaus JW, Stupfel M. Alveolar dead space as an index of distribution of blood flow in pulmonary capillaries. *J Appl Physiol* 1957;10:335–348.

THE LUNG: Scientific Foundations
edited by R.G. Crystal, J.B. West et al.
Raven Press, Ltd., New York © 1991.

CHAPTER 5.3.2.1

Structural Biology of Hemoglobin

Christian Bauer

Hemoglobin is the major protein of the red blood cells that allows vertebrates to transport oxygen from the lungs to the tissues and that helps the return transport of carbon dioxide from the tissues to the lung. Hemoglobin is a protein tetramer consisting of 574 amino acids and has a relative molecular weight of about 64,500. The junior partner of hemoglobin is named *myoglobin* because it occurs in striated and smooth muscle as well as in most vertebrate hearts. Myoglobin is a protein monomer consisting of 153 amino acids and has a relative molecular weight of about 17,800. Both hemoglobin and myoglobin consist of a protein part, the *globin,* and of a component that binds oxygen, the *heme* group. The heme and the globin of hemoglobin, but not of myoglobin, interact with each other in that the protein controls the oxygen-binding properties of the heme, which, in turn, reports the absence or presence of oxygen to its protein environment (1).

Oxygen is a nonpolar molecule, and therefore its solubility in the polar water phase of the extra- and the intracellular space of the human body is very poor. The heme group, to which oxygen binds, is harbored within the protein part of myoglobin or hemoglobin. The term *heme* refers to a complex of a metal ion (e.g., Fe, Co, Cd, Mg, Mn) chelated in a porphyrin ring; the porphyrin is protoporphyrin IX. Heme, however, is customarily used in reference to the iron complex of such chelates. In turn, porphyrins are cyclic tetrapyrroles in which the four pyrrole rings are attached through four methene bridges labeled α, β, γ, and δ (Fig. 1). The central iron atom is kept in place by a complex formation between the four nitrogens of the porphyrin ring that additionally carries side chains helping the heme group to obtain the correct orientation within the protein part of myoglobin or hemoglo-

bin. The red color of blood and muscle is due to the fact that the complex consisting of iron and porphyrin carries a number of conjugated double bonds. Because of these spectral properties of the heme group, **our** blood has a red color when fully oxygenated and turns purple upon removal of oxygen. The fact that the heme group is literally embedded in the globin or protein part of hemoglobin and myoglobin is biologically very important because an iron can exist in two states of valency: (i) ferrous iron, carrying two positive charges, and (ii) ferric iron, carrying three positive charges, as in iron oxide or rust. Normally, ferrous iron, even if bound within the heme group, reacts with oxygen irreversibly to yield ferric heme. When embedded in the folds of the globin chain, ferrous heme is protected in such a way that its reaction with oxygen is reversible; this type of situation does not occur under any other circumstances. One of the mechanisms that enables heme to reversibly combine with oxygen is due to the linkage of iron within the protein to the amino acid histidine, which donates a negative charge and thus enables the iron to form a loose bond with oxygen. It follows from these facts that the interaction between the protein part and the heme group is of major importance for reversible linkage of oxygen with the heme group. Therefore, we will now turn to the protein part of hemoglobin, which provides a secure environment for the heme group.

GENERAL TERMINOLOGY OF PROTEIN BIOCHEMISTRY

It is customary to speak of the primary, secondary, tertiary, and quaternary structure of proteins. *Primary structure* refers to the amino acid sequence, which is the important determinant of the folding of a protein in three dimensions (2). The term *secondary structure* refers to the local conformation of the polypeptide chain, such as the α-*helix* or the β-*pleated* sheet; some

C. Bauer: Department of Physiology, University of Zürich, CH-8057 Zurich, Switzerland.

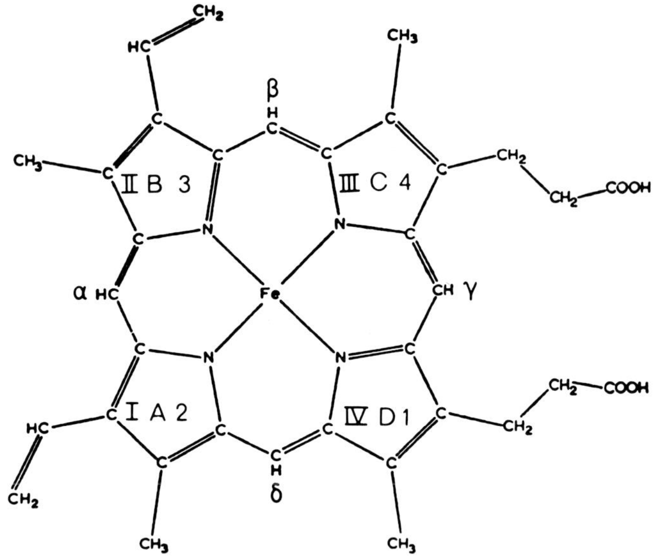

FIG. 1. Structure of heme, that is, of iron-protoporphyrin IX. Four pyrrole rings are linked by methene bridges to form a tetrapyrrole ring. Four methyl, two vinyl, and two propionate side chains are attached to the tetrapyrrole ring, thus forming protoporphyrin IX. The insertion of the ferros form of iron finally yields heme. (From ref. 1.)

fibrous proteins, such as myosin, are in the form of an α-helix, whereas others, such as silk fibroin, are in the form of a β-pleated sheet. One helix or coil consists of 3.6 amino acids per turn, with the side groups of the residues oriented externally in a radial fashion. Helical segments exhibit a periodic pattern of polar and nonpolar residues, the former in the interior and the latter in the exterior position. The *tertiary structure,* the next higher level of organization of a protein, is generated spontaneously because it represents a folding state with the least possible energy and therefore maximal stability (2). The stability of the tertiary structure is largely governed by hydrophobic interactions between the hydrocarbon side chains of the polypeptide. These hydrophobic side chains interact in a thermodynamically favorable way in that they turn away from the surrounding water phase and associate with each other, thus leading to the conformational nucleus of the tertiary structure. After completion of the conformational fold, the amino acids with strong hydrophobic side chains (e.g., valine, leucine, isoleucine, phenylalanine) are therefore clustered in the interior of the protein while the hydrophilic side chains (e.g., aspartate, glutamate, serine, threonine) lie at the surface of the molecule, where they form hydrogen bonds with the surrounding water molecules. The tertiary conformation of a protein can be further stabilized by hydrogen bonds (e.g., between the hydroxyl group of a tyrosine side chain and the keto group of the peptide bond) as well as by electrostatic interactions, such as those that occur in salt bridges [e.g., between the

amino group (NH_3^+) of lysine and the carboxyl group (COO^-) of glutamate]. Polymeric proteins, such as hemoglobin, have an additional degree of organization, namely, the *quaternary structure,* in which several subunits (polypeptide chains) assemble to form a functional unit. The subunits are usually held together by weak, noncovalent bonds such as hydrophobic interactions and hydrogen bonds. The amino acid side chains that are engaged in these bonds form clusters on the surface of the respective subunit and can therefore be regarded as recognition sites for subunit association.

MOLECULAR ANATOMY OF HEMOGLOBIN

Hemoglobin consists of four polypeptide chains: two identical α-subunits with 141 amino acids and two identical β-subunits with 146 amino acids. A comparison of the primary structure of the α- and β-subunits of hemoglobin and of myoglobin is given in Fig. 2. A detailed comparison of the amino acid sequence of the hemoglobin of many vertebrates has led to the conclusion that the present-day hemoglobins with optimized oxygen-binding properties have evolved by a number of gene duplications from an ancient homotetramer, consisting of β-like subunits, that was present some 450 million years ago (3,4). The adaptive evolution of the structure of hemoglobin is highlighted by the fact that the amino acids responsible for cooperative oxygen binding and heme fixation are invariant throughout the jawed vertebrates (3–5). This conservation of functionally important amino acid residues is reflected in the structure of the globin gene, in which the exons of the genes correspond with structural domains in the protein (6–8). As in myoglobin, the secondary structure of α- and β-subunits of hemoglobin is characterized by a high content of α-helices (about 75%). The length of these helices varies between 7 and 23 amino acids. The β- and α-subunits possess a total of 8 and 7 helices, respectively. In myoglobin, the number of α-helices is the same as the number of β-subunits. Despite the fact that only 25 of the 153 amino acids of myoglobin are found at the same position in the hemoglobin subunits, all three polypeptide chains have a surprisingly similar tertiary structure (9,10). This strongly indicates that the overall conformation depends upon only a few amino acids in key positions: those forming the hydrophobic nucleus (leucine, isoleucine, valine) and the ones engaged in heme binding (9,11).

The helices are designated A through H, starting from the amino end; the nonhelical segments that lie between the helices are named AB, BC, CD, and so on. The nonhelical parts at the N-terminus and the C-terminus of the protein chain are called NA and HC.

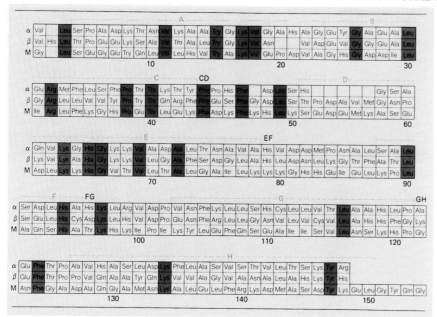

FIG. 2. Primary structure of the α- and β-subunits of human hemoglobin and of horse myoglobin. Invariant positions are indicated by gray shading. The dashed lines with letters indicate the helices A to H.

The α-subunits differ from the β-subunits in that the latter ones were shown to have eight helical segments, lettered A through H, whereas the residues making up the D helix of the β-subunit are absent in the α-subunit (Fig. 2). Amino acid residues within each helical segment are numbered from the amino end: A_1, A_2, CD_1, and so on. Accordingly, amino acid residues in polypeptide chains of various hemoglobins and of myoglobin can be assigned helical designations. For example, the heme-linked histidine F8 is amino acid number 8 in helix F.

The surface of the α- and β-subunits has nonpolar patches that allow them to form the $α_2β_2$-tetramer. The four subunits are joined by a total of six contacts, four of which are unique as a result of the symmetrical architecture of hemoglobin: $α_1β_1 = α_2β_2$; $α_1β_2 = α_2β_1$; $α_1α_2$ and $β_1β_2$. The four subunits are held together via hydrophobic interactions and by hydrogen bonds, as well as by electrostatic interactions of salt bridges. These noncovalent interactions allow the subunits to move relative to each other without requiring much energy to do so, a prerequisite for the functionally important change of the quaternary conformation upon the reversible interaction of oxygen with the heme group. Among the contacts between the subunits, only the most extensive one, the $α_1β_1$-contact, remains the same upon oxygen binding while all the other contacts change.

The surface of the hemoglobin tetramer is studded with many polar residues that are all hydrated and that therefore contribute to the high solubility of hemoglobin, which, in turn, allows a dense packing of hemoglobin within red blood cells, each of which contains 300 million molecules of tetrameric hemoglobin and four times as many oxygen-binding sites. Thus, the fact that our blood can transport 70 times more oxygen in the bound compared to the dissolved form is a direct consequence of the high solubility of hemoglobin, which, in turn, is related to the high proportion of polar side chains on the surface of the molecule.

THE INTERACTION OF HEME WITH GLOBIN

As was mentioned above, the prosthetic group of hemoglobin is ferro-protoporphyrin IX, commonly known as *heme*. High-resolution x-ray studies have provided precise information on the details of the linkage between heme and globin. The heme is wedged into a pocket or cleft between the helices E and F, with its hydrocarbon side chains buried deep in the hydrophobic interior of the cleft and with its polar propionated side chains oriented towards the hydrophilic surface of the subunit. The heme iron is covalently linked to the imidazole nitrogen of the "proximal" histidine F8, the only covalent bond of heme with globin. Inside the cleft, the position of the heme is further stabilized by a large number of contacts between the protoporphyrin ring and the hydrophobic side chains consisting of about 20 amino acid residues (Figs. 3 and 4). The entirety of these interactions yields a high degree of complementarity between the structure of the heme and the orientation of the hydrophobic side chains (12–14). There is one more interesting feature connected with the structure of the heme pocket that deserves mention: At its entrance are conveniently located two positively charged lysyl residues (lysine E1 and lysine FG2) that are essential for the reduction of the oxidized hemoglobin (methemoglobin), which has ferriheme

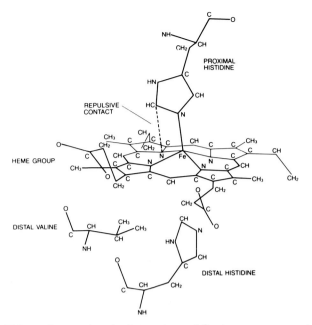

FIG. 3. Stereochemical structure of the heme group and surrounding amino acids. The only covalent bond between the heme and the globin is between the heme iron and the amino acid at the top, called the *proximal histidine* (F8). The proximal histidine is the principal path for communication between the heme and the rest of the molecule. The repulsive contact (*dashed line*) is typical for the deoxy state, where the iron protrudes above the porphyrin and may be hindered from returning to a centered position by the repulsive forces between one corner of the proximal histidine and one of the porphyrin nitrogen atoms. (From ref. 35.)

(Fe^{3+}) instead of ferroheme (Fe^{2+}). Because methemoglobin cannot bind oxygen, it must be reduced back to ferrohemoglobin by enzyme systems—the most important of which is cytochrome b_5, also a heme protein. Cytochrome b_5 carries acid groups around the entrance to its heme pocket. Combination between the two complementarily charged parts at the opening of the heme pocket allows hemoglobin and cytochrome b_5 to bring their respective heme groups close enough so that an electron can be transferred from the cytochrome b_5 onto the ferric heme (15,16).

BINDING OF OXYGEN TO THE HEME IRON

The first observation that provided evidence for an oxygen-induced change in the conformation of hemoglobin was made by Haurowitz (17) in 1938. Haurowitz observed that when crystals of horse deoxyhemoglobin were exposed to oxygen, extensive disintegration of the hemoglobin crystals took place. This observation provided strong evidence that oxygenation causes a dramatic change in the overall structure of hemoglobin, and it also provided a strong

incentive for Max Perutz to examine the three-dimensional structure of deoxyhemoglobin and oxyhemoglobin by using the technique of x-ray diffraction and Fourier summation (11,16,18,19). Before describing the main changes of the hemoglobin structure when it switches from the oxy to the deoxy conformation, let us first briefly look at the binding of oxygen to the heme iron that provides the crucial trigger mechanism for the conformational change of the globin part of hemoglobin.

Diatomic or molecular oxygen is bound to the iron atom by an end-on geometry with an Fe–O–O angle of about 155°; that is, the oxygen is tilted away from the axis perpendicular to the heme plane (see Fig. 5, 6 and ref. 16). As can be seen from Fig. 1, the iron

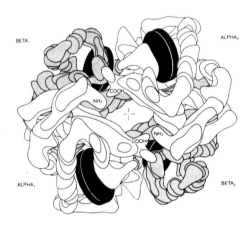

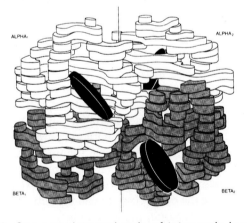

FIG. 4. One complete molecule of tetrameric hemoglobin is made up of four subunits, each of which consists of one polypeptide chain and one heme. The α-subunit consists of 141 amino acids and seven helices. The β-subunit is 146 amino acids long and has eight helices. The four subunits are arranged at the vertexes of a tetrahedron around an axis of twofold symmetry. The dark disks represent the heme groups, each of which lies in a separate pocket at the surface of the molecule. The overall structure of tetrameric hemoglobin is roughly spherical (6.5 × 5.5 × 5.0 nm). (From ref. 35.)

atom occupies the center of the porphyrin ring. The electronic configuration of ferrous iron is as follows: $1s^2\ 2s^2\ 2p^6\ 3s^2\ 3p^6\ 3d^6$. The outermost $3d$ electrons determine the physicochemical properties of the heme iron, such as *visible spectra* and the *ionic radius*. Iron in deoxyhemoglobin is five-coordinated with the four pyrrole nitrogens of porphyrin and the imidazole nitrogen of the proximal histidine. In this state, one of the six $3d$ electrons is forced to pair with one of the other five electrons that are on energetically equivalent orbitals. This results in a state with four unpaired electrons in the d orbitals of the metal ion. However, in oxyhemoglobin the iron is six-coordinated, leading to a state where the electrons are all paired; that is, there are no unpaired electrons in oxyhemoglobin. This pairing of the electrons leads to a reduction of magnetic moment or spin state in oxyhemoglobin compared to that in deoxyhemoglobin, which also explains the difference of the visible spectra between oxy- and deoxyhemoglobin (1,9).

THE TRIGGER MECHANISM INDUCING THE CONFORMATIONAL CHANGE IN HEMOGLOBIN

The spin changes accompanying the binding of oxygen give rise to stereochemical changes in the heme itself, which is the key to the conformational changes of hemoglobin, a prerequisite for cooperativity of oxygen binding and allosteric effects such as the Bohr effect. The main feature of the trigger mechanism that leads to these changes in the overall structure of hemoglobin is a relative movement of the heme iron when oxygen is bound or released.

In oxyhemoglobin, where the iron is in the low-spin configuration, the iron lies in the plane of the porphyrin ring; moreover, the distance from the iron to the porphyrin nitrogens is the shortest possible. In deoxyhemoglobin the ligand site is vacant, making the iron five-coordinated; as a result of the electronic changes, the iron is pushed and pulled out of the porphyrin plane toward the proximal histidine by about 0.6 Å. Thus, in deoxyhemoglobin the bond between the iron atom and the imidazole of the proximal histidine is under increased strain. In addition, the four pyrrole rings tilt about their methene bridges, making the porphyrin domed toward the proximal histidine. In summary, the subtle electronic changes that accompany the reaction of heme iron with oxygen leads to a reorientation of the heme iron when oxygen is bound or removed: The bond between the imidazole nitrogen is shortened in deoxyhemoglobin compared to that in oxyhemoglobin, by about 0.6 Å; in addition, the porphyrins are domed or ruffled in deoxyhemoglobin but not in oxyhemoglobin (1,9,19). These changes of the electronic configu-

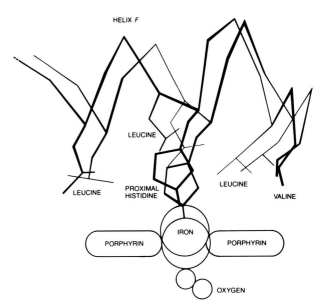

FIG. 5. The triggering mechanism for the switch from the T to the R structure of hemoglobin is a movement of the heme iron by about 0.6 Å into the plane of the porphyrin. Once the iron is in the heme plane, it can readily combine with oxygen. The movement of the heme iron leads to a displacement of the proximal histidine and helix F. These movements are transmitted to the contacts between the subunits and promote the transition of the T structure towards the R structure. (From ref. 35.)

ration are transmitted to the protein, as shown in Fig. 5. The most marked differences between the two structures are found at the C termini and the reactive cysteine F9β. In deoxyhemoglobin the hydroxyls of tyrosine HC2 and the carbonyls of valine FG5 form a hydrogen bond. Furthermore, the pocket between helices F and H is fully occupied by the side chain of tyrosine HC2, which allows no room for the side chain of cysteine F9. When oxygen binds to the heme group with the resulting change in the iron geometry, the pocket between helices F and H becomes narrower by 1.8 Å in the α-subunit and by 1.5 Å in the β-subunit (1,9). In addition, there is a lengthening of the bond between the hydroxyls of tyrosine HC2 and the carbonyls of valine FG5. The narrowing of the pocket, accompanied by the lengthening of the bond, leads to displacement of the tyrosine out of the pocket and pulls the C termini with it so that the Tyr and the C termini can no longer have electrostatic interactions with their respective counterparts (Fig. 6).

EFFECTS OF OXYGEN BINDING ON THE QUATERNARY STRUCTURE OF HEMOGLOBIN

Before entering into considerations of how the stereochemistry of the heme is transmitted to the entirety of

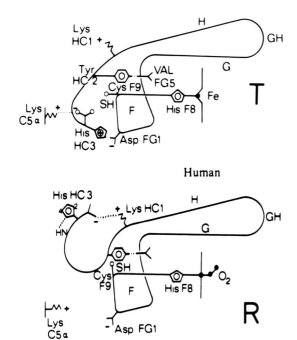

FIG. 6. In deoxyhemoglobin the β-subunits form extra bonds that are broken in oxyhemoglobin. These extra bonds are (i) between tyrosine HC2 and valine FG5 and (ii) between histidine HC3, aspartate FG1, and lysine C5 of the α-subunits. The trigger mechanism shown in Fig. 5 leads to a structural rearrangement and to a rupture of these bonds when oxygen is bound to the heme iron. (From ref. 9.)

the globin, it is necessary to introduce some of the terminology that is used in connection with the different properties of deoxy- and oxyhemoglobin. Deoxyhemoglobin is said to be in the *T state*, and oxyhemoglobin is considered to be in the *R state*. T stands for "tense," and R stands for "relaxed"; this nomenclature stems from a paper by Monod et al. (20) in which they put forward a general theory of allosteric enzymes, of which hemoglobin is a case in point (20). In this terminology the T state of hemoglobin has a low oxygen affinity whereas the R state of hemoglobin has an oxygen affinity that is about 150 times higher than that of the T structure (21). The transition between these conformational states is induced by the tiny movement of the heme iron when oxygen is bound or removed; this transition has dramatic consequences for the overall structure of hemoglobin (22,23).

The α- and β-subunits of hemoglobin form a tetrahedron having a twofold or dyad axis of symmetry. This axis runs down a water-filled cavity in the center of the molecule. On transition from the deoxy to the oxy structure, two αβ-dimers making up half of the tetrahedron move relative to each other along the $\alpha_1\beta_2$-contact, which is, from considerations of symmetry, identical to the $\alpha_2\beta_1$-interface. In contrast, the contacts between the α_1- and β_1-subunits and between the

α_2- and β_2-subunits are identical in oxyhemoglobin and deoxyhemoglobin (Fig. 7). The most interesting changes that occur in hemoglobin upon the binding or the release of oxygen occur in the $\alpha_1\beta_2$- and $\alpha_2\beta_1$-contacts. These contacts are dovetailed so that a turn of the C helix by one subunit fits into a V-shaped groove formed by the α-carbon of valine FG5 of the other subunit. The dovetailing and the respective hydrogen donor and acceptor sites are constructed in such a way that only two relative positions of the two subunits are stable. This is the structural basis for the two-state model that explains most of the physiological properties of hemoglobin (22,23). The cooperativity of oxygen binding is the direct consequence of the fact that hemoglobin can assume the two alternative structures just described: the liganded R structure whose oxygen affinity is high and the deoxy T structure whose oxygen affinity is lowered by molecular constraints such as salt bridges and the binding of organic phosphates (23). In order to provide a structural correlate for these allosteric effects on hemoglobin function, we will now briefly look at the difference between oxy- and deoxyhemoglobin with respect to their interactions with organic phosphates, protons, and carbon dioxide.

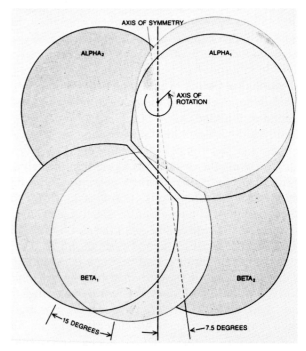

FIG. 7. Schematic diagram illustrating the change in quaternary structure that accompanies ligation of hemoglobin. On going from the T structure to the R structure, one pair of subunits rotates with respect to the other pair of subunits. If one dimer consisting of $\alpha_1\beta_1$ is held fixed, the other turns by 15° about an off-center axis and also shifts along it. The axis of symmetry rotates by 7.5°, while the twofold symmetry is preserved. (From ref. 35.)

INTERACTION OF HEMOGLOBIN WITH ORGANIC PHOSPHATES

The erythrocytes of humans and most other mammals (ruminants are a notable exception) have a very high concentration of the glycolytic intermediate 2,3-diphosphoglycerate (DPG). Its concentration within the red blood cell is normally about 5 mmol per liter of packed erythrocytes, equivalent to the concentration of tetrameric hemoglobin. DPG has a total of five titratable groups and carries about 3.5 negative charges at physiologic pH values. It binds to deoxyhemoglobin much more tightly than to oxyhemoglobin, in a 1:1 molar ratio (24). Accordingly, linkage equations can be written, similar to those for the oxygen-linked protons and oxygen-linked carbamino formation. The net reaction is as follows:

$$Hb_4\ (DPG) + 4O_2 \rightleftharpoons Hb_4(D_2)_4 + DPG$$

DPG is either bound to the central cavity or is deoxygenated hemoglobin to form a number of positively charged residues. The binding is electrostatic; in human hemoglobin, it includes the N-terminal α-amino group of the β-subunit, the imidazole groups of histidine H21(143)β and histidine NA2(2)β, and the ε-amino group of lysine EF6(82)β (25). The DPG binding site in deoxyhemoglobin is constructed to make it complementary to the phosphate, both sterically and electrostatically (Fig. 8).

In oxyhemoglobin, on the other hand, the EF and H segments of the β-subunits are too close together and the NA segments are too far apart to permit a snug fit; this results in a loss of complementarity and an ejection of the DPG molecule, with a drop in the affinity constant of DPG and hemoglobin that amounts to two orders of magnitude at physiological pH, temperature, and salt concentration (26). Interestingly, human fetal hemoglobin ($\alpha_2\gamma_2$) has a lower affinity for DPG than does adult human hemoglobin ($\alpha_2\beta_2$), a fact that can quantitatively account for the higher oxygen affinity of fetal blood compared to that of adult blood (26). The low affinity of fetal hemoglobin for DPG is caused mainly by the substitution histidine H21(143)β → serine, which reduces the cationic DPG binding groups from eight to six per tetramer; however, the changed conformation of the N-terminal segment, as well as the resultant increase in the distance of valine NA1(1)γ from the dyad axis of symmetry, may also contribute (27,28). Therefore, the high oxygen affinity of human fetal blood is the direct effect of a slight molecular modification in fetal, as compared to adult, hemoglobin. This is an interesting example of an oxygen-carrying protein in which new functions are created with very few amino acid exchanges at strategically important parts of the molecule (28). Other examples include the molecular adaptation of hemoglobin to hypoxia in a bird, namely the bar-headed goose (28,29), and in an adult mammal, namely the llama (26).

PROTON BINDING AND SALT BRIDGES

Salt bridges are defined as hydrogen bonds between oppositely charged ions, such as a positively charged guanidium side chain of arginine and a negatively charged carboxyl side chain of aspartic acid. The rearrangement of the quaternary structure that occurs upon oxygen binding leads to an increase in distance between the partners that form the salt bridges in deoxyhemoglobin, a fact commonly and illustratively referred to as the *breakage of the salt bridges*. What are

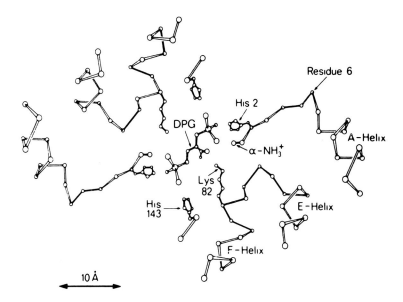

FIG. 8. The binding of negatively charged DPG to human deoxyhemoglobin. The stereochemistry of the polyanion DPG complements the basic residues of the central cavity to form salt bridges, thus stabilizing the T structure of human hemoglobin. (From ref. 25.)

the functional consequences of this disruption of the electrostatic forces that stabilize deoxyhemoglobin? The answer to this question can be derived by the fact that the apparent pK value of the respective partners (e.g., guanidium of arginine and carboxylate of aspartic acid) rises when a salt bridge is formed and drops when it is broken. Therefore, the likelihood for a proton to be set free in solution is higher in oxyhemoglobin than in deoxyhemoglobin. This difference in proton binding between oxy- and deoxyhemoglobin is the basis for the dependency of the oxygen affinity of hemoglobin upon pH, also known as the *Bohr effect*. Quantitatively, one has to account for about 2.0 H$^+$ that are set free upon oxygenation at neutral pH, in the absence of DPG, according to the following reaction:

$$Hb_4(H)_2 + 4O_2 \rightleftharpoons Hb_4(O_2)_4 + 2H^+$$

Protons are liberated upon oxygen binding from the following pairs of salt bridges: One pair lies between trapped chloride ions and valines NA1(1)α, another pair between histidines HC3(146)β and aspartates FG1(94)β, another pair between valines NA1(1)β and DPG, and finally one between histidines H21(143) and DPG (9,30). The sum of the changes in the apparent pK of these groups gives rise to the *alkaline Bohr effect* (pH effect on oxygen affinity) and to the difference in proton binding between oxy- and deoxyhemoglobin (*Haldane effect*). It follows from these interactions that both the Bohr effect and the Haldane effect must be smaller in the absence of DPG than in its presence, which is indeed found experimentally.

DIFFERENCES IN CARBAMINO FORMATION IN OXY- AND DEOXYHEMOGLOBIN

Carbon dioxide can directly bind to the unprotonated forms of amino groups according to the following reactions:

$$Hb-NH_3 \rightleftharpoons Hb-NH_2 + H^+$$

$$Hb-NH_2 + CO_2 \rightleftharpoons Hb-NH\,COO^- + H^+$$

The complex that is generated between the electron-poor carbon atom of CO$_2$ and the electron-rich amino group is named a *carbamino complex*. It can, in principle, be formed at the ϵ-amino groups of lysine residues and at the N-terminal α-amino groups. At physiological pH, almost all of the carbamino complexes are found at the terminal α-amino groups, which is due to the fact that only the unprotonated form of the amino group is able to accept CO$_2$. The ϵ-amino groups of the lysine residues have a pK of about 9, whereas the pK of the α-amino terminals is close to 7. Because carbamino formation can only proceed when the amino group is unprotonated, one can easily calculate that in

the physiological pH range, less than 1% of the ϵ-amino groups, but 50% of the α-amino groups, are available for the reaction with CO$_2$.

It has been known for some time that deoxyhemoglobin binds more CO$_2$ as carbamate than does oxyhemoglobin (31,32). Furthermore, it became apparent that about 80% of this oxygen-linked carbamate is confined to the β-subunits at physiological pH (33). The reason for the difference in the oxygen-linked carbamate formation between the N termini of the α- and β-subunits is twofold: (i) The pK value of the N-terminal α-amino groups of the α-subunits (valine NA1) H increases with deoxygenation from 7.0 to 7.8, thereby inhibiting carbamate formation, whereas the pK value of the terminal α-amino group of the β-subunit remains more or less constant at around 7.0, irrespective of the degree of oxygenation (30). (ii) The carbamate formed at the N-terminal α-amino group of the β-subunits (valine NA1) H is stabilized by positively charged groups that are found in the direct neighborhood of the N termini of the β-subunits in deoxyhemoglobin. During the process of oxygenation, these positively charged groups swing away with a consec-

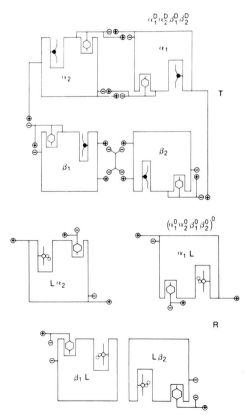

FIG. 9. Diagrammatic representation of the quaternary configuration of deoxyhemoglobin **(top)** and oxyhemoglobin **(bottom)**. Intrasubunit and intersubunit salt bridges (electrostatic interactions) are broken upon oxygenation, which also leads to an expulsion of DPG. (From ref. 22.)

utive decrease in stabilizing forces and release of CO_2 from the carbamino binding sites. On the basis of crystallographic results, it was proposed that the interaction that stabilizes the carbamate formed at the N termini of the β-subunits is a salt bridge between the carbamate anion and the ε-amino group of lysine EF6(82)β in deoxyhemoglobin and thus further contributes to the much stronger formation of oxygen-linked carbamate at the β-subunits (34).

SUMMARY

The change in quaternary configuration is shown diagrammatically in Fig. 9. As the four heme groups are successively populated by oxygen molecules, the inter- and intrasubunit bonds successively break. DPG, CO_2, and protons are released mainly after the main switch from the deoxygenated T structure to the oxygenated R structure, which occurs after the binding of the third oxygen molecule (16). Therefore, all the interactions with heterotropic ligands stabilize the T structure of hemoglobin, which leads to a macroscopic decrease in the oxygen affinity if the concentration of one or more of these cofactors is increased. The T→ R conformational switch is not only the basis for the modulation of the oxygen affinity by heterotropic ligands but is also the basis for the cooperativity of oxygen binding (i.e., the heme–heme interaction).

REFERENCES

1. Perutz MF. Regulation of oxygen affinity of hemoglobin. Influence of structure of the globin on the heme iron. *Annu Rev Biochem* 1979;48:327–386.
2. Jaenicke R. Folding and association of proteins. *Prog Biophys Mol Biol* 1987;49:117–237.
3. Goodman M. Decoding the pattern of protein evolution. *Prog Biophys Mol Biol* 1981;38:105–164.
4. Goodman M, Weiss ML, Czelusniak J. Molecular evolution above the species level: branching pattern, rates and mechanisms. *Syst Zool* 1982;31:376–399.
5. Lehmann H, Huntsman RG. *Man's haemoglobins.* Amsterdam: North-Holland, 1974.
6. Eaton WA. The relationship between coding sequences and function of haemoglobin. *Nature* 1980;284:183–185.
7. Gilbert W. DNA sequencing and gene structure. *Science* 1981;214:1305–1312.
8. Go M. Correlation of DNA exonic regions with protein structural units in haemoglobin. *Nature* 1981;291:90–92.
9. Perutz MF. Molecular anatomy, physiology, and pathology of hemoglobin. In: Stamatoyannopoulos G, Nienhuis AW, Leder P, Majerus PW, eds. *The molecular basis of blood disease.* Philadelphia: WB Saunders, 1987;127–178.
10. Kendrew JC. The three-dimensional structure of a protein molecule. *Sci Am* 1961;205:96–110.
11. Fermi G, Perutz MF, Shaanan B, Fourme R. The crystal structure of human deoxyhemoglobin at 1.74 Å resolution. *J Mol Biol* 1984;175:159–174.
12. Muirhaed H, Cox JM, Mazzarella L, Perutz MF. Structure and function of haemoglobin. III. A three dimensional Fourier synthesis of human deoxy-haemoglobin at 5.5 Å resolution. *J Mol Biol* 1967;28:117–156.
13. Perutz MF, Muirhaed H, Cox JM, Goaman LCG. Three dimensional Fourier synthesis of horse oxyhaemoglobin at 2.8 Å resolution: the atomic model. *Nature* 1968;219:131–139.
14. Dickerson RE, Geis I. *Hemoglobin: structure and function.* Menlo Park, CA: Benjamin/Cummings, 1983.
15. Gacon G, Lostanlen D, Labie D, Kaplan JC. Interaction between cytochrome b5 and hemoglobin: involvement of β66 (E10) and β95 (FG2) lysyl residues of hemoglobin. *Proc Natl Acad Sci USA* 1980;77:1917–1921.
16. Bunn HF, Forget BG. *Hemoglobin: molecular, genetic and clinical aspects.* Philadelphia: WB Saunders, 1986.
17. Haurowitz F. Das Gleichgewicht zwischen Hämoglobin und Sauerstoff. *Hoppe-Seyler's Z Physiol Chem* 1938;254:266–274.
18. Shaanan B. Structure of human oxyhaemoglobin at 2.1 Å resolution. *J Mol Biol* 1983;171:31–59.
19. Perutz MF. Hemoglobin structure and respiratory transport. *Sci Am* 1978;239:92–125.
20. Monod J, Wyman J, Changeux JP. On the nature of allosteric transitions: a plausible model. *J Mol Biol* 1965;12:88–118.
21. Imai K. *Allosteric effects in haemoglobin.* Cambridge, England: Cambridge University Press, 1982.
22. Perutz MF. Stereochemistry of cooperative effects in haemoglobin. *Nature* 1970;228:726–739.
23. Perutz MF. Nature of haem–haem interaction. *Nature* 1972;237:495–499.
24. Benesch R, Benesch RE. Intracellular organic phosphates as regulators of oxygen release by haemoglobin. *Nature* 1969;221:618–622.
25. Arnone A. X-ray diffraction study of binding of 2,3-diphosphoglycerate to human deoxyhemoglobin. *Nature* 1972;237:146–149.
26. Bauer C, Rollema HS, Till HW, Braunitzer G. Phosphate binding by llama and camel haemoglobin. *J Comp Physiol* 1980;136:67–70.
27. Frier JA, Perutz MF. Structure of human fetal deoxyhaemoglobin. *J Mol Biol* 1977;112:97–112.
28. Perutz MF. Species adaptation in a protein molecule. *Mol Biol Evol* 1983;1:1–28.
29. Rollema HS, Bauer C. The interaction of inositol pentaphosphate with the hemoglobins of highland and lowland geese. *J Biol Chem* 1979;254:12038–12043.
30. Perutz MF, Muirhaed H, Mazzarella L, Crowther RA, Greer J, Kilmartin JV. Identification of residues responsible for the alkaline Bohr effect in haemoglobin. *Nature* 1969;222:1240–1243.
31. Kilmartin JV, Rossi-Bernardi L. Interaction of hemoglobin with hydrogen ions, carbon dioxide and organic phosphates. *Physiol Rev* 1973;53:836–890.
32. Perrella M, Bresciani D, Rossi-Bernardi L. The binding of CO_2 to human hemoglobin. *J Biol Chem* 1975;250:5413–5418.
33. Bauer C, Baumann R, Engels U, Pacyna B. The carbon dioxide affinity of various human hemoglobins. *J Biol Chem* 1975;250:2173–2176.
34. Arnone A. X-ray studies of the interaction of CO_2 with human deoxyhemoglobin. *Nature* 1974;247:143–144.
35. Perutz MF. Hemoglobin structure and respiratory transport. *Sci Am* 1978;239:68–83.

THE LUNG: Scientific Foundations
edited by R.G. Crystal, J.B. West et al.
Raven Press, Ltd., New York © 1991.

CHAPTER 5.3.2.2

Oxygen–Hemoglobin Dissociation Curve

Robert M. Winslow and Luigi Rossi-Bernardi

The relationship between the fractional saturation of hemoglobin with oxygen and oxygen partial pressure, P_{O_2}, under equilibrium conditions is the familiar oxygen equilibrium curve (OEC) of hemoglobin (Fig. 1). Its position is often represented by the value P_{50}, the P_{O_2} at half-saturation. If oxygen affinity increases, the OEC shifts left (reduced P_{50}). If oxygen affinity decreases, the OEC shifts right (increased P_{50}). The principal physiologic effectors of hemoglobin function within the red cell, the molecules which cause such shifts, are H^+, 2,3-diphosphoglycerate (2,3-DPG), and CO_2. Other effectors, Cl^- and adenosine triphosphate (ATP), also decrease O_2 affinity, but their physiologic roles are minor. The OEC is very sensitive to temperature.

The sigmoid shape of the hemoglobin OEC is of great importance because it allows the normal loading and unloading of oxygen under physiologic conditions (1). Myoglobin, isolated α and β chains of hemoglobin, and $\alpha\beta$ subunits bind oxygen with such high affinity that no effective oxygen release could occur at tissue sites. This is illustrated in Fig. 1, which compares the equilibrium curves for hemoglobin and myoglobin under identical conditions. In the human alveolus the oxygen tension is about 90 torr and in resting tissues it is about 40 torr. It is apparent from Fig. 1 that at 40 torr, hemoglobin can release about 23% of its oxygen load. If myoglobin were the respiratory pigment in blood, P_{O_2} in the tissues would have to reach about 16 torr before an equivalent amount of O_2 could be released. Since the oxygen affinity of α or β hemoglobin chains (or of $\alpha\beta$ dimers) is approximately that of myoglobin, we can see that the tetrameric structure of hemoglobin is necessary for its suitably low oxygen affinity.

Although hemoglobin also acts as a buffer inside the red cell, the reciprocal transport of the respiratory gases, O_2 and CO_2, between tissues and lungs is its main function. The molecular properties underlying these functions are the cooperative binding of oxygen to heme sites, the Bohr effect, and the interactions of small molecules which alter oxygen binding. All these properties are closely interrelated with extraordinary intricacy.

EQUILIBRIUM MODELS

Empirical Description: Hill Model

Early physiologists observed the sigmoid nature of the OEC and concluded that oxygen binding increased during progressive oxygenation. They felt that this reflected interaction between heme sites so that oxygen binding to one site made binding at the next site more likely. They called this phenomenon "cooperativity."

Hill's empirical equation (see ref. 1),

$$\log\left(\frac{Y}{1-Y}\right) = n\log(p) + k \qquad [1]$$

relates hemoglobin saturation (Y) to oxygen tension (p). The constant k is the y-axis intercept. When plotted according to this equation, the major portion of the OEC falls on a straight line with slope (n) proportional to the degree of cooperativity. It was found that n for hemoglobin was about 3 and that n for myoglobin, devoid of cooperativity, was 1. This mathematical model provides no information about the mechanism of O_2 binding, but the use of Hill's parameter, n, as an index of cooperativity has persisted in the literature.

R. M. Winslow: Blood Research Department, Letterman Army Institute of Research, Presidio of San Francisco, San Francisco, California 94129.

L. Rossi-Bernardi: Via Selice Poggi 14, Milano 20131, Italy.

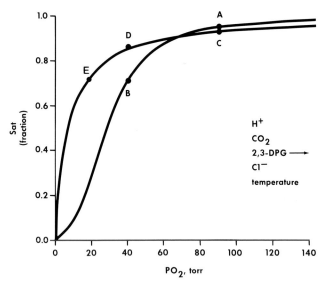

FIG. 1. The normal whole-blood oxygen equilibrium curve. P_{50} is the P_{O_2} at which hemoglobin is half-saturated with O_2. The principal effectors that alter the position and shape of the curve are indicated. Note that while both the hemoglobin and myoglobin curves allow saturation of about 95% at normal P_{AO_2} (points A and C), hemoglobin unloads 23% of its O_2 (point B) and myoglobin only 7% (point D) at 40 torr. In order for myoglobin to deliver 23% of bound O_2, a venous P_{O_2} of about 16 torr would result in this example (point E).

Partially Liganded Intermediates: Adair Model

A more general approach to the quantitation of the oxygenation of hemoglobin was made by Adair (2), who recognized that hemoglobin was made up of four subunits, each of which could bind a single O_2 molecule. He derived equations for the stepwise oxygenation of hemoglobin:

$$Hb(O_2)_i + O_2 \rightarrow Hb(O_2)_{i+1} \qquad [2]$$

where i ranges from 0 to 3, and the association equilibrium constants for the reactions could be represented as

$$K_i = \frac{[Hb(O_2)_{i+1}]}{[Hb(O_2)_i][O_2]} \qquad [3]$$

Combining the four resulting equations, we obtain

$$Y =$$

$$\frac{K_1 p + K_2 K_2 p^2 + K_1 K_2 K_3 p^3 + K_1 K_2 K_3 K_4 p^4}{1 + 4(K_1 p + K_1 K_2 p^2 + K_1 K_2 K_3 p^3 + K_1 K_2 K_3 K_4 p^4)}$$

$$[4]$$

where Y is the fractional saturation of hemoglobin with oxygen, the Ks are the equilibrium constants for the individual combinations of O_2 with hemoglobin, and p

is the partial pressure of O_2. Equation 4 is usually simplified by combining the equilibrium constants:

$$Y = \frac{a_1 p + 2a_2 p^2 + 3a_3 p^3 + 4a_4 p^4}{4(1 + a_1 p + a_2 p^2 + a_3 p^3 + a_4 p^4)} \qquad [5]$$

The new parameters (a's) are called "Adair parameters."

One difficulty with the Adair scheme is that it is too general: Unique values of the a's are difficult to determine experimentally, and therefore the Ks are nearly impossible to determine because of the high degree of interdependence among the parameters (3,4). In addition, the model is structure-independent, and thus it is of little help in conceptualizing structure–function relationships. Nevertheless, it is possible to describe the OEC by the Adair parameters, and this has practical utility even if the values are not unique.

Using experimentally derived values for the Adair parameters of human blood (5), the concentration of each of the partially liganded intermediates can be calculated. As shown in Fig. 2, the concentration of $Hb(O_2)_3$ is very low at all saturation levels. This is consistent with the notion that molecules undergo a conformational switch when the third O_2 binds, such that binding of the fourth O_2 is almost instantaneous.

Unless the affinities of the α- and β-chain O_2-binding sites are identical, the scheme proposed by Adair is an oversimplification, since a variety of intermediate molecules is possible (Fig. 3). Low-temperature quenching techniques have been developed by Perrella and Rossi-Bernardi (6) which verify the presence and amounts of partially liganded intermediates. The in-

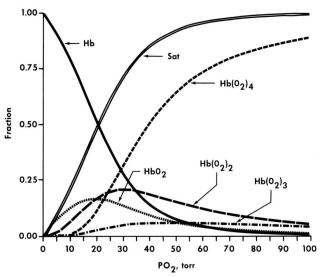

FIG. 2. Partially liganded O_2 intermediates calculated from the "Adair" parameters for the stepwise oxygenation of hemoglobin (Eq. 4). Note that the triply ligated species, $Hb(O_2)_3$, is predicted to be present in very small quantities.

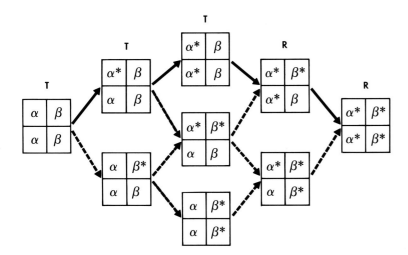

FIG. 3. The possible structural varieties of partially liganded oxygenation intermediates, assuming that α and β heme sites have unique affinities for O_2. The α_2-cooperon model suggests the preferred path shown with solid arrows. In this case, the transition from the tense (T) conformation to the relaxed (R) conformation occurs as the third O_2 is bound, so the fourth binds almost simultaneously.

termediates shown in Fig. 3 are, in fact, present, and their concentrations are in general agreement with the predictions from the Adair model (7). However, these conclusions are based on experiments carried out with hemoglobin–CO reactions and not with red blood cells, and whether or not they can be generalized to oxygenation of red blood cells is not yet clear.

Allosteric Effectors: Two-State Model

Since the elucidation of the exact structure of hemoglobin, several mechanistic theories for the influence of the allosteric effectors (e.g., H^+, 2,3-DPG, CO_2, and Cl^-) have been proposed (8). Monod et al. (9) proposed the most successful of these, based on the structural work of Bolton and Perutz (10), who described two conformations for hemoglobin, corresponding to deoxy- and oxyhemoglobin.

According to the two-state model, hemoglobin can exist in either R (relaxed) or T (tense) conformation, each with its unique oxygen affinity. The equilibrium constants for their reactions with oxygen are K_R and K_T. The ratio of these constants,

$$C = K_T/K_R \quad [6]$$

is about 0.01 for human hemoglobin A; that is, the affinity of molecules in the R conformation is much greater than the affinity of those in the T conformation. The constant C is characteristic of a given hemoglobin structure. The essence of the allosteric theory is that the equilibrium between the two conformations in the deoxy state,

$$Hb^R \leftrightarrow Hb^T \quad [7]$$

given by the allosteric constant,

$$L = [Hb]_T/[Hb]_R \quad [8]$$

is influenced by a number of other molecules or "al-losteric effectors." These small molecules react with hemoglobin at nonheme sites in such a way as to stabilize the T conformation. Thus, the overall reactivity of a mixture of R and T hemoglobin molecules toward oxygen will depend on the position of the R–T equilibrium. Monod et al. (9) related the allosteric constant L to Po_2 (p) and to the fractional saturation of hemoglobin with oxygen (Y):

$$Y = \frac{LK_Tp(1 + K_Tp)^3 + K_Rp(1 + K_Rp)^3}{L(1 + K_Tp)^4 + (1 + K_Rp)^4} \quad [9]$$

Of fundamental importance in this model is that the T state is physically constrained by salt and hydrogen bonds to a much greater degree than is the R state. With successive oxygenation of the heme groups, some of these bonds break and the stability of the T structure decreases; as a result the molecules undergo a transition to the R state, accompanied by the release of the constraints and an increase in oxygen affinity. For deoxyhemoglobin the equilibrium is almost entirely on the T side. It is the shift from T to R during oxygenation which accounts for cooperativity. For normal hemoglobin, most of the molecules probably shift from T to R between binding of the second and third oxygen molecules; hence the OEC is steepest in its middle portion (maximal value of Hill's parameter, n; see Eq. 1).

Although the two-state model may not apply in all circumstances, it has been very useful in explaining certain properties of some abnormal hemoglobins. Many of them can be viewed as structural alterations that affect the value of L by favoring either the T (low affinity) or R (high affinity) conformation.

Subunit Heterogeneity: The α_2-Cooperon Model

Experiments using concentrated hemoglobin (11,12) and whole blood (4) showed that when the data were analyzed according to the Adair scheme, the parameter a_3 (see Eq. 5) becomes undeterminable and tends to zero or even negative values. This prompted the formulation of a third model, which is really a special case of the two-state model (13,14). This model proposes chain heterogeneity for the T-state tetramer, such that O_2 binds preferentially to the α chain. Interaction between α chains may lead to cooperativity within the T state. But when the quaternary transition to the R state occurs, affinities of both α and β chains for O_2 are equal.

The α_2-cooperon model introduces a new parameter, γ, that defines the chain interactions in the T state. When γ is greater than 1, interaction is positive; when it is less than 1, interaction is negative. When γ equals 1, α chains are independent of each other. Mathematically, the α_2-cooperon model can be written as

$$Y = \frac{L(K_T p + \gamma K_T^2 p^2) + 2K_R p(1 + K_R p)^3}{L(1 + 2K_T p + \gamma K_T^2 p^2) + 2(1 + K_R p)^4} \quad [10]$$

Note that this expression has four parameters, like the Adair equation (Eq. 4).

The α_2-cooperon model suggests an explanation for the low population of triply ligated intermediates of oxygenation (i.e., zero value of a_3). Thus, binding of the first two O_2 molecules would be to the two α chains, because the affinity of the β sites is negligible in the T state. For the third O_2 to bind, the molecule must switch to the R state, where the affinity of both β sites is high and the population of molecules with only one β site saturated is very low (Fig. 3).

Structural information about the basis of chain heterogeneity has been gained from the study of site-directed mutants. Perutz (15) proposed that the distal histidine (E7) acts as a "gate" to allow ligand entry to the heme pocket only when it swings out. In the α chain, a hydrogen bond forms between N_ϵ of histidine E7 and the O_2 molecule. When histidine E7 is replaced by glycine, free access is given to the heme pocket. The result is that O_2 affinity and kinetic constants are unchanged for β, but the O_2 affinity is reduced 14-fold in myoglobin and 8-fold in α chains (16). This is interpreted to mean that the rate of movement of histidine E7 is so fast in β as to not restrict entry of ligand into the heme pocket. In contrast, the stabilization of O_2 by histidine E7α accounts for the relatively higher affinity for O_2 by the α chain than by the β chain.

The Bohr Effect

Bohr et al. (17) observed that the position of the blood OEC along the abscissa was affected by changes in P_{CO_2}. That is, when pH was lowered (or P_{CO_2} raised), the oxygen affinity of the blood decreased (increased P_{50}). The separate effects of H^+ and CO_2 have now been elucidated (18). They are qualitatively similar, but the effect of H^+ (now properly called the "pH Bohr effect") is much stronger than the CO_2 effect in lowering oxygen affinity.

According to the two-state model of hemoglobin function, H^+ shifts the R–T equilibrium toward T, stabilizing that structure. The stereochemical interpretation of this phenomenon is that H^+ participates in opening and closing salt bridges involving the carboxy-terminal residues. The pK values of the imidazoles of histidine HC3(146)β and of valine NaI(1)α are lowered in oxyhemoglobin as a result of the rupture of the salt bridges in which they participate. This change in pK leads to a release of protons during the transition from T to R. Experiments with mutant and chemically modified hemoglobins suggest that these groups account for about two-thirds of the alkaline Bohr effect (19).

2,3-DPG

The normal intracellular constituent 2,3-DPG (and, to a lesser extent, ATP) is very important in the regulation of the blood OEC (20). 2,3-DPG is present in normal human red blood cells and is a metabolic intermediate in the glycolytic pathway. Under conditions of diminished oxygen availability (such as anemia or hypoxia), its concentration increases and the blood OEC moves to the right. If arterial oxygenation is normal, this facilitates transfer of oxygen to the tissues. The regulatory mechanisms that govern the concentration of 2,3-DPG are not completely understood, but alkalosis in response to hyperventilation is probably an important factor (21).

The effect of 2,3-DPG can be explained in terms of the two-state theory of hemoglobin function. 2,3-DPG can bind to deoxyhemoglobin in a molar ratio of 1:1; by doing this, it further constrains the T conformation, leading to a further shift of the R–T equilibrium toward T and a lowering of oxygen affinity. Salt bridges involving the free amino groups of valine NAl(1)β and the imidazoles of histidine H21(143)β are probably the most important binding sites (22). In deoxyhemoglobin, 2,3-DPG lies in the central cavity of the molecule and is coordinated to the groups mentioned above, as well as to the α-amino groups of lysine EF6(82)β. On transition to the R structure, the valines move apart, the H helices move together, and 2,3-DPG drops out. Like the effects of the other salt bridges in the deoxy structure, 2,3-DPG increases the alkaline Bohr effect.

CO_2 Binding

Finally, CO_2 can bind to the α-amino groups of the amino-terminal amino acids with a resultant decrease of oxygen affinity (18). This binding is diminished in

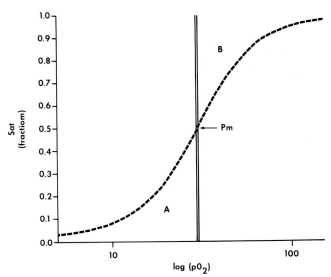

FIG. 4. Symmetry of oxygen binding. The median ligand concentration (P_m) is defined graphically as the P_{O_2} at which a vertical line passes through the curve such that area A is equal to area B. Reduced cooperativity would be manifest by clockwise rotation of the curve about P_m.

the presence of 2,3-DPG, since both 2,3-DPG and CO_2 can bind to the β-chain amino-terminal amino group. Such competition does not occur for the α-chain amino-terminus, since 2,3-DPG does not bind there.

SYMMETRY

Graphically (Fig. 4), a symmetrical OEC is one in which the area above the curve from its central point to infinite P_{O_2} is equal to the area below the curve from 0 to its central point (23). The P_{O_2} at which these two areas are equal to the median ligand pressure, P_m; for a symmetrical curve, $P_{50} = P_m$. To quantitate this concept, Allen et al. (24) defined symmetry as the condition $K_1K_4 = K_2K_3$, where the Ks are the Adair constants (Eq. 4). Roughton et al. (3) showed that for a symmetrical OEC, the "Wyman factor" (W) should approximate 1:

$$W = (a_1/a_3)^2 a_4 \qquad [11]$$

Weber (25) investigated symmetry for hemoglobin solutions and defined a descriptive parameter $A = \ln(K_1K_4/K_2K_3)$. This parameter has a positive value when $K_1K_4 > K_2K_3$, and it has a negative value when $K_1K_4 < K_2K_3$. Weber proposed that positive values of A are associated with efficient unloading of O_2 from hemoglobin but that negative values are better for scavenging oxygen in the lung. He calculated positive values of A, ranging from 0.44 for purified hemoglobin to 4.59 for hemoglobin with maximally reduced oxygen affinity.

In contrast, using the best whole-blood data avail-

able to them, Roughton et al. (3) concluded that W for whole blood is about 85, a value that did not seem to be consistent with any known model of hemoglobin function. More recent data suggest that W for whole blood is about 9 (26). Given the errors in the determination of the parameters, this is probably not significantly different from 1 and is consistent with the notion that within the red cell, very little triply ligated hemoglobin is present, probably because it is almost completely in the high-affinity (R) conformation. Calculation of Weber's parameter for whole blood gives a value of 2.16 (26). This positive value is consistent with Weber's hypothesis that the human blood system is geared towards efficient O_2 release in tissues. Experimental confirmation will await systematic studies of the effect of manipulation of the OEC on tissue oxygenation.

THE OEC AND OTHER DETERMINANTS OF OXYGEN TRANSPORT

It is clear that the oxygen-binding behavior of hemoglobin can affect overall oxygen transport, because certain genetic alterations in the molecule may lead to polycythemia (27). Furthermore, an extreme left-shift in the OEC caused by severe respiratory alkalosis was an essential feature in oxygen transport on the summit of Mt. Everest (28). The effect of reduced O_2 affinity has been shown by a number of authors to improve O_2 delivery to tissues when arterial oxygenation is adequate (29).

Experimental demonstration that changes in the position or shape of the OEC may affect oxygen transport in humans has been difficult, and therefore theoretical studies of the problem have been based on simplified models of hemoglobin oxygenation (30–32). Other known red blood cell properties that affect oxygen transport include (a) the rates of binding of physiologic ligands (O_2, CO_2, H^+, 2,3-DPG), (b) buffering capacity, (c) the barrier to diffusion presented by the red blood cell membrane, (d) the layer of unstirred plasma immediately surrounding it, and (e) the hematocrit-dependent blood viscosity (33).

O_2 and CO_2 Diffusion

Oxygen, CO_2, and hemoglobin interact in a very complex way in blood to regulate the position and shape of the OEC. This interaction can be appreciated by a classical analysis of the diffusive transfer of O_2 and CO_2 in the pulmonary capillary (34). The actual mechanisms are discussed in greater detail elsewhere in this book.

The flux of O_2 into the pulmonary capillary blood is proportional to the diffusing capacity of the lung and is also proportional to the difference in alveolar and capillary O_2 concentrations:

$$\frac{d(O_2)_i}{dt} = \frac{100}{V_c} \times \frac{D_L O_2}{60} \times (P_A O_2 - P_c O_2) \quad [12]$$

where V_c is the volume of capillary blood, $D_L O_2$ is the diffusing capacity for O_2 in the lung, $P_A O_2$ is the alveolar $P O_2$, and $P_c O_2$ is the pulmonary capillary $P O_2$.

The components of $D_L O_2$ are

$$\frac{1}{D_L O_2} = \frac{1}{D_M O_2} + \frac{1}{\theta O_2 \times V_c} \quad [13]$$

where $D_M O_2$ is the membrane component of the diffusing capacity and θO_2 is the reaction rate with hemoglobin (35). θO_2 is dependent on the hemoglobin concentration. Changes in total CO_2 follow an equation analogous to that for O_2:

$$\frac{d(CO_2)_i}{dt} = \frac{100}{V_c} \times \frac{D_L CO_2}{60} \times (P_c CO_2 - P_A CO_2) \quad [14]$$

where the definition of $D_L CO_2$ is parallel to that of $D_L O_2$. CO_2 affects O_2 affinity of blood in two ways: as an allosteric effector of the hemoglobin–O_2 reaction, and by its effect on intracellular pH (the Bohr effect). The second is of greater physiologic importance.

This brief overview description of the major acid–base reactions that occur in the blood demonstrates the multitude of effects that determine the actual *in vivo* shape and position of the OEC. H^+, perhaps the strongest physiologic effector, is regulated by $P CO_2$ and the buffering capacity of hemoglobin. Buffering by hemoglobin, in turn, is determined by hemoglobin concentration and the degree of O_2 saturation. O_2 saturation is determined by the $P O_2$ and O_2 affinity of hemoglobin, and so on. Exact quantitation of these multiple effects in the determination of gas exchange by blood is extremely difficult.

2,3-DPG/Hb Molar Ratio

An increase in 2,3-DPG is usually thought to augment O_2 delivery by a right-shift of the OEC, but probably only in normoxia (sea level). At altitude, because of the diffusion limitation of O_2 uptake in the lung, decreased O_2 affinity seems to limit uptake. Whether or not this is offset by tissue unloading remains to be seen, because too few data are available to indicate how low venous $P O_2$ can drop under hypoxic conditions. At this point it seems that the 2,3-DPG effect is a sea-level mechanism that is not suited to O_2 delivery at altitude. In addition to its role as an allosteric effector of the hemoglobin–O_2 reactions, 2,3-DPG also lowers intracellular pH because of its effect on the Donnan equilibrium. Thus it also contributes to the Bohr effect (36).

Hematocrit

Guyton et al. (37) carried out an extensive investigation of the effect of the hematocrit on hemodynamics in the denervated dog and suggested that there is an "optimal hematocrit" for O_2 transport that balances viscosity against O_2 carrying capacity. In general, increased hematocrit will increase the vascular resistance to flow, requiring an increased blood pressure and left atrial filling pressure until eventually a new equilibrium among these parameters is reached. Phlebotomy studies in patients with very high hematocrits demonstrate that polycythemia probably contributes to ventilation/perfusion mismatch and arterial desaturation (38).

PHYSIOLOGIC IMPLICATIONS OF THE OEC

The traditional view is that shifting the OEC to the right facilitates oxygen unloading in tissue sites. However, in certain situations the opposite could be true. For example, Barcroft et al. (39) believed that increased O_2 affinity was important in the adaptation to high altitude. His reasoning was based on analogy with the placental circulation, where fetal blood has a higher affinity than that of the mother. Chemical modification of hemoglobin to increase its affinity conveys superior survival on hypoxic rats (40), and mutant hemoglobins with increased affinity may precondition subjects to hypoxia (41). On the summit of Mt. Everest, the P_{50} of whole blood was found to be about 19 torr, protecting arterial saturation (28).

The interaction of the various physiologic effects is illustrated by the experimental determination that arterial desaturation may occur during extreme hypoxic exercise (42). This desaturation might be prevented by increasing the oxygen affinity of the blood by decreasing 2,3-DPG/Hb. If arterial oxygenation is normal, particularly at rest, the level of 2,3-DPG may be relatively unimportant. It is slightly more important during exercise, but it becomes critical in hypoxia.

The rate of O_2 uptake by red blood cells has not been adequately studied because of the difficulties in measurement. The importance of the layer of unstirred plasma surrounding the cell membrane *in vivo* is still not appreciated (43). It appears, however, that the reaction of O_2 with hemoglobin itself is not rate-limiting.

REFERENCES

1. Hill AV. The possible effects of the aggregation of the molecules of hemoglobin on its oxygen dissociation curve. *J Physiol (Lond)* 1910;40:4–7.
2. Adair GS. The hemoglobin system. VI. The oxygen dissociation curve of hemoglobin. *J Biol Chem* 1925;63:529–545.

3. Roughton FJW, DeLand EC, Kernohan JC, Severinghaus JW. Some recent studies of the oxyhemoglobin dissociation curve of human blood under physiological conditions and the fitting of the Adair equation to the standard curve. In: Astrup P, Rorth M, eds. *Oxygen affinity of hemoglobin and red cell acid base status.* Copenhagen: Munksgaard, 1972;73–83.

4. Winslow RM, Swenberg ML, Berger RL, Shrager RI, Luzzana M, Samaja M, Rossi-Bernardi L. Oxygen equilibrium curve of normal human blood and its evaluation by Adair's equation. *J Biol Chem* 1977;252(7):2331–2337.

5. Winslow RM, Samaja M, Winslow NJ, Rossi-Bernardi L, Shrager RI. Simulation of the continuous O_2 equilibrium curve over the physiologic range of pH, 2,3-diphosphoglycerate, and pCO_2. *J Appl Physiol* 1983;54(2):524–529.

6. Perrella M, Rossi-Bernardi L. Measurement of CO_2 equilibria: the chemical-chromatographic methods. In: Antonini E, Rossi-Bernardi L, Chiancone E, eds. *Methods in enzymology.* New York: Academic Press, 1981;487–495.

7. Perrella M. Intermediate compounds between hemoglobin and CO under equilibrium and kinetic conditions. In: *Symposium on oxygen binding heme proteins.* Pacific Grove, CA: Asilomar, 1988;PVI-8.

8. Antonini E, Brunori M. *Hemoglobin and myoglobin in their reactions with ligands.* New York: Elsevier, 1971.

9. Monod J, Wyman J, Changeaux J. On the nature of allosteric transitions: a plausible model. *J Mol Biol* 1965;12:88–118.

10. Bolton W, Perutz MF. Three dimensional Fourier synthesis of horse deoxyhemoglobin at 2 Angstrom units resolution. *Nature (Lond)* 1970;228:551–552.

11. Gill SJ, DiCera E, Doyle ML, Bishop GA, Robert CH. Oxygen binding constants for human hemoglobin tetramers. *Biochemistry* 1987;26:3995–4002.

12. Robert CH, Fall L, Gill SJ. Linkage of organic phosphates to oxygen binding in human hemoglobin at high concentrations. *Biochemistry* 1988;27:6835–6843.

13. Brunori M, Coletta M, DiCera E. A cooperative model for ligand binding to biological macromolecules as applied to oxygen carriers. *Biophys Chem* 1986;23:215–222.

14. DiCera E, Robert CH, Gill SJ. Allosteric interpretation of the oxygen-binding reaction of human hemoglobin tetramers. *Biochemistry* 1987;26:4003–4008.

15. Perutz MF. Myoglobin and haemoglobin: role of distal residues in reactions with haem ligands. *TIBS* 1989;14:42–44.

16. Olson JS, Mathews AJ, Springer BA, Egeberg KD, Sligar SG, Tame J, Renaud JP, Nagai K. The role of the distal histidine in myoglobin and haemoglobin. *Nature* 1988;336:265–266.

17. Bohr C, Hasselbalch KA, Krogh A. Uber einen in biologischer Bezeihung wichtigen Einfluss, den die Kohlensaurespannung des Blutes auf dessen Saurstoffbindung. *Skand Arch Physiol* 1904;16:402–412.

18. Kilmartin JV, Rossi-Bernardi L. Interaction of hemoglobin with hydrogen ions, carbon dioxide, and organic phosphates. *Physiol Rev* 1973;53(4):836–890.

19. Kilmartin JV, Fogg J, Rossi-Bernardi L. Identification of the high and low affinity CO_2-binding sites of human haemoglobin. *Nature* 1975;256:759–761.

20. Benesch R, Benesch RE. The effect of organic phosphates from the human erythrocyte on the allosteric properties of hemoglobin. *Biochem Biophys Res Commun* 1967;26:162–167.

21. Lenfant C, Sullivan K. Adaptation to high altitude. *N Engl J Med* 1971;284(23):1298–1309.

22. Arnone A. X-ray diffraction study of binding of 2,3-diphosphoglycerate to human deoxyhemoglobin. *Nature* 1972;237:146–149.

23. Wyman J. Linked functions and reciprocal effects in hemoglobins: a second look. In: Anfinson CB, Anson ML, Edsall JT, Richards FM, eds. *Advances in protein chemistry.* New York: Academic Press, 1964;223–286.

24. Allen DW, Guthe KF, Wyman J. Further studies on the oxygen equilibrium of hemoglobin. *J Biol Chem* 1950;187:393–410.

25. Weber G. Asymmetric ligand binding by haemoglobin. *Nature* 1982;300:603–607.

26. Winslow RM, Winslow NJ, Samaja M. Determination of the Adair parameters for the oxygen equilibrium curve of whole human blood by analysis of the temperature effect. 1990;in press.

27. Winslow RM, Anderson WF. The hemoglobinopathies. In: Stansbury JB, ed. *The metabolic basis of inherited disease,* 5th ed. New York: McGraw-Hill, 1982;1666–1710.

28. Winslow RM, Samaja M, West JB. Red cell function at extreme altitude on Mount Everest. *J Appl Physiol* 1984;56(1):109–116.

29. Woodson RD, Wranne B, Detter JC. Effect of increased blood oxygen affinity on work performance of rats. *J Clin Invest* 1973;52:2717–2724.

30. Neville JR. Altered haem–haem interaction and tissue-oxygen supply: a theoretical analysis. *Br J Haematol* 1976;34:387–395.

31. Bencowitz HZ, Wagner PD, West JB. Effect of change in P50 on exercise tolerance at high altitude: a theoretical study. *J Appl Physiol* 1982;53(6):1487–1495.

32. Willford DC, Hill EP, Moores WV. Theoretical analysis of optimal P50. *J Appl Physiol* 1982;52:1043–1048.

33. Winslow RM. A model for red cell O_2 uptake. *Int J Clin Monit Comput* 1985;2:81–93.

34. Wagner PD. Diffusion and chemical reaction in pulmonary gas exchange. *Physiol Rev* 1977;57(2):257–312.

35. Roughton FJW, Forster RE. Relative importance of diffusion and chemical reaction rates in determining rate of exchange of gases in the human lungs with special reference to tissue diffusing capacity of pulmonary membrane and volume of blood in the lung capillaries. *J Appl Physiol* 1957;11(2):290–302.

36. Samaja M, Winslow RM. The separate effects of H^+ and 2,3-DPG on the oxygen equilibrium curve of human blood. *Br J Haematol* 1979;41:373–381.

37. Guyton AC, Jones CE, Coleman TG. *Cardiac output and its regulation,* 2nd ed. Philadelphia: WB Saunders, 1973.

38. Winslow RM, Monge CC, Brown EG, Klein HG, Sarnquist F, Winslow NJ. The effects of hemodilution on O_2 transport in high altitude polycythemia. *J Appl Physiol* 1985;59:1495–1502.

39. Barcroft J, Binger CA, Bock AV, Doggart JH, Forbes HS, Garrop G, Meakins JC, Redfield AC. Observations upon the effect of high altitude on the physiological processes of the human body carried out in the Peruvian Andes chiefly at Cerro de Pasco. *Philos Trans R Soc Lond Ser B* 1923;211:351–480.

40. Eaton JW, Skelton TD, Berger E. Survival at extreme altitude: protective effect of increased hemoglobin–oxygen affinity. *Science* 1974;185:743–744.

41. Hebbel RP, Eaton JW, Kronenberg RS, Zanjani ED, Moore LG, Berger E. Human llamas. Adaptation to altitude in subjects with high hemoglobin oxygen affinity. *J Clin Invest* 1978;62:593–600.

42. Dempsey JA, Hanson PG, Henderson KS. Exercise-induced arterial hypoxemia in healthy human subjects at sea level. *J Physiol* 1984;355:161–175.

43. Vandegriff K, Olson JS. Morphological and physiological factors affecting the oxygen uptake and release by red blood cells. *J Biol Chem* 1984;259:12619–12627.

THE LUNG: Scientific Foundations
edited by R.G. Crystal, J.B. West et al.
Raven Press, Ltd., New York © 1991.

CHAPTER 5.3.2.3

Carbon Dioxide

Robert A. Klocke

Respiratory gases are relatively insoluble in aqueous solutions, and specialized systems have evolved to transport oxygen and carbon dioxide in blood. Heme proteins bind oxygen reversibly and are responsible for essentially all oxygen transport in mammals. In contrast, CO_2 is transported in several different modes. These forms interact, and their relative contributions to overall transport are a function of P_{CO_2}, hydrogen ion and 2,3-diphosphoglycerate (2,3-DPG) concentrations, and the degree of oxygen saturation of hemoglobin.

The CO_2 dissociation curve describes the summed contributions of all pathways of CO_2 transport as a function of CO_2 tension. The CO_2 dissociation curve is relatively steep in comparison to the O_2 dissociation curve. Consequently, large volumes of CO_2 can be exchanged with relatively small alterations in blood P_{CO_2}. This has profound implications on acid–base balance and pulmonary gas exchange. Small changes in blood P_{CO_2} minimize oscillations in blood acid–base balance. The hydrogen ion concentration of blood at rest varies only 10% between arterial and mixed venous values. The steep slope of the CO_2 dissociation curve also permits continued excretion of CO_2, albeit with lesser efficiency, despite abnormal distribution of pulmonary ventilation and blood flow (1,2). In contrast, oxygen exchange is more susceptible to alteratons in $\dot{V}_A/\dot{Q}$ matching.

PATHWAYS OF CO_2 TRANSPORT

Most of the CO_2 in blood exists in the form of bicarbonate ion. CO_2 also is transported in a physically dissolved state in blood, and it is bound to amino groups

R. A. Klocke: Departments of Medicine and Physiology, State University of New York at Buffalo, Buffalo, New York 14214.

of proteins as carbamate compounds. The latter achieves increased importance because the quantity of CO_2 carried in the carbamate state varies with oxygenation of the hemoglobin molecule.

CO_2 in Solution

Although CO_2 has an aqueous solubility approximately 20 times that of oxygen, CO_2 dissolved in physical solution accounts for only 5% of the CO_2 content of arterial or venous blood (3). Nevertheless, dissolved CO_2 plays a pivotal role in CO_2 transport and exchange. Access to the bicarbonate and carbamate pools is achieved only through dissolved CO_2. Furthermore, molecular CO_2 is lipid-soluble and can cross cell membranes. Exchange of CO_2 in both the lung and peripheral tissues occurs via diffusion of molecular CO_2 across the vascular endothelium. CO_2 diffuses across the pulmonary membrane so rapidly that limitation of the process can only be demonstrated in an isolated lung under nonphysiologic conditions (4). The diffusing capacity of the lung for CO_2 is so great that it cannot be measured *in vivo* (5).

Bicarbonate Pathway

Hydration of CO_2 produces carbonic acid (H_2CO_3), which is almost completely ionized to hydrogen and bicarbonate ions because the pK of carbonic acid ($\sim$3.8) is considerably lower than blood pH (3):

$$CO_2 + H_2O \rightleftharpoons H_2CO_3 \rightleftharpoons H^+ + HCO_3^- \qquad [1]$$

Equation 1 includes two processes. The first step is the hydration of CO_2 to carbonic acid, and the second step is the ionization of carbonic acid to bicarbonate. Bicarbonate ion can further dissociate into hydrogen and carbonate ions:

$$HCO_3^- \rightleftharpoons H^+ + CO_3^{2-} \qquad [2]$$

However, little carbonate is formed because the pK of this reaction (>10.0) is well above body pH (6). Carbonic acid, usually considered a weak acid, is actually as strong an acid as lactic acid, a substance usually considered a serious threat to acid–base balance. This misconception results from the combination of the hydration and dissociation steps in Eq. 1 to calculate a single apparent dissociation constant, K_a'. Rearranged in its logarithmic form, this yields the familiar Henderson–Hasselbalch equation expressing the relation between HCO_3^-, CO_2, and pH in plasma:

$$pH = pK_a' + \log\left(\frac{[HCO_3^-]}{s \cdot P_{CO_2}}\right) \qquad [3]$$

where s is the solubility of CO_2 in plasma, equal to 0.0307 mM/mmHg at 37°C (7), and pK_a' is 6.10. This latter value varies slightly with experimental conditions (8).

The hydration of CO_2 to H_2CO_3, the first step in Eq. 1, occurs naturally at a very slow rate, but carbonic anhydrase in blood catalyzes this reaction sufficiently to complete the process during passage through the peripheral capillaries. The reverse reaction, the dehydration of H_2CO_3 to CO_2, occurs during pulmonary excretion and similarly requires catalysis. Carbonic anhydrase is present within the cell in high concentrations (3) but is virtually absent from plasma (9,10). Carbonic anhydrase is localized to the capillary endothelium of the lung (11–13) and other organs (14), but the quantity of enzyme present is limited.

Human erythrocytes contain two isoenzymes of carbonic anhydrase, both approximately 30 kDa in size. Carbonic anhydrase I is a low-activity enzyme that is inhibited by anions (15). A concentration of only 6 mM chloride ion is sufficient to deplete its activity by 50%. Thus, it appears that this isoenzyme is relatively incapable of catalyzing reactions of CO_2 in vivo, leading Maren et al. (15) to speculate that it serves an entirely different, unknown function. The second isoenzyme, carbonic anhydrase II, has high catalytic activity and is markedly resistant to anion inhibition (15). Human carbonic anhydrase II is comprised of 259 amino acids (16) and has only moderate homology (less than two-thirds of amino acid residues) with carbonic anhydrase I. Red blood cells from most mammals contain similar high and low activity enzymes, but erythrocytes from the ox, cow, sheep, and dog only contain a single high-activity form (17).

All isoenzymes of carbonic anhydrase, regardless of species, have a single zinc atom that is essential for biochemical activity (18). Activity is lost with binding of an unsubstituted —SO_2NH_2 group of aromatic sulfonamides to the zinc ion. Acetazolamide is the most common of these inhibitors and has some clinical use-

fulness. A third isoenzyme, carbonic anhydrase III, has been isolated from various tissues, especially red muscle (19). This isoenzyme is more resistant to inhibition by sulfonamide derivatives, but its activity is reduced compared to that of the two other isoenzymes. It is not present in blood, and its physiologic function in other tissues is unknown.

Carbamate Compounds

Carbon dioxide and hydrogen ions reversibly bind to uncharged amino groups of proteins:

$$R\text{—}NH_2 + H^+ \rightleftharpoons R\text{—}NH_3^+ \qquad [4]$$

$$R\text{—}NH_2 + CO_2 \rightleftharpoons R\text{—}NHCOOH \qquad [5]$$

where R represents the protein moiety and R—NHCOOH is a carbamic acid (3). Under in vivo circumstances, carbamic acids dissociate completely to release protons and form carbamate ions, R—NHCOO$^-$. Because both protons and molecular CO_2 compete for uncharged amino groups, the formation of carbamate compounds is markedly pH-dependent and increases with decreasing acidity. Transport of CO_2 as carbamates is also influenced by P_{CO_2} and the pK of the amino groups in question. The pK values of α-amino groups, the amino groups present at the N-terminus of blood proteins, lie within the physiologic range of pH (20,21). Therefore, these frequently exist in the uncharged R—NH$_2$ form and are available to bind CO_2. In contrast, ϵ-amino groups, located throughout the protein chains, have a pK well above the physiologic pH range. Thus, the vast majority of ϵ-amino groups are bound to hydrogen ions and therefore cannot bind CO_2. The decreased ability of the ϵ-amino groups to bind CO_2 is offset to some extent by their greater concentration. There are five-fold more ϵ-amino than α-amino groups present on plasma proteins (20); this ratio rises to 15:1 for the hemoglobin molecule (21). Not all amino groups, especially those of the ϵ-amino variety, are able to bind CO_2, possibly the result of structural configuration of the protein molecules.

The concentration of carbamates in plasma is approximately 0.6 mM, and binding of CO_2 to α-amino groups accounts for 60% of this quantity. Plasma carbamates have no appreciable role in CO_2 exchange. The steep slope of the CO_2 dissociation curve minimizes changes in pH and P_{CO_2} between arterial and venous blood. These relatively small variations do not produce significant change in plasma carbamate concentration as blood traverses the lung or peripheral tissues. As a result, plasma carbamate concentration remains at a fixed concentration and does not contribute to CO_2 exchange.

Carbamate formation by ϵ-amino groups of hemoglobin is absent under *in vivo* circumstances because the pK of these groups is sufficiently high to preclude CO_2 binding. In contrast, binding of CO_2 to α-amino groups of hemoglobin is an important factor in CO_2 exchange. The total concentration of hemoglobin-carbamates in blood is relatively low, but reduced hemoglobin binds substantially more CO_2 as carbamate than does the oxygenated molecule (22). The difference in bound CO_2 between the reduced and oxygenated heme proteins, termed "oxylabile carbamate," leads to a greater role for carbamates in gas exchange than suggested by their concentration. Thus, release of oxygen by hemoglobin in the tissues is accompanied by increased binding of CO_2 to α-amino groups. Conversely, oxygenation of hemoglobin in the lung promotes release of CO_2 bound as carbamate. Earlier calculations indicated that this synergistic behavior accounted for 27% of all CO_2 excreted in the lungs (23). However, these computations were based on data obtained with dialyzed solutions of hemoglobin. Following the description of binding 2,3-DPG to hemoglobin (24,25), Bauer (26) demonstrated that addition of 2,3-DPG to reduced hemoglobin solutions decreased the total CO_2 content, presumably the result of reduction in oxylabile binding. Direct measurements of carbamate binding to hemoglobin demonstrated that oxylabile carbamate binding is inversely related to 2,3-DPG concentration (27).

The mechanism of interaction between 2,3-DPG and CO_2 binding was determined by Bunn and Briehl (28) utilizing naturally occurring variants of hemoglobin. Their work demonstrated that carbamate formation was inhibited by electrostatic binding of 2,3-DPG to the N-terminal amino groups of the β chains of hemoglobin. The α chains of hemoglobin do not bind 2,3-DPG, and organic phosphates do not affect carbamate formation at these portions of the molecule (29). Direct measurements of carbamate binding to the α and β chains of hemoglobin indicate that both chains participate equally in oxylabile carbamate formation at physiologic P_{CO_2} in the presence of 2,3-DPG (29).

In view of the demonstrated effect of organic phosphates on oxylabile carbamate formation, previous estimates of the role of this pathway in CO_2 exchange must be revised. Bauer and Schroder (30) estimate that oxylabile carbamate accounts for only 10% of total CO_2 exchange, appreciably lower than the earlier estimates of 27% (23). The exact contribution will not be constant under all circumstances and may be affected by the type of hemoglobin involved. The contribution of oxylabile carbamate to fetal CO_2 exchange is estimated to be 19% of the total because the γ chain of fetal hemoglobin is less likely to bind 2,3-DPG at the site of carbamate formation (30). It is difficult to determine the exact role of carbamate in CO_2 exchange based on extrapolation of *in vitro* data, but there is good evidence that its importance is considerably less than previously estimated.

CO₂ DISSOCIATION CURVE

Despite the physiologic importance of the CO_2 dissociation curve, there is a paucity of recent data in the literature describing the relationship between total CO_2 content and CO_2 tension of blood. The most comprehensive information is provided by the original data of Christiansen et al. (31), which were published in 1914 (Fig. 1, left panel). Fortunately, these investigators performed experiments on freshly drawn human blood, thereby avoiding depletion of 2,3-DPG, an important cofactor in carbamino formation which was unknown at the time. These data demonstrated that the CO_2 content at any given P_{CO_2} was greater in reduced blood than in oxygenated blood. This feature of CO_2 transport is usually referred to as the "Haldane effect," named after one of the three discoverers.

Substantial advances were made by Peters and co-workers (32–34) following the description of the Haldane effect. Peters (32) demonstrated that the CO_2 dissociation curve was linear when plotted on logarithmic axes (Fig. 1, right panel). The slope of this relationship is profoundly affected by the hemoglobin concentration of blood (33). Hemoglobin is the major nonbicarbonate buffer of blood and is essential to buffer the protons released by the ionization of carbonic acid to bicarbonate ion. The linear nature of the logarithmic expression of the dissociation curve also permits definition of the curve by measurement of a single experimental point and the hemoglobin concentration (34).

Visser (35) derived an empirical equation for the dissociation curve from the Van Slyke–Sendroy nomogram (36). This calculation is based on hemoglobin concentration, oxygen saturation, and plasma pH. The constants in this equation have been modified recently by Douglas et al. (37) to provide the best fit to more recent data. Plasma CO_2 content is calculated from the Henderson–Hasselbalch equation, and blood CO_2 content is computed from the empirical relation

$$[CO_2]_{blood} = [CO_2]_{plasma} \times \left(1 - \frac{0.0289[Hb]}{(3.352 - 0.456S_{O_2})(8.142 - pH)}\right) \quad [6]$$

where [Hb] is hemoglobin concentration in g/dl, S_{O_2} is fractional oxygen saturation, and pH is the plasma pH. Although an empirical relation is less satisfactory than an equation based on a theoretical construct, this approach is quite satisfactory from a practical standpoint. The absolute quantity of CO_2 present in blood is of secondary importance. The crucial physiologic value is the slope of the CO_2 dissociation curve, since

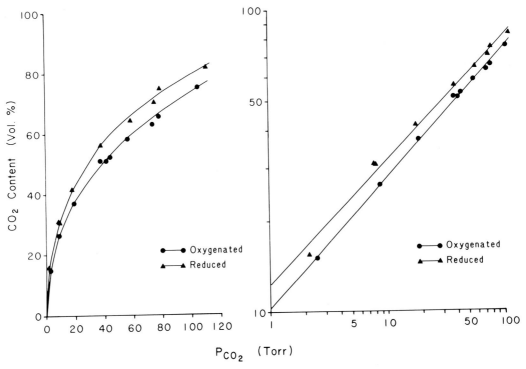

FIG. 1. Carbon dioxide dissociation curve of human blood in linear (*left panel*) and logarithmic (*right panel*) form. (From ref. 3; data originally from ref. 31.)

this determines the efficacy of CO_2 exchange (2). As McHardy (38) has pointed out, the slope of the CO_2 dissociation curve is essentially constant over a wide variety of circumstances, provided that blood hemoglobin concentration is taken into account. Thus, calculations of arterial–venous content differences and other parameters of gas exchange are correct regardless of the mathematic form of the dissociation curve utilized as long as the appropriate slope is chosen.

Plasma–Erythrocyte Interactions

Total CO_2 content is not distributed uniformly in blood. The total quantity of CO_2 contained in all forms in the plasma is twice as great as that of the red cells. However, this circumstance is only achieved when CO_2 equilibrates with whole blood. Plasma isolated and later equilibrated with CO_2 has only 20% of the CO_2 content of plasma separated from erythrocytes after equilibration with CO_2. This increased CO_2 capacity of plasma is a consequence of three characteristics of erythrocytes: (i) a large internal buffering capacity, (ii) the presence of intracellular carbonic anhydrase, and (iii) the ability to exchange bicarbonate and chloride ions across the erythrocyte membrane.

Buffering Capacity

The buffering power of plasma per se is provided by plasma proteins. The minimal concentrations of other

plasma conjugate buffer pairs provide essentially no buffering. However, plasma proteins have only one-eighth of the buffering power of intracellular hemoglobin (3). This is a consequence of lower concentration (i.e., one-half that of intracellular hemoglobin) and substantially less buffering capacity per unit weight. The ionization of carbonic acid not only produces bicarbonate ions but also liberates an identical number of hydrogen ions. Without buffering, these protons would produce a lethal level of blood acidity. Hemoglobin is an excellent buffer and is present in much higher concentration than any other nonbicarbonate buffer in blood. As a result, most hydrogen ions produced by ionization of carbonic acid to bicarbonate are buffered by hemoglobin within the red blood cell. The majority of the CO_2 content present in the plasma has been buffered previously by hemoglobin within the erythrocyte.

If plasma is separated from blood prior to equilibration with CO_2, the loss of the buffering capacity provided by hemoglobin substantially reduces the quantity of CO_2 contained in plasma. Failure to buffer hydrogen ions produced by the ionization of carbonic acid shifts the equilibrium of Eq. 1 to the left, thereby decreasing sequestration of CO_2 in the form of bicarbonate. Although buffering can occur outside of the blood in the tissues, this does not occur during pulmonary gas exchange. Exchange and buffering are essentially complete during capillary transit in the lung, and the relatively small volume of pulmonary parenchyma does not add significantly to the buffering provided by blood during gas exchange.

Distribution of Bicarbonate

The quantity of bicarbonate carried within the erythrocyte is substantially less than that transported in plasma: Only one-third of blood bicarbonate is carried intracellularly. Several factors are responsible for this difference. First, the plasma volume of blood is greater than erythrocyte volume in an approximate ratio of 0.55/0.45. Second, bicarbonate ion is transported in aqueous solution, and the fraction of water in plasma (0.94) is much greater than that of the intracellular milieu (0.72) because of the high concentration of hemoglobin in the intracellular space (39). Third, the Donnan effect, resulting from restriction of negatively charged hemoglobin molecules to the interior of the erythrocyte, leads to a lower intracellular concentration of diffusible anions such as bicarbonate (40).

Despite the lower bicarbonate content of erythrocytes, the red blood cells are essential for almost all bicarbonate transport. As CO_2 enters blood in the tissues, the large intracellular buffering capacity favors formation of bicarbonate inside erythrocytes. Intracellular ionization of carbonic acid to bicarbonate is further facilitated by the presence of large quantities of carbonic anhydrase within the red blood cells. Although this intracellular ionization of carbonic acid occurs rapidly, carbonic acid's uncatalyzed formation from CO_2 occurs quite slowly. Some buffering can occur within the plasma, but minimal CO_2 is hydrated to form carbonic acid during the short period of capillary transit. The overwhelming majority of bicarbonate formation occurs within the cell, and there is subsequent buffering of the protons released in the ionization reaction. These factors lead to rapid increase in intracellular bicarbonate concentration, which tends to shift Eq. 1 to the left as a result of a mass action effect, thereby impeding formation of more bicarbonate. However, a transport system contained within the erythrocyte membrane facilitates the rapid exchange of intracellular bicarbonate ions for extracellular chloride ions, thereby shuttling bicarbonate ions produced within the erythrocyte into the plasma (41). The exchange of anions is coupled so that transmembrane potential is not altered. This is essential, considering the large number of ions exchanged during CO_2 transport. If coupling did not occur, electrical potentials would be established which would prevent movement of bicarbonate. This facilitated transport is essential to permit rapid exchange of bicarbonate across the cell membrane during the short period of capillary transit. Even though the majority of bicarbonate is carried within the plasma, it is almost exclusively formed within the red cell. The entire process is reversed in the lungs as bicarbonate is converted to molecular CO_2, the only form of CO_2 that can cross the alveolar–capillary barrier.

The exchange of bicarbonate and chloride had been thought to occur via passive diffusion of anions across channels in the erythrocyte membrane (42). However, demonstration of saturation kinetics and pH dependence of chloride self-exchange across erythrocyte membrane led to the concept of facilitated transport of these anions (43). Cabantchik and Rothstein (44,45) isolated a protein (molecular weight 95 kDa) that mediates the exchange. There are 800,000 to 1,200,000 molecules of this protein, termed "Band 3 protein," in the erythrocyte membrane (41). A variety of anions are transported by this carrier, but bicarbonate and chloride ions exhibit the fastest rates of exchange by far. The actual mechanism involved in the exchange has not been elucidated completely, but the exchange is characterized by 1:1 bidirectional anion flux, probably associated with a conformational change in the Band 3 protein structure (41).

Haldane Effect

The influence of oxygenation on the CO_2 dissociation curve, the Haldane effect, receives far less attention than the converse relationship, the effect of carbon dioxide on the O_2 dissociation curve of blood. The latter, termed the "Bohr effect," is responsible for only 2% of total O_2 exchange in the tissues (46). However, the lesser-acknowledged Haldane effect accounts for almost one-half of resting CO_2 exchange. Although considerable reevaluation of the mechanisms of the Haldane effect has taken place in the last two decades (3,26,27), there has been no evidence presented which decreases its importance.

Oxygen-dependent exchange of CO_2 occurs via both the carbamate and bicarbonate pathways and is a function of pH, P_{CO_2}, and the concentration of 2,3-DPG (26,27). The relative contributions of these two pathways are shown in Fig. 2. Under conditions of eucapnia and normal 2,3-DPG concentration, the Haldane effect becomes more prominent with increasing pH, reaching a maximal value under normal acid–base conditions. The relative importance of the carbamate pathway in this process increases with greater alkalinity because carbamate formation is promoted at higher pH (21), and reduced 2,3-DPG binding at higher pH (47) leads to greater carbamate formation. The contribution of the bicarbonate pathway peaks in the physiologic range of pH, but it decreases at higher pH as a result of increasing prominence of carbamates. With oxygenation, oxylabile Bohr protons are released from the hemoglobin molecule (48). However, the carbamate reaction consumes protons, thereby leaving fewer of

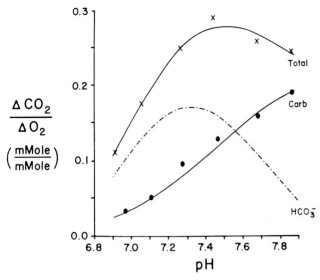

FIG. 2. The magnitude and components of the Haldane effect at physiologic P_{CO_2} (42.5 mmHg) in erythrocyte suspensions. Relative contributions of the carbamate and bicarbonate pathways to the total Haldane effect are labeled. (From ref. 27.)

TABLE 1. *Contributions of different pathways to CO_2 transport and exchange*[a]

	Arterial content		Arterial–venous difference	
	ml/dl blood	Percent of total	ml/dl blood	Percent of total
Plasma				
Dissolved CO_2	1.51	3.1	0.20	4.7
Bicarbonate	30.01	62.1	2.07	48.7
Carbamate	0.67	1.4	0.00	0.0
Total CO_2 content	32.19	66.6	2.27	53.4
Erythrocyte				
Dissolved CO_2	0.93	1.9	0.16	3.8
Bicarbonate	12.58	26.0	1.29	30.3
Carbamate	2.67	5.5	0.53	12.5
Total CO_2 content	16.18	33.4	1.98	46.6

[a] Data taken from ref. 3. Concentrations are expressed in ml/dl of blood. Arterial pH and P_{CO_2} are 7.40 and 40.0 mmHg, respectively. Corresponding venous values are 7.37 and 46 mmHg.

the Bohr protons to combine with bicarbonate ion to form CO_2.

Gas exchange would occur without a functioning Haldane effect despite the fact that one-half of CO_2 excretion normally occurs by this mechanism (49). The price of this loss would be (a) greater changes in arterial–venous parameters and (b) tissue hypercarbia and altered acid–base balance.

Arterial–Venous CO$_2$ Differences

The relative distribution of CO_2 in the plasma and erythrocytes of arterial blood is listed in Table 1. As noted in the table, plasma has twice the CO_2 content of the red blood cells, and the vast majority of this content exists as bicarbonate. As noted previously, however, the majority of the bicarbonate in plasma was formed within the erythrocyte and then entered the plasma in exchange for chloride ion. The relative contributions of each form of CO_2 during resting gas exchange also are listed in Table 1. In contrast to their lesser contributions to the overall CO_2 content of 5.0% and 6.9%, respectively, dissolved CO_2 and carbamate account for 8.4% and 12.5% of CO_2 excreted in the lungs. The fraction of CO_2 generated in the lungs via the carbamate pathway occurs entirely within the erythrocyte. The contributions of the three pathways of CO_2 transport to overall gas exchange are not fixed but will, instead, depend upon the conditions prevailing during exchange. Compromise of one pathway is accompanied by a compensatory increase in excretion via the other pathways (50).

ACKNOWLEDGMENTS

The author appreciates the assistance of Marsha Barber, Anne Coe, and Barbara Klocke in the preparation of this manuscript. This work was supported by grant HL-34323 from the National Heart, Lung and Blood Institute.

REFERENCES

1. West JB. Ventilation–perfusion inequality and overall gas exchange in computer models of the lung. *Respir Physiol* 1969; 7:88–110.
2. West JB. Effect of slope and shape of dissociation curve on pulmonary gas exchange. *Respir Physiol* 1969;8:66–85.
3. Klocke RA. Carbon dioxide transport. In: Farhi LE, Tenney SM, eds. *Handbook of physiology, Section 3: The respiratory system, vol. IV: Gas exchange.* Bethesda, MD: American Physiological Society, 1987;173–197.
4. Effros RM, Mason G, Silverman P. Role of perfusion and diffusion in $^{14}CO_2$ exchange in the rabbit lung. *J Appl Physiol* 1981;51:1136–1144.
5. Hyde RW, Puy RJM, Raub WF, Forster RE. Rate of disappearance of labeled carbon dioxide from the lungs of humans during breath holding: a method for studying the dynamics of pulmonary CO_2 exchange. *J Clin Invest* 1968;47:1535–1552.
6. Edsall JT. Carbon dioxide, carbonic acid, and bicarbonate ion: physical properties and kinetics of interconversion. In: Forster RE, Edsall JT, Otis AB, Roughton FJW, eds. *CO2: chemical, biochemical, and physiological aspects.* Washington, DC: NASA, SP-188, 1969;15–27.
7. Austin WH, Lacombe E, Rand PW, Chatterjee M. Solubility of carbon dioxide in serum from 15 to 38°C. *J Appl Physiol* 1963;18:301–304.
8. Rispens P, Dellebarre CW, Eleveld D, Helder W, Zijlstra WG. The apparent first dissociation constant of carbonic acid in plasma between 16 and 42.5°. *Clin Chim Acta* 1968;22:627–637.
9. Maren TH. Carbonic anhydrase: chemistry, physiology, and inhibition. *Physiol Rev* 1967;47:595–781.

10. Hill EP. Inhibition of carbonic anhydrase by plasma of dogs and rabbits. *J Appl Physiol* 1986;60:191–197.

11. Effros RM, Chang RSY, Silverman P. Acceleration of plasma bicarbonate conversion to carbon dioxide by pulmonary carbonic anhydrase. *Science* 1978;199:427–429.

12. Klocke RA. Catalysis of CO_2 reactions by lung carbonic anhydrase. *J Appl Physiol* 1978;44:882–888.

13. Crandall ED, O'Brasky JE. Direct evidence for participation of rat lung carbonic anhydrase in CO_2 reactions. *J Clin Invest* 1978;62:618–622.

14. O'Brasky JE, Crandall ED. Organ and species differences in tissue vascular carbonic anhydrase activity. *J Appl Physiol* 1980;49:211–217.

15. Maren TH, Rayburn CS, Liddell NE. Inhibition by anions of human red cell carbonic anhydrase B: physiological and biochemical implications. *Science* 1976;191:469–472.

16. Henderson LE, Henriksson D, Nyman PO. Primary structure of human carbonic anhydrase C. *J Biol Chem* 1976;251:5457–5463.

17. Carter MJ. Carbonic anhydrase: isoenzymes, properties, distribution, and functional significance. *Biol Rev* 1972;47:465–513.

18. Keilin D, Mann T. Carbonic anhydrase. Purification and nature of the enzyme. *Biochem J* 1940;34:1163–1176.

19. Holmes RS. Mammalian carbonic anhydrase isoenzymes: evidence for a third locus. *J Exp Zool* 1976;197:289–295.

20. Gros G, Forster RE, Lin L. The carbamate reaction of glycylglycine, plasma, and tissue extracts evaluated by a pH stopped flow apparatus. *J Biol Chem* 1976;251:4398–4407.

21. Gros G, Rollema HS, Forster RE. The carbamate equilibrium of α- and ε-amino groups of human hemoglobin at 37°C. *J Biol Chem* 1981;256:5471–5480.

22. Ferguson JKW, Roughton FJW. The direct chemical estimation of carbamino compounds of CO_2 with haemoglobin. *J Physiol (Lond)* 1934;83:68–86.

23. Rossi-Bernardi L, Roughton FJW. The specific influence of carbon dioxide and carbamate compounds on the buffer power and Bohr effects in human haemoglobin solutions. *J Physiol (Lond)* 1967;189:1–29.

24. Benesch R, Benesch RE. The effect of organic phosphates from the human erythrocyte on the allosteric properties of hemoglobin. *Biochem Biophys Res Commun* 1967;26:162–167.

25. Chanutin A, Curnish RR. Effect of organic and inorganic phosphates on the oxygen equilibrium of human erythrocytes. *Arch Biochem Biophys* 1967;121:96–102.

26. Bauer C. Reduction of the carbon dioxide affinity of human haemoglobin solutions by 2,3-diphosphoglycerate. *Respir Physiol* 1970;10:10–19.

27. Klocke RA. Mechanism and kinetics of the Haldane effect in human erythrocytes. *J Appl Physiol* 1973;35:673–681.

28. Bunn HF, Briehl RW. The interaction of 2,3-diphosphoglycerate with various human hemoglobins. *J Clin Invest* 1970;49:1088–1095.

29. Perrella M, Kilmartin JV, Fogg J, Rossi-Bernardi L. Identification of the high and low affinity CO_2-binding sites of human haemoglobin. *Nature* 1975;256:759–761.

30. Bauer C, Schröder E. Carbamino compounds of haemoglobin in human adult and foetal blood. *J Physiol* 1972;229:457–471.

31. Christiansen J, Douglas CG, Haldane JS. The absorption and dissociation of carbon dioxide by human blood. *J Physiol* 1914;48:244–277.

32. Peters JP. Studies of the carbon dioxide absorption curve of human blood. III. A further discussion of the form of the absorption curve plotted logarithmically, with a convenient type of interpolation chart. *J Biol Chem* 1923;56:745–750.

33. Peters JP, Bulger HA, Eisenman AJ. Studies of the carbon dioxide absorption curve of human blood. IV. The relation of the hemoglobin content of blood to the form of the carbon dioxide absorption curve. *J Biol Chem* 1924;58:747–768.

34. Peters JP, Bulger HA, Eisenman AJ. Studies of the carbon dioxide absorption curve of human blood. V. The construction of the CO_2 absorption curve from one observed point. *J Biol Chem* 1924;58:769–771.

35. Visser BF. Pulmonary diffusion of carbon dioxide. *Phys Med Biol* 1960;5:155–166.

36. Van Slyke DD, Sendroy J. Studies of gas and electrolyte equilibria in blood. XV. Line charts for graphic calculation by the Henderson–Hasselbalch equation and from calculation of plasma CO_2 content from whole blood content. *J Biol Chem* 1928;79:781–789.

37. Douglas AR, Jones NL, Reed JW. Calculation of whole blood CO_2 content. *J Appl Physiol* 1988;65:473–477.

38. McHardy GJR. The relationship between the differences in pressure and content of carbon dioxide in arterial and venous blood. *Clin Sci* 1967;32:299–309.

39. Altman PL, Dittmer DS, eds. *Blood and other body fluids.* Bethesda, MD: Federation of American Societies for Experimental Biology, 1971;19.

40. Reeves RB. Temperature-induced changes in blood acid–base status: Donnan r_{Cl} and red cell volume. *J Appl Physiol* 1976;40:762–767.

41. Knauf PA. Anion transport in erythrocytes. In: Andreoli TE, Hoffman JF, Fanestil DD, Schultz SG, eds. *Physiology of membrane disorders,* 2nd ed. New York: Plenum Press, 1986;191–220.

42. Passow H. Passive ion permeability of the erythrocyte membrane. *Prog Biophys Mol Biol* 1969;19:425–467.

43. Gunn RB, Dalmark M, Tosteson CD, Wieth JO. Characteristics of chloride transport in human red blood cells. *J Gen Physiol* 1973;61:185–206.

44. Cabantchik ZI, Rothstein A. The nature of the membrane sites controlling anion permeability of human red blood cells as determined by studies with disulfonic stilbene derivatives. *J Member Physiol* 1972;10:311–330.

45. Cabantchik ZI, Rothstein A. Membrane proteins related to anion permeability of human red blood cells. I. Localization of disulfonic stilbene binding sites in proteins involved in permeation. *J Membr Biol* 1974;15:207–226.

46. Hill EP, Power GG, Longo LD. Mathematical simulation of pulmonary O_2 and CO_2 exchange. *Am J Physiol* 1973;224:904–917.

47. Garby L, DeVerdier C-H. Affinity of human hemoglobin A to 2,3-diphosphoglycerate. Effect of hemoglobin concentration and of pH. *Scand J Clin Lab Invest* 1971;27:345–350.

48. Perutz MF, Muirhead H, Mazzarella L, Crowther RA, Greer J, Kilmartin JV. Identification of residues responsible for the alkaline Bohr effect in haemoglobin. *Nature* 1969;222:1240–1243.

49. Grant BJB. Influence of Bohr–Haldane effect on steady state gas exchange. *J Appl Physiol* 1982;52:1330–1337.

50. Cain SM, Otis AB. Carbon dioxide transport in anesthetized dogs during inhibition of carbonic anhydrase. *J Appl Physiol* 1961;16:1023–1028.

THE LUNG: Scientific Foundations
edited by R.G. Crystal, J.B. West et al.
Raven Press, Ltd., New York © 1991.

CHAPTER 5.3.2.4

Kinetics of Oxygen and Carbon Dioxide Reactions

Masaji Mochizuki

There are important interactions between the kinetics of the O_2 and CO_2 reactions in blood. As a consequence of the Bohr effect, the oxygenation rate of the red blood cell (RBC) is influenced by CO_2 diffusion. Conversely, CO_2 diffusion is influenced by oxygenation of hemoglobin (Hb) through the Haldane effect. In addition, the buffering reaction of plasma proteins is accelerated by carbonic anhydrase contained in the lung capillaries. Inevitably, the intracellular diffusion of O_2 and CO_2 is affected by these complicated reactions (1). Analysis of the fundamental relationships between the various parameters of the O_2 and CO_2 reactions is necessary to explain the overall gas exchange in the lung.

OXYGEN REACTIONS WITH HEMOGLOBIN AND RED BLOOD CELLS

The oxygenation rate of Hb is generally faster than that of the RBC. However, the former rate decreases as O_2 saturation of Hb proceeds, becoming comparable to the diffusion rate at high levels of O_2 saturation. Thus, for evaluating the oxygenation rate of the RBC it is necessary to add a term for the oxygenation rate of Hb to the differential equation for diffusion.

Oxygenation of Hemoglobin

The rate of oxygenation of Hb (2,3) is proportional to the difference in partial pressure (i.e., energy per unit volume) between the free and bound states of O_2 molecules. Let Po_2^* be the partial pressure of bound O_2 which corresponds to O_2 saturation (So_2) on the O_2

M. Mochizuki: Nishimaruyama Hospital, Geriatric Respiratory Research Center, 064 Sapporo/Chuo-Ku, Japan.

dissociation curve and which is referred to as the "O_2 back-pressure" (4). Designating the reaction rate constant by $F_s$ox, the change in bound O_2 molecules is given by $F_s$ox$\cdot(Po_2 - Po_2^*)$. $F_s$ox is a function of So_2 and approaches zero as So_2 increases to unity. Furthermore, in the RBC it is a little higher than in dilute Hb solution and is given (5,6) by

$$F_s\text{ox} = 2.09\cdot(1 - So_2)^{2.02} \quad (\text{sec}^{-1}\cdot\text{torr}^{-1}) \quad [1]$$

Oxygenation of the RBC

The oxygenation rate of the RBC measured in the early stages of the reaction depends on the convective conditions of suspension (7–12): The higher the flow rate of the suspension, the greater the oxygenation rate. However, in the extracellular Po_2 range of 90–110 torr, the half-time is in the range of 40–60 msec at 37°C (5,13,14). Two examples of the So_2–time curve for human RBCs measured in the rapid flow apparatus are shown in Fig. 1 (5). The RBC suspension was prepared by mixing 5 ml blood with 2 liters of a phosphate buffer solution. To observe the oxygenation rate, the suspension was mixed with the same amount of buffer solution with high Po_2. The RBC concentration in the observation tube had a fractional hematocrit of 0.56×10^{-3}, and the flow rate through the observation tube was about 42 cm·sec^{-1}. The oxygenation rate was proportional to the difference between O_2 back-pressure and extracellular Po_2. The rate constant ($F_c$ox), however, approached zero as So_2 increased to unity and was given by the following hyperbolic function of $F_s$ox:

$$F_c\text{ox} = \frac{0.025\cdot F_s\text{ox}}{0.025 + F_s\text{ox}} \quad (\text{sec}^{-1}\cdot\text{torr}^{-1}) \quad [2]$$

From a theoretical study of $F_c$ox (15), 0.025 is consid-

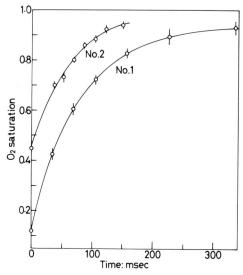

FIG. 1. Change in fractional O_2 saturation during oxygenation of RBCs at 37°C. Po_2 (torr) in RBC suspension is 9 (No. 1) and 24 (No. 2), and that in buffer solution is 205 before mixing. Pco_2 (torr) in RBC suspension is 55 (No. 1) and 74 (No. 2), and that in buffer solution is 40 (5,6).

ered to be the diffusion rate constant within and across the RBC membrane.

Deoxygenation of Hb and RBCs

The deoxygenation rate of Hb in RBC suspensions has hitherto been mainly measured by adding dithionate to the suspension (1,2,12,16); this gives a half-time of 15–50 msec at a temperature range of 15–20°C. However, to estimate the deoxygenation rates for human Hb and RBCs under physiologic conditions, it is necessary to make measurements at 37°C, using N_2 gas to change the Po_2 in Hb solution and RBC suspension. According to our measurements (17), the half-time of the change in So_2 of Hb ranges from 2 to 2.5 msec and depends not only on the So_2 level but also on the reaction time. Thus, the consistent relationship observed between So_2 and F_sox is not observed between So_2 and the rate constant for deoxygenation.

The deoxygenation rate of the RBC is considerably slower than that of Hb (17), suggesting that the deoxygenation of the RBC is limited mainly to O_2 diffusion within and across the RBC membrane. The rate constant F_cdeox was in the range of 0.02 and 0.03 $sec^{-1} \cdot torr^{-1}$, regardless of the So_2 level. The deoxygenation rate measured using dithionate (12) was much faster than that obtained with N_2 gas, and it increased with increasing dithionate concentration. Thus, it is probable that the transfer rate across the RBC boundary is significantly influenced by chemical reactions in the extracellular fluid.

OXYGEN DIFFUSION IN THE RBC

The transfer rate across the RBC boundary can be estimated only by comparing the measured So_2–time curve with the theoretical curve obtained from the diffusion equation. To increase the accuracy of the approximation, a two-dimensional diffusion equation for a disk model was adopted (6,15). In this section, O_2 solubility and the diffusion coefficient in the RBC are described first. Next, the permeability of O_2 across the RBC boundary—that is, the transfer coefficient (η) for O_2 (4)—is introduced. Finally, the reaction rate factor for deoxygenation of O_2Hb within the RBC is evaluated using the η value (18).

Solubility and Diffusion Coefficient of Oxygen in the RBC

The Hb concentration in the RBC is estimated to be about 35 $g \cdot dl^{-1}$, and the water content is approximately 70%. Thus, O_2 solubility in the RBC might be expected to be lower than in plasma, but this is not so. For example, in the bovine RBC the Bunsen's absorption coefficient (i.e., solubility per atmosphere) for O_2 is 0.026 atm^{-1} at 38°C (19), whereas in the plasma it is 0.0209 atm^{-1}.

The diffusion coefficient for O_2 in Hb solution with a concentration of 35.5 $g \cdot dl^{-1}$ at 25°C is about 3.3×10^{-6} $cm^2 \cdot sec^{-1}$ (20). Using the temperature dependency of the coefficient in aqueous solution, 2.5% per degree over a range of 25–37°C (21), the diffusion coefficient in the RBC at 37°C is estimated to be in the order of 4.3×10^{-6} $cm^2 \cdot sec^{-1}$. The diffusion coefficients for N_2 and CO in Hb solution with a concentration of 32 $g \cdot dl^{-1}$ at 20°C are equal to 3.6×10^{-6} $cm^2 \cdot sec^{-1}$ (22), which is compatible with the diffusion coefficient for O_2. Thus, assuming the O_2 solubility per torr in the RBC to be 0.31×10^{-4} $torr^{-1}$ [i.e., the same as that in water at 37°C (19)], the diffusion constant (diffusion coefficient × solubility) for O_2 in the RBC is estimated to be 1.43×10^{-10} $cm^2 \cdot sec^{-1} \cdot torr^{-1}$ (15).

In a dilute Hb solution, O_2 diffusion is usually facilitated by the motion of Hb molecules (23). However, when Hb concentration exceeds 30 $g \cdot dl^{-1}$, the molecules are in contact with each other, making the movement of Hb unlikely (20,24).

Diffusion Equation for Oxygenation in the RBC

Let r and z be variables for distance in the radial and vertical direction, respectively, in the disk RBC model, and let Pco_2 be the partial pressure of free O_2 molecules in the RBC under the experimental conditions to be modeled. Designating the O_2 solubility and diffusion coefficient in the RBC by $\alpha_c O_2$ and $D_c O_2$, respectively, the diffusion equation is given by (15)

$$\alpha_c \cdot \frac{\partial P_c}{\partial t} = \alpha_c \cdot D_c \cdot \left(\frac{\partial^2 P_c}{\partial r^2} + \frac{1}{r} \frac{\partial P_c}{\partial r} + \frac{\partial^2 P_c}{\partial z^2} \right) \quad [3]$$

$$- F_s ox \cdot (P_c - P^*) \quad [3]$$

where t is time. The second term represents the chemical reaction rate. For simplicity, the subscript O_2 is omitted. Let a be the radius of the model, and let b be half the model thickness. Taking the origin at the center ($r = 0$ and $z = 0$), the boundary conditions are written as follows:

$$(\partial P_c / \partial r)_{r=0} = (\partial P_c / \partial z)_{z=0} = 0 \quad [4]$$

$$\alpha_c \cdot D_c \cdot (\partial P_c / \partial r)_{r=a} = \eta \cdot (P_e - P_{c,r=a}) \quad [5]$$

$$\alpha_c \cdot D_c \cdot (\partial P_c / \partial z)_{z=\pm b} = \eta \cdot (P_e - P_{c,z=\pm b}) \quad [6]$$

where P_e is the PO_2 in the extracellular fluid.

After converting the differential form to the difference form, the PO_2 in the RBC is computed alternately for the r- and z-direction by using the alternating-direction implicit method (25). Starting the computation from the initial $P_c O_2$ and $S O_2$ values given by the experimental conditions, the change in $P_c O_2$ ($\Delta P_c O_2$) in individual segments of the RBC is first computed. Then, the change in $S O_2$ (ΔS) is obtained from the following equation:

$$\Delta S = F_s ox \cdot \Delta P_c O_2 \cdot \Delta t / N \quad [7]$$

where Δt is a time increment and N is the O_2 capacity of the RBC. Adding ΔS of Eq. 7 to $S O_2$ at the preceding time, $S O_2$ at the new time is obtained. To calculate $P O_2^*$, Hill's equation for the O_2 dissociation curve is used, where the equilibrium constant K is derived from the intracellular pH (pH_c) as follows (18):

$$\log K = 1.68 \cdot (pH_c - 7.17) - 3.555 \quad [8]$$

Furthermore, setting $S O_2$ at the new time in Eq. 1, the new $F_s ox$ is estimated. Setting the new $P O_2^*$ and $F_s ox$ together with the new $P_c O_2$ in Eq. 3, the difference equation is solved for the next step. Iterating the above procedure, the $S O_2$–time curve is computed. When the measuring system is closed, the extracellular $P O_2$ ($P_e O_2$) is corrected by adding its change ($\Delta P_e O_2$) to that of the preceding time increment. $\Delta P_e O_2$ is computed from $\overline{\Delta P_c O_2}$, the average of $\Delta P_c O_2$, as follows:

$$\Delta P_e O_2 = \frac{\text{Ht}(N \cdot \overline{\Delta S} + \alpha_c O_2 \cdot \overline{\Delta P_c O_2})}{\alpha_e O_2 \cdot (1 - \text{Ht})} \quad [9]$$

where $\overline{\Delta S}$ is the average change in $S O_2$, Ht is the fractional hematocrit, and $\alpha_e O_2$ is O_2 solubility per torr in extracellular fluid.

The oxygenation rate of the RBC measured by flow methods increases with increasing flow velocity (7–12). Assuming that the diffusion rate inside the RBC membrane is not influenced by convection, the flow dependency of the reaction can probably be ascribed to the dependency of the transfer coefficient, η, on the flow rate. During diffusion of gas across a heterogeneous interface, a gap in partial pressure is thought to occur as a result of the difference in energy per gas molecule between the RBC membrane and the extracellular fluid (26). Since η represents the relationship between the transfer rate and the gap in partial pressure (4), it is probable that η is influenced by the change in energy of gas molecules in extracellular fluid due to convection.

The curves in Fig. 1 show the numerical solution of Eq. 3 obtained when $a = 3.5 \times 10^{-4}$ cm, $b = 0.8 \times 10^{-4}$ cm, and $\eta O_2 = 2.5 \times 10^{-6}$ cm·sec^{-1}·torr^{-1} (5,6). Good agreement between the theoretical and experimental $S O_2$–time curves suggests the validity of the equations and the parameter values used.

Diffusion Equation for Deoxygenation in the RBC

The theoretical $S O_2$–time curve during deoxygenation of the RBC is obtained by solving a diffusion equation similar to Eq. 3 except for the term $F_s ox$. The same boundary conditions as shown for Eqs. 4–6 are used together with $\eta O_2 = 2.5 \times 10^{-6}$ cm·sec^{-1}·torr^{-1}. Since the deoxygenation rate constant ($F_s deox$) of hemoglobin in the RBC is difficult to obtain from the measured $S O_2$–time curve, it is determined by comparing the computed $S O_2$–time curve with the measured curve. From this, it is suggested that $F_s deox$ is in the order of 0.3 sec^{-1}·torr^{-1} in an $S O_2$ range of 0.96–0.74 (18).

CARBON DIOXIDE DIFFUSION IN THE RBC

The activity of carbonic anhydrase in the RBC is so high that the rates of CO_2 hydration and dehydration are about 13,000 times those in carbonic anhydrase-free solution (27), where the time constant is about 7.6 sec (28). Thus, the CO_2 reaction rate in the RBC is expected to be mainly limited by CO_2 and HCO_3^- diffusion within and across the RBC membrane. When a certain amount of CO_2 enters the RBC, part of it is hydrated and a new equilibrium state is established between PCO_2, HCO_3^-, and pH. Furthermore, the shift of HCO_3^- ions across the RBC membrane causes a change in PCO_2 in the RBC. Thus, mathematical equations to calculate the equilibration processes between PCO_2, HCO_3^- concentration, and pH resulting from the diffusion of CO_2 and HCO_3^- ions must be derived before solving the simultaneous diffusion equations for CO_2 and HCO_3^-

Changes in P_{CO_2}, HCO_3^-, and pH in the RBC Resulting from CO_2 Diffusion and HCO_3^- Shift

The equilibration processes in the RBC between P_{CO_2}, $(HCO_3^-)_c$, and pH_c are calculated using two relations: (i) the Henderson–Hasselbalch equation and (ii) the relation between $(HCO_3^-)_c$ and pH_c, or the buffer line (29). For simplicity the subscript CO_2 is omitted in the following treatment. From the Henderson–Hasselbalch equation at two equilibrium states [i.e., P_c, $(HCO_3^-)_c$, pH_c and $P_c + \Delta P_c$, $(HCO_3^-)_c + \Delta(HCO_3^-)_c$, $pH_c + \Delta pH_c$], the following relation is derived:

$$\Delta pH_c = \log\left(1 + \frac{\Delta(HCO_3^-)_c}{(HCO_3^-)_c}\right) - \log\left(1 + \frac{\Delta P_c}{P_c}\right) \quad [10]$$

The relation between ΔpH_c and $\Delta(HCO_3^-)_c$ is given using a buffer value β_c, expressed in $mmol \cdot liter(RBC)^{-1} \cdot pH_c^{-1}$ (30), by

$$\Delta(HCO_3^-)_c = \beta_c \cdot \Delta pH_c \quad [11]$$

Because $\beta_c < 0$, when HCO_3^- ions are dehydrated and their concentration decreases, pH_c turns alkaline. Conversely, when CO_2 is hydrated, pH_c turns acidic. When P_c is increased by $\Delta P_c'$ through CO_2 diffusion, this increase is partly offset by the hydration reaction. Let s_c be the molar CO_2 solubility per torr in RBC, 0.0262 $mmol \cdot liter(RBC)^{-1} \cdot torr^{-1}$ (19). Then, the resultant change in $P_c CO_2$ after hydration, ΔP_c, is given by

$$\Delta P_c = \Delta P_c' - \frac{\Delta(HCO_3^-)_c}{s_c} \quad [12]$$

where $\Delta(HCO_3^-)_c$ is the increase in $(HCO_3^-)_c$ due to the hydration reaction. Thus, from Eqs. 10–12 the following relation, which will be referred to as the "modified Henderson–Hasselbalch equation," is derived for $\Delta(HCO_3^-)_c$:

$$\log\left(1 + \frac{\Delta P_c' - \Delta(HCO_3^-)_c/s_c}{P_c}\right)$$
$$= -\frac{\Delta(HCO_3^-)_c}{\beta_c} + \log\left(1 + \frac{\Delta(HCO_3^-)_c}{(HCO_3^-)_c}\right) \quad [13]$$

Since all the parameters in Eq. 13 except $\Delta(HCO_3^-)_c$ are known, this can be evaluated and ΔP_c and ΔpH_c subsequently evaluated from Eqs. 12 and 11, respectively. When $(HCO_3^-)_c$ increases by the hydration of CO_2, HCO_3^- ions move out of the RBC, thereby decreasing $(HCO_3^-)_c$. Let $\Delta(HCO_3^-)_c'$ be the decrease in $(HCO_3^-)_c$ caused by the HCO_3^- shift. Then, further hydration of CO_2 molecules occurs to counter the fall in $(HCO_3^-)_c$, thereby decreasing P_{CO_2}. However, since $(HCO_3^-)_c$ increases, ΔpH_c becomes negative

from Eq. 11; that is, pH_c becomes more acidic. Thus, the following equation is derived:

$$\log\left(1 + \frac{\Delta P_c}{P_c}\right)$$
$$= \frac{s_c \cdot \Delta P_c}{\beta_c} + \log\left(1 + \frac{\Delta(HCO_3^-)_c' - s_c \cdot \Delta P_c}{(HCO_3^-)_c'}\right) \quad [14]$$

where $\Delta P_c CO_2$ and $\Delta(HCO_3^-)_c'$ have negative values. When the inward HCO_3^- shift occurs (from the extracellular fluid into the RBC), dehydration of HCO_3^- results, turning pH_c alkaline and increasing P_{CO_2}.

In CO_2 diffusion, β_c is an important parameter for computation of the change in HCO_3^-. From the measured CO_2 dissociation curve, β_c is given by a function of pH_c in a P_{CO_2} range of 20–60 torr (18,31):

$$\beta_c = -62.03 + 41.43 \cdot (pH_c - 7.17) + \quad [15]$$
$$92.04 \cdot (pH_c - 7.17)^2 \quad (mmol \cdot liter(RBC)^{-1} \cdot pH_c^{-1})$$

β_c given by Eq. 15 is fairly close to the value obtained in a laked Hb solution using a titration method (32).

Eqs. 13 and 14 are the fundamental equations for solving two simultaneous diffusion equations for CO_2 and HCO_3^-. Their validity was proved experimentally by measuring the change in P_{CO_2} caused by CO_2 diffusion and HCO_3^- shift in RBC suspensions (29).

CO_2 and HCO_3^- Diffusions in the RBC

The HCO_3^- shift across the RBC membrane determined by measuring pH or Cl^- in filtered extracellular fluid (33,34) gave half-times in the range of 0.1–0.12 sec. Subsequently, Piiper (35) measured the CO_2 diffusion rate in the RBC using the filtration technique and found the half-time to be about 0.04 sec. Constantine et al. (36) also measured the CO_2 diffusion rate combining a P_{CO_2} electrode with a rapid flow apparatus, where the half-time ranged from 0.04 to 0.11 sec. More recently, Niizeki et al. (37) measured the CO_2 diffusion rate with pH-sensitive fluorescence (38,39) in a stopped-flow method. The half-time was about 0.08 sec in the inward direction. In general, the diffusion rate in an RBC suspension is influenced by flow conditions; in addition, the half-time depends on the hematocrit. Taking the differences in experimental conditions into account, the spread of measured rates seems reasonable.

As reported by previous investigators (33,34), the HCO_3^- shift across the RBC boundary is slower than the CO_2 diffusion. Since the HCO_3^- shift accompanies CO_2 diffusion, permeability of HCO_3^- across the RBC membrane cannot be measured unless carbonic anhydrase activity in the RBC is entirely abolished. Klocke (40) measured the rate of HCO_3^- shift in an

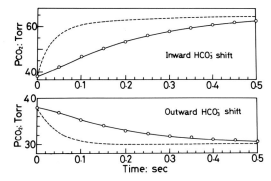

FIG. 2. PCO$_2$–time curve during the secondary CO$_2$ diffusion following the HCO$_3^-$ shift. The experimental conditions are shown in Table 1. The plotted points are the mean experimental values (41), and the curves represent computed extracellular (*solid line*) and intracellular (*broken line*) PCO$_2$ (43). The computation was made with ηHCO$_3^-$ = 5 × 10^{-4} and 7 × 10^{-4} cm·sec^{-1} for the inward and outward HCO$_3^-$ shifts, respectively, and with ηCO$_2$ = 2.5 × 10^{-6} cm·sec^{-1}·torr^{-1} (43).

RBC suspension with a hematocrit of 0.67 after inhibiting the carbonic anhydrase activity with acetazolamide, and he obtained a half-time of 0.07 sec. When dehydration of HCO$_3^-$ occurs in the intact RBC, the increase in intracellular HCO$_3^-$ concentration during the inward HCO$_3^-$ shift is delayed. In addition, since CO$_2$ diffusion out of the RBC is restricted by resistance of the RBC membrane (see below), the rate of HCO$_3^-$ shift is thought to be reduced by the presence of carbonic anhydrase. Thus, the half-time *in vivo* is expected to be longer than the figure of 0.07 sec measured by Klocke (40). Niizeki et al. (41) measured the change in extracellular pH caused by the HCO$_3^-$ shift using the same method as in the measurement of CO$_2$ diffusion. The experimental conditions are shown in Table 1. The fractional hematocrit in the observation chamber is 0.074, and the measured half-time is in the range of 0.13–0.15 sec, regardless of the direction of the shift, as shown in Fig. 2. The measured rate is comparable with the previous data (34,42). The solid and broken curves in Fig. 2 illustrate the changes in PCO$_2$ obtained from the numerical solution (see below) of simultaneous diffusion equations for CO$_2$ and

HCO$_3^-$ in the disk RBC model (43). The PCO$_2$–time curve was obtained when ηCO$_2$ = ηO$_2$, or 2.5 × 10^{-6} cm·sec^{-1}·torr^{-1}, and when ηHCO$_3^-$ = 5 × 10^{-4} and 7 × 10^{-4} cm·sec^{-1} in inward and outward HCO$_3^-$ shifts, respectively. Good agreement between the measured and computed curves suggests the validity of the η values used. Furthermore, this evidence suggests that resistance of the RBC membrane is mainly ascribed to a gap in partial pressure caused by heterogeneity in energy per gas molecule at the interface (26) rather than by resistance across a stagnant boundary layer (9,12), since CO$_2$ is about 24 times more soluble in plasma than O$_2$ at 37°C (19).

Constantine et al. (36) reported that CO$_2$ diffusion in the RBC was significantly retarded by resistance at the RBC membrane. Till then, the resistance had been considered negligible in view of the rapidity of diffusion resulting from the high CO$_2$ solubility. Chow et al. (44) measured the permeability of HCO$_3^-$ by recording the change in pH of an RBC suspension during the Jacobs–Stewart cycle reaction (45) and reported that the permeability of HCO$_3^-$ across the RBC membrane at 37°C was about 2.2 × 10^{-4} cm·sec^{-1}. This value is fairly close to the permeability of Cl$^-$ (42) but is about half the ηHCO$_3^-$ value (43). As will be described later in the calculation of the curve in Fig. 2, the transfer rate of HCO$_3^-$ across the RBC interface is expressed by multiplying ηHCO$_3^-$ by γ·(HCO$_3^-$)$_e$ − (HCO$_3^-$)$_c$, where γ is the ratio of (HCO$_3^-$)$_c$ to (HCO$_3^-$)$_e$ at equilibrium. When permeability is determined by dividing the transfer rate of HCO$_3^-$ by the difference, (HCO$_3^-$)$_e$ − (HCO$_3^-$)$_c$/γ, it corresponds to γ·ηHCO$_3^-$ [i.e., 2–4 × 10^{-4} cm·sec^{-1}, which coincides well with the permeability reported by Chow et al. (44)].

Reaction Rate of Carbamino Formation

The rate of carbamino formation of human deoxygenated Hb was measured by Forster et al. (46) with a rapid flow apparatus using a PCO$_2$ electrode and by Kernohan and Roughton (47), who observed the change in temperature caused by the reaction. The lat-

TABLE 1. *Experimental conditions before mixing, in a stopped-flow method for measuring the HCO$_3^-$ shift*

Parameters	Inward shift		Outward shift	
	Suspension	Solution	Suspension	Solution
Fractional hematocrit	0.140	0	0.148	0
(HCO$_3^-$)$_p$ (mmol·liter(plasma)$^{-1}$)	7.0	40.0	38.2	2.0
(HCO$_3^-$)$_c$ (mmol·liter(RBC)$^{-1}$)	5.0	—	21.2	—
Cl$^-$ (mM)	148.0	110.0	110.0	148.0
pH	6.86	7.67	7.65	6.45
PCO$_2$ (torr)	38.4	38.4	38.4	38.4

ter investigators measured the reaction rate only at an early stage (i.e., within the first 8 msec); furthermore, since no precise information on the final temperature level is given, the half-time cannot be estimated from their report. Forster et al. (46) inactivated carbonic anhydrase in the reacting solutions by adding acetazolamide to give a concentration of 1.1 mM, and the Hb concentration following mixing was about 4 mM. The Hb solution was initially equilibrated at P_{CO_2} close to 0, and then it was mixed with a high P_{CO_2} solution. The change in P_{CO_2} in solution was almost exponential, and the half-time was about 10 msec, regardless of the pH in the mixed solution. Thus, carbamate formation is a little slower than the oxygenation and deoxygenation reactions of Hb, but it is significantly faster than these reactions in the RBC.

Diffusion Equations for CO_2 Reactions

CO_2 diffusion is always accompanied by diffusion of HCO_3^-. Thus, two diffusion equations for CO_2 and HCO_3^- have to be solved simultaneously (43). More particularly, in a closed system such as the one used in the flow method, extracellular P_{CO_2} and HCO_3^- concentration should be computed together with their concentrations in the RBC. In principle, the CO_2 reaction in the RBC is assumed to be so fast that it is completed within 1 msec. Thus, unlike the equation for O_2 diffusion (Eq. 3), the differential equations for CO_2 and HCO_3^- contain no chemical reaction term. However, the changes in P_{CO_2} and HCO_3^- concentration resulting from diffusion are corrected at each time increment immediately after solving the differential equations, using the modified Henderson–Hasselbalch equations (Eqs. 13 and 14). To increase the accuracy of the approximation, the following two-dimensional differential equations are solved simultaneously using the same disk model as used in Eq. 3:

$$\frac{\partial P_c}{\partial t} = D_c CO_2 \cdot \left(\frac{\partial^2 P_c}{\partial r^2} + \frac{1}{r} \frac{\partial P_c}{\partial r} + \frac{\partial^2 P_c}{\partial z^2} \right) \quad [16]$$

$$\frac{\partial (HCO_3^-)_c}{\partial t} = D_c HCO_3^- \cdot \left(\frac{\partial^2 (HCO_3^-)_c}{\partial r^2} \right.$$
$$\left. + \frac{1}{r} \frac{\partial (HCO_3^-)_c}{\partial r} + \frac{\partial^2 (HCO_3^-)_c}{\partial z^2} \right) \quad [17]$$

where $D_c CO_2$ and $D_c HCO_3^-$ are intracellular diffusion coefficients for CO_2 and HCO_3^-, being 0.34×10^{-6} and 0.14×10^{-6} cm$^2 \cdot$sec^{-1}, respectively. These values are estimated from the CO_2 diffusion rate in a thin layer of Hb solution (39). For solving Eqs. 16 and 17, equations similar to Eqs. 4–6 are applied to the boundary conditions. Let ηHCO_3^- (cm$\cdot$sec^{-1}) be the transfer coefficient for HCO_3^- The transfer rates of HCO_3^-

across the outer boundary are expressed by the following equations:

$$D_c HCO_3^- \cdot (\partial (HCO_3^-)_c / \partial r)_{r=a} \quad [18]$$

$$= \eta HCO_3^- (\gamma \cdot (HCO_3^-)_e - (HCO_3^-)_{r=a}) \quad [19]$$

$$D_c HCO_3^- \cdot (\partial (HCO_3^-)_c / \partial z)_{z=\pm b}$$

$$= \eta HCO_3^- \cdot (\gamma \cdot (HCO_3^-)_e - (HCO_3^-)_{z=\pm b})$$

where $(HCO_3^-)_e$ is extracellular HCO_3^- concentration and γ is a function of pH in the RBC. In human blood it is given (18) by the following equation, regardless of O_2 saturation:

$$\gamma = 0.5 - 0.47 \cdot (pH_c - 7.17)$$
$$- 0.76 \cdot (pH_c - 7.17)^2 \quad [20]$$

The changes in extracellular dissolved CO_2 content and HCO_3^- during a time increment are calculated at the end of the respective diffusion process by dividing the quantities diffusing in and out of the RBC by the extracellular fluid volume, according to a formula similar to Eq. 9. When there is abundant carbonic anhydrase in the extracellular fluid, the CO_2 reaction rapidly equilibrates. In this case, the changes in the extracellular P_{CO_2} and HCO_3^- ($\Delta P_e CO_2$ and $\Delta (HCO_3^-)_e$) are corrected at the end of each time increment using the modified Henderson–Hasselbalch equation similar to Eqs. 13 and 14.

The computations of Eqs. 16 and 17 are made using the alternating-direction implicit method (25). To increase the accuracy of the solving procedure, the time increment is made less than 1 msec for the first 10 msec, but at later stages it is maintained at 2 msec. For computing the overall CO_2 reaction processes, the following steps are required: (a) Solve the CO_2 diffusion equation, Eq. 16; (b) correct the changes in P_{CO_2} and pH_c in the RBC by using Eq. 13, correct β_c by using Eq. 15, and correct γ by using Eq. 20; (c) correct $P_e CO_2$; (d) solve the HCO_3^- diffusion equation, Eq. 17; (e) correct $\Delta (HCO_3^-)_c$ by using Eq. 14; and (f) when abundant carbonic anhydrase is present in the extracellular fluid, correct $\Delta P_e CO_2$ and $\Delta (HCO_3^-)_e$ simultaneously.

**OVERALL OXYGEN
AND CARBON DIOXIDE REACTIONS**

The Bohr and Haldane effects result in O_2 and CO_2 diffusion and HCO_3^- shift. When pH_c is reduced, the energy of the O_2 bound to Hb rises (Bohr effect) in parallel with that of free O_2 in contact with Hb molecules. As a result of the new P_{O_2} gradient, outward O_2 diffusion occurs, reducing S_{O_2} (Bohr off-shift). When pH_c increases, the energies of bound and free O_2 in the RBC are simultaneously reduced, causing inward O_2 diffusion (Bohr on-shift). Furthermore, when Hb is oxygenated in the RBC, H^+ ions are released from Hb in exchange for K^+, resulting in dehydration of HCO_3^-; in addition, CO_2 molecules are released from carbamate. These reactions increase intracellular P_{CO_2}, causing outward CO_2 diffusion. When S_{O_2} is lowered in the RBC, inward CO_2 diffusion occurs, to increase the CO_2 content in the RBC. Physiologically, the contribution of the Haldane effect amounts to 25–27% of the whole CO_2 output in the lung. It is important to estimate the overall reaction rates of O_2 and CO_2 in the capillary blood.

Calculation of the Changes in P_{O_2} Resulting from the Bohr Effect

The change in $P_{O_2}^*$ resulting from the Bohr effect is evaluated from Hill's equation using K obtained from Eq. 8. The pH_c value relating to K is obtained from the diffusion equations for CO_2 and HCO_3^-. Let $\Delta P_{O_2}^*$ be the change in $P_{O_2}^*$ resulting from the Bohr effect. The P_{cO_2} after the change in pH_c, $P_{cO_2}(i)$, is given by adding $\Delta P_{O_2}^*$ to the preceding P_{cO_2}, $P_{cO_2}(i - 1)$, as given by

$$P_{cO_2}(i) = P_{cO_2}(i - 1) + \Delta P_{O_2}^* \quad [21]$$

Equation 21 states that the changes in P_{cO_2} and $P_{O_2}^*$ occur simultaneously. After the CO_2 diffusion is computed, pH_c and $P_{O_2}^*$ are corrected. Furthermore, after correcting P_{cO_2} by using Eq. 21, the O_2 diffusion equation (Eq. 3) is solved to obtain ΔS resulting from the Bohr effect.

Calculation of Changes in P_{CO_2} and HCO_3^- Content Resulting from the Haldane Effect

Let HE (mmol·liter(RBC)$^{-1}$) be the decrease in content of free CO_2 in the RBC caused by deoxygenation of the fully oxygenated RBC. If no dehydration of HCO_3^- occurred in the RBC during a deoxygenation process ($\Delta S < 0$), P_{cCO_2} would drop by as much as $HE \cdot \Delta S / s_c$. Following deoxygenation, however, HCO_3^- is dehydrated, decreasing $(HCO_3^-)_c$ and moderating the P_{CO_2} drop. Let $\Delta(HCO_3^-)_c$ be the amount of dehydrated HCO_3^-. Then, ΔP_{cCO_2}, the net change in P_{cCO_2}, is derived by subtracting $\Delta(HCO_3^-)_c/s_c$ from $HE \cdot \Delta S/s_c$:

$$\Delta P_{cCO_2} = (HE \cdot \Delta S - \Delta(HCO_3^-)_c)/s_c \quad [22]$$

where $\Delta(HCO_3^-)_c < 0$. Let C_m (mmol·liter(RBC)$^{-1}$) be the carbamate CO_2 component of HE. When H^+ ions are bound to Hb molecules as a result of deoxygenation, hydration of CO_2 occurs in the RBC to counter the decrease in H^+ concentration. Thus, $(HCO_3^-)_c$ is initially increased by $-(HE - C_m) \cdot \Delta S$. However,

since this increase is diminished (by dehydration) by $\Delta(HCO_3^-)_c$, the net $(HCO_3^-)_c$ change is given by

Net $(HCO_3^-)_c$ change

$$= -(HE - C_m) \cdot \Delta S + \Delta(HCO_3^-)_c \quad [23]$$

Let β_c^* (< 0; mmol·liter(RBC)$^{-1}$·pH_c^{-1}) be the buffer value for the Haldane effect. The change in pH_c caused by the Haldane effect is given by

$$\Delta pH_c = \Delta(HCO_3^-)_c/\beta_c^* \quad [24]$$

Thus, the relation between pH_c, P_cCO_2, and $(HCO_3^-)_c$ following the O_2 reactions is expressed from Eqs. 22–24 and is similar to Eq. 13 (18):

$$\log\left(1 + \frac{HE \cdot \Delta S - \Delta(HCO_3^-)_c}{s_c \cdot P_c}\right) = \frac{\Delta(HCO_3^-)_c}{\beta_c^*}$$
$$+ \log\left(1 - \frac{(HE - C_m) \cdot \Delta S - \Delta(HCO_3^-)_c}{(HCO_3^-)_c}\right)$$
$$[25]$$

The change in CO_2 content resulting from the Haldane effect, $-HE \cdot \Delta S$, must be equal to the CO_2 quantity diffusing in and out of the RBC caused by the same effect. Thus, the optimum β_c^* value is determined by comparing the computed CO_2 diffusion quantity with the $HE \cdot \Delta S$ value set in the initial conditions of the diffusion equations. The resulting β_c^* is -44 mmol·liter(RBC)$^{-1}$·pH_c^{-1}. The relationships between the parameters obtained from Eq. 25 are illustrated in Fig. 3, where $P_{CO_2} = 40$ torr. The net $(HCO_3^-)_c$ change [i.e., $-(HE - C_m) \cdot \Delta S + \Delta(HCO_3^-)_c$] and ΔpH_c are linearly related to ΔS, and ΔP_{cCO_2} is also almost linear against ΔS.

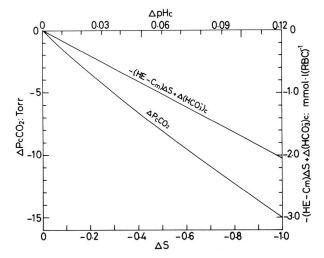

FIG. 3. Relationship between the changes in S, P_{CO_2}, and HCO_3^- in the RBC caused by the Haldane effect during deoxygenation. $P_{CO_2} = 40$ torr. The parameter values are calculated from Eq. 25, where $\beta_c^* = -44$ mmol·liter(RBC)$^{-1}$·pH_c^{-1}.

Calculation of the Change in P_{CO_2} and HCO_3^- in Plasma

The buffering reaction of plasma proteins is accelerated by carbonic anhydrase contained in the capillary wall (48–50). The rate of acceleration is thought to depend not only on carbonic anhydrase activity but also on the difference in energy between H^+ ions bound to plasma proteins and free H^+ ions in the surrounding fluid. The difference in the amount of H^+ combined with plasma proteins at two equilibria is equal to the difference in HCO_3^- content in separated plasma. Let $\Delta(HCO_3^-)_p$ be the change in HCO_3^- content in separated plasma. Then, the rate of the buffering reaction is formulated by using $\Delta(HCO_3^-)_p$. Furthermore, $(HCO_3^-)_p$ is linearly related to pH in separated plasma (pH_e) (51), as shown by the buffer line of separated plasma, whose slope, or buffer value β_p, is -7 mmol·liter(plasma)$^{-1}$·pH_e^{-1} (52). Let pH_p^* be hypothetical pH in the fluid equilibrated with H^+ ions bound to plasma proteins. Then, the reaction rate is treated as being proportional to the difference between the actual and hypothetical pH in the extracellular fluid, $pH_e - pH_p^*$. Since the product of β_p and $pH_e - pH_p^*$ corresponds to $\Delta(HCO_3^-)_p$ during the equilibration process, the rate of the change in $\Delta(HCO_3^-)$ is expressed by a reciprocal of the time constant, $1/T$. That is, $\Delta(HCO_3^-)_p$ resulting from carbonic anhydrase in the capillary wall is given by

$$\Delta(HCO_3^-)_p/\Delta t = \beta_p \cdot (pH_e - pH_p^*)/T \quad [26]$$

Starting from the initial pH_p^* value, pH_p^* ($i = 0$), pH_p^* at the ith time increment is successively given by

$$pH_p^*(i) = pH_p^*(i - 1) + \Delta(HCO_3^-)_p(i)/\beta_p \quad [27]$$

pH_e in Eq. 26 is evaluated from extracellular P_{CO_2} (P_eCO_2) and $HCO_3^-{}_e$ using the Henderson–Hasselbalch equation. Thus, $\Delta(HCO_3^-)_p$ is obtained by successive steps from Eq. 26. Adding $\Delta(HCO_3^-)_p$ of Eq. 26 along with $\Delta(HCO_3^-)_e$ (resulting from CO_2 diffusion and HCO_3^- shift) to $(HCO_3^-)_e$ of the preceding time increment, the value of $(HCO_3^-)_e$ for the new iterative time is calculated. The T value obtained by comparing the computed CO_2 exchange rate in the lung with the measured data (18) was about 0.1 sec.

Changes in P_{O_2}, P_{CO_2}, and HCO_3^- Resulting from the Bohr and Haldane Effects

By solving the simultaneous diffusion equations for O_2, CO_2, and HCO_3^- successively and repeatedly for every time increment (18), the changes in P_{O_2}, P_{CO_2}, and HCO_3^- in the RBC and extracellular fluid, caused by the Bohr and Haldane effects, are evaluated. Then,

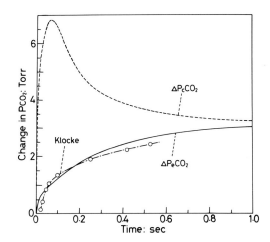

FIG. 4. Changes in intra- and extracellular P_{CO_2} in RBC suspension, with Ht = 0.025, during the Haldane effect. The initial P_{O_2} values in RBCs and surrounding solution are 10 and 165 torr, respectively. The initial P_{CO_2} is 41 torr in both. The plotted points are the P_{CO_2} values measured by Klocke (53).

by adding each change to the respective value in the preceding time increment, all the parameters are evaluated over the entire reaction time. An example of the change in extracellular P_{CO_2} resulting from the Haldane effect is shown in Fig. 4 (18,53). The fractional hematocrit is 0.025. Initially, P_cO_2 and P_eO_2 are 10 and 165 torr, respectively, but P_cCO_2 and P_eCO_2 are equally 40 torr. The solid curve shows P_eCO_2, and the broken curve shows P_cCO_2. Immediately after mixing, S_{O_2} rises from 0.08 to 0.83, and P_cCO_2 shows a high initial peak of about 6.8 torr. Following the initial increase in P_cCO_2, P_eCO_2 increases as outward CO_2 diffusion proceeds. The plotted points are the measured P_eCO_2 (53), showing good agreement with the computed curve.

Such good agreement was also observed between the computed and measured changes in S_{O_2} during the Bohr shift (18,54,55). The rate of the Bohr off-shift decreases as the S_{O_2} level is lowered. When the hematocrit is 0.015, the half-time at $S_{O_2} = 0.6$ is 0.2 sec, and in the S_{O_2} range between 0.85 and 0.93, the half-time falls in the range of 0.12–0.16 sec.

SUMMARY

The diffusion rates of O_2, CO_2, and HCO_3^- in the RBC are considered in order to obtain a numerical solution for overall gas-exchange processes. Furthermore, the relations between the changes in P_{O_2}, S_{O_2}, P_{CO_2}, HCO_3^- concentration, and pH resulting from the HCO_3^- shift and the Bohr and Haldane effects are derived.

1. The oxygenation rate of hemoglobin decreases as

S_{O_2} increases and is approximately proportional to the square of $(1 - S_{O_2})$. The oxygenation rate of the RBC is significantly lower than that of hemoglobin at low levels of S_{O_2}, suggesting that a gap in partial pressure exists at the interface surrounding the RBC membrane.

2. CO_2 diffusion in the RBC accompanies the HCO_3^- shift, and vice versa. For instance, when HCO_3^- ions enter the RBC, P_{CO_2} rises as a result of the dehydration reaction, causing outward CO_2 diffusion. The relationship between the changes in pH, P_{CO_2}, and HCO_3^- concentration in the RBC resulting from the HCO_3^- shift is derived from (a) the Henderson–Hasselbalch equations at two different equilibrium states and (b) the relation of the buffer line. The rate of carbamate formation is so high compared with that of CO_2 diffusion that it can be disregarded. From the computed and measured diffusion rates in the RBC, the transfer rate for CO_2 per unit difference in partial pressure at the interface (i.e., the transfer coefficient) is found to be identical to that for O_2. Since CO_2 is about 20 times more soluble than O_2, the origin of the difference in partial pressures is ascribed to the difference in energy per molecule of gas in the RBC membrane and gas in extracellular fluid.

3. The change in partial pressure of free O_2 in the RBC resulting from the Bohr effect is treated as occurring in parallel with that of O_2 molecules bound to hemoglobin, and it depends on intracellular pH. The changes in P_{CO_2} and HCO_3^- concentration in the RBC caused by the Haldane effect are given by the modified Henderson–Hasselbalch equation, in which the buffer value is about 70% of the slope of the usual CO_2 buffer line in the RBC. The computed rates of the Bohr and Haldane effects are compatible with the experimental data obtained by other investigators, verifying the validity of the equations and parameters used.

ACKNOWLEDGMENT

The author would like to express his sincere thanks to Dr. Ann Silver, Cambridge, England, for her painstaking work in revising the manuscript.

REFERENCES

1. Roughton FJW. Transport of oxygen and carbon dioxide. In: Fenn WO, Rahn H, eds. *Handbook of physiology, Section 3: Respiration, vol 1*. Washington, DC: American Physiological Society 1964;767–825.
2. Gibson QH, Kreuzer F, Meda E, Roughton FJW. The kinetics of human haemoglobin in solution and in the red cell at 37°C. *J Physiol* 1955;129:65–89.
3. Mochizuki M, Nakamura K, Oyama Y. Study on the oxygenation velocity of human hemoglobin. *Jpn J Physiol* 1966;16:519–527.
4. Mochizuki M, Fukuoka J. The diffusion of oxygen inside the red cell. *Jpn J Physiol* 1958;8:206–224.
5. Mochizuki M. Study on the oxygenation velocity of the human red cell. *Jpn J Physiol* 1966;16:635–648.
6. Kagawa T, Mochizuki M. Numerical solution of partial differential equation describing oxygenation rate of the red blood cell. *Jpn J Physiol* 1982;32:197–218.
7. Koyama T, Mochizuki M. A study on the relationship between the oxygenation velocity of the red blood cell and the flow velocity in a rapid flow method. *Jpn J Physiol* 1969;19:534–546.
8. Kutchai H, Staub NC. Steady-state, hemoglobin-facilitated O_2 transport in human erythrocytes. *J Gen Physiol* 1969;53:576–589.
9. Coin JT, Olsen JS. The rate of oxygen uptake by human red blood cells. *J Biol Chem* 1979;254:1178–1190.
10. Rotman H, Ikeda I, Chiu CS, et al. Resistance of red blood cell membrane to oxygen uptake. *J Appl Physiol* 1980;49:306–310.
11. Huxley VH, Kutchai H. The effect of red cell membrane and a diffusion boundary layer on the rate of oxygen uptake by human erythrocytes. *J Physiol* 1981;316:75–83.
12. Yamaguchi K, Nguyen-Phu D, Scheid P, Piiper J. Kinetics of O_2 uptake and release by human erythrocytes studied by a stopped-flow technique. *J Appl Physiol* 1985;58:1215–1224.
13. Roughton FJW. Diffusion and chemical reaction velocity as joint factors in determining the rate of uptake of oxygen and carbon monoxide by the red blood corpuscle. *Proc R Soc Lond [Biol]* 1932;CXI:1–36.
14. Forster RE, Roughton FJW, Kreuzer F, Briscoe WA. Photocolorimetric determination of rate of uptake of CO and O_2 by reduced human red cell suspensions at 37°C. *J Appl Physiol* 1957;11:260–268.
15. Mochizuki M. *Graphical analysis of oxygenation and CO combination rates of the red cells in the lung*. Tokyo: Hirokawa, 1975.
16. Sirs JA. The egress of oxygen from human HbO_2 in solution and in the erythrocyte. *J Physiol* 1967;189:461–473.
17. Mochizuki M. On the velocity of oxygen dissociation of human hemoglobin and red cell. *Jpn J Physiol* 1966;16:649–657.
18. Mochizuki M, Kagawa T. Numerical solution of partial differential equations describing the simultaneous O_2 and CO_2 diffusions in the red blood cell. *Jpn J Physiol* 1986;36:43–63.
19. Opitz E, Bartels H. Gasanalyse. In: *Hoppe–Seyler/Thierfelder, Handbuch der physiologisch- und pathologisch-chemischen Analyse*, vol 2. Berlin: Springer-Verlag, 1955;305–309.
20. Klug A, Kreuzer F, Roughton FJW. The diffusion of oxygen in concentrated haemoglobin solutions. *Helv Physiol Acta* 1956;14:121–128.
21. Gertz KH, Loeschcke HH. Bestimmung der Diffusions-Koeffizienten von H_2, O_2, N_2 und He in Wasser und Blutserum bei konstant gehaltener Konvektion. *Z Naturforsch* 1954;9b:1–9.
22. Longmuir IS, Roughton FJW. The diffusion coefficients of carbon monoxide and nitrogen in haemoglobin solutions. *J Physiol* 1952;118:264–275.
23. Kreuzer F. Facilitated diffusion of oxygen and carbon dioxide. In: Fahri LE, Tenny SM, eds. *Handbook of physiology, Section 3, The respiratory system: vol 4. Gas exchange*. Bethesda, MD: American Physiological Society, 1987:89–111.
24. Perutz M. Submicroscopic structure of the red cell. *Nature* 1948;161:204–205.
25. Douglas J Jr, Rachford HH Jr. On the numerical solution of heat conduction problems in two and three space variables. *Trans Am Math Soc* 1956;82:421–439.
26. Mochizuki M. Relationship between the transfer rate and the gap in partial pressure of gas molecules at a heterogeneous interface. *Jpn J Physiol* 1988;38:591–605.
27. Kernohan JC, Forrest WW, Roughton FJW. The activity of concentrated solutions of carbonic anhydrase. *Biochim Biophys Acta* 1963;67:31–41.
28. Roughton FJW. Some recent work on the chemistry of carbon dioxide transport by the blood. *Harvey Lectures* 1943;39:96–142.
29. Shimouchi A, Mochizuki M, Niizeki K. Change in PCO_2 in red cell suspension following bicarbonate shift. *Jpn J Physiol* 1984;34:1015–1027.
30. Van Slyke DD, Wu H, McLean FC. Studies of gas and electrolyte equilibria in the blood. V. Factors controlling the electrolyte

and water distribution in the blood. *J Biol Chem* 1923;106:765–849.

31. Tazawa H, Mochizuki M, Tamura M, Kagawa T. Quantitative analyses of the CO_2 dissociation curve of oxygenated blood and the Haldane effect in human blood. *Jpn J Physiol* 1983;33:601–618.

32. Siggaard-Andersen O. Oxygen-linked hydrogen ion binding of human hemoglobin. Effects of carbon dioxide and 2,3-diphosphoglycerate. I. Studies on erythrolysate. *Scand J Clin Lab Invest* 1971;27:351–360.

33. Dirken MNJ, Mook HW. The rate of gas exchange between blood cells and serum. *J Physiol* 1931;73:349–360.

34. Luckner H. Über die Geschwindigkeit des Austausches der Atemgase im Blut. *Pflugers Arch* 1939;241:753–781.

35. Piiper J. Geschwindigkeit des CO_2-Austausches zwischen Erythrocyten und Plasma. *Pflugers Arch* 1964;278:500–512.

36. Constantine HP, Craw MR, Forster RE. Rate of the reaction of carbon dioxide with human red blood cells. *Am J Physiol* 1965;208:801–811.

37. Niizeki K, Mochizuki M, Uchida K. Rate of CO_2 diffusion in the human red blood cell measured with pH-sensitive fluorescence. *Jpn J Physiol* 1983;33:635–650.

38. Lübbers DW, Opitz N. Die pCO_2/pO_2-optode; eine neue pCO_2-bzw. pO_2-Messsonde zur Messung des pCO_2 oder pO_2 von Gasen und Flüssigkeiten. *Z Naturforsch* 1975;30c:532–533.

39. Uchida K, Mochizuki M, Niizeki K. Diffusion coefficients of CO_2 molecule and bicarbonate ion in hemoglobin solution measured by fluorescence technique. *Jpn J Physiol* 1983;33:619–634.

40. Klocke RA. Rate of bicarbonate–chloride exchange in human red cells at 37°C. *J Appl Physiol* 1976;40:707–714.

41. Niizeki K, Mochizuki M, Kagawa T. Secondary CO_2 diffusion following HCO_3^- shift across the red blood cell membrane. *Jpn J Physiol* 1984;34:1003–1013.

42. Tosteson DC. Halide transport in red blood cells. *Acta Physiol Scand* 1959;46:19–41.

43. Kagawa T, Mochizuki M. Numerical solution of partial differential equations for CO_2 diffusion accompanying HCO_3^- shift in red blood cells. *Jpn J Physiol* 1984;34:1029–1047.

44. Chow EIH, Crandall ED, Forster RE. Kinetics of bicarbonate–chloride exchange across the human red blood cell membrane. *J Gen Physiol* 1976;68:633–652.

45. Jacobs MH, Stewart DR. The role of carbonic anhydrase in certain ionic exchanges involving the erythrocyte. *J Gen Physiol* 1942;25:539–552.

46. Forster RE, Constantine HP, Craw MR, et al. Reaction of CO_2 with human hemoglobin solution. *J Biol Chem* 1968;213:3317–3326.

47. Kernohan JC, Roughton FJW. Kinetics of carbamino compound formation in red cells and in hemoglobin solutions. In: Forster RE, et al., eds. *CO_2: chemical, biochemical and physiological aspects.* Washington, DC: NASA, 1968;61–64.

48. Effros RM, Chang RSY, Silverman P. Acceleration of plasma bicarbonate conversion to carbon dioxide by pulmonary carbonic anhydrase. *Science* 1978;199:427–429.

49. Klocke RA. Catalysis of CO_2 reactions by lung carbonic anhydrase. *J Appl Physiol* 1978;44:882–888.

50. Bidani A, Mathew SJ, Crandall ED. Pulmonary vascular carbonic anhydrase activity. *J Appl Physiol: Respir Environ Exercise Physiol* 1983;55:75–83.

51. Van Slyke DD, Hastings AB, Hiller A, Sendroy J Jr. Studies of gas and electrolyte equilibria in blood. XIV. The amounts of alkali bound by serum albumin and globulin. *J Biol Chem* 1928;79:769–780.

52. Takiwaki H, Mochizuki M, Niizeki K. Relationship between hematocrit and CO_2 contents in whole blood and true plasma. *Jpn J Physiol* 1983;33:567–578.

53. Klocke RA. Mechanism and kinetics of the Haldane effect in human erythrocytes. *J Appl Physiol* 1973;35:673–681.

54. Nakamura T, Staub NC. Synergism in the kinetic reactions of O_2 and CO_2 with human red blood cells. *J Physiol* 1964;173:161–177.

55. Forster RE, Steen JB. Rate limiting processes in the Bohr shift in human red cells. *J Physiol* 1968;196:541–562.

THE LUNG: Scientific Foundations
edited by R.G. Crystal, J.B. West et al.
Raven Press, Ltd., New York © 1991.

CHAPTER 5.3.2.5

Acid–Base Physiology

Norman L. Jones

This chapter will present an approach to acid–base physiology that is based on classical concepts of physical chemistry; this must be stated at the outset because in some respects it will seem to differ from the standard or conventional approach to the topic as taught during the last 50 years. The contrasts between these two general approaches will be highlighted, but it may help the reader to have an appreciation of the way the field developed from the earliest years of this century.

HISTORY (1)

Towards the end of the last century, the Law of Mass Action was already well understood; it states that the velocity of a chemical reaction is proportional to the active concentrations (or "activities") of the reactants. In a reaction that may proceed in either direction, such as

$$A + B \rightleftharpoons C + D$$

with rate constants for both the forward (k_1, $A + B \rightarrow C + D$) and reverse (k_2, $C + D \rightarrow A + B$) reactions, the concentrations of reactants will change until equilibrium is reached, when

$$k_1[A][B] = k_2[C][D]$$

or

$$k_1/k_2 = [C][D]/[A][B]$$

The term k_1/k_2 is the equilibrium constant, K_c. Considering an acid HA in solution, "dissociation" occurs in the reaction

$$HA \rightleftharpoons H^+ + A^-$$

and at equilibrium

$$K_a = [H^+][A^-]/[HA]$$

K_a is known as the dissociation constant for the acid. If the acid is "strong" (i.e., strongly dissociates to A^- and H^+), K_a is very large and $[A^-]$ is much higher than $[HA]$. The Law of Mass Action was rewritten by L. J. Henderson in 1909 (1,2) in terms of the hydrogen ion concentration:

$$[H^+] = K_a \times [HA]/[A^-] \qquad [1]$$

For carbonic acid he derived the following equation, now known as "Henderson's equation":

$$[H^+] = K \times [CO_2]/[HCO_3^-] \qquad [2]$$

Using the convention introduced by S. P. L. Sørensen in 1909 (1), in which $[H^+]$ was expressed by pH, where p is the negative power of 10, K. A. Hasselbalch rearranged Eq. 1 in 1917 (1) to obtain

$$pH = pK + \log([A^-]/[HA]) \qquad [3]$$

where $pH = -\log[H^+]$ and $pK = -\log K$.[1] Hasselbalch applied the equation to the CO_2 system (Eq. 2) to obtain

$$pH = pK + \log([HCO_3^-]/[CO_2]) \qquad [4]$$

The "Henderson–Hasselbalch equation" has provided the basic description for pH changes in plasma in standard teaching ever since. When methods for the measurement of P_{CO_2} became available, $[CO_2]$ was replaced by P_{CO_2}; from Eq. 2 we obtain

$$[H^+] = 24 P_{CO_2}/[HCO_3^-] \qquad [5]$$

N. L. Jones: Department of Medicine, McMaster University, Hamilton, Ontario L8N 3Z5, Canada.

[1] Note that when $[A^-] = [HA]$, $pH = pK + \log 1$; thus pK is the pH at which HA is half dissociated.

where [H$^+$] is in nEq/liter, PCO$_2$ is in mmHg, and [HCO$_3$$^-$] is in mEq/liter, and from Eq. 4 we obtain

$$pH = 6.1 + \log([HCO_3^-]/0.0301 PCO_2) \qquad [6]$$

Because the PCO$_2$ of arterial plasma is regulated by alveolar ventilation, it is used to indicate the respiratory component of an acid–base state, and [HCO$_3$$^-$] is used to quantify the nonrespiratory, or "metabolic," contribution to [H$^+$] (3,4). Although Eqs. 5 and 6 are accurate mathematical descriptions of the equilibrium relationships between these variables, conceptually they have been used also to "describe" the "control" of the system. For example, Pitts (5) emphasized that "regulation of the concentrations of the components of this one buffer pair fixes the hydrogen ion concentration and thereby determines the ratios of all the other buffer pairs." However, for this concept to be valid, both PCO$_2$ and [HCO$_3$$^-$] should be capable of acting independently, without significant influence from other systems influencing acid–base control.

Early on, one basic flaw to an approach based on the carbonic acid–bicarbonate system alone was recognized to be the independent and direct effect of PCO$_2$ on [HCO$_3$$^-$]; changes in [HCO$_3$$^-$] could not be used quantitatively to indicate "metabolic" changes alone. Several approaches were used to overcome this difficulty, culminating in the graphical approach of Siggaard-Andersen (7), based on titration studies of plasma, along with the methodological approach of Astrup (8), which normalized PCO$_2$ to 40 mmHg. These advances led to the concept of "base excess," (9) the excess [HCO$_3$$^-$] in arterial plasma in which respiratory changes had been allowed for. Although solidly based for plasma, having been established by *in vitro* titrations, the approach seemed not to hold when applied to whole blood, or to plasma changes in studies where the "titrations" were carried out *in vivo*. Schwartz and Relman (10), on the basis of such studies, criticized the concept of base excess, beginning what Bunker (11) termed "The Great Transatlantic Acid–Base Debate," which centered on the validity of *in vitro* relationships applied to *in vivo* situations. Astrup and Severinghaus (1) recount that the debate was resolved by using *in vitro* data based on whole blood having a hemoglobin concentration of 5 g/dl. However, other experts advocated an approach that used the expected *in vivo* behavior for "pure" disorders (12).

The importance of strong (i.e., fully dissociated) ions on [H$^+$] was appreciated early; their contribution may be expressed in the difference between the concentrations of anions and cations. In plasma, cations predominate and exert a basic, or alkalizing, effect; for this reason, Singer and Hastings in 1948 (13) termed the cation–anion difference the "buffer base." More recently, the concept has reemerged as a central independent variable in the physicochemical approach, known as the strong ion difference ([SID]) (14–16).

The effect of strong ions other than Na$^+$, K$^+$, and Cl$^-$ is conventionally expressed as the "anion gap"—the anion concentration that is not explained by the inorganic anions and bicarbonate ([Na$^+$] + [K$^+$] − [Cl$^-$] − [HCO$_3$$^-$]). The "normal" anion gap is taken as 17 mEq/liter; a value in excess represents "unmeasured anions," such as lactate or ketones.

THE PHYSICOCHEMICAL SYSTEMS APPROACH (15)

A systems approach to acid–base identifies the systems that contribute to [H$^+$], leading to the recognition of (a) independent variables and parameters (those not altered by changes outside the system in question) and (b) dependent variables (those that are influenced not only by the independent variable within the system but also by changes in other systems). The behavior of the systems may then be described in a series of equations in which the independent variables are specified. In the equations below, concentration will usually be expressed in mEq/liter instead of the more acceptable SI unit of mmol/liter, but this is to emphasize that equivalent ionic charge is the dominant quantity from an acid–base point of view.

Water

Body fluids may be considered as dilute aqueous solutions; in pure water there is a small dissociation expressed in the reaction

$$H_2O \rightleftharpoons H^+ + OH^-$$

(or, more correctly, $2H_2O \rightleftharpoons H_3O^+ + OH^-$).

The extent of the dissociation is defined by applying the Law of Mass Action:

$$K_w = [H^+][OH^-]/[H_2O] \qquad [7]$$

In this equation, [H$_2$O] in pure water is 55 mol/liter, and because [H$^+$] and [OH$^-$] are 10^{-7} Eq/liter or less, [H$_2$O] may be taken as constant and

$$K_w' = [H^+][OH^-]$$

where K_w', the ion product for water, is $K_w \times$ [H$_2$O]. In pure water, H$^+$ and OH$^-$ are the only ions and are equal in concentration:

$$[H^+] = [OH^-]$$

This equation expresses the concept of neutrality. At 25°C, K_w' has a value of 1.008×10^{-14} Eq$^2 \cdot$liter^{-2};

this is usually rounded off to 1.0×10^{-14}; thus, since

$$K'_w = [H^+][OH^-] = 10^{-14}$$

we obtain

$$[H^+] = [OH^-] = 10^{-7}$$

At 25°C, neutral $[H^+]$ is 10^{-7}, or pH = 7.0. However, at other temperatures, neutral $[H^+]$ will not be 10^{-7} Eq/liter; this has important implications in comparative physiology and in hypothermia. In body fluids at 37°C, $K'_w = 4.4 \times 10^{-14}$ and

$$[H^+] = (4.4 \times 10^{-14})/[OH^-] \quad Eq/liter \quad [8]$$

Thus at 37°C, neutral $[H^+]$ will be the square root of 4.4×10^{-14}, or 2.1×10^{-7} (a pH of 6.68).

Strong Electrolytes

Strong ions are fully dissociated in aqueous solutions; they may be defined as having K values (Eq. 1) that are greater than 10^{-4} (strong acids) or less than 10^{-12} (strong bases). This allows us to ignore K for strong electrolytes, because a strong acid HA exists only as H^+ and A^-, and a strong base BOH exists only as B^+ and OH^-; they are both "fully dissociated."

An acid tends to increase the $[H^+]$ of an aqueous solution, and a base tends to decrease it; this concept may be simpler to understand than the conventional definition independently proposed by Brønsted and Lowry in 1923 (1)—that an acid is a proton (H^+) donor and a base is a proton acceptor. The difficulty with the Brønsted–Lowry definition is that an ion may behave as an acid or a base, depending on the circumstance; for example, HCO_3^- can act as a proton donor (to form CO_3^{2-} and H^+) or as a proton acceptor (when it forms CO_2 and H_2O). In body fluids the main strong ions are Na^+, K^+, and Cl^-; if these were the only ions present, $[H^+]$ would be determined only by the Law of Electrical Neutrality and the dissociation of water. This law states that in any system the net charge must be zero; thus in a solution of Na^+, K^+, and Cl^- in water,

$$[Na^+] + [K^+] + [H^+] - [Cl^-] - [OH^-] = 0$$

Because $[OH^-]$ is equal to $K'_w/[H^+]$ (Eq. 8),

$$[Na^+] + [K^+] + [H^+] - [Cl^-] - K'_w/[H^+] = 0$$

The effects of the strong ions may be lumped into a term that expresses the net negative or positive charge that they exert, the "strong ion difference" ([SID]), where [SID] in plasma is normally $[Na^+] + [K^+] - [Cl^-]$; other strong ions, such as lactate or ketones, will also contribute to [SID], since they may be present

in concentrations as high as 30 mEq/liter; other strong inorganic (Ca^{2-}, Mg^{2-}, SO_4^{2-}) and organic ions (glutamate, aspartate) are always in insignificant concentration and generally are ignored.

The last equation may be rewritten

$$[SID] + [H^+] + K'_w/[H^+] = 0$$

In this system the independent variable is [SID] and the dependent variables are $[H^+]$ and $[OH^-]$. In normal plasma, $[Na^+]$ is 140 mEq/liter, $[K^+]$ is 4 mEq/liter, and $[Cl^-]$ is 104 mEq/liter; thus the normal [SID] is around 40 mEq/liter. If we assume for didactic purposes that there are no other electrolytes in plasma, $[OH^-]$ would also be close to 40 mEq/liter, or 4×10^{-2} Eq/liter; from Eq. 8,

$$[H^+] = 4.4 \times 10^{-14}/4 \times 10^{-2} \quad Eq/liter$$

$$= 1.1 \times 10^{-12} \quad Eq/liter$$

or a pH of 11.96. The calculation indicates the power of strong ions to influence $[H^+]$ and also indicates the importance of weak electrolytes and of the CO_2 system to the control of $[H^+]$, because with these systems in plasma, $[H^+]$ is 4×10^{-8} (i.e., a pH of 7.4).

Weak Electrolytes

Weak acids, which will be termed A_{tot} (or total weak acids), constitute the buffers that exist in a partially dissociated state [HA, H^+, and A^- (Eq. 1) are all present in significant amounts] in the body pH range; the extent to which they are dissociated is determined by the dissociation constant, K_a; they have K_a values between 10^{-4} and 10^{-12}. However, only weak electrolytes with a K_a that is close to the neutral $[H^+]$ (2.1×10^{-7} at 37°C) can be effective as buffers. The K_a of the imidazole group of histidine molecules in proteins is virtually identical to the neutral $[H^+]$ of water, making it very important in this respect, as discussed later. Buffer systems include plasma proteins ($K_a = 3 \times 10^{-7}$), proteins and phosphates in cells ($K_a = 5.5 \times 10^{-7}$), and hemoglobin in red cells. In hemoglobin the imidazole groups are closely associated with iron atoms; changes in the electron structure of the iron atoms associated with the release of oxygen makes the imidazole groups less acidic. For oxygenated Hb, K_a is 2.5×10^{-7}, but for fully reduced Hb it is 6.3×10^{-9}.

For plasma proteins at 37°C,

$$[H^+] \times [A^-] = (3 \times 10^{-7}) \times [HA] \quad Eq/liter \quad [9]$$

In addition to their K_a, the effectiveness of buffers in any site is dependent on their total concentration ($[A_{tot}]$). Although the proportion of weak acid that is dissociated, or ionized, may vary, the sum of the dissociated (A^-) and undissociated (HA) forms remains constant as defined by the Law of Conservation of Mass:

$$[HA] + [A^-] = [A_{tot}] \quad Eq/liter \qquad [10]$$

In this system, $[A_{tot}]$ is the independent variable and K_a is the parameter; [HA], $[H^+]$, and $[A^-]$ are dependent variables. In plasma, $[A_{tot}]$ represents the ionic equivalent of the plasma proteins and may be obtained by multiplying the protein content (g/liter) by 0.24. Thus at a normal total protein of 70 g/liter, $[A_{tot}]$ equals 17 mEq/liter, composed of $[A^-]$ at about 15 mEq/liter and [HA] of 2 mEq/liter.

It should be noted that although plasma proteins behave as weak acids, this is a relative term, because they are about 90% (15/17) dissociated at normal plasma pH. Also, abnormal proteins in some types of myeloma may carry a net positive charge within the body pH range and thus act to increase the net pK attributable to proteins in plasma.

Carbon Dioxide

The CO_2 system acts mainly through variations in its total content brought about by variations in P_{CO_2} and $[H^+]$. The system incorporates two components; the first reaction is the hydration of CO_2, namely,

$$CO_2 + H_2O \rightleftharpoons H_2CO_3$$

and the second is the dissociation of carbonic acid, namely,

$$H_2CO_3 \rightleftharpoons HCO_3^- + H^+$$

We may apply the Law of Mass Action to these reactions:

$$K_{a1}[H_2CO_3] = [CO_2] \times [H_2O]$$

and

$$K_{a2}[H_2CO_3] = [H^+] \times [HCO_3^-]$$

Combining these two equations and solving for $[H^+]$ yields

$$[H^+] = K_{a2}[CO_2][H_2O]/K_{a1}[HCO_3^-]$$

This equation contains two constants (K_{a1}, K_{a2}) and a virtual constant ($[H_2O]$), which may all be incorporated into one constant (K_a') (the "apparent" ionization constant) to obtain

$$[H^+] = K_a'[CO_2]/[HCO_3^-]$$

$[CO_2]$ is the concentration of dissolved CO_2, and may be derived from the P_{CO_2} and the solubility constant

for CO_2 (3.01×10^{-5} Eq/liter/mmHg); the equation may then be rewritten

$$[H^+] = K_a' \times 3.01 \times 10^{-5} P_{CO_2}/[HCO_3^-] \quad Eq/liter$$

Because K_a' is 7.94×10^{-7} we may use one constant, K_c:

$$[H^+] = K_c \times P_{CO_2}/[HCO_3^-]$$

where

$$K_c = (7.94 \times 10^{-7}) \times (3.01 \times 10^{-5})$$
$$= 2.4 \times 10^{-11} \qquad [11]$$

Thus

$$[H^+] = (2.4 \times 10^{-11}) \times P_{CO_2}/[HCO_3^-] \quad Eq/liter$$

If P_{CO_2} is expressed in torr and $[HCO_3^-]$ in mEq/liter, we obtain

$$[H^+] = 24 \times P_{CO_2}/[HCO_3^-] \quad nEq/liter$$

(Henderson's equation). In this equation, P_{CO_2} is the independent variable of the CO_2 system, with $[H^+]$ and $[HCO_3^-]$ both being dependent.

The Henderson–Hasselbalch equation may be derived from Eq. 11:

$$pH = 6.1 + \log[HCO_3^-]/0.301 P_{CO_2}$$

Throughout the rest of this chapter, Eq. 11 will be used to quantify the effect of the CO_2 sytem. At a normal $P_{a}CO_2$ of 40 mmHg, if H^+ is 40 mEq/liter, then $[HCO_3^-]$ is 24 mEq/liter.

The reactions just described are all assumed to be in equilibrium, and by the time blood or other body fluids have been sampled and analyzed, they will have reached equilibrium. However, the hydration of CO_2 in simple solution is a slow process, having a half-reaction time of about 40 sec. The process is accelerated by the enzyme carbonic anhydrase, which reduces the half-reaction time to much less than a second. These facts are important because carbonic anhydrase is virtually absent from plasma but has high activity in erythrocytes, vascular endothelium, and other tissues such as the kidneys and lungs (17,18). In some situations where large volumes of CO_2 are transported, such as in exercise, it is likely that the CO_2 system in circulating plasma is never in equilibrium (19). Also, a number of drugs, including sulfonamides and some diuretics, inhibit the activity of the enzyme. In these situations, measurement of acid–base variables in plasma may not reflect their true state in the body.

Bicarbonate itself dissociates into H^+ and carbonate ion:

$$HCO_3^- \rightleftharpoons H^+ + CO_3^{2-}$$

Because the K_a for this reaction is 6×10^{-11}, the equilibrium equation is

$$[H^+] = (6 \times 10^{-11})[HCO_3^-]/[CO_3^{2-}] \quad \text{Eq/liter} \quad [12]$$

all three variables in this equation may be considered as dependent on changes in the CO_2 and other systems. At a normal $[H^+]$ and $[HCO_3^-]$, CO_3^{2-} is about 4×10^{-5} Eq/liter.

Interaction Between Systems

The Law of Electrical Neutrality must be satisfied when all systems are in equilibrium; this requires us to sum all the charges contributed by the ions in all systems; for water we have $[H^+]$ and $[OH^-]$; for the strong ions we have the net positive charge of $[SID]$; for weak acids we have $[A^-]$; for the CO_2 system we have $[HCO_3^-]$, together with $[CO_3^{2-}]$ from bicarbonate dissociation. Thus

$$[SID] + [H^+] - [HCO_3^-] - [CO_3^{2-}]$$
$$- [A^-] - [OH^-] = 0 \quad [13]$$

Note that Eq. 13 is not used to calculate $[H^+]$ and $[OH^-]$ in plasma; this would be absurd, because measurements of $[SID]$, $[HCO_3^-]$, and $[A^-]$ are all milliequivalent quantities with measurement errors of at least 1% and also because $[H^+]$ and $[OH^-]$ in body fluids are in microequivalents or less. The equation is just one of the requirements, or a constraint, that has to be fulfilled in quantifying the effects of all the variables that we normally consider in electrolyte physiology. The calculated $[H^+]$ and $[OH^-]$ have to simultaneously satisfy *all* the equations in which they appear as dependent variables. The linkage between the variables is shown schematically in Fig. 1.

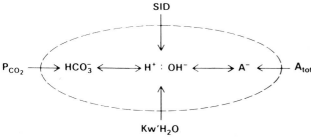

FIG. 1. The acid–base system. The arrows indicate the influence that variables may exert on each other, with single-headed arrows indicating the effect of the independent variables [SID], P_{CO_2}, and [A_{tot}] on the dependent variables [H^+], [OH^-], [HCO_3^-], [A^-], and (not shown) [CO_3^-]. Dependent variables are enclosed by the dashed ellipse, to indicate that they will *all* be influenced by a change in any one of the independent variables (5).

Computation

To fully quantify all the interactions described above, six equations (Eqs. 8–13) may be solved simultaneously, given the parameters and the independent variables. As a further definition of independent variables, notice that they only appear once in the series: $[SID]$ (Eq. 13), [A_{tot}] (Eq. 9), and P_{CO_2} (Eq. 11). The dependent variables appear in more than one equation: $[H^+]$, $[HCO_3^-]$, $[A^-]$, $[CO_3^{2-}]$, and $[OH^-]$. It may be helpful to list the equations again:

$$[H^+] \times [OH^-] = K_w' \quad [8]$$

(water dissociation)

$$[H^+] \times [A^-] = K_a \times [HA] \quad [9]$$

(weak acid dissociation)

$$[A_{tot}] = [HA] + [A^-] \quad [10]$$

(total weak acid content)

$$[H^+] \times [HCO_3^-] = K_c \times P_{CO_2} \quad [11]$$

(CO_2 equilibrium)

$$[H^+] \times [CO_3^{2-}] = K_3 \times [HCO_3^-] \quad [12]$$

(bicarbonate dissociation)

$$[H^+] + [SID] - [A^-] - [HCO_3^-] \quad [13]$$
$$- [CO_3^{2-}] - [OH^-] = 0$$

(electrical neutrality)

The equations are readily solved by a calculator program, for given values of $[SID]$, $[A_{tot}]$, and P_{CO_2} in plasma. The program may be modified, through changes in parameters (K_w', K_a, K_c, and K_3, values for which have already been given above, for plasma at 37°C), to define the acid–base state in any other tissue (interstitial fluid, red cells, muscle, etc.) or any other condition (temperature, osmolality, etc.). Also, the equations may be combined into a single expression, which appears extremely complex (because it is a fourth-order polynomial) but which is easily handled by computer:

$$[H^+]^4 + a[H^+]^3 + b[H^+]^2 - e[H^+] - d = 0$$

where

$$a = [SID] + K_a$$
$$b = K_a([SID] - [A_{tot}]) - K_w' - (K_c \cdot P_{CO_2})$$
$$c = K_a(K_w' + [K_c \cdot P_{CO_2}]) - (K_3 \cdot K_c \cdot P_{CO_2})$$
$$d = K_a \cdot K_c \cdot K_3 \cdot P_{CO_2}$$

In this expression, $[H^+]$ is the only unknown variable. Although it may be solved for $[H^+]$ in situations where

[H$^+$] is difficult to measure directly (e.g., muscle), as pointed out above it has no application to the routine assessment of plasma acid–base status where [H$^+$] may be measured accurately. A close concordance between measured [H$^+$] and [H$^+$] calculated with the equation has provided a validation of the general approach.

"The Conventional Approach" Reexamined

Before considering normal and abnormal acid–base physiology in light of the approach just described, some contrasts will be drawn between it and the standard approach used for at least the last 50 years. The relationships expressed in the equations above have their roots in the classical physical chemistry of the 1920s to 1940s, and thus they do not describe anything new; many readers will certainly find difficulty in identifying how the concepts have changed. First, there is a rigorous definition of the systems with their dependent and independent components, enabling us to readily identify the mechanisms by which changes in [H$^+$] are brought about. Second, measurement of "base excess" and the "anion gap" is not required, being replaced by the variables [SID] and [A$^-$]. Third, interactions between changes in cells and extracellular fluid may be understood and quantified. In addition, the new approach forces us to question a number of the earlier concepts, including (a) the use of the Henderson equation to imply that [H$^+$] is controlled by changes in [HCO$_3$$^-$], (b) the concept of protons being produced or removed, and (c) concepts that imply that [HCO$_3$$^-$] may be produced, removed, retained (by kidneys), or administered.

From a practical standpoint, the approach outlined above may be useful with the help of graphs such as those shown Fig. 2, or by solving the equations to obtain all the variables that satisfy the measured arterial [H$^+$] and PCO$_2$. To further analyze the problem, plasma electrolytes will yield a measured inorganic [SID] ([Na$^+$] + [K$^+$] − [Cl$^-$]) that may be compared to true or total [SID], the value that satisfies [H$^+$] and PCO$_2$, to evaluate the possible effects of other strong ions. If there is a difference between the inorganic [SID] and total [SID], this indicates the presence of unmeasured ions, such as lactate or ketoacids. This is an exercise that is similar to the calculation of anion gap, with the advantage that [A$^-$] is treated as a variable rather than as a constant. Because [H$^+$], [OH$^-$], and [CO$_3$$^{2-}$] are micromolar or less, Eq. 13 may be contracted to

$$[SID] - [HCO_3^-] - [A^-] = 0$$

In practical terms, this allows the effects of the independent measured variables ([SID], PCO$_2$, and [A$_{tot}$]) to be evaluated and enables us to identify whether any unmeasured strong anions are exerting an important effect.

CONTROL OF THE INTERNAL ENVIRONMENT

Variation Between Mechanisms Controlling [H$^+$] in Body Fluid Compartments

Because of variations in the relative magnitude of the independent variables, systems involved in control of acid–base status exert differing effects in different fluid compartments and different tissues (Fig. 3).

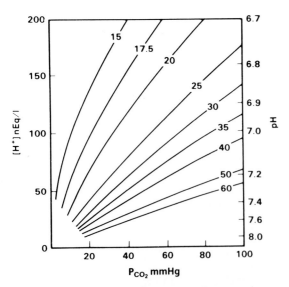
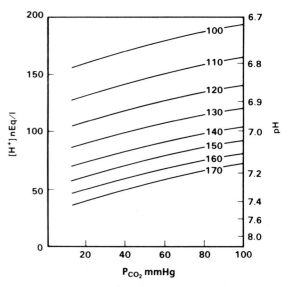

FIG. 2. Graphs showing the influence of PCO$_2$ and [SID] on plasma [H$^+$] (**left-hand panel**) and intracellular [H$^+$] (**right-hand panel**); [A$_{tot}$] is assumed constant at 20 mEq/liter for plasma and 200 mEq/liter for intracellular fluid. Isopleths are for different values of [SID] in mEq/liter (5).

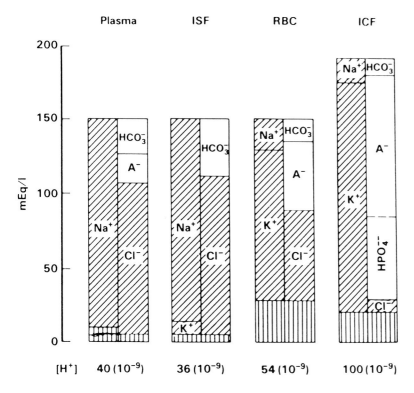

FIG. 3. Gamble diagrams (22) describing differences in normal ionic status in plasma, interstitial fluid (ISF), red blood cells (RBC), and intracellular (muscle) fluid (ICF). Strong ion concentrations are indicated by diagonal hatching; cations are in the left-hand bars, and anions are on the right; electrical neutrality is shown by the equal height of the two bars; the difference between the vertical hatched bars is [SID], occupied by [HCO$_3^-$] and [A$^-$]. Concentration of H$^+$ is too low to be distinguished; [H$^+$] is shown below the respective histograms (5).

In intracellular fluid there is a large [SID] (dominated by a high [K$^+$]), accompanied by large protein and phosphate concentrations (A$_{tot}$) that minimize the effects of reductions in [SID] resulting from falls in [K$^+$] or accumulation of organic strong ions such as La$^-$. Although P_{CO_2} in tissues is high and increased by metabolism, [HCO$_3^-$] is low. Changes in P_{CO_2} influence [H$^+$] much less than in plasma; this may be appreciated by comparing the slopes of the iso-[SID] lines for plasma with those for intracellular fluid (see Fig. 2). It follows that control of intracellular [H$^+$] is achieved through (a) buffering by A$_{tot}$, (b) exchange of strong ions with extracellular fluid, thereby changing [SID], and (c) diffusion of CO$_2$ down its pressure gradient.

In interstitial fluid, and all fluids that are ultrafiltrates of plasma (lymph, cerebrospinal fluid, etc.), the virtual absence of protein means that the weak acid system plays no part, and [H$^+$] is only influenced by changes in [SID] and P_{CO_2}.

In plasma the balance between the systems is also towards [SID], but large variations in P_{CO_2} may effect large and rapid changes in arterial [H$^+$].

In erythrocytes, all three systems have similar weighting because [SID] and [A$_{tot}$] are high, and P_{CO_2} is in equilibrium with the P_{CO_2} of the surrounding plasma; mathematically, the situation is probably the most complex to handle because K_a is influenced by the state of oxygenation.

These considerations emphasize the importance of fluid and ion shifts between the different body compartments. "Communication" between compartments from an acid–base point of view results mainly through the transfer of strong ions and CO$_2$ and, to a lesser extent, water; the molecules making up A$_{tot}$ do not move readily. Thus, the analysis of acid–base control mechanisms can never be completely separated from the mechanisms that control ionic and water balance, osmolality, circulating blood volume, systemic arterial pressure, and even left ventricular output.

What Is Being Controlled? The Alphastat Hypothesis

For many years, partly because of the difficulty in studying changes within tissues and partly because of the complexity of the interactions, acid–base physiology has concentrated on plasma ionic status. The effects of experimental and clinical perturbations on tissue function are now better understood. Marked changes in biochemical and physiological function accompany increases in [H$^+$] in the liver, red cells, brain, and muscle; membrane function is impaired, responses to hormones are blunted, and enzyme activity is usually inhibited. Because of such findings there has been an implicit acceptance of the concept of intracellular [H$^+$] control. However, a study of the effects of temperature in a variety of animals and systems suggested to Rahn et al. (23) that regulatory mechanisms were geared toward maintaining a constant protein ionization state. Rahn et al. (23) emphasized the close parallelism, shown in Fig. 4, between temperature effects on tissue pH and on the pK of the imidazole group of

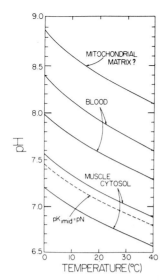

FIG. 4. Relationship of pH to body temperature in animal blood, muscle, and mitochondrial matrix. The effect of temperature on neutral pH (pN) of water is the same as for the pK of the imidazole dissociation reaction. (From ref. 25.)

histidine in peptide chains [the pK of imidazole is very close to "neutral" pH (6.68 at 37°C)], and they suggested that regulation served to protect the fractional dissociation of the imidazole —NH group:

$$\begin{array}{ccc} H & & H \\ | & & | \\ {}^+HN-C-NH & \rightleftharpoons H^+ + & N=C-NH \\ | \quad\quad | & & | \quad\quad | \\ HC=\!\!=\!\!=C\, - & & HC=\!\!=\!\!=C\, - \end{array}$$

Rahn et al. (23) termed the fractional dissociation "alpha," and they called the control the "alphastat." Subsequent work has strengthened their arguments; furthermore, the close involvement of imidazole groups in enzyme regulation, receptor function, and the operation of membrane pores and ion "pumps" neatly explains several mechanisms by which the physiological effects of acid–base perturbations, previously explained by changes in [H$^+$], are brought about (24). The reader is referred to the illuminating book by Hochachka and Somero (25) for the wide implications of the alphastat theory in comparative physiology and biochemistry.

Relationships Between Intracellular and Extracellular Acid–Base Status

In clinical acid–base work the data are obtained mainly from arterial and peripheral venous blood samples by analyzing plasma; intracellular measurements are not obtained, even in the case of erythrocytes. Probably in the perfect world we would be able to measure in-

tracellular [H$^+$], and the technique of nuclear magnetic resonance offers great promise in this regard (26). Although intracellular [H$^+$] is of great interest, in view of its influence on cellular metabolic processes, it is likely that large variations exist between different tissues in different clinical situations, and the concept of whole-body intracellular [H$^+$] is probably an abstraction. Experimental studies in animals and humans have been devised to establish the magnitude of intracellular fluid (ICF) changes relative to those of extracellular fluid (ECF), but they are only a partial answer to the problem for two reasons. First, most experimental studies have made "external" changes and followed internal [H$^+$]; however, in many situations the disturbance originates in the cells, and the reflected changes in plasma may bear only a limited relation to the intracellular changes. Second, the studies have often examined the intracellular responses to changes in [H$^+$] or [HCO$_3^-$] in plasma without distinguishing the independent variables that were manipulated to bring about the initial disturbance.

Studies in which arterial P_{CO_2} has been raised or lowered have shown that ICF [H$^+$] is well defended in a range of arterial P_{CO_2} between 40 and 80 mmHg (27); this is readily explained in terms of the differences in [SID] and [A$_{tot}$] between ICF and ECF as may be appreciated by noting the differences in the slopes of the relationship between P_{CO_2} and [H$^+$] at constant [SID] (Fig. 2). Studies of metabolic acidosis and alkalosis have similarly shown good defense of ICF [H$^+$] but have suggested that the defense against alkalosis is much less effective than that against acidosis (28). The reason for this apparent difference probably lies in the different extent to which changes in ECF [SID] are capable of influencing ICF [SID].

The Role of Erythrocytes in Acid–Base Control

Erythrocytes have already been mentioned at several points in this chapter, which will have suggested some important functions for them in responding to sudden changes in ions or P_{CO_2} and helping to maintain plasma and thus ECF conditions relatively constant. They have a number of unique properties that facilitate this function. First, their intracellular fluid composition lies between that of ICF and plasma (Fig. 3); [K$^+$] is not as high as in ICF, but [Na$^+$] and [Cl$^-$] are higher, though still well below plasma; [SID] is 60 mEq/liter compared to 42 mEq/liter in plasma and 130 mEq/liter in ICF. Second, hemoglobin provides a high [A$_{tot}$] of 60 mEq/liter, which compares with 20 mEq/liter in plasma and 200 mEq/liter in ICF. Third, the two forms of hemoglobin provide a variable K_a (see above) which enables reduced Hb to function as a more effective buffer of venous acidity (29). Fourth, the presence of carbonic anhydrase enables the hydration of CO_2 to proceed at a very rapid rate. Fifth, the carbamino reaction (29) is an additional mechanism to enable an increase in CO_2 carriage without a comparable increase in $[H^+]$. Lastly, a number of membrane transport systems enable ion exchange between the plasma and erythrocyte while at the same time controlling erythrocyte volume. A full discussion of these properties is beyond the scope of this chapter, but some mention of the processes that are influenced by erythrocytes is appropriate.

As blood flows through active tissues, O_2 dissociates from hemoglobin and there will be a tendency for erythrocyte $[H^+]$ to decrease. This will have two effects: (i) The influx of CO_2 along its pressure gradient is accommodated without much change in $[H^+]$ and (ii) an electrical charge difference will influence Cl^- to move into the cell, tending to increase plasma [SID] and leading to a rise in plasma $[HCO_3^-]$. As CO_2 hydration proceeds rapidly under the influence of carbonic anhydrase in the red blood cell, CO_2 production and hydration serve to increase P_{CO_2} in the cell. At the same time, carbamino CO_2 is rapidly formed; this reaction is facilitated by the reduction of Hb, which allows the $-NH_2$ groups associated with the terminal valine molecules of the beta chain of deoxyhemoglobin to undergo the reaction

$$HbNH_2 + CO_2 \rightleftharpoons HbNHCOOH \rightleftharpoons HbCOO^- + H^+$$

A number of factors influence this reaction, including $[H^+]$, and estimates of the proportion of CO_2 carried in this form have varied between 10% and 30% of the total CO_2 in venous blood. In addition to these reactions associated with the reduction of hemoglobin and carriage of CO_2 in venous blood, the erythrocyte is available to modulate rapid changes in plasma ion concentrations. This may be especially important when increases in $[K^+]$ occur; movement of K^+ into erythrocytes acts to minimize the increase in plasma $[K^+]$ with its potentially lethal effects.

The Role of the Kidneys (20,21)

The kidneys influence acid–base status mainly by changing the [SID] of the plasma flowing through them. From the ultrafiltrate of plasma in the glomerulus, Na^+ reabsorption in the tubules is an active, energy-requiring process that lowers both $[Na^+]$ and osmolality in the tubular fluid, leading to water reabsorption, which in the distal tubule is under the control of vasopressin. Chloride reabsorption is partly electrically mediated and partly an active process, related to adenosinetriphosphatase (ATPase)-driven ion pumps on the membrane of renal tubular cells. If Cl^- is less rapidly reabsorbed than Na^+, urine $[Cl^-]$ will increase

relative to $[Na^+]$; urine [SID] will fall, leading to an increase in urine $[H^+]$. If Na^+ is less rapidly reabsorbed than Cl^-, the opposite will be the case. In the tubular lumen, a fall in [SID] and an increase in $[H^+]$ will tend to increase P_{CO_2}, because the tubule is a partly "closed" system and also because the removal of CO_2 by the renal capillary blood flow may not keep pace with its production; however, $[HCO_3^-]$ will tend to fall in parallel with the increase in $[Cl^-]$, and when urine pH has fallen to less than 6, urine $[HCO_3^-]$ will be very small. The excretion of Cl^- in excess of Na^+ and K^+ may thus be seen as an important way to control plasma [SID] and $[H^+]$. However, when $[H^+]$ has increased because of accumulation of organic ions such as lactate, a choice is available to the renal tubular cells: excretion of the La^- or of Cl^-, or of both. Because the reabsorption of strong organic anions is not as efficient as for Cl^-, Cl^- is reabsorbed in preference to lactate, leaving a very high urine $[La^-]$ and low $[Cl^-]$ (30). In this situation the kidney defends itself against too low a urine pH, which seldom drops to below 4.5; it can do this by excreting more water and Na^+, if they are available, and by secreting ammonia and phosphates. Ammonia is produced in renal tubular cells from glutamine, which is metabolized to $2NH_4^+$ and the alpha ketoglutarate^{2-} ion; this allows reabsorption of Na^+ or excretion of Cl^- without an increase in urine $[H^+]$; both effects will tend to increase plasma [SID]. Because NH_4^+ and HPO_4^- secretion have a limited capacity, the importance of adequate Na^+ and water delivery to the distal tubule in an organic acidosis is obvious. It should be remembered that the kidneys normally are able to adjust to ranges of water excretion between 0.5 and 25 liters/day and to ranges of sodium between 0.05 and 25 g/day.

Ventilation in Acid–Base Control

P_{CO_2} in arterial plasma is mainly controlled by changes in ventilation as expressed in the alveolar ventilation equation $P_{aCO_2} = 0.863 \dot{V}_{CO_2}/\dot{V}_A$, where $\dot{V}_{CO_2}$ is the metabolic production of CO_2, conventionally expressed in ml STPD/min and $\dot{V}_A$ is the alveolar ventilation expressed in liters BTPS/min. The equation is useful practically as well as conceptually, because neither metabolic rate nor ventilation needs to be measured in order to assess the adequacy of breathing in relation to the demands of metabolism; an arterial P_{CO_2} of 80 mmHg, for example, indicates that alveolar ventilation is half that required to maintain a P_{CO_2} of 40 mmHg at the current metabolic rate. However, this general statement may not hold for P_{CO_2} in other body tissues, and it may also not hold if the activity of carbonic anhydrase is impaired. In tissues and venous blood, P_{CO_2} is largely controlled by the balance between metabolism and blood flow. Also, the extent to which arterial P_{CO_2} reflects the adequacy of ventilation is dependent on carbonic anhydrase activity in allowing rapid equilibration of P_{CO_2} between pulmonary capillary blood and alveolar gas, and it will thus be affected by carbonic anhydrase inhibition. These two caveats excepted, arterial P_{CO_2} represents the balance between body CO_2 production and breathing.

The alveolar ventilation equation expresses the combined effects of changes in $\dot{V}_A$ and metabolism on P_{CO_2}. In patients with severely impaired ventilatory capacity, respiratory failure may be worsened by changes in $\dot{V}_{CO_2}$ accompanying fever or changes in diet. In most patients presenting with an increase in P_{CO_2}, a number of factors may contribute to underventilation, including inefficient gas exchange, leading to dead-space ventilation ($\dot{V}_D$) (see Chapter 5.3.4), increased work of breathing (Chapter 5.1.2.8), impaired respiratory muscle strength and endurance (Chapter 5.1.1.6), and disorders of respiratory control (Chapter 5.4.12).

The ventilatory responses to acid–base disorders of nonrespiratory origin are extremely important in [H^+] control, particularly because they may act very rapidly. Although peripheral chemoreceptors in the carotid bodies do respond to changes in their pH, the response of central medullary chemoreceptors is more important in the relatively long-term responses to acid–base disorders. The dominant factor is the cerebrospinal fluid (CSF) [H^+], and because CSF is protein-free the CSF P_{CO_2} and [SID] are the two important variables in its control.

CLINICAL DISORDERS OF ELECTROLYTE AND ACID–BASE PHYSIOLOGY

Having identified which variables are capable of independent action and which are dependent on the result of more than one reaction, we may approach the primary clinical disorders in terms of conditions that are associated with abnormalities in [SID], [A_{tot}], and P_{CO_2} in arterial plasma. The primary changes are almost invariably modified by "adaptive" changes that, to be effective, also have to involve independent variables—changes in ventilation leading to changes in P_{CO_2}, and movement of strong ions into cells or urine to modify [SID], for example.

In the approach to disorders used below, the classification will be based on the initiating abnormality in independent variables or systems and will use a graphical approach to their description (Figs. 5 and 6). Examples (Table 1) will also be presented to demonstrate typical findings in clinical disorders; the normal acid–base state is presented as example 1 in this table.

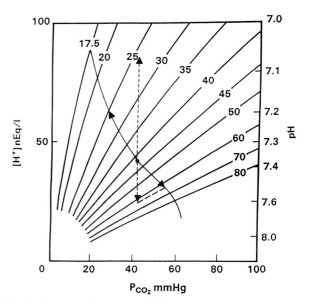

FIG. 5. Changes in plasma [H^+] that accompany changes in [SID], showing the effect of the reductions in P_{CO_2} that usually occur in metabolic acidosis and metabolic alkalosis. The solid upward arrow indicates the change seen with a reduction in [SID] from 42 to 25 mEq/liter, with a fall in P_{aCO_2} to 20 mmHg, [H^+] of 63 nEq/liter (pH 7.23); dashed vertical line shows that if the reduction in P_{aCO_2} had not occurred, [H^+] would be 90 (pH 7.05). The curvature in the solid line indicates that effectiveness in this adaptation lessens with increasing severity of acidosis (5). Also shown are the decreases in plasma [H^+] associated with increase in [SID]; these are lessened by increases in P_{aCO_2}. The curvature indicates the limited effect of increases in P_{aCO_2} in metabolic alkalosis (5), and the dashed line shows the change that would occur if P_{CO_2} did not change.

Primary Decrease in Plasma [SID]

Theoretically, [SID] may be reduced in several ways to produce a "metabolic acidosis":

1. Reduction in [Na^+]. Hyponatremia often may present without a fall in [SID] because loss of Na^+ is paralleled by a loss of Cl^-. However, the fall in [Na^+] rarely exceeds the reduction in [Cl^-], and [SID] is reduced; this may occur in diarrhea, water intoxication, inappropriate antidiuretic hormone (ADH) secretion, and renal tubular defects.
2. Increase in [Cl^-] (example 2, Table 1) occurs in renal failure, in ureterosigmoidostomy, and with administration of chloride.
3. Metabolic production of strong anions occurs in lactic acidosis (example 3, Table 1) and in diabetic ketoacidosis (example 4, Table 1).
4. Ingestion of strong anions (or their precursors) such as salicylates, glycolate in ethylene glycol poisoning, and formate in methanol poisoning.
5. Accumulation of strong ions normally excreted, such as SO_4^{2-} in renal failure.

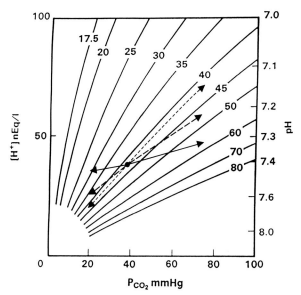

FIG. 6. Changes in plasma [H⁺] that accompany changes in $P_a co_2$: the increase in [H⁺] resulting from increases in $P_a co_2$, showing the usual increase in [SID] that occurs in acute respiratory acidosis (*dashed line*) and in chronic states (*solid line*) (5); and the decrease in [H⁺] resulting from decreases in $P_a co_2$, occurring acutely (*dashed arrow*) and chronically (*solid line*), compared to change expected in absence of changes in [SID] (5). (From ref. 16.)

Reduction in [SID] will tend to increase [H⁺] to an extent indicated by the vertical line in Fig. 5. However, a number of changes take place to minimize this potential effect. First, as mentioned above, reductions in [SID] may be offset by adaptations tending to increase [SID]; for example, in diabetic acidosis, dehydration may lead to an increase in [Na⁺], and increased Cl⁻ excretion in urine may help to reduce plasma [Cl⁻]; both changes will offset the effects of the increase in

plasma strong ketoacid concentration. Of course, these adaptive changes may not be available, in uremic acidosis, for example. Measurement of urine electrolyte excretion may be helpful in assessing the role of the kidneys in an acidosis. Second, a tendency for [H⁺] to increase leads to an association of weak acids (plasma proteins, A_{tot}) and thus to a reduction in [A⁻], which may amount to 3–4 mEq/liter but is seldom more except in very severe acidosis. Third, increases in [H⁺] will stimulate breathing, leading to a decrease in $P co_2$ and increase in CO_2 output by the lungs. The effectiveness of this response is dependent on the ventilatory capacity, the efficiency of pulmonary gas exchange, and the integrity of ventilatory control reflexes. If none of these adaptive mechanisms is impaired, the increase in [H⁺] expected for a given reduction in [SID] is shown in the upper part of Fig. 5, which may be used to identify the adequacy of the responses; the expected fall in $P co_2$ is 12 mmHg for a 10 mEq/liter decrease in [SID], but in severe acidosis the fall may be as little as 6 mmHg, as indicated by the convexity of the curve in Fig. 5. The ventilatory response is often described in terms of the fall in $P co_2$ related to the fall in [HCO₃⁻]; a fall of 10 mEq/liter in [HCO₃⁻] is usually accompanied by a fall of 12 mmHg in $P_a co_2$ (examples 2–4, Table 1; Table 2) (32,33).

Primary Increase in [SID]

An increase in [SID] tends to reduce [H⁺] and is conventionally termed a "metabolic alkalosis." The causes of a widened [SID] may be classified as follows:

1. Increase in [Na⁺]. This is an unusual cause of an alkalosis, because most conditions tending to increase [Na⁺] also increase [Cl⁻] without much of a change in [SID]; excess alkali ingestion, transfusions, peni-

TABLE 1. *Acid–base variables in clinical disorders*[a]

Example	Na⁺	K⁺	Cl⁻	Other[b]	SID	A_{tot}	A⁻	$P co_2$	HCO₃⁻	H⁺	pH
1	140	5.0	103	0	42	20	17	40	25	40	7.40
2	135	3.0	116	0	22	15	13	21	9	59	7.23
3	134	4.0	110	10	18	16	13	16	5	78	7.11
4	133	5.5	103	11	24	21	18	17	6	68	7.17
5	136	2.4	80	0	58	15	14	52	44	30	7.52
6	140	4.0	102	0	42	10	9	36	33	28	7.55
7	140	5.0	102	0	43	21	17	60	26	60	7.22
8	140	4.0	92	0	52	18	15	75	37	52	7.28
9	139	3.5	107	2	33	17	15	25	18	35	7.45
10	132	6.0	98	(5)	35	21	18	40	17	60	7.22
11	140	5.0	104	(4)	37	21	16	80	21	94	7.03
12	142	3.0	89	0	56	18	16	70	40	42	7.38
13	136	4.0	105	(3)	31	19	17	16	14	30	7.53

[a] See text for diagnoses. Units are mEq/liter, except for $P co_2$ (mmHg), H⁺ (nEq/liter), and pH (units).
[b] "Other" refers to other strong anions: lactate in examples 3, 9, and 11; ketones in 10; lactate and ketones combined in 4; and salicylate in 13.

TABLE 2. Clinical disorders of electrolyte and acid–base physiology

Disorder	Primary change	Adaptation	Final P_{CO_2}:[H^+]	P_{CO_2}:[HCO_3^-]
Respiratory acidosis	Acute rise in P_{CO_2}	Δ[SID] = 0.1 ΔP_{CO_2}	Δ[H^+] = 0.7 ΔP_{CO_2}	Δ[HCO_3^-] = 0.1 ΔP_{CO_2}
	(chronic)	Δ[SID] = 0.35 ΔP_{CO_2}	Δ[H^+] = 0.25 ΔP_{CO_2}	Δ[HCO_3^-] = 0.35 ΔP_{CO_2}
Respiratory alkalosis	Acute fall in P_{CO_2}	Δ[SID] = 0.2 ΔP_{CO_2}	Δ[H^+] = 0.8 ΔP_{CO_2}	Δ[HCO_3^-] = 0.2 ΔP_{CO_2}
	(chronic)	Δ[SID] = 0.35 ΔP_{CO_2}	Δ[H^+] = 0.5 ΔP_{CO_2}	Δ[HCO_3^-] = 0.35 ΔP_{CO_2}
Metabolic acidosis	Mild fall in [SID]	ΔP_{CO_2} = Δ[SID]	ΔP_{CO_2} = 1.2 Δ[H^+]	
				P_{CO_2} = 1.5[HCO_3^-] + 8
	(severe)	ΔP_{CO_2} = 0.5 Δ[SID]	ΔP_{CO_2} = 0.6 Δ[H^+]	
Metabolic alkalosis	Mild rise in [SID]	ΔP_{CO_2} = 0.7 Δ[SID]	ΔP_{CO_2} = 0.8 Δ[H^+]	
				P_{CO_2} = 0.9[HCO_3^-] + 15
	(severe)	ΔP_{CO_2} = 0.4 Δ[SID]	ΔP_{CO_2} = 0.5 Δ[H^+]	

cillin and carbenicillin therapy, and dehydration with urinary loss of chloride (contraction alkalosis) may predispose to this state.

2. Increases in [K^+] are self-limiting, because the toxic effects of hyperkalemia occur before an important increase in [SID] can occur.

3. Reduction in [Cl^-] (example 5, Table 1) is the factor underlying most increases in [SID]. Losses of Cl^- may be from the kidneys and identified by a high urine Cl^- excretion (''saline unresponsive''), or they may be from the gut (''saline responsive'') (4)—as in pyloric stenosis, vomiting, and gastric aspiration; in diarrhea due to villous adenoma of the colon; in diuretic therapy in severe K^+ depletion and the Bartter syndrome; with mineralocorticoids in primary aldosteronism and in Cushing's syndrome; and due to ingested mineralocorticoids such as licorice and carbenoxalone.

Increases in [SID] tend to lower [H^+], and if no adaptation occurred the change in [H^+] is described by the lower part of Fig. 5. The adaptations to an increase in [SID] may be considered in terms similar to those seen in low [SID] states; retention of Cl^- by the kidneys is usually seen in patients with normal renal function, and sometimes movement of Na^+ into ICF may play a small part. Although theoretically [H^+] may be partly defended by dissociation of weak acids, with an increase in [A^-], this is very limited (1 mEq/liter or less). Decreases in plasma [H^+] are usually accompanied by a reduction in ventilatory responsiveness, and P_{aCO_2} rises (on average) by 0.7 mmHg for each 1 mEq/liter increase in [SID] (Fig. 5; example 5, Table 1; Table 2) (33,34). In some conditions of metabolic alkalosis, severe loss of K^+ may occur with Cl^- in the kidneys; this leads to depletion of intracellular [K^+] and a fall in ICF [SID]—an intracellular acidosis complicating the extracellular alkalosis. It is possible that in some cases this leads to

respiratory muscle weakness and a greater-than-expected increase in P_{aCO_2}.

Primary Increase in [A_{tot}]

Normally, [A_{tot}] is provided by the plasma proteins without a significant contribution from other weak acids. Theoretically, [A_{tot}] may increase if plasma proteins or other weak acids (such as phosphate) increase; however, increases of more than 2 or 3 mEq/liter are rare, and other features of the causal condition dominate any acid–base effects. Because they act as weak acids, their effect is similar to a reduction in [SID]— a metabolic acidosis. Increases in plasma proteins, as in myelomatosis, have variable effects depending on the class of globulin involved, as a result of varying isoelectric points; most have isoelectric points similar to that of albumin, have a pk of around 6.5, and thus act as weak acids, but the gamma-G class have an isoelectric point that is higher (35) (see below).

Primary Decrease in [A_{tot}]

Reductions in plasma protein concentration will reduce [A_{tot}], leading to a fall in [A^-]; the effects are comparable to increases in [SID] of equimolar size— a metabolic alkalosis (example 6, Table 1). Quantitatively, the effect may be assessed by multiplying the total protein concentration in g/liter by 0.24 ([A_{tot}]) and by taking 0.9 of this value as [A^-], with A_{tot} being about 90% dissociated in most situations. This value may then be added to [Cl^-] and [HCO_3^-] to identify the presence of any unmeasured anions. There is one major exception to this rule-of-thumb; where a large increase in gamma-G paraproteins has occurred, as in multiple myeloma, they act as weak bases because of the divalent amino acids lysine and arginine, whose isoelectric points are close to pH 9.0. They exert a weak positive charge in the plasma pH range, and $[A_{tot}]$ and $[A^-]$ will appear falsely low in their presence.

Primary Increase in Carbon Dioxide Pressure

By definition, an elevated P_aCO_2 indicates alveolar hypoventilation and ventilatory failure; when it is not due to a metabolic alkalosis, it is termed a "respiratory acidosis." Some of the causes are as follows: severe airway obstruction; severe pulmonary fibrosis; thoracic cage deformity; respiratory muscle weakness, alone or as part of a neuromuscular disorder; drugs that depress the respiratory center; and pathology affecting the brainstem.

The potential effect of an increase in P_aCO_2 on plasma $[H^+]$ may be seen by referring to Fig. 5 and moving to the right along the normal [SID] isopleth. Similarly, it may be seen that the effect of an increase in P_aCO_2 may be minimized by an increase in [SID]. Virtually the only mechanism that is effective and also tolerated is a reduction in plasma $[Cl^-]$ (36). Acutely, this occurs through a shift of Cl^- into erythrocytes; over a longer time, excretion of Cl^- in excess of Na^+ and K^+ in urine leads to a fall in plasma $[Cl^-]$. As a rule-of-thumb, $[Cl^-]$ falls acutely by 1 mEq/liter (example 7, Table 1; Table 2)—and in chronic states, by 3–4 mEq/liter—for each 10-mmHg increase in P_aCO_2 (example 8, Table 1; Table 2) (37); these changes are associated with increases in $[HCO_3^-]$ that are similar to the reductions in $[Cl^-]$; changes in $[A^-]$ are inconsequential. The effectiveness of increases in [SID] in limiting increases in $[H^+]$ may be appreciated by looking at Fig. 5; this figure may also be used to assess the presence of an added metabolic acidosis (increase in [SID] less than expected for the rise in P_aCO_2) or metabolic alkalosis (increase in [SID] greater than expected). In the recovery from ventilatory failure, the resolution of the [SID] changes is also time-dependent; if the reduction in P_aCO_2 is rapid, there will be a delay in the increase in $[Cl^-]$ ("post-hypercapnic metabolic alkalosis").

Primary Reduction in Carbon Dioxide Pressure

Reductions in P_aCO_2 are secondary to ventilation, being higher than usual for a given carbon dioxide production. When the reduction in P_aCO_2 is the primary disturbance and is not secondary to a metabolic acidosis, the condition is termed "respiratory alkalosis"; conditions that may give rise to this situation include: mechanical overventilation; drug poisoning (salicylate); hypoxemia (altitude, pulmonary gas-exchange defects); voluntary or psychogenic hyperventilation; pulmonary vascular disease; brainstem disorders, such as Cheyne–Stokes breathing; and imbalance of hormones (progesterone, thyroxine).

Reductions in P_aCO_2 tend to reduce $[HCO_3^-]$ in plasma; but unless a change occurs in [SID], this reduction will be quite limited and a marked fall in $[H^+]$ will result, especially in acute hyperventilation. The extent of this effect may be judged by moving to the left along a constant [SID] isopleth in Fig. 6. Reductions in [SID] minimize the fall in $[H^+]$, and they are due to two main mechanisms: (i) retention of Cl^- through a fall in its renal excretion and (ii) a small accumulation of La^- resulting from the stimulation of glycolysis in erythrocytes and liver (38). In example 9 of Table 1, a 15-mmHg fall in P_aCO_2 was accompanied by (a) an increase in $[Cl^-]$ to 107 mEq/liter and (b) an increase in $[La^-]$ by 2 mEq/liter. Retention of Cl^- tends to characterize chronic states of hyperventilation, but increases in $[La^-]$ may occur very rapidly. These adaptive changes are associated with (a) increases in $[H^+]$ towards normal (Fig. 6) and (b) a fall in $[HCO_3^-]$. The usual reduction in total [SID] resulting from an increase in both $[Cl^-]$ and $[La^-]$ accompanying an acute fall in P_aCO_2 amounts to only 1–2 mEq/liter for each 10-mmHg fall in P_aCO_2, increasing to 3–4 mEq/liter when hyperventilation is sustained for several days (4) (Table 2). The reductions in P_aCO_2 and $[H^+]$ in hyperventilation are accompanied by a rather surprising increase in $[CO_3^{2-}]$, setting the stage for a combination with Ca^{2+}, hypocalcemia, and tetany.

Mixed Acid–Base Disorders

The typical major acid–base abnormalities resulting from a single underlying problem are usually easy to assess and quantify. However, not infrequently a multiple problem may occur; usually the initiating disorder is straightforward, but the expected adaptations are inefficient or absent, resulting from a coexisting impairment of function. Of great importance from this point of view is the presence of renal dysfunction or impairment of ventilatory capacity. Usually, such situations have to be considered within the clinical context and need to be identified by the unexpected response to the primary disorder. For example, a patient may present with an obvious acidosis resulting from poor diabetic control, but with a P_aCO_2 that is higher than expected in response to the reduction in [SID]; the reason for a poor ventilatory response is usually impaired breathing capacity resulting from airflow obstruction or weak respiratory muscles (see example 10, Table 1). Poor renal function may lead to an inappropriate response; for example, in chronic respiratory failure the kidneys may be unable to excrete Cl^-, adding a metabolic acidosis to the respiratory acidosis.

Urine analysis, including electrolytes and pH, may be invaluable in assessing these situations (39).

Complicated Acid–Base Disturbances

1. Double metabolic acidosis—two or more reasons for a reduction in [SID]. This situation may occur with lactic or renal acidosis complicating diabetic acidosis (example 3, Table 1), in severe diarrhea complicating a renal tubular disorder, and in several toxic acidoses, including alcohol poisoning.

2. Respiratory acidosis and metabolic acidosis. In addition to renal failure mentioned above, respiratory failure may be accompanied by hypoxemic lactic acidosis (example 11, Table 1). This combination is also seen following cardiac arrest, in pulmonary edema treated with morphia, and in several types of poisoning.

3. Respiratory acidosis and metabolic alkalosis. This combination may be secondary to diuretic and steroid therapy in a patient with chronic respiratory failure (example 12, Table 1). A less common cause is a metabolic alkalosis associated with intracellur hypokalemia, with secondary respiratory muscle weakness.

4. Metabolic alkalosis and respiratory alkalosis. This combination carries a high mortality and may be encountered in ill postoperative patients undergoing nasogastric aspiration and mechanical ventilation, for example.

5. Metabolic acidosis and metabolic alkalosis. Obviously, this combination might result in very little disturbance in plasma $[H^+]$, and the clinical features are more likely to be due to disturbances in fluid balance or to intracellular acidosis; the combination may be seen whenever severe vomiting complicates a metabolic acidosis.

6. Metabolic acidosis and respiratory alkalosis. This should be suspected where the fall in $P_{a}CO_2$ is greater than expected for the degree of [SID] fall, and it is usually caused by additional respiratory stimulation, as in salicylate poisoning (example 13, Table 1), by cerebrovascular disease, and by drugs that depress carbonic anhydrase activity (several diuretics, anticonvulsants, and antibiotics).

Therapeutic approaches to acid–base disturbances are beyond the scope of this chapter, but if they are approached in the context of manipulation of independent variables (mainly water, strong ions, and ventilation), they may usually be defined quite simply and logically.

ACKNOWLEDGMENTS

I am indebted to Dr. Clive Kearon for his careful reading of the manuscript and critical suggestions as well as to Dr. Peter Stewart and many colleagues for numerous discussions.

REFERENCES

1. Astrup P, Severinghaus JW. *History of acid–base physiology.* Stockholm: Munksgaard, 1986.
2. Henderson LJ. The theory of neutrality regulation in the animal organism. *Am J Physiol* 1908;21:427–448.
3. Cogan MG, Rector FC. Acid–base disorders. In: Brenner BM, Rector FC, eds. *The kidney,* 3rd ed. Philadelphia: WB Saunders, 1986;457–517.
4. Narins RG, Jones ER, Stom MC, Rudnick MR, Bastl CP. Diagnostic strategies in disorders of fluid, electrolyte and acid-base homeostasis. *Am J Med* 1982;72:496–520.
5. Pitts RF. The role of ammonia production and excretion in regulation of acid–base balance. *N Engl J Med* 1971;284:32–38.
6. Davenport HW. *The ABC of acid–base chemistry,* 5th ed. Chicago: University of Chicago Press, 1969.
7. Siggaard-Andersen O. The acid–base status of blood. *Scand J Clin Lab Invest [Suppl]* 1973;15:70.
8. Astrup P. A simple electrometric technique for the determination of carbon-dioxide tension in blood and plasma, total content of carbon-dioxide in plasma, and bicarbonate content in 'separated' plasma at a fixed carbon-dioxide tension (40 mmHg). *Scand J Clin Lab Invest* 1966;8:33–43.
9. Jorgensen K, Astrup P. Standard bicarbonate, its clinical significance, and new method for its determination. *Scand J Clin Lab Invest* 1957;9:122–132.
10. Schwartz WB, Relman AS. A critique of the parameters used in evaluation of acid-base disorders. *N Engl J Med* 1963;268:1382–1388.
11. Bunker JP. The great trans-Atlantic acid–base debate. *Anesthesia* 1965;26:591–594.
12. Brackett NC Jr, Cohen JJ, Schwartz WB. Carbon dioxide titration curve of normal man. *N Engl J Med* 1969;272:6–12.
13. Singer RB, Hastings AB. An improved clinical method for the estimation of disturbances of the acid–base balance of human blood. *Medicine (Baltimore)* 1948;27:223–242.
14. Stewart PA. *How to understand acid–base. A quantitative acid–base primer for biology and medicine.* New York: Elsevier/North-Holland, 1981.
15. Stewart PA. Modern quantitative acid–base chemistry. *Can J Physiol Pharmacol* 1983;61:1444–1461.
16. Jones NL. *Blood gases and acid–base physiology,* 2nd ed. New York, Thieme Medical Publishers, 1987.
17. Rossing TH, Maffeo N, Fencl V. Acid–base effects of altering plasma protein concentration in human blood *in vitro. J Appl Physiol* 1986;61:2260–2265.
18. Crandall ED, Obrasky JE. Direct evidence for participation of rat lung carbonic anhydrase in CO_2 reactions. *J Clin Invest* 1978;62:618–622.
19. Bidani A, Crandall ED, Forster RE. Analysis of post-capillary pH changes *in vivo* after gas exchange. *J Appl Physiol* 1978;44:770–781.
20. Arruda JAL, Kurtzman NA. Relationship of renal sodium and water transport to hydrogen ion secretion. *Annu Rev Physiol* 1978;40:43–66.
21. Koeppen BM, Steinmetz PR. Basic mechanisms of urinary acidification. *Med Clin North Am* 1983;67:753–770.
22. Gamble JL. *Chemical anatomy, physiology and pathology of extracellular fluid.* Cambridge, MA: Harvard University Press, 1949.
23. Rahn H, Reeves RB, Howell BJ. Hydrogen ion regulation, temperature, and evolution. *Am Rev Respir Dis* 1975;112:165–172.
24. Somero GN. Protons, osmolytes, and fitness of internal milieu for protein function. *Am J Physiol* 1986;251:R197–R213.
25. Hochachka PW, Somero GN. *Biochemical adaptation.* Princeton, NJ: Princeton University Press, 1984.
26. Gadian DG. *NMR and its applications to living systems.* Oxford: Clarendon Press, 1982.

27. Adler S. The simultaneous determination of muscle cell pH using a weak acid and a weak base. *J Clin Invest* 1972;51:256–265.

28. Tizianello A, de Ferrari G, Gurreri G, Acquarone N. Effects of metabolic alkalosis, metabolic acidosis and uraemia on whole-body intracellular pH in man. *Clin Sci Mol Med* 1977;52:125–135.

29. Roughton FJW. Transport of oxygen and carbon dioxide. In: *Handbook of physiology, Section 3: Respiration, vol 1.* Washington, DC: American Physiological Society, 1964;767–825.

30. McKelvie RS, Lindinger MI, Heigenhauser GJF, Sutton JR, Jones NL. Renal response to exercise-induced lactic acidosis. *Am J Physiol* 1989;257:R102–R108.

31. Nattie EE. Ionic mechanisms of cerebrospinal fluid acid–base regulation. *J Appl Physiol: Respir Environ Exercise Physiol* 1983;54:3–12.

32. Fulop M. The ventilatory response in severe metabolic acidosis. *Clin Sci Mol Med* 1976;50:367.

33. van Ypersele de Strihou C, Franz A. The respiratory response to chronic metabolic alkalosis and acidosis in disease. *Clin Sci Mol Med* 1973;45:439–448.

34. Tuller MA, Medhi F. Compensatory hypoventilation and hypercapnia in primary metabolic alkalosis. *Am J Med* 1971; 50:281–290.

35. De Troyer A, Stolarczyk A, Zegers de Beyl D, Stryckmans P. Value of anion-gap determination in multiple myeloma. *N Engl J Med* 1977;296:858–860.

36. Giebisch G, Berger L, Pitts RF. The extrarenal response to acute acid–base disturbances of respiratory origin. *J Clin Invest* 1955;34:231–245.

37. Brackett NC, Wingo CF, Muren O, Solano JT. Acid–base response to chronic hypercapnia in man. *N Engl J Med* 1969; 280:124–130.

38. Eldridge F, Salzer J. Effect of respiratory alkalosis on blood lactate and pyruvate in humans. *J Appl Physiol* 1967;22:461–468.

39. Battle DC, Hizon M, Cohen E, Gutterman C, Gupta R. The use of the urinary anion gap in the diagnosis of hyperchloremic metabolic acidosis. *N Engl J Med* 1988;318:594–599.

THE LUNG: Scientific Foundations
edited by R.G. Crystal, J.B. West et al.
Raven Press, Ltd., New York © 1991.

CHAPTER 5.3.2.6

Carbon Monoxide Effects on Oxygen Transport

P. E. Haab and W. Y. Durand-Arczynska

Carbon monoxide, CO, is not an ubiquitous gas in the atmosphere. As a product of incomplete combustion, CO is most commonly found in oxygen-poor environments such as caves and mines, as well as in tobacco smoke, automobile engine exhaust, and many industrial effluents. As early as the 17th century (1), CO had been recognized as a potentially life-threatening toxic gas; since the end of the last century, this toxicity has been recognized to be due to the very high affinity of CO for oxygen carrier proteins, mainly hemoglobin.

CO is constantly produced in minute amounts by living organisms through the catabolism of hemoglobin when protoporphyrin transforms to bilirubin (2,3). It is worth noting that CO can also be consumed, that is, oxidized to CO_2 in the heart and skeletal muscle (4). However, the production, albeit very small (about 0.5 ml/hr), is always much larger than the consumption, and CO elimination is an important function of the respiratory system. Normally the blood CO concentration does not exceed 1–2% of the blood CO-carrying capacity, and consequently it does not interfere with blood O_2 transport. However, when CO is taken up by the lungs from inspired air, CO-bound hemoglobin, HbCO, can easily increase to levels that impair O_2 transport in the blood for two reasons: It decreases the concentration of the functional hemoglobin, an effect often called "CO anemia," and it increases the O_2 affinity of the functional, not CO-bound hemoglobin. In addition, CO is exchanged in the periphery as easily as in the lung and thus can bind to extravascular proteins such as myoglobin and cytochromes (5). There-

fore it can also interfere with the transport and respiratory functions of those proteins.

Since CO acts primarily as a competitor for O_2, this chapter will attempt to consider its potential effects on the various steps of the O_2 pathway from the inspired air to the mitochondria. These steps are best visualized by the classical cascade diagram (6), where the O_2 partial pressure (P_{O_2}) of the different media are represented: inspired air, alveolar air, arterial blood, venous blood, and tissue. The diagram is presented in Fig. 1 in its usual form, with the addition of the possible roles of CO. In steady-state the O_2 flux, $\dot{V}_{O_2}$, is identical for each step and is defined by the general ohmic equation:

$$\dot{V}_{O_2} = G \cdot \Delta P_{O_2}$$

where G is a conductance and ΔP_{O_2} is equivalent to a driving force for the O_2 flux, $\dot{V}_{O_2}$. It will be seen that CO can alter the conductances of each step except maybe that of the first one. Thus CO toxicity is reflected by the fact that it lowers the P_{O_2} of the arterial, venous, and tissue media. It is the aim of this chapter to describe how CO creates hypoxic states—that is, how it affects alveolar ventilation (first step), alveolar–capillary diffusion and pulmonary functional inhomogeneity (second step), blood transport (third step), and tissue oxygenation (fourth step). This simplified view of the O_2 transfers has the didactic advantage of yielding a general view of the toxic effects of CO. Obviously the emphasis will be on the effect of CO on O_2 transport by the blood, since hemoglobin is the site of the major competition between O_2 and CO. It has been impossible to quote many important contributions, but the reader is referred to excellent recent reviews (7,8) showing a rebirth of interest for CO physiology and pharmacology as well as the general acceptance of the mechanism of CO toxicity (7).

P. E. Haab and W. Y. Durand-Arczynska: Department of Physiology, University of Fribourg, CH-1700 Fribourg, Switzerland.

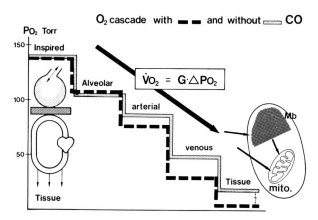

FIG. 1. Anticipated effects of CO on the oxygen partial pressure (P_{O_2}) cascade from inspired air (normoxia at sea level) to the mitochondria (mito.). Mb, myoglobin.

THE INSPIRED TO ALVEOLAR STEP

This step is defined quantitatively by the relationship

$$\dot{V}_{O_2} = G_{IA} \cdot (P_{I}O_2 - P_{A}O_2) \approx \dot{V}_A (P_{I}O_2 - P_{A}O_2)$$

where the inspired to alveolar conductance, G_{IA}, is essentially the alveolar ventilation, $\dot{V}_A$. Thus for a given metabolic rate and a given $P_{I}O_2$, $P_{A}O_2$ depends only upon $\dot{V}_A$; since $\dot{V}_A$ is influenced by the oxygen-sensitive carotid and aortic chemoreceptors, the question of the CO sensitivity of these O_2 receptors will be discussed here. CO anemia has often been used experimentally in an attempt to dissociate the effects of the arterial O_2 content from arterial $P_{a}O_2$ on chemoreceptors. Considerable controversy has surrounded the findings: About half a century ago, Comroe and Schmidt (9) showed that perfusion of the carotid body with HbCO-containing blood did not stimulate the carotid bodies, thus demonstrating the prevalent role of $P_{a}O_2$; Chiodi et al. (10) showed, in humans, that carboxemia did not elicit increases in ventilation, and Duke et al. (11) found no increase in the impulse frequency of the carotid body chemoreceptor even with very high levels of CO in the blood perfusing the chemoreceptors. Later on, these results were contradicted, but recent work by Lahiri et al. (12) has confirmed the results of the earlier studies. The carotid bodies have a high O_2 consumption but an even higher perfusion; thus the oxygen extraction is low, a feature that protects them from anemia, whether due to reduced hemoglobin concentration or to HbCO. Lahiri et al. (13) have recently reported that the aortic bodies differ from the carotid bodies in that they do have some sensitivity to CO, probably because the relative degree of overperfusion is less pronounced in those receptors than in the carotid bodies. This finding is consistent with the idea that stimulation of the chemoreceptors is related to the tissue P_{O_2}, although the ultimate mechanism of chemotransduction is still a matter of debate.

In summary, the carotid bodies appear to be more important than the aortic chemoreceptors for the regulation of the ventilatory drive but are not CO-sensitive, whereas the aortic chemoreceptors are more susceptible to the effects of CO but exert their influence more on the cardiovascular system. This is why the alveolar P_{O_2} level may be considered as almost identical with and without CO as indicated in Fig. 1.

THE ALVEOLAR TO ARTERIAL STEP

The magnitude of the alveolar to arterial P_{O_2} difference depends upon the potential effects of (a) alveolar–capillary diffusion limitation, (b) the maldistribution of the alveolar ventilation to the pulmonary perfusion and (c) the pulmonary venous admixture. These three factors must be analyzed, taking account of the fact that HbCO in the blood makes the oxygen equilibrium curve (OEC) more hyperbolic in shape (see next section). As a result, CO creates a left shift of the lower part and a flattening of the upper part of the OEC of functional hemoglobin. Such a flattening favors diffusional equilibration in the lung. Because diffusional limitation occurs only in hypoxia and/or with heavy exercise, no CO effect on this factor is expected. However, the flattening of the OEC amplifies the effects of $\dot{V}_A/\dot{Q}$ maldistribution and shunt, and even small amounts of carboxemia impair pulmonary oxygen transport in normoxia (14,15). On the other hand, in hypoxia it has been shown that the ideal alveolar to arterial P_{O_2} difference is augmented by a factor of 4 when HbCO is raised from 0% to 30% (16). Thus, CO must be considered an important factor in the lowering of $P_{a}O_2$.

THE ARTERIAL TO VENOUS STEP

Convectional transport of oxygen defines the magnitude of this step, which depends upon the product of the cardiac output, $\dot{Q}$, times the capacitance coefficient for O_2 of the circulating blood, $\beta_b O_2$. Thus the $\dot{Q} \cdot \beta_b O_2$ product is the arteriovenous conductance of the transfer equation for O_2:

$$\dot{V}_{O_2} = Q \cdot \beta_b O_2 (P_{a}O_2 - P_{v}O_2)$$

The coefficient $\beta_b O_2$ is the slope of the OEC expressed as O_2 content, C_{O_2}, per unit change of P_{O_2}: $\beta_b O_2 = \Delta C_{O_2}/\Delta P_{O_2}$. Obviously, because of the curvilinearity of the OEC, $\beta_b O_2$ is not a constant and varies with P_{O_2} in a manner that depends upon the shape of the OEC and upon the Hb concentration of the blood. Because CO reduces the O_2 capacity of the functional

Hb and because it hyperbolizes its equilibrium curve, CO has the general effect of decreasing the average value of $\beta_{b}O_2$ in the range covered by the arteriovenous difference, thereby decreasing the arteriovenous conductance. Consequently, as long as $\dot{V}O_2$ is maintained, CO induces a fall in the value of $P_{v}O_2$ because the possible increase in cardiac output as well as the increase in hematocrit observed in chronic CO exposure (17) only partially corrects for the fall in $\beta_{b}O_2$ (18). In muscles exercising near their maximal working capacity, CO may reduce the O_2 consumption and then the drop in $P_{v}O_2$ represented in Fig. 1 may not prevail (19,20).

Before describing more closely how CO changes the shape of the OEC, a brief description of the CO binding with O_2 carrier proteins in general will be presented.

CO Affinity for O_2 Carrier Proteins

Table 1 gives values from the literature for the partial pressures of CO and O_2, which saturate 50% of the capacity of three hemoproteins: hemoglobin, myoglobin, and cytochrome oxidase aa$_3$. These partial pressures, known as P_{50}, are the reciprocals of the affinities of the corresponding gases at half-saturation; thus the relative affinity of CO as compared to that of O_2 is given by the ratio $P_{50}O_2/P_{50}CO$, called M^*. CO binds chemically, like O_2, to the divalent iron atom of the heme in all three hemoproteins; however, the affinities differ, greatly depending on the hemoprotein. For Hb, CO has an affinity 200–250 times larger than that of O_2—for myoglobin, 20–25 times—whereas for cytochrome aa$_3$, the relative affinity is about unity or even less.

CO has an intrinsic affinity for isolated heme rings which is about 1500 times larger than that of O_2 (21), a feature that appears to be related to the more stable linear form of the CO–Fe^{2+} bond compared with the naturally bent form of the O_2–Fe^{2+} bond. When the hemes are located in the globin molecules, there are structural constraints (namely, those due to the distal histidine) that have relatively small effects on the O_2 binding but large effects on CO binding because CO must then also bind in a so-called "bent mode." Thermodynamically, this mode of binding significantly reduces the intrinsic affinity of CO for the heme.

The $P_{50}CO$ of the three hemoproteins are of the same order of magnitude (Table 1), which suggests that the structural constraints for the CO binding are similar for the three proteins. Thus, the larger differences in their CO–O_2 relative affinities result mainly from the large differences exhibited by their $P_{50}O_2$, with the value for Hb being one and two orders of magnitude greater than for myoglobin and for cytochrome aa$_3$, respectively. This may be due to differences in the chemical structure of the protein part of the hemoproteins or due to the effects of molecules that, when bound to the protein, modify the oxygen affinity more than the CO affinity. For instance, when hemoglobin is enclosed in erythrocyte, molecules present in the intracellular environment can modify the equilibria. Molecules binding to the Fe^{2+} atom of the heme ring are called "homotropic ligands" (O_2, CO, NO), whereas those binding to the chains are called "heterotropic ligands." Heterotropic ligands such as H$^+$, CO_2, Cl$^-$, and 2,3-diphosphoglycerate found in the intracellular space modify Hb affinity for the homotropic ligand in a manner that is remarkable but not very different for O_2 and for CO.

TABLE 1. *Values of $P_{50}O_2$, $P_{50}CO$, and M^* for hemoglobin, myoglobin, and cytochromes aa$_3$ in various mammalian species[a]*

Hemoproteins	Allostery	$P_{50}O_2$ (torr)	$P_{50}CO$ (torr)	M^* ($P_{50}O_2/$ $P_{50}CO$)
Human hemoglobin A (blood *in vitro*)	+	26.7(36)	0.125(27)	215[b]
Umbilical cord blood	+	21(56)	0.122(56)	175(56)
Sheep hemoglobin B (blood *in vitro*)	+	37.9(32)	0.210(32)	180(32)
Myoglobin	−	1.3(58) 2.3(39) 5.3(59)	0.05–0.2[c]	25(60) 20(47)
Cytochromes aa$_3$	−	0.07(47) 0.5–0.6(61)	1[d]	0.1–0.5(63)

[a] Numbers inside parentheses are reference numbers.
[b] Calculated from refs. 27 and 36.
[c] Calculated with the values of $P_{50}O_2$ and of M^*.
[d] Calculated from ref. 62.

CO Affinity for Whole Blood

Methodological Aspects

Carbon monoxide equilibrium curves (COECs) are more difficult to measure than OECs because blood equilibration with known gas mixtures, tonometry, takes much more time with CO than with O_2. An efficient tonometer should quickly equilibrate blood samples with the desired gas without damaging the formed blood elements. The rate constant of tonometric equilibration is proportional to the surface area of blood–gas interface and the efficiency of blood stirring in the tonometer, and it is inversely proportional to the blood capacitance for the equilibrating gas (i.e., the product of the blood volume in the tonometer and the capacitance coefficient β_b of that gas). Because CO has a capacitance coefficient 200–250 times larger than that of O_2, extremely long times may be required to attain equilibrium. Consequently, during prolonged equilibration, preservation of the biochemical integrity of blood may become a major difficulty. On the other hand, since CO tends to make the OEC hyperbolic, long tonometry duration may also be required for O_2 equilibrations with low oxygen tensions. Although remarkably rapid instruments have recently been developed for the measurement of OEC (22), such instruments do not exist for COEC.

Remarkable progress has been made in the measurement of hemoglobin O_2 and CO saturations. Modern four-wavelength spectrophotometers provide rapid measurements of HbO_2, HbCO, methb, and Hbtot, but it is important to ensure that the reference spectrum used corresponds to that of the Hb of the measured blood. Gasometry has also made rapid progress thanks to its coupling to high-precision gas chromatography.

Very few COEC curves have been obtained in recent years, and our present-day information relies mainly on data obtained before the effects of heterotropic ligands such as 2,3-diphosphoglycerates were known. However, the effects of the heterotropic ligands have been studied on the OEC modified by the presence of HbCO (23,24).

CO Equilibrium Curve and CO–O_2 Relative Affinity

The pioneering studies of Douglas et al. (25) early in this century established that the COEC had a shape very similar to that of the OEC, and that $P_{50}CO$ was about 220 times smaller than $P_{50}O_2$. These investigators used a very ingenious colorimetric method based on the visual comparison of the pink color of HbCO with that of carmine solutions. Their results led them to believe that COEC and OEC were isomorphous and that the curves could be made to coincide by multi-plying the abscissa of the COEC by a single factor of 220. This factor, the CO–O_2 relative affinity factor M^*, was therefore considered as saturation-independent. This last feature was questioned as early as 1928 by Barcroft (26), who thought that the COEC was more sigmoidal than the OEC, a feature that was confirmed in 1958 by Joels and Pugh (27) and by Roughton (28). According to these investigators, a variation of M^* from 120 to 225 from low to high saturation is possible in human blood at constant P_{CO_2} (40 torr) and pH (7.4). Explained in terms of the intermediate compounds hypothesis of Adair, the equilibrium constant of the first monomer of the tetrameric Hb molecule appears to be only 120 times larger for CO than for O_2 (28), whereas for the other monomers the affinity ratio is much higher. This also means that the heme–heme interaction is larger for CO as is the value of Hill's coefficient n. In terms of the more recent two-state allosteric model of Wyman, Monod, and Changeux, the saturation dependency of M^* indicates that the T state of Hb has a smaller CO–O_2 relative affinity than the R state. The above statements remain purely descriptive, and the cause of the greater sigmoidicity of whole-blood COEC is not yet completely understood; however, in hemoglobin solutions, preferential binding of CO to the Hb β chains provides a clue (29), since those chains could have a lower affinity for CO (30).

Haldane (25) has defined a CO–O_2 relative affinity factor that he called M for the conditions where blood is exposed to and contains O_2 and CO simultaneously. This factor may be thought of as the ratio of the apparent equilibrium constants for CO (L_{CO}) and for O_2 (K_{CO}):

$$L_{CO} = [HbCO]/[Hb] \cdot [CO], \quad K_{O_2} = [HbO_2]/[Hb] \cdot [O_2]$$

from which it follows that

$$L_{CO}/K_{O_2} = HbCO \cdot P_{O_2}/HbO_2 \cdot P_{CO} = M$$

Haldane found that, as long as P_{O_2} and P_{CO} were large enough to fully saturate hemoglobin, the value of M was independent of the relative amounts of HbCO and HbO_2. This is often called Haldane's "first law." Because Haldane believed that COEC and OEC were isomorphous, he also proposed that his first law be applicable when P_{CO} and P_{O_2} do not fully saturate Hb. This has been called Haldane's "second law." Since it is now established that the CO–O_2 relative affinity, M^*, is lower at lower saturation, Haldane's M is also expected to decrease at low Hb saturation and even more so the larger the HbCO. Whereas Haldane's first law has been amply verified, his second law is considered of limited value (31), although measurements of M in desaturation are scarce. Joels and Pugh (27) also observed that, at full saturation, M and M^* were not identical, a disparity that Roughton (28) attempted to explain by the fact that the chemical definition of

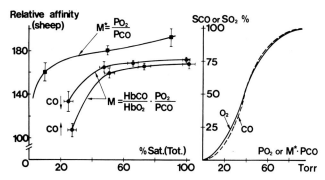

FIG. 2. Right: Superposition of O_2 (——) and CO (---) equilibrium curves of sheep blood with HbB, showing the greater sigmoidicity of the CO equilibrium curve. **Left**: CO–O_2 relative affinity factors M^* and M as a function of total saturation, HbCO + HbO$_2$. For M, the lower curve corresponds to a higher HbCO/HbO$_2$ ratio than does the higher curve.

M involves more equilibrium constants than does that of M^*.

Measured values of M^* and M in sheep blood are presented in Fig. 2 as a function of total Hb saturation (HbCO + HbO$_2$). Because the effects of 2,3-diphosphoglycerate on the value of M are not completely elucidated, ovine blood with hemoglobin type B (HbB) (32) was used. Sheep blood is known to be devoid of 2,3-diphosphoglycerate, and ovine HbB does not bind this phosphate. Values of M were obtained for blood tonometered with high (upper curve for M, Fig. 2) and low (lower curve for M, Fig. 2) P_{O_2}/P_{CO} ratios. M^* is much lower at low saturation, confirming the non-isomorphism of the equilibrium curves. The values of M are constant for the saturation range from 50% to 100% and are independent of the P_{O_2}/P_{CO} ratio, confirming both of Haldane's laws in this saturation range. However, below 50% saturation M starts to decline; the richer in CO the blood is, the greater the decline. These observations are not in accordance with Haldane's second law but must be regarded as a consequence of the greater sigmoidicity of the COEC. Finally, the data of Fig. 2 also point out that the values of M and M^* are species-dependent. In adult human blood, M has been found to be equal to (33), or about 7% higher than (27), M^* (see Table 1).

Effects of CO on Position and Shape of the Oxygen Equilibrium Curve

In 1912, Douglas et al. (25) and Haldane (34) discovered and studied quantitatively the fact that HbCO in blood induces a hyperbolization of the OEC. In doing so, they elucidated one of the most important features of CO toxicity: In addition to reducing the amount of functional hemoglobin available for O_2, CO augments

the O_2 affinity of this hemoglobin and consequently reduces the blood O_2 partial pressure and the driving force for O_2 diffusion to peripheral tissues. They have very clearly shown that tissue oxygenation is hindered more by a decrease in functional Hb through CO anemia than by a reduction of equal percentage of the hemoglobin concentration (i.e., simple anemia).

In 1912, Haldane (34) proposed a procedure for computing the hyperbolization of the OEC by HbCO based on the assumed validity of his two laws. Later on, Roughton and Darling (35) proposed a simplification of Haldane's calculation. Their method relies on the fact that the total saturation of Hb, HbO$_2$ + HbCO, is determined by a partial pressure of O_2, P_{O_2}, equal to the sum of the blood P_{O_2} + MP_{CO}, which can be read on a normal OEC. The interesting feature of this procedure is that although (like in Haldane's procedure) M is considered a constant, knowledge of its exact value is not required.

The Roughton–Darling method gives fairly good agreement with experimental results for HbCO levels up to 60%, and it remains a useful tool today. However, since it is now well established that neither M^* nor M is constant, some divergence between computed and measured OEC can be expected, mainly in the low saturation range (<50%). This has been confirmed with the newly developed techniques for rapid recording of the OEC by Okada et al. (31) and by Zwart et al. (24). Such methods are appropriate for measuring OEC in the presence of HbCO, since the CO binding to Hb is stable enough to rule out the risk of CO dissociating during the procedure (23,24,31,35). Recent investigators have generally found that measured OEC corresponded fairly well with the prediction made by Roughton and Darling as long as total saturation of Hb is between 50% and 100%—that is, as long as M can be considered saturation-independent as depicted in Fig. 2. For lower saturations, the OEC lies to the left of the predicted one as a result of the decrease of M.

Figure 3 illustrates the hyperbolizing effects of CO, redrawn mostly after Zwart et al. (24) but in full accordance with data of Okada et al. (31) and of Hlastala et al. (23).

Figure 3A represents the O_2 saturation versus P_{O_2} for different concentrations of HbCO: 0%, 20%, 40%, and 60%, corresponding to the curves 1, 2, 3, and 4, respectively. It is seen that the curves of the HbCO-containing bloods are progressively left-shifted. Figure 3B represents the effect of the same HbCO concentrations on the O_2 content versus P_{O_2} relationships. These curves, important for the analysis of gas exchange, show the simultaneous decrease in O_2 capacity and OEC hyperbolization; each curve intersects the normal curve at a progressively lower P_{O_2} as HbCO increases. On such curves the term "left shift" may be misleading, since it applies only to the part below

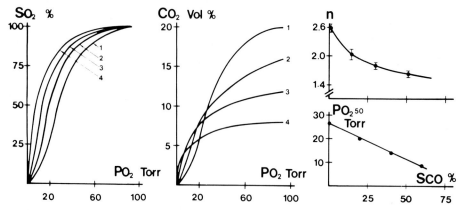

FIG. 3. Effect of various HbCO concentrations on the O_2 equilibrium curve of human blood. Curves 1, 2, 3, and 4 correspond to HbCO concentrations of 0%, 20%, 40%, and 60%, respectively.

the point of intersection; above this point, in contrast, the curves are right-shifted. Because of this, the effects of the left-shifted OEC on tissue oxygenation are most pronounced in hypoxia.

Figure 3C shows that $P_{50}O_2$ drops linearly with HbCO (lower part) and that the Hill coefficient, n, falls in an exponential manner with HbCO (upper part). This draws attention to the fact that even small amounts of HbCO have an influence on OEC and that the variability of normal P_{50} depends critically upon the HbCO concentrations in normal individuals (36). The progressive decrease in n is indicative of a loss of the cooperative allosteric function of the tetrameric Hb molecule when partially bound to CO.

THE BLOOD TO TISSUE STEP

CO Effect on Capillary to Mitochondria O_2 Transport

To reach the site of its consumption, O_2 must first be detached from hemoglobin and move out of the erythrocytes to proceed through various tissue components (such as capillary wall, interstitial space, and cell membranes) to its final destination, the mitochondria. Hence, it must overcome many resistances in series, which, by analogy to what has been proposed in the lung (37), can be classified into two types: (i) a blood resistance, including a chemical component due to off-rate kinetics of deoxygenation, and (ii) a tissular resistance. Overcoming of the second type of resistance may be facilitated in contractile tissues by the carrier-assisted transport of myoglobin (38,39). Thus, after the blood resistance, two resistances in parallel, corresponding to simple and facilitated diffusion, respectively, must be considered. Carbon monoxide may affect the value of the overall conductance for O_2 of the blood to tissue path by way of its competition with O_2 on hemoglobin and myoglobin.

The overall blood-to-tissue conductance may be written as a general transfer equation:

$$\dot{V}_{O_2} = D_{tiss} (P_{\bar{c}}O_2 - P_{tiss}O_2)$$

where: D_{tiss}, the apparent tissue diffusing capacity, is a lumped parameter comprising the above-mentioned resistances; $P_{\bar{c}}O_2$ is the mean capillary P_{O_2}; and $P_{tiss}O_2$ is the tissue P_{O_2} in the immediate vicinity of the mitochondria. In real organs, the $P_{\bar{c}}O_2-P_{tiss}O_2$ difference (and, consequently, the value of D_{tiss}) is defined not only by diffusion but also by factors such as shunts and uneven distribution of blood flow, which are not affected by CO. However, when $\dot{V}_{O_2}$ is large, the diffusion limitation may become predominant and the adverse effects of CO may become more evident.

Recently, Wagner and co-workers have provided evidence that diffusion limitation may be the major determinant of maximal oxygen consumption in humans (40) as well as in isolated muscle perfused *in situ* (41). It has been shown in smokers that $\dot{V}_{O_2}max$ is reduced by about 1% per % HbCO (42); isolated muscles working in normoxia but with 60% HbCO have an oxygen consumption 16% lower than in hypoxia (20), whereas the same preparation working at maximal aerobic capacity exhibits a 25% reduction in $\dot{V}_{O_2}max$ when perfused with hypoxemic blood containing 30% HbCO as compared to hypoxia with no CO (19). At rest, however, CO does not induce any change in $\dot{V}_{O_2}$ in normoxic humans (18) or in hypoxic dogs (16). Recent studies performed on myocardial cells in culture showed that the growth rate and the beating rate of muscle cells were not affected by the addition of up to 20% CO to the incubation gas; in contrast, the growth rate of nonmuscle cells was paradoxically reduced in the presence of CO, even when the O_2 concentration was maintained at a normal level (43). These observations suggest an adaptation of the metabolism of the cardiac cells in culture. *In vivo*, however, the myocardial O_2 consumption has been shown to undergo a small decrease under the influence of CO (44).

Quantitative analysis of different effects of CO on $\dot{V}O_2$max is difficult because of their simultaneous occurrence. First, the left shift of the OEC must certainly play a role in diminishing the driving forces for O_2 diffusion through tissues that contain no myoglobin. However, no proportionality is expected between this effect and HbCO concentration, since the left shift does not increase linearly with CO concentration (Fig. 3B). Second, the off-rate reaction kinetics of oxygen are expected to be slower in the presence of CO, and the role of this factor has been suspected to be important (45). The O_2 off-rate is known to depend upon the absolute concentration of HbO_2 and upon capillary PO_2, both of which are reduced in the presence of CO. Third, the well established myoglobin carrier function (39) is complex because it depends on its degree of oxygenation. On normoxic isolated cardiac myocytes, myoglobin-facilitated O_2 diffusion does not contribute to the overall O_2 transfer. When myoglobin is completely blocked by H_2O_2 (46) or by CO (47), 30–50% of the O_2 transfer is suppressed. Myoglobin binds CO with a relative CO–O_2 affinity of 20–25 (Table 1) and has been shown to be only 20–30% O_2 saturated in maximally working muscles, where it acts as an O_2 redistributor and thus as a PO_2 buffer (48). Therefore, relatively large reductions of $\dot{V}O_2$max resulting from the presence of MbCO must be predicted.

CO Binding to Mitochondrial Cytochrome C Oxidase

The chemical structure of the cytochrome C oxidase allows a reversible binding of CO with the metal ligand of its heme (49,50). Although this property has been widely exploited for chemical analysis, its physiological implications for the mitochondrial function has been less studied. Cytochrome aa_3 binds CO in vivo and in vitro, and one of the consequences of this binding is the oxidation of CO to CO_2 (4,51). Recently, it has been shown that CO combustion is entirely dependent on the reaction with cytochrome C oxidase (52). This phenomenon could be involved in the tolerance developed for low levels of inhaled CO.

A further consequence of the CO binding cytochrome aa_3 could be the inhibition of the mitochondrial electron transfer (i.e., cellular respiration). Recent studies performed on brain tissue of rats in vivo showed modifications of the oxidative metabolism associated to CO exposure even at low CO/O_2 ratio (53). The results were obtained in fluorocarbon-circulated rats, a condition that prevents the decline of O_2 delivery related to carboxyhemoglobin formation. In these conditions, CO caused an increase of phosphocreatine

and adenosine diphosphate (ADP) concentrations with no modification of $\dot{V}O_2$, indicating a change in the overall efficiency of the oxidative phosphorylation. It must be pointed out that all these experiments have been performed with gases containing at least 1% CO, which produce a higher PCO than those encountered in most CO intoxications in humans. In summary, the above observations point to the fact that it is difficult to impede mitochondrial oxygen consumption with CO in concentrations that are otherwise incompatible with life.

CARBON MONOXIDE EFFECTS ON THE FETUS

The effect of CO on fetal oxygenation has been of great epidemiological importance since the discovery of retarded fetal growth when mothers smoke cigarettes during pregnancy (54). Thorough review of the subject can be found (55), and the topic is only briefly treated here. CO is suspected to create a tissue hypoxia in the fetus to a degree that is not compensated by a secondary increase in hematocrit. In addition, the developing fetus has a high metabolic rate, a large blood O_2 extraction ratio, and arterial PO_2 levels similar to those of an adult climbing near the summit of Mt. Everest. Hence, it is very likely to be susceptible to adverse effects of CO.

The CO–O_2 relative affinity factor M is 180 in umbilical cord blood (33), a value that is 20% lower than in adult maternal blood. Because the value of $P_{50}O_2$ of umbilical cord blood is also about 20% lower than that of adult blood, it appears that the smaller value of fetal M results entirely from the augmented affinity of fetal blood for O_2 without any change in its CO affinity (56). This interpretation requires confirmation, since it means that O_2 and CO affinities are not regulated the same way by the organic phosphates. The M value of 180 can be used to predict the ratio of CO concentration in maternal and fetal bloods when mother and fetus are in diffusional equilibrium. This ratio, calculated by Longo (55), should be very close to unity. Experimentally, a ratio of 1.1 is found, with the 10% difference being easily explained by the higher fetal hematocrit and/or by absence of maternal–fetal equilibrium. Before the need for a special correction of spectrophotometric HbCO measurements was recognized (57), it was believed that HbCO was always 4–6% higher in umbilical cord blood than in maternal blood. The HbCO level in maternal blood of cigarette smokers can reach levels of up to 10–12%, depending on the number of cigarettes consumed per day. It remains unclear how much O_2 consumption of the fetus may be impaired by this carboxemia, but many studies have pointed out the potential dangers of left-shifted OEC for the fetal development.

ACKNOWLEDGMENTS

The authors thank S. C. Hempleman for helpful discussion of the manuscript, and they thank Mrs. Y. Schütz for secretarial assistance. The authors' research was supported by grants of the Swiss National Foundation and of the Swiss Association of Cigarette Manufacturers.

REFERENCES

1. Moray R. A relation of persons killed with subterraneous damps. *Philos Trans R Soc Lond [A] Math Phys Sci* 1665;1:44–45.
2. Coburn RF, Williams WJ, Forster RE. Effect of erythrocyte destruction on carbon monoxide production in man. *J Clin Invest* 1964;43:1098–1103.
3. Coburn RF, Blakemore WS, Forster RE. Endogenous carbon monoxide production in man. *J Clin Invest* 1964;42:1172–1178.
4. Fenn WO, Cobe DM. The burning of carbon monoxide by heart and skeletal muscle. *Am J Physiol* 1932;102:393–401.
5. Coburn RF. The carbon monoxide body stores. *Ann NY Acad Sci* 1970;174:11–22.
6. Haab P. Systématisation des échanges gazeux pulmonaires. *J Physiol (Paris)* 1982;78:108–119.
7. Coburn RF, Forman HJ. Carbon monoxide toxicity. In: *Handbook of physiology, Section 3: The respiratory system, vol IV—Gas exchange.* Bethesda, MD: American Physiological Society, 1987;439–456.
8. Longo LD, Hill EP. Carbon monoxide uptake and elimination in fetal and maternal sheep. *Am J Physiol* 1977;232(3):H324–H330.
9. Comroe JH Jr, Schmidt CP. The part played by reflexes from the carotid body in the chemical regulation of respiration in the dog. *Am J Physiol* 1938;121:75–97.
10. Chiodi H, Dill DB, Comsolazio F, Horvath SM. Respiratory and circulatory response to acute carbon monoxide poisoning. *Am J Physiol* 1941;134:683–693.
11. Duke HN, Green JH, Neil E. Carotid chemoreceptor impulse activity during inhalation carbon monoxide mixtures. *J Physiol (Lond)* 1952;118:520–527.
12. Lahiri S, Mulligan E, Nishino T, Mokashi A, Davies RO. Relative responses of aortic body and carotid body chemoreceptors to carboxyhemoglobinemia. *J Appl Physiol: Respir Environ Exercise Physiol* 1981;50:580–586.
13. Lahiri S, Penney DG, Mokashi A, Albertine KH. Chronic CO inhalation and carotid body catecholamines: testing of hypotheses. *J Appl Physiol* 1989;67(1):239–242.
14. Ayres SM, Giannelli S. Effects of small amounts of carboxyhemoglobin on oxygen transport. *J Clin Invest* 1966;45:983.
15. Brody JS, Coburn RF. Effects of elevated carboxyhemoglobin on gas exchange in the lung. *Ann NY Acad Sci* 1970;255–260.
16. Savoy J, Michoud M-C, Robert M, Geiser J, Haab P, Piiper J. Comparison of steady state pulmonary diffusing capacity estimates for O$_2$ and CO in dogs. *Respir Physiol* 1980;42:43–59.
17. Fisher JW. Pharmacologic modulation of erythropoietin production. *Annu Rev Pharmacol Toxicol* 1988;28:101–122.
18. Ayres SM, Giannelli S Jr, Meuller H. Myocardial and systemic response to carboxyhemoglobin. *Ann NY Acad Sci* 1970;174:268–293.
19. Haab PE, Hogan MC, Bedout DE, Gray A, Wagner PD, West JB. Limitation of O$_2$ uptake in working muscle due to the presence of carbon monoxide in blood. *FASEB J* 1988;2:A760.
20. King CE, Dodd SL, Cain SM. O$_2$ delivery to contracting muscle during hypoxic or CO hypoxia. *J Appl Physiol* 1987;63:726–732.
21. Collman JP, Brauman JI, Halbert TR, Suslick KS. Nature of O$_2$ and CO binding to metalloporphyrins and heme proteins. *Proc Natl Acad Sci USA* 1976;73:3333–3337.
22. Duvelleroy MA, Buckles RG, Rosenkaimer S, Tung C, Laver MB. An oxyhemoglobin dissociation analyzer. *J Appl Physiol* 1970;28:227–233.
23. Hlastala MP, McKenna HP, Franada RL, Detter JC. Influence of carbon monoxide on hemoglobin–oxygen binding. *J Appl Physiol* 1976;41:893–899.
24. Zwart A, Kwant G, Oeseburg B, Zijlstra WG. Human whole-blood oxygen affinity: effect of carbon monoxide. *J Appl Physiol: Respir Environ Exercise Physiol* 1984;57:14.
25. Douglas CG, Haldane JS, Haldane JBS. The laws of combination of haemoglobin with carbon monoxide and oxygen. *J Physiol Lond* 1912;44:275–304.
26. Barcroft J. *The respiratory function of the blood. Haemoglobin,* Part II. London: Cambridge University Press, 1928.
27. Joels N, Pugh LGCE. The carbon monoxide dissociation curve of human blood. *J Physiol (Lond)* 1958;142:63–77.
28. Roughton FJW. The equilibrium of carbon monoxide with human hemoglobin in whole blood. *Ann NY Acad Sci* 1970; 174:177–188.
29. Lau PW, Asakura T. Comparative study of oxygen and carbon monoxide by hemoglobin. *J Biol Chem* 1980;255:1617–1622.
30. Perrella M, Sabbioneda L, Samaja M, Rossi-Bernardi L. The intermediate compounds between human hemoglobin and carbon monoxide at equilibrium and during approach to equilibrium. *J Biol Chem* 1986;261:8391–8396.
31. Okada Y, Tyuma I, Ueda Y, Sugimoto T. Effect of carbon monoxide on equilibrium between oxygen and hemoglobin. *Am J Physiol* 1976;230:471–475.
32. Maendly C. Affinité relative de l'oxygène et du monoxyde de carbone pour le sang de mouton (Hb B) en fonction du taux de saturation de l'hémoglobine. Thèse, Université de Lausanne, 1989.
33. Engel RR, Rodkey FL, O'Neal JD, Collison HA. Relative affinity of human fetal hemoglobin for carbon monoxide and oxygen. *Blood* 1969;33(1):37–45.
34. Haldane JBS. The dissociation of oxyhemoglobin in human blood during partial CO-poisoning. *J Physiol (Lond)* 1912; 45:XXII.
35. Roughton FJW, Darling RC. The effect of carbon monoxide on the oxyhemoglobin dissociation curve. *Am J Physiol* 1944; 51:17–31.
36. Winslow R, Morissey J, Berger R, Smith P, Gibson C. Variability of oxygen affinity of normal blood: an automated method of measurement. *J Appl Physiol* 1978;45:289–297.
37. Forster RE, Roughton FJW, Cander L, Briscoe WA, Kreuzer F. Apparent pulmonary diffusing capacity for CO at varying alveolar O$_2$ tensions. *J Appl Physiol* 1957;II:277.
38. De Koning J, Hoofd LJC, Kreuzer F. Oxygen transport and the function of myoglobin. Theoretical model and experiments in chicken gizzard smooth muscle. *Pflügers Arch* 1981;389:211–217.
39. Wittenberg BA, Wittenberg JP. Transport of oxygen in muscle. *Annu Rev Physiol* 1989;51:857–878.
40. Roca J, Hogan MC, Story D, Bedout DE, Haab P, Gonzalez R, Ueno O, Wagner PD. Evidence for tissue diffusion limitation of VO$_2$max in normal humans. *J Appl Physiol* 1989;67(1):291–299.
41. Hogan MC, Roca J, Wagner PD, West JB. Limitation of maximal O$_2$ uptake and performance by acute hypoxia in *in situ* dog muscle. *J Appl Physiol* 1988;65(2):815–821.
42. Hirsch GL, Sue DY, Wasserman K, Robinson TE, Hansen JE. Immediate effects of cigarette smoking on cardiorespiratory responses to exercise. *J Appl Physiol* 1985;58(6):1975–1981.
43. Nag AC, Chen KC, Cheng M. Effects of carbon monoxide on cardiac muscle cells in culture. *Am J Physiol* 1988;255:C291–C296.
44. Adams JD, Erickson HH, Stone HL. Myocardial metabolism during exposure to carbon monoxide in the conscious dog. *J Appl Physiol* 1973;34:238–242.
45. Rose CP, Goresky CA. Limitations of tracer oxygen uptake in the canine coronary circulation. *Circ Res* 1985;56:57–70.
46. Cole RP. Skeletal muscle function in hypoxia: effect of alteration of intracellular myoglobin. *Respir Physiol* 1983;53:1–14.

47. Wittenberg BA, Wittenberg JB. Myoglobin-mediated oxygen delivery to mitochondria of isolated cardiac myocytes. *Proc Natl Acad Sci USA* 1987;84:7503–7507.

48. Honig CR, Frierson JL, Gayeski TEJ. Anatomical determinants of O_2 flux density at coronary capillaries. *Am J Physiol* 1989;256:H375–H382.

49. Chance B, Erecinska M. Mitochondrial response to carbon monoxide toxicity. *Ann NY Acad Sci* 1970;174:193–204.

50. Wilson DF, Miyata Y. Reaction of CO with cytochrome c oxidase. Titration of the reaction site with chemical oxidant and reductant. *Biochim Biophys Acta* 1977;461:218–230.

51. Breckenridge B. Carbon monoxide oxidation by cytochrome oxidase in muscle. *Am J Physiol* 1953;173:62–69.

52. Young LJ, Caughey WS. Mitochondrial oxygenation of carbon monoxide. *Biochem J* 1986;239:225–227.

53. Piantadosi CA, Lee PA, Sylvia AL. Direct effects of CO on cerebral energy metabolism in bloodless rats. *J Appl Physiol* 1988;65(2):878–887.

54. Bureau MA, Shapcott D, Berthiaume Y, Monette J, Blouin D, Blanchard P, Begin R. Maternal cigarette smoking and fetal oxygen transport: a study of P50,2,3-diphosphoglycerate, total hemoglobin, hematocrit, and type F hemoglobin in fetal blood. *Pediatrics* 1983;72:22–26.

55. Longo LD. The biological effects of carbon monoxide on the pregnant woman, fetus, and newborn infant. *Am J Obstet Gynecol* 1977;129:69–103.

56. Schuwey D, Tempini A, Haab P. Carbon monoxide dissociation curve of human umbilical cord blood. *Adv Exp Med Biol* 1989;232:in press.

57. Cornelissen PJH, Van Woensel CLM, Van Oel WC, De Jong PA. Correction-factors for hemoglobin derivatives in fetal blood as measured with the "IL 282" CO-oximeter. *Clin Chem* 1983;29(8):1555.

58. Wittenberg BA, Wittenberg JB. Oxygen pressure gradients in isolated cardiac myocytes. *J Biol Chem* 1985;260:6548–6554.

59. Gayeski TE, Honig CR. Intracellular oxygen pressure in individual cardiac myocytes in dog, cat, rabbit, ferret, and rat. *Am J Physiol* 1990;in press.

60. Coburn RF, Mayers LB. Myoglobin O_2 determined from measurements of carboxymyoglobin in skeletal muscle. *Am J Physiol* 1971;220(1):66–74.

61. Wilson DF, Rumsey WL. Factors modulating the oxygen dependence of mitochondrial oxidative phosphorylation. *Adv Exp Med Biol* 1988;222:121–131.

62. Wohlrab H, Ogunmola GB. Carbon monoxide binding studies of cytochrome a3 hemes in intact rat liber mitochondria. *Biochemistry* 1971;10:1103–1106.

63. Piantadosi CA, Sylvia AL, Jobsis Vandervliet FF. Differences in brain cytochrome responses to carbon monoxide and cyanide in vivo. *J Appl Physiol* 1987;62:1277–1284.

THE LUNG: Scientific Foundations
edited by R.G. Crystal, J.B. West et al.
Raven Press, Ltd., New York © 1991.

CHAPTER 5.3.3

Diffusion

Peter Scheid and Johannes Piiper

On its way to the mitochondria, the oxygen is brought by convection into the alveolar airspace, and convection with blood delivers it to the various tissues. But the tissue separating gas from blood in the lung, the alveolocapillary membrane, must be penetrated by *diffusion*. This tissue membrane thus constitutes a diffusive barrier for O_2 uptake in the lung, and likewise for CO_2 excretion or exchange of any other gas.

The resistance to gas exchange offered by the barrier is kept very small, largely because the membrane is exceedingly thin, on average a fraction of 1 μm, just enough to warrant mechanical stability, and extremely large, 50–100 m^2 or about 50 times the external body surface area. This geometry is made possible by the placement of the lung inside the body cavity and by formation of many parallel units, about 300 million alveoli. Other types of gas exchange organ have been developed in vertebrate classes other than mammals (1). Although small, the diffusive resistance for O_2 uptake may become measurable under various conditions, leading to reduction in arterial partial pressure and saturation of O_2, and it is the aim of this chapter to review the factors that govern diffusion in the lung and that lead to *diffusion limitation* of alveolar gas exchange.

When two media, for example, the alveolar gas space and the capillary blood space, have contact through a separating membrane, gas molecules will migrate across the barrier, and the physical laws of diffusion predict that an *equilibrium* is reached when the partial pressures of the gas species are identical in both spaces. In the lung, the blood is moving, and when it comes into the first contact with the membrane, there

will be, in general, no such equilibrium. However, gas exchange across the alveolocapillary membrane aims at attaining this equilibrium—a process called *equilibration*. Attainment of an equilibrium state of gas exchange in the lung is judged from the blood at the end of the capillary contact, that is, the *end-capillary blood*: equality of alveolar and end-capillary partial pressure indicates attainment of an equilibrium, and vice versa. Since the composition of end-capillary blood is normally similar to that in arterial blood, these statements hold for arterial blood as well.

This is the belief today, which is based on the generally accepted assumption that passive diffusion governs alveolar gas exchange. The existence of specific carrier mechanisms for oxygen and carbon monoxide, for example, P450, which would facilitate their transfer across the tissue barrier (2), has not been substantiated in later experiments (3,4).

A number of authors over the last 20 years have claimed that the P_{CO_2} in arterial blood may be lower than that in alveolar gas, even when an equilibrium is attained. This finding, which would have severe consequences for the analysis of alveolar gas exchange, has not been verified in later studies (5).

We analyze in the following sections alveolar gas exchange and derive models that allow a quantitative assessment of diffusion limitation. In doing so, we start from simple models that apply to the unrealistic ideal situation only but allow a particularly clear view into the basic parameters governing gas exchange. We discuss experimental methods, based on these simple models, to estimate the pulmonary diffusing capacity D, a quantitative measure of the diffusive conductance of the barrier. Thereafter, we turn to methods of estimating D in real lungs, in which regional heterogeneity of ventilation, diffusion, and perfusion exert a significant influence on gas exchange.

P. Scheid and J. Piiper: Institute for Physiology, Ruhr University, Bochum, and Department of Physiology, Max Planck Institute for Experimental Medicine, D-3400 Göttingen, Federal Republic of Germany.

DIFFUSING CAPACITY

In the simplest model we describe the alveolocapillary membrane by a homogeneous barrier of some thickness (1) and area (A). The laws of diffusion predict that a steady transfer of gas through the membrane ($\dot{M}$) will occur down a partial pressure difference (ΔP) across the membrane:

$$\dot{M} = d\alpha \frac{A}{l} \Delta P, \qquad [1]$$

where d and α are the diffusivity and solubility of the gas in the study within the membrane material.

In real lungs, neither the geometric (A, l) nor the physical parameters (d, α) can independently be determined, and they are normally lumped together,

$$D = d\alpha \frac{A}{l}, \qquad [2]$$

so that

$$\dot{M} = D \, \Delta P. \qquad [3]$$

This equation, applied to alveolocapillary gas transfer, is usually regarded as the definition of the *pulmonary diffusing* capacity D. Its physical meaning is that of a conductance (transfer rate divided by driving pressure difference). Equation 3 describes the overall effective diffusing capacity even though the component factors are neither known nor regionally constant throughout the lung.

Application of the apparently simple Eq. 3 to real lungs is complex, largely because ΔP is not constant along the pulmonary capillary. This calls for introducing the diffusion/perfusion model.

DIFFUSION/PERFUSION MODEL AND EQUILIBRATION COEFFICIENT

Model

The model of Fig. 1 is appropriate to describe alveolocapillary transfer of any gas species (6). It represents one alveolus (partial pressure, PA) separated from a capillary (blood flow $\dot{Q}$) by a barrier (diffusing capacity D). When we assume the lung to be homogeneous, that is, built of identical such alveolar units, then D and $\dot{Q}$ can be assumed to represent the values for the total lung.

Below the model in Fig. 1A is the partial pressure profile in capillary blood (Pc) along the capillary for the case that gas is taken up into blood (mixed venous partial pressure P$\bar{\text{v}}$ lower than PA). The gas flow across a small segment of the barrier (dD) into blood follows

the driving ΔP (= PA − Pc) and leads to an increase in Pc by dPc. Since the driving ΔP diminishes along the capillary, so does the rate of increase in Pc. The important value of the end-capillary, or the arterial partial pressure (Pa) depends on both diffusion and perfusion (4):

$$\frac{P_A - P_a}{P_A - P\bar{v}} = e^{-D/\dot{Q}\beta}. \qquad [4]$$

The left-hand side of this equation represents the *equilibration deficit* (PA − Pa) relative to the "entrance difference" (PA − P$\bar{\text{v}}$). This relative equilibration deficit is dependent on a single coefficient, the *equilibration coefficient*, D/$\dot{Q}\beta$, which contains D and $\dot{Q}$ and the *capacitance coefficient* β.

This parameter β is the slope of the relation between content C and partial pressure P of the gas in the study (Fig. 1B). For inert gases, β equals the physical solubility α; for O_2, CO_2, CO, and NO, β is the slope of the respective blood binding curve (7). For gases with chemical binding, in particular for O_2, β is nearly constant, independent of P, only in the hypoxic range (Fig. 1B). Note that Eq. 4 is applicable for (nearly) constant β only; it is thus valid for inert gases, for CO_2 and for O_2 in hypoxia.

Sometimes the (mean) capillary transit time or *contact time* (t_c) is considered in alveolocapillary equilibration. Since t_c equals the ratio of pulmonary capillary volume (Vc) and flow ($\dot{Q}$),

$$\frac{D}{\dot{Q}\beta} = \frac{D}{Vc \cdot \beta} t_c. \qquad [5]$$

It follows that t_c, independent of Vc, is not sufficient to replace $\dot{Q}$. Moreover, it is confusing to regard "too short a transit time" as a factor separate from "too high a cardiac output" in producing equilibration deficit.

Diffusion Limitation

With large values of D/$\dot{Q}\beta$, Pa reaches PA, and the equilibration deficit of Eq. 4 is zero (Fig. 1C). In this situation, there is no diffusion limitation, since a further increase of D, thereby increasing D/$\dot{Q}\beta$, will not raise Pa any further. On the other hand, as D/$\dot{Q}\beta$ is reduced, an equilibration deficit develops (Fig. 1C) up to the limit, where Pa remains at P$\bar{\text{v}}$ and the (relative) equilibration deficit is unity. This is the case of strongest diffusion limitation.

D/$\dot{Q}\beta$ and the equilibration deficit can thus be used to quantify diffusion limitation Ldiff:

$$L_{diff} = e^{-D/\dot{Q}\beta}. \qquad [6]$$

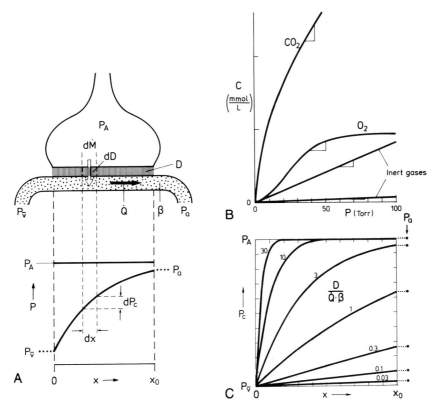

FIG. 1. Diffusion/perfusion model and capillary–alveolar equilibration. **A:** Model and partial pressure profile. **B:** Blood CO_2 and O_2 dissociation curves, and solubility lines of an inert gas with low solubility and one with medium solubility. **C:** Equilibration profiles for various values of the equilibration coefficient, $D/\dot{Q}\beta$. (Modified from ref. 4.)

A value of $L_{diff} = 0.6$ would mean that 60% more gas could be transferred if $D/\dot{Q}\beta$ could be raised to infinity and, likewise, that the relative equilibration deficit is 0.6 (4).

It is thus not D alone, but the combination $D/\dot{Q}\beta$, that determines the diffusion limitation. Figure 2 represents a plot of L_{diff} against $D/\dot{Q}\beta$.

Physical Properties of Gases

Let us look at the defining Eq. 2 to identify the factors determining $D/\dot{Q}\beta$:

$$\frac{D}{\dot{Q}\beta} = \frac{d}{\beta/\alpha}\frac{A/l}{\dot{Q}}. \qquad [7]$$

Since A/l and $\dot{Q}$ are identical for all gases, differences between them are reflected in (a) the diffusivity in the barrier (d) and (b) the solubility ratio (β/α).

For most inert gases, β/α is close to unity; but for gases chemically bound in blood, β/α is much greater than unity and varies with P. The range for β or α among gases is much wider than that for d.

The resulting $D/\dot{Q}\beta$ values for various gases in human lungs are indicated in Fig. 2.

Inert gases exhibit a rather high $D/\dot{Q}\beta$ and are in general not diffusion limited. This is true for soluble and insoluble, as well as for low-mass and high-mass, gases. It may not always be true at exercise or in lung pathology.

Carbon monoxide (CO) and *nitrous oxide* (NO) transfer are strongly diffusion limited due to the very high β/α.

For *oxygen* (O_2), the $D/\dot{Q}\beta$ value varies largely with P_{O_2} according to the shape of the blood O_2 dissociation curve. The maximum value, at a P_{O_2} around 20 torr for human blood, is about 170 times the value at P_{O_2} higher than 200 torr, where β is virtually equal to the physical solubility. In the hypoxic range, β may safely be considered as constant, and the diffusion/perfusion model thus applied. Furthermore, β for O_2 depends on all the factors that affect the O_2 dissociation curve, like temperature, pH, P_{CO_2}, and O_2 capacity. In particular, the venoarterial changes of pH and P_{CO_2} (physiological Bohr effect) should be considered.

Also, for *carbon dioxide* (CO_2), β varies with partial pressure, but much less than for O_2. With P_{CO_2} increasing from 20 to 60 torr, β decreases by a factor of 2.

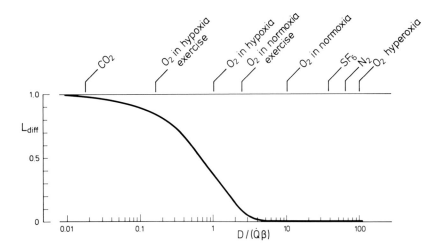

FIG. 2. Diffusion limitation L_{diff}, as a function of the equilibration coefficient $D/\dot{Q}\beta$. Estimated $D/\dot{Q}\beta$ values for various gases in normal human lungs are indicated on the top. (Modified from ref. 4.)

ADDITIONAL COMPONENTS OF THE GAS EXCHANGE RESISTANCE

We have treated the alveolocapillary membrane in the diffusion/perfusion model as a single barrier, uniform and homogeneous. In real lungs, however, the membrane in each alveolus is composed of multiple layers of irregular thickness: the alveolar epithelium with its alveolar surface lining, the interstitium, and the endothelium. The analysis remains nonetheless valid, and D constitutes the effective diffusive conductance of this composite and irregular barrier.

There are, however, other factors on either side of this membrane which provide an additional resistance to gas transfer and which may give rise to diffusion limitation: incomplete mixing in alveolar gas and diffusion in plasma and red cells, as well as chemical reaction with hemoglobin and ionic exchange across the red cell membranes. Although the relative importance of these additional components in limiting gas exchange has not yet been identified, recent progress warrants some general remarks.

Alveolar Gas: Stratified Inhomogeneity

Incomplete mixing of tidal with lung resident gas gives rise to concentration gradients in the alveolar gas, termed *stratified inhomogeneity*. Inert gases have been employed to estimate its significance for O_2 and CO_2 transfer, and a quantitative estimate of the stratified diffusive resistance has been attempted on the basis of simple models. In one of them, all resistance to gas mixing is concentrated into a uniform "gas-filled membrane," which divides the alveolar space into a proximal and a distal compartment. The membrane is characterized by a conductance, G_{mix}, which has the same dimensions as the pulmonary diffusing capacity D (8).

Several methods have been used to estimate G_{mix} by employing gases of different molecular mass and hence of different diffusivity (9). The main result is that G_{mix} in most cases appears to be substantially larger than D; that is, the stratificational resistance is much smaller than that of the alveolocapillary membrane. Hence, incomplete alveolar gas mixing does not appear to limit alveolar gas exchange to an appreciable degree. That is not to say that stratification cannot become important under certain experimental conditions or in pathological states.

Pulmonary Capillary Blood: Diffusion and Reaction Rate

Blood and Membrane Components of D

In the diffusion/perfusion model, the blood was assumed to be in perfect equilibrium in any segmental element of the blood capillary; that is, no transfer resistances were assumed to be present in blood. Several steps may, however, limit attainment of this equilibrium: diffusion in the plasma, across the red cell membrane, and within it; reaction rate with hemoglobin (Hb), particularly for O_2 and CO; and $CO_2/HCO_3^-/H^+$ equilibration, requiring carbonic anhydrase and ion exchange across the red cell membrane (10). These factors are expected to add to the overall gas transfer resistance, particularly for gases chemically bound in blood.

There are several ways to account for this blood resistance in a quantitative way (4). Particularly instructive is to treat it as a resistance in series with that of the alveolocapillary membrane. The total lung diffusing capacity D_L can thus be divided into the diffusing capacity of the membrane, D_M, and that of the blood, θV_c, where θ is the exchange capacity per unit capillary blood volume and V_C is the capillary blood volume. This leads to the formula (11)

$$\frac{1}{D_L} = \frac{1}{D_M} + \frac{1}{\theta V_C},$$ [8]

since the inverse of a conductance (diffusing capacity) constitutes a resistance. This formula was first applied to analyze CO transfer and was later extended to the analysis of O_2 and CO_2 exchange (4).

The model of Eq. 8 does not attempt to differentiate the blood resistance into its components, plasma and red cells, which would be of particular interest for O_2 and CO with their high blood capacitance (β). Since this capacitance resides mainly in the red cells, the plasma can be regarded as a capacitance-free resistive layer surrounding the red cells in the capillary. It can then be allotted to the (resisting) alveolocapillary membrane, and D_M in Eq. 8 can be regarded to consist of the combined conductances of the (resting) tissue membrane and the (moving) plasma layer.

Capillary Hematocrit

The second term in Eq. 8 pertains to red cells alone, and this is evidenced by introducing the red cell-specific quantities using the hematocrit (hct),

$$\theta_{ery} = \frac{\theta}{hct}$$ [9]

and

$$V_{ery} = V_C \cdot hct.$$ [10]

Since the solubility in plasma is small compared with effective solubility in red cells, the capacitance coefficient per unit red cell volume, β_{ery}, is related to β by hct:

$$\beta_{ery} = \frac{\beta}{hct}.$$ [11]

Since red cell flow $\dot{Q}_{ery}$ equals $hct \cdot \dot{Q}$,

$$\dot{Q}\beta = \dot{Q}_{ery} \cdot \beta_{ery}.$$ [12]

Equations 9–12 can then be introduced with Eq. 5 into Eq. 8 to yield the (inverse of the) equilibration coefficient,

$$\frac{\dot{Q}\beta}{D_L} = \frac{\dot{Q}\beta}{D_M} + \frac{\beta_{ery}}{\theta_{ery}} \cdot \frac{1}{t_{ery}}.$$ [13]

Experimental evidence suggests capillary hematocrit to be smaller than that in larger vessels, and Eq. 13 may be used to discuss effects of membrane and blood in lung gas equilibration (4).

In the one limiting case of predominant membrane diffusion limitation,

$$\frac{\dot{Q}\beta}{D_L} = \frac{\dot{Q}\beta}{D_M},$$ [14]

independent of hematocrit or of how fast the red cells traverse the capillary. What matters is the net flow of pulmonary capillary blood or red cells, which must equal that in the pulmonary artery.

With predominant limitation in blood,

$$\frac{\dot{Q}\beta}{D_L} = \frac{\beta_{ery}}{V_{ery}} \cdot \frac{1}{t_{ery}}.$$ [15]

This equation predicts equilibration to depend on red cell-specific quantities, β_{ery} and V_{ery}, which are basic properties of red cells, independent of the flow conditions, and on the red cell contact time t_{ery}, as the decisive parameters. In the general case of a mixed limitation, both red cell flow and red cell contact time determine equilibration.

In dog lungs, D_{O_2} and D_{CO} are found to be proportional to hct; that is, $\dot{Q}\beta/D_L$ is independent of hct (4). This could mean either predominant blood limitation or D_M to be proportional to hct, for example, only areas adjacent to red cell being utilized for gas transfer (12). In any case, neither the equilibration coefficient nor the equilibration deficit would depend on hematocrit. In human patients, D_{CO} has been found to increase less than in proportion with hemoglobin concentration, suggesting combined limitation by membrane and blood.

Specific O_2 Exchange Conductance of Blood and Red Cells

To experimentally determine θ_{O_2} has been a particular problem, and several methods have been employed (4,13). Nearly all techniques are burdened by artifacts deriving from O_2 transport limitation in the buffer fluid surrounding the red cells in the stopped-flow or continuous-flow apparatus. These artifacts may be minimized when O_2 release from red cells is measured into buffer solution of sufficiently high dithionite concentration (14,15) or when O_2 exchange kinetics are studied with thin whole blood layers exposed directly to a gas phase (16).

The question has further been addressed as to what might limit O_2 exchange of red cells (13). Experimental evidence suggests that it is mainly diffusion of O_2, probably with a small contribution by facilitated transport of hemoglobin. Convection by the mechanical mixing of the red cell content while it moves seems to contribute insignificantly. Reaction of O_2 with Hb appears to be fast enough to prevent any major limitation of O_2 exchange by reaction, at least between 10 and 90% O_2 saturation (4).

The value of θ_{O_2} is found to be O_2 saturation dependent with a maximum in the middle range. When using the higher values, that are probably less affected by artifacts, together with estimates of D_L and V_c (4), one can estimate the contribution of blood to the total O_2 exchange resistance to be 6% or less. This estimate suggests that the main resistance to O_2 uptake from alveolar gas to pulmonary capillary blood resides outside the red cells. This lends support to the appropriateness of the diffusion/perfusion model.

DETERMINATION OF PULMONARY DIFFUSING CAPACITY

A number of different methods have been devised to assess diffusion limitation in the lung and to estimate D. These may be grouped into steady-state and unsteady-state methods.

Steady-State Methods

In these methods, steady-state conditions are attained before measurements of gas exchange are being made. Steady state means that none of the variables entering analysis displays variations in time during the measuring period.

Diffusing Capacity for O_2

The basic relationship of Eq. 4 may be solved for D:

$$D_{O_2} = \dot{Q}\beta_{O_2} \cdot \ln \left[\frac{P_A - P\bar{v}}{P_A - P_a} \right]_{O_2}. \qquad [16]$$

Experimentally, $\dot{Q}$ may be obtained from the direct Fick principle, measuring O_2 uptake, $\dot{M}_{O_2}$, and the arteriovenous O_2 content difference. Partial pressures of O_2 must, furthermore, be measured in alveolar gas and in arterial and mixed venous blood. For alveolar gas, it is appropriate to use the ideal-alveolar value.

Application of Eq. 16 and of the diffusion/perfusion model requires the O_2 dissociation curve to be straight, so that β is constant, independent of P. This condition is met with sufficient accuracy for measurements in hypoxia. If this condition, on the other hand, is not met with enough accuracy, the Bohr integration procedure may be applied instead of Eq. 16 as a mathematical variant in the diffusion/perfusion model (4).

Diffusing Capacity for CO

For CO, whose transfer has a strong diffusion limitation (see Fig. 2), $P_a \approx P\bar{v}$ and Eq. 16 simplifies to (4):

$$D_{CO} = \frac{\dot{M}_{CO}}{(P_A - P\bar{v})_{CO}}. \qquad [17]$$

This equation becomes even simpler when $P\bar{v}$ can be assumed as zero (nonsmokers, no preceding exposure to CO).

Unsteady-State Methods

In these methods an existing equilibrium for gas exchange is disturbed in a stepwise manner, and the time course of the approach to a new steady state is observed (usually by measuring P_A). The time course of approach is determined not only by conductances but also by capacitances (proportional to volumes).

The simplest lung model (model I, Fig. 3) is represented by constant convective ($\dot{Q}\beta$) and diffusive conductances (D) and a single capacitance [$V_A\beta g$; V_A, compartment volume; βg, capacitance coefficient in the gas phase (7)]. The time course of approach of P_A to $P\bar{v}$ is monoexponential in this case. This model is commonly used for breath-holding experiments. Model II (Fig. 3) depicts the situation realized in rebreathing between an alveolar compartment and a bag. In this case, the time course of changing P_A toward $P\bar{v}$ is biexponential (17), and the slower component is mostly used for evaluation. Distinct from these "enclosed" methods is an "open" method in which a sudden step change, for example, of inspired gas composition, is imposed during open-circuit breathing (model III, Fig. 3).

When in the experimental situation underlying the models of Fig. 3, lung (P_A) or bag gas (P_R) is continuously recorded, an apparently straight portion is seen in the semilog plots of the difference of P_A (or P_R) and its asymptotic value, after completion of initial mixing and before blood recirculation. The slope of this straight part yields the rate constant k, which is related to the total conductance G for each model (4), as we now outline.

Breath-Holding (Single-Breath) Methods

In the well-known single-breath D_{CO} method, a mixture containing about 0.3% is inspired (from RV to TLC) and expired after 10 sec of breath-holding. In terms of our analysis, the rate constant k is obtained from the CO concentration (partial pressure) ratio before/after breath-hold, $F_{CO}(0)/F_{CO}(t)$, and the breath-hold time t:

$$k_{CO} = \frac{\ln[F_{CO}(0)/F_{CO}(t)]}{t}; \qquad [18]$$

and D_{CO} is calculated therefrom as

$$D_{CO} = V_A \cdot \beta g \cdot k_{CO}. \qquad [19]$$

The initial CO value, $F_{CO}(0)$, is usually calculated from

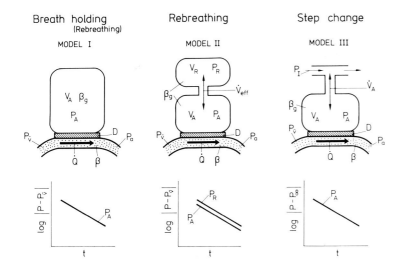

FIG. 3. Models for determination of D using non-steady-state methods. **Upper row:** Models. **Lower row:** Semilogarithmic plots of partial pressures, their slopes (s) being proportional to the exponential rate constants k ($= s \cdot \ln 10 = 2.3s$). In model II, equilibration is biexponential and k corresponds to the slower component, which determines the kinetics of the latter part of the equilibration. (Modified from ref. 4.)

the dilution of a poorly soluble gas (He). The single-breath curve may also be analyzed using several values of P_A along with a slow continuous expiration (single-exhalation method).

Rebreathing Methods

In most applications of the rebreathing principle to determine D_{CO}, it is assumed that rebreathing leads to complete homogenization of lung and rebreathing bag gas. In this case, the model is the same as for single-breath D_{CO} except that the effective volume, from which CO is absorbed, is the total lung and bag volume ($V_A + V_R$) instead of alveolar volume (V_A). In this case, the whole time course of lung or bag CO concentrations can be used for determination of k_{CO}:

$$k_{CO} = - \frac{d \ln(P_{CO})}{dt}. \qquad [20]$$

Since in practice an effective ventilation high enough not to limit CO uptake is difficult to achieve, its limiting effect may be taken into account according to model II of Fig. 3. The equation for calculating D_{CO} for model II is (4)

$$D_{CO} = V_A \cdot \beta_g \cdot k_{CO} \left[1 + \frac{V_R/V_A}{1 - k_{CO} \, V_R/\dot{V}_{eff}} \right]. \qquad [21]$$

V_A and $\dot{V}_{eff}$ are determined from insoluble inert gas dilution and mixing kinetics, respectively.

Unlike for CO, the equilibration kinetics for O_2 depends on blood perfusion $\dot{Q}$ as well, just as is the case in the steady-state methods. For O_2, the rebreathing relationship in model II is therefore slightly more complex (4):

$$
D_{O_2} = - \dot{Q}\beta \ln \left\{ 1 - k_{O_2} \frac{V_A \beta_g}{\dot{Q}\beta} \right.
$$
$$
\left. \times \left[1 + \frac{V_R/V_A}{1 - k_{O_2} \, V_R/\dot{V}_{eff}} \right] \right\}. \qquad [22]
$$

For the volumes V_A and V_R, the mean values between end-inspiration and end-expiration should be used. The total (apparatus + lung) dead space is considered as part of the (non-gas-exchanging) V_R.

In animal experiments, the mixed venous P_{O_2} (required for determination of k_{O_2}) can be measured directly in blood samples; in humans, $P\bar{v}_{O_2}$ is mostly determined by a separate rebreathing maneuver. Determination of $P\bar{v}_{O_2}$ is facilitated by the use of isotopes.

Cardiac output in Eq. 22 may be obtained by independent measurement, for example, by the Fick principle. It is possible, however, to determine $\dot{Q}$ during the rebreathing maneuver from the kinetics of uptake of a soluble inert gas (4).

Step Change of Inspired Gas

In its first application, after a step change of inspired gas from room air to 0.1–0.2% CO in air (or vice versa), the wash-in and wash-out of CO were recorded and compared to N_2 wash-out. Later, the method was also used to estimate functional lung heterogeneity (4).

Use of Isotopes

In rebreathing and breath-holding experiments, test gases containing stable, naturally occurring rare isotopes of C and O have proved to be better suited than the normal, abundant isotopes. The isotopes C ^{18}O (18) and ^{13}CO are useful because the resolving power of mass spectrometers built for continuous recording of respired gases is insufficient for distinguishing ^{12}C ^{16}O from ^{14}N ^{14}N (both with mass number 28) (19). Another advantage is that in smokers $P\bar{v}$ for the naturally abundant ^{12}C ^{16}O may not be negligible, whereas $P\bar{v}$ for CO containing a rare isotope is effectively zero.

The use of stable O_2 isotopes (^{18}O—^{16}O, ^{18}O—^{18}O) is of particular interest, because it offers important advantages. (a) Since mixed venous P_{O_2} for the isotopes can be assumed to be zero, an important source of error due to difficulties in determination of $P\bar{v}$, the asymptote for O_2 equilibration is eliminated. (b) When there is an equilibrium of the abundant isotope ($^{32}O_2$), the gas–blood transfer of a rare isotope ($^{34}O_2$ or $^{36}O_2$) occurs in accordance with a constant $\beta = C\bar{v}_{O_2}/P\bar{v}_{O_2}$, provided the P_{O_2} for the rare isotope is small compared with that of the abundant isotope. This condition was met in a number of studies using breath-holding and rebreathing (cf. ref. 4). A very good agreement between the D_{O_2} values for $^{16}O_2$ and $^{18}O_2$ was achieved in exercising humans (20). For determination of pulmonary D_{CO_2}, the use of rare isotopes appears to be obligatory (21,22).

Relations Among Gases: O_2, CO, CO_2, and NO

Relationship Between D_{O_2} and D_{CO}

In the analysis of diffusion limitation, CO is often used as the test gas because of its very high β, and thus its low $D/\dot{Q}\beta$, value, resulting in strong diffusion limitation for this gas (see Fig. 2). The concentration of CO and the time of exposure are small enough to render such procedures harmless for the subject.

A value for (the only interesting) D_{O_2} can be obtained from D_{CO}, since the ratio D_{O_2}/D_{CO} should be equal to the ratio $(d\cdot\alpha)_{O_2}/(d\cdot\alpha)_{CO}$ (see Eq. 2), which is 1.23. Simultaneous determination by rebreathing of D_{O_2} and D_{CO} confirmed this ratio (20). Other studies yielded smaller or larger experimental ratios, which could be caused, for example, by functional lung heterogeneities (4).

Diffusing Capacity for NO

Not only is the hemoglobin affinity of nitric oxide (NO) even higher than that of CO, but hemoglobin reacts even faster with this gas than with O_2. This would render NO more suitable as a test gas in the study of diffusion limitation. Problems derive, however, from the instability and toxicity of the gas, and very low concentrations and special analytical techniques with high sensitivity (chemiluminescent NO analyzers, mass spectrometers) are required.

The experimental ratios of D_{NO}/D_{CO} in breath-holding humans (23,24) and rebreathing dogs (25) have yielded values between 3 and 5.3, whereas the NO/CO ratio of $d\cdot\alpha$ is estimated at only about 2.0. This would indeed indicate some reaction limitation for CO, reducing D_{CO} but not D_{NO}.

Diffusing Capacity for CO_2

CO_2 is usually not regarded in the study of alveolar diffusion limitation because the high solubility of CO_2 in the tissue would predict much higher D_{CO_2} than D_{O_2}, ruling out the development of diffusion limitation. Experimental values of D_{CO_2} are in fact three to five times higher than those for O_2 (4).

Nonetheless, the ratio D_{CO_2}/D_{O_2} is substantially smaller than that expected for pure diffusion from the ratio $(d\cdot\alpha)_{CO_2}/(d\cdot\alpha)_{O_2}$ of 20. This may be due to the presence of functional lung heterogeneities, to CO_2 reaction and exchange processes in blood (10,13), or to technical problems (4).

Calculations based on the equilibration coefficient $D/\dot{Q}\beta$ suggest a slight diffusion limitation for CO_2 at rest, contributing to the $(P_a - P_A)_{CO_2}$ difference about 0.2 torr. In heavy exercise, this limitation is expected to increase substantially, leading to an arterial–alveolar P_{CO_2} difference of about 7 torr. Thus, in heavy exercise or with reduced D_L, CO_2 may be even more impaired than O_2 (26).

DIFFUSION LIMITATION IN THE PRESENCE OF FUNCTIONAL LUNG INHOMOGENEITY

Functional Lung Heterogeneity and Gas Exchange

Diffusion limitation leads to arterial deoxygenation, or more precisely to alveolar–arterial P_{O_2} differences. Is it then necessary to go through the trouble of analyzing D for estimating the extent of diffusion limitation? Would the relative equilibration deficit of Eq. 4 not be better suited, since it constitutes the parameter of physiologic relevance? That this is not so is due to the fact that other factors impinge on the $(P_A - P_a)_{O_2}$ difference, predominantly functional lung heterogeneities and shunt, and their effects, impairment of gas exchange (see Chapter 5.3.4), are difficult to separate from diffusion limitation.

The idealized diffusion/perfusion model considered so far assumes that all parameters relevant for gas exchange are homogeneously distributed; for example, the allotment of D to $\dot{Q}$ or to $\dot{Q}\beta$ must be the same in any lung unit. Equality of P_A in these units requires, moreover, homogeneous distribution of alveolar ventilation ($\dot{V}_A$) to $\dot{Q}$ (or $\dot{Q}\beta$). In real lungs, both $D/\dot{Q}$ and $\dot{V}_A/\dot{Q}$ are inhomogeneously distributed, and this results in regional variations of P_A and P_a, yielding ($P_A - P_a$) differences, even for gases that are not diffusion limited (inert gases).

Effects of Lung Heterogeneities on the Determination of D

The various methods described to estimate D may be expected to have different sensitivities to functional inhomogeneities (4). Thus, unlike unsteady-state methods, the steady-state methods do not depend on alveolar lung volume (V_A), and its regional inhomogeneity does not affect steady-state D. The higher ventilation in rebreathing may be expected to homogenize lung gas and thus abolish the effects of $\dot{V}_A/\dot{Q}$ inhomogeneity. However, in markedly underventilated lung regions, this goal cannot be achieved in practice.

Since uptake of CO (and NO) in lungs is predominantly diffusion limited, regional inhomogeneity of $\dot{Q}$ does not affect D_{CO} determined with either steady-state or unsteady-state methods (provided $\dot{Q}$ in ventilated alveoli is not too small).

Estimation of Diffusion Limitation in Inhomogeneous Lungs

How can we then differentiate the impairment to gas exchange induced by inhomogeneity and diffusion limitation? This may be a relevant question even though gas exchange impairment in diseased lungs mostly results in a combined impairment (27). The idea is to account for functional inhomogeneity when estimating D.

One way of doing this is to elaborate the simple diffusion/perfusion model by the addition of two more compartments, alveolar dead space and shunt. The resulting three-compartment model is that underlying the ideal-alveolar air concept (28,29), which attributes all $\dot{V}_A/\dot{Q}$ heterogeneity to alveolar dead space ventilation.

A second way is to estimate independently the $\dot{V}_A/\dot{Q}$ heterogeneity by the study of inert gases of a wide range of blood solubility using a 50-compartment lung model (multiple inert gas elimination technique, MIGET; see Chapter 5.3.4). When Pa_{O_2}, *predicted* on the basis of this analysis, is compared with the Pa_{O_2} actually *measured* in the same lung, a lower measured than predicted Pa_{O_2} can be attributed to the existence of diffusion limitation (30). It must be noted, however, that even MIGET constitutes only an approximation to the situation in real lungs and so is the diffusion limitation estimated from the (predicted − measured) Pa_{O_2} difference.

Hammond and Hempleman (31) have estimated diffusion limitation from this Pa_{O_2} difference by assigning to each of the 50 $\dot{V}_A/\dot{Q}$ compartments a value of D until this difference disappeared. In this method, it is important how D is distributed to the various compartments since this determines the compartment values of the equilibration coefficient, $D/\dot{Q}\beta$. Hammond and Hempleman (31) have allotted D in proportion to either $\dot{Q}$ or $\dot{V}_A$, and their results did not differ much. But any intermediate distribution may likewise be warranted, resulting in different regional distributions of $D/\dot{Q}\beta$. It

is important to note that the estimated value of D depends on the (arbitrary) mode of its distribution.

There are a number of reasons to assume $D/\dot{Q}\beta$ inhomogeneity in lungs, partly independent of $\dot{V}_A/\dot{Q}$ inhomogeneity. (a) D may vary with the thickness of the air–blood barrier, with the capillary radius and length, and with the hematocrit (because only the barrier adjacent to red cells is effective in gas exchange). (b) $\dot{Q}$ varies according to flow resistance in both the capillary and the arterial and venous vessels. Pulsatile flow means temporal variations of blood flow, which have effects similar to spatial $D/\dot{Q}\beta$ inhomogeneity. (c) β varies with hematocrit and with O_2 saturation of hemoglobin (which depends on alveolar P_{O_2}). It follows from the discussion of Eq. 13 that regional variations in red cell flow are expected to affect alveolar O_2 uptake when there is a diffusion limitation due to the alveolar membrane (and plasma layer); when the red cell exchange capacity is limiting, on the other hand, regional variations in red cell contact time affect O_2 uptake. Particularly large effects are expected where changes in several parameters occur concurrently. For example, a short capillary would have a small D, large $\dot{Q}$ (due to small resistance), and high β (high hematocrit due to unequal distribution of red cells and plasma at asymmetric branchings).

The combined effects of $\dot{V}_A/\dot{Q}$ and $D/\dot{Q}$ inhomogeneities have been analyzed in theory (32). Recently, Yamaguchi et al. (33) have extended the model underlying MIGET by 50 $D/\dot{Q}$ compartments assigned to each $\dot{V}_A/\dot{Q}$ compartment (50 × 50 model) and have used the exchange data of inert gases as well as of O_2 to determine independently $\dot{V}_A/\dot{Q}$ and $D/\dot{Q}$ distributions and to estimate diffusion limitation therefrom.

DIFFUSION LIMITATION UNDER VARIOUS CONDITIONS

In this section we briefly review the evidence that exists for diffusion limitation in alveolar lungs under various conditions. The evidence depends largely on the techniques used for assessment. For values for D_{O_2} and D_{CO}, see Chapter 5.6.2.1 and reviews by Piiper and Scheid (34) and Cerretelli and di Prampero (35).

Rest and Exercise in Normoxia

There is general agreement that alveolar O_2 uptake in healthy human subjects in *normoxia at rest* is not diffusion limited. The measured alveolar-to-arterial P_{O_2} difference (AaD_{O_2}) of about 10 torr can readily be accounted for by $\dot{V}_A/\dot{Q}$ heterogeneity (30).

In *exercise*, the AaD_{O_2} increases (30,36), and Dempsey et al. (37) found that in highly trained runners at short exercise bouts Pa_{O_2} decreases below 75 torr, in two cases down to 60 torr, with AaDo$_2$ values in excess of 40 torr.

Is this impairment of gas exchange with normoxic exercise due to $\dot{V}A/\dot{Q}$ heterogeneity or to developing diffusion limitation? Despite early belief, recent experimental evidence obtained with MIGET suggests $\dot{V}A/\dot{Q}$ heterogeneity to increase with exercise (28,36,38). Comparison of predicted with measured Pa$_{O_2}$ reveals a significant contribution by diffusion limitation in severe normoxic exercise (30,36).

Hypoxia

The simple diffusion/perfusion model predicts diffusion limitation to be present in hypoxia. The reason is the increase in β (steeper part of the O$_2$ dissociation curve) and $\dot{Q}$, which yields diminished values of the D/$\dot{Q}\beta$ ratio (6).

An attempt has been made by Wagner and his colleagues to determine diffusion limitation in hypoxia at rest and during exercise and to separate, by using MIGET, the AaDo$_2$ under these conditions from those attributable to $\dot{V}A/\dot{Q}$ heterogeneity. In acute hypoxic exposure, induced by either reduced inspired O$_2$ fraction (39) or reduced barometric pressure (30,40), and in chronic exposure to simulated altitude equivalent to Mt. Everest (41), the diffusion limitation increases at rest. This is revealed when the *relative* equilibration deficit for O$_2$, (PA − Pa)/(PA − P$\overline{v}$), is considered, which increases with hypoxia, due to decreasing PA − P$\overline{v}$ (steeper O$_2$ dissociation curve) at largely unaltered AaDo$_2$ [or (PA − Pa)$_{O_2}$]. These studies also show a further increase of diffusion limitation with exercise in hypoxia, concurrent with an exercise-induced increase in $\dot{V}A/\dot{Q}$ heterogeneity.

Lung Disease

There is evidence to suggest that patients with interstitial lung disease (cryptogenic fibrosing alveolitis or idiopathic pulmonary fibrosis, sarcoidosis, scleroderma, asbestosis) display diffusion limitation as O$_2$ uptake is increased with exercise (42–44). In chronic obstructive pulmonary disease (COPD), there is no evidence for diffusion limitation at exercise (42). Except for the study of Lockwood et al. (43), these results were based on MIGET comparing predicted with measured Pa$_{O_2}$. The results are readily explained since all patients showed evidence for reduced DL at rest. That the COPD patients did not reveal diffusion limitation may be due to their strong ventilation limitation as a result of severe airflow obstruction.

There is thus evidence for both normal and diseased subjects that pulmonary O$_2$ uptake may become diffusion limited at extreme exercise levels even in normoxia. In healthy humans, this becomes particularly evident when the subjects are well trained so that the large O$_2$ demand stresses the functional reserves of the lung. With diseased lungs, this functional lung capacity is reached at moderate O$_2$ uptake levels already, so that lung diffusion becomes the rate-limiting step in the O$_2$ supply to the tissues at moderate work levels.

REFERENCES

1. Piiper J, Scheid P. Oxygen exchange in the metazoa. In: Gilbert DL, ed. *Oxygen and living processes.* New York: Springer, 1981;150–176.
2. Gurtner G, Peavy H, Summer W, Burns B. Physiological evidence for the presence of specific O$_2$, CO carrier in the lung and placenta. *Prog Respir Res* 1975;8:166–176.
3. Meyer M, Lessner W, Scheid P, Piiper J. Pulmonary diffusing capacity for CO independent of alveolar CO concentration. *J Appl Physiol* 1981;51:571–576.
4. Scheid P, Piiper J. Blood gas equilibration in lungs and pulmonary diffusing capacity. In: Chang HK, Paiva M, eds. *Respiratory physiology, an analytical approach.* New York: Marcel Dekker, 1989;453–497.
5. Piiper J. Blood–gas equilibrium of carbon dioxide in lungs: a continuing controversy. *J Appl Physiol* 1986;60:1–8.
6. Piiper J, Scheid P. Model for capillary–alveolar equilibration with special reference to O$_2$ uptake in hypoxia. *Respir Physiol* 1981;46:193–208.
7. Piiper J, Dejours P, Haab P, Rahn H. Concepts and basic quantities in gas exchange physiology. *Respir Physiol* 1971;13:292–304.
8. Adaro F, Piiper J. Limiting role of stratification in alveolar exchange of oxygen. *Respir Physiol* 1976;26:195–206.
9. Scheid P, Piiper J. Intrapulmonary gas mixing and stratification. In: West JP, ed. *Pulmonary gas exchange,* vol 1, *Ventilation, blood flow, and diffusion.* New York: Academic Press, 1980;87–130.
10. Bidani A, Crandall ED. Quantitative aspects of capillary CO$_2$ exchange. In: Chang HK, Paiva M, eds. *Respiratory physiology, an analytical approach.* New York: Marcel Dekker, 1989;371–419.
11. Roughton FJW, Forster RE. Relative importance of diffusion and chemical reaction rates in determining rate of exchange of gases in the human lung, with special reference to true diffusing capacity of pulmonary membrane and volume of blood in the lung capillaries. *J Appl Physiol* 1957;11:291–302.
12. Federspiel WJ. Pulmonary diffusing capacity: implications of two-phase blood flow in capillaries. *Respir Physiol* 1989;77:119–134.
13. Klocke RA. Kinetics of pulmonary gas exchange. In: West JB, ed. *Pulmonary gas exchange,* vol 1, *Ventilation, blood flow, and diffusion.* New York: Academic Press, 1980;173–218.
14. Coin JT, Olson JS. The rate of oxygen uptake by human red blood cells. *J Biol Chem* 1979;254:1178–1190.
15. Yamaguchi K, Nguyen-Phu D, Scheid P, Piiper J. Kinetics of O$_2$ uptake and release by human erythrocytes studied by a stopped-flow technique. *J Appl Physiol* 1985;58:1215–1224.
16. Heidelberger E, Reeves RB. Theta (θ) for oxygen and its saturation dependence determined with a new whole blood thin-layer technique. *Fed Proc* 1987;46:1427.
17. Adaro F, Scheid P, Teichmann J, Piiper J. A rebreathing method for estimating pulmonary Do$_2$: theory and measurements in dog lungs. *Respir Physiol* 1973;18:43–63.
18. Wagner PD, Mazzone RW, West JB. Diffusing capacity and anatomic dead space for carbon monoxide (C^{18}O). *J Appl Physiol* 1971;31:847–852.
19. Scheid P. Respiratory mass spectrometry. In: Laszlo G, ed. *Measurement in clinical respiratory physiology.* London: Academic Press, 1983;131–166.
20. Meyer M, Scheid P, Riepl G, Wagner HJ, Piiper J. Pulmonary

diffusing capacities for O_2 and CO measured by a rebreathing technique. *J Appl Physiol* 1981;51:1643–1650.

21. Piiper J, Meyer M, Marconi C, Scheid P. Alveolar–capillary equilibration kinetics of $^{13}CO_2$ in human lungs studied by rebreathing. *Respir Physiol* 1980;42:29–41.

22. Schuster K-D. Kinetics of pulmonary CO_2 transfer studied by using labeled carbon dioxide C ^{16}O ^{18}O. *Respir Physiol* 1985;60:21–37.

23. Guénard H, Varène N, Vaida P. Determination of lung capillary blood volume and membrane diffusing capacity in man by the measurements of NO and CO transfers. *Respir Physiol* 1987;70:113–120.

24. Borland CDR, Higenbottam TW. A simultaneous single breath measurement of pulmonary diffusing capacity with nitric oxide and carbon monoxide. *Eur Respir J* 1989;2:56–63.

25. Piiper J, Schuster K-D, Mohr M, Schulz H, Meyer M. Pulmonary diffusing capacity for carbon monoxide and nitric oxide. In: Mochizuki M, Honig CR, Koyama T, Goldstick TK, Bruley DF, eds. *Oxygen transport to tissue*, vol 10. New York: Plenum Press, 1988;491–495.

26. Wagner PD, West JB. Effects of diffusion impairment of O_2 and CO_2 time courses in pulmonary capillaries. *J Appl Physiol* 1972;33:62–71.

27. West JB. *Pulmonary pathophysiology—the essentials*. Baltimore: Williams & Wilkins, 1982.

28. Rahn H. A concept of mean alveolar air and the ventilation-blood flow relationships during pulmonary gas exchange. *Am J Physiol* 1949;158:21–30.

29. Riley RL, Cournand A. "Ideal" alveolar air and the analysis of ventilation–perfusion relationships in the lungs. *J Appl Physiol* 1949;1:825–847.

30. Torre-Bueno JR, Wagner PD, Saltzman HA, Gale GE, Moon RE. Diffusion limitation in normal humans during exercise at sea level and simulated altitude. *J Appl Physiol* 1985;58:989–995.

31. Hammond MD, Hempleman SC. Oxygen diffusing capacity estimates derived from measured $\dot{V}A/\dot{Q}$ distributions in man. *Respir Physiol* 1987;69:129–142.

32. Piiper J. Variations of ventilation and diffusing capacity to perfusion determining the alveolar–arterial O_2 difference: theory. *J Appl Physiol* 1961;16:507–510.

33. Yamaguchi K, Kawai A, Mori M, Takasugi T, Umeda A, Yokoyama T. Continuous distributions of ventilation and gas conductance to perfusion in the lungs. In: Piiper J, Goldstick TK, Meyer M, eds. *Oxygen transport to tissue*, vol 12. New York: Plenum Press, 1990.

34. Piiper J, Scheid P. Blood–gas equilibration in lungs. In: West JB, ed. *Pulmonary gas exchange*, vol 1, *Ventilation, blood flow, and diffusion*. New York: Academic Press, 1980;131–171.

35. Cerretelli P, di Prampero PE. Gas exchange in exercise. In: Farhi LE, Tenney SM, eds. *Handbook of physiology*, sec 3, vol 4, *Gas exchange*. Bethesda: American Physiological Society, 1987;297–339.

36. Hammond MD, Gale GE, Kapitan KS, Ries A, Wagner PD. Pulmonary gas exchange in humans during exercise at sea level. *J Appl Physiol* 1986;60:1590–1598.

37. Dempsey JA, Hanson PG, Henderson KS. Exercise-induced arterial hypoxaemia in healthy human subjects at sea level. *J Physiol* 1984;355:161–175.

38. Gale GE, Torre-Bueno JR, Moon RE, Saltzman HA, Wagner PD. Ventilation–perfusion inequality in normal humans at sea level and simulated altitude. *J Appl Physiol* 1985;58:978–988.

39. Hammond MD, Gale GE, Kapitan KS, Ries A, Wagner PD. Pulmonary gas exchange in humans during normobaric hypoxic exercise. *J Appl Physiol* 1986;61:1749–1757.

40. Wagner PD, Gale GE, Moon RE, Torre-Bueno JR, Stolp BW, Saltzman HA. Pulmonary gas exchange in humans exercising at sea level and simulated altitude. *J Appl Physiol* 1986;61:260–270.

41. Wagner PD, Sutton JR, Reeves JT, Cymerman A, Groves BM, Malconian MK. Operation Everest II: pulmonary gas exchange during a simulated ascent of Mt. Everest. *J Appl Physiol* 1987;63:2348–2359.

42. Wagner PD. Ventilation–perfusion inequality and gas exchange during exercise in lung disease. In: Dempsey JA, Reed CE, eds. *Muscular exercise and the lung*. Madison: The University of Wisconsin Press, 1976;345–356.

43. Lockwood DNJ, Clark RJ, Jones HA, Hughes JMB. Exercise hypoxaemia in fibrosing alveolitis: $\dot{V}/\dot{Q}$ mismatch or diffusion defect? *Thorax* 1988;43:850P.

44. Eklund A, Broman L, Broman M, Holmgren A. $\dot{V}/\dot{Q}$ and alveolar gas exchange in pulmonary sarcoidosis. *Eur Respir J* 1989;2:135–144.

THE LUNG: Scientific Foundations
edited by R.G. Crystal, J.B. West et al.
Raven Press, Ltd., New York © 1991.

CHAPTER 5.3.4

Ventilation–Perfusion Relationships

John B. West and Peter D. Wagner

HISTORICAL BACKGROUND

Most of the hypoxemia and carbon dioxide retention seen in patients with lung disease is caused by mismatching of ventilation and blood flow within the lung. The importance of the ratio of ventilation to blood flow in determining gas exchange in any lung region was first recognized over 70 years ago. However, developing a comprehensive and quantitative appreciation of the effects of ventilation–perfusion inequality on pulmonary gas exchange has proved to be very demanding, and it has only been in the last few years that many important aspects have been clarified.

From a historical point of view, we can identify three phases in the advance of knowledge in this difficult area. This first was the recognition that the gas exchange which takes place in any lung unit is determined not only by the ventilation or the blood flow, but by the ratio of one to another. Perhaps Krogh and Lindhard (1) were the first to state this specifically. In 1917 they wrote, "if the different lobes of the lungs are not equally dilated during inspiration the air in them must obtain a different composition and this must be true both with respect to O_2 and CO_2 during normal breathing and with regard to other gases during special mixing respirations." They then added in a footnote, "Unless, indeed, the circulation through each lobe should be in proportion to its ventilation." Shortly after this, Haldane (2) recognized that ventilation–perfusion inequality could cause hypoxemia, but, unfortunately, he also stated that carbon dioxide retention would not occur. This was an important misconception that still surfaces from time to time, even in the thickest textbooks of respiratory medicine.

The second phase began in the late 1940s following the upsurge of interest in respiratory physiology which occurred during World War II. Fenn et al. (3) and Riley and Cournand (4) tackled the qualitative relationships between ventilation, blood flow, and gas exchange. Because these depend on the nonlinear oxygen and carbon dioxide dissociation curves, they introduced graphical analysis of these relationships which were not amenable to algebraic manipulation. The third phase began in the mid-1960s when Kelman (5–7) and Olszowka and Farhi (8) introduced computer procedures to describe the oxygen and carbon dioxide dissociation curves. This stimulated the development of numerical techniques for describing the gas-exchange behavior of distributions of ventilation–perfusion ratios (9). Shortly after this, the multiple inert-gas elimination technique was introduced (10,11), which allowed distributions of ventilation–perfusion ratios to be recovered from normal subjects and patients with various types of lung disease. The extensive use of this technique has greatly clarified both the physiological aspects and the clinical implications of ventilation–perfusion inequality over the last 15 years. Readers who want a more extensive discussion of the topic than can be accommodated in the space available here are referred to more extensive reviews (12,13).

GAS EXCHANGE IN A SINGLE LUNG UNIT

Basic Equation

The Po_2, Pco_2, and Pn_2 in any gas-exchanging unit of the lung are uniquely determined by three major factors: (i) ventilation–perfusion ratio, (ii) composition of inspired gas, and (iii) composition of mixed venous blood. Additional minor factors alter the "chemical" status of the blood and therefore the shapes or positions of the O_2 and CO_2 dissociation curves. These

J. B. West and P. D. Wagner: Department of Medicine, University of California–San Diego, La Jolla, California 92093-0623.

include the temperature, hemoglobin, hematocrit, and acid–base status of the blood.

The ventilation–perfusion ratio equation is derived as follows. The amount of CO_2 lost from alveolar gas per minute is given by

$$\dot{V}_{CO_2} = \dot{V}_A \cdot P_{A CO_2} \cdot K$$

where $\dot{V}_{CO_2}$ is CO_2 output, $\dot{V}_A$ is alveolar ventilation, $P_{A CO_2}$ is alveolar P_{CO_2}, K is a constant, and the inspired gas contains no CO_2.

The amount of CO_2 lost from capillary blood per minute is given by

$$\dot{V}_{CO_2} = \dot{Q}(C_{\bar{v}CO_2} - C_{c'O_2})$$

where $\dot{Q}$ is blood flow, $C_{\bar{v}CO_2}$ is mixed venous CO_2 content, and $C_{c'CO_2}$ is CO_2 content of end-capillary blood. Under steady-state conditions these are the same. Therefore

$$\dot{V}_A \cdot P_{A CO_2} \cdot K = \dot{Q}(C_{\bar{v}CO_2} - C_{c'CO_2})$$

or

$$\frac{\dot{V}_A}{\dot{Q}} = \frac{C_{\bar{v}CO_2} - C_{c'CO_2}}{P_{A CO_2} \cdot K}$$

This equation looks simple, but this is deceptive, because when the P_{CO_2} rises as the ventilation–perfusion ratio is decreased, the alveolar P_{O_2} falls. Because of the consequent fall in O_2 saturation, the relationship between P_{CO_2} and CO_2 content in the blood is altered. Thus, the alveolar P_{O_2} is an implicit variable in the equation. This is the reason why it was only possible to solve the equation graphically using the O_2–CO_2 diagram until the advent of numerical analysis by computer.

Oxygen–Carbon Dioxide Diagram

Although this is no longer used to obtain quantitative information about the effects of ventilation–perfusion inequality, it is still conceptually valuable. A simple introduction to this complex topic is given elsewhere (14). Figure 1 shows P_{O_2} and P_{CO_2} plotted on the x and y axes, respectively (15). If the lung is breathing air, the inspired point, I, has a P_{O_2} of 150 mmHg and a P_{CO_2} of 0 mmHg. The composition of normal mixed venous blood is shown as $\bar{v}$, with the P_{O_2} and P_{CO_2} being 40 and 45 mmHg, respectively. The line joining the inspired and mixed venous points is called the ''ventilation–perfusion line,'' and it shows all possible combinations of P_{O_2} and P_{CO_2} in a lung that has the given values for inspired gas and mixed venous blood. The normal ventilation–perfusion ratio of approximately 1 results in a P_{O_2} of 100 mmHg and a P_{CO_2} of 40 mmHg. As the ventilation–perfusion ratio is in-creased, the P_{O_2} rises and the P_{CO_2} falls, so that eventually the composition of inspired gas is reached. In contrast, as the ventilation–perfusion is decreased, the P_{O_2} falls and the P_{CO_2} rises slightly. Eventually, these values approach those of mixed venous blood. If we assume that there is no difference in partial pressure between alveolar gas and end-capillary blood, the line also shows the values for both of these. The O_2–CO_2 diagram can also be used to show the effects of changing the ventilation–perfusion ratio on other variables, including (a) the O_2 and CO_2 concentrations and pH of end-capillary blood and (b) P_{N_2} values (16). Figure 2 is similar to Fig. 1, except that it shows the two respiratory exchange ratio (R) lines and the ideal point (17) (see below).

Effect of Changing the Ventilation–Perfusion Ratio

Figure 3 shows the changes in P_{O_2} and P_{CO_2}, as well as in the O_2 concentration of the effluent blood, as the ventilation–perfusion ratio is raised from zero to infinity. The unit is assumed to be breathing air, and it is supplied with mixed venous blood having a P_{O_2} and P_{CO_2} of 40 and 45 mmHg, respectively. Note that there is little change in the P_{O_2} and P_{CO_2} until the ventilation–perfusion ratio exceeds 0.2, and that the O_2 concentration rises little when the ratio exceeds 1.

Effect of Changing the Inspired Oxygen Concentration

The inspired O_2 concentration is frequently raised when treating patients with severe hypoxemia. The rise in arterial P_{O_2} depends on the distribution of ventilation–perfusion ratios and, especially, on the amount of blood going to units with very low ventilation–perfusion ratios. This is clarified by Fig. 4. Here the inspired O_2 fraction ($F_{I O_2}$) is increased from 0.14 to 1.0, the barometric pressure is 760 mmHg, and the $P_{\bar{v}O_2}$ and $P_{\bar{v}CO_2}$ are assumed to remain at 40 and 45 mmHg, respectively, to clarify the principles involved. In practice the $P_{\bar{v}O_2}$ will generally increase. Note that units with ventilation–perfusion ratios of 1 or more have high end-capillary O_2 concentrations regardless of the inspired P_{O_2}. Units with ventilation–perfusion ratios of 0.1 increase their end-capillary O_2 concentration rapidly as the inspired P_{O_2} is increased, whereas alveoli with ventilation–perfusion ratios of 0.01 and less show little response when the $F_{I O_2}$ is less than 0.5. This means that distributions with substantial amounts of blood flow to units in the range of 0.01–0.001 may show a relatively small increase in arterial P_{O_2} unless the $F_{I O_2}$ is raised to very high levels.

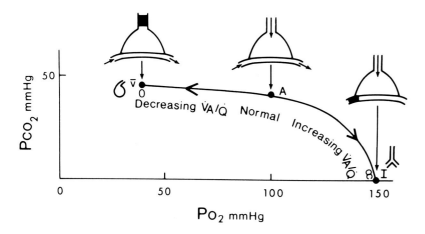

FIG. 1. Oxygen–carbon dioxide diagram showing a ventilation–perfusion ratio ($\dot{V}_A/\dot{Q}$) line. The P_{O_2} and P_{CO_2} of a lung unit move along this line from the mixed venous point, $\bar{v}$, to the inspired gas point, I, as its ventilation–perfusion ratio is increased. A, alveolar gas for a lung unit with a normal ventilation–perfusion ratio. (From ref. 15.)

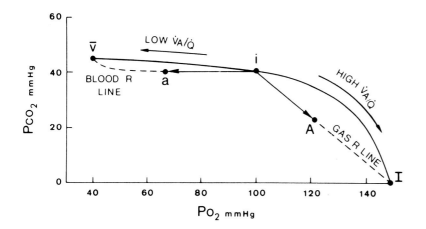

FIG. 2. Diagram similar to Fig. 1, showing the points for ideal gas, i; arterial blood, a; alveolar gas, A; and expired gas, E. Note that the points lie on the blood and gas R (respiratory exchange ratio) lines. (From ref. 15.)

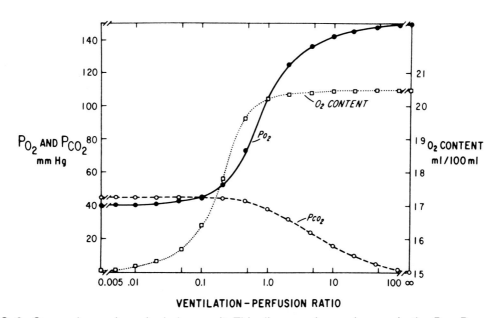

FIG. 3. Gas exchange in a single lung unit. This diagram shows changes in the P_{O_2}, P_{CO_2}, and end-capillary O_2 content in a lung unit as its ventilation–perfusion ratio is increased. Hemoglobin concentration is 14.8 g/dl. (From ref. 17.)

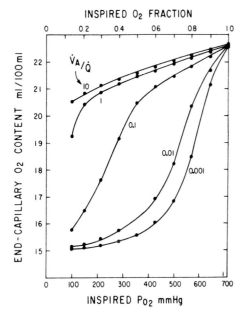

FIG. 4. Changes in the O_2 content of end-capillary blood as the inspired PO_2 is increased. The PO_2 and PCO_2 of mixed venous blood are assumed to remain at 40 and 45 mmHg, respectively. $\dot{V}_A/\dot{Q}$ is the ventilation–perfusion ratio. (From ref. 17.)

Effect of Changing the Composition of Mixed Venous Blood

The importance of the PO_2 and PCO_2 of the mixed venous blood in determining the arterial PO_2 and PCO_2 is often overlooked. For example, a patient with myocardial infarction and decreased cardiac output may have a very low mixed venous PO_2, which therefore exaggerates his arterial hypoxemia. In contrast, a patient with asthma after bronchodilator therapy may have an abnormally high cardiac output, which leads to a higher arterial PO_2 than would be expected from the amount of ventilation–blood-flow mismatching.

Figure 5 shows how the PO_2 of mixed venous blood affects the end-capillary PO_2 of lung units having different ventilation–perfusion ratios. Note that for an alveolus with a normal ventilation–perfusion ratio of 1.0, the end-capillary PO_2 increases from approximately 44 to 128 mmHg (i.e., more than 80 mmHg) as the mixed venous PO_2 is increased from 10 to 60 mmHg. For abnormally high or low ventilation–perfusion ratios, the change in end-capillary PO_2 is less.

Effect of Changing the Inspired PO_2 on the Ventilation–Perfusion Ratio

The last three sections have examined the role of the three major determinants of gas exchange in single lung units: ventilation–perfusion ratio, composition of inspired gas, and composition of mixed venous blood.

However, it is worth noting that changes in the inspired PO_2 can alter the ventilation–perfusion ratio.

There are two important mechanisms. One is that hypoxic vasoconstriction normally reduces the blood flow of poorly ventilated units as their alveolar PO_2 decreases (18,19). Increasing the inspired oxygen releases this vasoconstriction. Animal studies shed some light on the extent to which this occurs. Barer et al. (20) indicated that this mechanism chiefly affects alveoli that have a PO_2 of less than 100 mmHg. These include (a) units with ventilation–perfusion ratios of less than approximately 1.0 when the inspired gas is air and (b) units with ratios of less than 0.1 when 50% O_2 is inspired. However, Grant et al. (21) showed that the mechanism may operate over a larger range of alveolar PO_2 values, at least up to 150 mmHg. They also found that the vasoconstriction that occurs in response to a local decrease in PO_2 can, at best, restore the local PO_2 halfway back to its original level, and that this feedback efficiency is most effective in the alveolar PO_2 range of 70–90 mmHg.

The other mechanism that can change the ventilation–perfusion ratio of a lung unit when an enriched O_2 mixture is breathed is gradual collapse of units with very low ventilation–perfusion ratios. This phenomenon was analyzed by Dantzker et al. (22), who showed that poorly ventilated units may have a much lower expired, as compared to inspired, alveolar ventilation. When the ventilation–perfusion ratio is reduced to a "critical" value, there is no expired alveolar ventilation at all, and all the inspired gas is taken up by the blood. If the ventilation–perfusion ratio is reduced to an even lower level, more gas is absorbed by

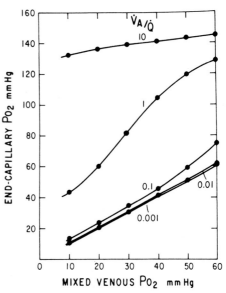

FIG. 5. Changes in the alveolar and end-capillary PO_2 as the PO_2 of the mixed venous blood is increased. (From ref. 17.)

the blood than is delivered during inspiration. Such a unit is inherently unstable and may collapse. The critical ventilation–perfusion ratio depends on the inspired O_2 concentration, and it rises dramatically as this approaches 100%. In other words, at these high inspired O_2 fractions, increasing numbers of lung units are vulnerable. This inherent instability of units with very low ventilation–perfusion ratios during enriched O_2 breathing has been seen to a small extent in normal subjects (11). However, it is particularly evident in patients with acute respiratory failure where breathing high concentrations of oxygen may cause collapse of many lung units (17).

GAS EXCHANGE IN A THREE-COMPARTMENT MODEL: TRADITIONAL ASSESSMENT OF VENTILATION–PERFUSION INEQUALITY

Because ventilation–perfusion inequality is the most common cause of hypoxemia and CO_2 retention, much effort has been devoted by physicians and physiologists to determining the degree of inequality in individual patients. By far the most extensive information can be obtained using the multiple inert-gas elimination technique, which is described below. However, because of its complexity, this method can only be used in large centers. In this section we look briefly at some of the traditional ways of assessing ventilation–perfusion inequality.

Arterial P_{O_2}

This is often a useful measure of the amount of ventilation–perfusion inequality, with its chief merits being simplicity and ease of measurement. However, the arterial P_{O_2} can be considerably altered by the level of ventilation, as well as by other causes of hypoxemia such as shunts and, possibly, diffusion impairment.

Arterial P_{CO_2}

This is of little value in assessing the amount of ventilation–perfusion inequality because it is so sensitive to the level of ventilation. Even lungs with grossly mismatched ventilation and blood flow can still decrease the arterial P_{CO_2} by increasing the ventilation to the alveoli. Nevertheless, it is important to appreciate that ventilation–perfusion inequality must increase the arterial P_{CO_2} unless the ventilation to the alveoli increases (see later).

Alveolar–Arterial P_{O_2} Difference

This index has the advantage that it is less sensitive to the level of ventilation. Figure 2 clarifies how an al-

veolar–arterial P_{O_2} difference develops in the presence of ventilation–perfusion inequality.

Suppose that initially a lung has no ventilation–perfusion inequality. The P_{O_2} and P_{CO_2} of the alveolar gas and arterial blood will then be represented by i, known as the "ideal point." This is at the intersection of the gas and blood respiratory exchange ratio (R) lines. These lines show all possible compositions of alveolar gas and arterial blood that are consistent with the overall respiratory exchange ratio (carbon dioxide output/oxygen uptake) of the whole lung. In other words, a lung in which $R = 0.8$ would have to have its mixed alveolar gas point, A, located somewhere on the line joining points i and I. A similar statement can be made for the arterial point, a.

When ventilation–perfusion inequality is imposed on the lung, both the alveolar gas and arterial blood points diverge away from the ideal point, i, along the appropriate gas and blood R lines. The more extreme the degree of inequality, the further the divergence. As a result, the horizontal distance between the points A and a—that is, the mixed alveolar–arterial P_{O_2} difference—is a useful measure of the degree of ventilation–perfusion inequality.

In practice, the composition of point A cannot usually be obtained because it represents the composition of mixed expired gas excluding the anatomic dead-space gas. Since most diseased lungs empty sequentially (poorly ventilated alveoli empty last), a post-dead-space sample is not representative of all mixed expired gas. For this reason, a more useful index is the P_{O_2} difference between ideal alveolar gas and arterial blood—that is, the horizontal distance between points i and a. The ideal alveolar P_{O_2} is calculated from the alveolar gas equation:

$$P_{O_2} = P_{I_{O_2}} - \frac{P_a CO_2}{R} + \left(P_a CO_2 \cdot F_I CO_2 \cdot \frac{1 - R}{R} \right)$$

This assumes that the ideal alveolar P_{CO_2} is the same as that of arterial blood, a reasonable assumption for clinical purposes because the line along which point a moves is so nearly horizontal (Fig. 2). Note that this ideal alveolar–arterial P_{O_2} difference is caused by units situated on the ventilation–perfusion ratio line between points i and v; that is, units with abnormally low ventilation–perfusion ratios.

Physiologic Shunt

This can be looked upon as a further refinement of the (ideal) alveolar–arterial P_{O_2} difference (4,23), and it has the advantage of being even less affected by the level of ventilation. Because of the nonlinear shape of the O_2 dissociation curve, a given pattern of ventilation–perfusion inequality causes a larger alveolar–arterial P_{O_2} difference the higher the ventilation. This is because the O_2 dissociation curve is relatively flat at its upper end, so that a small addition of blood with a low O_2 concentration from units with very low ventilation–perfusion ratios (Fig. 1) results in a marked decrease in arterial P_{O_2}. This disadvantage does not apply to the physiologic shunt, which is therefore less sensitive to the level of ventilation.

To calculate the physiologic shunt, we pretend that all of the leftward movement (Fig. 2) of the arterial point, a, away from the ideal point, i (the hypoxemia), is caused by the addition of mixed venous blood, v, to ideal blood, i. This is not as unreasonable as it might at first seem, because units with very low ventilation-perfusion ratios put out blood that has essentially the same composition as that of mixed venous blood (Fig. 3). In practice, the shunt equation is used in the following form:

$$\frac{\dot{Q}_{PS}}{\dot{Q}_T} = \frac{C_iO_2 - C_aO_2}{C_iO_2 - C_{\bar{v}}O_2}$$

where $\dot{Q}_{PS}$ refers to physiologic shunt, $\dot{Q}_T$ is total blood flow through the lungs, and C_iO_2, C_aO_2, and $C_{\bar{v}}O_2$ refer, respectively, to the O_2 concentrations of ideal, arterial, and mixed venous blood. The O_2 concentration of ideal blood is calculated from the ideal P_{O_2} and the O_2 dissociation curve. The normal value for the physiologic shunt is less than 5%.

Physiologic Dead Space

We have seen that both the "ideal" alveolar–arterial P_{O_2} difference and the physiologic shunt chiefly reflect the amount of blood flow going to lung units with abnormally low ventilation–perfusion ratios (4,23). In contrast, the physiologic dead space is a measure of the amount of ventilation going to lung units with abnormally high ventilation–perfusion ratios. To obtain physiologic dead space, we pretend that all the movement of the alveolar point, A, away from the ideal point, i, is caused by the addition of inspired gas, I, to ideal gas (Fig. 2). Again, this is not as unreasonable as it may first appear, because units with very high ventilation–perfusion ratios behave very much like point I. As pointed out earlier, it is usually impossible to obtain a sample of pure mixed expired alveolar gas, A. In practice, therefore, we collect mixed expired gas and measure its composition, E. This contains a contribution from the anatomic dead space which therefore moves its composition further towards point I. The Bohr equation is used in the form

$$\frac{V_{D_{phys}}}{V_T} = \frac{P_aCO_2 - P_ECO_2}{P_aCO_2}$$

where $V_{D_{phys}}$ is physiologic dead space, V_T is tidal volume, P_ECO_2 is mixed expired P_{CO_2}, and again we use the fact that the P_{CO_2} in ideal gas and arterial blood are virtually the same.

The physiologic dead space as measured in this way includes the anatomic dead space, and there is also a contribution from the instrumental dead space of the valve box which can be subtracted. In normal lungs, the value of the physiologic dead space is approximately 30% of the tidal volume at rest. It is less on exercise and consists almost completely of anatomic dead space.

Limitations of These Traditional Indices

It is important to appreciate that these simple measures of ventilation–perfusion inequality may vary even though the degree of mismatching of ventilation and blood flow remains unchanged. For example, it can be shown in lung models that if we fix the distribution of ventilation–perfusion ratios but increase the total ventilation going to the alveoli, calculated physiologic dead space increases and physiologic shunt decreases (9). Opposite changes occur if the total pulmonary blood flow is increased. Again, if the inspired oxygen concentration rises, the calculated physiologic shunt decreases even though there is no change in the matching of ventilation and blood flow.

This unfortunate behavior of these indices can lead to misinterpretations in the clinical setting. For example, suppose a patient with hypoxemia after a myocardial infarction shows an increase in physiologic shunt. This could be caused by increasing edema interfering with the distribution of ventilation. However, it could also be explained by a return of the cardiac output from depressed levels. Another example is a patient with asthma who shows a decrease in physiologic dead space after treatment. This might indicate a better matching of ventilation and blood flow in the lung, but it could equally well be explained by a decrease in total ventilation. There is no satisfactory explanation of why the indices behave in this way. After all, they are relatively crude "as if" models of what must be a continuous distribution of ventilation–perfusion ratios in the lung.

GAS EXCHANGE IN DISTRIBUTIONS OF VENTILATION–PERFUSION RATIOS

Up to this point we have considered gas exchange in a single lung unit as well as in simple three-compartment models of the lung. The latter are important because they have traditionally been used to obtain indices of ventilation–perfusion inequality. However, it was recognized many years ago that real lungs must contain distributions of ventilation–perfusion ratios, although the prospect of determining their gas-exchange behavior was daunting because this involved nonlinear, interdependent O_2 and CO_2 dissociation curves. The breakthrough came with the application of numerical analysis which allowed the gas exchange in any number of compartments of a distribution to be analyzed and which also allowed the resulting behavior of the distribution to be computed. These advances not only allowed many difficult questions about gas exchange in distributions of ventilation–perfusion ratios to be answered, but also paved the way for recovering distributions from real lungs in normal subjects and patients with lung disease (see next section).

Plotting a Distribution

It is not immediately clear how best to portray a distribution of ventilation–perfusion ratios, and various attempts have been made (24,25). Experience has shown that the most informative distribution is one in which both ventilation and blood flow on the vertical axis are plotted against ventilation–perfusion ratio on the horizontal axis, as shown in Fig. 6 (26). This is a logarithmic normal distribution first used in this context by Rahn and co-workers (27,28). Its advantages are that it is one of the simplest distributions in which

the dispersion can be characterized by a single parameter (log standard deviation), that negative values which would be physiologically meaningless cannot exist, and that there is some evidence that the normal lung has such a distribution (24). In models such as these, the degree of ventilation–perfusion inequality can be increased by simply raising the log standard deviation.

Gas-Exchange Behavior of Distributions

Suppose that we have a log normal distribution of ventilation–perfusion ratios as shown in Fig. 6, and that the dispersion is suddenly increased while everything else remains unchanged. What happens to gas exchange? It can easily be shown that this "pure" ventilation–perfusion inequality reduces both the O_2 uptake and CO_2 output of the lung (9). In other words, the lung becomes less efficient as a gas exchanger. The relative impairment of O_2 and CO_2 transfer depends on the type of distribution. However, it is important to emphasize that both gases are affected. In practice, this situation cannot last long because the lung must increase the O_2 uptake and CO_2 output to the levels required by steady-state metabolism of body tissues. This occurs as a result of changes in the P_{O_2} and P_{CO_2} of the arterial and mixed venous blood. Figure 7 shows conceptual "stages" in the changes that occur in gas exchange.

In stage zero, ventilation and blood flow are well

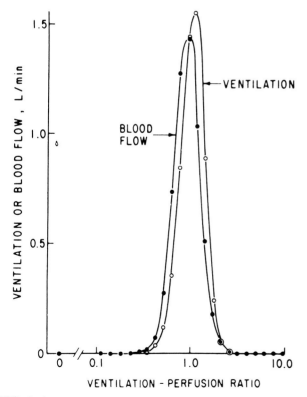

FIG. 6. Log normal distribution of ventilation–perfusion ratios. The dispersion is determined by the log standard deviation. (From ref. 26.)

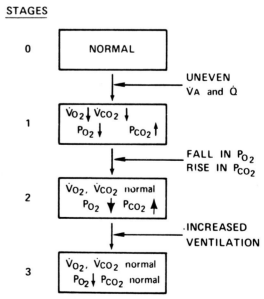

FIG. 7. Conceptual stages of pulmonary gas exchange after introducing ventilation–perfusion inequality—in a log normal distribution, for example. See text for details. $\dot{V}_A$ = alveolar ventilation, $\dot{Q}$ = blood flow, $\dot{V}_{O_2}$ = O_2 uptake, $\dot{V}_{CO_2}$ = CO_2 output. (From ref. 17.)

matched, or, if there is some mismatching as is the case in the normal lung, it is trivial from the point of view of overall gas exchange. Some disturbance then occurs which mismatches ventilation and blood flow, thus causing O_2 uptake and CO_2 output to fall and also causing arterial P_{O_2} to fall and arterial P_{CO_2} to rise (stage 1). This must be transient because the lung must restore the O_2 uptake and CO_2 output to satisfy the demands of the metabolizing tissues. This is done by a fall in P_{O_2} and rise in P_{CO_2} of both arterial and mixed venous blood. The decrease in mixed venous P_{O_2} increases the amount of oxygen that can be loaded by the blood in its passage through the pulmonary capillaries, and the unloading of carbon dioxide is similarly assisted. We then have stage 2, in which the O_2 uptake and CO_2 output have been returned to normal, but there is an abnormally low P_{O_2} and high P_{CO_2} in both arterial and mixed venous bloods. This stage is compatible with continuous steady-state gas exchange. It is seen in many patients with advanced chronic obstructive lung disease, for example.

An additional stage 3 may occur, particularly in mild disease. The chemoreceptors are reluctant to see the arterial P_{CO_2} rise, and they respond by increasing the ventilation to the alveoli until the arterial P_{CO_2} is returned to normal. This increase in ventilation improves the arterial P_{O_2} to some extent but does not return it to normal. The reason why a lung with ventilation–perfusion inequality can return the arterial P_{CO_2}, but not the arterial P_{O_2}, to normal levels by an increase in ventilation to the alveoli is the different shapes of the O_2 and CO_2 dissociation curves. This is clearly demonstrated in lung models of this kind. Thus a common end result as shown in stage 3 consists of a normal O_2 uptake, normal CO_2 output, and normal arterial P_{CO_2} but decreased arterial P_{O_2}. This is the situation seen in many patients with moderate chronic obstructive lung disease, and it is even seen in patients with relatively advanced asthma.

The stages shown in Fig. 7 are conceptual and usually do not occur sequentially. For example, a patient who gradually develops chronic obstructive lung disease will not show an increased arterial P_{CO_2} that is then returned to normal. Rather, as the disease progresses, the ventilation to the alveoli is increased to hold the arterial P_{CO_2} normal. Also, some patients do not make the transition from stage 2 to stage 3, or some of those who have made it will revert from stage 3 back to stage 2. The usual reason is that these patients have a high work of breathing and they "elect" to allow their arterial P_{CO_2} to increase rather than accept the penalty of increasing their ventilation in the face of the large effort and oxygen cost.

Patients in stage 2 are sometimes described as "hypoventilating." This term is used by people who define the adequacy or inadequacy of alveolar ventilation by whether it maintains a normal arterial P_{CO_2}. Thus "hypoventilation" in this context really simply means an increased arterial P_{CO_2}. This can be confusing terminology because most patients with ventilation–perfusion inequality and an increased arterial P_{CO_2} have more air than normal going to their alveoli. We prefer to restrict the term "hypoventilation" to patients whose CO_2 retention is caused by a true reduction in ventilation, as in barbiturate intoxication. The basic cause of the CO_2 retention in a patient with chronic obstructive lung disease is the inefficiency of gas exchange and therefore CO_2 elimination resulting from ventilation–perfusion inequality.

What other options does a diseased lung have for improving the arterial P_{O_2} and P_{CO_2} in the presence of ventilation–perfusion inequality? One is to increase the total pulmonary blood flow. It can be shown that in a lung with ventilation–perfusion inequality, increasing cardiac output raises the arterial P_{O_2}. The reason for this can be seen by referring back to Fig. 5, where we saw that a rise in mixed venous P_{O_2} improves the end-capillary P_{O_2} of lung units. Since an increase in cardiac output will raise the P_{O_2} of mixed venous blood (other things being equal), this will have a salutary effect on the arterial value. Thus, as mentioned earlier, the hypoxemia of a patient with myocardial infarction may be exaggerated by his reduced cardiac output.

Another option for improving the arterial P_{O_2} in the presence of ventilation–perfusion inequality is to raise the inspired P_{O_2}. The effectiveness of this will depend on the distribution of ventilation–perfusion ratios. As shown in Fig. 4, lung units with very low ventilation–perfusion ratios show little improvement in the end-capillary O_2 content until the inspired P_{O_2} reaches very high levels. This means that a diseased lung which has substantial amounts of blood flow going to units with extremely low ventilation–perfusion ratios may show little change in the arterial P_{O_2} until the inspired oxygen fraction is very high. Interestingly, the alveolar–arterial P_{O_2} difference of such a lung may continue to increase as the inspired P_{O_2} is raised up to a certain maximum and then decrease at the highest inspired P_{O_2} levels.

In practice, ventilation–perfusion inequality always reduces the gas-exchange efficiency of the lung and interferes with the uptake of oxygen, elimination of carbon dioxide, and the transfer of any other gas, including the anesthetic gases. However, it is of interest that Evans et al. (29) have made a theoretical analysis of the conditions under which ventilation–perfusion inequality impairs pulmonary gas exchange, and they have been able to find a theoretical distribution where mismatching of ventilation and blood flow actually improves the transfer of a hypothetical gas. However, the characteristics of this gas are such that this would never be seen in practice.

MULTIPLE INERT GAS ELIMINATION TECHNIQUE

Introduction

The preceding section used theoretical modeling to compute the effects of nonuniform $\dot{V}_A/\dot{Q}$ distribution on overall parameters of gas exchange—in particular, arterial and expired P_{O_2} and P_{CO_2}. It is possible to move in the reverse direction—that is, to use measured parameters of overall gas exchange (such as arterial and expired gas concentrations) to estimate the qualitative and quantitative features of the $\dot{V}_A/\dot{Q}$ distribution present in any circumstance. This can be done because $\dot{V}_A/\dot{Q}$ distribution is the principal determinant of overall gas exchange for any given set of boundary conditions (i.e., inspired and mixed venous gas concentrations) for any particular gas (of known hemoglobin association properties and physical solubility). The major question becomes, How closely can the $\dot{V}_A/\dot{Q}$ distribution be approximated by such an approach? The answer is that the broad features of the distribution can be reliably determined if a sufficient number of gases of different hemoglobin association and/or solubilities can be studied (30–32). One approach has been to study the overall gas-exchange response (arterial P_{O_2} in particular) to increases in $F_{I_{O_2}}$ (24,33,34). Limited approximations to the $\dot{V}_A/\dot{Q}$ distribution can be obtained because the response to increasing $F_{I_{O_2}}$ depends on the $\dot{V}_A/\dot{Q}$ ratios of the gas-exchange units present. Drawbacks of this approach are (a) the sequential nature of the method, such that systematic or random changes in the $\dot{V}_A/\dot{Q}$ distribution interfere with the internal consistency of the data, (b) the well-known effects of increased $F_{I_{O_2}}$ on $\dot{V}_A/\dot{Q}$ inequality itself through release of hypoxic vasoconstriction and/or absorption atelectasis (22,35) which changes the $\dot{V}_A/\dot{Q}$ distribution as it is being measured, and (c) the potential diffusion limitation of O_2 transport across the alveolar wall which cannot be delineated from the effects of $\dot{V}_A/\dot{Q}$ inequality.

On the other hand, forcing the lung to simultaneously eliminate a number of inert gases of different solubilities overcomes all of these drawbacks, especially if the inert gases are kept in the parts per million range. Based on earlier work by Kety (36) and Farhi and co-workers (37–39), the multiple inert-gas elimination technique (MIGET) was developed as a means of estimating the $\dot{V}_A/\dot{Q}$ distribution (10,30,40).

Principles of the MIGET

If an inert gas (defined here as a gas that obeys Henry's law—i.e., showing a linear relationship between par-

tial pressure and concentration in blood) is dissolved in 5% dextrose or normal saline and then infused at a constant rate into a peripheral vein, a steady state of gas exchange across the lung is reached within a few minutes. In any single gas-exchange unit in that lung, the relationships amongst the alveolar (P_A), endcapillary ($P_{c'}$), and mixed venous ($P_{\bar{v}}$) partial pressures is given by Eq. 1 (10,36,37):

$$\frac{P_A}{P_v} = \frac{P_{c'}}{P_{\bar{v}}} = \frac{\lambda}{\lambda + \dot{V}_A/\dot{Q}} \qquad [1]$$

In this expression, $\dot{V}_A/\dot{Q}$ is the value of the $\dot{V}_A/\dot{Q}$ ratio of the lung unit in question and λ is the blood–gas partition coefficient of the gas being infused. Equation 1 is derived from simple mass balance considerations on the assumption of (a) a steady state of gas exchange in the lungs, (b) continuous ventilatory and circulatory movement of gas and blood through the lungs, and (c) alveolar–end-capillary diffusion equilibration of partial pressure for the gas, well-argued on both theoretical (41,42) and experimental grounds (43).

If Eq. 1, describing events in a single lung unit, is now applied to each lung unit present and the results summed to represent total lung gas exchange, we have as a result:

$$E \equiv \frac{P_{\overline{EXP}}}{P_{\bar{v}}} = \sum_{j=1}^{j=N} \dot{V}_{A_j} \cdot \left(\frac{\lambda}{\lambda + \dot{V}_A/\dot{Q}_j}\right) \qquad [2]$$

$$R \equiv \frac{P_{\overline{art}}}{P_{\bar{v}}} = \sum_{j=1}^{j=N} \dot{Q}_j \cdot \left(\frac{\lambda}{\lambda + \dot{V}_A/\dot{Q}_j}\right) \qquad [3]$$

Here, $P_{\overline{EXP}}$ is mixed expired and $P_{\overline{art}}$ mixed arterial inert-gas partial pressure, and $\dot{V}_{A_j}$ and $\dot{Q}_j$ are, respectively, fractional alveolar ventilation and blood flow of the jth lung unit, of which there are N in the entire lung. We have coined the terms "retention" (R) and "excretion" (E) to define the associated partial pressure ratio. Note that Eqs. 2 and 3 can include unventilated "shunt" units of $\dot{V}_A/\dot{Q} = 0$ and unperfused "dead-space" units of $\dot{V}_A/\dot{Q} = \infty$ without disturbing the arithmetic involved. The variables R, E, and λ can all be measured experimentally during a steady state produced by a continuous inert gas infusion, so that for Eq. 2 the single conceptual unknown is the relationship, unit by unit, between $\dot{V}_A$ and $\dot{V}_A/\dot{Q}$. Similarly for Eq. 3, given the above measured data, the single unknown is the relationship between $\dot{Q}$ and $\dot{V}_A/\dot{Q}$. In fact, because $\dot{V}_A = \dot{Q} \cdot \dot{V}_A/\dot{Q} \cdot (\dot{Q}_T/\dot{V}_{E_T})$, where $\dot{V}_A/\dot{Q}$, $\dot{Q}$, and $\dot{V}_A$ are as defined, and $\dot{Q}_T$ and $\dot{V}_{E_T}$ are, respectively, total lung blood flow and ventilation, Eqs. 2 and 3 are actually not independent and merely reflect the same $\dot{V}_A/\dot{Q}$ distribution viewed from opposite sides of the blood–gas barrier.

Although complicated, the relationship, unit by unit, between $\dot{V}_A$, $\dot{Q}$, and $\dot{V}_A/\dot{Q}$ (i.e., the $\dot{V}_A/\dot{Q}$ distribution) can be determined mathematically from measurements of R, E, λ, $\dot{Q}_T$, and $\dot{V}_{ET}$ (30,44,45) using Eqs. 2 and 3. While in theory such a computation could be made from measurements using a single gas of known λ, it turns out that simultaneous infusion of six to eight gases whose λ values are widely scattered from very low ($\lambda \approx 0.001$) to very high ($\lambda \approx 100$) is necessary to obtain enough data to usefully define the $\dot{V}_A/\dot{Q}$ distribution.

The mathematical details of how the $\dot{V}_A/\dot{Q}$ distribution is recovered from such data are beyond the scope of this chapter but are described elsewhere (30,44,45). So, too, is the important consideration of the quantitative information content of the method (31,46,47). Several approaches to using the retention and excretion data have been tried (30,48,52), but the best accepted and most useful is that based on a multicompartment approach with enforced smoothing (30,44).

Measurement Aspects

The MIGET is applied by first dissolving six different gases in a single bag of dextrose (or saline) under sterile conditions. First, a gas mixture of 20% sulfur hexafluoride (SF$_6$, $\lambda \approx 0.005$), 20% cyclopropane ($\lambda \approx 0.5$), and 60% ethane ($\lambda \approx 0.1$) is bubbled into the dextrose bag and shaken to enhance dissolution of the gases. After removing any residual gas bubbles, small amounts of liquid enflurane ($\lambda \approx 2$), diethyl ether ($\lambda \approx 12$), and acetone ($\lambda \approx 300$) are injected into the bag (2 ml/liter, 0.5 ml/liter, and 6 ml/liter of dextrose, respectively). The solution is then infused at a rate equal to about 1/3000 of the minute ventilation into a peripheral vein for about 20–30 min, at which time mixed venous blood, arterial blood, and mixed expired gas are simultaneously sampled (5–7 ml blood per sample, 15–30 ml gas). An equilibration process is used to extract the test gases out of the blood samples (40), and their concentrations in all three samples are measured by gas chromatography (flame ionization for the hydrocarbons and electron capture for SF$_6$). Similar procedures are used to measure λ for each gas (40). Total expired ventilation is recorded conventionally and by means of mass balance, total pulmonary blood flow is calculated from R, E, λ, and $\dot{V}_{ET}$.

If the mathematical approach of Evans and Wagner (30) is followed, these data are then used to estimate the $\dot{V}_A/\dot{Q}$ distribution by a linear least-squares regression method with smoothing (53).

From the recovered distribution that is based only on the inert gas data, the expected values for arterial P_{O_2} and P_{CO_2} can be computed as indicated in the preceding section of this chapter, and they can be compared to simultaneously measured values.

Information Content of the MIGET

A remarkable amount of information can be derived from this method:

1. A qualitative and quantitative description of the $\dot{V}_A/\dot{Q}$ distribution pattern can be obtained by plotting $\dot{V}_A$ and $\dot{Q}$ against $\dot{V}_A/\dot{Q}$, compartment by compartment.

2. One can obtain parameters such as principal moments, describing the degree of $\dot{V}_A/\dot{Q}$ mismatch in terms that permit statistical inference regarding effects of manipulation or therapy.

3. One can assess the compatibility of the inert gas data with the basic conceptual model behind the MIGET: that the lung acts as a collection of distinct gas-exchange units (each governed by its own $\dot{V}_A/\dot{Q}$ ratio) arranged in either parallel or series networks. This assessment is based on the residual sum of squares between the measured data and the least-squares best fit by the above model. The use of this information is well-illustrated in application of the method to the avian lung (54,55).

4. One can detect indications of diffusion limitation of the inert gases through the differential behavior of high- and low-molecular-weight gases in the mixture. Thus, enflurane and SF$_6$ have severalfold greater molecular weights than do the other gases. Such diffusion limitation would be evident by a preferential retention of enflurane and SF$_6$ after allowing for differences in λ. Such is rarely, if ever, observed—even in the lung of species with large gas-exchange cavities, such as the alligator (56).

5. One can determine the diffusion limitation of O$_2$ exchange across the alveolar wall. In the absence of such limitation, the arterial P_{O_2} predicted by MIGET (see above) statistically agrees with that actually measured. In the presence of such limitation, the predicted arterial P_{O_2} is systematically greater than that measured (57–60).

6. Finally, this method enables one to partition the causes of hypoxemia into intrapulmonary factors ($\dot{V}_A/\dot{Q}$ mismatch, shunt, diffusion limitation) and extrapulmonary factors (altered cardiac output, metabolic rate, inspired P_{O_2} and ventilation) in a quantitative manner, and it also enables one to predict how changes in extrapulmonary factors would alter arterial P_{O_2}. These concepts will be illustrated below.

Patterns of $\dot{V}_A/\dot{Q}$ Inequality in Health and in Common Disease States

Normal Subjects (Fig. 8)

The amount of mismatch is minimal in young, normal subjects (20- to 30-year age range). Using the most

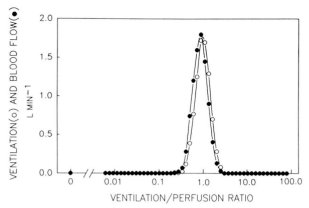

FIG. 8. Distribution of ventilation–perfusion ratios in an upright, young, normal subject. There is little inequality evident and, in particular, no areas of very low or very high ventilation–perfusion ratio. Shunt is absent.

common parameter, the second moment of the distribution about its mean on a log scale ("LOG SD"), the 95% upper confidence limit is at a LOG SD of 0.6 (61) and the usual range is 0.3–0.4. This is a minor degree of mismatch, with perfect homogeneity giving a LOG SD of 0, and the most severe forms of inequality seen in patients with respiratory distress syndromes yielding values of 2–2.5. A LOG SD of 0.3 is consistent with an alveolar–arterial difference of about 5 torr (9), as commonly found in normals. In addition to the low LOG SD, the curves are log normal in shape, are centered on a $\dot{V}_A/\dot{Q}$ ratio of about 1.0, and do not contain lung units of low $\dot{V}_A/\dot{Q}$ (<0.1), shunt ($\dot{V}_A/\dot{Q} = 0$), or high $\dot{V}_A/\dot{Q}$ (>10). In general, there is more mismatch than expected on just gravitational grounds (11), indicating probably some intraregional $\dot{V}_A/\dot{Q}$ inequality as well.

The $\dot{V}_A/\dot{Q}$ distribution of normal, older subjects remains to be determined beyond a few anecdotal measurements (11); however, it is likely to reflect increasing heterogeneity with age, consistent with the well-known progressive reduction in arterial P_{O_2} (62).

Asthma (Fig. 9)

There are many reports of $\dot{V}_A/\dot{Q}$ measurements in asthmatics, ranging from patients in clinical remission (63) all the way to patients in status asthmaticus (64). In between, there are data on patients with chronic symptomatic asthma (61) and on patients with acute, severe asthma (65,66). The main observations from these and other studies can be condensed into the following general conclusions:

1. $\dot{V}_A/\dot{Q}$ mismatch is very commonly present in patients in *all* of the above clinical circumstances.
2. $\dot{V}_A/\dot{Q}$ mismatch is often typically reflected by a

pattern in which a distinct population of low $\dot{V}_A/\dot{Q}$ ratio units exists separate from units with normal $\dot{V}_A/\dot{Q}$ ratios—the "bimodal" pattern (63) (Fig. 9).

3. Shunting ($\dot{V}_A/\dot{Q} = 0$) is notably absent until patients develop the most severe level such as status asthmaticus (64).

4. Across the spectrum of activity, the arterial P_{O_2} is accurately predicted by the $\dot{V}_A/\dot{Q}$ pattern, confirming $\dot{V}_A/\dot{Q}$ mismatch rather than shunt or diffusion limitation as the mechanism of hypoxemia.

5. Despite considerable $\dot{V}_A/\dot{Q}$ inequality, hypoxemia is often attenuated by the presence of a higher-than-normal cardiac output that preserves P_aO_2 due to maintenance of mixed venous P_{O_2} (63).

6. Acute administration of bronchodilators to patients with naturally occurring asthma fails to improve $\dot{V}_A/\dot{Q}$ relationships despite simultaneous restoration of airflow rates (63). This strongly suggests airway mucus and/or edema, rather than bronchoconstriction, causes the $\dot{V}_A/\dot{Q}$ mismatch.

7. The correlation between airflow rates and $\dot{V}_A/\dot{Q}$ mismatch is almost nonexistent, even in a single patient over time (66), further suggesting that bronchoconstriction is relatively unimportant to $\dot{V}_A/\dot{Q}$ relationships and that gas exchange is determined by events in the most peripheral airways poorly reflected by flow rate data. As a corollary, there is only a weak association between severity of $\dot{V}_A/\dot{Q}$ mismatch and clinical severity of asthma (63,64,66,67).

8. Finally, sequential measurements over time in chronic symptomatic asthmatics reveal considerable week-by-week variability in $\dot{V}_A/\dot{Q}$ inequality, mostly unrelated to clinical symptoms or airflow rate changes (61).

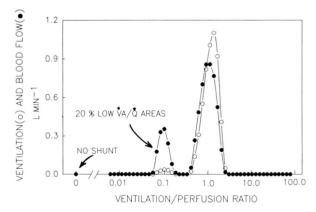

FIG. 9. An example of the distribution of ventilation–perfusion ratios in an asthmatic subject. Note the separate population of areas of low ventilation–perfusion ratio distinct from the main mode. The size of the low $\dot{V}_A/\dot{Q}$ mode varies considerably among individuals, but it commonly comprises about 20% of the cardiac output as indicated. Shunt is notably absent in most patients with asthma.

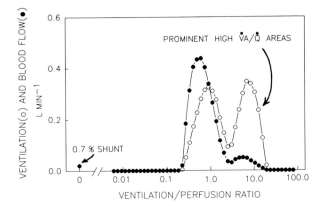

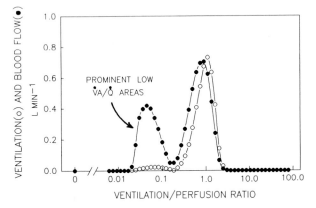

FIG. 10. Typical patterns of ventilation–perfusion ratios in patients with chronic obstructive pulmonary disease (COPD). **Upper panel:** Pattern typical of a patient with type A presentation (hyperinflation, well-preserved blood gases, and evidence of pathological emphysema). **Lower panel:** Pattern typical of a patient with type B presentation (chronic bronchitis). The type A patient usually shows areas of abnormally high ventilation–perfusion ratio as indicated, but no areas of extremely low ventilation–perfusion ratio. As in this example, right-to-left shunts are minimal. The type B patient, on the other hand, commonly has areas of abnormally low ventilation–perfusion ratio as shown, but, again, generally no shunting.

Chronic Obstructive Pulmonary Disease (COPD) (Fig. 10)

Several reports of $\dot{V}_A/\dot{Q}$ distribution in COPD have been published, with most of them focusing on the question of $\dot{V}_A/\dot{Q}$ distribution pattern and its relationships to underlying pathology and clinical manifestations (43,67,68). Patients corresponding to the Burrows et al. (69) stereotype of the "emphysematous" patient (pink puffer, type A) and the "chronic bronchitic" patient (blue bloater, type B) have received special attention. To date, data support the finding of areas of abnormally high $\dot{V}_A/\dot{Q}$ ratios in type A patients (43,67,68). Very few such patients fail to show such areas, but many type B patients also have high $\dot{V}_A/\dot{Q}$

units. Type A patients rarely have abnormally low $\dot{V}_A/\dot{Q}$ areas, but type B patients do commonly, but by no means universally, possess such low $\dot{V}_A/\dot{Q}$ areas. As in asthma (see above), true shunting ($\dot{V}_A/\dot{Q} = 0$) is rarely observed (43).

The pathological basis of these $\dot{V}_A/\dot{Q}$ changes is speculative, but the most likely hypothesis to explain high $\dot{V}_A/\dot{Q}$ areas is continued ventilation of the enlarged and putatively hypoperfused air spaces produced by emphysematous digestion of the associated alveolar walls. Competing hypotheses such as microvascular obstruction or the phenomenon of "auto-positive end-expiratory pressure" (auto-PEEP) due to hyperinflation remain to be excluded. The most likely cause of the low $\dot{V}_A/\dot{Q}$ areas in type B patients appears to be peripheral airway obstruction with mucus/edema (or distortion of bronchioles), such as hypothesized for asthma (see above). It is, however, difficult to explain the absence of low $\dot{V}_A/\dot{Q}$ areas in perhaps one-third of the type B patients. The presence of high $\dot{V}_A/\dot{Q}$ areas in the type B patient is consistent with occult emphysema, often found at postmortem examination.

$\dot{V}_A/\dot{Q}$ inequality is the sole basis for hypoxemia in COPD, and there is no evidence of O_2 diffusion limitation at rest or even during exercise (43,68). There is also no evidence for impaired diffusive gas mixing as might have been expected in the presence of large emphysematous air spaces. This conclusion is based on the observation that in patients with COPD there is no systematically increased retention of high-molecular-weight inert gases (see above) (43).

Interstitial Pulmonary Fibrosis (IPF) (Fig. 11)

Despite the huge variety of pathological causes of fibrosis, patients with advanced disease show remarkably similar $\dot{V}_A/\dot{Q}$ patterns (70) characterized by a relatively modest amount of $\dot{V}_A/\dot{Q}$ inequality manifest by areas of very low and of zero $\dot{V}_A/\dot{Q}$ ratio. Typically, only 10–20% of the cardiac output perfuses such abnormal regions, and the remainder of the $\dot{V}_A/\dot{Q}$ distribution lies within the normal range of $\dot{V}_A/\dot{Q}$ ratios. Accordingly, the usually very low arterial P_{O_2} requires additional explanation; and using the MIGET (71), it has been noted that due to subnormal values of cardiac output, the mixed venous P_{O_2} is often reduced, even at rest. This explains how a modest amount of $\dot{V}_A/\dot{Q}$ mismatch can produce quite severe hypoxemia [identical conclusions are reached in pulmonary edema caused by heart failure from myocardial infarction (72)]. Note that it is the converse of what is often seen in asthma, as noted above.

At rest, there is little evidence that the well-known reduction in (carbon monoxide) diffusing capacity in IPF results in diffusion limitation of alveolar–capillary

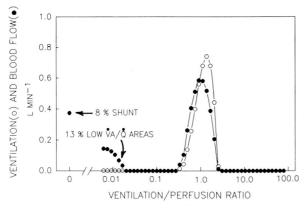

FIG. 11. The typical pattern of $\dot{V}_A/\dot{Q}$ inequality in patients with interstitial pulmonary fibrosis. Such patients have relatively small amounts of $\dot{V}_A/\dot{Q}$ inequality, usually consisting of areas of very low or zero ventilation–perfusion ratio as shown. In this example, a total of only 21% of the cardiac output is associated with unventilated or essentially unventilated areas, but this is sufficient to produce moderately severe hypoxemia as discussed in the text.

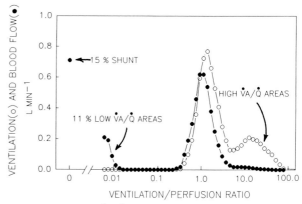

FIG. 12. A typical $\dot{V}_A/\dot{Q}$ pattern in a patient (75) with the adult respiratory distress syndrome (ARDS). Abnormalities throughout the $\dot{V}_A/\dot{Q}$ range are evident, with shunting, areas of abnormally low ventilation–perfusion ratio, and areas of abnormally high ventilation–perfusion ratio. Although this is typical, some patients do not show areas of either high or low ventilation–perfusion ratio. Most, however, will exhibit some degree of right-to-left shunting.

exchange of O_2: there is sufficient reserve in transit time that even with a reduced diffusing capacity, alveolar–end-capillary O_2 equilibrium is reached at rest (71). However, on exercise, there is now good evidence that the further hypoxemia commonly observed in such patients is actually partially due to O_2 diffusion limitation, although even here it should be stressed that only about 15% of the total alveolar–arterial P_{O_2} difference is due to this process (71). The remaining 85% is still the result of $\dot{V}_A/\dot{Q}$ mismatch, and it is especially important to note that the mixed venous P_{O_2} in IPF often falls to very low values (<20 torr) during exercise, accentuating the hypoxemia ascribed to $\dot{V}_A/\dot{Q}$ inequality.

Adult Respiratory Distress Syndrome (ARDS) (Fig. 12)

The $\dot{V}_A/\dot{Q}$ patterns published in this conglomeration of syndromes, generally confined to seriously ill patients on ventilators, take several different forms, as might be expected in such complex situations (73–75). True shunts ($\dot{V}_A/\dot{Q} = 0$) are almost always observed and likely reflect (a) alveoli flooded with exudate, (b) alveoli filled with cellular debris, (c) atelectasis, or (d) right-to-left shunt through a patent foramen ovale. Of course, more than one explanation could account for any given patient's pattern. Areas of low $\dot{V}_A/\dot{Q}$ are sometimes seen as well (75), but this is by no means as common as are shunts. It would seem that such low $\dot{V}_A/\dot{Q}$ areas may reflect relatively transient events with alveoli on their way to becoming completely unventilated (or becoming normally ventilated during recovery). The pathological basis for such low $\dot{V}_A/\dot{Q}$ areas

is speculative but may lie in partial alveolar filling, distal airway partial obstruction, or local reductions in lung compliance.

Areas of high $\dot{V}_A/\dot{Q}$ are also commonly seen, and most often these correlate with (a) the level of alveolar pressure imposed by the ventilator and (b) the mechanical properties of the lungs. As shown in dogs (76), high inflation pressures and/or PEEP causes compliant lung regions to be hyperinflated, which, by alveolar capillary compression, reduces blood flow and increases the $\dot{V}_A/\dot{Q}$ ratio. Consequently, the appearance of high $\dot{V}_A/\dot{Q}$ areas may warn of impending barotrauma.

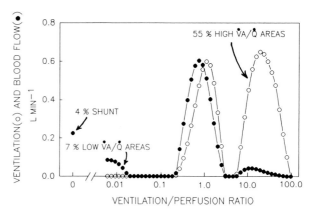

FIG. 13. Example of the distribution of ventilation–perfusion ratios in a patient with severe pulmonary embolus. The dominant abnormality is the appearance of a population of lung units with abnormally high ventilation–perfusion ratios—in this example, comprising more than 50% of the total alveolar ventilation. As in many patients with embolism, areas of low and zero $\dot{V}_A/\dot{Q}$ are also seen, as discussed in the text.

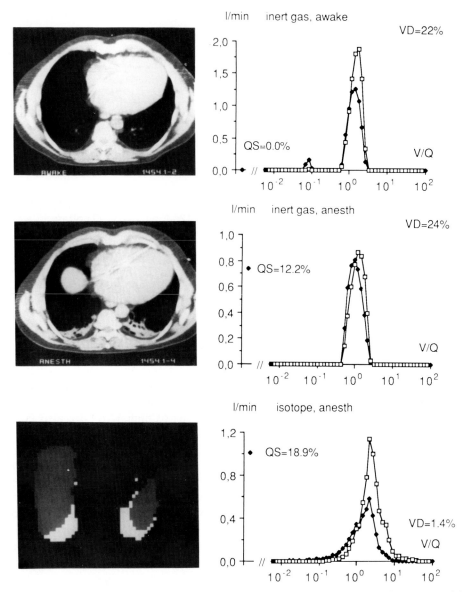

FIG. 14. Effects of anesthesia. The **top left panel** is a transverse computed tomographic (CT) image showing well-expanded lungs without areas of atelectasis, and the **top right panel** shows the associated essentially normal $\dot{V}_A/\dot{Q}$ distribution. The **middle left panel** shows in the same patient at the same thoracic level a transverse CT image exhibiting dependent atelectasis (white irregular areas dorsally within the lung fields), the **middle right panel** shows the associated $\dot{V}_A/\dot{Q}$ distribution exhibiting a 12% shunt, but otherwise no abnormality. The **lower left panel** is the single photon emission computed tomography (SPECT) scan images from this patient, and the lighter-tone areas at the base reflect areas that are perfused but not ventilated. The simultaneously measured $\dot{V}_A/\dot{Q}$ distribution under these conditions **(lower right panel)** shows a 19% shunt. These three approaches to examining the effects of anesthesia confirm that anesthesia produces shunting which is essentially confined to the dependent areas and which is the result of atelectasis. (From ref. 92.)

Another possibility for the presence of high $\dot{V}_A/\dot{Q}$ areas is pulmonary arterial microvascular obstruction or frank (macroscopic) pulmonary embolus (see below).

Because most patients with ARDS are treated with high F_IO_2 values, much of their $\dot{V}_A/\dot{Q}$ inequality is not evident from measurement of arterial PO_2 (see above); moreover, a particular benefit of using the MIGET in these patients is that the $\dot{V}_A/\dot{Q}$ distribution can be determined equally well at all F_IO_2 values, since the methodology is independent of F_IO_2. Also, since many ARDS patients are hemodynamically unstable, the MIGET is a valuable tool in the understanding of how sudden changes in cardiac output affect pulmonary gas exchange; furthermore, the MIGET assists in answering questions concerning intrapulmonary versus extrapulmonary determinants of gas exchange.

Pulmonary Embolism (PE) and Primary Pulmonary Hypertension (PPH) (Fig. 13)

Limited data are available in these diseases, which are difficult to study because of their acute and often severe nature. There is no question but that $\dot{V}_A/\dot{Q}$ inequality develops acutely from the mechanical obstruction of pulmonary arteries in PE (77–79) and must contribute to any hypoxemia observed. As expected, the $\dot{V}_A/\dot{Q}$ pattern is characterized by the appearance of high $\dot{V}_A/\dot{Q}$ areas (78), as shown also in animal models of the disease (80,81). Additional changes are often observed, however, and one report (79) has pointed to an association between the development of radiologically determined atelectasis and intrapulmonary shunts, with both appearing to increase in the days following the embolic event. It is not clear whether this is due to (a) reduced expansion occasioned by chest pain, (b) impaired surfactant function in embolized areas, or (c) infarction, but simple, acute hyperinflation has been effective (82) in reversing hypoxemia in some patients. It is of considerable interest (and currently unexplained) that the degree of $\dot{V}_A/\dot{Q}$ mismatch and the level of hypoxemia appear to bear little relation to the percentage obstruction of the vascular bed (83). Finally, other explanations for hypoxemia, such as diffusion limitation of O_2 uptake, are not supported by the close agreement between arterial P_{O_2} predicted from the MIGET and that measured simultaneously. Consequently, early in PE, hypoxemia (when present) is presumed to be due to just $\dot{V}_A/\dot{Q}$ mismatch produced by the embolus; later in the process, however, scattered atelectasis appears to play a role, causing shunt and hence further hypoxemia.

In PPH, the principal observation is only modest amounts of $\dot{V}_A/\dot{Q}$ mismatch (84), but in the presence of a usually substantially reduced cardiac output, there is often considerable hypoxemia because of the low mixed venous P_{O_2}.

General Anesthesia (Fig. 14)

Abnormal gas exchange has long been known to develop during anesthesia (85,86), but its full extent was not appreciated until the MIGET was brought to bear on the problem. This is because the usually high $F_{I}O_2$ and concurrent use of nitrous oxide (which increases alveolar O_2 concentration) (87) maintain arterial P_{O_2} at above-normal levels.

Using the MIGET, even young patients with normal lungs develop $\dot{V}_A/\dot{Q}$ abnormalities characterized essentially by development of shunt (88). Hedenstierna

et al. (89) have shown that this correlates, patient by patient, with the development of dependent atelectasis (detected by computed tomography), and that these areas are perfused but unventilated (detected by radionuclide imaging). However, the cause-and-effect relationships (at the level of changes of lung mechanical properties) between gas exchange and changes in lung volume and/or chest wall shape remain to be elucidated, as does the possible role of increased intrathoracic blood volume as a factor reducing gas volume and thus promoting atelectasis (90).

Patients with moderate COPD undergoing surgery for nonpulmonary diseases have also been studied by the MIGET. The magnitude of the $\dot{V}_A/\dot{Q}$ inequality that is seen in such patients following induction of general anesthesia (prior to surgery) is astounding (91), and it is much greater than that found in normal subjects during anesthesia. Presumably, this is multifactorial and includes such phenomena as (a) interference to hypoxic vasoconstriction by anesthetic agents and (b) lung mechanical effects, such as in normal subjects. It is of interest that the $\dot{V}_A/\dot{Q}$ changes appear within minutes of induction and do not progress (91). Whether they can be prevented by particular ventilatory strategies remains to be determined.

REFERENCES

1. Krogh A, Lindhard J. The volume of the dead space in breathing and the mixing of gases in the lungs of man. *J. Physiol (Lond)* 1917;51:59–90.
2. Haldane JS. *Respiration.* New Haven, CT: Yale University Press, 1922.
3. Fenn WO, Rahn H, Otis AB. A theoretical study of the composition of alveolar air at altitude. *Am J Physiol* 1946;146:637–653.
4. Riley RL, Cournand A. "Ideal" alveolar air and the analysis of ventilation-perfusion relationships in the lungs. *J Appl Physiol* 1949;1:825–847.
5. Kelman GR. Digital computer subroutine for the conversion of oxygen tension into saturation. *J Appl Physiol* 1966;21:1375–1376.
6. Kelman GR. Calculation of certain indices of cardiopulmonary function using a digital computer. *Respir Physiol* 1966;1:335–343.
7. Kelman GR. Digital computer procedure for the conversion of P_{CO_2} into blood CO_2 content. *Respir Physiol* 1967;3:111–116.
8. Olszowka AJ, Farhi LE. A system of digital computer subroutines for blood gas calculation. *Respir Physiol* 1968;4:270–280.
9. West JB. Ventilation–perfusion inequality and overall gas exchange in computer models of the lung. *Respir Physiol* 1969;7:88–110.
10. Wagner PD, Saltzman HA, West JB. Measurement of continuous distributions of ventilation–perfusion ratios: theory. *J Appl Physiol* 1974;36:588–599.
11. Wagner PD, Laravuso RB, Uhl RR, West JB. Continuous distributions of ventilation–perfusion ratios in normal subjects breathing air and 100% O_2. *J Clin Invest* 1974;54:54–68.
12. West JB, Wagner PD. Pulmonary gas exchange. In: West JB, ed. *Bioengineering aspects of the lung.* New York: Marcel Dekker, 1977.
13. West JB, Wagner PD. Ventilation–perfusion relationships. In: West JB, ed. *Pulmonary gas exchange. Ventilation, blood flow and diffusion,* vol 1. New York: Academic Press, 1980.

14. West JB. *Ventilation/bloodflow and gas exchange,* 5th ed. Oxford: Blackwell Scientific Publications; Philadelphia: Lippincott, 1990.

15. West JB. *Respiratory physiology—the essentials,* 4th ed. Baltimore: Williams & Wilkins, 1990.

16. Rahn H, Fenn WO. *A graphical analysis of the respiratory gas exchange.* Washington, DC: American Physiological Society, 1955.

17. West JB. State of the art. Ventilation–perfusion relationships. *Am Rev Respir Dis* 1977;116:919–943.

18. Rodman DM, Voelkel NF. Regulation of vascular tone. In: Crystal RA, West JB, eds. *The lung: scientific foundations.* New York: Raven Press, 1990.

19. Archer SL, McMurtry IF, Weir EK. Mechanisms of acute hypoxic and hyperoxic changes in pulmonary vascular reactivity. In: Weir EK, Reeves JT, eds. *Pulmonary vascular physiology and pathophysiology.* New York: Marcel Dekker, 1989.

20. Barer GR, Howard P, Shaw JW. Stimulus–response curves for the pulmonary vascular bed to hypoxia and hypercapnia. *J. Physiol (Lond)* 1970;211:139–155.

21. Grant BJB, Davies EE, Jones HA, Hughes JMB. Local regulation of pulmonary blood flow and ventilation–perfusion ratios in the coati mundi. *J Appl Physiol* 1976;40:216–228.

22. Dantzker DR, Wagner PD, West JB. Instability of lung units with low $\dot{V}_A/\dot{Q}$ ratios during O_2 breathing. *J Appl Physiol* 1975;38:886–895.

23. Riley RL, Cournand A. Analysis of factors affecting partial pressures of oxygen and carbon dioxide in gas and blood of lungs: theory. *J Appl Physiol* 1951;4:77–101.

24. Lenfant C, Okubo T. Distribution function of pulmonary blood flow and ventilation–perfusion ratio in man. *J Appl Physiol* 1968;24:668–679.

25. Gomez DM, Briscoe WA, Cumming G. Continuous distribution of specific tidal volume throughout the lung. *J Appl Physiol* 1964;19:683–692.

26. West JB. *Pulmonary pathophysiology—the essentials,* 3rd ed. Baltimore: Williams & Wilkins, 1987.

27. Rahn H. A concept of mean alveolar air and the ventilation–blood flow relationships during pulmonary gas exchange. *Am J Physiol* 1949;158:21–30.

28. Farhi LE, Rahn H. A theoretical analysis of the alveolar-arterial oxygen difference with special reference to the distribution effect. *J Appl Physiol* 1955;7:699–703.

29. Evans JW, Wagner PD, West JB. Conditions for reduction of pulmonary gas transfer by ventilation–perfusion inequality. *J Appl Physiol* 1974;36:533–537.

30. Evans JW, Wagner PD. Limits on $\dot{V}_A/\dot{Q}$ distributions from analysis of experimental inert gas elimination. *J Appl Physiol* 1977;42:889–898.

31. Ratner ER, Wagner PD. Resolution of the multiple inert gas method for estimating $\dot{V}_A/\dot{Q}$ maldistribution. *Respir Physiol* 1982;49:293–313.

32. Kapitan KS, Wagner PD. Information content of multiple inert gas elimination measurements. *J Appl Physiol* 1987;63(2):861–868.

33. Briscoe WA. A method for dealing with data concerning uneven ventilation of the lung and its effect on gas transfer. *J Appl Physiol* 1959;14:291–298.

34. Briscoe WA, Cree EM, Filler J, Houssay HEJ, Cournand A. Lung volume, alveolar ventilation and perfusion interrelationships in chronic pulmonary emphysema. *J Appl Physiol* 1960; 15:785–795.

35. Lenfant C. Effect of high F_1 of measurement of ventilation–perfusion distribution in man at sea level. *Ann NY Acad Sci* 1965;21:797–808.

36. Kety S. The theory and applications of the exchange of inert gas at the lungs and tissues. *Pharmacol Rev* 1951;3:1–41.

37. Farhi LE. Elimination of inert gas by the lung. *Respir Physiol* 1967;3:1–11.

38. Farhi LE, Yokoyama T. Effects of ventilation–perfusion inequality on elimination of inert gases. *Respir Physiol* 1967;3:10–12.

39. Yokoyama T, Farhi LE. The study of ventilation–perfusion ratio distribution in the anesthetized dog by multiple inert gas washout. *Respir Physiol* 1967;3:166–176.

40. Wagner PD, Naumann PF, Laravuso RB. Simultaneous measurement of eight foreign gases in blood by gas chromatography. *J Appl Physiol* 1974;36:600–605.

41. Forster RE. Exchange of gases between alveolar air and pulmonary capillary blood: pulmonary diffusing capacity. *Physiol Rev* 1957;37:391–452.

42. Wagner PD. Diffusion and chemical reaction in pulmonary gas exchange. *Physiol Rev* 1977;57:257–312.

43. Wagner PD, Dantzker DR, Dueck R. Clausen JL, West JB. Ventilation–perfusion inequality in chronic obstructive pulmonary disease. *J Clin Invest* 1977;59:203–216.

44. Olszowka AJ, Wagner PD. Numerical analysis in gas exchange. In: West JB, ed. *Pulmonary gas exchange,* vol 1. New York: Academic Press, 1980;263–306.

45. Wagner PD. Calculation of the distribution of ventilation–perfusion ratios from inert gas elimination data. *Fed Proc* 1982;41:136–139.

46. Kapitan KS, Wagner PD. Linear programming analysis of $\dot{V}_A/\dot{Q}$ distributions: Limits on central moments. *J Appl Physiol* 1986;60(5):1772–1781.

47. Kapitan KS, Wagner PD. Linear programming analysis of $\dot{V}_A/\dot{Q}$ distributions: average distribution. *J Appl Physiol* 1987; 62(4):1356–1362.

48. Hlastala MP, Robertson HT. Inert gas elimination characteristics of the normal and abnormal lung. *J Appl Physiol* 1978; 44:258–266.

49. Neufeld GR, Williams JJ, Klineberg PL, Marshall BE. Inert gas a–v differences: a direct reflection of $\dot{V}/\dot{Q}$ distribution. *J Appl Physiol* 1978;44:277–283.

50. Poon C-S, Golestani C. Recovery of $\dot{V}_A/\dot{Q}$ distributions by discrete deconvolution. In: *Proceedings of the IEEE Conference on Frontiers in Engineering and Computer Health Care 7th,* 1985.

51. Stewart WE, Mastenbrook SM Jr. Parametric estimation of ventilation–perfusion ratio distributions. *J Appl Physiol* 1983;55:37–51.

52. Hendricks FFA, Van Zomeren B, Kroll K, Wise ME, Quanier PHH. Distributions of $\dot{V}_A/\dot{Q}$ in dog lungs obtained with the 50 compartment and the log normal approach. *Respir Physiol* 1979;38:267–282.

53. Lawson CL, Hanson RJ. *Solving least squares problems.* New Jersey: Prentice–Hall, 1974;160–164, 190.

54. Powell FL, Wagner PD. Measurement of continuous distributions of ventilation–perfusion in non-alveolar lungs. *Respir Physiol* 1982;48(2):219–232.

55. Powell FL, Wagner PD. Ventilation–perfusion inequality in avian lungs. *Respir Physiol* 1982;48:233–241.

56. Powell FL, Gray AT. Ventilation–perfusion relationships in alligators. *Respir Physiol* 1989;78:83–94.

57. Torre-Bueno J, Wagner PD, Saltzman HA, Gale GE, Moon RE. Diffusion limitation in normal humans during exercise at sea level and simulated altitude. *J Appl Physiol* 1985;58(3): 989–995.

58. Hammond MD, Gale GE, Kapitan KS, Ries A, Wagner PD. Pulmonary gas exchange in humans during exercise at sea level. *J Appl Physiol* 1986;60(5):1590–1598.

59. Hammond MD, Gale GE, Kapitan KS, Ries A, Wagner PD. Pulmonary gas exchange in humans during normobaric hypoxic exercise. *J Appl Physiol* 1986;61(5):1749–1757.

60. Wagner PD, Gale GE, Moon RE, Torre-Bueno J, Stolp BW, Saltzman HA. Pulmonary gas exchange in humans exercising at sea level and simulated altitude. *J Appl Physiol* 1986;60(1):260–270.

61. Wagner PD, Hedenstierna G, Bylin G. Ventilation–perfusion inequality in chronic asthma. *Am Rev Respir Dis* 1987;136:605–612.

62. Raine JM, Bishop JM. A–a difference in O_2 tension and physiological dead space in normal man. *J Appl Physiol* 1963;18:284–288.

63. Wagner PD, Dantzker DR, Iacovoni VE, Tomlin WC, West JB. Ventilation–perfusion inequality in asymptomatic asthma. *Am Rev Respir Dis* 1978;118:511–524.

64. Rodriguez-Roisin R, Ballester E, Roca J, Torres A, Wagner PD.

Mechanisms of hypoxemia in patients with status asthmaticus requiring mechanical ventilation. *Am Rev Respir Dis* 1989;139: 732−739.

65. Ballester E, Reyes A, Roca J, Guitart R, Wagner PD, Rodriguez-Roisin R. Ventilation−perfusion mismatching in acute severe asthma: effects of salbutamol and 100% oxygen. *Thorax* 1989;44:258−267.

66. Roca J, Ramis LI, Rodriguez-Roisin R, Ballester E, Montserrat JM, Wagner PD. Serial relationships between ventilation−perfusion inequality and spirometry in acute severe asthma requiring hospitalization. *Am Rev Respir Dis* 1988;137:1055−1061.

67. Marthan R, Castaing I, Manier G, Guenard H. Gas exchange alterations in patients with chronic obstructive lung disease. *Chest* 1985;87:470−475.

68. Dantzker DR, D'Alonzo GE. The effect of exercise on pulmonary gas exchange in patients with severe chronic obstructive pulmonary disease. *Am Rev Respir Dis* 1986;134:1135−1139.

69. Burrows B, Fletcher CM, Heard BE, Jones NL, Wootliff JS. The emphysematous and bronchial types of chronic airways obstruction. A clinicopathological study of patients in London and Chicago. *Lancet* 1966;1:830−835.

70. Wagner PD, Dantzker DR, Dueck R, dePolo JL, Wasserman K, West JB. Distribution of ventilation−perfusion ratios in patients with interstitial lung disease. *Chest* 1976;69:256.

71. Wagner PD. Ventilation−perfusion inequality and gas exchange during exercise in lung disease. In: Dempsey JA, Reed CW, eds. *Muscular exercise and the lung.* Madison, WI: University of Wisconsin Press, 1977;345−356.

72. Bencowitz HZ, Le Winter MM, Wagner PD. Effect of sodium nitroprusside on ventilation−perfusion mismatching in heart failure. *J Am Coll Cardiol* 1984;4(5):918−922.

73. Dantzker DR, Brook LJ, Dehart P, Lynch JP, Weg JG. Ventilation−perfusion distributions in the ARDS. *Am Rev Respir Dis* 1979;120:1039−1052.

74. Gerdeaux M, Lemaire F, Matamis D, Lampton N, Teisseire B, Harf A. Distribution des rapports ventilation−perfusion dans le syndrome de detresse respiratoire aigue de l'adulte. *Presse Med* 1984;13:1315−1318.

75. Lemaire F, Harf A, Teisseire BP. Oxygen exchange across the acutely injured lung. In: Zapol WM, Falke KJ, eds. *Acute respiratory failure,* vol 17. New York: Marcel Dekker, 1985, 521−554.

76. Dueck R, Wagner PD, West JB. Effects of PEEP on gas exchange in dogs with normal and edematous lungs. *Anesthesiology* 1977;47:359−366.

77. D'Alonzo, Bower JS, DeHart P, Dantzker DR. Case reports.

The mechanisms of abnormal gas exchange in acute massive pulmonary embolism. *Am Rev Respir Dis* 1983;128:170−172.

78. Manier G, Castaing Y, Guenard H. Determinants of hypoxemia during the acute phase of pulmonary embolism in humans. *Am Rev Respir Dis* 1985;132:332−338.

79. Huet F, Lemaire F, Brun-Buisson C, et al. Hypoxemia in acute pulmonary embolism. *Chest* 1985;88(6):829−836.

80. Dantzker DR, Wagner PD, Tornabene VW, Alazarki NP, West JB. Gas exchange after pulmonary thromboembolization in dogs. *Circ Res* 1978;42:92−103.

81. Young I, Mazzone RW, Wagner PD. Identification of functional lung unit in the dog by graded vascular embolization. *J Appl Physiol* 1980;49(1):132−141.

82. Wilson JE, Pierce AK, Johnson RL, et al. Hypoxemia in pulmonary embolism: a clinical study. *J Clin Invest* 1971;50:481−491.

83. Wagner PD. Mechanisms of hypoxemia in pulmonary embolism. *Appl Cardiopulm Pathophysiol* 1987;1:63−71.

84. Dantzker DR, Bower JS. Mechanisms of gas exchange abnormality in patients with chronic obliterative pulmonary vascular disease. *J Clin Invest* 1979;64:1050−1055.

85. Bendixen HH, Hedley-Whyte J, Laver MB. Impaired oxygenation in surgical patients during general anesthesia with controlled ventilation. *N Engl J Med* 1963;269:991−996.

86. Nunn JF. Factors influencing the arterial oxygen tension during halothane anesthesia with spontaneous ventilation. *Br J Anaesth* 1964;36:327−341.

87. Farhi LE, Olszowka AJ. Analysis of alveolar gas exchange in the presence of soluble inert gases. *Respir Physiol* 1968;5:53−67.

88. Rehder K, Knopp TJ, Sessler AD, Didier EP. Ventilation−perfusion relationship in young healthy awake and anesthetized-paralyzed man. *J Appl Physiol* 1979;47:745−753.

89. Hedenstierna G, Strandberg A, Tokics L, Lundquist H, Brismar B. Correlation of gas exchange impairment to development of atelectasis during anesthesia and muscle paralysis. *Acta Anaesthesiol Scand* 1986;30:183−191.

90. Hedenstierna G, Strandberg A, Brismar B, Svensson L, Tokics L. Functional residual capacity, thoraco-abdominal dimensions and central blood volume during general anesthesia with muscle paralysis and mechanical ventilation. *Anesthesiology* 1985;62:247−254.

91. Dueck R, Young I, Clausen J, Wagner PD. Identification of functional lung unit in the dog by graded vascular embolization. *J Appl Physiol* 1980;49(1):132−141.

92. Tokics L, Hedenstierna G, Svensson L, et al. Location of shunt in anaesthetized−paralyzed man. *J Appl Physiol* 1990; in press.

THE LUNG: Scientific Foundations
edited by R.G. Crystal, J.B. West et al.
Raven Press, Ltd., New York © 1991.

CHAPTER 5.4.1

Neural Organization and Rhythm Generation

Curt von Euler

CONTROL OF BREATHING BEHAVIOR

Breathing—that is, pumping air in and out to match the prevailing metabolic needs—may appear as a fairly simple, unsophisticated motor act not worthy much attention. However, at a closer look it becomes apparent that breathing is a fairly complex behavior which can exhibit a variety of patterns under different conditions. The generation and adaptive control of the breathing movements is governed by a multitude of intricate neural mechanisms. These seem to be hierarchically organized to adapt the magnitude of ventilation and time parameters of the respiratory movements to match optimally the whole spectrum of bodily activities and the ever-changing energy requirements as well as the many nonmetabolic behavioral demands on the breathing apparatus. For these purposes, many different parts of the central nervous system are involved besides the bulbar respiratory mechanisms, (a) different cerebral cortical areas, (b) amygdalar nuclei, (c) hypothalamic and other limbic areas, and (d) mesencephalic, (e) pontine, and (f) cerebellar structures. The process of breathing engages motoneuron pools, with their internuncial sensorimotor integrating mechanisms, from the level of cranial nerve V all the way down to the upper lumbar segments.

All the respiratory muscles have different mechanical actions on the chest and provide variable, condition-dependent contributions to the breathing movements. Their coordination and adjustments to trunk movements and postural activities require neural mechanisms capable of immediate automatic compensations for any changes in muscle length, direction of muscle forces, and other factors of chest wall mechanics. However, the mechanics of the ventilatory

pump and its muscular components are far from being clearly understood. A detailed knowledge of the mechanics of the system is a prerequisite for a full understanding of the system's neural control.

Many studies of the control of respiration have focused largely on (a) the pumping activity of the main inspiratory muscles and (b) the regulation of this activity by chemoreceptive and mechanoreceptor reflexes. The motor synergy for breathing includes not only the main and accessory pumping muscles but also, very importantly, pharyngeal, laryngeal, genioglossus, and alae nasi muscles controlling the patency of the upper airways, as well as the smooth muscles of the trachea and bronchial tree.

The basic rhythm generation and pattern control in breathing have many features in common with corresponding mechanisms for locomotion and probably also for mastication. For example, the central pattern generator (CPG) for breathing, like those for locomotion and mastication, is capable of generating a basic rhythmic pattern even in the complete absence of all extrinsic reflexes and feedback loops, provided that it receives sufficiently strong tonic excitatory "drive" inputs. As a matter of fact, "fictive breathing" (in analogy with "fictive locomotion") in completely paralyzed and deafferented preparations has been studied in many laboratories. Unique for breathing is that it is the only skeletal muscle activity which is continuous from birth to death. This life-dependent feature is probably reflected by an organization securing maximal endurance and reliance.

For optimal performance during all conditions and in all situations that humans are able to cope with, the controllers for ventilatory magnitude and breathing pattern need continuous recalibrations and readjustments by a multitude of reflexes, feedback circuits, integrating mechanisms, and inputs from higher central structures. Among these, feedforward mechanisms seem to play important roles in adapting the systems

C. von Euler: Nobel Institute for Neurophysiology, Karolinska Institutet, S-104 01 Stockholm, Sweden.

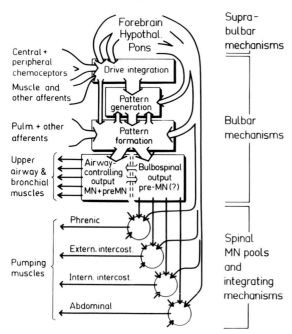

FIG. 1. The main features of the functional organization of the neural control of breathing discussed in the text. Emphasis is placed on (a) the mechanisms for drive integration, pattern generation, and pattern formation and (b) their influences on the two main output systems for the airway-controlling and pumping muscles. The scheme further emphasizes the great influences originating from forebrain and other suprabulbar structures, and it also indicates the importance of the internuncial networks of the bulbar, airway-controlling, and spinal pump-muscle-controlling motoneuron (MN) pools. Hypothal., hypothalamus; Pulm., pulmonary; Extern. intercost., external intercostal; Intern. intercost., internal intercostal. (From ref. 4.)

to anticipated changes in metabolic rate—as, for instance, at the initiation of exercise (1,2). These mechanisms, largely under the supervision of cortical and other forebrain structures, are prerequisites for the great adaptability of the mammalian (especially the human) respiratory control system. The cortical supervision of most motor acts in humans involves not only the conscious but also the subconscious control of performance of automatized movements. This seems to be true also for breathing (cf. refs. 3 and 4).

Thus, just as when dealing with the control of locomotion, it seems both justified and conceptually advantageous to discuss separately (a) the mechanisms for the basic rhythmic *pattern generation,* (b) the mechanisms for the adaptive control of breathing and optimal *pattern formation,* and (c) the set of mechanisms for the ventilatory *drive integration.* Most likely, there is a great deal of overlap and interaction existing between these three sets of mechanisms (see Fig. 1). This chapter will deal mainly with the mechanisms for the basic respiratory pattern generation. But before going into any details of the neural organization un-

derlying this function, we will consider briefly some aspects of adaptive pattern formation and drive integration in the control of breathing behavior.

Comments on Adaptive Control and Pattern Formation—Aims and Compromises

Much work on the control of breathing rests upon the tacit assumption of a simple reflexogenic control; that is, changes in ventilation are taken as reflecting corresponding changes in certain ventilatory stimuli. This "stimulus–response" hypothesis approach has a certain attraction because it seems capable of explaining the ventilatory responses to the most-studied ventilatory stimuli such as hypoxia, hypercapnia, and acidemia (although it fails to explain exercise hyperpnea) and because it lends itself to descriptions by proportional control system models. However, the control of breathing cannot be dealt with adequately merely in terms of a set of reflexes integrated by a "respiratory center." On the contrary, breathing should be regarded as a complex behavior, governed by a multitude of control systems hierarchically arranged to regulate ventilation and the pattern of breathing so as to meet optimally the prevailing metabolic needs and the various nonchemostatic demands on the respiratory apparatus. The view that ventilation is governed by an optimization policy such that the net costs of breathing are minimized even when chemical and nonchemical demands are in conflict further implies a minimum work rate criterion in the control of the different respiratory pattern variables under various conditions (see, e.g., refs. 5 and 6). This suggests the importance of complex sensorimotor integrations in the control of breathing allowing the integrating mechanisms to also adapt the system to trunk movements and changes in posture and to other demands on the muscles of the trunk during various laborious muscular activities and exercises. The breathing muscles and their motor control circuitries are engaged also in the control of posture and movements of the trunk as well as in several somatovisceral reflexes and expulsive motor acts. In these functions, inspiratory and expiratory muscles may operate synergistically, whereas in breathing they act as antagonists (3,7). Thus, breathing, like all complex motor behaviors, needs to be governed by continuous information from many types of receptors located in the muscles, joints, and skin as well as from intracentral efferent–afferent comparators utilizing feedback of "efferent-copy" information (3).

In humans, one of the most important nonchemostatic employments of the breathing apparatus is for voice production and speech. When utilizing breathing for these purposes, the supreme control of the rate and volume of inhalation before an utterance, and of the duration and rate of exhalation during vocalization, is taken over by forebrain mechanisms according to the specific requirements for phrasing, loudness, and articulation (8–10). This may lead to certain compromises with respect to the precision of the chemostatic regulation when the control for speech purposes is given highest "priority."

The breathing apparatus is being utilized also for other homeostatic purposes (especially for temperature regulation), which may cause some rivalry. Modern homeostasis research focuses its attention on regulation towards what is optimal for the whole organism in each prevailing situation rather than on constancy in all conditions of each factor of the internal milieu.

Although breathing continues through all sleep states, the respiratory control mechanisms are strongly influenced also by the sleep-cycle pattern (see, e.g., ref. 11). In slow-wave sleep, for instance, the breathing pattern is fairly regular, with approximately linear relationships between P_{CO_2} and ventilation. In this sleep state, breathing appears to be regulated mainly by the bulbar control mechanisms for chemostatic purposes. In rapid eye movement (REM) sleep, on the other hand, there is no longer a linear relationship between P_{O_2} and ventilation. The switch to REM sleep is associated with a dramatic increase in variability of rate and depth of breathing. Hence, one may see a marked hyperpnea with a series of rapid breaths or apneic pauses (or both), concomitant with clusters of rapid eye movements. It is as if there were sudden changes in the tonic drive for ventilation, giving rise either to increased ventilation (mainly by faster rates) or to momentary pauses, or to both, in irregular alternations. Hobson and Steriade (11) suggest that the networks responsible for the respiratory patterns are of similar design and are located in close approximation to the "sleep-cycle clock." It is therefore, they argue, not surprising that the respiratory system shows such dramatic state dependency. It may even be that some neurons, especially those in the pontine parabrachial–Kölliker/Fuse complex, are common to both systems.

The respiratory system is engaged in many other forebrain influenced functions and emotional reactions (see chapter 5.4.9). In the awake state, these influences constitute important, although very variable, additional drives for ventilation beyond the immediate metabolic needs. These "wakefulness drives" act as an excitatory "noise" causing considerable variations in the blood gas levels. Merely closing the eyes causes changes in the breathing pattern as well as in the ventilatory CO_2 responsiveness (12).

The data mentioned above suggest that the different challenges on the breathing apparatus from chemostatic and nonchemostatic functions may at times be competing and result in compromises from both sides, depending on which purpose is given priority in each situation (cf. ref. 4).

Comments on Drive Integration

The generation and control of a behavior depends not only on the anatomical and functional connectivity of the pattern-generating network but also on the excitatory tonic drive inputs to this network. This is certainly true also for breathing. In the absence of drive inputs, apnea ensues. This tonic activity derives, to an important extent, from the peripheral and central chemoreceptors but also derives from many other peripheral and central sources. These drive inputs seem to be integrated by the structures in, as well as adjacent to, the paragigantocellular nucleus—that is, the "apnea" region of Budzinska et al. (13; cf. ref. 14).

Students of the neural control of respiration have paid relatively little attention to those mechanisms that serve to mediate and integrate the different drive inputs. Recent results suggest that the lateral paragigantocellular and preolivar nuclei (NPGL and NPO) are involved in these functions. A focal, cold block (20°C) applied unilaterally within these areas causes strong depression or apnea (13,15). Neurons of these areas are characterized by tonic discharge patterns without significant respiratory modulation. They receive converging afferents of several different modalities from peripheral and central chemoreceptors and from low- and high-threshold mechanoreceptors in muscles, joints, and skin, including nociceptors. In addition, many of these neurons receive direct inputs from the "defense and alarm" areas in the posterior hypothalamus (16; T. Pantaleo, J. Mitra, N. Prabhakar, Y. Yamamoto, M. Runold, N. S. Cherniack, and C. von Euler, *to be published*). The lack of respiratory modulation of the neurons of this "apnea region" in the rostral ventrolateral regions of the medulla oblongata may explain why these neurons have not been recognized as forming vital parts of the respiratory control system. This "apnea region" seems to be involved also in the cardiovascular control. However, the respiratory drive integrating functions can be selectively depressed or blocked within these structures without any concomitant blood pressure effects.

In addition to the aggregate drive effects on the whole respiratory control system, there seem to exist pathways mediating some drive-specific influences on different parts of the respiratory motor system. For instance, the peripheral chemoreceptors exert relatively stronger effects on the upper-airway muscles than on the pumping muscles (17,18). Likewise, initiation of exercise causes a relatively stronger recruitment of the expiratory motor systems as compared to an isoventilatory effect of CO_2 stimulation (19).

THE BASIC RHYTHM-GENERATING MECHANISMS

General Properties of Rhythm-Generating Mechanisms

One of the most challenging problems of the neurosciences of today concerns the question of how networks of neurons are constructed to generate animal behavior. To reach an understanding of how a neural network operates to generate a simple behavior (such as an alternating motor activity in breathing or locomotion) and how it may fail as a result of disease or injury, it is necessary to acquire knowledge both on the overriding principles of neuronal functions and on how these principles are implemented by the individual building blocks, i.e. the neurons and synapses in the particular network. Although knowledge of *anatomical* connectivity is essential, it is not enough; neural network operation depends critically also upon the synaptic and cellular properties, many of which are inherently nonlinear. Neurons not only are simple integrators of synaptic inputs but also possess a variety of intrinsic properties that enable them to transform the synaptic input signals into complex activity patterns. Synaptic properties are far more diverse than merely being excitatory or inhibitory (see, e.g., ref. 20).

Intrinsic properties of nerve cells can be altered in many ways—for example, by alterations of the ionic conductances by neuromodulators. Acting on surface receptors, these neuromodulators may cause changes in the kinetics of certain ion channels either by direct actions or by way of second-messenger induction. These effects can be strong enough to provide a neuron with new intrinsic properties not present in the absence of the modulator. Examples of properties that may be modulator-induced are: altered excitability properties, altered input–output relations with different firing patterns and bursting activities, and postinhibitory rebound.

As Getting (20) emphasized, the flow of activity within the circuit must also be defined quantitatively—for example, by assessing the temporal sequence of states of activity of the circuit elements using such criteria as membrane potential, membrane conductance, firing frequency, the onset and termination of firing, or "integrated" activity across a set of neurons. It is important to keep in mind that the *functional* connectivity within a neural network, and thus its operation, is under dynamic control according to the prevailing tasks but is within the constraints of its *anatomical* organization. This provides possibilities not only for adaptive control of the output activity of the network but also for it to generate *different* behaviors during different conditions. This implies that

a separate neural network is not necessary for each behavior or for each behavioral modification, such as breathing for gas exchange, breathing for the purpose of speech and singing, or breathing for thermoregulatory panting. Certain inputs to a network may be both *instructive* and *permissive* in that they may reorganize the functional interactions within the network to fit the task at hand and to activate the network to perform the task (20).

The *functional* connectivity, and thus the operation of the network, can be altered by modulation of synaptic efficiency (depression, facilitation, potentiation, reflex reversal), which, in turn, may depend on the pattern of transmission in that synapse or on the activity in another pathway, either by direct action of the second pathway (as in presynaptic inhibition) or by the influence of a more remotely released neuromodulator substance. Task-dependent alterations of reflex operation have been well documented, for example, for the proprioceptive control of leg movements during the different phases of the step cycle (21) and for the low-threshold, slowly adapting pulmonary stretch receptors' action during different phases of the breathing cycle providing (a) *facilitation* of inspiratory activity during the course of the inspiratory phase and (b) the terminating *inhibition* of this activity at inspiratory off-switch (19). By the latter effect the afferent input from these receptors causes cycle shortening of the inspiratory phase when acting in this phase. The same afferent input arriving during the expiratory phase causes lengthening of this phase by different phase-dependent central mechanisms.

Characteristics of the Generated Motor Output Pattern

During normal eupneic breathing, the expiratory muscles participate minimally. Expiration in these conditions is largely a passive event driven by the elastic recoil forces accumulated during the act of inspiration. However, during the first part of expiration the inspiratory muscles are being activated again. This postinspiration inspiratory activity (PIIA) counteracts the initially strong elastic recoil and brakes the rate of exhalation in the first part of expiration (see, e.g., refs. 22 and 23).

The inspiratory motor activity—as revealed, for example, by recording the neural activity from the phrenic or external intercostal nerves—is characterized by a sudden onset followed by a "ramp"-shaped increase in discharge rate progressing at a more or less steady rate until it is terminated or switched off.

Following the inspiratory off-switch, there is often a fairly marked PIIA, which continues in a declining manner during the first part of expiration. During the second part of expiration, there is no activity in the inspiratory muscles; moreover, the expiratory muscles are being recruited only in case of increased ventilatory drives (24,25). Expiratory motor activity is generally not recruited until the PIIA has ceased. Thus, as proposed by Richter and co-workers (26–29; see also ref. 7), the expiratory phase may be subdivided into two subphases: (i) E-phase I, characterized by the presence of PIIA; and (ii) E-phase II, which either is "silent" or, in conditions of increased ventilatory drive, exhibits active expiratory motor activity.

The inspiratory motor output to the external intercostal and parasternal muscles exhibits patterns which are grossly similar to those of the phrenic nerve, although, in quiet breathing, the onset of the intercostal and parasternal inspiratory activity may be delayed relative to the phrenic activity. These differences in synchrony tend to disappear with increasing ventilatory drive and vary with postural demands.

The activity patterns of the "airway-controlling muscles" are somewhat different from those of the main "pump muscles." For instance, the upper-airway dilator muscles are generally activated significantly earlier (sometimes several hundred milliseconds) than the main pump muscles (see, e.g., ref. 17). It has been suggested that this temporal difference in onset between the airway dilator muscles and the pump muscles is a result of a brief active inhibition of the premotor neurons for the pump muscles delaying the onset of inspiration in order to allow the airways to be dilated before any negative intrathoracic pressure is created. The neural phase of inspiration should therefore probably be measured from the earliest onset of the upper-airway dilation rather than from the onset of the phrenic or intercostal activity. The brief interval between the onset of the upper-airway activity and the pump muscle activity—or, differently expressed, the short period of "withheld" activation of the pump muscles—might be regarded as a "moment of preparation" before the commencement of the act of inhalation. The neurophysiology of the control of movements offers many examples of such brief preparatory acts of inhibition; these inhibitory actions are especially evident in the postural adjustments which occur just prior to intended limb movements and which are necessary for maintenance of equilibrium (30). Abolishing the preparatory delay of the onset of inspiratory activity of the pump muscles might lead to problems involving upper-airway obstruction.

The Anatomical Organization of Respiration-Related Neuronal Populations in the Medulla Oblongata

The central pattern generator for automatic breathing, along with its main output system of premotor neurons,

is located in the lower brainstem, probably within the medulla oblongata. This location, in close approximation to the motoneuron pools for the upper-airway and bronchial muscles, is at a considerable distance from the spinal motoneuron pools for the volume driving muscles. This organization, which appears to contrast with the spinal localization of the CPGs for locomotion, reflects the phylogenetic origin of large parts of the respiratory apparatus from the branchial structures (see, e.g., ref. 7). This arrangement forms the basis for the close cooperation between the airway-controlling and the volume driving muscles in breathing, as well as in many nonrespiratory reflexes (e.g., expulsory) and in behavioral functions involving vocalization.

In addition to the brainstem motoneurons for the different airway-controlling muscles, the lower brainstem contains several groups of neurons with respiration-related (RR) discharge patterns. These are grossly organized in two main aggregates of neurons: One is located dorsomedially in medulla in the region of the nuclear complex of the tractus solitarius (NTS). This group is known as the "dorsal respiratory group" (DRG). It should be noted that this group not only encompasses the ventrolateral part of NTS (as is often implied) but also encompasses neurons of the dorsolateral and medial aspects of NTS (31). The second group of RR neurons constitutes a longitudinal column of neurons in a more ventral and lateral region of the medulla oblongata, extending from its rostral to its caudal border. Traditionally, this group of neurons is referred to as the "ventral respiratory group" (VRG) despite the fact that it is situated at a level only about half the distance between the dorsal and ventral aspects of the medulla and is not reaching down to the chemoreceptive structures of the ventral surface of medulla.

The DRG contains mainly inspiration-related (IR) cells, of which about half or more are bulbospinal neurons referred to as "R-alpha neurons" (32). The axons of most of these neurons cross the midline just rostral to the obex before they descend to the contralateral side of the spinal cord. Most of these are supposed to make contact with the spinal motoneurons of the inspiratory muscles, namely, the diaphragm and the external intercostals. It now appears, however, that these neurons may not form such homogeneous groups with respect to their connections with the various spinal motoneurons as hitherto believed (cf., e.g., refs. 33 and 34). The bulbospinal premotor neurons does not seem to be involved in the pattern generation. Antidromic activation of these neurons does not seem to influence the phase switching and rhythmic pattern (35).

There are also propriobulbar IR interneurons with similar, augmenting discharge patterns. Characteristic for the DRG are also the R-beta neurons (32). These neurons receive both an augmenting IR input, apparently derived from the same source as that which exits the R-alpha neurons, and a direct input from the pulmonary stretch receptor afferents. The precise functional role of the R-beta neurons remains obscure. It has been believed by many that they feed into the off-switch mechanism, but there is no direct evidence for that view. In the DRG there is also another group of second-order pulmonary stretch receptor sensory neurons. These do not receive other RR inputs, and thus their discharge patterns only reflect the degree of lung inflation. These neurons are known as "pump cells" or "P-neurons."

The DRG further contains different types of IR neurons, such as propriobulbar "inspiratory-ramp" interneurons, "early inspiratory" or "early-burst" neurons, and "late-onset IR" neurons. These types of neurons are found also in the VRG. Present in the DRG are also a small group of early-peak-decrementing expiration-related (ER) neurons or postinspiration (PI)-related neurons.

The VRG can be subdivided into three main parts:

1. The caudal part, known as "nucleus retroambigualis" (NRA), contains mainly ER neurons, the majority of which are bulbospinal expiratory premotor neurons. Their axons cross the midline just caudal to the obex before descending on the contralateral side to the motoneuron pools for the expiratory intercostal and abdominal muscles. It has been claimed that they largely lack medullary axon collaterals and that they are not involved in pattern-generating mechanisms (36).

2. The intermediate part, denoted "nucleus paraambigualis" (because it parallels the ambiguus nucleus), contains mainly IR neurons, including both (a) bulbospinal inspiratory premotor neurons and (b) propriobulbar interneurons of the various types present also in the DRG.

3. The most rostral part of VRG largely coincides with "nucleus retrofacialis" (NRF). This part includes a dense population of ER neurons known as the "Bötzinger complex" (31,37–43). The Bötzinger complex consists of several functional types of ER neurons; some of these are pharyngeal and laryngeal motoneurons, whereas some are interneurons (42,43). Intracellular recordings from Bötzinger neurons have shown (a) waves of inhibitory postsynaptic potentials during inspiration and (b) an augmenting number of excitatory postsynaptic potentials during expiration (42). These ER neurons differ from the neurons with similar discharge patterns located in the caudal, retroambigual part of the VRG with respect to the postsynaptic effects induced by stimulation of laryngeal afferents (42). Apart from the Bötzinger complex, NRF contains a variety of RR neurons, some of which are laryngeal and pharyngeal motoneurons (42,43).

A few ER neurons have been encountered ventromedial to the NRF fairly close to the rostral area of the ventral surface of medulla (43). The location of these neurons within, or close to, a part of the "apnea area" of Budzinska et al. (13) suggests the possibility that they are involved in the central chemoceptive system (43). Onimaru and Homma (44), in their *in vitro* preparation of neonatal rat brain stem, have encountered both RR neurons (especially a type of preinspiratory ones) and tonically firing neurons; both types of neuron are ventral to the Bötzinger complex.

The DRG and VRG seem to have somewhat different pattern-forming and output functions. The DRG appears to be involved more in the reflex and central control of timing, whereas the VRG seems to be more strongly involved in the control of inspiratory amplitude (45–47). In addition, the threshold for active expiration appears to be controlled by structures in the dorsolateral medulla outside the DRG and VRG (48).

Further rostrally in the parabrachial and Kölliker/Fuse nuclei in rostral pons, there are groups of neurons with RR discharge patterns of several different phase relations to the respiratory cycle. These groups of neurons have important excitatory and pattern-modulating effects on breathing. However, these rostral pontine mechanisms do not seem to be critically involved in the most basic respiratory rhythm generation itself and will not be discussed further in this context.

Concepts on the Functional Organization of the Pattern-Generating Mechanisms

At the present state of our knowledge, the CPG for breathing cannot be defined in terms of any circumscribed region of the VRG or DRG or any other anatomically specified bulbar structure. Rather, the CPG seems to have a great deal of redundancy, or "degeneracy," and to consist of parallel, self-sustaining oscillating networks organized as a set of coupled oscillators (47,49) arranged fairly widespread in the medulla, probably to secure continuous operation under all conditions. This view is corroborated by the experience of several investigators that it is difficult to abolish rhythmic activity by focal lesions or focal cold blocks within the VRG or DRG, respectively (7,45,46,50): Lesioning of *one* circuit in a multioscillatory system would not seriously impair rhythmogenesis but could change the pattern by shifting the leader oscillator (49).

It would seem likely, although still quite uncertain, that the neurons constituting the building blocks of the basic pattern generator for breathing, along with its different part mechanisms, can be found within the DRG and VRG (including the retrofacial nucleus, as well as the Bötzinger complex and the RR neurons ventral thereof). New types of RR neurons at new locations may still be discovered, however.

Some recent concepts on the operation of the pattern generator are based largely on (a) the relationships between the patterns of excitatory and inhibitory postsynaptic activity (EPSPs and IPSPs) and the discharge patterns of different types of RR neurons and (b) the relationships between the motor output patterns during the different phases of the breathing cycle and the reflex perturbations of these functions (22,23,26,28, 29,42,43,51,52; see also ref. 7). Information on synaptic interactions between RR neurons has been obtained also by means of cross-correlations of simultaneously recorded spike trains from pairs of RR neurons (see, e.g., refs. 47 and 53–55).

The available data have suggested excitatory and inhibitory synaptic interconnections with a preponderance of inhibitory interactions between the various types of RR propriobulbar neurons. This, in turn, has led to several hypotheses that the respiratory pattern-generating networks are designed on the principle of neurons interacting largely through inhibitory synaptic connections in parallel with excitatory, mainly drive-dependent inputs (cf., e.g., refs. 20 and 56). The classical view, however, that rhythm generation in breathing depends on reciprocal inhibition between two symmetrical populations of inspiratory and expiratory premotor neurons forming inspiratory and expiratory "half-centers" has, for several reasons, been found untenable in their proposed form (7,26,36,56).

Instead, the respiratory cycle has been regarded as consisting of *three* phases: (i) the inspiratory phase; (ii) the postinspiratory phase or expiratory phase I (E-phase I) characterized by the reappearance of some declining inspiratory activity, the postinspiration inspiratory activity (PIIA); and (iii) the expiratory phase II (E-phase II), during which expiratory motor activity may be recruited in conditions of increased drive for ventilation (7,26,28,29,51). In this model, each cycle phase is considered to reflect a *state* of the oscillating network, rather than a particular configuration of the motor output (28). Four sequentially activated submechanisms are considered to define the three phases and to be causally involved in the phase transitions. These submechanisms are those generating (a) the sudden onset of, as well as a progressive increase in, inspiratory ramp, known as the "central inspiratory activity" (CIA), (b) the termination of the inspiratory activity (i.e., the inspiratory "off-switch" mechanisms), (c) the events of the early part of E-phase I such as the PIIA and the laryngeal adductor activation, and (d) the E-phase II and the expiratory motor output (7).

For this operation, the following six types of neuron (see Fig. 2) have been proposed as the main neuronal

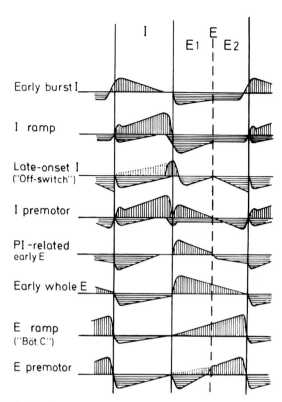

FIG. 2. Excitatory and inhibitory activity patterns of main types of inspiration- and expiration-related neurons in medulla during inspiratory (I) and expiratory (E) phases (E_1 and E_2 denote subdivisions of this phase). PI, postinspiration; Böt. C., Bötzinger complex. See text for further explanation. Vertical hatching represents excitatory synaptic activity and discharge rate; horizontal hatching denotes synaptic inhibition. During main part of inspiratory phase, late-onset neurons receive an augmenting excitation but are kept silent by an inhibition that may emanate from early-burst neurons. (Modified from ref. 7.)

building elements constituting the most basic rhythm-generating network (7,28,56):

1. "Early inspiratory interneurons," or "early-burst interneurons" (57). These are characterized by an early onset, often somewhat prior to that of the phrenic nerve activity, a rapidly attained peak, and a subsequent declining activity reaching zero level at a variable time during the last part of the inspiratory phase.

2. "Inspiratory-ramp interneurons." These are characterized by (a) a sudden onset of, as well as a ramp-like progressive increase in, firing rate during the course of inspiration and (b) a fairly abrupt termination.

3. "Late-onset inspiratory interneurons," or putative "off-switch neurons." These are characterized by firing patterns starting late in the inspiratory phase. Their discharge peak appears to coincide with the transition from inspiration to expiration.

4. "Early expiratory interneurons," or "postin-

spiration (PI)-related interneurons." These are characterized by a rapid onset and a rapidly attained peak of discharge at the transition from the inspiratory to the expiratory phase corresponding to the irreversible stage 2 of the inspiratory off-switch. Thereafter, their discharge rate declines at a variable rate towards the end of E-phase I.

5. "Early-peak whole expiratory interneurons." These have a discharge pattern similar to that of the PI-related neurons but continue in a declining manner for the whole expiratory phase.

6. "Expiratory-ramp interneurons." These are characterized by a ramp-like augmenting discharge pattern during the whole phase of expiration.

As mentioned above, the inspiratory and expiratory bulbospinal premotor neurons, also shown in Fig. 2, do not seem to participate in the basic rhythm-generating networks.

The Submechanisms of the Pattern Generator: Possible Neural Correlates

The Ramp Generation

The inspiratory trajectory of the spirogram usually approximates that of the "central inspiratory activity", as reflected by the inspiratory-ramp interneurons in the medulla and by the bulbospinal inspiratory premotor neurons. Following a fairly rapid onset, the rate of increase of their discharge pattern changes proportionally to the drive input. At conditions with stable drive influence, the inspiratory trajectory is usually not far from linear (58), with fairly small breath-to-breath variations; the corresponding scatter in the durations of the inspiratory phases is relatively greater (59). It is important to understand, however, that there are many conditions during which the efferent phrenic nerve activity is not representative of the ramp generator or CIA (see ref. 7).

The great stability of the time course of the inspiratory trajectory during constant conditions suggests that the CIA generation is the result of a well-controlled balance between self-excitatory and self-inhibitory processes, a balance that would depend on the strength of the drive inputs and reflex perturbations (see, e.g., refs. 56, 59, and 60). This view is further supported by the finding that both excitatory and inhibitory postsynaptic potentials determine the trajectory of membrane depolarization, as well as the discharge pattern, of both the inspiratory-ramp interneurons (26,47,51) and the inspiratory bulbospinal premotor neurons. Thus the augmenting postsynaptic pattern of EPSPs is damped somewhat by a simultaneous, mainly declining pattern of IPSPs probably derived from the "early inspiratory neurons" (26,55).

The termination of the inspiratory-ramp neuron discharge at the end of inspiration, as well as the subsequent early expiratory phase, E-phase I, is associated with a rapidly rising deep wave of hyperpolarization of these neurons which then declines towards the end of E-phase I. During E-phase II, they exhibit a new wave of augmenting postsynaptic inhibition which terminates abruptly at transition from E-phase II to inspiration. This sudden termination seems to give rise to a postinhibitory rebound excitation providing the sudden-burst onset of the inspiratory ramp activity (51).

These ramp inspiratory interneurons seem to provide the augmenting ramp-like inspiratory discharge pattern both to the bulbospinal inspiratory premotor neurons and to the R-beta neurons (61).

The Inspiratory "Off-Switch" Functions

The inspiratory activity is being terminated when it either has reached an intensity sufficient with respect to the corresponding tidal volume or has proceeded for an adequate duration of time, or both, as "deemed adequate" under the prevailing condition by the respiratory controller. This "judgment" seems to be expressed in terms of progressively increasing activities attaining a centrally controlled threshold, the off-switch threshold. This threshold is not a fixed one but is, instead, subject to adaptive control, the level of which is one of the important means by which depth and rate of breathing are regulated (7,62). There seems to be general agreement that this occurs when the threshold has been attained by combined actions of two (or more) progressively increasing inputs to the inspiratory off-switch mechanisms: (i) a centrally generated inspiration-related activity and (ii) the increasing afferent volume-related input from the lungs (and chest wall). In the absence of such cyclic afferent input (e.g., by withholding inflation in inspiration), the first-mentioned input alone is responsible for the attainment of the off-switch threshold (62–64).

The nature of this central activity is debated. It has been postulated that it reflects a corollary activity of the inspiratory ramp neuron activity (i.e., the CIA) which in this way contributes to, or triggers off, its own termination (7,62,65). Alternatively, this input may derive from some other integrator operating in parallel with, but independent of, the inspiratory ramp or CIA integrator, providing a time-related attainment of the off-switch threshold (50,66).

However, not only the off-switch threshold but also the timing of the off-switch event shows significant drive dependence after vagotomy. The proposed "timing integrator" would, therefore, have to be dependent on the chemical, thermal, and other drive inputs in a manner similar to that of the CIA integrator. Thus, the hypothesis of a separate timing integrator, in addition to the intensity-related CIA integrator, implies that the off-switch mechanisms consist of two fairly similar integrating mechanisms operating in parallel. So far, there is no conclusive evidence proving or disproving either of these two hypotheses. However, the fact that the off-switch excitability is continuously and progressively increasing during the course of the inspiratory phase (7,62) definitely precludes a timing device acting through trigger signals. The occasional occurrence of what appears as discrepancies between the timing of the inspiratory termination and the corresponding level of inspiratory phrenic activity cannot be taken as evidence against the first alternative because, as mentioned above, it is only under certain well-controlled experimental conditions that the efferent phrenic activity reliably represents the CIA. Thus, even if the off-switch operation is controlled by a corollary activity of the CIA generator, there are many different factors that may give rise to changes in the amplitude of the phrenic nerve activity at which inspiratory termination occurs (7,62).

With respect to the possible neural correlates to the inspiratory off-switch mechanisms, it has been postulated that the Stage 1 reversible off-switch events (63,64) correspond closely to the discharge of the late-onset inspiratory neurons, also referred to as the "putative off-switch neurons" by Feldman and Cohen (67). Their onset and time–activity profile is strongly influenced by pulmonary stretch receptor inputs: Lung inflation causes facilitation, resulting in an earlier onset and steeper rate of rise of firing, whereas withholding lung inflation causes disfacilitation and later onset. Analyses of membrane potential changes and the patterns of EPSPs and IPSPs of these neurons have revealed that they receive a ramp-like increase of EPSPs during the entire process of inspiration, but this excitatory input is counteracted by an initially strong but decrementing postsynaptic inhibitory activity that starts off and reaches its peak at the very beginning of the inspiratory phase and then declines. The time course of this IPSP activity seems to correspond to that of the discharge rate of the early inspiratory ("early-burst") interneurons (26) (see Fig. 2).

It has been suggested (26,28) that the long delay between the start of inspiration and the neural discharge late in inspiration is a result of the fact that neurons receive an initially strong and gradually declining barrage of IPSPs, probably deriving from the early inspiratory interneurons, counteracting the augmenting pattern of EPSPs during the inspiratory phase so as to prevent the neurons from discharging until late in inspiration. It would seem that this declining inhibitory power provides the progressively increasing excitability of the off-switch. This would imply that the firing

threshold of the late-onset neurons constitutes the off-switch threshold. The facilitation of the late-onset inspiratory neurons in response to lung inflation, which mimics the inhibition of the early inspiratory neurons to the same stimulus, is providing the off-switch function with its well-known dependence on lung inflation (i.e., the Hering–Breuer inflation reflex).

The late-onset inspiratory neurons should probably not be regarded as a special class of R-beta neurons (68; cf. also ref. 69), since their modulation by lung inflations may be derived secondarily from the early inspiratory neurons. According to Orem (69), these neurons do not participate in the inhibition of inspiratory activity in behavioral arrest of breathing.

The final, irreversible Stage 2 off-switch (28,55, 63,64) might be executed by the early expiratory PI-related neurons (28), probably in combination with early whole expiratory neurons which may have the capacity to keep the CIA inhibited during the whole expiratory phase, although at a declining power (7,55,60,70).

E-Phase I

This phase is characterized by the postinspiration inspiratory activity and the activity of the underlying early expiratory PI-related interneurons. Their declining discharge pattern during E-phase I might be caused by an augmenting input IPSPs probably derived from ramp expiratory interneurons. During E-phase II these neurons receive a progressively increasing postsynaptic inhibition. During inspiration they receive an initially strong and declining postsynaptic inhibition (28) as depicted in Fig. 2. Such neurons are found in DRG and in VRG, as well as in the population of ER neurons of the Bötzinger complex which have been shown to inhibit IR neurons in the DRG and VRG (37,38, 41,42,71).

The time–activity profile of the PI-related expiratory interneurons is modulated by pulmonary stretch receptor input (67,72): Lung inflation during E-phase I causes (a) a slowing of the rate of decline of discharge and (b) prolongation of this phase. Conversely, preventing inflation from occurring during the phase of inspiration causes a more rapid decline in the firing rate of these cells, associated with a shortening of this phase.

The PI-related interneurons have been postulated to have important roles in the rhythm-generating network by suppressing (or "gating") the inputs to the system from the drive-integrating mechanisms in the ventral rostrolateral structures of medulla. This "gating" effect might serve to prevent a too-early onset of active expiration. The strong "release" of expiratory activity by focal cooling (20°C) of certain structures in dorsal medulla (48) may be due to blocking this gating activity.

E-Phase II

The inhibitory activity that depresses the various inspiration-promoting influences and reflexes during the expiratory phase acts not only during the E-phase I but also during practically the entire expiratory phase, although with a declining power. This inhibitory activity, which has been referred to as the "central inspiratory inhibition" (CII) (70), seems to control the whole expiratory duration. The rate of decay of this inhibition is slowed down by lung inflations, resulting in prolonged expiratory duration, and is accelerated by inspiration-facilitating reflexes (e.g., those mediated by some rapidly adapting pulmonary reflexes). Extensive studies of the time course of the declining inhibitory power of CII and its reflex perturbations (70; cf. also refs. 7 and 60) have shown that it is more closely related to the time course of the early-peak whole expiratory neurons than to that of the PI-related ones. It therefore does not seem likely that the control of the CII and the whole expiratory duration depends on the PI-related neurons or on augmenting E-phase-II-related neurons. Rather, it would seem that this effect is mediated by the early-peak whole expiratory neurons (47). These types of ER neurons receive postsynaptic inhibition during the phase of inspiration. The pattern of postsynaptic inhibition observed in some of these ER neurons seems to correspond to the discharge pattern of inspiratory-ramp interneurons, whereas in other ER neurons the pattern of IPSPs was similar to the firing pattern of early-onset inspiratory neurons. Furthermore, it has been reported that IR neurons of the VRG and DRG send inhibitory projections to ER neuron populations (36). Similarly, early-onset inspiratory neurons appear to project to the contralateral ER neurons of the NRA group (73).

SUMMARY

The correlative data described above suggest that the decremental postsynaptic inhibition of the ER neurons (except the PI-related ones) during inspiration is caused by the early inspiratory ("early-burst") neurons, which also would seem likely candidates for the cause of the decremental inhibition of the late-onset inspiratory neurons and their modulation by lung inflations.

The early inspiratory neurons seem to mediate strong inhibition on the population of expiratory premotor neurons in the caudal VRG (55). At the onset of expiration these neurons are inhibited by a strong wave of postsynaptic inhibition that declines during the course of the expiratory phase. This inhibition is possibly mediated by the early expiratory PI-related neurons and by other early-peak whole expiratory neurons. Their declining discharge rate during the inspiratory phase seems to mirror the increasing activity of inspiratory-ramp interneurons; the latter may inhibit the former (55). It is further suggested that the postsynaptic inhibition during E-phase I of the various IR neurons, as well as during E-phase I of the expiratory premotor neurons, is caused by the early expiratory PI-related neurons.

Thus, according to this hypothesis, the early- and the late-onset inspiratory neurons, together with the early expiratory PI-related neurons, can be regarded as key elements in the rhythm-generating network (23,28,29).

Although there is no conclusive evidence that the neurons of the Bötzinger complex are critically involved in the basic pattern generation, they seem to play important roles in the control of the breathing pattern by exerting inhibitory effects on inspiratory activity and, possibly, by contributing to the off-switch mechanisms (13). Furthermore, these neurons may be involved in the central regulation of the expiratory motor output (40,42,43).

The above considerations on possible neural correlates to the different submechanisms and the functional connectivity of the basic CPG for breathing have been subjected to model simulations by Botros and Bruce (56). Their quantitative results have indicated the feasibility of most of the qualitative concepts mentioned above. However, as stated above, there is no conclusive evidence as to the actual functional involvement of any of these neurons in the pattern-generating networks. More investigations are required in order to discern the anatomical interconnections and functional connectivity and interactions under different conditions between the different types of respiration-related neurons as discussed earlier in this chapter.

So far, there is little conclusive evidence that pacemaker cells are involved in mammalian central pattern generators for breathing. However, participation of such elements can, by no means, be excluded. On the basis that some respiration-like rhythmic activity continues in *in vitro* preparations of neonatal rat brain stem in a Cl^--free medium or a medium containing antagonists to the inhibitory neurotransmitters GABA or glycine, it has been suggested that this rhythmic activity is independent of Cl^--dependent synaptic inhibitors but may depend on the fact that those neurons have pacemaker properties (44,66,74). However, all respiration-related neurons in the DRG and VRG (including Bötzinger complex) that have been well studied with intracellular techniques have shown firing patterns that depend on postsynaptic modulations of membrane potentials and membrane conductances.

Nevertheless, it does not seem unlikely that unstable or bistable membrane properties, electrical coupling, and local circuit mechanisms influencing only parts of neurons may be involved (cf. ref. 75).

REFERENCES

1. DiMarco AF, Romaniuk JR, Euler C von, Yamamoto Y. Immediate changes in ventilation and respiratory pattern associated with onset and cessation of locomotion in the cat. *J Physiol (Lond)* 1983;343:1–16.
2. Eldridge FL, Millhorn DE, Waldrop TG. Exercise hyperpnea and locomotion: parallel activation from the hypothalamus. *Science* 1981;211:844–846.
3. Euler C von. On the role of proprioceptors in perception and execution of motor acts with special reference to breathing. In: Pengelly LD, Rebuck AS, Campbell EJM, eds. *Loaded breathing.* Ontario: Longman Canada Ltd, 1974;139–149.
4. Euler C von. Introduction: forebrain control of breathing behaviour. In: Euler C von, Katz-Salamon M, eds. *Respiratory psychophysiology.* Wenner-Gren International Symposium Series, vol 50. Basingstoke: Macmillan Press, 1988;1–14.
5. Yamashiro SM, Daubenspeck JA, Lauritsen TN, Grodins FS. Total work rate of breathing optimization in CO_2 inhalation and exercise. *J Appl Physiol* 1975;38:702–709.
6. Poon CS. Optimal control of ventilation in hypercapnia and exercise: an extended model. In: Benchetrit G, Baconnier P, Demongeot J, eds. *Concepts and formalizations in the control of breathing.* Manchester: Manchester University Press, 1987;119–131.
7. Euler C von. Brainstem mechanisms for generation and control of breathing pattern. In: Cherniack NS, Widdicombe JG, eds. *Handbook of physiology. The respiratory system, vol 2: control of breathing.* Bethesda, MD: American Physiological Society, 1986;1–67.
8. Bunn JC, Mead J. Control of ventilation during speech. *J Appl Physiol* 1971;31:870–872.
9. Phillipson EA, McClean PA, Sullivan CE, Zamel N. Interaction of metabolic and behavioral respiratory control during hypercapnia and speech. *Am Rev Respir Dis* 1978;117:903–909.
10. Leanderson R, Sundberg J, Euler C von. Role of diaphragmatic activity during singing: a study of transdiaphragmatic pressures. *J Appl Physiol* 1987;62:259–270.
11. Hobson JA, Steriade M. The neuronal basis of behavioral state control. In: Mountcastle V, ed. *Handbook of physiology, section 1. The nervous system: intrinsic regulatory systems of the brain.* Bethesda, MD: American Physiological Society, 1986;701–823.
12. Asmussen E. Regulation of respiration: "the black box." *Acta Physiol Scand* 1977;99:85–90.
13. Budzinska K, Euler C von, Kao FF, Pantaleo T, Yamamoto Y. Effects of graded focal cold block in rostral areas of the medulla. *Acta Physiol Scand* 1985;124:329–430.
14. Schlaefke ME. Central chemosensitivity: a respiratory drive. *Rev Physiol Biochem Pharmacol* 1981;90:171–244.
15. Adams M, Chonan T, Cherniack NS, Euler C von. Effects on respiratory pattern of focal cooling in the medulla of the dog. *J Appl Physiol* 1988;65:2004–2010.
16. Arita H, Kogo N, Koshiya N. Morphological and physiological properties of caudal medullary expiratory neurons of the cat. *Brain Res* 1987;401:258–266.
17. Haxhiu MA, Lunteren E van, Mitra J, Cherniack NS. Responses and chemical stimulation of upper airway muscles and diaphragm in awake cats. *J Appl Physiol* 1984;56:397.
18. Cherniack NS. Potential role of optimization in alveolar hypoventilation and respiratory instability. In: Euler C von, Lagercrantz H, eds. *Neurobiology of the control of breathing.* New York: Raven Press, 1987;45–50.
19. DiMarco AF, Euler C von, Romaniuk JR, Yamamoto Y. Positive feedback facilitation of external intercostal and phrenic inspiratory activity by pulmonary stretch receptors. *Acta Physiol Scand* 1981;113:375–386.
20. Getting PA. Emerging principles governing the operation of neural networks. *Annu Rev Neurosci* 1989;12:185–204.
21. Forssberg H, Grillner S, Rossignol S. Phase dependent reflex reversal during walking in chronic spinal cats. *Brain Res* 1975;85:103–107.
22. Richter DW, Camerer H, Meesman M. Röhrig N. Studies on the synaptic interconnection between bulbar respiratory neurones of cats. *Pflugers Arch* 1979;380:245–257.
23. Richter DW, Ballantyne D, Remmers JE. The differential organization of medullary post-inspiratory activities. *Pflugers Arch* 1987;410:420–427.
24. Bertrand F, Hugelin A, Vibert JF. A stereologic model of pneumotaxic oscillator based on spatial and temporal distributions of neuronal bursts. *J Neurophysiol* 1974;37:91–107.
25. Camerer H, Richter DW, Röhrig N, Meesmann M. Lung stretch receptor inputs to R-alpha-neurones: a model for "respiratory gating." In: Euler C von, Lagercrantz H, eds. *Central nervous control mechanisms in breathing.* Wenner-Gren International Symposium Series, vol 32. Oxford, England: Pergamon Press, 1979;261–266.
26. Richter DW. Generation and maintenance of the respiratory rhythm. *J Exp Biol* 1982;100:93–107.
27. Richter DW, Ballantyne D. A three phase theory about the basic respiratory pattern generator. In: Schlaefke ME, Koepchen HP, See WR, eds. *Central neurone environment and the control systems of breathing and circulation.* Berlin: Springer-Verlag, 1983;164–174.
28. Richter DW, Ballantyne D, Remmers JE. How is the respiratory rhythm generated? *News Physiol Sci* 1986;1:109–112.
29. Lawson EE, Richter DW, Bischoff AM. Intracellular recordings of respiratory neurons in the lateral medulla of the piglet. *J Appl Physiol* 1989; in press.
30. Nashner LM. Organization and programming of motor activity during posture control. In: Granit R, Pompeiano O, eds. *Reflex control of posture and movement. Progress in Brain Research,* vol 50. Amsterdam: Elsevier, 1979;177–184.
31. Pantaleo T, Corda M. Expiration-related neurons in the region of the retrofacial nucleus: vagal and laryngeal inhibitory influences. *Brain Res* 1985;359:343–346.
32. Baumgarten R von, Kanzow E. The interaction of two types of inspiratory neurons in the region of the tractus solitarius of the cat. *Arch Ital Biol* 1958;96:361–373.
33. Aoki M, Mori S, Kawahara K, Watanabe H, Ebata N. Generation of spontaneous respiratory rhythm in high spinal cats. *Brain Res* 1980;202:51–63.
34. Aoki M, Fujito Y, Kurosawa Y, Kawasaki H, Kosaka I. Descending inputs to the upper cervical inspiratory neurons from the medullary respiratory neurons and the raphe nuclei in the cat. In: Sieck GC, Gandevia SC, Cameron WE, eds. *Respiratory muscles and their neuromotor control.* New York: Raven Press, 1987;73–82.
35. Feldman JL, McCrimmon DR, Speck DF. Effect of synchronous activation of medullary inspiratory bulbo-spinal neurones on phrenic nerve discharge in cat. *J Physiol (Lond)* 1984;347:241–254.
36. Merrill EG. Is there reciprocal inhibition between medullary inspiratory and expiratory neurones? In: Euler C von, Lagercrantz H, eds. *Central nervous control mechanisms in breathing.* Wenner-Gren International Symposium Series, vol 32. Oxford: Pergamon Press, 1979;239–254.
37. Lipski J, Merrill EG. Electrophysiological demonstration of the projection from expiratory neurones in rostral medulla to contralateral dorsal respiratory group. *Brain Res* 1980;197:521–524.
38. Merrill EG, Lipski J, Kubin L, Fedorko L. Origin of the expiratory inhibition of nucleus tractus solitarius inspiratory neurones. *Brain Res* 1983;263:43–50.
39. Fedorko L, Merrill EG. Axonal projections from the rostral expiratory neurones of the Bötzinger complex to medulla and spinal cord in the cat. *J Physiol (Lond)* 1984;350:487–496.
40. Bongianni F, Fontana G, Pantaleo T. Effects of electrical and chemical stimulation of the Bötzinger complex on respiratory activity in the cat. *Brain Res* 1988;445:254–261.
41. Bianchi AL, Barilot JC, Grélot L. Pattern of excitability of respiratory neurons in the region of the retrofacial nucleus. In:

Euler C von, Lagercrantz H, eds. *Neurobiology of the control of breathing*. New York: Raven Press, 1987;149–155.

42. Bianchi AL, Grélot L, Iscoe S, Remmers JE. Electrophysiological properties of rostral medullary respiratory neurones in the cat: an intracellular study. *J Physiol (Lond)* 1988;407:293–310.

43. Grélot L, Bianchi AL, Iscoe S, Remmers JE. Expiratory neurones of the rostral medulla: anatomical and functional correlates. *Neurosci Lett* 1988;89:140–145.

44. Onimaru H, Homma I. Respiratory rhythm generator neurons in medulla of brainstem–spinal cord preparation from newborn rat. *Brain Res* 1987;403:308–384.

45. Budzinska K, Euler C von, Kao FF, Pantaleo T, Yamamoto Y. Effects of graded focal cold block in the solitary and para-ambigual regions of the medulla in the cat. *Acta Physiol Scand* 1985;124:317–328.

46. Morin-Surun M, Champagnat E, Boudinot E, Denavit-Saubié M. Differentiation of two respiratory areas in the cat medulla using kainic acid. *Respir Physiol* 1984;58:323–334.

47. Lindsey BG, Segers LS, Shannon R. Functional associations among simultaneously monitored lateral medullary respiratory neurons in the cat. II. Evidence for inhibitory actions of expiratory neurons. *J Neurophysiol* 1987;57:1101–1117.

48. Budzinska K, Euler C von, Kao FF, Pantaleo T, Yamamoto Y. Release of expiratory muscle activity by graded focal cold block in the medulla. *Acta Physiol Scand* 1985;124:341–351.

49. Vibert JF, Villard MF, Caille D, Foutz AS, Hugelin A. Does a multioscillator system control respiratory frequency independently of ventilation? In: Benchetrit G, Baconnier P, Demongeot J, eds. *Concepts and formalizations in the control of breathing*. Manchester: Manchester University Press, 1987;377–388.

50. Speck DF, Feldman JL. The effect of microstimulation and microlesions in the dorsal and ventral respiratory groups in medulla of cat. *J Neurosci* 1982;2:744–757.

51. Ballantyne D, Richter DW. Post-synaptic inhibition of bulbar inspiratory neurones in the cat. *J Physiol (Lond)* 1984;348:67–88.

52. Ballantyne D, Richter DW. The non-uniform character of expiratory synaptic activity in expiratory bulbospinal neurones of the cat. *J Physiol (Lond)* 1986;370:433–456.

53. Feldman JL, Speck DF. Interactions among inspiratory neurons in dorsal and ventral respiratory groups in cat medulla. *J Neurophysiol* 1983;49:472–490.

54. Hilaire G, Monteau R, Bianchi AL. A cross-correlation study of interactions among respiratory neurons of dorsal, ventral and retrofacial groups in cat medulla. *Brain Res* 1984;302:19–31.

55. Segers LS, Shannon R, Saporta S, Lindsey BG. Functional associations among simultaneously monitored lateral medullary respiratory neurons in the cat. I. Evidence for excitatory and inhibitory actions of inspiratory neurons. *J Neurophysiol* 1987;57:1078–1100.

56. Botros SM, Bruce EN. Neural network implementation of a three-phase model of respiratory rhythm generation. Submitted for publication, 1990.

57. Merrill EG. Finding a respiratory function for the medullary respiratory neurons. In: Bellairs R, Gray EG, eds. *Essays on the nervous system*. Oxford: Clarendon Press, 1974;451–486.

58. Milic-Emili J. Spirometric and airway occlusion waveform. In: Euler C von, Lagercrantz H, eds. *Central nervous control mechanisms in breathing*. Wenner–Gren International Symposium Series, vol 32. Oxford: Pergamon Press, 1979;185–193.

59. Bruce EN, Euler C von, Yamashiro SM. Reflex and central chemoceptive control of the time course of inspiratory activity. In: Euler C von, Lagercrantz H, eds. *Central nervous control mechanisms in breathing*. Wenner–Gren Center International Symposium Series, vol 32. Oxford: Pergamon Press, 1979;177–184.

60. Cohen MI. Neurogenesis of respiratory rhythm in the mammal. *Physiol Rev* 1979;59:1105–1173.

61. Madden KP, Remmers JE. Short time scale correlations between spike activity of neighboring respiratory neurons of nucleus tractus solitarius. *J Neurophysiol* 1982;48:749–760.

62. Euler C von, Trippenbach T. Excitability changes of the inspiratory 'off-switch' mechanism tested by electrical stimulation in nucleus parabrachialis in the cat. *Acta Physiol Scand* 1976;97:175–188.

63. Younes MK, Remmers JE, Baker J. Characteristics of inspiratory inhibition by phasic volume feedback in cats. *J Appl Physiol* 1978;45:80–86.

64. Remmers JE, Baker Jr JP, Younes MK. Graded inspiratory inhibition: the first stage of inspiratory "off-switching." In: Euler C von, Lagercrantz H, eds. *Central nervous control mechanism in breathing*. Wenner–Gren International Symposium Series, vol 32. Oxford: Pergamon Press, 1979;195–201.

65. Bradley GW, Euler C von, Marttila I, Roos B. A model of the central and reflex inhibition of inspiration in the cat. *Biol Cybern* 1975;19:105–116.

66. Feldman JL, Smith JC, McCrimmon DR, Ellenberger HH, Speck DF. Generation of respiratory pattern in mammals. In: Cohen AH, Rossignol S, Grillner S, eds. *Neural control of rhythmic movements in vertebrates*. New York: John Wiley & Sons, 1988;73–100.

67. Feldman JL, Cohen MI. Relation between expiratory duration and rostral medullary expiratory neuronal discharge. *Brain Res* 1978;141:172–178.

68. Cohen MI, Feldman JL. Discharge properties of dorsal medullary inspiratory neurones: relation to pulmonary afferent and phrenic efferent discharge. *J Neurophysiol* 1984;51:753–776.

69. Orem J. The activity of late inspiratory cells during the behavioral inhibition of inspiration. *Brain Res* 1988;458:224–230.

70. Knox CK. Reflex and central mechanisms controlling expiratory duration. In: Euler C von, Lagercrantz H, eds. *Central nervous control mechanisms in breathing*. Wenner–Gren International Symposium Series, vol 32. Oxford: Pergamon Press, 1979;203–216.

71. Bianchi AL, Barillot JC. Respiratory neurons in the region of the retrofacial nucleus: pontile, medullary, spinal and vagal projections. *Neurosci Lett* 1982;31:277–282.

72. Remmers JE, Richter DW, Ballantyne D, Bainton CR, Klein JP. Reflex prolongation of stage I of expiration. *Pflugers Arch* 1986;407:190–198.

73. Long S, Duffin J. The neuronal determinants of respiratory rhythm. *Prog Neurobiol* 1986;27:101–182.

74. Smith JC, Feldman JL. *In vitro* brainstem–spinal cord preparations for study of motor systems for mammalian respiration and locomotion. *J Neurosci Methods* 1987;21:321–333.

75. Grillner S, Wallén P, Dale N, Brodin L, Buchanan J, Hill R. Transmitters, membrane properties and network circuitry in the control of locomotion in lamprey. *Trends Neurosci* 1987;10:34–41.

THE LUNG: Scientific Foundations
edited by R.G. Crystal, J.B. West et al.
Raven Press, Ltd., New York © 1991.

CHAPTER 5.4.2

Cellular Aspects of Peripheral Chemoreceptor Function

Salvatore J. Fidone, Constancio Gonzalez, Bruce Dinger, Angela Gomez-Niño, Ana Obeso, and Katsuaki Yoshizaki

The carotid bodies are small, highly vascularized organs located near the bifurcations of the common carotid arteries. The specialized parenchymal tissue of these arterial chemoreceptors consists of groups or lobules of type I (glomus) cells, which are synaptically innervated by afferent fibers of the carotid sinus nerve (CSN), a branch of the IXth cranial nerve (Fig. 1). The type I cell–afferent nerve terminal complexes are enveloped by slender cytoplasmic processes of type II cells, whose inconspicuous cytoplasm resembles that of Schwann cells. It is on this morphological basis that a glial-like function has been assigned to type II cells in the carotid body. Type I cells, in contrast, display a cytoplasmic composition rich in organelles, including an extensive endoplasmic reticulum, numerous mitochondria, and a variety of dense- and clear-cored synaptic vesicles. The afferent fiber component within the cell lobules consists of specialized bouton and calyciform nerve terminals directly apposed to the type I cells. The morphological relationship between the nerve endings and type I cells fits the criteria established for chemical synapses transmitting centripetally (see ref. 1). However, centrifugal and reciprocal synaptic structures have also been described, suggesting that afferent fibers can modulate type I cell activity via a complex interchange at the synaptic level.

Based upon his meticulous studies of the "glomus caroticum" during the 1920s, De Castro (2,3) concluded that in response to an appropriate natural stimulus, "glomus cells excite the nerve endings through products of their metabolism to produce the conse-

quent reflexes. . . ." This basic notion that the type I cell is the primary transducer, releasing excitatory substances to activate the apposed sensory terminals, has served as a foundation for more than six decades of scientific research on the carotid body. The recent demonstration of the stimulus-evoked release of multiple neurotransmitter agents by type I cells, including acetylcholine (ACh), dopamine (DA), norepinephrine (NE), and the neuropeptides substance P (SP) and met-enkephalin (ME), has bolstered support for De Castro's fundamental hypothesis. Progress made in the past decade has also helped to elucidate some of the mechanisms involved in the chemotransduction of multiple natural stimuli (hypoxia, hypercapnia, low pH) by the type I cell–afferent nerve terminal complex.

In the present chapter, we will focus on the present state of knowledge of chemotransduction and chemotransmission in the carotid body. Although our discussions are limited to this organ, cautious extrapolations may also be made to the mechanisms of chemoreception in the aortic bodies, which are located on large vessels near the heart. Although some historical and background information is included in each section of this chapter, our focus is primarily on those recent findings which serve to illustrate and emphasize what we perceive to be the most salient current issues and ideas relevant to carotid body function. More comprehensive presentations can be found elsewhere (1,4).

SENSORY TRANSDUCTION IN PERIPHERAL CHEMORECEPTORS

Plurimodal Chemoreceptors

It is relevant to the issue of transduction by carotid body type I cells to consider how a single sensory re-

---

S. Fidone, C. Gonzalez, B. Dinger, A. Gomez-Niño, A. Obeso, and K. Yoshizaki: Department of Physiology, University of Utah School of Medicine, Salt Lake City, Utah 84108.

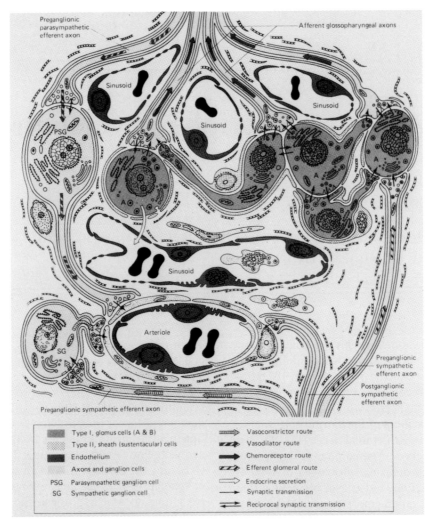

FIG. 1. Cellular, neural, and vascular architecture of the carotid body. (From ref. 115.)

ceptor can respond to multiple stimuli (for the carotid body, these include low O_2, elevated CO_2, decreased pH, osmolarity, temperature, and perhaps others). Important lessons for scientists studying arterial chemoreceptors may be learned from recent findings reported for the plurimodal olfactory and gustatory chemoreceptors, which show that multiple stimuli activate second-messenger-generating enzymes to produce cyclic AMP and/or cyclic GMP (5–7). These cyclic nucleotides depolarize the receptor cell membranes by directly modulating the conductance of specialized potassium channels (8–10). But not all odorants and gustatory stimuli utilize these classical second messengers in the sensory transduction process. Thus, while herbaceous odorants stimulate olfactory adenylate cyclase, putrid odors may not involve second messengers (6). Likewise, sucrose and amino acids activate adenylate cyclase in taste cells (5,11), but taste responses to Na^+ and Li^+ salts are blocked by Na^+ channel blockers (12). Acids, which taste sour, de-

polarize receptor cells by a hydrogen-ion block of K^+ channels (13,14). Because the carotid body is also sensitive to multiple chemical stimuli, it may also utilize diverse transduction mechanisms. Indeed, as described below, at least two distinct transduction mechanisms are likely utilized by the carotid body in responding to hypoxic versus hypercapnic/acidic stimuli, yet both finally elevate intracellular calcium and evoke the release of putative neurotransmitters from the type I cells.

Low O_2 Transduction by the Carotid Body

The oxygen dependence of cellular energy metabolism forms the foundation for the "metabolic hypothesis" of chemoreception, which attempts to explain the sensitivity of the carotid body to low O_2. It proposes that hypoxia lowers the production and content of ATP in the carotid body, which ultimately leads to the release of excitatory transmitters (see ref. 1). The increase in CSN activity produced by metabolic poisons and uncouplers of oxidative metabolism is consistent with such a metabolic basis for hypoxic chemotransduction. Support for this notion also came from early spectrometric and fluorometric studies, which showed that type I cells might contain a cytochrome oxidase with a very low affinity for oxygen, such that it is already reduced by 10–40% at a Po_2 of 140 torr and is completely reduced at a Po_2 of 7–9 torr (15). However, later experiments were unable to confirm the existence of this specialized cytochrome (16,17).

In a recent series of experiments relevant to the metabolic hypothesis, we studied directly the energy metabolism of the carotid body. Exposure of rabbit carotid bodies *in vitro* to a moderate low-O_2 stimulus, which had no effect on ATP levels in the superior cervical ganglion, significantly depressed the content of ATP in the glomus tissue (18). This low-O_2 stimulus also increased the uptake of the glucose analogue $[^3H]$-2-deoxyglucose ($[^3H]$-2DG) by the carotid body, and in autoradiographic studies we identified the type I cells as the primary site of glucose metabolism in this organ (19). Cyanide (10^{-4} M) decreased the ATP content of the carotid body and induced a corresponding increase in the release of the putative neurotransmitter, DA, as well as causing excitation of the CSN (18).

Although the data cited above are consistent with increased energy utilization by carotid body type I cells under conditions of reduced ambient O_2, they do not identify the transducing mechanism(s) within the tissue which is responsible for triggering this increased metabolism. In other nervous tissues, physiological stimulation has been shown to increase $[^3H]$-2DG uptake as a consequence of activation of the Na–K pump, which acts to restore ionic gradients following membrane depolarization (20). In the carotid body, we have found that ouabain, an inhibitor of Na,K-ATPase, eliminates the increased $[^3H]$-2DG uptake associated with hypoxia (*unpublished observations*). These findings suggest that metabolic activation of the carotid body by low O_2, leading to a decrease in tissue ATP content, is the consequence of membrane depolarization. It is noteworthy that the ability of cyanide to depress ATP levels is not mimicked by other uncoupling agents [dinitrophenol (DNP) and carbonyl cyanide *m*-chlorophenyl hydrazone (CCCP)] which also act as chemostimulants (21). Thus, the metabolic changes initiated by hypoxia appear to be secondary to antecedent transductive events which induce depolarization of type I cells without initially disturbing mitochondrial ATP production.

The notion that type I cells are depolarized by natural stimuli has received additional support from recent neurochemical and electrophysiological experiments by Obeso et al. (21,22), who demonstrated a Ca^{2+} dependence for $[^3H]$catecholamine ($[^3H]$CA) release from the carotid body. They showed that more than 95% of the release evoked by hypoxia was blocked in Ca^{2+}-free superfusion media and that nitrendipine, an organic blocker of voltage-dependent Ca^{2+} channels, inhibited 87% of the $[^3H]$CA release evoked *in vitro* by moderate hypoxic stimuli (22). These findings suggest that the stimulus-evoked release of CA from the carotid body follows depolarization of the type I cells and Ca^{2+} entry via voltage-dependent Ca^{2+} channels. Experiments demonstrating $^{22}Na^+$ influx (23) and $[^3H]$CA release (24) by veratridine also suggest the presence of voltage-dependent Na^+ channels in type I cells which may be directly involved in membrane depolarization.

Until recently, relatively little was known about the electrical properties of type I and type II cells in the carotid body. Early microelectrode studies reported that type I cells were inexcitable (see ref. 25), but the low resting potentials reported suggested that electrode impalement may have routinely damaged these small cells. This interpretation has now been supported by three separate laboratories using whole-cell patch-clamp studies of dissociated type I cells, in which action potentials and time-dependent voltage-gated ionic currents have been demonstrated following the establishment of ultra-high-resistance seals ($>1 \times 10^9$ ohm). In these studies, Duchen et al. (26), Urena et al. (27), and Hescheler et al. (28,29) patch-clamped cells dissociated from adult rabbit carotid bodies or cultured embryonic tissue and independently observed voltage-dependent inward currents consisting of a fast inactivating, tetrodotoxin (TTX)-sensitive Na^+ current and a slowly inactivating Ca^{2+} current which was blocked by Co^{2+} and Cd^{2+}. The depolarizing actions of these Na^+ and Ca^{2+} channels were countered by voltage-dependent K^+ currents which activated and inactivated more slowly. The full activation of the K^+ current was found to be dependent on the presence of Ca^{2+} in the bathing solution, suggesting that at least part of the K^+ conductance is Ca^{2+}-dependent, a finding common to many types of excitable cells (e.g., see ref. 30). The smaller type II cells of the carotid body did not generate action potentials, and depolarization of these cells applied via the whole-cell patch-clamp technique evoked only slowly activating K^+ currents (26,27).

Although there has been general agreement regarding many of the electrophysiological properties of the type I cells, the role of specialized membrane channels in the chemotransduction of hypoxic stimuli remains controversial. Diverse views have been set forth with respect to the initial effects of low-O_2 stimuli on the biophysics of these cells. Lopez-Lopez et al. (31,32) and Hescheler et al. (28,29) compared membrane currents in control (normoxic) versus hypoxic bathing media and reported that the K⁺ conductance of type I cells was reversibly reduced by 28–50% at P_{O_2} levels below 100 torr (see Fig. 2). In contrast, hypoxia did not alter the Na⁺ and Ca²⁺ currents in type I cells (28,31,32), and K⁺ currents in type II cells or in dispersed septal neurons were also unaffected by hypoxia (31). Furthermore, in the current-clamp mode, Lopez-Lopez et al. (31) reported that hypoxia increased the rate of spontaneous depolarization and the frequency of action potential generation. These effects suggest that decreased ambient O₂ inactivates some K⁺ channels, resulting in an increase of cell input resistance and a rapid spontaneous depolarization (pacemaker potential). Lopez-Lopez et al. (31) concluded that both the increased firing frequency and action potential size induced by low O₂ should enhance the entry of Ca²⁺, thereby leading to neurotransmitter release from type I cells during hypoxia.

In similar experiments, Biscoe and Duchen (33) found that cyanide (CN⁻), a classical chemostimulant, produced a hyperpolarization of type I cells and decreased action potential frequency. These investigators also reported that CN⁻ reduced the Ca²⁺ current and increased a Ca²⁺-dependent K⁺ current, which was 60% inhibited by 2 mM Co²⁺ (26). These findings are not in agreement with those of Lopez-Lopez et al. (31), and they call into question the notion that hypoxia and CN⁻ stimulate chemoreceptors via the same mechanism. In more recent publications, Biscoe et al. (34,35) have used intracellular Ca²⁺ fluorescent dyes to measure changes in free cytoplasmic Ca²⁺ under different stimulus conditions. As expected, they found that CN⁻ produced a rise in Ca²⁺ᵢ when the cells were bathed in normal Ca²⁺, and "in six out of eleven prepa-

rations, the response was still present soon after removal of Ca²⁺ₒ, but was smaller than control. In the remainder, Ca²⁺ᵢ fell rapidly on removal of Ca²⁺ₒ and no increase could be seen in response to CN⁻" (34). On the basis of these findings with CN⁻, these investigators proposed an intracellular origin for the Ca²⁺ which was responsible for the observed rise in free cytoplasmic Ca²⁺. They suggested that the electrophysiological responses of type I cells to hypoxia are not central to the transduction process (35). As additional support for their hypothesis, they offer the fact that TTX does not block the increase in Ca²⁺ᵢ produced by hypoxia. In this context, it should be mentioned that it is well established that acetylcholine depolarizes adrenomedullary cells, generates action potentials, and promotes a secretory response totally dependent on extracellular Ca²⁺; yet TTX, an established blocker of action potentials, only moderately reduces this secretory response (36). Similarly in the carotid body, Rocher et al. (37) recently showed that the CA release evoked by hypoxia is only moderately decreased by TTX. Additionally, in proposing an intracellular source for the increase in free cytoplasmic Ca²⁺, Biscoe et al. (34,35) suggested that mitochondria release Ca²⁺ upon stimulation by CN⁻ or hypoxia, which assumes that type I cell mitochondria are uniquely specialized to this task; under physiological conditions, mitochondria in other cells do not play a role in the control of cytoplasmic free Ca²⁺ (38,39).

One possible interpretation, supported by two independent research groups (28,29,31,32), implicates the electrical properties of type I cells in the O₂ transduction process, and this interpretation is in line with findings reported for other secretory cells. The alter-

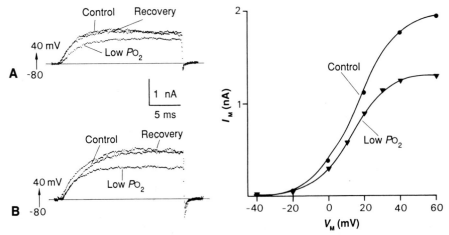

FIG. 2. Effect of lowering P_{O_2} from 150 mmHg on K⁺ currents in the absence of internal ATP and Ca²⁺. Response to test solutions with 110 mmHg (low P_{O_2}) (**A**) and 10 mmHg (low P_{O_2}) (**B**). Recovery traces were recorded 3 min after restoration of normal (150 mmHg) P_{O_2}. (**C**) Current–voltage (I_M–V_M) curves for control (●; P_{O_2} = 150 mmHg) and test (▼; P_{O_2} = 10 mmHg) solutions. Current amplitude was measured at the end of the 20-msec voltage steps. (From ref. 32. Copyright 1988 by the AAAS.)

native proposal by Biscoe and co-workers (33–35) is also supported by electrophysiological data as well as by measurements of intracellular Ca^{2+}. It is hoped that further experimentation will permit a resolution of these conflicting sets of data and reveal the actual transductive cascade of events in the hypoxic response by the type I cells.

Transduction of High CO_2 and Low pH

Torrance and co-workers (40) were the first to propose that the ability of the carotid body to respond to increased CO_2 resided within cellular elements containing carbonic anhydrase, the enzyme which combines CO_2 with water to form carbonic acid. This hypothesis was based upon the ability of acetazolamide, an inhibitor of the enzyme, to depress the CO_2 response recorded from the CSN. These investigators also showed that another carbonic anhydrase inhibitor, benzolamide, which is less effective in crossing cell membranes, was also less effective in inhibiting the CO_2-evoked activity. This suggested that the enzyme was located intracellularly within carotid body elements, but its exact distribution amongst type I cells, type II cells, or afferent nerve terminals was unknown at that time. Recent histochemical studies have demonstrated that the enzyme is localized to the type I cells of the organ, as expected (41,42). It has also been found that acetazolamide causes a 50% reduction in the release of CA evoked by high P_{CO_2} (Gonzalez et al., *unpublished observations*). These observations clearly reinforce the notion that type I cells act as transducer elements for CO_2 stimuli, and they emphasize the likelihood that increased intracellular H^+ ion concentration in type I cells is the common event in the response to CO_2 and pH. This interpretation received further support from recent experiments showing that elevation of intracellular pH in the carotid body evokes the release of CA. In these studies, the metabolic uncouplers DNP and CCCP were used as protonophores to allow H^+ ions to come into electrochemical equilibrium across the mitochondrial and cytoplasmic membranes (21). Assuming a plasma membrane potential of -60 mV, the intracellular pH under these conditions will tend to move to 6.4. However, biochemical assay showed that ATP levels in these carotid bodies were unchanged in the presence of DNP and CCCP, apparently due to the use of only moderate concentrations of these drugs (21), which thereby only partially uncoupled mitochondrial oxidative phosphorylation. Thus, the activation of type I cells and CA release could not be attributed to a decreased high-energy phosphate potential.

Although these experiments established intracellular pH as an important determinant of type I cell activity, they did not reveal the mechanism(s) linking H^+ ions to transmitter release. Further experimentation with the uncouplers and the CO_2 stimulus, however, showed that the evoked CA release was inhibited by about 80% in the absence of extracellular Ca^{2+} (Gonzalez et al., *unpublished observations*), indicating that Ca^{2+} entry is coupled to increased H^+ concentration. The participation of voltage-sensitive Ca^{2+} channels in this process appeared unlikely because the uncouplers are purported not to modify membrane potential (43). And, in fact, it was found that the Ca^{2+} channel antagonist nisoldipine failed to inhibit CA release evoked by high P_{CO_2} or DNP (Gonzalez et al., *unpublished observations*). Thus, in response to these stimuli, Ca^{2+} appears to enter via alternate pathways which may be coupled to elevated intracellular H^+ concentration. Depolarization by acidic stimuli seems unlikely because although it has been reported that on lowering pH the O_2-sensitive K^+ current is reduced (31), recent findings by the same investigators (*personal communication*) show an identical pH-dependent reduction of the Na^+ and Ca^{2+} currents.

A plausible mechanism for elevation of intracellular $[Ca^{2+}]$ in response to an H^+ load was proposed by Gonzalez et al. (44), who showed that ethyl isopropyl amiloride (EIPA), a compound which blocks Na^+–H^+ exchange across the cell membrane, inhibits DNP-induced CA release by 55%. The implication that Na^+ enters cells in response to elevated $[H^+]$ supports the notion that Ca^{2+} gains access to the cell via the Na^+–Ca^{2+} exchange mechanism common to a great variety of cells, including squid axons and neuroblastoma cells, where under resting conditions it contributes to the low (10^{-7} M) internal $[Ca^{2+}]$ (see ref. 45). In this exchange system, however, the direction of net Ca^{2+} flux can be reversed depending on the electrochemical gradients for both Na^+ and Ca^{2+} across the plasma membrane. Gonzalez et al. (44) have therefore proposed that an acidic load is followed by activation of the Na^+–H^+ exchanger (see ref. 43), which moves Na^+ in and H^+ out of the cell; as a consequence, the concentration of intracellular Na^+ increases, which, in turn, reverses the extrusion of Ca^{2+}, thereby initiating the critical increase in $[Ca^{2+}]_i$ (see ref. 45) necessary for transmitter release. Direct evidence in support of this scheme is currently unavailable; however, it may be possible to test this hypothesis by evaluating Na^+ and Ca^{2+} fluxes in type I cells.

CHEMICAL TRANSMISSION BETWEEN TYPE I CELLS AND AFFERENT NERVE TERMINALS

The elegant studies of De Castro (3) and Heymans et al. (46) described the salient structural and sensory properties of the arterial chemosensory tissue of the mammalian carotid body; these studies set the stage for contemporary research on chemotransmission by suggesting that type I (glomus) cells excite closely apposed afferent nerve terminals by releasing transmitter agents in response to natural stimuli. This fundamental tenet of carotid body physiology has endured numerous challenges for more than half a century, and today, following the discoveries of multiple neurotransmitter agents in type I cells, it has emerged as a central theme in research on arterial chemoreception. Current views hold that chemosensation very probably involves the concerted actions of multiple neuroactive agents, and that each of these agents plays a role in the generation and/or modulation of the chemosensory response. Although there is little consensus regarding the complex synaptic events which occur between type I cells and afferent terminals, considerable progress has been made through the utilization of increasingly more powerful neurochemical and electrophysiological techniques and the development of greatly refined experimental preparations. The present discussion focuses on recent experimental evidence which is relevant to the functional roles of biogenic amines (DA, NE, and ACh) and neuropeptides (enkephalins, SP) in chemoreception.

Dopamine

Biochemical Studies

DA is the predominant carotid-body CA in many species and is abundant in all, and its localization to the type I cells is firmly established (see ref. 1). Its synthetic and rate-limiting enzyme, tyrosine hydroxylase (TH), has been measured in several species, and the presence of L-aromatic amino acid decarboxylase, although not directly assayed, is inferred from the fact that the in vitro carotid body is able to synthesize DA from dihydroxyphenylalanine (dopa) (47). The mechanisms for DA uptake and catabolism in the carotid body have been recently characterized (48), and the presence of dopaminergic receptors (D-2) on the sensory nerve endings as well as on the type I cells has also been described (49–51).

Numerous studies have characterized the metabolism of DA in the carotid body, particularly as it relates to natural and pharmacological stimuli. Short-term low P_{O_2} stimulation in vivo is accompanied by a decrease in carotid-body DA content (52); also, in vitro incubation of carotid bodies previously exposed to hypoxic conditions in vivo reveals an increase in [^{3}H]DA synthesis from [^{3}H]tyrosine (53,54). Long-term exposure to hypoxia produces a marked increase in DA content despite an accompanying increase in DA turnover, in-

dicating that synthesis exceeds utilization (55,56). Induction of TH in the carotid body is also observed in response to hypoxia (57–59). Perhaps the most convincing data implicating DA involvement in the response of the carotid body to natural stimuli have been obtained from the in vitro preparation, where studies with both the rabbit and cat carotid bodies (54,60) have demonstrated that low-P_{O_2}-induced release of DA is proportional to both the stimulus intensity and the neural response recorded from the CSN. Shaw et al. (61) have recently confirmed these observations in the rat. The Ca^{2+} dependency of the low-O_2 response is such that DA release is reduced by more than 90% in Ca^{2+}-free media, although CSN activity is reduced by only 50%, suggesting either (a) the involvement of other transmitters or mechanisms in the chemoresponse or (b) the existence of a safety factor for nerve impulse generation arising from convergence and summation of sensory potentials at branch points of afferent fibers (see ref. 60 for discussion). Besides low P_{O_2}, a combination of low pH and high P_{CO_2} has also been shown to increase DA release in proportion to CSN activity (62,63), and the Ca^{2+} dependency of this response has also been demonstrated (unpublished observations). In addition to natural stimuli, pharmacological chemostimulants of CSN activity (e.g., nicotine, cyanide, metabolic uncouplers, and 2-deoxyglucose) are also known to increase DA release in a dose-dependent manner (21,64–66).

Pharmacological Studies

Although the pharmacological action of exogenously administered DA has been shown to be inhibitory to CSN discharge, some important findings in these studies suggest that such exogenous DA may have multiple effects on the carotid body. In the cat preparation in vivo, for instance, although the principal action of DA is to depress CSN discharge, there is commonly observed a delayed excitatory rebound from DA depression that is especially pronounced at higher doses of DA (67,68). In these studies and in another by Nishi (69), it was shown that dopaminergic blockers, including spiroperidol, α-flupenthixol, and haloperidol, converted the inhibitory action of DA into excitation. Okajima and Nishi (70), also studying the cat, reported that intracarotid injections of DA produced inhibition followed by excitation, depending on the dose and interval between DA injections. In the in vitro cat carotid-body preparation, Zapata (71) made a detailed study of DA actions on the chemoreceptor activity of the CSN, and he reported that of 88 DA injections, 27 (31%) produced pure excitatory effects and 29 (33%) produced pure inhibitory effects. For 16 injections (18%) he observed inhibition followed by excitation, and for the remaining 16 injections (18%) there was no effect. He also found that the excitatory response was slower in onset and longer in duration, and in all the preparations which exhibited an inhibitory response, repeated injections of DA transformed the inhibition into excitation.

In their initial studies of this problem, Donnelly et al. (72) observed that haloperidol potentiated the *in vivo* response to hypoxia, and they concluded that DA had an inhibitory role in the cat carotid body. However, these same investigators (73) later reported that superfusion of the *in vitro* cat carotid-body preparation with haloperidol nearly abolished basal CSN activity, and they consequently proposed that DA might actually play an excitatory role. They attributed their earlier findings to vascular effects. DA consistently produces excitation *in vitro* in the carotid body of the rabbit (74–77), whereas DA actions *in vivo* in this animal are similar to those observed in the cat, producing mostly inhibition of CSN activity (78; also Monti-Bloch and Eyzaguirre, *personal communication*).

Leitner et al. (76), working with carotid bodies excised from reserpinized rabbits, found that the basal (normoxic) chemoreceptor discharge was very low (about one-sixth of that in nonreserpinized animals) and that the response to low P_{O_2} was very slow in onset and low in amplitude. Superfusion of these reserpinized organs with relatively high concentrations of DA (100 μM) (see ref. 74) led to activation of the CSN and partial restoration of the response to hypoxia. In a later publication using normal, unreserpinized rabbit carotid bodies *in vitro* (74), these investigators confirmed an excitatory action for DA at any concentration of this CA that produced a CSN response. At 10 μM DA, only four of nine trials yielded CSN activation (the remainder showed no change in neural activity), whereas at 100 μM and higher concentrations, powerful excitation was consistently observed. On the other hand, neither haloperidol nor (+)butaclamol (each at 0.5 μM) blocked the responses to 100 μM DA (unfortunately, results with lower DA concentrations were not reported) or to hypoxia, but in some trials these blockers produced a reduction in the response to high P_{CO_2} which lasted more than 5 min after exposure to the drug. It should be noted that hypoxic and hypercapnic media similar to that used by Leitner and Roumy (74) have been shown to have very different effects on DA release (8-fold versus 0.5- to 1-fold increase above control release with low O_2 versus high CO_2, respectively; ref. 60 and *unpublished observations*). Thus, use of the dopaminergic blockers at 0.5 μM was effective only when the concentration of DA in the intraglomic milieu was low. In a later paper, Leitner and Roumy (75) extended their study with reserpinized carotid bodies to the cat, with results identical to those for the rabbit. They further observed that

α-methyl-*p*-tyrosine pretreatment produced effects on the hypoxic response which were similar to those of reserpine, and they found also that this drug markedly reduced the response to high CO_2.

From these experiments, Leitner and Roumy (75) concluded that DA does more than simply inhibit CSN activity. Vascular effects must be considered when dealing with dopaminergic agents (79), and it must be conceded that the carotid-body vasculature is likely exposed to the overflow of released DA at concentrations set by the prevailing P_{O_2} and P_{CO_2}–pH and by other stimulants. Furthermore, DA receptors (D-2) in the carotid body are located both on the type I cells (presynaptic autoreceptors?) and on the sensory nerve endings [postsynaptic (49,51)]. This is pertinent to the studies described earlier in which exogenously administered DA evoked complex responses that were characterized early in the experiment by rapid inhibition followed by slow excitation but that later evolved into purely excitatory responses with repeated administration of DA. Such responses might be expected if the two populations of DA receptors mentioned above corresponded to inhibitory presynaptic autoreceptors and excitatory postsynaptic receptors. For the brain, in fact, according to Siggins (80), "... it is reasonable to expect that the 'lowest dose' response of neurons to bath-applied transmitters might reflect more presynaptic mechanisms than the response to higher transmitter concentrations. There is now evidence that presynaptic receptors might be the most sensitive to neurotransmitters. ... Extrasynaptic (spare) receptors might also be expected to be exposed to lower transmitter levels and therefore to be more sensitive than subsynaptic receptors." In accord with these ideas, considerable evidence suggests that presynaptic autoreceptors inhibit DA release in the brain (see ref. 81).

In recent experiments we have tested the possibility that DA autoreceptors located on type I cells in the carotid body modulate the release of DA. Figure 3 shows the [^{3}H]CA release from rabbit (Fig. 3A) and cat (Fig. 3B) carotid bodies and also shows the effects of D-2 receptor antagonists. Moderate doses of the butyrophenone, spiperone, caused a marked elevation of the basal [^{3}H]CA release from rabbit carotid bodies incubated in media equilibrated with 100% O_2. Furthermore, in the presence of spiperone the [^{3}H]CA release evoked by superfusion media equilibrated with 10% O_2 was elevated by 264% ± 29% ($\bar{X}$ ± SEM; $p < 0.001$, compared to [^{3}H]CA release in the absence of the drug). High-pressure liquid chromatography (HPLC) analysis showed that the increased [^{3}H]CA release was almost exclusively [^{3}H]DA. Experiments with a similar D-2 receptor antagonist, haloperidol, in cat carotid bodies have provided similar results (Fig. 3B). These new findings suggest that the process of

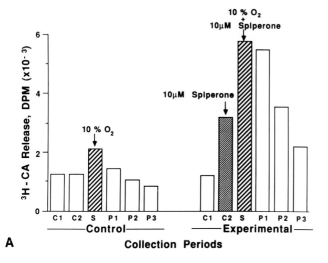

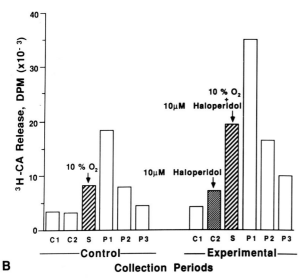

FIG. 3. The time course of basal and stimulus evoked [³H]catecholamine ([³H]CA) release from rabbit (**A**) and cat (**B**) carotid bodies. Each bar represents the [³H]CA release during a 10-min superfusion period *in vitro.* Basal [³H]CA release was evaluated in media equilibrated with 100% O_2. The left side of each panel shows the excess [³H]CA release evoked by an exposure to media equilibrated with 10% O_2. In a second stimulus cycle (shown by the right side of each panel), the effects of spiperone (**A**) or haloperidol (**B**) were evaluated under basal and stimulus conditions. See text for explanation.

DA release from type I cells is continuously modulated via feedback inhibition mediated by D-2 autoreceptors. Consequently, the ability of exogenously applied DA to inhibit CSN activity could result from its actions at inhibitory autoreceptors that may be more accessible and/or sensitive to dopaminergic drugs. In fact, in a much earlier publication, Llados and Zapata (82) showed that following the application of spiperone, DA became an excitatory agent in the cat carotid body (Fig. 4). Although the available data fall short of proving that endogenous DA directly excites CSN termi-

nals, they are nonetheless suggestive; at the very least they demonstrate the difficulties inherent in the pharmacological approach to the problem of chemotransmission.

Norepinephrine

The early studies of NE actions in the carotid body (reviewed in refs. 1, 83, and 84) established that this CA produced hyperventilation; they also established that this effect was mediated by the carotid body, because it was abolished after CSN transection. The NE effects were mimicked by isoproterenol and blocked by propranolol, thereby implicating β-adrenergic receptor mediation. More recently (85), it has been shown that isoproterenol activates CSN activity throughout the entire physiological range of blood P_{O_2} and P_{CO_2}. Folgering et al. (86) reported similar findings in the rabbit and cat and also showed that $β_1$-antagonists depress the response to hypoxia. However, because these studies were conducted *in vivo,* the possibility that the drug effects were mediated by changes in blood flow in the carotid body rather than by direct actions on type I cells and/or nerve endings could not be eliminated. In addition, the apparent absence of stimulus-induced changes in NE turnover and utilization (see ref. 1) have further hampered conceptual progress with regard to the function of this CA in chemoreception.

Recent experiments, however, have reexamined the possible role of NE in chemoreception by measuring the release of CAs (synthesized from [³H]tyrosine) from carotid bodies superfused *in vitro.* Gomez-Niño et al. (87) used chronically sympathectomized rabbit carotid bodies to eliminate the sympathetic (NE-containing) nerve terminals from the chemosensory tissue. Their results showed that although only a small percentage of the release evoked by hypoxia was due to [³H]NE (the remainder was largely [³H]DA plus its metabolite, [³H]DOPAC), its absolute concentration in the superfusion media was nonetheless approximately doubled by the stimulus. Shaw et al. (61) confirmed these results using rat carotid bodies *in vitro,* and they further showed that the release of NE was Ca^{2+}-dependent, suggesting that as with DA release, the secretion of NE in response to hypoxia may be initiated by membrane depolarization. In other experiments, Gomez-Niño et al. (87) demonstrated that while hypoxia evoked the release of DA and NE approximately in proportion to their content in the rabbit carotid body (DA/NE ≃ 10), the release of CA in response to 50 μM nicotine was comprised of >90% NE. The finding that nicotine evokes the preferential release of NE suggests the existence of differential mechanisms for the mo-

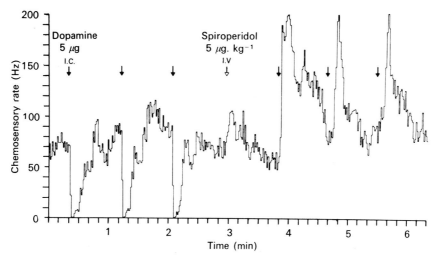

FIG. 4. Changes in chemosensory activity elicited by 5 μg dopamine hydrochloride (*solid arrows*) injected at approximately 1-min intervals, before and after spiroperidol (5 μg·kg⁻¹) (*open arrow*). *Ordinate:* Frequency of carotid nerve discharges, in hertz (impulses per second). *Each horizontal trace:* Frequency counted for 1-sec period. (From ref. 82.)

bilization of CAs in the carotid body, as discussed below.

Cholinergic Receptor Coupling to Catecholamine Release

The finding that nicotine evokes a unique profile of NE and DA release raises fundamental questions regarding the role played by endogenous ACh and cholinergic receptors in chemoreception. Eyzaguirre and co-workers (83,88), who championed ACh as the chemosensory transmitter more than 20 years ago, demonstrated that natural stimuli evoked the release of an ACh-like substance from the cat carotid body. More recently, receptor binding experiments using the nicotinic ligand alpha-bungarotoxin (α-BGT) and the muscarinic ligand quinuclidinylbenzilate (QNB) have revealed cholinergic receptor populations in cat and rabbit carotid bodies (89,90). The results of these studies can be summarized as follows: (a) Nicotinic sites are approximately 10 times more abundant in the carotid body of the cat than in that of the rabbit; (b) muscarinic receptor density in the rabbit is nearly double that in the cat; (c) chronic CSN-denervation does not modify either the number of α-BGT or QNB binding sites; and (d) chronic sympathectomy of the carotid body (10–14 days prior removal of the superior cervical ganglion) in the cat reduces by about 50% the number of α-BGT binding sites (the number of QNB binding sites remains unchanged), whereas in the rabbit about 50% of the QNB binding sites are lost with sympathectomy. Thus, chronic sympathectomy in each species halves the density of the dominant cho-

linergic receptor subtype (because of the very small number of α-BGT binding sites in the rabbit carotid body, the binding of this ligand was not assessed in sympathectomized rabbits). Such species differences for cholinergic receptor subtypes are not unique to the carotid body; the adrenal medulla also manifests species differences with regard to both (a) the relative density of nicotinic versus muscarinic receptors and (b) the purported functional roles of these receptor subtypes in the carotid body (91). However, it is important to note that in the carotid body, αBGT may not bind to the "classical" nicotinic receptor site, because we have observed (*unpublished observations*) that at saturation, binding α-BGT reduces the nicotine-induced release of CA by only 50%, whereas mecamylamine and hexamethonium block this release by more than 95%. This point notwithstanding, there is nonetheless a good correlation between (a) the density of α-BGT binding in the cat and rabbit and (b) the potency of nicotine in increasing both CA release and CSN discharge (77). It thus appears that whichever receptor molecule binds α-BGT in the carotid body, it has a density comparable to that of the "classical" nicotinic receptor.

The different pharmacological effects of cholinergic drugs in the cat versus rabbit carotid body appear to be related to the relative proportions of nicotinic versus muscarinic receptors in these species. In the cat, ACh is a potent stimulant of CSN activity both *in vivo* and *in vitro,* and its effectiveness is reduced in Ca^{2+}-free and/or high-Mg^{2+} superfusion media (83,92). Likewise, nicotine promotes release of CA from the cat carotid body in a Ca^{2+}-dependent manner (22), and mecamylamine completely blocks this nicotine-induced release (*unpublished observations*) and also blocks the accompanying CSN discharge (see ref. 84). Muscarinic agonists, on the other hand, do not modify basal CSN activity in the cat (84); their effect on CA release is unknown. In the rabbit carotid body, nicotine only weakly increases CSN activity and CA release, and mecamylamine completely blocks this response (87; also, *unpublished observations*). In contrast, muscarinic agonists markedly reduce both the basal and nicotine-evoked release of CA (93), as well as the basal and nicotine-induced increase in CSN activity in the rabbit carotid body (94; also, *unpublished observations*). In summary, cholinergic receptors in the cat carotid body are primarily nicotinic, and nicotine (as well as ACh) activates both CA release and CSN discharge; in the rabbit, however, muscarinic receptors dominate and muscarinic agonists (as well as ACh) depress both CA release and CSN discharge.

In spite of the wealth of available data, the precise physiological role of ACh in chemotransmission remains ill-defined. Although some evidence indicates that ACh is released from type I cells, there are no data to show that it can directly excite the sensory nerve terminals. For one thing, most, if not all, cholinergic receptors in both the rabbit and cat carotid body are located on the presynaptic element (i.e., the type I cells); any receptors on the postsynaptic element (i.e., the sensory nerve endings) are not revealed in studies which compare [^{125}I]-αBGT (or [^{3}H]QNB) binding in normal versus CSN-denervated organs (89,90). However, it must be conceded that while αBGT binds to nicotinic receptors on skeletal muscle end-plates, its high-affinity binding sites in central and peripheral nervous tissues may not be equivalent to functional nicotinic receptors. On the other hand, some insights pertinent to chemotransmission in the carotid body may be obtained from a consideration of the profile of CA release induced by nicotine in the cat versus rabbit carotid bodies. In the cat carotid body, nicotine evokes the release of NE and DA in amounts proportional to their nearly equal stores in the tissue (*unpublished observations*). On the other hand, as mentioned earlier, nicotine induces a markedly preferential release of NE over DA from the rabbit carotid body (87), despite the fact that the NE content in this organ is very low in comparison to the DA content (see ref. 1). Consequently, the small nicotine-evoked CSN discharge in the rabbit correlates better with the release of DA than with the release of NE. Taken together, these findings point to an important coupling between cholinergic and catecholaminergic systems in the carotid body, and they are consistent with a prominent role for DA in chemotransmission.

The Role of Opiate and Tachykinin Peptides in Chemotransmission

Opiate Peptides

The enkephalins have been localized to the type I cells, where they appear to be co-stored with CA in dense-cored granules (95). Short-term exposure to hypoxia reduces enkephalin levels in the rabbit carotid body by 40–50%, as does chronic sensory or sympathetic denervation of the organ. These findings suggest that opioid peptides are released from type I cells by natural stimuli and that their metabolism may be regulated by the neural innervation to the organ (96). Opioid peptide processing in the carotid body is unusual: Nearly 80% of opioid activity is in the form of Met- and Leu-enkephalins (ME, LE), whereas only 20% is contained in precursor molecules (97). These findings are correlated with significant levels of carboxypeptidase E in the carotid body; interestingly, denervation of the organ reduces the levels of this processing enzyme by about 50%. Also, the sensory and sympathetic innervation to the carotid body appear to exert long-term control over opioid levels through regulation of the processing of higher-molecular-weight precursor molecules (R. Rigual, *unpublished observations*).

Kirby and McQueen (98) reported that the chemodepressant actions of opioids on cat chemoreceptors *in vivo* are mediated by a delta-type receptor; this is consistent with the finding that ME, which exhibits its greatest affinity toward delta receptors, is the most abundant peptide in the carotid body. McQueen's group has found that opioid agonists depress the response to hypoxia, although under normoxic conditions opioid antagonists have little effect on basal CSN activity. Monti-Bloch and Eyzaguirre (99) observed similar effects *in vitro*. These results suggest that the opioid peptides are effective modulators of CSN activity only when the receptor is activated, which agrees with the finding that delta-receptor antagonists increase chemoreceptor sensitivity to hypoxia (98). Monti-Bloch and Eyzaguirre (99) also found that 10^{-6} M ME markedly depressed the excitatory action of ACh in the cat carotid body, and we have found (*unpublished observations*) that this opioid peptide inhibits the nicotine-induced release of CA. This latter observation suggests that type I cell function may be directly influenced by endogenous opioid peptides. The possibility that these peptides also act at other sites, such as on sensory or sympathetic nerve terminals, has not yet been explored. In this regard, studies on the autoradiographic localization of delta receptors in the carotid body, as well as on the effects of opiates on second messenger levels and ionic conductances in type I cells, should be of great interest. Finally, Kummer and co-workers (100) have observed in guinea-pig carotid bodies that type I cells exhibit dynorphin-like immunoreactivity; however, the ID_{50} for dynorphin-induced chemosensory inhibition is about 70 times higher than that for ME (98).

Substance P

The presence of SP in intraglomic sensory fibers as well as type I cells has recently been confirmed, and this peptide is sometimes found to coexist with dynorphin (101,102). In addition, Prabhakar et al. (103) have demonstrated the coexistence of the related tachykinin, neurokinin A, in type I cells. As shown for the opiates, acute exposure of awake rabbits to hypoxia reduces carotid body SP by 40% (96); however, in anesthetized, artificially ventilated cats, hypoxia elevates the levels of SP (103). In rabbits, chronic CSN denervation (12–14 days) results in a marked increase in SP, but chronic sympathectomy (also 12–14 days) fails to change basal SP levels (96). The results of this latter study emphasize the dual regulatory control over carotid body neurotransmitters via the sensory and sympathetic innervation to the organ, and they are reminiscent of those previously reported for regulation of carotid body TH levels (58).

With some exceptions, there is general agreement regarding the actions of SP and its antagonists on CSN activity. Prabhakar et al. (104,105) confirmed the excitatory action of SP earlier described by McQueen's group (106), but they further made the important observation that SP antagonists blocked the response to hypoxia, thereby raising great expectations for this peptide as the candidate primary neurotransmitter in the carotid body. With their *in vitro* cat carotid-body preparation, Monti-Bloch and Eyzaguirre (99) observed that SP had a mixed excitatory/inhibitory effect (depending on dose) on the response to low Po_2. In addition, McQueen and Evrard (107) have recently reported that certain SP antagonists have no effect on the hypoxic response of the carotid body *in vivo*. Prabhakar and co-workers (105,108) have emphasized the need for adequate doses (in addition to continuous infusions of the antagonist) to inhibit the excitatory effects of SP and hypoxia. McQueen (106) also showed that SP inhibited the ACh-evoked response from the cat CSN *in vivo*, but this response was augmented *in vitro* (99).

The mechanism of action of SP in the carotid body remains uncertain, and assumptions that it produces its effects exclusively at the type I cell–nerve terminal complex via specific neurotransmitter receptors may

be premature. It needs to be recalled that SP is a potent vasodilator in many vascular beds, and that tachyphylaxis develops rapidly with repeated injections of this peptide (109). Also, in the adrenal medulla, two different actions have been described for SP: While on the one hand it inhibits the nicotine-evoked release of CA, at the same time it attenuates the desensitization of this nicotinic secretory response (110). Marley (111) has suggested that this latter effect may be of physiological importance in maintaining secretion of CA under conditions of prolonged stress. Finally, Prabhakar et al. (112) have made the uniquely important observation that SP increases the oxygen consumption of isolated mitochondria, suggesting an intracellular site of action for this peptide.

PERSPECTIVES

At one time or another, the arterial chemoreceptors of the mammalian carotid body have been considered to be either primary or secondary sensory receptors. As primary receptors, natural stimuli would be expected to act principally on the sensory nerve terminals; as secondary receptors, the site of stimulus transduction should be a preneural element (e.g., the type I cells) that would drive the CSN afferent fibers through release of an excitatory transmitter(s). Although the available data on chemotransduction processes do not unequivocally rule out a primary receptor role for the afferent nerve endings, it must be conceded that the sum total of biophysical and neurochemical data clearly demonstrates mechanisms inherent in the type I cells, which are capable of transducing changes in ambient Po_2 into Ca^{2+}-dependent transmitter release. Furthermore, the recent histochemical data showing carbonic anhydrase localization to type I cells, combined with the demonstration that an H^+–Na^+ exchanger and extracellular Ca^{2+} are involved in the release of CAs evoked by elevated Pco_2 (decreased pH), also constitute a plausible mechanism for type I cell transduction of these stimuli as well. Further investigation is clearly required, however, to confirm these hypotheses and to extend our knowledge with respect to how feedback (modulatory) effects of released neurotransmitters can modify the ongoing chemotransductive process.

The precise role of each of the biogenic amines and neuropeptides in mediating transmission between type I cells and afferent nerve terminals remains a challenging problem. Compelling and conclusive evidence does not exist in favor of any single substance as the chemosensory transmitter in the carotid body, despite the striking correlation between (a) natural stimuli-induced changes in putative transmitter synthesis and release and (b) the associated chemosensory afferent discharge—a correlation which is particularly striking for the transmitter candidate, DA. A chronic weakness in the arguments implicating any such transmitter candidate has been the lack of convincing pharmacological evidence showing that specific antagonists are able to block both the response to the applied transmitter and the response to natural stimuli. However, it needs to be noted that this time-worn criticism is recognized in other synaptic systems as the expected result when comparing the efficacy of antagonist blockade of exogenous versus endogenous transmitter actions (see refs. 113 and 114). Although current data describing putative neurotransmitter actions in the carotid body do not establish an unequivocal causal relationship between transmitter release and the genesis of CSN discharge, it is inescapable that substances which are known to be released by the type I cells during stimulation and which have clearly demonstrated effects on modulating chemoreceptor discharge—and for which receptor populations have been described and localized within the chemosensory apparatus—must be recognized (at least) as participating in the chemoresponse. The important questions with respect to transduction and transmission in the carotid body are, first, Which of these several putative neurotransmitters play a truly significant and immediate participatory role in the chemoresponse? and, second, What other agents or mechanisms in addition to candidate transmitters also participate in the chemoresponse, and what is their role?

REFERENCES

1. Fidone SJ, Gonzalez C. Initiation and control of chemoreceptor activity in the carotid body. In: Fishman AP, ed. *Handbook of physiology, Section 3: The respiratory system*, vol II, Part I. Bethesda, MD: American Physiological Society, 1986;247–312.
2. De Castro F. Sur la structure et l'innervation de la glande intercarotidienne (glomus caroticum) de l'homme et des mammifères, et sur un nouveau système d'innervation autonome du nerf glossopharyngien. *Trab Lab Invest Biol Univ Madrid* 1928;25:331–380.
3. De Castro F. Sur la structure et l'innervation du sinus carotidien de l'homme et des mammifères. Nouveaux faits sur l'innervation et la fonction du glomus caroticum. Etudes anatomiques et physiologiques. *Trab Lab Invest Biol Univ Madrid* 1940;32:297–384.
4. Eyzaguirre C, Fitzgerald RS, Lahiri S, Zapata P. Arterial chemoreceptors. In: Shepherd JJ, Abboud FM, eds. *Handbook of physiology, Section 2: The cardiovascular system*, vol II. Bethesda, MD: American Physiological Society, 1983;Chapter 16.
5. Lancet D, Striem B, Pace U, Zehavi U, Naim M. Adenylate cyclase and GTP binding protein in rat sweet taste transduction. *Soc Neurosci Abstr* 1987;13:361.
6. Sklar PB, Anholt RH, Snyder SH. The odorant-sensitive adenylate cyclase of olfactory receptor cells. *J Biol Chem* 1986;261:15538–15543.
7. Pace U, Hanski E, Salomon Y, Lancet D. Odorant-sensitive adenylate cyclase may mediate olfactory reception. *Nature* 1985;316:255–258.
8. Tonosaki K, Funakoshi M. Cyclic nucleotides may mediate taste transduction. *Nature* 1988;331:354–356.
9. Nakamura T, Gold GH. A cyclic nucleotide-gated conductance in olfactory receptor cilia. *Nature* 1987;325:442–444.
10. Avenet P, Hofmann F, Lindemann B. Transduction in taste receptor cells requires cAMP-dependent protein kinase. *Nature* 1988;331:351–354.
11. Kalinoski DL, LaMorte V, Brand JG. Characterization of a taste-stimulus sensitive adenylate cyclase from the gustatory epithelium of the channel catfish, *Ictalurus punctatus*. *Soc Neurosci Abstr* 1987;13:1405.
12. Heck GL, Mierson S, diSimone JA. Salt taste transduction occurs through an amiloride-sensitive sodium transport pathway. *Science* 1984;223:403–405.
13. Kinnamon SC, Roper SC. Membrane properties of isolated mudpuppy taste cells. *J Gen Physiol* 1988;91:351–372.
14. Sugimoto K, Teeter JH. Voltage-dependent and chemically-modulated ionic currents in isolated taste receptor cells of the tiger salamander. *Soc Neurosci Abstr* 1987;13:1404.
15. Mills E, Jobsis FF. Mitochondrial respiratory chain of carotid body and chemoreceptor response to changes in oxygen tension. *J Neurophysiol* 1972;35:405–428.
16. Acker H, Eyzaguirre C. Spectrophotometric studies on carotid body tissue. In: Ribeiro JA, Pallot DJ, eds. *Chemoreceptors in respiratory control*. London: Croom Helm, 1987;69–75.
17. Acker H, Dufau E, Huber J, Sylvester D. Indications to an NADPH oxidase as a possible pO₂ sensor in the rat carotid body. *FEBS Lett* 1989;256:75–78.
18. Obeso A, Almaraz L, Gonzalez C. Correlation between adenosine triphosphate levels, dopamine release and electrical activity in the carotid body: support for the metabolic hypothesis of chemoreception. *Brain Res* 1985;348:64–68.
19. Obeso A, Gonzalez C, Dinger B, Fidone S. Metabolic activation of carotid body glomus cells by hypoxia. *J Appl Physiol* 1989;67:484–487.
20. Mata M, Find DJ, Gainer H, Smith CB, Davidsen L, Savaki H, Schwartz WJ, Sokoloff L. Activity-dependent energy metabolism in rat posterior pituitary reflects sodium pump activity. *J Neurochem* 1980;24:213–215.
21. Obeso A, Almaraz L, Gonzalez C. Effects of cyanide and uncouplers on chemoreceptor activity and ATP content of the cat carotid body. *Brain Res* 1989;481:250–257.
22. Obeso A, Fidone S, Gonzalez C. Pathways for calcium entry into type I cells: significance for the secretory response. In: Ribeiro JA, Pallot DJ, eds. *Chemoreceptors in respiratory control*. London: Croom Helm, 1987;91–97.
23. Sato M, Yoshizaki K, Koyano H. Veratridine stimulation of sodium influx in carotid body cells from newborn rabbits in primary culture. *Brain Res* 1989;504:132–135.
24. Rocher A, Obeso A, Herreros B, Gonzalez C. Activation of the release of dopamine in the carotid body by veratridine. Evidence for the presence of voltage-dependent Na⁺ channels in type I cells. *Neurosci Lett* 1988;94:274–278.
25. Eyzaguirre C, Monti-Bloch L, Hayashida Y, Baron M. Biophysics of the carotid body receptor complex. In: Acker H, O'Regan RG, eds. *Physiology of the peripheral arterial chemoreceptors*. Amsterdam: Elsevier, 1983;59–87.
26. Duchen MR, Caddy KWT, Kirby GC, Patterson DL, Ponte J, Biscoe TJ. Biophysical studies of the cellular elements of the rabbit carotid body. *Neuroscience* 1988;26:291–311.
27. Urena J, Lopez-Lopez J, Gonzalez C, Lopez-Barneo J. Ionic currents in dispersed chemoreceptor cells of the mammalian carotid body. *J Gen Physiol* 1989;93:979–999.
28. Hescheler J, Delpiano MA, Acker H, Pietruschka F. Ionic currents on type-I cells of the rabbit carotid body measured by voltage-clamp experiments and the effect of hypoxia. *Brain Res* 1989;486:79–88.
29. Hescheler J, Delpiano MA. Ionic currents on carotid body type-I cells and the effect of hypoxia and NaCN. In: Eyzaguirre C, Fidone SJ, Fitzgerald RS, Lahiri S, McDonald DM, eds. *Arterial chemoreception*. New York: Springer-Verlag, 1990;in press.
30. Marty A, Neher E. Potassium channels in cultured bovine adrenal chromaffin cells. *J Physiol* 1985;367:117–141.

31. Lopez-Lopez J, Gonzalez C, Urena J, Lopez-Barneo J. Low Po_2 selectively inhibits K channel activity in chemoreceptor cells of the mammalian carotid body. *J Gen Physiol* 1989;93:1001–1015.

32. Lopez-Barneo J, Lopez-Lopez JR, Urena J, Gonzalez C. Chemotransduction in the carotid body: K^+ current modulated by Po_2 in type I chemoreceptor cells. *Science* 1988;241:580–582.

33. Biscoe TJ, Duchen MR. Electrophysiological responses of dissociated type I cells of the rabbit carotid body to cyanide. *J Physiol* 1989;413:447–468.

34. Biscoe TJ, Duchen MR, Eisner DA, O'Neill SC, Valdeolmillos M. Measurements of intracellular Ca^{2+} in dissociated type I cells of the rabbit carotid body. *J Physiol (Lond)* 1989;416:421–434.

35. Biscoe TJ, Duchen MR. The cellular basis of transduction in carotid chemoreceptors. *Am J Physiol* 1990;in press.

36. Rubin RP. *Calcium and cellular secretion*. New York: Plenum Press, 1982.

37. Rocher A, Obeso A, Gonzalez C, Herreros B. Presence and significance of tetrodotoxin sensitive sodium channels in carotid body chemoreceptor cells. *Soc Neurosci Abstr* 1988;14:836.

38. Carafoli E. Intracellular calcium homeostasis. *Annu Rev Biochem* 1987;56:395–433.

39. Somlyo AP, Himpens B. Cell calcium and its regulation in smooth muscle. *FASEB J* 1989;3:2266–2276.

40. Hanson MA, Nye PCG, Torrance RW. The exodus of an extracellular bicarbonate theory of chemoreception and the genesis of an intracellular one. In: Belmonte C, Pallot D, Acker H, Fidone S, eds. *Arterial chemoreceptors. Proceedings of the 6th international meeting*. Leicester, England: Leicester University Press, 1981;403–416.

41. Rigual R, Iniguez C, Carreres J, Gonzalez C. Carbonic anhydrase in the carotid body and the carotid sinus nerve. *Histochemistry* 1985;82:577–580.

42. Ridderstrale Y, Hanson MA. Histochemical localization of carbonic anhydrase in the cat carotid body. *Ann NY Acad Sci* 1984;429:398–400.

43. Grinstein S, Cohen S. Cytoplasmic $[Ca^{++}]$ and intracellular pH in lymphocytes. Role of membrane potential and volume-activated Na^+/H^+ exchange. *J Gen Physiol* 1987;89:185–213.

44. Gonzalez C, Rocher A, Obeso A, Lopez-Lopez JR, Lopez-Barneo J, Herreros B. Ionic mechanisms of the chemoreception process in type I cells of the carotid body. In: Eyzaguirre C, Fidone SJ, Fitzgerald RS, Lahiri S, McDonald DM, eds. *Arterial chemoreception*. New York: Springer-Verlag, 1990;in press.

45. Blaustein MP. Calcium transport and buffering in neurons. *Trends Neurosci* 1988;11:438–443.

46. Heymans C, Bouckaert JJ, Dautrebande L. Sinus carotidien et reflexes respiratoires; sensibilite des sinus carotidiens aux substances chimiques. Action stimulante respiratoire reflexe du sulfure de sodium, du cyanure de potassium, de la nicotine et de la lobeline. *Arch Int Pharmacodyn Ther* 1931;40:54–91.

47. Fidone SJ, Gonzalez C. Catecholamine synthesis in rabbit carotid body *in vitro*. *J Physiol (Lond)* 1982;333:69–79.

48. Gonzalez E, Rigual R, Fidone SJ, Gonzalez C. Mechanisms for termination of the action of dopamine in carotid body chemoreceptors. *J Auton Nerv Syst* 1987;18:249–259.

49. Dinger B, Gonzalez C, Yoshizaki K, Fidone S. [^3H]spiroperidol binding in normal and denervated carotid bodies. *Neurosci Lett* 1981;21:51–55.

50. Goldman WF, Eyzaguirre C. The effects of dopamine on glomus cell membranes in the rabbit. *Brain Res* 1984;321:337–340.

51. Mir AK, McQueen DS, Pallot DJ, Nahorski SR. Direct biochemical and neuropharmacological identification of dopamine D-2 receptors in the rabbit carotid body. *Brain Res* 1984;291:273–283.

52. Hanbauer I, Hellstrom S. The regulation of dopamine and noradrenaline in the rat carotid body and its modification by denervation and by hypoxia. *J Physiol (Lond)* 1978;282:21–34.

53. Fidone SJ, Gonzalez C, Yoshizaki K. Effects of hypoxia on catecholamine synthesis in rabbit carotid body *in vitro*. *J Physiol (Lond)* 1982;333:81–91.

54. Rigual R, Gonzalez E, Gonzalez C, Fidone S. Synthesis and release of catecholamines by the cat carotid body *in vitro*. Effects of hypoxic stimulation. *Brain Res* 1986;374:101–109.

55. Hanbauer I, Karoum F, Hellstrom S, Lahiri S. Effects of hypoxia lasting up to one month on the catecholamine content in rat carotid body. *Neuroscience* 1981;6:81–86.

56. Pequignot JM, Cottet-Emard JM, Dalmaz Y, Peyrin L. Dopamine and norepinephrine dynamics in rat carotid body during long-term hypoxia. *J Auton Nerv Syst* 1987;21:9–14.

57. Gonzalez C, Kwok Y, Gibb JW, Fidone SJ. Effects of hypoxia on tyrosine hydroxylase activity in rat carotid body. *J Neurochem* 1979;33:713–719.

58. Gonzalez C, Kwok Y, Gibb JW, Fidone S. Reciprocal modulation of tyrosine hydroxylase activity in rat carotid body. *Brain Res* 1979;172:572–576.

59. Hanbauer I, Lovenberg W, Costa E. Induction of tyrosine 3-mono-oxygenase in carotid body of rats exposed to hypoxic conditions. *Neuropharmacology* 1977;16:277–282.

60. Fidone SJ, Gonzalez C, Yoshizaki K. Effects of low oxygen on the release of dopamine from the rabbit carotid body *in vitro*. *J Physiol (Lond)* 1982;333:93–110.

61. Shaw K, Montague W, Pallot DJ. Biochemical studies on the release of catecholamines from the rat carotid body *in vitro*. *Biochim Biophys Acta* 1989;1013:42–46.

62. Rigual R, Gonzalez E, Fidone S, Gonzalez C. Effects of low pH on synthesis and release of catecholamines in the cat carotid body *in vitro*. *Brain Res* 1984;309:178–181.

63. Rigual R, Gonzalez E, Gonzalez C, Jones L, Fidone S. A comparative study of the metabolism of catecholamines in the rabbit and cat carotid body. In: Ribeiro JA, Pallot DJ, eds. *Chemoreceptors in respiratory control*. London: Croom helm, 1987;124–134.

64. Obeso A, Almaraz L, Gonzalez C. Correlation between adenosine triphosphate levels, dopamine release and electrical activity in the carotid body: support for the metabolic hypothesis of chemoreception. *Brain Res* 1985;348:64–68.

65. Obeso A, Almaraz L, Gonzalez C. Effects of 2-deoxy-D-glucose on *in vitro* cat carotid body. *Brain Res* 1986;371:25–36.

66. Rigual R. Efectos de la estimulacion natural sobre el metabolismo de catecolaminas en el cuerpo carotideo de gato. PhD thesis, Universidad de Valladolid, Valladolid, Spain, 1984.

67. Docherty RJ, McQueen DS. Inhibitory action of dopamine on cat carotid chemoreceptors. *J Physiol (Lond)* 1978;279:425–436.

68. Zapata P, Llados F. Blockade of carotid body chemosensory inhibition. In: Acker H, Fidone S, Pallot D, Eyzaguirre C, Lubbers DW, Torrance RW, eds. *Chemoreception in the carotid body*. Berlin: Springer-Verlag, 1977;152–159.

69. Nishi K. A pharmacologic study on a possible inhibitory role of dopamine in the cat carotid body chemoreceptor. In: Acker H, Fidone S, Pallot D, Eyzaguirre C, Lubbers DW, Torrance RW, eds. *Chemoreception in the carotid body*. Berlin: Springer-Verlag, 1977;145–151.

70. Okajima Y, Nishi K. Analysis of inhibitory and excitatory actions of dopamine on chemoreceptor discharges of carotid body of cat *in vivo*. *Jpn J Physiol* 1981;31:695–704.

71. Zapata P. Effects of dopamine on carotid chemo- and baroreceptors *in vitro*. *J Physiol (Lond)* 1975;244:235–251.

72. Donnelly DF, Smith EJ, Dutton RE. Neural response of carotid chemoreceptors following dopamine blockade. *J Appl Physiol: Respir Environ Exercise Physiol* 1981;50:172–177.

73. Nolan WF, Donnelly DF, Smith EJ, Dutton RE. Haloperidol-induced suppression of carotid chemoreception *in vitro*. *J Appl Physiol* 1985;59:814–820.

74. Leitner LM, Roumy M. Effects of dopamine superfusion on the activity of rabbit carotid chemoreceptors *in vitro*. *Neuroscience* 1985;16:431–438.

75. Leitner LM, Roumy M. Chemoreceptor response to hypoxia and hypercapnia in catecholamine depleted rabbit and cat carotid bodies *in vitro*. *Pflugers Arch* 1986;406:419–423.

76. Leitner LM, Roumy M, Verna A. *In vitro* recording of che-

moreceptor activity in catecholamine-depleted rabbit carotid bodies. *Neuroscience* 1983;10:883–891.

77. Monti-Bloch L, Eyzaguirre C. A comparative physiological and pharmacological study of cat and rabbit carotid body chemoreceptors. *Brain Res* 1980;193:449–470.

78. Docherty RJ, McQueen DS. The effects of acetylcholine and dopamine on carotid chemosensory activity in the rabbit. *J Physiol London* 1979;288:411–423.

79. Starke K. Presynaptic α-autoreceptors. *Rev Physiol Biochem Pharmacol* 1987;107:74–146.

80. Siggins GR. Monoamines and message transduction in central neurons. In: Magistretti PJ, Morrison JH, Reisine PD, eds. *Transduction of neuronal signals.* Geneva, Switzerland: FESN, 1986;61–67.

81. Chesselet MF. Presynaptic regulation of neurotransmitter release in the brain: facts and hypothesis. *Neuroscience* 1984;12:347–375.

82. Llados F, Zapata P. Effects of dopamine analogues and antagonists on carotid body chemosensors *in situ. J Physiol (Lond)* 1978;274:487–499.

83. Eyzaguirre C, Zapata P. A discussion of possible transmitter or generator substances in carotid body chemoreceptors. In: Torrance RW, ed. *Arterial chemoreceptors.* Oxford, England: Blackwell, 1968;213–251.

84. McQueen DS. Pharmacological aspects of putative transmitters in the carotid body. In: Acker H, O'Regan RG, eds. *Physiology of the peripheral arterial chemoreceptors.* Amsterdam: Elsevier, 1984;149–195.

85. Lahiri S, Pokorski M, Davies RO. Augmentation of carotid body chemoreceptor responses by isoproterenol in the cat. *Respir Physiol* 1981;44:351–364.

86. Folgering H, Ponte J, Sadig T. Adrenergic mechanisms and chemoreception in the carotid body of the cat and rabbit. *J Physiol (Lond)* 1982;325:1–21.

87. Gomez-Niño A, Cheng GF, Yoshizaki K, Gonzalez C, Dinger B, Fidone S. Regulation of the release of dopamine and norepinephrine from rabbit carotid body. In: Eyzaguirre C, Fidone SJ, Fitzgerald RS, Lahiri S, McDonald DM. *Arterial chemoreception.* New York: Springer-Verlag, 1990;in press.

88. Eyzaguirre C, Koyano H, Taylor JR. Presence of acetylcholine and transmitter release from carotid body chemoreceptors. *J Physiol (Lond)* 1965;178:463–476.

89. Dinger B, Gonzalez C, Yoshizaki K, Fidone S. Localization and function of cat carotid body nicotinic receptors. *Brain Res* 1985;339:295–304.

90. Dinger BG, Hirano T, Fidone SJ. Autoradiographic localization of muscarinic receptors in rabbit carotid body. *Brain Res* 1986;367:328–331.

91. Livett BG. Chromaffin cells and chromaffin granules. In: Adelman G, ed. *Encyclopedia of neuroscience.* Boston: Birkhauser, 1987;239–242.

92. Eyzaguirre C, Fidone S, Nishi K. Recent studies on the generation of chemoreceptor impulses. In: Purves MJ, ed. *The peripheral arterial chemoreceptors.* London: Cambridge University Press, 1975;175–194.

93. Dinger BG, Almaraz L, Fidone SJ. Nicotinic and muscarinic-induced release of dopamine in cat and rabbit carotid body. *Soc Neurosci Abstr* 1985;11:745.

94. Monti-Bloch L, Eyzaguirre C. A comparative physiological and pharmacological study of cat and rabbit carotid body chemoreceptors. *Brain Res* 1980;193:449–470.

95. Kobayashi S, Uchida T, Okashi T, et al. Immunocytochemical demonstration of the co-storage of noradrenaline with Met-enkephalin-Arg 6-Phe 7 and Met-enkephalin-Arg 6-Gly 7-Leu 8 in the carotid body chief cells of the dog. *Arch Histol Jpn* 1983;46:713–722.

96. Hanson G, Jones L, Fidone S. Physiological chemoreceptor stimulation decreases enkephalin and substance P in the carotid body. *Peptides* 1986;7:766–769.

97. Rigual RJ, Diliberto EJ, Sigafoos J, Gonzalez C, Viveros OH. Proenkephalin-derived peptides in the carotid body. In: Eyzaguirre C, Fidone SJ, Fitzgerald RS, Lahiri S, McDonald D, eds. *Arterial chemoreception.* New York: Springer-Verlag, 1990;in press.

98. Kirby GC, McQueen DS. Characterization of opioid receptors in the cat carotid body involved in chemosensory depression *in vivo. Br J Pharmacol* 1986;88:889–898.

99. Monti-Bloch L, Eyzaguirre C. Effects of methionine-enkephalin and substance P on the chemosensory discharge of the cat carotid body. *Brain Res* 1985;338:297–307.

100. Colombo M, Kummer W, Heym C. Immunohistochemistry of opioid peptides in guinea pig paraganglia. *Exp Brain Res* 1987;16:67–72.

101. Kummer W. Retrograde neuronal labelling and double-staining immunohistochemistry of tachykinin and calcitonin gene-related peptide-immunoreactive pathways in the carotid sinus nerve of the guinea pig. *J Auton Nerv Syst* 1988;23:131–141.

102. Cuello AC, McQueen DS. Substance P: a carotid body peptide. *Neurosci Lett* 1980;17:215–219.

103. Prabhakar NR, Landis SC, Kumar GK, Mullikin-Kilpatrick D, Cherniack NS, Leeman S. Substance P and neurokinin A in the cat carotid body: localization, exogenous effects and changes in content in response to arterial pO_2. *Brain Res* 1989;481:205–214.

104. Prabhakar NR, Runold M, Yamamoto Y, Langercrantz M, von Euler C. Effects of substance P antagonist on the hypoxia-induced carotid chemoreceptor activity. *Acta Physiol Scand* 1984;121:301–303.

105. Prabhakar NR. Mechanisms of action of tachykinins in the carotid body: evidence for possible extra- and intracellular effects of the peptides. In: Eyzaguirre C, Fidone SJ, Fitzgerald RS, Lahiri S, McDonald D, eds. *Arterial chemoreception.* New York: Springer-Verlag, 1990;in press.

106. McQueen DS. Effects of substance P on carotid chemoreceptor activity in the cat. *J Physiol (Lond)* 1980;302:31–47.

107. McQueen DS, Evrard Y. Effects of selective antagonists on responses of cat carotid body chemoreceptors to hypoxia and almitrine. In: Eyzaguirre C, Fidone SJ, Fitzgerald RS, Lahiri S, McDonald D, eds. *Arterial chemoreception.* New York: Springer-Verlag, 1990;in press.

108. Prabhakar NR, Mitra J, Cherniack NS. Role of substance P in hypercapnic excitation of carotid chemoreceptors. *J Appl Physiol* 1987;63:2418–2425.

109. von Euler VS, Pernow B. *Substance P.* New York: Raven Press, 1977.

110. Boska P, Livett BG. Desensitization to nicotinic cholinergic agonists and K^+ agents that stimulate catecholamine secretion in isolated chromaffin cells. *J Neurochem* 1984;42:607–617.

111. Marley PD. Desensitization of the nicotinic secretory response of adrenal chromaffin cells. *Trends Pharmacol Sci* 1988;9:102–107.

112. Prabhakar NR, Runold M, Kumar GF, Cherniack NS, Scarpa A. Substance P and mitochondrial oxygen consumption: evidence for a direct intracellular role for the peptide. *Peptides* 1989;10:1003–1006.

113. Campbell G. Cotransmission. *Annu Rev Pharmacol Toxicol* 1987;27:51–70.

114. Gershon MD. The identification of transmitters to smooth muscle. In: Bulbring E, Brading AF, Jones AW, Tomita T, eds. *Smooth muscle.* Baltimore: Williams & Wilkins, 1970;496–524.

115. Williams PL, Warwick R, eds. *Gray's anatomy.* Philadelphia: WB Saunders, 1980.

THE LUNG: Scientific Foundations
edited by R.G. Crystal, J.B. West et al.
Raven Press, Ltd., New York © 1991.

CHAPTER 5.4.3

Physiologic Responses:

Peripheral Chemoreflexes

Sukhamay Lahiri

RESPIRATION AND FEEDBACK HOMEOSTASIS

Cellular respiration involves O_2 consumption and oxidation of organic food material to produce CO_2 and H^+, among other products. Molecular species of the gases O_2 and CO_2 are transported by the respiratory system through the airways and across the lung alveoli in a measured way so that extracellular and intracellular homeostasis of O_2 and CO_2 and associated $[H^+]$ are maintained. This goal is accomplished through the operation of negative feedback mechanisms, developed by natural evolution. Respiratory feedback involves reflex action, the essential elements of which are: sensors (chemoreceptors), controller (central nervous system), and effectors (respiratory muscles). Among the sensors are peripheral chemoreceptors (carotid and aortic bodies), the only organs that continuously monitor oxygen tension in the arterial blood. They also monitor arterial CO_2 tension and $[H^+]$ and send signals to the brainstem through the sensory fibers.

The chemoreflex not only controls respiratory muscles for ventilation but also controls those of the upper and lower airways and of cardiovascular systems. The respiratory and cardiovascular reflexes are precisely integrated in the sensorimotor areas of the brainstem for unimpaired transport of respiratory gases. This chapter will deal primarily with the characteristics of peripheral chemoreceptor function with respect to the control of ventilation and of airways. Earlier and more

detailed reviews on peripheral chemoreceptors and chemoreflexes appeared in 1983 and 1986 (1–3).

Peripheral Chemoreceptors

The discharges of the peripheral chemoreceptors are an expression of chemoreception, the cellular and molecular mechanisms of which are not known despite a great deal of research and despite an accumulation of a large amount of facts since its discovery half a century ago (see refs. 1–3 for reviews). One possible reason for the uncertainty is that all the observations may not apply to a single mechanism subserving chemosensory response. A common working model of oxygen chemoreception is that upon excitation by hypoxia, glomus cells of carotid and aortic bodies mobilize and release granular vesicles containing neurotransmitters which then act on the excitable cell membrane to generate propagated action potentials. However, the neurotransmitter for the hypoxia response has not been identified. Blockade of the receptors for the putative neurotransmitters does not block the chemosensory effect of hypoxia. Accordingly, it is a reasonable suggestion that more than one oxygen-sensitive mechanism is involved: One leads directly to membrane depolarization and initiates propagated action potential, and the other leads to the release of neuromodulators (e.g., acetylcholine, catecholamines, neuropeptides, ATP) that strongly influence neural discharge.

Two relatively independent oxygen-sensitive processes could account for the failure of the antagonists to block the effect of hypoxia on the chemosensory discharge. The initiation of the two processes could still involve the same oxygen-sensitive reaction (or a

S. Lahiri: Department of Physiology, University of Pennsylvania School of Medicine, Philadelphia, Pennsylvania 19104.

similar one) at two different sites. The plausible mechanisms will not be reviewed here, but it is worthy of consideration that chemosensing involving neurotransmitters may be too slow a process to explain the rapid chemosensory responses to natural stimuli (4). It is necessary, however, to describe here the characteristics of the chemosensory functions which are the bases of the respiratory chemoreflexes.

Characteristics of Chemosensory Discharge

A common characteristic of the *in vivo* and *in vitro* carotid body preparation is that its sensory discharge pattern is irregular, independent of external stimuli. The pattern is more bursty for aortic chemoreceptors (5). The physiologic meaning of the pattern is unknown. As expected, the frequency of discharge to a given stimulus level and the maximal frequency vary with the fiber size (diameter) and fiber myelination (1).

Responses to O_2 and CO_2 Stimuli

The same chemoreceptor afferent fiber is stimulated by both hypoxia and hypercapnia (and H^+), with the effect of one being augmented by the other (2). A similar relationship is found in the whole carotid sinus nerve (2), even though new fibers are recruited as stimulus strength increases.

Threshold Stimulus

The response to P_aCO_2 is linear, and the activity can be reduced to near zero at a sufficiently low arterial PCO_2 if arterial Po_2 is kept constant, with this threshold P_aCO_2 being lower at a lower P_aO_2 (see refs. 1 and 3 for reviews).

Saturation Response

Chemoreceptor activity achieves a plateau with hypercapnia; the lower the P_aO_2, lower the P_aCO_2 at which the same plateau is reached. However, whether the same maximal response to PCO_2 is reached at all values of P_aO_2 is unclear. Fitzgerald and Lahiri (3) reported that the maximal activity was lower at higher levels of P_aO_2. However, it appears that at a sufficiently high P_aCO_2 the same maximal activity can be reached during hyperoxia and hypoxia (6). Pulses of CO_2–saline (PCO_2 = 250 torr) injections into the carotid sinus area elicit similar maximal responses at high and low Po_2 (S. Lahiri et al., *unpublished observations*).

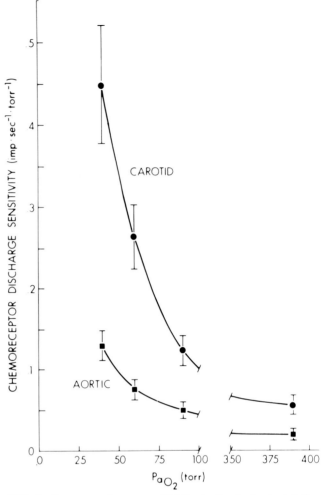

FIG. 1. Summary (mean ± SEM) of effect of arterial Po_2 levels on slopes of CO_2 response curves of aortic and carotid chemoreceptor activities (*n* = 15 each). Note that sensitivity of carotid chemoreceptors to the stimuli is significantly greater than those of aortic chemoreceptors. (From ref. 40.)

Stimulus Interaction

The foregoing characteristics of carotid chemoreceptor responses to O_2 and CO_2 manifest a cooperative phenomenon that is reminiscent of CO_2–H^+-dependent binding of O_2 by a hemoglobin molecule. This resemblance suggested and supported the chromophore hypothesis of O_2 chemoreception (see ref. 4). However, it is possible to eliminate O_2 chemoreception without blocking CO_2 chemoreception by the administration of metabolic inhibitors of oxidative phosphorylation to the carotid body (see refs. 1–3 and 7) and by exposing the cat to chronic hyperoxia (8).

Stimulus interaction in aortic chemoreceptors is considerably less than that in carotid chemoreceptors (Fig. 1). This distinction presumably occurs because aortic chemoreceptors are far less sensitive to CO_2 (see ref. 3).

H^+ Stimulus

The stimulatory effect of CO_2 seems to be mostly due to increases in intracellular H^+ levels (see refs. 1 and 2). A delay in the rise of intracellular $[H^+]$ due to blockade of intracellular carbonic anhydrase and in an increase in chemoreceptor discharge during the sudden onset of hypercapnia has been taken to suggest that it is the cellular H^+ which is the stimulus species and that molecular CO_2 is inert. However, the increment in intracellular $[H^+]$ due to hypercapnia does not fully account for the augmented chemosensory discharge.

Application of metabolic acidosis only slowly increases carotid chemosensory discharge (see ref. 3) and shows relatively little effect on aortic chemoreceptors.

Dynamic Chemosensory Responses

The onset of hypercapnia is normally followed by a sharp increase in the chemosensory discharge, but the steady-state effect is less than the peak discharge (see ref. 3). Withdrawal of hypercapnia is followed by an undershoot of carotid chemoreceptor activity. The total magnitude of these dynamic responses to CO_2 is augmented by hypoxia (see refs. 1 and 3).

The onset of hypoxia is not usually followed by an overshoot in chemoreceptor activity, although the withdrawal of hypoxia often produces an undershoot (T. Nishino and S. Lahiri, unpublished observations; R. W. Torrance and P. G. Nye, personal communication). Normal respiratory rhythm causes reciprocal oscillations of arterial PO_2 and PCO_2 which are more closely monitored by carotid body chemoreceptors than by aortic chemoreceptors partly because of its high blood flow (see ref. 1) and partly because of its greater sensitivity to CO_2. These normal oscillations of chemosensory afferent discharge are potentially critical in sensorimotor integration in the brainstem and efferent output to the target organ (see later).

There is another type of chemosensory rhythm (10- to 12-sec duration) of unknown origin, particularly prominent in the aortic chemoreceptors (unpublished observations). These oscillations may be related to swings in arterial blood pressure and sympathetic nerve activity.

Depressant Effect of Hypoxia on Chemoreceptors

It is not an uncommon experience that activity of the chemosensory afferents disappears during hypoxia. Some of this activity is restored upon reoxygenation (see ref. 9). Also, carotid chemoreceptor activity diminishes from a peak during severe hypoxia. Reoxygenation first increases this activity before restoring the normal response. These patterns indicating a depressant effect of hypoxia are seen more often in the aortic chemoreceptors (unpublished observations). Thus, a minimal concentration of oxygen is needed to support the chemosensory response to hypoxia. In any case, this phenomenon may contribute to ventilatory depression during moderate to severe hypoxia. However, the depressant effect on ventilation after an initial stimulation is presumably mainly central.

Arterial Blood Pressure

Experimentally induced hypotension down to 60 torr during normoxia does not excite carotid chemoreceptors. Hypoxia, however, increases the sensitivity to hypotension. Aortic chemoreceptors, on the other hand, are stimulated by hypotension even during normoxia (1,3).

Anemia

A reduction of red blood cell concentration and O_2 content down to 50% of normal does not stimulate carotid chemoreceptors during normoxia but does excite aortic chemoreceptors (1,3). Accordingly, a decrease in O_2 content due to an increase in P_{50} (5,7), other factors being equal, could stimulate aortic, but not carotid, chemoreceptors.

Carboxyhemoglobinemia

Carboxyhemoglobinemia decreases O_2 content, increases O_2 affinity, and makes the O_2–hemoglobin dissociation curve hyperbolic. Accordingly, carboxyhemoglobinemia is ordinarily expected to lower tissue PO_2 and excite the chemoreceptors. Aortic (but not carotid) chemoreceptors are stimulated by carboxyhemoglobinemia during normoxia (see ref. 3 for reviews). Hence, it is reasonable to infer that carboxyhemoglobinemia does not lower carotid chemoreceptor tissue PO_2 but does lower aortic chemoreceptor PO_2. This inference is consistent with the recent observations that chronic inhalation of low concentration of CO ($PCO = 0.5$ torr at $P_IO_2 = 150$ torr), which increases hematocrit from 42% to 75%, did not increase catecholamine content of the carotid body (10), nor did it stimulate the growth of carotid body glomus cells (11), unlike chronic hypoxia ($P_IO_2 = 70$ torr) (see refs. 1 and 2). Clearly, the increase in hematocrit shows that carboxyhemoglobinemia caused hypoxia of erythroprotein-producing tissue which led to the release of erythroprotein. Any possible effect of molecular CO on a hypothetical chromophore protein (6,12), to diminish erythropoietic effects, was not obvious at the low concentration of CO and a low CO:O$_2$ ratio.

Chemoreflexes

Ventilation

Several characteristics of peripheral chemoreflex controlling breath-by-breath respiration in the anesthetized cat are illustrated in Fig. 2. The left-hand panel shows oscillations of carotid body tissue Po_2 synchronous with respiration in the cat breathing air (P_IO_2 = 150 torr). Carotid chemoreceptor activity (single fiber) tracked the arterial blood gas (Po_2 and Pco_2) oscillations. The right-hand panel shows the effect of lowering inspired Po_2. Carotid body tissue Po_2 declined following the changes in end-tidal Po_2, whereas carotid chemoreceptor activity increased promptly in a reciprocal fashion. Ventilation increased breath by breath following the chemosensory discharge.

Steady-state ventilatory response to hypoxia resembles those of peripheral chemoreceptors. Most of the chemoreflex response is due to carotid chemosensory input, with aortic chemoreceptor input producing a negligible effect in the cat (3). Also, unilateral denervation of carotid body only marginally affects chemoreflex stimulation of ventilation by hypoxia (see ref. 3). After bilateral denervation, hypoxia depresses ven-

tilation in the anesthetized animals (3,13–15). CO$_2$, however, continues to stimulate ventilation through central chemoreception mechanism.

The O$_2$–CO$_2$ stimulus interaction observed in the carotid chemoreceptor activity is reflected in the ventilatory responses in humans and animals (see refs. 3 and 16 for reviews; see also ref. 17).

Respiratory-Cycle-Dependent Chemoreflex

The effect of chemoreceptor afferent input on the efferent respiratory output is dependent on the cyclic gating and sensitivity changes of brainstem respiratory neurons (see ref. 18 for review). The inspiratory neurons become more responsive when they are disinhibited (see refs. 18 and 19) during inspiration. During expiration the same chemoreceptor stimulation further inhibits these neurons and prolongs expiration (18,20,21). Lipski et al. (22) concluded that the Botzinger group of expiratory neurons are stimulated by chemoreceptor input and that these neurons are responsible for the inhibition of nucleus tractus solitarius inspiratory cells during expiration. The caudal expiratory neurons mediate the chemosensory effect on the spinal neurons controlling intercostal muscles.

According to the cyclic events, the ventilatory effect would depend on the timing of the chemosensory input (see ref. 16 for review).

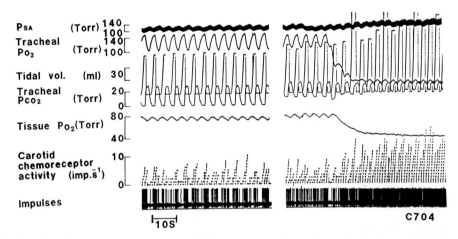

FIG. 2. Carotid chemoreceptor and ventilatory responses to hypoxia in the anesthetized cat. Tracings from top to bottom are: arterial blood pressure (P_{SA}), tracheal Po_2 (P_TO_2) showing end-tidal Po_2, tidal volume (V_T), tracheal Pco_2 (P_TCO_2), carotid body tissue Po_2, carotid chemoreceptor activity, and carotid chemoreceptor impulses. Left-hand panel shows the parameters during normoxia. Note oscillations in the carotid body tissue Po_2 with each breath, and also note a corresponding oscillation in the chemosensory activity. Right-hand panel shows the effects of onset of hypoxia. Lowering of tracheal Po_2 was promptly followed by a decline in the carotid body tissue Po_2 and a reciprocal rise in the chemosensory activity and tidal volume in parallel, beginning with an augmented breath. Note that every fourth breath was an augmented breath and that there was an increase in the breath frequency. The oscillations in the chemosensory activity diminished partly because of decreased oscillations in the blood gas stimuli as reflected in the carotid body tissue Po_2. (From S. Lahiri and I. A. Silver, *unpublished data.*)

Responses to Transient Stimulus

Transient excitatory stimuli are often applied to test chemoreflex responses. These responses will obviously depend on the timing of the chemosensory input and can be variable. Transient withdrawal of a stimulus has also been used, but the reflex response may not always be seen unless all the excitatory input is diminished or eliminated at once, the reason being that the bilateral sensory input shows overlap and occlusion in the central integrative system.

Response to Prolonged Stimulus

Prolonged stimulation of carotid sinus nerves over several breaths or minutes augments phrenic nerve activity that often outlasts the actual period of stimulation. The effects have been studied extensively by Eldridge and Millhorn (see ref. 18 for review) and have been variously termed "afterdischarge," "memory," and "potentiation" in the respiratory control system. The effect develops rapidly but decays only slowly. The mechanism probably involves central neurotransmitters but has not been precisely established. The significance of the effects is to prevent abrupt large changes in respiration following withdrawal of the chemosensory stimulus and, hence, to stabilize breath-to-breath respiration. However, it does not prevent periodic breathing with apnea in the newcomers at high altitude. Clearly, the phenomenon is expressed only under certain boundary conditions.

Plasticity of Chemoreflex

It is well known that the integrative function of the central nervous system manifests plasticity. An increased chemosensory input over a long period can further increase synaptic output of the respiratory control system, as seen in high-altitude adaptation (9,13,19). The initial augmentation could attenuate after a further lapse of time at high altitude (3,9,19).

Peripheral Chemoreflex and Breathing Stability

Peripheral chemosensory input can contribute to breathing instability during hypoxia because of its rapid speed of response and alinear gain, relative to the central chemoreceptors (see ref. 23 for review). This fact becomes evident particularly during sleep at high altitude. Those with high chemosensitivity are predisposed to periodic breathing with apnea in contrast to those with blunted chemosensitivity (23). Also, carotid chemoreceptor denervation eliminates peri-

odic breathing in anesthetized cats (see ref. 3 for review). However, recent work showing that periodic breathing occurs in chemodenervated ponies during sleep raises new questions (H. V. Forster, *personal communication*). Also, the role of afterdischarge and memory in periodic breathing is not clearly established (see ref. 18 for review).

The state of wakefulness, however, can fluctuate and influence breathing stability.

Airways

Chemoreflex Control Through the Autonomic Nervous System

The muscles of upper (nose, pharynx, and larynx) and lower airways must function in coordination with those for ventilation in order to achieve normal respiration. The muscles of the airways are primarily innervated by parasympathetic cholinergic nerves (24,25). Sympathetic innervation is sparse, but yet there is evidence for alpha- and beta-adrenergic control of the airway muscle (26). Neural impulses release small granular vesicles and neurotransmitters which activate alpha and beta receptors of the parasympathetic ganglion cell membranes, as well as beta receptors of the airway smooth muscle cells (27), without mediation of neuromuscular synapse. The process is apparently slower than those that control respiratory muscles of diaphragm and chest wall involving neuromuscular junction.

Several types of mechanoreceptor which are strategically placed in the airways send afferent input to the brainstem (6). The sensory fibers from the peripheral and central chemoreceptors also supply appropriate input. The sensorimotor integration in the central nervous system leads to efferent outflow to the respiratory (smooth and skeletal) muscles.

The role of peripheral chemoreflex in the control of airway function has started to receive more attention recently. Widdicombe (28) recorded efferent vagal activity to trachea and lungs, and more recently Mitchell et al. (29) identified inspiratory rhythm in airway smooth muscle tone in the cat and showed that carotid chemoreceptor stimulation caused, in parallel with phrenic nerve discharge, an increased tracheal tension that was blocked by atropine. They concluded that the major excitory input to airway arises from cholinergic parasympathetic nerves controlled by the central activity related to respiratory neurons. It is interesting to note that sympathetic nerve activity also shows inspiratory rhythm in the cat (30,31). Baker and Don (32) reported that catecholamines released from sympathetic nerves inhibit parasympathetic-ganglion-me-

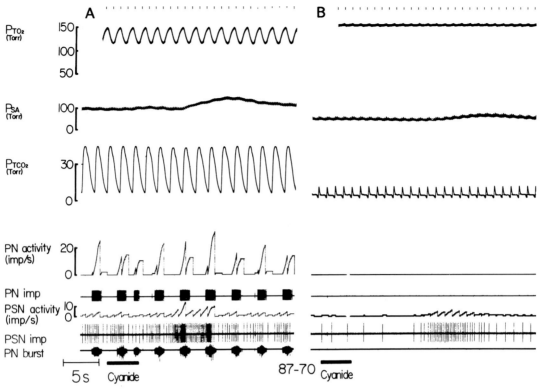

FIG. 3. Relationship between chemoreflex stimulation of phrenic nerve and sympathetic nerve activities in the anesthetized cat. Tracings from top to bottom are: tracheal P_{O_2} (P_{TO_2}), systemic arterial pressure (P_{SA}), tracheal P_{CO_2} (P_{TCO_2}), single phrenic nerve (PN) activity and impulses, preganglionic sympathetic nerve (PSN) activity and impulses, and phrenic nerve (PN) burst from a nerve bundle. **A:** Note that the PSN manifested rhythmic discharges in parallel with PN rhythm. Peripheral chemoreceptor stimulation by cyanide (50 µg, intravenous) increased PSN discharges in two respects: The activity increased before the increase in PN discharges, but peak response coincided with those of PN discharges. **B:** Hyperventilation of the cat with air which lowered end-tidal P_{CO_2} and raised end-tidal P_{O_2} eliminated both PN-bundle and single-fiber discharge. Cyanide injection excited the PSN without a PN response. Thus the PSN chemoreflex was independent of the brainstem inspiratory neuron response. (From ref. 31.)

diated airway tone. The interaction of the sympathetic and parasympathetic nerves in airway control is further influenced by cardiopulmonary mechanoreceptors in the spontaneously breathing animal (see refs. 25 and 28 for reviews). It seems that the major role of the sympathetic nerves is to modulate the dominant parasympathetic control of the airway.

Whether there is a preferential chemoreceptor drive to upper airway relative to respiratory pump muscle has been studied (see ref. 33 for review). A selective distribution was found in the anesthetized animals, preferring cranial over the spinal motor pathway. However, a proportional distribution was found in the decerebrate, unanesthetized cats. Thus, anesthesia apparently exerts differential effects in the central nervous system.

Although it has not been worked out as clearly, it is assumed that the autonomic outflow to the airway muscles are gated and controlled in the same way as chemoreceptor input to the respiratory neurons (29). New

observations testing this assumption are needed, particularly in view of the observation that certain sympathetic nerve discharge can be excited by carotid chemoreceptor stimulation independent of stimulation of phrenic nerve responses (31). An example is shown in Fig. 3.

Dependence of Chemoreceptor Function on the Oxygen Environment

Peripheral chemoreceptor response to hypoxia increases during chronic exposure despite respiratory alkalosis (see ref. 34–36). In fact, the inevitable alkalosis may be an important antecedent for carotid body hypertrophy, enhanced synthetic activity, and augmented chemosensory response. The response is obviously initiated by some process of oxygen sensing by the carotid body cells, separate from the acute sensory response, but the mechanism of effects needs to be elaborated.

Higher oxygen levels in the environment than at sea level alter carotid chemoreceptor activity (8) and chemoreflex response (37,38). Chronic exposure of newborn kittens to 210 torr of inspired Po_2 levels diminished ventilatory response to hypoxia (39), and chronic exposure of adult cats to 350 torr for 14 days specifically diminished carotid chemoreceptors response to hypoxia. Exposure to inspired Po_2 levels of 710 torr for 2–3 days attenuated the response more severely (8), but the mechanism of effect has not been elucidated. A role of oxygen free radical is suspected. Brief but severe hyperbaric oxygen pressure (HBO) appears to attenuate ventilatory response to hypoxia (37,38). However, hyperoxia also changes pulmonary mechanics and consequently leads to breathing pattern changes, causing ventilatory limitations (36). A role of chemoreflex in the altered ventilatory response to hypoxia after a short exposure to hyperbaric oxygenation has not been established. A longer exposure at lower levels of HBO may be needed for the peripheral chemoreceptors to show the effects.

SUMMARY

The peripheral chemoreceptors are the only oxygen sensors that initiate chemoreflexes. Oxygen biology of these processes at systemic, cellular, and molecular levels is only partially known. The chemosensory responses to O_2 are modulated not only by blood gas composition but also by several other blood-borne factors such as temperature, osmolarity, and humoral substances (see refs. 1 and 3 for review). The sensory output of the peripheral chemoreceptors monitoring the arterial blood gases may not always be clearly manifested in the efferent output because of gating, memory, plasticity, and other processing and integrating mechanisms in the central nervous system.

ACKNOWLEDGMENTS

I wish to thank Ms. Valerie Johnson, Ms. Wendy Patriquin, and Mr. Anil Mokashi for their help with the preparation of the manuscript. This work was supported, in part, by grants HL-19737, HL-43413, and NS-21068.

REFERENCES

1. Eyzaquirre C, Fitzgerald RS, Lahiri S, Zapata P. Arterial chemoreceptors. In: Shepherd JT, Abboud FM, eds. *Handbook of physiology, Section 2: The cardiovascular system, vol 3—Peripheral circulation and oxygen blood flow.* Bethesda, MD: American Physiological Society, 1983;557–621.
2. Fidone SJ, Gonzalez C. Initiation and control of chemoreceptor activity in the carotid body. In: Cherniack NS, Widdicombe JG, eds. *Handbook of physiology, Section 3: The respiratory system, vol 2—Control of breathing.* Bethesda, MD: American Physiological Society, 1986;247–312.
3. Fitzgerald RS, Lahiri S. Reflex responses to chemoreceptor stimulation. In: Cherniack NS, Widdicombe JG, eds. *Handbook of physiology, Section 3: The respiratory system, vol 2—Control of breathing.* Bethesda, MD: American Physiological Society, 1986;313–362.
4. Lahiri S. Chemical modification of carotid body chemoreception by sulphhydryls. *Science* 1981;212:1065–1066.
5. Lahiri S, Mulligan E, Nishino T, Mokashi A. Aortic body chemoreceptor responses to changes in PCO_2 and PO_2 in the cat. *J Appl Physiol* 1979;47:858–866.
6. Lahiri S. Oxygen linked response of carotid chemoreceptors. In: Reivich M, Coburn R, Lahiri S, Chance B, eds. *Tissue hypoxia and ischemia.* New York: Plenum Press, 1976;185–202.
7. Shirahata M, Andronikou S, Lahiri S. Differential effects of oligomycin on carotid chemoreceptor responses to O_2 and CO_2 in the cat. *J Appl Physiol* 1987;63:2084–2092.
8. Lahiri S, Mulligan E, Andronikou S, Mokashi A. Carotid body chemosensory function in prolonged normobaric hyeroxia in the cat. *J Appl Physiol* 1987;62:1924–1931.
9. Lahiri S, Smatresk NS, Mulligan E. Responses of peripheral chemoreceptors to natural stimuli. In: Acker H, O'Regan RG, eds. *Physiology of the peripheral arterial chemoreceptors.* Amsterdam: Elsevier, 1983;221–256.
10. Lahiri S, Penney DG, Mokashi A, Albertine KH. Chronic CO inhalation and carotid body catecholamines: testing of hypothesis. *J Appl Physiol* 1989;67:239–242.
11. Sherpa AK, Albertine KH, Penney DG, Thompkins B, Lahiri S. Chronic CO exposure stimulates erythropoiesis but not glomus cell growth. *J Appl Physiol* 1989;67:1383–1387.
12. Goldberg MA, Dunning SP, FranklinBurn H. Regulation of erythropoietin gene: evidence that oxygen sensor is a heme protein. *Science* 1988;242:1412–1415.
13. Weill JV, Vizek M. Ventilatory response to hypoxia in high-altitude acclimatization. In: Lahiri S, Forester RE, Davis RO, Pack AI, eds. *Chemoreceptor and reflexes in breathing.* New York: Oxford University Press, 1989;199–207.
14. Anthonisen NR, Easton PA. Carbon dioxide effects on the ventilatory responses to sustained hypoxia. *J Appl Physiol* 1988;64(4):1451–1456.
15. Lahiri S, Edelman NH, Cherniack NS, Fishman AP. Role of carotid chemoreflex in respiratory acclimatization to hypoxemia in goat and sheep. *Respir Physiol* 1981;46:367–382.
16. Cunningham DJC, Robbins PA, Wolff CB. Integration of respiratory response to changes in alveolar partial pressures of CO_2 and O_2 and arterial pH. In: *Handbook of physiology, Section 3: The respiratory system, vol 2—Control of breathing.* Bethesda, MD: American Physiological Society, 1986;475–528.
17. Daristotle L, Bisgard GE. Central and peripheral chemoreceptor ventilatory interaction in awake goats. *Respir Physiol* 1989;76:383–392.
18. Eldridge F, Millhorn D. Oscillation, gating and memory in the respiratory control system. In: Cherniack NS, Widdicombe JG, eds. *Handbook of physiology, Section 3: The respiratory system, vol 2—Control of breathing.* Bethesda, MD: American Physiological Society, 1986;475–528.
19. Lahiri S, Gelfand R. In: Hornbein T, ed. *Regulation of breathing.* New York: Marcel Dekker, 1981;773–843.
20. Lipski J, McAllen RM, Syper KM. The carotid chemoreceptor input to the respiratory neurons of the nucleus of the tractus solitarius. *J Physiol* 1977;296:797–810.
21. Ballantyne D, Lawson EE, Lalley PM, Richter DW. How arterial chemoreceptor activity influences the respiratory rhythm. In: Lahiri S, Forster R, Davies RO, Pack AI, eds. *Chemoreceptors and reflexes in breathing.* New York: Oxford University Press, 1989;332–342.
22. Lipski J, Trzebski A, Chodobska J, Kruk P. Effects of carotid chemoreceptor excitation on medullary expiratory neurons in cats. *Respir Physiol* 1984;57:279–291.
23. Cherniack NS, Longobardo GS. Abnormalities in respiratory rhythm. In: Cherniack NS, Widdicombe JG, eds. *Handbook of physiology, Section 3: The respiratory system, vol 2—Control*

of breathing. Bethesda, MD: American Physiological Society, 1986;729–749.

24. Nadel JA. Autonomic regulation of airway smooth muscle. In: Nadel JA, ed. *Physiology and pharmacology of the airways.* New York: Marcel Dekker, 1980;217–258.

25. Burnstock G. Autonomic neural control mechanisms with special reference to the airways. In: Kaliner MA, Barnes PJ, eds. *The airways.* New York: Marcel Dekker, 1988;1–22.

26. Barnes PJ. Adrenergic regulation of airway function. In: Kaliner MA, Barnes PJ, eds. *The airways.* New York: Marcel Dekker, 1988;57–86.

27. Barnes PJ. Cell surface receptors in airway smooth muscle. In: Coburn R, ed. *Airway smooth muscle in health and disease.* New York: Plenum Press, 1989;77–97.

28. Widdicombe J, Sant'Ambrogio G, Mathews OP. Nerve receptors of the upper airway. In: Mathews OP, Sant'Ambrogio G, eds. *Respiratory function of the upper airway.* New York: Marcel Dekker, 1988;193–232.

29. Mitchell RA, Herbert DA, Baker DG. Inspiratory rhythm in airway muscle tone. *J Appl Physiol* 1985;58:911–920.

30. Preiss G, Kirchman F, Polosa C. Patterning of sympathetic preganglionic neuron firing by the central respiration drive. *Brain Res* 1975;87:363–374.

31. Huang W, Lahiri S, Mokashi A, Sherpa AK. Relationship between sympathetic and phrenic nerve responses to peripheral chemoreflex in the cat. *J Auton Nerv Syst* 1988;25:95–105.

32. Baker DG, Don H. Catecholamines abolish vagal but not acetylcholine tone in the intact cat trachea. *J Appl Physiol* 1987;63:2490–2498.

33. Iscoe SD. Central control of the upper airway. In: Mathews OP, Sant'Ambrogio G, eds. *Respiratory function of the upper airway.* New York: Marcel Dekker, 1990;in press.

34. Lahiri S. Oxygen biology of the peripheral chemoreceptors. In: Lahiri S, Cherniack NS, Fitzgerald RS, eds. *Oxygen biology of adaptation: organ to organelle.* New York: 1990;in press.

35. Bisgard GE, Busch MA, Forster HV. Ventilatory acclimatization to hypoxia is not dependent upon central hypocapnic alkalosis. *J Appl Physiol* 1986;60:1011–1015.

36. Vizek M, Pickett C, Weil JV. Increased carotid body hypoxic sensitivity during acclimatization to hypobaric hypoxia. *J Appl Physiol* 1987;60:2403–2410.

37. Arieli R, Kerem D, Melamed Y. Hyperoxic exposure affects the ventilatory response to hypoxia in awake rats. *J Appl Physiol* 1988;64(1):181–186.

38. Torbati D, Mokashi A, Lahiri S. Effects of acute hyperbaric oxygenation on respiratory control in cats. *J Appl Physiol* 1990;67:2351–2356.

39. Hanson MA, Kumar P, Williams BA. The effects of chronic hypoxia upon the development of respiratory chemoreflexes in the newborn kitten. *J Physiol (London)* 1989;411:563–574.

40. Lahiri S, Mokashi A, Mulligan E, Nishino T. Comparison of aortic acid and carotid chemoreceptor responses to hypercapnia and hypoxia. *J Appl Physiol* 1981;51:55–61.

THE LUNG: Scientific Foundations
edited by R.G. Crystal, J.B. West et al.
Raven Press, Ltd., New York © 1991.

CHAPTER 5.4.4

Hypoxic Depression of Breathing

Norman H. Edelman and Judith A. Neubauer

MANIFESTATIONS OF HYPOXIC DEPRESSION IN THE INTACT SUBJECT

The ventilatory response to acute hypoxic hypoxia has been studied extensively and is generally considered to be well characterized. An immediate response (seconds) is mediated by the peripheral chemoreceptors and is followed in seconds to minutes by a steady lower plateau, which reflects the peripheral and central chemoreceptor response to the associated lowering of CO_2 tension. As the time of observation is extended, the characteristics of the ventilatory response to hypoxia become more difficult to define both phenomenologically and mechanistically. These include: a secondary decline in ventilation (minutes), often called the "roll-off" (especially prominent in neonates); a subsequent increase in ventilation (days), best characterized as acclimatization to altitude; and, ultimately, an often profound loss of ventilatory responsiveness to hypoxia (years). It is the thesis of this discussion that for all but the immediate response to hypoxia there is potential for modulation of the ventilatory response to hypoxia by the largely depressant effects of brain hypoxia on the ventilatory control system. The concept, although not new, has only been recently integrated into the conceptual framework of respiratory control theory in order to explain various physiologic or pathophysiologic phenomena. A few of these phenomena are described below.

The neonatal (about 1–5 days post-partum) response to inhalation of an hypoxic gas, in a variety of animals, is quite distinct from that in the more mature animal. The initial hyperventilation is quickly (about 5 min) followed by a decline in ventilation which returns to baseline or even below (1,2). A portion of the declining phase of this "biphasic" response seems to be related to the neonate's propensity to reduce metabolic rate during hypoxia, but it persists even after metabolic rate is controlled (1,3). Although a few investigators maintain that the declining ventilatory phase reflects a decline in peripheral chemoreceptor activity with time (4), the majority ascribe the decline to the depressant effects of central nervous system hypoxia. The evidence for this idea comes from several sources.

First and simplest, the sudden inhalation of oxygen during the secondary depressed stage of the response results in immediate further depression of ventilation even in the absence of hypocapnia (5). This is taken to show that sudden diminution of peripheral chemoreceptor activity reveals an underlying depression of output from control circuits. Second, the phenomenon has been substantially ameliorated by administration of antagonists of both adenosine (6) and endogenous opioids (7). Third, the phenomenon has been diminished or ameliorated by a high pontine section of the neuraxis (8,9). This observation is taken to signify that not only is the depressant phase of the neonatal response to hypoxia mediated by the central nervous effects of hypoxia but that, in addition, the central nervous effects of hypoxia are mediated by a discrete region of the diencephalon. Finally, in anesthetized neonates, some (but not all) studies show no decline in peripheral chemoreceptor output over the period of time associated with the biphasic response to hypoxia (1,10).

A similar (although less dramatic) phenomenon has been demonstrated in unanesthetized adult mammals, including humans. Within 15–30 min after the onset of isocapnic hypoxia, a decline in ventilation equal to 25–40% of the peak response is noted (11). If the subject is allowed to breathe room air for 15 min or O_2 for 5 min, full responsiveness to hypoxia returns. Lesser pe-

N. H. Edelman and J. A. Neubauer: Division of Pulmonary and Critical Care Medicine, Department of Medicine, University of Medicine and Dentistry of New Jersey—Robert Wood Johnson Medical School, New Brunswick, New Jersey 08903.

riods of "recovery" are associated with levels of responsiveness to renewed hypoxia which are closer to those observed during the decline phase of the initial experiment. These observations are consistent with the idea that brain hypoxia results in elaboration of depressant neuroeffectors which, at appropriate levels, reduce ventilatory output. The relatively slow and oxygen-dependent nature of the "recovery" period is consistent with the time and environment required for metabolism or dissipation of these neural depressant molecules. In partial support of this idea, the "roll-off" phenomenon in adults is ameliorated by administration of antagonists of adenosine (12) but not by endogenous opioids (13). Furthermore, the administration of somatostatin (which blocks peripheral chemoreception) to unanesthetized humans converts the ventilatory response to hypoxia to one of pure depression approximately 25 min after onset of hypoxia (14).

Familial dysautonomia (Riley–Day syndrome) is an uncommon heritable disorder that is characterized by a variety of defects in sensation and autonomic nervous function. We studied it to determine whether the sensory defects included impairment of chemoreception (15). We observed a response to hypoxia which was strikingly similar to the neonatal biphasic response. Increased ventilation quickly was reduced to baseline or below; subsequent inhalation of oxygen resulted in profound further depression of respiratory output, frequently characterized by prolonged apneic periods. An additional characteristic of these subjects was an inability to maintain blood pressure during inhalation of the hypoxic gas mixture. We interpreted these data as signifying an intact chemoreceptor response to hypoxia (whether it was "normal" or not was difficult to ascertain) with an exaggerated central nervous depressant response, perhaps due to inadequate blood pressure control that resulted in decreased brain blood flow, thereby causing decreased O_2 delivery to the brain.

Severe anemia is commonplace—especially in the setting of modern medicine, which includes (a) long-term support of functionally anephric patients and (b) chemotherapy with agents that suppress bone marrow function. We postulated that severely limited O_2-carrying capacity of arterial blood would enhance the central depressant component of the integrated ventilatory response to hypoxia (16). The model was that of the unanesthetized goat repeatedly bled to various hemoglobin concentrations. The response to brief transient hypoxia (several breaths of N_2) was taken to reflect peripheral chemoreceptor function, whereas the response to more prolonged inhalation of a hypoxic gas mixture was taken to reflect the sum of (a) peripheral chemoreceptor stimulation by hypoxia and (b) the dynamically slower depression of respiratory output attributable to central nervous system hypoxia. We observed that the response to transient hypoxia was

enhanced by anemia, a phenomenon that could be attributed to the increased sympathetic tone in these animals. In contrast, the response to more prolonged hypoxia was depressed in direct relation to the severity of the anemia produced. We thus concluded that anemia allows enhanced expression of the depressant effect on ventilation of central nervous system hypoxia by further limiting O_2 delivery to the brain during inhalation of a hypoxic gas mixture.

It is generally agreed that the ventilatory response to isocapnic hypoxia is depressed during sleep, and there is evidence that this phenomenon is more pronounced in rapid eye movement (REM) sleep as compared to slow-wave sleep (17). The mechanisms are unclear, since it has not been possible to do the necessary invasive studies (e.g., recording output from the carotid body) in unanesthetized sleeping animals. The simplest explanation is that reduced responsiveness to hypoxia reflects the generalized reduction of responsiveness to respiratory stimuli during sleep. However, our recent studies suggest that when the effects of sleep on respiratory system mechanical properties and upon brain blood flow are taken into account, a reduction in intrinsic responsiveness of respiratory neuronal output to a CO_2 stimulus cannot be demonstrated during either sleep stage (18). Thus, the mechanism for reduced responsiveness to hypoxia during sleep remains unclear. In an attempt to assess the role of brain hypoxia, we (19) administered carbon monoxide to awake and sleeping animals on the assumption that this compound would produce tissue hypoxia without stimulating the peripheral chemoreceptors. In the range studied (blood carboxyhemoglobin levels to 35%), there were no effects on ventilation in awake animals but there was measurable depression of ventilation with associated hypercapnia in animals during slow-wave and REM sleep. We postulate that in the absence of the "waking stimulus" and other nonspecific stimuli to breathing present in the awake animal, the sleeping animal is able to manifest depression of respiratory output due to brain hypoxia.

CHARACTERISTICS OF THE VENTILATORY RESPONSE TO BRAIN HYPOXIA: HYPERPNEA IN UNANESTHETIZED ANIMALS

The nature of the ventilatory response to brain hypoxia is strongly state-dependent. In unanesthetized, peripherally chemodenervated animals, inhalation of a hypoxic gas mixture (10–16% O_2) results in hyperpnea, which is usually manifest as an intense tachypnea with relatively slight hypocapnia (20). Unanesthetized goats given carbon monoxide to breathe manifest the same response at carboxyhemoglobin levels of about 40–60% (21,22). Similar responses are observed as a result of restriction of brain blood flow (23) and injection of sodium cyanide into sinoaortic denervated animals (24). Enhancement of certain respiratory reflexes during brain hypoxia in unanesthetized animals has also been demonstrated. We (25) have shown (a) an increased response to CO_2 of the respiratory phasic genioglossal electromyogram and (b) an intensification of the Hering–Breuer reflex. On the other hand, during inhalation of carbon monoxide by unanesthetized goats, there is no enhancement of ventilatory responsiveness to hypoxic hypoxia or hypercapnia. Under virtually all experimental conditions to date, hypoxia results in depression of respiratory phasic activity in the majority of expiratory muscles operating on the thoracic pump.

We and others explain enhancement of respiratory activity by brain hypoxia in unanesthetized animals by reference to the selective vulnerability of the neuraxis to hypoxia (25,26). A rostral-to-caudal progression of sensitivity has been demonstrated with measurable impairment of certain cortical functions of unanesthetized animals in the presence of carboxyhemoglobin levels as low as 10%. Furthermore, cortical influences on respiratory output are largely inhibitory, especially on the potent rate-facilitating function of the diencephalon. Thus, we interpret the excitatory respiratory effects of brain hypoxia in unanesthetized animals as being due to depression of cortical function with consequent disinhibition of diencephalic and perhaps other excitatory influences. Tachypnea is not seen in anesthetized animals because the respiratory modulating effects of both the cortex and diencephalon are largely lost.

CHARACTERISTICS OF CENTRAL HYPOXIC DEPRESSION

We have found that the depressant action of brain hypoxia is best demonstrated in a model of the anesthetized, peripherally chemodenervated cat with arterial P_{CO_2} and blood pressure maintained constant (27,28). Progressive tissue hypoxia is produced by inhalation of carbon monoxide. In this system, there is a highly reproducible sequence of events which correlates with reduction in O_2 content of arterial blood. Respiratory depression produced in this way is characterized by an early reduction of the peak amplitude of the time-averaged phrenic neurogram followed by a reduction in burst frequency of the neurogram occurring only after the peak amplitude has been reduced by approximately 50% (29). Complete silence of the phrenic neurogram usually occurs when O_2 content in arterial blood has been reduced by about 50%. In this model, this corresponds to an O_2 tension at the surface of the medulla of about 13 torr. During this period of phrenic

silence, the ability of the respiratory control system to respond to adequate stimuli appears to remain completely intact. The response of the phrenic neurogram to inhalation of CO_2 equals or exceeds that in the control state (28), and the response to electrical stimulation of the carotid sinus nerve is unchanged (30).

If tissue hypoxia is allowed to progress beyond this period of phrenic silence, phasic activity of the phrenic neurogram resumes when O_2 content in arterial blood is lowered by 80–85% of the control value (31). The activity observed in this phase resembles gasping in that it is characterized by high-amplitude bursts of short duration with relatively longer and not entirely regular intervening periods (32). This activity continues to the limits of stability of the preparation—that is, to the point where depression of cardiac output prevents maintenance of arterial blood pressure. The gasping period, although reversible with subsequent oxygenation, appears to be one in which various respiratory neuronal functions are impaired. Thus, there is little or no response of the phrenic neurogram to inhalation of CO_2 or carotid sinus nerve stimulation. In addition, in our recent studies we have shown that the gasping period is associated with an abrupt rise in the extracellular potassium ion concentration in respiratory neural pools, implying that ionic pumps of cellular membranes are no longer capable of maintaining normal gradients (33). These observations are consistent with the proposal by St. John et al. (34) that a separate respiratory pattern generator is responsible for gasping. That is, much of the "normal" responsiveness of the respiratory controller appears to have been abolished while a more simple or "primitive" pattern generator, highly resistant to the effects of tissue hypoxia, is uncovered, probably by disinhibition (i.e., the inactivation of a normally strong inhibitory influence upon the gasping pattern generator).

The depressant response to brain hypoxia seems to be a generalized characteristic of the central respiratory controller, since outputs other than that of the phrenic nerve behave similarly but have, however, different apparent vulnerabilities. In sharp contrast to the unanesthetized animal, progressive hypoxia by inhalation of carbon monoxide in anesthetized animals results in depression of output from the hypoglossal nerve, with silencing of the phasic activity in this nerve occurring well before silencing of the phrenic neurogram (35). As indicated earlier, phasic expiratory muscle activity is silenced by hypoxia under virtually all conditions and is lost very early in the course of progressive hypoxia (36).

On the other hand, depression of central nervous motor output is not a uniform response to hypoxia if one considers outputs other than those associated with phasic respiratory activity. Single-fiber recordings from the preganglionic cervical sympathetic nerve have demonstrated different populations of nerves: Some increase firing frequency with hypoxia, whereas others decrease it (37). When time-averaged whole-nerve recordings are made from the preganglionic cervical sympathetic nerve, the phasic respiratory-synchronous activity declines in parallel with the activity of the phrenic bursts during progressive hypoxia (38). However, the time component of output in the sympathetic nerve increases to the limits of the model (i.e., cardiovascular collapse during very severe hypoxia). The increase of tonic sympathetic activity in the blood-pressure-controlled deafferented animal suggests either that decreased oxygenation of brain tissue directly stimulates central sympathetic neurons or that selective vulnerability within the central sympathetic neural network results in a disinhibition of these neurons.

MECHANISMS OF HYPOXIC DEPRESSION OF RESPIRATORY OUTPUT

Various mechanisms have been proposed as general explanations of depression of respiratory neuronal output due to brain hypoxia. These include: (a) direct depression of neuronal function due to substrate (O_2) limitation; (b) an inhibitory "reflex" involving higher (than brain stem) mechanisms; (c) brain hemodynamic response to tissue hypoxia resulting in overperfusion of medullary chemosensitive areas with depression of their output in relation to the consequent reduction of tissue CO_2 tension; and (d) alteration of the balance of excitatory and inhibitory neuroeffectors such that inhibition of respiratory output is favored.

Inadequate Availability of O_2

This is the most straightforward mechanistic suggestion that has been raised. However, there are strong arguments against it as an explanation for the respiratory depression associated with moderate brain hypoxia (i.e., reductions in O_2 content of arterial blood, ranging from 20% to 60%). To begin with, generally more severe hypoxia has been required to deplete brain tissue of high-energy phosphate molecules, the source of energy for neural transmission (39). In *in vivo* preparations, severe depression of output to phrenic silence is associated with completely preserved responsiveness to adequate stimuli such as hypercapnia and carotid sinus nerve stimulation (28,30). These findings suggest that tissue hypoxia has silenced the unstimulated motor neuronal pool by membrane hyperpolarization rather than by the membrane depolarization which would be expected with inadequate substrate for neuronal energy metabolism. Direct evidence of hypoxia-induced hyperpolarization of med-

ullary respiratory neurons from intracellular recordings is lacking. However, one group has found that the latency for antidromic stimulation of most medullary neurons is increased by hypoxia, suggesting that these neurons are hyperpolarized (40).

In vitro preparations have provided insight into the neuronal responses to hypoxia. By recording intracellularly and extracellularly from CA1 neurons in hippocampal slices and assessing excitability by orthodromic stimulation via Schaffer collateral fibers, a sequence of neuronal events may be observed during progressive hypoxia (41). Initially, CA1 neurons hyperpolarize, with the duration and amplitude of hyperpolarization increasing with more prolonged hypoxic exposure. After 5–12 min of complete O_2 deprivation, hyperpolarization is followed by progressive depolarization that eventually becomes irreversible. In addition, excitatory postsynaptic potentials were found to be less vulnerable to hypoxia than were inhibitory postsynaptic potentials, suggesting that CA1 neurons retain an ability to be excited while hyperpolarized.

Taken together, these studies suggest that depression of respiratory output due to moderate brain hypoxia reflects neuronal hyperpolarization rather than the depolarization which would be expected to result from substrate limitation of energy metabolism. It is our belief that hyperpolarization reflects increased influence of inhibitory neuroeffectors. The potential neuroeffectors involved are discussed later.

Higher Brain Centers

The suggestion that brain hypoxia stimulates the higher brain centers which then depress respiratory output is based upon the observation that stimulation of most cortical regions that influence respiratory activity results in depression of output (42). In addition, decortication augments ventilation in hypoxic cats (26). Since the cortex generally acts to inhibit diencephalic facilitatory areas, the latter observation may simply reflect a disinhibited diencephalon. However, more recent studies in neonates suggest that a hypoxia-sensitive suprapontine inhibitory center exists. In these studies, hypoxic depression of breathing was attenuated in fetal lambs and newborn rabbits after mid-collicular transection (8,9).

Brain Blood Flow

The vasodilatory action of hypoxia on the brain vasculature is substantial—with the greatest effect being evident in the brain stem (43)—and is not associated with an increase in tissue metabolic rate (44). Thus, it has been proposed that washout of tissue CO_2 at the site of the central chemoreceptor may be a mechanism for depression of breathing during brain hypoxia. When responses of ventral medullary surface pH and ventilation to progressive carboxyhemoglobinemia and hypoxic hypoxia were assessed in anesthetized, peripherally chemodenervated cats, it was found that medullary alkalosis did occur, was greatest during mild hypoxia, and was associated with respiratory depression (45). However, the alkalosis was only transient and replaced by acidosis (probably reflecting the brain's great propensity for anaerobic glycolysis) if the hypoxia was prolonged or made more severe.

A similar biphasic extracellular fluid pH response to brain hypoxia has been recently shown to occur in the newborn piglet (46). These findings suggest that hyperperfusion of ventral medullary chemoreceptors with washout of CO_2 may play a role in hypoxic ventilatory depression, especially with mild brain hypoxia. The effect is unlikely to persist into the steady state and thus has the potential for significance in transient or periodic phenomena. One such state is represented by REM sleep. In this state, there is considerable hyperperfusion (47,48) unaccompanied by increase in aerobic metabolism (48), which is exaggerated by hypoxia (19). An inverse relation between brain blood flow and phasic respiratory output during REM sleep has been demonstrated in sleeping goats, and inhalation of carbon monoxide produced hypercapnia during REM sleep in the same model (48).

Modulation of Neuroeffector Balance

Mild to moderate brain hypoxia has been associated with a reduction in the synthesis or release of excitatory neurotransmitters such as acetylcholine (49), aromatic monoamines (50), and the amino acids glutamate and aspartate (51). Correspondingly, an increase in synthesis or release of a variety of inhibitory neuroeffectors has been demonstrated. These include gamma-aminobutyric acid (GABA), adenosine, β-alanine, taurine, endogenous opioids, and lactate (27,51–56). Although the synthesis of acetylcholine and the monoamines appears to be quite sensitive to reductions in tissue O_2 tension, it is experimentally difficult to assess the respiratory effects of the modulation of these molecules. Accordingly, most existing data address the role of increase in depressant neurotransmitters as agents of hypoxic depression of respiratory output through neuronal hyperpolarization.

Endogenous opioids are central respiratory depressants that are often elaborated in response to physiological stresses (57). A depressant effect upon respiratory output by endogenous opioids during hypoxia has been convincingly demonstrated for neonatal animals. Several studies have shown that the

apnea which follows severe asphyxia in neonates is reversible by infusion of the specific opioid antagonist, naloxone (56,58). In addition, the depressant phase of the biphasic response of the mammalian neonate to hypoxia is attenuated by pretreatment with naloxone (7).

In contrast, a role for endogenous opioids in hypoxic depression of respiratory output is difficult to demonstrate in adult animals. In adult humans, the secondary decline of ventilation after 15–30 min of isocapnic hypoxia is not influenced by naloxone (13), and no increase in cerebrospinal fluid (CSF) endorphins was found in goats exposed to arterial Po_2 values of 30 torr for 2.5 hr (59). In the anesthetized deafferented cat, endogenous opioids seem to mediate only a small portion of hypoxic respiratory depression (60). However, a somewhat greater role has been found in dogs (61).

Adenosine levels in brain tissue are readily increased by hypoxia in relation to degree of O_2 deprivation (54). Adenosine decreases evoked neuronal activity *in vitro* (62), and there is good evidence that exogenously administered adenosine or more stable analogues may cause profound depression of respiration in both adult and neonatal animals (63,64).

In one study, systemically administered aminophylline (an adenosine antagonist, although it has other actions relevant to respiratory control) attenuated the depressant phase of the biphasic respiratory response to hypoxia in intact neonatal piglets (6). However, the effect was solely on respiratory frequency. In another study on piglets which involved recording of the phrenic electroneurogram of vagotomized ventilated animals, aminophylline pretreatment had no effect on the phrenic response to hypoxia (65). In the latter study, frequency was not affected by hypoxia. Taken together, these studies suggest that elaboration of adenosine plays, at best, only a partial role in the depressant phase of the biphasic ventilatory response of the neonate to hypoxia by an action solely on mechanisms setting respiratory rate.

Similarly, only the frequency component of the secondary decline of the adult human response to isocapnic hypoxia was blocked by pretreatment with theophylline (12). Furthermore, in anesthetized adult animals, theophylline does little to prevent depression of respiratory output during hypoxia but does eliminate depression of respiratory output in the posthypoxic phase (66,67).

During normoxia, GABA (or any of its analogues) applied to the brain in various ways is a potent inhibitor of respiration (1,68–70). GABA is widely distributed in the brain and has important tonic effects; thus, GABA antagonists applied in sufficient concentrations cause seizures. GABA has been shown to accumulate in the brain during hypoxia in adult and neonatal mammals as well as in lower vertebrates (52,53,71). Hypoxia produces increases in extracellular GABA concentrations by both increased production and impairment of re-uptake systems (55).

We directly tested whether GABA antagonism could reverse hypoxic respiratory depression in our model of the deafferented cat exposed to progressive hypoxia by carbon monoxide inhalation (72). Minute phrenic activity that had been reduced by 73% during hypoxia was fully restored by bicuculline administration. The effect was primarily that of a restoration of the reduced amplitude of bursts in the phrenic neurogram. Accordingly, we have postulated that GABA may be the principal inhibitory neurotransmitter responsible for hypoxic depression of respiratory output.

Lactic Acid

The brain manifests an early and intense Pasteur effect when exposed to hypoxia, resulting in significant production of lactic acid. When medullary surface pH is measured during progressive tissue hypoxia in the anesthetized cat, a strong correlation exists between the decrease in pH and the decline in respiratory output (45). Since medullary acidosis is generally considered to be a respiratory stimulant, this correlation seems, at first, to be paradoxical. However, there is a considerable amount of experimental data supporting the notion that most neurons decrease their excitability in the presence of extracellular acidosis (73–75). Although neurons at the surface of the ventrolateral medulla which serve a chemoreceptor function may be an exception to this generalization, even among these neurons there is far less response to metabolic acidosis than to hypercapnic acidosis. Most convincingly, when brain lactate production is blocked by pretreatment of the anesthetized cat with dichloroacetate, respiratory depression with progressive tissue hypoxia is blocked until the hypoxia is severe (27). Thus, the net effect of brain lactic acidosis in this model seems to be respiratory depression.

Many mechanisms may be proposed for the depressant effect of lactic acidosis on respiratory output. For example, acidosis decreases calcium ion influx into cells by inhibiting slow inward Ca^{2+} membrane channels (76) and Na^+–Ca^{2+} exchange (77). However, the most attractive to us is the potential effect on GABA metabolism. The key synthetic enzyme for GABA synthesis, glutamic acid decarboxylase, has a pH optimum of 7.0, whereas the key enzyme for GABA degradation, GABA transaminase, has a pH optimum of 8.0 (78). Thus, acidosis should favor accumulation of GABA.

CONCLUSION

The mechanisms by which brain hypoxia modulates ventilation are clearly multiple. We feel that all respiratory manifestations of brain hypoxia reflect depression of neuronal activity (with the exception of effects on brain blood flow), and we recognize the evidence to the contrary provided by midcollicular sections in the neonate. In the unanesthetized state, brain hypoxia causes tachypnea, probably by depression of cortical function with disinhibition of diencephalic facilitatory influences. In the anesthetized state, we recognize three general types of respiratory effects of brain hypoxia. Type I occurs with mild hypoxia, tends to be transient, and can be related to CO_2 washout of chemoreceptor tissues by increased brain blood flow. It is probably only of importance in nonsteady states such as may be found in REM sleep. Type II occurs with moderate hypoxia. It appears to reflect elaboration of inhibitory neuroeffectors (principally GABA) causing hyperpolarization of respiratory neurons with decreased output. Neuronal integrity is preserved, and responsiveness to adequate stimuli such as hypercapnia remains intact. Type III occurs with severe hypoxia, causes limitation of substrate availability, and causes impairment of neuronal function. The transition between Type II and Type III hypoxia appears to be associated with gasping respiratory activity. Current evidence is consistent with the idea that the gasping oscillator is separate from the eupneic oscillator, is extremely hypoxia-resistant, and is normally under strong inhibitory influences which are released only by severe tissue hypoxia.

It would appear that Type II hypoxic depression of ventilation is an important part of the neonatal response to hypoxia and is a less important but desirable part of the adult response as well. Pathophysiological conditions that impair O_2 delivery to the brain during hypoxia, such as anemia and autonomic dysfunction, are associated with enhanced manifestations of hypoxic depression.

What remains to be explained is the adaptive value of Type II hypoxic depression. Why should the organism have in place a mechanism unassociated with neuronal dysfunction which reduces ventilatory activity during hypoxia? The answer may be both general and specific. From a general point of view, it must be noted, as pointed out by Hochachka (79), that augmentation of respiration or circulation is not always the best strategy for survival in the face of a hypoxic challenge. The turtle survives submersion in water equilibrated with nitrogen for days to weeks by reduction of metabolic rate (80). To the extent possible, available energy is used to maintain ionic gradients across cell membranes, the hallmark of life.

A more specific clue may be found in the fact that

hypoxic depression of respiration is most pronounced in the neonate. This suggests that it may play an important adaptive role *in utero*. Consideration of the physiology of life *in utero* makes the adaptive value clear. The mature fetus must have sufficiently developed respiratory reflexes, including the response to hypoxia, to survive extrauterine life after birth. On the other hand, *in utero* a brisk ventilatory response to hypoxia is maladaptive. The respiratory movements do not improve oxygenation, and they deplete O_2 stores of the body. Thus, a mechanism which dampens or eliminates the ventilatory response to hypoxia in late gestation and which is lost soon after birth has protective value. The endogenous opioid system that is readily activated by hypoxia early in extrauterine life but is quickly dissipated within days seems to fit this description.

ACKNOWLEDGMENT

This work was supported by National Heart, Lung and Blood Institute Research Grant HL 16022.

REFERENCES

1. Blanco CE, Hanson MA, Johnson P, Rigatto H. Breathing pattern of kittens during hypoxia. *J Appl Physiol* 1984;56:12–17.
2. Haddad GG, Mellins RB. Hypoxia and respiratory control in early life. *Annu Rev Physiol* 1984;46:629–643.
3. Saetta M, Mortola JP. Interaction of hypoxic and hypercapnic stimuli on breathing pattern in the newborn rat. *J Appl Physiol* 1987;62:506–512.
4. Bureau MA, Lamarche J, Foulon P, Dalle D. The ventilatory response to hypoxia in the newborn lamb after carotid body denervation. *Respir Physiol* 1985;60:109–119.
5. Holtby SG, Berezanski DJ, Anthonisen NR. Effect of 100% O_2 on hypoxic eucapnic ventilation. *J Appl Physiol* 1988;65:1157–1162.
6. Darnall RA. Aminophylline reduces hypoxic ventilatory depression: possible role of adenosine. *Pediatr Res* 1985;19:706–710.
7. DeBoeck C, van Raempts P, Rigatto H, Chernick V. Naloxone reduces decrease in ventilation induced by hypoxia in newborn infants. *J Appl Physiol* 1984;56:1507–1511.
8. Dawes GS, Gardner WN, Johnston BM, Walker DW. Breathing in fetal lambs: the effect of brainstem section. *J Physiol (Lond)* 1983;335:535–553.
9. Martin-Body RL, Johnston BM. Central origin of the hypoxic depression of breathing in the newborn. *Respir Physiol* 1988;71:25–32.
10. Lawson EE, Long WW. Central origin of biphasic breathing pattern during hypoxia in newborns. *J Appl Physiol* 1983;55:483–488.
11. Easton PA, Slykerman LJ, Anthonisen NR. Ventilatory response to sustained hypoxia in normal adults. *J Appl Physiol* 1986;61:906–911.
12. Easton PA, Anthonisen NR. Ventilatory response to sustained hypoxia after pretreatment with aminophylline. *J Appl Physiol* 1988;64:1445–1450.
13. Kagawa S, Stafford MJ, Waggener TB, Severinghaus JW. No effect of naloxone on hypoxia-induced ventilatory depression in adults. *J Appl Physiol* 1982;52:1030–1034.
14. Maxwell DL, Clahal P, Nolop KB, Hughes JMB. Somatostatin inhibits the ventilatory response to hypoxia in humans. *J Appl Physiol* 1986;60:997–1002.
15. Edelman NH, Cherniack NS, Lahiri S, Richards E, Fishman AP. The effects of abnormal sympathetic nervous function upon the ventilatory response to hypoxia. *J Clin Invest* 1970;49:1153–1165.
16. Santiago TV, Edelman NH, Fishman AP. The effect of anemia on the ventilatory response to transient and steady-state hypoxia. *J Clin Invest* 1975;55:410–418.
17. Santiago TV, Scardella AT, Edelman NH. Determinants of the ventilatory responses to hypoxia during sleep. *Am Rev Respir Dis* 1984;130:179–182.
18. Parisi RA, Edelman NH, Santiago TV. Central respiratory chemosensitivity during sleep is a function of cerebrovascular CO_2 response. *Am Rev Respir Dis* 1989;139:A84.
19. Santiago TV, Neubauer JA, Edelman NH. Correlation between ventilation and brain blood flow during hypoxic sleep. *J Appl Physiol* 1986;60:295–298.
20. Miller MJ, Tenney SM. Hypoxia-induced tachypnea in carotid-deafferented cats. *Respir Physiol* 1975;23:31–39.
21. Doblar D, Santiago TV, Edelman NH. Correlation between ventilatory and cerebrovascular responses to inhalation of CO. *J Appl Physiol* 1977;43:455–462.
22. Santiago TV, Edelman NH. Mechanism of the ventilatory response to carbon monoxide. *J Clin Invest* 1976;57:977–986.
23. Chapman RW, Santiago TV, Edelman NH. Effects of graded reduction of brain blood flow on ventilation in unanesthetized goats. *J Appl Physiol* 1979;47:104–111.
24. Jansen AH, Chernick V. Respiratory response to cyanide in fetal sheep after peripheral chemodenervation. *J Appl Physiol* 1974;36:1–5.
25. Hutt DA, Parisi RA, Santiago TV, Edelman NH. Brain hypoxia preferentially stimulates genioglossal EMG responses to CO_2. *J Appl Physiol* 1989;66:51–56.
26. Tenney SM, Ou LC. Ventilatory response of decorticate and decerebrate cats to hypoxia and CO_2. *Respir Physiol* 1976;29:81–92.
27. Neubauer JA, Simone A, Edelman NH. Role of brain lactic acidosis in hypoxic depression of respiration. *J Appl Physiol* 1988;65:1324–1331.
28. Melton JE, Neubauer JA, Edelman NH. CO_2 sensitivity of cat phrenic neurogram during hypoxic respiratory depression. *J Appl Physiol* 1988;65:736–743.
29. Yu QP, Neubauer JA, Melton JE, Wasicko MJ, Li JK-J, Krawciw N, Edelman NH. Effect of brain hypoxia on the dynamic characteristics of the peak and frequency of phrenic nerve [Abstract]. *FASEB J* 1988;2(5):A1508.
30. Parisi RA, Melton JE, Wasicko MJ, Neubauer JA, Yu QP, Edelman NH. Phrenic responsiveness to carotid sinus nerve stimulation during progressive brain hypoxia [Abstract]. *FASEB J* 1988;2(5):A1507.
31. Melton JE, Wasicko MJ, Neubauer JA, Edelman NH. Patterns of phrenic depression during progressive brain hypoxia [Abstract]. *FASEB J* 1988;2(4):A510.
32. St John WM, Knuth KV. A characterization of the respiratory pattern of gasping. *J Appl Physiol* 1981;50:984–993.
33. Melton JE, Oyer LM, Neubauer JA, Edelman NH. Brain extracellular [K^+] homeostasis during hypoxic respiratory depression. *FASEB J* 1989;3(3):A251.
34. St John WM, Bledsoe TA, Tenney SM. Characterization by stimulation of medullary mechanisms underlying gasping neurogenesis. *J Appl Physiol* 1985;58:121–128.
35. Wasicko MJ, Neubauer JA, Melton JE, Harangozo AM, Edelman NH. The effect of progressive brain hypoxia on the respiratory activity of the hypoglossal nerve [Abstract]. *Fed Proc* 1987;46:1418.
36. Fregosi RF, Knuth SL, Ward DK, Bartlett D Jr. Hypoxia inhibits abdominal expiratory nerve activity. *J Appl Physiol* 1987;63:211–220.
37. Rohlicek CV, Polosa C. Hypoxic responses of sympathetic preganglionic neurons in sino-aortic-denervated cats. *Am J Physiol* 1983;244(*Heart Circ Physiol* 13):H681–H686.
38. Wasicko MJ, Melton JE, Neubauer JA, Krawciw N, Edelman NH. Cervical sympathetic and phrenic nerve responses to progressive brain hypoxia. *J Appl Physiol* 1990;68:53–58.
39. Siesjo BK, Nilsson L. The influence of arterial hypoxemia upon

labile phosphates and upon extracellular and intracellular lactate and pyruvate concentration in the rat brain. *Scand J Clin Lab Invest* 1971;27:83–96.

40. Bianchi AL, St John WM. Changes in antidromic latencies of medullary respiratory neurons in hypercapnia and hypoxia. *J Appl Physiol* 1985;59:1208–1213.

41. Fujiwara N, Higashi H, Shimoji K, Yoshimura M. Effects of hypoxia on rat hippocampal neurones *in vitro*. *J Physiol (Lond)* 1987;384:131–151.

42. Smith WK. Respiratory effects of cortical stimulation. *J Neurophysiol* 1938;1:55–68.

43. Neubauer JA, Edelman NH. Non-uniform brain blood flow response to hypoxia in unanesthetized cats. *J Appl Physiol* 1984;57:1803–1808.

44. Artu AA, Michenfelder JD. Canine cerebral metabolism and blood flow during hypoxemia and normoxic recovery from hypoxemia. *J Cereb Blood Flow Metab* 1981;1:277–283.

45. Neubauer JA, Santiago TV, Posner MA, Edelman NH. Ventral medullary pH and ventilatory responses to hyperperfusion and hypoxia. *J Appl Physiol* 1985;58:1659–1668.

46. Brown DL, Lawson EE. Brain stem extracellular fluid pH and respiratory drive during hypoxia in newborn pigs. *J Appl Physiol* 1988;64:1055–1059.

47. Reivich M, Isaacs G, Evarts E, Kety SS. The effect of slow-wave sleep and REM sleep on regional cerebral blood flow in cats. *J Neurochem* 1968;15:301–306.

48. Santiago TV, Guerra E, Neubauer JA, Edelman NH. Correlation between ventilation and brain blood flow during sleep. *J Clin Invest* 1984;73:497–506.

49. Gibson GE, Shimada M, Blass JP. Alterations in acetylcholine synthesis and in cyclic nucleotides in mild cerebral hypoxia. *J Neurochem* 1978;31:757–760.

50. Davis JN, Carlsson A. Effect of hypoxia on monoamine synthesis, levels and metabolism in rat brain. *J Neurochem* 1973;21:783–790.

51. Erecinska M, Nelson D, Wilson DF, Silver IA. Neurotransmitter amino acids in the CNS. I. Regional changes in amino acid levels in rat brain during ischemia and reperfusion. *Brain Res* 1984;304:9–22.

52. Iversen K, Hedner T, Lundborg P. GABA concentrations and turnover in neonatal rat brain during asphyxia and recovery. *Acta Physiol Scand* 1983;118:91–94.

53. Wood JD, Watson WJ, Drucker AJ. The effect of hypoxia on brain gamma-aminobutyric acid levels. *J Neurochem* 1968;15:603–608.

54. Winn HR, Rubio R, Berne RM. Brain adenosine concentration during hypoxia in rats. *Am J Physiol* 1981;241:H235–H242.

55. Hagberg H, Lehmann A, Sandberg M, Nystrom B, Jacobson I, Hamberger A. Ischemia-induced shift of inhibitory and excitatory amino acids from intra- to extracellular compartments. *J Cereb Blood Flow Metab* 1985;5:413–419.

56. Chernick V, Craig RJ. Naloxone reverses neonatal depression caused by fetal asphyxia. *Science* 1982;216:1252–1253.

57. Santiago TV, Edelman NH. Opioids and breathing. *J Appl Physiol* 1985;59:1675–1685.

58. Grunstein MM, Hazinski TA, Schleuter MA. Respiratory control during hypoxia in newborn rabbits: implied action of endorphins. *J Appl Physiol* 1981;51:122–130.

59. Freedman A, Scardella AT, Edelman NH, Santiago TV. Hypoxia does not increase CSF or plasma beta-endorphin activity. *J Appl Physiol* 1988;64:966–971.

60. Neubauer JA, Posner MA, Santiago TV, Edelman NH. Naloxone reduces ventilatory depression of brain hypoxia. *J Appl Physiol* 1987;63:699–706.

61. Schaeffer JI, Haddad GG. Ventilatory response to moderate and severe hypoxia in adult dogs: role of endorphins. *J Appl Physiol* 1988;65:1383–1388.

62. Dunwiddie TV, Haas HL. Adenosine increases synaptic facilitation in the *in vitro* rat hippocampus: evidence for a presynaptic site of action. *J Physiol London* 1985;369:365–377.

63. Eldridge FL, Millhorn DE, Kiley JP. Respiratory effects of a long-acting analog of adenosine. *Brain Res* 1984;301:273–280.

64. Lagercrantz H, Yamamoto Y, Fredholm BB, Probhakas NR, Euler C von. Adenosine analogues depress ventilation in rabbit neonates. Theophylline stimulation of respiration via adenosine receptors? *Pediatr Res* 1984;18:387–390.

65. Long WA, Lawson EE. Neurotransmitters and biphasic respiratory response to hypoxia. *J Appl Physiol* 1984;57:213–222.

66. Nissley FP, Melton JE, Neubauer JA, Edelman NH. Effect of adenosine antagonism on phrenic nerve output during brain hypoxia [Abstract]. *Fed Proc* 1986;45:1046.

67. Millhorn DE, Eldridge FL, Kiley JP, Waldrop TG. Prolonged inhibition of respiration following acute hypoxia in glomectomized cats. *Respir Physiol* 1984;57:331–340.

68. Kneussl MP, Pappagianopoulos P, Hoop B, Kazemi H. Reversible depression of ventilation and cardiovascular function by ventriculocisternal perfusion with gamma-aminobutyric acid in dogs. *Am Rev Respir Dis* 1986;133:1024–1028.

69. Yamada KA, Hamosh P, Gillis RA. Respiratory depression produced by activation of GABA receptors in hindbrain of cat. *J Appl Physiol* 1981;5:1278–1286.

70. Bennett JA, McWilliam PN, Shepheard SL. Gamma-aminobutyric acid-mediated inhibition of neurones in the nucleus tractus solitarius of the cat. *J Physiol (Lond)* 1987;392:417–430.

71. Lutz PL, Edwards R, McMahon PM. Gamma-aminobutyric acid concentrations are maintained in anoxic turtle brain. *Am J Physiol* 1985;249(*Regul Integrative Comp Physiol* 18):R372–R374.

72. Melton JE, Neubauer JA, Edelman NH. GABA antagonism reverses hypoxic respiratory depression in the cat. *J Appl Physiol* 1989; in press.

73. Balestrino M, Somjen GG. Concentration of carbon dioxide, interstitial pH and synaptic transmission in hippocampal formation of the rat. *J Physiol (Lond)* 1988;396:247–266.

74. Jodkowski JS, Lipski J. Decreased excitability of respiratory motoneurons during hypercapnia in the acute spinal cat. *Brain Res* 1986;386:296–304.

75. Mitchell RA, Herbert DA. The effect of carbon dioxide on the membrane potential of medullary respiratory neurons. *Brain Res* 1974;75:345–349.

76. Irisawa H, Sato R. Intra- and extracellular actions of proton on the calcium current of isolated guinea pig ventricular cells. *Circ Res* 1986;59:348–355.

77. Philipson KD, Bersohn MM, Nishimoto AY. Effects of pH on Na^+–Ca^{++} exchange in canine cardiac sarcolemmal vesicles. *Circ Res* 1982;50:287–293.

78. Wu J-Y. Purification, characterization, and kinetic studies of GAD and GABA-T from mouse brain. In: Roberts E, Chase T, Tower D, eds. *GABA in nervous system function*. New York: Raven Press, 1976;7–55.

79. Hochachka PW. Defense strategies against hypoxia and hypothermia. *Science* 1986;231:234–241.

80. Ultsch GR, Jackson DC. Long-term submergence at 3°C of the turtle, *Chrysemys picta belli* in normoxic and severely hypoxic water. I. Survival, gas exchange, and acid–base status. *J Exp Biol* 1982;96:11–28.

THE LUNG: *Scientific Foundations*
edited by R.G. Crystal, J.B. West et al.
Raven Press, Ltd., New York © 1991.

CHAPTER 5.4.5

Central Chemoreceptors

Neil S. Cherniack

The capacity to respond to altered levels of arterial P_{CO_2} by compensatory changes in ventilation is essential to acid–base homeostasis and normal body function. Deviations of P_{CO_2} from its usual value of 40 torr in the arterial blood produce significant physiological effects (1–7). Besides augmenting the activity of motor nerves supplying the muscles that drive the respiratory pump, hypercapnia also reflexly heightens the activity of cranial nerves, thereby diminishing the resistance to flow in the upper airways and enhancing the respiratory modulation of the discharge of sympathetic and parasympathetic nerves (8). Decreases in arterial P_{CO_2} reduce this nervous discharge and, during sleep and/or anesthesia, regularly cause apnea (5).

When this response is absent, as in certain patients with alveolar hypoventilation, ventilation decreases; this results in hypercapnia and hypoxia, which lead to pulmonary hypertension and heart failure (9).

Some of the reflex effects of changing CO_2 levels originate from stimulation of the peripheral chemoreceptors (the carotid body and, to a lesser extent, the aortic body), but the bulk of the ventilatory response to CO_2 remains following peripheral chemoreceptor denervation and is, therefore, assumed to arise from chemoreceptors within the brain (1,3,10,11,68). Because of the physiological importance of these "central chemoreceptors," much time and effort has been expended in attempting to identify their exact location and mechanism of action (6,7). Although physiological studies have narrowed the site of the central chemoreceptors to the medulla, exactly where in the medulla they are remains elusive.

Central chemoreceptors have not been anatomically differentiated from other tissues, nor have their connections to other areas of the brain been histologically tracked. Because the anatomical relationship of the central chemoreceptors is uncertain, precise data cannot be obtained on P_{CO_2} or pH changes in their microenvironment. Nonetheless, from experiments performed both *in vivo* and *in vitro*, much information concerning the operation of central chemoreceptors can be inferred.

METHODS OF STUDYING CENTRAL CHEMORECEPTORS

In vivo studies of central chemoreceptors are frequently carried out in animals in which the peripheral chemoreceptors have been denervated, since these receptors are also sensitive to CO_2 (12,13). In some of these studies the medulla has been separately perfused. Peripheral chemoreceptors affect more than respiration, and their denervation distorts normal physiology to a certain extent (3). Hence, a number of investigators have attempted to study central chemoreceptors in the intact subject, taking advantage of the difference in the time course of the response of peripheral and central chemoreceptors to CO_2 stimulation (14). Although peripheral chemoreceptor discharge immediately mimics the temporal profile of changes in arterial P_{CO_2}, when CO_2 is inhaled, ventilation increases for a much longer period of time (often for more than 10 or 15 min) after both arterial CO_2 and peripheral chemoreceptor discharge reach steady levels (15,16). This temporal dissociation has been believed to reflect the time required for arterial CO_2 to equilibrate with P_{CO_2} in the brain. Because changes in P_{CO_2} measured in the blood of the venous effluent from the brain approximate the time course of the changes in ventilation rather well, it was thought that the central chemoreceptors were located near the venous side of the circulation and that its CO_2 stimulus would be affected by cerebral blood flow. More recent studies

N. S. Cherniack: Department of Medicine, Case Western Reserve University School of Medicine, Cleveland, Ohio 44106.

suggest that changes in medullary P_{CO_2} can occur quite rapidly and have led to the proposal that the slower increase in ventilation arterial P_{CO_2} is to process the signal from the central chemoreceptor (17). While this conjecture complicates somewhat the conclusions reached from time course studies about the location and stimulus to the central chemoreceptors, the finding in these studies that the central chemoreceptors contribute 70–80% of the total ventilatory response to CO_2 has been confirmed by studies using other techniques, such as injections of CO_2 or other acids into the vertebral arteries or the cerebrospinal fluid, or by studies employing isolated perfusion of the brain *in vivo* with solutions containing different partial pressure of CO_2 (1,3,6,13).

CO_2 can influence respiration indirectly as well by stimulating chemoreceptors by its actions on cerebral blood flow, its direct effects on smooth and skeletal muscle, and its effects on the myocardium (by altering rates of catecholamine secretion), all of which complicate *in vivo* studies (see, e.g., refs. 18 and 19).

A number of *in vitro* methods have recently been developed to better elucidate the mechanism of CO_2 stimulation. These methods include (a) preparations of the isolated brain and spinal cord of the newborn rat and (b) slices of tissue from different regions of the medulla (20,21). These preparations allow extracellular and intracellular nerve recordings to be made in situations where the neuronal environment can be controlled with much greater precision than *in vivo*. However, normal interconnections among neurons are disrupted in slice preparations. In addition, in slice preparations it is difficult to know what the normal function of a given nerve cell is, because of the heterogeneity of the structure and function in the mammalian medulla. Although these problems are less severe where neuronal recordings can be correlated to recordings made from the proximal stubs of the phrenic nerve, results may be distorted because this preparation depends on the use of the immature rat.

CHARACTERISTICS OF THE CO₂ RESPONSE

The afferent discharge of peripheral chemoreceptors increases linearly as arterial P_{CO_2} is raised (10,11). Since the afferent activity of the central chemoreceptors has not yet been directly measured because its location is uncertain, inferences have been made about the characteristics of the afferent response from studies of respiratory motor output.

In both intact and peripherally chemodenervated anesthetized animals, there is no ventilation and no phasic respiratory nerve or neuronal activity until P_{CO_2} in the arterial blood reaches some minimum level (the

apneic threshold) (1,3,22). Thereafter, responses are linearly related to change in arterial P_{CO_2} until P_{CO_2} reaches a very high value (often exceeding 100 torr). Thereafter, no further increase occurs, and there may even be a decline in response with further hypercapnia (see Fig. 1). Cranial nerves innervating upper airway muscles and cervical spinal nerves and accessory muscles like the sternohyoid show a similar pattern with a threshold, a linear portion, and then a plateau, but the exact P_{CO_2} values for the threshold and the plateau differ among nerves, as shown in Fig. 2 (23). Rather than consisting of three roughly linear segments, some investigators believe P_{CO_2} responses are better represented by convexly curvilinear, or even S-shaped, curves.

In awake subjects it may be difficult to demonstrate an apneic threshold for CO_2 because ventilation continues, albeit at a minimum level, in many conscious subjects as P_{CO_2} is lowered. However, with passive hyperventilation, obvious respiratory activity is rather easily eliminated even during wakefulness (3). However, CO_2 may have respiratory actions even when there is no clearly demonstrable respiratory activity. For instance, anesthetized animals made apneic by hyperventilation can be made to respire spontaneously by the administration of hypoxic gases to lower arterial P_{O_2}. Even though P_{CO_2} was too low before hypoxia to affect breathing, hyperventilation of these animals even more after hypoxia allows apnea to reoccur. This suggests that even very low levels of P_{CO_2} can stimulate central chemoreceptors, but whether this discharge produces respiratory activity depends on the level of other excitatory inputs to the respiratory neurons.

Sears et al. (24) have suggested that the apneic threshold for expiratory neurons may be lower than for inspiratory neurons, so that as P_{CO_2} is raised from subthreshold values, breathing begins with expiratory firing. The reverse—that is, the initial activity being inspiratory rather than expiratory—was reported to occur when hypoxia was the stimulus to incite respiration in the apneic animals.

Regions of the brain rostral to the medulla can affect respiratory response when the central chemoreceptor is stimulated. For example, decerebration generally accentuates the CO_2 response of the hypoglossal nerve (which supplies the tongue) whereas decerebration inhibits it (25).

The increased ventilation produced by inhaled CO_2 varies considerably in conscious humans. Reported responses have varied from 1 to 8 liter/min/torr P_{CO_2}, which may reflect the effects of other internal and external stimuli on respiratory neurons rather than an actual variability in the sensitivity of central chemoreceptors (1,3). Anesthesia and sleep depress the increase in phrenic nerve activity caused by hypercap-

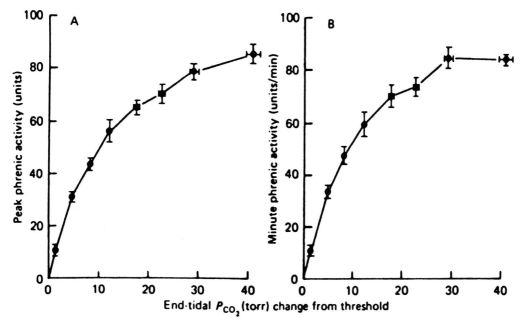

FIG. 1. Increases over apneic threshold of end-tidal CO_2. **A:** Peak tidal phrenic nerve activity. **B:** Neural minute phrenic nerve activity. (From ref. 22.)

nia, but not as much as they reduce the responses to CO_2 of cranial nerves or motor nerves supplying the accessory respiratory muscles (5). In rapid eye movement (REM) sleep, the effect of stimuli originating in the brain may become sufficiently large so as to mask the effects of central chemoreceptor stimulation and eliminate any consistent effect on ventilation of hypercapnia (5).

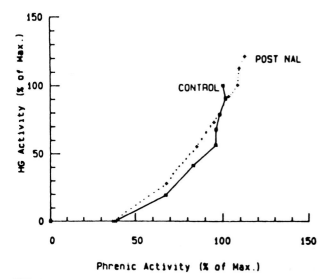

FIG. 2. Average data from eight cats showing the relationship between phrenic nerve activity and hypoglossal (HG) activity before and after naloxone (NAL) infusion. Note that hypoglossal activity starts after phrenic activity but that it plateaus later. (From ref. 23.)

Lack of certainty concerning the exact stimulus to the central chemoreceptors may also contribute to the apparent variability of CO_2 responses. For example, changes in cerebral blood flow may alter the P_{CO_2} stimulus to central chemoreceptors so that venous P_{CO_2} of the brain or P_{CO_2} in the cerebrospinal fluid may better reflect (as opposed to P_{CO_2} of the arterial blood) the actual stimulus to the central chemoreceptors (26).

In intact animals, it is clear that the respiratory responses to P_{CO_2} depend on the presence or absence of other respiratory inputs. The apneic threshold, but not CO_2 responsivity (defined here as the change in ventilation divided by the change in arterial P_{CO_2}), is affected by acidosis and by alkalosis. With acidosis the ventilation achieved at any given P_{CO_2} is greater than it is normally, whereas with alkalosis it is less. Hypoxia, on the other hand, alters CO_2 responsivity but has smaller effects on apneic threshold. Hypoxia increases CO_2 sensitivity, and the effect is magnified until P_{O_2} is lowered to very low levels (probably to about 30–40 torr), as shown in Fig. 3 (27). This effect requires the presence of peripheral chemoreceptors. Some of the changes in CO_2 response with hypoxia occur by O_2 and CO_2 interaction at the carotid body. Afferent activity from the carotid body in response to CO_2 increases with hypoxia. Other studies suggest that peripheral chemoreceptor output may interact with central chemoreceptor output in the central nervous system (28). It is also possible that hypoxia might somehow directly alter the responses of the central chemoreceptor by altering cerebral blood flow or by depressing the activity of medullary respiratory neu-

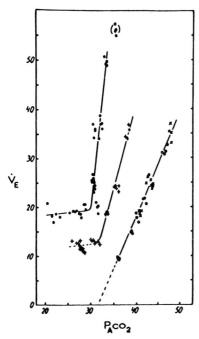

FIG. 3. Ventilation ($\dot{V}_E$) as a function of $P_{A}CO_2$ at steady-state Pa_{O_2} of 37 (●), 47 (+), and 169 (×) in conscious humans. (From ref. 71.)

rons (29). It is also of interest that central chemoreceptor output may affect peripheral chemoreceptor activity. Efferent nerves with an inhibitory action have been described running between the medulla and the carotid body. Hypocapnia has been said to enhance this inhibitory action.

There is probably little effect of the central chemoreceptors on the ventilatory response to exercise. In most studies in which it has been examined, exercise has been reported to have no effect on CO_2 responsivity, although an increase in responsivity has been observed in some recent experiments. All observers agree that exercise lowers the apneic threshold (30).

Arterial P_{CO_2} levels and brain pH levels (to a much smaller extent) oscillate during a breath, falling with inspiration and rising with expiration. These oscillations, which increase in magnitude with higher metabolic rates, may be signals used by the brain to match ventilation with metabolism during exercise. These arterial P_{CO_2} oscillations are known to increase peripheral receptor discharge more than steady (nonoscillatory) increases in P_{CO_2} (31). It is not known whether pH oscillations observed on the surface of the medulla have any effect at all on central chemoreceptor discharge. It is probable, however, that central chemoreceptors play an important role in a process of fine-tuning which allows arterial P_{CO_2} to be virtually unchanged even with large changes in metabolic rate.

Central chemoreceptors have also a substantial stabilizing effect on respiratory activity (32). The relative

slowness of the respiratory response to CO_2 that occurs in the absence of peripheral chemoreceptors prevents abrupt changes in respiratory activity from occurring. If peripheral chemoreceptors are left intact, ablation of most CO_2 responsivity by medullary lesions increases tendencies for periodic breathing with recurrent apneas.

LOCATION OF CENTRAL CHEMORECEPTORS

Studies carried out in the past 30 years have established that the pH of the cerebrospinal fluid can significantly alter respiration. Acidic pH levels excite breathing, whereas alkaline pH levels inhibit it (6). These findings seemed to indicate that central chemoreceptors receive information from cerebrospinal fluid and that some or all are placed superficially in the medulla.

Experiments from different groups of investigators have provided evidence indicating that the cells in the medulla that are responsive to CO_2 are located in its ventrolateral portion within a millimeter of the surface (4,6,7). Two groups of investigators have presented the initial evidence that these ventral cells were the central chemoreceptors (33–35). Application of acidic solutions or respiratory stimulants like lobelline to the ventral medullary surface, in these studies, augmented breathing and excited respiratory responses to CO_2, whereas topical applications of local anesthetics abolished respiratory responses to inhaled CO_2.

Three areas could be identified on the ventral surface which seemed to be important in central chemoreceptor sensitivity (4,34). The rostral area (which extended from the pontine–medullary border to the rostral hypoglossal rootlets) and the caudal area (which spanned the distance from the caudal hypoglossal rootlets to the medullary spinal junction) were believed to mark regions in which central chemoreceptors or their endings were located. These chemoreceptor zones extended about 1 mm deep. The two chemosensitive regions were separated by an intervening intermediate area through which chemoreceptor fibers traveled into the interior of the medulla. Acids applied on the intermediate area in these studies did not stimulate respiration.

These observations were supported by subsequent studies that demonstrated strong effects of bilateral focal cooling (in discrete areas of the ventral surface) on the apneic threshold to CO_2 (36). Using thermodes with 1- to 2-mm² cooling plates, it could be shown that cooling this surface from 37°C to 20°C produced a progressive increase in the P_{CO_2} required to initiate respiration in the anesthetized cat. This degree of cooling was enough to interfere with synaptic trans-

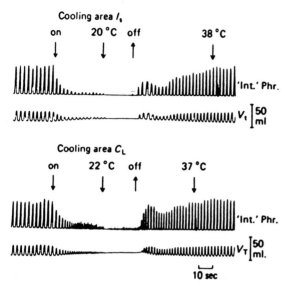

Cooling area I_s

on   20 °C   off   38 °C

'Int.' Phr.

V_t | 50 ml

Cooling area C_L

on   22 °C   off   37 °C

'Int.' Phr.

V_T | 50 ml.

10 sec

FIG. 4. Effects of focal cooling of intermediate areas **(upper trace)** and caudal areas **(lower trace)** of ventral atrial medullary surface on tidal phrenic activity (Int Phr) and tidal volume (V_T) in spontaneously breathing cat after bilateral vagotomy. (From ref. 36.)

mission but not with fiber transmission or cell function (Fig. 4). The greatest effects of cooling on breathing were observed in the intermediate area. Greater cooling could produce apnea, but even then breathing could be reinstituted by raising arterial P_{CO_2} levels. In these studies, surface cooling had little or no effect on the phrenic nerve response to hypoxia and did not alter the effect of pulmonary stretch receptor stimulation on breathing. Differences in respiration were also observed on cooling rostral and ventral areas. Cooling the caudal area tended to diminish the amplitude of phrenic nerve excursion but often increased respiratory rate. This acceleration of rate was not observed in the rostral area, where rate slowed as surface temperature was lowered. Changes like those produced by cooling occurred with the topical application of local anesthetics. Similar differences in the effects of cooling on rostral and caudal areas of the ventral medullary surface have been reported in rabbits by Homma et al. (37). Areas close to the surface where temperature reduction causes apnea have also been reported in dogs and rats (21,38). In cats, unilateral intramedullary cooling of the nucleus paragigantocellularis lateralis abolished all respiratory responses to CO_2 even if arterial CO_2 was considerably raised. This suggested that afferent signals from the central chemoreceptors synapse in neurons in this nucleus (see Fig. 5) (39). Coagulation of the ventral surface of cats subsequently allowed to recover produced chronic elevation in P_{CO_2} and markedly depressed responses to inhaled CO_2 and to hypoxia (40).

Interventions at the ventral surface which alter res-

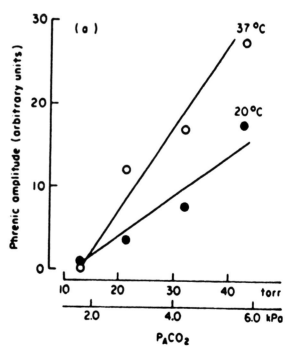

FIG. 5. Effect of CO_2 on tidal phrenic activity at 37°C and during unilateral cooling to 20°C of nucleus paragigantocellularis lateralis. (From ref. 39.)

piration, like cooling, frequently also affect other physiological responses. Besides depressing respiratory responses to CO_2, cooling the intermediate area also eliminates the respiratory excitation caused by irritant receptor stimulation and prolongs the apnea caused by stimulating J receptors (receptors in the airway supplied by unmyelinated vagal fibers) (34,36,41,42). Intermediate area cooling also blocks the tracheal constriction and decreases the sympathetic nerve activity induced by CO_2 inhalation. It also depresses the formation of tracheal secretion elicited by irritant receptor stimulation at the carina and prevents the tracheal constriction arising from mechanical probing of the carina (43,44).

Systemic blood pressure is frequently reduced by intermediate area cooling (Fig. 6) (45–47). Independent studies have demonstrated that the region near the ventrolateral medullary surface is populated by a group of vasomotor neurons which are largely responsible for resting vasomotor tone. These vasomotor neurons have been divided into rostral (epinephrine-producing) pressor neurons and caudal (norepinephrine-producing) depressor neurons (48–50). The rostral pressor neurons project to preganglionic vasomotor neurons in the intermediolateral column of the spinal cord, and they modulate the baroreceptor reflex; the caudal groups have an inhibitory effect on the rostral group, but they also project to the hypothalamus where they modulate the release of vasopressin. The vasomotor neurons in the ventral medulla receive connections

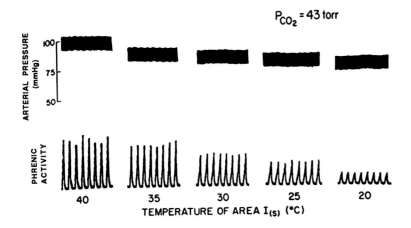

FIG. 6. Effect of graded cooling of intermediate area $I_{(S)}$ on integrated phrenic nerve activity and arterial blood pressure in a cat. End-tidal P_{CO_2} was kept constant at 43 mmHg. (From ref. 7.)

from many areas of the brain, including regions that contain high concentrations of respiratory-related neurons, such as the nucleus tractus solitarius and the hypothalamic defense areas.

These vasomotor neurons can be affected by the surface application of a variety of substances, including nicotine, phenobarbital, glycine, and gamma-aminobutyric acid (51). Surface areas from which the rostral pressor neurons can be affected overlap the rostral and intermediate respiratory chemosensitive areas, whereas the caudal depressor area overlaps the caudal chemosensitive area.

The possibility that these vasomotor neurons might be responsible in some way for the respiratory effects observed from the ventral medulla has occurred to many investigators. Loeschcke et al. (52) reported almost 30 years ago that these vasomotor neurons in the ventral medulla were more deeply placed than the respiratory chemoreceptors. More recent experiments have shown a clear spatial separation of the locations in the ventral medulla from which respiratory and vasomotor effects can be elicited. Areas of the surface from which respiratory and vasomotor effects can be produced by N-methyl-D-aspartate and other glutamate agonists can be distinguished in cats (53). Agonists to different glutamate receptor subtypes have different relative effects on breathing and blood pressure. In an elegant experiment in which kainate and other glutamate agonists were microinjected into the ventral medullary surface (VMS), McAllen (54) has conclusively shown that the areas from which respiratory and vasomotor effects can be elicited from the ventral medulla are distinct and easily separable.

Another proposal is that neurons in the ventral medulla act on breathing and blood pressure by producing an excitatory input that is necessary for both vasomotor and respiratory activity (7). This does not seem to be entirely correct, because areas of the ventral medulla can produce either pressor or depressor responses and also because cooling of the ventral medulla does not prevent (a) the respiratory excitation produced by stimulation of somatic afferents or (b) the tachypnea caused by heating the hypothalamus or the whole body (55,56). Nonetheless, many neurons in the VMS seem to respond to multiple inputs, including hypercapnia, peripheral chemoreceptor stimulation, and input from the hypothalamus and somatic afferents.

Thus, it seems established that the regions near the VMS contain neurons that respond to CO_2 and can be considered to be central chemoreceptors. What remains uncertain is whether these neurons also respond to hypoxia and whether there are chemosensitive neurons located in other areas of the brain.

Interventions that involve either surface applications of agents or cooling can affect the respiratory response to hypoxia (34,36,57). In some studies these effects on hypoxic response have occurred only with larger interventions, whereas other studies have shown effects on hypoxic response in proportion to the effects on CO_2. It would not be surprising if the central chemoreceptors, like the peripheral ones, respond to more than one stimulus. Peripheral chemoreceptors can be excited by hypoxia and CO_2 as well as by temperature, mechanical, and osmotic changes (13). It is of interest that one group of investigators has evidence indicating the presence of hypoxia-sensitive neurons in the rostral ventrolateral medulla that control cerebral blood flow (58).

CO_2 may excite cells outside the ventral medulla. For example, it has been suggested that acids applied at the VMS could reach other areas of the medulla through the bloodstream (59).

A number of studies have shown that microinjection of CO_2-containing solutions directly depress the activity of respiratory neurons (see, e.g., ref. 60). Arita and co-workers (61,62) have shown that intravertebral artery injections of solutions equilibrated with 100% CO_2 can excite neurons in both the ventral and dorsal medulla. In many instances this excitation correlates with local decreases in extracellular pH and with increases in phrenic nerve activity. Studies with brain slices indicate that even after synaptic transmission is prevented by reducing the calcium and increasing the magnesium ion concentrations of the bathing fluids, high levels of CO_2 or acid solutions can depolarize neurons in slices of dorsal as well as ventral medulla, even though the number of neurons stimulated in dorsal locations is usually less (20). These studies usually involve the use of severely acidic and/or hypercapnic solutions and are difficult to relate to normal physiology. Also, in slices it is difficult to know whether the neurons excited have a respiratory function.

At the present time it seems reasonable to conclude that the ventral medulla contains central chemoreceptors, but so may other areas of the brain. Again, there is an analogy to peripheral chemoreceptors. Chemoreceptors sensitive to hypoxia in the carotid and aortic body have been repeatedly reported to be present in the thorax and in the abdomen.

MECHANISMS INVOLVED IN THE RESPONSE OF THE CENTRAL CHEMORECEPTORS

It has been argued for many years whether CO_2 and H^+ act independently as respiratory stimulants or whether all of the effects of CO_2 on breathing are secondary to pH changes induced by CO_2 either intra- or extracellularly (4,6,7,63). Many studies have been based on the assumption that there is some site corresponding to the location of the central chemoreceptors where changes in pH account for ventilation changes whether they were caused by CO_2 inhalation or by systemic acid infusion.

No such extracellular site has yet been identified. If only the pH changes in the arterial blood are considered, H^+ and P_{CO_2} appear to operate as separate stimuli, because the effect of CO_2 is much greater than can be explained by the changes in blood pH that it produces.

The cerebrospinal fluid (CSF) or brain extracellular fluid (ECF) may be more similar to the environment of central chemoreceptors than the blood (4,68). The pH of brain ECF, as well as that of CSF, is actively regulated and varies considerably from pH values in the blood (4,27). Generally, CO_2 inhalation produces greater effects on pH of brain fluids than does the infusion of acid into the bloodstream. Studies that have measured changes in both blood and bulk CSF pH find that neither pH change by itself accounts for breathing changes brought about by CO_2 or acids. These studies have suggested that central chemoreceptors were at some site that could be influenced both by the CSF and by the blood (27).

Recent studies by Ahmad and Loeschcke (17) and by Millhorn et al. (31) show that pH near the ventral medulla, measured by flat electrodes applied gently to the surface, changes far more rapidly than pH in the bulk CSF (away from the surface). However, inhaled CO_2 has a much greater effect on breathing than do blood-infused acids or acids applied to the exterior of the brain in relation to the pH changes measured at the VMS (63).

Because CO_2 crosses cell membranes with much greater ease than do hydrogen ions, these observations have led to the revival of the old hypothesis that intracellular pH, rather than the pH outside the cells, is the actual stimulus to central chemoreceptors. Cell structure is, however, quite complex, and pH in the cell interior is not uniform. Even if internal pH does specify respiratory responses, we will need to know the crucial intracellular site.

It is highly likely that pH changes by themselves do not generate action potentials but that, instead, a series of intermediary steps are triggered which involve neurotransmitters. Many neurotransmitters exert excitatory effects on respiration when applied to the VMS or when microinjected into the ventral medulla and may, in addition, alter respiratory responses to CO_2. These agents include glutamate, tachykinins, and serotonin, However, it is not clear whether the agents act at the central chemoreceptors or downstream from them. Neurons containing these substances are present in the medulla, as are cells containing the appropriate receptors.

Dev and Loeschcke (64) have proposed that H^+ alters respiratory discharge by inhibiting the metabolism of acetylcholine in the synapse. Like other enzymes, the activity of acetylcholine esterase, which degrades acetylcholine, is pH-sensitive. Cholinergic agents stimulate breathing when applied to the VMS, as do antagonists to acetylcholine esterase (e.g., physiostigmine). Dev and Loeschcke (64) found that atropine, a muscarinic receptor antagonist, blocked the response to CO_2. This has recently been confirmed by Nattie (cited in ref. 65; see also ref. 66), who, using more specific antagonists, showed that the M2 muscarinic binding site was the pertinent receptor. It is of interest that Loeschcke postulated that the weaker effects of infused acid (rather than those of CO_2) on breathing were accounted for by the greater difficulty of H^+ in accessing the synapse.

Studies of cold-blooded animals provide clues that may be useful in understanding the principles of central receptor operation. At 37°C, respiration seems to be regulated so that blood pH is maintained at about 7.4. However, in cold-blooded animals the pH, which is maintained by breathing, becomes more alkaline as the animal is cooled and more acidic when temperature is raised above 37°C (67). At each of these temperatures,

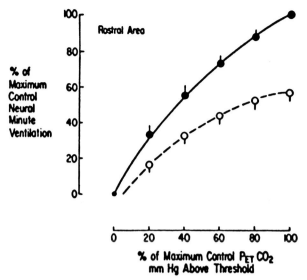

FIG. 7. Average responses to CO₂ before (●) and after (○) application of diethylpyrocarbonate to rostral ventrolateral medulla in six cats. (From ref. 69.)

because of temperature-dependent changes in dissociation constants, the H^+/OH^- ratio remains the same. If breathing is, in fact, adjusted to keep this ratio fixed, then it is conceivable that pH changes affect breathing by altering the degree of dissociation of some moiety present in crucial proteins. With the pH changes, electrostatic forces might alter some receptor protein and initiate the cellular events that would lead ultimately to increased respiratory activity. Reeves (68) has proposed that pH changes the dissociation of imidazole–histidine groups in key proteins, thereby eliciting physiological effects. On the other hand, temperature does not affect imidazole dissociation, since the pK of imidazole is similar to that of the fluid with which it is in contact.

Nattie (69,70), in an intriguing series of experiments, has examined the effects of diethylpyrocarbonate (DEPC), which alters the dissociation of imidazole on the respiratory responses to inhaled CO₂ in cats and rabbits. He demonstrated in both species that DEPC depressed respiratory response to CO₂ but did not alter the response to hyoxia (Fig. 7). In cats, DEPC effects were greatest when it was applied to the rostral chemosensitive area of the ventral medulla, and they were reversed by a specific antagonist.

Thus, although there is overwhelming evidence that neurons near the ventral medulla surface are crucial to the central response to CO₂, it remains controversial whether other cells in the central nervous sytem also contribute to *in vivo* responses to CO₂. The cellular mechanisms that allow respiratory responses to CO₂ are still unclear, but a number of different neurochemicals, including acetylcholine, appear to be involved.

REFERENCES

1. Longobardo GS, Cherniack NS, Gothe B. Factors affecting respiratory system stability. *Ann Biomed Eng* 1989;17:377–396.
2. Cunningham DJC. The control system regulating breathing in man. *Q Rev Biophys* 1974;6:433–483.
3. Lloyd BB, Jukes MGM, Cunningham DJC. The relation between alveolar oxygen pressure and the respiratory response to carbon dioxide in man. *Q J Exp Physiol* 1958;43:214–227.
4. Loeschcke HH. Review lecture: central chemosensitivity and the reaction theory. *J Physiol (Lond)* 1982;332:1–24.
5. Cherniack NS. Respiratory dysrhythmias during sleep. *N Engl J Med* 1981;305:325–330.
6. Bruce EN, Cherniack NS. Central chemoreceptors. *J Appl Physiol* 1987;62:389–402.
7. Millhorn DE, Eldridge FL. Role of ventrolateral medulla in regulation of respiratory and cardiovascular systems. *J Appl Physiol* 1986;61:1249–1263.
8. Cherniack NS. The central nervous system and respiratory muscle coordination. *Chest* 1990;97(3,suppl):525–575.
9. Wolkove N, Altose MD, Kelsen SG, Cherniack NS. Respiratory control abnormalities in alveolar hypoventilation. *Am Rev Respir Dis* 1980;122:163–167.
10. Lahiri S, Delaney RG. Stimulus interaction in the responses of carotid body chemoreceptor single afferent fibers. *Respir Physiol* 1975;24:249–266.
11. Fitzgerald RS, Dehyhani GA. Neural responses of the cat carotid and aortic bodies to hypercapnia and hypoxia. *J Appl Physiol* 1982;52:596–601.
12. Berkenbosch A, Heeringa J, Olievier CN, Kruyt EW. Artificial perfusion of the ponto-medullary region of cats. A method for separation of central and peripheral effects of chemical stimulation of ventilation. *Respir Physiol* 1979;37:347–364.
13. Fitzgerald RS, Lahiri S. Reflex responses to chemoreceptor stimulation. In: Cherniack NS, Widdicombe J, eds. *Handbook of physiology, Section 3; vol II: Control of breathing*. Bethesda, MD: American Physiological Society, 1986;313–362.
14. Dejours P. Approaches to the study of arterial chemoreceptors. In: Torrance RW, ed. *Arterial chemoreceptors*. Oxford, England: Blackwell, 1968;41–48.
15. Gelfand R, Lambertsen CJ. Dynamic respiratory responses to abrupt change of inspired CO₂ at normal and high PO₂. *J Appl Physiol* 1973;35:903–913.
16. Gelfand R, Lambertsen CJ. CO₂-related ventilatory response dynamics: how many components? In: Whipp BJ, Wiberg DM, eds. *Modelling and the control of breathing*. New York: Elsevier, 1983;301–308.
17. Ahmad HR, Loeschcke HH. Fast bicarbonate–chloride exchange between brain cells and brain extracellular fluid in respiratory acidosis. *Pflugers Arch* 1982;395:293–299.
18. Lambertsen CJ, Semple SJG, Smyth MS, Gelfand R. H⁺ and PCO₂ as chemical factors in respiratory and circulatory control. *J Appl Physiol* 1961;16:473–484.
19. Schnader JY, Juan G, Howell S, Fitzgerald R, Roussos C. Arterial CO₂ partial pressure affects diaphragmatic function. *J Appl Physiol* 1985;58:823–829.
20. Harada Y, Kuno M, Wang YZ. Differential effects of carbon dioxide and pH in central chemoreceptors in the rat respiratory center *in vitro*. *J Physiol (Lond)* 1985;368:679–693.
21. Onimaru H, Homma I. Respiratory rhythm generator neurons in medulla of brain stem–spinal cord preparation from newborn rat. *Brain Res* 1987;403:380–384.
22. Eldridge FL, Gill-Kumar P, Millhorn DE. Input–output relationships of central neural circuits involved in respiration in cats. *J Physiol (Lond)* 1981;311:81–95.
23. Overholt JL, Mitra J, van Lunteren E, Prabhakar NR, Cherniack NS. Naloxone enhances the response to hypercapnia of spinal and cranial respiratory nerves. *Respir Physiol* 1988;4:299–310.
24. Sears TA, Berger AJ, Phillipson EA. Reciprocal and onic activation of inspiratory and expiratory motor neurons by chemical drive. *Nature* 1982;299:728–730.
25. Mitra J, Prabhakar NR, Haxhiu MA, Cherniack NS. Comparison of the effects of hypercapnia on phrenic and hypoglossal

activity in anesthetized decerebrate and decorticate animals. *Brain Res Bull* 1986;17:181–187.

26. Neubauer JA, Strumpf DA, Edelman NH. Regional medullary blood flow during isocapnic hyperpnea in anesthetized cats. *J Appl Physiol* 1983;55:447–452.

27. Dempsey JA, Forster HV. Mediation of ventilatory adaptations. *Physiol Rev* 1982;62:262–308.

28. Edelman NH, Epstein PE, Lahiri S, Cherniack NS. Ventilatory responses to transient hypoxia and hypercapnia in man. *Respir Physiol* 1973;17:302–314.

29. Cherniack NS, Edelman NH, Lahiri S. Hypoxia and hypercapnia as respiratory stimulants and depressants. *Respir Physiol* 1970;11:113–126.

30. Poon CS. Ventilatory control in hypercapnia and exercise: optimization hypothesis. *J Appl Physiol* 1986;64:1481–1491.

31. Millhorn DE, Eldridge FL, Kiley JP. Oscillation of medullary extracellular fluid pH caused by breathing. *Respir Physiol* 1984;55:193–203.

32. Cherniack NS, Longobardo GS. Cheyne–Stokes breathing: an instability in physiological control. *N Engl J Med* 1973;288:952–957.

33. Mitchell RA, Loeschcke HH, Severinghaus JW, Richardson BW, Massin WH. Regions of respiratory chemosensitivity on the surface of the medulla. *Ann NY Acad Sci* 1963;109:661–681.

34. Schlaefke ME. Central chemosensitivity: a respiratory drive. *Rev Physiol Biochem Pharmacol* 1981;90:171–249.

35. Schlaefke ME, See WR, Herker A. Response of neurons in the ventral medullary surface to alterations of H^+ in concentration in the cerebrospinal fluid. *Pflugers Arch* 1975;359:49.

36. Cherniack NS, Euler C von, Homma I, Kao FF. Graded changes in central chemoreceptor input by local temperature changes on the ventral surface of medulla. *J Physiol (Lond)* 1979;287:191–211.

37. Homma I, Isobe A, Iwase M, Kanamaru A, Sibuya M. Two different types of apnea induced by focal cold block of ventral medulla in rabbits. *Neurosci Lett* 1988;87:41–45.

38. Adams EM, Chonan T, Cherniack NS, Euler C von. Effects on respiratory pattern of focal cooling in the medulla of the dog. *J Appl Physiol* 1988;65:2004–2010.

39. Budzinska K, Euler C von, Kao FF, Panaleo T, Yamamoto Y. Effects of graded focal cold block in rostral areas of medulla. *Acta Physiol Scand* 1985;124:329–340.

40. Schlaefke ME, See WR, Herker-See A, Loeschcke HH. Respiratory response to hypoxia and hypercapnia after elimination of central chemosensitivity. *Pflugers Arch* 1979;381:241–248.

41. Mitra J, Prabhakar NR, Haxhiu MA, Cherniack NS. The effects of hypercapnia and cooling of the ventral medullary surface on capsaicin induced respiratory reflexes. *Respir Physiol* 1985;60:377–385.

42. Millhorn DE, Kiley JP. Effect of graded cooling of intermediate areas on respiratory response to vagal input. *Respir Physiol* 1984;58:51–64.

43. Deal EC Jr, Haxhiu MA, Norcia MP, van Lunteren E, Cherniack NS. Cooling the intermediate area of the ventral medullary surface affects tracheal responses to hypoxia. *Respir Physiol* 1987;69:335–345.

44. Haxhiu MA, Deal EC Jr, Norcia MP, van Lunteren E, Mitra J, Cherniack NS. Influence of the ventrolateral medulla on reflex tracheal constriction. *J Appl Physiol* 1986;61:791–796.

45. van Lunteren E, Mitra J, Prabhakar NR, Haxhiu MA, Cherniack NS. Ventral medullary surface inputs to cervical sympathetic respiratory oscillations. *Am J Physiol* 1987;252:R1032–R1038.

46. Millhorn DE. Neural respiratory and circulatory interaction during chemoreceptor stimulation and cooling of the ventral medulla in cat. *J Physiol (Lond)* 1986;370:217–231.

47. Lioy F, Hanna BP, Polosa C. Cardiovascular control by medullary surface chemoreceptor. *J Auton Nerv Syst* 1981;3:1–7.

48. Ciriello J, Caverson MM, Polosa C. Function of the ventrolateral medulla in the control of the circulation. *Brain Res Rev* 1986;11:359–391.

49. Ross CA, Ruggiero DA, Park DH, Joh TH, Sved AF, Fernandez-Pardal J, Saavedra JM, Reis DJ. Tonic vasomotor control by the rostral ventral medulla: effect of electrical or chemical stimulation of the area containing L_1 adrenaline neurons on arterial pressure, heart rate, and plasma catecholamines and vasopressin. *J Neuro Sci* 1984;4:274–294.

50. Granata AR, Kumada M, Reis DJ. Sympatho-inhibition by A_1-noradrenergic neurons is mediated by neurons in the C_1 area of the rostral medulla. *J Auton Nerv Syst* 1988;14:387–395.

51. Guertzenstein PG, Silver A. Fall in blood pressure produced from discrete regions of the ventral surface of the medulla by glycine and lesions. *J Physiol (Lond)* 1974;242:489–503.

52. Loeschcke HH, Lattre JD, Schlaefke ME, Trouth CO. Effects on respiration and circulation of electrically stimulating the ventral surface of the medulla oblongata. *Respir Physiol* 1970;10:184–197.

53. Mitra J, Prabhakar NR, Overholt J, Cherniack NS. Respiratory and vasomotor effects of excitatory amino acids on ventral medullary surface. *Brain Res Bull* 1987;18:681–684.

54. McAllen RM. Location of neurons with cardiovascular and respiratory function at the ventral surface of the cat's medulla. *Neuroscience* 1986;18:43–49.

55. Millhorn DE, Eldridge FL, Waldrop TG. Effects of medullary area $I_{(S)}$ cooling on respiratory response to muscle stimulation. *Respir Physiol* 1982;49:41–48.

56. See WR, Schlaefke ME, Loeschcke HH. Role of chemical afferents in the maintenance of rhythmic respiratory movements. *J Appl Physiol* 1983;54:453–459.

57. Millhorn DE, Eldridge FL, Waldrop TG. Effects of medullary area $I_{(S)}$ cooling on respiratory response to chemoreceptor inputs. *Respir Physiol* 1982;49:23–39.

58. Reis DJ. Central neural control of cerebral circulation and metabolism. In: Mackenzie ET, Seylaz J, Bes A, eds. *LERS Monograph Series*, vol 2. New York: Raven Press, 1984;91–119.

59. Lipscomb WT, Boyarsky LL. Neurophysiological investigations of medullary chemosensitive areas of respiration. *Respir Physiol* 1972;16:362–376.

60. Mitchell RA, Herbert DA. Effect of carbon dioxide on the membrane potential of medullary respiratory neurons. *Brain Res* 1974;75:345–349.

61. Arita H, Kogo W, Ichikawa K. Rapid and transient excitation of respiration mediated by central chemoreceptors. *J Appl Physiol* 1988;64:1369–1375.

62. Ichikawa K, Kuwana S, Arita H. ECF pH dynamics with the ventrolateral medulla: a microelectrode study. *J Appl Physiol* 1989;64:193–198.

63. Shams H. Differential effects of CO_2 and H^+ as central stimuli of respiration in the cat. *J Appl Physiol* 1985;58:357–364.

64. Dev NB, Loeschcke HH. Topography of the respiratory and circulatory responses to acetylcholine and nicotine of the ventral surface of the medulla oblongata. *Pflugers Arch* 1979;379:19–27.

65. Wood J, Mega A, Goritski W. Rostral ventrolateral medulla muscarinic receptor involvement in central ventilatory chemosensitivity. *J Appl Physiol* 1989;66:1462–1470.

66. Nattie E, Aihua L. Fluorescent microbead localization and 4-D, AMP microinjection that decrease baseline and CO_2 sensitive phrenic output. *Neurosci Abstr* 1989;15(2):471.6.

67. Burton RF. The role of imidazole ionizations in the control of breathing. *Comp Biochem Physiol* 1986;83A:333–336.

68. Reeves RB. An imidazole alphastat hypothesis for vertebrate acid–base regulation: tissue carbon dioxide content and body temperature in bullfrogs. *Respir Physiol* 1972;14:219–236.

69. Nattie EE. Diethylpyrocarbonate (an imidazole binding substance) inhibits rostral VLM CO_2 sensitivity. *J Appl Physiol* 1986;61:843–850.

70. Nattie EE. Diethylpyrocarbonate inhibits rostral ventrolateral medullary H^+ sensitivity. *J Appl Physiol* 1988;64:1600–1609.

71. Nielsen M, Smith H. Studies on the regulation of respiration in acute hypoxia. *Acta Physiol Scand* 1952;24:293–313.

THE LUNG: *Scientific Foundations*
edited by R.G. Crystal, J.B. West et al.
Raven Press, Ltd., New York © 1991.

CHAPTER 5.4.6

Cerebrospinal Fluid and the Control of Ventilation

Homayoun Kazemi

Fluids bathing the brain have been of interest to scientists since the early part of the 20th century, and their clinical relevance has become more apparent in the past two to three decades. This interest in cerebral fluids is, to a large extent, a result of the fact that cerebral fluids may well reflect what is happening in brain cells, which are otherwise not readily accessible. The cerebrospinal fluid (CSF) has been studied most extensively; more recently, new approaches have allowed for assessment of brain extracellular fluid (ECF).

Composition of cerebral fluids has profound effects on ventilation, cardiovascular function, cerebral blood flow, and mental status (1,2). The role of cerebral fluids in central control of ventilation has been the subject of studies and speculation since 1905, when Haldane and Priestley (3) proposed that the ventilatory response to CO_2 was through changes in "brain acidity." Leusen's experiments in the 1950s showed that changing the CSF pH was associated with changes in ventilation in anesthetized dogs who underwent ventriculocisternal perfusion (VCP) (4). In these seminal experiments, Leusen showed that making the CSF acid increased ventilation and that making CSF alkaline decreased ventilation. A decade later, Pappenheimer et al. (5) showed that in the unanesthetized goat, brain interstitial fluid $[H^+]$ was the single determinant of ventilation in the steady state. Their work suggested that the H^+-sensitive areas were in the medulla, at some finite distance below the ventral medullary surface. A number of other studies have suggested that there are at least three specific chemosensitive areas

on the ventral medullary surface that are sensitive to H^+ concentration in their environment and that abolition of these areas leads to disappearance of the central ventilatory response to H^+ (6) (Fig. 1). It is important to point out, however, that no specific anatomical structures have been identified at the central "chemosensitive areas," which are "physiological" and "biochemical" functioning areas that modulate the central ventilatory drive. Since fluids bathing these areas have profound effects on ventilation, their ionic composition and pH have been of interest to many investigators.

Before embarking on a discussion of cerebral fluid composition and its effect on ventilation, it is necessary to emphasize that composition of all cerebral fluids may not be the same and that acid–base status of the CSF obtained from the lumbar region may be different from that in the cisterna magna or the brain ECF. Thus, conclusions on central ventilatory drive based on ionic composition and $[H^+]$ in lumbar or cisternal CSF need to be interpreted with caution (7). To appreciate changes in cerebral fluid composition and its effects on ventilation, it is appropriate to begin with a brief discussion of normal CSF physiology and anatomy.

CSF ANATOMY AND PHYSIOLOGY

CSF is secreted in the central nervous system by the choroid plexus and brain tissue itself. It is a protein-free fluid that surrounds the brain and the subarachnoid and ventricular system. The choroid plexus is responsible for two-thirds of the fluids secreted, and the other one-third comes from brain cells (8). CSF is continuously formed and reabsorbed. Its flow is from the lateral ventricles towards the third and fourth ventri-

H. Kazemi: Pulmonary and Critical Care Unit, Department of Medicine, Harvard Medical School, Massachusetts General Hospital, Boston, Massachusetts 02114.

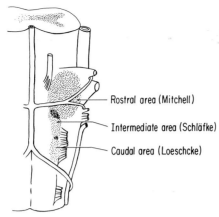

FIG. 1. Location of chemosensitive areas on the ventral surface of the medulla. (Modified from ref. 6.)

cles and then over the cerebral cortex into the arachnoid villi. The normal volume of CSF is approximately 140 ml in humans, and about one-fifth of that is found in the cerebral ventricles. The CSF production rate in humans is approximately 0.5% of its volume per minute, with a turnover rate of 2–3 hr. The normal composition of the CSF in humans is given in Table 1.

A number of factors are responsible for the differences in electrolyte composition and acid–base values in cerebral fluids as compared to those in plasma. These factors include: the brain blood barrier, the nature of brain blood vessels, and the mechanisms of CSF formation. The brain–blood barrier has several components, including the brain capillary endothelium, choroid plexus, pia–glia membranes, and the arachnoid membranes. Each part of the membrane with its own permeability and transport characteristics contributes to the separation of CSF from brain and from blood. The composition of the CSF is regulated by movement of substances across these membranes with specific transport mechanisms. The significant aspect of the brain–blood barrier as a whole and of the

brain capillaries in particular is the fact that they contain a number of enzymes and carrier transport proteins that are important in the regulation of CSF composition. They contain Na^+,K^+-ATPase, Na^+–H^+ exchange mechanisms, anion exchange protein (Cl^-–HCO_3^- exchange), and Na^+-coupled chloride transport.

The choroid plexus is important in CSF composition, since it is a major source of CSF production. The choroid plexus is composed of microvilli and a core containing capillaries and fenestrated endothelial cells with loose connective tissue in between. The cells of the choroid plexus are also endowed with a number of ionic pumps and transport systems that are similar to those in the brain capillaries. Furthermore, cells of the choroid plexus also contain abundant quantities of carbonic anhydrase, which catalyzes the CO_2 hydration reaction.

CSF is secreted as an ultrafiltrate of the plasma and has a Na^+ and Cl^- concentration similar to that of plasma. The cisternal CSF, however, has (a) a Cl^- concentration that is about 10–15 mEq higher than that of the nascent CSF and (b) a HCO_3^- concentration that is 10–15 mEq lower than that of the nascent CSF (11). Exactly where this transformation takes place is not clear, but there are chloride-concentrating mechanisms that reside on the CSF side of the CSF–blood barrier and that allow for the increase in chloride and the fall in bicarbonate.

CSF H^+ AND IONIC REGULATION

There are differences in the ionic composition, pH, and P_{CO_2} between blood and plasma (Table 1). These differences for ions are maintained by active regulation of cerebral fluid composition. The CSF under normal conditions has a positive charge of 4–6 mV compared to plasma (12). Using the Nernst equation and this potential difference, one can calculate the expected concentration for different ions in the CSF. Comparing the calculated differences by the Nernst equation for different ions to the measured differences shows that the ions in the CSF are actively regulated. The normal measured CSF/plasma ratio for the major ions is 0.99 for Na^+, 0.65 for K^+, 1.44 for Cl^-, 0.44 for Ca^{2+}, and 1.22 for Mg^{2+}.

Mechanisms of "regulating" $[H^+]$ in the central nervous system (CNS) have been evaluated, and recently the concept has been put forth that $[H^+]$ in the cerebral fluids depends on dissociation of strong ions and that it is the strong ion difference (SID) which ultimately determines the $[H^+]$ (13). The difference between cations and anions in the cerebral fluids determines what the $[HCO_3^-]$ will be, and in the classical Henderson

TABLE 1. *Acid–base and electrolyte composition of plasma and CSF in humans[a]*

	Plasma	CSF		
Sodium (mmol/kg H_2O)	150	147		
Potassium (mmol/kg H_2O)	4.6	2.9		
Magnesium (mmol/kg H_2O)	3.2	4.5		
Calcium (mmol/kg H_2O)	2.4	1.2		
Chloride (mmol/kg H_2O)	99	113		
Bicarbonate (mmol/kg H_2O)	27	23		
pH	7.40	7.33	7.35	(C)
P_{CO_2} (mmHg)	41	49	47	(C)
Osmolarity (mosm/liter)	289	289		
Protein (mg/100 ml)	6800	28		

[a] Data are from refs. 9 and 10.
All values are for lumbar CSF. P_{CO_2} and pH are also given for cisternal CSF (C).

equation the relationship between P_{CO_2} and $[HCO_3^-]$ determines the $[H^+]$:

$$[H^+] = K \frac{P_{CO_2}}{[HCO_3^-]}$$

Changes in $[H^+]$ can be brought about by changing P_{CO_2} and/or bicarbonate, and the latter depends on the SID.

P_{CO_2}

The partial pressure of CO_2 is a key determinant of $[H^+]$ of cerebral fluids. The CSF P_{CO_2} depends on (a) P_{CO_2} in the arterial blood, (b) brain blood flow, (c) brain CO_2 production ($\dot{V}_{CO_2}$), and (d) brain CO_2 dissociation curve. The mean CSF P_{CO_2} is about 4–11 mmHg higher than arterial P_{CO_2} (14), and this gradient is relatively well maintained in respiratory acidosis and alkalosis in the steady state.

$[HCO_3^-]$ and $[H^+]$ Regulation

In the past three decades a number of theories have been advanced on regulation of CSF $[HCO_3^-]$ and $[H^+]$. They include the concepts of (a) simple diffusion along electrochemical gradients, (b) H^+ and HCO_3^- pumps at the blood–CSF barrier, (c) electrochemical disequilibrium at the blood–CSF barrier, with movement of H^+ toward the negatively charged capillary wall (Wien effect), (d) the interaction with brain cells whose metabolic activities influence CSF $[H^+]$ and $[HCO_3^-]$ (2,15), and (e) the direct contributions of HCO_3^- from both blood and brain to CSF $[H^+]$ and $[HCO_3^-]$ regulation (16). Experimental evidence for or against these theories has been presented, but none can adequately explain all the variations in CSF acid–base balance in a variety of acid–base perturbations. The major difficulty resides in the assumption that HCO_3^- is an "independent" variable. Namely, a molecule of HCO_3^-, either as HCO_3^- or as $CO_2 + H_2O$, can move from blood to CSF and increase CSF $[HCO_3^-]$ by one molecule. However, this is incorrect because HCO_3^- differs from other completely dissociated ions, such as Na^+, Cl^-, and K^+, because bicarbonate is in dynamic equilibrium with CO_2 and H_2O (i.e., $H^+ + HCO_3^- \rightleftarrows CO_2 + H_2O$), and its concentration can change readily. It thus becomes "dependent" on the fixed anions and cations (i.e., the strongly dissociated "independent" ions). It is the difference between strong cations and anions which determines $[HCO_3^-]$.

SID and H^+ Regulation

In a new approach to acid–base analysis in physiological solutions, Stewart (13) derived equations to describe the solutions $[H^+]$, $[OH^-]$, and $[HCO_3^-]$ based on electroneutrality, conservation of mass, and dissociation of weak electrolytes. In such a solution— and cerebral fluids are such solutions (17)—$[H^+]$, $[OH^-]$, and $[HCO_3^-]$ are the "dependent" variables; furthermore, their concentrations are determined by the P_{CO_2}, the SID, the concentration of weak acids and bases, and the dissociation constants of these acids and bases. In the cerebral fluids, in addition to the P_{CO_2}, the SID is the other major determinant of the "dependent" variables. The SID is the difference between (a) the "fixed" cations Na^+, K^+, Mg^{2+}, and Ca^{2+} and (b) the "fixed" anions Cl^-, PO_4^{3-}, and lactate. Therefore, in this setting to maintain electroneutrality, SID for all practical purposes equals $[HCO_3^-]$. Bicarbonate concentration cannot be changed without changing one or more of the independent variables. Therefore, cerebral fluid $[H^+]$ and $[HCO_3^-]$ regulation, regardless of the systemic acid–base perturbation, becomes dependent on changes in P_{CO_2} and SID (18).

ROLE OF CHLORIDE

Since regulation of ionic composition, and specifically SID, is the key to H^+ and HCO_3^- content of the CSF, the mechanisms of ion transport and regulation in the CNS become of particular relevance. Of the various strongly dissociated ions, chloride is the most significant in regulation of CSF acid–base status. Na^+ concentration in the CSF is kept constant in a variety of conditions (19,20), most probably because of its role as an "osmoregulator"; thus, brain cell volume is kept relatively constant. The other cations are also well regulated and kept constant despite major alterations in their plasma concentration (15). Chloride, whose concentration varies considerably in CSF in acid–base distress, becomes the variable ion in determining SID in cerebral fluids. In metabolic and respiratory acid–base disorders there is a reciprocal relationship between CSF $[Cl^-]$ and $[HCO_3^-]$ (19). These reciprocal changes are seen not only in bulk CSF but also in brain ECF (21).

Regulation of Chloride

Ionic regulation of cerebral fluids is a dynamic process that includes movement of ions to and from blood as well as to and from brain. Entry or exit of ions into the CSF can be directly from blood or through the choroid plexus.

Flux of chloride into the CSF from blood—in particular, relative to that for Na^+—is of importance to CSF SID. Cl^- is freely diffusible from blood into most tissues except the CNS (5). There are at least three mechanisms for Cl^- transport: (i) passive movement related to transepithelial concentration differences and electrical gradients (Na^+,K^+-ATPase-mediated system), (ii) carrier-mediated electrically neutral Cl^- movement coupled to Na^+ transport, and (iii) carrier-mediated anion exchange (Cl^-–HCO_3^- exchange). All these transport mechanisms are involved in regulation of CSF [Cl^-].

Na^+,K^+-ATPase is present in the choroid plexus, brain capillaries, and brain cells. It is important in (a) CSF formation, (b) Na^+ movement from blood to CSF, and (c) K^+ efflux from CSF. By extruding Na^+ from cells and allowing K^+ into cells, Na^+,K^+-ATPase facilitates Na^+–Cl^- cotransport and Na^+–H^+ exchange. Using the specific inhibitor of Na^+,K^+-ATPase, ouabain, it has been shown that CSF formation is reduced (22), K^+ entry increased (23), and H^+ homeostasis adversely affected during hypercapnia (24). ATPase activity also facilitates Na^+–H^+ exchange across cerebral membranes. Na^+–H^+ exchange can be inhibited by amiloride. Amiloride inhibits two different Na^+ transport mechanisms across membranes: At lower concentrations (10^{-6}–10^{-7} M) it interferes with a conductive Na^+ pore (25), and at higher concentrations (10^{-3} M) it inhibits Na^+,K^+-ATPase (26). In the CNS, amiloride reduces CSF formation (27), and in respiratory acidosis it reduces the degree of pH compensation in the CSF (28). Thus, the Na^+–H^+ exchange is an important event in the maintenance of ionic homeostasis in cerebral fluids (29,30). The role of Na^+–H^+ exchange is depicted schematically in Fig. 2, where (a) Na^+ enters the cells from blood, (b) Na^+,K^+-ATPase allows for lowering of intracellular Na^+, creating a gradient for Na^+ entry as intracellular Na^+ rises, (c) SID is increased, (d) CO_2 is hydrated,

forming HCO_3^- and H^+, and (e) H^+ thus formed is then exchanged for Na^+ with blood.

Na^+-coupled electrically neutral Cl^- transport is another major mechanism for cerebral fluid ionic regulation, since inhibitors of this transport system, furosemide and bumetanide, significantly reduce Cl^- entry into the CSF from blood (31) and, in hypercapnia, prevent the expected bicarbonate rise in the CSF (32). This transport mechanism most likely resides on the luminal (blood) side of brain capillaries (33). Inhibitors of Na^+-coupled Cl^- transport lead to reduction in CSF formation (34). The Na^+-coupled Cl^- transport may be stimulated by cyclic AMP, and in many tissues the relative transport system is 1:1:2 for $Na^+:K^+:Cl^-$ (35). A model for Na^+-coupled Cl^- transport and direct anion exchange from blood to CSF is depicted in Fig. 3. The role of Na^+,K^+-ATPase is to reduce intracellular [Na^+], which then creates a Na^+ gradient and facilitates Cl^- entry into the cell coupled to Na^+ entry.

Anion Exchange (Cl^-–HCO_3^- Exchange)

Anion exchange has been studied most extensively in red blood cells, where the carrier is an asymmetric, 95,000-dalton protein known as band 3 (36). This protein is present in the CNS in the neuroglial cells (37). The action of anion exchange is thought to be like a ping-pong model, with one-for-one exchange of Cl^- and HCO_3^- (38).

The Cl^-–HCO_3^- exchange is important in regulation of cerebral fluid SID. Using specific inhibitors of anion exchange (namely, the disulfonic stilbene family of agents such as DIDS and SITS), it has been shown

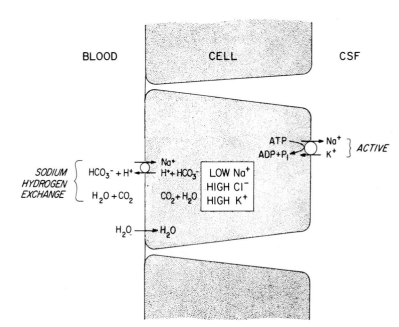

FIG. 2. Model of Na^+–H^+ exchange from blood to CSF and its relation to CO_2 hydration. Na^+ is transported out of the cell by Na^+,K^+-ATPase, thereby reducing intracellular [Na^+] and allowing sodium to enter the cell along its gradient in exchange for H^+. Change in strong ion difference leads to CO_2 hydration in the cell. (From ref. 2.)

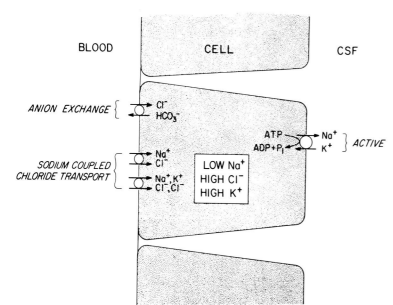

FIG. 3. Schematic presentation of Na^+-coupled Cl^- transport from blood to CSF. There is $Cl^- - HCO_3^-$ exchange across the cell membrane. Na^+ is transported out of the cell by utilizing Na^+, K^+-ATPase, and this lowers the intracellular $[Na^+]$. The Na^+ gradient thus created is used to transport Cl^- into the cell. (From ref. 2.)

that CSF pH compensation in hypercapnia is less effective than without the inhibitors (39) and that there is less of a rise in CSF HCO_3^-. In normocapnia, anion exchange inhibition also causes a reduction in CSF $[Cl^-]$ anion exchange (40). This suggests that anion exchange contributes to the rise in bulk CSF $[Cl^-]$ as compared to nascent CSF and may be the key mechanism for changing the composition of nascent CSF to that of bulk CSF in the cisterna magna.

CARBONIC ANHYDRASE AND IONIC COMPOSITION

Carbonic anhydrase catalyzes the reaction $CO_2 + H_2O \rightleftharpoons HCO_3^- + H^+$ and is found in abundance in many tissues (41). In the CNS, glia cells and the choroid plexus contain carbonic anhydrase in high concentrations (42). The carbonic anhydrase inhibitor, acetazolamide, when given intraventricularly or intravenously, reduces CSF formation (43); during hypercapnia, acetazolamide reduces the rise in CSF $[HCO_3^-]$, and CSF pH compensation is less complete (30). Inhibition of carbonic anhydrase alters ion fluxes across the choroid plexus into the CSF, with reduced Cl^- entry being the major event (44). Carbonic anhydrase in the CNS not only is important for the formation of HCO_3^- locally but also is probably important in anion exchange across cerebral membranes.

CSF AND BRAIN ECF

Cerebral fluids are formed continuously, and their ionic composition and pH are well regulated. Much of the data on cerebral fluids are based on studies on bulk

CSF in the cisterna magna or in the lumbar region. The brain interstitial fluid (ISF) and the ECF of brain tissue may have a composition different from that of the CSF. The general principles of ionic homeostasis discussed earlier in this chapter apply to both ISF and brain ECF, but the exact composition in any given setting may be different from one fluid compartment to another. Using brain surface electrodes, it has been shown that acute changes in arterial blood acid–base status are reflected rapidly in cerebral cortical surface ECF but not in the cisternal CSF (21,45). In many instances there is a significant "lag" between changes in brain ISF and ECF on one side and bulk CSF on the other (46).

Cerebral fluids are electrolyte solutions with little protein and no inherent buffer capacity. Their composition depends on exchanges with blood through the blood–CSF barrier and through the choroid plexus. Furthermore, the fluids surround the brain tissue, a highly metabolically active organ; the composition of these fluids is influenced by the activity of the brain and spinal cord.

BRAIN AND CEREBRAL FLUID COMPOSITION

Brain influences the cerebral fluid composition through several mechanisms. First, CSF P_{CO_2} is in equilibrium with brain tissue P_{CO_2} (14). Brain tissue P_{CO_2} is determined by the arterial P_{CO_2}, brain CO_2 production, and brain blood flow. Changes in any of these will change brain P_{CO_2} and thus CSF P_{CO_2}.

Second brain is an active metabolic organ; as part of its metabolic processes, it produces organic acids, primarily lactate and pyruvate. Depending on its state of oxygenation, brain lactate production will vary. The normal CSF lactate is relatively low at less than 2 mM (47,48). During hypoxia and hypocapnia (47–49), or when brain blood flow is reduced (50), there is a significant increase in brain lactate production. This increase in brain lactate is then reflected by a rise in CSF lactate. The increase in CSF lactate is usually matched by an equal reduction in CSF [HCO_3^-]. In hypocapnia, brain lactate increases when arterial P_{CO_2} is about 20 mmHg, at which time brain blood flow has also fallen significantly (51).

Because lactate level is low in the CSF, reduction in lactate does not play a major role in CSF ionic homeostasis; in hypercapnia, however, CSF lactate is reduced further (47). Change in CSF lactate content, particularly when it is increased, is one of the mechanisms involved in regulation of CSF [H^+] and electrolyte balance.

Cerebral fluids have no inherent buffering capacity, but the brain cells that they surround do. The whole-brain CO_2 dissociation curve, an index of the brain's buffering capacity, is slightly below that of blood but greater than skeletal muscle, cardiac muscle, and lung tissue (2). The brain CO_2 dissociation curve shifts as the function of prevailing P_{CO_2}. It shifts to the left during hypercapnia and to the right during hypocapnia (52,53). These shifts in brain CO_2 dissociation curve are associated with concurrent changes in CSF [HCO_3^-] in the same direction (53).

The cells in the brain responsible for regulation of acid–base status are the glia cells that contain (a) carbonic anhydrase, which is needed for CO_2 hydration, (b) Na^+,K^+-ATPase, which is required in electrolyte exchange, and (c) a Na^+–H^+ exchange system.

Brain intracellular pH has been measured by several indirect techniques, and these techniques all have shown better intracellular pH regulation in the brain than in blood during hyper- and hypocapnia. Direct measurement of brain intracellular pH by nuclear magnetic resonance (NMR) spectroscopy has recently shown that brain intracellular pH compensates rapidly and better than blood during hypercapnia (54). Results of all these studies show that brain cells have the ability to regulate their intracellular acid–base environment and that in the process they contribute to regulation of cerebral fluid composition. Brain cells further influence CSF composition by their metabolism of ammonia and certain related amino acid neurotransmitters which will be detailed later in relation to ventilatory control.

CSF ACID–BASE BALANCE IN ACID–BASE DISORDERS

Numerous studies in humans and animals have shown that in systemic acid–base disorders there are also changes in CSF [H^+] and [HCO_3^-]; however, in all instances, for any given change in plasma [H^+] and [HCO_3^-] there is less of a change in CSF [H^+] and [HCO_3^-]. The change in CSF [HCO_3^-] is equal to 30–40% of the change in plasma [HCO_3^-] in metabolic acidosis and alkalosis and 65–95% in respiratory acidosis and alkalosis (15).

Respiratory Acidosis

The rise in arterial P_{CO_2} in respiratory acidosis is rapidly reflected in brain and CSF P_{CO_2}, because CO_2 is freely diffusible across membranes. CSF pH becomes acidic during hypercapnia, and there is then variable compensation in both magnitude and rapidity. This variability in pH compensation is also associated with a variable increase in CSF [HCO_3^-]. With hypercapnia, the initial increase in CSF [HCO_3^-], in the first 2–4 hr, is faster than that in the plasma, but in time the changes in CSF [HCO_3^-] may become similar to those in arterial plasma (16,20,52,55). The fast response of CNS [HCO_3^-] increase probably represents HCO_3^-–Cl^- exchange between blood and brain ECF as well as between brain ECF and glia cells. Studies measuring other ions in the CSF during hypercapnia have shown that [Na^+] and [K^+] are well maintained, but there is an equal and reciprocal relationship between CSF [Cl^-] and [HCO_3^-] (19,20).

The mechanisms of bicarbonate increase in the CSF during hypercapnia fall into two broad categories: (i) contribution of [HCO_3^-] from plasma and (ii) local formation of [HCO_3^-] in the CNS (16). The final CSF [HCO_3^-] will obviously depend on the P_{CO_2} and SID. The HCO_3^- formed within the CNS is by hydration of CO_2. It is P_{CO_2}-dependent and is catalyzed by carbonic anhydrase present in the choroid plexus and glia cells. Carbonic anhydrase inhibition limits the rise in CSF [HCO_3^-] in hypercapnia. The bicarbonate increase is also limited if Na^+,K^+-ATPase is inhibited, because the H^+ formed in the CO_2 hydration reaction cannot be exchanged across the brain–blood barrier for Na^+. [HCO_3^-] increase in the CNS is also impeded in hypercapnia if the Cl^-–HCO_3^- exchange carrier protein is inhibited by such agents as DIDS and SITS. Therefore, the local increase in CNS [HCO_3^-] in hypercapnia is a multifaceted event beginning with CO_2 hydration and requiring specific enzymes and ionic pumps to establish its final concentration.

Brain ammonia and certain amino acid neurotransmitters, such as glutamate and gamma-aminobutyric acid (GABA), are also altered in hypercapnia and have independent effects on central ventilatory drive.

The central drive of ventilation in chronic respiratory acidosis is diminished; and the higher the CSF

$[HCO_3^-]$, the smaller the slope of the CO_2–ventilatory-response curve (55).

Respiratory Alkalosis

CSF acid–base balance in respiratory alkalosis has been studied extensively, particularly because of the respiratory adaptation to high altitude. With a fall in P_{CO_2} in respiratory alkalosis, CSF pH becomes alkaline, and over several hours to days it returns toward normal. The degree of alkalinity is less than that in blood, but CSF pH remains slightly more alkaline compared to the CSF pH when P_{CO_2} was normal. CSF $[HCO_3^-]$ falls rapidly with the fall in P_{CO_2}, and the rapidity of the fall is P_{CO_2}-dependent. An important contributor to the reduction in CSF $[HCO_3^-]$ in hypocapnia is the concurrent increase in CSF lactate (56). The rise in CSF lactate accounts for approximately one-third of the fall in CSF $[HCO_3^-]$. The CSF lactate increase comes from brain tissue (47), and brain lactate increases significantly when P_{CO_2} is less than 20 mmHg (51). Presence of hypoxia accentuates the lactate increase. The fall in CSF $[HCO_3^-]$ in experimentally induced respiratory alkalosis depends on the concurrent fall in plasma $[HCO_3^-]$ in the first 2–4 hr, but eventually CSF $[HCO_3^-]$ falls regardless of plasma $[HCO_3^-]$ (57,58).

In high-altitude acclimatization, CSF pH becomes alkaline during the first few hours; by 24 hr, CSF pH becomes less alkaline but does not change any further for as long as 10 days (59). Long-term natives of high altitude also have slightly more alkaline CSF pH than do lowlanders (60).

There is some experimental evidence to suggest that despite an alkaline cisternal CSF pH in hypocapnia, the brain ISF may be acidic, which could account for continued hyperventilation seen in these subjects (61).

Metabolic Acidosis and Alkalosis

In metabolic acid–base disorders, the changes in CSF $[H^+]$ and $[HCO_3^-]$ are in the same direction as those in plasma $[H^+]$ and $[HCO_3^-]$, but much less so. The ratio of change in CSF $[HCO_3^-]$ to that in plasma $[HCO_3^-]$ is 0.3–0.4 in metabolic acidosis and alkalosis (15), and thus the cerebral fluid environment is better "protected." This better protection of CSF pH is seen (in humans) in diabetic ketoacidosis and lactic acidosis (62,63) as well as in experimentally induced metabolic acidosis and alkalosis (64,65). In acute metabolic acidosis and alkalosis there can be small changes in CSF pH in the same direction as those in blood pH, but often there is no change in cisternal CSF pH (66,67). However, brain surface electrodes show rapid changes in brain ECF pH with acute systemic infusion of alkali

or acids, but these changes are not reflected in the cisternal CSF (21,45).

Two factors are important in determining the changes in CSF ionic homeostasis in metabolic acid–base disorders. One is the change in P_{CO_2}, and the other is movement of HCO_3^- or H^+ across the blood–brain barrier. The rise or fall in CSF $[HCO_3^-]$ in metabolic acid–base disorders is P_{CO_2}-dependent. If P_{CO_2} is kept constant, CSF $[HCO_3^-]$ remains constant or changes very little (68). The impermeability of the blood–brain barrier to HCO_3^- has been questioned lately, and there is evidence that there is a finite but limited entry of HCO_3^- from plasma into the CNS, approximately 16% of a bolus injected intraarterially on the first pass through brain (18). Molecular CO_2 has an entry rate of over 89% on the first pass. The other evidence in favor of permeability of the membranes to H^+ is the shift in brain ECF pH in acid or alkaline direction immediately following systemic injection of an alkaline or acid solution (21). As for other electrolytes in the CSF, K^+ and Na^+ are kept constant in metabolic acidosis and alkalosis, and changes in $[HCO_3^-]$ are matched by those in $[Cl^-]$ in the opposite direction (19).

In terms of central control of ventilation, the changes in cisternal CSF pH cannot account for the hyperventilation of acidosis, nor can they account for the hypoventilation of alkalosis. In humans there is a linear relationship between plasma $[HCO_3^-]$ and the change in P_{CO_2} in metabolic acidosis and alkalosis (69). The slope of the line is 0.7—that is, a 0.7-mmHg change in P_{CO_2} for every 1-mEq/liter change in $[HCO_3^-]$. The peripheral chemoreceptors have a role in increasing or decreasing ventilation when blood pH is lowered or raised. However, the steady-state ventilatory adaptation to metabolic acid–base disturbances remains relatively unchanged after peripheral chemodenervation (67,70). Since the cisternal CSF pH change cannot account for the continued hyper- or hypoventilation of metabolic acidosis or alkalosis, it has been suggested that central respiratory drive is encountering the $[H^+]$ at some other site. This could be at some location in the midbrain whose ECF pH is different from that of the cisternal CSF pH, possibly at higher centers or through different mechanisms.

NEUROTRANSMITTERS, BRAIN METABOLISM, AND CENTRAL CONTROL OF BREATHING

Metabolic activities of brain cells are important to central ventilatory drive and to ionic composition and pH homeostasis in cerebral fluids. The brain generates some ammonia as part of its normal metabolism, and some of the CO_2 it produces is "fixed" into the Kreb's cycle intermediates and, ultimately, into certain amino acids such as glutamate, glutamine, and GABA. Ammonia can act as an H^+ buffer, and the amino acids glutamate and GABA are important neurotransmitters that modulate central ventilatory drive. Brain ammonia increases in acute and chronic hypercapnia and is related to the P_{CO_2} increase (71). The increase in brain ammonia is probably from within brain cells; moreover, the increase helps buffer H^+ by the reaction $NH_3 + H^+ \rightarrow NH_4^+$, thereby increasing SID and allowing for more HCO_3^- to be formed. This contribution to buffering, however, is relatively small (30). But since ammonia is a central respiratory stimulant (72), it helps increase the central drive in hypercapnia where it is otherwise depressed because of the compensatory CNS $[HCO_3^-]$ increase.

More importantly, the increase in brain ammonia is associated with a reduction in alpha-ketoglutarate and glutamic acid content and an increase in glutamine via the "detoxification" pathway of ammonia:

$$\text{Alpha-ketoglutarate} + NH_3 \rightleftharpoons \text{Glutamic acid}$$

$$+ NH_3 \underset{\text{Glutaminase}}{\overset{\substack{\text{Glutamine} \\ \text{synthetase}}}{\rightleftharpoons}} \text{Glutamine}$$

The enzyme glutamine synthetase is found only in glia cells, the same cells that are so essential to CO_2 hydration, HCO_3^- formation, and Na^+–H^+ exchange in maintaining CNS acid–base balance.

Hypercapnia is associated with increases in brain glutamine and reductions in brain glutamate and aspartate (73,74) as well as increases in GABA. These changes are important in several ways. By reducing certain acids, the H^+ load in the brain is decreased. But of greater significance is the fact that aspartate, glutamate, and GABA are neurotransmitters that have profound effects on central ventilatory drive. Thus in the process of CO_2 fixation in the brain, certain amino acid neurotransmitters are altered. GABA and glutamate have been studied most extensively in terms of central drive of ventilation, with glutamate being an excitatory neurotransmitter and GABA being an inhibitory one (75). The metabolism of GABA is closely related to that of glutamate. Glutamate is formed by amidation of alpha-ketoglutarate; and then, by addition of another NH_3, glutamine is formed. Glutamine is a neutral amino acid, but it is the pool from which both glutamate and GABA are derived for neurotransmission:

$$\text{Glutamine} \xrightarrow{\text{Glutaminase}}$$

$$\text{Glutamate} \underset{\text{synthetase}}{\overset{\text{Glutamine}}{\longrightarrow}} \text{Glutamine}$$

$$\text{Glutamine} \longrightarrow \text{Glutamate} \xrightarrow{\substack{\text{Glutamic acid} \\ \text{decarboxylase (GAD)}}}$$

$$\text{GABA} \xrightarrow{\text{GABA-T}} \text{Glutamine}$$

Both neurotransmitters are then cycled back to glu-

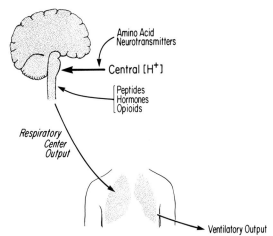

FIG. 4. The central chemical drive of ventilation is critically dependent on $[H^+]$ in the cerebral fluids, which act at a site on or near the ventral surface of the medulla. The H^+ effect is modulated by certain amino acid neurotransmitters, such as GABA and glutamate, whose concentration is dependent on H^+ and "CO_2 fixation" in the brain. The respiratory center output is also modified by a number of other central agents such as neuropeptides, hormones, and opioids.

tamine as shown in the above reactions. Central application of GABA depresses ventilation by decreasing inspiratory drive (76–78), and the site of action appears to be on the ventral surface of the medulla in the intermediate area (79). Glutamate given centrally increases ventilation (80), again by acting primarily on the ventral medullary surface. When endogenous glutamate in the brain is increased by inhibiting glutamine synthetase, again there is increased inspiratory drive and minute ventilation (81). Therefore, CO_2 fixation and H^+ homeostasis in the brain are associated with changes in these two neurotransmitters that modulate the central ventilatory drive and, depending upon which one is increased, either augment or diminish the central ventilatory effects of H^+ (Fig. 4). Their site of action appears to be in the region of H^+-"chemosensitive" areas on the ventral surface of the medulla. The mechanisms of action of these neurotransmitters have not been entirely elucidated; however, they may be through opening of the Cl^- channels on cell membranes (82), involving the ion that is also so important in determining cerebral fluid electrolyte composition.

VENTILATORY CONTROL

Ionic composition and $[H^+]$ of cerebral fluids are important in the central control of breathing (1,4). The exact site of action of the H^+ central stimulus has been controversial, but some site within the CNS is H^+-responsive (83). How H^+ acts and brings about neuronal discharge is not clear. Recent evidence suggests that H^+, whether of "metabolic" or "respiratory" origin, stimulates ventilation through cholinergic mechanisms, with acetylcholine as the neurotransmitter (84). The site of action of acetylcholine has been suggested to be through the M_1 receptors in the rostral area on the ventral surface of the medulla (85).

Whether it is truly the H^+ content or another variable that influences central drive of ventilation is the subject of much discussion. Reeves (86) has suggested that it is the protein charge state that is being regulated; that is, the fractional dissociation of the imidazole moiety of histidine (alpha-imidazole) is the regulated variable. Regulation of alpha-imidazole (alphastat) would maintain protein charge states and enzymatic functions constant and would do the same to the OH^-/ H^+ ratio in the intra- and extracellular compartments. The alphastat regulation has been shown experimentally to hold true for the central chemical drive of ventilation (87). Furthermore, inhibiting the alpha-imidazole on the ventral surface of the medulla with a specific binder, diethyl pyrocarbonate, abolishes the H^+ central ventilatory drive (88), providing more evidence in support of the alphastat hypothesis. This is an attractive concept that could explain both (a) the central drive of ventilation and (b) cerebral fluid ionic composition.

REFERENCES

1. Leusen IR. Regulation of cerebrospinal fluid composition with reference to breathing. *Physiol Rev* 1972;52:1–56.
2. Kazemi H, Johnson DC. Regulation of cerebrospinal fluid acid–base balance. *Physiol Rev* 1986;66:953–1037.
3. Haldane JS, Priestley JG. The regulation of the lung ventilation. *J Physiol (Lond)* 1905;32:224–266.
4. Leusen IR. Chemosensitivity of the respiratory center. Influence of changes in the H^+ and total buffer concentrations in the cerebral ventricles on respiration. *Am J Physiol* 1954;176:45–51.
5. Pappenheimer JR, Fencl V, Heisey SR, Held D. Role of cerebral fluids in control of respiration as studied in unanesthetized goats. *Am J Physiol* 1965;208:436–450.
6. Dermietzel R. Central chemosensitivity, morphological studies. In: Loeschke HL, ed. *Acid–base homeostasis of the brain extracellular fluid and the respiratory control system*. Stuttgart: Thieme Edition/Publishing Sciences Group, 1976;52–66.
7. Dempsey JA, Forster HV. Mediation of ventilatory adaptations. *Physiol Rev* 1982;62:262–346.
8. Cserr HF. Physiology of the choroid plexus. *Physiol Rev* 1971;51:273–311.
9. Katzman R, Pappius HM. *Brain electrolytes and fluid metabolism*. Baltimore: Williams & Wilkins, 1973.
10. Van Heijst ANP, Maas AHJ, Visser BF. Comparison of the acid–base balance in cisternal and lumbar cerebrospinal fluid. *Pflugers Arch* 1966;287:242–246.
11. Ames S III, Sakanoue M, Endo S. Na^+, K^+, Ca^{++}, Mg^{++}, and Cl^- concentrations in choroid plexus fluid and cisternal fluid compared with plasma ultrafiltrate. *J Neurophys* 1964;27:672–681.
12. Held D, Fencl V, Pappenheimer JR. Electrical potential of cerebrospinal fluid. *J Neurophysiol* 1964;27:942–959.
13. Stewart PA. *How to understand acid–base balance. A quantitative acid–base primer for biology and medicine*. New York: Elsevier, 1981.
14. Ponten U, Siesjo BK. Gradients of CO_2 tension in the brain. *Acta Physiol Scand* 1966;67:129–140.
15. Fencl V. Acid–base balance in cerebral fluids. In: Cherniack NS, Widdicombe JG, eds. *Handbook of physiology, Section 3, part I: the respiratory system—control of breathing*. Baltimore: Williams & Wilkins Co. and Am Physiol Soc 1986;115–140.
16. Hasan FM, Kazemi H. Dual contribution theory of regulation of CSF HCO_3^- in respiratory acidosis. *J Appl Physiol* 1976;40:559–567.
17. Nattie EE. Ionic mechanisms of cerebrospinal fluid acid–base regulation. *J Appl Physiol* 1983;54:3–12.
18. Johnson DC, Hoop B, Kazemi H. Movement of CO_2 and HCO_3^- from blood to brain in dogs. *J Appl Physiol* 1983;54:989–996.
19. Javaheri S, Kazemi H. Electrolyte composition of cerebrospinal fluid in acute acid–base disorders. *Respir Physiol* 1981;45:141–151.
20. Nattie EE, Edwards WH. CSF acid–base regulation and ventilation during acute hypercapnia in the newborn dog. *J Appl Physiol* 1981;50:566–574.
21. Ahmad HR, Loeschcke HH. Fast bicarbonate–chloride exchange between brain cells and brain extracellular fluid in respiratory acidosis. *Pflugers Arch* 1982;395:293–299.
22. Vates TS, Bonting SL Jr, Oppelt WW. Na–K activated adenosine triphosphatase formation of cerebrospinal fluid in the cat. *Am J Physiol* 1964;206:1165–1172.
23. Bronsted HE. Transport of glucose, sodium, chloride and potassium between the cerebral ventricles and surrounding tissues in cats. *Acta Physiol Scand* 1970;79:523–532.
24. Kazemi H, Choma L. H^+ transport from CNS in hypercapnia and regulation of CSF HCO_3^-. *J Appl Physiol* 1977;42:667–672.
25. Benos DJ. Amiloride: A molecular probe of sodium transport in tissues and cells. *Am J Physiol* 1982;242:C131–C145.
26. Soltoff SP, Mandel LJ. Amiloride directly inhibits the Na,K-ATPase activity of rabbit kidney proximal tubules. *Science* 1983;220:957–958.
27. Davson H, Segal MB. The effects of some inhibitors and accelerators of sodium transport on the turnover of $^{22}Na^+$ in the cerebrospinal fluid and the brain. *J Physiol (Lond)* 1970;209:131–150.
28. Javaheri S, Weyne J. Effect of amiloride on cisternal fluid $[HCO_3^-]$ in acute respiratory acidosis. *Respir Physiol* 1984;58:101–110.
29. Maren TH. Bicarbonate formation in cerebrospinal fluid: role in sodium transport and pH regulation. *Am J Physiol* 1972;222:885–899.
30. Wichser J, Kazemi H. CSF bicarbonate regulation in respiratory acidosis and alkalosis. *J Appl Physiol* 1975;38:504–511.
31. Johnson DC, Singer S, Hoop B, Kazemi H. Chloride flux from blood to CSF: inhibition by furosemide and bumetanide. *J Appl Physiol* 1987;63:1591–1600.
32. Johnson DC, Frankel HM, Kazemi H. Effect of furosemide on cerebrospinal fluid composition. *Respir Physiol* 1984;56:301–308.
33. Betz AL. Sodium transport from blood to brain: inhibition by furosemide and amiloride. *J Neurochem* 1983;41:1158–1164.
34. Reed DJ. The effect of furosemide on cerebrospinal fluid flow in rabbits. *Arch Int Pharmacodyn Ther* 1969;178:324–330.
35. Haas M, McManus TJ. Bumetanide inhibits (Na + K + 2Cl) cotransport at a chloride site. *Cell Physiol* 1983;14:C235–C240.
36. Cabantchik ZI, Knauf PA, Rothstein A. The role of membrane protein evaluated by the use of 'probes'. The anion transport system of the red blood cell. *Biochim Biophys Acta* 1978;515:239–299.
37. Kimelberg HK, Biddlecome S, Bourke RS. SITS-inhibitable Cl^- transport and Na^+-dependent H^+ production in primary astroglial cultures. *Brain Res* 1979;173:111–124.
38. Furuya W, Tarshis T, Law FY, Knauf PA. Transmembrane effects of intracellular chloride on the inhibitory potency of extracellular H2DIDS. *J Gen Physiol* 1984;83:657–681.
39. Javaheri S, Weyne J. Effects of 'DIDS', an anion transport blocker, on CSF $[HCO_3^-]$ in respiratory acidosis. *Respir Physiol* 1984;57:365–376.
40. Frankel H, Kazemi H. Regulation of CSF composition—block-

ing chloride–bicarbonate exchange. *J Appl Physiol* 1983;55:177–182.

41. Maren TH. Carbonic anhydrase: chemistry, physiology, and inhibition. *Physiol Rev* 1967;47:595–781.

42. Giacobini E. A cytochemical study of the localization of carbonic anhydrase in the nervous system. *J Neurochem* 1962;9:169–177.

43. Vogh BP. The relation of choroid plexus carbonic anhydrase activity to cerebrospinal fluid formation: study of three inhibitors in cat with extrapolation to man. *J Pharmacol Exp Ther* 1980;213:321–331.

44. Maren TH, Broder LE. The role of carbonic anhydrase in anion secretion into cerebrospinal fluid. *J Pharmacol Exp Ther* 1970;172:197–202.

45. Javaheri S, Clendening A, Papadakis N, Brody JS. Changes in brain surface pH during acute isocapnia metabolic acidosis and alkalosis. *J Appl Physiol* 1981;51:276–281.

46. Kiley JP, Eldridge FL, Milhorn DE. The roles of medullary extracellular and cerebrospinal fluid pH in control of respiration. *Respir Physiol* 1985;59:117–130.

47. Kazemi H, Valenca LM, Shannon DC. Brain and cerebrospinal fluid lactate concentration in respiratory acidosis and alkalosis. *Respir Physiol* 1969;6:178–186.

48. Plum F, Posner JB. Blood and cerebrospinal fluid lactate during hyperventilation. *Am J Physiol* 1967;212:864–870.

49. Severinghaus JW, Mitchell RA, Richardson BW, Singer MM. Respiratory control at high altitude suggesting active transport regulation of CSF pH. *J Appl Physiol* 1963;18:1155–1166.

50. Shannon DC, Kazemi H, Croteau N, Parsons EF. Cerebral acid–base changes during reduced cranial blood flow. *Respir Physiol* 1970;8:385–396.

51. Weyne J, Demeester G, Leusen IR. Effects of carbon dioxide, bicarbonate and pH on lactate and pryuvate in brain of rats. *Pfluger Arch* 1970;314:292–311.

52. Arieff AI, Kerian A, Massry SG, DeLima J. Intracellular pH of brain: alterations in acute respiratory acidosis and alkalosis. *Am J Physiol* 1976;230:804–812.

53. Kazemi H, Shannon DC, Carvallo-Gil E. Brain CO_2 buffering capacity in respiratory acidosis and alkalosis. *J Appl Physiol* 1967;22:241–246.

54. Nishimura M, Johnson DC, Hitzig BM, Okunieff P, Kazemi H. Effects of hypercapnia on brain pHi and phosphate metabolite regulation by ^{31}P-NMR. *J Appl Physiol* 1989;66(5):2181–2188.

55. Jennings DB, Davidson JSD. Acid–base and ventilatory adaptation in conscious dogs during chronic hypercapnia. *Respir Physiol* 1984;58:377–393.

56. Van Vaerenbergh PJ, Demeester G, Leusen I. Lactate in cerebrospinal fluid during hyperventilation. *Arch Int Physiol Biochim* 1965;73:738–747.

57. Kazemi H, Javaheri S. Interaction between P_{CO_2} and plasma HCO_3^- in regulation of CSF HCO_3^- in respiratory alkalosis and metabolic acidosis. *Adv Exp Med Biol* 1978;99:173–183.

58. Pelligrino DA, Dempsey JA. Dependence of CSF on plasma bicarbonate during hypocapnia and hypoxemic hypocapnia. *Respir Physiol* 1976;26:11–26.

59. Dempsey JA, Forster HV, Gledhill N, DoPico GA. Effects of moderate hypoxemia and hypocapnia on CSF [H$^+$] and ventilation in man. *J Appl Physiol* 1974;38:665–674.

60. Blayo MC, Vergnes MJP, Pocidalo JJ. pH, P_{CO_2} and P_{O_2} of cisternal cerebrospinal fluid in high altitude natives. *Respir Physiol* 1973;19:298–311.

61. Fencl V, Gabel RA, Wolfe D. Composition of cerebral fluids in goats adapted to high altitude. *J Appl Physiol* 1979;47:508–513.

62. Marks Jr CE, Goldring RM, Vecchione JJ, Gordon EE. Cerebrospinal fluid acid–base relationships in ketoacidosis and lactic acidosis. *J Appl Physiol* 1973;35:813–819.

63. Ohman JL, Marliss EB, Aoki TT, Munichoodappa CS, Khanna VV, Kozak GP. The cerebrospinal fluid in diabetic ketoacidosis. *N Engl J Med* 1971;284:283–290.

64. Fencl V, Vale JR, Brock JR. Cerebral blood flow and pulmonary ventilation in metabolic acidosis and alkalosis. *Scand J Clin Lab Invest [Suppl]* 1968;102(8):B22.

65. Irsigler GB, Stafford MJ, Severinghaus JW. Relationship of CSF

pH, O_2, and CO_2 responses in metabolic acidosis and alkalosis in humans. *J Appl Physiol* 1980;48:355–361.

66. Bureau MA, Ouellet G, Begin R, Gagnon N, Geoffroy L, Berthiaume Y. Dynamics of the control of ventilation during metabolic acidosis and its correction. *Am Rev Respir Dis* 1979;119:933–939.

67. Javaheri S, Herrera L, Kazemi H. Ventilatory drive in acute metabolic acidosis. *J Appl Physiol* 1979;46:913–918.

68. Pavlin EG, Hornbein TF. Distribution of H$^+$ and HCO$_3^-$ between CSF and blood during metabolic alkalosis in dogs. *Am J Physiol* 1975;228:1141–1144.

69. Javaheri S, Kazemi H. Metabolic alkalosis and hypoventilation in humans. *Am Rev Respir Dis* 1987;136:1011–1016.

70. Steinbrook RA, Javaheri S, Gabel RA, Donovan JC, Leith DE, Fencl V. Respiration of chemodenervated goats in acute metabolic acidosis. *Respir Physiol* 1984;56:51–60.

71. Weyne J, VanLeuven F, Kazemi H, Leusen IR. Selected brain amino acids and ammonium during chronic hypercapnia in conscious rats. *J Appl Physiol* 1978;44:333–339.

72. Wichser J, Kazemi H. Ammonia and ventilation: site and mechanism of action. *Respir Physiol* 1974;20:393–406.

73. Folbergrova J, Ponten U, Siesjo BK. Patterns of changes in brain carbohydrate metabolites, amino acids and organic phosphates at increased carbon dioxide tensions. *J Neurochem* 1974;22:1115–1125.

74. Weyne J, VanLeuven F, Leusen IR. Glutamate and glutamine in the brain: influence of acute P_{CO_2} changes in normal rats and in rats under sustained hypercapnia or hypocapnia. *Life Sci* 1973;12:211–218.

75. Toleikis JR, Frazier DT. Effects of L-glutamate and GABA on the response of expiratory neurons to mechanical loads. *J Neurosci Res* 1982;7:443–452.

76. Hedner J, Hedner T, Wessberg P, Johason J. An analysis of the mechanism by which gamma-aminobutyric acid depresses ventilation in the rat. *J Appl Physiol* 1984;56:849–856.

77. Kneussl M, Pappagianopoulos P, Hoop B, Kazemi H. Reversible depression of ventilation and cardiovascular function by ventriculo cisternal perfusion with gamma-aminobutyric acid in dogs. *Am Rev Respir Dis* 1986;133:1024–1028.

78. Yamada KA, Hamosh P, Gillis RA. Respiratory depression produced by activation of GABA receptors in hindbrain of cat. *J Appl Physiol* 1981;51:1278–1286.

79. Yamada KA, Norman WP, Hamosh P, Gillis RA. Medullary ventral surface GABA receptors affect respiratory and cardiovascular function. *Brain Res* 1982;248:71–78.

80. Chiang CH, Pappagianopoulos P, Hoop B, Kazemi H. Central cardiorespiratory effects of glutamate in dogs. *J Appl Physiol* 1986;60:2056–2062.

81. Hoop B, Systrom DM, Shih VE, Kazemi H. Central respiratory effects of glutamine synthesis inhibition in dogs. *J Appl Physiol* 1988;65:1099–1109.

82. Harris RA, Allan AM. Functional coupling of gamma-aminobutyric acid receptors to chloride channels in brain membranes. *Science* 1985;228:1108–1110.

83. Bledsoe SW, Hornbein TF. Central chemosensors and the regulation of their chemical environment. In: Hornbein TF, ed. *Regulation of breathing*. New York: Marcel Dekker, 1981;347–428.

84. Burton MD, Johnson DC, Kazemi H. CSF acidosis augments ventilation through cholinergic mechanisms. *J Appl Physiol* 1989;66(6):2562–2572.

85. Nattie EE, Wood J, Mega A, Goritski E. Rostral ventrolateral medulla muscarinic receptor involvement in central ventilatory chemosensitivity. *J Appl Physiol* 1989;66(3):1462–1470.

86. Reeves RB. An imidazole alphastat hypothesis for vertebrate acid–base regulation: tissue carbon dioxide content and body temperature in bullfrogs. *Respir Physiol* 1972;14:219–236.

87. Hitzig BM. Temperature-induced changes in turtle CFS pH and central control of ventilation. *Respir Physiol* 1982;49:205–222.

88. Nattie EE, Mills JW, Ou LC. Pirenzepine prevents diethyl pyrocarbonate inhibition of central CO_2 sensitivity. *J Appl Physiol* 1988;65(5):1962–1966.

THE LUNG: *Scientific Foundations*
edited by R.G. Crystal, J.B. West et al.
Raven Press, Ltd., New York © 1991.

CHAPTER 5.4.7

Neurotransmission and Regulation of Respiration

David E. Millhorn, Douglas A. Bayliss, Jeffery T. Erickson, Eve A. Gallman, Caroline L. Szymeczek, Maria F. Czyzyk-Krzeska, and Jay B. Dean

The primary task of brainstem networks that regulate respiration is maintenance of homeostasis regardless of the metabolic demands of the organism. Accomplishment of this task requires continuous and precise signaling among an immense number of neurons involved in a variety of activities such as (a) integration of sensory information, (b) generation and maintenance of respiratory rhythm, and (c) transmission of electrical signals to the muscles of respiration. The most crucial element in achieving coordinated activity in such a complex sensorimotor system is transmission of impulses from one neuron to another (i.e., cell-to-cell communication). Neurons communicate with each other and with nonneural target cells (e.g., muscle) at special sites of contact called the *synapse*. The synapse consists of the *presynaptic* terminal of one neuron (the presynaptic neuron), the receptive membrane of the target cell (the postsynaptic cell), and the narrow space separating them (the synaptic cleft). It is at the synapse that an electrical impulse that has reached the presynaptic terminal is converted into a chemical signal and then converted back again to an electrical impulse on the membrane of the postsynaptic cell. The chemical messengers or molecules that mediate transmission of signals across the synaptic cleft are referred to as *neurotransmitters*.

We should like to emphasize at the outset that research on chemical transmission in the nervous system is still in its infancy. Although many chemical messengers have now been identified and much is now known about the cellular and molecular framework of the chemical transmission and signal transduction, there is relatively little information concerning the identity and action(s) of neurotransmitters that mediate specific physiological responses, including those associated with respiration. We have chosen to devote a major portion of this chapter to a discussion of synaptic transmission and how newly identified synaptic mechanisms might function in regulation of respiration. In addition, we shall discuss the biochemical and functional classification of chemical messengers and the concept of "coexistence" of multiple messengers in individual neurons. We conclude the chapter with a review of the chemical neuroanatomy (i.e., transmitter and peptide content) of sensory ganglia and brainstem areas traditionally associated with regulation of respiration. We shall offer examples of how chemical messengers identified in these areas might affect cellular activity and respiration.

MOLECULAR AND CELLULAR MECHANISMS OF CHEMICAL SYNAPTIC TRANSMISSION

There are three primary events associated with synaptic transmission: (i) transmitter *release,* (ii) transmitter–receptor *interaction,* and (iii) signal *transduction.* Here we shall give a brief account of the molecular and cellular mechanisms associated with each of these events.

Transmitter Release

Early electron-microscopic studies of the synapse showed that the presynaptic terminal contains two

---

D. E. Millhorn, D. A. Bayliss, J. T. Erickson, E. A. Gallman, C. L. Szymeczek, M. F. Czyzyk-Krzeska, and J. B. Dean: Department of Physiology, University of North Carolina, Chapel Hill, North Carolina 27599.

types of morphologically distinct *synaptic vesicles* clustered near the membrane: (i) small clear spherical vesicles and (ii) large dense-core vesicles (1–3). The concept of "quantal" release of transmitter that evolved from electrophysiological studies of the neuromuscular junction (see ref. 4) led to speculation that synaptic vesicles might be vehicles for transmitter release. Differential cell fractionation studies showed that synaptic vesicles actually contain transmitter molecules (5) and that procedures that caused prolonged release of transmitter from the terminal also caused depletion of presynaptic vesicles (6). Moreover, electron micrographs showed that vesicles actually rupture in the vicinity of the synapse (7).

The work of Katz and Miledi (8) revealed that the divalent ion Ca^{2+} plays an essential role in transmitter release. These workers discovered that the presence of Ca^{2+} in the extracellular fluid surrounding the synapse was required for transmitter release. There is now convincing evidence that Ca^{2+} enters the presynaptic terminal via voltage-gated Ca^{2+} channels and facilitates transmitter release by acting as a second messenger to induce phosphorylation of a protein, synapsin I, associated with the synaptic vesicles. Greengard (9) has shown that the dephosphorylated form of synapsin I binds to synaptic vesicles and prevents them from fusing with the synaptic membrane. Once phosphorylated, synapsin I alters its binding to the vesicle, thus allowing it to fuse with the membrane and discharge its contents into the synaptic cleft. Greengard (9) has also shown that the phosphorylation of synapsin I requires (a) increased Ca^{2+} concentration in the terminal and (b) activation of Ca^{2+}/calmodulin-dependent protein kinase.

Once released, the transmitter diffuses across the synaptic cleft and binds to the extracellular domain of a receptor protein. The binding of a transmitter to its receptor is the initial event that leads to an alteration in the activity of the postsynaptic cell.

Transmitter–Receptor Interaction

Released transmitter binds to a specific recognition molecule on the surface of the target cell and initiates a series of events that lead ultimately to altered electrical activity and, in some cases, to a change in the phenotype of the target cell (i.e., activity-dependent regulation of gene expression) (see ref. 10). There are basically two types of postsynaptic receptors: (i) receptors that mediate their effects *directly* by acting as a ligand-gated ion channel (i.e., an ionophore) and (ii) receptors that mediate their effects *indirectly* via a molecular linkage with a guanine nucleotide-binding protein (G protein). It is important to recognize that the cellular effects that result from transmitter–receptor

binding are "receptor-specific," not "transmitter-specific." By this we mean that the "activated" receptor, via its molecular linkage with certain other membranous and cytoplasmic macromolecules, actually determines the effect of transmitter–receptor binding on cellular activity. This is particularly evident in cases where there are multiple receptor subtypes for a given transmitter molecule. For example, at least six different serotonin (5-HT) receptor subtypes (5-HT$_{1A-D}$, 5-HT$_2$, and 5-HT$_3$) have been identified (11); when activated by 5-HT, some mediate depolarization whereas others mediate hyperpolarization. Thus, the same transmitter molecule initiates a different response depending on the receptor subtype activated. Multiple receptor subtypes have been identified for acetylcholine, the biogenic amines, and many of the amino acid transmitters.

Transmitter (Ligand)-Gated Receptor–Ion-Channel Complex

A number of *receptor–ion-channel complexes* have been identified in the nervous system. These complexes are characterized by an extracellular domain and an extensive hydrophobic membrane-spanning region that functions (once activated) as an ion channel. At rest, the receptor does not permit passage of ions. Transmitter binding activates the receptor and leads to a conformational change in the membrane-spanning region that permits ions to pass through the membrane. This type of receptor is ideally suited for rapid signaling. The most widely studied of these are (a) the nicotinic acetylcholine (ACh) receptor and (b) receptors for excitatory (L-glutamate) and inhibitory (GABA) amino acid transmitters.

Nicotinic ACh receptors are found at the neuromuscular junction, in neurons in sympathetic and parasympathetic ganglia, and, perhaps, in discrete regions of the central nervous system (12,13). Cloning studies have revealed that the nicotinic receptor is a pentamer made from four membrane-spanning subunits (α_2, β, γ, δ) that are arranged in a rosette to define a central channel which allows passage of certain cations when activated by ACh (12,14). The receptor is activated by the binding of two ACh molecules in the extracellular domain (N terminal), one molecule becomes bound to each of the two α subunits. When the membrane is near resting potential, the activated channel favors inward movement of Na^+; this leads to rapid depolarization of the cell. This receptor plays an essential role in regulation of respiration; it is located at the neuromuscular junction of respiratory muscle and mediates synaptic signals between the motor nerve and muscles of respiration.

Certain amino acid receptors also function as ligand-gated ion channels. Perhaps the most extensively studied of these are the family of receptors that mediate the neuronal effects of L-glutamate. Four glutamate-receptor subtypes have been identified in the nervous system (see ref. 15). Three of these receptors are named for the high-affinity agonist action of N-methyl-D-aspartate (NMDA), quisqualate (Q), and kainate (K). The fourth subtype is classified by the antagonist action of L-2-aminophosphonobutyric acid. The NMDA, Q, and K glutamate receptors have been studied most extensively. Electrophysiological studies revealed that fast monosynaptic depolarization is mediated by the Q and K receptors (see ref. 15). Thus, the Q and K receptors are excellent candidates for fast signaling. The NMDA receptor, on the other hand, appears to mediate slower depolarizing events and has been implicated in a number of functions such as (a) neuronal plasticity, (b) learning and memory, (c) burst firing, and (d) generation of rhythmic activity.

In recent years the NMDA receptor has been one of the "hottest" topics in neurobiology. Although the molecular structure of the NMDA structure is not fully elucidated, there is considerable information concerning the physiological and pharmacological characteristics of this receptor. For instance, it is now known that the glutamate/NMDA-binding site is located on the extracellular domain (see ref. 15). In addition, an allosteric binding site for glycine has also been identified on the extracellular domain of the receptor (16). Binding of glycine to this site enhances the action of L-glutamate (or NMDA). Conductance of cations through the NMDA-receptor channel is modulated by intracellular Mg^{2+} that acts in a voltage-dependent manner at a site on the inside of the channel (17). At normal resting membrane potential, Mg^{2+} blocks the open channel. As the membrane depolarizes, Mg^{2+} moves out of the channel, thereby allowing passage of cations. A site on the inside of the NMDA-receptor channel which binds certain psychoactive drugs (e.g., phencyclidine) has also been discovered. Thus, the NMDA receptor is more complex than most transmitter-gated channels.

The diverse temporal characteristics of the glutamate-receptor subtypes suggest that they mediate a variety of neural activities, some of which may be crucial for control of respiration; among these activities are (a) fast monosynaptic signaling (Q and K receptors), (b) long-term alterations in neuronal activity, and (c) bursting activity (NMDA receptor). For example, involvement of the NMDA receptor in generation of rhythmic bursting activity in spinal-cord locomotor circuits (18) certainly makes this receptor an attractive candidate for mediating respiratory-related rhythms (19). In addition, there is evidence that a non-NMDA receptor is involved in mediating respiratory drive to the phrenic motor neurons in the spinal cord (20).

Gamma-aminobutyric acid (GABA) is normally associated with inhibitory signaling in the nervous system. GABA mediates its effects through the $GABA_A$ and $GABA_B$ receptors. The $GABA_A$ receptor is an ionophore that is distinguished from the $GABA_B$ receptor, a G-protein-linked complex, by its ability to bind bicuculline (21). The $GABA_A$ receptor consists of α and β subunits that form a channel when the receptor is activated. The transmitter detection/binding site is situated on the extracellular domain of the β subunit. The activated receptor increases conductance for Cl^- across the membrane (see ref. 21). The direction of Cl^- movement across the membrane depends on membrane potential. At resting membrane potential, the electrochemical gradient for Cl^- is near zero and there is no net movement of Cl^- into the cell despite the fact that Cl^- concentration is approximately 10 times higher on the outside of the cell. Depolarization of the membrane (e.g., by the action of an excitatory receptor) when $GABA_A$ is activated leads to movement of Cl^- into the cell; this tends to counteract the effect on membrane potential of movement of depolarizing cations into the cell. In this sense the $GABA_A$ receptor serves to stabilize the membrane. Another distinguishing factor of the $GABA_A$ receptor is an allosteric binding site for benzodiazepines (e.g., diazepam) on the α subunit (22). Binding to this site facilitates conductance of Cl^- through the "activated" channel. Much of the fast inhibitory signaling in respiratory-related circuits may be mediated by GABA via the $GABA_A$ receptor (23).

G-Protein-Linked Receptors

A number of transmitters, including the biogenic amines (dopamine, norepinephrine, epinephrine, serotonin, and histamine), ACh (via the muscarinic receptor), GABA (via the $GABA_B$ receptor), and certain peptides, activate receptors that alter the activity of the target cell indirectly via their linkage with intramembranous and cytoplasmic macromolecules. Several G-protein-linked receptors have now been cloned, and their neuropeptide and amino acid sequences have been determined (24,25). Findings from cloning studies revealed that the molecular structures of these receptors (e.g., the $5\text{-}HT_{1a}$ and $5\text{-}HT_{1c}$ receptors and alpha-adrenergic receptor) are remarkably similar; they consist of an extracellular domain (amino terminus), seven membrane-spanning regions, and an intracellular domain (carboxy terminus). The second or third membrane-spanning segment appear to participate in transmitter recognition and binding. The third cytoplasmic domain (between the sixth and seventh membrane-spanning regions) "links" the receptor to a G protein that is involved in signal transduction (see below).

The important distinction between transmitter-gated receptor–channel complexes (discussed above) and G-protein-coupled receptors is that the latter mediates its effects *indirectly* via biochemical intermediaries. It is now generally accepted that transmitter binding alters the molecular configuration of the receptor in the membrane, which, in turn, activates a cascade of reactions (i.e., signal transduction) that leads to altered activity of the target cell.

Signal Transduction

The signal that results from the binding of the transmitter to the receptor on the outer surface of the membrane is transmitted into the cell via a membrane-bound heterotrimeric complex called the *G protein* (26,27). The sequence of events involved in transmembrane signal transduction has been elucidated largely through the efforts of Gilman (27) and Rodbell (28). Briefly, transmitter binding to the receptor activates the G protein, which then binds to guanosine triphosphate (GTP) on the cytoplasmic surface of the membrane. The G-protein–GTP complex activates adenylate cyclase (AC), a membrane-bound enzyme that repeatedly catalyzes the formation of adenosine 3',5'-monophosphate (cyclic AMP, also known as cAMP) from adenosine triphosphate (ATP). This sequence of events is depicted in Fig. 1.

A number of different species of G proteins have now been identified. Two of these are named for their ability to stimulate (G_s) and inhibit (G_i) AC activity. Increased AC activity and accumulation of cAMP activates a specific protein kinase (cAMP-dependent protein kinase) that leads to phosphorylation of existing proteins (9). Proteins phosphorylated by the "second messenger" action of cAMP (and other second messenger systems) represent a final common pathway in signal transduction by which transmitter–receptor binding leads to an alteration in cell function. For ex-

ample, phosphorylation of a channel protein might alter ionic conductance through the channel and thereby change the electrical activity of the cell.

A relatively new concept also depicted in Fig. 1 is that proteins phosphorylated by second messengers might act as transcription factors to regulate expression of certain genes (10,29,30). In this scenario the phosphorylated protein interacts with a specific nucleotide sequence on the gene (i.e. response element, re) to either enhance or repress its transcription. Thus, a change in synaptic activity might alter gene expression via a second messenger system and thereby change the phenotype of the target cell. This phenomenon, which is referred to as "activity-dependent regulation of gene expression," might offer explanations for long-lasting alterations or changes in the "state of activity" of respiratory drive that may occur as the result of changing environmental or pathological conditions. For example, the phemonenon of respiratory acclimatization to chronic hypoxia might be explained by such a mechanism. Here the increased synaptic input from the carotid body chemoreceptors during hypoxia might lead to activation of a second messenger system and phosphorylation of existing nuclear proteins; this, in turn, might activate gene expression for some unknown protein. This newly synthesized protein (e.g., a channel protein) functions to enhance the state of excitability of the target cell. If altered gene expression were involved in such a response, one would expect the "enhancement" of activity to continue for some time after removal of the initial stimulus. Such is the case with acclimatization to hypoxia; the facilitated respiration persists for days after return to normoxic conditions.

In addition to cAMP-dependent protein kinase second messenger system, three other second messenger systems have been identified and characterized: (i) guanine 3', 5'-monophosphate (cGMP)-dependent protein kinase, (ii) inositol trisphosphate-protein kinase C, and (iii) Ca^{2+} calmodulin-dependent protein kinase. A

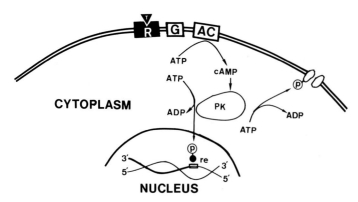

FIG. 1. Model of a cell containing a G-protein-linked receptor. The binding of transmitter to receptor activates a specific G protein which, in turn, activates adenylate cyclase (AC). The activated AC causes accumulation of cAMP via a specific protein kinase. Proteins phosphorylated by this system can lead to changes in conductance of ions through the membrane or can act as transcription factors to alter gene expression for certain proteins. re, response element.

TABLE 1. *Neuroactive peptides found in mammalian nervous tissue (listed alphabetically)*

Adrenocorticotropin	Melanocyte-stimulating
Angiotensin II	hormone (MSH)
Bombesin	Motilin
Bradykinin	Neurokinin A
Calcitonin gene-related	(substance K)
peptide (CGRP)	Neuropeptide tyrosine
Cholecystokinin (CCK)	(NPY)
Corticotropin-releasing	Neurophysin
hormone	Neurotensin
β-Endorphin	Oxytocin
(Leucine)-enkephalin	Prolactin
(Methionine)-enkephalin	Secretin
Galanin	Sleep peptide
Gastrin	Somatostatin
Glucagon	Substance P
Growth hormone	Thyrotropin-releasing
Growth-hormone-	hormone (TRH)
releasing hormone	Vasoactive intestinal
Insulin	peptide (VIP)
Luteinizing hormone	Vasopressin

number of excellent reviews on second messenger systems and signal transduction are available (9,27,31–33).

CHEMICAL MESSENGERS

Since the establishment of chemical transmission as the primary means by which neurons communicate with each other (see ref. 34 for historical account of chemical transmission), considerable effort has been devoted to identifying chemical substances involved in synaptic transmission. The first messengers identified were small-molecular-weight compounds such as ACh, the biogenic amines (i.e., dopamine, norepinephrine, epinephrine, serotonin, and histamine), and certain amino acids (e.g., glutamate, aspartate, GABA, and glycine). Because these compounds meet most of the established criteria for acceptance as a neurotransmitter (35), they are generally referred to as "classical" neurotransmitters. During the present decade there has been an unprecedented growth of transmitter candidates, due primarily to the inclusion of an entire new class of compounds, the *neuropeptides,* as potential neurotransmitters (36). To date, approximately 30 peptides ranging in size from a few to more than 40 amino acids have been identified in neurons of the peripheral and central nervous systems. A list of peptides that have been identified in the mammalian nervous system is provided in Table 1.

Identification of Chemical Messengers in Neurons

Largely as a result of findings from immunohistochemical mapping studies, much is known about distribu-tions of classical neurotransmitters and peptides in the nervous system (see ref. 37). Two important observations were made. First, transmitters and peptides are not distributed randomly but instead show precise distribution patterns in the nervous system which are well conserved in animals of the same species and, to a large extent, in different species. Second, most brain areas or nuclei are not homogeneous in terms of transmitter and peptide content but instead contain a wide variety of these compounds. A classic example is nucleus tractus solitarii (NTS), a major integrative area for autonomic regulation, where cell bodies and fibers contain most of the classical neurotransmitters and many of the identified peptides.

Although much is now known about the distributions of chemical messengers in various regions of the nervous system (including those messengers traditionally associated with respiration), little is known concerning the role of these compounds in mediating specific functions. Experiments of this type are technically very difficult to perform. They require (a) intracellular recordings *in vivo* to verify the functional characteristics of the cell and (b) injection of the cell with a dye. The chemical messenger in the electrophysiologically characterized dye-filled neuron must then be determined from a number of candidates. Moreover, as we shall discuss below, many neurons contain multiple messengers that may be released under different circumstances. This exacerbates the problem of identifying the chemical messenger that actually mediates the function. Successful experiments of this type have been rare.

Information about *possible* involvement of a transmitter or peptide as a candidate for mediating certain functions is accomplished by combining immunohistochemistry and axonal tracing (38). This approach requires that the axonal tracer be placed into the terminal fields (for retrograde tracing) or near the soma (for anterograde tracing) of the pathway of interest. After adequate time for transport, the animal is sacrificed, and the tracer-labeled neurons are analyzed immunohistochemically to identify the messenger(s). This approach has been used successfully to determine the chemical nature of specific pathways. Thus, transmitter "candidates" for mediating certain responses have been identified. Figure 2 shows neurons in the region of nucleus paragigantocellularis of the ventral medulla (an area associated with regulation of both the respiratory and cardiovascular systems) which are retrogradely labeled with Fluoro-Gold dye (Fig. 2B and D) that had been injected into the spinal cord. A number of the retrogradely labeled cells also showed positive immunostaining for somatostatin (SOM) (Fig. 2A) and cholecystokinin (CCK) (Fig. 2C). These findings show that SOM- and CCK-immunoreactive neurons in the ventral medulla project to the spinal cord. An obvious

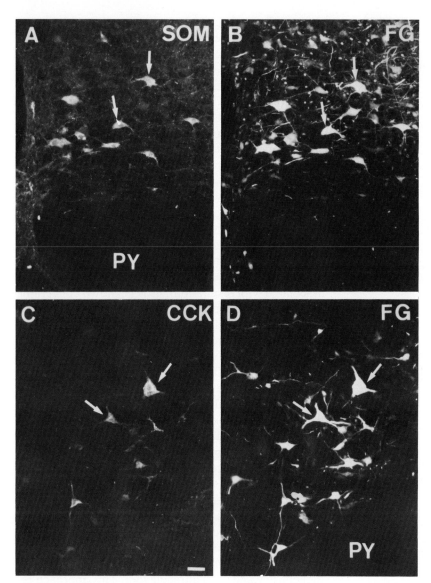

FIG. 2. Illustration of the use of immunohistochemistry and axonal labeling to identify the projection sites of peptide-containing neurons in the ventral medulla in the region of nucleus paragigantocellularis. The arrows in **A** and **B** show cells that are somatostatin (SOM)-immunoreactive and contain Fluoro-Gold (FG), a retrogradely transported dye, that had been injected previously into the cervical region of the spinal cord. The arrows in **C** and **D** indicate cholecystokinin (CCK)-immunoreactive neurons that contain FG that had been injected into the cervical spinal cord. The bar in panel C is equal to 50 μm. PY indicates the pyramidal tract.

limitation to this approach is that it does not provide information about the *function* of the tracer-labeled neurons.

New techniques have been developed in recent years which provide a means to study the molecular substrate of chemical messengers and receptors. One such technique, *in situ* hybridization, has proven to be extremely useful in studying gene expression at the single-cell level, even in heterogeneous tissue such as brain (39). Briefly, this technique involves the use of either DNA or RNA "probes," complementary to the mRNA of the protein of interest. The probe is labeled with a radioactive isotope and applied to thinly cut tissue sections. The sections are exposed to radiographic emulsion (1–3 weeks) and then examined with a microscope equipped with light- and dark-field capabilities. Cells that express the mRNA of interest are labeled with silver grains as a result of hybridization

of the mRNA with the probe. Recent work from our laboratory showing cells in sensory ganglia (petrosal and nodose) associated with regulation of respiration that express mRNA for neuropeptides is shown in Fig. 3. Cells with a low concentration of the mRNA of interest contain fewer silver grains than do those with a higher concentration of the mRNA.

In situ hybridization and other molecular techniques offer the possibility to quantitate gene expression for mRNA that encodes for (a) peptides, (b) transmitter synthesizing enzymes, and (c) receptor proteins, and thus these techniques provide tremendous opportunity for elucidating transmitter- and receptor-mediated effects during different physiological, pathological, and developmental states. In this regard, our laboratory has recently begun studying gene expression for neuropeptides in brainstem respiratory areas during development. We found that the peptide phenotype of

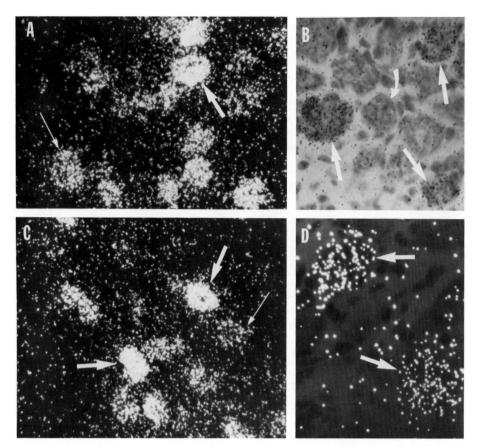

FIG. 3. Dark (**A,C,D**)- and light (**B**)-field photomicrographs of cell bodies in the nodose ganglion (**A,B**) and petrosal ganglion (**C,D**) in which *in situ* hybridization with radioactive oligo-DNA probes was used to detect several different peptides. The clusters of silver grains are over cells that contain mRNA that encode for substance P/neurokinin A (preprotachykinin A; ppTA) in the nodose ganglion (**A,B**), calcitonin gene-related peptide (CGRP) (**C**), and somatostatin (**D**) in the petrosal ganglion. The cellular resolution of this technique is evident in **B**, where the silver grains (*black dots*) are over the cells indicated by straight arrows. The curved arrow in **B** shows a cell that does not contain ppTA mRNA. The thick arrows in **A** and **C** indicate cells that have a high concentration of mRNA for ppTA (**A**) and CGRP (**C**). Thin arrows show cells that have relatively less mRNA for these peptides. The magnification in **A** and **C** is 100×, in **B** it is 200×, and in **D** it is 400×.

many cells changes during the first weeks following birth. For instance, SOM and its mRNA are present in neurons of the hypoglossal nucleus in rats at birth and then disappear by the end of the first month. Thyrotropin-releasing hormone (TRH) mRNA, on the other hand, is not present (or is present only at very low levels) in cells of the medullary raphe nuclei at birth and increases gradually during the first 3–4 weeks after birth (40,41). Thus, the peptide phenotype of many neurons in the brainstem nuclei associated with regulation of respiration is not "set" at birth but, instead, changes during the first few weeks after birth. The significance of "programmed" gene expression for peptides is unknown but may be related either to some trophic effect or to changing function of these neurons.

Coexistence of Multiple Transmitters in Individual Neurons

An important finding from immunohistochemical mapping studies was that the distributions of many transmitters and peptides often overlap in various regions of the nervous system. This observation led to speculation that individual neurons might contain more than one transmitter species, thereby challenging the "one-neuron–one-transmitter" theory of chemical transmission (often referred to as *Dale's law*). There is now direct evidence from immunohistochemical studies that neurons in many regions of the nervous system, including those involved in regulation of respiration, often contain a classical neurotransmitter and one or more peptide; in some instances, they contain

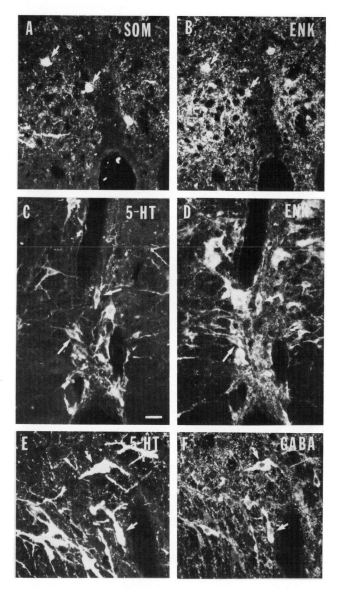

FIG. 4. Photomicrographs of single cells (*arrows*) that contain immunoreactivities for both somatostatin (SOM) (**A**) and enkephalin (ENK) (**B**) in the commissural region of nucleus tractus solitarii. The arrows in **C** and **D** indicate neurons in the region of nucleus raphe obscurus/pallidus that show immunostaining for both serotonin (5-HT) and ENK. The arrows in **E** and **F** designate individual neurons in the region of nucleus raphe magnus cells that contain immunoreactivities for both 5-HT and GABA. The bar in **C** is equal to 50 μm.

two classical neurotransmitters (see refs. 42–44). In addition, there are instances where individual neurons contain two peptides but no classical neurotransmitter. Examples of coexistence situations in respiratory-related areas of the brainstem are shown in Fig. 4. Individual neurons that contain immunostaining for two peptides, SOM (Fig. 4A) and enkephalin (ENK) (Fig. 4B), in nucleus tractus solitarii are indicated by arrows (45). Colocalization of the classical neurotransmitter

serotonin (5-HT) (Fig. 4C) and ENK (Fig. 4D) (46) and coexistence of two classical neurotransmitters, 5-HT (Fig. 4E) and GABA (Fig. 4F) (47), in the ventrolateral aspect of the medulla oblongata (an area associated with both respiratory and cardiovascular regulation) are also shown.

Coexistence of multiple messengers in individual neurons has complicated efforts to elucidate the transmitters and/or peptide that mediate certain responses. Although the functional significance of coexistence remains unknown, a number of interesting possibilities have been suggested (42,44). Perhaps the most attractive of these are those in which a coexisting peptide modulates the effects of a classical transmitter or another peptide. For example, a population of neurons in the medullary raphe nuclei that contain the classical neurotransmitter 5-HT also contain two peptides, TRH and substance P (SP). Hökfelt et al. (48) proposed a model to illustrate how the coexisting peptides might modulate the effects of the classical transmitter. When released alone, 5-HT acts (a) postsynaptically to alter the activity of the target neuron and (b) presynaptically via an "autoreceptor" to inhibit its own release. When co-release is achieved, SP interacts with the "autoreceptor" to prevent 5-HT from inhibiting its own release. Co-released TRH, on the other hand, potentiates the action of 5-HT via a postsynaptic receptor. In both cases the coexisting peptide serves to modulate (or enhance) the effect of the classical transmitter. We recently proposed this model to explain the long-lasting facilitation of respiration (hours) that is evoked by brief (10 min) stimulation of raphe obscurus (49). Electrical stimulation of raphe obscurus at a rate of 15 Hz or higher leads to prolonged release of 5-HT in the NTS (*unpublished observations*). The role of SP in mediating this release is unclear at this time. Similar models have been proposed to explain the functional significance of other coexistence situations (42,43).

How is differential release of coexisting transmitters and peptides achieved, and how might co-released messengers mediate physiological effects? The substrate for co-release appears to involve differential "packaging" of transmitters and peptides in presynaptic vesicles; small clear vesicles are believed to contain exclusively the low-molecular-weight transmitter, whereas large dense-core vesicles contain both the classical transmitter and peptides (50). It has been hypothesized that frequency of depolarization of the presynaptic terminal may somehow encode for differential release. In this model the small clear vesicles containing the classical transmitter are released at low rates of depolarization of the terminal, whereas both small and large vesicles are released at higher frequencies of depolarization. The most convincing support for frequency-dependent differential release of coexisting messengers comes from work on parasympathetic neurons that innervate the salivary gland and contain both ACh and vasoactive intestinal peptide (VIP). Low-frequency stimulation evokes release of ACh, which leads to salivary secretions and a transient increase in blood flow (51). High-frequency stimulation, on the other hand, causes release of both ACh and VIP, which, in turn, mediates salivary secretions and *prolonged* increase in blood flow in the salivary gland. Pretreatment with drugs that antagonize ACh receptors (e.g., atropine) blocks the salivary secretions but not the prolonged increase in blood flow. These findings indicate that coexisting messengers in the parasympathetic neurons that innervate the salivary gland are released differentially: ACh mediates salivary secretions and has a short-lasting effect on blood flow, whereas VIP mediates the prolonged increases in blood flow. It is unknown whether messengers that are colocalized in other systems are released in a similar manner.

Peptides as Transmitters

Whether or not all identified neuropeptides function as transmitters remains unclear. Even if a peptide were to serve as a transmitter, its role would probably differ from that of the low-molecular-weight transmitter. This notion is based on differences in the biosynthesis of peptides and classical transmitters. Classical transmitters are synthesized at the site of release by specific enzymes (52) that are produced in the soma and transported to the axon terminals, where they repeatedly synthesize transmitters from readily available substrate. Localization of the synthesizing enzyme at the site of release is ideal for rapid and continuous signaling. Peptides, on the other hand, are the products of gene expression and must therefore be synthesized in the cell body and transported to the site of release. Once released, they are enzymatically degraded by peptidases in the synaptic cleft. Released peptides can only be replaced in the synaptic terminal by transport of newly synthesized peptide. This process may take hours to days. Thus, peptides are not logical candidates for mediating continuous, rapid signals. Peptides appear to be more suited for modulating the effects of other messengers (as discussed above for coexisting peptides).

Although peptides are not ideal candidates for long-term rapid signaling, there is growing evidence that some of the identified peptides may function as a neurotransmitter. For example, several lines of evidence suggest that substance P, an 11-amino-acid tachykinin peptide derived from preprotachykinin A (ppTA) gene, serves a transmitter function in primary sensory afferents (53). In fact, there is growing evidence that SP-containing neurons may transmit primary sensory sig-

nals from the carotid body O_2 chemoreceptors to brainstem respiratory networks. This is based on findings that SP and ppTA mRNA (see Fig. 3 above) are located in primary sensory neurons in the petrosal ganglion that project to NTS (54–56), that SP is released during hypoxia (57), and that the carotid chemoreceptor response to hypoxia is attenuated by SP antagonists (58). The cellular and respiratory effects of other peptides are discussed below.

CHEMICAL MESSENGERS AND REGULATION OF RESPIRATION

Because of its remarkable diversity, the respiratory control system is perhaps the most complex of the autonomic regulatory systems. Respiratory neurons are engaged in a wide variety of activities that range from primary sensory afferent signaling, rhythm generation, and subsequent transmission of motor signals to the skeletal muscles that produce ventilation and to the smooth muscles that control airway caliber. In addition, respiratory neurons and networks mediate long-lasting alterations in respiratory "drive" in response to certain physiological and pathological conditions (e.g., chronic hypoxia). It seems likely therefore that these diverse functions may require different modes of chemical signaling. This implies that different chemical messengers (transmitters and peptides) might be involved in regulation of respiration. For example, the continuous rapid signaling in primary sensory afferent fibers is probably mediated by a fast-acting messenger such as an excitatory amino acid, acting via a transmitter-gated channel, whereas input from intracranial sources that modulate respiration (e.g., during the wake–sleep cycle) is probably slower and might involve either a monoamine or peptide transmitter acting via a G-protein-linked receptor.

Here we shall give a brief description of recent work to identify and characterize chemical messengers in sensory ganglia and certain brainstem networks involved in regulation of respiration. Our intent is not to provide an exhaustive review of this material but, instead, to provide an overview of some of the more interesting findings concerning (a) cellular localization of transmitter substances and (b) the effects of these compounds on cellular activity and respiration.

Sensory Neurons: The Nodose and Petrosal Ganglia

The inferior sensory ganglia, petrosal and nodose, of the glossopharyngeal and vagus nerves contain the cell bodies of visceral afferent fibers that convey sensory information from receptors of various modality (e.g., carotid sinus and aortic chemo- and baroreceptors; pulmonary and atrial mechanoreceptors; and gastrointestinal receptors) to second-order neurons in the nucleus of the solitary tract. Numerous peptides have been identified in fibers that innervate peripheral organs and project centrally to NTS (59,60). Immunohistochemical studies revealed that a number of peptides, including SP, neurokinin A, calcitonin gene-related peptide (CGRP), SOM, VIP, and CCK, are present in neurons located in the petrosal and nodose ganglia (54,59). In addition, neuropeptide tyrosine (NPY) mRNA (55,56) as well as tyrosine hydroxylase (the rate-limiting enzyme for catecholamine biosynthesis) and its mRNA (61) have been identified in cells of the petrosal ganglion.

In situ hybridization studies have been performed to determine whether neurons in the petrosal and nodose ganglia contain the molecular substrate (i.e., mRNA) for these peptides (55,56). Findings from these studies were, for the most part, consistent with immunohistochemical results with one notable exception: No evidence for CCK gene expression was found in either the petrosal or nodose ganglia. The immunohistochemical evidence for CCK in these ganglia (59) is inconclusive because CCK antibodies show significant cross-reactivity with CGRP, suggesting that CCK positive immunoreactivity may, in fact, represent CGRP. Thus, it appears unlikely that sensory neurons in these ganglia in most species (guinea pig may be an exception) contain CCK.

Other than the experiments described above suggesting a possible role for SP in mediating the respiratory response to stimulation of O$_2$ receptors in the carotid body, there is little or no information concerning the functional significance of peptides in these ganglia. It is unlikely that peptides are involved in moment-to-moment transmission of sensory information, a function more likely to involve a fast-acting neurotransmitter such as an excitatory amino acid. There is indirect evidence which suggests that L-glutamate might be the transmitter in primary sensory afferents in the carotid sinus (62) and vagus nerves (63). Moreover, receptors for excitatory amino acids exist in the NTS (64), the termination site for primary sensory afferents in the nodose and petrosal ganglia. Although amino acids appear to be the best candidates for fast excitatory transmission in respiratory sensory afferent fibers, to date there is no direct evidence that this is the case. Additional research using new innovative approaches is needed to identify and elucidate the action of transmitters and peptides in these sensory neurons.

Major Respiratory-Related Areas (Nuclei) in the Medulla Oblongata

Respiratory-related neurons are located, for the most part, in two regions of the medulla: nucleus tractus solitarii and a rather diffuse area in the ventral medulla that includes nucleus ambiguus, nucleus paragigantocellularis, and the raphe nuclei. Here we shall give a brief overview of the chemical neuroanatomy of these areas. Space limitations prevent us from providing an in-depth account of all transmitters and peptides found in respiratory-related areas. Instead, we shall attempt to illustrate the diversity of chemical messengers in these areas and provide examples of how some of the identified messengers in these areas affect neuronal activity and respiration. Precise maps showing transmitter and peptide distributions in these areas are available elsewhere (37).

Nucleus Tractus Solitarii

The NTS is located in the dorsomedial region of the medulla oblongata just lateral to the fourth ventricle and dorsal to the motor nucleus of the vagus nerve. The caudal half of NTS receives afferent synaptic input from chemo- and mechanoreceptors involved in regulation of the respiratory and cardiovascular systems, whereas the rostral half of the nucleus is innervated, for the most part, by afferents from sensory receptors in the gastrointestinal tract. In addition, the NTS receives input from various areas of the central nervous system that are involved in regulation of autonomic function. The NTS is generally considered as the major autonomic (including respiration) regulatory region in the brain. A number of anatomically and functionally distinct subdivisions (subnuclei) of NTS have been identified. The regions most often associated with regulation of respiration are the commissural, medial, and ventrolateral subnuclei.

Biochemical and immunohistochemical approaches have been used to identify a variety of transmitters and peptides in NTS. In fact, NTS is one of the most chemically heterogeneous areas in the brain; many of the classical transmitters and most of the identified peptides (see Table 1) have been identified in cell bodies and fibers in NTS (see refs. 37 and 65). Because of the importance of NTS in integration of sensory inputs, a number of immunohistochemical studies have been performed to identify transmitters and peptides in *fibers* that innervate NTS. Kalia et al. (66) reported that subnuclei believed to be involved in respiratory and cardiovascular regulation showed moderate densities of fibers containing ENK, SOM, and SP immunoreactivity. Maley and Elde (67) found that punctate varicosities (presumed terminals) in NTS that contain SP, ENK, and 5-HT were most numerous. These workers also found that the distribution patterns for these messengers often "overlapped," suggesting that they may coexist in the same fibers. Recent immunohistochemical studies have verified that 5-HT and SP immunoreactivities often coexist within single fibers in NTS (68). The source of these fibers is believed to be 5-HT/SP cell bodies in the medullary raphe complex.

Immunohistochemical studies revealed that cell bodies in NTS also contain a wide variety of transmitters and peptides in subnuclei traditionally associated with respiration (commissural, medial, and ventrolateral). For instance, noradrenergic (the A2 cell group), adrenergic (the C2 cell group), and 5-HT cells have been identified in the caudal half of NTS (see ref. 37). The C3 group of adrenaline-containing cells and the A2 group of noradrenergic neurons are located just outside the borders of NTS. The NTS also contains a large distribution of somata that show immunostaining for the amino acid transmitters, especially glutamate and GABA (69). In addition to these classical transmitters, a variety of peptides such as ENK, SOM, SP, VIP, neurokinin A, neurotensin, angiotensin II, and CCK have been identified in NTS. Moreover, there is increasing evidence that a number of these compounds coexist in the same neuron. An example of coexistence of SOM- and ENK-like immunoreactivities in cells in the commissural region of NTS is shown in Fig. 2A and B. Autoradiographic studies have revealed the existence of receptors in NTS for a number of these substances. The reader should consult the *Handbook of Chemical Neuroanatomy* for a more complete description of the location of classical transmitters, peptides, and receptors in NTS (37).

The chemical heterogeneity of NTS has made it very difficult to identify chemical messengers within this important autonomic regulatory nucleus that might be involved in regulation of respiration. One approach that has been used to attempt to gain information of this type is to administer the "candidate" transmitter directly into NTS and measure the respiratory response. Several classical transmitters and peptides identified in perikarya or fibers in NTS have been tested this way. One interesting example involves the tripeptide TRH. When applied to a rat brain slice preparation, TRH was found to modulate membrane excitability in such a way so as to induce rhythmic bursting in neurons of NTS (70). When administered to intact rat, TRH induced a marked tachypnea (71). These findings suggest that TRH may have a stimulatory effect on neurons responsible for generation of respiratory rhythm. SOM, on the other hand, has been shown to have a depressant effect on respiratory rhythm (72). SOM was also found to depress the excitability of neurons in NTS by augmentation of a voltage-dependent outward current (I_M) (73).

The respiratory effects of several other peptides found in NTS have also been measured. For instance, iontophoretic application of angiotensin II onto respiratory-related neurons in NTS in intact cat either stimulated or had no effect on their spontaneous firing activity (74). However, when administered systemically to animals in which peripheral respiratory receptors had been denervated, angiotensin II caused inhibition of spontaneous ventilation (75). The reason for this discrepancy is unclear. In other experiments, CCK was shown to inhibit bursting activity in respiratory neurons (76) whereas neurotensin caused stimulation of single-unit activity in NTS that was accompanied by apneustic breathing in cats (77).

These are but a sampling of studies that have been performed to attempt to identify a potential respiratory role for chemical messengers that have been identified in NTS. We should like to emphasize that these findings should not be misconstrued to mean that the exogenously administered substance, simply because it evoked a respiratory response, is actually involved as a respiratory transmitter. These data should only be interpreted to mean that the administered substance either stimulates, inhibits, or has no effect on respiration.

Nucleus Ambiguus (NA)

Nucleus ambiguus has long been associated with regulation of respiration. Neurons in NA show respiratory rhythmicity and project to spinal-cord respiratory motor neurons and to parasympathetic ganglia in the airways. In comparison to NTS, there have been relatively few studies to identify the role of transmitters and peptides in control of breathing. Immunohistochemical studies have identified a number of classical transmitters (glutamate, GABA, 5-HT, and norepinephrine) and peptides (SP, TRH, ENK, CGRP, neurotensin, and SOM) in cell bodies and/or fibers in NA. It seems likely that many more transmitters and peptides will be identified as more studies focus on this small cylindrical nucleus. The reader should refer to ref. 37 for immunohistochemical and biochemical maps of classical transmitters and peptides in NA.

Ventrolateral Medulla (VLM)

The ventrolateral medulla is a relatively nondescript area that encompasses several nuclei and cell groups that have been implicated in regulation of respiration and other autonomic systems. The VLM has been studied extensively in recent years, and the distributions of transmitters and peptides have been mapped (see ref. 37). This area is dominated by several prominent catecholamine-containing and 5-HT-containing cell groups. A large adrenergic group (C_1) is located rostrally and a noradrenergic group (A_1) caudally in the VLM. The majority of 5-HT-containing cells are found in the raphe nuclei, a narrow structure located on the midline of the medulla. Many of the C_1 epinephrine-containing neurons project to the intermediolateral sympathetic column of spinal cord and are thought to be involved in regulation of blood pressure (78). Several recent studies revealed that epinephrine in the C_1 group coexists with NPY (79), SP (80), and ENK (81). ENK has also been shown to coexist with norepinephrine in the A_1 group (81). The function of A_1 norepinephrine cells is unknown.

The 5-HT neurons in the medullary raphe complex project to the both the dorsal and ventral horns of the spinal cord and to other regions of the brain stem. In recent years, 5-HT in the medullary raphe complex has been shown to coexist with GABA (47,82) and several different peptides, including SP, TRH, and ENK (see refs. 42 and 46). Examples of coexistence of 5-HT with ENK and GABA are shown in Fig. 2. The use of retrograde labeling with immunohistochemistry revealed that 5-HT/GABA and 5-HT/ENK neurons in VLM project to the spinal cord (46,82). In addition, there is now evidence that 5-HT neurons in the region of raphe obscurus that contain SP- and/or TRH-like immunoreactivities project to the phrenic motor nucleus (83) and NTS (68). That 5-HT neurons in medullary raphe nuclei might play a role in respiration is indicated by findings from studies in which electrical stimulation of raphe obscurus was found to have a facilitatory effect on phrenic activity that lasts for hours following cessation of the stimulus (49). This response is blocked by pretreating the animal with the 5-HT receptor antagonist methysergide.

SUMMARY

Although much is known concerning the chemical neuroanatomy of respiratory-related areas of the medulla, little is known about the identity of transmitters and peptides that are involved in mediating specific respiratory responses. Much of the difficulty in obtaining information of this type is attributed to the heterogeneity of transmitter and peptide content of these areas as well as to the recent finding that multiple messengers often coexist in individual neurons. Because of space limitations, we concentrated our discussion of chemical messengers on nucleus tractus solitarius, nucleus ambiguus, and the ventrolateral aspect of the medulla oblongata. Information concerning the chemical nature of other respiratory areas in the brain stem (e.g., parabrachial nucleus in the pons; hypoglossal nucleus; and vagal motor nucleus hypothalamus) is found elsewhere (37).

ACKNOWLEDGMENTS

The authors acknowledge the assistance of Luisa Klingler in preparation of this chapter. Research from the authors' laboratory was supported by Grants HL33831 and AHA 881108. DEM is a Career Investigator of the American Lung Association. DAB is supported by a graduate fellowship from Glaxo Pharmaceutical Company, Research Triangle Park, North Carolina. DAB, JTE, EAG, and CLS receive doctoral scholarships from Glaxo Pharmaceutical Company. JBD was supported by a NRSA fellowship and is currently supported by a Parker B. Francis Fellowship.

REFERENCES

1. Palade GE. Electron microscope study of the cytoplasm of neurones. *Anat Record* 1954;118:335–336.
2. De Robertis EDP. Submicroscopic changes of the synapse after nerve section in the acoustic ganglion of the guinea pig. An electron microscope study. *J Biophys Biochem Cytol* 1956;2:503–512.
3. Palay SL. Synapses in the central nervous system. *J Biochem Biophys Cytol [Suppl]* 1956;2:193–201.
4. Katz B. *The release of transmitter substance*. Liverpool: Liverpool University Press, 1969.
5. Whitaker VP. Origin and function of synaptic vesicles. *Ann NY Acad Sci* 1971;183:21–32.
6. Jones SF, Kwanbunbumpen S. The effects of nerve stimulation and hemicholinum on synaptic vesicles at the mammalian neuromuscular junction. *J Physiol* 1970;215:31–50.
7. Hubbard JI, Kwanbunbumpen S. Evidence for the vesicle hypothesis. *J Physiol* 1968;194:407–420.
8. Katz B, Miledi R. The timing of calcium action during neuromuscular transmission. *J Physiol* 1967;189:535–544.
9. Greengard P. Neuronal phosphoproteins—mediators of signal transduction. *Mol Neurobiol* 1987;1:81–119.
10. Laufer R, Changeux JP. Activity-dependent regulation of gene expression in muscle and neuronal cells. *Mol Neurobiol* 1989;3:1–53.
11. Peroutka SJ. 5-Hydroxytryptamine receptor subtypes. *Annu Rev Neurosci* 1988;11:45–60.
12. Changeux JP. The acetylcholine receptor: an "allosteric" membrane protein. *Harvey Lect* 1981;75:85–254.
13. Schmidt JS, Hunt S, Polz-Tejera G. Nicotinic receptors of the central and autonomic nervous system. In: Essman WB, ed. *Neurotransmitter, receptors and drug action*. New York: SP Medical and Scientific Books, 1980;1–45.
14. Numa S, Noda M, Takahashi T, et al. Molecular structure of the nicotinic acetylcholine receptor. *Cold Spring Harbor Symp* 1983;49:9–25.
15. Cotman CW, Iversen LL. Excitatory amino acids in the brain—focus on NMDA receptors. *Trends Neurosci* 1987;7:273–279.
16. Johnson JW, Ascher P. Glycine potentiates the NMDA response in cultured mouse brain neurons. *Nature* 1987;325:529–531.
17. Nowak L, Bregestoviski P, Ascher P, et al. Magnesium gates glutamate-activated channels in mouse central neurons. *Nature* 1984;307:462–465.
18. Wallen P, Grillner S. N-Methyl-D-aspartate receptor-induced inherent oscillatory activity in neurons active during fictive locomotion in lamprey. *J Neurosci* 1987;7:2745–2755.
19. Foutz AS, Champagnat J, Denavit-Saubie. N-Methyl-D-aspartate (NMDA) receptors control respiratory off-switch in cat. *Neurosci Lett* 1988;87:221–226.
20. Liu G, Smith JC, Feldman FL. Role of excitatory amino acids in transmission of respiratory drive to phrenic motor neurons. I: kainate and quisqualate receptors [Abstract]. *Soc Neurosci* 1988;14:938.
21. Bormann J. Electrophysiology of $GABA_A$ and $GABA_B$ receptor subtypes. *Trends Neurosci* 1988;11:112–116.
22. Schofield PR, Darlison MG, Fujita N, et al. Sequence and functional expression of the $GABA_A$ receptor shows a ligand-gated receptor superfamily. *Nature* 1987;328:221–227.

23. Haji A, Connelly C. Schultz SA, Wallace J, Remmers JE. Post-synaptic actions of inhibitory neurotransmitters on bulbar respiratory neurons. In: von Euler C, Lagercrantz H. eds. *Neurobiology of control of breathing*. New York: Raven Press, 1986;187–194.

24. Kobilka BK, Frielle T, Collins S, et al. An intronless gene encoding a potential member of the family of receptors coupled to guanine nucleotide regulatory proteins. *Nature* 1987;329:75–79.

25. Julius D, MacDermott AB, Axel R, Jessel TM. Molecular characterization of a functional cDNA encoding the serotonin 1c receptor. *Science* 1988;241:558–564.

26. Rodbell M, Birnbaumer L, Pohl SL, Krans HMJ. The glucagon sensitive adenyl cyclase system in plasma membranes of rat liver. *J Biol Chem* 1971;246:1877–1882.

27. Gilman AG. G proteins: transducers of receptor generated signals. *Annu Rev Biochem* 1987;56:615–649.

28. Rodbell M. The role of hormone receptors and GTP-regulatory proteins in membrane transduction. *Nature* 1980;284:17–22.

29. Maniatis T, Goodbourn S, Fischer JA. Regulation of inducible and tissue-specific gene expression. *Science* 1987;236:1237–1244.

30. Atchinson ML. Enhancers: mechanisms of action of cell specificity. *Annu Rev Cell Biol* 1988;4:127–153.

31. Berridge MJ. Inositol trisphosphate and idacylglycerol: two interacting second messengers. *Nature* 1987;312:315–321.

32. Nishizuka Y. Studies and perspectives of protein kinase C. *Science* 1986;233:305–312.

33. Schulman H. The multifunctional Ca^{2+}/calmodulin-dependent protein kinase. In: Greengard P, Robinson GA, eds. *Advances in second messenger and phosphoprotein research*, vol 22. New York: Raven Press, 1988.

34. Millhorn DE, Bayliss DA, Erickson JT, et al. Cellular and molecular mechanisms in chemical synaptic transmission. *Am J Physiol (Lung Cell Mol Physiol)* 1989;257:L289–310.

35. Bloom FE. Neurotransmitters: past, present, and future directions. *FASEB J* 1988;2:32–41.

36. Snyder S. Brain peptides as neurotransmitters. *Science* 1980;209:976–983.

37. Björklund A, Hökfelt T, Kuhar M, eds. *Handbook of chemical neuroanatomy*, vols 2–4. Amsterdam: Elsevier, 1984–1985.

38. Hökfelt T, Skagerberg G, Skirboll L, Björklund A. Combination of retrograde tracing and neurotransmitter histochemistry. In: Björklund A, Hökfelt T, eds. *Handbook of chemical neuroanatomy*, vol 1. Amsterdam: Elsevier, 1983;228–285.

39. Uhl GR. *In situ hybridization in brain*. New York: Plenum Press, 1986.

40. Millhorn DE, Seroogy K, Bayliss DA. Programmed gene expression for neuropeptides in brainstem nuclei during development. *Proc Int Union Physiol Sci* 1989;XVII:233.

41. Millhorn DE, Szymeczek CL, Erickson JT, Bayliss DA, Seroogy K. Chemical neuroanatomy of brainstem and spinal cord: gene expression and development. In: Haddad G, Farber J, eds. *Developmental neurobiology of breathing*. New York: Marcel Dekker, 1989; in press.

42. Hökfelt T, Millhorn DE, Seroogy K, et al. Coexistense of peptides with classical neurotransmitters. *Experientia* 1987;43:768–779.

43. Hökfelt T, Meister B, Melander M, et al. Coexistence of multiple messengers: new aspects on chemical transmission. In: Costa E, ed. *Fidia Research Foundation neuroscience award lectures*, vol 2. New York: Raven Press, 1988;61–114.

44. Millhorn DE, Hökfelt T. Chemical messengers and their coexistence in individual neurons. *News Physiol Sci* 1988;3:1–5.

45. Millhorn DE, Hökfelt T, Terenius L, et al. Somatostatin- and enkephalin-like immunoreactivities are frequently colocalized in neurons in the caudal brain stem of rat. *Exp Brain Res* 1987;67:420–428.

46. Millhorn DE, Hökfelt T, Verhofstad AAJ, Terenius L. Individual cells in the raphe nuclei of the medulla oblongata in rat that contain immunoreactivities for both serotonin and enkephalin project to the spinal cord. *Exp Brain Res* 1989;75:536–542.

47. Millhorn DE, Hökfelt T, Seroogy K, Verhofstad AAJ. Extent of colocalization of serotonin and GABA in neurons of the ventral medulla oblongata in rat. *Brain Res* 1988;461:169–174.

48. Hökfelt T, Johansson O, Goldstein M. Chemical anatomy of the brain. *Science* 1981;225:477–481.

49. Millhorn DE. Stimulation of raphe (obscurus) nucleus causes long-term potentiation of phrenic nerve activity in cat. *J Physiol (Lond)* 1986;381:169–179.

50. Fried G, Terenius L, Hökfelt T, Goldstein M. Evidence for the differential localization of noradrenaline and neuropeptide Y (NPY) in neuronal storage vesicles isolated from rat vas deferens. *J Neurochem* 1985;5:450–458.

51. Lundberg J, Hökfelt T. Coexistence of peptides and classical neurotransmitters. *Trends Neurosci* 1983;6:325–333.

52. Siegel G, Albers RW, Agranoff BW, Katzman R. *Basic neurochemistry*, 3rd ed. Boston: Little, Brown and Co., 1981.

53. Pernow B. Substance P. *Pharmacol Rev* 1983;35:85–141.

54. Kummer W. Retrograde neuronal labelling and double-staining immunohistochemistry of tachykinin- and calcitonin gene-related peptide-immunoreactive pathways in the carotid sinus nerve of the guinea pig. *J Auton Nerv Syst* 1988;23:131–141.

55. Millhorn DE, Czyzyk-Krzeska M, Bayliss D, Seroogy K. Gene expression for neuropeptides in primary sensory neurons of the petrosal and nodose ganglia. In: Koepchen HP, ed. *Cardiorespiratory and motor coordination*. Berlin: Springer-Verlag, 1989; in press.

56. Czyzyk-Krzeska M, Seroogy K, Bayliss D, Millhorn DE. Identification of messenger RNA (mRNA) for peptides in neurons of the petrosal ganglion. In: Acker H, Trzebski A, O'Regan RC, eds. *Chemoreceptors and chemoreceptor reflexes*. London: Plenum Press, 1989; in press.

57. Lindefors N, Yamamoto Y, Pantaleo T, et al. *In vivo* release of substance P in the nucleus tractus solitarii increases during hypoxia. *Neurosci Lett* 1986;69:94–97.

58. Prabhakar NR, Runold M, Yamamoto Y, et al. Effect of substance P antagonist on the hypoxia-induced carotid chemoreceptor activity. *Acta Scand Physiol* 1984;121:301–303.

59. Helke CJ, Hill KM. Immunocytochemical study of neuropeptides in vagal and glossopharyngeal afferent neurons in the rat. *Neuroscience* 1988;26:539–551.

60. Gillis RA, Helke CJ, Hamilton BL, et al. Evidence that substance P is a neurotransmitter of baro- and chemoreceptor afferents in nucleus tractus solitarius. *Brain Res* 1980;181:476–481.

61. Katz DM, Black IB. Expression and regulation of catecholaminergic traits in primary sensory neurons: relationship to target innervation *in vivo*. *J Neurosci* 1986;6:983–989.

62. Housley GD, Sinclair JD. Localization by kainic acid lesions of neurones transmitting the carotid chemoreceptor stimulus for respiration in rat. *J Physiol (Lond)* 1988;406:99–114.

63. Guynet PG, Filtz TM, Donaldson SR. Role of excitatory amino acids in rat vagal and sympathetic baroreflexes. *Brain Res* 1987;407:272–284.

64. Miller BD, Felder RB. Excitatory amino acid receptors intrinsic to synaptic transmission in nucleus tractus solitarii. *Brain Res* 1988;456:333–343.

65. Leslie RA (with critique by Palkovits M). Neuroactive substances in the dorsal vagal complex of the medulla oblongata: nucleus of the tractus solitarius, area postrema, and dorsal motor nucleus of the vagus. *Neurochem Int* 1985;7:191–218.

66. Kalia M, Fuxe K, Hökfelt T, et al. Distribution of neuropeptide immunoreactive nerve terminals within the subnuclei of the nucleus of the tractus solitarius of the rat. *J Comp Neurol* 1984;222:409–444.

67. Maley B, Elde R. Immunohistochemical localization of putative neurotransmitters within the feline nucleus tractus solitarii. *Neuroscience* 1982;7:2469–2490.

68. Thor KB, Helke CJ. Serotonin- and substance P-containing projections to the nucleus tractus solitarii of the rat. *J Comp Neurol* 1987;265:275–293.

69. Ottersen OP, Storm-Mathesin J. Neurons containing or accumulating transmitter amino acids. In: Björklund A, Hökfelt T, Kuhar MJ, eds. *Handbook of chemical neuroanatomy*, vol 3. Amsterdam: Elsevier, 1984;141–246.

70. Dekin MS, Richerson GB, Getting PA. Thyrotropin-releasing hormone induces rhythmic bursting in neurons of the nucleus tractus solitarius. *Science* 1985;229:67–69.

71. Hedner J, Hedner T, Wessberg P, et al. Effects of TRH and TRH analogues on the central regulation of breathing in the rat. *Acta Physiol Scand* 1983;117:427–437.

72. Harfstrand A, Fuxe K, Kalia M, Agnati LF. Somatostatin induced apnoea: prevention by central and peripheral administration of the opiate receptor blocking agent naloxone. *Acta Physiol Scand* 1985;125:91–95.

73. Jacquin T, Champagnat J, Madamba S, et al. Somatostatin depresses excitability in neurons of the solitary tract complex through hyperpolarization and augmentation of I_M, a non-inactivating voltage-dependent outward current blocked by muscarinic agonists. *Proc Natl Acad Sci USA* 1988;85:948–952.

74. Sessle BJ, Henry JL. Angiotensin II excites neurones in cat solitary tract nuclei which are involved in respiration and related reflex activities. *Brain Res* 1987;407:163–167.

75. Borison HL, Hubbard JI, McCarthy LE. Central respiratory inhibition by angiotensin II in anesthetized cats. *J Pharmacol Exp Ther* 1988;247:781–790.

76. Morin MP, De Marchi J, Champagnat J, et al. Inhibitory effect of cholecystokinin octapeptide on neurons in the nucleus tractus solitarius. *Brain Res* 1983;265:333–338.

77. Morin-Surun MP, Marlot D, Kessler JP, Denavit-Saubie M. The excitation by neurotensin of nucleus tractus solitarius neurons induces apneustic breathing. *Brain Res* 1986;384:106–113.

78. Ross CA, Ruggiero DA, Joh TH, et al. Adrenalin synthesizing neurons in the rostral ventrolateral medulla: a possible role in tonic vasomotor control. *Brain Res* 1983;273:356–361.

79. Everitt JE, Hökfelt T, Terenius L, et al. Differential co-existence of neuropeptide Y (NPY)-like immunoreactivity with catecholamines in the central nervous system of the rat. *Neurosci* 1984;11:443–462.

80. Lorenz RG, Saper CB, Wong DL, et al. Co-localization of substance P- and phenylethanolamine-*N*-methyltransferase-like immunoreactivity in neurons of ventrolateral medulla that project to the spinal cord: potential role in control of vasomotor tone. *Neurosci Lett* 1985;55:255–260.

81. Ceccatelli S, Millhorn DE, Hökfelt T, Goldstein M. Evidence for the occurrence of an enkephalin-like peptide in adrenaline and noradrenaline neurons of the rat medulla oblongata. *Exp Brain Res* 1989;74:631–640.

82. Millhorn DE, Hökfelt T, Seroogy K, et al. Immunohistochemical evidence for colocalization of gamma-aminobutyric acid (GABA) and serotonin in neurons of ventral medulla oblongata projecting to the spinal cord. *Brain Res* 1987;410:179–185.

83. Holtman JR, Norman WP, Skirboll L, et al. Evidence for 5-hydroxytryptamine, substance P and thyrotropin-releasing hormone in neurons innervating the phrenic motor nucleus. *J Neurosci* 1984;4:1064–1071.

THE LUNG: Scientific Foundations
edited by R.G. Crystal, J.B. West et al.
Raven Press, Ltd., New York © 1991.

CHAPTER 5.4.8

Reflexes from the Airway, Lung, Chest Wall, and Limbs

Giuseppe Sant'Ambrogio and Franca B. Sant'Ambrogio

REFLEXES FROM THE UPPER AIRWAY

General Considerations

It has been known since the 19th century that chemical, mechanical, and thermal irritation of the upper airway gives rise to changes in the pattern of breathing. Lately, much attention has been paid to this portion of the respiratory tract that, because of its location, can play an important role in the maintenance of an optimal environment for both tracheobronchial tree and gas-exchange zone.

The Nose

The most common response to strong odors and irritants such as ammonia and cigarette smoke is apnea. Apnea can also be elicited by water. This reflex is part of the so-called "diving response" (which can be initiated by water on the face or inside the nose) and also affects the larynx, lower airway, and the cardiovascular system (1).

Bradycardia and vasoconstriction (in most vascular beds, with the exclusion of cerebral and coronary circulations) accompany the apneic response. The effect on systemic blood pressure varies among species (1).

Another important reflex effect of mechanical or irritative stimulation of the nasal cavity is laryngeal closure, which can be considered as an additional protective mechanism that prevents noxious agents from entering the lower airway (2).

G. Sant'Ambrogio and F. B. Sant'Ambrogio: Department of Physiology and Biophysics, The University of Texas Medical Branch, Galveston, Texas 77550.

As in the case of other upper-airway reflexes, nasal stimulation generally leads to stronger responses in newborns than in adults (3). For example, mechanical stimulation or cold water instillation into the nasal cavity in newborn rabbits can even cause death. This hyperresponsiveness has been viewed as a contributing factor in the sudden infant death syndrome (3).

Receptors other than olfactory endings involved in the above responses have fibers in the ethmoidal branches of the trigeminal nerve.

The effect of mechanical or irritant stimulation of the nose on the tracheobronchial smooth muscle is controversial. In fact, whereas bronchodilation seems to be a more common response, in some cases bronchoconstriction has been observed. The possible stimulation of the pharynx and/or larynx in addition to the nasal mucosa could explain the discrepancy (1).

Trigeminal afferents contribute to the maintenance of upper-airway patency; negative pressure in the nasal cavity increases the activity of the genioglossus (4) and the hypoglossal nerves (5).

An interesting and common reflex that can be evoked by mechanical and chemical irritations of the nose is sneezing. It is characterized by a deep inspiration, followed by a forced expiration against a closed glottis and a constricted pharynx. In the following phase, a blast of air is expelled through the mouth and nose as glottis and pharynx are suddenly reopened. Sneezing can also be elicited from sites other than the nose; even a bright light can trigger this reflex. Moreover, at variance with cough, it cannot be performed voluntarily (6).

Airflows at room temperature through the nose have an inhibitory effect on breathing in anesthetized rabbits and cats (7). Inhibition of ventilation due to the cooling effect of air through the nose has been demonstrated also in humans by McBride and Whitelaw (8) and Burgess and Whitelaw (9). The pharynx, and perhaps even the larynx, might also be involved in this response.

Moreover, cooling of the nasal cavity can induce bronchoconstriction in humans and experimental animals (1) and can inhibit the activity of the alae nasi muscle (10).

Cold receptors have indeed been found in the nasal cavity of cats (11) and rats (12) and are likely candidates for the reflex effects of nasal cooling.

The Pharynx

Reflex responses attributed to stimulation of the pharynx include: bronchodilation, hypertension, tachycardia, laryngeal abduction, and mucus secretion in the lower airway; the afferent and efferent pathways for these reflexes have not been clearly established (1).

Pharyngeal reflexes may also be important for the regulation of pharyngeal patency; topical anesthetization of the pharynx and glottis increases pharyngeal resistance in human subjects during sleep (13).

In newborns, instillation of water into the pharynx elicits apnea followed by bradycardia; in some cases also cough is present (14). However, the involvement of the larynx in these responses cannot be ruled out and seems indeed very probable.

One of the most important pharyngeal responses elicited by mechanical stimulation is the aspiration reflex (6). It consists of several rapid strong inspiratory efforts that, unlike sneezing and coughing, are not followed by expiratory efforts. Endings responsible for this reflex are in the epipharynx, and the corresponding fibers are in the glossopharyngeal nerve (1).

Swallowing is another reflex that can be elicited from the pharynx; its physiological importance is obvious. During swallowing, diaphragm and abductor laryngeal muscles are inhibited while the thyroarytenoid, the main adductor laryngeal muscle, is activated (15).

The Larynx

The larynx has multiple functions: It has a unique role in vocalization, plays a crucial part in airway defense and in the maintenance of upper-airway patency, and participates in the initial phases of deglutition.

The reflexogenic importance of the larynx is properly represented by the richness of its afferent supply: For example, in the superior laryngeal nerve of the cat there are about 2200 afferent myelinated fibers distributed over a few square centimeters (16), whereas the whole cervical vagus nerve, which innervates the considerably larger area of the tracheobronchial tree, as well as other thoracic and abdominal viscera, has only 3000 myelinated afferent fibers (17).

The superior laryngeal nerve provides the most important sensory supply to the larynx, whereas the recurrent laryngeal nerve has only a minor role (18).

Reflexes arising from the larynx are very powerful and can override opposite influences from other sources. For instance, electrical stimulation of the superior laryngeal nerve blocks the increase in ventilation caused by carotid chemoreceptor input (19).

Reflexes Arising from Respiratory-Related Events

During inspiration, the larynx is subjected to negative transmural pressure as air flows in the craniocaudal direction and abductor (posterior cricoarytenoid) muscles are active; during expiration, the reverse happens and the activity of adductor muscles predominates.

Recording from the peripheral cut end of the superior laryngeal nerve discloses a well-defined respiratory modulation that increases during inspiration. Single-fiber recordings have led to the description of three general types of respiratory-modulated receptors: one mainly or only affected by pressure (mostly negative pressure), another influenced by the action of the laryngeal muscles or by the tracheal pull, and a third one stimulated only by the decrease in laryngeal temperature due to airflow (20).

Negative pressure in the upper airway decreases respiratory frequency as a result of an increase in both inspiratory and expiratory times (21,22). Apnea is a rare occurrence in adult animals but is rather common in newborns (14,23).

Positive pressure seems to be a less important stimulus than negative pressure, and its effects are variable and generally opposite to those occurring with negative pressure (21).

Negative pressure increases the activity of the genioglossus, posterior cricoarytenoid, and alae nasi; all these muscles have a dilating action on the upper airway (Fig. 1). Positive pressure has opposite effects; in fact, it decreases the activity of the genioglossus muscle (24).

Stimulation of laryngeal afferents can also modify cardiovascular functions: Distortion of laryngeal structures, negative pressure, and stimulation of the central cut end of the superior laryngeal nerve cause arrhythmia or even cardiac arrest (24).

Airflow per se does not change the pattern of breathing in anesthetized adult animals, but it prolongs expiratory time and decreases tidal volume in newborn animals (23,25,26). These inhibitory influences on ventilation are entirely due to the cooling effect of airflow and are abolished by laryngeal denervation.

A decrease in laryngeal temperature of about 10°C reduces the increase in posterior cricoarytenoid muscle activity that occurs during upper-airway occlusion

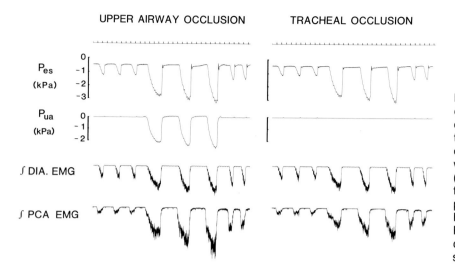

FIG. 1. Effect of upper-airway and tracheal occlusions on the activity of the diaphragm and the posterior cricoarytenoid muscle. Traces are: time, in seconds; esophageal (P_{es}) and upper-airway (P_{ua}) pressures, in kiloPascals (kPa); integrated electromyographic activity of the diaphragm (∫DIA. EMG); and posterior cricoarytenoid muscle (∫PCA EMG). Note the greater activation of the PCA during upper-airway occlusions as compared to during tracheal occlusions. (Modified from ref. 22.)

(27), suggesting that laryngeal cooling increases upper-airway resistance.

The bronchoconstrictive effect of cold air and the contribution of the larynx to this response are controversial. Boushey et al. (28) did not find in cats any effect of laryngeal cooling on bronchomotor tone, whereas Jammes et al. (29) found in the same species at laryngeal temperatures below 15°C a marked increase in lower-airway resistance. Cold-induced bronchospasm does not usually occur in healthy humans; nevertheless, the possibility exists of a role of the larynx in eliciting the bronchoconstriction seen in asthmatic subjects during cold air breathing (30,31).

Laryngeal receptors specifically stimulated by cooling have been described (32). They are stimulated during inspiration as long as the inspiratory airflow decreases laryngeal temperature.

Stimulation of cold receptors and/or inhibition of laryngeal mechanoreceptors as a result of cooling (24) could account for the responses described above. L-Menthol, a specific stimulant of laryngeal cold receptors without effect on laryngeal mechanoreceptors (33), has strong inhibitory influences on breathing in animals showing similar responses to upper-airway cooling. These observations suggest that stimulation of cold receptors is the main factor in the apneic response seen with laryngeal cooling in newborn animals (*unpublished observations*).

Effects of Mechanical and Chemical Irritation

Mechanical irritation of the laryngeal mucosa induces slowing and deepening of breathing, cough, laryngeal adduction, bronchoconstriction, and, less often, apnea and bradycardia (1,28,34). In unanesthetized dogs (34), apnea and bradycardia are absent when laryngeal stimulation is performed during wakefulness but occur during sleep.

Reflexes similar to those induced by mechanical irritation follow laryngeal insufflation of chemical irritants such as ammonia, phenyldiguanide, and veratridine (2,28), though cough is not as frequent as with mechanical stimulation (28). There are marked species differences in the response to irritants; in fact, capsaicin induces apnea and an increase in arterial systemic blood pressure in rats but not in dogs (35).

The purpose of these reflexes seems obvious for some (i.e., slowing of breathing, cough, and laryngeal closure) but not for others (i.e., bronchoconstriction).

In anesthetized dogs, two puffs of cigarette smoke in the larynx induce a consistent, but relatively mild, bradypnea that lasts only as long as the stimulus is applied (36). Other studies with cigarette smoke in the upper airway (see above) show vigorous responses [i.e., apnea, bradycardia, and peripheral vasoconstriction (19,28,37)]; these differences might be accounted for by a more prolonged exposure to the stimulus or by involvement of other regions of the upper airway, possibly the nose.

Distilled water is also a powerful laryngeal irritant: It causes hypoventilation, sometimes apnea (especially in newborn animals), bradycardia (19,38,39), swallowing (39), cough (40), and peripheral vasoconstriction (19). As for mechanical stimulation of the larynx, instillation of water in the adult dog elicits cough during wakefulness but elicits apnea and bradycardia during sleep (34) (Fig. 2). Sleeping and anesthetized animals therefore seem to behave similarly. Moreover, newborns are more vulnerable than adults to this type of stimuli (41). Recently, a water reflex has been demonstrated also in preterm infants (42). The effective stimulus for the laryngeal water-induced reflexes is the lack of, or reduction in, concentration of chloride ions (or other small permeant anions) in the test solutions. Receptors specifically activated by the same stimulus have indeed been identified (39).

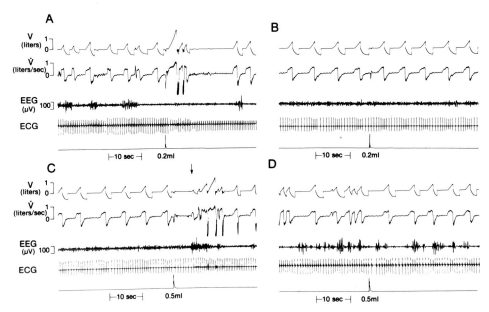

FIG. 2. Responses to laryngeal injection of water in the isolated larynx of a dog breathing spontaneously through a tracheostomy. Traces are: inspiratory volume (V; above 0 line), airflow ($\dot{V}$; inspiration upwards), electroencephalogram (EEG), electrocardiogram (ECG), and stimulus marker. During wakefulness **(A)**, 0.2 ml of water causes an immediate expiration followed by cough; apnea and bradycardia occur only as a secondary response to cough. The same type of stimulus during slow-wave sleep **(B)** causes only a brief expiration. During slow-wave sleep **(C)** a larger stimulus (0.5 ml of water) causes arousal followed by cough, whereas during rapid eye movement sleep **(D)** it causes only transient bradycardia. (From ref. 34.)

Hypercapnic, but not hypoxic, mixtures reduce respiratory frequency with no effects on cardiovascular functions (43). When the CO_2 concentration is raised above 5%, also tidal volume is decreased (43,44).

Switching from Nasal to Oral Breathing

Normal subjects at rest breathe through the nose; when higher levels of ventilation are attained, as in exercise, breathing is diverted to the oral passage, which offers a lower flow resistance. The switching from nasal to oral breathing is accomplished by raising the soft palate. Breathing is actually switched from an exclusive nasal route to an oronasal route: The relative amount of air flowing through each of the two is regulated by the relative resistance of the two passages arranged in parallel; this airflow is dependent on the position of the tongue and the soft palate (Fig. 3).

Direct measurements in humans (45) have determined that the transition from nasal to oronasal breathing during an exercise of moderate intensity (916 kgm/min) occurs at an average ventilation of 35.4 liters/min. On passing to oronasal breathing, while maintaining a constant intensity of exercise, ventilation increases to 44.1 liters/min. The same investigators have estimated that there is a decrease in alveolar P_{CO_2} of 2.8 mmHg

when switching from nasal to oronasal breathing during exercise. Therefore, during nasal breathing there is a significant degree of alveolar hypoventilation.

Multiple factors have been suggested as determinants of the nasal-to-oronasal switching: (a) threshold stimulation of nasal pressure or flow receptors and (b) activation of respiratory muscle proprioceptors due to the inspiratory loading that intervenes with nasal breathing.

In infants the larynx has a more cranial position than in adults, and the epiglottis is much closer to the soft palate; therefore the oral cavity has a better separation from the rest of the upper airway. Infants are often said to be "obligatory" nose breathers, but this qualification should not be taken very strictly (46). For sure they are, to a greater extent than adults, preferential nose breathers. It is interesting to note that newborns, unlike adults, have a lower resistance across the nasal passage than across the oral passage (47), which makes nose breathing energetically advantageous. The greater difficulty of newborns to switch to oral breathing cannot be attributed to mechanical factors, since normalized oral resistance is similar to that of adults. Neural mechanisms have been suggested for the difficulty of the newborn to breathe through the mouth (47).

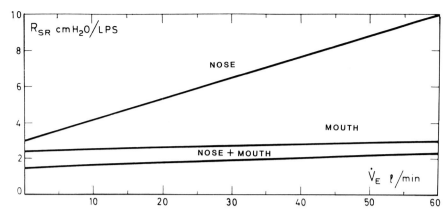

FIG. 3. Relationship between flow resistance of the respiratory system (R_{SR}, in cmH$_2$O· liter^{-1}·sec) and minute ventilation ($\dot{V}_e$, in liter·min^{-1}) when breathing through the nose, the mouth, and both nose and mouth. (Modified from ref. 45.)

REFLEX INFLUENCES FROM THE TRACHEOBRONCHIAL TREE AND THE LUNGS

Afferent Activity from the Tracheobronchial Tree and the Lungs

There is an afferent activity with a clear and fixed temporal relationship to respiratory movements, and there is also an afferent activity that does not show a clear respiratory modulation. The former activity is carried by myelinated fibers (at least in adult animals), mostly within the vagus nerves, whereas the latter activity is carried by nonmyelinated vagal fibers (48).

The activity showing a respiratory modulation originates from two different types of receptor. The slowly adapting receptors (SARs) exhibit a steady rate of discharge with regular interspike intervals during maintained lung inflation at constant transpulmonary pressure. The rapidly adapting receptors (RARs) show, in the same condition, a rapidly fading activity with irregular interspike intervals. During the respiratory cycle, SARs change their firing rate in a regular fashion, whereas RARs have an irregular bursting activity, with interspike intervals randomly distributed. SARs are about 10 times more numerous than RARs; the conduction velocity of their respective fibers has approximately the same value, consistent with their myelinated nature. Both types of receptor are found in extra- and intrapulmonary airways, with a higher concentration in the larger ones. SARs are located within the tracheobronchial smooth muscles, and RARs are located within the more superficial mucosal layers (48).

Our knowledge of the afferent sympathetic supply to the respiratory structure is still very fragmentary. Action potentials evoked by lung manipulation have been recorded from nerves associated with the stellate ganglion (49). Recently, a respiratory modulated activity has been found in the myelinated fibers of the higher thoracic white rami communicantes of dogs (50).

Another category of vagal endings associated with the lung parenchyma and the airways has an activity without a distinct respiratory modulation carried by nonmyelinated fibers that constitute the majority of the vagal afferents. The properties of these receptors are generally studied by administering extraneous substances such as capsaicin and phenyldiguanide (51). On the basis of their circulatory accessibility, two groups of C-fiber receptors are distinguished: (i) "pulmonary," stimulated with shorter latencies after injection of excitatory substances into the pulmonary circulation, and (ii) "bronchial," reached with shorter delays following administration into the systemic circulation. Another difference between the two groups is the greater mechanosensitivity of the "pulmonary" endings. These latter receptors correspond to the J-receptors described by Paintal (52).

Vagal Influences on the Breathing Pattern

The administration of aerosols of topical anesthetics (lidocaine, bupivacaine, etc.) exerts a blocking action unequivocally limited to the afferents of the respiratory structures. In humans, either awake or anesthetized, local anesthesia of the airways does not change the pattern of breathing, even when the Hering–Breuer inflation reflex is abolished or greatly reduced (53). On the contrary, in anesthetized dogs (53) and rabbits (54) the pattern of breathing changes markedly: Tidal volume and inspiratory duration increase, whereas the expiratory duration is unaffected. In anesthetized animals, vagotomy introduces further increases in tidal volume and in cycle duration. In both humans and experimental animals, cough in response to chemical and mechanical irritation can be blocked more easily and consistently than can the Hering–Breuer inflation apnea. These results seem to imply that in humans, unlike in experimental animals, no influences related to airway distension or motion are at work in the regulation of breathing, at least at rest.

Similar observations on the pattern of breathing at rest have been made after direct blockade of the vagus nerves. In conscious humans, no changes have been detected with block of this nerve at its entrance into the skull, or, in anesthetized subjects, with block in its cervical tract (55,56). In conscious animals (57–59), blocking of the cervical vagus nerve causes an increase in tidal volume and in the duration of both inspiration and expiration. These results, essentially similar to those with aerosol anesthesia, suggest that the effects of vagotomy or vagal block are mostly contributed by airway endings. They also suggest that this afferent activity is not effective in humans during quiet breathing. Nevertheless, activity from airway SARs has been identified in humans breathing at eupneic levels, both by the "collision" technique (60) and by direct recording from vagal filaments (61).

Even if vagal block and airway anesthesia do not modify breathing during eupnea, they do compromise respiratory function as indicated by the lack of important defensive mechanisms such as cough. Furthermore, different studies have disclosed that airway anesthesia enhances the ventilatory response to hypercapnia in humans (53,62), but not ventilatory response to hypoxia (63). The observation that the ventilatory response to hypercapnia is similarly enhanced after SO_2 block of SARs (64) would suggest the involvement of airway stretch receptors in the ventilatory response to hypercapnia.

In anesthetized animals the duration of the respiratory cycle and tidal volume appear to be regulated by two mechanisms (65): (i) the volume feedback from the lung related to SAR activity and (ii) bulbopontine mechanisms. A volume threshold, corresponding to a given SAR activity, must be reached for switching-off inspiration. Moreover, the volume threshold decreases with time from the beginning of inspiration; that is, larger volumes are required to switch-off inspirations of shorter durations. In the absence of volume feedback, the duration of inspiration is regulated only by bulbopontine mechanisms. The duration of expiration would be dependent on the duration of the preceding inspiration. The existence of this inverse relationship between cycle duration and tidal volume allows for an increase in both rate and depth of respiration as the drive to breathe increases. Without vagal afferents,

ventilation could increase only through changes in tidal volume.

This model, however, does not satisfy all the experimental results. A V_T–T_I relationship could not be verified either in conscious animals (66–68) or in awake or anesthetized humans (67). This relationship could not be established even when vagotomy produced a decrease in respiratory rate and an increase in tidal volume (67). It was therefore concluded that "the dependence of T_I on V_T is not sufficient to account for the role of the Hering–Breuer reflex in the regulation of breathing pattern" (67).

An increase of lung volume above functional residual capacity diminishes ventilatory activity in anesthetized animals and humans by prolonging expiration (69) and also by shortening inspiration (70). This vagal reflex aggravates the mechanical disadvantage introduced by the shift toward an inspiratory position and the consequent shortening of inspiratory muscles. However, in conscious humans the situation is reversed: Inspiratory activity is stimulated (71), maintaining a normal level of CO_2. The diaphragm remains active in conscious human subjects breathing at positive pressure, even when inspiration could be completely passive according to the volume–pressure diagram of the relaxed respiratory system. These findings indicate, once more, that the vagal influences, known as Hering–Breuer inflation reflex, are not operational, at least in isolation, in the conscious subject. In humans, lung volume increases whenever they stand up; therefore, an active inflation reflex would work against their respiratory function. Humans, at variance with other species, seem therefore particularly well equipped for defending their ventilation during postural changes.

Another feature of vagal influences on breathing is that all the inspiratory muscles are uniformly affected. The maintenance of such a coordinated action should contribute to a displacement of the chest wall along its passive configuration. In the absence of vagal influences, the respiratory muscles acting on the chest wall can be differentially activated. In fact, resistive loads applied after sectioning the vagus nerves increase the activity of inspiratory intercostal motor units while that of the diaphragm is inhibited (72,73).

Vagal influences also affect expiratory muscles (74,75). In anesthetized animals, vagal reflexes activate the abdominal muscles when lung volume is increased either by positive-pressure breathing or by posture (75). The endings responsible for these reflexes have been identified with SARs. These vagal influences represent a mechanism for keeping rather constant the end-expiratory volume during postural changes. Observations consistent with this view have also been obtained in human subjects (76). In fact, whereas abdominal muscle activity was absent in su-

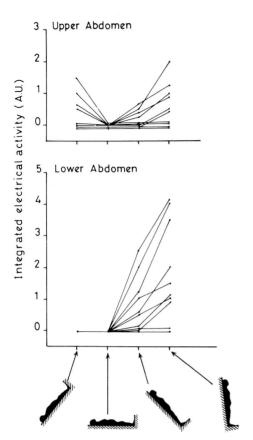

FIG. 4. Changes in tonic electrical activity in the upper and lower portions of the external oblique in 10 normal naive subjects in supine, 45° head-up, standing, and 45° head-down positions. The integrated activity is expressed in arbitrary units (A.U.). (From ref. 76.)

pine individuals, it was present in most of them when standing. This activity prevails in the dependent regions of the abdomen, where the hydrostatic pressure is greater; this increased hydrostatic pressure suggests the participation of proprioceptive muscle reflexes, expected to be stronger in the regions subjected to a greater stretch (Fig. 4).

Vagal afferents, besides exerting inhibitory influences on respiration, promote facilitatory effects. In fact, they are capable of initiating inspiration (77), prolonging inspiration, and increasing tidal volume (78), as well as augmenting the rate at which the inspiratory activity is increased (79).

Inspiratory-initiating reflex responses have been demonstrated in rabbits artificially ventilated and exposed to SO_2 inhalation to block the Hering–Breuer inflation reflex. Under control conditions (i.e., previous to SO_2 exposure), the inspiratory discharge of the phrenic nerve occurred invariably during the ventilator expiratory pause; after SO_2 block, however, the inspiratory burst could be triggered by the ventilator. This "locking" effect between ventilator and phrenic

nerve was attributed to a reflex originating from RARs (77).

RARs are generally thought to be responsible for the augmented breaths that occur spontaneously with an irregular periodicity in many species. Both chemical and mechanical factors play a role in the elicitation of augmented breaths. This has been demonstrated by the elegant experiments of Glogowska et al. (78). These investigators found that an augmented breath could be triggered by injecting potassium cyanide (KCN) into the carotid artery only when the injections were administered at sufficient intervals after a spontaneously occurring augmented breath. The investigators reasoned that the increase in lung compliance caused by the augmented breath removed a mechanical stimulus that constituted an essential factor for triggering a sigh. In fact, they saw that in artificially ventilated animals (in which the deeper breaths, as seen through the phrenic bursts, could not affect lung compliance), KCN injections could always induce a "neural" augmented breath.

Facilitatory vagal influences have been found to be active during normal tidal breaths (79). For example, it was shown that the rate of increase of the electrical activity of inspiratory nerves is greater during unoccluded breaths than during occluded efforts. This facilitation has a greater influence on the intercostal muscles than on the diaphragm; in fact it was suggested that "the functional significance of this reflex may be to serve in the regulation of the relative contribution of the different respiratory muscles to different-size tidal volume" (80).

Coleridge and Coleridge (51,81) have described the presence of C-fiber receptors in the tracheobronchial airways. The activity of these receptors is sparse and irregular during both spontaneous and artificial respiration. They seem to have a prevalent chemosensitive function and are activated by many substances produced, released, and catabolized within the lung (histamine, bradykinin, and some of the prostaglandins of the F and E series). Injection of bradykinin into bronchial arteries causes bronchoconstriction, bradycardia, and hypotension together with apnea followed by rapid and shallow breathing. Even more interest has been dedicated in the last several years to the pulmonary C-fiber receptors and their reflex effects. These endings, on the basis of their circulatory accessibility, have been presumed to be located between alveolar walls and pulmonary capillaries (juxtapulmonary capillary receptors). In general, pulmonary C-fiber receptors show a greater response to mechanical events than do bronchial C-fiber receptors. Moreover, during spontaneous breathing, pulmonary C-fiber receptors have some rhythmic activity that virtually disappears with artificial ventilation with the chest open. Of great interest are the observations that many stimuli affecting the pulmonary circulation (such as pulmonary congestion, edema, and microembolism, all of which have clinical relevance) excite these endings. Moreover, they have been implicated in the mechanisms that limit the intensity of exercise (J-reflex). The reflex responses attributed to these receptors have been mostly established by administering substances such as phenyldiguanide and capsaicin into the right heart. Reflex responses elicited by these challenges include apnea, followed by rapid and shallow breathing, laryngeal constriction, and bronchoconstriction. Pulmonary C-fiber endings are stimulated by prostaglandins, especially those of the E series, but remain virtually unaffected by histamine, serotonin, or bradykinin (51).

Bronchopulmonary C-fibers have been alleged to be sensitive to CO_2 and have been considered as possible sensors of CO_2 in mixed venous blood and thus implicated in exercise hyperpnea. However, a study by Coleridge and Coleridge (82) revealed only a very small increase in both bronchial and pulmonary C-fiber receptors when end-tidal CO_2 of a vascularly isolated lung was raised from 19 to 30 mmHg. CO_2 either inhaled or added to the mixed venous blood evokes a vagally mediated hyperpnea. Recent data (83) seem to support a role of C-fiber receptors in this response. In fact, evidence in favor of a CO_2/H^+ sensitivity of pulmonary C-fiber receptors has been provided by experiments in which lactic acid and acetic acid administered into the right atrium caused a vagally mediated tachypnea. However, this remains a very controversial issue that undoubtedly will stimulate and necessitate further investigation.

Pisarri et al. (84) have recently presented evidence that supports a role of C-fiber receptors in shortening the duration of expiration (i.e., an excitatory input to the control of breathing rate that opposes the inhibitory input from SARs).

Persistent inspiratory muscle activity has been recorded in the earlier portion of expiration in both anesthetized and unanesthetized animals and humans (85–87). This inspiratory activity provides a mechanism whereby the passive return of the respiratory system toward its resting position is opposed and retarded, effectively prolonging expiratory duration. The combined action of this postinspiratory activation of inspiratory muscles and the neurally regulated laryngeal resistance provides a controlled braking of expiratory flow through a change in the effective elastance and resistance of the respiratory system. When ventilation increases, the postinspiratory activity of the inspiratory muscles decreases, allowing a faster expiration. The regulation of this braking mechanism depends on vagal feedback from respiratory structures (88).

Experimental data suggest a different role of extrapulmonary and intrapulmonary vagal reflexes. Whereas distension of extrapulmonary airways (trachea and main-stem bronchi) leads only to transitory changes in breathing pattern, inflation of the lung introduces long-lasting alterations of the breathing pattern (89,90). Agostoni et al. (91) have obtained evidence that supports an altogether different role of bronchial and tracheal stretch receptors. The input from the former would activate the inspiratory "off-switch" mechanism that terminates inspiration, whereas input from the latter would delay its activation. Moreover, bronchial input inhibits the postinspiratory discharge of the diaphragm, whereas tracheal input promotes it. These results could be interpreted as being dependent on different central connections of the afferents from the two regions.

A more general consideration on the role of vagal afferents can be based on the observation that the work of breathing increases when the vagus nerves are blocked (92). This could depend, in part, on changes in the breathing pattern and, in part, on the lack of a proper adjustment between airway resistance and dead space normally attained through the regulation of tracheobronchial smooth muscles (93).

Sympathetic Afferents

Sympathetic afferents having either excitatory or inhibitory influences on respiration have been described. Banister et al. (94) reported that, in dogs, phosgene or ammonia inhaled through a tracheostomy elicited apnea followed by rapid and shallow breathing when the vagi were intact, whereas it elicited a marked tachypnea with only a modest increase in tidal volume after cervical vagotomy. This response disappeared after removal of the stellate ganglia. On the other hand, Kostreva et al. (95) found that electrical stimulation of sympathetic afferents inhibits phrenic and intercostal activity.

In summary, the functional role of sympathetic afferents is not yet clear, but some of the experimental data suggest that it is only of secondary importance. Shannon (96) found that dorsal rhyzotomy of the first thoracic roots, which contain sympathetic afferents, does not modify the pattern of breathing.

SOMATIC REFLEXES

Reflexes from Intercostal Afferents

We distinguish three types of reflex originating from intercostal muscle receptors: (i) segmental reflexes that involve motor effects limited to the same intercostal segment of the afferent input activating the reflex; (ii) intersegmental intercostal reflexes that involve spinal respiratory motoneurons located in segments other than the one of the afferent input; and (iii) supraspinal intercostal reflexes in which supraspinal motoneurons (e.g., laryngeal or hypoglossal), medullary respiratory neurons, or projection to the cerebellum, pons, or higher structures is involved (97).

Segmental Reflexes

Experiments based on selective electrical stimulation of different intercostal muscle afferents have shown that those originating from primary (group I) and secondary (II) muscle spindle endings are monosynaptically connected to the alpha motoneurons of the same segment and lead to the depolarization of these motoneurons (98,99). Group I afferents are additionally connected to contralateral alpha motoneurons of the same and nearby spinal levels. Intercostal muscle spindle afferents have been found to impinge only on the same functional type of motoneurons; that is, inspiratory motoneurons are depolarized only by afferents from inspiratory intercostals. A characteristic feature of the intercostals is that their muscle spindles do not inhibit the antagonist intercostals. This arrangement provides the intercostal muscles with a mechanism of segmental autogenic facilitation that regulates the muscle contraction to obtain the "desired" change in length (i.e., volume in the case of the respiratory system). The demand for a given length change is transmitted to the muscle spindle through the activation of gamma motoneurons that results in a given change of length of the fusimotor fiber. Because of a synchronous activation of the alpha and gamma motoneurons, change in a mechanical load (e.g., increase in respiratory resistance) to the contracting muscle leads to compensatory adjustments in the activity of alpha motoneurons. In short, the system operates as a load compensator.

Intercostal muscles do have Golgi tendon organs which (similarly to other skeletal muscles), when activated, produce an autogenic inhibition on their respective homonymous alpha motoneurons of the same segment.

Intersegmental Reflexes

Well documented are the facilitatory influences that originate from internal and external intercostal muscle receptors of the lower thoracic segments (T9–T13) and impinge upon phrenic motoneurons (100–102). The reflex can be elicited by deformation of the lower rib cage (as during a strong diaphragmatic contraction); furthermore, this reflex can be considered as a load-compensating response from the diaphragm, which lacks its own autogenic facilitation (*vide infra*).

Supraspinal Reflexes

The observations that intercostal muscle afferents can influence cranial motoneurons and modify respiratory rhythmicity are a clear indication that they project to supraspinal centers. Group I and II afferents from the external intercostals of the 4th–8th thoracic segments and the abdominal muscles inhibit laryngeal abductor motoneurons (posterior cricoarytenoid) and both inspiratory and expiratory neurons of the medulla. The overall effect of these influences is that of shortening inspiration and prolonging expiration (103–107).

Reflexes from Diaphragmatic Receptors

The preponderance of Golgi tendon organs seems to be a characteristic of the diaphragmatic afferent innervation (108). In keeping with this feature, autogenic inhibition appears to be the dominant segmental reflex influence, whereas segmental facilitatory reflexes have not been found (72,108). Intersegmental and supraspinal reflexes originating from diaphragmatic afferents have yet to be demonstrated.

As mentioned above, an increase in lung volume, obtained by positive-pressure breathing, by subatmospheric pressure applied around the chest wall, or by changing posture from horizontal to upright, enhances inspiratory activity in conscious individuals (71) (Fig. 5). Similar effects have been verified in patients with a spinal transection at the lower cervical levels (109). In these cases only cranial (vagal) and cervical (phrenic) afferents can be implicated as possible sources of a reflex response. It must be noted that this response occurs in a direction opposite to that expected from known vagal (Hering–Breuer inflation inhibition) and myotatic (lung inflation should shorten inspiratory muscle fibers) reflex influences. Its almost immediate onset is not compatible with chemoreceptor influences. The observation that the inspiratory aug-

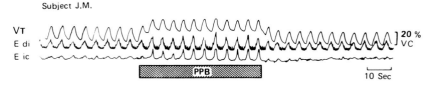

FIG. 5. Effect of positive-pressure breathing (PPB) on tidal volume (V_T), diaphragm (E_{DI}), and intercostal (E_{IC}) activity. (From ref. 123.)

mentation occurs without any change in breathing rate would suggest a major role for diaphragmatic segmental reflexes. Fryman and Frazier (110) found that cats, vagotomized and with a transection at the lower cervical spinal levels, responded with a longer diaphragmatic discharge to the application of lower-body negative pressure. This response could be abolished by cervical dorsal rhizotomy.

The diaphragm is made up by two distinct portions: costal and crural (111). Both portions contribute to lung expansion; however, the costal diaphragm expands the lower rib cage, whereas the crural diaphragm does not. Considering the different segmental levels of the motor and sensory innervation of these two regions of the diaphragm and their functional independence in some nonrespiratory acts (swallowing, vomiting, defecation), it seems reasonable to see the possibility of some change in their respective activities in the course of respiration that could modify chest-wall configuration.

Costovertebral Joint Afferents

Rib movements, which do not involve intercostal muscles, inhibit inspiration and prolong expiration (112). These reflex responses originate from costovertebral joint afferents that project to brainstem respiratory neurons.

General Considerations

Although all the above-described reflex influences from the chest wall have been unequivocally documented, their overall functional role in the regulation of breathing does not seem to be of major importance. Actually, experiments on animals, both anesthetized and decerebrated, in which various respiratory parameters were examined before and after thoracic and/or cervical dorsal rhizotomy, have revealed only minor changes, if any, in breathing pattern and gas exchange (96,113).

The extensive morphological and functional results obtained by Duron (114,115) support the view that both external and internal intercostal muscles primarily function as postural muscles (at least in quiet breathing), and their extensive proprioceptive innervation would thus reflect this function. Only the diaphragm and the interchondral portion of the intercostals function as truly respiratory muscles, being active also during quiet breathing; however, their proprioceptive innervation is far less than that of the external and the internal intercostals. These observations and conclusions are entirely consistent with the results of dorsal rhizotomy.

CHANGES IN VENTILATION ELICITED FROM LIMB MUSCLES AND JOINTS

Both passive and active movements of the limbs cause an increase in ventilation. Joint receptors (116) and muscle proprioceptors (117,118) have been implicated as the afferents responsible for these responses thought to constitute an important factor in the hyperpnea of exercise. The increase in ventilation has been found to be largely independent of vagal influences both with induced limb movements in anesthetized animals (119) and with actual exercise in awake animals (57). According to an analysis by Agostoni and D'Angelo (119), passive and active limb movements increase ventilation and modify the pattern of breathing by displacing the V_T–T_I relationship to the left (off-switch threshold reduced at any given inspiratory duration), lowering the T_E–T_I relationship with T_E being shortened more than T_I and increasing the inspiratory "drive" (V_T/T_I). Similar results were found after vagotomy. All these results, in the absence of any blood-gas change, could be attributed to purely neurogenic stimuli. The time course of the alterations in timing and pattern of breathing at the onset and termination of the exercise indicated the presence of both a slow and a fast component of the neurogenic drive. The slow component could be attributed to the activation of reverberating neural circuits activated by stimuli originating from the limbs.

Electrical stimulation of muscle and cutaneous nerves could, in some experiments on anesthetized cats (120), induce a synchronous activation of the diaphragmatic discharge. These results indicate the presence of peripheral inputs possibly responsible for locking respiratory frequency in response to stepping or pedaling rate in exercising humans and animals (121). It must, however, be recognized that such a relationship has not been unequivocally established (122).

ACKNOWLEDGMENT

The work of G. and F. B. Sant'Ambrogio is supported by NIH grant HL-20122.

REFERENCES

1. Widdicombe JG. Reflexes from the upper respiratory tract. In: Cherniack NS, Widdicombe JG, eds. *Handbook of physiology, Section 3: The respiratory system, vol II—Control of breathing, Part 1.* Bethesda, MD: American Physiological Society, 1986;363–394.
2. Szereda-Przestaszewska M, Widdicombe JG. Reflex effects of chemical irritation of the upper airways on the laryngeal lumen in cats. *Respir Physiol* 1973;18:107–115.
3. Wealthall SR. Factors resulting in a failure to interrupt apnea. In: Bosma JF, Showacre J, eds. *Development of upper respiratory anatomy and function. Implications for sudden infant*

death syndrome. Washington, DC: U.S. Government Printing Office, 1975;212–225.

4. Mathew OP, Abu-Osba YK, Thach BT. Influence of upper airway pressure changes on genioglossus muscle respiratory activity. *J Appl Physiol* 1982;52:438–444.

5. Hwang J-C, St. John WM, Bartlett D Jr. Afferent pathways for hypoglossal and phrenic responses to changes in upper airway pressure. *Respir Physiol* 1984;55:341–354.

6. Korpas J, Tomori Z. *Cough and other respiratory reflexes*. Basel: Karger, 1979.

7. Garcia Ramos J. On the integration of respiratory movements. III. The fifth nerve afferents. *Acta Physiol Latinoam* 1960;10:104–113.

8. McBride B, Whitelaw WA. A physiological stimulus to upper airway receptors in humans. *J Appl Physiol* 1981;51:1189–1197.

9. Burgess KR, Whitelaw WA. Reducing ventilatory response to carbon dioxide by breathing cold air. *Am Rev Respir Dis* 1984;129:687–690.

10. Eccles R, Tolley NS. The effect of a nasal airflow stimulus upon human alae nasi e.m.g. activity. *J Physiol* 1987;394:78P.

11. Glebovsky VD, Bayev AV. Depressing effect of carbon dioxide on excitation of nasal cavity cold receptors in cats. *Sechenov Physiol J USSR* 1986;72:595–605.

12. Tsubone H. Nasal 'flow' receptors of the rat. *Respir Physiol* 1989;75:51–64.

13. DeWeese EL, Sullivan TY. Effects of upper airway anesthesia on pharyngeal patency during sleep. *J Appl Physiol* 1988; 64:1346–1353.

14. Davies AM, Koenig JS, Thach BT. Characteristics of upper airway chemoreflex prolonged apnea in human infants. *Am Rev Respir Dis* 1989;139:668–673.

15. Miller AJ. Deglutition. *Physiol Rev* 1982;62:129–184.

16. DuBois FS, Foley JO. Experimental studies on the vagus and spinal accessory nerves in the cat. *Anat Rec* 1936;64:285–307.

17. Agostoni A, Chinnock JE, de Burg Daly M, Murray JG. Functional and histological studies of the vagus nerve and its branches to the heart, lungs and abdominal viscera in the cat. *J Physiol* 1957;135:182–205.

18. Wyke BD, Kirchner JA. Neurology of the larynx. In: Hinchcliffe R, Harrison D, eds. *Scientific foundations of otolaryngology*. William Heinemann Medical Books, 1976;546–574.

19. Angell-James JE, Daly M de B. Some aspects of upper respiratory tract reflexes. *Acta Otolaryngol* 1975;79:242–252.

20. Sant'Ambrogio G, Mathew OP, Fisher JT, Sant'Ambrogio FB. Laryngeal receptors responding to transmural pressure, airflow and local muscle activity. *Respir Physiol* 1983;54:317–330.

21. Mathew OP, Abu-Osba YK, Thach BT. Influence of upper airway pressure changes on respiratory frequency. *Respir Physiol* 1982;49:223–233.

22. Sant'Ambrogio FB, Mathew OP, Clark WD, Sant'Ambrogio G. Laryngeal influences on breathing pattern and posterior cricoarytenoid muscle activity. *J Appl Physiol* 1985;58:1298–1304.

23. Fisher JT, Mathew OP, Sant'Ambrogio FB, Sant'Ambrogio G. Reflex effects and receptor responses to upper airway pressure and flow stimuli in developing puppies. *J Appl Physiol* 1985;58:258–264.

24. Mathew OP, Sant'Ambrogio FB. Laryngeal reflexes. In: Mathew OP, Sant'Ambrogio G, eds. *Respiratory function of the upper airway*. New York: Marcel Dekker, 1988;259–302.

25. Al-Shway SF, Mortola JP. Respiratory effects of airflow through the upper airways in newborn kittens and puppies. *J Apply Physiol* 1982;53:805–814.

26. Mathew OP, Anderson JW, Sant'Ambrogio FB, Sant'Ambrogio G. Laryngeal cooling and breathing pattern in newborn puppies. *Physiologist* 1989;32:228.

27. Mathew OP, Sant'Ambrogio FB, Sant'Ambrogio G. Effects of cooling on laryngeal reflexes in the dog. *Respir Physiol* 1986;66:61–70.

28. Boushey HA, Richardson PS, Widdicombe JG. Reflex effects of laryngeal irritation on the pattern of breathing and total lung resistance. *J Physiol (Lond)* 1972;224:501–513.

29. Jammes Y, Barthelemy P, Delpierre S. Respiratory effects of cold air breathing in anesthetized cats. *Respir Physiol* 1983; 54:41–54.

30. Deal EC Jr, McFadden ER Jr, Ingram RH Jr, Breslin FJ, Jaeger JJ. Airway responsiveness to cold air and hyperpnea in normal subjects and in those with hay fever and asthma. *Am Rev Respir Dis* 1980;121:621–628.

31. Tal A, Pasterkamp H, Serrette C, Leahy F, Chernick V. Response to cold air hyperventilation in normal and in asthmatic children. *J Pediatr* 1984;104:516–521.

32. Sant'Ambrogio G, Mathew OP, Sant'Ambrogio FB, Fisher JT. Laryngeal cold receptors. *Respir Physiol* 1985;59:35–44.

33. Sant'Ambrogio FB, Anderson JW, Sant'Ambrogio G. Effect of L-menthol on laryngeal cold receptors. *Physiologist* 1989;32:167.

34. Sullivan CE, Murphy E, Kozar LF, Phillipson EA. Waking and respiratory responses to laryngeal stimulation in sleeping dogs. *J Appl Physiol* 1978;45:681–689.

35. Palecek F, Mathew OP, Sant'Ambrogio FB, Sant'Ambrogio G. Cardiorespiratory responses to inhaled irritants. *Inhal Toxicol* 1989;in press.

36. Lee LY, Morton RF. Reflex bradypnea elicited by cigarette smoke inhaled through an isolated larynx. *Respir Physiol* 1988;73:301–310.

37. Angell-James JE, Daly M de B. Nasal reflexes. *Proc R Soc Med* 1969;62:1287–1293.

38. Johnson P, Salisbury DM, Storey AT. Apnea induced by stimulation of sensory receptors in the larynx. In: Bosma JF, Showacre J, eds. *Development of upper respiratory anatomy and function*. Washington, DC: U.S. Government Printing Office, 1975;160–178.

39. Boggs DF, Bartlett D Jr. Chemical specificity of a laryngeal apneic reflex in puppies. *J Appl Physiol* 1982;53:455–462.

40. Storey AT. Laryngeal initiation of swallowing. *Exp Neurol* 1968;20:359–365.

41. Harding R. Function of the larynx in the fetus and newborn. *Annu Rev Physiol* 1984;46:645–659.

42. Davies AM, Koenig JS, Thach BT. Upper airway chemoreflex responses to saline and water in preterm infants. *J Appl Physiol* 1988;64:1412–1420.

43. Boushey HA, Richardson PS. The reflex effects of intralaryngeal carbon dioxide on the pattern of breathing. *J Physiol (Lond)* 1973;228:181–191.

44. Lee L-Y, Morton RF, McIntosh MJ, Turbek JA. An isolated upper airway preparation in conscious dogs. *J Appl Physiol* 1986;60:2123–2127.

45. Saibene F, Mognoni P, Rotondo G. Respirazione per via nasale od orale nella iperventilazione da lavoro. *Riv Med Aeronaut Spaz* 1969;32:329–339.

46. Rodenstein DO, Perlmutter N, Stanescu DC. Infants are not obligatory nose breathers. *Am Rev Respir Dis* 1985;131:343–347.

47. Mortola JP, Fisher JT. Mouth and nose resistance in newborn kittens and puppies. *J Appl Physiol* 1981;51:641–645.

48. Sant'Ambrogio G. Information arising from the tracheobronchial tree of mammals. *Physiol Rev* 1982;62:531–569.

49. Holmes R, Torrance RW. Afferent fibers of the stellate ganglion. *Q J Exp Physiol* 1959;44:271–281.

50. Kostreva DR, Zuperku EJ, Hess GL, Coon RL, Kampine JP. Pulmonary afferent activity recorded from sympathetic nerves. *J Appl Physiol* 1975;39:37–40.

51. Coleridge JCG, Coleridge HM. Afferent vagal C-fibre innervation of the lungs and airways and its functional significance. *Rev Physiol Biochem Pharmacol* 1984;99:1–110.

52. Paintal AS. Mechanism of stimulation of type J pulmonary receptors. *J Physiol (Lond)* 1969;203:511–532.

53. Cross BA, Guz A, Jain SK, Archer S, Stevens J, Reynolds F. The effect of anesthesia of the airway in dog and man: a study of respiratory reflexes, sensation and lung mechanics. *Clin Sci* 1976;50:439–454.

54. Jain SK, Trenchard D, Reynolds F, Noble MIM, Guz A. The effect of local anesthesia of the airway on respiratory reflexes in the rabbit. *Clin Sci* 1973;44:519–538.

55. Guz A, Noble MIM, Trenchard D, Cochrane HL, Makey AR. Studies on the vagus nerve in man: their role in respiratory and regulatory control. *Clin Sci* 1964;27:293–304.

56. Guz A, Noble MIM, Widdicombe JG, Trenchard D, Mushin

WW. The effect of bilateral block of vagus and glossopharyn-geal nerves on the ventilatory response to CO_2 of conscious man. *Respir Physiol* 1966;1:206–210.

57. Phillipson EA, Hickey RF, Bainton CR, Nadel JA. Effect of vagal blockade on regulation of breathing in conscious dog. *J Appl Physiol* 1970;29:475–479.

58. Remmers JE, Bartlett D Jr, Putnam MD. Changes in the respiratory cycle associated with sleep. *Respir Physiol* 1976;28:227–238.

59. Derksen FJ, Robinson NE, Stick JA. Techique for reversible vagal blockade in the standing conscious pony. *Am J Vet Res* 1981;42:523–525.

60. Guz A, Trenchard D. Pulmonary stretch receptor activity in man: a comparison with dog and cat. *J Physiol (Lond)* 1971;213:329–343.

61. Langrehr D. Receptor-afferenzen in halsvagus des menschen. *Klin Wochenschr* 1964;42:239–244.

62. Sullivan TY, Yu PL. Airway anesthesia effects on hypercapnic breathing patterns in humans. *J Appl Physiol* 1983;55:368–376.

63. Sullivan TY, De Weese EL. Lack of effect of airway anesthesia on hypoxic ventilation. *J Appl Physiol* 1985;58:1698–1702.

64. Davies A, Dixon M, Callanan D, Huszczuk A, Widdicombe JG, Wise JCM. Lung reflexes in rabbits during pulmonary stretch receptor block by sulphur dioxide. *Respir Physiol* 1978;34:83–101.

65. Clark FJ, von Euler C. On the regulation of depth and rate on breathing. *J Physiol (Lond)* 1972;222:267–295.

66. Gautier H. Pattern of breathing during hypoxia or hypercapnia of the awake or anesthetized cat. *Respir Physiol* 1976;27:193–206.

67. Gautier H, Gaudy JH. Changes in ventilatory pattern induced by intravenous anesthetic agents in human subjects. *J Appl Physiol* 1978;45:171–176.

68. Gautier H, Bonora M, Gaudy JH. Breuer–Hering inflation reflex and breathing pattern in anesthetized humans and cats. *J Appl Physiol* 1981;51:1162–1168.

69. Widdicombe JG. Respiratory reflexes in man and other mammalian species. *Clin Sci* 1961;21:163–170.

70. D'Angelo E, Agostoni E. Tonic vagal influences on respiratory duration. *Respir Physiol* 1975;24:287–302.

71. Mead J. Implications of internal loading to breathing in man. *Acta Neurobiol Exp* 1973;33:343–354.

72. Sant'Ambrogio G, Widdicombe JG. Respiratory reflexes acting on the diaphragm and inspiratory intercostal muscles of the rabbit. *J Physiol (Lond)* 1965;108:766–799.

73. Corda M, Eklund G, von Euler C. External intercostal and phrenic alpha motor responses to changes in respiratory load. *Acta Physiol Scand* 1965;63:391–400.

74. Bishop B. Diaphragm and abdominal muscle responses to elevated airway pressure in the cat. *J Appl Physiol* 1967;22:959–965.

75. Davies A, Sant'Ambrogio FB, Sant'Ambrogio G. Control of postural changes of end expiratory volume (FRC) by airways slowly adapting mechanoreceptors. *Respir Physiol* 1980;41:211–216.

76. De Troyer A. Mechanical role of the abdominal muscles in relation to posture. *Respir Physiol* 1983;53:341–353.

77. Davies A, Sant'Ambrogio FB, Sant'Ambrogio G. Onset of inspiration in rabbits during artificial ventilation. *J Physiol (Lond)* 1981;318:17–23.

78. Glogowska M, Richardson PS, Widdicombe JG, Winning AJ. The role of the vagus nerves, peripheral chemoreceptors and other afferent pathways on the genesis of augmented breaths in cats and rabbits. *Respir Physiol* 1972;16:179–196.

79. Bartoli A, Cross BA, Guz A, Huszczuk A, Jefferies R. The effect of varying tidal volume on the associated phrenic motoneurone output: studies of vagal and chemical feedback. *Respir Physiol* 1975;25:135–155.

80. DiMarco AF, von Euler C, Romaniuk JR, Yamamoto Y. Positive feedback facilitation of external intercostal and phrenic inspiratory activity by pulmonary stretch receptors. *Acta Physiol Scand* 1981;113:375–386.

81. Coleridge HM, Coleridge JCG. Impulse activity in afferent vagal C-fibers with endings in the intrapulmonary airways of the dogs. *Respir Physiol* 1977;29:143–150.

82. Coleridge HM, Coleridge JCG, Banzett RB. Effect of CO_2 on afferent vagal endings in the canine lung. *Respir Physiol* 1978;34:135–141.

83. Trenchard D. CO_2/H^+ receptors in the lungs of anesthetized rabbits. *Respir Physiol* 1986;63:227–240.

84. Pisarri TE, Yu J, Coleridge HM, Coleridge JCG. Background activity in pulmonary vagal C-fibers and its effect on breathing. *Respir Physiol* 1986;64:29–43.

85. Gautier H, Remmers JE, Bartlett D Jr. Control of the duration of expiration. *Respir Physiol* 1973;18:205–221.

86. Petit JM, Milic-Emili J, Delhez L. Role of the diaphragm in breathing in conscious normal man: an electromyographic study. *J Appl Physiol* 1960;15:1101–1106.

87. Agostoni E, Sant'Ambrogio G, Del Portillo Carrasco H. Electromyography of the diaphragm in man and transdiaphragmatic pressure. *J Appl Physiol* 1960;15:1093–1097.

88. Remmers JE, Bartlett D Jr. Reflex control of expiratory airflow and duration. *J Appl Physiol* 1977;42:80–87.

89. Lloyd TC Jr. Effects of extrapulmonary airway distension on breathing in anesthetized dogs. *J Appl Physiol* 1979;46:890–896.

90. Rao SV, Sant'Ambrogio FB, Sant'Ambrogio G. Respiratory reflexes evoked by tracheal distension. *J Appl Physiol* 1981;50:421–427.

91. Agostoni E, Citterio G, Piccoli S. Reflex partioning of inputs from stretch receptors of bronchi and thoracic trachea. *Respir Physiol* 1985;60:311–328.

92. Zechman FW Jr, Salzano J, Hall FG. Effect of cooling the cervical vagi on the work of breathing. *J Appl Physiol* 1958;12:301–304.

93. Widdicombe JG, Nadel JA. Airway volume, airway resistance, and work and force of breathing: theory. *J Appl Physiol* 1963;18:863–868.

94. Banister J, Fegler G, Hebb C. Initial respiratory responses to the intratracheal inhalation of phosgene or ammonia. *Q J Exp Physiol* 1949;35:233–250.

95. Kostreva DR, Hopp FA, Zuperku EJ, Igler FO, Coon RL, Kampine JP. Respiratory inhibition with sympathetic afferent stimulation in the canine and primate. *J Appl Physiol* 1978;44:718–724.

96. Shannon R. Effects of thoracic dorsal rhizotomies on the respiratory pattern in anesthetized cats. *J Appl Physiol* 1977;43:20–26.

97. Sant'Ambrogio G, Remmers JE. Reflex influences acting on the respiratory muscles of the chestwall. In: Roussos C, Macklem PT, eds. *The thorax*, Part A. New York: Marcel Dekker, 1985;531–594.

98. von Euler C, Peretti G. Dynamic and static contributions to the rhythmic gamma activation of primary and secondary spindle endings in external intercostal muscle. *J Physiol (Lond)* 1966;187:501–516.

99. Kirkwood PA, Sears TA. Monosynaptic excitation of mononeurons from secondary endings of muscle spindles. *Nature* 1974;252:243–244.

100. Decima EE, von Euler C, Thoden U. Intercostal to phrenic reflexes in the spinal cat. *Acta Physiol Scand* 1969;75:568–579.

101. Decima EE, von Euler C. Intercostal and cerebellar influences on efferent phrenic activity in the decerebrate cat. *Acta Physiol Scand* 1969;76:148–158.

102. Decima EE, von Euler C. Excitability of phrenic motoneurons to afferent input from lower intercostal nerves in the spinal cat. *Acta Physiol Scand* 1969;75:580–591.

103. Remmers JE. Inhibition of inspiratory activity by intercostal muscle afferents. *Respir Physiol* 1970;10:358–383.

104. Remmers JE. Extra-segmental reflexes derived from the intercostal afferents: phrenic and laryngeal responses. *J Physiol (Lond)* 1973;233:45–62.

105. Remmers JE, Tsiaras WG. Effects of lateral cervical cord lesions on the respiratory rhythm of anesthetized decerebrate cats after vagotomy. *J Physiol (Lond)* 1973;233:63–64.

106. Remmers JE, Martilla I. Action of intercostal muscle afferents

on the respiratory rhythm of anesthetized cats. *Respir Physiol* 1975;24:31–41.

107. Remmers JE. Functional role of inspiratory terminating reflex from intercostal muscle spindles. In: Duron B, ed. *Respiratory centres and afferent sysrtems*, vol 59. Paris: INSERM, 1976;183–191.

108. Corda M, von Euler C, Lennerstrand G. Proprioceptive innervation of the diaphragm. *J Physiol (Lond)* 1965;178:161–177.

109. Banzett RB, Inbar GF, Brown R, Goldman M, Rossier A, Mead J. Diaphragm electrical activity during negative lower torso pressure in quadriplegic men. *J Appl Physiol* 1981;51:654–659.

110. Fryman DL, Frazier DT. Diaphragm afferent modulation of phrenic motor drive. *J Appl Physiol* 1987;62:2436–2441.

111. De Troyer A, Sampson M, Sigrist S, Macklem PT. Action of costal and crural parts of the diaphragm on the rib cage in dog. *J Appl Physiol* 1982;53:30–39.

112. Shannon R. Respiratory pattern changes during costovertebral joint movement. *J Appl Physiol* 1980;48:862–867.

113. Speck DF, Weber CL. Thoracic dorsal rhizotomy in the anesthetized cat: maintenance of eupneic breathing. *Respir Physiol* 1979;38:347–357.

114. Duron B. Postural and ventilatory functions of intercostal muscles. *Acta Neurobiol Exp* 1973;33:355–380.

115. Duron B. Intercostal and diaphragmatic muscle endings and afferents. In: Hornbein TF, ed. *Regulation of breathing*, Part I. New York: Marcel Dekker, 1981.

116. Flandrois F, Lacour JR, Islas-Maroquin J, Charlot J. Limb mechanoreceptors inducing the reflex hyperpnea of exercise. *Respir Physiol* 1967;2:335–343.

117. Gautier H, Lacaisse A, Dejours P. Ventilatory response to muscle spindle stimulation by succinylcholine in cats. *Respir Physiol* 1969;7:383–388.

118. Carcassi AM, Concu A, Decandia M, Onnis M, Orani GP, Piras MB. Respiratory responses to stimulation of large fibers afferent from muscle receptors in cats. *Pflugers Arch* 1983;399:304–314.

119. Agostoni E, D'Angelo E. The effect of limb movements on the regulation of depth and rate of breathing. *Respir Physiol* 1976;27:33–52.

120. Iscoe S, Polosa C. Synchronization of respiratory frequency by somatic afferent stimulation. *J Appl Physiol* 1976;40:138–148.

121. Paulev PE. Respiratory and cardiac responses to exercise in man. *J Appl Physiol* 1971;30:165–172.

122. Kay JDS, Strange Petersen E, Vejby-Christensen H. Breathing in man during steady-state exercise on the bicycle at two pedalling frequencies and during treadmill walking. *J Physiol (Lond)* 1975;251:645–656.

123. Green M, Mead J, Sears TA. Muscle activity during chest wall restriction and positive pressure breathing in man. *Respir Physiol* 1978;35:283–300.

THE LUNG: Scientific Foundations
edited by R.G. Crystal, J.B. West et al.
Raven Press, Ltd., New York © 1991.

CHAPTER 5.4.9

Behavioral Control of Breathing

John Orem

Behavioral control of breathing can be defined narrowly as voluntary control or broadly as control of the respiratory apparatus for purposes other than ventilation of the lung. The broader definition leads to consideration of responses such as sneezing, coughing, straining, swallowing, laughing, and crying. In each of these responses, as in the case of voluntary control, we would like to know how and where control occurs. The possible sources of influence on the respiratory system are many and comprise all levels of the neuraxis (1–12). In some cases, these influences may be exerted at both brainstem and spinal levels of the respiratory system (1–3). Immunohistochemical studies reveal that spinal and brainstem respiratory motoneurons are contacted by terminals that use many different neurotransmitters. The latter include serotonin, substance P, thyrotropin-releasing hormone, norepinephrine, and gamma-aminobutyric acid (GABA) (13,14). Thus, there are many possibilities for behavioral control, and the problem is to determine which of the many possible sources of influence control which area(s) of the respiratory system during any behavioral respiratory response.

VOLUNTARY CONTROL

As shown in the following text, several authors propose that voluntary control of breathing involves projections which bypass the neurons of the pons and medulla and which engage directly, or through local interneurons, the motoneurons that innervate the muscles of respiration (see Fig. 1). Thus, they suggest that there is a dual control of respiratory musculature: The signals producing automatic breathing arise in the pontomedullary respiratory areas and are conducted to the

spinal cord by pathways within the ventrolateral quadrants, whereas voluntary control arises from forebrain structures and is conducted to the spinal cord by the corticospinal and rubrospinal pathways within the dorsolateral quadrants. There is ample evidence that destruction of corticofugal fibers can result in the loss of voluntary control of respiration (see refs. 15 and 16 for reviews), but the evidence that corticospinal rather than corticobulbar fibers are responsible for this control is not conclusive.

Evidence of separate control comes primarily from neurological cases, and the interested reader should consult Plum and Leigh (16) for an excellent review of these. Here, discussion is restricted to those cases that have been cited to support the notion of a separation of voluntary and automatic systems up to the level of respiratory motoneurons.

Meyer and Herndon (17) have described a patient with bilateral infarction of the pyramids and the adjoining ventromedial medulla who breathed spontaneously and regularly but who was unable to control his breathing voluntarily. This case is cited as evidence that voluntary and automatic pathways are separate until the two are integrated finally at the level of spinal respiratory motoneurons (e.g., see ref. 18, p. 219). Yet the lesion of the pyramids and the nearby medulla may have interrupted pathways from the cortex to the medulla as well as pathways from the cortex to the spinal cord. If such were the case, then the inability to control breathing voluntarily could have resulted from lesions of those fibers that link the cortex with the automatic system. Indeed, the patient's pharyngeal and hypoglossal motor paralysis make it clear in this case that some corticobulbar fibers were interrupted by the infarction. The motoneurons for these muscles are within (nucleus ambiguus for the pharynx) or near (the hypoglossal nucleus) the regions that comprise the automatic system. Thus, in this case, corticospinal and corticobulbar fibers were interrupted by the infarction.

J. Orem: Department of Physiology, Texas Tech University Health Sciences Center, Lubbock, Texas 79430.

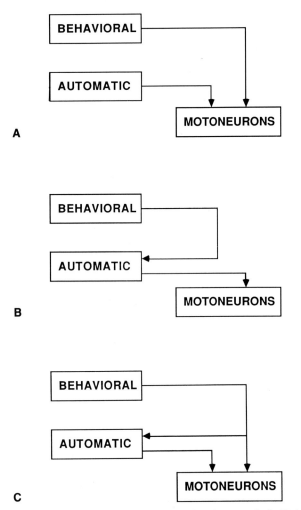

FIG. 1. Possible modes of behavioral control. **A:** Behavioral control involves direct control of respiratory motoneurons. **B:** Behavioral control occurs through control of the automatic system within the pons and medulla. **C:** Behavioral control occurs both through direct control of respiratory motoneurons and through control of the automatic system. As shown in this chapter, depending upon the behavior, there are different modes of control.

Lesions of the ventrolateral columns of the upper cervical cord (wherein travel fibers from the brainstem automatic system), or lesions of parts of the brainstem automatic system itself, can produce a syndrome (Ondine's curse) in which breathing persists in wakefulness but fails in sleep. To Plum in 1970 (15), this seemed strong evidence of separate voluntary and automatic pathways through and below the medulla. He reasoned that breathing was maintained in wakefulness by functional voluntary pathways but that it failed in sleep with the loss of voluntary activity. Yet, the waking vital capacities (i.e., the maximal voluntary efforts) of almost all patients with Ondine's curse are reduced. This suggests, as Plum and Leigh (16) have noted, that all voluntary effort is not mediated by corticospinal fibers and that some of this effort may be mediated by corticobulbar fibers that engage the automatic system.

This, in turn, suggests that breathing in these patients is maintained in wakefulness by corticospinal and corticobulbar voluntary pathways. The idea that breathing is maintained in wakefulness by inputs to the respiratory system from higher centers related to voluntary control has profound implications—so profound as to justify a brief discussion here of the wakefulness stimulus for breathing.

It has been known for many years that wakefulness stimulates breathing. This knowledge came from the study of normal subjects as well as from the study of patients having Ondine's curse (19–21).

The concept of the wakefulness stimulus for breathing has been invoked repeatedly to explain various respiratory phenomena; however, little is known of the nature of this stimulus. It seems not to act exclusively through the metabolic control system, because breathing is stimulated in wakefulness even when chemical stimuli are absent or not detected adequately (22). It seems also to affect some parts of the respiratory system more than others. In particular, there is evidence that the wakefulness stimulus affects the muscles of the upper airways preferentially, but how this occurs is not known. Indeed, the origin, form, and site of action of the wakefulness stimulus are not known. Stimulation of regions of the brainstem related to arousal results in activation of respiratory muscles [preferentially that of upper-airway respiratory muscles (23)], but it is not known whether or how these regions mediate the wakefulness stimulus. For example, their involvement, if any, in producing the wakefulness stimulus may be either by direct activation of brainstem respiratory areas or by indirect activation of voluntary (behavioral) systems that, in turn, activate brainstem respiratory areas.

Plum's interpretation (15) of the wakefulness stimulus is straightforward and elegant: There are separate systems for automatic and voluntary control of breathing; in sleep, inputs from the voluntary system are lost; these inputs comprise the wakefulness stimulus.

Recent studies of brainstem respiratory neurons during sleep and during the behavioral control of breathing have extended the theory of dual respiratory control: It has been postulated that there are separate components for the automatic and behavioral systems, respectively. In this theory (24), these components are not separate at the gross anatomic level. Indeed, the cells forming the two components coexist in clusters within brainstem respiratory areas. Their separateness arises instead from the differing synaptic relations of the cells: The cells of the automatic system are interrelated closely and are consequently unresponsive to nonrespiratory inputs; in contrast, the cells of the behavioral system integrate respiratory and nonrespiratory inputs and act to modify respiratory output. In this theory, the wakefulness stimulus comprises the host of nonrespiratory inputs reflected in the activity of the latter cells—inputs that are related to the behavioral exigencies of wakefulness. The evidence of this theory is addressed in the following section ("Learned Behavioral Respiratory Responses").

Some experimental evidence supports the idea that voluntary control bypasses the automatic system and engages respiratory motoneurons directly. Aminoff and Sears' study (25) of intercostal nerve activity in the anesthetized and paralyzed cat is sometimes cited as evidence of separate voluntary and automatic pathways (e.g., see ref. 18, p. 216). In that study, Aminoff and Sears showed short-latency responses in the internal intercostal (expiratory) nerves to stimulation of the motor cortex. Transection of the ventrolateral quadrants of the spinal cord abolished intercostal-nerve respiratory activity below the transection but left intact the response to cortical stimulation. Transection of the dorsolateral columns abolished the excitatory response of the internal intercostal nerve to cortical stimulation, but rhythmic respiratory activity continued. The authors report, also, however, that the inhibition of external intercostal inspiratory activity evoked by cortical stimulation was reduced but not blocked by transections of the dorsolateral columns. They conclude that this residual inhibition could have resulted from corticofugal inhibition of brainstem inspiratory neurons. Thus, this study showed that cortical stimulation excites expiratory intercostal nerves and inhibits inspiratory intercostal nerves. The excitation, but not the inhibition, could be blocked by lesions of the dorsolateral quadrant. It is, of course, impossible to know the functional significance of these findings in the anesthetized and paralyzed cat, but they demonstrate, nevertheless, cortical influences that bypass the automatic system and engage segmental expiratory motoneurons.

LEARNED BEHAVIORAL RESPIRATORY RESPONSES

Cats have been trained to stop inspiration in response to a conditioning stimulus (26). Whether this learned response is identical to the voluntary responses demonstrated by humans is unclear. Accordingly, the neural mechanisms of these responses are referred to as the "mechanisms of behavioral control."

In a series of experiments in the intact, unanesthetized cat trained to perform a respiratory response, Orem and co-workers (27–29) have recorded the activity of single brainstem respiratory neurons. Their initial interest was to determine whether behavioral control occurred within the brainstem automatic system—that is, whether the activity of the cells of the automatic system changed to produce the behavioral response. This seems, in fact, to be the case, but the results are complex. They found that some respiratory cells were inactivated and others were activated when inspiration was inhibited behaviorally (see Figs. 2 and 3). Whether a respiratory cell was activated or inactivated was related to the nature of the cell's spontaneous activity: If a cell had a strong and consistent respiratory signal, it was inactivated during the behavioral respiratory response. This was true regardless of the type of respiratory cell—that is, regardless of whether it was an inspiratory, expiratory, or phase-spanning cell. In contrast, activated cells were a subset of those respiratory cells having weak and inconsistent respiratory signals.

The strength and consistency of the respiratory activity of a cell were quantified with an effect-size statistic, η^2 (30). The value of the statistic reflects directly the degree to which the afferents driving the cell have a respiratory form (or, inversely, the degree to which the afferents to the cell have a nonrespiratory form). In the behavioral control studies, all high-η^2-valued respiratory cells were inactivated during the response; respiratory cells that were activated had low-η^2-valued activity. One interpretation of these cells is that the low-η^2-valued cells that are activated form an interface between nonrespiratory inputs and high-η^2-valued cells. According to this interpretation, behavioral control is effected through activation of the low-η^2-valued cells that, in turn, inhibit the high-η^2-valued cells (see Fig. 4).

As discussed in the previous section, it has been proposed (24,27) that cells forming the automatic sys-

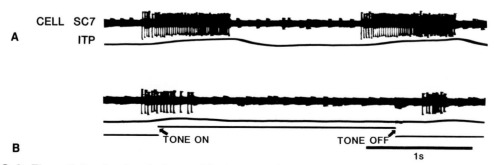

FIG. 2. The activity of an inspiratory cell in the medulla during behavioral inhibition of inspiration. **A:** Control activity of the cell and intratracheal pressure (ITP). Negative pressures (inspiration) are signaled by upward deflections. **B:** Activity of the cell when, in response to the tone (conditioning stimulus), the animal stopped inspiring. (Adapted from ref. 29.)

CELL C10

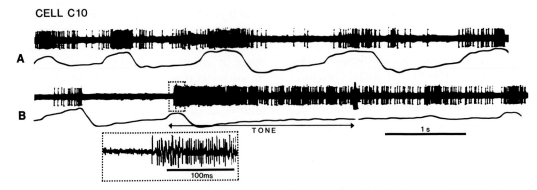

FIG. 3. Activity of an inspiratory cell that was activated when inspiration was inhibited behaviorally. **A:** Shows spontaneous activity of this cell and intratracheal pressure. Inspiration is signaled by an upward deflection. Note that the breath-to-breath variability in the activity of the cell gives the cell its low η^2 value. **B:** The conditioning stimulus is presented, and inspiration is stopped behaviorally. The cell is activated intensely during the behavioral inhibition. The insert below shows a high-speed tracing of the onset of the activation and corresponds to the boxed area shown in tracing **B.** (From ref. 27.)

tem and cells forming the behavioral system coexist in clusters within brainstem respiratory areas. In this theory, the low-η^2-valued cells act as the behavioral-state system whereas the high-η^2-valued cells are the cells of the respiratory oscillator or its output. This theory is based on three results: (i) The η^2 statistic applied to the analysis of brainstem respiratory activity reveals that the signal strength and consistency of respiratory activity differ greatly among respiratory cells. The low-η^2-valued cells seem to integrate many inputs having nonrespiratory forms, whereas the high-η^2-valued cells are apparently interrelated closely—perhaps to form an oscillator such as that modeled by Richter et al. (31). (ii) Studies of brainstem respiratory neurons during wakefulness and non-rapid eye movement (NREM) sleep have revealed that high-η^2-valued cells are affected little whereas low-η^2-valued cells are affected greatly by sleep (32). This finding, combined with the interpretation given in point "i" above, leads

to the principle that the effect of sleep on a respiratory neuron is proportional to the amount of nonrespiratory activity of the neuron. (iii) Experiments on behavioral control show that high-η^2-valued cells are inactivated when inspiration is inhibited and that some low-η^2-valued cells are activated intensely.

The validity of this theory remains to be determined, but it is clear that behavioral control occurs within the automatic system of the brainstem—a fact that does not preclude the possibility of simultaneous behavioral control at the levels of brainstem and spinal respiratory motoneurons.

CONTROL DURING SNIFFING, SNEEZING, AND COUGHING

Batsel and co-workers (33–35) have demonstrated that medullary respiratory neurons participate in sneezing

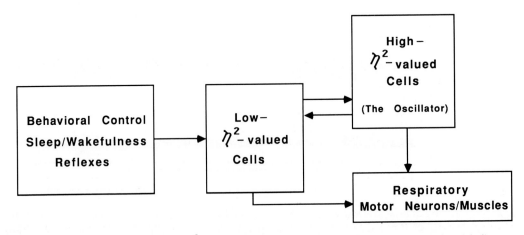

FIG. 4. Hypothesized role of low-η^2-valued cells as an interface between behavioral influences and the cells of the oscillator.

and in the aspiration reflex. Mechanical stimulation of the nasal mucosa of the lightly anesthetized cat causes caudal expiratory neurons to be activated intensely in association with the expiratory thrusts of sneezing. The same expiratory neurons are involved in (a) coughing, (b) sneezing, and (c) the increased expiratory effort elicited by an imposed resistance to expiration. Ethmoidal nerve stimulation, too, can elicit sneezing. Applied at a rate of approximately 35 Hz, this stimulation produces an apnea or depression of inspiration followed by a series of active and augmenting expiratory efforts. The majority of medullary expiratory neurons show time-locked responses to these stimuli. The latencies of these responses (which can be elicited, in some cases, during inspiration) vary from approximately 5 msec to 25 msec. With continuation of the stimulation, expiratory thrusts are produced in association with bursts of activity of the expiratory neurons. During these bursts, instantaneous discharge frequencies can exceed 400 Hz.

Sniffing can be elicited in anesthetized cats by mechanical stimulation of the nasopharyngeal mucosa during expiration. The sniff reflex is a brief, rapid activation of the diaphragm; bulbar inspiratory neurons are activated intensely, and expiratory neurons are inhibited during this response (33). Inspiratory neurons of the dorsal respiratory group are particularly responsive to this stimulation: They are activated at shorter latencies than are the ventral respiratory group inspiratory neurons, and they respond preferentially to stimulation of the ipsilateral nasopharyngeal mucosa. These results of Batsel have been confirmed recently (36), but contrasting with them are the results of a recent study showing that brainstem expiratory neurons are inactive during expiratory responses elicited by stimulation of the superior laryngeal nerve or cold-water infusion into the larynx in anesthetized, vagotomized, paralyzed, and ventilated cats (37).

CONTROL DURING STRAINING, VOMITING, AND SWALLOWING

There are behaviors during which the activity of inspiratory neurons in the brainstem is dissociated from the activity of inspiratory muscles such as the diaphragm. Rhythmic straining, similar to that occurring in conscious dogs during defecation, can be induced in the decerebrate dog by distention of the rectum (38–41). This behavior comprises cocontraction of the diaphragm, the adductors of the glottis, and the abdominal muscles. Recordings of respiratory neurons within the dorsal- and ventral-medullary respiratory groups from approximately 2 mm rostral to 4–6 mm caudal to the obex showed that expiratory, but not inspiratory, cells tended to have activity patterns associated with straining. Thus, in this case there is activation of the dia-

phragm, but brainstem inspiratory cells (many identified as bulbospinal cells) must not mediate the activation. Fukuda and Fukai (38–41) propose that there is a reflex straining center in the Kölliker–Fuse nucleus and that neurons within this area of the pons produce the command signals that control rhythmic straining. The command to the diaphragm, they propose, descends to the level of the phrenic nucleus through pathways that bypass the bulbospinal inspiratory neurons, whereas the command to expiratory muscles occurs by way of bulbospinal expiratory neurons.

The evidence of pontine involvement in rhythmic straining comes from transection, stimulation, and recording experiments that show (a) that rhythmic straining is eliminated by partial cuts in the rostrolateral pons (the region of the Kölliker–Fuse nucleus), (b) that rhythmic straining can be induced by stimulation of an area of the Kölliker–Fuse nucleus, and (c) that within the Kölliker–Fuse nucleus, there are neurons that respond to stimulation of pelvic afferents and that discharge synchronously with rhythmic straining (some of the latter neurons discharged spontaneously in phase with some part of the respiratory cycle).

Vomiting, like straining, involves coactivation of the diaphragm (and the external intercostal muscles) and the abdominal muscles in a rhythmic pattern (retching) that culminates in a prolonged expulsive phase. Recordings of caudal brainstem expiratory neurons during vomiting show that they are activated synchronously with either the abdominal muscle activity or the activity of the internal intercostal muscles (the latter are activated between the bursts of diaphragmatic and abdominal activity) (42). Although this evidence indicates that, as in straining, caudal brainstem expiratory neurons may mediate activation of the abdominal and internal intercostal muscles, cutting of the axons of these caudal neurons by midline transection from C_1 to the obex did not eliminate the activation of the abdominal muscles during vomiting. Thus, inputs other than those arising from caudal expiratory neurons may activate the abdominal muscles during vomiting.

During the expulsive phase of vomiting, there is strong contraction of the costal diaphragm but relaxation of the periesophageal diaphragm. The relaxation of the periesophageal diaphragm is not reflexive in response to esophageal distention but depends, instead, on unknown central mechanisms (43). Preliminary studies (44) suggest that medullary, bulbospinal inspiratory neurons may not mediate diaphragmatic or external intercostal activation during either the retching or expulsive phases of vomiting. A study of 16 bulbospinal inspiratory neurons revealed that most did not have activity patterns that could account for the activity of the phrenic nerve during vomiting (44).

Swallowing (as do vomiting, sniffing, and straining)

involves control of respiratory muscles for a nonrespiratory function. There is evidence of control of brainstem respiratory neurons during swallowing. Sumi (45) recorded inspiratory and expiratory neurons rostral to the obex and found that inspiratory and expiratory cells were either activated or inhibited during swallows. The contrasting behavior of different inspiratory neurons is not surprising in view of the complex behavior of respiratory musculature during swallowing. For example, during swallowing, costal diaphragmatic activity may be unaffected, but the crural diaphragm is inhibited to allow passage of the bolus (46). Similarly, during the expulsive phase of vomiting and during eructation, costal diaphragmatic fibers are activated, but crural fibers are inhibited (46). If these responses are organized at the brainstem level, some inspiratory neurons should be activated while others are inhibited during swallowing, vomiting, and eructation. Although Sumi (45) found this to be the case, another group of investigators (47) recorded 424 inspiratory neurons in the dorsal and ventral respiratory group and found that none were inhibited during crural inhibition elicited by distention of the distal esophagus or during spontaneous swallowing. These investigators concluded that inhibition of the crural diaphragm during swallowing is mediated by pathways that do not include the inspiratory neurons of the dorsal and ventral respiratory groups.

CONCLUSION

The simple generalization that behavioral control of the respiratory system occurs, or does not occur, through control of the brainstem automatic respiratory system cannot be made. Expiratory efforts in sneezing, vomiting, coughing, and straining are mediated, at least in part, by some brainstem expiratory neurons, but an expiratory effort elicited by superior laryngeal nerve stimulation can occur independently of these neurons. Similarly, the behavioral control of inspiratory muscles involves medullary inspiratory neurons in some, but not other, cases. Brainstem inspiratory neurons are inhibited during behavioral apneas and activated during the sniff reflex but are not activated during the diaphragmatic activation associated with straining and vomiting, and it is questionable whether some are inhibited to produce the inactivation of the crural diaphragm during swallowing.

It is apparent, also, that for none of the behavioral responses discussed here is there anything approaching a thorough study of all known brainstem respiratory areas. The data on straining (38–41) are perhaps most complete in that they relate to both medullary and pontine respiratory groups. Furthermore, a model based on these data proposes that there is a center within the Kölliker–Fuse nucleus that produces, through control of brainstem and spinal respiratory neurons, the coactivation of various muscles to produce rhythmic straining. The theory of a cough center has its proponents (e.g., see ref. 48), but, in general, the data have been insufficient to warrant the development of models (such as that of Fukada and Fukai for straining).

In those cases in which behavioral control occurs within brainstem respiratory areas, there is the issue of the mechanism for this control. In the abstract, the issue is one of how afferents having a nonrespiratory form modify the system that produces rhythmic respiration—an issue that is more complex than it appears. For example, in a recent model, based on results from intracellular recordings (49,50), generation of the rhythm relies greatly on inhibitory interactions among the cells of the network (31), and inspiratory cells are inhibited by late inspiratory, postinspiratory, and expiratory neurons. It could be then that behavioral inhibition of inspiration occurs by activation of one or all of these types of inspiratory–inhibitory cells. To investigate this possibility, Orem and Brooks (29) recorded the activity of the expiratory cells in the region of the retrofacial nucleus in cats trained to stop inspiration behaviorally. Although these cells are reported to be inhibitory to inspiratory neurons in the brainstem and to phrenic motoneurons (51,52), they were inactive during the response and thus could not be the cause of it (see also ref. 53 for another case in which inspiration is inhibited when these cells are not activated). Similarly, late inspiratory cells, like the expiratory cells, are unlikely to cause the behavioral inhibition of inspiration, because they are either inactive or discharge only weakly during this response (28). Such evidence suggests that cells that have inspiratory–inhibitory actions during eupnea may not be involved in the behavioral inhibition of inspiration.

This result is understandable if, as models and intracellular studies suggest (31), these late-onset inspiratory cells and retrofacial expiratory cells are inhibited during the early phases of inspiration. Inhibited cells are difficult to excite, but excited cells can be inhibited. Thus, inspiratory cells can be inhibited prematurely, but the inhibition is unlikely to come from cells that stop that phase normally and that are inhibited in the early parts of the phase. This led Orem (27) to the conclusion that stopping inspiration prematurely would be most readily achieved by activation of inhibitory cells other than those integral to the close network of respiratory cells that produce within one another rigid sequences of inhibitory and excitatory postsynaptic potentials.

Orem has proposed (a) that low-η^2-valued cells act as the interface between nonrespiratory afferents and the closely interrelated cells of the oscillator and (b) that some low-η^2-valued cells act as inhibitory cells during the behavioral inhibition of inspiration. It is certain that the activity of these cells contains a large nonrespiratory component and that some cells are activated intensely when inspiration is stopped behaviorally, but their inhibitory role is not proven.

ACKNOWLEDGMENTS

Alma Wood, Etta Powell, and Judith Keeling assisted in the preparation of this chapter. This work was supported by Grant HL 21257 from the National Heart, Lung, and Blood Institute.

REFERENCES

1. Bassal M, Bianchi AL. Effets de la stimulation des structures nerveuses centrales sur les activités respiratoires efférentes chez le chat. I. Réponses à la stimulation corticale. *J Physiol (Paris)* 1981;77:741–757.
2. Bassal M, Bianchi AL. Effets de la stimulation des structures nerveuses centrales sur les activités respiratoires efférentes chez le chat. II. Réponses à la stimulation sous-corticale. *J Physiol (Paris)* 1981;77:759–777.
3. Bassal M, Bianchi AL, Dussardier M. Effets de la stimulation des structures nerveuses centrales sur l'activite des neurones respiratoires chez le chat. *J Physiol (Paris)* 1981;77:779–795.
4. Eldridge FL, Millhorn DE, Waldrop TG. Exercise hyperpnea and locomotion: parallel activation from the hypothalamus. *Science* 1981;211:844–846.
5. Harper RM, Frysinger RC. Suprapontine mechanisms underlying cardiorespiratory regulation: implications for the Sudden Infant Death Syndrome. In: Harper RM, Hoffman JH, eds. *Sudden infant death syndrome: risk factors and basic mechanisms.* New York: PMA Publishing, 1988;399–414.
6. Harper RM, Frysinger RC, Terreberry RR, Marks JD, Zhang J-X, Ni HF. Suprapontine control of respiratory activity. In: Sieck GC, Gandevia SC, Cameron WE, eds. *Respiratory muscles and their neuromotor control.* New York: Alan R Liss, 1987;93–101.
7. Lipski J, Bektas A, Porter R. Short latency input to phrenic motoneurons from sensorimotor cortex in the cat. *Exp Brain Res* 1986;61:280–290.
8. Lutherer LO, Williams JL. Stimulating fastigial nucleus pressor region elicits patterned respiratory responses. *Am J Physiol* 1986;250:R418–R426.
9. Marks JD, Frysinger RC, Harper RM. State-dependent respiratory depression elicited by stimulation of the orbital frontal cortex. *Exp Neurol* 1987;95:714–729.
10. Reis DJ, McHugh PR. Hypoxia as a cause of bradycardia during amygdala stimulation in monkey. *J Appl Physiol* 1968;214:601–610.
11. Williams JL, Robinson PJ, Lutherer LO. Inhibitory effects of cerebellar lesions on respiration in the spontaneously breathing, anesthetized cat. *Brain Res* 1986;399:224–231.
12. Zhang J-X, Harper RM, Ni H. Cryogenic blockade of the central nucleus of the amygdala attenuates aversively conditioned blood pressure and respiratory responses. *Brain Res* 1986;386:136–145.
13. Holtman JR. Immunohistochemical localization of serotonin- and substance P-containing fibers around respiratory muscle motoneurons in the nucleus ambiguus of the cat. *Neuroscience* 1988;26:169–178.
14. Holtman JR, Norman WP, Skirboll L, Dretchen KL, Cuello C, Visser TJ, Hökfelt T, Gillis RA. Evidence for 5-hydroxytryptamine, substance P and thyrotropin-releasing hormone in neurons innervating the phrenic motor nucleus. *J Neurosci* 1984;4:1064–1071.
15. Plum F. Neurological integration of behavioral and metabolic control of breathing. In: Porter R, ed. *Breathing: Hering-Breuer Centenary Symposium.* London: Churchill, 1970;159–175.
16. Plum F, Leigh RJ. Abnormalities of central mechanisms. In: Hornbein TF, ed. *Regulation of breathing,* part II. New York: Marcel Dekker, 1981;989–1067.
17. Meyer JS, Herndon RM. Bilateral infarction of the pyramidal tract in man. *Neurology* 1962;12:637–642.
18. Mitchell RA, Berger AJ. Neural regulation of respiration. *Am Rev Resp Dis* 1975;111:206–224.
19. Plum F, Swanson AG. Abnormalities in central regulation of respiration in acute and convalescent poliomyelitis. *Arch Neurol Psychiatry* 1958;80:267–285.
20. Severinghaus JW, Mitchell RA. Ondine's curse—failure of respiratory center automaticity while asleep. *Clin Res* 1962;10:122.
21. Fink BR, Katz R, Reinhold H, Schoolman A. Suprapontine mechanisms in regulation of respiration. *Am J Physiol* 1962;202:217–220.
22. Sullivan CE, Kozar LF, Murphy E, Phillipson EA. Primary role of respiratory afferents in sustaining breathing rhythm. *J Appl Physiol* 1978;45:11–17.
23. Orem J, Lydic R. Upper airway function during sleep and wakefulness: experimental studies on normal and anesthetized cats. *Sleep* 1978;1:49–68.
24. Orem J. The nature of the wakefulness stimulus. In: Suratt P, Remmers JE, eds. *Sleep and respiration.* New York: Alan R Liss, 1990; in press.
25. Aminoff MJ, Sears TA. Spinal integration of segmental, cortical and breathing inputs to thoracic respiratory motoneurons. *J Physiol (Lond)* 1971;215:557–575.
26. Orem J, Netick A. Behavioral control of breathing in the cat. *Brain Res* 1986;366:238–253.
27. Orem J. Inspiratory neurons that are activated when inspiration is inhibited behaviorally. *Neurosci Lett* 1987;83:282–286.
28. Orem J. The activity of late inspiratory cells during the behavioral inhibition of inspiration. *Brain Res* 1988;458:224–230.
29. Orem J, Brooks EG. The activity of retrofacial expiratory cells during behavioral respiratory responses and active expiration. *Brain Res* 1986;374:409–412.
30. Orem J, Dick T. Consistency and signal strength of respiratory neuronal activity. *J Neurophysiol* 1983;50:1098–1107.
31. Richter DW, Ballantyne D, Remmers JE. How is the respiratory rhythm generated? A model. *NIPS* 1986;1:109–112.
32. Orem J, Osorio I, Brooks E, Dick T. Activity of respiratory neurons during NREM sleep. *J Neurophysiol* 1985;54:1144–1156.
33. Batsel HL, Lines AJ Jr. Bulbar respiratory neurons participating in the sniff reflex in the cat. *Exp Neurol* 1973;39:467–481.
34. Batsel HL, Lines AJ. Neural mechanisms of sneeze. *Am J Physiol* 1975;229:770–776.
35. Price WH, Batsel HL. Respiratory neurons participating in sneeze and in response to resistance to expiration. *Exp Neurol* 1970;29:554–570.
36. Jakuš J, Tomori Z, Stránsky A. Activity of bulbar respiratory neurones during cough and other respiratory tract reflexes in cats. *Physiol Bohemoslov* 1985;34:127–136.
37. Jodkowski JS, Berger AJ. Influences from laryngeal afferents on expiratory bulbospinal neurons and motoneurons. *J Appl Physiol* 1988;64:1337–1345.
38. Fukuda H, Fukai K. Postural change and straining induced by distension of the rectum, vagina and urinary bladder of decerebrate dogs. *Brain Res* 1986;380:276–286.
39. Fukuda H, Fukai K. Location of the reflex centre for straining elicited by activation of pelvic afferent fibres of decerebrate dogs. *Brain Res* 1986;380:287–296.
40. Fukuda H, Fukai K. Ascending and descending pathways of reflex straining in the dog. *Jpn J Physiol* 1986;36:905–920.
41. Fukuda H, Fukai K. Discharges of bulbar respiratory neurons during rhythmic straining evoked by activation of pelvic afferent fibers in dogs. *Brain Res* 1988;449:157–166.
42. Miller AD, Tan LK, Suzuki I. Control of abdominal and expi-

ratory intercostal muscle activity during vomiting: role of ventral respiratory group expiratory neurons. *J Neurophysiol* 1987;57:1854–1866.

43. Miller AD, Lakos SF, Tan LK. Central motor program for relaxation of periesophageal diaphragm during the expulsive phase of vomiting. *Brain Res* 1988;456:367–370.

44. Miller AD, Tan LK, Lakos SF. Activity of inspiratory neurons in the dorsal and ventral respiratory groups during fictive vomiting. *Soc Neurosci Abstr* 1987;13:1638.

45. Sumi T. The activity of brain-stem respiratory neurons and spinal respiratory motoneurons during swallowing. *J Neurophysiol* 1963;26:466–477.

46. Monges H, Salducci J, Naudy B. Dissociation between the electrical activity of the diaphragmatic dome and crura muscular fibers during esophageal distension, vomiting and eructation. An electromyographic study in the dog. *J Physiol (Paris)* 1978; 74:541–554.

47. Altschuler SM, Davies RO, Pack AI. Role of medullary inspiratory neurons in the control of the diaphragm during oesophageal stimulation in cats. *J Physiol (Lond)* 1987;391:289–298.

48. Kase Y. Antitussive agents and their sites of action. *Trends Pharmacol Sci* 1980:237–239.

49. Ballantyne D, Richter DW. Postsynaptic inhibition of bulbar inspiratory neurons in the cat. *J Physiol (Lond)* 1984;348:67–87.

50. Richter DW. Generation and maintenance of the respiratory rhythm. *J Exp Biol* 1982;100:93–107.

51. Merrill EG. One source of the expiratory inhibition of phrenic motoneurones in the cat. *J Physiol (Lond)* 1982;332:79p.

52. Merrill EG, Lipski J, Rubin L, Fedorko L. Origin of the expiratory inhibition of nucleus tractus solitarius inspiratory neurons. *Brain Res* 1983;263:43–50.

53. Pantaleo T, Corda M. Expiration-related neurons in the region of the retrofacial nucleus: vagal and laryngeal inhibitory influences. *Brain Res* 1985;359:343–346.

THE LUNG: Scientific Foundations
edited by R.G. Crystal, J.B. West et al.
Raven Press, Ltd., New York © 1991.

CHAPTER 5.4.10

Integration of Ventilatory and Cardiovascular Control Systems

Hazel M. Coleridge, John C. G. Coleridge, and David Jordan

The circulatory system of vertebrates links gas exchange at the level of the external environment with gas exchange at the level of the individual cell. The overall rate of external gas exchange and the constancy of the internal milieu with respect to respiratory gases depend critically on integrated changes in ventilation and perfusion at the respiratory exchange surfaces. Hence the neural mechanisms that couple respiratory exchange and blood flow are of vital importance. These neural integrating mechanisms include the control networks in the brainstem that regulate ventilatory and cardiovascular function, descending pathways from suprapontine levels that converge on the brainstem networks, and a variety of afferent inputs, most notably from sensory endings in the ventilatory and cardiovascular systems themselves, that reach the brainstem networks in the cranial and spinal nerves. These neural mechanisms, central and peripheral, are the topic of the present chapter. We do not deal in detail with the central respiratory or cardiovascular control networks themselves, nor do we give a detailed account of the sensory receptors that provide the centers with information; rather, we deal with the neural mechanisms that ensure the functional integration of the two control systems. The purely mechanical interactions such as the rhythmic ventilatory variations in venous return, cardiac output, and pulmonary blood volume induced by operation of the thoracic pump are outside the scope of this chapter. A comprehensive account of both mechanical and neural interactions between the ventilatory and cardiovascular systems is given by Daly (1). Space permits no more than a general treatment of many topics, and at several points in the text the reader is referred to review articles that provide a more extensive bibliography than is possible here.

In fish, as well as in mammals, the respiratory networks appear to play the dominant role in integrating the two systems. This dominance probably arises because ventilation is entirely dependent on the medullary neurons that provide rhythmic drive to the respiratory muscles, whereas the circulatory system, though dependent on neural mechanisms for its fine-tuning, is inherently autonomous. In the dogfish, gill movements and heart rate are coordinated by rhythmic, respiratory-related bursts of firing in vagal cardiomotor efferents (2). In mammals, a ventilatory rhythm can be detected in the various motor outflows to the cardiovascular system, and the baroreceptor reflex, perhaps the most important reflex concerned with cardiovascular regulation, is subject to a pronounced respiratory modulation. Moreover, cardiovascular function is strongly affected by reflexogenic input from the upper and lower respiratory tract, as well as by input from the carotid body chemoreceptors, evoked by changes in arterial P_{O_2}, P_{CO_2}, and pH.

We begin by reviewing the central interactions involved in ventilatory–cardiovascular integration, dealing with interactions at the level of the medulla, an area in which integration of ventilatory and cardiovascular control mechanisms is most complex and flexible. In the medulla a respiratory modulation is imposed on cardiovascular reflexes, partly by central inspiratory cells and partly by feedback from pulmonary stretch receptors. Numerous potential sites for ventilatory–cardiovascular integration also exist at

H. M. Coleridge and J. C. G. Coleridge: Cardiovascular Research Institute and Department of Physiology, University of California San Francisco, San Francisco, California 94143.

D. Jordan: Department of Physiology, Royal Free Hospital School of Medicine, University of London, London, England NW3 2PF.

higher levels of the central nervous system, in the cerebellum, hypothalamus, orbital cortex, and cingulate gyrus. These suprapontine mechanisms are dealt with more briefly.

INTEGRATION IN THE MEDULLA

Within the medulla are two groups of neurons that fire with a respiratory rhythm (see Chapter 5.4.1): a "dorsal respiratory group" located in the ventrolateral subnucleus of the solitary tract, and a "ventral respiratory group" consisting of a longitudinal strip of neurons associated with nucleus retroambigualis and nucleus ambiguus. The medulla also contains the vagal motoneurons supplying the heart and airways, several groups of bulbospinal premotor sympathetic neurons supplying the heart and resistance vessels, and the central terminations of afferent fibers from the lungs, airways, heart, and great vessels. Together, these provide the basic neural substrate for cardiorespiratory integration. They also represent sites at which descending pathways from more rostral brain areas modify ventilatory and cardiovascular function and, most importantly, at which central inspiratory neurons influence the motor centers controlling cardiovascular function and interact with cardiovascular afferent inputs.

Before we discuss the interactions between ventilatory and cardiovascular control mechanisms at the medullary level, it seems important to draw attention to the often expressed view that investigation of cardiorespiratory interactions is hampered by outmoded notions of separate and specific medullary "centers" controlling the two systems. According to this view, the specificity of the neurons grouped in the so-called medullary respiratory and cardiovascular "centers" is virtually always relative, and, even within the two major respiratory neuron groups, neurons whose function is dedicated solely to ventilation are comparatively rare (3). Koepchen (3) argues that the division of medullary neurons into localized and specific respiratory and cardiovascular "centers" results from the particular approaches used by individual investigators, and that virtually the only neurons whose function can be exclusively assigned to a particular system are the motor neurons whose axons leave the central nervous system. Koepchen suggests that the use of the term "interaction" in this context harks back to the concept of "central irradiation," which implies that central or reflex influences of major concern to one system have a secondary influence by irradiation on the other—hence his preference for the term "linkage" rather than "interaction." Certainly, the further the central control systems are traced rostrally, the less it is possible to distinguish between them, and the more "linkage" appears preferable to "interaction" as the appropriate descriptive term.

Such arguments might lead one to question the utility of attempting to trace the central pathways of ventilatory and cardiovascular reflex arcs and to define the precise location and mechanism of central and reflex interactions. They also appear to refute the suggestion that the ventilatory networks of the medulla play a dominant role in ventilatory–cardiovascular integration, inferring instead that a common pattern is imposed on both systems. Nevertheless, the presence of respiratory rhythms in the cardiovascular motor outflows from the medulla and spinal cord, combined with the pronounced central inspiratory modulation of cardiovascular reflexes, suggests that for all practical purposes the central respiratory networks are dominant. Hence, even allowing for the possibility that integration depends more on the complexity of the links between medullary relay neurons than on the exclusive character of their individual inputs, there seems at present to be no alternative but to search the brainstem for specific sites of interaction along the central pathways. In the present chapter we adhere to this more conventional view.

The mechanisms by which central inspiratory drive and baroreceptor and pulmonary stretch receptor input interact to influence vagal cardiomotor output have been investigated in some detail. The little that is known about the corresponding central and reflex interactions with sympathetic cardiovascular motoneuron output suggests that the interactive effects on vagal cardiomotor output serve as a paradigm for the medullary integration of the ventilatory and cardiovascular control systems as a whole.

Integration Within the Nucleus of the Solitary Tract

Termination of Sensory Inputs

The sites of termination of afferent fibers originating in the lungs and cardiovascular system were first delineated by tracing degenerating axons after the appropriate peripheral nerve had been sectioned; more recent studies have employed neuronal tracer substances such as horseradish peroxidase or labeled amino acids. Terminations of axons of the vagus, aortic depressor, and carotid sinus nerves were found to be generally confined to the nucleus of the tractus solitarius and its immediate vicinity, although endings were also identified in other brainstem nuclei of secondary importance (for references, see ref. 4). Detailed analysis of these central projections is complicated by the fact that each of the three nerves contains axons from more than one type of sensory receptor. The termination of afferents of known function has been explored only recently, in electrophysiological studies using antidromic mapping techniques (4). Extracellular recordings have been made from the cell bodies of single afferent fibers in the nodose (Xth) and petrosal (IXth) ganglia of cats and rabbits, the type of afferent being deduced from the pattern of activity and the response to ventilatory or cardiovascular maneuvers. The central sites of termination of individual slowly and rapidly adapting pulmonary stretch receptors, arterial baroreceptors, and carotid chemoreceptors have been identified by serial microstimulation of their axons within the brainstem.

These studies provide some evidence of topographical organization of the different types of afferent within the nucleus tractus solitarius. However, there is also much overlapping of central terminals—a feature that could provide the anatomical substrate for ventilatory–cardiovascular interactions within the nucleus. Most investigators report that slowly adapting pulmonary stretch receptors project ipsilaterally, mainly to the medial subnucleus of the solitary tract, with a less dense projection to lateral and ventrolateral subnuclei (5,6). The projection of rapidly adapting receptors is distinct from, and significantly more caudal than, that of slowly adapting receptors, with the densest innervation being to the ventral parts of the medial subnucleus and to both the ipsi- and contralateral commissural nuclei (7). Carotid chemoreceptors terminate predominantly in the medial, dorsomedial, and commissural subnuclei of the solitary tract, with a much less dense innervation of the lateral regions (8). By contrast, baroreceptor afferents from the aortic arch or carotid sinus project mainly to the lateral subnuclei on the ipsilateral side, with less dense projections to the medial and commissural regions of the nucleus (8,9).

The terminals of superior laryngeal nerve afferents and other pulmonary afferents traveling in the vagus nerve appear to be restricted mainly to the nucleus tractus solitarius, and both vagal and sympathetic cardiac afferents project to this nucleus (10,11). The precise sites of termination of these afferents have not yet been determined.

Presynaptic Interactions

Interaction between the central terminals of pulmonary and cardiovascular afferents, leading to a decrease in the amount of transmitter released by one set of terminals (presynaptic depolarization), is a possible mechanism for ventilatory–cardiovascular integration. Indeed, axo-axonal synapses, which form the anatomical basis of such presynaptic interactions, have been demonstrated by electron microscopy in parts of the nucleus tractus solitarius (12). Such inhibitory presynaptic interactions have been shown to occur between the terminals of slowly adapting stretch receptors and those of superior laryngeal nerve afferents in the solitary tract nucleus (13,14), and they have been confirmed by direct intracellular recordings from the stretch receptor terminals (15). However, baroreceptor afferents do not appear to be subject to a presynaptic ventilatory influence (13,15)—either from pulmonary afferents or from central inspiratory neurons—even though the cardiac effects of both baroreceptor and chemoreceptor stimulation are clearly inhibited by central inspiratory drive and by feedback from slowly adapting stretch receptors (16,17). This suggests that the ventilatory modulation of baroreceptor and chemoreceptor reflex bradycardia occurs at a later site along the reflex pathway.

Postsynaptic Interactions

The respiratory modulation of vagal cardiomotor output could be explained by convergence of excitatory input (e.g., from arterial baroreceptors) and inhibitory input (e.g., from central inspiratory drive and pulmonary stretch receptors) upon relay neurons in the solitary tract nucleus. However, the balance of evidence from studies involving extracellular recording from solitary tract neurons during stimulation of the aortic depressor, carotid sinus, and vagus nerves suggests that convergence in the solitary nucleus proper is rare, and that when convergence does occur it is only between excitatory inputs (for references, see ref. 4). In one such study, afferent inputs were engaged more selectively by stimulating the central cut ends of small cardiac and pulmonary vagal branches in the thorax (18). Results indicated that although some solitary tract neurons received convergent inputs from cardiac and pulmonary afferents, the inputs were segregated according to conduction velocity, so that myelinated and nonmyelinated fibers never converged on the same neuron. This observation may have important implications for reflex interactions.

The degree of convergent interaction on a given neuron may be seriously underestimated by extracellular recordings, however, especially when interactive effects are subliminal or inhibitory. More substantial evidence has been obtained in experiments involving intracellular recordings (19,20). Although it remains clear from these more sophisticated studies that solitary tract neurons receiving convergent inputs from aortic, carotid sinus, and vagal afferent fibers are not in the majority, convergence does occur. Moreover, similar interactions may occur at neurons outside the solitary tract proper (for references, see ref. 4). Nevertheless, investigators who were successful in recording intracellularly from large numbers of solitary tract neurons could find no evidence that either central inspiratory drive or volume-related feedback from pulmonary stretch receptors inhibited the activity of solitary tract neurons receiving excitatory input from carotid sinus nerve afferents (20). Again, this suggests that the major ventilatory modulation of cardiovascular reflexes occurs relatively late in the central reflex pathway.

Integration in the Vicinity of Vagal Cardiomotor Neurons

Extracellular and intracellular recordings from vagal cardiomotor neurons in cats and rabbits provide unequivocal evidence of ventilatory and cardiovascular interaction at the level of the motoneurons themselves (for references, see refs. 21 and 22). In anesthetized cats and rabbits, species commonly used for recording central nervous activity, vagal tone is low or absent, so that vagal motoneurons with ongoing activity are rare and may not be representative of the population of vagal cardiomotor neurons as a whole. Attempting to obtain a more representative sample, Spyer and co-workers (23–25) recorded activity from neurons that were excited antidromically by electrical stimulation of the cardiac vagal branches. Such cardiac vagal motoneurons were located in the nucleus ambiguus of the cat and in both the nucleus ambiguus and dorsal vagal nucleus of the rabbit. The motoneurons received a bilateral excitatory input from the aortic and carotid sinus baroreceptors, which was manifest either as a pulsatile rhythm in the few neurons that discharged spontaneously or as an evoked discharge in response to electrical stimulation of the aortic or carotid sinus nerves in otherwise inactive neurons. Feedback from pulmonary stretch receptors was kept at a minimum in these experiments by ventilating the lungs rapidly at small tidal volumes, so that central inspiratory rhythm was dissociated from the cycling of the respiratory pump.

Iontophoretic application of excitant amino acids was used to raise neuronal excitability and cause otherwise silent cells to discharge. At all levels of excitability the neurons were found to maintain a central respiratory rhythm, firing predominantly or exclusively in the expiratory phase. Not only were they rarely active in inspiration, they were often unaffected by stimulation of the aortic or carotid sinus nerves during this phase of the ventilatory cycle. However, when the activity of the cardiomotor neurons was increased by further application of excitant amino acids, a pulse-related rhythm was present during both inspiration and expiration, and stimulation of the carotid sinus nerve was now effective in inspiration. This suggests that although vagal cardiac motoneurons receive barore-

ceptor signals throughout the respiratory cycle, they are normally subject to a phasic inhibition by central inspiratory drive, which decreases their excitability during inspiration and acts as a final gate that blocks baroreflex bradycardia during this phase of the cycle.

This hypothesis is supported by the results of experiments in which the membrane events underlying the phasic changes in vagal cardiomotor activity were demonstrated by intracellular recordings (26). These showed that vagal cardiomotor neurons are relatively hyperpolarized in inspiration and, in addition, are relatively depolarized (and may fire action potentials) in the immediate postinspiratory phase. The inspiratory waves of hyperpolarization were converted to waves of depolarization by Cl^- injection, confirming that the cells received inhibitory input during central inspiration. Membrane input resistance was at a minimum in inspiration, thus decreasing the effectiveness of any excitatory input, including that from baroreceptors and chemoreceptors, during this phase of the cycle. Input resistance increased to a maximum in the immediate postinspiratory phase.

The inhibitory influence of inspiration on vagal cardiomotor neurons was explored further in experiments in which multibarreled glass micropipettes were used to record neuronal activity extracellularly during iontophoresis of various transmitter agonists and antagonists (27). Acetylcholine, as well as the inhibitory amino acids gamma-aminobutyric acid (GABA) and glycine, inhibited the motoneurons, the inhibitory effects being antagonized by atropine, bicuculline, and strychnine, respectively (27). Moreover, the ongoing activity of the vagal cardiomotor neurons was increased by atropine and bicuculline, suggesting a tonic release of acetylcholine and GABA in the vicinity of the cells. These two transmitter antagonists had somewhat different effects, however, the respiratory modulation of neuronal activity being abolished by atropine but unaffected by bicuculline.

Thus, vagal cardiomotor neurons appear to receive at least two tonically active inhibitory inputs: one related to central inspiratory drive and mediated by muscarinic acetylcholine receptors, the other of nonrespiratory origin and mediated by GABA receptors. The neurons may also receive an excitatory input from propriobulbar postinspiratory neurons that discharge in the immediate postinspiratory period (see ref. 22).

The central sites at which pulmonary stretch receptor input interacts with baroreceptor and chemoreceptor reflex arcs to inhibit vagal cardiomotor output have not yet been determined. Indirect evidence from reflex studies in cats suggests that the action of stretch receptor feedback is proximal to the motoneuron, because the inhibitory influence of lung inflation on cardiovascular reflex bradycardia varies with the origin of the reflex (28). Thus, compared with the bradycardia obtained with lungs at end-expiratory volume, a moderate lung inflation reduced chemoreceptor-evoked bradycardia by 83%, baroreceptor-evoked bradycardia by 44%, and cardiac receptor-evoked bradycardia by 12%; it had no effect at all on the vagal bradycardia induced by chemical stimulation of pulmonary C fibers (see below). It seems reasonable to conclude, therefore, that although pulmonary stretch receptor input exerts its major inhibitory action on the central pathways of cardiovascular reflexes distal to the nucleus of the solitary tract (20), it does not act directly on the cardiomotor neurons themselves. These reflex inhibitory effects of pulmonary stretch receptors appear to be less pronounced than those of central inspiratory drive (17).

Respiratory Modulation of Sympathetic Outflow

That sympathetic nerve activity commonly has a pronounced respiratory rhythm, activity being maximal in inspiration, was first noted more than 50 years ago by Adrian et al. (29). By the same token, the vasomotor effects of the baroreceptor reflex vary with the phase of respiration, baroreflex vasodilation being most pronounced in expiration (30). The temporal relationship between impulse activity in sympathetic nerve branches and central inspiratory drive (assessed from the phrenic neurogram) has been analyzed in several recent studies, in most of which the feedback from slowly adapting pulmonary stretch receptors was eliminated by cutting the vagus nerves. A majority of sympathetic cardiomotor (31) and vasoconstrictor fibers, including those in the cervical and renal sympathetic nerves (31,32) and in skin and skeletal muscle nerves (33), discharge maximally in time with central inspiratory drive. The remaining sympathetic cardiomotor and vasoconstrictor fibers either discharge maximally in expiration or do not display any respiratory rhythm at all. The inspiratory modulation of the majority of fibers is followed by a sharp decrease in discharge in the immediate postinspiratory phase (31,32). A similar temporal relationship has been observed between central inspiratory discharge and the activity of sympathetic preganglionic neurons in the upper thoracic spinal cord (34,35) and of sympathetic premotor neurons in the subretrofacial nucleus of the medulla (36).

The abrupt postinspiratory decrease in discharge is a relatively constant feature of spinal sympathetic neurons that discharge maximally in inspiration, and also of the corresponding medullary sympathetic premotor neurons (36). It is thought by some to be evidence of an active inhibition by propriobulbar postinspiratory neurons (for discussion, see refs. 31 and 35). It is tempting to regard this phasic excitatory–inhibitory modulation of sympathetic motor and premotor neu-

rons as a mirror image of the inhibitory–excitatory changes demonstrated by intracellular recordings from vagal cardiomotor neurons (26).

Reflex experiments in dogs have shown that the central inspiratory drive to cardiac sympathetic motoneurons contributes to the inspiratory suppression of baroreceptor and chemoreceptor reflex bradycardia (37). They have also shown that, whereas input from pulmonary stretch receptors reinforces the inhibitory effects of central inspiratory drive on vagal cardiomotor output, it opposes the effects of central inspiratory drive on sympathetic vasomotor tone (for references, see ref. 1). Most exeriments designed to examine the central coupling between inspiratory events and sympathetic neuronal activity have been carried out in vagotomized animals. In a study in which the vagus nerves were left intact, Lipski et al. (34) observed an increase in the antidromic response latency of 8 of 13 spinal sympathetic neurons during normal tidal lung inflation, suggesting the phasic operation of a reflex inhibitory feedback. Nevertheless, this feedback has somewhat complex effects in its interaction with other reflex inputs. Thus, increasing feedback from pulmonary stretch receptors can overcome the vasoconstriction evoked by stimulating carotid chemoreceptors, but not that evoked by the unloading of arterial baroreceptors (38). Again this suggests that pulmonary stretch receptor input interacts with cardiovascular reflex arcs at sites proximal to the final common path.

INTEGRATED RESPONSES
FROM ROSTRAL BRAIN AREAS

Integrated changes in ventilatory and cardiovascular function can be evoked by electrical or pharmacological stimulation of many sites outside the brainstem, but only a brief account can be given here. The cerebellum has been suggested as a possible site for such extramedullary integration (39), although the patterns of ventilatory and cardiovascular response evoked by stimulating cerebellar sites vary widely with experimental circumstances and are difficult to interpret in functional terms. Complex patterns of ventilatory–cardiovascular response of a thermoregulatory nature are organized in the preoptic region of the anterior hypothalamus (40). The central and peripheral pathways for integrated thermoregulatory responses are beyond the scope of the present chapter; they are reviewed in detail by Hensel (41).

It has been known for many years that coupled ventilatory and cardiovascular responses can be evoked by electrical stimulation of the cerebral cortex. The distribution of these cortical areas is described by Kaada (42), who summarizes the early studies. Descending pathways from cortex to medulla have a powerful influence on the medullary control networks and, in addition, produce somatic and behavioral effects. For example, electrical or chemical activation of a longitudinal strip of neurons stretching from the level of the amygdala through the hypothalamus and midbrain to the medulla can evoke a stereotyped combination of effects called an "alerting" or "defense" response, which comprises (if the animal is unanesthetized) defensive behavior, with pupillary dilation and piloerection on the back and tail, accompanied by hyperventilation, increases in arterial blood pressure and heart rate, and vasoconstriction in most vascular beds but vasodilation in the hind limb. The defense response evoked from a small area of the perifornical hypothalamus within this general region, known as the "hypothalamic defense area," has been particularly well studied (for references, see ref. 43).

In contrast, stimulation of the orbitoinsulotemporal and anterior cingulate cortex often evokes a "playing dead" reaction, characterized by cessation of movement, reduction in skeletal muscle tone, and apparent analgesia, accompanied by apnea in expiration and profound bradycardia (see refs. 42 and 43). Kaada (42) has called these cortical regions "vagal zones" because they receive projections of the vagus nerve, and because the ventilatory and cardiovascular components of the "playing dead" reaction resemble those evoked by stimulating vagal afferents. A transitory response that is similar in many respects to the "playing dead" reaction is evoked in anesthetized animals when pulmonary C fibers are stimulated by injection of chemicals into the right atrium (44,45).

All mammalian species are thought to be capable of responding to threatening situations with either an alerting or a "playing dead" reaction, the type of response apparently depending on how the threat is perceived. In conscious animals, "playing dead" or "fear paralysis" occurs most often in threatening situations that appear inescapable. The response is reduced by habituation and is therefore more common in young animals, although in some species (e.g., rabbit) it prevails throughout adult life.

The descending pathways by which output from these suprapontine mechanisms affect the medullary networks controlling ventilatory and cardiovascular output have been studied only for the defense response. Stimulation of the defense area affects ventilation by both direct and indirect pathways to medullary respiratory neurons (46). It inhibits nucleus tractus solitarius neurons that receive baroreceptor inputs (47), and it activates sympathetic premotor neurons in the ventrolateral medulla (48). There is also evidence that axons from the defense area project to sympathetic preganglionic neurons in the spinal cord (49). The excitability of cardiovascular motor neurons

may also be influenced by cortically evoked changes in central inspiratory drive, by mechanisms described above.

Finally, stimulation of sites in the posterior hypothalamus (the "subthalamic locomotor region") and the mesencephalon can elicit organized locomotor activity and matching ventilatory and cardiovascular adjustments. These sites are thought to engage the central pathways for the exercise response (50,51), which will be discussed below.

INTEGRATED RESPONSES INVOLVING PERIPHERAL REFLEX MECHANISMS

Afferent nerve endings that signal mechanical and chemical changes in the ventilatory and cardiovascular systems themselves play a vital part in ventilatory–cardiovascular integration. In fish, mechanoreceptors in the gill arches provide feedback related to gill movement; in mammals, low-threshold stretch receptors provide feedback related to cyclic changes in lung volume. In both fish and mammals, arterial baroreceptors and chemoreceptors signal changes in arterial blood pressure and blood gases: In fish these sensory endings are associated with gill arch arteries, and in mammals they are associated with the surviving remnants of the branchial arch arteries.

Afferents arising from the ventilatory and cardiovascular systems are of two main types: those subserving regulatory reflexes and those subserving protective or defensive reflexes. Regulatory reflexes are subject to a continuous input from low-threshold sensory endings whose impulse frequency increases and decreases as their stimulus (e.g., pressure or volume) varies around a control or resting setpoint. Reflexes triggered by slowly adapting pulmonary stretch receptors and arterial baroreceptors clearly fall into this category. Defense reflexes, on the other hand, are triggered by input from nerve endings whose activity is sparse or even absent under normal conditions but increases in response to potentially harmful stimuli. A variety of sensory nerve endings that innervate all levels of the respiratory tract of mammals subserve protective airway reflexes, and they trigger dramatic combinations of ventilatory and cardiovascular effects. Afferents subserving protective reflexes include endings of nonmyelinated fibers (C fibers) in the intrathoracic airways and endings in the upper airways, larynx, nares, and muzzle area. Reflexes involving arterial chemoreceptors could be included in either category. Although chemoreceptor activity in mammals at sea level is relatively low under normal conditions, small changes in firing above and below the baseline level appear to exert a measurable influence on ventilation; in this sense, carotid chemoreceptors have a regulatory function. Chemoreceptor activity increases greatly, however, and provides a strong reflex drive to ventilation in hypoxia and asphyxia, which are only occasional hazards for most mammals; in this sense, chemoreceptors have a protective function.

For most of the interactions discussed here, only the input and output segments of the reflex arcs have been investigated, but results of even this partial analysis give some indication of the complexity of the interactions at the level of the medulla. The integrative effects of input from the respiratory tract on the cardiovascular system must be considered in terms of the specific sensory inputs that evoke them, because the motor outputs to the heart and resistance vessels are engaged in different combinations according to the type of airway afferent involved and the level of the respiratory tract from which the input arises. These integrative effects are also influenced by the activity of the central respiratory networks. In addition, not only does sensory input from lung mechanoreceptors influence the operation of the baroreceptor reflex, but baroreceptor input influences ventilation. Finally, although carotid chemoreceptors exert powerful reflex effects on the cardiovascular system, the expression of these effects is influenced by central respiratory activity and by secondary reflexes from the respiratory tract; moreover, the carotid chemoreflex potentiates the cardiovascular effects of certain airway reflexes.

In considering the integrated responses involving peripheral reflex mechanisms, we deal almost exclusively with afferent inputs traveling in the cranial nerves. Input from the respiratory tract (including the larynx) and from the arterial chemoreceptors and baroreceptors reaches the brainstem in the IXth and Xth cranial nerves; input from the nares and muzzle region travels in the Vth cranial nerve. Nevertheless, integrated ventilatory and cardiovascular responses can also be triggered by sensory input from the heart, lungs, and intrathoracic blood vessels that travels in sympathetic nerve branches to the spinal cord. In general, this spinal visceral input has received less attention than the corresponding input in the cranial nerves, and less is known about its significance, although the sensation of pain from cardiovascular structures has been shown to depend on the integrity of this spinal pathway (11). Nociceptive input in somatic sensory nerves can also evoke integrated patterns of ventilatory and cardiovascular response, which, again, are often associated with the sensation of pain. Input from thermal receptors in the skin also evokes integrated responses (41). Finally, afferent input from exercising muscle contributes to the accompanying changes in ventilatory and cardiovascular function. Space permits us to deal only with the last of these spinal inputs.

Cardiovascular Effects Associated with Pulmonary Stretch Receptor Input

By far, the greatest volume of input traveling to the brainstem in the vagus nerves originates in slowly adapting pulmonary stretch receptors. Their rhythmic waxing and waning discharge evoked by the normal volume excursions of the lung has conspicuous effects not only on breathing and bronchomotor tone (see Chapters 5.4.8 and 5.1.2.1.2) but also on the cardiovascular system: An increase in pulmonary stretch receptor input promotes a combination of tachycardia and systemic vasodilation, and it modulates the operation of both baroreceptor and chemoreceptor reflexes.

Effects on Heart Rate

That stimulation of slowly adapting pulmonary stretch receptors evokes tachycardia has been confirmed repeatedly, both by moderate lung inflation from zero transpulmonary pressure and by electrical stimulation of the cut central end of pulmonary vagal branches at the threshold intensity for ventilatory changes. In 1860, Einbrodt (see ref. 1) showed that ventilation of the lungs at high transpulmonary pressures (25–30 mmHg) evoked bradycardia, an effect now known to be due to stimulation of lung C fibers (see below). In 1871, Hering (see ref. 1) found that inflation with more moderate pressures caused tachycardia, and he concluded that tachycardia was evoked by the receptors responsible for the inflation-inhibitory "selbeststeuerung" reflex. The tachycardia is attributed entirely to inhibition of vagal cardiomotor tone; it is not accompanied by positive inotropic effects (52).

The inspiratory increase in stretch receptor discharge in each ventilatory cycle causes a phasic inhibition of vagal cardiomotor output (provided that this output is initially high) and adds a reflex component to sinus arrhythmia (17,53). Phasic input from pulmonary stretch receptors also contributes to the inspiratory-phase-related inhibition of baroreceptor and chemoreceptor reflex bradycardia (16,17,54). When the cardiac component of the arterial baroreflex is assessed in human subjects by the neck suction method, the reflex effects on heart period are examined during the expiratory phase, often during a brief voluntary breath-holding at functional residual capacity (55). Even though central inspiratory drive might be expected to increase during breath-holding, the concomitant reduction of pulmonary stretch receptor input allows a significant potentiation of the bradycardic response.

Effects on Vascular Resistance

Although input from pulmonary stretch receptors reinforces the effects of central inspiratory drive on heart rate, it opposes the effects of central inspiratory drive on peripheral vascular resistance. Thus, stretch receptors inhibit sympathetic vasoconstrictor output, whereas central inspiratory drive excites it (see above). That large lung inflations caused reflex systemic vasodilation was known for many years. Evidence for major involvement of slowly adapting stretch receptors was lacking, however, until Daly et al. (56) showed, in dogs whose systemic circulation was perfused at constant flow, that sympathetic α-adrenergic vasoconstrictor tone decreased when the lungs were inflated by small increments of pressure between zero and a few cmH_2O and increased when pressure was reduced. Sympathetic tone was also reduced when the lungs were inflated cyclically at increasing tidal volumes in the eupneic range. Since the vasodilation was abolished by denervating the lungs, it was reflex in origin. Since slowly adapting stretch receptors are the only pulmonary afferents whose impulse discharge would increase and decrease within these volume ranges, their input must have been responsible. The vasodilation involved cutaneous, splanchnic, and muscle vascular beds, but it had the net effect of redistributing cardiac output in favor of voluntary muscle—a response that could be beneficial in exercise (57).

During normal breathing there is little doubt that the vasoconstrictor influence of central inspiratory drive predominates; sympathetic preganglionic vasoconstrictor discharge increases in inspiration, and a voluntary deep breath causes vasoconstriction in the fingers and forearm of human subjects (see ref. 33). Thus although stimulation of pulmonary stretch receptors in anesthetized animals was found to inhibit the inspiratory increase in sympathetic vasoconstrictor output, this effect was thought to be largely a consequence of reflex inhibition of central inspiratory activity (58). Even so, when ventilation is stimulated reflexly by engagement of carotid body chemoreceptors, the resulting increase in pulmonary stretch receptor input overcomes the combined vasoconstrictor influence of central inspiratory drive and the chemoreceptors themselves, thus promoting vasodilation as well as tachycardia (59). When the systemic circulation of dogs was artificially perfused with asphyxic blood, the primary reflex cardiovascular effects of carotid body stimulation (bradycardia and systemic vasoconstriction—see below) occurred only if the lungs were kept at expiratory volume. When stretch receptors were activated by phasic lung inflation, the cardiovascular responses to chemoreceptor stimulation were no longer apparent, and the net effects were tachycardia and vasodilation. Inhibition of α-adrenergic vasoconstrictor output continued for as long as feedback from stretch receptors in the artificially ventilated lungs remained intact (59). This combination of tachycardia and vasodilation would promote an increase in blood flow to match the increase in ventilation. The reflex vasodilator action of pulmonary stretch receptors is not invariably prepotent, however, because increasing stretch receptor input has little effect on the vasoconstriction evoked when arterial baroreceptors are unloaded (38).

Arterial Baroreceptor–Ventilatory Interactions

Just as ventilatory inputs have reflex cardiovascular effects, so sensory inputs from the cardiovascular system can influence respiratory control mechanisms. It was known for many years that abrupt increases in systemic arterial pressure inhibit breathing and airway smooth muscle tone, but, because large changes in pressure appeared to be required to evoke the inhibitory effects, their physiological significance was uncertain. Recently, however, changes in carotid sinus pressure within the range of commonly observed arterial pressure fluctuations have been found, in anesthetized dogs, to have measurable reflex effects on ventilation and bronchomotor tone. Thus, relatively small reductions of sinus pressure caused respiratory frequency to increase and tidal volume to decrease, with an overall increase in minute ventilation (60). In addition, small stepwise increases and decreases in carotid sinus pressure above and below the normal setpoint have been shown to induce reciprocal changes in tracheal smooth muscle tone, in addition to the conventional effects on arterial blood pressure and heart rate (61). Carotid baroreceptors were subsequently found to exert a corresponding inhibitory influence on total lung resistance. When sinus pressure was held at normotensive levels, cooling the carotid sinus nerves to block baroreceptor input caused an increase in tracheal tone. Taken together, these experiments provide clear evidence that arterial baroreceptors exert a tonic inhibitory influence on ventilation and bronchomotor tone at normal levels of arterial blood pressure. Although the functional significance of these baroreceptor–ventilatory reflexes remains obscure, they are yet another example of the close coupling between cardiovascular and ventilatory control during the operation of regulatory reflexes.

Cardiovascular Responses Associated with Defense Reflexes from the Lower Airways

The afferent vagal input responsible for triggering defense reflexes from the lower airways and lungs is carried predominantly in nonmyelinated C fibers (conduction velocities of less than 2.5 m/sec). Although nonmyelinated afferent fibers greatly outnumber myelinated ones in the pulmonary and bronchial branches of the vagus nerve and their endings are distributed throughout the intrathoracic airways, their total input to the medullary centers under normal conditions is extremely low. When stimulated, these respiratory C fibers evoke reflex responses involving close interaction between ventilatory and cardiovascular control systems—having marked effects not only on breathing, bronchomotor tone, and bronchosecretion but also on heart rate and vascular tone (62).

C fibers whose endings are immediately accessible to chemicals injected into the bronchial circulation have been designated "bronchial C fibers," and those closer to the gas-exchange region, immediately accessible to chemicals injected into the pulmonary circulation, have been designated "pulmonary C fibers" (63). Pulmonary C fibers are probably responsible for the potent cardiovascular depressor effects evoked by stimuli applied to the lungs. Brodie and Russell (64) showed that a profound bradycardia and systemic vasodilation were evoked either by administering irritant chemicals directly to the intrapulmonary airways or by injecting them into the pulmonary circulation; similar effects were obtained by stimulating the central ends of fine vagal branches ("alveolar nerves") at the lung roots. In fact, the reflex cardiac effects of stimulating pulmonary C fibers were indicated even earlier by Einbrodt's observation that bradycardia could be evoked by large lung inflations.

Electroneurographic studies in dogs and cats have established that pulmonary C fibers are indeed polymodal in character, and that the C fibers stimulated promptly by injection of chemicals into the pulmonary circulation are also stimulated by large inflations of the lungs (62). The inflation threshold pressure for the afferent response is approximately 10 cmH$_2$O, which is similar to the threshold pressure for the cardiac depressor effects. The cardiovascular effects of stimulating pulmonary C fibers by large lung inflations have been studied in open-chest dogs, in which one lung was vascularly isolated and inflated at transpulmonary pressures of up to 30 cmH$_2$O (for references, see ref. 65). In these preparations, unilateral lung inflation evoked bradycardia, decreased cardiac contractility, decreased cardiac output, and peripheral vasodilation. [Although rapidly adapting airway receptors with myelinated fibers are also stimulated by large lung inflations, their reflex cardiovascular influence, if any, is unknown. It is certain, however, that they do not evoke vasodilation. Thus lung deflation or collapse, which is a strong and selective stimulus to rapidly adapting receptors, causes vasoconstriction, not vasodilation (56).]

When irritant chemicals such as capsaicin are injected into the right atrium or pulmonary artery, pulmonary C fibers are stimulated and evoke a characteristic combination of ventilatory and cardiovascular effects known as the "pulmonary chemoreflex." Such injections evoke a combination of bradycardia, systemic hypotension, and apnea, followed by prolonged rapid, shallow breathing (for references, see ref. 62). The bradycardia may involve several seconds of complete asystole followed by variable periods of atrioventricular (A-V) conduction block; it is accompanied by a negative inotropic effect. The vascular effects include reflex withdrawal of sympathetic α-adrenergic vasoconstrictor tone in abdominal viscera, skin, and hind limb muscle (66,67). Stimulation of pulmonary C fibers also evokes a profound and widespread depression of the somatic motor system, manifest as a loss of voluntary muscle tone and an inhibition of spinal reflexes (44,45,65).

This combination of effects, evoked by bolus injections of irritant chemicals into the pulmonary circulation, may seem no more than a pharmacological curiosity or the evolutionary survival of a primitive, protective reflex. In fish, whose respiratory exchange surface is more immediately accessible to the environment, an equivalent of the pulmonary chemoreflex, including apparent loss of muscle tone, can be produced by adding chemical irritants to the surrounding water (68). In mammals, chemical threats to the respiratory exchange surface proper must be relatively rare outside the laboratory, although they may occur on exposure to toxic gases. Inhalation of a single breath of cigarette smoke through a tracheal tube in dogs stimulates pulmonary C fibers (69) and produces the combined ventilatory and cardiovascular effects of the pulmonary chemoreflex (70).

The reflex vasodilator influence of pulmonary C fibers extends to the coronary circulation, and an active reflex coronary vasodilation can be evoked in anesthetized dogs by injection of capsaicin into the right atrium (71,72). The effects are abolished by denervation of the lung. In this case, withdrawal of sympathetic vasoconstrictor tone is only a minor factor, the major effect being by activation of the vagal muscarinic coronary vasodilator pathway first described by Feigl (for references, see ref. 71). Although there can be no doubt that autoregulation is the prevailing mechanism by which coronary blood flow increases, this reflex mechanism was found to be surprisingly effective even at low coronary perfusion pressures and in the presence of considerable metabolic vasodilation (71).

Stimulation of bronchial C fibers can also cause bradycardia: Indeed, selective engagement of bronchial C fibers by delivery of bradykinin aerosols to the lower airways sometimes evokes a dramatic decrease in heart rate (73). In general, however, effects of bronchial C fibers on the cardiovascular system are weaker than those of pulmonary C fibers (62). Thus, selective stimulation of bronchial C fibers by injection of small doses of bradykinin into the bronchial circulation can have marked excitatory effects on airway smooth muscle and submucosal gland secretion, with only minor effects on heart rate. There is little or no evidence that bronchial C fibers evoke reflex changes in vasomotor tone. Bronchial C fibers have a higher threshold to inflation and are stimulated less consistently than pulmonary C fibers by inflation, but with very large inflations they may contribute to the resulting bradycardia (62,65).

Cardiovascular Responses Associated with Defense Reflexes from the Upper Airways

Sneezing, coughing, and laryngeal spasm, accompanied by bronchoconstriction and increased airway secretion, are the immediate ventilatory responses that protect the upper airways from the entry of liquids, solid particles, or irritant gases. Other disturbances can also occur, accompanied by characteristic changes in cardiovascular function. Thus, chemical or mechanical stimulation of the nasal passages or larynx often evokes a combination of apnea, bradycardia, and systemic vasoconstriction (for references, see ref. 1). The initial apnea and bradycardia are comparable to those of the pulmonary chemoreflex, but when breathing resumes it is slow and deep rather than rapid and shallow; moreover, effects on sympathetic vasoconstrictor outflow are opposite in sign. The afferent input from the nasal passages travels in the maxillary branch of the trigeminal nerve, and that from the larynx travels in the superior laryngeal branch of the vagus nerve; both myelinated and nonmyelinated afferent fibers are probably involved. Since the reflex ventilatory and cardiovascular responses to stimulation of these two upper-airway sensory areas have important features in common, they will be considered together (74). Cardiac effects are due to increased vagal cardiomotor discharge and are abolished by atropine. Although cardiac output decreases, arterial pressure may change very little because of the compensating vasoconstriction. Blood flow in splanchnic, cutaneous, and muscle vascular beds decreases, but flow in the carotid artery is well maintained (75). The combination of reflex ventilatory and cardiovascular responses to stimulation of the upper airways bears a strong resemblance to the immediate reflex effects of underwater immersion, and studies of the reflex responses to stimulation of the nose and larynx are thought to throw light on the ventilatory and cardiovascular reflex phenomena of breath-hold diving (for references, see ref. 76).

Even though this combination of ventilatory and cardiovascular responses is undoubtedly protective in origin, effects are not always benign. Bradycardia and variable changes in arterial pressure evoked by clinical manipulations in the nasal cavities and larynx have sometimes led to cardiovascular collapse and even death (for references, see ref. 74). The reflexes are conveniently studied in anesthetized animals by passing water at room temperature through the nares or larynx (74), and in this way the neural interactions that lead to severe cardiac depression have been identified. The reflex bradycardia evoked by nasal or laryngeal stimulation is a function of the reflex apnea, being supported not only by cessation of central inspiratory drive but also by withdrawal of phasic input from slowly adapting stretch receptors. In the laboratory the bradycardia can be terminated by rapidly inflating the lungs during the period of apnea, and it is significantly less if upper-airway defense reflexes are evoked while the lungs are artificially ventilated. However, if apnea is prolonged and results in asphyxia, the bradycardia may be potentiated by input from carotid body chemoreceptors (see below). It has been suggested that such potentiation of vagal cardiomotor activity may be responsible for lethal arrhythmias leading to crib deaths in infants (74). In these circumstances, restoration of breathing movements can be lifesaving, by increasing pulmonary stretch receptor input and inhibiting vagal cardiomotor effects.

Cardiovascular Effects of Arterial Chemoreceptors

The carotid body chemoreceptors represent a special case in reflex ventilatory and cardiovascular interactions, because although they have powerful effects on each system, the effects are manifest in different circumstances (reviewed in ref. 77). The cardiovascular effects of stimulating carotid chemoreceptors are best demonstrated by injecting cyanide into a carotid artery or by perfusing the carotid bodies with hypoxic blood in animals whose lungs are ventilated at constant rate and tidal volume. Reflex decreases in heart rate and cardiac contractility result from increasing vagal and decreasing sympathetic cardiomotor activity (78,79). Systemic vascular resistance increases, with a reduction of blood flow in the splanchnic and limb vascular beds (59,78). There is, in addition, a vagal muscarinic vasodilation of the coronary vascular bed (80,81).

Aortic chemoreceptors also evoke systemic vasoconstriction. They have little, if any, effect on ventilation, and their influence on heart rate is disputed, some investigators reporting that selective stimulation causes bradycardia, others tachycardia (for references, see refs. 77 and 82). However, the location of the aortic bodies makes them difficult to investigate.

The bradycardia and systemic vasoconstriction of the carotid chemoreceptor reflex are rarely seen in freely breathing mammals (although there are some species differences) and are not seen in human subjects (77,82). Bradycardia can be evoked briefly in spontaneously breathing dogs when the chemoreceptors are stimulated abruptly by bolus injections of cyanide into the carotid artery, but it is not pronounced unless the injection is delivered in expiration, a phase at which the stimulus has little effect on ventilatory drive (54). If, instead of being exposed to a brief stimulus, the isolated carotid bodies are perfused with hypoxic blood, the resulting reflex hyperventilation increases pulmonary stretch receptor input, which causes reflex tachycardia and systemic vasodilation (59,77,78).

Integrated Responses at High Altitude

Emphasis on the role of the carotid chemoreceptors in the hyperventilation of hypoxia has led to neglect of their role in cardiovascular regulation. The reflex hyperpnea of high-altitude hypoxia activates a secondary reflex from pulmonary stretch receptors that contributes to the masking of primary carotid chemoreflex effects on the cardiovascular system. This secondary reflex serves a useful function at high altitude, because any influence that would reduce cardiac output would be prejudicial to survival. In most mammalian species, systemic hypoxia increases heart rate and cardiac output and reduces peripheral resistance. Moreover, the primary cardiovascular effects of the carotid chemoreflex are opposed, not only by feedback from pulmonary stretch receptors but also by the effects of local hypoxia on the heart and resistance vessels (for references, see ref. 82).

Diving Reflexes

Major cardiovascular reflex effects attributable to input from carotid chemoreceptors are seen only when the central drive to breathing is suppressed. For example, if prolonged apnea is evoked by passing water through the nasal cavities or larynx or by stimulating the central end of the superior laryngeal nerve, excitation of carotid-body chemoreceptors by injection of cyanide greatly accentuates the vagal bradycardia but fails to stimulate ventilation (74,83). This vagal cardiodepressor effect is much greater than could be accounted for by the additive effects of upper-airway and carotid-body stimulation, and asystole may last for many seconds. Potentiation of the vagal cardiomotor component of nasal and laryngeal reflexes by carotid body input is particularly striking in diving mammals (84).

In diving and underwater swimming, the suppression of central inspiratory drive is triggered by input from sensory receptors in the muzzle region. In these circumstances, carotid chemoreceptor effects on the cardiovascular system become prepotent and represent vital physiological adjustments (for references, see ref. 76). When ventilation is arrested, chemore-

ceptor reflex bradycardia and muscarinic vasodilation of the coronary vessels protect cardiac function in the face of dwindling oxygen supplies, and chemoreceptor reflex vasoconstriction helps to preserve those oxygen supplies for the most essential vascular circuits. The cardiovascular effects of carotid body stimulation are pronounced in diving mammals, and in harbor seals the bradycardia of simulated dives is abolished if the carotid bodies are perfused with blood of high arterial O_2 and normal CO_2 content (85). The reflex bradycardia appears to be crucial to survival, because during simulated dives seals rapidly succumb if the bradycardia is abolished by atropine (82).

Integrated Responses in Exercise

Integration of ventilatory and cardiovascular activity with metabolic demand is vital if the constancy of the respiratory gases in blood and interstitial fluid is to be maintained. These integrative mechanisms have been studied repeatedly in muscular exercise, and it is clear that the link between exercise and the matching changes in ventilation and circulation involves both descending central drive and peripheral reflex input. Investigators have gone to considerable lengths to show that both central and peripheral integrative mechanisms are effective when engaged in isolation. Arguments as to the relative importance of central and peripheral mechanisms in the integrated ventilatory and cardiovascular responses to exercise appear to be fruitless, especially since it is very likely that other ventilatory and cardiovascular reflex mechanisms contribute to the fine-tuning of these integrated responses.

The presence of a "central drive" to breathing, heart rate, and arterial pressure that is proportional to conscious muscular effort and independent of feedback from contracting muscles has been demonstrated in humans (86). A central drive has also been demonstrated in cats during spontaneous exercise (walking or running on a treadmill) and during the muscular movements produced by electrical stimulation of the subthalamic locomotor region of the hypothalamus (50). In the latter experiments the combination of locomotor, ventilatory, and cardiovascular changes was clearly the result of stimulating hypothalamic relay cells on the descending pathway from the motor cortex (rather than the result of stimulating fibers of passage), because similar effects were produced by injecting the GABA antagonist picrotoxin into the same region. Effects were shown to be independent of feedback from contracting muscles.

The presence of a sustained peripheral drive to breathing, heart rate, and arterial pressure originating in the exercising muscles has been demonstrated in anesthetized cats in which the cut peripheral ends of ventral nerve roots (L7–S1) were stimulated electrically (87). The cardiovascular response includes an increase in cardiac contractility and a decrease in blood flow to resting muscle, skin, and gut (for references, see ref. 88). The ventilatory and cardiovascular effects are abolished by cutting the dorsal roots supplying the exercising muscle.

Input from the sensory receptors responsible for these integrated effects is transmitted to the spinal cord in small myelinated fibers and C fibers (groups III and IV afferents, respectively), the magnitude of the input correlating well with the degree of muscle contraction (89). Group III afferents are mechanoreceptors that signal the force of contraction; group IV afferents are stimulated by metabolites released by ischemic muscle. Both groups are stimulated in a concentration-dependent fashion by small increases in interstitial potassium, but the significance of this effect to the integrated reflex responses is unclear, because it adapts rapidly.

CONCLUSIONS

Integration of ventilatory and cardiovascular function is accomplished with great flexibility by numerous groups of neurons between cortex and medulla, as well as by a series of complex ventilatory and cardiovascular reflex interactions. Our understanding of the mechanisms underlying this integration is based necessarily on studies of isolated components in anesthetized animals; hence, results must be interpreted with caution. Studies of interactions at the level of the medullary control networks provide a clear description of the central mechanism of sinus arrhythmia. The site at which central inspiratory neurons inhibit vagal cardiomotor output and influence the vagal motor pathways of the baroreceptor and chemoreceptor reflexes has been identified, and the role of acetylcholine as the central inhibitory transmitter has been established. The mechanism by which central inspiratory neurons increase sympathetic cardiomotor and vasoconstrictor output has been investigated less fully, but the evidence obtained so far suggests that it is the excitatory counterpart of the mechanism by which these neurons modulate vagal output.

Reflex interactions have been studied more extensively. They often give rise to integrated patterns of response with obvious functional utility. Thus when ventilation increases in exercise or at high altitude the augmented input from pulmonary stretch receptors has a beneficial influence on cardiovascular function. Recent studies by Daly and others provide a clue to the central sites of this reflex interaction, although the medullary neurons and transmitters have not been identified. In diving and underwater swimming the reflex inhibition of central inspiratory drive and the reflex excitation of sympathetic vasoconstrictor output combine to reduce cardiac function and constrict nonessential vascular circuits, an integrated response that is crucial to survival. The central pathways are unknown. Other examples of integrated ventilatory–cardiovascular responses appear, by contrast, to be in the nature of temporizing reactions to potentially harmful events. Such responses include the combination of apnea, bradycardia, and vasoconstriction evoked as a first line of defense from the upper airways when gas exchange is threatened by inhalation of solids and liquids, and the profoundly depressor pulmonary chemoreflex evoked when nociceptive stimuli threaten the respiratory exchange surface itself. Again, the central pathways remain to be explored.

The links between ventilatory and cardiovascular control are most evident in exercise. Experimental simulation of exercise in humans and anesthetized animals has shown that the two control systems are linked by paths descending from the cortex and by reflex input to the spinal cord. These central and reflex mechanisms are independently effective, suggesting a redundancy of integrative mechanisms—a redundancy not uncommon in physiological control systems. Until we understand the underlying organizational principles, however, it seems more prudent to consider this duplication of mechanisms as a reflection of the functional importance of the integrative response and as a means of ensuring that the interactions between ventilation and cardiovascular function in exercise are accomplished smoothly.

REFERENCES

1. Daly M de B. Interactions between respiration and circulation. In: Cherniack NS, Widdicombe JG, eds. *Handbook of physiology, Section 3: The respiratory system, vol II—Control of breathing, Part 2.* Bethesda, MD: American Physiological Society, 1986;529–594.
2. Satchell GH. The reflex co-ordination of the heart beat with respiration in the dogfish. *J Exp Biol* 1960;37:719–731.
3. Koepchen HP. Respiratory and cardiovascular "centres": functional entirety or separate structures? In: Schlafke ME, Koepchen HP, See WR, eds. *Central neurone environment.* Berlin: Springer-Verlag, 1983;221–237.
4. Jordan D, Spyer KM. Brainstem integration of cardiovascular and pulmonary afferent activity. *Prog Brain Res* 1986;67:295–314.
5. Donoghue S, Garcia M, Jordan D, Spyer KM. The brain-stem projections of pulmonary stretch afferent neurones in cats and rabbits. *J Physiol (Lond)* 1982;322:353–363.
6. Berger AJ, Averill DB. Projection of single pulmonary stretch receptors to solitary tract region. *J Neurophysiol* 1983;49:819–830.
7. Davies RO, Kubin L. Projection of pulmonary rapidly adapting receptors to the medulla of the cat: an antidromic mapping study. *J Physiol (Lond)* 1986;373:63–86.
8. Donoghue S, Felder RB, Jordan D, Spyer KM. The central projections of carotid baroreceptors and chemoreceptors in the cat: a neurophysiological study. *J Physiol (Lond)* 1984;347:397–409.
9. Donoghue S, Garcia M, Jordan D, Spyer KM. Identification and

brain-stem projections of aortic baroreceptor afferent neurones in nodose ganglia of cats and rabbits. *J Physiol (Lond)* 1982; 322:337–352.

10. Kalia M, Mesulam MM. Brain stem projections of sensory and motor components of the vagus complex in the cat. II. Laryngeal, tracheobronchial, pulmonary, cardiac and gastrointestinal branches. *J Comp Neurol* 1980;193:467–508.

11. Foreman RD, Blair RW. Central organization of sympathetic cardiovascular response to pain. *Annu Rev Physiol* 1988;50:607–622.

12. Kalia M, Richter D. Morphology of physiologically identified slowly adapting lung stretch receptor afferents stained with intra-axonal horseradish peroxidase in the nucleus of the tractus solitarius of the cat. II. An ultrastructural analysis. *J Comp Neurol* 1985;241:521–535.

13. Rudomin P. Presynaptic inhibition induced by vagal afferent volleys. *J Neurophysiol* 1967;30:964–981.

14. Barillot J-C. Depolarisation presynaptique des fibres sensitives vagales et laryngees. *J Physiol (Paris)* 1970;62:273–294.

15. Richter DW, Jordan D, Ballantyne D, Meesmann M, Spyer KM. Presynaptic depolarization in myelinated vagal afferent fibres terminating in the nucleus of the tractus solitarius in the cat. *Pflugers Arch* 1986;406:12–19.

16. Koepchen HP, Wagner P-H, Lux HD. Uber die Zusammenhange zwischen zentraler Erregbarkeit, reflektorischem Tonus und Atemrhythmus bei der nervosen Steuerung der Herzfrequenz. *Pflugers Arch* 1961;273:443–465.

17. Potter EK. Inspiratory inhibition of vagal responses to baroreceptor and chemoreceptor stimuli in the dog. *J Physiol (Lond)* 1981;316:177–190.

18. Bennett JA, Goodchild CS, Kidd C, McWilliam PN. Neurones in the brain stem of the cat excited by vagal afferent fibres from the heart and lungs. *J Physiol (Lond)* 1985;369:1–15.

19. Donoghue S, Felder RB, Gilbey MP, Jordan D, Spyer KM. Postsynaptic activity evoked in the nucleus tractus solitarius by carotid sinus and aortic nerve afferents in the cat. *J Physiol (Lond)* 1985;360:261–273.

20. Mifflin SW, Spyer KM, Withington-Wray DJ. Baroreceptor inputs to the nucleus tractus solitarius in the cat: postsynaptic actions and the influence of respiration. *J Physiol (Lond)* 1988; 399:349–367.

21. Jordan D, Spyer KM. Central neural mechanisms mediating respiratory–cardiovascular interactions. In: Taylor EW, ed. *Neurobiology of the cardiorespiratory system.* Manchester: Manchester University Press, 1987;322–341.

22. Spyer KM, Jordan D. Electrophysiology of the nucleus ambiguus. In: Hainsworth R, McWilliam PN, Mary DASG, eds. *Cardiogenic reflexes.* Oxford: Oxford University Press, 1987;237–249.

23. McAllen RM, Spyer KM. Two types of vagal preganglionic motoneurones projecting to the heart and lungs. *J Physiol (Lond)* 1978;282:353–364.

24. McAllen RM, Spyer KM. The baroreceptor input to cardiac vagal motoneurones. *J Physiol (Lond)* 1978;282:365–374.

25. Jordan D, Khalid MEM, Schneiderman N, Spyer KM. The location and properties of preganglionic vagal cardiomotor neurones in the rabbit. *Pflugers Arch* 1982;395:244–250.

26. Gilbey MP, Jordan D, Richter DW, Spyer KM. Synaptic mechanisms involved in the inspiratory modulation of vagal cardio-inhibitory neurones in the cat. *J Physiol (Lond)* 1984;356:65–78.

27. Jordan D, Gilbey MP, Richter DW, Spyer KM, Wood LM. Respiratory–vagal interactions in the nucleus ambiguus of the cat. In: Bianchi AL, Denavit-Saubie M, eds. *Neurogenesis of central respiratory rhythm.* Lancaster: MTP Press, 1985;370–378.

28. Daly M de B, Kirkman E. Differential modulation by pulmonary stretch afferents of some reflex cardioinhibitory responses in the cat. *J Physiol (Lond)* 1989;417:323–341.

29. Adrian ED, Bronk DW, Phillips G. Discharges in mammalian sympathetic nerves. *J Physiol (Lond)* 1932;74:115–153.

30. Seller H, Langhorst P, Richter D, Koepchen HP. Uber die Abhangigkeit der pressoreceptorischen Hemmung des Sympathicus von der Atemphase und ihre Auswirkung in der Vasomotorik. *Pflugers Arch* 1968;302:300–314.

31. Bainton CR, Richter DW, Seller H, Ballantyne D, Klein JP. Respiratory modulation of sympathetic activity. *J Auton Nerv Syst* 1985;12:77–90.

32. Preiss G, Kirchner F, Polosa C. Patterning of sympathetic preganglionic neuron firing by the central respiratory drive. *Brain Res* 1975;87:363–374.

33. Janig W, Sundlof G, Wallin BG. Discharge patterns of sympathetic neurons supplying skeletal muscle and skin in man and cat. *J Auton Nerv Syst* 1983;7:239–256.

34. Lipski J, Coote JH, Trzebski A. Temporal patterns of antidromic invasion latencies of sympathetic preganglionic neurons related to central inspiratory activity and pulmonary stretch receptor reflex. *Brain Res* 1977;135:162–166.

35. Gilbey MP, Numao Y, Spyer KM. Discharge patterns of cervical sympathetic preganglionic neurones related to central respiratory drive in the rat. *J Physiol (Lond)* 1986;378:253–265.

36. McAllen RM. Central respiratory modulation of subretrofacial bulbospinal neurones in the cat. *J Physiol (Lond)* 1987;388:533–545.

37. Davis AL, McCloskey DI, Potter EK. Respiratory modulation of baroreceptor and chemoreceptor reflexes affecting heart rate through the sympathetic nervous system. *J Physiol (Lond)* 1977;272:691–703.

38. Daly M de B, Ward J, Wood LM. Modification by lung inflation of the vascular responses from the carotid body chemoreceptors and other receptors in dogs. *J Physiol (Lond)* 1986;378:13–30.

39. Bradley DJ, Pascoe JP, Paton JFR, Spyer KM. Cardiovascular and respiratory responses evoked from the posterior cerebellar cortex and fastigial nucleus in the cat. *J Physiol (Lond)* 1987;393:107–121.

40. Pleschka K, Kuhn P, Nagai M. Differential vasomotor adjustments in the evaporative tissues of the tongue and nose in the dog under heat load. *Pflugers Arch* 1979;382:255–262.

41. Hensel H. *Thermoreception and temperature regulation.* New York: Academic Press, 1981.

42. Kaada BR. Cingulate, posterior orbital, anterior insular and temporal pole cortex. In: Field J, Magoun HW, Hall VE, eds. *Handbook of physiology, Section 1: Neurophysiology, vol II.* Washington, DC: American Physiological Society, 1960;1345–1372.

43. Jordan D. Autonomic changes in affective behavior. In: Loewy AD, Spyer KM, eds. *Central regulation of autonomic functions.* Oxford: Oxford University Press. 1990;in press.

44. Ginzel KH, Eldred E, Sasaki Y. Comparative study of the actions of nicotine and succinylcholine on the monosynaptic reflex and spindle afferent activity. *Int J Neuropharmacol* 1969;8:515–533.

45. Paintal AS. The mechanism of excitation of type J receptors, and the J reflex. In: Porter R, ed. *Breathing: Hering–Breuer centenary symposium.* London: Churchill, 1970;59–71.

46. Ballantyne D, Jordan D, Spyer KM, Wood LM. Synaptic rhythm of caudal medullary expiratory neurones during stimulation of the hypothalamic defence area of the cat. *J Physiol (Lond)* 1988;405:527–546.

47. Mifflin SW, Spyer KM, Withington-Wray DJ. Baroreceptor inputs to the nucleus tractus solitarius in the cat: modulation by the hypothalamus. *J Physiol (Lond)* 1988;399:369–387.

48. Lovick TA, Smith PR, Hilton SM. Spinally projecting neurones near the ventral surface of the medulla in the cat. *J Auton Nerv Syst* 1984;11:27–33.

49. Saper CB, Loewy AD, Swanson LW, Cowan WM. Direct hypothalamoautonomic connections. *Brain Res* 1976;117:305–312.

50. Eldridge FL, Millhorn DE, Kiley JP, Waldrop TG. Stimulation by central command of locomotion, respiration and circulation during exercise. *Respir Physiol* 1985;59:313–337.

51. Mitchell JH. Cardiovascular control during exercise: central and reflex neural mechanisms. *Am J Cardiol* 1985;55:34D–41D.

52. Greenwood PV, Hainsworth R, Karim F, Morrison GW, Sofola OA. Reflex inotropic responses of the heart from lung inflation in anaesthetized dogs. *Pflugers Arch* 1980;386:199–205.

53. Anrep GV, Pascual W, Rossler R. Respiratory variations of the heart rate. II. The central mechanism of the respiratory arrhythmia and the interrelations between the central and the reflex mechanisms. *Proc R Soc Lond [Biol]* 1936;119:218–230.

54. Gandevia SC, McCloskey DI, Potter EK. Inhibition of baro-

receptor and chemoreceptor reflexes on heart rate by afferents from the lungs. *J Physiol (Lond)* 1978;276:369–381.

55. Hainsworth R, Al-Shamma YMH. Cardiovascular responses to stimulation of carotid baroreceptors in healthy subjects. *Clin Sci* 1988;75:159–165.

56. Daly M de B, Hazzledine JL, Ungar A. The reflex effects of alterations in lung volume on systemic vascular resistance in the dog. *J Physiol (Lond)* 1967;188:331–351.

57. Daly M de B, Robinson BH. An analysis of the reflex systemic vasodilator response elicited by lung inflation in the dog. *J Physiol (Lond)* 1968;195:387–406.

58. Gerber U, Polosa C. Effects of pulmonary stretch receptor afferent stimulation on sympathetic preganglionic neuron firing. *Can J Physiol Pharmacol* 1978;56:191–198.

59. Angell-James JE, Daly M de B. Cardiovascular responses in apnoeic asphyxia: role of arterial chemoreceptors and the modification of their effects by a pulmonary vagal inflation reflex. *J Physiol (Lond)* 1969;201:87–104.

60. Brunner MJ, Sussman MS, Greene AS, Kallman CH, Shoukas AA. Carotid sinus baroreceptor reflex control of respiration. *Circ Res* 1982;51:624–636.

61. Schultz HD, Pisarri TE, Coleridge HM, Coleridge JCG. Carotid sinus baroreceptors modulate tracheal smooth muscle tension in dogs. *Circ Res* 1987;60:337–345.

62. Coleridge JCG, Coleridge HM. Afferent vagal C fibre innervation of the lungs and airways and its functional significance. *Rev Physiol Biochem Pharmacol* 1984;99:1–110.

63. Coleridge HM, Coleridge JCG. Impulse activity in afferent vagal C-fibres with endings in the intrapulmonary airways of dogs. *Respir Physiol* 1977;29:125–142.

64. Brodie TG, Russell AE. On reflex cardiac inhibition. *J Physiol (Lond)* 1900;26:92–106.

65. Kaufman MP, Cassidy SS. Reflex effects of lung inflation and other stimuli on the heart and circulation. In: Scharf SM, Cassidy SS, eds. *Heart–lung interactions in health and disease.* New York: Marcel Dekker, 1989;339–363.

66. Brender D, Webb-Peploe MM. Vascular responses to stimulation of pulmonary and carotid baroreceptors by capsaicin. *Am J Physiol* 1969;217:1837–1845.

67. Cassidy SS, Ashton JH, Wead WB, Kaufman MP, Monsereenusorn Y, Whiteside JA. Reflex cardiovascular responses caused by stimulation of pulmonary C-fibers with capsaicin in dogs. *J Appl Physiol* 1986;60:949–958.

68. Satchell GH. The J reflex in fish. In: Paintal AS, Gill-Kumar P, eds. *Respiratory adaptations, capillary exchange and reflex mechanisms.* Delhi: University of Delhi, 1977;432–441.

69. Lee L-Y, Kou YR, Frazier DT, et al. Stimulation of vagal pulmonary C-fibers by a single breath of cigarette smoke in dogs. *J Appl Physiol* 1989;66:2032–2038.

70. Lee L-Y, Beck ER, Morton RF, Kou YR, Frazier DT. Role of bronchopulmonary C-fiber afferents in the apneic response to cigarette smoke. *J Appl Physiol* 1987;63:1366–1373.

71. Clozel JP, Roberts AM, Hoffman JIE, Coleridge HM, Coleridge JCG. Vagal chemoreflex coronary vasodilation evoked by stimulating pulmonary C-fibers in dogs. *Circ Res* 1985;57:450–460.

72. Ordway GA, Pitetti KH. Stimulation of pulmonary C fibres decreases coronary arterial resistance in dogs. *J Physiol (Lond)* 1986;371:277–288.

73. Coleridge HM, Coleridge JCG, Roberts AM. Rapid shallow breathing evoked by selective stimulation of airway C fibres in dogs. *J Physiol (Lond)* 1983;340:415–433.

74. Angell-James JE, Daly M de B. Some aspects of upper respiratory tract reflexes. *Acta Otolaryngol (Stockh)* 1975;79:242–252.

75. Angell-James JE, Daly M de B. Reflex respiratory and cardiovascular effects of stimulation of receptors in the nose of the dog. *J Physiol (Lond)* 1972;220:673–696.

76. Butler PJ, Jones DR. The comparative physiology of diving in vertebrates. *Adv Comp Physiol Biochem* 1982;8:179–364.

77. Daly M de B, Ward J, Wood LM. The peripheral chemoreceptors and cardiovascular-respiratory integration. In: Taylor EW, ed. *Neurobiology of the cardio-respiratory system.* Manchester: Manchester University Press, 1987;342–368.

78. Daly M de B, Scott MJ. An analysis of the primary cardiovascular reflex effects of stimulation of the carotid body chemoreceptors in the dog. *J Physiol (Lond)* 1962;162:555–573.

79. Hainsworth R, Karim F, Sofola OA. Left ventricular inotropic responses to stimulation of carotid body chemoreceptors in anaesthetized dogs. *J Physiol (Lond)* 1979;287:455–466.

80. Hackett JG, Abboud FM, Mark AL, Schmid PG, Heistad DD. Coronary vascular responses to stimulation of chemoreceptors and baroreceptors. Evidence for reflex activation of vagal cholinergic innervation. *Circ Res* 1972;31:8–17.

81. Ito BR, Feigl EO. Carotid chemoreceptor reflex parasympathetic coronary vasodilation in the dog. *Am J Physiol* 1985;249:H1167–H1175.

82. Coleridge JCG, Coleridge HM. Chemoreflex regulation of the heart. In: Berne RM, ed. *Handbook of physiology, Section 2: The cardiovascular system, vol I—The heart.* Bethesda, MD: American Physiological Society, 1979;653–676.

83. Daly M de B, Korner PI, Angell-James JE, Oliver JR. Cardiovascular–respiratory reflex interactions between carotid bodies and upper-airways receptors in the monkey. *Am J Physiol* 1978;234:H293–H299.

84. Elsner R, Angell-James JE, Daly M de B. Carotid body chemoreceptor reflexes and their interactions in the seal. *Am J Physiol* 1977;232:H517–H525.

85. Daly M de B, Elsner R, Angell-James JE. Cardiorespiratory control by carotid chemoreceptors during experimental dives in the seal. *Am J Physiol* 1977;232:H508–H516.

86. Goodwin GM, McCloskey DI, Mitchell JH. Cardiovascular and respiratory responses to changes in central command during isometric exercise at constant muscle tension. *J Physiol (Lond)* 1972;226:173–190.

87. McCloskey DI, Mitchell JH. Reflex cardiovascular and respiratory responses originating in exercising muscle. *J Physiol (Lond)* 1972;224:173–186.

88. Mitchell JH, Kaufman MP, Iwamoto GA. The exercise pressor reflex: cardiovascular effects, afferent mechanisms, and central pathways. *Annu Rev Physiol* 1983;45:229–242.

89. Kaufman MP, Rybicki KJ. Discharge properties of group III and IV muscle afferents: their responses to mechanical and metabolic stimuli. *Circ Res* 1987;61(Suppl):I-60–I-65.

THE LUNG: Scientific Foundations
edited by R.G. Crystal, J.B. West et al.
Raven Press, Ltd., New York © 1991.

CHAPTER 5.4.11

Periodic Breathing

Michael C. K. Khoo

The purpose of this chapter is to review the current state of our knowledge about (a) periodic breathing (PB) and (b) the stability of ventilatory control. This is an area that has received substantial input from engineering science (particularly the fields of control theory and signal analysis). A substantial portion of the chapter is thus devoted to elucidating the concepts and quantitative methodology that allow us to understand in detail why and how oscillatory behavior arises in certain conditions. Methods for characterizing ventilatory oscillations are surveyed, and the relationship between PB and apnea is also examined. Since length restrictions do not permit a truly comprehensive treatise on such a rich subject, we recommend that the reader refer also to a number of reviews that have appeared in the literature recently (1–3).

CLINICAL DESCRIPTION

PB is characterized by repetitive cyclic variations in minute ventilation, such that periods of hyperpnea alternate with periods of hypopnea or apnea on a fairly predictable basis. In classical Cheyne–Stokes respiration (CSR), which may be regarded as an exaggerated form of PB, apnea is generally present during the hypopneic phases. In CSR, the breathing phase that follows the end of an apnea contains breaths that gradually wax and wane in amplitude until the next period of apnea occurs (1,4). In another form of PB, commonly referred to as "cluster breathing," the apnea in each cycle ends with a large breath that is greater in amplitude than, or comparable to, the breaths that follow. The duration of the apnea is usually longer than the breathing phase—unlike CSR, where the opposite

occurs. This pattern has also been termed "Biot periodic breathing" (5). However, it should be cautioned that, in some reports (4,6), "Biot breathing" is used synonymously with ataxic breathing, which is characterized by breath clusters and relatively long apneas with no definite periodicity. At the other end of the spectrum, one may include the following in a broad definition of PB: periodic fluctuations in ventilation and breathing pattern that are not immediately apparent unless analyzed with signal processing techniques (7–12).

The ventilatory fluctuations in PB are accompanied by dynamic changes in blood gases and several cardiovascular and neurologic parameters. During the hyperpneic phases, arterial P_{CO_2} (Pa_{CO_2}) peaks while arterial O_2 saturation (Sa_{O_2}) and pH attain their lowest values; the reverse situation occurs during the apneic or hypopneic phases (13,14). Cardiac output and cerebral blood flow oscillate in phase, whereas heart rate fluctuations occur out of phase, with the changes in ventilation (15). Cardiac arrhythmias generally occur during the hyperpneic phase of CSR; during the apneic phase, signs of neurologic depression are often present (15). However, the accompanying changes in systemic blood pressure are variable: Blood pressure may increase or decrease during apnea (16). PB can be abolished by CO_2 inhalation or administration of respiratory stimulants, such as theophylline and caffeine (15). In most cases, inhalation of hyperoxic mixtures can also eliminate PB. However, there have been reports that ventilatory fluctuations or apnea persists in patients with cardiovascular ailments (17) and in normals during sleep (18). It has also been observed that O_2 administration can prolong the duration of the associated apneas (19).

UNDERLYING MECHANISMS

Uncertainty surrounding the causal relationships between the fluctuations in ventilation during CSR and

M. C. K. Khoo: Biomedical Engineering Department, University of Southern California, Los Angeles, California 90089.

the associated variations in several cardiorespiratory parameters has fueled substantial debate over the pathogenesis of this phenomenon since the late nineteenth century. Broadly speaking, one may divide the postulated mechanisms for PB into three categories. These are individually examined below.

Cardiovascular Factors

The earliest accounts of CSR emphasized the close association between this form of disordered breathing and heart disease (16). The observation of concomitant fluctuations in blood pressure led Pembrey (20) to the hypothesis that delays in the transport of oxygenated blood from the lungs to the brain were responsible for CSR. Klein (21) showed that circulation times in patients with CSR were approximately twice as long as those found in normals. Subsequently, Pryor (22) also found prolonged circulation times in patients with congestive heart failure who exhibited CSR. Guyton et al. (23) induced CSR in anesthetized dogs by artificially lengthening the carotid arteries and thus prolonging the heart-to-brain transport delay. However, only one-third of their animals developed CSR spontaneously despite the imposition of extremely long circulation times that ranged from 2 to 5 minutes. It is therefore possible that CSR was induced in these animals as a direct result of neurologic damage caused by this highly invasive intervention.

Severe hypotension induced in animal preparations has been shown to produce oscillations in blood pressure; these are commonly referred to as "Mayer waves," which lead to respiratory oscillations (24,25). These blood pressure oscillations and concomitant oscillations in phrenic discharge may persist despite the elimination of blood gas fluctuations through artificial ventilation (24). These results indicate that an instability in baroreflex control can affect respiratory control as well.

Neurogenic Factors

The earliest report of CSR by Cheyne documented the presence of both heart disease and brain lesions. Traube (26) suggested that diminished blood flow to the brain, whether or not this resulted from heart failure, produced CSR through a reduction in medullary sensitivity. However, failed attempts at inducing CSR through medullary damage led Marckwald (27) to conclude that the respiratory fluctuations reflected an intrinsic oscillation generated within the brainstem reticular formation. Subsequent studies (14,28,29) pointed to associations between CSR and a wide variety of supramedullary lesions, found anywhere from the cortical regions of the cerebral hemispheres down

to the pons. Thus, it has been hypothesized that PB results from the unmasking of a central oscillator which is normally inhibited by supramedullary influences. This belief is supported by the study of Preiss et al. (24), in which phrenic oscillations in anesthetized, paralyzed cats persisted despite the abolition of ventilatory, blood gas, and blood pressure fluctuations.

Significant increases in the ventilatory sensitivity to CO_2 and the apneic threshold for CO_2 were reported in patients with chronic neurologic lesions who exhibited CSR (14,30). Brown and Plum (14) postulated that the increased chemosensitivity was responsible for the hyperventilatory phases of CSR, whereas the elevated apneic threshold allowed posthyperventilation apnea to occur subsequent to the hyperpneic phase. Later, North and Jennett (31) found elevated apneic thresholds but failed to detect any significant change in chemosensitivity in patients with acute brain damage and CSR.

Instability in Respiratory Control

Plum and Leigh (32) have contended that the frequent association of prolonged circulatory delay with CSR does not necessarily imply a direct causal relationship. To support this argument, they cite the small incidence of CSR in patients with advanced rheumatic heart disease, in which circulation time is increased but little neurologic damage is found. In their previous studies (14,33), the authors noted that the patients with heart disease who exhibited CSR also had some form of neurologic damage. On the other hand, results from other studies have not supported this association between cardiovascular disease and neurologic abnormality (34).

Observations of PB in healthy subjects cannot be completely accounted for by either the "cardiogenic" or "neurogenic" theories. The frequent occurrence of PB in healthy mountaineers, particularly during sleep, was initially reported by Mosso (35). This observation has been confirmed by subsequent studies performed at various levels of acclimatization (8,36–39). Douglas and Haldane (40), performing a number of experiments on themselves, showed that PB could be easily induced by forced hyperventilation or by rebreathing hypoxic gas that had been scrubbed of CO_2 content. PB has also been reported in normoxic healthy adults during sleep (18,41–45). Numerous studies have documented the appearance of PB in apparently healthy infants ranging in age from 1 day to 40 weeks (46,47).

Taken together, the preceding observations support the proposal by Douglas and Haldane (40) that PB is "a phenomenon analogous to the 'hunting' often produced by the governor of an engine; and what is remarkable is not that it should occur, but that its occurrence should be so unusual under normal conditions." The underlying notion is that arterial blood gases are constantly being regulated by a dynamic control system that, when perturbed sufficiently under certain conditions, can become unstable and exhibit oscillatory behavior. It is currently accepted that this instability hypothesis can account for most of the observations of PB in disease and health (1–3,15,46,47). Furthermore, the hypothesis establishes a common underlying mechanism for clinically defined PB and the ventilatory oscillations that are found in normal spontaneous breathing. In the sections that follow, the basic properties of control systems are summarized, and the conditions that can lead to oscillatory behavior are closely examined.

QUANTITATIVE ANALYSIS OF PERIODIC BREATHING

Homeostatic Regulation by Negative Feedback

Feedback plays a fundamental role in homeostasis at all levels in the hierarchy of biological processes (48–50). Since natural feedback systems are generally complex, an understanding of how negative feedback works is best achieved by first examining a simple technological control system. A common application of negative feedback may be found in the thermostat-based temperature control system of a home. This system may be broken down into three major components: (i) the heating/cooling device, which forms the controller and actuator for the system; (ii) the space within the building being heated/cooled, which represents the controlled system or "plant"; and (iii) the temperature sensor, which is the feedback element in this case. The temperature within the building is the variable being controlled here. The performance of this control system is based on how closely the temperature inside the building can be constrained to approximate the desired temperature that the occupant has set. This desired temperature represents the "set-point" of the control system.

Let us suppose that the desired temperature and the original temperature in the building are both 70°F. Warming of the building by the midday sun slowly raises the temperature inside. If the thermal sensor is not present or not functioning, the controller would have no means of "knowing" that the building temperature has changed; consequently, the cooling element would continue to remove heat at the same rate. Under such conditions, a control system is said to be operating without feedback and is referred to as an "open-loop" system. However, with the thermal sensor installed and functioning, the new temperature is

transduced into a voltage, which is "fed back" to the controller and compared to the set-point. The difference between actual and desired temperatures is converted into an increase in the actuating signal. As a result, the cooling element is driven harder and the rate of heat removal is increased. As the temperature change is halted and then reversed, the actuating signal and consequently the rate of heat removal are also adjusted. In this way, the effect of the external disturbance (i.e., heating by the sun) is offset by automatic adjustment of the input signal to the controller. Such a system is termed a "closed-loop" control system. Since the corrective action taken by the controller is opposite in direction to the effect of the external disturbance, this closed-loop system is said to operate with "negative" feedback. If the corrective action were to be carried out in the same direction as the effect of the disturbance (i.e., with "positive" feedback), the result would be a progressively unstable situation.

Homeostatic control of arterial blood gases is achieved through the chemoreflexes. The feedback sensors in this case are the chemoreceptors located in the medulla and the carotid bodies. The controller consists of (a) the respiratory center in the medulla and (b) the diaphragm and chest wall muscles, while the plant is composed of the lungs and body tissues. A rise in $P_{a_{CO_2}}$ is sensed by the chemoreceptors and then the information is relayed back to the controller, which corrects for the disequilibrium by increasing ventilation and consequently increasing the rate of elimination of CO_2.

Differences Between Engineering and Biological Control Systems

Although there are many similarities between the thermostat and the respiratory chemostat, there is a fundamental difference. In the former, there is an explicit set-point (e.g., 70°F) that is selected, depending on the comfort level desired by the user. In the respiratory system, there is no explicit reference input that the feedback signal may be compared to and no specific organ that is assigned the task of such a comparator. Instead, the operating equilibrium point is determined by the constraints exerted by the controller on the plant, and vice versa. To better understand this, let us consider the steady-state properties of the plant, which may be described mathematically by

$$PA_{CO_2} = k\dot{V}_{CO_2}/(\dot{V}_E - \dot{V}_D)$$ [1]

where $\dot{V}_{CO_2}$, $\dot{V}_E$, and $\dot{V}_D$ represent the metabolic production rate of CO_2, minute ventilation, and dead space ventilation, respectively, and k is a constant. The inverse proportionality between alveolar P_{CO_2}

(PA_{CO_2}) and $\dot{V}_E$ implies that PA_{CO_2} will be decreased by hyperventilation. On the other hand, the CO_2 controller behaves in the following way:

$$\dot{V}_E = H(Pa_{CO_2} - I) \qquad [2]$$

Here, as Pa_{CO_2} increases, ventilatory drive increases proportionately. The constant of proportionality, H, in this relationship represents the CO_2 response slope, while I reflects the apneic threshold. We will assume that PA_{CO_2} is equal to Pa_{CO_2} in the steady state. Since the controller and plant are coupled to each other, the steady-state operating values of $\dot{V}_E$ and PA_{CO_2} (or Pa_{CO_2}) must satisfy both Eq. 1 and Eq. 2. Thus, it is possible to compute these values by simultaneous solution of the above two equations.

Another feature that distinguishes a biological control system from an engineering control system is that the former usually contains nonlinear components. The gas exchanger represented by Eq. 1 is a simple example of a nonlinear component. Using calculus of variations, it can be deduced that the change in PA_{CO_2} (δPA_{CO_2}) that would accompany a small departure in $\dot{V}_E$ ($\delta \dot{V}_E$) from the equilibrium value is given by

$$\delta PA_{CO_2} = -k\dot{V}_{CO_2}\delta\dot{V}_E/(\dot{V}_E - \dot{V}_D)^2 \qquad [3]$$

Therefore, referring to the small change in PA_{CO_2} that would be produced by a small change in $\dot{V}_E$ as the gain of the plant, the magnitude of this gain, G, is given by the expression

$$G = k\dot{V}_{CO_2}/(\dot{V}_E - \dot{V}_D)^2 \qquad [4a]$$

By substituting Eq. 1 into Eq. 4a, we may rewrite the latter in the following form:

$$G = PA_{CO_2}^2/k\dot{V}_{CO_2} \qquad [4b]$$

In a similar way, it can be deduced that the controller gain, defined as the change in ventilatory drive produced by a small change in Pa_{CO_2}, is equal to H. Whereas the controller gain is constant, the gain of the nonlinear controlled system varies, depending on the values of $\dot{V}_E$ and PA_{CO_2} at which the control system is operating. Another important feature that should be noted from the above analysis is the negativity of the plant gain. This negativity means that an increase in ventilation would result in a decrease in PA_{CO_2}. Therefore, in contrast to the simple thermostat system, the negative feedback necessary for stable respiratory control is embedded in the inherent characteristics of the plant.

Stability Analysis of a Simple Dynamic Model

The analysis presented in the preceding section was highly simplistic in that attention was limited to only steady-state considerations. Dynamic properties and time delays were completely ignored. In the case of the respiratory control system, time lags are present in the process of gas exchange, the transmission of the humoral stimuli from the pulmonary capillaries to the sites of the chemoreceptors, the neural transmission and processing of the feedback information, and the activation of the respiratory muscles to produce airflow. As a step upwards in complexity, we perform a dynamic analysis that takes into consideration the most important delay: the time taken for blood to be transported from the lungs to the chemoreceptors. The model of respiratory control is schematized in Fig. 1. For simplicity, the "controller" now includes the chemoreceptors. Using a time scale based on breaths of uniform duration, we assume that the processes represented by the plant and controller take less than 1 breath for completion. Blood from the lungs takes N_D breaths to reach the chemoreceptors. Ventilation results from the summation of the chemoreflex-mediated ventilatory drive and a "nonchemical" drive, which incorporates all other extraneous influences (e.g., changes in the level of wakefulness, voluntary influences on breathing, and random phasic changes in drive).

Let us consider the effect of a transient ventilatory disturbance on the model shown in Fig. 1. A simple but realistic perturbation is a sigh. We can represent the effect of this disturbance on ventilation in the following way:

$$\delta\dot{V}_E(i) = \delta\dot{V}_c(i) + \delta\dot{V}_n(i) \qquad [5]$$

where $\delta\dot{V}_E(i)$, $\delta\dot{V}_c(i)$, and $\delta\dot{V}_n(i)$ represent the respective changes in ventilation, chemical drive, and nonchemical drive at the ith breath. To simulate the ventilatory effect of a sigh, $\delta\dot{V}_n(i)$ is assigned a positive value only at the first breath but set equal to zero in subsequent breaths. The change in ventilation produces a corresponding change in alveolar P_{CO_2}:

$$\delta PA_{CO_2}(i) = -G\delta\dot{V}_E(i) \qquad [6]$$

where G represents the magnitude of plant gain, which we will assume constant for this calculation. After a transport delay of N_D breaths, the change in alveolar P_{CO_2} is reflected by an equal change in arterial P_{CO_2} at the site of the chemoreceptors:

$$\delta Pa_{CO_2}(i + N_D) = \delta PA_{CO_2}(i) \qquad [7]$$

The controller responds to the change in arterial P_{CO_2} by altering chemical drive proportionally:

$$\delta\dot{V}_c(i + N_D) = H\delta Pa_{CO_2}(i + N_D) \qquad [8]$$

Using Eqs. 5 through 8, one can easily compute the time course of the changes produced by a sigh for given values of G, H, and N_D. Case 1 in Table 1 shows the results of such a computation for the situation where G, H, and N_D are assigned the values of 0.5, 1, and 2,

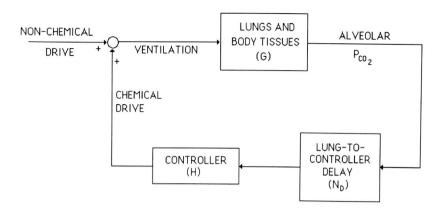

FIG. 1. Simplified closed-loop model of the respiratory chemoreflex system.

respectively. Initially (prior to breath no. 1), $\delta\dot{V}_E$ and δPA_{CO_2} are both zero, implying that the system is originally operating in a state of equilibrium. At breath no. 1, a sigh occurs, thereby increasing ventilation by 1000 (arbitrary) units. Applying Eq. 6, we find that the effect on the lungs is to lower PA_{CO_2} by 500 (arbitrary) units in the same breath. Since it takes 2 breaths for the change in PA_{CO_2} to appear as a change in Pa_{CO_2} at the chemoreceptors, the sigh does not affect the controller until breath no. 3, when the drop in Pa_{CO_2} is sensed by the chemoreceptors and produces a corresponding drop in $\dot{V}_E$, consistent with Eq. 8. This produces a rise in PA_{CO_2} of 500 units above the original equilibrium value, and this change consequently affects $\dot{V}_E$ another 2 breaths later. The calculation is repeated for several consecutive breaths. In this case, successive changes in $\dot{V}_E$ and PA_{CO_2} are progressively attenuated and the system eventually returns to its original equilibrium state.

In Case 2 of Table 1, the calculation is repeated with controller gain, H, doubled, but with no change in the other parameters. The increase in controller gain is sufficient to ensure that successive changes in $\dot{V}_E$ and PA_{CO_2} are not attenuated. Consequently, a sustained oscillation with periodicity of 4 breaths is produced. Case 3 shows that a sustained oscillation will also result if the plant gain magnitude (G) is doubled instead of controller gain. As in Case 2, the period of the oscillation is 4 breaths, which is twice as large as the lung-to-chemoreceptor delay.

TABLE 1. *Changes (shown in arbitrary units) in minute ventilation ($\delta\dot{V}_E$) and alveolar P_{CO_2} (δPA_{CO_2}) induced by a hyperventilatory breath in the closed-loop model of Fig. 1[a]*

Breath no.	Case 1		Case 2		Case 3		Case 4		Case 5	
	$\delta\dot{V}_E$	δPA_{CO_2}	$\delta\dot{V}_E$	δPA_{CO_2}	$\delta\dot{V}_E$	δPA_{CO_2}	$\delta\dot{V}_E$	δPA_{CO_2}	$\delta\dot{V}_E$	δPA_{CO_2}
1	1000	−500	1000	−500	1000	−1000	1000	−700	1000	−700
2	0	0	0	0	0	0	0	−210	0	−210
3	−500	250	−1000	500	−1000	1000	−700	427	0	−63
4	0	0	0	0	0	0	−210	275	0	−19
5	250	−125	1000	−500	1000	−1000	427	−216	−700	484
6	0	0	0	0	0	0	275	−257	−210	292
7	−125	63	−1000	500	−1000	1000	−216	74	−63	132
8	0	0	0	0	0	0	−257	203	−19	53
9	63	−31	1000	−500	1000	−1000	74	9	484	−323
10	0	0	0	0	0	0	203	−139	292	−302
11	−31	16	−1000	500	−1000	1000	9	−48	132	−183
12	0	0	0	0	0	0	−139	83	53	−92
13	16	−8	1000	−500	1000	−1000	−48	58	−323	199
14	0	0	0	0	0	0	83	−41	−302	271
15	−8	4	−1000	500	−1000	1000	58	−53	−183	209
16	0	0	0	0	0	0	−41	12	−92	127
17	4	−2	1000	−500	1000	−1000	−53	41	199	−101
18	0	0	0	0	0	0	12	4	271	−220
19	−2	1	−1000	500	−1000	1000	41	−28	209	−212
20	0	0	0	0	0	0	4	−11	127	−153

[a] Values are computed using Eqs. 5 through 9 in Cases 1, 2, and 3. In Cases 4 and 5, Eqs. 5, 7, 8, and 9 are used with damping index (b) set equal to 0.3. Controller and plant gains: (i) Case 1: $G = 0.5$, $H = 1$; (ii) Case 2: $G = 0.5$, $H = 2$; (iii) Case 3: $G = 1$, $H = 1$; (iv) Case 4: $G = 1$, $H = 1$; (v) Case 5: $G = 1$, $H = 1$. In all cases, N_D is set equal to 2, except Case 5 where N_D is 4.

The preceding calculations were performed for a highly idealized situation. Aside from the circulatory delay, the next most significant time lag would be that associated with CO_2 exchange in the lungs and tissues. Significant CO_2 stores exist in the alveolar spaces and tissues of the lungs. These present a damping effect on any abrupt ventilatory changes, and a finite time is necessary for the ventilatory change to be fully reflected in terms of a corresponding change in alveolar P_{CO_2}. To take this factor into account in our simple model, we substitute the following for Eq. 6:

$$\delta P_{ACO_2}(i) = b\delta P_{ACO_2}(i-1) - G(1-b)\delta\dot{V}_E(i) \quad [9]$$

where b represents a damping index, which increases as the degree of damping increases. Also, since $b = 0$ represents the case with no damping, Eq. 6 may be considered a special case of Eq. 9. Equation 9 implies that ventilatory changes at a given breath affect P_{ACO_2} not only in the same breath but in future breaths as well. As a result, changes in P_{ACO_2} will lag behind changes in $\dot{V}_E$.

The results for a situation similar to Case 3, where $G = 1$, $H = 1$, and $N_D = 2$, is presented as Case 4 (Table 1). The only difference here is the inclusion of damping with b set equal to 0.3. Whereas the previous case went into sustained oscillation, this case with damping results in an oscillation that decays in amplitude. Furthermore, it can be seen that the changes that occur here are considerably less abrupt than the changes shown in Table 1. The average period of the oscillation, deduced from consecutive ventilatory peaks or consecutive ventilatory troughs, is 4.5 breaths. This is 0.5 breath longer than the period exhibited by the same system without damping. Thus, damping exerts a stabilizing influence and also increases the effective time lag around the loop, thereby prolonging the period of the decaying oscillation.

In Case 5 (Table 1), the parameters (including b) are given the same values as Case 4, except that N_D is increased to 4 breaths. The sigh at breath no. 1 provokes a damped oscillation with an average period of 8.5 breaths. Careful analysis will reveal that the amplitude of one cycle to the next is reduced by 50%, which is less than the reduction of 60% demonstrated by Case 4. Therefore, although the same value of b is used in this calculation, the *effective* degree of damping achieved here is less than that exhibited by Case 4, where N_D is half as long. Thus, prolongation of the circulatory delay makes the system less stable.

The preceding calculations demonstrate a number of important points about closed-loop stability. Firstly, stability is affected not only by changes in controller gain but also by changes in plant gain. Secondly, feedback regulation often results in "hunting" or oscillatory behavior as the controller attempts to correct for deviations from an existing equilibrium point. However, the corrective action occurs too late; instead of offsetting the original disturbance, the corrective action itself creates one. Thirdly, because of the importance of timing, shorter delays enhance stability in a closed-loop system.

Loop Gain and System Stability

In Cases 2 and 3 (Table 1), which show sustained oscillation, a common feature may be noted. In both instances, the product of the controller gain and magnitude of plant gain equals 1. On the other hand, in Case 1 (where the system is stable), this product is less than 1. The product of the gains of all components in the loop of a closed-loop control system is termed the "loop gain." For the system to be stable, the magnitude of its loop gain must be less than 1. The loop gain therefore provides a quantitative index of the propensity for instability in negative feedback systems.

When dynamic characteristics are incorporated into the components of a closed-loop system (as in Cases 4 and 5), the definition of loop gain becomes more complicated. Phase delays as well as gain magnitudes must be taken into consideration in the computation of loop gain. For this purpose, it is generally most convenient mathematically to deduce loop gain from the amplitude and phase response of the system to small sinusoidal perturbations (48–50). A number of recent studies (51–54) have employed this approach to determine the stability characteristics of different models of respiratory control. These studies have been useful in identifying the factors most important for the initiation of PB.

Limitations of Linear Stability Analysis

As mentioned earlier, because of the nonlinearity of the plant equation, G is not constant but depends on the operating value of P_{ACO_2} (see Eq. 4b). Therefore, an implicit assumption in our preceding computations is that G remains close to its original value despite the occurrence of fluctuations in P_{ACO_2}. This kind of analysis effectively linearizes all components in the closed-loop system and is strictly valid only for determining the local stability characteristics in the immediate vicinity of the operating point being studied. As such, the computations shown in Table 1 must be considered highly approximate solutions for the response to a large ventilatory disturbance such as a sigh (see Fig. 2).

Nonlinearities become progressively more important as the amplitude of an oscillation grows. Low values of P_{aCO_2} that fall below the apneic threshold lead to cessation of breathing. On the other hand, high values of P_{aCO_2} or low values of P_{aO_2} are bounded by mixed venous values that do not change as much.

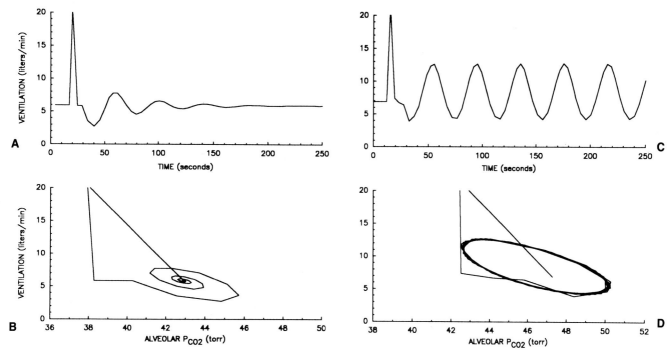

FIG. 2. Responses of a computer model of respiratory control (refs. 61 and 62) to a hyperventilatory sigh. Lower (**B, D**) panel displays responses in terms of the ventilation–PA_{CO_2} state-plane where time is not shown. **A, B**: Damped oscillatory response of a stable system. **C, D**: Sustained oscillations of a marginally stable system, where orbital stability is maintained as a consequence of system nonlinearity.

These limits prevent the swings in ventilation and blood gases from becoming indefinitely large. At the same time, a loop gain of magnitude 1 or greater ensures that the oscillation does not decay. Thus, with the appropriate combination of parameters, a stable large-amplitude oscillation, or a "limit cycle," can be produced. In some nonlinear closed-loop systems, certain parameter combinations can lead to complex oscillatory patterns or chaotic behavior (55).

Computer Models of Periodic Breathing

Several investigators have taken the alternative approach of using analog or digital computers to study the stability characteristics of respiratory control models (56–62). The general procedure has been to model respiratory control as a system of coupled differential equations that are solved numerically by finite difference methods. This approach circumvents the need for assuming linearity, thus allowing stability characteristics to be explored over a wide range of parameter variations. A discussion highlighting the differences between some of these PB models may be found in a recent review (3).

Examples of respiratory stability analysis by computer simulation of a recent model (61,62) are shown

in Fig. 2. As in our previous simple calculations (Table 1), we examine the stability of the response to a sigh. However, in this case, the effects of system nonlinearities are fully accounted for. In Fig. 2A (upper panel), a large sigh leads to a damped oscillatory response in $\dot{V}_E$. In the lower panel (Fig. 2B), the same response is displayed with $\dot{V}_E$ plotted against concurrent values of PA_{CO_2}. The sigh displaces $\dot{V}_E$ and PA_{CO_2} far from the original equilibrium point, but these variables eventually spiral back (in an anti-clockwise direction) towards their original values. In Fig. 2C, the loop gain is increased by increasing plant gain only. One may note the change in equilibrium point prior to the disturbance (lower panel of Fig. 2D). The post-sigh response is now a sustained oscillation, which takes the form of a closed ellipse in the $\dot{V}_E$–PA_{CO_2} state plane. In both cases, the fluctuations in $\dot{V}_E$ and PA_{CO_2} are quite large, and therefore the assumptions inherent in linear stability analysis would not be valid.

Comparison of Model Predictions with Empirical Data

Significant differences exist between the various mathematical models of PB, in terms of level of complexity as well as in the details of implementation. However, all have been successful in reproducing some, if not most, of the characteristics of PB. A comparison between model predictions and empirical data is outlined below.

Oscillations occur when circulatory delays are increased two- to threefold to simulate congestive heart failure (51,53,57,58). The simulated periodicities of approximately 1–1.5 min in duration are similar in magnitude to the periodicities noted in patients with heart failure who have CSR. In general, a doubling of circulatory delay leads to a doubling of the oscillation cycle time.

Hypoxia also induces PB by increasing peripheral gain (51,53,58); these models predict that the frequency of incidence and strength of the oscillations increase with growing severity of hypoxia. Taking into account the rise in cardiac output and the lowering of the lung washout time constant for O_2 (due to steeper slope of the O_2 dissociation curve in hypoxia), a decrease in cycle time with increasing acute hypoxia is also predicted (51). These predictions are consistent with the observations of Waggener et al. (37) that the intensity of ventilatory oscillations increases with altitude, whereas cycle time decreases.

Animal experiments have demonstrated that interventions that enhance the relative importance of peripheral drive also increase the incidence of PB, a result consistent with model predictions (51,52,59). Examples of such interventions are (a) central drive depression by focal cooling of the medulla (63) and (b) augmentation of carotid chemoreceptor sensitivity by blocking dopamine receptors (25).

An increase in the apneic threshold (i.e., rightward shift of the CO_2 response line) raises the operating level of Pa_{CO_2} and lowers alveolar ventilation (see Eq. 4b). This increases plant gain and therefore promotes respiratory instability. This mechanism for instability has been demonstrated in Fig. 2B as well as by several other models (51,58,64,65). The increase in apneic threshold has been reported in normals during sleep (1,18,44,66) as well as in awake patients with supramedullary lesions (14,31). Both groups show increased incidence of PB. It is believed that the rightward shift of the CO_2 response line reflects the removal of nonspecific stimuli to the respiratory center arriving from supramedullary sources (32). On the other hand, a leftward shift of the CO_2 response line, which occurs with increased levels of vigilance or during acclimatization, lowers plant gain and leads to greater stability in the breathing pattern. This result has been confirmed in sleep and acclimatization studies (18,39,64).

Inhalation of hypercapnic or hyperoxic mixtures depresses plant gain and therefore eliminates or attenuates PB (51,52,59,62). This is consistent with most experimental and clinical studies of PB (15,25,46,63), although some researchers have reported the persistence of PB despite O_2 administration (17–19). One possible explanation for the latter is that O_2 inhalation tends to increase oscillation cycle time and thus lengthen the duration of apnea, which, in turn, could act to offset the reduction in plant gain.

A decrease in lung stores for CO_2 and O_2 reduces the degree of damping, thereby increasing plant gain. This explains the increased incidence of PB in subjects that are in the supine position relative to those that are seated, since the horizontal posture leads to a reduction in FRC (15).

Passive hyperventilation of anesthetized dogs (67) and subjects during sleep (66) has been shown to produce transient PB after an initial period of apnea. This result has been simulated in several models (51,56,58).

Substantial differences in hypercapnic and hypoxic sensitivities exist between individuals. It follows from the instability hypothesis that the incidence of PB should be higher in subjects with larger chemosensitivities. A number of studies on humans have indeed demonstrated strong statistical correlations between incidence of PB and hypoxic or hypercapnic sensitivities (36,39,65). Data from the study of Chapman et al. (65) also suggest that a stronger degree of hypercapnic–hypoxic interaction (augmentation of CO_2 sensitivity by hypoxia) may promote greater susceptibility to PB.

VENTILATORY OSCILLATIONS, PERIODIC BREATHING, AND APNEA

Relationship Between PB and Ventilatory Oscillations

It is natural to infer from the instability hypothesis that clinically defined PB represents the class of ventilatory oscillations that have grown to sufficiently large amplitudes to be visually distinguishable from random fluctuations in breathing pattern. A recent study of hypoxia-induced PB in sleeping normals has demonstrated close correspondence between the incidence of visually identified PB and the incidence of oscillations in ventilatory pattern as detected by spectral analysis (65). In another study (37), strength and incidence of ventilatory oscillations in healthy volunteers were found to increase with increasing altitude; at the same time, the incidence of PB with apnea also increased, with the apnea taking up a progressively larger fraction of the PB cycle. Carley and Shannon (53,68) computed loop gains of normal subjects at different levels of hypoxia and found that these were significantly correlated with the corresponding strengths of ventilatory oscillations provoked by transient challenges of a hypercapnic mixture. A continuum of oscillations of different strengths was observed, ranging from virtually no oscillation at a loop gain magnitude of about 0.2 to frank PB at a loop gain magnitude of about 1.2.

Quantitative Measures of Oscillation Strength

While most clinical studies merely report the presence or absence of oscillatory behavior and, in some cases, cycle duration, the "strength" of ventilatory oscillation can provide additional information about the stability of the system. Several different methods have been used to quantify "strength" of oscillatory ventilation. Some researchers have employed standard Fourier or spectral analysis techniques to detect and identify significant ventilatory oscillations (9,11,60,69). In these studies, strength is quantified in terms of the power contained in the band of frequencies that span the fundamental frequency of the oscillation being studied. In comb-filtering, the strength of an oscillation of particular cycle time is given by the average power of the specific band-pass filter in the comb that contains the frequency of the oscillation in question (7,8,12,45).

The "strength index" defined by Waggener et al. (37) is simple and useful for quantifying the strength of PB or oscillatory patterns that can be visually identified. One of two definitions of this strength index (M) is used, depending on whether the oscillation includes apnea. For nonapneic oscillations, M is given by the difference between maximum ($\dot{V}_{Emax}$) and minimum ventilation ($\dot{V}_{Emin}$) in a given cycle, divided by the sum of $\dot{V}_{Emax}$ and $\dot{V}_{Emin}$:

$$M = (\dot{V}_{Emax} - \dot{V}_{Emin})/(\dot{V}_{Emax} + \dot{V}_{Emin}) \quad [10]$$

For this definition, M varies from zero when ventilation is uniform to unity when $\dot{V}_{Emin}$ becomes zero (i.e., apnea just begins to occur). In the idealized situation where the modulation in $\dot{V}_E$ is sinusoidal, Eq. 10 represents simply the ratio of the oscillation amplitude to the average ventilation calculated over all breaths of the cycle. For PB with apnea, strength is defined as

$$M = T_c/(T_c - T_a) \quad [11]$$

where T_c and T_a represent the cycle time and duration of apnea, respectively. It can be seen that Eq. 11 extends the range of values for M above unity. Starting with unity when apneic duration is zero (i.e., apnea just begins to appear), M increases as the ratio of apneic duration to total cycle duration increases.

Classification Based on Breathing Pattern

Careful analysis of ventilatory oscillations has revealed differences not only in cycle duration and strength but also in the pattern of distribution of these changes in $\dot{V}_E$ into tidal volume and breath duration

components. In infants, Waggener et al. (70) have found that oscillations with shorter cycle times are due more to tidal volume changes, whereas changes in breath duration are more important in the slower oscillations. In both adults (8) and infants (12), two broad categories of ventilatory oscillations have been distinguished, based on the relative phases of their constituent oscillations. The first group consists of "compensating" oscillations, in which increases in tidal volume are accompanied by increases in breath duration, so that the resulting fluctuations in $\dot{V}_E$ are smaller than those of its components. The other category contains "reinforcing" oscillations, where the constituent oscillations in tidal volume and breath duration are out of phase. In some subjects, PB tends to be associated with reinforcing oscillations (8,11), but this result has not been consistently observed (12,70). The underlying causes of these two different classes of oscillations are still unknown.

Periodic Apnea Resulting from High-Loop-Gain Instability

According to the instability hypothesis, repetitive episodes of apnea are produced when an oscillation has grown to a sufficiently large amplitude that its hypoventilatory portions attain zero ventilation. With further growth in amplitude, the apneic fraction of the oscillatory cycle duration would increase. This view is consistent with the definition of oscillation strength given by Eq. 11. Evidence in support of this mechanism of apnea production has been provided by Waggener et al. (70), who demonstrated by comb-filtering that the vast majority of periodic apneas seen in premature infants coincide with the minimum phase of the dominant ventilatory oscillation.

Since the apneic duration must be less than the cycle time of an oscillation, it follows that long apneas can only be produced by oscillations with long cycle durations. Waggener's study of premature infants revealed two major groups of oscillations: (i) high-frequency oscillations with cycle times ranging from 12 to 40 sec and (ii) low-frequency oscillations with cycle times of 44–90 sec. Long apneas (10 sec or greater) were related to the minimum phase of the slower oscillations, whereas short apneas were produced by high-frequency oscillations or a combination of both kinds of oscillations occurring simultaneously. It is reasonable to believe that the short apneas and high-frequency oscillations were mediated by the peripheral chemoreflex loop. The origin of the low-frequency oscillations is unclear, although it has been suggested that they reflect dynamic behavior of the central chemoreflex (47). However, this possibility is somewhat unlikely based on the results of most PB models, which suggest that the central chemoreflex is extremely stable (51,52,54,59). For oscillatory behavior to be mediated by the medullary chemoreceptors, there would have to be substantial increases in circulatory delay, chemoreceptor response rate, or controller gain.

Periodic Sleep Apnea

The onset of sleep brings about the reduction of a potent nonchemical drive to breathe, often referred to as the "wakefulness stimulus" (44,71). As mentioned earlier, this withdrawal of nonspecific input to the respiratory center causes a shift of the hypercapnic response line to the right, raising the apneic threshold (18,44,66). Consequently, the operating level of alveolar ventilation falls and Pa_{CO_2} is increased. Together with a reduction in metabolic rate, these changes lead to an increase in plant gain (see Eq. 4b). However, at the same time, hypercapnic and hypoxic sensitivities are depressed. Therefore, loop gain is increased if the plant gain increase is larger than the controller gain decrease (64). Using hypercapnic response data from Bulow's classic study (18), Khoo has recently demonstrated in a computer model that loop gain is increased in the light stages of sleep but depressed in slow-wave sleep (61,62). The enhancement in loop gain is greater when there is a larger increase in apneic threshold or less depression in controller gain. These model predictions are consistent with the results of most sleep studies performed on adult humans (44). Some studies have also shown that subjects with higher hypercapnic and hypoxic sensitivities in wakefulness are more likely to develop PB with apnea during sleep (36,39,65).

The process of the wakefulness stimulus withdrawal in itself constitutes a large disturbance to the respiratory chemoreflexes. Furthermore, the increase in apneic threshold allows apnea to occur with lower levels of hyperventilation (66). Thus, the magnitude and rate of withdrawal are important factors that can initiate PB during the transition from wakefulness to light sleep. Sleep researchers have noted a greater tendency for PB to occur in subjects who fall asleep abruptly (18,44).

In cases where loop gain is greatly depressed as a result of substantial reduction in chemoresponsiveness during sleep (e.g., in patients with primary alveolar hypoventilation syndrome), a different kind of "instability" may appear. Rapid withdrawal of wakefulness drive would lead to apnea. Since there is little or no chemoresponsiveness, there is insufficient drive to terminate the apnea. Consequently, blood gases deteriorate to the point where an arousal is triggered, restoring the wakefulness drive to some extent. Breathing is reinitiated with large inspiratory drives in the initial breaths because of the poor blood gas levels. As blood gases return to normal, drowsiness may set in again and the next transition to sleep occurs. Recent model simulations show that this type of instability can lead to repetitive large fluctuations in ventilation and arterial blood gases with periodicities that are longer than those reported in high-loop-gain PB (61,62,72). In a situation of low loop gain, the respiratory control system is also more susceptible to being affected by external influences. Therefore, respiratory oscillations secondary to oscillations in other organ systems may appear.

Periodic Breathing and Obstructive Sleep Apnea

The loss of wakefulness stimulus that accompanies sleep also leads to a general reduction in tonic activity of the upper-airway muscles (44). Thus, airway resistance is generally higher during sleep than in wakefulness. This may account for part of the decrease in chemoresponsiveness that accompanies sleep (64). As in the case of the respiratory muscles, during sleep the tone of the upper-airway muscles becomes highly dependent on chemoreceptor inputs. It has been hypothesized (73,74) that obstructive apneas are caused by differences in the pattern of activation of the respiratory muscles and upper-airway muscles by chemical drive: The generation of negative pressures by the respiratory muscles at the times when the tone of the upper-airway muscles is diminished leads to upper-airway collapse. Using a mathematical model, Longobardo et al. (73) have shown that central apneas produced by PB tend to promote the occurrence of obstructive apneas. By aggravating the fluctuations in blood gases, the obstructive apneas perpetuate PB and central apnea. Studies in patients with hypersomnia–sleep apnea syndrome (74) and CSR (75) support this hypothesis. A combination of upper-airway obstruction and failure of early arousal may produce prolonged apnea with life-threatening consequences (76).

Other Mechanisms of Apnea

It has been demonstrated in anesthetized animals (77) and awake humans (78) that the abrupt removal of any drive that produces active hyperventilation leads not to apnea but, instead, to a more gradual decay in ventilation. This phenomenon, termed the "neural afterdischarge," seems to be attenuated by hypoxia (79) and absent altogether in patients with certain types of brain lesions (32). The difficulty in achieving apnea with this mechanism intact suggests that it may be structurally or functionally impaired in subjects that have PB with apnea (2). This hypothesis has important

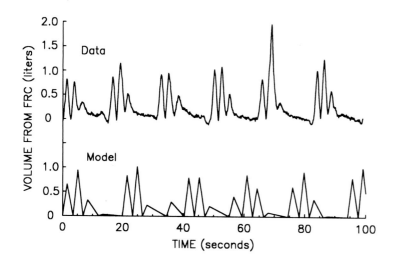

FIG. 3. Comparison of "cluster breathing" pattern obtained from a healthy subject exposed acutely to 11,000-ft altitude (*upper tracing*) with model simulation which incorporates an inverse relationship between tidal volume and expiratory duration. See text for details.

clinical implications and needs to be ascertained in future studies.

It has been suggested that some central apneas may not be "true" apneas but are actually prolonged expirations (2,80). These may occur because the net excitatory input to the expiratory off-switch is insufficient to raise off-switch excitability to the threshold level necessary to terminate the expiratory phase (2). In infants, it has been postulated that "prolonged expiratory apnea" may result from alveolar atelectasis with consequent disturbance of the lung stretch receptors (81). Since this mechanism can lead to long periods in which no fresh air enters the lungs, its importance as a potential life-threatening disorder should not be underestimated (81). An illustration of how a mild manifestation of this mechanism may interact with a high-loop-gain instability is shown in Fig. 3 (lower tracing). Here, the model of Khoo (61,62) is used to simulate PB at high altitude. The simple assumptions embodied in this example are as follows: (a) Greater volume removal during expiration leads to larger reduction of expiratory duration; (b) inspiratory duration remains constant; and (c) mean inspiratory flow reflects ventilatory drive. The fluctuating chemical drive leads to barely perceptible breaths that start at around 13, 67, and 86 sec on the time axis displayed in Fig. 3. These breaths are associated with prolonged expiratory phases by virtue of assumption "a." Consequently, initiation of the breaths that immediately follow is delayed. By the time these prolonged expirations terminate, the build-up in CO_2 and hypoxia induces large initial breaths. These abrupt transitions from expiratory "apnea" to high inspiratory drives are commonly noted in the cluster breathing patterns produced by hypoxia, as exemplified by the upper tracing of Fig. 3. Variability in cycle duration of the oscillation is also produced. It is interesting to note that the oscillations in both model prediction and data segment are of the "reinforcing" kind (i.e., tidal volume and

breath duration oscillate out-of-phase with each other). In contrast, Brusil et al. (8) have observed that the wax-and-wane patterns of CSR are generally of the "compensating" variety.

Although numerous questions remain at the present time, it is clear that much of our current knowledge about the stability of respiratory control has resulted from the application of mathematical modeling techniques to empirical data on PB. It is envisaged that the continued interaction between modeling and careful experimentation will be fruitful in addressing many of the unresolved issues.

ACKNOWLEDGMENT

This work was supported, in part, by NIH Grant RR-01861.

REFERENCES

1. Cherniack NS, Longobardo GS. Abnormalities in respiratory rhythm. In: Fishman AP, ed. *Handbook of physiology—the respiratory system II.* Bethesda, MD: American Physiological Society, 1987;729–749.
2. Younes M. The physiologic basis of central apnea and periodic breathing. *Curr Pulmonol* 1989;10:265–326.
3. Khoo MCK, Yamashiro SM. Models of control of breathing. In: Chang HK, Paiva M, eds. *Respiratory physiology: an analytical approach,* New York: Marcel Dekker, 1989;799–829.
4. Specht H, Fruhmann G. Incidence of periodic breathing in 2000 subjects without pulmonary or neurological disease. *Bull Physiopathol Respir* 1972;8:1075–1083.
5. Webber CL, Speck DF. Experimental Biot periodic breathing in cats: effects of changes in PIO_2 and $PICO_2$. *Respir Physiol* 1981;46:327–344.
6. Plum F, Posner JB. *Diagnosis of stupor and coma.* Philadelphia: FA Davis, 1980;25–32.
7. Brusil PJ. Statistical analysis of natural breathing patterns in supine man. PhD thesis, Harvard University, Cambridge, MA, 1973.
8. Brusil PJ, Waggener TB, Kronauer RE, Gulesian P. Methods for identifying respiratory oscillations disclose altitude effects. *J Appl Physiol* 1980;48:545–556.

9. Fleming PJ, Levine MR, Long AM, Cleave JP. Postneonatal development of respiratory oscillations. *Ann NY Acad Sci* 1988;533:305–313.

10. Goodman L. Oscillatory behavior of ventilation in resting man. *IEEE Trans Biomed Eng* 1964;11:81–93.

11. Hathorn MKS. Analysis of periodic changes in ventilation in new-born infants. *J Physiol (Lond)* 1978;285:85–99.

12. Waggener TB, Frantz ID III, Stark AR, Kronauer RE. Oscillatory breathing patterns leading to apneic spells in infants. *J Appl Physiol* 1982;52:1288–1295.

13. Anthony AJ, Cohn AE, Steele JM. Studies on Cheyne–Stokes respiration. *J Clin Invest* 1932;11:1321–1341.

14. Brown HW, Plum F. The neurological basis of Cheyne–Stokes respiration. *Am J Med* 1961;30:849–861.

15. Dowell AR, Buckley CE III, Cohen R, Whalen RE, Sieker HO. Cheyne–Stokes respiration: a review of clinical manifestations and critique of physiological mechanisms. *Arch Intern Med* 1971;127:712–726.

16. Eyster JAE. Clinical and experimental observations upon Cheyne–Stokes respiration. *J Exp Med* 1906;8:565–613.

17. Greene AJ. Clinical studies of respiration. IV. Some observations on Cheyne–Stokes respiration. *Arch Intern Med* 1933;52:454–463.

18. Bulow K. Respiration and wakefulness in man. *Acta Physiol Scand* 1963;59(Suppl 209):1–110.

19. Motta J, Guilleminault C. Effects of oxygen administration on sleep-induced apneas. In: Guilleminault C, Dement WC, eds. *Sleep apnea syndromes*. New York: Alan R Liss, 1978.

20. Pembrey MS. Observations on Cheyne–Stokes respiration. *J Pathol Bacteriol* 1908;12:258–266.

21. Klein O. Untersuchungen uber das Cheyne–Stokesche Atsmungsphanomen. *Verh Dtsch Ges Inn Med* 1930;42:217–222.

22. Pryor WW. Cheyne–Stokes respiration in patients with cardiac enlargement and prolonged circulation time. *Circulation* 1951;4:233–238.

23. Guyton AC, Crowell JW, Moore JW. Basic oscillating mechanism of Cheyne–Stokes breathing. *Am J Physiol* 1956;187:395–398.

24. Preiss G, Iscoe S, Polosa C. Analysis of a periodic breathing pattern associated with Mayer waves. *Am J Physiol* 1975;228:768–774.

25. Lahiri S, Hsiao C, Zhang R, Mokashi A, Nishino T. Peripheral chemoreceptors in respiratory oscillations. *J Appl Physiol* 1985;58:1901–1908.

26. Traube L. Zur Theorie des Cheyne–Stokes 'schen Atsmungsphanomen. *Berlin Klin Wschr* 1874;11:185–209.

27. Marckwald M. *The movements of respiration and their innervation in the rabbit* (Haig TA, translator). London: Blackie & Son, 1888.

28. Talbert OR, Currens JH, Cohen ME. Cheyne-Stokes respiration: Clinical, experimental and pathological observations with emphasis on the role of the nervous system. *Trans Am Neurol Assoc* 1954;79:226–228.

29. North JB, Jennett S. Abnormal breathing patterns associated with acute brain damage. *Arch Neurol* 1974;31:338–344.

30. Heyman A, Birchfield RI, Sieker HO. Effects of bilateral cerebral infarction on respiratory center activity. *Neurology* 1958;8:694–700.

31. North JB, Jennett S. Response of ventilation and of intracranial pressure during rebreathing of carbon dioxide in patients with acute brain damage. *Brain* 1976;99:169–182.

32. Plum F, Leigh RJ. Abnormalities of central mechanisms. In: Hornbein TF, ed. *Regulation of breathing, part II*. New York: Marcel Dekker, 1981;989–1067.

33. Plum F, Brown HW. The effect on respiration of central nervous system disease. *Ann NY Acad Sci* 1963;109:915–931.

34. Lange RL, Hecht H. The mechanism of Cheyne–Stokes respiration. *J Clin Invest* 1962;41:42–52.

35. Mosso A. *Life of man on the high Alps*. London: T Fisher-Unwin, 1898.

36. Lahiri S, Maret K, Sherpa MG. Evidence of high altitude sleep apnea on ventilatory sensitivity to hypoxia. *Respir Physiol* 1983;52:281–301.

37. Waggener TB, Brusil PJ, Kronauer RE, Gabel RA, Inbar GF. Strength and cycle time of high-altitude ventilatory patterns in unacclimatized humans. *J Appl Physiol* 1984;56:576–581.

38. West JB, Peters RM Jr, Aksnes G, Maret KH, Milledge JS, Schoene RB. Nocturnal periodic breathing at altitudes of 6,300 and 8,050 m. *J Appl Physiol* 1986;61:280–287.

39. White DP, Gleeson K, Pickett C, Rannels AM, Cymerman A, Weil JV. Altitude acclimatization: influence on periodic breathing and chemoresponsiveness during sleep. *J Appl Physiol* 1987;63:401–412.

40. Douglas CG, Haldane JS. The causes of periodic or Cheyne–Stokes breathing. *J Physiol (Lond)* 1909;38:401–419.

41. Webb P. Periodic breathing during sleep. *J Appl Physiol* 1974;37:899–903.

42. Lugaresi EA, Coccagna G, Cirignotta P, Farnetti P, Gallassi R, Di Donato G, Verucchi P. Breathing during sleep in man in normal and pathological conditions. In: Fitzgerald RS, Gautier H, Lahiri S, eds. *The regulation of respiration during sleep and anesthesia*. New York: Plenum Press, 1977.

43. Cherniack NS. Respiratory dysrhythmias in sleep. *N Engl J Med* 1981;305:325–330.

44. Phillipson EA, Bowes G. Control of breathing during sleep. In: Fishman AP, ed. *Handbook of physiology—the respiratory system II*. Bethesda, MD: American Physiological Society, 1987.

45. Pack AI, Silage DA, Millman RP, Knight H, Shore ET, Chung DC. Spectral analysis of ventilation in elderly subjects awake and asleep. *J Appl Physiol* 1988;64:1257–1267.

46. Shannon DC, Carley DW, Kelly DH. Periodic breathing: quantitative analysis and clinical description. *Pediatr Pulmonol* 1988;4:98–102.

47. Waggener TB. The relationship between abnormalities in respiratory control and apnea in infants. *Respir Care* 1986;31:622–627.

48. Grodins FS. *Control theory and biological systems*. New York: Columbia University Press, 1963.

49. Milhorn HT Jr. *The application of control theory to physiological systems*. Philadelphia: WB Saunders, 1966.

50. Jones RW. *Principles of biological regulation: an introduction to feedback systems*. New York: Academic Press, 1973.

51. Khoo MCK, Kronauer RE, Strohl KP, Slutsky AS. Factors inducing periodic breathing in humans: a general model. *J Appl Physiol* 1982;53:644–659.

52. Nugent ST, Finley JP. Periodic breathing in infants: a model study. *IEEE Trans Biomed Eng* 1987;34:482–485.

53. Carley DW, Shannon DC. A minimal mathematical model of human periodic breathing. *J Appl Physiol* 1988;65:1400–1409.

54. ElHefnawy A, Saidel GM, Bruce EN. CO_2 control of the respiratory system: plant dynamics and stability analysis. *Ann Biomed Eng* 1988;16:445–461.

55. Glass L, Beuter A, Larocque D. Time delays, oscillations, and chaos in physiological control systems. *Math Biosci* 1988;90:111–125.

56. Horgan JD, Lange DL. Analog computer studies of periodic breathing. *IRE Trans Biomed Eng* 1962;9:221–228.

57. Milhorn HT Jr, Guyton AC. An analog computer analysis of Cheyne–Stokes breathing. *J Appl Physiol* 1965;20:328–333.

58. Longobardo GS, Cherniack NS, Fishman AP. Cheyne–Stokes breathing produced by a model of the human respiratory system. *J Appl Physiol* 1966;21:1839–1846.

59. Nugent ST, Tan GA, Finley JP. A nonlinear model study of periodic breathing in infants. *Proc 9th Annu Conf IEEE EMBS* 1987;4:1108–1110.

60. Revow M, England SJ, O'Beirne H, Bryan AC. A model of the maturation of respiratory control in the newborn infant. *IEEE Trans Biomed Eng* 1989;36:414–423.

61. Khoo MCK. A model for respiratory variability during non-REM sleep. In: Swanson GD, Grodins FS, Hughson RL, eds. *Respiratory control: modelling perspective*. New York: Plenum Press, 1990;327–336.

62. Khoo MCK. Modeling the effect of sleep state on respiratory stability. In: Khoo MCK, ed. *Modeling and parameter estimation in respiratory control*. New York: Plenum Press, 1990; in press.

63. Cherniack NS, von Euler C, Homma I, Kao FF. Experimentally

induced Cheyne–Stokes breathing. *Respir Physiol* 1979;37:185–200.

64. Cherniack NS. Sleep apnea and its causes. *J Clin Invest* 1984;73:1501–1506.

65. Chapman KR, Bruce EN, Gothe B, Cherniack NS. Possible mechanisms of periodic breathing during sleep. *J Appl Physiol* 1988;64:1000–1008.

66. Dempsey JA, Skatrud JB. A sleep-induced apneic threshold and its consequences. *Am Rev Respir Dis* 1986;133:1163–1170.

67. Cherniack NS, Longobardo GS, Levine OR, Mellins R, Fishman AP. Periodic breathing in dogs. *J Appl Physiol* 1966;21:1847–1854.

68. Carley DW, Shannon DC. Relative stability of human respiration during progressive hypoxia. *J Appl Physiol* 1988;65:1389–1399.

69. Nugent ST, Finley JP. Spectral analysis of periodic and normal breathing in infants. *IEEE Trans Biomed Eng* 1983;30:672–675.

70. Waggener TB, Stark AR, Cohlan BA, Frantz ID III. Apnea duration is related to ventilatory oscillation characteristics in newborn infants. *J Appl Physiol* 1984;57:536–544.

71. Fink BR. Influence of cerebral activity in wakefulness on regulation of breathing. *J Appl Physiol* 1961;16:15–20.

72. Pack AI. Sleep state and periodic ventilation. In: Khoo MCK, ed. *Modeling and parameter estimation in respiratory control*. New York: Plenum Press, 1990; in press.

73. Longobardo GS, Gothe B, Goldman MD, Cherniack NS. Sleep apnea considered as a control system instability. *Respir Physiol* 1982;50:311–333.

74. Onal E, Lopata M. Periodic breathing and the pathogenesis of occlusive sleep apneas. *Am Rev Respir Dis* 1982;126:676–680.

75. Alex CG, Onal E, Lopata M. Upper airway occlusion during sleep in patients with Cheyne–Stokes respiration. *Am Rev Respir Dis* 1986;133:42–45.

76. Guilleminault C. Sleep-related respiratory function and dysfunction in postneonatal infantile apnea. In: Culbertson JL, Krous HF, Bendell RD, eds. *Sudden infant death syndrome: medical aspects and psychological management*. Baltimore: Johns Hopkins University Press, 1988;94–120.

77. Eldridge FL. Maintenance of respiration by central neural feedback mechanisms. *Fed Proc* 1977;36:2400–2404.

78. Tawadrous FD, Eldridge FL. Posthyperventilation breathing patterns after active hyperventilation in man. *J Appl Physiol* 1974;37:353–356.

79. Holtby SG, Berezanski DJ, Anthonisen NR. The effect of 100% oxygen on hypoxic eucapnic ventilation. *J Appl Physiol* 1988;65:1157–1162.

80. Sanders MH, Rogers RM, Pennock BE. Prolonged expiratory phase in sleep apnea: a unifying hypothesis. *Am Rev Respir Dis* 1985;131:401–408.

81. Southall DP. Role of apnea in the sudden infant death syndrome: a personal view. *Pediatrics* 1988;80:73–84.

THE LUNG: Scientific Foundations
edited by R.G. Crystal, J.B. West et al.
Raven Press, Ltd., New York © 1991.

CHAPTER 5.4.12

Dyspnea

Kieran J. Killian and E. J. M. Campbell

Whenever a new discovery is reported to the scientific world, they say first, "It is probably not true." Thereafter, when the truth of the new proposition has been demonstrated beyond question they say, "Yes, it is true, but it is not important." Finally, when sufficient time has elapsed to fully evidence its importance, they say, "Yes, surely it is important, but it is no longer new."

Montaigne

Discomfort in the act of breathing occurs in health and in many forms of disease affecting the lungs, heart, or neuromuscular systems. When breathing discomfort is experienced at a level of activity where it is not expected, dyspnea is said to be present. Clinically, severity is inversely related to the intensity of activity that precipitates it; when breathing discomfort is experienced while climbing stairs, walking, or at rest, increasing severity is inferred. Thus the circumstances under which it occurs are essential components to its recognition. Dyspnea arises under many different circumstances, and because it is associated with diverse physiological changes, there has been a natural curiosity to discover whether there is some common underlying mechanism (often called the cause). Breathlessness, shortness of breath, and dyspnea are some of the expressions used to describe this discomfort. The variable use of these terms leads to confusion, but adopting a narrow definition is presently unhelpful because common usage has established that the definitions are practically synonymous and also because we do not yet have sufficient understanding to base our terminology on anything more fundamental. Thus dyspnea is used throughout this chapter as referring to discomfort experienced with, as well as associated with, the act of breathing. By contrast, the disorders giving rise to dyspnea are both well known and ac-

cepted. This results in the use of terms such as cardiac and respiratory dyspnea, fostering the notion that dyspnea is somehow uniquely related to its etiology. In the last 20 years there has been progress in defining the anatomy, physiology, and psychophysics of dyspnea and in elucidating the mechanisms of its generation.

HISTORY

The present understanding of dyspnea began with clinical observation and evolved with advances in the chemical and neural control of breathing, advances in the ability to measure the mechanics of breathing, and advances in sensory physiology, and it continues with the application of psychophysics in the interaction of all these elements.

Dyspnea and Clinical Observation

In his book entitled *Pathology and Diagnosis of Diseases of the Chest*, C. J. B. William (1) described dyspnea:

> Dyspnea, difficult or disordered breathing, is the most important general symptom of diseases of the chest, inasmuch as it implies more or less interruption to the due performance of some part of the great function of the chest respiration. Dyspnea may be caused by circumstances affecting any one or more of the several elements concerned in the function of respiration: viz. the blood in the lungs, the air, the machinery of respiration by which these are brought together, and the nervous system through which the impression which prompts the respiratory act is conveyed from the lung to the medulla, and thence to the muscles which move the machinery.

Thus, the multiple nature of dyspnea was identified from an early stage, but exploration was often confined to single processes and was unidimensional.

K. J. Killian and E. J. M. Campbell: Department of Medicine, McMaster University Medical Center, Hamilton, Ontario L8N 3Z5, Canada.

Dyspnea and Chemical Control

Pfluger (2) noted that hypoxemia and hypercarbia resulted in dyspnea but considered oxygen the dominant contributor. Dyspnea was ascribed to the lack of free oxygen in the tissues, particularly in the medulla oblongata. Miescher-Rusch (3), appreciating that alveolar P_{CO_2} was closely controlled, noted that any rise resulted both in accelerated breathing and in dyspnea. Haldane and Smith (4) found that breathing in a closed chamber resulted in dyspnea when CO_2 levels rose by 3% but not until oxygen dropped to 14%. Hydrogen ion as a common stimulus to respiratory activity and dyspnea was introduced by Winterstein (5). Meakins (6), representing the culmination of this period, stated that dyspnea is produced by two causes: want of oxygen and carbon dioxide retention.

Dyspnea and Neural Reflexes

Cullen et al. (7) were unhappy with chemical changes in the blood as the cause of breathlessness, arguing that hydrogen ion, oxygen, and carbon dioxide remain largely unchanged in blood during and following exercise, making these factors less tenable as the mechanisms giving rise to dyspnea. Harrison et al. (8) went on to show that breathing is stimulated by vagally mediated reflexes, by reflexes arising in the central vessels (induced by increased pressure), and by muscular movements. The role of reflexes in dyspnea was raised by Harrison (9) and by Gesell and Moyer (10). Christie (11) summarized the understanding of this period:

> Though the conditions under which dyspnea occurs are various and manifold, giving rise to an impression of complexity, the fundamental causes are few and relatively simple. They consist of chemical and reflex disturbances. Chemical disturbance would seem to be of minor importance. Dyspnea is usually reflex in origin.

Dyspnea and Mechanics

Ventilation expressed relative to ventilatory capacity and its relationship to dyspnea was recognized by Means in the 1920s (12) and was popularized by Cournand and co-workers in the 1930s (13,14). The mechanical characteristics of the respiratory system were outlined by Rohrer in the 1920s (15), and in the 1940s Rahn et al. (16) made it possible to measure the forces and impedances involved in the act of breathing in living subjects. The mechanical work of breathing in patients with heart failure was found to be twice as much at rest and three to four times as much during exercise as that found in normal subjects (17). The work of breathing in patients with emphysema was found to be

similarly increased (18). Marshall et al. (19) suggested that dyspnea was related to transpulmonary pressure and not to work. Although consensus as to the particular mechanical factor giving rise to breathlessness did not emerge, the idea that mechanics are important persists to the present day.

Dyspnea and Oxygen Cost of Breathing

Oxygen cost of breathing increases when ventilation is increased and when the impedance to the action of the respiratory muscles is increased (20–23), McIlroy (24) concluded that dyspnea occurred when the respiratory muscles incur an oxygen debt.

Dyspnea and Length–Tension Inappropriateness

Campbell and Howell (25) suggested that an imbalance in the relationship between tension and displacement in respiratory muscle might be the neurophysiological mechanism giving rise to dyspnea. Tension mediated by tendon organs, as well as length (volume or flow) mediated by muscle spindles and joint receptors, is transmitted to the central nervous system. The central processing of these signals provides a viable neurophysiological mechanism for the sensation. At the time of Campbell and Howell's report (1963), gamma efferent motor activity to intrafusal muscle fibers (spindles) was considered as a possible primary motor innervation to muscle. The increase in spindle discharge resulting from the stretching of the nuclear bag would cause afferent fiber stimulation and would increase alpha motoneuron activity reflexly. Alpha motor activity acted as a follow-up to the length servo system. Later, Campbell (26,27) substituted length–length for length–tension. According to this view, an imbalance between programmed length change and achieved length change would trigger dyspnea.

Summary

There is general agreement with regard to the following: (a) Hypoxemia, hypercapnia, and increased hydrogen ion concentration cause dyspnea; (b) increasing ventilation as a consequence of reflex activity arising in the muscles, lungs, and/or central vessels causes dyspnea; and (c) heart, lung, and neuromuscular disorders cause dyspnea. The dyspneic victims of poliomyelitis and other neurological disorders had an equally viable causality. While understanding cause is important, the missing link is mechanism, and this remains inadequately explained by respiratory muscle work, transpulmonary pressure, oxygen debt, hypoxemia, hypercarbia, acidemia, or increased ventilation.

The theory of length–tension inappropriateness and subsequently length–length inadequacy provided an explanation for dyspnea, but in its simple form it did not account for the dyspnea of increased ventilation in the absence of mechanical or neuromuscular defects.

SENSORY PHYSIOLOGY

The emergence of interest in sensory mechanisms was an inevitable consequence of this evolution in understanding. Conscious sensation (light, sound, taste, olfaction, touch, muscular forces, and movement, and presumably more complex sensory experiences such as discomfort with breathing) is initiated by physical stimuli that gain entry to the nervous system by acting on sensory receptors. The magnitude of the stimuli results in a graded alteration in the receptors that are transformed into a graded firing frequency in afferent nerves. The afferent nerve relays the conditions at the proximal receptors, coded by firing frequency, to the central nervous system. Central impression of the condition of peripheral receptors is formulated; then this information is interpreted in light of experience and learning, resulting in conscious sensation (28).

Stimulus → Receptor →

Afferent nerve → Central impression

Central impression → Experience/learning →

Attention → Consciousness

Quality of Sensation

The simple scheme outlined above provides the fundamental units of sensory processes. However, most sensations are compound (rather than discrete) functions of a given receptor or sets of receptors operating alone. Compound sensations involve multiple different types of receptors, each operating in a systematic fashion. The quality of a given sensation is related to the specific receptors stimulated, the magnitude of stimulation, and the conditions simultaneously occurring in other sets of sensory receptors activated by the same or related stimuli. Quality is multidimensional and involves the stimulation of multiple receptor types. Quantity is often unidimensional and involves a specific receptor type.

BASIC SENSORY NEUROANATOMY OF RESPIRATORY SENSATION

Dyspnea reaches consciousness through the sensory infrastructure of the respiratory system. Receptors, route of afferent feedback, and central processing form the infrastructure of all respiratory sensations, including dyspnea.

RECEPTORS

Vagal receptors (irritant, stretch, and J receptors)
Chemoreceptors (peripheral and central receptors)
Muscular receptors (tendon organs, muscle spindles, and joint and skin receptors)
Central collateral discharge (efferent copy) receptors
Upper-airway receptors

Pulmonary Sensory Mechanisms

There are receptors in the walls of airways, in lung parenchyma, and around capillaries. They respond to a variety of stimuli, both chemical and mechanical. Afferent impulses travel by means of vagal and sympathetic pathways. These receptors have been extensively studied and reviewed in recent publications (29). Although stimulation of these receptors modifies breathing, it is uncertain whether they are themselves sentient. It seems more likely that sensation is generated by the reflex motor consequences of their stimulation. Irritation of the trachea, presumably by stimulation of vagal receptors, does produce a crude visceral sensation, but it is distinguishable from dyspnea.

Chemoreceptors

Peripheral and central chemoreceptors respond to hypoxemia, hypercapnia, and changes in hydrogen ion concentration, and their stimulation causes dyspnea. These receptors have been extensively studied and reviewed in recent publications (30,31). Their stimulation results in increased respiratory muscle activity and in activation of muscular and pulmonary receptors, making it difficult to isolate the sensation resulting from chemoreceptor activation alone from that generated by muscular and/or pulmonary receptors. Total neuromuscular blockade provides an opportunity to isolate chemoreceptor activity from its motor consequences. Neuromuscular blockade to the point of apnea results in an inevitable increase in chemoreceptor activity but is not accompanied by dyspnea (32). The results of these studies oppose the idea that chemoreceptor activity results in discomfort directly. Dyspnea appears to be a consequence of muscular activation and not a direct consequence of chemoreceptor activity.

Muscular Receptors

The proprioceptive properties of muscle in general are shared by respiratory muscle. Tendon organs are mechanically stimulated by the tension developed by muscle; then the tension is transduced into a neural firing frequency and is transmitted to the central nervous system by afferent nerves, yielding a sensation of tension. Muscle spindles and joint receptors are mechanically stimulated by the extent and velocity of muscle contraction. The displacement achieved is transduced into a neural firing frequency and transmitted to the central nervous system by afferent peripheral nerves (33–36), yielding a sensation of displacement. Free nerve endings within muscle are mechanically and chemically stimulated. Following overuse of muscle, structural damage or leakage of cellular contents stimulates these receptors, thereby yielding a sensation of pain.

Humans are thus capable of consciously perceiving a variety of sensations during muscular activity—tension, displacement, interrelationship between tension and displacement (impedance, resistance, elastance), and their derivatives in the time domain (34,35,37–39). The quality of muscular sensation is determined primarily by the varying inputs from these different kinds of receptors and their interrelationships.

Central Collateral Discharge (Efferent Copy) Receptors

Interneurons high in the central nervous system act as receptors that transduce the intensity of motor output to muscle. These interneurons transmit the intensity of motor command to the sensory cortex, yielding a sensation of effort—the intensity of the motor command (40–45).

Upper-Airway Receptors

Receptors in the nose, nasopharynx, oropharynx, and larynx have been recently reviewed by Widdicombe (46). These receptors have received little attention, but reflexes arising within the upper airway are multiple, highly complex, and important in speech and in stabilizing the patency of the upper airway. Afferent activity travels via the trigeminal, glossopharyngeal, hypoglossal, and vagal nerves. Their stimulation can contribute to conscious sensation; irritation, pressure, and flow can be sensed, but their role in sensing external respiratory loads remains controversial.

RESPIRATORY SENSATIONS

The availability of psychophysical techniques initiated an era for the study of respiratory sensations in which the physical stimulus, sensory response, sensory receptors, and their afferent neural pathways constituted the ingredients. These studies have been recently reviewed (47–49).

The Sensation of Loaded Breathing

The sensation of loaded breathing deserves special attention because increases in mechanical load are common to most clinical conditions in which dyspnea occurs and because of the light shed on basic mechanisms. Campbell et al. (50) and Bennett et al. (51) showed that humans can detect small added loads to breathing (elastic and resistive). They reasoned that a change in pressure, volume, or flow alone could not explain detection because pressure, volume, and flow change during the course of normal breathing and are not appreciated as a change in load. They concluded that the most likely explanation was a change in the relationship between pressure and volume (elastance) and pressure and flow (resistance). Both pressure (tension) and volume (displacement) are mechanical stimuli amenable to transduction by known sensory receptors activated by respiratory muscle activity. These simple psychophysical experiments on load detection paved the way for studies on other respiratory sensations.

During the 1960s the neuroanatomy of respiratory load detection received attention with the introduction of reliable threshold detection and discrimination techniques. By comparing load detection applied at the mouth and at the trachea, with and without airway anesthesia, and with and without vagal blockade, in patients with complete spinal blockade at various levels, it became possible to define the neuroanatomy of load detection with classical neurophysiological techniques.

These studies showed the following: (a) Load detection bears a relatively fixed relationship to the magnitude of the background load (52); (b) load detection at the mouth deteriorates in patients with airflow limitation but is similar when expressed as a fraction of background load, suggesting that upper-airway receptors are unlikely to be the primary receptors (53–55); (c) load detection is unaffected by vagal blockade (56); (d) load detection is unaffected by local anesthesia to the airway (57); (e) load detection is preserved as long as any respiratory muscle is capable of sustaining ventilation as with high spinal neuromuscular blockade (58–60); and (f) load detection is virtually abolished when the respiratory muscles are inactive (passive ventilation) (61). These studies, while refuting some of the other popular alternatives, support the concept of inappropriateness, which was introduced by Campbell and his colleagues. The primary receptors, tendon organs (tension), and spindles (displacement—volume and flow) relay the afferent information, and the interrelationship is centrally processed.

Dimensions of Respiratory Sensation

In the early 1970s, Bakers and Tenney (62) showed that humans can directly estimate the magnitude of volume, ventilation, and respiratory pressures using open magnitude scaling. These studies were followed by a variety of similar studies and established that humans can consciously perceive the magnitude of external loads (55,63), the magnitude of internal loads (64), the magnitude of respiratory pressures (65), the magnitude of volume (66–68), and the magnitude of effort (40,43,45).

These studies were accompanied by others investigating the neurophysiological mechanism through which these sensory events were perceived. Complete agreement has not yet emerged, but the following is a broad consensus. Volume changes are probably sensed through muscle spindles and joint receptors, similar to position sense in peripheral limb movement (66–69). Tension is sensed through tendon organs. The sensation of effort is sensed by efferent copy by collateral discharge. Sherrington's (39) opposition to a separate sense of effort (sense of willed motor command) has been largely refuted; tension and effort are accepted as separate sensory events. The idea that humans can sense the intensity of the motor command to muscle in general (35,36) and respiratory muscle in particular (40,43,45) is reasonably accepted.

ASSESSMENT OF DYSPNEA

Having reviewed some of the basic mechanisms in the generation of respiratory sensations, we will now consider these mechanisms in the context of dyspnea. The assessment of dyspnea requires the following: (a) We must come to the realization that dyspnea is a sensation; (b) the sensation results from the stimulation of sensory receptors activated by the act of breathing; (c) the quality of dyspnea depends on the conditions of stimulation in all receptor types stimulated under the conditions in which it is experienced; (d) assessment of dyspnea requires basic understanding of the principles of psychophysics which are used to their greatest advantage when we can control or measure the intensity of stimulation of specific receptor types. Thus, knowledge of these receptors and the conditions of their stimulation is a prerequisite to fundamental understanding. However, for practical purposes we are presently limited to measuring the conditions of their stimulation (exercise, hypoxemia, hypercapnia, loaded breathing) and can make only crude approxi-

mations regarding the intensity of specific receptor stimulation.

The stimuli and receptors important in the generation of dyspnea are singled out against this background of understanding, which includes (a) knowledge of the common clinical and physiological conditions under which dyspnea occurs and (b) knowledge of a viable neurophysiological mechanism that is in agreement with the known properties of the sensory system. Hypotheses are then (a) forwarded, (b) tested using established psychophysical techniques, and (c) refuted, modulated, or accepted, based on experimental results. This approach has only recently been applied to the problem of dyspnea.

The first problem with this approach is isolation of the stimulus or stimuli. Whereas we often measure the conditions of stimulation (i.e., the intensity of an added load, the magnitude of ventilation), these events are remote from the proximal receptors stimulated. Receptor stimulation can be crudely approximated in the following manner:

Motor command: Motor command can be approximated by expressing the activity of the muscle as a percentage of maximum achievable activity. The rationale for this approach is simple. If the activity generated with maximal effort represents recruitment of all motor units, then expressing the actual activity measured as a proportion of maximal activity gives a measurement of motor command relative to maximal as long as the conditions of operation are the same.

$$\frac{Motor\ command}{Maximum\ motor\ command} \rightarrow \frac{Tension}{Maximum\ tension} \rightarrow$$

$$\frac{Rate\ of\ displacement}{Maximum\ rate\ of\ displacement}$$

Tension: Tension can be approximated by measuring pressure.

Displacement: Displacement can be approximated by measuring volume and its time derivatives (flow).

Although the approach is simple, there are problems associated with it. The conversion of tension to pressure involves complex mechanical considerations; pressure results from the recruitment of various respiratory muscles such that receptor stimulation is remote; the velocity and extent of inspiratory muscle shortening and volume are not synonymous. Despite these problems, this approach provides an understanding of how the intensity of dyspnea varies in a number of clinical settings. The sensation of dyspnea is clarified by formally identifying how the various factors (exercise, hypercapnia, hypoxemia, neuromuscular weakness, etc.) alter the stimulation of the various sensory receptors. The roles of exercise, mechanical load, hypoxemia, hypercapnia, and acidemia readily fall in place. Dyspnea emerges as a sensory experience whose quality varies with the stimulus conditions at the various sensory receptors. The intensity of stimulation at each receptor, along with interrelationships in time and between each other, thus determines the overall quality and intensity of dyspnea.

In the common clinical conditions under which dyspnea is experienced, the mechanical state of the respiratory system is confined to a limited number of conditions. (a) The impedance to the action of the respiratory muscles is increased; this can be sensed by the increased effort, increased inspiratory muscle tension, and the relationship between tension and displacement (inappropriateness). (b) Breathing is increased; this can be sensed by increased effort, tension, and displacement. (c) The respiratory muscles are weak; this can be sensed by the increased effort required to sustain ventilation. The mechanical events result in the stimulation of a variety of sensory receptors, and often all three major primary receptor types (effort, volume, pressure) are stimulated simultaneously.

Motor output to the respiratory muscles is controlled to meet the metabolic demands imposed by the varying needs for oxygen uptake, carbon dioxide output, and hydrogen ion homeostasis. The greatest demands occur during muscular activity, particularly exercise. In meeting the required ventilation, the motor output is dependent not only on metabolic demand but also on the strength and condition (perfusion and metabolic support) of the respiratory muscles. The sensory consequences are further modified by the duration, frequency, and intensity of respiratory muscle activity and by the evolution of fatigue.

Mechanical efficiency of the respiratory muscles, the operating conditions of the respiratory muscle (length, extent, velocity of contraction), the impedance imposed by the chest cage/lungs, and the efficiency of gas exchange are independent contributors to the various receptors that are stimulated. The interdependent interaction of these processes and their effects on sensory structures provide the background for the mechanistic evaluation of dyspnea and are illustrated in Fig. 1.

Chest Tightness

Some patients complain of a sensation of chest tightness. The circumstance under which this sensation most commonly occurs is bronchoconstriction. During bronchoconstriction, the following events occur: (i) The lungs are hyperinflated, and inspiratory muscles are shortened and thus weakened; (ii) the lungs and inspiratory muscles work with a mechanical disadvantage; (iii) inspiratory resistance and dynamic elastance are increased; and (iv) ventilation is frequently increased, possibly due to (a) irritant receptor firing, contributing to alveolar hyperventilation, and (b) inhomogeneous lungs, contributing to dead space ventilation. This is associated with an inability to take a deep breath. The global quality is thus interdependent on a variety of sensory events. Individual analysis of the dimensions shows that (a) effort is increased, (b) tension is increased as a result of a mechanical disadvantage and a high inspiratory impedance, (c) impedance is increased, and (d) inspiratory muscles are weak. All these sensory dimensions can be individually perceived and have discrete sensory mechanisms. Their interrelationships and intensities determine the overall sensory experience.

Need to Breathe

Patients occasionally report that their need to breathe exceeds the current level of their breathing and that they are unable to breathe as much as they perceive is appropriate. This perceptual experience occurs in normal subjects after very short high-intensity exercise (e.g., climbing three to four flights of stairs rapidly) and is associated with a transient rise in P_{CO_2}. Although it is tempting to suggest a link with chemoreceptor activity, the primary and secondary processing remain ill-defined and the mechanism responsible for this perception remains unknown. Acute airflow limitation is another common circumstance in which this sensory experience can occur. Effort is increased, but hyperinflation commonly limits the muscular response in that the forces generated are limited by mechanical disadvantages.

Inappropriateness

Behavioral learning contributes additional dimensions to respiratory sensation. During the course of repeated respiratory activity, the relationships between the intensities of the primary sensations are learned. Just as we are aware of the amount of peripheral muscular effort involved in walking and climbing stairs, we are at least potentially aware of the respiratory muscle effort required to breathe. Although we are normally unaware of respiratory effort, this reaches consciousness when it becomes substantial or changes. We are aware of the amount of effort, tension, and displacement expected with both peripheral and respiratory muscles under the common circumstances in which they are used. When there are changes in (a) the effort required to generate a given ventilation, (b) the tension required to generate a given ventilation, (c) the effort required to generate a given tension, and (d) the ventilation required to perform a given activity, the abnormal quan-

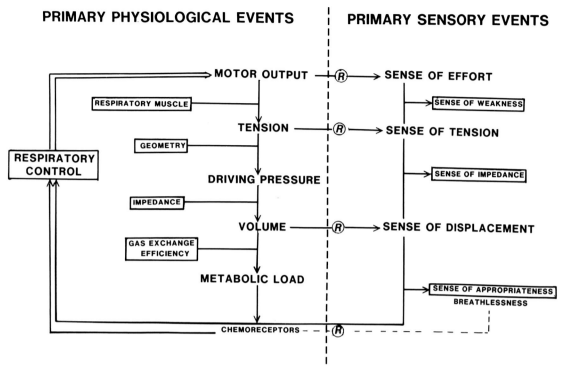

FIG. 1. Schematic representation of the interdependent interaction of physiological processes and their effects on sensory receptors.

titative relationships between these dimensions are readily recognized and reach consciousness. Inappropriateness between any or all of these dimensions is readily detected and contributes to respiratory sensation. Patients may sense inappropriateness at a time when discomfort is not a major concern. Inappropriateness and dyspnea are not synonymous.

THE MEASUREMENT OF DYSPNEA

The final issue we will consider is measurement of the intensity of dyspnea. A variety of techniques have been used. Some are indirect, such as the Medical Research Council questionnaire, in which no stimulus is applied but the intensity of dyspnea is inferred from either (a) limitation in functional capacity or (b) various modifications of behavior resulting from associated breathing discomfort. Measurement of disability and handicap resulting from dyspnea has resulted in the use of a variety of questionnaires based on the comparison of responses found in discrete population groups; these types of questionnaire are widely used in experimental psychology. While it might be argued that these techniques measure the intensity of dyspnea, they are not classical psychophysical techniques in which a stimulus is applied and the sensory response rated. We will not address these techniques, but they should be recognized as a measurement of disability

and handicap and are quite different from psychophysical techniques in which the conditions of stimulation are varied systematically in order to induce the sensation with the subsequent measurement of the sensory response.

Psychophysics is the quantitative study of the relationship between a stimulus and the conscious sensory response and is dependent on the interaction of all the processes already described. These quantitative studies describe, in a unique fashion, the operation of the system as a whole. Psychophysical techniques provide a bridge between (a) the wealth of knowledge related to the act of breathing and (b) the sensations experienced with breathing. Their utility is dependent on understanding the techniques, their limitations, and their attributes, and a knowledge of respiratory and neurophysiology is required.

Recognition and scaling of dyspnea is traditionally based on the intensity of functional activity (such as rest, walking, or stairclimbing) that is required to produce discomfort in the act of breathing. Measurement takes place in the physical domain by quantifying the stimulus required (e.g., one flight of stairs) to reach a defined criterion state. The criterion state, though not precisely defined, tacitly assumes dyspnea sufficiently severe to stop the patient from continued activity. The tolerance of the individual for discomfort is thus an inherent component. This approach to the measurement of dyspnea is essentially similar to the psychophysical measurement of sensory intensity using the techniques introduced and popularized by Fechner in the 1850s (70). These scales have ordinal properties, have considerable practical utility, and form the conceptual basis of the assessment of dyspnea during the routine interrogation of patients.

The fundamental process involved in making a direct measurement is the "matching" of one continuum (number continuum being one specific example) to another while conforming to preset rules. The rules and the independent continuum define a "scale." Scales are classified by preset rules: nominal, to distinguish one object or event from another; ordinal, to rank objects or events in order of magnitude; interval, to determine equality and magnitude of differences in objects or events while preserving rank order; and ratio, to determine ratio relationships.

Stevens (71–76) made the initially controversial observation that there is no fundamental reason why sensory intensity cannot be scaled directly. Stevens showed that sensations varying in intensity (sound, light, lifted weights, etc.) can be scaled ("open-magnitude scaling") by matching the perceived magnitude to a variety of continuums (numbers, other sensory stimuli, "cross-modality matching") while observing the preset rule of ratio relationships. Open-magnitude scaling has distinct limitations in that it describes the increase in sensory magnitude as the stimulus increases. True zero and absolute magnitude may be defined for an individual, but a direct comparison between individuals or in the same individual across time is not possible. This technique is successful in measuring the quantitative effects of various stimulus characteristics (frequency of breathing, duration of stimulation, etc.) on perceptual magnitude by comparing the differences in sensory magnitude with changing stimulus characteristics.

To estimate absolute sensory intensity and to compare intensity between individuals, category scaling techniques (a visual analogue scale is a category scale with an infinite number of categories) were introduced. When formally compared to validated open-magnitude scales, the ratio of the increase in sensory magnitude relative to the ratio increase in physical magnitude is systematically reduced and is thus invalid. The reasons for this remain inadequately explained. However, despite the lack of validity there is considerable practical utility.

The Borg scale deserves special attention because of its widespread use and its utility. In describing sensory intensity in everyday life, simple descriptive terms are used, such as "slight," "moderate," and "severe." Borg formally measured the precision of these descriptors by noting (a) their locality in a stimulus range from zero to maximum intensity and (b)

their variability in the different populations. Borg then went on to address the ratio properties of these descriptive terms relative to each other (quantitative semantics). Knowing both (a) the validated psychophysical relationship and (b) the localities of these descriptors and their ratio properties relative to each other, he constructed a scale. By tagging the simple descriptive terms to specific numbers from 0 to 10, he constructed a scale with both ratio properties and properties of absolute intensity. This scale has proved remarkably easy to use in practice, is readily understood by people of diverse educational backgrounds, is used in several languages, and is used for patients with a variety of disorders, in a manner expected from their known pathophysiological relationships (77–81). Utility is well established.

Incremental exercise can be used as a condition of stimulation resulting in dyspnea. The condition of stimulation can be easily standardized and systematically applied by expressing the work as a percentage of maximum expected capacity using normal predicted capacity. The Borg scale can be used by each individual to estimate the intensity of dyspnea at comparable levels of stimulation. When applied to large numbers of subjects with widely varying severity of lung impairment, the intensity of dyspnea can be compared under comparable working conditions (work expressed as a percentage of predicted capacity for all subjects, both normal and impaired). This is of practical clinical utility in that these individuals should be capable of achieving their expected capacity. Disability can be measured as the reduction in their work capacity, and the limiting symptom can be identified. Symptom handicap can be quantified by abstracting the intensity of dyspnea at various percentages of predicted capacity and then comparing these with normal subjects. This approach, while variable in individual subjects, is extremely useful in mean responses from groups where response bias can be minimized.

In Fig. 2 we see the results of this approach applied to a large group of subjects with varying impairments of ventilatory capacity and varying degrees of inspiratory muscle strength as assessed by maximum inspiratory pressure. The intensity of dyspnea increased as respiratory muscle strength decreased, both in normal subjects and in patients at all levels of ventilatory impairment; this illustrates the importance of respiratory muscle strength and pulmonary impairment in the generation of dyspnea. Using these approaches, normal standards can be established. At maximum exercise the intensity of dyspnea was not systematically increased in the impaired group because all subjects exercised to a similar limiting symptom intensity. Many of these subjects were primarily limited by leg fatigue. All subjects were limited by leg fatigue and/or

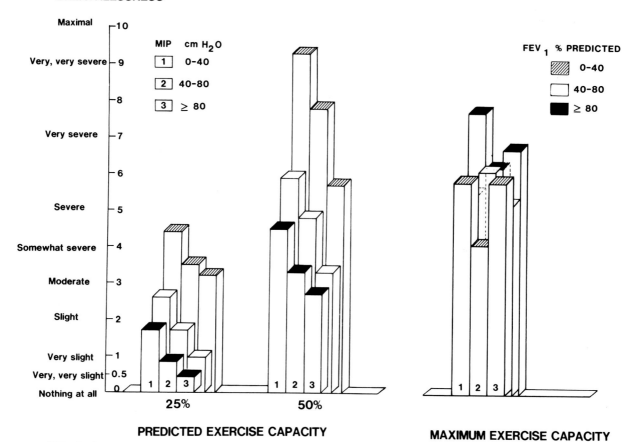

BREATHLESSNESS

FIG. 2. Perceived magnitude of dyspnea experienced during exercise on a cycle ergometer in 550 subjects, at 25%, 75%, and maximum capacity.

dyspnea, and both normal subjects and patients with lung impairment exercised to the same limiting intensity of 7 ("very severe") on the Borg scale. Tolerance varied from subject to subject, but 90% of patients continued to exercise until the limiting symptom intensity exceeded 5 ("severe"). Only 20% exercised until symptom intensity was perceived as "maximal."

Similar approaches can be used with loading (resistive or elastic), induced bronchoconstriction, and stimulated breathing (hypoxemia and/or hypercapnia), but these are best used to establish mechanism.

In summary, the causes of dyspnea have been well recognized for many years. Traditionally, approaches to its investigation and management have been largely confined to the identification and amelioration of these causative factors. However, dyspnea is a sensory experience and can only be fully understood with a knowledge of the sensory mechanisms. By understanding the mechanisms, approaches to both investigation and management can be improved. The quality of the sensory experience of dyspnea is formed from more than one source of information. Effort, tension,

and displacement are the most important sources and account for qualitative differences. Of these sources, the intensity of dyspnea appears to be most closely related to respiratory muscle effort.

ACKNOWLEDGMENT

This work was supported by the Medical Research Council, Canada.

REFERENCES

1. William CJB. Examination of chest through functions. In: London WCJB, ed. *Pathology and diagnosis of diseases of the chest.* 1840.
2. Pfluger E. On the causes of respiratory movement and of dyspnea and apnea. In: J West, ed. *Translations in repiratory physiology.* Stroudsburg, Pennsylvania: Dowden, Hutchinson and Ross Inc., 1975;404–434.
3. Miescher-Rusch F. Bemerkungen zur Lehre von den Atembewegungen (Notes on the theory of respiratory movements). In: Fenn WO, Rahn H, eds. *Handbook of Physiology, Vol 1.* Baltimore, Md.: American Physiological Society, 1964;1–62.

4. Haldane JS, Smith JL. Carbon dioxide and regulation of breathing. In: Haldane JS, Priestley JG, eds. *Respiration*. Oxford: Clarendon Press, 1935;16–42.

5. Winterstein H. The regulation of breathing by the blood. In: J West, ed. *Translations in respiratory physiology*. Stroudsburg, Pennsylvania: Dowden, Hutchinson and Ross Inc., 1975;529–548.

6. Meakins JM. The cause and treatment of dyspnea in cardiovascular disease. *B Med J* 1923;1:1043–1055.

7. Cullen GE, Harrison TR, Calhoun JA, Wilkins WE, Tims MM. Regulation of dyspnea of exertion to oxygen saturation and acid-base condition of the blood. *J Clin Invest* 1931;10:807.

8. Harrison TR, Harrison WG, Calhoun JA, Marsh JP. Congestive heart failure. XVII. The mechanism of dyspnea on exertion. *Arch Int Med* 1932;50:690–720.

9. Harrison TR. *Failure of the Circulation*. Baltimore, Md: Williams and Wilkins, 1935.

10. Gesell R, Moyer C. Effect of sensory nerve stimulation on costal and abdominal breathing in anaesthetized dog. *Q J Exp Physiol* 1935;25:1.

11. Christie R. Dyspnea. *Q J Med* 1938;7:421–454.

12. Means JH. Dyspnea. *Medicine Monogr*, Vol 5. Baltimore, Md.: Williams and Wilkins, 1924.

13. Cournand A, Brock HJ, Rappaport L, Richards DW. Disturbance of action of respiratory muscles as a contributing cause of dyspnea. *Arch Intern Med* 1936;57:1008–26.

14. Cournand A, Richards DW. Pulmonary insufficiency. *Am Rev Tuberc* 1941;44:26–41.

15. Rohrer F. The Physiology of Respiratory Movements. In: J West, eds. *Translations in Respiratory Physiology*. Stroudsburg, Pennsylvania: Dowden, Hutchinson and Ross, Inc., 1975;93–170.

16. Rahn H, Otis AB, Chadwick LE, Fenn WO. Pressure–volume diagram of the thorax and lung. *Am J Physiol* 1946;146:161–178.

17. Marshall R, McIlroy MB, Christie RV. The work of breathing in mitral stenosis. *Clin Sci* 1954;13:137–146.

18. Cherniack RM, Snidal DP. The effect of obstruction to breathing on the ventilatory response to CO_2. *J Clin Invest* 1956;35:1286–1290.

19. Marshall R, Stone RW, Christie RV. The relationship of dyspnoea to respiratory effort in normal subjects, mitral stenosis and emphysema. *Clin Sci* 1954;13:625.

20. Cournand A, Richards DW, Bader RA, Bader ME, Fishman AP. The oxygen cost of breathing. *Trans Assoc Am Physiol* 1954;67:162–173.

21. Campbell EJM, Westlake EK, Cherniack RM. Simple methods of estimating oxygen consumption and efficiency of the muscles of breathing. *J Appl Physiol* 1957;11(2):303–308.

22. Campbell EJM, Westlake EK, Cherniack RM. The oxygen consumption of the respiratory muscles of young male subjects. *Clin Sci* 1959;18:55–62.

23. Bartlett RG, Brubach HF, Specht H. Oxygen cost of breathing. *J Appl Physiol* 1958;14:413–424.

24. McIlroy MB. Dyspnea and the work of breathing in diseases of the heart and lungs. *Prog Cardiovasc Dis* 1958;1:284–297.

25. Campbell EJM, Howell JBL. The sensation of breathlessness. *Br Med Bull* 1963;19:36–40.

26. Campbell EJM. The relationship of the sensation of breathlessness to the act of breathing. In: Howell JBL, Campbell EJM, eds. *Breathlessness*. Oxford: Blackwell Scientific Publications, 1966;55.

27. Campbell EJM. *The respiratory muscles and the mechanics of breathing*. Chicago: Year Book Publishers, 1958.

28. Schmidt RF. *Fundamentals of sensory physiology*. New York: Springer-Verlag, 1981.

29. Coleridge HM, Coleridge JCG. Reflexes evoked from tracheobronchial tree and lungs. In: Geiger SR, Widdicombe JD, Cherniack NS, Fishman AP, eds. *Handbook of physiology, section 3: respiratory system*, vol II, part I. Bethesda, MD: American Physiological Society, 1986;395–429.

30. Fidone SJ, Gonzales C. Initiation and control of chemoreceptor activity in the carotid body. In: Geiger SR, Widdicombe JG, Cherniack NS, Fishman AP, eds. *Handbook of physiology, section 3: the respiratory system*, vol II, part I. Bethesda, MD: American Physiological Society, 1986;247–312.

31. Fitzgerald RS, Lahiri S. Reflex responses to chemoreceptor stimulation. In: Geiger SR, Widdicombe JG, Cherniack NS, Fishman AP, eds. *The handbook of physiology, section 3: the respiratory system*, vol II, part I. Bethesda, MD: American Physiological Society, 1986;313–362.

32. Campbell EJM, Freedman S, Clark TJH, Robson JG, Norman J. The effect of muscular paralysis induced by tubocurarine on the duration and sensation of breath-holding. *Clin Sci* 1967;20:223–231.

33. Gandevia SC, McCloskey DI. Joint sense, muscle sense, and their combination as position sense, measured at the distal interphalangeal joint of the middle finger. *J Appl Physiol* 1976;260:387–407.

34. Matthews PBC. Evolving views on the internal operation and functional role of the muscle spindle. *J Physiol* 1981;320:1–30.

35. Matthews PBC. Where does Sherrington's "muscular sense" originate? Muscles, joints, corollary discharge? *Annu Rev Neurosci* 1982;5:189–218.

36. McCloskey DI. Kinesthetic sensibility. *Physiol Rev* 1978;58:763–820.

37. Burgess PR, Wei JY, Clark FJ, Simon J. Signalling of kinesthetic information by peripheral sensory receptors. *Annu Rev Neurosci* 1982;5:171.

38. Roland PE, Ladegaard-Pederson H. A quantitative analysis of sensations of tension and kinaesthesia in man. Evidence for peripherally originating muscular sense and for a sense of effort. *Brain* 1977;100:671–692.

39. Sherrington CS. The muscular sense. In: Shafer EA, ed. *Textbook of physiology*, vol 12. Edinburgh: TJ Pentland, 1900;1002–1025.

40. Campbell EJM, Gandevia SC, Killian KJ, Mahutte CK, Rigg JRA. Changes in the perception of inspiratory resistive load during partial curarization. *J Physiol* 1980;309:93–100.

41. Gandevia SC. The perception of motor commands or effort during muscular paralysis. *Brain* 1982;105:151–195.

42. Gandevia SC, McCloskey DI. Sensation of heaviness. *Brain* 1977;100:345–354.

43. Gandevia SC, Killian KJ, Campbell EJM. The effect of respiratory muscle fatigue on respiratory sensations. *Clin Sci* 1981;60:463–466.

44. Gandevia SC, McCloskey DI. Changes in motor commands, as shown by changes in perceived heaviness, during partial curarization and peripheral muscle anaesthesia in man. *J Physiol (Lond)* 1977;272:673–689.

45. Killian KJ, Gandevia SC, Summers E, Campbell EJM. Effect of increased lung volume on perception of breathlessness, effort and tension. *J Appl Physiol* 1984;57:686–691.

46. Widdicombe JG. Reflexes from the upper respiratory tract. In: Geiger SR, Widdicombe JG, Cherniack NS, Fishman AP, eds. *Handbook of physiology, section 3: the respiratory system*, vol II, part I. Bethesda, MD: American Physiological Society, 1986;363–394.

47. Killian KJ, Campbell EJM. Dyspnea and exercise. *Annu Rev Physiol* 1983;45:465–479.

48. Killian KJ, Campbell EJM. Dyspnea. In: Roussos C, Macklem PT, eds. *The Thorax*, part B. New York: Marcel Dekker, 1985;787–828.

49. Zechman FW Jr, Wiley RL. Afferent inputs to breathing: respiratory sensation. In: Geiger SR, Widdicombe JG, Cherniack NS, Fishman AP, eds. *Handbook of physiology, section 3: the respiratory system*, vol II, part I. Bethesda, MD: American Physiological Society, 1986;449–474.

50. Campbell EJM, Freedman S, Smith PS, Taylor ME. The ability of man to detect added elastic loads to breathing. *Clin Sci* 1961;20:223–231.

51. Bennett ED, Jayson MIV, Rubenstein D, Campbell EJM. The ability of man to detect added non-elastic loads to breathing. *Clin Sci* 1962;23:155–162.

52. Wiley RL, Zechman FE Jr. Perception of added airflow resistance in humans. *Respir Physiol* 1966;2:73–87.

53. Burki NK. Effects of added inspiratory loads on load detection thresholds. *J Appl Physiol* 1981;50:162–164.

54. Burki NK, Mitchell K, Chaudhary BA, Zechman FW. The ability of asthmatics to detect added resistive loads. *Am Rev Respir Dis* 1978;117:71–75.

55. Gottfried SB, Altose MD, Kelsen SG, Fogarty CM, Cherniack NS. The perception of changes in airflow resistance in normal subjects and patients with chronic airways obstruction. *Chest* 1978;73:286–288.

56. Guz A, Noble MIM, Widdicombe JG, Trenchard D, Mushin WW, Makey AR. The role of vagal and glossopharyngeal afferent nerves in respiratory sensation, control of breathing and arterial pressure regulation in conscious man. *Clin Sci* 1966;30:161–170.

57. Burki NK, Davenport PW, Safdar F, Zechman FW. The effects of airway anesthesia on magnitude estimation of added inspiratory resistive and elastic loads. *Am Rev Respir Dis* 1983;127:2–4.

58. Eisele J, Trenchard D, Burki N, Guz A. The effect of chest wall block on respiratory sensation and control in man. *Clin Sci* 1968;35:23–33.

59. Noble MIM, Eisele JH, Trenchard D, Guz A. Effect of selective peripheral nerve blocks on respiratory sensations. In: Porter R, ed. *Breathing: Hering–Breuer Centenary Symposium (Ciba Found Symp)*. London: Churchill, 1970;233–246.

60. Zechman FW, O'Neill R, Shannon R. Effect of low cervical cord lesion on detection of increased airflow resistance in man. *Physiologist* 1967;10:356.

61. Killian KJ, Mahutte CK, Campbell EJM. Resistive load detection during passive ventilation. *Clin Sci* 1980;59:493–495.

62. Bakers JHCM, Tenney SM. The perception of some sensations associated with breathing. *Respir Physiol* 1970;10:85–92.

63. Killian KJ, Mahutte CK, Campbell EJM. Magnitude scaling of externally added loads to breathing. *Am Rev Respir Dis* 1981;123:12–15.

64. Burdon JGW, Juniper EF, Killian KJ, Hargreave FE, Campbell EJM. Perception of breathlessness in asthma. *Am Rev Resp Dis* 1982;126:825–828.

65. Stubbing DG, Ramsdale EH, Killian KJ, Campbell EJM. Psychophysics of inspiratory muscle force. *J Appl Physiol* 1983;54:1216–1221.

66. Stubbing DG, Killian KJ, Campbell EJM. The quantification of respiratory sensations by normal subjects. *Respir Physiol* 1981;44:251–260.

67. Wolkove N, Altose MD, Kelsen SG, Kondapalli PG, Cherniack NS. Perception of changes in breathing in normal human subjects. *J Appl Physiol* 1981;50:78–83.

68. Gliner JA, Folinsbee LJ, Horvath SM. Accuracy and precision of matching inspired lung volume. *Percept Psychophysiol* 1981;29:511–515.

69. Salamon M, von Euler C, Franzen O. Perception of mechanical factors in breathing. Presented at the International Symposium on "Physical Work and Effort," Wenner-Gren Center, Stockholm, 1975.

70. Fechner GT. *Elemente der Psychophysik*. Leipzig: Breitkopf und Hartel, 1860. Volume 1 available in English translation as *Elements of psychophysics*. New York: Holt, Rinehart and Winston, 1966.

71. Stevens SS. On the theory of scales of measurement. *Science* 1946;103:677–680.

72. Stevens SS. Mathematics, measurement and psychophysics. In: Stevens SS, ed. *The handbook of experimental psychology*. New York: John Wiley & Sons, 1951;1–49.

73. Stevens SS. On the psychophysical law. *Psychol Rev* 1957;64:153–181.

74. Stevens SS. Measurement, psychophysics and utility. In: Churchman CW, Ratoosh P, eds. *Measurement: definition and theories*. New York: John Wiley & Sons, 1959;18–63.

75. Stevens SS. Ratio scales, partition scales and confusion scales. In: Gulliksen H, Messick S, eds. *Psychological scaling: theory and applications*. New York: John Wiley & Sons, 1960;49–66.

76. Stevens SS. In: Stevens G, ed. *Psychophysics. Introduction to its perceptual, neural, and social prospects*. New York: Wiley–Interscience, 1975.

77. Borg G. The perception of muscular work. *Publications of the Umea Research Library* 1960;5:1–27.

78. Borg G. On quantitative semantics in connection with psychophysics. *Educational and Psychological Research Bulletin, University of Umea* 1964;3:1–7.

79. Borg G, Hosman J. The metric properties of adverbs. *Reports from the Institute of Applied Psychology of the University of Stockholm* 1970;7:1–7.

80. Borg G, Lindblad I. The determination of subjective intensities in verbal descriptions of symptoms. *Reports from the Institute of Applied Psychology of the University of Stockholm* 1976;75:1–22.

81. Borg G. A category scale with ratio properties for intermodal and interindividual comparisons. In: Geissler HS, Petzold P, eds. *Psychophysical judgment and the process of perceptions. Proceedings of the 22nd international congress of psychology*. Amsterdam: North-Holland, 1980;25–34.

THE LUNG: *Scientific Foundations*
edited by R.G. Crystal, J.B. West et al.
Raven Press, Ltd., New York © 1991.

CHAPTER 5.5.1.1

Intracellular Respiration

Tak Yee Aw and Dean P. Jones

Cellular respiration is relevant to lung function because this process establishes the work load for the lungs. The primary role of cellular respiration is to produce ATP; the machinery for this process and its regulation resides principally within the mitochondria. Thus, an understanding of organismic respiration and its regulation requires knowledge of the mitochondrial respiratory components and their regulation in the diverse, specialized cells throughout the body. In this discussion we summarize the ubiquitous components of the respiratory apparatus, the plasticity of mitochondrial function in muscle and other specialized tissues, and the optimization of function by changes in protein composition and spatial distribution.

COMPONENTS OF THE RESPIRATORY APPARATUS OF CELLS

The fundamental events and components of ATP production and O_2 utilization are common to all tissues (Fig. 1). Diverse nutrients are converted by digestion and intermediary metabolism to common substrates for oxidation. This oxidation provides the energy to establish an electrochemical proton gradient (Δp) across the mitochondrial inner membrane. The Δp drives the accumulation of precursors for substrate oxidation, synthesis of ATP, export of products, and maintenance of osmotic stability.

Supply of Oxidizable Substrates

Dietary carbohydrates, fats, and proteins supply most of the substrates for cellular energy production. Carbohydrates and some amino acids are converted to

three-carbon units (e.g., pyruvate), whereas fats and other amino acids are converted to two-carbon acetyl units. Mitochondria contain systems to convert pyruvate and hydrocarbon chains to acetyl-CoA and to oxidize acetyl-CoA to CO_2. These systems directly supply the reducing equivalents to the mitochondrial electron transport chain and are of primary importance in supporting mitochondrial ATP production.

Oxidation of acetyl-CoA to CO_2 is catalyzed by the enzymes of the citric acid cycle. The reducing equivalents from this oxidation are transferred through four dehydrogenases: Three of these reduce NAD^+ to NADH, and the other reduces ubiquinone to ubiquinol. The enzymes that are involved in the production of NADH are isocitrate, α-ketoglutarate, and malate dehydrogenases. The other, succinate dehydrogenase, contains a flavin coenzyme and does not require NAD^+ for function.

Other dehydrogenases such as glutamate, pyruvate, aldehyde, α-glycerol phosphate, and fatty acyl-CoA dehydrogenases also transfer electrons into the electron transfer chain through NADH and ubiquinone. The contributions of these reactions to the supply of reducing equivalents are usually small relative to the electron supply from the citric acid cycle.

Several factors affect the turnover of the cycle. The most important are availability of NAD^+, rate of acetyl-CoA production, mitochondrial ADP and ATP concentrations, and utilization of citric acid cycle intermediates for other biosynthetic processes (1). Under some conditions, flux through the cycle is rate-limited by condensation of acetyl-CoA and oxaloacetate. Because oxidations of NADH and ubiquinol are coupled to synthesis of ATP, regulation must also occur at the level of the dehydrogenases (2).

Electron Transfer Components

Oxidizable substrates supply reducing equivalents for reduction of O_2 to water through a series of electron

T.Y. Aw and D.P. Jones: Department of Biochemistry and Winship Cancer Center, Emory University, Atlanta, Georgia 30322.

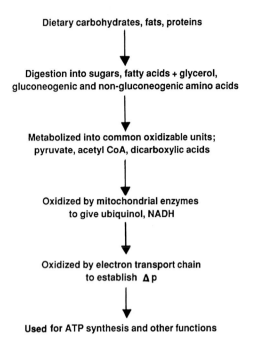

Dietary carbohydrates, fats, proteins

↓

Digestion into sugars, fatty acids + glycerol,
gluconeogenic and non-gluconeogenic amino acids

↓

Metabolized into common oxidizable units;
pyruvate, acetyl CoA, dicarboxylic acids

↓

Oxidized by mitochondrial enzymes
to give ubiquinol, NADH

↓

Oxidized by electron transport chain
to establish Δp

↓

Used for ATP synthesis and other functions

FIG. 1. Conversion of dietary nutrients into usable energy forms. Energy sources from the diet are digested into common molecules, such as sugars, fatty acids, and amino acids, prior to absorption and presentation to cells via the circulatory system. Subsequent reactions in intermediary metabolism, which occur principally within mitochondria, convert the carbon chains to two- or three-carbon units. These units are oxidized to supply the energy for establishment of a proton-motive force, which is used for ATP synthesis, exchange of nutrients and products, and maintenance of osmotic stability.

transfer complexes in the mitochondrial inner membrane. These complexes catalyze three successive redox reactions in which NADH plus ubiquinone produce NAD^+ plus ubiquinol, ubiquinol plus two oxidized cytochrome c produce ubiquinone plus two reduced cytochrome c, and two reduced cytochrome c plus $\frac{1}{2}O_2$ produce oxidized cytochrome c plus H_2O. The overall process uses ubiquinone and cytochrome c catalytically and results in oxidation of NADH by O_2.

Each of the complexes functions as a proton transporter in which there is an obligate movement of protons out of the mitochondrial matrix in response to flow of electrons toward the terminal acceptor, O_2 (3). The energy available from the oxidation reactions is captured in the form of an electrochemical proton gradient (Δp) across the inner membrane. This Δp provides the energy to drive ATP synthesis from ADP and P_i by coupling the reaction to movement of protons down the electrochemical proton gradient.

The Δp has two components, a chemical gradient (ΔpH) and an electrical potential ($\Delta \psi$). The chemical gradient is the difference in concentration of protons between the matrix space and the cytoplasm. The concentration of protons is commonly expressed as pH so that the chemical term is given as a ΔpH. The matrix

pH is often in the range of 7.6–7.8, whereas the cytoplasmic pH is 6.8–7.2. It remains unclear whether the extruded protons are in rapid equilibrium with the cytoplasmic aqueous phase; if the transported protons remain sequestered in or near the inner membrane, the chemical term cannot be accurately determined by measuring the pH in the bulk phase.

The energy available from ΔpH as measured from the bulk phase is insufficient to drive ATP synthesis under prevailing conditions in the cell. Through the function of multiple transport systems, the energy available from oxidation also maintains a large electrical potential across the inner membrane. This potential is about 160 mV and is negative inside, and it drives positively charged particles into the matrix that supplies most of the energy needed for ATP synthesis.

ATP Synthesis

The enzyme that synthesizes ATP from ADP and P_i, ATP synthase, is an electrogenic proton transporter that utilizes energy from the Δp. From *in vitro* studies, the enzyme appears to function in three different modes. Under usual conditions, the Δp formed by electron transfer is sufficient to synthesize ATP. Without electron transfer, such as occurs during anoxia and with mitochondrial inhibitors, the ATPase can generate Δp by hydrolyzing ATP from glycolysis. The ATPase can also function as an uncoupled ATP hydrolase when the membrane cannot maintain the pH gradient, such as occurs in the presence of uncouplers of oxidative phosphorylation. Recent evidence indicates that control mechanisms exist to prevent the second mode during short-term anoxia in rat hepatocytes (4), and it is not yet clear whether this mode is important under physiological conditions. The third mode is physiologically important only in heat production by brown fat but also can occur under some toxicological and pathological conditions.

Mitochondrial Metabolite and Ion Transport Systems

Because the $\Delta \psi$ across the inner membrane is highly negative on the inside, metabolic anions would be effectively excluded from the matrix if special carrier mechanisms did not exist to couple anion movement with that of other ions. Similarly, cations would be accumulated to high concentrations if the membrane was permeable to cations or if ion-coupled efflux mechanisms did not exist. Consequently, compartmentation of metabolites and ions across the inner membrane must be tightly controlled and is crucial to respiratory function. The steady flow of essential substrates (e.g., P_i, citric acid cycle intermediates, ADP) into the mitochondrial compartment, along with extrusion of products (e.g., ATP), is achieved by specific porter systems that are driven by components of the Δp.

ΔpH-Dependent Electroneutral Transporters

Pyruvate is primarily transported by an electroneutral proton-compensated transport system that functions as either an H^+-symporter or an OH^--antiporter. Phosphate transport also occurs by an electroneutral mechanism. These systems accumulate pyruvate and P_i in the matrix according to the ΔpH across the inner membrane. Thus, both of these systems directly use energy from the Δp. The dicarboxylate and tricarboxylate carriers catalyze electroneutral exchange of P_i for citric acid cycle intermediates; thus the distributions of these anions are also indirectly dependent on ΔpH. The dicarboxylate carriers exchange L-malate, succinate, or fumarate for P_i while the tricarboxylate carrier functions as an antiporter exchanging citrate, isocitrate, and phosphoenolpyruvate for malate.

$\Delta\psi$-Dependent Transport Systems

Some systems catalyze transport that is dependent upon $\Delta\psi$ and result in net charge movement across the inner membrane. These systems can establish a potential (electrogenic movement) or can move charged species according to an existing potential (electrophoretic movement).

The adenine nucleotide transporter catalyzes the exchange of matrix ATP^{4-} for cytosolic ADP^{3-} (5), which allows electrophoretic movement of a negative charge out of the matrix. This is the major mechanism for supply of ADP that is needed for oxidative phosphorylation and for supply of ATP to the cytoplasm. The contribution of the transporter to the energetics of ATP synthesis is important because the resulting decrease in ATP concentration and increase in ADP concentration account for up to one-third of the total energy needed for ATP synthesis. The electrophoretic exchange of glutamate plus a proton in exchange for aspartate allows for the unidirectional entry of glutamate into the mitochondria. Regulation of this system can control the direction of movement of electrons via the malate–aspartate shuttle between mitochondrial and cytoplasmic NAD^+/NADH pools. The mitochondrial uptake of Ca^{2+}, which is critical for regulation of many mitochondrial and cytoplasmic functions (2), also occurs by an electrophoretic uptake mechanism. Thus, the energy available from the mitochondrial $\Delta\psi$ is of general importance for mitochondrial function and regulation.

TABLE 1. *Relative contributions of organs to total body O_2 consumption*

Tissue	Weight (kg)	Basal $\dot{V}O_2$ (ml/min/kg)	Percentage of total O_2 consumption
Heart	0.3	90	10.8
CNS	1.5	33	19.8
Liver	1.7	44	29.9
Kidneys	0.3	62	7.2
Skeletal muscle	30	1.7 (at rest)	20.4

HETEROGENEITY OF MITOCHONDRIA

Although the principal components of the mitochondrial oxidative phosphorylation system are the same in different tissues, the maximal O_2 consumption rate, respiratory control characteristics, mitochondrial morphology, and mitochondrial distribution vary. A consideration of these heterogeneities is worthwhile because the mitochondria are dynamic entities that change characteristics in response to various physiological and pathological stimuli.

In most differentiated cell types, the requirement for continuous energy supply to support uninterrupted function is met by specific associations of mitochondria with energy-requiring systems. Because energy demand varies with work load, there is no "normal" O_2 consumption rate; instead, there is a range of O_2 consumption rates (Table 1). Changes in function can have a marked effect on the relative contributions of different tissues to the total O_2 consumption by the body. For instance, following ingestion of a meal, the basal metabolic rate increases from about 250 ml/min up to 350 ml/min. Much of this increase is attributable to increased O_2 consumption in the gastrointestinal tract, and the functional demand on the lung is increased by the need for O_2 in the intestine. The largest effect of this type occurs in skeletal muscle, where the O_2 consumption rate can be increased to over 70 ml/min/kg, or over 2100 ml/min for all of the muscle. Under these conditions, cardiac output must also increase, but it is the large increase in O_2 consumption by the skeletal muscle that is the major determinant of the functional demand on the lung.

Variations in energy needs and other functional demands are associated with differences in mitochondrial respiratory components and their regulation. This is apparent in a comparison of heart muscle, renal proximal tubules, and liver parenchyma. In the muscle, cells must undergo a rhythmic contraction. This requires cyclical changes in mitochondrial shape and in cellular oxygenation. The cells have features to accommodate these unique demands; that is, the mitochondria exist as networks, or reticulae (6–8), and have the O_2-binding protein, myoglobin, to dampen oscillations in cellular oxygenation (9,10). In contrast, proximal tubule cells do not undergo rapid changes in shape but have specialized adaptations to function, such as a heterogeneity in distribution wherein mitochondria are concentrated in the basal region of the cells juxtaposed to the highly energy-requiring Na^+,K^+-ATPase (11). In liver, where plasma membrane ATP utilization represents a considerably lower fraction of the total cell requirement, mitochondria are distributed in apparent clusters throughout the cytoplasm surrounding the central nucleus (12).

Mitochondria differ considerably in protein composition. They vary qualitatively in contents of enzymes and transporters (e.g., 25-hydroxycholecalciferol 1α- and steroid 7α-hydroxylases, cytochrome P-450$_{scc}$, carbonic anhydrase, pyruvate carboxylase, Na^+/Ca^{2+} antiporter) and quantitatively in the amounts of common enzymes and transporters (e.g., NADH, succinate, glutamate dehydrogenases, adenine nucleotide transporter). Genetic and molecular biological studies show that tissue-specific isozymes also exist for ubiquitous components such as the adenine nucleotide transporter, cytochrome c, and cytochrome c oxidase (13,14).

Heterogeneity of mitochondria in tissues is apparent at the morphological level. Volume density of mitochondria in different human tissues varies up to 100-fold. Furthermore, mitochondria differ between tissues in their size, shape, inner membrane appearance, buoyant density, and staining properties (6,15,16). Differences in mitochondrial structure and composition also occur in different cells of the same cell type. In liver, the mitochondria are larger and more densely packed in periportal cells than in centrilobular cells (17). Periportal cells have higher activities of enzymes of fatty acid β-oxidation, citric acid cycle, respiratory chain, gluconeogenesis, and ureogenesis (18). The extent to which similar gradients in oxidative capacities occur from arteriolar to venular ends of capillaries in other tissues is presently unclear.

OPTIMIZATION OF MITOCHONDRIAL STRUCTURE AND FUNCTION

Mitochondrial function may be optimized by control of enzyme contents and activities per unit volume of mitochondria, volume percent of mitochondria in cells, and spatial distribution of mitochondria in cells. Regulation of mitochondrial enzyme and transport functions is frequently considered in terms of ATP needs and ADP availability. Although this is a reasonable first approximation, it does not account for the differences in regulation to accommodate the large range of respiratory responses that occur in different tissues. A more correct description is that regulation occurs at several sites (Fig. 2), especially those involving (a) generation and utilization of Δp and (b) volume regulation. Regulation of generation of Δp involves control of electron flow into the electron transport chain at the NAD^+-linked dehydrogenases (2) as well as out of the chain at cytochrome c oxidase (13). Several of the important NAD^+-linked dehydrogenases are regulated by Ca^{2+} (2), and cytochrome c oxidase contains regulatory subunits (19). Regulation of utilization of Δp occurs at electrophoretic transport systems, including the adenine nucleotide transporter, Glu/Asp exchanger, and Ca^{2+} uniporter (20). Regulation also occurs at the H^+/K^+ exchanger that functions in volume regulation (21) and at the P_i uptake system to prevent P_i loading during short-term anoxia (20). Variations in control at different sites could result in significant differences in respiratory function without qualitative changes in the mitochondria.

In addition to changes in regulation, adaptive changes in mitochondria can occur in response to physiological challenges. These changes serve to adjust function toward some optimal state, and they include changing volume density, enzymatic and transport activities per unit mass, and spatial distribution within cells.

Changes in volume density are associated with altered aerobic work capacity; greater mitochondrial density provides a greater maximal ATP production. This does not always hold, since impaired mitochondrial function can necessitate increased density to maintain function. Change in volume density also occurs in response to development and differentiation, exercise conditioning, starvation, chronic hypoxia, changes in diet, and pharmacological agents (22–24).

Altered expression of enzyme and transport activities per unit mitochondrial volume also occurs during acclimatization to different physiological states. Thyroxin administration and recovery from hyperthyroidism result in changes in cytochrome oxidase and citrate synthase (25). Urea cycle enzymes are increased by high-protein diets (26) and by starvation (27). Chronic hypoxia causes a decrease in mitochondrial enzymes (28), whereas exercise conditioning results in increases in these enzymes (29). Thus, alterations in the composition of enzymes and transport systems provide another mechanism for cells to optimize energy production.

A final cellular mechanism to optimize cellular energetics involves spatial redistribution of mitochondria. Evolution of complex multicellular organisms required acquisition of a cellular respiratory apparatus with high energy output. The corresponding requirement for a high O_2 input provided a primary driving force for evolution of respiratory and circulatory sys-

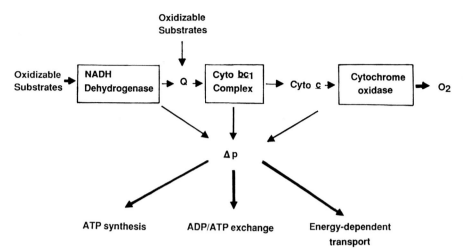

FIG. 2. Sites of regulation of mitochondrial function. Reactions leading to generation and utilization of Δp are both regulated, as indicated by the thicker arrows. In addition to limitation in supply of oxidizable substrates, as in starvation, transfer of electrons can be limited by control of NAD^+-linked dehydrogenases. This occurs by Ca^{2+}-dependent mechanisms and can effectively control the energy available for establishing the Δp from substrate oxidations. Regulation of electron transfer to O_2 also appears to occur at cytochrome oxidase; the details of regulation at this site are unclear and may involve coordinate regulation with earlier sites in the pathway, such as with NADH dehydrogenase. The Δp provides the energy for several functions, including ATP synthesis, ADP/ATP exchange, and the energy-dependent uptake of precursors and intermediates for oxidative phosphorylation. Regulation occurs at these energy-utilizing processes, but it is not clear whether separate regulatory mechanisms occur for each or whether common mechanisms exist.

tems to minimize diffusional limitations for O_2 from the atmosphere into the cells.

Mitochondrial Distribution and Cellular Oxygenation

Resistances to O_2 delivery occur at many sites in the transit from air to mitochondria, and the relative importance of these sites in rate limitation is different under different conditions (30,31). At the cellular level, mitochondrial density and heterogeneous distribution of mitochondria are also important determinants of the O_2 concentration required to maintain cellular ATP production. This distribution of mitochondria appears to represent a balance between (a) the need to have high ATP-producing power at sites of high ATP demand (tendency to increase clustering) and (b) the need to adequately oxygenate the cells at physiological blood Po_2 (tendency to decrease clustering).

Morphometric studies show that mitochondria within cells have a defined distribution that is frequently cell-specific; morphometric techniques are available to analyze these spatial inhomogeneities (8,32), and application of these techniques is needed to describe intracellular distribution. In fetal, neonatal, and cultured cells, mitochondria are present at relatively low densities and are not extensively clustered

(33,34). The O_2 concentration requirements for these cells are similar to those for isolated mitochondria (33), indicating that significant O_2 concentration gradients occur only under extremely low concentrations (<1 μM, < 0.76 torr). Thus, diffusion into these cells would not be limiting unless the blood Po_2 is very low or the path length is increased, such as occurs in solid tumors (35).

In contrast, cardiac myocytes, proximal tubule cells, and hepatocytes from adult rats require much higher O_2 concentrations to maintain mitochondrial function. In heart cells, at least four factors are involved in the diffusional limitation of oxygenation: (i) an extracellular unstirred layer, (ii) diffusion within the aqueous cytoplasm with an effective diffusion coefficient that is 4- to 10-fold lower than that in water, (iii) high mitochondrial density (creating a transcellular O_2 gradient due to O_2 consumption), and (iv) nonhomogeneous distribution of mitochondria (10). Of these effects, the latter three were found to be quantitatively more important in isolated cells, but the resistance to diffusion at the plasma membrane/capillary surface (36) is likely to be relatively more important in intact heart than reflected in cellular studies. In proximal tubule cells and hepatocytes, mitochondria are present in large aggregates or clusters (11). This increases the local O_2 consumption rate and enhances intracellular gradients in the vicinity of the clusters (37,38).

Gradients of ATP
and the Creatine Phosphate Shuttle

Clustering of mitochondria allows inclusion of higher ATP-producing power at sites of high ATP demand than would be possible with uniform distribution. The proximity of mitochondria to sites of high ATP utilization presupposes that a limitation of ATP supply occurs under some conditions. Studies of subcellular ATP supply in hepatocytes under various ATP-limiting conditions showed that ATP concentration gradients can occur in the aqueous cytoplasm (39). Thus, proximity to mitochondria provides a preferential access to ATP under conditions of limited production. This optimization of distribution of mitochondria is apparent in proximal tubule cells. A significant proportion of the total cellular O_2 consumed by the kidney is utilized to support ion and solute absorption. Aggregates of mitochondria and the Na^+, K^+-ATPase are uniquely colocalized to the basal regions of the renal proximal tubular cells (11), in which the transport activities predominate. Similarly, the neuronal synaptic terminals are focal points of O_2 consumption, mitochondrial clustering, and energy utilization for signal transmission (40).

In heart, the association of three apparent subpopulations of mitochondria with the myofibrils, sarcolemmal membrane, and the nucleus fulfills the energy requirement for contraction, membrane ion transport, and DNA replication (41,42). These associations may have a functional significance, but this has not been demonstrated experimentally. A similar association of mitochondria with specific structures and functions occurs in skeletal muscle.

Another mechanism to optimize energy supply that is especially important in cardiac and skeletal muscle involves the high-energy compound, creatine phosphate. Creatine is phosphorylated by ATP and the mitochondrial creatine kinase at the outer surface of the inner membrane. Diffusion of creatine phosphate to the contractile elements, along with hydrolysis by a different creatine kinase associated with myosin ATPase, releases ATP in the immediate vicinity of ATP consumption (43). This coordinate sequence of phosphorylation and dephosphorylation of creatine by the respective mitochondrial and myofibrillar kinases provides a means to minimize diffusion limitations of ATP and facilitate energy transfer.

The spatial separation of mitochondria and glycolytic enzymes provides another mechanism to optimize ATP supply. Several examples are known in which mitochondria and glycolytic enzymes have different and apparently complementary distributions, allowing preferential utilization of ATP from these two sources for different functions (44). In vascular smooth muscle, energy required for contractile activities comes from oxidative phosphorylation, whereas that required for Na^+ and K^+ transport comes from glycolysis (45). In rat cardiac muscle (46) and in cultured chick embryo ventricular cells (47), maintenance of contraction and delay of contracture are primarily responsive to mitochondrially produced ATP. Under varied conditions of glycolytic flux, the brain hexokinase alternates between association with the cytosol and the mitochondrial membrane. In the latter case, this allows preferential utilization by the enzyme of mitochondrially produced ATP (48). These examples indicate that spatial redistribution of energy-supplying systems can supplement changes in mitochondrial density and enzyme induction to optimize energy supply.

Function of Myoglobin (Mb)

In vitro studies have shown that Mb facilitates O_2 diffusion in solution by providing an alternate diffusing species, MbO_2, that is functionally equivalent to O_2 (49). Mb is found in high concentrations in heart and skeletal muscle and could, in principle, function to facilitate O_2 diffusion from the capillary to the mitochondria. However, studies designed to establish this function by chemically inactivating O_2 binding of Mb do not distinguish between a function of Mb in O_2 diffusion and other aspects of O_2 supply. Studies performed with perfused dog heart (50) as well as those on O_2 dependence of oxidation of mitochondrial cytochrome *a* in both isolated, quiescent and contracting cardiac myocytes (51), showed that elimination of functional myoglobin by oxidation to metMb did not alter the O_2 requirement and oxygenation characteristics of the mitochondria. These latter findings suggest that Mb may function as a temporary O_2 reservoir (9) to support mitochondrial oxygenation during contraction phases when supply from capillaries is impaired. This possible function is supported by the observation that diffusion limitation of O_2 is not likely to occur only in heart and skeletal muscle, yet myoglobin is largely restricted to these tissues.

Compartmentation of cell structures and metabolic processes also occurs in the mitochondrial matrix (52). Metabolic systems exist either as stable multifunctional proteins and multienzyme complexes or as sequential complexes of enzymes (52). Several studies in disruptive liver mitochondria show that the metabolic enzymes of the citric acid cycle are complexed in sequential, nonrandom arrangement. This interacting complex, termed a *metabolon*, is associated with the inner membrane. The complex functions to allow metabolite channeling, that is, catalysis of a sequence of reactions by different enzymes in which the intermediates are not in equilibrium with the bulk phase (52). Several mitochondrial NAD^+-coupled dehydrogenases can bind Complex I and couple NADH generation directly to NADH oxidation by the respiratory chain. The evolution of such specific interaction of enzymatic activities overcomes the problem of solvation of metabolic intermediates and provides a mechanism to optimize electron transport and its regulation.

STRUCTURAL AND FUNCTIONAL LIMITS TO CELLULAR RESPIRATION

Most cells and tissues have a reserve capacity for function that allows enhanced activity under physiological or pathological challenge. For highly energy-requiring processes, this is associated with high volume density of mitochondria and, in some tissues, with extensive clustering of mitochondria. The increased volume density and clustering can increase the O_2 concentrations required for function, but the magnitude of an O_2 concentration gradient is also determined by the respiration rate. When O_2 consumption rate is low, the cellular O_2 concentration requirement is low, but it is enhanced upon increased respiratory activity. For instance, in isolated cardiac myocytes, electrical stimulation of quiescent cells results in a two- to threefold increase in O_2 consumption rate and a similar increase in the O_2 concentration required for half-maximal respiration (53). Similar changes in renal proximal tubule cells occur upon stimulation of transport functions (37). Because increases in respiratory rate of up to fivefold can occur in heart muscle and kidneys and up to about 40-fold in skeletal muscle, diffusion limitations can be much more severe under conditions of maximal function. Thus, tissues with high mitochondrial volume density and clustering are inherently more susceptible to O_2 deficiency, and this susceptibility is increased by higher functional demands.

In addition to this general difference in susceptibility, data accumulated over the years on the effects of hypoxia on functions of mitochondria and various pathways of intermediary and drug metabolism indicate that different metabolic pathways are selectively vulnerable to varying degrees of O_2 deficiency (54). For example, the order of sensitivities for O_2-dependent drug metabolizing reactions is as follows: monoamine oxidation $\approx$ glucuronidation (fasted) > cytochrome P-450 > glucuronidation (fed) $\approx$ methylation > sulfation > NAD^+-linked oxidations (55). The half-maximal oxidation of cytochrome oxidase in many adult mammalian cells is around 3.5 μM O_2 (54); this means that failure of mitochondrial function can occur at a relatively high O_2 concentration compared to that for isolated mitochondria. Many reactions that are secondarily dependent on O_2 (i.e., those dependent on ATP) are vulnerable over the same O_2 concentration range.

Studies of activities of different ATP-requiring systems in cells show that some are much more sensitive to ATP depletion, and hence to O_2 limitation, than others. For instance, the order of sensitivities for ATP-dependent reactions in hepatocytes is as follows: Na^+,K^+-ATPase > transsulfuration $\approx$ ATP sulfurylase > GSH synthesis (39,56). The order of these sensitivities is determined both by the K_m values of the enzymes for ATP and by the site of localization of the enzymes in the cells relative to the mitochondria. Depending on whether changes in enzymic activities cause irreversible injury, the differential sensitivities of the O_2- and ATP-dependent enzymes to O_2 availability could directly affect cell survival.

Metabolic Suppression

All mammalian cells can survive some period of severe O_2 deficiency without irreversible injury. This nonlethal hypoxic period in which cells function with reduced metabolic and respiratory capacity is termed *neahypoxia* (55) and is distinct from the aerobic state and the irreversible pathological hypoxic conditions. The critical changes in mitochondrial function during neahypoxia have recently been delineated in isolated hepatocytes (4,20). Short-term anoxia elicits protective mechanisms to selectively preserve the mitochondrial Δp despite substantial decreases in cellular ATP concentrations (4). The energy required for maintenance of Δp is not derived from reversal of the ATP synthase reaction and glycolytically produced ATP (4). Rather, there is inhibition of specific ion transport systems and the ATP synthase activity (4,20). Such selective inhibition of ion transport allows cells to preserve mitochondrial homeostasis and allows for facile recovery upon reoxygenation.

Similar responses of metabolic suppression may occur in other tissues, such as the kidneys, where inhibition of transport functions protects against anoxic injury (57). The heart exhibits a response termed the "stunned myocardium," in which an anoxic/ischemic episode results in inhibition of mitochondrial respiratory functions and reversible cessation of contractile activities (58). Suppression of synaptic function protects neurons from anoxic injury (59), and the postanoxic suppression of cellular respiratory rate found in feline brain (60) may also be a consequence of endogenous mechanisms to prolong survival time. The full details of these mechanisms to regulate respiratory function are not clear, but the consequences are certain to affect organismic O_2 demand and are directly relevant to the amount of O_2 delivery that must be supplied by the lungs.

SUMMARY AND CONCLUSIONS

A primary determinant of the required function for lungs is the tissue O_2 consumption rate, which is primarily due to mitochondrial activity. Mitochondria are present at different volume densities and have distinct morphologies and metabolic and transport properties in different tissues. O_2 consumption by mitochondria can be affected by several factors, and it is likely that differences occur in regulatory characteristics in different tissues. In addition, mitochondria are distributed heterogeneously in cells, often being associated in apparent clusters adjacent to sites of high ATP utilization. All of these parameters are under physiological control; that is, volume densities, metabolic and transport activities, and subcellular distributions are modulated by factors such as exercise conditioning, hypoxia, and nutrition. Thus, the demand upon the lungs to supply O_2 is not a simple function of mitochondrial content; rather, it entails a summation of O_2 utilization by diverse systems, each with its own customized ATP-producing devices that are adapted to the unique functional requirements of the different tissues.

REFERENCES

1. Williamson JR. Mitochondrial function in the heart. *Annu Rev Physiol* 1979;41:485–506.
2. Denton RM, McCormack JG. On the role of the calcium transport cycle in heart and other mammalian mitochondria. *FEBS Lett* 1980;119:1–8.
3. Mitchell P. Vectorial chemistry and the molecular mechanics of chemiosmotic coupling: power transmission by protocity. *Biochem Soc Trans* 1976;4:399–430.
4. Andersson BS, Aw TY, Jones DP. Mitochondrial transmembrane potential and pH gradient during anoxia. *Am J Physiol* 1987;252:C349–C355.
5. Klingenberg M, Heldt HW. The ATP/ADP translocation in mitochondria and its role in intracellular compartmentation. In: Sies H, ed. *Metabolic compartmentation*. London: Academic Press, 1982;101–122.
6. Cowdry EV. The mitochondrial constituents of protoplasm. In: *Contributions to embryology*, vol 8. Washington, DC: Carnegie Institution of Washington, 1918;39.
7. Kirkwood SP, Munn EA, Brooks GA. Mitochondrial reticulum in limb skeletal muscle. *Am J Physiol* 1986;251:C395–C402.
8. Kayar SR, Hoppeler H, Mermod L, Weibel ER. Mitochondrial size and shape in equine skeletal muscle: a three-dimensional reconstruction study. *Anat Rec* 1988;222:333–339.
9. Millikan GA. Muscle hemoglobin. *Physiol Rev* 1939;19:503–523.
10. Jones DP, Kennedy FG. Analysis of intracellular oxygenation of isolated adult cardiac myocytes. *Am J Physiol* 1986;250:C384–C390.
11. Sjostrand FS, Rodin J. The ultrastructure of the proximal convoluted tubules of the mouse kidney as revealed by high resolution electron microscopy. *Exp Cell Res* 1953;4:426–456.
12. Jones DP, Aw TY. Mitochondrial distribution and O_2 gradients in mammalian cells. In Jones DP, ed. *Microcompartmentation*. Boca Raton, FL: CRC Press, 1988;37–53.
13. Kadenbach B, Reinmann A, Stroh A, Huther F-J. Evolution of cytochrome c oxidase. In: King TE, Mason HS, Morrison M, eds. *Oxidases and related redox systems*. New York: Alan R. Liss, 1988;653–668.
14. Powell SJ, Medd SM, Runswick MJ, Walker JE. Two bovine genes for mitochondrial ADP/ATP translocase expressed differences in various tissues. *Biochemistry* 1989;28:866–873.
15. Fawcett DW. *The cell*, 2nd ed. Philadelphia: WB Saunders, 1981;410–485.
16. Novikoff AB. Mitochondria (chondriosomes). In: Brachet J, Mirsky AE, eds. *The cell, vol 2: Biochemistry, physiology, morphology*. New York: Academic Press, 1961;299–421.
17. Loud AV. A quantitative stereological description of the ultrastructure of normal rat liver parenchymal cells. *J Cell Biol* 1968;37:27–46.
18. Jungermann K. Metabolic zonation of carbohydrate metabolism in the liver. In: Lemasters JJ, Hackenbrock CR, Thurman RG, Westerhoff HV, eds. *Integration of mitochondrial function*. New York: Plenum Press, 1988;561–579.
19. Kadenbach B. Regulation of respiration and ATP synthesis in higher organisms: hypothesis. *J Bioenerg Biomembr* 18:39–54.
20. Aw TY, Andersson BS, Jones DP. Mitochondrial transmembrane ion distribution during anoxia. *Am J Physiol* 1987;252:C356–C361.
21. Garlid KD. Mitochondria volume control. In: Lemasters JJ, Hackenbrock CR, Thurman RG, Westerhoff HV, eds. *Integration of mitochondrial function*. New York: Plenum Press, 1988;259–278.
22. Lang CA, Herbener GH. Quantitative comparison of the mitochondrial populations in the livers of newborn and weanling rats. *Dev Biol* 1972;29:176–182.
23. Hoppeler H, Luthi P, Claassen H, Weibel ER, Howald H. The ultrastructure of the normal human skeletal muscle. *Pflugers Arch* 1973;344:217–232.
24. Saltin B, Gollnick PD. Skeletal muscle adaptability: significance for metabolism and performance. In: Peachey LD, Adrian RH, eds. *Handbook of physiology, Section 10: Skeletal muscle*. Washington DC: American Physiological Society, 1983;555–631.
25. Sillau AH. Changes in soleus muscle capillarity, oxidative capacity and fiber composition in rats recovering from hyperthyroidism. *Pflugers Arch* 1985;404:67–72.
26. Schmike RT. Adaptive characteristics of urea cycle enzymes in the rat. *J Biol Chem* 1962;237:459–468.
27. Schmike RT. Differential effects of fasting and protein free diets on levels of urea cycle enzymes in rat liver. *J Biol Chem* 1962;237:1921–1924.
28. MacDougall JD. Structural changes in muscle with chronic hypoxia. In: Sutton JR, Houston CS, Coates G, eds. *Hypoxia. The tolerable limits*. Indianapolis: Benchmark Press, 1988;93–98.
29. Williams RS. Regulation of mitochondrial biogenesis by contractile activity in skeletal muscle: recent advances and directions for future research. In: Benzi G, Packer L, Siliprandi N, eds. *Biochemical aspects of physical exercise*. Amsterdam: Elsevier, 1986;171–180.
30. Weibel E. *The pathway for oxygen*. Boston: Harvard University Press, 1984.
31. Denison D. Where and how hypoxia works. In: Heath D, ed. *Aspects of hypoxia*. Liverpool: Liverpool University Press, 1986;235–245.
32. Eisenberg BR. Quantitative ultrastructure of mammalian skeletal muscle. In: Peachey LD, Adrian RH, eds. *Handbook of physiology, Section 10: Skeletal muscle*. Washington, DC: American Physiological Society, 1983;73–112.
33. Aw TY, Jones DP. Respiratory characteristics of neonatal rat hepatocytes. *Pediatr Res* 1987;21:492–496.
34. Jones DP, Aw TY, Lincoln BL, Bonkovsky HL. Oxygen concentration requirement for mitochondrial function in rat hepatocyte decreases dramatically during 2 days in primary culture. *Physiologist* 1987;30:123.
35. Sutherland RM, Durand RE. Radiation response of multicell spheroids—an *in vitro* tumor model. *Curr Top Radiat Res* 1976;11:87–139.
36. Honig CR, Gayeski TEJ, Federspiel W, Clark A, Clark P. Muscle O_2 gradients from hemoglobin to cytochrome: new concepts, new complexities. *Adv Exp Med Biol* 1984;169:23–28.
37. Aw TY, Wilson E, Hagen TM, Jones DP. Determinants of mitochondrial O_2 dependence in kidney. *Am J Physiol* 1987;253:F440–F447.

38. Jones DP. Effect of mitochondrial clustering on O_2 supply in hepatocytes. *Am J Physiol* 1984;247:C83–C89.
39. Aw TY, Jones DP. ATP concentration gradients in cytosol of liver cells during hypoxia. *Am J Physiol* 1985;249:C385–C392.
40. Rohlicek CV, Polosa C. Hypoxic responses of sympathetic preganglionic neurons in the acute spinal cat. *Am J Physiol* 1981;241:H679–H683.
41. Palmer JW, Tandler B, Hoppel CL. Biochemical properties of subsarcolemmal and interfibrillar mitochondria isolated from rat cardiac muscle. *J Biol Chem* 1977;252:8731–8739.
42. McNutt NS, Fawcett DW. Myocardial ultrastructure. In: Lunger GA, Brady AJ, eds. *The mammalian myocardium.* New York: John Wiley & Sons, 1984;1.
43. Bessman SP, Carpenter CL. The creatine–creatine phosphate energy shuttle. *Annu Rev Biochem* 1985;54:831–862.
44. Lynch RM, Paul RJ. Functional compartmentation of carbohydrate metabolism. In: Jones DP, ed. *Microcompartmentation.* Boca Raton, FL: CRC Press, 1988;17–35.
45. Lynch RM, Paul RJ. Compartmentation of glycolytic and glycogenolytic metabolism in vascular smooth muscle. *Science* 1983;222:1344–1346.
46. Bricknell DL, Davies PS, Opie LH. A relationship between adenosinetriphosphate, glycolysis and ischemic contracture in the isolated rat heart. *J Mol Cell Cardiol* 1980;13:941–945.
47. Barry WH, Pober J, Marsh JD, Frankel SR, Smith TM. Effects of graded hypoxia on contraction of cultured chick embryo ventricular cells. *Am J Physiol* 1980;239:H651–H657.
48. Wilson JE. Brain hexokinase, the prototype ubiquitous enzyme. *Curr Top Cell Regul* 1980;16:1–54.
49. Wittenberg BA. Myoglobin in isolated adult rat heart cells. In: Caughey WS, ed. *Biochemical and clinical aspects of oxygen.* New York: Academic Press, 1979;35–50.
50. Cole RP, Wittenberg BA, Caldwell PRB. Myoglobin function in the isolated fluorocarbon-perfused dog heart. *Am J Physiol* 1978;234:H567–H572.
51. Jones DP, Kennedy FG. Intracellular O_2 gradients in cardiac myocytes. Lack of a role for myoglobin in facilitation of intracellular O_2 diffusion. *Biochem Biophys Res Commun* 1982;105:419–424.
52. Srere PA. Complexes of sequential metabolic enzymes. *Annu Rev Biochem* 1987;56:89–124.
53. Jones DP, Kennedy FG, Aw TY. Intracellular O_2 gradients and the distribution of mitochondria. In: Sutton JR, Houston CS, Coates G, eds. *Hypoxia: the tolerable limits.* Indianapolis: Benchmark Press, 1988;59–69.
54. Jones DP, Aw TY, Kennedy FG. Isolated hepatocytes as a model for the study of cellular hypoxia. In: Harris RA, Cornell NW, eds. *Isolation, characterization and use of hepatocytes.* New York: Elsevier, 1983;323–332.
55. Jones DP, Kennedy FG, Andersson BS, Aw TY, Wilson E. When is a mammalian cell hypoxic? Insights from studies of cells vs mitochondria. *Mol Physiol* 1985;8:473–482.
56. Shan X, Aw TY, Shapira R, Jones DP. O_2 dependence of glutathione synthesis in isolated hepatocytes. *Toxicol Appl Pharmacol* 1989;101:261–270.
57. Brezis M, Rosen S, Silva P, Epstein FH. Transport-dependent anoxic cell injury in the isolated perfused rat kidney. *Am J Pathol* 1984;116:327–341.
58. Braunwald E, Kloner RA. The stunned myocardium: prolonged postischemic ventricular dysfunction. *Circulation* 1982;66:1146–1149.
59. Rothman SM. Synaptic activity mediates death of hypoxic neurons. *Science* 1983;220:536–537.
60. Gibson GE, Freeman GB, Mykytyn V. Selective damage in striatum and hippocampus with in vitro anoxia. *Neurochem Res* 1988;113:329–335.

THE LUNG: Scientific Foundations
edited by R.G. Crystal, J.B. West et al.
Raven Press, Ltd., New York © 1991.

CHAPTER 5.5.1.2

Aerobic and Anaerobic Mechanisms

Kent Sahlin

Hydrolysis of ATP is the immediate energy source for practically all energy-requiring processes in the cell:

$$ATP \leftrightarrow ADP + \text{inorganic phosphate} + \text{energy} \quad [1]$$

Regeneration of ATP occurs through a reversal of reaction 1, along with a transformation of energy-rich chemical substances into compounds with less energy. This is achieved by sequences of chemical reactions whereby the change in free energy is partially trapped in the synthesis of ATP. The ATP–ADP cycle (Fig. 1) constitutes a basic feature of energy metabolism in all cells and functions as an intermediate between the energy-utilizing and the energy-consuming processes.

During the transition from rest to exercise, the rate of ATP utilization can increase more than 100 times and corresponds to a utilization of the whole muscle store of ATP in about 2–3 sec. In order to maintain the ATP content approximately constant, which is necessary for cellular homeostasis, the rate of ATP regeneration must equal the rate of ATP utilization. Because of the unique ability to change the metabolic demands, skeletal muscle is faced with intricate problems related to fuel homeostasis and metabolic regulation.

The ultimate process for ATP formation in aerobic cells is the oxidation of different substrates, with O_2 being the final electron acceptor. The efficiency in transforming stored chemical energy into work can be calculated from the O_2 utilization and the caloric coefficient for oxygen. The mechanical efficiency during bicycling is about 24% when calculated from the exercise-induced increase in whole-body O_2 uptake and about 34% when calculated from the O_2 uptake by the leg muscles (1). In contrast, during static contractions the mechanical efficiency is zero, since no external work is performed.

For a limited period of time, ATP can also be produced through non-oxygen-requiring processes. Some species have evolved a high ability to survive for a prolonged period under anaerobic conditions (2); one of the most remarkable is the turtle, which can survive for 12 weeks during anoxic conditions at 3°C (3).

The present chapter will focus on the aerobic and anaerobic mechanisms of energy production in human skeletal muscle during exercise. Factors such as adaptation to training and influence of fiber-type heterogeneity will not be discussed but have been reviewed elsewhere (4,5).

MAXIMUM RATES OF AEROBIC AND ANAEROBIC ENERGY PRODUCTION *IN VIVO* AND *IN VITRO*

During two-leg exercise, O_2 utilization can increase to more than 100 ml·min^{-1}·kg^{-1} muscle. A major determinant of the maximal aerobic capacity ($V_{O_2}max$) during exercise under normoxic conditions is the cardiac output which sets an upper limit of the capacity to transport O_2 to the tissues. It has been estimated that exercise with only 10 kg of muscle is sufficient to elicit an average person's maximal O_2 uptake (6). The maximum local aerobic capacity of the muscle cell is therefore not utilized during two-leg exercise. However, during exercise with small muscle groups it is possible to increase the O_2 utilization to a level where the lim-

K. Sahlin: Department of Clinical Physiology, Karolinska Institute, Huddinge University Hospital, S-141 86 Huddinge, Sweden.

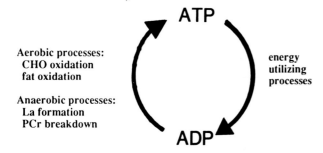

FIG. 1. The ATP–ADP cycle. CHO, carbohydrate; La, lactate; PCr, phosphocreatine.

itation is determined by the maximal aerobic capacity of the muscle. Studies of one-leg knee extension have revealed that O_2 uptake can increase to about 0.8 liter/ min or to more than 300 ml $O_2 \cdot min^{-1} \cdot kg^{-1}$ muscle, which corresponds to an 80-fold increase from the value at rest (6). During these conditions, the aerobic ATP production *in vivo* is much higher than *in vitro* estimates of maximal oxidative potential obtained from measurements of maximal enzyme activities, isolated mitochondria, or muscle homogenates (Table 1). These data demonstrate that the *in vitro* methods are inadequate to assess the true maximum metabolic flux in the aerobic metabolism.

Several lines of evidence suggest that the maximum rate of ATP formation obtainable from the oxidation of fatty acids is considerably lower than that from carbohydrate (CHO) oxidation (for a full discussion see ref. 12). Thus, it has been shown that tissue homogenates (11) and isolated mitochondria (5) can oxidize pyruvate at a higher rate than palmitate. Furthermore, it is known that ultradistance running, which results

in a depletion of the body storage of carbohydrates, will cause a decline in the power output to 50% of V_{O_2}max simultaneously with a decrease in the respiratory change ratio (decreasing to about 0.7), indicating mainly oxidation of fatty acids (13). It has been discussed that oxidation of fatty acids is limited by the capacity to transport the fuel to the site of utilization (12). The presence of a large intracellular triglyceride store (Table 2) that is utilized during exercise (4) does, however, suggest that utilization of fat during exercise is limited by additional factors other than transport. *In vitro* data indicate that reduction of the mitochondrial redox state can inhibit the β-oxidation of fatty acids in isolated liver mitochondria (14) and is thus a potential mechanism for the control of fat utilization.

The anaerobic processes for energy formation [i.e., mainly lactate formation and phosphocreatine (PCr) utilization] can proceed in the absence of O_2, and the maximal rate of ATP formation by these processes *in vivo* is two to three times higher than for the aerobic processes (Table 1).

SUBSTRATE STORES IN HUMANS

CHOs are stored as glycogen both in muscle and liver and can maintain the energy demand during exercise for about 1–2 hr if these are the sole energy substrate available (Table 2). In contrast, fat is present abundantly as triglycerides both in adipose tissue and in muscle. The high amount of available fat ensures that this is not a limiting factor for the exercise. In this context it should be pointed out that oxidation of 1 g of fat provides about nine times more energy than does

TABLE 1. *Maximum* in vivo *and in vitro* *capacity for ATP formation*

	Calculated maximum rate of ATP formation ($mmol \cdot kg^{-1}$ wet wt. $\cdot min^{-1}$ at 35°C)	Conditions	Reference
Phosphocreatine breakdown			
In vivo	120[a]	Electrical stimulation at 50 Hz	7
In vitro	200[b]	V_{max} of CK[c]	8
Anaerobic glycolysis			
In vivo	73[d]	Electrical stimulation at 50 Hz	7
In vitro	130–191[b]	Trained–untrained; V_{max} of PFK[c]	9
Aerobic ATP formation			
In vivo	80[d]	One-leg knee extension	6
In vitro	26–58[b]	Untrained–trained; V_{max} of KGDH[c]	9
In vitro	14–22[b]	Isolated mitochondria	10
In vitro	3[b]	Muscle homogenate	11

[a] Recalculated from dry weight to wet weight, assuming 3.3 liters H_2O/kg dry weight.
[b] Recalculated to 35°C (using $Q_{10} = 2$).
[c] CK, creatine kinase; PFK, phosphofructokinase; KGDH, ketoglutarate dehydrogenase.
[d] Calculated from O_2 utilization, assuming 6 mol ATP per mol O_2.

TABLE 2. *Substrate stores in humans*[a]

Process	Concentration (mmol/kg)	Available energy (mol ATP)[b]	Exercise (min)[c]
ATP hydrolysis (muscle)	6	0.02[d]	0.02
PCr breakdown (muscle)	19	0.29	0.4
Anaerobic glycolysis of muscle glycogen			
Ischemic conditions	80	0.56[e]	0.8
Free circulation	80	2.4[f]	3.3
Carbohydrate oxidation (glucosyl units)			
Leg muscle glycogen	80	44	60
Liver glycogen	300	19	25
Extracellular glucose	5	2.5	3
Fat oxidation			
Adipose tissue TG	>90%	7180	9567
Leg muscle TG	14	86	115
Extracellular FFA	0.3	0.5	0.7

[a] TG, triglycerides; FFA, free fatty acids; PCr, phosphocreatine.

[b] Values have been calculated by assuming a leg muscle weight of 15 kg, a fat depot of 15 kg, and a V_{O_2}max of 4.0 liters/min.

[c] Exercise (min) corresponds to the time to fatigue during exercise at 70% of V_{O_2}max, provided that this is the sole substrate for ATP formation.

[d] Only a small fraction of the ATP store (about 20%) can be utilized during exercise: $6 \times 0.2 \times 15$.

[e] Calculated from an assumed maximal lactate accumulation of 25 mmol/kg and 1.5 mol of ATP per mol of lactate.

[f] Theoretical value assuming that all of the muscle glycogen is converted to lactate.

oxidation of 1 g of CHO, partly as a result of the storage of water together with CHO. It is thus of physiological advantage to store energy as fat during conditions of intermittent access to food.

The oxygen requirements for formation of ATP varies between different substrates, being about 10% higher for free fatty acid (0.18 mol O_2/mol ATP) than for glycogen (0.16 mol O_2/mol ATP). From such basic metabolic characteristics, one would teleologically expect that the strategy during hypoxic conditions would be to switch from fat to CHO oxidation. Experimental evidence is available to suggest that a decrease in O_2 availability does exert such an effect (15,16). The control mechanism whereby this is achieved is not known.

Because of the limited store of PCr and the accumulation of lactic acid, the amount of ATP that can be produced through anaerobic processes during ischemic conditions is rather limited (about 60 mmol ATP/kg muscle). This corresponds to 15–20 sec of maximal activity or to 70 sec of exercise at 70% of V_{O_2}max (Table 2). Formation of ATP through anaerobic processes is therefore of great importance during short bursts of high-intensity exercise or during ischemic

conditions but is negligible in terms of energy equivalents during sustained exercise.

SUBSTRATE UTILIZATION DURING EXERCISE

Aerobic Processes

The type of fuels utilized during exercise is determined by exercise intensity, exercise duration, training status, and substrate availability. The major part of the energy demand at rest and during low-intensity exercise is covered by oxidation of fat, whereas oxidation of CHO is required during exercise at higher intensities. The preferential use of fat during conditions of low metabolic rates may be related to the metabolic characteristics of mitochondria, since the increase in ADP required to obtain half-maximal respiratory rates in isolated mitochondria is lower during oxidation of fat than during oxidation of CHO (5).

Anaerobic Processes

During sustained exercise at low or moderate intensities the rate of pyruvate oxidation is similar to the rate of glycolysis, but at higher intensities the catabolism of CHO is incomplete and lactic acid is formed and accumulates in the body fluids (Fig. 2). Accumulation of lactate in muscle and blood begins at about 50–70% of V_{O_2}max (Fig. 2); at 100% of V_{O_2}max, 10–20% of the total energy production is provided through glycolysis with subsequent lactate formation (17).

Accumulation of lactate in blood is accompanied by an increased ventilation and CO_2 excretion. The exercise intensity when blood lactate and ventilation increase disproportionally to the increase in intensity and V_{O_2} has been termed the "anaerobic threshold" or the "lactate threshold" (for references see ref. 21) and is widely used in exercise physiology to define the training status of subjects. The average marathon running speed has been shown to be closely related to the running speed at the lactate threshold (22) and implies a high prognostic value of this parameter for performance. Because of the noninvasiveness of ventilatory measurements, assessment of the lactate threshold by this technique would be advantageous. Controversy does, however, exist regarding the cause of the increase in ventilation, and evidence exists that a high blood lactate is not necessarily related to an increased ventilation (23). Changes in respiratory parameters may therefore not always correctly reflect the blood lactate level.

It has been argued that the increased blood lactate concentration during submaximal exercise is not due to an increased production but that a decreased re-

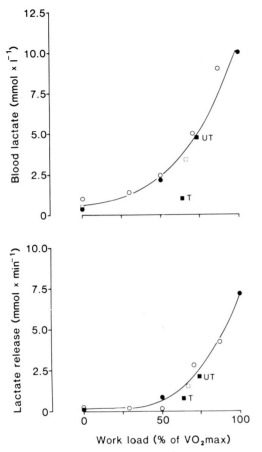

FIG. 2. Blood lactate and lactate release from the working leg during cycling for 3–20 min at different intensities. Lactate release was calculated from the difference in concentration between femoral venous and arterial blood, multiplied by the leg blood flow. Symbols indicate the mean value from the following studies: ref. 17 (●), ref. 18 (○), ref. 19 (□), and ref. 20 (■). T, endurance-trained subjects; UT, untrained subjects.

moval of lactate is a major factor involved (24). This conclusion was based on data from tracer studies using ^{14}C-labeled lactate (for references see ref. 24). However, it has recently been pointed out that this technique cannot fully separate lactate metabolism from that of pyruvate (25). Consequently, the quantitative importance of a "lactate shuttle" where a large fraction of produced lactate is removed in lactate-utilizing tissues (24) is questionable.

The idea that lactate accumulation in blood corresponds to an increased production and thus corresponds to a breakpoint in metabolism is supported by the parallel increase in lactate release as calculated from the product of leg blood flow and arteriovenous lactate difference (Fig. 2).

PCr is classically regarded as a buffer of high-energy phosphate, which can maintain the cellular ATP concentration approximately constant despite fluctuating energy demands. During maximal short-term exercise

the muscle content of PCr can be almost completely depleted, and the corresponding amount of energy corresponds to about 0.29 mol ATP (Table 2).

Although the classical view of PCr as a high-energy phosphate buffer seems to be valid, it is clear that changes occur in the PCr level also under other conditions. Thus, it has been shown that PCr decreases during submaximal exercise and that the extent of the decrease is related to the intensity of the exercise (26,27). The decline in PCr occurs at the onset of exercise and is maintained practically constant during the exercise (26).

Oxygen Deficit

The difference between the steady-state O_2 uptake and the actual O_2 uptake at the onset of exercise has been termed the "O_2 deficit." The O_2 deficit is known to be proportional to the exercise intensity (28) and is a classical way to estimate the total anaerobic energy utilization. In addition to the anaerobic processes that correspond to about 90% of the incurred O_2 deficit (29), the desaturation of the O_2 stores in blood and muscle is included in O_2 deficit (about 10% of O_2 deficit) (29). During maximal running, O_2 deficit amounts to 3.2–8.5 liters (29); during maximal bicycling, it amounts to about 6 liters (30). These values are in agreement with the estimated formation of ATP by the anaerobic processes (29). Hypoxia induced either by hypobaria (30) or by reducing the fraction of O_2 in inspired air (29) increases O_2 deficit during submaximal exercise but not during maximal exercise (30,31).

During submaximal exercise the O_2 deficit is incurred during the first 3 min of exercise and is largely independent of the exercise duration (32). Furthermore, O_2 deficit seems to be closely related to the metabolic rate at steady state and independent of the way this point is reached. Thus the same O_2 deficit and anaerobic energy utilization was reached after slow transition from rest to exercise at a certain intensity as after a direct transition (33,34). These studies and others (35) suggest that O_2 deficit and anaerobic energy utilization at the onset of exercise is not due to a mismatch between the O_2 delivery and the tissue demand of O_2 but is, instead, a consequence of metabolic regulation at a cellular level (see below).

CELLULAR MECHANISMS
FOR THE METABOLIC CONTROL
OF AEROBIC AND ANAEROBIC METABOLISM

A detailed account of the intricate control of the energetic cellular processes is outside the scope of the present chapter, and for an in-depth review the reader is referred to other textbooks or reviews (12,36,37).

The relative concentrations of the adenine nucleotides are of major importance for the control of the energetic processes and are determined by the energy potential of the system as well as by the adenylate kinase reaction, which is considered to be close to equilibrium:

$$2 \text{ ADP} \leftrightarrow \text{AMP} + \text{ATP} \qquad [2]$$

The total cellular concentrations (including both the free and bound portions) of AMP, ADP, and ATP are in many tissues related to each other approximately as 1:10:100. The cellular concentration of ATP remains fairly constant during most physiological conditions, but because of the large difference in concentration a small decrease in ATP will result in a large relative increase in ADP and in an even more pronounced increase in the relative concentration of AMP (due to the square root of ADP in the mass-action ratio and to the low absolute concentration of AMP).

Evidence exists that a large portion of the cellular ADP in muscle is bound to proteins and does not take part in the enzymatic reactions (38). Increases in free ADP, which is the metabolic active form of ADP, could thus occur despite the absence of an observed increase in total ADP. Currently, free ADP in muscle is usually calculated from the mass-action ratio of the creatine kinase reaction (39,40) and from free AMP from the mass-action ratio of the adenylate kinase reaction (reaction 2):

$$\text{PCr} + \text{free ADP} + \text{H}^+ \leftrightarrow \text{creatine} + \text{ATP} \qquad [3]$$

By this method, free ADP in resting cat muscle has been calculated as 0.3 and 14 μM (39) for fast-twitch and slow-twitch muscles, respectively; these figures imply that 99% or more of the total ADP content is protein-bound or otherwise unavailable. This is considerably higher than 50–80%, which was obtained from actual measurements (38). Considering the major importance of the adenine nucleotides in cellular energetics (see below), further research is required in this area.

Although the exact values of calculated free ADP and free AMP are uncertain, it is clear that the ratio Cr/PCr reflects the changes in the free ADP during conditions of stable pH and thus could serve as an important index of cellular energetics.

Metabolic Control of Cellular Respiration

Early studies on isolated mitochondria have shown that ADP is an important regulator of mitochondrial respiration (41). These studies indicate a kinetic control of oxidative phosphorylation by the cytosolic free ADP. Other studies on intact tissues have, however, shown that at least two of the three ATP-producing steps in the respiratory chain are reversible (for references see ref. 12), implying a near-equilibrium control by the involved substrates and products. This model would suggest that mitochondrial respiration is enhanced by increases in ADP and that factors such as the redox state, O_2 tension, and P_i concentration are of additional importance (42). Others have come to a similar conclusion by using a kinetic model (43) or a model based on irreversible thermodynamics (44).

In intact skeletal muscle a relation has been observed between the decrease in PCr (26,27) and the rate of O_2 consumption during exercise. These data and others (40,43) suggest that the adenine nucleotide control is important *in vivo* in skeletal muscle. Similar results have been obtained in saline-perfused cardiac tissue (45). In contrast, cardiac muscle has a constant PCr level during conditions of increasing metabolic rate *in vivo* (46). This indicates that the adenine nucleotide control is less important, and it was suggested that the redox state of mitochondrial NADH could be an important factor in the control of cardiac cellular respiration *in vivo* (46). Subsequent studies on isolated liver mitochondria have demonstrated that V_{O_2} depends on the levels of both NAD(P)H and extramitochondrial ADP over a wide range of respiratory rates (47), supporting the view that the redox state of mitochondria is an important regulator of mitochondrial respiration.

The contraction process is intimately linked to increases in cytosolic Ca^{2+}, which are likely transmitted to the mitochondria. Because several of the NADH-producing reactions in the tricarboxylic acid cycle are activated by Ca^{2+} (36), Ca^{2+}-signaling might be a mechanism whereby the mitochondria senses an increased energy demand. This mechanism would bypass or attenuate the stimulation by ADP and reduce the associated metabolic perturbations (i.e., the activation of glycolysis).

PCr Utilization

As discussed above, breakdown of PCr is catalyzed by creatine kinase, and because of the high enzymatic activity the reaction is likely to be close to equilibrium under most conditions. An increase in both free ADP and H^+, both of which are products of ATP hydrolysis (reaction 1), is a factor that will promote breakdown of PCr. An activation of aerobic energy production through an increase in free ADP will therefore, through the creatine kinase equilibrium, result in a breakdown of PCr. A breakdown of PCr is therefore not necessarily a sign of anaerobiosis but could instead be a reflection of an increased energy turnover and activation of aerobic metabolism.

The combination of ATP hydrolysis (reaction 1) and

rephosphorylation of ADP by PCr (reaction 3) will result in a release of inorganic phosphate (P_i). The cellular concentration of P_i in resting cat muscle determined by nuclear magnetic resonance is about 3 mM in fast-twitch muscle and 10 mM in slow-twitch muscle (39). During maximal exercise when the whole PCr store is depleted, P_i can increase with about 10–15 mM. The increase in cellular P_i will exert metabolic influence through activation of oxidative phosphorylation, glycogenolysis, and glycolysis (see below).

Control of Glycogenolysis

The initial step of glycogen breakdown to glucose-1-phosphate is a nonequilibrium reaction and is catalyzed by glycogen phosphorylase:

$$\text{glycogen } (n) + P_i \leftrightarrow \text{glucose-1-phosphate}$$
$$+ \text{ glycogen } (n-1)$$

where n shows the number of glucose units and P_i is inorganic phosphate. The control of glycogenolysis is exerted by different mechanisms involving enzyme transformation, allosteric regulation, and substrate regulation. Phosphorylase exists in two interconvertible forms, phosphorylase a and phosphorylase b, of which phosphorylase b is active only in the presence of AMP or IMP. Transformation of phosphorylase b to phosphorylase a is achieved by a hormonal mechanism involving epinephrine and cyclic AMP as well as by a Ca^{2+}-dependent mechanism that links the fuel supply to the contraction process. In contrast to glycogen, which is present in a saturating concentration, the cellular level of P_i is within the range where it influences the activity of both phosphorylase a and phosphorylase b (48). Thus increases in P_i which occur in contracting muscle as a result of the breakdown of PCr (see above) will be an important factor for the activation of glycogenolysis (48). Both phosphorylase b and phosphorylase a are activated by AMP, but the concentration of AMP required to activate phosphorylase b is much higher than the cellular level (49); the physiological significance is therefore questionable. In contrast, the activity of phosphorylase a is influenced by a low concentration of AMP (49), thus providing a link between the ATP demand and the activation of glycogenolysis.

Control of Glycolysis

Glycogenolysis is the flux-generating step of glycolysis from glycogen and thus controls the rate of hexosephosphate formation from glycogen. The rate of glycolysis (breakdown of glucose units to pyruvate) is, however, largely controlled by phosphofructokinase (PFK), which catalyzes a nonequilibrium reaction. The characteristic feature of PFK control is the allosteric inhibition by ATP (for references see refs. 12 and 37), which can be attenuated by a number of metabolites (such as AMP, ADP, P_i, hexosephosphates, and cyclic AMP) and potentiated by H^+ and citrate. Although a large amount of information about the control of the enzyme *in vitro* is available, present models cannot satisfactorily explain a 1000- to 2000-fold increase in the glycolytic rate during contraction (50). Current hypotheses suggest that factors closely linked to the contraction, such as increases in Ca^{2+} (51) or transient increases in AMP and ADP (52), control both phosphorylase and glycolysis during exercise.

INFLUENCE OF O_2 AVAILABILITY ON CELLULAR ENERGETIC PROCESSES

Oxygen is the ultimate electron acceptor in the respiratory chain and is essential for the cellular energetic processes. Despite the importance of the oxidative processes in the generation of ATP, there is practically only one cellular reaction that utilizes molecular O_2, namely, the cytochrome c oxidase. Although aerobic cells require O_2 for the maintenance of life, an O_2 tension only slightly higher than those at which cells function is toxic (53), probably due to the formation of free radicals.

There is little doubt that contracting muscle is hypoxic during exercise at workloads exceeding the Vo_2max or during sustained static contractions where the intramuscular pressure impairs the local blood flow. Whether the lactate formation during submaximal exercise is due to cellular hypoxia has, however, been discussed extensively. Part of the controversy exists for the following reasons: (a) Investigators have extrapolated results from animal experiments where a small muscle group with a high aerobic potential has been investigated (24,54–56) to humans working with a large muscle mass; (b) hypoxia at the cellular level can be defined in different ways. It is often stated or implied that unless cellular respiration is reduced, cellular metabolism (including lactate formation) is not affected by Po_2. There is no evidence to support this axiom, which probably stems from the function of glycolysis as an ATP source when oxidative processes are insufficient. An alternative view advanced by Wilson et al. (42) is that a decrease of tissue Po_2 has an impact on metabolism before cellular respiration is impaired. In fact, there are theoretical reasons as well as experimental evidence to believe that the imbalance between the formation and oxidation of pyruvate is a consequence of the necessity to stimulate aerobic energy production (see above) and that the availability of O_2 plays a major role in this process.

The critical intracellular P_{O_2} (P_{O_2}crit) for respiration is usually defined as the P_{O_2} at which O_2 availability limits electron transport and oxidative phosphorylation. The respiration in isolated mitochondria has been shown to have an O_2 affinity (K_m) of 0.05–0.5 μM or 0.04–0.4 torr (57), depending on the respiratory rate and the metabolic state, and should correspond to a P_{O_2}crit of about 0.15–1.5 torr. Measurements have been made of the O_2 saturation of myoglobin in freeze-clamped contracting dog gracilis muscle (58). This technique enables calculations of the tissue P_{O_2} with a subcellular resolution. From these studies it was concluded that P_{O_2}crit in vivo is about 0.5 torr (58) and thus on the same order as for isolated mitochondria. It was concluded that the lactate formation in this muscle during submaximal contractions, when the minimal P_{O_2} was about 1.5–3 torr, could not be due to an O_2 limitation of respiration or metabolism and that the concept of anaerobic threshold does not apply to red muscle (55,59).

In contrast to these data where P_{O_2}crit appears to be similar in isolated mitochondria and intact tissue, studies of the redox state of the respiratory chain have shown that the P_{O_2}crit is quite different in isolated mitochondria and in hepatocytes (60). Thus, intact cells required about one order of magnitude higher O_2 concentration (11 torr) than did isolated mitochondria (0.6 torr) to obtain the same reduction state of cytochrome a_3 (60), and the major reason for this difference was considered to be the clustering and uneven distribution of mitochondria (60,61). An important difference between the studies on myoglobin saturation in contracting dog muscle (55,58,59) and the work by Jones and co-workers (60,61) is that the former group defined P_{O_2}crit as the O_2 tension where respiration was diminished, whereas Jones and co-workers (60,61) studied the O_2 dependence of the redox state of the respiratory chain.

In human studies it has been shown that the P_{O_2} of femoral venous blood during bicycle exercise at $\dot{V}_{O_2}$max decreases to about 17 torr (62) and that P_{O_2} in human gastrocnemius muscle decreases to about 7 torr during exercise to fatigue (63), which is within the region where an effect on the redox state of the respiratory chain in intact cells has been observed (60). Because of O_2 gradients between femoral venous blood and the mitochondria of the contracting muscle and also because of a lack of homogeneity within the muscle, P_{O_2} can probably reach lower values in certain intracellular loci. More specific methods are therefore required to assess the P_{O_2} in the working muscle cell in humans.

Many studies have shown that alterations of the O_2 availability have an effect on the cellular metabolism during submaximal exercise (50). A reduction of O_2 supply during submaximal exercise results in (a) ele-

vated lactate concentrations in blood (16,30,31) and in muscle (16,30), (b) decreased PCr levels (16,30,63,64), (c) increased deamination of AMP to IMP (65), (d) accumulation of glucose and glucose-6-phosphate in muscle (66), and (e) an increased O_2 deficit (30,31). In contrast to cellular respiration, which is not dependent on P_{O_2} during submaximal exercise, cellular metabolism shows a clear O_2 dependency.

Evidence has been presented that cellular respiration, in addition to being dependent upon P_{O_2}, is dependent upon the cytosolic phosphorylation potential (ATP/ADP × P_i) and the mitochondrial redox state (42). Adaptive changes in the mitochondrial redox state (increase in NADH/NAD$^+$) and the cytosolic phosphorylation potential (increase in ADP × P_i/ATP) could thus maintain cellular respiration during conditions of increased metabolic rate or decreased O_2 availability. According to this view, the increased lactate production during submaximal exercise should be regarded more as a regulatory phenomenon than as a necessary supplementation of the ATP production.

A sensitive index of mitochondrial availability of O_2 would be the reduction state of the NAD–NADH redox couple and/or the respiratory chain. A state of O_2 deficiency would be characterized by an increased reduction of mitochondrial NAD and respiratory chain. Surface fluorescence measurements of NADH in intact dog skeletal muscle showed an oxidation of NADH during contractile activity despite lactate formation and despite prevailing anoxic conditions (54). Subsequent measurements with more specific techniques using laser fluorimetry have shown a reduction [i.e., increase in NAD(P)H] of both slow-twitch and fast-twitch muscles during tetanic contractions (67).

Recent studies of the isolated dog gracilis muscle have shown that during submaximal work there is an oxidation of cytochrome oxidase (obtained by near-infrared measurements) despite an increased release of lactate (56). These results are consistent with the findings by Connett et al. (55), where under similar experimental conditions the oxygen saturation of myoglobin was maintained high during the contraction despite an increased formation of lactate. From these data it can be inferred that increased formation of lactic acid can occur by mechanisms other than through decreased O_2 availability. However, the results cannot be extrapolated to humans exercising with a large muscle group, where the conditions regarding O_2 supply, metabolic flux, and cellular oxidative and glycolytic capacity are vastly different.

Recently, quantitative measurements have been made of NADH in human skeletal muscle under a variety of conditions (16,27,68–70). It was shown that when the blood supply to the muscle was occluded, muscle NADH increased rapidly and reached a plateau after about 10 min at about two- to threefold the initial

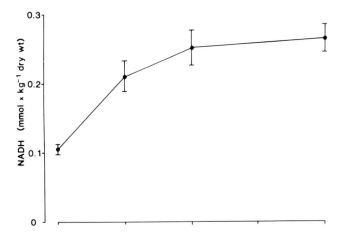

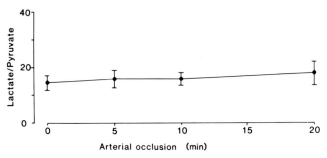

FIG. 3. Muscle content of NADH and lactate/pyruvate ratio at rest and during arterial occlusion. Values are means ± SEM ($n = 4$). Values are from ref. 68.

value (Fig. 3). The increase in NADH occurred despite unchanged values of lactate/pyruvate. The lactate/pyruvate ratio is classically used as a measure of cytosolic redox state, and the results therefore suggest that the increase in NADH did not occur in the cytosol but, instead, within the mitochondria. These data are consistent with studies of the oxygenation of human skeletal muscle during ischemia by near-infrared monitoring of the redox state of cytochrome oxidase (71) and by usage of O_2 probes (72), where it was shown that the local O_2 store is depleted after 4–5 min of ischemia. Static contraction resulted in a twofold increase in NADH within 5 sec (69), which is consistent with the expected rapid depletion of the O_2 store (2–3 sec) at this contraction force. When the contraction was sustained to fatigue, muscle lactate and lactate/pyruvate ratio increased. These studies and others (for references see refs. 50 and 69) show that changes in muscle NADH primarily reflect the changes in the mitochondrial compartment and thus could be used as a marker of tissue O_2 availability.

The influence of submaximal and maximal dynamic exercise on the relationship between muscle NADH and lactate has been investigated in subjects performing incremental bicycle exercise (27). At low exercise

intensities (40% V_{O_2}max) muscle NADH decreased, whereas at higher intensities (75% and 100% V_{O_2}max) NADH increased above the value at rest (Fig. 4), which suggests that the O_2 availability was limiting for the respiratory chain. The increase in NADH coincided with lactate accumulation in both muscle and blood. The decrease in NADH during low-intensity exercise was not accompanied by changes in either muscle or blood lactate and is consistent with data from isolated mitochondria, where an increase of ADP in the presence of sufficient substrate and O_2 results in an oxidation of mitochondrial NADH (41). Further studies have shown that submaximal exercise during conditions of respiratory hypoxia (11% of O_2 in inspired air) results in increased muscle levels of both lactate and NADH as well as decreases in PCr, as compared with normoxic exercise (16). These metabolic changes occurred despite similar rates of oxygen consumption and are consistent with the idea that reduced levels of P_{O_2} result in adaptive changes in mitochondrial redox state and cytosolic free ADP and P_i (related to the decrease in PCr) in order to maintain a constant cellular respiration.

These data obtained from humans exercising with a large muscle mass demonstrate that the availability of O_2 at the cellular level plays a major role in the energetic processes. However, this conclusion does not

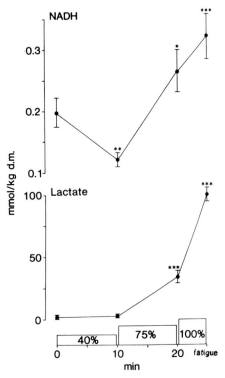

FIG. 4. Muscle contents of lactate and NADH during cycling at different intensities (40%, 75%, and 100% of V_{O_2}max). Values are means ± SEM ($n = 4$). The upper part of the figure and the lactate values are from ref. 27.

exclude that other factors are of additional importance. Furthermore, the relative importance of O_2 availability for the control of cellular energetics will presumably be dependent upon the working muscle mass as well as upon the oxidative and glycolytic potential of the tissue.

SUMMARY

The mechanisms and significances of aerobic and anaerobic ATP formation in human skeletal muscle have been described in the present chapter. Signals of major importance for the control of the energetic processes are Ca^{2+}, ADP, AMP, P_i, and the mitochondrial redox state (Fig. 5). Increases in Ca^{2+}, ADP, AMP, and P_i are intimately linked to the contraction process and the energy demand and ensure that the rate of ATP formation equals the rate of ATP utilization. Further control of the different pathways is achieved through substrate activation, feedback inhibition, and allosteric regulation; some of the mechanisms for these are presented in Fig. 5.

At low metabolic rates the rate of glycolysis is balanced by an equal rate of pyruvate oxidation, and there is no accumulation of pyruvate or lactate in the tissues despite a large increase in the glycolytic rate. At higher metabolic rates when either the availability of O_2 is limited or the maximal aerobic capacity of the tissue is approached, formation of pyruvate exceeds the pyruvate oxidation; as a result, lactate accumulates. The metabolic signals to turn on pyruvate formation (glycogenolysis and glycolysis) and pyruvate oxidation (Krebs cycle and mitochondrial respiration) are, to some extent, similar (i.e., increases in ADP, P_i, and Ca^{2+}). The imbalance between these processes (i.e., lactate formation) at higher exercise intensity or during O_2 limitations is probably related to both a decreased sensitivity of pyruvate oxidation to these signals (due to limitation in O_2 concentration or aerobic capacity) and a retained sensitivity of glycolysis to these signals.

From the discussion above, it is clear that lactate formation and PCr breakdown are not necessarily related to anaerobiosis, and the term "anaerobic threshold" may therefore be misleading. However, the lactate threshold (or anaerobic threshold) is related to work intensity when formation of ATP occurs, to an increasing extent, through non-oxygen-requiring processes; therefore the lactate threshold does indicate an important breakpoint in metabolism. Both theoretical reasons and experimental evidence suggest that a decrease in tissue O_2 availability does have metabolic consequences (e.g., PCr breakdown and enhanced glycolysis) before cellular respiration is impaired. These metabolic changes reflect the adaptation of the tissue

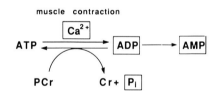

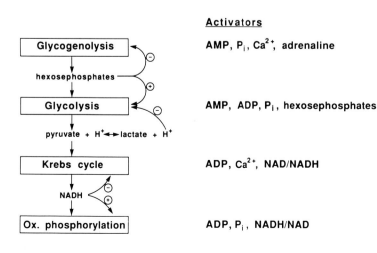

FIG. 5. Top: Schematic diagram illustrating the initial changes during muscle contraction resulting in increased levels of Ca^{2+}, free ADP, free AMP, and inorganic phosphate (P_i). **Bottom:** Major metabolic pathways involved in the formation of ATP through oxidation of carbohydrates. Some of the most important control mechanisms are shown.

to an increased metabolic rate or to a decreased availability of O_2.

ACKNOWLEDGMENTS

Financial support from the Swedish Medical Research Council (grant 8671) and the Swedish Research Council of Sports Medicine is gratefully acknowledged.

REFERENCES

1. Jorfeldt L, Wahren J. Leg blood flow during exercise in man. *Clin Sci* 1971;41:459–473.
2. Hochachka PW. *Living without oxygen.* Cambridge, MA: Harvard University Press, 1980.
3. Jackson DC, Heisler N. Plasma ion balance of submerged anoxic turtles at 3°C: the role of calcium lactate formation. *Respir Physiol* 1982;49:8–15.
4. Saltin B, Gollnick PD. Skeletal muscle adaptability: significance for metabolism and performance. In: Peachey LD, Adrian RH, Geiger SR, eds. *Handbook of physiology, Section 10: Skeletal muscle.* Bethesda, MD: American Physiological Society, 1983;555–632.
5. Gollnick PD, Riedy M, Quintinskie JJ, Bertocci LA. Differences in metabolic potential of skeletal muscle fibres and their significance for metabolic control. *J Exp Biol* 1985;115:191–199.
6. Andersen P, Adams RP, Sjøgaard G, Saltin B. Dynamic knee extension as model for study of isolated exercising muscle in humans. *J Appl Physiol* 1985;59:1647–1653.
7. Hultman E, Sjöholm H. Substrate availability. In: Knuttgen HG, Vogel JA, Poortmans J, eds. *Biochemistry of exercise*, vol 13. Champaign, IL: Human Kinetics Publishers, 1983;63–75.
8. Thorstensson A, Sjödin B, Karlsson J. Enzyme activities and muscle strength after "spring training" in man. *Acta Physiol Scand* 1975;94:313–318.
9. Blomstrand E, Ekblom B, Newsholme EA. Maximum activities of key glycolytic and oxidative enzymes in human muscle from differently trained individuals. *J Physiol* 1986;381:111–118.
10. Wibom R, Hultman E. Mitochondrial ATP production rate in needle biopsy samples of human muscle. *Am J Physiol*, in press.
11. Ivy JL, Withers RT, Van Handel PJ, Elgers DH, Costill DL. Muscle respiratory capacity and fiber type as determinants of the lactate threshold. *J Appl Physiol* 1980;48:523–527.
12. Newsholme EA, Leech AR. *Biochemistry for the medical sciences.* Chichester: John Wiley & Sons, 1983.
13. Davies CTM, Thompson MW. Aerobic performance of female marathon and male ultramarathon athletes. *Eur J Appl Physiol* 1979;41:233–245.
14. Latipää PM, Kärki TT, Hiltunen JK, Hassinen IE. Regulation of palmitoylcarnitine oxidation in isolated rat liver mitochondria. Role of the redox state of NAD(H). *Biochim Biophys Acta* 1986;875:293–300.
15. Jones NL, Robertson DG, Kane JW, Hart RA. Effect of hypoxia on free fatty acid metabolism during exercise. *J Appl Physiol* 1972;33:733–738.
16. Katz A, Sahlin K. Effect of decreased oxygen availability on NADH and lactate contents in human skeletal muscle during exercise. *Acta Physiol Scand* 1987;131:119–128.
17. Katz A, Broberg S, Sahlin K, Wahren J. Muscle ammonia and amino acid metabolism during dynamic exercise in man. *Clin Physiol* 1986;6:365–379.
18. Jorfeldt L, Juhlin-Dannfelt A, Karlsson J. Lactate release in relation to tissue lactate in human skeletal muscle during exercise. *J Appl Physiol* 1978;44:350–352.
19. Broberg S, Sahlin K. Adenine nucleotide degradation in human skeletal muscle during prolonged exercise. *J Appl Physiol* 1990;in press.
20. Jansson E, Kaijser L. Substrate utilization and enzymes in skel-

etal muscle of extremely endurance-trained men. *J Appl Physiol* 1987;62:999–1005.
21. Jones NL, Ehrsam RE. The anaerobic threshold. *Exerc Sport Sci Rev* 1981;10:49–83.
22. Sjödin B, Jacobs I. Onset of blood lactate accumulation and marathon running performance. *Int J Sports Med* 1981;2:23–26.
23. Davis HA, Gass GC. Thie anaerobic threshold as determined before and during lactic acidosis. *Eur J Appl Physiol* 1981;47:141–149.
24. Brooks GA. Anaerobic threshold; review of the concept and directions for future research. *Med Sci Sports Exerc* 1985;17:22–31.
25. Sahlin K. Lactate production cannot be measured with tracer techniques. *Am J Physiol* 1987;252:E439–E440.
26. Hultman E, Bergström J, McLennan Anderson N. Breakdown and resynthesis of phosphorylcreatine and adenosine triphosphate in connection with muscular work in man. *Scand J Clin Lab Invest* 1967;19:56–66.
27. Sahlin K, Katz A, Henriksson J. Redox state and lactate accumulation in human skeletal muscle during dynamic exercise. *Biochem J* 1987;245:551–556.
28. Karlsson J. Lactate and phosphagen concentrations in working muscle of man. *Acta Physiol Scand [Suppl]* 1971;358:7–72.
29. Medbø JI, Mohn A-C, Tabata I, Bahr R, Vaage O, Sejersted OM. Anaerobic capacity determined by maximal accumulated O_2 deficit. *J Appl Physiol* 1988;64:50–60.
30. Linnarsson D, Karlsson J, Fagraeus L, Saltin B. Muscle metabolites and oxygen deficit with exercise in hypoxia and hyperoxia. *J Appl Physiol* 1974;36:399–402.
31. Knuttgen HG, Saltin B. Oxygen uptake, muscle high-energy phosphates, and lactate in exercise under acute hypoxic conditions in man. *Acta Physiol Scand* 1973;87:368–376.
32. Schneider EG, Robinson S, Newton JL. Oxygen debt in aerobic work. *J Appl Physiol* 1968;25:58–62.
33. Sahlin K, Ren JM, Broberg S. Oxygen deficit at the onset of submaximal exercise is not due to an inadequate oxygen delivery. *Acta Physiol Scand* 1988;134:175–180.
34. Ren JM, Broberg S, Sahlin K. Oxygen deficit is not affected by the rate of transition from rest to submaximal exercise. *Acta Physiol Scand* 1989;135:545–548.
35. Hansen E. Über die Sauerstoffschuld bei körperlicher Arbeit. *Arbeitsphysiologie* 1935;8:151–171.
36. Hansford RG. Control of mitochondrial substrate oxidation. *Curr Top Cell Regul* 1980;10:217–278.
37. Hofman E. The significance of phosphofructokinase to the regulation of carbohydrate metabolism. *Rev Physiol Biochem Pharmacol* 1976;75:1–68.
38. Seraydarian K, Mommaerts WFHM, Wallner A. The amount and compartmentalization of adenosine diphosphate in muscle. *Biochim Biophys Acta* 1962;65:443–460.
39. Meyer RA, Brown TR, Kushmerick MJ. Phosphorus nuclear magnetic resonance of fast- and slow-twitch muscle. *Am J Physiol* 1985;248:C279–C287.
40. Dudley GA, Tullson PC, Terjung RL. Influence of mitochondrial content on the sensitivity of respiratory control. *J Biol Chem* 1987;262:9109–9114.
41. Chance B, Williams GR. Respiratory enzymes in oxidative phosphorylation. III. The steady state. *J Biol Chem* 1955;217:409–427.
42. Wilson DF, Erecinska M, Drown C, Silver IA. Effect of oxygen tension on cellular energetics. *Am J Physiol* 1977;233:C135–C140.
43. Chance B, Leigh JS, Kent J, McCully K. Metabolic control principles and ^{31}P NMR. *Fed Proc* 1986;45:2915–2920.
44. Meer R, Akerboom PM, Groen AK, Tager JM. Relationship between oxygen uptake of perifused rat-liver cells and the cytosolic phosphorylation state calculated from indicator metabolites and a redetermined equilibrium constant. *Eur J Biochem* 1978;84:421–428.
45. Ingwall JS. Phosphorous nuclear magnetic resonance spectroscopy of cardiac and skeletal muscles. *Am J Physiol* 1982;242:H729–H744.
46. Balaban RS, Kantor HL, Katz LA, Briggs RW. Relation be-

tween work and phosphate metabolite in the *in vivo* paced mammalian heart. *Science* 1986;232:1121–1123.

47. Koretsky AP, Balaban RS. Changes in pyridinenucleotide levels alter oxygen consumption and extramitochondrial phosphates in isolated mitochondria: a ^{31}P-NMR and NAD(P)H fluorescence study. *Biochim Biophys Acta* 1987;893:398–408.

48. Chasiotis D, Sahlin K, Hultman E. Regulation of glycogenolysis in human muscle at rest and during exercise. *J Appl Physiol* 1982;53:708–715.

49. Aragon JJ, Tornheim K, Lowenstein JM. On a possible role of IMP in the regulation of phosphorylase activity in skeletal muscle. *FEBS Lett* 1980;117(Suppl):K56–K64.

50. Katz A, Sahlin K. Regulation of lactic acid production during exercise. *J Appl Physiol* 1988;65:509–518.

51. Wilkie DR, Dawson MJ, Edwards RHT, Gordon RE, Shaw D. ^{31}P NMR studies of resting muscle in normal human subjects. In: Pollack GM, Suai H, eds. *Contractile mechanisms in muscle.* New York: Plenum Press, 1984;333–346.

52. Sahlin K. Metabolic changes limiting muscle performance. In: Saltin B, ed. *Biochemistry of exercise*, vol 16. Champaign, IL: Human Kinetics Publishers, 1986;323–343.

53. Gerschman R. Biological effects of oxygen. In: Dickens F, Neil E, eds. *Oxygen in the animal organism.* Oxford: Pergamon Press, 1964;475–494.

54. Jöbsis FF, Stainsby WN. Oxidation of NADH during contractions of circulated mammalian skeletal muscle. *Respir Physiol* 1968;4:292–300.

55. Connett RJ, Gayeski TEJ, Honig CR. Lactate accumulation in fully aerobic, working dog gracilis muscle. *Am J Physiol* 1984;246:H120–H128.

56. Stainsby WN, Brechue WF, O'Drobinak DM, Barclay JK. Oxidation/reduction state of cytochrome oxidase during repetitive contractions. *J Appl Physiol* 1989;67:2158–2162.

57. Chance B. Reaction of oxygen with the respiratory chain in cells and tissues. *J Gen Physiol* 1965;49:163–188.

58. Gayeski TEJ, Connett RJ, Honig CR. Minimum intracellular P_{O_2} for maximum cytochrome turnover in red muscle *in situ.* *Am J Physiol* 1987;252:H906–H915.

59. Connett RJ, Gayeski TEJ, Honig CR. Lactate efflux is unrelated to intracellular P_{O_2} in working red muscle *in situ.* *Am J Physiol* 1986;61:H402–H408.

60. Kennedy FG, Jones DP. Oxygen dependence of mitochondrial function in isolated cardiac myocytes. *Am J Physiol* 1986;250:C374–C383.

61. Jones DP. Intracellular diffusion gradients of O_2 and ATP. *Am J Physiol* 1986;250:C663–C675.

62. Pirnay F, Lamy M, Dujardin J, Deroanne R, Petit JM. Analysis of femoral venous blood during maximum muscular exercise. *J Appl Physiol* 1972;33:289–292.

63. Bylund-Fellenius A-C, Walker PM, Elander A, Holm S, Holm J, Scherstén T. Energy metabolism in relation to oxygen partial pressure in human skeletal muscle during exercise. *Biochem J* 1981;200:247–255.

64. Idström JP, Harihara Subramanian V, Chance B, Scherstén T, Bylund-Fellenius A-C. Oxygen dependence of energy metabolism in contracting and recovering rat skeletal muscle. *Am J Physiol* 1985;248:H40–H48.

65. Sahlin K, Katz A. Hypoxemia increases the accumulation of IMP in human skeletal muscle during submaximal exercise. *Acta Physiol Scand* 1989;136:199–203.

66. Katz A, Sahlin K. Effect of hypoxia on glucose metabolism in human skeletal muscle during exercise. *Acta Physiol Scand* 1989;136:377–382.

67. Duboc D, Muffat-Joly M, Renault G, Degeorges M, Toussaint M, Pocidalo J-J. *In situ* NADH laser fluorimetry of rat fast- and slow-twitch muscles during tetanus. *J Appl Physiol* 1988;64:2692–2695.

68. Sahlin K. NADH and NADPH in human skeletal muscle at rest and during ischaemia. *Clin Physiol* 1983;3:477–485.

69. Henriksson J, Katz A, Sahlin K. Redox state changes in human skeletal muscle after isometric contraction. *J Physiol* 1986;380:441–451.

70. Sahlin K. NADH and lactate in human skeletal muscle during short-term intense exercise. *Pflugers Arch* 1985;403:193–196.

71. Hampson NB, Piantadosi CA. Near infrared monitoring of human skeletal muscle oxygenation during forearm ischemia. *J Appl Physiol* 1988;64:2449–2457.

72. Bonde-Petersen F, Lundgaard JS. Gas tensions (O_2, CO_2, Ar and N_2) in human muscle during static exercise and occlusion. In: Knuttgen HG, Vogel JA, Poortmans J, eds. *Biochemistry of exercise*, vol 13. Champaign, IL: Human Kinetics Publishers, 1983;781–786.

THE LUNG: *Scientific Foundations*
edited by R.G. Crystal, J.B. West et al.
Raven Press, Ltd., New York © 1991.

CHAPTER 5.5.2.1

Mitochondria and Microvascular Design

H. Hoppeler, O. Mathieu-Costello, and S. R. Kayar

STRUCTURAL DETERMINANTS OF OXYGEN FLOW IN MUSCLE

During strenuous physical activity a major fraction of the cardiac output is directed to active skeletal muscles to satisfy the oxygen demand created by skeletal muscle mitochondria supplying ATP to activated myofibrils. The distribution of blood flow among and within active muscles is achieved by neuronal and local control mechanisms as well as by metabolic factors (1–3). Using the radioactive microsphere method, it has been shown in rats running at or close to their aerobic maximum ($\dot{V}_{O_2}max$) that the skeletal muscle capillary bed is able to accommodate blood flows as high as 320 $ml \cdot min^{-1} \cdot 100 g^{-1}$ of muscle tissue (4). In humans, perfusion rates of skeletal muscles during maximal voluntary activation are reported to be around 250 $ml \cdot min^{-1} \cdot 100 g^{-1}$, with oxygen consumption rates as high as 35 ml $O_2 \cdot min^{-1} \cdot 100 g^{-1}$ (5). Unfortunately, these very high blood flows and aerobic metabolic rates cannot nearly be approached in isolated contracting muscle preparations (6). This has made the design of experiments probing into the limitations of oxygen flow in muscle tissue under well-controlled experimental conditions rather difficult.

The size of the capillary bed and the rate at which blood flows through it are by no means the sole determinants of mitochondrial oxygen supply. It is evidently a necessary condition that a sufficient number of oxygenated erythrocytes pass muscle tissue. However, erythrocyte spacing and the time for oxygen un-

H. Hoppeler: Institute of Anatomy, University of Berne, CH-3000 Berne, Switzerland.

O. Mathieu-Costello: Department of Medicine, University of California, San Diego, School of Medicine, La Jolla, California 92093-10623.

S. R. Kayar: Department of Physiology, Robert Wood Johnson Medical School, Piscataway, New Jersey 08854.

loading from erythrocytes must also be respected (7–9). Furthermore, provision must be made that tissue diffusion distances and conditions are such that even mitochondria farthest away from capillaries are adequately supplied with oxygen (10).

The first investigator to model oxygen supply to muscle tissue was August Krogh (11). He essentially considered straight and parallel capillaries supplying a tissue cylinder in which oxygen consumption and the effective diffusion coefficient for oxygen were distributed homogeneously from the erythrocytes to the very edge of this tissue cylinder. Despite the fact that virtually all the simplifying assumptions that Krogh made have subsequently been proven to be much oversimplified or even wrong, his analysis is still much in use today. The reason for the continued popularity of Krogh's model is that there is currently no alternative model that would allow one to incorporate all the complexities of tissue oxygen supply, both functional and structural, which have been uncovered in over 70 years of research effort since Krogh published his milestone paper. The present chapter aims at exploring available knowledge on the many factors influencing oxygen flow to mitochondria in exercising muscle tissue. The emphasis will be on structural aspects. This is done in an attempt to identify the building blocks used in the construction of different types of muscle tissue capable of coping with the very wide range of energetic demands imposed on a muscle's respiratory system by the sustained use of the contractile machinery.

MITOCHONDRIA COMPRISE THE CELLULAR OXYGEN SINK

Mitochondria are the major site of cellular oxygen consumption. They are bound by a continuous outer membrane, and a complexly folded inner membrane (containing mainly the enzymes of the respiratory chain) subdivides the mitochondrial interior into a matrix and

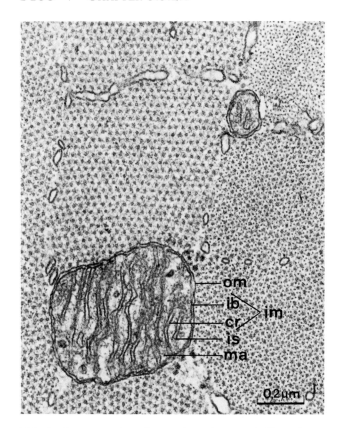

FIG. 1. Cross-section of a portion of a muscle fiber showing two mitochondria. A continuous outer membrane (om) is visible; also visible is the inner membrane (im), which can be subdivided into cristae (cr) and inner boundary membrane (ib). The inner membrane separates the matrix (ma) from the intermembrane space (is).

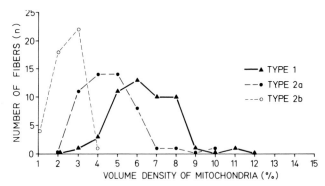

FIG. 2. Histogram of the distribution of mitochondrial volume densities in histochemically identified single human muscle fibers (M. vastus lateralis). For each fiber type, 50 fibers were analyzed. (Adapted from ref. 19.)

an intermembrane space (Fig. 1). The matrix houses most enzymes of the citric acid cycle as well as the mitochondrial DNA and ribosomes. An electrochemical gradient is established across the inner membrane by enzymes of the respiratory chain, and this drives the mitochondrial ATP synthetase also located in the inner membrane. Contacts between the inner and outer membrane serve as entry points for nuclear-coded proteins (12), and most of the traffic of small solutes and ions in and out of mitochondria is controlled by a number of transport and exchange systems (13,14).

Mitochondrial ultrastructure is found to be highly variable when different cell types such as muscle fibers, hepatocytes, astrocytes, fat cells, or steroid-synthesizing cells are compared (14). This diversity of mitochondrial internal structure is poorly understood. It seems to reflect primarily the metabolic functions *other* than ATP synthesis performed by mitochondria in these tissues. In skeletal muscle, mitochondria appear to be structurally quite uniform and of the cristae type (Fig. 1). Their major task is to rephosphorylate ADP to ATP for the myosin heads and calcium pumps involved in muscle contraction. Their close apposition

to parts of the sarcoplasmic reticulum has been taken as structural evidence for their role in calcium regulation (15). When skeletal muscle mitochondria are analyzed ultrastructurally, it is found that the surface density of their inner mitochondrial membranes (i.e., the surface area of inner mitochondrial membrane per unit volume of mitochondria) ranges from 20 to 40 $m^2 \cdot cm^{-3}$. The packing density of the inner mitochondrial membranes is apparently not related either to body size or to aerobic capacity of animals or muscles (16). It has further been established both by structural (17) and biochemical (18) techniques that changes of muscle aerobic capacity brought about by exercise training or chronic electrical stimulation have no effect on mitochondrial morphology. From this it becomes apparent that mitochondrial internal structure is quite invariant in skeletal muscle tissue of most mammalian species even when muscle tissue oxidative capacity varies manifold.

This constancy of mitochondrial internal ultrastructure has the convenient implication that muscle oxidative capacity can be described morphologically by estimating the relative space taken up by this organelle in a muscle fiber or in muscle tissue—the mitochondrial volume density. In human vastus lateralis, individual muscle fibers may contain as little as 1% mitochondria in some type IIB fibers or as much as 13% mitochondria in some type I fibers (19) (Fig. 2). Considerably larger mitochondrial volume densities are found in small mammals, particularly in continuously active skeletal muscles, such as the diaphragm [35% mitochondria in the shrew diaphragm (20)].

In order to understand the functional implication of the diversity of mitochondrial contents in various fibers, muscles, and species, we should ideally know how much oxygen could be used by a given quantity of mitochondria under defined condition of maximal activity. The biochemical approach to this problem, using isolated mitochondria or muscle homogenates, has not led to satisfactory results. This is not only because tissue and mitochondria integrity has to be disrupted before the necessary biochemical assays can be carried out, but also because the observed oxygen consumption rates are largely dependent on external conditions, such as the choice of substrates (21). Because the local microconditions for mitochondria working *in situ* (in an intact animal running at $\dot{V}O_2$max) are not known, these conditions cannot be replicated in the test tube. To overcome some of these problems, we have recently used a novel approach to seek information on *in situ* maximal oxygen consumption of muscle mitochondria. We have first measured $\dot{V}O_2$max in animals varying greatly in their aerobic performance capacity. We have then determined the volume of mitochondria in their entire skeletal musculature by a statistical sampling procedure (16,22). From these two estimates, a lower boundary for average mitochondrial oxygen consumption under *in vivo* conditions of $\dot{V}O_2$max could be calculated. The two major assumptions made were that all oxygen is taken up by skeletal muscle mitochondria and that all mitochondria are active simultaneously. The rather surprising results of these calculations indicated that mitochondrial oxygen consumption at $\dot{V}O_2$max was invariant (close to 5 ml $O_2 \cdot min^{-1} \cdot cm^{-3}$ of mitochondria) among all species analyzed (16,22,23). Still to be tested is whether this apparently invariant operational characteristic of mitochondria remains conserved when muscle or whole-animal oxidative capacity is changed by experimental procedures such as endurance exercise, cold exposure, or hypoxia.

In conclusion, it appears that both the structure and the function of skeletal muscle mitochondria are invariant among mammalian species and among muscles varying widely in oxidative capacity. For the sake of the ensuing discussion, we will therefore assume that local muscle oxidative capacity is adequately characterized by mitochondrial volume or volume density. If muscle oxidative capacity is varied between animals or muscles, this occurs through adding or taking away mitochondrial volume while the rate at which mitochondria operate remains constant.

DISTRIBUTION OF MITOCHONDRIA IN MUSCLE CELLS

Interfibrillar Versus Subsarcolemmal Mitochondria

Clearly, mitochondria are not scattered randomly in muscle fibers. When fibers are cut transversely and examined by electron microscopy, it is common to find clusters of mitochondrial profiles directly beneath the fiber sarcolemma, particularly near capillaries (Fig. 3).

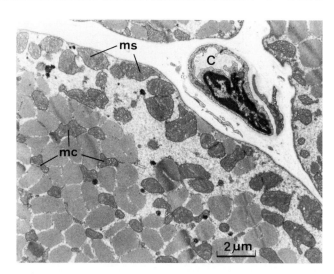

FIG. 3. Subsarcolemmal mitochondria (ms) are clustering beneath the sarcolemma close to a capillary (C). Interfibrillary mitochondria (mc) are distributed between myofibrils.

The interpretation comes immediately to mind that these mitochondria are accumulating where diffusion distances from capillaries are particularly short. Muscle fiber types that are highly oxidative in their metabolism typically have greater densities of subsarcolemmal mitochondria than do fiber types that depend more heavily on glycolytic metabolism (19). In muscles trained for endurance exercise, there is an increase in total mitochondrial content of muscle fibers, with a greater relative increase in the subsarcolemmal mitochondria than in the mitochondria distributed farther into the fiber, between the myofibrils (24,25). This has led to the speculation that subsarcolemmal and interfibrillar mitochondria are two biochemically distinct populations. In support of this speculation, Palmer et al. (26) and Krieger et al. (27) found that when muscle fibers were homogenized and differentially treated to extract separately the subsarcolemmal from interfibrillar mitochondria, the two groups of mitochondria had differing metabolic rates. However, Matlib et al. (28) have argued that these differing metabolic rates are actually an artifact of the extraction procedures. Thus while there is some basis for considering that the mitochondria near capillaries may be functionally different from mitochondria farther from capillaries, the direct biochemical demonstration of this is currently equivocal.

Gradients Across the Fiber Width

In a variety of muscles, mitochondria have been demonstrated to be distributed in a gradient that is highest near capillaries, slightly lower between capillaries at the fiber border, and decreasing with distance toward estimates of P_{O_2} in transverse sections of muscle fibers have shown that P_{O_2} gradients are indeed small (34).

Gradients Along the Fiber Length

It would be tempting to speculate that if mitochondrial distribution is partly dictated by tissue P_{O_2} and diffusion distances from capillaries, then there should be a systematic shift in mitochondrial density along a muscle fiber, in the direction of blood flow in the adjacent capillaries. A rigorous attempt at finding such a gradient has not yet been reported. In a transverse section of a muscle fiber and its surrounding capillaries as viewed by electron microscopy, the observer is unable to detect whether the capillaries have been sectioned near their arteriolar or venular ends. A random section of muscle is expected to contain an unbiased sample of capillaries cut at all possible levels along their length. Consequently, the studies of gradients in mitochondrial distribution across the fiber width are averaging any longitudinal gradients, if they indeed existed. However, a longitudinal gradient in mitochondria would be expected only on the assumption of a longitudinal gradient in tissue P_{O_2}, such as proposed in the classic Krogh model (11). There is a growing body of evidence that capillary blood flow heterogeneity, both within one capillary and between capillaries, is great enough that a systematic decline in tissue P_{O_2} along a fiber does not exist (35,36).

Mitochondrial Connectivity

Sections of muscle, whether longitudinal or transverse to the fibers, show profiles of mitochondria that are roughly circular or ovoid and of varying length (Fig. 3). One therefore automatically imagines that these profiles represent sections of spherical or cylindrical objects in three dimensions. Mitochondria that have been isolated from homogenized muscle samples are indeed spherical (21). However, close inspection of the internal structure of these isolated muscle mitochondria reveals that they are swollen and may have lost a small amount of outer membrane. These changes suggest that they have been broken during isolation and have reformed into spheres (21).

Three-dimensional reconstructions and scanning electron microscopy have shown that muscle mitochondria *in situ* may actually be quite complex in shape and variable in size (Fig. 5) (37–40). It appears that both complexity and size of individual mitochondria increase with the total density of mitochondria in a muscle fiber (37,40). Some isolated spherical and cylindrical mitochondria have been found in the subsarcolemmal region of certain muscle fibers (38), and in deeper regions in muscle fibers with a density of less

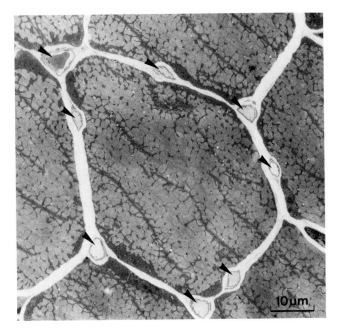
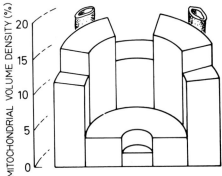

FIG. 4. Diagrammatic representation of the pattern of distribution of mitochondrial volume density across muscle fibers as well as with regard to capillaries. Arrows in top panel indicate capillaries. (From ref. 30.)

the fiber center (Fig. 4) (29,30). Such observations lead one again to the appealing notion that mitochondrial location is related to mitochondrial function. One may reason that if diffusion distances for oxygen or other metabolic substrates from capillaries to mitochondria were a critical factor to mitochondrial metabolism, then all mitochondria should be located near capillaries. Conversely, if the distances for exchanging high-energy phosphate compounds between mitochondria and myofibrils were critical to muscle work rate, then mitochondria should be distributed uniformly between the myofibrils. The actual distribution of mitochondria in muscle is intermediate to these two cases; this has been interpreted as an indication that mitochondrial distribution reflects a balance between these opposing demands (31,32). Mathematical modeling has suggested that when mitochondrial peak density is at an intermediate location in muscle fibers, the tissue P_{O_2} will be nearly constant across the fiber (33). Direct

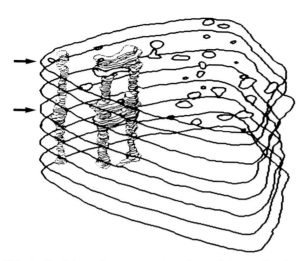

FIG. 5. Serial-section reconstruction of two mitochondria in a single equine muscle fiber. Profiles of all mitochondria contained in the fiber are drawn on the top section. The arrows indicate the position of the z-bands in the fiber. (From ref. 40.)

than 5% (40). In fibers of around 10% mitochondrial density, mitochondria may have relatively simple cylindrical forms in the A-band region of fiber sarcomeres, but these are often interlinked by transverse portions in the I-band region of a sarcomere (Fig. 5). At the Z-band, short cylindrical portions of mitochondria are found, which may interconnect the more complex portions of two adjacent I-bands (Fig. 5) (40). It has been reported that in a muscle of over 20% mitochondrial density (rat diaphragm), all mitochondrial material appears to be interconnected into a single reticulum (37). This contention is difficult to substantiate for technical reasons. Three-dimensional reconstructions of membrane-bound organelles such as mitochondria, using ultrathin sections, are problematic. It is quite possible that apposing membranes of adjacent mitochondria might not be detected as separate membranes in some cases. This would lead to an overestimation of the size and complexity of mitochondria. In muscle fibers of moderate to high mitochondrial density, three-dimensional reconstructions appear to show that there are interconnections between portions of mitochondria which in single sections one would have separated into subsarcolemmal and interfibrillar mitochondria (39,40).

The significance of the size and shape of mitochondria with respect to their metabolism is totally unknown. It has been hypothesized that the transverse portions of mitochondria facilitate the diffusion of oxygen from capillaries deep into muscle fibers, by virtue of the high oxygen solubility of their lipid-rich membranes (41). However, the reconstructions of mitochondria suggest that the greater axis of mitochondrial

connectivity is longitudinal to the muscle fibers (40). There is no obvious hypothesis as to how this orientation of mitochondria parallel to capillaries would be related to metabolism. It seems logical that mitochondrial shape and size must also face some constraints imposed by placing mitochondria between cylindrical, contracting myofibrils.

Mitochondria and Substrate Stores

Metabolic substrate stores in the form of lipid droplets and glycogen granules are visible in electron micrographs of muscle. Lipid droplets, which are usually found directly apposed to mitochondria, increase in muscles with endurance exercise training (42) and disappear following an extended bout of endurance exercise (43) (Fig. 6). Glycogen granules may be found in the interfibrillar spaces throughout a muscle fiber, but wherever there are large accumulations of subsarcolemmal mitochondrial profiles, there are often also large accumulations of glycogen granules (Fig. 6). These subsarcolemmal glycogen stores also selectively disappear following one extended bout of endurance

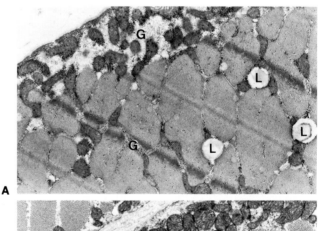
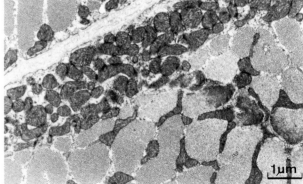

FIG. 6. Cross-sections of muscle fibers obtained from biopsies taken before (**A**) and after (**B**) a 100-km run. It is evident that most of the glycogen (G) and lipid (L) contained in the fibers has disappeared in the post-run biopsy. (From ref. 43.)

exercise (43) as well as when subsarcolemmal mitochondria are catabolized during several weeks of extreme high altitude trekking (44). We are drawn once again to the suggestion that mitochondrial location relative to the stores of metabolic substrates must play an important role by facilitating mitochondrial function (45,46).

The distribution of mitochondria in rat soleus muscle was found to be different in animals subjected to a high-intensity, short-duration form of exercise training when compared to that in untrained controls and animals subjected to a lower-intensity, long-duration form of training (47). The control and endurance-trained muscles had the usual distribution of mitochondria in transverse sections of fibers—that is, relatively higher mitochondrial density near capillaries, and decreasing density toward the fiber center. The high-intensity, short-duration-exercised muscles had a uniform distribution of interfibrillar mitochondria across transverse sections of fibers. These differing mitochondrial distributions were interpreted to reflect differing substrate sources: The control and endurance-exercised muscles were thought to rely heavily on blood-borne fuels and oxygen; whereas the high-intensity, short-duration-exercised muscles were hypothesized to be using primarily glycogen stored within the fibers. Thus while there are numerous indications that mitochondrial distribution may be significant to mitochondrial metabolism, there is a possibility that the diffusion distance for oxygen is not the *only*—maybe not even the *primary*—determinant.

ARE CAPILLARIES MATCHED TO MITOCHONDRIA?

Estimating Capillarity

Because of its importance for muscle blood–tissue transfer, capillarity has been one of the most commonly measured variables in skeletal muscles after a variety of experimental conditions. In his pioneering work, Krogh (11) estimated muscle capillarity by simply counting the number of capillary sections per unit cross-sectional area of muscle. This measurement, commonly called "capillary density" (i.e., number of capillaries per square millimeter), is still widely used in the literature. It provides an estimate of the area of tissue per capillary in muscle transverse section (1/ "capillary density") from which the radius of the tissue cylinder associated with each capillary, the classic "Krogh cylinder," can be calculated. In this approach as mentioned above, capillaries are considered as straight tubes running perpendicular to the fiber axis, and the contribution of tortuosity and branching to capillary length is not taken into account. Another fre-

quently used estimate of muscle capillarity is the number of capillaries per number of fibers, or capillary-to-fiber ratio, $N_N(c,f)$, which avoids the effect of tissue preparation on fiber size and, therefore, on capillary "density." Plyley and Groom (48) considered muscle vascular supply on the basis of individual fibers and fiber types. They introduced the estimate of the number of capillaries around a fiber, CAF, and the sharing factor, SF, which is the number of fibers sharing one capillary, $SF = CAF/N_N(c,f)$. The drawback of capillary-to-fiber ratios is that they do not incorporate information on either capillary geometry or diffusion distances.

Gray and Renkin (49) pointed out the importance of normalizing data to sarcomere length when comparing capillary density and fiber size, and therefore diffusion distances, in different muscles. Unfortunately, this source of variation has generally been disregarded. Several methods have been proposed to quantify the heterogeneity of capillary spacing and the distribution of diffusion distances in muscles (50–53). So far, all these methods for quantifying capillarity have been based on measurements on transverse sections only and have not incorporated the contribution of capillary geometry.

In recent years, efforts were made to quantify the geometry of the capillary network in muscles. Capillary geometry is best estimated after tissue vascular perfusion fixation *in situ,* to avoid capillary collapsing and muscle fiber kinking in immersion fixed material (54). Capillary length per fiber volume, $J_V(c,f)$, is to be preferred to capillary number per unit cross-sectional area of muscle fiber, since it takes into account capillary branching and tortuosity. Also, two important estimates of a muscle potential for O_2 delivery—capillary volume per unit volume of fiber, $V_V(c,f)$, and capillary surface available for exchange per unit fiber volume, $S_V(c,f)$—are related to $J_V(c,f)$ by the following equations (55):

$$V_V(c,f) = a(c) \cdot J_V(c,f) \qquad [1]$$

$$S_V(c,f) = b(c) \cdot J_V(c,f) \qquad [2]$$

where $a(c)$ and $b(c)$ are the mean area and perimeter of capillary cross-sections, respectively. The radius (R) of the Krogh cylinder can be approximated as

$$R[\pi \cdot J_V(c,f)]^{-1/2} \qquad [3]$$

The estimation of capillary orientation, which is necessary to estimate $J_V(c,f)$, is a difficult morphometric problem because there is partial anisotropy of the capillary network in muscles. Capillaries run mostly parallel to the muscle fibers, but they can show various degrees of tortuosity and branching. For perfectly anisotropic capillaries (no tortuosity, no branching),

J_V(c,f) is related to capillary counts per fiber sectional area in transverse section, $Q_A(0)$, by the equation

$$J_V(c,f) = Q_A(0) \qquad [4]$$

For randomly oriented (perfectly isotropic) capillaries, the following equation is used:

$$J_V(c,f) = 2 \cdot Q_A(0) \qquad [5]$$

For partially oriented capillaries, we have

$$J_V(c,f) = c(K,0) \cdot Q_A(0) \qquad [6]$$

where $c(K,0)$ is an anisotropy coefficient that varies from 1 to 2, depending on the degree of anisotropy of capillaries (Eqs. 4 and 5). Mathieu et al. (56) proposed a model-based method to estimate capillary anisotropy coefficient, $c(K,0)$, and length per fiber volume, J_V(c,f), in muscles, using a set of sections taken both parallel and transverse to the muscle fiber axis. The model, a Fisher axial distribution of capillary segment orientations, has been validated in muscles with widely differing capillary geometries, such as cat extended soleus muscle (56), rat solei fixed at different sarcomere length (57), pigeon flight muscle (58), and rat heart (59). It can be seen from Eq. 6 that simply counting capillaries per fiber sectional area in transverse section, as is commonly done, would underestimate muscle capillarity [i.e., J_V(c,f)] by as much as 100%, if muscle capillaries were perfectly isotropic. Until recently, the amount of capillary tortuosity actually found in skeletal muscles has been a matter of controversy. Using vascular microcorrosion casts, Potter and Groom (60) showed a substantial degree of capillary tortuosity in shortened muscles. It has been demonstrated that capillary tortuosity (a) is a direct function of sarcomere length and (b) can contribute as much as 70% to total capillary length per volume of muscle fiber in shortened muscles, within physiological sarcomere length (57,61,62). Sarcomere length needs to be taken into account when estimates of capillary density (49) and geometry (57) are compared between muscles.

Because it is free of O_2 carriers, the space between capillaries and muscle fibers is an important component in the diffusion pathway from blood to muscle mitochondria. Unfortunately, the preservation of intercellular spaces during the histological preparation of muscle tissue is unreliable. Capillary length estimates are therefore best determined by using the fiber volume as a reference space, rather than by using muscle volume, to avoid variation resulting from the preparation procedure.

The finding of a change in capillary geometry with muscle shortening has important implications for the modeling of blood tissue transfer in muscle. Obviously, the vascular geometry found in shortened muscles represents a substantial departure from the assumption of straight vessels running parallel to the muscle fibers.

In shortened muscles, capillarity is substantially underestimated by simply counting capillary number per fiber cross-sectional area. In addition, Ellis et al. (63) pointed out that the increased tortuosity tends to provide a more uniform capillary supply to the muscle fibers. Opposite to the Krogh approach, the Hill geometry (64) considers the inward diffusion of O_2 into a tissue cylinder (the muscle fiber in this case) from a uniform peripheral O_2 supply. Such a model, although likely not completely achieved in most muscles, can be a closer approximation of the geometry of blood–tissue exchange in shortened muscles than can the Krogh cylinder (63).

The Local Comparison; Capillary Supply and Fiber Types

Romanul (65) and Nishiyama (66) first reported that the number of capillaries surrounding individual muscle fibers is proportionate to the fiber oxidative capacity. Taking into account capillary sharing by adjacent muscle fibers in the estimate of fiber-type vascular supply in mixed muscles, Gray and Renkin (49) found that capillary densities (capillary number/fiber cross-sectional area) for red fibers were twice those of white fibers in the same muscles. The capillary-to-fiber ratio revealed smaller differences, illustrating the dependence of capillary density on fiber size (49). There is substantial heterogeneity of intercapillary distances in the supply of individual fiber types (51,53). Mean differences in capillary density are primarily related to fiber size, with the CAF showing little difference among individual fiber types (48,67).

Comparing Muscles

Red muscles generally have a higher capillary density than do white muscles (68). As for capillarity and fiber types, large differences in capillary density between muscles are primarily related to size difference and to relative proportion of fiber types. Plyley and Groom (48) found no systematic difference between red and white muscles with respect to both capillary-to-fiber ratio and CAF. Myrhage (69) found a positive correlation between fiber size and the number of surrounding capillaries in different muscle, and he observed large differences between muscles with respect to the number of capillaries surrounding individual fiber types. Large differences between studies in terms of capillary number/fiber cross-sectional area in different muscles have been attributed to possible technical artifacts (fiber shrinkage during fixation; incomplete staining; or filling of the capillary bed) (48).

It has been a source of controversy as to whether or not capillary tortuosity is larger in red than in white muscles. Stingl (70) found strongly undulated capillaries both in red and white muscles. Several reports suggested a more tortuous course of capillaries, thereby suggesting an increased blood volume and surface available for exchange per capillary in red muscles (65,71,72). When sarcomere length was taken into account, there was no systematic difference in capillary tortuosity between rat muscles, with almost a threefold difference in capillary density (number per fiber cross-sectional area ranging from 880 to 3260 mm^{-2}) (73).

Comparing Animals

It has been known since Krogh's work that capillary number per muscle cross-sectional area is (a) larger in warm-blooded animals than in cold-blooded ones and (b) larger in smaller animals than in larger ones (11). Large scatter in the data and discrepancy between studies have characterized interanimal comparisons of muscle capillarity and oxidative capacity. As much as a threefold difference was found in capillary number per fiber cross-sectional area in muscles of different animals with similar mitochondrial densities (55). Maxwell et al. (74) found a very poor correlation between muscle capillarity and oxidative capacity in various muscles from different animals. When capillarity was compared in different muscles (locomotor, diaphragm, and heart) ranging from those of shrew to those of cattle (mitochondrial volume density range: 1–40%), a strong correlation was found between capillary and mitochondrial density (55,75).

In a study on adaptive variation, "athletic" animals such as horses and dogs were compared to "sedentary" animals such as steers and goats (76). It was found that athletic animals had both a 2.5-fold higher $\dot{V}o_2$max and a 2.5-fold larger skeletal muscle mitochondrial volume. Capillary length was found to be only 1.7-fold larger in the athletic animals. However, this difference was complemented by a 1.7-fold larger systemic hemoglobin concentration. It was reasoned that this combination of two structural adaptations (more capillaries and more erythrocytes) contributed to the match between capillary O_2 delivery and mitochondrial O_2 demand.

There has been increasing evidence that capillarity in glycolytic muscles is related to metabolite supply and/or removal rather than to O_2 delivery (77). Differences in capillary geometry have been found between animals and/or muscles. However, capillary tortuosity differences are found between mammals but are not related systematically to body size, animal athletic ability, or mitochondrial density (62). Highly tortuous capillaries were found in shortened muscles of mouse and alligator, with more than a 30-fold difference in capillary density (78). A different capillary arrangement and a larger degree of capillary anisotropy were found in the highly aerobic flight muscle of the pigeon, compared to that of mammal and pigeon hindlimb (78).

Varying the Supply: Hypoxia

There has been considerable discrepancy in the literature as to the effect of chronic exposure to hypoxia on muscle capillarity (79). Banchero (79) pointed out the effect of body size on fiber cross-sectional area (and, therefore, on capillary density) when comparing muscle capillarity, since there is often retarded growth at high altitudes when compared to that at sea level. When body weight was taken into account, there was no effect of chronic hypoxia per se on capillary number per fiber cross-sectional area (79). Exposure to both cold and hypoxia induced a fiber-type transformation from fast-twitch glycolytic (FG) to fast-twitch oxidative–glycolytic (FOG) and also increased the number of capillaries around each fiber type (80). Despite the absence of change in capillary number after exposure to hypoxia alone, there was still the possibility of an increased capillary tortuosity and branching, yielding an increased capillary surface area available for exchange. However, when sarcomere length was taken into account, capillary anisotropy was not systematically different in skeletal muscles of mice native to 3800 m when compared to that of sea-level mice (82), nor was it systematically different in sea-level rats kept at the same altitude of 3800 m for 5 months when compared to that of sea-level controls (83).

The response of muscle oxidative capacity and fiber size to chronic exposure to hypoxia have also been controversial, possibly because of differences in preparation, animal activity, and/or level of hypoxia (e.g., moderate versus extreme altitude). Earlier studies reported an increase in muscle oxidative capacity and mitochondrial density after high-altitude hypoxia (83). Recent data indicate a decrease in mitochondrial volume at extremely high altitudes (44,85).

Mathieu-Costello et al. (86) found no difference in fiber cross-sectional area in muscles of animals chronically exposed to an altitude of 3800 m, confirming earlier reports that hypoxia alone, especially at moderate altitude, may not be severe enough to induce a reduction in fiber size. There is evidence of muscle-wasting at extremely high altitudes (44,84), and this could result in apparent increase in capillary density.

Varying the Demand: Training

It is well known that the augmented muscle oxidative capacity induced by increased physical activity is accompanied by an increased capillary-to-fiber ratio

(68,87). Considerable scatter in the data and discrepancies between studies of muscle capillary "density" after endurance training have also been attributed to preparation artifacts and methodological difficulties (54). Poole et al. (61) found no change in capillary tortuosity, at various measured sarcomere lengths, in soleus muscle of rats after an endurance-training protocol that produced a 35% increase in citrate synthase activity. In the same study, capillary length per fiber volume, $J_V(c,f)$, was closely correlated with fiber aerobic capacity, whereas capillary number per fiber cross-sectional area was not (61). A correlation between muscle capillarity and oxidative capacity was found in predominantly glycolytic muscles transformed into aerobic muscles by chronic electrical stimulation, but not in non-stimulated glycolytic or purely oxidative muscles (77). There is qualitative evidence that muscle capillary tortuosity might be increased after chronic electrical stimulation (88), although the study of capillary geometry at various measured sarcomere lengths has not yet been carried out in response to this experimental manipulation.

CONCLUSION

When muscles with broad differences in oxidative capacity are compared, there is clearly a relationship between fiber mitochondrial content and the size of the capillary network, either between animals or after experimental manipulations. However, individual data show considerable scatter, possibly related to (a) methodological difficulties in assessing muscle capillarization or (b) differences between muscles, animals, and/or experimental conditions between studies. One factor that has been identified to affect the capillary–mitochondria relationship is systemic hemoglobin content. Additional factors such as blood-flow patterns and heterogeneity, as well as the role of capillaries for functions other than O_2 supply, need to be taken into account when comparing capillarity and O_2 demand in muscles. From a methodological perspective, it is possible to account for capillary geometry in estimates of muscle capillarization. The application of appropriate methodology will be an important tool for improving both the estimation and the modeling of blood–tissue transfer capacity in muscles.

ACKNOWLEDGMENTS

The excellent technical assistance of L. Tüscher, B. Krieger, and R. M. Fankhauser in the preparation of this manuscript is gratefully acknowledged. Experimental work related to the topic of this review has been supported for many years by grants of the Swiss National Science Foundation, the U.S. National Science Foundation, and the U.S. National Institutes of Health.

REFERENCES

1. Joyner WL, Davis HJ. Pressure profile along the microvascular network and its control. *Fed Proc* 1987;46:266–269.
2. Segal SS, Duling BR. Flow control among microvessels coordinated by intracellular conduction. *Science* 1987;234:868–870.
3. Björnberg J, Maspers M, Mellander S. Metabolic control of large-bore arterial resistance vessels, arterioles, and veins in cat skeletal muscle during exercise. *Acta Physiol Scand* 1989;135:83–94.
4. Laughlin MH, Armstrong RB. Muscular blood flow distribution patterns as a function of running speed in rats. *Am J Physiol* 1982;243:296–306.
5. Andersen P, Saltin B. Maximal perfusion of skeletal muscle in man. *J Physiol (Lond)* 1985;366:233–249.
6. Hoppeler H, Hudlicka O, Uhlmann E. Relationship between mitochondria and oxygen consumption in isolated cat muscles. *J Physiol (Lond)* 1987;385:661–675.
7. Tyml K. Red cell perfusion in skeletal muscle at rest and after mild and severe contractions. *Am J Physiol* 1987;252:H485–H493.
8. Tyml K, Ellis GC, Safranyos RG, Fraser S, Groom AC. Temporal and spatial distribution of red blood cell velocity in capillaries of resting skeletal muscle, including estimates of red cell transit times. *Microvasc Res* 1981;22:14–31.
9. Vandegriff KD, Olson JS. Morphological and physiological factors affecting oxygen uptake and release by red blood cells. *J Biol Chem* 1984;259:12619–12627.
10. Kayar SR, Banchero N. Distribution of capillaries and diffusion distances in guinea pig myocardium. *Pflügers Arch* 1983;396:350–352.
11. Krogh A. The number and distribution of capillaries in muscle with calculations of the oxygen pressure head necessary for supplying the tissue. *J Physiol (Lond)* 1919;52:409–415.
12. Hartl FU, Pfanner N, Nicholson DW, Neupert W. Mitochondrial protein import. *Biochim Biophys Acta* 1989;988:1–45.
13. Diwan JJ. Mitochondrial transport of K and Mg. *Biochim Biophys Acta* 1989;895:155–166.
14. Tzagoloff A. *Mitochondria*. New York: Plenum Press, 1982; Chapters 2 and 9.
15. Carafoli E. Intracellular calcium homeostasis. *Annu Rev Biochem* 1987;56:395–433.
16. Hoppeler H, Lindstedt SL. Malleability of skeletal muscle tissue in overcoming limitations: structural elements. *J Exp Biol* 1985;115:355–364.
17. Hoppeler H, Lüthi P, Claassen H, Weibel ER, Howald H. The ultrastructure of the normal human skeletal muscle. A morphometric analysis on untrained men, women, and well-trained orienteers. *Pflügers Arch* 1973;344:217–232.
18. Davies KJA, Packer L, Brooks GA. Exercise bioenergetics following sprint training. *Arch Biochem Biophys* 1982;215:260–265.
19. Howald H, Hoppeler H, Claassen H, Mathieu O, Straub R. Influence of endurance training on the ultrastructural composition of the different muscle fiber types in humans. *Pflügers Arch* 1985;403:369–376.
20. Hoppeler H, Mathieu O, Krauer R, Claassen H, Armstrong RB, Weibel ER. Design of the mammalian respiratory system. VI. Distribution of mitochondria and capillaries in various muscles. *Respir Physiol* 1981;44:87–111.
21. Schwerzmann K, Hoppeler H, Kayar SR, Weibel ER. Oxidative capacity of muscle and mitochondria: correlation of physiological, biochemical and morphometric characteristics. *Proc Natl Acad Sci USA* 1989;86:1583–1587.
22. Hoppeler H, Jones JH, Claassen H, Lindstedt SL, Longworth KE, Taylor CR, Straub R, Lindholm A. Relating maximal oxygen consumption to skeletal muscle mitochondria in horses. In: Gillespie JR, Robinson NE, eds. *Equine exercise physiology II*. ICEEP Publications. Ann Arbor, MI: Edwards Brothers, 1987; 278–289.

23. Hoppeler H, Turner DL. Plasticity of aerobic scope: adaptation of the respiratory system in animals, organs and cells. In: Wieser W, Gnaiger E, eds. *Energy transformations in cells and organisms.* Stuttgart: Georg Thieme Verlag, 1989;116–122.

24. Müller W. Subsarcolemmal mitochondria and capillarization of soleus muscle fibers in young rats subjected to an endurance exercise. A morphometric study of semithin sections. *Cell Tissue Res* 1976;174:367–389.

25. Rösler KM, Conley KE, Claassen H, Howald H, Hoppeler H. Transfer effects in endurance exercise: adaptations in trained and untrained muscles. *Eur J Appl Physiol* 1985;54:355–362.

26. Palmer JW, Tandler B, Hoppel CL. Biochemical differences between subsarcolemmal and interfibrillar mitochondria from rat cardiac muscle: effects of procedural manipulations. *Arch Biochem Biophys* 1985;236:691–713.

27. Krieger DA, Tate CA, McMillin-Wood J, Booth FW. Populations of rat skeletal muscle mitochondria after exercise and immobilization. *J Appl Physiol* 1980;48:23–28.

28. Matlib MA, Rebmann D, Ashraf M, Rouslin W, Schwartz A. Differential activities of putative subsarcolemmal and interfibrillar mitochondria from cardiac muscle. *J Mol Cell Cardiol* 1981;13:163–170.

29. Rakusan K, Tomanek RJ. Distribution of mitochondria in normal and hypertrophic myocytes from the rat heart. *J Mol Cell Cardiol* 1986;18:299–305.

30. Kayar SR, Hoppeler H, Essen-Gustavsson B, Schwerzmann K. The similarity of mitochondrial distribution in equine skeletal muscles of differing oxidative capacity. *J Exp Biol* 1988;137:253–263.

31. Weibel ER. *The pathway for oxygen: structure and function in the mammalian respiratory system.* Cambridge, MA: Harvard University Press, 1984.

32. Kayar SR, Banchero N. Volume density and distribution of mitochondria in myocardial growth and hypertrophy. *Respir Physiol* 1987;70:275–286.

33. Tonellato PJ, Zhang Z, Greene AS. Oxygen distribution in a complex tissue model. In: *36th Annual Conference of the Microcirculatory Society,* New Orleans, March 18–19, 1989;73.

34. Gayeski TEJ, Honig CR. O₂ gradients from sarcolemma to cell interior in red muscle at maximal $\dot{V}O_2$. *Am J Physiol* 1986;251:H789–H799.

35. Ellsworth ML, Popel AS, Pittman RN. Assessment and impact of heterogeneities of convective oxygen transport parameters in capillaries of striated muscle: experimental and theoretical. *Microvasc Res* 1988;35:341–362.

36. Gayeski TEJ, Honig CR. Intracellular P_{O_2} in long axis of individual fibers in working dog gracilis muscle. *Am J Physiol* 1988;254:H1179–H1186.

37. Bakeeva LE, Chentsov YS, Skulachev VP. Mitochondrial framework (reticulum mitochondriale) in rat diaphragm muscle. *Biochim Biophys Acta* 1978;501:349–369.

38. Ogata T, Yamasaki Y. Scanning electron-microscopic studies on the three-dimensional structure of mitochondria in the mammalian red, white and intermediate muscle fibers. *Cell Tissue Res* 1985;241:251–256.

39. Kirkwood SP, Munn EA, Brooks GA. Mitochondrial reticulum in limb skeletal muscle. *Am J Physiol* 1986;251:C395–C402.

40. Kayar SR, Hoppeler H, Mermod L, Weibel ER. Mitochondrial size and shape in equine skeletal muscle: a three-dimensional reconstruction study. *Anat Rec* 1988;222:333–339.

41. Longmuir IS. Channels of oxygen transport from blood to mitochondria. In: Kovach AGB, Dora E, Kessler M, Silver IA, eds. *Oxygen transport to tissue. Advances in Physiological Science,* vol 25. Elmsford, NY: Pergamon Press, 1981;19–22.

42. Hoppeler H, Howald H, Conley KE, Lindstedt SL, Claassen H, Vock P, Weibel ER. Endurance training in humans: aerobic capacity and structure of skeletal muscle. *J Appl Physiol* 1985;59:320–327.

43. Kayar SR, Hoppeler H, Howald H, Claassen H, Oberholzer F. Acute effects of endurance exercise on mitochondrial distribution and skeletal muscle morphology. *Eur J Appl Physiol* 1986;54:578–584.

44. Hoppeler H, Kleinert E, Schlegel C, Claassen H, Howald H, Cerretelli P. Muscular exercise at high altitude. II. Morphological adaptation of skeletal muscle to chronic hypoxia. *Int J Sports Med* 1990;11,S2:53–59.

45. Reichmann H, Hoppeler H, Mathieu-Costello O, von Bergen F, Pette D. Biochemical and ultrastructural changes of skeletal muscle mitochondria after chronic electrical stimulation in rabbits. *Pflügers Arch* 1985;404:1–9.

46. Hoppeler H. Exercise-induced ultrastructural changes in skeletal muscle. *Int J Sports Med* 1986;7:187–204.

47. Kayar SR, Conley KE, Claassen H, Hoppeler H. Capillarity and mitochondrial distribution in rat myocardium following exercise training. *J Exp Biol* 1986;102:189–199.

48. Plyley MJ, Groom AC. Geometrical distribution of capillaries in mammalian striated muscle. *Am J Physiol* 1975;228:1376–1383.

49. Gray SD, Renkin EM. Microvascular supply in relation to fiber metabolic type in mixed skeletal muscles of rabbits. *Microvasc Res* 1978;16:404–425.

50. Loats JT, Sillau AH, Banchero N. How to quantify skeletal muscle capillarity. In: Silver IA, Erecinska M, Bicher HI, eds. *Oxygen transport to tissue—III.* New York: Plenum Press, 1978;41–48.

51. Renkin EM, Gray SD, Dodd LR, Lia BD. Heterogeneity of capillary distribution and capillary circulation in mammalian skeletal muscles. In: Bachrach AJ, Matzen M, eds. *Symposium on O₂ transport. Underwater physiology.* Proceedings of the 7th Symposium. Bethesda, MD: Undersea and Hyperbaric Medical Society. 1981;465–474.

52. Kayar SR, Archer PG, Lechner AJ, Banchero N. Evaluation of the concentric-circles method for estimating capillary–tissue diffusion distances. *Microvasc Res* 1982;24:342–353.

53. Egginton S, Turek Z, Hoofd LJC. Differing patterns of capillary distribution in fish and mammalian skeletal muscle. *Respir Physiol* 1988;74:383–389.

54. Zumstein A, Mathieu O, Howald H, Hoppeler H. Morphometric analysis of the capillary supply in skeletal muscles of trained and untrained subjects—its limitations in muscle biopsies. *Pflügers Arch* 1983;397:277–283.

55. Hoppeler H, Mathieu O, Weibel ER, Krauer R, Lindstedt SL, Taylor CR. Design of the mammalian respiratory system. VIII. Capillaries in skeletal muscles. *Respir Physiol* 1981;44:129–150.

56. Mathieu O, Cruz-Orive LM, Hoppeler H, Weibel ER. Estimating length density and quantifying anisotropy in skeletal muscle capillaries. *J Microsc* 1983;131:131–146.

57. Mathieu-Costello O. Capillary tortuosity and degree of contraction or extension of skeletal muscle. *Microvasc Res* 1987;33:98–117.

58. Mathieu-Costello O, Durand CM. Capillary supply of bird flight muscle. *Fed Proc* 1985;44:638.

59. Poole DC, Mathieu-Costello O, West JB. Analysis of capillary geometry in rat sub-epicardium and sub-endocardium. *Am J Physiol* 1990(in press).

60. Potter RF, Groom AC. Capillary diameter and geometry in cardiac and skeletal muscle studied by means of corrosion casts. *Microvasc Res* 1983;25:68–84.

61. Poole DC, Mathieu-Costello O, West JB. Capillary tortuosity in rat soleus muscle is not affected by endurance training. *Am J Physiol* 1989;256:H1110–H1116.

62. Mathieu-Costello O, Hoppeler H, Weibel ER. Capillary tortuosity in skeletal muscles of mammals depends on muscle contraction. *J Appl Physiol* 1989;66:1436–1442.

63. Ellis CG, Potter RF, Groom AC. The Krogh cylinder geometry is not appropriate for modelling O₂ transport in contracted skeletal muscle. *Adv Exp Med Biol* 1983;159:253–268.

64. Hill AV. The diffusion of oxygen and lactic acid through tissues. *Proc R Soc B* 1928;104:39–96.

65. Romanul FCA. Capillary supply and metabolism of muscle fibers. *Arch Neurol* 1965;12:497–509.

66. Nishiyama A. Histochemical studies on the red, white and intermediate muscle fibers of some skeletal muscles. II. The capillary distribution on three types of fibers of some skeletal muscles. *Acta Med Okayama* 1965;19:191–198.

67. Egginton S, Ross HF. Planar analysis of tissue capillary supply in *Morone saxatilis* muscle. *J Physiol (Lond)* 1989;53.

68. Hudlicka O. Effect of training on macro- and microcirculatory

changes in exercise. In: Hutton RS, ed. *Exercise and sport sciences reviews,* vol 5. Santa Barbara, CA: Journal Publishing Affiliates, 1977;181.

69. Myrhage R. Capillary supply of the muscle fibre population in hindlimb muscles of the cat. *Acta Physiol Scand* 1978;103:19–30.

70. Stingl J. Arrangement of the vascular bed in the skeletal muscles of the rabbit. *Folia Morphol (Praka)* 1969;17:257.

71. Ranvier L. Note sur les vaisseaux sanguins et la circulation dans les muscles rouges. *Arch Physiol Norm Pathol* 1874;6:446–450.

72. Andersen P, Kroese AJ. Capillary supply in soleus and gastrocnemius muscle of man. *Pflügers Arch* 1978;375:245–249.

73. Mathieu-Costello O, Potter RF, Ellis CG, Groom AC. Capillary configuration and fiber shortening in muscles of the rat hindlimb: correlation between corrosion casts and stereological measurements. *Microvasc Res* 1988;36:40–55.

74. Maxwell LC, White TP, Faulkner JA. Oxidative capacity, blood flow, and capillarity of skeletal muscles. *J Appl Physiol* 1980;49:627–633.

75. Hoppeler H, Kayar SR. Capillarity and oxidative capacity of muscles. *News Physiol Sci* 1988;3:113–116.

76. Conley KE, Kayar SR, Rösler K, Hoppeler H, Weibel ER, Taylor CR. Adaptive variation in the mammalian respiratory system in relation to energetic demand. IV. Capillaries and their relationship to oxidative capacity. *Respir Physiol* 1987;69:47–64.

77. Hudlicka O, Hoppeler H, Uhlmann E. Relationship between the size of the capillary bed and oxidative capacity in various cat skeletal muscles. *Pflügers Arch* 1987;410:369–375.

78. Mathieu-Costello O. Capillary configuration in contracted muscles: comparative aspects. *Adv Exp Med Biol* 1988;227:229–236.

79. Banchero N. Cardiovascular responses to chronic hypoxia. *Annu Rev Physiol* 1987;49:465–476.

80. Jackson CGR, Sillau AH, Banchero N. Fiber composition and capillarity in growing guinea pigs acclimated to cold and cold plus hypoxia. *Proc Soc Exp Biol Med* 1987;185:101–106.

81. Appell H-J. Capillary density and patterns in skeletal muscle. III. Changes of the capillary pattern after hypoxia. *Pflügers Arch* 1978;377(Suppl):210.

82. Mathieu-Costello O. Muscle capillary tortuosity in high altitude mice depends on sarcomase length. *Resp Physiol* 1989;76:289–302.

83. Poole DC, Mathieu-Costello O. Skeletal muscle capillary geometry: adaptation to chronic hypoxia. *Resp Physiol* 1989;77:21–30.

84. Hudlicka O. Growth of capillaries in skeletal and cardiac muscle. *Circ Res* 1982;50:451–461.

85. Ward MP, Milledge JS, West JB. *High altitude medicine and physiology.* London: Chapman & Hall, 1989.

86. Mathieu-Costello O, Poole DC, Logemann RB. Muscle fiber size and chronic exposure to hypoxia. *Adv Exp Med Biol* 1989;248:305–311.

87. Saltin B, Gollnick PD. Skeletal muscle adaptability: Significance for metabolism and performance. In: Peachy LD, Adrian RH, Geigerleds SR, eds. *Handbook of physiology, Section O: Skeletal muscle.* Baltimore: Williams & Wilkins, 1983;555–631.

88. Dawson JM, Hudlicka O. The effect of long-term activity on the microvasculature of rat glycolytic skeletal muscle. *Int J Microcirc Clin Exp* 1989;8:53–69.

THE LUNG: Scientific Foundations
edited by R.G. Crystal, J.B. West et al.
Raven Press, Ltd., New York © 1991.

CHAPTER 5.5.2.2

Oxygen Transfer from Blood to Mitochondria

F. Kreuzer, Z. Turek, and L. Hoofd

One of the central tasks of the microcirculation is to deliver an adequate amount of O_2 to ensure a proper function of the terminal oxidase of the respiratory chain in the mitochondria. Thus, during steady state, the amount of O_2 released from the microvasculature must equal the amount of O_2 consumed by the mitochondria. This O_2 delivery or supply is so essential because more than 95% of the energy generated by the body normally originates via aerobic pathways, and so urgent because the entire O_2 store of the body would support resting needs for less than 5 min. In this chapter we describe the pathway of O_2 from its delivery by the microvasculature to its consumption in the mitochondria for skeletal and cardiac muscle. In view of the limited space available, the coverage has to be restricted to the essential points and the references must be condensed to the most central and recent papers, other references often being subsumed in citing review articles.

MICROVASCULAR ARCHITECTURE

Microvascular arrangement varies according to structure and function of an organ or tissue. Terminal arterioles empty directly into capillaries, which run parallel to the muscle fibers and often cross connect with one another, thus forming a network. Precapillary sphincters are the final smooth muscle cells guarding the entrance to the capillary network and functionally represent the local control site for blood flow into the exchange area (1). Microcirculation may be arranged in repeating modules or units consisting of approximately 15 capillaries supplied by a common arteriole. Capillary blood flow is intermittent while all or not all capillaries may be perfused at rest. There are no anatomic arteriovenous anastomoses but possibly preferential channels across large capillaries. The most important morphologic data for skeletal and cardiac muscles are summarized in Weibel (2) and Rakusan (3).

EXPERIMENTAL ASSESSMENT OF OXYGEN PARTIAL PRESSURE (P_{O_2}) OF STRIATED MUSCULAR TISSUE

The propagation of O_2 from the capillaries into the tissue must result in an O_2 field in the tissue. Silver (4), using his P_{O_2} microelectrode, mapped this field on and in rat cerebral cortex and found a P_{O_2} distribution as expected from the histologic electrode track in relation to the microvascular pattern. Numerous subsequent studies with various kinds of electrode, however, failed to provide such rather regular P_{O_2} profiles. When stepwise penetrating the tissue or measuring along the surface, usually very irregular P_{O_2} profiles are obtained. The various P_{O_2} values then are plotted as percentages of their frequencies, providing a P_{O_2} histogram or, when being summed up, a cumulative P_{O_2} histogram, indicating the range and the peak P_{O_2} values in the tissue (5,6). Figure 1 shows the P_{O_2} histograms of six organs including skeletal and cardiac muscles (6). Numerous other P_{O_2} histograms have been obtained with surface or needle P_{O_2} electrodes. The P_{O_2} profiles measured in tissue are the result of the interference of the P_{O_2} field in the tissue and the electrode diffusion field and are affected by the local consequences of pressure and impalement in the tissue (review of P_{O_2} electrodes in refs. 5, 7, and 8). Some representative P_{O_2} values, obtained with surface or needle microelectrodes, for skeletal and cardiac muscles are listed in Table 1. Knowledge of the order of magnitude of these "normal" normoxic P_{O_2} values will be im-

F. Kreuzer, Z. Turek, and L. Hoofd: Department of Physiology, University of Nijmegen, NL-6500 HB Nijmegen, The Netherlands.

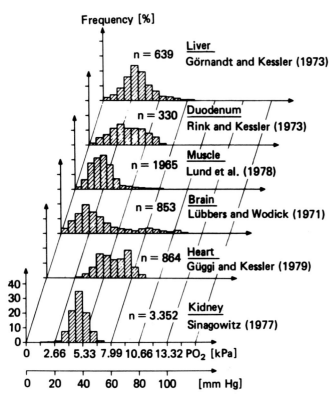

FIG. 1. P_{O_2} histograms in different organs. (From ref. 6.)

of the cylinder. The mathematical relationships developed by Krogh's mathematician Erlang and later by Kety (18) permit the calculation of the P_{O_2} field in this tissue (5,19). In spite of its oversimplifications (numerous assumptions; see ref. 20), the Krogh model remains a valuable approach to assess the general properties of O_2 transport. The most critical location in the tissue cylinder with respect to O_2 supply is at the periphery of the venous end of the cylinder (lethal corner). Scheid and Piiper (21) calculated the maximum P_{O_2} gradient from the artery to that point with a formula expressing this gradient as the sum of the diffusive and perfusive (convective) O_2 transfer resistances.

Effect of Axial Diffusion

Axial diffusion, which is neglected in the Krogh model, lowers the P_{O_2} in normoxic tissue, particularly at the arterial end of the cylinder, and increases it at the venous end; that is, it renders the axial gradient in the tissue somewhat less steep. This effect is minimized by increasing capillary flow velocity. It may be effective mostly in venous hypoxia due to the steepened axial gradient in this condition (review in ref. 20).

The Value of Krogh's O_2 Diffusion Coefficient K

The coefficient K is assumed homogeneous and isotropic in the Krogh model, although its effective value may be influenced by several factors and there must be local differences according to structure and components of the tissue. Homer et al. (22) found that O_2 diffuses twice as fast along muscle fibers as perpendicularly to the fiber axis. Ellsworth and Pittman (23) noted in hamster muscles a linear correlation between the physical O_2 diffusion coefficient D_{O_2} and the percentage of transverse cross-sectional area occupied by oxidative fibers. Popel et al. (24) noted in hamster retractor muscle that K of the arteriolar wall and tissue is 10 times higher in perfused than in unperfused tissue; that is, K is a function of the perfusion conditions and

portant for a subsequent evaluation of various models of O_2 transport in tissue.

MODELING APPROACH TO O_2 TRANSPORT TO TISSUE

The Krogh Model

Thinking about O_2 supply to tissues started long before a realistic experimental approach as described above became possible. The decisive breakthrough for a theoretical approach is due to Krogh (17) with his model of a tissue cylinder around a central capillary running parallel to resting muscle fibers (centrifugal divergent model), assuming no O_2 flux at the periphery

TABLE 1. Experimental striated muscle tissue P_{O_2} (in torr) obtained from P_{O_2} electrode measurements

	Heart			Skeletal muscle			
				Resting		Working	
Method	Range		Mean	Range	Mean	Range	Mean
Surface P_{O_2} electrodes	20–70 (6)			2–65 (12)	16–39 (12)	20–45 (14)	28 (14)
	35–55 (9)		45.1 (9)				
Needle P_{O_2} microelectrodes	0–90 (10)	Peak	15–20 (10)	0–110 (13)	20–39 (13)	15–30 (15)	
	0–13 (11)		6.9 (11)				
P_{O_2} from cryomicrospectroscopic MbO_2 (for comparison)	1.5–10 (16)	Median	5 (16)			1.3–11.4 (16)	

might be a regulated variable. Due to this high K, intracapillary resistance would become dominant and the rate of loss of O_2 from arterioles should be 10 times larger than expected.

Effect of Facilitated O_2 Diffusion

The possible physiological significance of O_2 diffusion facilitated by hemoglobin (Hb) or myoglobin (Mb) has been reviewed recently by Kreuzer and Hoofd (25). Oxymyoglobin (MbO$_2$) diffusion in muscle flattens both axial and radial Po$_2$ profiles; that is, it raises tissue Po$_2$ particularly at the venous end of the capillary and at the periphery of the tissue cylinder.

Resistance of Capillary Wall and Red Blood Cell (RBC) Membrane

It is widely accepted that these two membranes do not offer any extra resistance to O_2 diffusion (for RBC membrane see ref. 26). The capillary wall accordingly is mostly included in the tissue mass and RBC membrane in the RBC interior.

The Determinants of Tissue Po$_2$

Kety (18) and Rakusan (3) examined how the determinants of O_2 supply to tissue affect tissue Po$_2$ in the Krogh model when they are manipulated independently. In Fig. 2 (3), the steep course of oxygen consumption M, blood flow F, and arterial oxygen concentration C shows a strong effect on Po$_2$. Krogh radius R becomes important when it increases, whereas capillary radius r and K become influential only when they decrease to very low values.

The Hill and Solid Cylinder Models

Whereas the centrifugal divergent Krogh model deals with a tissue cylinder around a single capillary, in the centripetal convergent models the O_2 is supplied to a solid cylinder from a homogeneous peripheral sheet of blood (27) or, more realistically, from a certain number of peripheral capillaries (solid cylinder model). In comparison with the Krogh model, the Hill model provides higher Po$_2$ values in all radial positions. Rakusan et al. (28) compared the Krogh model with various symmetric solid cylinders and found that the Po$_2$ profiles were similar. Groom et al. (29) suggested that for the maximally contracted muscle the Hill model would be more applicable as a dense network of folded capillaries around the individual muscle fibers forms an almost continuous layer of blood around the muscle fibers.

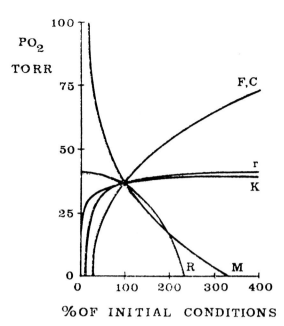

FIG. 2. Changes in myocardial oxygen pressure as a result of changes in individual oxygen determinants. M, myocardial O_2 consumption; F, myocardial blood flow; C, arterial O_2 concentration; R, tissue cylinder radius; r, capillary radius; K, Krogh's O_2 diffusion coefficient. (From ref. 3.)

Piiper and Scheid (30) compared the Krogh and solid cylinder models and found that the differences indeed largely reside in the respective geometries (circumferences and cumulative cross-sectional areas). The radial Po$_2$ profiles are steeper close to the capillary and flatten only with larger distance from the capillary in the Krogh model. The Krogh model as one extreme situation passes into the solid cylinder model as the number of capillaries and the capillary-to-fiber ratio increase. These authors did not include axial diffusion, diffusive interaction, and heterogeneity of various factors in their analysis.

All these models agree in that they assume an idealized (cylindrical) geometry and, with the exception of the original Hill model, the origination of O_2 from uniform sources, the capillaries. However, whereas in the Krogh cylinder mostly a single cylinder and capillary are considered (presuming homogeneity), the solid cylinder model admits the possibility of a differing number, distribution, and nature of capillaries (including interactions).

A Direct Empirical Approach

In view of the constraints (including a great number of assumptions; see ref. 12) in these idealized models, it may be preferable to adopt an approach that starts from the actual capillary locations and their respective supply areas. These cannot be circular as can be seen from the method of capillary domains developed by Hoofd et al. (31); such domains, geographic areas around the capillaries, cover the entire tissue surface area of a histologic section, resulting in irregular polygonal areas. When modeling such irregular areas as ellipsoidal O_2 supply regions, deviations from the Krogh model were marked (32). A whole histologic section covering several capillaries was modeled recently by superposition of source terms (33,34), taking into account the actual capillary locations. This method also permits calculation of the actual capillary O_2 supply areas, which coincide with the morphologic domains remarkably well for identical capillary P_{O_2} (34).

O_2 Diffusion Versus O_2 Supply

We have seen above that the P_{O_2} gradient from capillary blood to tissue depends on the sum of diffusive and perfusive resistances to O_2 transport. The question is which of these two resistances is mainly limiting. The Krogh and Hill models stipulate a limitation by diffusion. Cain (35), however, comparing anemic and hypoxic hypoxia in the dog, concluded that M was not limited by diffusion but by O_2 supply ($= Ca_{O_2} \times$ flow, where Ca_{O_2} is the arterial oxygen concentration) and that therefore the validity of mixed venous oxygen pressure $P\bar{v}_{O_2}$ as a measure of tissue O_2 supply is open to question.

According to Schumacker and Samsel (36), the Krogh model fails to fully predict O_2 supply dependency due to its basic limitations or assumptions. The $\dot{D}$/M relationship, where $\dot{D}$ is the oxygen delivery, was similar for anemic, hypoxic, and stagnant hypoxia as long as the intercapillary distance (ICD) was below 80 μm, but O_2 extraction was unrealistically high. This high O_2 extraction in the Krogh model may be due to assuming homogeneity of tissue and could be made realistic when assuming an O_2 shunt of 30%. With ICD above 80 μm, realistic O_2 extractions were predicted but now the critical point was higher for hypoxic hypoxia, indicating an effect of diffusion at large distance but leaving the overall decision between O_2 supply and diffusion limitation open.

Gutierrez et al. (37) found in experiments with low versus high flow in the rabbit hindlimb preparation perfused with blood that M is primarily limited by diffusion during hypoxemia and therefore venous oxygen pressure (Pv_{O_2}) is an accurate reflection of capillary oxygen pressure (Pc_{O_2}), thus supporting the Krogh diffusion theory of capillary exchange. This was confirmed by Hogan et al. (38) in isolated canine gastrocnemius muscle *in situ*, where M for maximal contraction was linearly related to Pv_{O_2} when Pc_{O_2} was

decreased in arterial hypoxemia. When comparing low flow–high Ca_{O_2} and high flow–low Ca_{O_2} at the same O_2 supply, the ratio M/Pv_{O_2} and thus tissue O_2 conductance (M/Pc_{O_2}; first law of Fick) are similar in these two conditions, while M is higher with low flow–high Ca_{O_2}; this confirms that normoxic maximal M is limited by O_2 diffusion in the peripheral tissue. It is, however, impossible to ascertain the location of this diffusive resistance from these experiments.

An Alternative Experimental Concept

Honig et al. (39) measured local MbO_2 saturation by cryomicrospectroscopy in maximally contracting dog gracilis muscle and deduced the corresponding P_{O_2} values from the MbO_2 dissociation curve; their measurements with a spatial resolution of 4 μm covered the intracellular regions beyond a distance of 3–5 μm from the capillary. In this and much subsequent work, this group found that intracellular P_{O_2} was only a few torr and evenly distributed, which they ascribed to Mb-facilitated O_2 diffusion; an apparent Km (P_{O_2} for half-maximal O_2 consumption) of 0.06 torr was similar to that in mitochondrial suspensions, and the perimitochondrial O_2 gradient was very low. There are no radial or axial tissue P_{O_2} gradients and therefore there is no lethal corner; that is, the tissue is "well stirred," tissue P_{O_2} is much lower than Pv_{O_2}, and the main P_{O_2} gradient occurs at the capillary level.

The same basic view was expressed by Groebe and Thews (40), Federspiel (41), and Wittenberg and Wittenberg (42) but contrasted with that of Jones (43), who ascribed intracellular O_2 gradients in myocytes to clustering of mitochondria with high O_2 consumption and an unstirred layer around the cells, while refuting any role of Mb-facilitated O_2 diffusion (44). Tamura et al. (45) showed that the curve of a plot of oxidized cytochrome aa_3 versus % MbO_2 ("coherence diagram") moves to the right (higher half-maximum value) as M increases. The corresponding P_{O_2} gradient between cytosol and mitochondria ("gradient coherence") therefore also increases with M from small values at low M to more than 10 torr at high M. Isolated cardiac myocytes may have a low M, whereas intact tissue is apt to have a higher M. Thus, discrepant results may be due to different viability of the *in vitro* cell preparations, and isolated cells are not identical to intact tissue where, furthermore, M can vary according to the state of activity.

Honig and his group suggested the following possible reasons for their O_2 diffusion barrier at the capillary level: (a) a 1-μm layer of deoxygenation nonequilibrium underneath the RBC membrane, resulting in a decreased O_2 release; (b) the layer of plasma–endothelium–interstitium with high flux density and no facilitation by hemoglobin; (c) a high O_2 flux density across the capillaries as against a low O_2 flux density across the mitochondria according to the differing respective surface areas (1:200); this argument, however, holds for all models; (d) short RBC transit time at exercise, leading to incomplete equilibration, decreased axial decline of capillary Po_2, and O_2 shunting (increased venous Po_2); (e) several aspects of a possible role of the RBC in creating an O_2 diffusion resistance at the capillary level have been considered by various authors (see ref. 46).

There is a striking difference between the cumulative myocardial Po_2 histograms obtained experimentally from Po_2 electrode studies and those derived by Honig's group. Turek et al. (47) tried to find the changes in various factors necessary to approach the Po_2 histograms of Honig and Gayeski (16) and found that manipulation of the input data is able to provide Po_2 profiles or Po_2 histograms more similar to either of these. One interesting finding was that inclusion of Michaelis–Menten kinetics of M (not considered by Honig's group) seems to be more apt to approach the flat Po_2 profiles measured by this group than does Mb-facilitated O_2 diffusion (being a central factor there).

Possible Effects of Stirring in Blood and Tissue

Stirring in plasma and of the RBC contents as well as in tissue might greatly enhance O_2 transport but no quantitative data amenable to a realistic estimation of these effects are available (25,48,49).

CAPILLARY DISTRIBUTION AND FLOW

Capillary Distribution

That precapillary O_2 loss is possible has been shown repeatedly but its estimates vary widely and are controversial so that it will not be considered further here.

Practically all variables in muscle may be heterogeneously distributed: $ICD = 2R = (CD)^{-1/2}$ (where CD is the capillary density), capillary length and diameter, blood flow, transit time, M, and oxyhemoglobin (HbO_2) and MbO_2 saturations and their respective Po_2 values.

Apart from technical, geometric, and histologic problems, counting capillaries to obtain CD is subject to at least two more problems: (a) open versus closed or functional versus nonfunctional capillaries; capillaries with or without RBC or with moving versus stationary RBC (50); (b) capillary length, cross section, and volume are neglected when simply counting capillaries.

Capillary density is, when considering only the open capillaries, a particularly important determinant of tissue Po_2 because R occurs squared in the Krogh–Erlang

equation. However, R is really important only where it increases (Fig. 2). There is a distinct effect of the capillary-to-fiber ratio on tissue Po_2 only when it increases from 1 to 2 (normal range in skeletal muscle); an increase of capillary-to-fiber ratio above 2 has a minimal effect (51). Thus, it may not be surprising that there is no agreement concerning a possible increase and effect of CD in hypoxia and exercise.

Capillary density may increase toward the venous side of the capillary, thus shortening R in the region where Pc_{O_2} is lowest. The Krogh cylinder therefore should be tapering toward the venule in the form of a cone (2,52).

Turek and Rakusan (53) showed that increased heterogeneity of R lowers mean tissue Po_2 (particularly at normoxia) and increases the percentage of anoxic tissue (particularly at hypoxia). The effects of heterogeneity can be compensated for by adaptation of local blood flow to local M, that is, by a more uniform ratio of these two variables (54). In the presence of an unequal distribution of the local capillary-to-fiber ratio, the ensuing interaction between capillaries can decrease the heterogeneity of tissue O_2 supply (55).

Mitochondrial Distribution

Muscular mitochondria occur preferentially subsarcolemmal and interfibrillar (56). Their density decreases with increasing distance from the capillary, rendering the Po_2 profile flatter and penetrating deeper into the cell (2). CD in general correlates well with mitochondrial density and M, an important adjustment since the Po_2 gradient in the tissue is proportional to M according to the Krogh–Erlang equation (49). Capillary length and blood volume are proportional to the O_2 flux necessary for maximal M (2).

Mainwood and Rakusan (57) showed that when the mitochondria are clustered around the capillaries, R shrinks from the anatomic value to that of the cluster and the required Po_2 gradient decreases accordingly. On the other hand, Jones (58) found that mitochondrial clustering results in a marked decrease of O_2 permeability.

Capillary Flow

The Krogh model assumes straight, parallel, and concurrent capillaries. Reeves and Rakusan (59) found 95% of cardiac capillaries to have concurrent flow. A number of alternative geometries have been proposed (reviews in refs. 20, 60, and 61). Countercurrent flow results in conical tissue regions. Countercurrent or asymmetric exchange may be most favorable, but the differences between various models in terms of tissue Po_2 are often surprisingly small or contradictory. The expected arteriovenous O_2 diffusion shunting with countercurrent flow has been found to be minor or negligible (62). If present (63), the concomitant veno-arterial back diffusion of CO_2 with resulting drop in pH may increase Pa_{O_2} (Bohr effect) particularly in hypoxia; in hyperoxia, Pa_{O_2} would be decreased by the O_2 diffusion shunt (64).

A large fraction of the total number of capillaries is perfused in resting skeletal muscle and blood flow rates in individual capillaries are very inhomogeneous (50,65) and often intermittent. This allows for a capillary reserve where the distribution of blood flow becomes a regulatory factor to maintain tissue P_{O_2} over a wide range of changes in O_2 supply and/or M (66).

Piiper et al. (67) noted that resting skeletal muscle perfusion inhomogeneity was even increased during contraction and relaxation; Renkin (68) and Tyml (69), however, found all capillaries open and a decreased flow heterogeneity during exercise. Duling (70) pointed out that heterogeneity during exercise may decrease, or increase at very high work load. Ellsworth et al. (71) noted a marked effect of heterogeneity on O_2 supply also with increased flow and high M. On the other hand, local flow heterogeneity in O_2 supply may be reduced due to intercapillary exchange, particularly with high flow (72).

Capillary Transit Time and O_2 Shunting

Whereas heterogeneous capillary spacing leads to variable radii of the tissue cylinders, variability of capillary transit time results in differing P_{O_2} patterns in various tissue cylinders. Capillaries with very long transit time imply almost stagnant blood with fast exhaustion of its O_2; capillaries with very short transit time lead to O_2 shunting. There must be an optimal transit time somewhere in between these extremes. Sarelius (73) observed that mean flow pathlength in different networks is twice anatomic capillary length; that is, actual transit time is longer than expected from anatomic measurements.

Gutierrez (74) suggested that nonequilibrium O_2 release from capillaries might lead to a Pv_{O_2} greater than Pc'_{O_2} (end-capillary P_{O_2}), that is, to functional arteriovenous O_2 shunting in hypoxic and anemic hypoxia. However, the effect of nonequilibrium becomes noticeable only when transit time is shorter than 0.5 sec (36). It seems that mean transit time is considerably longer than mean O_2 release time even with maximal muscular exercise. Gutierrez et al. (75) found Pv_{O_2} to be higher than tissue P_{O_2} in rabbit gracilis muscle when Pa_{O_2} was below 52 torr, possibly due to P_{O_2} gradients from RBC to tissue cells.

Capillary Hematocrit

The role of the capillary hematocrit in gas exchange remains poorly understood, also because practically nothing is known about the capillary hematocrit in resting and working muscles. It is generally accepted, however, that capillary hematocrit bears little relation to arterial hematocrit and is certainly much lower (down to 10%). It fluctuates in parallel with M and the contractile state of the arterioles, which suggests that it is a controlled variable in the regulation of tissue oxygenation (76). A decreased capillary hematocrit elicits a steeper P_{O_2} gradient along the capillary (77). Enhanced RBC spacing leads to decreased plasma P_{O_2}, which might limit O_2 transfer (78), but this does not seem to play an important role for tissue O_2 supply (79). Preferential flow channels with increased hematocrit and flow in skeletal muscle (to compensate for low capillary hematocrit) might result in functional arteriovenous O_2 shunting and in a higher Pv_{O_2} (80).

Venous P_{O_2} Versus Tissue P_{O_2}

Tenney (81) calculated that there is close agreement between venous P_{O_2} and mean tissue P_{O_2} for normal resting conditions but there are significant deviations when CD (82), M, Hb concentration, and cardiac output are altered. An appropriate increase in CD results in a venous P_{O_2} again being a good approximation of mean tissue P_{O_2} even in conditions deviating from normal resting condition. Misleadingly high venous P_{O_2} values occur particularly in the presence of functional arteriovenous O_2 shunting due to countercurrent flow, too short transit time or preferential flow channels, or to shock (83).

Capillary Regulation

There seems to be a common regulatory mechanism for functional hyperemia, hypoxic vasodilation, flow autoregulation, reactive hyperemia after vascular occlusion, and regulation of CD in skeletal muscle (84). The arterioles, innervated by the sympathetic nervous system, control the resistance and thus the flow, whereas the functional precapillary sphincters metabolically regulate the exchange by the capillaries, with a feedback from the more sensitive precapillary sphincters to the arterioles. The decreased P_{O_2} acts directly or indirectly by vasodilating metabolites on the smooth muscles of the sphincters. ICD decreases or CD increases in a linear fashion as Pa_{O_2} decreases from 120 to 20 torr. This autoregulation may be a self-protection against anoxia in the tissue (85). Capillary recruitment is due to increased RBC velocity and a more homogeneous flow rather than to opening of unperfused capillaries (86), and to a denser RBC spacing and pathlength recruitment. It leads to (a) decreased diffusion distance or increased interaction between diffusion fields; (b) decreased linear blood velocity due to increased total capillary surface area with increased transit time; (c) often decreased heterogeneity of CD and transit times with removal of the longest diffusion pathways and of the shortest and longest transit times (prevention of O_2 shunting and excessive O_2 extraction, respectively); and (d) an increased transcapillary O_2 conductance (85).

CAPILLARY BLOOD

Effect of Chemical Reactions Between Hb and O_2

Some authors found a moderate influence of a slowed release of O_2 from Hb on plasma or tissue Po_2 (see ref. 49). Increase in M enhances the Po_2 gradient between RBC and plasma (87). Other workers concluded that the contribution of chemical reactions is minor (88); O_2 diffusion within the RBC mainly is rate limiting for O_2 transfer.

Effect of O_2 Dissociation Curve

Turek et al. (89) have shown that the effect of a shift of the oxygen dissociation curve (ODC) depends on the level of oxygenation. High P_{50} (Po_2 for 50% saturation) increases and low P_{50} decreases Pv_{O_2} in normoxia and mild hypoxia, whereas the opposite holds in severe hypoxia. It is the local steepness of the ODC that determines this difference. A P_{50} inadequate for a particular oxygenation level can be compensated for by an increase in blood flow (90). The effect of a shift of the ODC on tissue oxygenation has been confirmed in many studies, though not always, but the effect of moderate shifts may often be of questionable practical significance (36,91). At normoxia, an increase in P_{50} (e.g., due to the Bohr effect) makes the capillary blood maintain a higher Po_2 toward the venous end of the capillary and renders the axial Po_2 profile flatter after the first third of capillary length (2).

OXYGEN CONSUMPTION

Critical Po_2 and Apparent Km

One of the many assumptions of the Krogh model is that M is of zero-order kinetics, that is, independent of Po_2 throughout. It is generally accepted that Km is very low in well-stirred mitochondrial suspensions (order of 0.05 torr). Longmuir (92) showed that M of cells depends on Po_2 up to considerably higher values

than expected from zero-order kinetics; he ascribed this to intracellular diffusion resistance. Liver slices *in vitro* follow Michaelis–Menten kinetics rather than zero-order kinetics (93), Km being about 100 times higher than in mitochondrial suspensions (94). Thus, one has to distinguish between "true" mitochondrial Km and "apparent" Km in tissues. The notion of an apparent Km is well established in the kinetics of immobilized enzymes, which are analogous to the situation of the enzymes in the mitochondria (e.g., ref. 95).

Wilson et al. (96) found that mitochondrial oxidative phosphorylation depends on Po_2 over the entire physiologic range of Po_2 but metabolic adjustments ensure a constant adenosine triphosphate (ATP) synthesis and M with decreasing Po_2; that is, there are no critical Po_2, no difference between isolated mitochondria and intact cells (97), and thus no appreciable effect of O_2 gradients. O_2 diffusion limitation of M is to be expected only in extreme O_2 lack. But since Km is linearly related to maximal oxygen consumption Mmax, O_2 dependency of M can be used to quantify the Po_2 gradient between mitochondria and extracellular medium (98).

Physiologic O_2 Supply Dependency

Isolated small muscles and muscle slices *in vitro* show O_2 supply dependency, presumably due to subcritical Po_2 values in the core (99). For a muscle *in situ*, Stainsby and Otis (100) found the same in the absence of flow autoregulation but a supercritical plateau with flow autoregulation. Autoregulation is very sensitive to experimental manipulations (101), which may explain some discrepant results. Autoregulation leads to redistribution of capillary blood flow to achieve a homogeneous local M/F or D/M and thus a more uniform tissue Po_2. Physiologic O_2 supply dependency means a condition where M increases with O_2 supply below a low critical threshold and there is a horizontal plateau above that critical threshold; the subcritical slope indicates optimal O_2 extraction (102,103). Decreases in O_2 supply do not lower M in the plateau region because O_2 extraction increases proportionately. However, when O_2 supply is reduced below the critical threshold, M falls because O_2 extraction no longer increases proportionately and thus cannot compensate for the reduction in O_2 supply (Fig. 3) (104).

Pathologic O_2 Supply Dependency

Powers et al. (105) found O_2 supply dependency of M over a wide range of O_2 supplies in adult respiratory distress syndrome (ARDS) patients during positive end-expiratory pressure (PEEP) and O_2 breathing. Pathologic O_2 supply dependency is characterized by a lower subcritical slope, a higher critical O_2 supply,

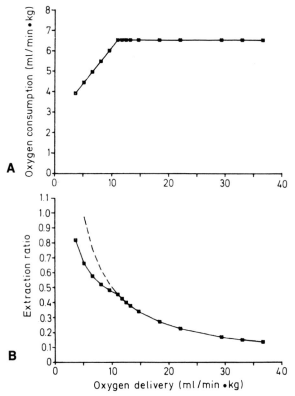

FIG. 3. Whole body O_2 consumption **(A)** and O_2 extraction ratio **(B)** versus O_2 delivery. Whole body O_2 consumption remains virtually constant at normal or high delivery but becomes limited by O_2 delivery below a critical threshold. O_2 extraction ratio increases asymptotically as delivery is reduced, until the critical extraction ratio is reached. When delivery is reduced further, extraction does not increase proportionally although further increases may occur. *Dashed line* in **B** shows the increase in extraction necessary to maintain O_2 consumption. (From ref. 104.)

a higher supercritical plateau (which may be slightly sloping) (106), or no plateau at all. The lower slope indicates a deficiency in O_2 extraction from the blood with ensuing increase in mixed-venous P_{O_2}. The underlying mechanisms for this deficiency are vascular microembolization, disruption of endothelial function resulting in a protein-rich permeability edema, and microvascular dysregulation by loss of autoregulation. Its consequences are a decrease in capillary reserve, an increase in capillary distances (loss of open capillaries and edema), a massive increase in heterogeneity of capillary distribution and flow, and an increase in capillary shunts. All this results in a derangement of the microvascular adaptability and in an impaired O_2 extraction from the blood with a consequent deficiency of O_2 supply to the tissue.

GENERAL CONCLUSION

Experimental determinations of tissue P_{O_2} are afflicted by great scattering of the results and remain contro-

versial among various investigators. Modeling attempts have led to divergent conclusions that are difficult to reconcile and sometimes deviate greatly from experimental results. A systematic comparison between experiments and modeling is still lacking (see also ref. 107). There remains much disagreement concerning the effects of the serial resistances to O_2 transport from the RBC to the mitochondria, in particular whether the main resistance resides at the capillary level or in the tissue. Although many single aspects of this problem have been investigated, there remains the need for an integrative concept that preferably should be based on the actual experimental situation and hopefully may provide a general total frame for modeling.

ACKNOWLEDGMENTS

The authors wish to thank Dr. K. Rakusan for valuable comments, B. E. M. Ringnalda and J. Evers for help in preparing the list of references, and A. Minke for typing the manuscript.

REFERENCES

1. Wiedeman MP. Architecture. In: *Handbook of physiology*, sec 2: *The cardiovascular system*, vol IV: *Microcirculation*, part 1. Bethesda: American Physiological Society, 1984;11–40.
2. Weibel ER. *The pathway of oxygen.* Cambridge MA: Harvard University Press, 1984.
3. Rakusan K. *Oxygen in the heart muscle.* Springfield IL: Charles C Thomas, 1971.
4. Silver IA. Some observations on the cerebral cortex with an ultramicro, membrane-covered, oxygen electrode. *Med Electron Biol Eng* 1965;3:377–387.
5. Lübbers DW. Exchange processes in the microcirculatory bed. In: Meessen H, ed. *Handbuch der allgemeinen Pathologie* III/7, *Mikrozirkulation.* Berlin: Springer-Verlag, 1977;411–476.
6. Kessler M, Höper J, Pohl U. Monitoring of local P_{O_2} in skeletal muscle of critically ill patients. In: Berk JL, ed. *Handbook of critical care*, 2nd ed. Boston: Little, Brown & Co, 1982;599–609.
7. Kreuzer F, Kimmich HP, Brezina M. Polarographic determination of oxygen in biological materials. In: Koryta J, ed. *Medical and biological applications of electrochemical devices.* London: Wiley, 1980;173–261.
8. Kreuzer F, Kimmich HP. Techniques using O_2 electrodes in respiratory physiology. In: Otis AB, ed. *Techniques in respiratory physiology*—part 1, P406. County Clare, Ireland: Elsevier Scientific Publishers Ireland Ltd, 1984;1–29.
9. Kessler M, Höper J. Signaloxidasen, Signalketten in Leber, Niere und Myokard. In: Kinne R, Acker H, Leniger-Follert E, eds. *Festschrift aus Anlass der Emeritierung von Prof. Dr. D. W. Lübbers*, Dortmund: Max Planck Institute for System Physiology, 1985;121–155.
10. Schuchhardt S. Myocardial oxygen pressure: mirror of oxygen supply. *Adv Exp Med Biol* 1985;191:21–35.
11. Whalen WJ, Nair P, Buerk D. Oxygen tension in the beating cat heart in situ. In: Kessler M, Bruley DF, Clark LC Jr, Lübbers DW, Silver IA, Strauss J, eds. *Oxygen supply.* Munich: Urban und Schwarzenberg, 1973;199–201.
12. Ehrly AM, ed. *Determination of tissue oxygen pressure in patients.* Oxford: Pergamon Press, 1983.
13. Lund N. Skeletal and cardiac muscle oxygenation. *Adv Exp Med Biol* 1985;191:37–43.
14. Boekstegers P, Heinrich R, Günderoth-Palmowski M, Grauer

W, Fleckenstein W, Schomerus H. Tissue P_{O_2} in isometrically contracting skeletal muscle of rats with portocaval anastomosis (PCA). *Adv Exp Med Biol* 1986;200:429–437.

15. Lash JM, Bohlen HG. Perivascular and tissue P_{O_2} in contracting rat spinotrapezius muscle. *Am J Physiol* 1987;252:H1192–H1202.

16. Honig CR, Gayeski TEJ. Comparison of intracellular P_{O_2} and conditions for blood–tissue O_2 transport in heart and working red skeletal muscle. *Adv Exp Med Biol* 1987;215:309–321.

17. Krogh A. The number and distribution of capillaries in muscles with calculations of the oxygen pressure head necessary for supplying the tissue. *J Physiol* 1919;52:409–415.

18. Kety SS. Determinants of tissue oxygen tension. *Fed Proc* 1957;16:666–670.

19. Opitz E, Schneider M. Über die Sauerstoffversorgung des Gehirns und den Mechanismus von Mangelwirkungen. *Ergeb Physiol* 1950;46:126–260.

20. Kreuzer F. Oxygen supply to tissues: the Krogh model and its assumptions. *Experientia* 1982;38:1415–1426.

21. Scheid P, Piiper J. Oxygen exchange at external and internal surfaces. In: Jones DR, Satchel GH, eds. *Oxygen: physiological adjustments to changes in its supply and demand*, vol 3, Queenstown NZ: Physiology Society of New Zealand, 1983;57–65.

22. Homer LD, Shelton JB, Dorsey CH, Williams TJ. Anisotropic diffusion of oxygen in slices of rat muscle. *Am J Physiol* 1984;246:R107–R113.

23. Ellsworth ML, Pittman RN. Heterogeneity of oxygen diffusion through hamster striated muscle. *Am J Physiol* 1984;246:H161–H167.

24. Popel AS, Pittman RN, Ellsworth ML. Rate of oxygen loss from arterioles is an order of magnitude higher than expected. *Am J Physiol* 1989;256:H921–H924.

25. Kreuzer F, Hoofd L. Facilitated diffusion of oxygen and carbon dioxide. In: Farhi LE, Tenney SM, eds. *Handbook of physiology—the respiratory system IV*. Bethesda: American Physiological Society, 1987;89–111.

26. Kreuzer F, Yahr WZ. Influence of red cell membrane on diffusion of oxygen. *J Appl Physiol* 1960;15:1117–1122.

27. Hill AV. The diffusion of oxygen and lactic acid through tissues. *Proc R Soc Lond [Biol]* 1928;104:39–96.

28. Rakusan K, Hoofd L, Turek Z. The effect of cell size and capillary spacing on myocardial oxygen supply. *Adv Exp Med Biol* 1984;180:463–475.

29. Groom AC, Ellis CG, Potter RF. Microvascular architecture and red cell perfusion in skeletal muscle. In: Hammersen F, Messmer K, eds. *Progress in applied microcirculation*, vol 5. Basel: Karger, 1984;64–83.

30. Piiper J, Scheid P. Cross-sectional P_{O_2} distribution in Krogh cylinder and solid cylinder models. *Respir Physiol* 1986;64:241–251.

31. Hoofd L, Turek Z, Kubat K, Ringnalda BEM, Kazda S. Variability of intercapillary distance estimated on histological sections of rat heart. *Adv Exp Med Biol* 1985;191:239–247.

32. Turek Z, Hoofd L, Rakusan K. Myocardial capillaries and tissue oxygenation. *Can J Cardiol* 1986;2:98–103.

33. Clark PA, Kennedy SP, Clark A Jr. Buffering of muscle tissue P_{O_2} levels by the superposition of the oxygen field from many capillaries. *Adv Exp Med Biol* 1989;248:165–174.

34. Hoofd L, Turek Z, Olders J. Calculation of oxygen pressures and fluxes in a flat plane perpendicular to any capillary distribution. *Adv Exp Med Biol* 1989;248:187–196.

35. Cain SM. Oxygen delivery and uptake in dogs during anemic and hypoxic hypoxia. *J Appl Physiol* 1977;42:228–234.

36. Schumacker PT, Samsel RW. Analysis of oxygen delivery and uptake relationships in the Krogh tissue model. *J Appl Physiol* 1989;67:1234–1244.

37. Gutierrez G, Pohil RJ, Strong R. Effect of flow on O_2 consumption during progressive hypoxemia. *J Appl Physiol* 1988;65:601–607.

38. Hogan MC, Roca J, West JB, Wagner PD. Dissociation of maximal O_2 uptake from O_2 delivery in canine gastrocnemius in situ. *J Appl Physiol* 1989;66:1219–1226.

39. Honig CR, Gayeski TEJ, Federspiel W, Clark A Jr, Clark P. Muscle P_{O_2} gradients from hemoglobin to cytochrome: new

concepts, new complexities. *Adv Exp Med Biol* 1984;169:23–38.

40. Groebe K, Thews G. Theoretical analysis of oxygen supply to contracted skeletal muscle. *Adv Exp Med Biol* 1986;200:495–514.

41. Federspiel WJ. A model study of intracellular oxygen gradients in a myoglobin-containing skeletal muscle fiber. *Biophys J* 1986;49:857–868.

42. Wittenberg BA, Wittenberg JB. Transport of oxygen in muscle. *Annu Rev Physiol* 1989;51:857–878.

43. Jones DP. Intracellular diffusion gradients of O_2 and ATP. *Am J Physiol* 1986;250:C663–C675.

44. Jones DP, Kennedy FG. Intracellular O_2 gradients in cardiac myocytes. Lack of a role for myoglobin in facilitation of intracellular O_2 diffusion. *Biochem Biophys Res Commun* 1982;105:419–424.

45. Tamura M, Hazeki O, Nioka S, Chance B. *In vivo* study of tissue oxygen metabolism using optical and nuclear magnetic resonance spectroscopies. *Annu Rev Physiol* 1989;51:813–834.

46. Kreuzer F. Critical oxygen supply to striated muscle: influence of various factors. In: Frank K, Kessler M, Harrison DK, eds. *Quantitative spectroscopy in tissue*. Berlin: Springer-Verlag, 1989; in press.

47. Turek Z, Olders J, Hoofd L, Egginton S, Kreuzer F, Rakusan K. P_{O_2} histograms in various models of tissue oxygenation in skeletal muscle. *Adv Exp Med Biol* 1989;248:227–237.

48. Hudson JA, Cater DB. An analysis of factors affecting tissue oxygen tension. *Proc R Soc Lond [Biol]* 1964;161:247–274.

49. Tenney SM. Tissue oxygenation. *Curr Pulm* 1987;8:299–327.

50. Damon DH, Duling BR. Distribution of capillary blood flow in the microcirculation of the hamster: an *in vivo* study using epifluorescent microscopy. *Microvasc Res* 1984;27:81–95.

51. Snyder GK. Model analysis of capillary growth and tissue oxygenation during hypoxia. *J Appl Physiol* 1988;65:2332–2336.

52. Batra S, Kuo C, Rakusan K. Spatial distribution of coronary capillaries: a–v segment staggering. *Adv Exp Med Biol* 1989;248:241–247.

53. Turek Z, Rakusan K. Lognormal distribution of intercapillary distance in normal and hypertrophic rat heart as estimated by the method of concentric circles: its effect on tissue oxygenation. *Pflügers Arch* 1981;391:17–21.

54. Rakusan K, Turek Z. The effect of heterogeneity of capillary spacing and O_2 consumption–blood flow mismatching on myocardial oxygenation. *Adv Exp Med Biol* 1985;191:257–262.

55. Egginton S, Turek Z, Hoofd L. Differing patterns of capillary distribution in fish and mammalian skeletal muscle. *Respir Physiol* 1988;74:383–396.

56. Romanul FCA. Capillary supply and metabolism of muscle fibers. *Arch Neurol* 1965;12:497–509.

57. Mainwood GW, Rakusan K. A model for intracellular energy transport. *Can J Physiol Pharmacol* 1982;60:98–102.

58. Jones DP. Effect of mitochondrial clustering on O_2 supply in hepatocytes. *Am J Physiol* 1984;247:C83–C89.

59. Reeves WJ, Rakusan K. Myocardial capillary flow pattern as determined by the method of coloured microspheres. *Adv Exp Med Biol* 1988;222:447–454.

60. Leonard EF, Jørgensen SB. The analysis of convection and diffusion in capillary beds. *Annu Rev Biophys Bioeng* 1974;3:293–339.

61. Acker H. Tissue oxygen transport in health and disease. In: Pallot DJ, ed. *Control of respiration*. London: Croom Helm Ltd., 1983;157–202.

62. Beek JHGM van, Elzinga G. Diffusional shunting of oxygen in saline-perfused isolated rabbit heart is negligible. *Pflügers Arch* 1987;410:263–271.

63. Harris PD. Movement of oxygen in skeletal muscle. *NIPS* 1986;1:147–149.

64. Kobayashi H, Pelster B, Piiper J, Scheid P. Significance of the Bohr effect for tissue oxygenation in a model with countercurrent blood flow. *Respir Physiol* 1989;76:277–288.

65. Renkin EM, Gray SD, Dodd LR, Lia BD. Heterogeneity of capillary distribution and capillary circulation in mammalian skeletal muscle. In: Bachrach AJ, Matzen MM, eds. *Underwater physiology VII*. Bethesda: Undersea Medical Society, 1981.

66. Granger JH, Goodman AH, Granger DN. Role of resistance

and exchange vessels in local microvascular control of skeletal muscle oxygenation in the dog. *Circ Res* 1976;38:379–385.

67. Piiper J, Pendergast DR, Marconi C, Meyer M, Heisler N, Cerretelli P. Blood flow distribution in dog gastrocnemius muscle at rest and during stimulation. *J Appl Physiol* 1985;58:2068–2074.

68. Renkin EM. Control of microcirculation and blood–tissue exchange. In: *Handbook of physiology*, sec 2: *The cardiovascular system*, vol IV: *Microcirculation*, part 1. Bethesda: American Physiological Society, 1984;627–687.

69. Tyml K. Red cell perfusion in skeletal muscle at rest and after mild and severe contractions. *Am J Physiol* 1987;252:H485–H493.

70. Duling BR. Coordination of microcirculatory function with oxygen demand in skeletal muscle. In: Kovách AGB, Hamar J, Szabó L, eds. *Cardiovascular physiology, microcirculation and capillary exchange*. Oxford: Pergamon Press, 1981;1–16.

71. Ellsworth ML, Popel AS, Pittman RN. Assessment and impact of heterogeneities of convective oxygen transport parameters in capillaries of striated muscle: experimental and theoretical. *Microvasc Res* 1988;35:341–362.

72. Wieringa PA, Stassen HG, Spaan JAE. One-dimensional model to illustrate the importance of intercapillary O_2 exchange with capillary flow heterogeneities. *Abstract ISOTT Meeting*, Ottowa, Ontario, Canada, 1988.

73. Sarelius IH. Cell flow path influences transit time through striated muscle capillaries. *Am J Physiol* 1986;250:H899–H907.

74. Gutierrez G. The rate of oxygen release and its effect on capillary O_2 tension: a mathematical analysis. *Respir Physiol* 1986;63:79–96.

75. Gutierrez G, Lund N, Acero AL, Marini C. Relationship of venous P_{O_2} to muscle P_{O_2} during hypoxemia. *J Appl Physiol* 1989;67:1093–1099.

76. Duling BR, Desjardins C. Capillary hematocrit—what does it mean? *NIPS* 1987;2:66–69.

77. Niimi H, Yamakawa T. Rheological factors influencing oxygen transfer in heart and brain. *Adv Exp Med Biol* 1985;191:523–532.

78. Federspiel WJ, Popel AS. A theoretical analysis of the effect of the particulate nature of blood on oxygen release in capillaries. *Microvasc Res* 1986;32:164–189.

79. Groebe K, Thews G. Effects of red cell spacing and red cell movement upon oxygen release under conditions of maximally working skeletal muscle. *Adv Exp Med Biol* 1989;248:175–185.

80. Boyle J III. Microcirculatory hematocrit and blood flow. *J Theor Biol* 1988;131:223–229.

81. Tenney SM. A theoretical analysis of the relationship between venous blood and mean tissue oxygen pressures. *Respir Physiol* 1974;20:283–296.

82. Sharan M, Jones MD Jr, Koehler RC, Traystman RJ, Popel AS. A compartmental model for oxygen transport in brain microcirculation. *Ann Biomed Eng* 1989;17:13–38.

83. Miller MJ. Tissue oxygenation in clinical medicine: an historical review. *Anesth Analg* 1982;61:527–535.

84. Granger HJ, Shepherd AP. Dynamics and control of the microcirculation. *Adv Biomed Eng* 1979;7:1–63.

85. Honig CR. *Modern cardiovascular physiology*. Boston: Little, Brown & Co, 1981.

86. Hudlicka O. Regulation of muscle blood flow. *Clin Physiol* 1985;5:201–229.

87. Mochizuki M, Kagawa T. The effect of deoxygenation rate of the erythrocyte on oxygen transport to the cardiac muscle. *Adv Exp Med Biol* 1978;94:169–174.

88. Hook C, Yamaguchi K, Scheid P, Piiper J. Oxygen transfer of red blood cells: experimental data and model analysis. *Respir Physiol* 1988;72:65–82.

89. Turek Z, Kreuzer F. Hoofd L. Advantage or disadvantage of a decrease of blood oxygen affinity for tissue oxygen supply at hypoxia. *Pflügers Arch* 1973;342:185–197.

90. Duvelleroy MA, Mehmel H, Laver MB. Hemoglobin–oxygen equilibrium and coronary blood flow: an analog model. *J Appl Physiol* 1973;35:480–484.

91. Schumacker PT, Long GR, Wood LDH. Tissue oxygen extraction during hypovolemia: role of hemoglobin P_{50}. *J Appl Physiol* 1987;62:1801–1807.

92. Longmuir IS. Respiration rate of bacteria as a function of oxygen concentration. *Biochem J* 1954;57:81–87.

93. Longmuir IS, Martin DC, Gold HJ, Sun S. Nonclassical respiratory activity of tissue slices. *Microvasc Res* 1971;3:125–141.

94. Buerk DG, Saidel GM. A comparison of two nonclassical models for oxygen consumption in brain and liver tissue. *Adv Exp Med Biol* 1978;94:225–232.

95. Engasser J-M. A fast evaluation of diffusion effects on bound enzyme activity. *Biochim Biophys Acta* 1978;526:301–310.

96. Wilson DF, Erecinska M, Drown C, Silver IA. The oxygen dependence of cellular energy metabolism. *Arch Biochem Biophys* 1979;195:485–493.

97. Wilson DF, Owen CS, Erecinska M. Quantitative dependence of mitochondrial oxidative phosphorylation on oxygen concentration: a mathematical model. *Arch Biochem Biophys* 1979;195:494–504.

98. Robiolio M, Rumsey WL, Wilson DF. Oxygen diffusion and mitochondrial respiration in neuroblastoma cells. *Am J Physiol* 1989;256:C1207–C1213.

99. Stainsby WN, Lambert CR. Determinants of oxygen uptake in skeletal muscle. *Exercise Sports Sci Rev* 1980;7:125–151.

100. Stainsby WN, Otis AB. Blood flow, blood oxygen tension, oxygen uptake, and oxygen transport in skeletal muscle. *Am J Physiol* 1964;206:858–866.

101. Durán WN, Renkin EM. Oxygen consumption and blood flow in resting mammalian skeletal muscle. *Am J Physiol* 1974;226:173–177.

102. Cain SM. Supply dependency of oxygen uptake in ARDS: myth or reality? *Am J Med Sci* 1984;288:119–124.

103. Kreuzer F, Cain SM. Regulation of the peripheral vasculature and tissue oxygenation in health and disease. *Crit Care Clin* 1985;1:453–470.

104. Schumacker PT, Cain SM. The concept of a critical oxygen delivery. *Intensive Care Med* 1987;13:223–229.

105. Powers SR Jr, Mannal R, Neclerio M, English M, Marr C, Leather R, Ueda H, Williams G, Custead W, Dutton R. Physiologic consequences of positive end-expiratory pressure (PEEP) ventilation. *Ann Surg* 1973;178:265–272.

106. Samsel RW, Schumacker PT. Determination of the critical O_2 delivery from experimental data: sensitivity to error. *J Appl Physiol* 1988;64:2074–2082.

107. Popel AS. Theory of oxygen transport to tissue. *Crit Rev Biomed Eng* 1989;17:257–321.

THE LUNG: Scientific Foundations
edited by R.G. Crystal, J.B. West et al.
Raven Press, Ltd., New York © 1991.

CHAPTER 5.5.2.3

Myoglobin and Oxygen Gradients

Carl R. Honig, Thomas E. J. Gayeski, and Karlfried Groebe

The objectives of this chapter are to (a) quantify the spatial distribution of resistances to diffusive O_2 transport, (b) explain the functions of myoglobin (Mb), and (c) identify the reserves of diffusive O_2 transport in Mb-containing muscles.

THE MECHANISM OF TISSUE O₂ TRANSPORT

Tissue O_2 transport in red muscle is described by Equation 1

$$\dot{V}_{O_2} \cong [Pcap_{O_2} - Pmb_{O_2}] \times C \qquad [1]$$

Eq. 1 states that O_2 flux is the product of a driving force times a conductance. A flux is a rate of production, consumption, or transport, whereas flux density is a diffusive flux normalized to the available surface area. *O_2 flux density* is a major determinant of O_2 transport (1,3–7). There are two diffusive fluxes in parallel within red myocytes: (i) a flux of free, dissolved O_2 and (ii) a flux of O_2 bound to the carrier protein Mb. The carrier-mediated flux, called *Mb-facilitated diffusion*, varies as the product of the PO_2 gradient (torr/μm), Mb concentration, Mb diffusivity, and the steepness of the Mb oxydissociation curve at the prevailing PO_2. The flux of free O_2 depends on the product of the PO_2 gradient, O_2 solubility, and O_2 diffusivity. The ratio of the facilitated flux to the free O_2 flux is about 3 in dog gracilis at the Mb P_{50} (about 5.3 torr). Since muscles work near the Mb P_{50} (2,6), the Mb-facilitated flux is dominant. Mb-facilitated diffusion promotes O_2 extraction from red cells by lowering PO_2 near the sarcolemma. The short diffusion path through plasma, en-

dothelium, and interstitium is devoid of an O_2 carrier. A large drop in driving force (i.e., ΔPO_2) is therefore required to deliver the flux through this carrier-free region (CFR).

Pmb_{O_2} in Eq. 1 is the PO_2 in equilibrium with Mb at loci remote from capillaries. Pmb_{O_2} is low relative to PO_2 in blood. Federspiel and Popel (1) defined $Pcap_{O_2}$ as the PO_2 in an individual red cell. It can also be defined as the mean along a capillary, or as the population mean for all capillaries in a specified volume of tissue (2,3). The difference between $Pcap_{O_2}$ and Pmb_{O_2} is the driving force for blood–tissue O_2 transport.

C, the factor of proportionality between the flux and the driving force, is a lumped conductance for O_2. C depends on red-cell-containing capillary surface area, $Pcap_{O_2}$, Pmb_{O_2}, and other factors (1,2,6). In particular, C in Eq. 1 subsumes red-cell transit time, a major determinant of O_2 extraction. (Transit time per se is considered in Fig. 6.) If $Pcap_{O_2}$ and Pmb_{O_2} are defined as population means, C is analogous to D_L, the diffusion capacity of the lung. Since C and D_L are empirical, multifactorial, and highly nonlinear, Eq. 1 is not a statement of Fick's law of diffusion. We shall see that adaptive change in C are a major component of the aerobic reserve (2,3,6–9).

INTRACELLULAR VERSUS EXTRACELLULAR RESISTANCE TO O₂ TRANSPORT

The PO_2 drop per unit length of diffusion path defines the PO_2 gradient (torr/μm). At any location, this gradient is directly proportional to the local resistance to oxygen diffusion, which varies along the diffusion path. There are four PO_2 drops to consider: (A) the ΔPO_2 from the interior to the surface of a red cell [this amounts to only 3–4 torr at maximal O_2 consumption ($\dot{V}_{O_2}$max) and will not be considered further (4)]; (B) the extracellular ΔPO_2 across the CFR (1,6,7); (C) the ΔPO_2 over the (on average) long diffusion path from

C. R. Honig and T. E. J. Gayeski: Departments of Physiology and Anesthesiology, University of Rochester, Rochester, New York 14642.

K. Groebe: Department of Physiology, University of Mainz, 6500 Mainz, West Germany.

sarcolemma to mitochondria (6,7,9–11); and (D) the ΔPo_2 around an individual mitochondrion (4,5,10). An estimate of these gradients can be obtained by considering the anatomy. As in a plumbing system, a large pressure gradient is required in order to drive a large flux through a small area. Conversely, a small gradient will suffice if the flux density is very low. Thus the greatest resistance to tissue O_2 transport is located where flux density is highest, and vice versa.

The same O_2 flux traverses the mitochondrial and capillary membranes. The aggregate surface area of external mitochondrial membranes is about 500 times greater than the aggregate surface area of red-cell-containing capillaries in red muscle. Since the O_2 flux density across mitochondrial membranes is extremely low, the calculated ΔPo_2 between cytosol and an individual mitochondrion is less than 0.05 torr at $\dot{V}o_2$max (4,5). In accord with those calculations, no perimitochondrial O_2 wells were observed in experiments with subcellular spatial resolution, in which a ΔPo_2 of 0.25 torr could have been detected (10). Wittenberg and Wittenberg (12) set an upper bound of 0.2 torr on the ΔPo_2 between Mb and cytochrome in isolated cardiac myocytes. They estimate that if unstirred layers had been taken into account, the actual ΔPo_2 would have been an order of magnitude less (12). Clark et al. (5) point out that large perimitochondrial drops in Po_2 are incompatible with Fick's law of diffusion, and that experiments purporting to show large drops can be accounted for by system heterogeneities. Thus, gradient D never limits $\dot{V}o_2$ in red muscle if any O_2 is available at all.

Gradient B should be greater than gradient D by roughly the ratio of the aggregate mitochondrial surface area to the aggregate red-cell-containing capillary surface area (~500:1). According to this logic, the ΔPo_2 across the 1- to 2-μm CFR should be on the order of 25 torr, or ~15–20 torr/μm at high $\dot{V}o_2$. Gradient B is large because of the extremely high flux density near red cells. For example, measurements of red-cell-containing capillary density and red-cell spacing in dog gracilis at $\dot{V}o_2$max indicate that the O_2 supply to four fibers, each 500 μm long, is delivered by only ~240 erythrocytes. The aggregate volume of these cells is ~16 pl versus 3200 pl of fiber volume. Since the flux density is highest and the conductance lowest in the CFR, the CFR behaves as a functional O_2 barrier. We emphasize that no anatomical barrier or unique diffusivity is required to account for this behavior.

Gradient C, the ΔPo_2 between sarcolemma and cell interior, is much less than gradient B because flux density becomes progressively smaller with distance from the red cell. Moreover, Mb-facilitated diffusion greatly increases the net O_2 conductance, particularly at high $\dot{V}o_2$ (2,6–9,13).

MATHEMATICAL MODELS

Recent models that take account of the high flux density at red cells and diffusion boundary layers predict a large ΔPo_2 across the CFR (1,6,7,14). In contrast, the calculated ΔPo_2 within myocytes is shallow when Mb-facilitated diffusion is considered at the Mb concentration and saturation actually observed in working red muscle (6,7,9). A model that formally links convective and diffusive transport is described in ref. 6. It takes account of flow, transit times, capillary density, capillary hematocrit, the CFR, and carrier-facilitated diffusion by hemoglobin (Hb) and Mb. The model was parameterized for values observed experimentally in dog gracilis to permit comparison of calculated and measured gradients in the same muscle. The diffusion problem is solved in three dimensions for the measured red-cell spacing. Results for a heavily working fiber are shown in Fig. 1A (6).

The apex of each peak in panel A represents Po_2 at the surface of a red cell. Three red cells abut a 50-μm myocyte. The ΔPo_2 across the 1.5-μm CFR is 30 torr, or 20 torr/μm. An additional 5-torr drop occurs within 3 μm of the sarcolemma immediately subjacent to the red cell, where O_2 enters at high flux density. The ΔPo_2 in the rest of the fiber is <4 torr despite diffusion paths of up to 22 μm in length. Though the capillaries are clustered, the Po_2 distribution in the bulk of the fiber volume is remarkably flat, and it is above the minimum Po_2 required for maximum $\dot{V}o_2$ (15). Because of Mb-facilitated diffusion, intracellular O_2 conductance is so high that the intracellular Po_2 distribution is not significantly altered by changing the positions of the three capillaries. If more capillaries are added, the Po_2 at the red-cell surface can be lower without compromising the flux or lowering $Pmbo_2$ because a smaller O_2 flux per red cell can be delivered by a smaller driving force. Though $Pmbo_2$ is not strongly dependent on the local capillary geometry, it is highly sensitive to the concentration of Mb, in accord with observations (8,11,13). For conditions in Fig. 1A, intracellular Po_2 would be zero 5–10 μm into the fiber if Mb were not present, even if $Pcapo_2$ were set equal to arterial Po_2. If the Mb concentration were higher, as in racing greyhounds, the increase in diffusive conductance would allow a larger $\dot{V}o_2$, a smaller driving force, or larger-diameter fiber.

A similar model has been used to calculate O_2 gradients in the long axis of the capillary and fiber (6). The fiber in Fig. 1B is served by four capillaries, each more than 20 μm from the plane of observation. Po_2 gradients in the capillary for conditions in Fig. 1 are about 0.1 torr/μm near the arterial end and 0.02 torr/μm near the venous end. In contrast, the calculated $Pmbo_2$ remote from the sarcolemma is almost uniform along the entire length of the fiber. Except for the im-

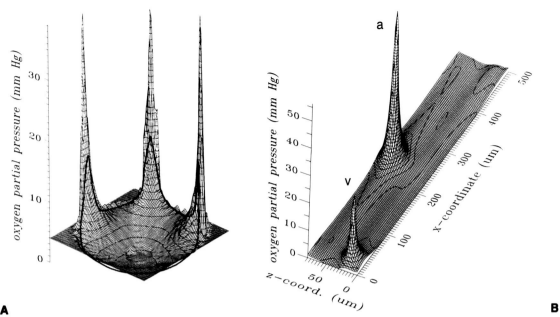

FIG. 1. A: Calculated P_{O_2} distribution around three capillaries in a heavily working red fiber. P_{O_2} contours are at intervals of 1 torr. **B:** P_{O_2} distribution in a plane that bisects the fiber along its axis. The plane is 20 μm from capillaries; a and v indicate a terminal arteriole and venule.

mediate surround of a terminal arteriole (a) and collecting venule (v), longitudinal gradients are $<10^{-3}$ torr/μm. Thus the calculated intracellular P_{O_2} is remarkably uniform despite the microvascular heterogeneities included in the model.

MEASURED Mb SATURATION AND P_{mbO_2}

Magnitude and Variability of Intracellular P_{O_2}

Mb saturation represents the instantaneous balance of all determinants of O_2 supply and demand. The spatial uniformity of this balance and the adequacy of intracellular P_{O_2} for cell metabolism must be judged from a probability distribution of measurements at various locations (2,15–18). The distributions in Fig. 2 were obtained by Mb cryospectroscopy of dog gracilis muscles, as described in reference 11. The filled circles, open circles, and triangles represent muscles frozen during twitch contraction at about 20%, 60%, and 100% of $\dot{V}_{O_2}$max, respectively. Each distribution is based on 50 randomly chosen cells from the same muscle. The cells were sampled near the lowest point of the shallow gradient from sarcolemma to cell interior. Median P_{mbO_2} in resting gracilis is typically 20–50 torr (15). Medians for the muscles in Fig. 2 are 13, 6.1, and 1.7 torr. The large fall in P_{mbO_2} as $\dot{V}_{O_2}$ increases must not be interpreted in a pejorative sense. On the contrary, low P_{mbO_2} is an adaptive response that maintains $P_{capO_2} - P_{mbO_2}$ as extraction increases and P_{capO_2}

falls (2,6,7,16,19). In heavy submaximal exercise, as in muscle 248, P_{mbO_2} is close to the Mb P_{50} of 5.3 torr. In this range the Mb-facilitated O_2 flux is substantial, a large reserve of diffusive conductance exists, and the remaining Mb O_2 store is well matched to the time scale of microvascular heterogeneities. It is of interest that the hearts of five species function at about a median Mb saturation of 60% (18).

The variabilities of Mb saturation and P_{mbO_2} change with $\dot{V}_{O_2}$. At 20% $\dot{V}_{O_2}$max there was little spatial variability of Mb saturation, but P_{mbO_2} ranged from 5 to 40 torr. The long upper tail of the P_{mbO_2} distribution reflects the shallow slope of the oxymyoglobin dissociation curve at saturations greater than 80% (refer to Fig. 5B). This shallow slope allows a large fall in P_{mbO_2} as $\dot{V}_{O_2}$ increases 50- to 100-fold from rest. Mb saturation (and hence the intracellular O_2 content) was lower and more variable near $\dot{V}_{O_2}$max, reflecting a more precarious balance between O_2 supply and demand. In contrast, P_{mbO_2} was almost uniform in the cell population because the steep slope of the oxymyoglobin dissociation curve acts as a P_{O_2} buffer. Uniformity of P_{mbO_2} was also promoted by diffusion of O_2 from cells in which P_{mbO_2} was high into cells in which it was low; see, for example, arrow at right in Fig. 3.

Relation to P_{O_2} in Blood

The arrows above the abscissa in Fig. 2 (bottom panel) denote P_{vO_2} in the gracilis effluent. Even at low $\dot{V}_{O_2}$

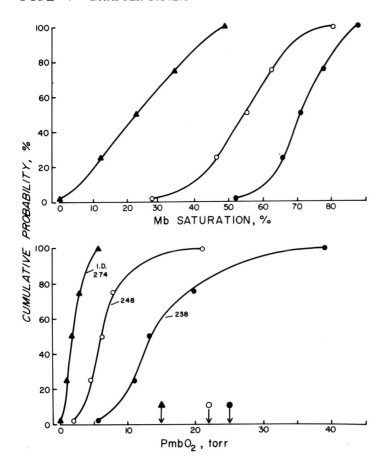

FIG. 2. Frequency distribution of Pmbo$_2$ and Mb saturation in muscle cells. Each ogive is based on a random sample of 50 cells. Muscles 238, 248, and 274 were frozen at about 20, 60, and 100% of V̇o$_2$max. Arrows indicate effluent venous Po$_2$ for each muscle. (From ref. 17.)

(filled circle), Pvo$_2$ exceeded Pmbo$_2$ in 90% of cells sampled; the difference between median Pmbo$_2$ and Pvo$_2$ was 8 torr. At V̇o$_2$max (triangle), Pvo$_2$ was triple the highest Pmbo$_2$ encountered and was almost nine times the median Pmbo$_2$. Pvo$_2$ can be interpreted as end-capillary Po$_2$ because arteriovenous diffusive shunting is negligible (20). The difference between Pvo$_2$ and Pmbo$_2$ is therefore a lower bound on the average driving force in Eq. 1. Comparable estimates of Pcapo$_2$ − Pmbo$_2$ have been obtained based on intracellular O$_2$ electrodes (21) and on the blood–tissue partition of CO (22). Low Pmbo$_2$ relative to blood confirms calculations like those in Fig. 1.

Relation to O$_2$ Dependence of Cell Metabolism

Intracellular Po$_2$ falls into three ranges (2,16): (i) The [O$_2$] saturates cytochrome a,a$_3$, and metabolism is independent of [O$_2$]. Resting red muscle falls in this range. (ii) The [O$_2$] is not sufficient to saturate the terminal oxidase, but the V̇o$_2$ is maintained by metabolic adaptations. Data of Wilson et al. (23) indicate that almost all values of Po$_2$ shown in Fig. 2 are in this adaptive range. (iii) The lower bound on the adaptive range defines the critical Po$_2$ for maintenance of V̇o$_2$

(16). This P$_{crit}$O$_2$ is 0.3–0.5 torr in red muscle at aerobic capacity, and it is substantially lower at physiological work rates (15). We emphasize that cell hypoxia is defined as O$_2$-limited V̇o$_2$ rather than O$_2$-modified metabolism (2,16).

V̇o$_2$ depends on three related drives: free O$_2$, redox state, and phosphorylation state (16,23,24). The higher the rate of cytochrome turnover, the greater the net effect of these drives. Because of the creatine kinase and adenylate kinase equilibria, the phosphorylation state changes progressively with V̇o$_2$. This modifies not only electron transport but also the Krebs cycle and mitochondrial redox, as well as glycolysis and cytosolic redox, at Pmbo$_2$ well above P$_{crit}$O$_2$ (2,16,23,24). Thus, intermediary metabolism must be profoundly modified to maintain V̇o$_2$ when Pmbo$_2$ is in the range required to defend the driving force, conductance, and transcapillary O$_2$ flux. Metabolic reserves therefore play an essential role in support of diffusive transport (2,16).

MEASURED INTRACELLULAR O$_2$ GRADIENTS

Data in Figs. 3 and 4 were collected with a 1.5- × 1.5-μm measuring diaphragm positioned at locations in-

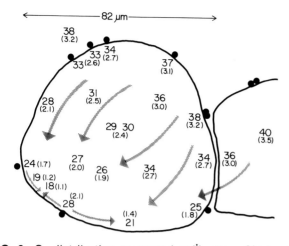

FIG. 3. O_2 distribution measured at $\dot{V}O_2$max. Circles indicate capillaries that contained red cells in the plane of cross-section. Numbers indicate Mb saturation and (in parentheses) Pmb_{O_2} at loci 5 and 25 μm from the sarcolemma, as well as at the center of the cell profile. Arrows show direction of O_2 flux.

dicated by the numerals. Reproducibility was within 3% saturation. The muscle used for Fig. 3 had exceptionally large cells, and its $\dot{V}O_2$ was the highest we have observed in random source dogs. Consequently, a Krogh model predicts steep intracellular gradients, with saturation greater than 50% 5 μm from the sarcolemma, and zero in about half the cell volume. Instead, intracellular gradients in the accessible portion of cell volume were shallow and no anoxic loci were found (11), in agreement with the calculated gradients in Fig. 1A. Note that the capillaries in Fig. 3 are clustered at upper right. The 20% ΔSat from upper right to lower left corresponds to 2 torr over 70 μm, or about 0.3 torr/μm. Recall that calculated extracellular gradients are two orders of magnitude larger. As in Fig. 1A, minimum Po_2 is not at the center of the cross-section when capillaries are asymmetrically spaced,

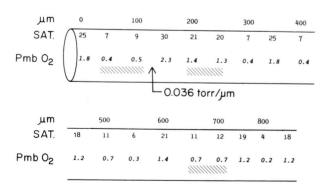

FIG. 4. Cell from muscle 274 showing Mb saturation and Pmb_{O_2} at 50-μm intervals. Shading indicates lengths over which differences are within error of measurement. Arrow indicates largest gradient observed. Probability distributions for this muscle are shown in Fig. 2. (From ref. 17.)

due to a Mb-facilitated flux into the region less favorably supplied.

Intercellular O_2 fluxes (ultimately derived from more remote capillaries) further minimize the influence of capillary spacing, $Pcapo_2$, and cell diameter; see, for example, the arrow at right in Fig. 3. The intercellular O_2 flux in gracilis muscle can be comparable in magnitude to O_2 flux from a capillary despite small intercellular gradients, because the area of the interface between adjacent cells is large relative to the interface between capillary and myocyte. Mb-facilitated redistribution of O_2 among myocytes should be more effective in voluntary exercise than during twitch contraction because, in the former, contracting fibers are contiguous to resting ones in which Pmb_{O_2} is high. Thus, the O_2 supply unit is not an individual capillary but rather a population of cells and capillaries with interactive diffusion fields.

Longitudinal gradients in a maximally working fiber are shown in Fig. 4 (17). Axial variability exhibited no orderly trend, and gradients did not exceed 0.04 torr/μm, in accord with the modeling data in Fig. 1B. No evidence of the drop in $Pcapo_2$ along the red-cell flow path was observed within the fiber. In particular, there was no evidence of anoxic loci at the venous ends of capillaries (so-called "lethal corners") predicted by Krogh-type models.

Mb partly accounts for the shallow intracellular gradients in Figs. 1, 3, and 4. At high $\dot{V}O_2$ the steep slope of the oxymyoglobin dissociation curve minimizes the drop in Pmb_{O_2} if Mb saturation falls. More important, the lower the Mb saturation and Pmb_{O_2}, the greater the concentration of available unbound carrier, and the larger the ratio of facilitated diffusion to free diffusion (8,13); see Fig. 5B. The Po_2 dependence of facilitated diffusion has important consequences for O_2 release from blood, as shown in Fig. 5A (6). Entry of O_2 at high Po_2 results in high Mb saturation and loss of carrier effectiveness near the sarcolemma; we emphasize that the depletion of unbound carrier is functional and that it is dependent on Po_2. The carrier-depleted region (CDR), like the CFR, impedes diffusive transport. Penetration of the CDR into the fiber depends on $Pcapo_2$ as shown in Fig. 5A. Near the arterial end of the capillary, penetration is relatively deep (4–5 μm). The CDR becomes thinner as $Pcapo_2$ falls (6). This behavior is admirably suited to the long cells and capillaries of skeletal muscle because longitudinal changes in the CDR, and hence in C, roughly compensate for the longitudinal drop in $Pcapo_2$ (6). The result is an almost uniform O_2 efflux along an individual capillary. This uniformity partly accounts for the small longitudinal gradients in Pmb_{O_2} in Fig. 1B and Fig. 4, as well as for the narrow range of the probability distribution of Pmb_{O_2} at high $\dot{V}O_2$.

Longitudinal gradients and heterogeneity of Pmb_{O_2}

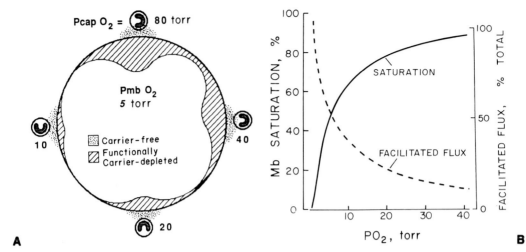

FIG. 5. A: Effect of decreasing Pcapo₂ on penetration of CDR into the fiber. Extent of CDR is exaggerated to illustrate the concept. **B:** Solid line is oxymyoglobin dissociation curve; dashed line indicates the influence of Po₂ on carrier-facilitated transport.

are further minimized by the arrangement of microvascular units. Each unit consists of a terminal arteriole and its sheaf of interconnected capillaries (25). The origins and terminations of the units are staggered. At any fiber cross-section, heterogeneity of Pcapo₂ and red-cell flux within or among microvascular units is integrated by convective interaction among capillaries, as well as by diffusive interactions among myocytes. Together the microvascular anatomy and the CDR create an almost uniform Pmbo₂ on the scale of a microvascular unit (17).

Spatial uniformity allows red cells in working muscle to release O₂ as though they were dipped in a solution of Mb. Consequently, extraction at any V̇o₂ depends mainly on red-cell flux, aggregate red-cell surface area, and the time available for O₂ release.

RED-CELL TRANSIT TIME

Release time for O₂ is identical to red-cell transit time, because O₂ in red cells does not equilibrate with O₂ in working red muscle (1,2,6–8,11,17,19). Transit time is the ratio of red-cell path length to red-cell velocity. Velocity varies directly with muscle blood flow and inversely with the aggregate cross-sectional area of the capillary bed. The expansion factor for capillary cross-sectional area is less than half that for blood flow (26). Consequently, exercise hyperemia increases velocities and shortens transit times (27). Fortunately, transit times also become more uniform (28). Higher V̇o₂ in the face of shorter transit times necessitates a fall in Pmbo₂ to maintain the driving force, and to increase the Mb-facilitated O₂ flux (2,6,7,17,19).

ROLE OF O₂ CONDUCTANCE

Perhaps the most astonishing feature of O₂ transport in red muscle is that V̇o₂ can increase two orders of magnitude despite shorter red-cell transit times and decreased driving force. The explanation is an enormous increase in C. A major determinant of C is the aggregate capillary surface area subjacent to red cells. Exercise hyperemia is accompanied by higher capillary hematocrit (27), along with entry of erythrocytes into a larger fraction of the capillary network (3,26,27). These changes decrease flux density at the capillary "bottleneck." The strong dependence of facilitation on Po₂ results in a CDR that matches C to O₂ extraction and V̇o₂ (Fig. 5). The reserve of facilitated diffusion is recruited automatically as V̇o₂ increases and Pmbo₂ falls (2,6–8). The resulting increase in conductance is essential for normal V̇o₂ in exercise (8,29).

INTEGRATION: THE O₂ RELEASE CURVE

A convenient tool for analysis of diffusive O₂ transport is offered in Fig. 6 based on a mathematical model developed by Federspiel (19). Recall that, to a first approximation, Pmbo₂ is spatially uniform on the scale of an individual capillary. Consequently, O₂ extraction can be modeled as the time required to release O₂ through a CFR into a Mb solution of known saturation. Movement along the abscissae gives the extraction; the ordinate is identical to capillary transit time in working red muscle because red cells do not equilibrate with tissue. Each isopleth is calculated for a fixed CFR and fixed Pmbo₂ (1, 5, or 20 torr).

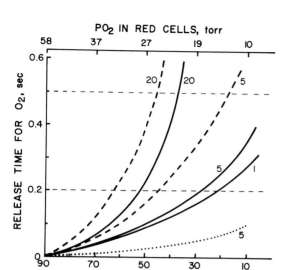

FIG. 6. O_2-release curves, based on model in ref. 19. Thickness of carrier-free region: Dotted curve represents 0-μm thickness; solid curves represent 1-μm thickness; and dashed curves represent 2-μm thickness. Numbers beside isopleths represent Pmb_{O_2}.

Role of Pmb_{O_2}

If Pmb_{O_2} were 20 torr, as in resting muscle, the release time for O_2 would approach an asymptote as $Pcap_{O_2}$ − Pmb_{O_2} approaches zero. Saturation could not be less than 40% if the CFR were 1 μm no matter how long a red cell resides in a capillary, and $\dot{V}_{O_2}$ would be severely limited. If, however, Pmb_{O_2} were 5 torr and the CFR were 1 μm, hemoglobin saturation would fall from 90% to 30% in only 200 msec and to 8% in 500 msec. Pmb_{O_2} *must* be well below values in blood to achieve high $\dot{V}_{O_2}$. Isopleths for Pmb_{O_2} of 1 and 5 torr are almost linear over the usual range of extraction, and the slopes are almost the same. Consequently, lowering Pmb_{O_2} from 5 torr to 1 torr produces a relatively small increase in extraction, at a cost of severe stress on the reserves of phosphorylation state and redox. It is of interest that a substantial population of cells near 1 torr is found only near $\dot{V}_{O_2}$max.

Role of Transit Time

Transit times measured at rest range from 500 to 4000 msec (30); the shortest transit times in heavy exercise are about 200 msec (28). If Pmb_{O_2} were 20 torr, release curves would approach an asymptote at about 500 msec. Consequently, heterogeneity of transit times would have almost no effect on O_2 extraction at rest. However, if Pmb_{O_2} were 5 torr, increasing transit time from 200 to 500 msec would increase extraction by about one-third. Thus, transit time and its variability

are major determinants of O_2 extraction from red cells in exercise.

Influence of CFR

If Pmb_{O_2} were 5 torr and a CFR did not exist, extraction would be virtually complete in only 200 msec (dotted curve, Fig. 6). If the CFR were 1 or 2 μm, end-capillary saturation would be 20% or 46%, respectively, at 200 msec. The CDR is not included in the model used to produce Fig. 6. The effect of a 1-μm change in the CFR gives a qualitative idea of the influence of the CDR on O_2 extraction and $\dot{V}_{O_2}$.

SUMMARY

Peripheral O_2 transport depends on microvascular geometry, red cell flux, functions of Mb, and intermediary metabolism. Interaction of these variables as a system largely accounts for the extraordinary expansion factor for $\dot{V}_{O_2}$ in red muscle (2,6,8,16).

ACKNOWLEDGMENTS

This research was supported by grant HLB03290 from the United States Public Health Service, as well as by grant GR887/1-1 from the Deutsche Forschungsgemeinschaft.

REFERENCES

1. Federspiel WJ, Popel AS. A theoretical analysis of the effect of the particulate nature of blood on oxygen release in capillaries. *Microvasc Res* 1986;32:164–189.
2. Honig CR, Connett RJ, Gayeski TEJ. O_2 transport and its interaction with metabolism; a systems view of aerobic capacity. *Med Sci Sport Exercise* 1990; in press.
3. Honig CR, Frierson JL, Gayeski TEJ. Anatomical determinants of O_2 flux density at coronary capillaries. *Am J Physiol* 1989;256:H375–H382.
4. Clark A Jr, Clark PAA. The end-points of the oxygen path: transport resistance in red cells and mitochondria. *Adv Exp Med Biol* 1986;200:43–47.
5. Clark A Jr, Clark PAA, Connett RJ, Gayeski TEJ, Honig CR. How large is the drop in PO_2 between cytosol and mitochondria? *Am J Physiol* 1987;252:C583–C587.
6. Groebe K. A versatile model of steady state O_2 supply to tissue. Application to skeletal muscle. *Biophys J* 1990;57:485–498.
7. Groebe K, Thews G. Theoretical analysis of oxygen supply to contracted skeletal muscle. *Adv Exp Med Biol* 1986;200:495–514.
8. Wittenberg BA, Wittenberg JB. Transport of oxygen in muscle. *Annu Rev Physiol* 1989;51:857–878.
9. Federspiel WJ. A model study of intracellular oxygen gradients in a myoglobin-containing skeletal muscle fiber. *Biophys J* 1986;49:857–868.
10. Gayeski TEJ, Honig CR. Shallow intracellular O_2 gradients and absence of perimitochondrial O_2 "wells" in heavily working red muscle. *Adv Exp Med Biol* 1986;200:487–494.
11. Gayeski TEJ, Honig CR. O_2 gradients from sarcolemma to cell

interior in a red muscle at maximal $\dot{V}O_2$. *Am J Physiol* 1986;251:789–799.

12. Wittenberg BA, Wittenberg JB. Oxygen pressure gradients in isolated cardiac myocytes. *J Biol Chem* 1985;260:6548–6554.

13. Kreuzer F, Hoofd L. Facilitated diffusion of oxygen and carbon dioxide. In: Farhi L, Tenney SM, eds. *Handbook of physiology, Section 3: The respiratory system, vol IV—gas exchange.* Bethesda, MD: American Physiological Society, 1987;89–111.

14. Hellums JD. The resistance to oxygen transport in the capillaries relative to that in the surrounding tissue. *Microvasc Res* 1977; 13:131–136.

15. Gayeski TEJ, Connett RJ, Honig CR. Minimum intracellular PO_2 for maximum cytochrome turnover in red muscle *in situ*. *Am J Physiol* 1987;252:H906–H915.

16. Connett RJ, Honig CR, Gayeski TEJ, Brooks GA. Defining hypoxia: a systems view of $\dot{V}O_2$, glycolysis, energetics, and intracellular PO_2. *J Appl Physiol* 1990; 68:833–842.

17. Gayeski TEJ, Honig CR. Intracellular PO_2 in long axis of individual fibers in working dog gracilis muscle. *Am J Physiol* 1988;254:H1179–H1186.

18. Gayeski TEJ, Honig CR. Intracellular PO_2 in individual cardiac myocytes in dog, cat, rabbit, ferret and cat. *Am J Physiol* 1990; in press.

19. Gayeski TEJ, Federspiel WJ, Honig CR. A graphical analysis of the influence of red cell transit time, carrier-free layer thickness, and intracellular PO_2 on blood–tissue O_2 transport. *Adv Exp Med Biol* 1988;222:25–35.

20. Honig CR, Gayeski TEJ. Precapillary O_2 loss and arteriovenous O_2 diffusion shunt are below limit of detection in myocardium. *Adv Exp Med Biol* 1989;247:591–599.

21. Whalen WJ. Intracellular PO_2 in heart and skeletal muscle. *Physiologist* 1971;14:69–82.

22. Coburn RF, Mayers LB. Myoglobin O_2 tension determined from measurements of carboxymyoglobin in skeletal muscle. *Am J Physiol* 1971;220:66–74.

23. Wilson DF, Erećinska M, Drawn C, Silver IA. The oxygen dependence of cellular energy metabolism. *Arch Biochem Biophys* 1979;195:485–493.

24. Connett RJ, Honig CR. Regulation of $\dot{V}O_2$ in red muscle: Do current biochemical hypotheses fit *in vivo* data? *Am J Physiol* 1989;256:R898–R906.

25. Lund N, Damon DN, Duling BR. Capillary grouping in hamster tibialis anterior muscle: flow patterns and physiological significance. *Int J Microcirc Clin Exp* 1987;5:359–372.

26. Honig CR, Odoroff CL, Frierson JL. Active and passive capillary control in red muscle at rest and in exercise. *Am J Physiol* 1982;243:H196–H206.

27. Klitzman B, Duling BR. Microvascular hematocrit and red cell flow in resting and contracting striated muscle. *Am J Physiol* 1979;237:H481–H490.

28. Honig CR, Odoroff CL. Calculated dispersion of capillary transit time: significance for oxygen exchange. *Am J Physiol* 1979; 237:H481–H490.

29. Cole RP. Myoglobin function in exercising skeletal muscle. *Science* 1982;216:523–525.

30. Sarelius IH, Duling BR. Direct measurement of microvessel hematocrit, red cell flux, velocity and transit time. *Am J Physiol* 1982;243:H1018–H1026.

THE LUNG: Scientific Foundations
edited by R.G. Crystal, J.B. West et al.
Raven Press, Ltd., New York © 1991.

CHAPTER 5.5.2.4

Control of Striated Muscle Blood Flow

Brian R. Duling

METABOLIC DEMANDS
AND VASCULAR ADAPTATION

The vasculature of striated muscle must be remarkably adaptive because it supplies a tissue whose major characteristic is change, both in the work that it does and in the metabolic activity that supports the work (1). A close coupling between vascular capacity and striated muscle function is manifest in the form of short-term adaptive processes operating over periods of minutes to hours, as well as in the form of chronic adaptations of the muscle phenotype and its associated vasculature, which can occur over periods of several days or more (2–4). The former processes are the subject of this chapter.

Figure 1 shows the results of the short-term adaptations of the vasculature. These are evident as changes in blood flow and in O_2 extraction from the blood, and they can be observed in a variety of striated muscle types (3,5–8). For each muscle type, a high degree of correlation between flow and oxygen consumption is observed over some portion of the metabolic range (Fig. 1A). The correlation tends to be tighter in cardiac than in skeletal muscle, and it is usually best in the intermediate ranges of muscle oxygen consumption. As is evident from the changes in the arteriovenous (A-V) O_2 difference (Fig. 1B), in the low end of the metabolic range the muscles tend to rely more heavily on changes in extraction, and in the high end they tend to rely more on changes in flow (8,9).

The details of the means by which O_2 extraction is augmented in the working muscle are beyond the scope of this review, but it should be noted that the process is multifactorial and reflects diverse vascular and extravascular changes. In general, it can be said that stri-

ated muscle alters O_2 extraction by adjustment of the longitudinal and radial P_{O_2} gradients that surround the exchange vessels. The key adaptations employed are: decreasing tissue P_{O_2} (10–12), increasing capillary density (9,13,14), increasing the homogeneity of perfusion of the available vasculature (14–16), and increasing capillary red blood cell content (17).

Intrinsic Regulation of Blood Flow in Striated Muscle

The vasculature of striated muscle is critical to every aspect of the regulation of the cardiovascular system, and an enormous number of neural, humoral, and paracrine regulatory mechanisms come to a focus on these tissues (18,19). The present chapter emphasizes the means by which the vascular supply adapts directly to the muscle's metabolic needs—that is, *intrinsic* or *local* regulation of flow as typified by such processes as autoregulation and functional hyperemia.

Figure 2 is a simple conceptual model of vascular metabolic control. The figure suggests the variety of processes that might be involved in the coupling of O_2 supply and O_2 demand. ATP hydrolysis by active muscle myofilaments produces several potent vasoactive products that are part of the feedback process. At the same time, the products of ATP hydrolysis are key signal molecules whose concentrations regulate diverse biochemical adaptations within the muscle (20,21); any of these processes are potentially a secondary source of vasodilator metabolites (e.g., M in Fig. 2).

The coupling between O_2 supply and O_2 demand is so tight that it is often assumed that O_2 itself plays a key role in the process. The involvement of O_2 might be *direct*; that is, it might occur via a reduction in smooth muscle P_{O_2}, which in some way causes smooth muscle relaxation and increased flow. This process contrasts with an *indirect* mechanism, in which there is a primary production of a vasodilator metabolite in

---

B. R. Duling: Department of Physiology, University of Virginia School of Medicine, Charlottesville, Virginia 22908.

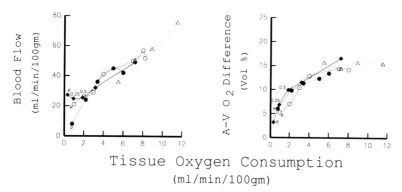

FIG. 1. Relations among blood flow, O$_2$ extraction, and metabolic rate in resting and stimulated striated muscles. The data were obtained from refs. 5–7 and represent both oxidative [cardiac, soleus, and extensor digitorum longus (EDL)] and glycolytic (gastrocnemius) fibers. In the case of the soleus and gastrocnemius, the minimum stimulus frequency was 1 Hz; in the case of the EDL, however, intermediate stimuli at 0.25 and 0.5 Hz were used. (◆) EDL, dog (5); (△) cardiac muscle, dog (7); (○) soleus, cat (6); (●) gastrocnemius, cat (6).

response to the altered supply–demand ratio. The metabolite (e.g., adenosine) then couples the altered striated muscle metabolism to a change in smooth muscle tone. Two arrows in Fig. 2 connect the O$_2$ source (capillary) to the muscle parenchyma: One arrow suggests that the metabolite's production might be associated with some alteration in mitochondrial oxidative phosphorylation (a common assumption), and the other arrow reflects the existence of the myriad other oxidative processes that might produce a vasoactive material (22,23) (Fig. 2, Oxygenase ?).

Criteria for Mediators of Metabolic Control

Much of the experimental work on this problem is of the "consistent with" variety, following a set of criteria clearly enunciated by Mellander and Johansson in 1968 (24). These criteria represent a set of *a priori* requirements that a mediator must meet if it is to be a viable candidate as a flow controller. For example,

venous levels of a proposed substance must rise during muscle work. Although such criteria were adequate in the formative periods of investigation, what must be sought at a time when the field is more mature are those criteria that are both necessary and sufficient to establish a cause-and-effect role for a proposed mediator.

In broadest terms, one can define two basic criteria. First, we must know the concentration of the presumed coupling molecule at the surface of the particular smooth muscle cells involved in the regulatory process. Second, the reactivity of those smooth muscle cells to the proposed mediator must be well-defined. Much of the lack of progress toward unequivocal definition of the controllers of flow has stemmed from a failure of the basic experimental designs to directly address one or the other, or both, of these criteria.

Basal Vascular Smooth Muscle Tone

Inherent in the regulatory scheme shown in Fig. 2 is a need for vascular smooth muscle tone, since this is

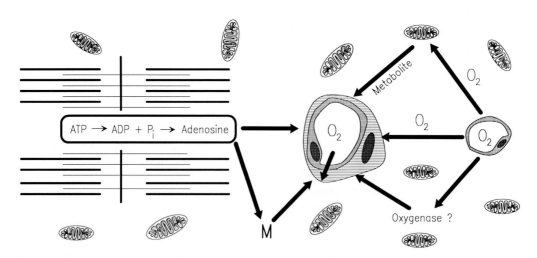

FIG. 2. Metabolic regulatory scheme for working striated muscle. The figure shows the source of O$_2$ (capillary), the site of control (arteriole), and the site of utilization of ATP (myofilaments). "Oxygenase ?" and "M" represent the yet-to-be-defined sites of action of either O$_2$ or cellular regulatory mechanisms that produce vasoactive metabolites.

the background against which all of the metabolically derived vasodilators must act. Several sources of tone are recognized, but their quantitative significance is imperfectly understood. Their importance to our understanding metabolic control stems from the fact that different sources of tone may interact differently with the metabolic control mechanisms (25,26).

Myogenic Mechanism

The stretch-induced contraction of the vessel wall, known as the "myogenic mechanism," is a major source of resting vasomotor tone (27–30). Although intrinsic in the vessel wall, it is now recognized that the "myogenic response" may be attributable to either the smooth muscle or the endothelium (31–33). Stretch-dependent ion channels exist in the surface membrane of smooth muscle and endothelial cells, as well as in that of other cell types (34,35). Thus, the simplest explanation of the myogenic response is that stretch deforms the cell membrane, of either endothelial cell or smooth muscle (or both), thereby inducing a change in calcium influx either through a change in membrane potential (36,37) or via a direct effect on calcium channels of the vascular smooth muscle cell membrane (38).

In addition to acting as a source of vasomotor tone, the myogenic mechanism also plays a more direct role in coupling flow to metabolism (28). In the working muscle, compression and release of the vasculature induces the myogenic response (39). Additionally, the stretch-sensitive mechanism serves to stabilize muscle blood flow in face of the hypertension of exercise (19,28).

Endothelin is a newly discovered product of the endothelial cell; it is an extremely potent vasoconstrictor (40) and may be a significant contributor to vasomotor tone. *In vivo* release has yet to be shown, but the proximity of the endothelium to the smooth muscle cell makes this peptide an ideal candidate for setting resting vasomotor tone, particularly in view of its long duration of action (41,42).

Neural and Humoral Mechanisms

Sympathetic nerves, acting via tonic release of norepinephrine, are a major source of resting vasomotor tone. The magnitude of their contribution to tone, as evidenced by the effect of chemical or surgical denervation, varies longitudinally along the vasculature, with diminishing effects in the smallest arterioles. This variation shows a strong correlation with a decrease in the density of innervation (18,43). Spontaneous and neurally induced vasomotor tone are supplemented by circulating hormones, especially catecholamines and

peptides (18,44,45). At present, it is impossible to define the components of tone resulting from each source. However, this will be an important concern for future work in the field, as the metabolic control mechanisms interact differently with different forms of vasomotor tone (25,26).

The various sources of vasomotor tone, acting on the smooth muscle cell, are overcome in working muscle groups by the actions of locally produced dilator metabolites, thereby automatically diverting flow to the working muscles from other regions of the vasculature (46). The particular case of metabolically induced dilation acting on neurally induced tone has been referred to as "functional sympatholysis" (46), a term that recognizes that metabolic events cause not only smooth muscle relaxation but diminished sympathetic neurotransmitter release as well (47).

MEDIATORS OF METABOLIC COUPLING

The details summarizing the complexities of the subject of local blood flow control may be found in a number of reviews (18,48–51); the literature is voluminous, and what follows represents only a summary of the basic aspects of the problem. In an effort to provide a framework for understanding, each mediator is presented in relation to the basic cellular process that might lead to its production.

Coupling Via Membrane Depolarization

Potassium

Potassium ions are released into interstitial fluid and venous blood as the direct result of striated muscle activation during cellular repolarization. Furthermore, potassium ion (at low to moderate concentration) is a good vasodilator, especially in microvessels (52–54). Both the rise in venous K^+ concentration with exercise and the vasomotor effect of K^+ are transient (52,55) and are thus easily missed in the evaluation of reactivity. Furthermore, since K^+ functions either as a dilator or as a constrictor, with differential effects on the large and small vessels (52), it is very difficult to evaluate its dilator capacity in an intact tissue.

In view of its transient behavior, it is apparent that K^+ can play little role in the regulation of steady-state exercise vasodilation. However, K^+ may play a key role in the initiation of the exercise response, since it can function as an ideal "early warning" dilator. Repolarization of a stimulated striated muscle leads directly to K^+ release, as well as to a vasodilation that anticipates (a) the accumulation of metabolically produced dilators and (b) the depletion of energy stores. Potassium's effect wanes early during sustained muscle work, and the steady-state flow response is then presumably determined by the actions of those molecules described below that more closely mimic the relation between O_2 supply and O_2 demand.

Coupling Via Oxidative Phosphorylation

Oxygen and Carbon Dioxide

The idea that the respiratory gases might be active participants in the regulatory process is attractive because venous oxygen saturation and Po_2 vary in inverse proportion to metabolic rate and because the average tissue Po_2 falls with the level of muscle work (5–7,9,10). The K_m for oxidative phosphorylation is less than 1 mmHg, and there is little evidence that O_2 falls to such low values in working muscles except under extreme conditions. Therefore, although there are other hypotheses (21), most current models of control assume (a) that oxidative phosphorylation, as the major O_2-consuming process, sets the tissue level of O_2 and (b) that other biochemical processes must ultimately couple flow and metabolism.

As mentioned above, O_2 might act either directly or indirectly in the regulatory process. For O_2 to act directly, the resistance vessels must be sensitive to O_2, and the smooth muscle contraction must vary with O_2 in the appropriate range. Both criteria have proved extremely difficult to establish to date (56,57). Direct measurements of smooth muscle surface Po_2 in the working muscle (58,59), and of hemoglobin O_2 saturation within the arteriolar blood (60,61), have helped to clarify this issue. These measurements show that the smooth muscle Po_2 is high, in the range of 20–50 mmHg.

Two factors have made it difficult to extrapolate existing Po_2 measurements to the smooth muscle of the arterioles in situ. First, the perivascular Po_2 decreases along the length of the resistance vessels, due to the diffusion of O_2 into the surrounding parenchyma. The resulting longitudinal decrement in O_2 is evident, both as a reduction in Po_2 (62) and a reduction in hemoglobin O_2 saturation (61). A second complicating factor in the estimation of the arteriolar smooth muscle Po_2 is the existence of a radial gradient across the arteriolar wall, equivalent to a few millimeters of mercury. This radial gradient could, in principle, provide a signal by which altered striated muscle metabolism is coupled to altered smooth muscle Po_2 (62). Unfortunately, these data cannot be extrapolated to predict the smooth muscle Po_2 in situ, since there is some uncertainty regarding the diffusion coefficient, which will have a determining influence on the magnitude of the radial gradient. There are reports that the O_2 diffusion coefficient across the microvessel wall is both unex-pectedly high (63) and unexpectedly low (13,64), and the differences in the magnitudes of the estimates are large enough to produce substantial differences in the estimates of the magnitude of the radial gradient. Clearly this is a problem in need of additional experimental work.

Defining the reactivity of the arterioles to O_2 has also led to equivocal or conflicting results. Hypoxic vascular smooth muscle does relax, but as mentioned above, the smooth muscle of the arteriolar wall is not hypoxic under normal circumstances (58,59). Thus, the idea has developed that other oxidative processes might be involved.

Small arteries and arterioles in vitro are reported to relax when the O_2 is varied within ranges that are far above what should limit oxidative phosphorylation (56,65,66). Unfortunately, it is difficult to draw any firm conclusions as to the physiological significance of the in vitro observations, since the responses of the in vitro vessels appear to be somewhat different from those in situ, particularly with regard to their stability (56).

The molecular basis for the oxygen sensitivity of the vessel wall is unknown, but the Po_2 range over which it occurs makes it unlikely that oxidative phosphorylation is involved. The role of arachidonic acid metabolites has been explored, with conflicting results (67,68). Recently, the O_2 reactivity of the arterioles in situ has been linked to a lipoxygenase, but apparently to one in the tissue rather than to one in the vessel wall (56).

The other respiratory gas, CO_2, is usually thought to be a relatively weak dilator based on the effects of alterations in arterial Pco_2 (69–71). However, it may be of more significance when acting in combination with O_2 (72). Furthermore, lacking direct measurements of the arteriolar smooth muscle Pco_2, the magnitude of the CO_2 stimulus is very poorly defined.

Reactivity to CO_2 is almost always tested by varying arterial CO_2, and substantial underestimation in the vascular smooth muscle CO_2 sensitivity may occur with such a diffusible gas. In most striated muscles, the arterioles and venules parallel one another down to levels of 20–100 μm, a pattern particularly striking in the heart (73). As a result, the effect of an alteration in the arterial level of CO_2 is likely to be damped as CO_2 diffuses from the arteriole either into the tissue or, by diffusive shunt, into the paralleling venules (73,74). To the degree that this happens, smooth muscle Pco_2 may be significantly lower than either arterial or venous Pco_2, and the sensitivity of the arterioles to CO_2 may be underestimated.

Lactate and Acetate

Most of the products or intermediates of oxidation either are poor dilators or are not released from muscles. Lactate ion itself is not a potent dilator, but the H^+ that usually accompanies its release is sufficiently potent to play a small role in striated muscle flow control (18,69). Acetate is released from working muscle and is a moderately potent dilator. Though not extensively studied, it might play a role in metabolic coupling (75).

Coupling Via ATP Hydrolysis

Adenosine

Adenosine typifies a class of dilators whose production is directly tied to tissue metabolic activity, and it is thus in an ideal position to couple flow and metabolism. Whereas the evidence for some role for adenosine is extensive, its exact quantitative importance remains in question (48,50,76,77). The strength of the adenosine hypothesis rests on the correlation between tissue adenosine levels and blood flow (48), but the correlation seems to depend on the tissue and the type of metabolic stress encountered. For example, blood flow and adenosine correlate strongly in the myocardium when it is subjected to beta-adrenoceptor stimulation, but the two variables are poorly coupled during elevated metabolic drive induced in the heart by paired pacing (78).

Because adenosine is a relatively labile molecule, the differences between concentrations at the smooth muscle surface and either venous blood or tissue samples may be large. In addition, a large component of intracellular adenosine artificially elevates estimates of interstitial concentration that are based on simple tissue samples (50,77). Furthermore, adenosine is rapidly taken up and degraded by endothelial cells, thus inducing major differences between either mean tissue or venous adenosine levels and the smooth muscle surface adenosine concentration (79–81). These facts have led to the development of involved sampling techniques for adenosine (82) and to complex arguments regarding the role of this substance in flow control (48,50,77). Recently, sophisticated analytical models have shown some promise in reconciling the diverse results (81).

Vascular reactivity to adenosine has also proved difficult to quantify appropriately. Adenosine reactivity increases along the vascular tree (83); as a result, if adenosine infusions are used to estimate *in vivo* reactivity, the averaged reactivity of all segments of the bed is measured, a value that is difficult to relate to the adenosine hypothesis. Furthermore, with a molecule that is metabolized so rapidly, and taken up by the endothelial cells so avidly, there is likely to be a great disparity between (a) its concentration in the ar-

terial and/or venous blood and (b) the concentration that actually reaches the smooth muscle cell.

ATP

The findings that suggest a role for ATP in the regulation of flow are less extensive than those for adenosine. ATP is a dilator and is released into the interstitium of working muscle (76). However, it has been argued that a large fraction of the ATP which is released originates in damaged tissue and would thus not be part of a normal regulatory process (84).

Inorganic Phosphate

Inorganic phosphate is a direct product of ATP hydrolysis and has been proposed as a mediator of striated muscle blood flow. Although it is released by working muscles, it has not been shown to be a particularly powerful dilator and thus probably contributes minimally to functional hyperemia (85).

Osmolality

The total solute concentration in the venous blood rises during muscle work (86). Furthermore, hypertonic solutions produce modest dilations (54,87). Thus, the hypertonicity produced by muscle work is likely to be a small but significant contributor to functional hyperemia, perhaps more in the transient state than in the steady state (71).

Is the Whole Greater than the Sum of the Parts?

Implicit in the design of many of the experiments on local control is the search for a particular mediator. In view of the large number of agents that have been shown to partially fulfill this role of mediator, it is conceivable that the problem of flow control has been solved. Simultaneous addition of mediators may lead to multiplicative, rather than additive, responses (87). Although this is not a particularly elegant outcome to the search, perhaps a careful study of the aggregate effects of all of the mediator candidates based on modern nonlinear systems analysis will clarify many of the quantitative issues in the field.

INTEGRATION OF VASOMOTOR RESPONSES

Importance of Distributed Vascular Resistance

In most striated muscles there is no single class of "resistance vessels," but rather a set of resistances distributed over several vessel branch orders, beginning with vessels of a few hundred microns in diameter and continuing into the capillaries (88,89). The consequence of this pattern of distributed resistance is that the control of blood flow may reside in vessels which are several centimeters or more away from a metabolically active tissue element.

A purely local response to a metabolic stimulus— that is, one in which metabolite production leads to the dilation of a microvessel segment immediately adjacent to an active parenchymal cell—can be shown to occur (58). However, in an intact system, with significant resistances in proximal and distal vascular segments, the effect of a change in arteriolar resistance will be strongly influenced by the distant vascular segments. This raises the need for the *conducted* and *flow-dependent* vasomotor phenomena, mechanisms which are described below and which can convert an isolated, metabolically induced vasodilation of an arteriole into a coordinated flow response that matches blood flow and metabolism.

Conducted Vasomotor Response

Elements comprising the arteriolar wall have been shown to be electrically (90), chemically (91), and functionally coupled (92). As a result, a metabolically induced dilation originating in a restricted vessel segment (58) can spread bidirectionally along the longitudinal axis of the vessel from the site of origin, with a length constant of approximately 2 mm (92). In addition, responses may spread from arteriole to venule (93).

This spread of vasomotor response has two effects. First, a sufficiently large vascular segment is dilated to produce an overall decrease in microvessel resistance, and thereby an increase in blood flow within the limited portion of the muscle supplied by the vessel. Second, the conducted vasomotor response contributes to flow homogeneity by inducing a metabolically related vasomotor response in more proximal segments of the vascular bed which might be out of the range of influence of the dilator metabolite. The response propagates into both the parent vessel and some portion of the adjacent daughter vessels arranged in parallel with the vessel in which the response originated. The result of this network connectivity is a more homogeneous functional dilation than might otherwise occur (92).

Flow-Dependent Dilation

The conducted vasomotor response has a length constant of approximately 2 mm; thus, vasomotor responses initiated at a particular site in a tissue can extend their influence over several millimeters. However, because of the distributed nature of vascular resistance, vessel segments many millimeters to many centimeters from the site of initiation of a local dilation must also respond to achieve the maximal blood flow of which the muscle is capable (94,95). A key element in integrating the function of these more proximal vessels into the overall local metabolic response is flow-dependent dilation.

When striated muscle is stimulated, the blood flow is augmented initially by local events; after a brief delay, the blood flow is further augmented by dilation of the feed arteries supplying the tissue dilate, even though these vessels would appear to be well beyond the influence of either vasodilator metabolites or conducted vasomotor responses (96–99). This secondary dilation of the feed vessels is independent of alteration in intravascular pressure and is apparently due to the effects of blood-induced shear stress on the endothelial cell surface (31,97,100), perhaps by a direct effect on the membrane potential (34). The process has been demonstrated in a wide range of vessel sizes, including resistance vessels (31,101).

The physiological significance of flow-dependent dilation remains to be shown, however, since it is inherently a positive feedback process. Increase of flow in a vessel, for whatever reason, would lead to flow-dependent dilation, a further increase in flow, and so on, until maximal dilation had been achieved. Because maximal dilation is not the inevitable result of any dilator stimulus, other forces must contravene (60). It is noteworthy in this regard that the myogenic response is also a positive feedback process, but with opposite sign. Also, the metabolic feedback mechanisms discussed previously are all negative feedback systems and would tend to dampen the positive feedback signals induced by either the flow-dependent or the myogenic response.

SUMMARY

The intrinsic control of striated muscle blood flow must be viewed in broader terms than has been the case in the past. First, inherent in the fact that resistance to flow is widely distributed along the vascular axis is a need for a consideration of flow control from a broad perspective. The entire vascular axis must be viewed as an integrated functional unit, rather than being viewed in terms of an isolated release of a dilator which acts solely on the smooth muscle in the immediate vicinity (the more common perception).

The integration of the local, conducted, and flow-dependent dilator mechanisms may take place as follows. First, activation of a striated muscle motor unit leads to production of dilators and reduction in tissue oxygen tension. These phenomena lead to a local vasodilation and trigger a conducted response that spreads, in a decremental fashion, several millimeters beyond the active motor units of the striated muscle. These two processes (i.e., direct local effects and conducted vasomotor responses) serve to distribute flow within muscle and thereby ensure a relatively homogeneous supply-to-demand ratio within the tissue and allow modification of distribution with minimal change in flow. As muscle demands become greater, and larger numbers of motor units are involved, the locally initiated increases in flow cause rising wall shear stress in the intermediate-sized vessels, which induces flow-dependent vasodilation and ultimately the maximal blood flow that the basic morphology of the vasculature allows (94,95).

ACKNOWLEDGMENTS

This work was supported by USPHS grants HL-12792 and HL-19242.

REFERENCES

1. Blomqvist C, Saltin B. Cardiovascular adaptations to physical training. *Annu Rev Physiol* 1983;45:169–189.
2. Langille BL, O'Donnell F. Reductions in arterial diameter produced by chronic decreases in blood flow are endothelium-dependent. *Science* 1986;231:405–407.
3. Hudlicka I, Airman T, Heilig A, Leberer E, Tyler KR, Pette D. Effects of different patterns of long-term stimulation on blood flow, fuel uptake and enzyme activities in rabbit fast skeletal muscles. *Pflügers Arch* 1984;402:306–311.
4. Saltin B, Gollnick P. Skeletal muscle adaptability: significance for metabolism and performance. In: Peachy LD, ed. *Handbook of physiology, Section 10: Skeletal muscle*. Bethesda, MD: American Physiological Society, 1983;555–631.
5. Belloni F, Phair R, Sparks H. The role of adenosine in prolonged vasodilation following flow-restricted exercise of canine skeletal muscle. *Circ Res* 1979;44:759–766.
6. Folkow B, Hlicka H. A comparison between "red" and "white" muscle with respect to blood supply, capillary surface area and oxygen uptake during rest and exercise. *Microvasc Res* 1968;1:1–14.
7. Knabb R, Ely S, Bacchus A, Rubio R, Berne R. Consistent parallel relationships among myocardial oxygen consumption, coronary blood flow, and pericardial infusate adenosine concentration with various interventions and α-blockade in the dog. *Circ Res* 1983;53:33–41.
8. Granger H, Goodman A, Granger D. Role of resistance and exchange vessels in local microvascular control of skeletal muscle oxygenation in the dog. *Circ Res* 1976;38:379–385.
9. Klitzman B, Damon DN, Gorczynski RJ, Duling BR. Augmented tissue oxygen supply during striated muscle contraction in the hamster. Relative contributions of capillary recruitment, functional dilation, and reduced tissue P_{O_2}. *Circ Res* 1982; 51:711–721.
10. Gayeski TE, Connett RJ, Honig CR. Oxygen transport in rest-work transition illustrates new functions for myoglobin. *Am J Physiol* 1985;248:H914–H921.
11. Proctor K, Damon D, Duling B. Tissue P_{O_2} and arteriolar responses to metabolic stimuli during maturation of striated muscle. *Am J Physiol* 1981;241:H325–H331.
12. Schubert R, Whalen W, Nair P. Myocardial P_{O_2} distribution:

relationship to coronary autoregulation. *Am J Physiol* 1978; 234:H361–H370.
13. Gayeski TE, Honig CR. O_2 gradients from sarcolemma to cell interior in red muscle at maximal V_{O_2}. *Am J Physiol* 1986; 251:H789–H799.
14. Tyml K. Capillary recruitment and heterogeneity of microvascular flow in skeletal muscle before and after contraction. *Microvasc Res* 1986;32:84–98.
15. Lindbom L, Arfors KE. Non-homogeneous blood flow distribution in the rabbit tenuissimus muscle. Differential control of total blood flow and capillary perfusion. *Acta Physiol Scand* 1984;122:225–233.
16. Renkin EM. Control of microcirculation and blood–tissue exchange. In: Renkin EM, Michel CC, eds. *Handbook of physiology, Section 2: The cardiovascular system, vol IV—Microcirculation, Part 2*. Bethesda, MD: American Physiological Society, 1984;627–688.
17. Klitzman B, Duling B. Microvascular hematocrit and red cell flow in resting and contracting striated muscle. *Am J Physiol* 1979;237:H481–H490.
18. Shepherd JT. Circulation to skeletal muscle. In: Shepherd JT, Abboud FM, eds. *Handbook of physiology, Section 2: The cardiovascular system, vol III—Peripheral circulation and organ blood flow, Part 1*. Bethesda, MD: American Physiological Society, 1983;319–370.
19. Rowell LB. *Human circulation during physical stress*. New York: Oxford University Press, 1986;416.
20. McGilvery RW, Murray TW. Calculated equilibria of phosphocreatine and adenosine phosphates during utilization of high energy phosphate by muscle. *J Biol Chem* 1974;249:5845–5850.
21. Wilson D, Erecinska M, Drown C, Silver I. The oxygen dependence of cellular energy metabolism. *Arch Biochem Biophys* 1979;195:485–493.
22. Duling B. Oxygen, metabolism, and microcirculatory control. In: Kaley G, Altura BM, eds. *Microcirculation, vol II*. Baltimore: University Park Press, 1978;401–429.
23. Hayaishi O, ed. *Molecular mechanisms of oxygen activation*. New York: Academic Press, 1974;678.
24. Mellander S, Johansson B. Control of resistance, exchange, and capacitance functions in the peripheral circulation. *Pharmacol Rev* 1968;20:117–196.
25. Jackson PA, Duling BR. Myogenic response and wall mechanics of arterioles. *Am J Physiol* 1989;257:1147–1155.
26. Meininger G, Trzeciakowski J. Vasoconstriction is amplified by autoregulation during vasoconstrictor-induced hypertension. *Am J Physiol* 1988;254:H709–H718.
27. Borgstrom P, Gestrelius S. Integrated myogenic and metabolic control of vascular tone in skeletal muscle during autoregulation of blood flow. *Microvasc Res* 1987;33:353–376.
28. Johnson P. The myogenic response. In: Bohr DF, Somlyo AP, Sparks HV, eds. *Handbook of physiology, Section 2: Cardiovascular physiology, vol II—Vascular smooth muscle*. Bethesda, MD: American Physiological Society, 1980;409–442.
29. Johansson B, Mellander S. Static and dynamic components in the vascular myogenic response to passive changes in length as revealed by electrical and mechanical recordings from the rat portal vein. *Circ Res* 1975;36:76–83.
30. Lombard JH, Chenoweth JL, Stekiel WJ. Nonneural vascular smooth muscle tone in arterioles of the hamster cheek pouch. *Microvasc Res* 1985;29:81–88.
31. Bevan J. Basal tone in resistance arteries: role of wall stretch, flow, and receptor specialization. In: Bevan JA, Majewski H, Maxwell RA, Story DF, eds. *Vascular neuroeffector mechanisms*. Washington, DC: IRL Press, 1988;1–14.
32. Rubanyi GM. Endothelium-dependent pressure-induced contraction of isolated canine carotid arteries. *Am J Physiol* 1988; 255:H783–H788.
33. Harder D. Pressure induced myogenic activation of cat cerebral arteries is dependent on an intact endothelium. *Circ Res* 1987;60:102–107.
34. Olesen S-P, Clapham DE, Davies PF. Haemodynamic shear stress activates a K^+ current in vascular endothelial cells. *Nature* 1988;331:168–170.

35. Sachs F. Baroreceptor mechanisms at the cellular level. *Fed Proc* 1987;46:12–16.

36. Harder DR. Pressure-dependent membrane depolarization in cat middle cerebral artery. *Circ Res* 1984;55:197–202.

37. Kirber M, Singer J, Walsh J. Stretch-activated channels in freshly dissociated smooth muscle cells. *Biophysics J* 1987; 51:252A.

38. Laher I, Van Breemen C, Bevan JA. Stretch-dependent calcium uptake associated with myogenic tone in rabbit facial vein. *Circ Res* 1988;63:669–772.

39. Mohrman D, Sparks H. Myogenic hyperemia following brief tetanus of canine skeletal muscle. *Am J Physiol* 1974;227:531–535.

40. Yanagisawa M, Inoue A, Ishikawa T, et al. Primary structure, synthesis, and biological activity of rat endothelin, an endothelium-derived vasoconstrictor peptide. *Proc Natl Acad Sci USA* 1988;85:6964–6967.

41. Clarke JG, Benjamin S, Larkin SW, Webb DG, Davies GJ, Maseri A. Endothelin is a potent long-lasting vasoconstrictor in men. *Am J Physiol* 1989;257:H2033–H2035.

42. Minkes RK, Kadowitz P. Influence of endothelin on systemic pressure and regional flow in the cat. *Eur J Pharmacol* 1989; 163:163–166.

43. Fleming BP. Innervation of the microcirculation. *J Reconstr Microsurg* 1988;4:237–240.

44. Hammer M, Skagen K. Effects of small changes of plasma vasopressin on subcutaneous and skeletal muscle blood flow in man. *Acta Physiol Scand* 1986;127:67–73.

45. Schmid P, Sharabi F, Phillips M. Peptides and blood vessels. In: Shepherd JT, Abboud FM, eds. *Handbook of physiology, Section 2: The cardiovascular system, vol III—Peripheral circulation and organ blood flow, Part 2.* Bethesda, MD: American Physiological Society, 1983;815–836.

46. Thompson LP, Mohrman DE. Blood flow and oxygen consumption in skeletal muscle during sympathetic stimulation. *Am J Physiol* 1983;245:66–71.

47. Shepherd JT, Vanhoutte PM. Local modulation of adrenergic neurotransmission in blood vessels. *J Cardiovasc Pharmacol* 1985;7(Suppl 3):167–178.

48. Berne RM, Rubio R. Coronary circulation. In: Berne RM, Sperelakis N, Geiger SR, eds. *Handbook of physiology, Section 2: The cardiovascular system, vol I—The heart.* Bethesda, MD: American Physiological Society, 1979;873–952.

49. Hudlicka O. Regulation of muscle blood flow. *Clin Physiol* 1985;5:201–229.

50. Olsson RA, Bugni W. Coronary circulation. In: Fozzard HA, ed. *The heart and cardiovascular system.* New York: Raven Press, 1986;987–1037.

51. Sparks H. Effect of local metabolic factors on vascular smooth muscle. In: Bohr DF, Somlyo AP, Sparks HV, eds. *The handbook of physiology, Section 2: The cardiovascular system, vol II—Vascular smooth muscle.* Bethesda, MD: American Physiological Society, 1980;475–513.

52. Duling B. Effects of potassium ion on the microcirculation of the hamster. *Circ Res* 1975;37:325–332.

53. Kjellmer I. The potassium ion as a vasodilator during vascular exercise. *Acta Physiol Scand* 1965;63:460–468.

54. Overbeck H, Molnar J, Haddy F. Resistance to blood flow through the vascular bed of the dog forelimb: local effects of sodium, potassium, calcium, magnesium, acetate, hypertonicity, and hypotonicity. *Am J Cardiol* 1961;8:533–541.

55. Mohrman D, Sparks H. Role of potassium ions in the vascular response to a brief tetanus. *Circ Res* 1974;35:384–390.

56. Jackson WF. Arteriolar oxygen reactivity: where is the sensor? *Am J Physiol* 1987;253:H1120–H1126.

57. Pittman RN. Influence of oxygen lack on vascular smooth muscle contraction. In: Vanhoutte PM, Leusen MD, eds. *Vasodilatation.* New York: Raven Press, 1981;181–192.

58. Gorczynski R, Duling B. Role of oxygen in arteriolar functional vasodilation in hamster striated muscle. *Am J Physiol* 1978; 235:H505–H515.

59. Lash JM, Bohlen HG. Perivascular and tissue P_{O_2} in contracting rat spinotrapezius muscle. *Am J Physiol* 1987;252:H1192–H1202.

60. Hester RL, Duling BR. Red cell velocity during functional hyperemia: implications for rheology and oxygen transport. *Am J Physiol* 1988;255:236–244.

61. Kuo L, Pittman RN. Effect of hemodilution on oxygen transport in arteriolar networks of hamster striated muscle. *Am J Physiol* 1988;254:H331–H339.

62. Duling B. Changes in microvascular diameter and oxygen tension induced by carbon dioxide. *Circ Res* 1973;32:370–376.

63. Popel AS, Pittman RN, Ellsworth ML. Rate of oxygen loss from arterioles is an order of magnitude higher than expected. *Am J Physiol* 1989;256:921–924.

64. Rose CP, Goresky CA. Limitations of tracer oxygen uptake in the canine coronary circulation. *Circ Res* 1985;56:57–71.

65. Busse R, Pohl U, Kellner C, Klemm U. Endothelial cells are involved in the vasodilatory response to hypoxia. *Pflügers Arch* 1983;397:78–80.

66. Pohl U, Dezsi L, Simon B, Busse R. Selective inhibition of endothelium-dependent dilation in resistance-sized vessels *in vivo. Am J Physiol* 1987;253:H234–H239.

67. Busse R, Forstermann U, Matsuda H, Pohl U. The role of prostaglandins in the endothelium-mediated vasodilatory response to hypoxia. *Pflügers Arch* 1984;401:77–83.

68. Jackson WF. Prostaglandins do not mediate arteriolar oxygen reactivity. *Am J Physiol* 1986;250:H1102–H1108.

69. Daugherty R Jr, Scott J, Dabney J, Haddy F. Local effects of O_2 and CO_2 on limb, renal and coronary vascular resistances. *Am J Physiol* 1967;213:1102–1110.

70. Gaebelein CJ, Ladd CM. Blood flow, P_{O_2}, P_{CO_2} and pH during progressive working contractions in a whole muscle group. *Eur J Appl Physiol* 1986;54:638–642.

71. Mohrman DE. Lack of influence of potassium or osmolality on steady-state exercise hyperemia. *Am J Physiol* 1982;242:H949–H954.

72. Mohrman DE, Regal RR. Relation of blood flow to V_{O_2}, P_{O_2}, and P_{CO_2} in dog gastrocnemius muscle. *Am J Physiol* 1988; 255:H1004–H1010.

73. Bassingthwaighte JB, Yipintsoi T, Knopp TJ. Diffusional arteriovenous shunting in the heart. *Microvasc Res* 1984;28:233–253.

74. Pittman R, Duling B. Effects of altered carbon dioxide tension on hemoglobin oxygenation in hamster cheek pouch microvessels. *Microvasc Res* 1977;13:211–224.

75. Steffen RP, McKenzie JE, Bockman EL, Haddy FJ. Changes in dog gracilis muscle adenosine during exercise and acetate infusion. *Am J Physiol* 1983;244:387–395.

76. Forrester T. Adenosine or adenosine triphosphate. In: Vanhoutte PM, Leusen I, eds. *Vasodilatation.* New York: Raven Press, 1981;205–229.

77. Schrader J, Deussen A. Free cytosolic adenosine sensitively signals myocardial hypoxia. In: Acker H, ed. *Oxygen sensing in tissues.* Berlin: Springer-Verlag, 1988;165–176.

78. Manfredi J, Sparks H. Adenosine's role in coronary vasodilation induced by atrial pacing and norepinephrine. *Am J Physiol* 1982;243:H536–H545.

79. Kroll K, Kelm MK, Burrig KF, Schrader J. Transendothelial transport and metabolism of adenosine and inosine in the intact rat aorta. *Circ Res* 1989;64:1147–1157.

80. Nees S, Herzog V, Becker BF, Bock M, Des Rosiers C, Gerlach E. The coronary endothelium: a highly active metabolic barrier for adenosine. *Basic Res Cardiol* 1985;80:515–529.

81. Wangler RD, Gorman MW, Wang CY, DeWitt DF, Chan IS, Bassingthwaighte JB, Sparks HV. Transcapillary adenosine transport and interstitial adenosine concentration in guinea pig hearts. *Am J Physiol* 1989;257:89–106.

82. Gidday JM, Hill HE, Rubio R, Berne RM. Estimates of left ventricular interstitial fluid adenosine during catecholamine stimulation. *Am J Physiol* 1988;254:H207–H216.

83. Harder DR, Belardinelli L, Sperelakis N, Rubio R, Berne RM. Differential effects of adenosine and nitroglycerin on the action potentials of large and small coronary arteries. *Circ Res* 1979; 44:176–182.

84. Bockman EL, Berne RM, Rubio R. Release of adenosine and lack of release of ATP from contracting skeletal muscle. *Pflügers Arch* 1975;355:229–241.

85. Hudlicka O, El Khelly F. Metabolic factors involved in regulation of muscle blood flow. *J Cardiovasc Pharmacol* 1985;7(Suppl 3):59–72.
86. Mellander S, Lundvall J. Role of tissue hyperosmolality in exercise hyperemia. *Circ Res* 1971;28 & 29(Suppl 1):I39–I45.
87. Skinner N Jr, Costin J. Interactions of vasoactive substances in exercise hyperemia: O_2, K^+, and osmolality. *Am J Physiol* 1970;219:1386–1392.
88. Bohlen H, Gore R, Hutchins P. Comparison of microvascular pressures in normal and spontaneously hypertensive rats. *Microvasc Res* 1977;13:125–130.
89. Chilian WM, Eastham CL, Marcus ML. Microvascular distribution of coronary vascular resistance in beating left ventricle. *Am J Physiol* 1986;251:H779–H788.
90. Hirst GD, Neild TO. An analysis of excitatory junctional potentials recorded from arterioles. *J Physiol* (*Lond*) 1978;280:87–104.
91. Sheridan J, Larson D. Junctional communication in the peripheral vasculature. In: Pitts JD, Finbow ME, eds. *Functional integration of cells in animal tissues*. British Society for Cell Biology Symposium 5. Cambridge, England: Cambridge University Press, 1982;263–283.
92. Segal SS, Damon DN, Duling BR. Propagation of vasomotor responses coordinates arteriolar resistances. *Am J Physiol* 1989;256:H832–H837.
93. Tigno XT, Ley K, Pries AR, Gaehtgens P. Venulo-arteriolar communication and propagated response. A possible mechanism for local control of blood flow. *Pflügers Arch* 1989;414:450–456.
94. Segal S, Duling B. Communication between feed arteries and microvessels in hamster cremaster muscle: segmental vascular responses are functionally coordinated. *Circ Res* 1986;59:283–290.
95. Rowell LB. Muscle blood flow in humans: how high can it go? *Med Sci Sports Exerc* 1988;20:97–103.
96. Holtz J, Forstermann U, Pohl U, Giesler M, Bassenge E. Flow-dependent, endothelium-mediated dilation of epicardial coronary arteries in conscious dogs: effects of cyclooxygenase inhibition. *J Cardiovasc Pharmacol* 1984;6:1161–1169.
97. Kaiser L, Sparks HV. Mediation of flow-dependent arterial dilation by endothelial cells. *Circ Shock* 1986;18:109–114.
98. Macho P, Hintze T, Vatner S. Regulation of large coronary arteries by increases in myocardial metabolic demands in conscious dogs. *Circ Res* 1981;49:594–599.
99. Pohl U, Holtz J, Busse R, Bassenge E. Crucial role of endothelium in the vasodilator response to increase flow *in vivo*. *Hypertension* 1986;8:37–44.
100. Bevan JA, Joyce EH, Wellman GC. Flow-dependent dilation in a resistance artery still occurs after endothelium removal. *Circ Res* 1988;63:980–985.
101. Smiesko V, Lang DJ, Johnson PC. Dilator response of rat mesenteric arterioles to increased blood velocity. *Am J Physiol* 1989;257:H1958–H1965.

THE LUNG: Scientific Foundations
edited by R.G. Crystal, J.B. West et al.
Raven Press, Ltd., New York © 1991.

CHAPTER 5.5.2.5

Heterogeneity of Blood Flow in Striated Muscle

M. Harold Laughlin

Although transcapillary diffusion from blood to tissue is the final step in oxygen transport from air to active muscle, convective transfer of oxygenated blood to, and appropriate distribution of blood among, skeletal-muscle capillaries is equally important. If blood flow and capillary exchange area are not matched, oxygen transport will be inadequate because of limitation of diffusion from blood to tissue. The relationship between capillary perfusion and capillary-exchange surface area in an organ is determined by the distribution of blood flow among the capillaries. Nonuniformity of blood-flow distribution among the exchange vessels of an organ (blood-flow heterogeneity) and/or other vascular heterogeneities can produce limitation of transport of oxygen and other small solutes (see Chapter 5.5.2.3). The purpose of this chapter is to summarize available information concerning (a) blood-flow heterogeneity in striated muscle and (b) the influence of blood-flow heterogeneity on O_2 transport to active striated muscle during normal locomotory exercise.

Discussion of blood-flow heterogeneity in muscle during exercise is preceded by (a) consideration of the types of blood-flow heterogeneity present in skeletal muscle and (b) definitions of terms to be used in this chapter. After discussion the magnitude and causes of blood-flow heterogeneity, the influence of blood-flow heterogeneity on oxygen transport to active muscle tissue is considered. Although data from many sources are incorporated in the discussion, the focus of this chapter is on blood flow to skeletal muscle during rhythmic dynamic exercise.

DEFINITION OF BLOOD-FLOW HETEROGENEITY

Nonuniformities of blood flow can be observed in the form of *spatial heterogeneity* (i.e., variations in flow among muscles or among regions within muscles, and/or flow variations among vessels within muscles or within regions of muscles) and/or in the form of *temporal heterogeneity* (i.e., variations in flow over time). The phrase "blood-flow heterogeneity" engenders different concepts among cardiorespiratory investigators (1) and is often associated with the techniques used to measure flow. This is because the type of blood-flow heterogeneity observed in a set of experiments is determined by the technique used to measure blood flow. Two general types of heterogeneity have been shown to exist in skeletal muscle under a variety of conditions: *gross blood-flow heterogeneity* and *microvascular blood-flow heterogeneity*. This chapter examines these two general types of blood-flow heterogeneity. The phrase "gross blood-flow heterogeneity" is used to refer to (a) differences in perfusion determined with techniques that measure flow to muscle groups, individual muscles, and/or bits of muscle of 0.2–1.0 g mass, expressed as volume flow per unit mass of tissue, and (b) differences in blood flow within and among muscles or in the distribution of cardiac output among tissues. The phrase "microvascular blood-flow heterogeneity" is used to refer to (a) variations in perfusion of microvessels recorded with *in vivo* microscopy (i.e., total inflow to a muscle is not distributed identically among the perfused vessels) and (b) variations in red blood cell (RBC) (and/or plasma) capillary transit times, velocities, and/or path lengths.

M. H. Laughlin: Departments of Veterinary Biomedical Sciences and Medical Physiology and Dalton Research Center, University of Missouri, Columbia, Missouri 65211.

GROSS BLOOD-FLOW HETEROGENEITY

Blood flow is not distributed uniformly among or within resting skeletal muscles (2–6). As will be discussed in detail below, this gross heterogeneity of blood flow seems to be due to the fact that blood flow in resting muscle is related to fiber-type composition of skeletal muscle (3,5). When skeletal muscles start to contract, due to electrical stimulation or initiation of exercise, blood-flow heterogeneity becomes more apparent and the causes of flow heterogeneity become more complex.

Figure 1 presents blood-flow data from the leg muscles of rats performing treadmill exercise at different speeds. These data demonstrate four examples of spatial blood-flow heterogeneity: (i) Blood flow varies among and within muscles before exercise [i.e., soleus flow is greater than all others, and flow in the red portion of the gastrocnemius (GR) is greater than flow in the white portion (GW)]; (ii) blood flow varies within and among muscles at all intensities of exercise; (iii) the relative amount of blood flow distributed to each muscle varies with exercise intensity; and (iv) flow varies among and within muscles as a function of exercise intensity. Similar results can be shown for thigh muscles of rats and in the extensor muscles of other species of mammal (2,7).

Muscle blood-flow distribution also changes with time during sustained treadmill exercise (8,9). For example, blood flows measured during the initial period of hyperemic responses often exceed the values measured later during sustained exercise (3,8). These variations in blood flow may be due to local metabolic and/or temperature effects or to changes in central hemodynamics. However, as discussed below, these influences seem to be superimposed upon the variations resulting from muscle-fiber-type composition, muscle fiber activity patterns, and mechanical factors.

DETERMINANTS OF GROSS BLOOD-FLOW HETEROGENEITY

Although a thorough accounting of the causes of blood-flow heterogeneity and the degree to which flow heterogeneity is physiologically modulated cannot be provided with the data presently available, some of the determinants of skeletal-muscle blood-flow heterogeneity have been established. The determinants of gross blood-flow heterogeneity include: (a) fiber-type composition of the muscle, (b) muscle fiber recruitment patterns within and among muscles, (c) mechanical factors associated with the type of contraction of the muscle (e.g., twitch contractions versus tetanic contractions) and the location of the muscle in relation to other muscles (i.e., deep versus superficial), and (d) vascular control mechanisms.

Muscle Fiber Type

Mammalian skeletal muscles are composed of fibers with different physiologic, morphologic, hemodynamic, and biochemical characteristics (10–12). Although it is clear that there is a continuum among fiber types for each characteristic, mammalian skeletal-muscle fibers can be divided into three general categories based upon contractile (often myofibrillar ATPase activity) and metabolic characteristics. One commonly used classification system is that proposed by Peter et al. (13). According to this system of nomenclature, the fibers are identified as slow-twitch oxidative (SO) (also known as type I), fast-twitch oxidative glycolytic (FOG) (also known as type IIa), and fast-twitch glycolytic (FG) (also known as type IIb). In general, the muscle fiber types are distributed within and among synergistic groups of extensor muscles in similar patterns in most mammalian species (9,14,15).

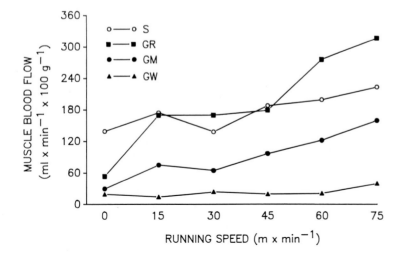

FIG. 1. Rat skeletal-muscle blood flow as a function of treadmill running speed. GR, GM, and GW are red, middle, and white portions of the gastrocnemius muscle, respectively, and S is the soleus muscle. (Data were taken from ref. 2.)

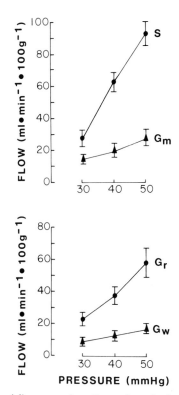

FIG. 2. Blood flow as a function of perfusion pressure in leg muscles of isolated, perfused rat hindquarters. Flows were measured during maximal papaverine vasodilation. S, soleus muscle; G_r, G_m, and G_w are red, middle, and white portions of the gastrocnemius muscle. Data are from Laughlin and Ripperger (19) and from unpublished data on groups of control rats. (From ref. 18.)

For example, the deepest muscle in an extensor muscle group is usually composed of a high proportion of SO fibers. The muscles adjacent to the deep SO muscles are usually composed of high proportions of SO and FOG fibers. In the remaining muscles of the group, the relative percentage of FOG fibers is seen to decrease as one goes from deep to superficial, whereas the percentage of FG fibers increases. The degree of stratification of fiber types among the muscles varies among species (14).

In studies of blood flow to resting and contracting skeletal muscle (*in situ*), it is common to observe a relationship between muscle fiber type and blood flow, with the red, high-oxidative muscles having higher blood flows (4,5,16). In addition, morphological evidence indicates that high-oxidative skeletal muscles (SO and FOG) have higher capillary densities (12,17). Thus, within a given species, the capacity of skeletal muscle for blood flow (expressed in ml/min/100 g) would be expected to be related to the fiber-type composition of the muscle. As shown in Fig. 2, we have found that blood flow to resting rat skeletal muscles during maximal papaverine-induced vasodilation is different in muscles composed of various fiber types

(18,19). Similarly, the highest blood flows attainable in rat skeletal muscles with treadmill exercise are linearly related to succinate dehydrogenase activity (oxidative capacity) of the muscles (3,7). These data indicate that one cause of muscle blood-flow heterogeneity within a muscle group, even with uniform vasodilator stimuli, is the relationship between muscle-fiber-type composition and blood-flow capacity of the skeletal-muscle vascular bed. Because of these factors, in the presence of maximal vasodilation, one would expect blood-flow distribution to be related to the distribution of fiber types within and among the muscles. This applies to a skeletal muscle or muscle group that is stimulated such that all fibers are active. Even if maximal exercise hyperemia is produced, blood flow will not be homogeneously distributed if the fiber-type composition of the muscle tissue is heterogeneous. Furthermore, in submaximal locomotory exercise gross blood-flow heterogeneity would be expected to be more extreme because the skeletal-muscle fibers are not uniformly activated to contract.

Muscle Fiber Recruitment Patterns

It is intuitively obvious that the most efficient method for O_2 transport to active muscle during exercise will result from increasing blood flow to the active skeletal muscles rather than increasing flow to all muscle tissue. This rationale predicts that, within a muscle that is not uniformly active during a bout of exercise, blood flow should be directed to the active muscle fibers. The data presented in Fig. 1 support this notion in that blood flow seems to follow muscle fiber recruitment patterns both within and among muscles (2,3). Consider the changes in blood flow seen in the different portions of the gastrocnemius muscle when the rats went from rest to walking at 15 m/min (Fig. 1). Blood flow increased to the red portion of the gastrocnemius muscle (GR) and decreased to the superficial white portion (GW). Blood flow remained high in the soleus muscle when the rats started to walk at 15 m/min (Fig. 1). We know from the work of Armstrong et al. (20) and Sullivan and Armstrong (21) that the muscle fibers in the GR region of the rat are recruited at this intensity of exercise whereas those in the GW are not. Thus, just as there appears to be sympathetic vasoconstriction of the vascular beds in inactive skeletal muscles and muscle groups [i.e., the arms during leg exercise (22,23)], there also appears to be increased vascular resistance and decreased blood flow to inactive fibers (GW) within active muscles of rats during exercise. These data suggest that the increased blood flow associated with exercise is directed specifically to the active muscle fibers within and among the muscles. When rats run at 75 m/min, all of the muscle fibers of the ankle extensor muscles should be active (21). As predicted by this hypothesis, blood flow is increased to all muscle tissue (Fig. 1), with the blood flows being greatest in the more oxidative muscle tissue. The data in Fig. 1 illustrate the interactions of the effects of muscle-fiber-type composition and muscle-fiber recruitment patterns upon blood-flow distribution patterns. Skeletal-muscle blood-flow distribution patterns are also related to muscle fiber type, expected muscle fiber recruitment patterns, and time during exercise in (a) rats during swimming (24), (b) miniature swine during treadmill exercise (7), and (c) horses and cattle during treadmill exercise (*unpublished observations*).

Type of Contraction

If a skeletal muscle is stimulated so that a maximal sustained tetanic contraction is produced, blood flow will cease. A hyperemia will only be seen upon relaxation of the tetanus [postexercise hyperemia (4)]. Although increases in time-averaged blood flow are observed with rhythmical twitch contractions and rhythmical tetanic contractions (5), the flow of arterial blood into the muscle is impeded during contraction whereas venous outflow occurs primarily during contraction (25). Thus, temporal blood-flow heterogeneity exists at all levels throughout the vascular beds of skeletal muscles during rhythmic contractions. Under these conditions the interactions among blood flow, the muscle's tension time index, and the time between contractions (diastole) are similar to those seen in the coronary circulation.

The magnitude of exercise hyperemia observed during muscle activity varies with the fiber-type composition of the muscle (5), in a manner that would be predicted from the blood-flow capacity measured in resting muscle as illustrated in Fig. 2. Thus, during uniform activation of a muscle group, the greatest flow is seen in the high-oxidative muscle tissue. In addition, the magnitude of the hyperemia varies with the type of contraction produced by the stimulation parameters. For example, Folkow and Halicka (16) compared the hyperemic responses to muscle contractions at various frequencies in the soleus (SO) and red gastrocnemius (FOG and FG) muscles of cats. They found that soleus blood flow increased linearly with frequency of stimulation up to frequencies of 6–8 Hz. At higher frequencies of stimulation, soleus flow was higher immediately after contraction stopped than during contraction. In the soleus muscle the highest flow recorded was 120 ml/min/g, measured after tetanic contraction. In the gastrocnemius muscle, as compared with the soleus, blood flow increased more rapidly as a function of increasing stimulation frequency. Peak blood flow for gastrocnemius muscle was about

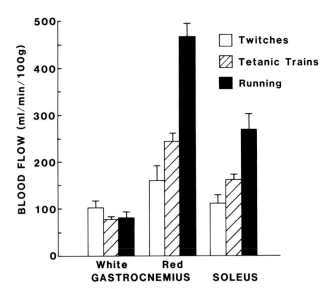

FIG. 3. Peak blood flow to three types of rat skeletal muscle during three different types of contractile activity. The data for muscles during twitch and tetanic stimulation conditions are from Mackie and Terjung (5), and those for running rats are from the 75-m/min running speeds of Laughlin and Armstrong (2). The blood-flow values for twitch-type stimulation were taken after 10 min of contraction, and those for tetanic stimulation were taken after 1 min of contraction (5). The perfusion pressure for all measurements was approximately 120 mmHg. (From ref. 18.)

50 ml/min/100 g for both twitch-type contractions and following tetanic contractions. These results demonstrated three differences between these two types of skeletal muscle: (i) SO muscle (soleus) had higher resting blood flow; (ii) SO muscle had a higher peak blood flow; and (iii) maximal blood flow was measured in the SO muscle between tetanic contractions, whereas the gastrocnemius muscle had similar peak flows following tetanic contractions and during twitch-type contractions.

The data presented in Fig. 3 are consistent with the notion that the magnitude of exercise hyperemia is related to the type of contractile activity performed by the muscles. Mackie and Terjung (5) determined stimulation parameters that produced the highest blood flow with each type of contraction. As can be seen in Fig. 3, twitch-type contractions produced greater blood flows than did tetanic trains or treadmill exercise in white gastrocnemius (85% FG fibers). In GR (30% SO, 60% FOG), blood flow was higher during rhythmic tetanic contractions than during twitch contractions, and locomotory exercise produced even higher blood flows than did tetanic contractions. Locomotory exercise also produced the highest blood flows in the soleus muscle. Thus, in high-oxidative skeletal muscle (SO and FOG), the type of muscle contraction performed determines the magnitude of the exercise hyperemia observed, whereas FG muscle appears to have similar peak flows during all types of rhythmic contractile activity.

Mechanical factors associated with the location of the muscle within muscle groups in relation to other muscles and/or to the pennation of the muscles may be responsible for the different effects of type of contraction on blood flow in the various types of muscle as illustrated in Fig. 3. These mechanical factors could affect blood flow in at least two ways: (i) increased resistance to blood flow as a result of mechanical interference during contraction or (ii) differences in the efficiency of the muscle pump in assisting perfusion of the muscle.

A sustained tetanic contraction stops blood flow by causing mechanical interference (26). During contraction, intramuscular pressure varies throughout muscles and muscle groups, with pressures being greatest deep in the muscle groups and lower in superficial areas (27,28). Some nonuniformity in blood-flow distribution may result from these variations in intramuscular pressure that would cause different degrees of interference with blood flow throughout the muscle. Mechanical effects of contraction may also be different in fusiform muscles (such as the soleus) as compared to pennate muscles (such as the gastrocnemius).

On the other hand, during rhythmic muscle activity the mechanical effects of muscle contraction upon veins combined with venous valves can counteract the mechanical interference with blood flow via the "muscle pump" effect. The increased intramuscular pressures generated by contraction of skeletal muscle result in compression of the veins, causing blood to flow out of the compressed segments. The venous valves and their orientation toward the heart allow blood to flow out of the compressed venous segments in only one direction. Rhythmical contractions cause a pumping action on the veins in that the kinetic energy imparted to the venous blood during muscle contraction causes blood to flow out of the veins during contraction (venous outflow); moreover, the vascular compartments are refilled from the capillaries and arteries during muscle relaxation (18,29,30). Thus, during rhythmic skeletal-muscle contractile activity, arterial inflow occurs during relaxation and venous outflow occurs during contraction, much as in the coronary circulation (18,25).

If we return to Fig. 3, it seems possible that the reason that muscle blood flows in high-oxidative muscle tissue are higher during rhythmic tetanic contraction (tetanic trains) than during twitch-type contraction is that the muscle pumping action during twitching is less efficient. It is also possible that the muscle pump is less effective in the white muscle tissue as a result of the superficial location of FG muscle (and the related lower tissue pressures during contraction) and/or

because the vascularity per gram of FG muscle is less. If one or both of these postulates are correct, lower muscle pump efficiency could be the reason that twitch contractions produce as much blood flow in white gastrocnemius muscle as do the other forms of contraction. These data suggest that any type of rhythmic muscle contraction can produce a similar amount of muscle pump contribution to perfusion in FG muscle. On the other hand, the data in Fig. 3 indicate that the situation is different for the high-oxidative muscle tissue. The SO and FOG muscle both appear to have peak blood flows during treadmill exercise. These higher flows may be partially the result of a more efficient muscle pumping action during normal muscle activity (18).

Blood-Flow Control

Chapter 5.5.2.4 discusses the control of blood flow in detail. Therefore, this chapter will only briefly focus on some examples of how flow control mechanisms can cause gross blood-flow heterogeneity. Although there is evidence that mechanisms for the control of vascular resistance vary as a function of skeletal-muscle fiber type, it is unlikely that the control mechanisms are totally different in different types of muscle. Rather, the relative importance of each control mechanism appears to differ among the vasculature in muscles composed of different fiber types. For example, considering central control of blood flow, the vasculature of SO muscle is less influenced by sympathetic alpha-adrenergic activity than is the vasculature of fast-twitch muscle (16,31–33), whereas fast muscles show greater vasodilation in response to epinephrine infusions (32).

Local control factors may also vary within and among skeletal muscles. For example, Mellander (34) has suggested that vascular resistance in muscles composed primarily of FG fibers may be influenced more by osmolarity than is vascular resistance in high-oxidative muscle, and Hilton et al. (35) proposed that K^+ may be an important factor in the control of blood flow in FG muscle but not in SO muscle. Also, we have found that dipyridamole produces decreases in vascular resistance in SO skeletal muscle and respiratory muscle of pigs during submaximal exercise but has no effect upon vascular resistance in fast-twitch skeletal-muscle tissue. These results suggest that SO and respiratory muscle release more adenosine during exercise than does fast skeletal muscle. In this regard, SO skeletal muscle and respiratory muscle appear similar to cardiac muscle (36).

Blood-flow heterogeneity within skeletal muscle cannot be completely explained by muscle fiber type, muscle fiber recruitment patterns, types of muscle contraction, and other mechanical effects. Piiper et al. (6) have shown that considerable blood-flow heterogeneity exists within resting and uniformly stimulated dog gastrocnemius muscle. Pendergast et al. (37) have reported similar amounts of heterogeneity within several skeletal muscles of dogs during treadmill exercise. The blood-flow heterogeneity described by these studies (6,37) does not appear to be related to muscle fiber type, recruitment order, or other known functional parameters. Also, considerable blood-flow heterogeneity has been demonstrated in the coronary vascular bed where the muscle is relatively uniform in composition, recruitment, and anatomical characteristics (38,39).

In conclusion, established sources of spatial heterogeneity within and among skeletal muscles include variations in (a) muscle-fiber-type composition, (b) vascularization and blood-flow capacity of the muscle, (c) muscle-fiber-type distribution patterns, (d) type of muscle construction (i.e., fusiform versus pennate muscles), and (e) location of the muscle within muscle groups. All of these structural sources of heterogeneity in skeletal muscle can influence blood flow and its distribution. Functional determinants of blood flow are superimposed upon the structural sources of blood-flow heterogeneity, including neural–humoral control mechanisms, local metabolic control mechanisms, and both temporal and spatial variations in muscle fiber activity patterns. Because of these factors (and perhaps other unknown factors), blood flow is normally distributed within and among skeletal muscles in a heterogeneous manner.

MICROVASCULAR BLOOD-FLOW HETEROGENEITY

The energy required for the transport of blood throughout the body is provided by the heart. Since the cardiovascular system of most mammals has a measurable maximal cardiac output, the cardiovascular system appears to be designed so that the needs of the body are met with a minimal amount of blood flow (cardiac output) (40). During exercise, oxygen consumption of the tissues of the body (in particular, within and among skeletal muscles) is not uniform. Therefore, a heterogeneous distribution of blood flow is the most efficient manner to transport the required amount of oxygen to a heterogeneous mass of muscle. Thus, gross blood-flow heterogeneity is not necessarily an indication of poor vascular function. In contrast, perfusion heterogeneity among exchange vessels resulting in poor matching between perfusion and exchange capacity is believed to cause limited transport of small solutes under many circumstances (1,38,41). Therefore an appreciation of the importance of blood-flow heterogeneity on oxygen transport requires the consideration of blood-flow heterogeneity at the microcirculatory level within muscles (and/or within the muscle samples).

Evidence that microvascular blood-flow heterogeneity exists under a variety of conditions has been obtained with several techniques, including indicator dilution, *in vivo* microscopy, and *in vitro* histological examination (42–49). The definition of microvascular blood-flow heterogeneity also varies among investigators, depending upon (a) the techniques used to investigate perfusion and (b) the interests of the investigator. Indeed, there is controversy about the definition of a perfused capillary. Honig et al. (44) define a perfused capillary as any capillary containing RBCs, whereas others define a perfused capillary as a capillary in which plasma and/or RBC movement is observed (42–44). Since our focus is on oxygen transport, in this chapter a perfused capillary is considered to be a capillary that contains moving RBCs.

Microvascular heterogeneity can be estimated from measurements of RBC and/or plasma velocity through individual exchange vessels. Perhaps the simplest example of microvascular blood-flow heterogeneity is the fact that both perfused and nonperfused capillaries can be observed in resting skeletal muscle. In fact, many capillaries are not perfused in resting skeletal muscle. Vasomotion has also been observed in resting muscle, so that the capillaries that are perfused or nonperfused change as a function of time. Furthermore, patterns of RBC flow in the perfused capillaries of resting skeletal muscle reveal variations in RBC velocities, total RBC fluxes, RBC transit times, and RBC path lengths (48,50,51). Damon and Duling (42) have shown that the number of RBCs per length of capillary varies not only in capillaries with RBC movement (flow) but in capillaries with no RBC movement as well.

Indicator dilution experiments also indicate that blood flow is not uniformly distributed in resting skeletal muscle (41,46,47). The pattern of venous outflow of intravascular indicators is influenced by the distribution of transit times through the large arteries and veins as well as by the distribution of capillary blood flows. Although indicator dilution data contain information about the degree of both gross blood-flow heterogeneity and microvascular blood-flow heterogeneity, the data can only be correctly interpreted if the curves can be deconvoluted to allow separation of these (gross and microvascular) effects (38,41). If experiments are carefully designed and appropriate models are applied, indicator dilution techniques can be used to study microvascular blood-flow heterogeneity at the whole-organ level (38,41).

EFFECTS OF MICROVASCULAR BLOOD-FLOW HETEROGENEITY ON OXYGEN TRANSPORT

The microcirculatory parameters that are known to show heterogeneity and that are most likely to have a significant impact on oxygen transport include: RBC transit time through the portion of the vascular bed that allows exchange; the number of RBCs per length of capillary; the relationship between RBC transit time and surface area available for gas exchange; microvascular oxygen content; and functional capillary density. If the exchange surface area is heterogeneously distributed, a matched, heterogeneous distribution of blood flow and RBC transit times would be most efficient for oxygen transport (efficient in that the largest amount of O_2 can be transported with the smallest amount of blood flow). Capillaries with the greatest exchange surface area should receive relatively greater flow (41,52). Thus, as is true for gross blood-flow heterogeneity, the presence of microvascular blood-flow heterogeneity is not necessarily a sign of poor vascular function.

RBC transit time is determined by both capillary length and by the route RBCs take through the bed (path length). If an RBC goes through branches or cross-connections between capillaries, its transit time and the capillary surface area to which the cell is exposed will be increased as compared to transit directly through the shortest path. Sarelius (50) painstakingly followed RBCs as they were carried through skeletal muscle microvascular beds and determined RBC path lengths. She found that the paths taken by RBCs as they pass through a branching capillary network in muscle are nonuniform. Furthermore, she determined that the mean RBC path length is longer than would be predicted from anatomical measurements of capillary lengths and capillary RBC velocities, and that measured RBC mean transit times are longer than capillary mean transit times estimated from the combination of indicator dilution techniques and histological estimates of capillarization. Indeed, Sarelius's measured RBC transit times (2–3 sec) indicate that exchange-vessel transit time may be an order of magnitude greater than the minimal time required for unloading O_2 from the RBC (50).

The location of the primary O_2 exchange area in the microvascular bed may also change as a function of total flow and/or RBC velocity. Under low flow conditions (resting muscle), some gas exchange occurs in the precapillary vessels (43,53). During intense exercise, the increased flux of blood through the vascular bed and decreased capillary transit times result in very little O_2 exchange at the precapillary level. Thus, the location within the microcirculation where gas exchange occurs will change with flow so that as flow increases, the region over which O_2 exchange occurs moves further toward the venous end of the exchange vessels.

CAUSES OF MICROVASCULAR BLOOD-FLOW HETEROGENEITY

The cause and potential controlling factors for microvascular blood-flow heterogeneity are currently of intense interest in the microcirculatory field. As with gross blood-flow heterogeneity, the causes of microvascular blood-flow heterogeneity can be divided into functional and anatomical elements.

Functional Control of Flow Distribution

Although vasomotion is commonly observed in resting striated muscle, the mechanisms responsible for vasomotion in the microcirculation and the control of capillary perfusion heterogeneity have yet to be established. Recruitment (perfusion) of nonperfused (or underperfused) exchange vessels appears to occur in association with the hyperemia observed at the initiation of exercise (44,54). This results in an increase in both (a) total blood flow to the muscle and (b) surface area available for transcapillary exchange. Control of capillary perfusion is generally considered to be located in the terminal arterioles (42–44,53,55). Honig et al. (44) proposed that vasomotor control of the density of perfused capillaries in skeletal muscle is an all-or-none type of control at the start of muscle contraction. They proposed that when a terminal arteriole dilates, all the capillaries located downstream are perfused. This conclusion was based upon (a) measurements of the number of capillaries containing RBCs in dog gracilis muscles quick-frozen under various conditions *in situ* and (b) the resulting definition of a perfused capillary as any capillary containing RBCs (44). As a result, considerable variation in RBC velocity, path length, etc., would not be detected with this method for the study of control of microvascular exchange area. The observations of Honig et al. (44) are consistent with the idea that vasodilation of skeletal-muscle vascular beds produces increased blood flow, increased functional capillary exchange area, and less spatial capillary flow heterogeneity (in that some unperfused capillaries become perfused).

The notion that the recruitment of unperfused capillaries (capillaries without RBCs and/or with nonmoving RBCs) resulting from vasodilation will result in less capillary flow heterogeneity is not uncommon (1,39,52,54). For example, Tyml (49) measured mean RBC velocity in capillary networks and found that the distribution of RBC velocities changed following contraction in frog skeletal muscle. However, there is also evidence that microvascular heterogeneity of blood flow is not altered by vasodilation or during active hyperemia.

Microvascular blood-flow heterogeneity may be as great in resting skeletal muscle as in vasodilated or active muscle (1,51). For example, Sarelius (50) reported that although adenosine-induced vasodilation caused a shift in the distribution of RBC mean transit times in mammalian striated muscle, neither RBC path lengths nor the distribution of RBC path lengths changed during vasodilation. In an in-depth analysis of the question of the potential control of microvascular blood-flow heterogeneity, Duling and Damon (1) found that the coefficient of variation (SD/mean) of RBC velocities in capillaries of striated muscles remains relatively constant over a sevenfold range of mean RBC velocities (see Table 2 of ref. 1). Table 2 of Duling and Damon's article (1) also documents the importance of distinguishing between absolute and relative dispersions of flow. That is, standard deviation of RBC velocity was related to mean RBC velocity, whereas the coefficient of variation was not. Duling and Damon (1) concluded that the increase in standard deviation of RBC velocity seen with increased capillary RBC velocity was predominantly the result of increased total flow through the muscle, not due to a change in the distribution of flow among the vessels.

If the vascular beds of muscle tissue consist of a large number of microvascular units composed of groups of capillaries connected to a single arteriole and if blood-flow heterogeneity within these vascular units is similar from one unit to the next, then microvascular blood-flow heterogeneity would be similar among various levels of vascular tone and levels of capillary recruitment. This hypothesis is attractive because it provides an explanation of the observation that microvascular blood-flow heterogeneity does not change with vasodilation. Consistent with the hypothesis that microvascular units consist of several capillaries (potentially interconnecting) in which blood flow is distributed in a heterogeneous manner are the reports of Gorczynski et al. (55), Klitzman et al. (53), and Damon and Duling (42). In these studies, perfused capillaries and nonperfused capillaries were often supplied by the same terminal arteriole. Also, Sarelius (50) observed that hyperemia is associated with recruitment of new capillary networks in hamster cremaster muscle. Similarly, Damon and Duling (51) presented data demonstrating that capillary perfusion heterogeneity is not controlled and does not decrease with increases in blood flow produced by vasodilation in hamster tibialis anterior muscles. Rather, Damon and Duling's data (51) suggest that microvascular units recruited via vasodilation have dispersions of capillary blood flows

similar to the microvascular units perfused under resting conditions (prior to vasodilation).

Anatomical Factors

The capillary beds of striated muscles have variations in: capillary lengths; capillary volumes; cross-connections between capillaries; vessel tortuosity; capillary permeabilities; and the extravascular environment (56–58). These anatomical nonuniformities may contribute to microvascular blood-flow heterogeneity. For example, Sarelius (50) proposed that variations in microvessel RBC velocities could result from the fact that successive segments along branching capillary networks have larger diameters. Thus, as the blood flows through the successive branches, velocity decreases with increasing cross-sectional area. It is also well known that frequent cross-connections exist between adjacent capillary segments (1). Blood flow through these cross-connections could also cause variations in flow along the capillaries. If the hypothesis of Duling and Damon (1)—that perfusion heterogeneity is relatively constant from one microvascular unit to the next—is correct, perfusion heterogeneity of exchange vessels may be primarily determined by anatomical factors. The only controlled variables may be the number of microvascular units perfused, the regional distribution of resistance throughout the vascular tree, and the total flow (total resistance) through the tissue.

SUMMARY

Blood-flow heterogeneity exists in skeletal muscle in at least two forms: (i) gross blood-flow heterogeneity within and among skeletal muscles and (ii) microvascular blood-flow heterogeneity within and among exchange vessels of skeletal muscles. Gross blood-flow heterogeneity is the result of (a) the relationship between blood flow and muscle-fiber-type composition, (b) muscle fiber distribution and recruitment patterns, (c) mechanical factors related to muscle contraction, and (d) physiologic factors responsible for controlling vascular resistance. Information available at this time indicates that the net effect of these factors, coupled with the blood-flow heterogeneity that results from their interaction, is a matching of blood flow (spatially) to the oxygen consumption and capillary exchange capacities present within and among skeletal muscles during exercise. In support of this notion, it has been demonstrated that capillary volume (or capillary RBC volume) is reasonably well matched to mitochondrial content of the associated muscle fibers (56–58). It appears that vascularization and capillary exchange capacity of skeletal muscle is matched to the tissue's biochemical oxidative capacity. If blood flow is distributed equally among the exchange vessels, then differences in blood flow from one area of muscle to another (gross flow heterogeneity) does not lead to limited O_2 transport. A heterogeneous distribution of blood flow is the most efficient manner to transport the required amount of oxygen to a heterogeneous mass of muscle in that the O_2 is transported with minimal blood flow. Therefore, blood-flow heterogeneity is not necessarily a sign of poor vascular function. However, further gross heterogeneity of blood flow within and/or among skeletal muscles, resulting from pathology, abnormal environments, or unusual stress, may cause limitations in oxygen transport.

Microvascular heterogeneity of blood flow within and among exchange vessels can exist within muscle tissue even when blood flow appears to be grossly homogeneous. Microvascular blood-flow heterogeneity is the result of anatomical factors in the microcirculation and physiological control mechanisms. Both the anatomical characteristics of the exchange vessels and the perfusion of these exchange vessels show considerable heterogeneity. To the extent that the number of perfused microvascular units is the result of the vascular tone of terminal arterioles (see Chapter 5.5.2.4), physiological control mechanisms are also determinants of microvascular blood-flow heterogeneity. However, there is evidence that the perfusion heterogeneity among the exchange vessels of microvascular units within skeletal muscles is relatively constant from one unit to the next. Thus, while it appears that the number of perfused microvascular units and total blood flow through the recruited units are controlled by physiologic mechanisms, the relative amount of microvascular heterogeneity may not be a controlled variable.

Microvascular blood-flow heterogeneity can result in limitation of oxygen transport, particularly if the exchange vessels and the connecting arteries and veins are of uniform structural dimensions. It is not clear whether the amount of microvascular heterogeneity that normally exists within skeletal muscle produces oxygen transport limitation. One major limitation to further understanding of the importance of vascular control in determining microvascular heterogeneity is that the muscles in which microvascular perfusion can be directly observed (with *in vivo* microscopy) are generally very thin muscles. These may or may not represent other types of muscle. The amount of heterogeneity within microvascular units may be different in muscles of varying fiber-type composition, in fusiform and pennate muscles, and/or in extensor versus flexor muscles. While it is likely that considerable heterogeneity exists in capillary perfusion within active skeletal muscles during locomotory exercise, a complete understanding of these phenomena within active skeletal muscles will not be obtained easily because of the technical limitations involved in applying available microcirculatory techniques to the observation of capillary perfusion in these muscles under these conditions.

ACKNOWLEDGMENTS

I thank my good friend and colleague R. B. Armstrong for our collaborative efforts and the numerous discussions we have had concerning the perfusion of skeletal muscle during exercise. I also thank Drs. J. F. Amann and M. Powers for scientific criticisms of this manuscript. This research was supported by NIH grants HL-36088 and HL-36531 and by Research Career Development Award HL-01774.

REFERENCES

1. Duling BR, Damon DH. An examination of the measurement of flow heterogeneity in striated muscle. *Circ Res* 1986;60:1–13.
2. Laughlin MH, Armstrong RB. Muscular blood flow distribution patterns as a function of running speed in rats. *Am J Physiol* 1982;243:H296–H306.
3. Laughlin MH, Armstrong RB. Muscle blood flow during locomotory exercise. *Exerc Sport Sci Rev* 1985;13:95–136.
4. Hudlicka O. *Muscle blood flow: its relation to muscle metabolism and function.* Amsterdam: Swets & Zeitlinger, 1973.
5. Mackie BG, Terjung RL. Blood flow to different skeletal muscle fiber types during contraction. *Am J Physiol* 1983;2245:H265–H275.
6. Piiper J, Pendergast DR, Marconi C, Meyer M, Heisler N, Cerretelli P. Blood flow distribution in dog gastrocnemius muscle at rest and during stimulation. *J Appl Physiol* 1985;58:2068–2074.
7. Armstrong RB, Delp MD, Goljan EF, Laughlin MH. Distribution of blood flow in muscles of miniature swine during exercise. *J Appl Physiol* 1987;62:1285–1298.
8. Laughlin MH, Armstrong RB. Rat muscles blood flow as a function of time during prolonged slow treadmill exercise. *Am J Physiol* 1983;244:H814–H824.
9. Armstrong RB, Laughlin MH. Blood flows within and among rat muscles as a function of time during high speed treadmill exercise. *J Physiol* 1983;344:189–208.
10. Burke RE. Motor units: anatomy, physiology and functional organization. In: Brooks VB, ed. *Handbook of physiology. Section 1: The nervous system.* Bethesda, MD: American Physiological Society, 1981;345–422.
11. Burke RE, Edgerton VR. Motor unit properties and selective involvement in movement. *Exerc Sport Sci Rev* 1975;3:31–81.
12. Saltin B, Gollnick PD. Skeletal muscle adaptability: significance for metabolism and performance. In: Peachey LD, Adrian RH, Geiger SR, eds. *Handbook of physiology. Section 10: Skeletal muscle.* Bethesda, MD: American Physiological Society, 1983;555–631.
13. Peter JB, Barnard RJ, Edgerton VR, Gillespie CA, Stemel KE. Metabolic profiles of three types of skeletal muscle in guinea pigs and rabbits. *Biochemistry* 1972;11;2627–2633.
14. Armstrong RB. Properties and distributions of the fiber types in the locomotory muscles of mammals. In: Schmidt-Neilsen K, Taylor CR, eds. *Comparative physiology: primitive mammals.* Cambridge, England: Cambridge University Press, 1980;243–254.
15. Collatos TC, Edgerton VR, Smith JL, Botterman BR. Contractile properties and fiber type compositions of flexors and extensors of elbow joint in cat: implications for motor control. *J Neurophysiol* 1977;40;1292–1300.
16. Folkow B, Halicka HD. A comparison between red and white muscle with respect to blood supply, capillary surface area and

oxygen uptake during rest and exercise. *Microvasc Res* 1968; 1:1–14.

17. Mia JV, Edgerton VR, Barnard RJ. Capillarity of red, white, and intermediate muscle fibers in trained and untrained guinea pigs. *Experientia* 1970;26:1222–1223.

18. Laughlin MH. Skeletal muscle blood flow capacity: role of muscle pump in exercise hyperemia. *Am J Physiol* 1987;253:H993–H1004.

19. Laughlin MH, Ripperger J. Vascular transport capacity of hindlimb muscles of exercise trained rats. *J Appl Physiol* 1987; 62:438–443.

20. Armstrong RB, Marum P, Saubert IV CW, Seeherman HW, Taylor CR. Muscle fiber activity as a function of speed and gait. *J Appl Physiol* 1977;43:672–677.

21. Sullivan TE, Armstrong RB. Rat locomotory muscle fiber activity during trotting and galloping. *J Appl Physiol* 1978;44:358–363.

22. Blair DA, Gloves WE, Roddie IC. Vasomotor response in the human arm during leg exercise. *Circ Res* 1961;9:264–274.

23. Bevegard BJ, Shepherd JT. Reaction in man of resistance and capacity vessels in forearm and hand to leg exercise. *J Appl Physiol* 1966;21:123–132.

24. Laughlin MH, Mohrman SJ, Armstrong RB. Muscular blood flow distribution patterns in the hindlimb of swimming rats. *Am J Physiol* 1984;246:H398–H403.

25. Folkow B, Gaskell P, Waaler BA. Blood flow through limb muscles during heavy rhythmic exercise. *Acta Physiol Scand* 1970;80:61–72.

26. Shepherd JT. Circulation to skeletal muscle. In: Shepherd JT, Abbond FM, eds. *Handbook of physiology. Section 2: The cardiovascular system, vol III—Peripheral circulation.* Bethesda, MD: American Physiological Society, 1983;319–370.

27. Kirkebo A, Wisnes A. Regional tissue fluid pressure in rat calf muscle during sustained contraction or stretch. *Acta Physiol Scand* 1982;114:551–556.

28. Petrofsky JS, Hendershot DM. The interrelationship between blood pressure, intramuscular pressure, and isometric endurance in fast and slow twitch skeletal muscle in the cat. *Eur J Appl Physiol* 1984;53:106–111.

29. Gray SD, Carlsson E, Staub NC. Site of increased vascular resistance during isometric muscle contraction. *Am J Physiol* 1967;213:683–689.

30. Pollack AA, Wood EH. Venous pressure in the saphenous vein at the ankle in man during exercise and changes in posture. *J Appl Physiol* 1949;1:649–662.

31. Gray SD. Responsiveness of the terminal vascular bed in fast and slow skeletal muscle to adrenergic stimulation. *Angiologica* 1971;8:285–296.

32. Hilton SM, Jefferies MG, Vrbova G. Functional specializations of the vascular bed of soleus. *J Physiol* 1970;206:545–562.

33. Laughlin MH, Armstrong RB. Adrenoreceptor effects on rat muscle blood flow during treadmill exercise. *J Appl Physiol* 1987;62:1465–1472.

34. Mellander S. Differentiation on fiber composition, circulation and metabolism in limb muscles of dog, cat, and man. In: Vanhoutte PM, Lenses I, eds. *Vasodilation.* New York: Raven Press, 1981;243–254.

35. Hilton SM, Hudlicka O, Marshall JM. Possible mediators of functional hyperemia in skeletal muscle. *J Physiol* 1978;282:131–147.

36. Laughlin MH, Klabunde RE, Delp MD, Armstrong RB. Effects of dipyridamole on muscle blood flow in exercising miniature swine. *Am J Physiol* 1989;257:H1507–H1515.

37. Pendergast DR, Krasney JA, Ellis A, McDonald B, Marconi C, Cerretelli P. Cardiac output and muscle blood flow in exercising dogs. *Respir Physiol* 1985;61:317–326.

38. Bassingthwaighte JB, Goresky CA. Modeling in the analysis of solute and water exchange in the microvasculature. In: Renkin EM, Michel CC, eds. *Handbook of physiology. Section 2: The cardiovascular system, vol IV—Microcirculation.* Bethesda, MD: American Physiological Society, 1984;549–626.

39. Rose CP, Goresky GA. Vasomotor control of capillary transit time heterogeneity in the canine coronary circulation. *Circ Res* 1976;39:541–554.

40. Rowell, LB. *Human circulation: regulation during physical stress.* New York: Oxford University Press, 1986;1–327.

41. Renkin EM. Control of microcirculation and blood–tissue exchange. In: Renkin EM, Michel CC, eds. *Handbook of physiology. Section 2: Cardiovascular system, vol IV—Microcirculation, part 2.* Bethesda, MD: American Physiological Society, 1984;627–687.

42. Damon DH, Duling BR. Distribution of capillary blood flow in the microcirculation of the hamster: an *in vivo* study using epifluorescent microscopy. *Microvasc Res* 1984;27:81–95.

43. Duling BR, Klitzman B. Local control of microvascular function: role in tissue oxygen supply. *Annu Rev Physiol* 1980;42:373–382.

44. Honig CR, Odoroff CL, Frierson JL. Active and passive capillary control in red muscle at rest and in exercise. *Am J Physiol* 1982;243:H196–H206.

45. Kjellmer I, Lindbjerg I, Prerovsky I, Tonnesen H. The relation between blood flow in an isolated muscle measured with the 135 Xe clearance and a direct recording technique. *Acta Physiol Scand* 1967;69:69–78.

46. Paradise NF, Swayze CR, Shin DH, Fox IJ. Perfusion heterogeneity is skeletal muscle using tritiated water. *Am J Physiol* 1971;220:1107–1115.

47. Sparks HV, Mohrman DE. Heterogeneity of flow as an explanation for the multi-exponential washout of inert gas from skeletal muscle. *Microvasc Res* 1977;13:181–184.

48. Tyml K, Groom AC. Regulation of blood flow in individual capillaries of resting skeletal muscle in frogs. *Microvasc Res* 1980;20:346–357.

49. Tyml K. Capillary recruitment and heterogeneity of microvascular flow in skeletal muscle before and after contraction. *Microvasc Res* 1986;32:84–98.

50. Sarelius IH. Cell flow path influences transit time through striated muscle capillaries. *Am J Physiol* 1986;250:H899–H907.

51. Damon DH, Duling BR. Evidence that capillary perfusion heterogeneity is not controlled in striated muscle. *Am J Physiol* 1986;248:H386–H392.

52. Renkin EM, Hudlicka O, Sheehan RM. Influence of metabolic vasodilation on blood tissue diffusion in skeletal muscle. *Am J Physiol* 1966;211:87–98.

53. Klitzman B, Damon DN, Gorczynski RJ, Duling BR. Augmented tissue oxygen supply during striated muscle contraction in the hamster: relative contributions of capillary recruitment, functional dilation and reduced tissue PO_2. *Circ Res* 1982; 51:711–721.

54. Granger HJ, Goodman AH, Granger DN. Role of resistance and exchange vessels in local microvascular control of skeletal muscle oxygenation in the dog. *Circ Res* 1976;38:379–385.

55. Gorczynski RJ, Klitzman B, Duling BR. Interrelations between contracting striated muscle and precapillary microvessels. *Am J Physiol* 1978;235:H494–H504.

56. Hoppeler H, Mathieu O, Weibel ER, Krauer R, Lindstedt SL, Taylor CR. Design of the mammalian respiratory system. VIII. Capillaries in skeletal muscle. *Respir Physiol* 1981;44:129–150.

57. Mathieu-Costello O. Capillary tortuosity and degree of contraction or extension of skeletal muscle. *Microvasc Res* 1987;33:98–117.

58. Conley KE, Kayer SR, Rosler K, Hoppler H, Weibel ER, Taylor CR. Adaptive variation in the mammalian respiratory system in relation to energetic demand. IV. Capillaries and their relationship to oxidative capacity. *Respir Physiol* 1987;69:47–64.

THE LUNG: *Scientific Foundations*
edited by R.G. Crystal, J.B. West et al.
Raven Press, Ltd., New York © 1991.

CHAPTER 5.5.2.6

Influence of Exercise Training on O_2 Delivery to Skeletal Muscles

R. B. Armstrong

A number of physiologic changes occur during exercise to increase O_2 and substrate delivery to, as well as metabolic product and heat removal from, the active skeletal muscles. Repeatedly challenging the O_2 delivery system through exercise training results in adaptations to the system that increase O_2 delivery and promote greater extraction of the O_2 by the active skeletal muscles. The purpose of this chapter is to summarize what is known about the effects of exercise training on O_2 delivery to skeletal muscles during exercise. The focus will be on training effects in human subjects; much of the available information is from animal models, however, so these data will be integrated in the discussion. To provide a basis for considering the influence of training on O_2 delivery to muscle, a brief outline of O_2 transport during exercise in normal, untrained subjects is first presented.

THE INFLUENCE OF EXERCISE ON O_2 DELIVERY TO SKELETAL MUSCLES

O_2 delivery to total skeletal muscle ($\dot{F}_{O_2M}$) is related to total muscle blood flow ($\dot{Q}_M$) and arterial oxygen content (C_{aO_2}) according to the equation

$$\dot{F}_{O_2M} = \dot{Q}_M \cdot C_{aO_2} \qquad [1]$$

The most important factor contributing to elevated $\dot{F}_{O_2M}$ during exercise is increased $\dot{Q}_M$, since there is little change in C_{aO_2} in the transition from rest to exercise (1–4). In a healthy man of average size (~70 kg) at rest, $\dot{Q}_M$ is about 1 liter·min^{-1} (Fig. 1), which is 15–20% of cardiac output (4–6). $\dot{Q}_M$ increases as a function of exercise intensity (7–10); during heavy exercise eliciting maximal O_2 consumption ($\dot{V}_{O_2}max$), $\dot{Q}_M$ is about 22–23 liters·min^{-1} (Fig. 1), representing approximately 85% of cardiac output (4,6).

Total muscle blood flow ($\dot{Q}_M$) is the difference between total cardiac output ($\dot{Q}_T$) and total flow to nonmuscular tissues ($\dot{Q}_{NM}$), or

$$\dot{Q}_M = \dot{Q}_T - \dot{Q}_{NM} \qquad [2]$$

As indicated above, in normal untrained subjects, $\dot{Q}_T$ increases about four- to fivefold from rest to exercise at $\dot{V}_{O_2}$ max (Fig. 1) (2,5,11). At the same time, absolute $\dot{Q}_{NM}$ decreases (Fig. 1) (4–6,12). At rest, approximately 83% of a $\dot{Q}_T$ of about 6 liters·min^{-1} is to nonmuscular tissues (4); during exercise at $\dot{V}_{O_2}max$, about 15% of $\dot{Q}_T$ (25 liters·min^{-1}) perfuses tissues other than skeletal muscle (Fig. 1) (4,6). Thus, in absolute terms, $\dot{Q}_{NM}$ decreases from rest to maximal exercise by about 25%, whereas $\dot{Q}_M$ increases by over 20-fold. The nonmuscular tissues showing the greatest attenuation in blood flow during exercise are those in the visceral organs (Fig. 1). Splanchnic blood flow is decreased about 77% in human subjects from rest to maximal exercise (1500 to 350 ml·min^{-1}) (4). In pigs and rats, splenic blood flow decreases from about 300 ml·min^{-1}·100 g^{-1} during preexercise to less than 10 ml·min^{-1}·100 g^{-1} during exercise at or near $\dot{V}_{O_2}max$ (9,10). On the other hand, some tissues other than skeletal muscle show increases in blood flow during exercise (e.g., heart), whereas others have no significant change in blood flow during relatively brief bouts of exercise at $\dot{V}_{O_2}max$ (e.g., brain). It is clear that the greatest contribution to the increase in $\dot{Q}_M$ during maximal exercise is the elevation in $\dot{Q}_T$ (about 88%), with the redistribution from the nonmuscular tissues making a smaller contribution (about 12%).

As described in Chapter 5.5.2.5, blood flow is het-

R. B. Armstrong: Department of Physical Education, University of Georgia, Athens, Georgia 30602.

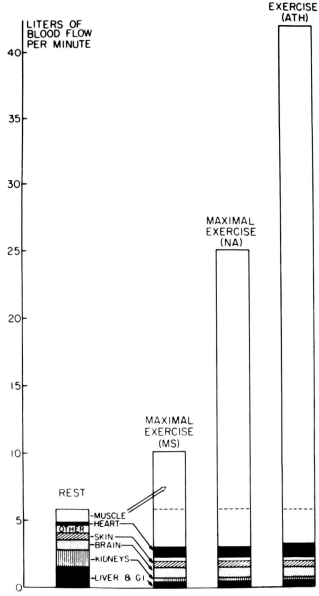

FIG. 1. Distribution of cardiac output at rest and during exercise at $\dot{V}O_2$max in patients with mitral stenosis (MS), normally active subjects (NA), and elite endurance-trained athletes (ATH). Distribution of cardiac output at rest is similar among the three groups. During maximal exercise, blood flow to nonmuscular tissues is similar in the three groups. GI, gastrointestinal tract. (From ref. 4.)

erogeneously distributed among and within muscles under most conditions. During both rest and exercise, blood flow is specifically directed to the active motor units in the muscles (8). If it is assumed that skeletal muscle comprises about 40% of body mass, estimated average muscle blood flow would increase from about 4 ml·min^{-1}·100 g^{-1} at rest ($\dot{Q}_M$ of 1 liter·min^{-1} in a 70-kg man) to about 82 ml·min^{-1}·100 g^{-1} during exercise at $\dot{V}O_2$max ($\dot{Q}_M$ of 23 liters·min^{-1}). In human subjects performing one-legged knee extension ex-

ercise, quadriceps muscle blood flow increases from less than 10 ml·min^{-1}·100 g^{-1} at rest to about 230 ml·min^{-1}·100 g^{-1} during intense exercise (13), so blood flow in active muscle may be much higher during exercise than indicated by the simple calculations for average muscle blood flow above. During walking in rats, blood flow to active high oxidative (slow and fast) fibers located in the deeper portions of large extensor muscles (i.e., gastrocnemius and vastus lateralis) increases two- to threefold over that at rest, whereas blood flow in the inactive superficial parts composed predominantly of fast glycolytic fibers in the same muscles decreases from 40 to 65% (7). During high-speed galloping in rats, blood flow in the red part of gastrocnemius muscle (467 ml·min^{-1}·100 g^{-1}) is about sevenfold higher than that in the white part of the same muscle (68 ml·min^{-1}·100 g^{-1}) (9).

Differences in magnitude of blood flow among muscles and muscle parts are dependent upon (a) differences in activity of the constituent motor units and (b) differences in vascular anatomy and responsivity to vasodilatory and vasoconstrictor influences (see Chapter 5.5.2.5). Although the degree of heterogeneity of blood flow within and among active human muscles is not known, conductance decreases in inactive muscles during exercise (6,14). For example, blood flow to the arm muscles is attenuated during bicycling exercise (12). In animals, blood flow is distributed within and among the active muscles in proportion to the oxidative capacity of the constituent motor units during maximal exercise (9,10), similar to the blood flow distribution patterns that occur during electrical stimulation of the muscles (15,16). Presumably the same patterns would be observed in human muscles, since some stratification of fiber types among and within muscles occurs in humans (17,18). Thus, $\dot{Q}_M$ represents the sum of blood flow to the active [$\dot{Q}(am)$] and inactive [$\dot{Q}(im)$] muscles according to the equation

$$\dot{Q}_M = \dot{Q}(am)_1 + \dot{Q}(im)_1 + \cdots + \dot{Q}(am, im)_n \quad [3]$$

This heterogeneity has undoubtedly led to much of the confusion in the literature about the magnitude of changes in muscle blood flow during exercise. Measurement of blood flow in one muscle or one group of muscles may not be representative of the $\dot{Q}_M$ under various conditions of rest and exercise.

There are also differences in the literature regarding the pattern of increases in blood flow in muscle expressed as a function of exercise intensity up to $\dot{V}O_2$max. Some investigators have reported that skeletal muscle blood flow does not increase further at exercise intensities above about 70% $\dot{V}O_2$max (19–21), whereas others have found that muscle blood flow increases up to $\dot{V}O_2$max (22–24). These differences again may be explained by the heterogeneity of blood flow among and within muscles. In animals, some muscles or muscle parts attain peak blood flows at even slow walking speeds, whereas others do not attain peak blood flows until the animal is running at $\dot{V}_{O_2}$max (7,9,10). Thus, different patterns of blood flow in muscles with increasing exercise intensity emerge, depending on which muscles or muscle groups are studied.

The biophysical factors that govern the increase in blood flow through the muscles during exercise can be appreciated by considering Poiseuille's law, which describes steady laminar flow of a Newtonian fluid through a cylindrical tube:

$$\dot{Q} = (P_i - P_o)\pi r^4 \cdot (8\eta l)^{-1} \qquad [4]$$

This equation indicates that flow is directly proportional to the pressure difference across the tube ($P_i - P_o$) and the fourth power of the radius (r) of the tube and is inversely related to the viscosity of the fluid (η) and the length of the tube (l). Since blood flow through a tissue involves flow of a non-Newtonian fluid that may be turbulent through a complex of tubes, it is more appropriate to simplify Eq. 4 to

$$\dot{Q}_M \propto (P_a - P_v)r \cdot (\eta l)^{-1} \qquad [5]$$

where P_a and P_v are the arterial and muscle venous pressures, respectively. With the exception of the variable l, each of these factors changes when the subject goes from rest to exercise. Mean arterial pressure, P_a, increases as a function of exercise intensity up to that eliciting $\dot{V}_{O_2}$max (3,10,11,25). Mean pressure in the aorta increases about 25 mmHg (or, about 28%) from rest to maximal exercise in human subjects (25). Also, during rhythmic exercise, there is a decrease in muscle P_v as a result of action of the "muscle pump" (26). The extent of this attenuation is not known. Laughlin (26) presented theoretical estimates from the measurements of muscle venous pressures reported by Folkow et al. (27), indicating that muscle venule pressures during the relaxation phase of rhythmic exercise would be -10 to -20 mmHg. During the contraction phase, venous pressures are high, decreasing or obliterating the difference between P_a and P_v. Ankle venous pressure in exercising human subjects appears to decrease by about 60 mmHg (about 70%) during walking exercise (28). Therefore, the ΔP across the capillary beds in the active skeletal muscles may increase by about 100% from rest to exercise.

Resistance (R) to blood flow in the muscles also decreases in the muscles during exercise as a result of various neural, metabolic, and myogenic vasodilatory influences on the arterioles, as discussed in detail in Chapter 5.5.2.4. Vasodilation of the arterioles in the muscles results in increased r in Eq. 5. Finally, viscosity (η) of the blood increases slightly during exercise because of loss of plasma volume ($\sim 10\%$) (2),

which minimally counters the effects of increased ΔP and r in elevating blood flow in the muscles.

According to Eq. 1, the factor other than $\dot{Q}_M$ that is important in determining O$_2$ delivery to skeletal muscle is C_aO_2, the O$_2$ content of the arterial blood. C_aO_2 is dependent upon hemoglobin (Hb) concentration and O$_2$ saturation of the Hb, according to the equation

$$C_aO_2 = O_2 \text{ saturation} \cdot 100^{-1} \cdot [\text{Hb}] \cdot 1.36 \qquad [6]$$

In most normal subjects, there is little change in C_aO_2 from rest to maximal exercise (2). During exercise at $\dot{V}_{O_2}$max, there is a slight fall in O$_2$ saturation of hemoglobin (~ 3–5%) as a result of the Bohr shift (from lowered pH and elevated temperature) (2), but this is countered by plasma water loss ($\sim 10\%$) resulting in an increase in [Hb]. Thus, during exercise in normal subjects, O$_2$ delivery to skeletal muscles increases as a function of muscle blood flow. It follows that muscle O$_2$ consumption ($\dot{V}_{O_2M}$) is determined by muscle blood flow ($\dot{Q}_M$) and O$_2$ extraction by the muscle ($C_aO_2 - C_vO_2M$), or

$$\dot{V}_{O_2M} = \dot{Q}_M \cdot (C_aO_2 - C_vO_2M) \qquad [7]$$

As pointed out above, C_aO_2 does not change significantly from rest to exercise at $\dot{V}_{O_2}$max. However, C_vO_2M progressively decreases with exercise intensity (2); for example, femoral venous O$_2$ content may decrease from about 10 ml O$_2 \cdot 100$ ml^{-1} at rest to less than 2 ml O$_2 \cdot 100$ ml^{-1} during intense exercise (29). It is apparent that the most important factor for increasing $\dot{V}_{O_2M}$ from rest to maximal exercise is the elevation in blood flow ($\dot{Q}_M$), which increases 10- to 20-fold (see discussion above) as compared with the approximately twofold increase in O$_2$ extraction.

THE INFLUENCE OF TRAINING ON O$_2$ DELIVERY TO MUSCLES

In the following sections, the effects of exercise training on O$_2$ delivery to the muscles will be considered under three general conditions: during rest; during submaximal exercise; and during intense exercise at or near $\dot{V}_{O_2}$max. The discussion will be restricted to training involving dynamic, rhythmic exercise.

During Rest

Under normal resting conditions, training does not appear to have any major effect on blood flow or O$_2$ delivery to the muscles (2,22,30). Thus, considering Eq. 1, training would not influence $\dot{Q}_M$ or C_aO_2 in the resting condition. Some highly trained endurance athletes (1,31) and trained animals (32) have a relative anemia resulting in attenuated C_aO_2; $\dot{V}_{O_2M}$ presumably is maintained through increased O_2 extraction in these individuals.

During the preexercise period there is a cardiovascular anticipatory response that includes elevated mean arterial pressure, heart rate, and muscle blood flow (33–35). Rats trained with moderate-intensity exercise have higher preexercise blood flows in several muscles than do untrained control animals (34); for example, blood flow in the deep red portion of the gastrocnemius muscle is 70% higher in the trained group (102 ml·min^{-1}·100 g^{-1}) than in the untrained group (60 ml·min^{-1}·100 g^{-1}) during the preexercise period. On the other hand, rats that have been conditioned to run on the treadmill at high intensities show elevated anticipatory preexercise blood flows specifically in muscles composed primarily of fast-twitch glycolytic fibers (35). Thus, it appears that with conditioning or training, blood flows increase in specific muscles or muscle parts during the preexercise period in anticipation of the impending exercise; this specificity is probably dependent on whether or not the constituent motor units were regularly activated during the preceding training sessions. "Priming" O_2 delivery to the motor units that will subsequently be active would seem to make biological sense. The mechanisms underlying these training-induced alterations in muscle blood flow are not known.

During Submaximal Exercise

There is some confusion in the literature about the effect of training on muscle blood flow during submaximal exercise. Although total muscle blood flow ($\dot{Q}_M$) has not been measured in human subjects, deduction indicates that $\dot{Q}_M$ is decreased when the same exercise intensity is performed after training. Thus, according to Eq. 2, total cardiac output ($\dot{Q}_T$) is unchanged (11,36,37), whereas total nonmuscle blood flow ($\dot{Q}_{NM}$) increases (4,5,11,36) and $\dot{Q}_M$ decreases. Most studies in which blood flow has been measured in active individual muscles (Xenon-133 clearance) or limbs (dye dilution or plethysmography) have shown that at a given exercise intensity, blood flow either is not changed by training (22,38,39) or is decreased (19,40–43). However, there is evidence that during moderate-intensity exercise, $\dot{Q}_M$ is distributed differently among and within muscles after training, so that the active high oxidative fibers receive elevated blood flows [$\dot{Q}(am)$]—and the inactive white fibers, reduced flows [$\dot{Q}(im)$]—according to Eq. 3 (Fig. 2). This has been demonstrated in rats using the radiolabeled microsphere technique (34); whether this occurs in human muscles remains to be seen, although the decreases in blood flow after training in the superficial parts of vastus lateralis muscles of human subjects measured with the Xenon-133 method reported by some investigators

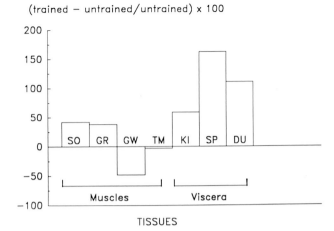

FIG. 2. Percent difference in tissue blood flows in endurance-trained and control rats during the 15th minute of running at a moderate treadmill speed (30 m·min^{-1}). Muscle tissues are: SO, soleus muscle (primarily slow-twitch oxidative fibers); GR, red portion of gastrocnemius (primarily fast-twitch oxidative fibers); GW, white portion of gastrocnemius (primarily fast-twitch glycolytic fibers); and TM, total hindlimb musculature. Visceral tissues are: KI, kidney; SP, spleen; and DU, duodenum. With the exception of TM, all blood flows were significantly different between groups ($p < 0.05$). (Data are from ref. 34.)

(19,40,42) could represent a similar training-induced redistribution of blood flow within the active muscles. An alternative explanation for the reported decreases in blood flow with training using the Xenon-133 clearance technique is that elevations in lipid content in the muscle fibers (44) attenuate removal of the lipophilic Xenon-133 from the muscle (11).

The mechanisms underlying the redistribution of blood flow in rat muscles after training are unknown. Considering Eq. 4, it is not clear what changes in the active red muscle to permit elevated blood flow after training. P_a, represented by mean arterial pressure, is not different during submaximal exercise after training (3,11,34). It is possible that training increases the efficiency of the muscle pump in the active muscles, which could lower P_v, but this remains speculative. It is probable that the major change occurs in regulation of the resistance arterioles, affecting the r term of Eq. 5. Decreased α_1-adrenergic influences, increased α_2- or β_2-adrenergic influences, or altered responsivity to local metabolic signals could contribute to increased vasodilation in the active muscles or muscle parts (for discussion of these factors in the control of muscle blood flow, see Chapter 5.5.2.4). One of the well-documented changes that accompanies training is a decrease in circulating norepinephrine during exercise at a given intensity (45,46).

Total muscle O_2 delivery ($\dot{F}_{O_2M}$) at a given submaximal exercise intensity should decrease after training because of the decrease in $\dot{Q}_M$, with no change in C_aO_2

(1,3) (Eq. 1), although O$_2$ delivery specifically to the active motor units in the muscles would be elevated with the increased blood flow as described above. $\dot{V}_{O_2}$ at a given submaximal exercise intensity is similar before and after training (4,11). Thus, the arteriovenous O$_2$ difference across the total musculature must be elevated because of the reduced $\dot{Q}_M$ discussed above. The elevated O$_2$ extraction may be related to the increase in capillary density in the muscles that occurs with training (47–51), which would maintain adequate capillary mean transit times in the active muscles in the face of increased blood flows and provide a greater capillary surface area for O$_2$ exchange. There is evidence that the increase in capillary density with training occurs specifically in the muscles and muscle parts that are active during the training sessions (52). The increased O$_2$ extraction could also be facilitated by the increased mitochondrial volume in the muscles (51), which would affect P_{O_2} gradients from capillaries to muscle fibers (see Chapter 5.5.2.3).

During Exercise at $\dot{V}_{O_2}$max

During exercise at $\dot{V}_{O_2}$max, total muscle blood flow ($\dot{Q}_M$) is increased after training, with little change occurring in blood flow to nonmuscular organs ($\dot{Q}_{NM}$) (4,53) (Fig. 1). Thus the increase in total cardiac output ($\dot{Q}_T$) is quantitatively equal to the elevation in $\dot{Q}_M$ (4).

Little is known about the effect of training on blood flow distribution among muscles during locomotory exercise at $\dot{V}_{O_2}$max. However, it appears that the increases in $\dot{Q}_M$ result from elevations in blood flow primarily to the active muscles [$\dot{Q}$(am)], from Eq. 3. For example, Musch et al. (53) found that average total blood flow in nine hindlimb muscles in foxhounds increased significantly (10%) with training, whereas there was no significant change in blood flow to tongue (presumably inactive muscle). Also, training of a relatively small muscle mass (e.g., one limb) results in clear elevations in muscle blood flow during heavy exercise of the trained muscles (54–56). During high-intensity exercise on a bicycle, there is a marked decrease in blood flow to the inactive arm muscles (12). Referring to Poiseuille's law (Eq. 5), the elevations in skeletal muscle blood flow during maximal exercise after training could result from increased pressure gradient across the muscle vascular beds ($P_a - P_v$) or from elevated cross-sectional area of the resistance vessel lumina (r). Training does not cause an alteration in arterial pressure during heavy exercise (3,4,11), but as discussed above, it is possible that after training there may be more efficient muscle pump action, which would decrease active muscle venous pressure (thus increasing [$P_a - P_V$]). Probably of more importance is an increase in the total cross-sectional area of the lumina of resistance vessels in the active muscles.

An increase in blood flow in a given muscle during maximal exercise after training could theoretically result from greater vasodilation of the same arterioles, or from vasodilation of a new population of arterioles associated with different motor units. According to the latter hypothesis, with training there is an increase in the aerobic power, so that a larger muscle mass participates in the exercise (57). With increased myocardial performance with training, the heart is able to pump a higher cardiac output while maintaining mean arterial pressure ($\bar{P}_a$) (4,57), so total conductance (C) is elevated according to the equation

$$C = \dot{Q}_T \cdot \bar{P}_a^{-1} \qquad [8]$$

Thus, after training, the cardiovascular system is able to maintain normal arterial pressure during exercise while perfusing a larger active muscle mass. It is probable that the increase in the number of active fibers occurs within already active muscles through recruitment of new motor units, as opposed to recruitment of new muscles.

The second hypothesis would hold that with training there is increased vasodilation of the same resistance vessels, which are associated with the same population of motor units that are active in both the untrained and trained conditions. Thus, instead of the increased blood flow going to additional motor units, blood flow is increased to the same muscle mass. The increases in myocardial performance would also support this hypothesis, since elevated $\dot{Q}_T$ with constant $\bar{P}_a$ would permit higher flow through the same vascular beds.

Several investigators have demonstrated that blood flow capacity is elevated in muscles after training, and that the muscles or muscle parts undergoing the adaptation differ depending on the training intensity. Mackie and Terjung (58) reported that high-speed treadmill training resulted in increased blood flow in parts of rat muscles composed of fast-twitch glycolytic fibers during *in situ* electrical stimulation with tetanic trains. Similarly, Sexton et al. (59) showed that high-speed treadmill training in rats results in increases in blood flow capacity in the resting hindlimb when the muscles are maximally vasodilated with papaverine (Fig. 3A). In a separate paper, these investigators (60) demonstrated that the elevated flow capacity in the hindlimb of the high-speed-trained rats was primarily localized in muscle parts composed of fast-twitch glycolytic fibers (Fig. 3B). On the other hand, Laughlin and Ripperger (61) reported that after moderate-intensity training, flow capacity is increased in both fast-twitch and slow-twitch rat muscles that are maximally vasodilated with papaverine. Total hindquarter flow capacity was elevated by about 50% with training (61), with the largest increases in flow capacity occurring in the fast oxidative muscle parts (about 200%).

Although similar peripheral adaptations presumably

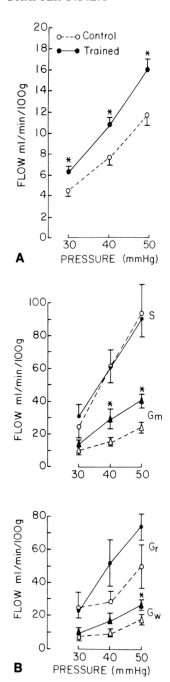

FIG. 3. Effects of high-intensity treadmill training program (in rats) on blood flow capacity of resting muscle maximally vasodilated with papaverine of total hindquarter **(A)** and individual muscles or muscle parts **(B)** as a function of perfusion pressure. Muscles or muscle parts in panel **B** are: S, soleus; G_m, middle part of gastrocnemius; G_r, red part of gastrocnemius; and G_w, white part of gastrocnemius (see legend for Fig. 2 for dominant fiber type in each of these muscles or muscle parts). Asterisks indicate that group means are different ($p < 0.05$). (From ref. 60.)

occur in human subjects with training (57), it seems clear that elevated muscle blood flows during maximal locomotory exercise in humans are dependent upon increased capacity of the heart to pump a higher cardiac output and maintain arterial pressure in the face of increased conductance in the muscles (4,54,57). The blood flow capacity of human skeletal muscle is considerably higher than is ever used during whole-body exercise (57,62); that is, during maximal whole-body exercise, when a relatively large muscle mass is involved, the blood flow capacity of the active muscles far surpasses the capacity of the heart to pump blood and maintain arterial pressure. Thus, peak quadriceps muscle blood flow during one-legged knee extension exercise may exceed 250 ml·min^{-1}·100 g^{-1}, but during two-legged bicycling, peak leg blood flow is only about 100 ml·min^{-1}·100 g^{-1} (57,63).

As pointed out above, some investigators have shown that with training there are increases in capillary density in the muscles (47–51). In guinea pigs the changes in capillarity appear to be associated specifically with the motor units that are recruited during the exercise training (52). The increased capillary volume in the muscles would maintain longer mean transit times in the face of elevated blood flows, as well as presenting a larger capillary surface area for exchange of O_2 with the surrounding muscle tissue (44). Sexton et al. (59) reported that the capillary filtration coefficient is increased by about 65% in rat muscle after high-speed treadmill training. Although this change could be due to a change in permeability to filtered fluid, it more likely resulted from an increase in capillary surface area. Similarly, Leinonen et al. (64) found that the capillary diffusion capacity in tibialis anterior muscle, as measured with ^{131}I clearance, was about 48% higher in endurance athletes than in sedentary control subjects.

Not all studies have demonstrated increases in capillary density with training. For example, endurance training in foxhounds resulted in a 28% increase in $\dot{V}_{O_2}$max and a 21% elevation in gastrocnemius muscle blood flow during treadmill exercise at $\dot{V}_{O_2}$max; however, the 12% increase in capillary density in the same muscle was not statistically significant (53,65). Similarly, several human studies have not found changes in capillary density with training (29,66,67). However, in these studies there were increases in muscle fiber diameter and in the capillary/fiber ratios.

During exercise at $\dot{V}_{O_2}$max, $\dot{V}_{O_2}$ of the muscles ($\dot{V}_{O_2M}$) is increased after training because of the elevated $\dot{Q}_M$ and an increase in O_2 extraction by the muscles, according to the equation

$$\dot{V}_{O_2M} = \dot{Q}_M \cdot (C_aO_2 - C_vO_2M) \qquad [9]$$

where C_vO_2M is the mean O_2 content of the venous blood leaving the muscles. Whereas C_aO_2 is not significantly affected by training (1,3), except in elite athletes, C_vO_2M is decreased (4,11,68), presumably through the increased capillary density (and associated elevations in capillary mean transit time and capillary surface area) in the muscle (4,44). In some species there is an associated increase in myoglobin in the trained muscles (69), although myoglobin does not appear to change in human muscle with training (44).

SUMMARY

Chronic exercise training increases the blood flow capacity of the muscles that are active during the exercise sessions. Following training, blood flows appear to be increased specifically in the active muscles or muscle parts during exercise, although total muscle blood flow is lower during exercise at submaximal intensities. During exercise at $\dot{V}o_2$max, total muscle blood flow is elevated after training. During intense exercise, the elevated muscle blood flow is provided by an increased cardiac output with little change in mean arterial pressure.

Training also increases the capillary volume of the active muscles, which facilitates O$_2$ exchange with the muscle during exercise by slowing the mean red cell capillary transit time and presenting a larger capillary surface exchange area.

Thus, the overall effect of exercise training on O$_2$ delivery to the muscle is to increase the blood flow to the active muscle fibers and to facilitate O$_2$ diffusion by increasing the volume and surface area of the exchange vessels.

REFERENCES

1. Ekblom B. Effect of physical training on oxygen transport system in man. *Acta Physiol Scand* 1969;328:5–45.
2. Åstrand PO, Rodahl K. *Textbook of work physiology.* New York: McGraw-Hill, 1970.
3. Musch TI, Haidet GC, Ordway GA, Longhurst JC, Mitchell JH. Dynamic exercise training in foxhounds I. Oxygen consumption and hemodynamic responses. *J Appl Physiol* 1985;59:183–189.
4. Rowell LB. *Human circulation regulation during physical stress.* New York: Oxford University Press, 1986.
5. Rowell LB. Human cardiovascular adjustments to exercise and thermal stress. *Physiol Rev* 1974;54:75–159.
6. Clausen JP. Circulatory adjustments to dynamic exercise and effect of physical training in normal subjects and in patients with coronary artery disease. *Prog Cardiovasc Dis* 1976;6:459–491.
7. Laughlin MH, Armstrong RB. Muscular blood flow distribution patterns as a function of running speed in rats. *Am J Physiol* 1982;243:H296–H306.
8. Laughlin MH, Armstrong RB. Muscle blood flow during exercise. *Exerc Sports Sci Rev* 1985;13:95–136.
9. Armstrong RB, Laughlin MH. Rat muscle blood flows during high speed locomotion. *J Appl Physiol* 1985;59:1322–1328.
10. Armstrong RB, Delp MD, Goljan EF, Laughlin MH. Distribution of blood flow in muscles of miniature swine during exercise. *J Appl Physiol* 1987;62:1285–1298.
11. Clausen JP. Effect of physical training on cardiovascular adjustments to exercise in man. *Physiol Rev* 1977;57:779–815.
12. Bevegård BS, Shepherd JT. Reaction in man of resistance and capacity vessels in forearm and hand to leg exercise. *J Appl Physiol* 1966;21:123.
13. Saltin B. Hemodynamic adaptations to exercise. *Am J Cardiol* 1985;55:42D–47D.
14. Bevegård BS, Shepherd JT. Regulation of the circulation during exercise in man. *Physiol Rev* 1967;47:178.
15. Folkow B, Halicka HD. A comparison between red and white muscle with respect to blood supply, capillary surface area and oxygen uptake during rest and exercise. *Microvasc Res* 1968;1:1–14.
16. Mackie BG, Terjung RL. Blood flow to different skeletal muscle fiber types during contraction. *Am J Physiol* 1983;245:H265–H275.
17. Edgerton VR, Smith JL, Simpson DR. Muscle fibre type populations of human leg muscles. *Histochem J* 1975;7:259–266.
18. Lexell J, Henriksson-Larsen K, Sjöström J. Distribution of different fibre types in human skeletal muscles. *Acta Physiol Scand* 1983;117:115–122.
19. Clausen JP, Trap-Jensen J. Effects of training on the distribution of cardiac output in patients with coronary artery disease. *Circulation* 1970;XLII:611–624.
20. Clausen JP, Lassen NA. Muscle blood flow during exercise in normal man studied by the ^{133}xenon clearance method. *Cardiovasc Res* 1971;5:245–254.
21. Pendergast JA, Krasney JA, Ellis A, McDonald B, Marconi C, Cerretelli P. Cardiac output and muscle blood flow in exercising dogs. *Respir Physiol* 1985;61:317–326.
22. Grimby G, Häggendal E, Saltin E. Local xenon 133 clearance from the quadriceps muscle during exercise in man. *J Appl Physiol* 1967;22:305–310.
23. Pirnay F, Marechal R, Radernecker R, Petit JM. Muscle blood flow during submaximum and maximum exercise on a bicycle ergometer. *J Appl Physiol* 1972;32:210–212.
24. Bonde-Peterson F, Henriksson J, Lundin B. Blood flow in thigh muscle during bicycling exercise in varying work rats. *Eur J Appl Physiol Occup Physiol* 1975;34:191–197.
25. Rowell LB, Brengelmann GL, Blackmon JR, Bruce RA, Murray JA. Disparities between aortic and peripheral pulse pressures induced by upright exercise and vasomotor changes in man. *Circulation* 1968;XXXVII:954–964.
26. Laughlin MH. Skeletal muscle blood flow capacity: role of muscle pump in exercise hyperemia. *Am J Physiol* 1987;253:H993–H1004.
27. Folkow B, Gaskell P, Waaler BA. Blood flow through limb muscles during rhythmic exercise. *Acta Physiol Scand* 1970;80:61–72.
28. Pollack AA, Wood EH. Venous pressure in the saphenous vein at the ankle in man during exercise and changes in posture. *J Appl Physiol* 1949;1:649–662.
29. Saltin B, Blomqvist G, Mitchell JH, Johnson RL Jr., Wildenthal K, Chapman CB. Response to submaximal and maximal exercise after bedrest and training. *Circulation* 1968;38(Suppl 7):1–78.
30. Hudlická O. Effect of training on macro- and microcirculatory changes in exercise. *Exercise Sport Sci Rev* 1977;181–230.
31. Grimby G, Saltin B. Physiological analyses of physically well-trained middle-aged and old athletes. *Acta Med Scand* 1966;179:513–526.
32. McKeever KH, Schurg WA, Convertino VA. Exercise training-induced hypervolemia in greyhounds: role of water intake and renal mechanisms. *Am J Physiol* 1985;248:R422–R425.
33. McArdle WD, Foglia GF, Patti AV. Telemetered cardiac response to selected running events. *J Appl Physiol* 1967;23:566–570.
34. Armstrong RB, Laughlin MH. Exercise blood flow patterns within and among rat muscles after training. *Am J Physiol* 1984;246:H59–H68.
35. Armstrong RB, Hayes DA, Delp MD. Blood flow distribution in rat muscles during preexercise anticipatory response. *J Appl Physiol* 1989;67:1855–1861.
36. Clausen JP, Klausen K, Rasmussen B, Trap-Jensen J. Central and peripheral circulatory changes after training of the arms or legs. *Am J Physiol* 1973;225:675–682.

37. Hartley LH, Grimby HG, Kilbom A, Nilsson NJ, Åstrand I, Bjure J, Ekblom B, Saltin B. Physical training in sedentary middle-aged and older men. III. Cardiac output and gas exchange at submaximal and maximal exercise. *Scand J Clin Lab Invest* 1969;24:335–344.

38. Klassen GA, Andrew GM, Becklake MR. Effect of training on total and regional blood flow and metabolism in paddlers. *J Appl Physiol* 1970;28:397–406.

39. Saltin B, Nazar K, Costill DL, Stein E, Jansson E, Essen B, Gollnick PD. The nature of the training response; peripheral and central adaptations to one-legged exercise. *Acta Physiol Scand* 1983;96:289–305.

40. Varnauskas E, Björntorp P, Fahlén M, Přerovský I, Stenberg J. Effects of physical training on exercise blood flow and enzymatic activity in skeletal muscle. *Cardiovasc Res* 1970;4:418–422.

41. Treumann F, Schroeder W. Trainingseinfluss auf Muskeldurchblutung und Herzfrequenz. *Z Kreislauff* 1968;57:1024–1033.

42. Bergman H, Björntorp P, Conradson TB, Fahlén M, Stenberg J, Varnauskas E. Enzymatic and circulatory adjustments to physical training in middle-aged men. *Eur J Clin Invest* 1973;3:414–418.

43. Saito M, Matsui H, Miyamura M. Effects of physical training on the calf and thigh blood flows. *Jpn J Physiol* 1980;30:955–959.

44. Saltin B, Gollnick PD. Skeletal muscle adaptability: significance for metabolism and performance. In: *Handbook of physiology, Section: Skeletal muscle.* Bethesda, MD: American Physiological Society, 1983;555–631.

45. Winder WW, Hagberg JM, Hickson RC, Ehsani AA, McLane JA. Time course of sympathoadrenal adaptation to endurance exercise training in man. *J Appl Physiol* 1978;45:370–374.

46. Péronnet F, Cleroux FJ, Perrault H, Cousineau D, DeChamplain J, Nadeau R. Plasma norepinephrine response to exercise before and after training in humans. *J Appl Physiol* 1981;51:812–815.

47. Andersen P, Henriksson J. Capillary supply of the quadriceps femoris muscle of man: adaptive response to exercise. *J Physiol (Lond)* 1977;270:677–690.

48. Brodal P, Ingjer F, Hermansen L. Capillary supply of skeletal muscle fibers in untrained and endurance-trained men. *Am J Physiol* 1977;232:H705–H712.

49. Ingjer F. Maximal aerobic power related to the capillary supply of the quadriceps femoris muscle in man. *Acta Physiol Scand* 1978;104:238–240.

50. Klausen K, Andersen LB, Pelle I. Adaptive changes in work capacity, skeletal muscle capillarization and enzyme levels during training and detraining. *Acta Physiol Scand* 1981;113:9–16.

51. Hoppeler H, Howald H, Conley K, Lindstedt L, Claassen H, Vock P, Weibel ER. Endurance training in humans: aerobic capacity and structure of skeletal muscle. *J Appl Physiol* 1985;59:320–327.

52. Mai JV, Edgerton VR, Barnard RJ. Capillary of red, white and intermediate muscle fibers in trained and untrained guinea-pigs. *Experientia* 1970;26:1222–1223.

53. Musch TI, Haidet GC, Ordway GA, Longhurst JC, Mitchell JH. Training effects on regional blood flow response to maximal exercise in foxhounds. *J Appl Physiol* 1987;52:1724–1732.

54. Klausen K, Niels HS, Clausen JP, Hartling O, Trap-Jensen J. Central and regional circulatory adaptations to one-leg training. *J Appl Physiol: Respir Environ Exerc Physiol* 1982;52:976–983.

55. Andersen P, Saltin B. Maximal perfusion of skeletal muscle in man. *J Physiol* 1985;366:233–249.

56. Saltin B, Kiens B, Savard G, Pederson PK. Role of hemoglobin and capillarization for oxygen delivery and extraction in muscular exercise. *Am J Physiol* 1986;128:21–32.

57. Saltin B. Capacity of blood flow delivery to exercising skeletal muscle in humans. *Am J Cardiol* 1988;62:30E–35E.

58. Mackie BG, Terjung RL. Influence of training on blood flow to different skeletal muscle fiber types. *J Appl Physiol: Respir Environ Exerc Physiol* 1983;55:1072–1078.

59. Sexton WI, Korthuis RJ, Laughlin MH. High-intensity exercise training increases vascular transport capacity of rat hindquarters. *Heart Circ Physiol* 1988;23:H274–H278.

60. Laughlin MH, Korthuis RJ, Sexton WL, Armstrong RB. Regional muscle blood flow capacity and exercise hyperemia in high-intensity trained rats. *J Appl Physiol* 1988;64:2420–2427.

61. Laughlin MH, Ripperger J. Vascular transport capacity of hindlimb muscles of exercise-trained rats. *J Appl Physiol* 1987;62:438–443.

62. Rowell LB. Muscle blood flow in humans: how high can it go? *Med Sci Sports Exerc* 1988;20:S97–S103.

63. Savard G, Kiens B, Saltin B. Limb blood flow in prolonged exercise: magnitude and implication for cardiovascular control during muscle work in man. *Can J Sport Sci* 1987;12:89S–101S.

64. Leinonen H, Salminen S, Peltokallio P. Capillary permeability and maximal blood flow in skeletal muscle in athletes and nonathletes measured by local clearances of ^{133}Xe and ^{131}I. *Scand J Clin Lab Invest* 1978;38:223–227.

65. Parsons D, Musch TI, Moore RL, Haidet GC, Ordway GA. Dynamic exercise training in foxhounds. II. Analysis of skeletal muscle. *J Appl Physiol* 1985;59:190–197.

66. Hermansen L, Wachtlová M. Capillary density of skeletal muscle in well trained and untrained men. *J Appl Physiol* 1971;30:860–863.

67. Pařizková J, Eiselt E, Šprynarová S, Wachtlová M. Body composition, aerobic capacity and density of muscle capillaries in young and old man. *J Appl Physiol* 1971;31:323–325.

68. Saltin B, Hartley LH, Kilbom A, Åstrand I. Physical training in sedentary middle-aged and older men. II. Oxygen uptake, heart rate and blood lactate concentration at submaximal and maximal exercise. *Scand J Clin Lab Invest* 1969;24:323–334.

69. Pattengale PK, Holloszy JO. Augmentation of skeletal muscle myoglobin by a program of treadmill running. *Am J Physiol* 1967;213:783–785.

THE LUNG: Scientific Foundations
edited by R.G. Crystal, J.B. West et al.
Raven Press, Ltd., New York © 1991.

CHAPTER 5.5.3.1

Cellular Effects

Guillermo Gutierrez

Decreases in O_2 supply set in motion adaptive mechanisms designed to maintain cellular activity at a minimum acceptable level. The failure of these mechanisms during hypoxia results in cellular dysfunction and can lead to irreversible cell damage. Cellular hypoxia, defined here as an O_2 limitation of mitochondrial adenosine triphosphate (ATP) production, can be produced by decreases in capillary perfusion (ischemia), arterial blood P_{O_2} (hypoxemia), or hemoglobin concentration (anemia).

The cellular response to hypoxia is heterogeneous and some cells tolerate hypoxia better than others. For example, skeletal muscle recovers normal function after 30 min of total ischemia (1), and irreversible damage does not occur in isolated hepatocytes until 2.5 hr of ischemia (2). However, hypoxic brain cells can be permanently damaged after 4–6 min (3,4). Among the possible mechanisms responsible for the development of irreversible hypoxic cellular injury are: (a) cellular energy depletion; (b) development of cellular acidosis; (c) increases in the concentration of metabolic products; (d) degradation of membrane phospholipids; (e) production of O_2-free radical species; and (f) cellular loss of adenine nucleotides.

METABOLIC ALTERATIONS

With abundant supply of O_2, the synthesis of ATP takes place by oxidative phosphorylation in the mitochondria. ATP is transported to the sites of energy utilization, such as the myofibrils and the membrane-associated ionic pumps, where it is hydrolyzed by the ATPases. This results in the liberation of energy and

the generation of adenosine diphosphate (ADP), inorganic phosphate (P_i), and H^+:

$$MgATP^{2-} \rightarrow MgADP^{1-} + P_i^{2-} + H^+ \qquad [1]$$

In the above equation, ADP and ATP are shown complexed with Mg^{2+}, their usual physiologic state. ADP, P_i, and H^+ are recycled in the mitochondria to produce ATP and CO_2.

With limited O_2 supply, the rate of aerobic ATP production falls behind the rate of ATP hydrolysis, resulting in the intracellular accumulation of ADP, P_i, and H^+. These metabolites behave as metabolic feedback signals, altering the pattern of substrate utilization by the cells and promoting the anaerobic synthesis of ATP. The anaerobic pathways of ATP production are glycolysis, the creatine kinase reaction, and the adenylate kinase reaction.

The Pasteur effect, defined as the preferential utilization of glucose as a metabolic substrate, is an early response to hypoxia (5). The metabolism of free fatty acids produces substantially more ATP than glucose. On the other hand, the number of ATP molecules produced per molecule of O_2 consumed is greater with glucose than with any other substrate. This becomes important in hypoxia when aerobic metabolism is limited by the availability of oxygen. In other words, by increasing glucose metabolism the hypoxic cell becomes a more efficient user of O_2.

The net consumption of glucose, as well as its clearance from arterial blood, increases during hypoxia. For example, myocytes normally utilize free fatty acids, such as palmitate, as the major substrate during the aerobic production of ATP. Palmitate represents approximately 60% of the total substrate metabolized, with glucose and lactate contributing approximately 11% and 29%, respectively. This pattern changes during cellular hypoxia, as the consumption of lactate ceases and that of glucose rises to 70–90% of the total substrate consumed (6).

G. Gutierrez: Pulmonary and Critical Care Division, University of Texas Health Science Center at Houston, Houston, Texas 77030.

The lower rate of fatty acid oxidation during hypoxia is related to a decrease in available ATP and also to impairments in the transport of long-chain fatty acids into the mitochondria. The latter occurs by the inhibition of the carnitine–acylcarnitine translocase enzyme system (7). Furthermore, the accumulation of long-chain acyl-CoA and acylcarnitine in the cytosol results in the inhibition of many enzymes (in particular, the Na^+, K^+-ATPases) and also hinders the mitochondrial production and transport of ATP (8).

Hypoxia depresses protein synthesis by inhibiting peptide chain elongation, resulting in the intracellular accumulation of most amino acids, with the exception of aspartate and glutamate (9). The concentrations of aspartate and glutamate decrease as they are transaminated with pyruvate to form alanine. Increases in alanine synthesis from pyruvate serve to moderate the formation of lactate during hypoxia.

ANAEROBIC SOURCES OF ENERGY

Glycolysis

The primary defense against the effects of hypoxia is the mobilization of anaerobic energy pathways—in particular, glycolysis, where glucose, or glycogen, is metabolized to lactate with the production of ATP. The overall reaction of glycolysis is

$$\text{Glucose} + 2\ \text{MgADP}^{1-} + 2\ P_i^{2-} \rightarrow$$
$$2\ \text{Lactate}^{1-} + 2\ \text{MgATP}^{2-} \quad [2]$$

An important regulator of glycolysis is phosphofructokinase (PFK), the enzyme that catalyzes the conversion of fructose-6-phosphate to fructose-1,6-bisphosphate. PFK is strongly inhibited by ATP and is activated by metabolites whose concentration increases with hypoxia: ADP, adenine monophosphate (AMP), and P_i. Consequently, glycolysis is stimulated when cellular requirements outpace the production of ATP.

Cellular acidosis is a major drawback of glycolysis as a source of ATP, since the production of one molecule of lactate generates one H^+. There is some argument with respect to the contribution of glycolysis to cellular acidosis. Some investigators maintain that glycolysis does not generate protons when cellular pH is at the physiologic level of 7.2 (10). It is generally agreed, however, that at low pH levels (pH ~6.2) the protonation of ADP^{1-} increases and one H^+ is formed per molecule of lactate generated. The reader is referred to the works of Gevers (10) and Mainwood and Renaud (11) for comprehensive discussions of intracellular acid–base balance during hypoxia.

The hydrolysis of ATP constitutes another important source of intracellular H^+ during hypoxia (see Eq. 1).

When mitochondrial function is limited by O_2 supply, the recycling of protons by oxidative phosphorylation declines and cytosolic H^+ concentration rises. Therefore, persistent hypoxia produces increasing levels of cellular acidosis, as protons generated by glycolysis and by the hydrolysis of ATP accumulate in the cytosol.

The Creatine Kinase Reaction

Organs with high metabolic demands, such as the brain, the heart, and skeletal muscle, have another anaerobic source of ATP in addition to glycolysis. This is the creatine kinase reaction, where phosphocreatine (PCr), a form of high-energy phosphate storage, is metabolized into ATP and creatine. The creatine kinase reaction also helps decrease the cytosolic concentration of ADP and H^+:

$$\text{PCr}^{2-} + \text{MgADP}^{1-} + H^+ \leftrightarrow \text{MgATP}^{2-} + \text{Creatine}$$
$$[3]$$

Under physiologic conditions the creatine kinase reaction is in equilibrium. Increases in ADP and H^+ during hypoxia will promote the formation of ATP and creatine, whereas the opposite occurs when the supplies of ATP rise. These changes can be measured *in vivo* with phosphorus-31 magnetic resonance spectroscopy (^{31}P-MRS) (12).

The creatine kinase reaction also participates in the transport of high-energy phosphates from the mitochondria to the ATPases. This is the phosphate energy shuttle (13), described in greater detail in Chapter 5.5.1.1.

The Adenylate Kinase Reaction

Increases in cytosolic ADP activate a third anaerobic source of energy, the adenylate kinase reaction:

$$\text{MgADP}^{1-} + \text{MgADP}^{1-} \rightarrow \text{MgATP}^{2-} + \text{MgAMP}$$
$$[4]$$

This reaction leads to the accumulation of AMP, which, in turn, is dephosphorylated to adenosine by 5'-nucleotidase (Fig. 1). Adenosine leaves the cell by facilitated diffusion across the membrane and acts as a potent vasodilator in most vascular beds, except in the renal vasculature, where it produces vasoconstriction (14). Recent data support the hypothesis that adenosine is not produced within the myocardial cells but that AMP is released into the interstitium, where it is rapidly dephosphorylated to adenosine (15). Whatever the mechanism involved, conversion of AMP to adenosine provides the cell with a metabolic feedback loop

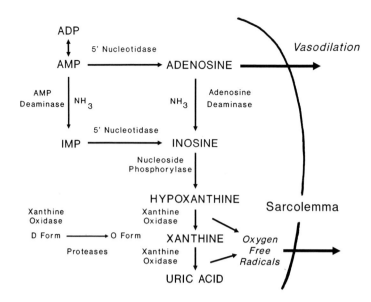

FIG. 1. The degradation pathway of adenine nucleotides. AMP can be dephosphorylated to adenosine or deaminated to IMP. These metabolites can undergo further catabolism to inosine and hypoxanthine. The formation of xanthine and uric acid by xanthine oxidase results in the generation of O_2 free radicals.

to counter hypoxia with increases in capillary flow (16).

The Catabolism of Adenine Nucleotides

As shown in Fig. 1, AMP also can be deaminated to inosine monophosphate (IMP) and ammonia (NH_3) by AMP deaminase. This reaction is important in skeletal muscle during periods of intense normoxic contraction. The formation of IMP helps to maintain a low intracellular AMP concentration, promoting further ATP formation by the adenylate kinase reaction (17). Furthermore, the AMP deaminase reaction also buffers intracellular protons by the production of NH_3. The activity of the AMP deaminase reaction is proportional to increases in H^+, AMP, and ADP concentrations (18).

IMP formation serves as the mechanism to prevent the loss of adenine nucleotides from the cell during hypoxia. ATP resynthesis during recovery takes place by the condensation of IMP and aspartate to succinyl-AMP (sAMP), a reaction catalyzed by the enzyme sAMP synthetase and requiring the use of energy in the form of guanosine triphosphate (GTP). sAMP is cleaved to AMP and fumarate by sAMP lyase. Alternatively, adenine nucleotides can be synthesized *de novo* from small molecule precursors, a slow process that may be inadequate as a source of ATP precursors during recovery from hypoxia.

The deamination of AMP may represent the first step towards the irreversible cellular loss of adenine nucleotides, as IMP is converted to inosine and then to hypoxanthine and xanthine. Intracellular adenosine also enters this degradation pathway by deamination to inosine in the adenosine deaminase reaction. The

relative contributions of the AMP deaminase and the 5′-nucleotidase reactions to the loss of adenine nucleotides during hypoxia are not well understood. Studies of these reactions in red blood cells have shown that the deamination of AMP to IMP is more sensitive to changes in P_i concentration, whereas the dephosphorylation of AMP to adenosine responds to changes in the intracellular concentration of AMP (19).

OTHER CELLULAR ALTERATIONS WITH HYPOXIA

Increases in Intracellular Calcium Concentration

The intracellular level of calcium is closely regulated by transport processes that maintain a 10,000:1 ratio of extracellular to intracellular concentrations. The entry of Ca^{2+} into the cell is controlled by voltage-dependent Ca^{2+} channels, whereas extrusion from the cell occurs by ATP-driven membrane Ca^{2+} pumps and by the Ca^{2+}–Na^+ exchanger (Fig. 2). The energy source of the Ca^{2+}–Na^+ exchanger is the transmembrane Na^+ gradient created by the Na^+, K^+-ATPase. Ca^{2+} is passively exchanged for Na^+, which, in turn, is pumped out of the cell by the energy-consuming Na^+, K^+-ATPase. Other mechanisms involved in the regulation of cytosolic free Ca^{2+} concentration are: (a) sequestration into the mitochondria and into the endoplasmic reticulum by ATP-driven pumps; (b) binding to intracellular proteins; and (c) attachment to the polar heads of the plasma membrane phospholipids.

Hypoxia results in intracellular Ca^{2+} overload by inhibiting ATP-driven membrane transport pumps and the Na^+–Ca^{2+} exchanger (20). Increasing cellular acidosis may be responsible for the latter, since H^+ takes

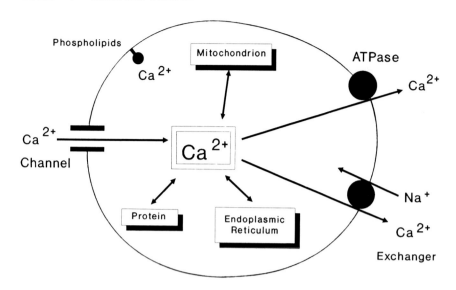

FIG. 2. Cellular mechanisms to regulate cytosolic free calcium concentration: influx through voltage-dependent channels; efflux by plasma membrane Ca^{2+} ATPases; Na^{+}–Ca^{2+} exchanger; sequestration in the mitochondria and the endoplasmic reticulum; binding to cytosolic proteins; and binding to polar heads of membrane phospholipids.

the place of Ca^{2+} as it is exchanged for Na^{+}. Increases in intracellular Ca^{2+} are a pivotal event in cellular dysfunction during hypoxia, since Ca^{2+} activated proteases can destroy the sarcolemma and the cytoskeleton (21). Furthermore, elevations in free Ca^{2+} heighten the activity of Ca^{2+}-dependent ATPases, at a time when the cellular ATP supply is critically low. The reader is referred to the work of Cheung et al. (22) for a thorough review on cellular Ca^{2+} dynamics during hypoxia.

Degradation of Membrane Phospholipids

The loss of membrane phospholipids with the accompanying disruption of membrane ionic gradients has been implicated in the production of irreversible hypoxic damage (23). Three possible mechanisms of membrane damage during hypoxia are: (i) the activation of phospholipases by Ca^{2+}; (ii) the inhibition of phospholipid resynthesis by an energy deficit; and (iii) physical alterations in the cell membrane, leading to mechanical rupture.

The degradation of membrane-bound phospholipids appears to be related to an influx of Ca^{2+} into the cell (24). Ca^{2+} stimulates phospholipases A_2 and C, and these enzymes are known to degrade membrane phospholipids. However, the importance of increased phospholipase activity in the process of membrane degradation during hypoxia has not been well established. It is argued that phospholipase A_2 activity already is maximal at normal levels of intracellular Ca^{2+} (25). Furthermore, increases in phospholipase C activity have not been shown to occur during hypoxia.

Another mechanism that results in cellular membrane damage during hypoxia is the inhibition of phospholipid synthesis. Membrane phospholipids are con-

tinuously broken down and resynthesized in a cycle of deacylation and reacylation. Reacylation of phospholipids is an energy-consuming reaction, and ATP depletion during hypoxia results in the inhibition of phospholipid synthesis. Decreases in cellular ATP concentration to 75% of normal levels produce increases in deacylation without corresponding increases in reacylation (26). This imbalance between the rate of synthesis and the rate of breakdown results in membrane damage and the accumulation of arachidonic acid, a precursor of membrane phospholipids. The metabolism of arachidonic acid, in turn, results in the production of prostaglandins and leukotrienes, substances that produce further cellular damage and profound alterations in microvascular control.

Cellular membrane damage during hypoxia also occurs by mechanical alterations produced by cellular edema. This mechanism results in membrane rupture by physical forces (27). Furthermore, there are reports of hypoxic alterations in vinculin, a protein that anchors the cellular membrane to the cytoskeleton (28). These physical alterations result in the extrusion of lipids from the membrane, and they also result in the degradation of these lipids by cytosolic phospholipases and O_2 free radicals.

Ionic Alterations in Hypoxia

Decreases in ATP concentration during hypoxia inhibit the energy-dependent Na^{+}–K^{+} pump, resulting in decreased K^{+} influx and a rise in the intracellular Na^{+} concentration (29). Hypoxia also produces a greater efflux of K^{+} from the cell by increasing K^{+} membrane conductance with the opening of ATP-dependent K^{+} channels (30). As previously discussed, decreases in Na^{+}–K^{+} exchange also produce a rise in intracellular

Ca^{2+} concentration, with the potential of further cellular damage. For a comprehensive discussion of this topic, the reader is referred to the review by Sayeed (31).

MECHANISMS OF CELLULAR DAMAGE DURING ISCHEMIA, HYPOXEMIA, AND REOXYGENATION

Failure of Respiratory Control

The transition from reversible to irreversible cellular damage is poorly understood. Chance et al. (32) proposed that irreversible injury occurs as the control of oxidative phosphorylation becomes unstable during severe hypoxia. According to this theory, ATP production can be characterized by a Michaelis–Menten-type reaction, where mitochondrial O_2 consumption (Vo_2) is a function of ADP concentration and Po_2. The transfer function of Vo_2 control appears to be hyperbolic, with its operating point located in the ascending portion of the curve (Fig. 3). The flat portion of this curve corresponds to maximal levels of Vo_2 and correspondingly high levels of ADP concentration. Decreases in cellular Po_2 shift the operating curve to the right, lowering the maximum Vo_2 attainable at a given ADP concentration. Severe hypoxia results in the accumulation of ADP, driving the operating point of the system towards the flatter portion of the hyperbola, an unstable position. Increasingly greater concentrations of ADP are required in order to maintain a given level of Vo_2, and eventually the system becomes unstable.

At that point, ATP production ceases and ADP is rapidly converted to AMP and adenosine, which are lost from the cell or deaminated to hypoxanthine.

Intracellular Acidosis

Acidosis impairs recovery from hypoxia by one, or several, of the following mechanisms: (a) loss of adenine nucleotides from the mitochondria by H^+ inhibition of the ATP–Mg/P_i carrier (33); (b) inhibition of the Na^+–Ca^{2+} exchanger, resulting in the intracellular sequestration of Ca^{2+}; (c) increases in the activity of AMP deaminase and the loss of adenine nucleotide precursors from the cell (34); (d) decreases in the nicotinamide adenine nucleotide (NAD) pool by the acid-catalyzed destruction of NADH (35); and (e) the conversion of intracellular P_i to its inhibitory diprotonated form (36).

On the other hand, cellular acidosis has been shown to have some beneficial effects during hypoxia (37). Decreases in ATP utilization have been demonstrated in ischemic heart (38) and skeletal muscle (39). It may be that mitochondrial ATPase inhibition by acidosis protects the cell by slowing the rate of ATP depletion.

Loss of Adenine Nucleotides

The replenishment of adenine nucleotides by *de novo* synthesis is a relatively slow process; therefore, the loss of ATP precursors from the hypoxic cell may impair recovery during reoxygenation. Furthermore, the relative compartmentalization of adenine nucleotides

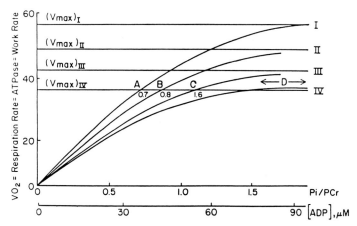

FIG. 3. Transfer function of ADP control of mitochondrial respiration. Horizontal lines represent decreasing levels of maximal ATP production (V_{max}) I through IV. Control curves A through D correspond to decreasing levels of mitochondrial oxygenation. The intersection of the control curve with the V_{max} line represents the operating point at a particular level of mitochondrial oxygenation and ATP production. The intersection of curve A and (V_{max})$_{IV}$ is in the stable (i.e., ascending) portion of the control curve. Increases in ATP production, (V_{max})$_I$, or declining oxygen levels (curve D) shift the operating point to the unstable (i.e., flat) portion of the control curve, also resulting in greater levels of ADP. (From ref. 32.)

in the cytosol and in the mitochondria may be important in the recovery process. Since acidosis favors the accumulation of adenine nucleotides in the cytosol, ATP production could be impaired upon reoxygenation if the mitochondrial adenylate pool is markedly diminished (33).

Production of Oxygen Radicals

Additional cellular damage has been shown to occur immediately after reoxygenation—the so-called "ischemia–reperfusion" paradox. This phenomenon appears to be mediated by O_2 free radicals generated during the catabolism of adenine nucleotides (40).

Increases in inosine concentration lead to the accumulation of hypoxanthine and the formation of xanthine and uric acid by the enzymatic action of xanthine oxidase. Under normoxic conditions, the D form of xanthine oxidase accounts for approximately 90% of the enzyme activity. During hypoxia, the enzyme is converted to its O form by the action of calcium activated proteases. The O form of the enzyme reduces O_2 instead of NAD, resulting in the generation of free oxygen radical species upon reoxygenation (41).

Neutrophil Accumulation

A temporal relationship exists between myocardial ischemia and neutrophil (polymorphonuclear neutrophil leukocyte, or PMN) accumulation (42), reaching a maximum after 24 hr of coronary occlusion and persisting for several days thereafter (43). The accumulation of PMNs creates an inflammatory response, with increased endothelial permeability and the release of proteolytic enzymes. PMN aggregation also results in microcirculatory disruption, characterized by the "no reflow" phenomenon, where capillaries become totally occluded by PMNs (44).

The course of PMN accumulation following a brief period of ischemia is rapid, reaching a peak after 6 hr of reperfusion (45). The accumulation of PMNs may play an important role in the pathogenesis of the myocardial ischemia–reperfusion injury. It is possible that PMN aggregation results in endothelial damage by generating O_2 free radical species in the xanthine oxidase reaction. This enzyme is species-specific (46) and appears to be absent in human myocytes (47). The role of PMNs in the ischemia–reperfusion injury has not been well established, and conflicting results have been found in animal preparations depleted of PMNs prior to an ischemic insult (48,49).

CELLULAR RESPONSES TO ISCHEMIA AND HYPOXEMIA

There are conflicting data on the effects of ischemia and hypoxemia on heart, brain, and skeletal muscle cells. In 1935, Tennant and Wiggers (50) showed that hypoxemia was less harmful to the heart than ischemia. These findings were corroborated by Neely and Grotyohann (51), who studied isolated rat heart preparations perfused at high flow and low Po_2 (hypoxemia) and compared them to preparations perfused at low flow and high Po_2 (partial ischemia). Glycolysis was enhanced in both groups during the first 5 min of hypoxia. This increase in glycolytic flux persisted in the hypoxemic group, but it decreased after 10 min of ischemia. Increased glycolytic flux resulted in a higher rate of lactate production during hypoxemia. However, because lactate and other metabolites were removed from the tissues by the bloodstream, the *accumulation* of lactate was 10 times lower during hypoxemia than during ischemia. Another finding of the study was a greater impairment of mechanical function in the ischemic hearts. This was attributed to the decrease in glycolytic flux and to lower levels of glycolytic ATP production during ischemia.

Subsequent experiments comparing the effect of total ischemia and partial ischemia on myocardial function showed better recovery by partially ischemic hearts upon reperfusion. It was concluded from these experiments that the removal of tissue lactate and the maintenance of intracellular pH are very important factors in maintaining glycolytic ATP production when O_2 supply is limited.

Opposite results have been reported regarding the effect of total and partial ischemia ("trickle" ischemia) on brain cellular function. Hossman and Kleihues (52) noted that 60 min of cerebral partial ischemia was worse than a similar period of total ischemia. This finding was verified by Nordstrom et al. (53) in rats subjected to bilateral carotid ligation for 30 min, followed by reperfusion. One group exposed to total ischemia was compared to another group where the cerebral blood flow was decreased by 90–95% of baseline. Total ischemia produced lower levels of lactate than partial ischemia. Furthermore, the rats exposed to total ischemia had higher levels of PCr and adenine nucleotides than those exposed to partial ischemia. These results imply that brain cells tolerate total ischemia better than partial ischemia. In subsequent experiments, Rehncrona et al. (54) demonstrated that hypoxemia is more harmful to the brain than total ischemia. The greater injury potential of hypoxemia or low-flow ischemia to the brain may be related to increases in glycolysis with the accumulation of intracellular lactate and H^+. It is hypothesized that lactate production during total ischemia is limited, since the substrate for glycolysis is restricted to the levels of available glycogen stores (4). On the other hand, with low-flow ischemia, or hypoxemia, the tissues are exposed to an abundant supply of glucose, resulting in continuing glycolysis and a greater degree of cellular acidosis. Furthermore, a trickling of oxygen may promote the continuous production of O_2 free radical species during the hypoxic period.

Results similar to those found in the brain have been reported in skeletal muscle by Gutierrez et al. using a blood-perfused rabbit hindlimb preparation (55). There was adequate recovery in the levels of PCr and P_i following reperfusion after 1 hr of total ischemia. Recovery of these metabolites did not occur after a similar period of severe hypoxemia ($Pao_2 < 10$ torr).

The apparent discrepancy between the effects of ischemia and hypoxemia on heart, brain, and skeletal muscle may be the result of different experimental designs. The isolated heart preparations were perfused with nonrecirculating Krebs–Henseleit bicarbonate buffer, whereas brain and muscle were exposed to recirculating blood with increasing levels of lactate. Moreover, recirculating blood could have carried other harmful substances released by hypoxic tissues, including prostaglandins, platelet aggregating factor, O_2 free radicals, phospholipases, etc. It does appear certain, however, that the intracellular accumulation of H^+, lactate, and other products of metabolism, such as inorganic phosphate, portends an unfavorable outcome during reoxygenation.

THERAPEUTIC STRATEGIES IN HYPOXIA

A number of agents have been tried in an effort to ameliorate the cellular effects of hypoxia. These agents fall in the categories of ATP precursors, O_2 radical scavengers, Ca^{2+}-channel blockers, components of the glycolytic pathway, and glucose.

It has been shown that ATP depletion contributes to the increase in cytosolic free Ca^{2+} in ischemic renal cells (56), whereas treatment with ATP-$MgCl_2$ improves mitochondrial function and reflow in ischemic liver (57). Possible mechanisms of action include the preservation of intracellular adenine nucleotide levels (58) and a direct vasodilatory effect on the microvasculature (59). The administration of nucleotide precursors, such as inosine (60) and adenosine (61), also has been shown to improve the recovery of ischemic myocardium.

There is a large body of literature showing the beneficial effects of O_2 free-radical scavengers and allopurinol, an inhibitor of the xanthine oxidase reaction, on cellular recovery from hypoxia (41,46). It has been proposed that endotoxin pretreatment also affords protection against the ischemia–reperfusion injury by increasing the production of endogenous catalase (62).

The use of Ca^{2+}-channel blockers, such as diltiazem, has been reported to protect myocardial cells from hypoxia by decreasing intracellular Ca^{2+} accumulation (63). On the other hand, the use of pyruvate and dichloroacetate, an activator of the enzyme pyruvate dehydrogenase, has met with disappointing results (64,65).

The role of exogenous glucose in the development of hypoxic cellular damage during hypoxia is controversial. Elevated glucose levels during hypoxia are detrimental to the brain (4) and spinal cord (66), most likely the result of intracellular lactate and H^+ accumulation. The threshold of injury for cerebral lactate concentration is approximately 25 mmol/kg (67). ATP resynthesis by the cerebral cortex during ischemic reperfusion is greatly impaired when blood glucose levels are greater than 12–13 mM (68), whereas insulin administration appears to confer a protective effect (69).

An opposite effect of glucose has been demonstrated in the hypoxic myocardium, where glucose administration appears to be of benefit (30,51). However, dogs given glucose after 6 min of cardiac arrest had greater mortality than a control group (70). It is possible that glucose administration may be beneficial in hemodynamically stable myocardial infarction; however, hyperglycemia should be avoided in low-cardiac-output states, where the possibility of brain ischemia exists. Resolution of this issue awaits carefully designed, prospective clinical studies.

CONCLUSIONS

The cellular response to hypoxia is a complex process composed of multiple physiologic, cellular, and molecular mechanisms. Some of these mechanisms help to maintain cellular energy production, whereas others produce cellular injury. The relative magnitude of these mechanisms determines whether the resumption of O_2 supply results in cellular death or in normal cellular function.

The transition from reversible to irreversible hypoxic injury appears to be related to the degree of cellular membrane damage and to the capacity of the mitochondria to resume ATP production. Advances in the therapy of myocardial infarction, respiratory failure, and cerebral stroke require greater understanding of these mechanisms.

ACKNOWLEDGMENT

This work was supported, in part, by National Institutes of Health grant HL41415-01.

REFERENCES

1. Sapega AA, Heppenstall RB, Chance B, Parks YS, Sokolow D. Optimizing tourniquet application and release times in extremity and surgery. A biochemical and ultrastructural study. *Bone Joint Surg* 1985;67:303–314.

2. Andersson BS, Aw TY, Jones DP. Mitochondria transmembrane potential and pH gradient during anoxia. *Am J Physiol* 1987;252:C349–C355.

3. Weinberger LM, Gibbon MN, Gibbon JH. Temporary arrest of the circulation to the central nervous system. *Arch Neurol Psychiatry* 1940;43:961–986.

4. Siesjo BK. Cell damage in the brain: a speculative synthesis. *J Cereb Blood Flow Metab* 1981;1:155–185.

5. Hochachka PW. Defense strategies against hypoxia and hypothermia. *Science* 1986;231:234–241.

6. Myears DW, Sobel BE, Bergmann SR. Substrate use in ischemic and reperfused canine myocardium: quantitative considerations. *Am J Physiol* 1987;253:H107–H114.

7. Pauly DF, Yoon SB, McMillin JB. Carnitine–acylcarnitine translocase in ischemia: evidence for sulfhydryl modification. *Am J Physiol* 1987;253:H1557–H1565.

8. Neely JR. Metabolic disturbances after coronary occlusion. *Hosp Pract* 1989;24:81–96.

9. Kao R, Rannels DE, Morgan HE. Effects of anoxia and ischemia on protein synthesis in perfused rat hearts. *Circ Res* 1976; 38(Suppl I):124–130.

10. Gevers W. Generation of protons by metabolic processes in heart cells. *J Mol Cell Cardiol* 1977;9:867–874.

11. Mainwood GW, Renaud JM. The effect of acid–base balance on fatigue of skeletal muscle. *Cancer J Physiol Pharmacol* 1985;63:403–416.

12. Gutierrez G, Pohil JP, Narayana P. Skeletal muscle O_2 consumption and energy metabolism during hypoxemia. *J Appl Physiol* 1989;66:2117–2123.

13. Bessman SP. The creatine–creatine phosphate energy shuttle. *Annu Rev Biochem* 1985;54:831–862.

14. Berne RM. Adenosine: an important physiological regulator. *News Physiol Sci* 1986;1:163–167.

15. Van Belle H, Goossens F, Wynants J. Formation and release of purine catabolites during hypoperfusion, anoxia, and ischemia. *Am J Physiol* 1987;252:H886–H893.

16. Wei HM, Kang YH, Merrill GF. Coronary vasodilation during global myocardial hypoxia: effects of adenosine deaminase. *Am J Physiol* 1988;58:H1004–H1009.

17. Whitlock DM, Terjung RL. ATP depletion in slow-twitch red muscle of rat. *Am J Physiol* 1987;253:C426–C432.

18. Dudley GA, Terjung RL. Influence of aerobic metabolism on IMP accumulation in fast-twitch muscle. *Am J Physiol* 1985; 248:C37–C42.

19. Bontemps F, Berghe GVD, Hers HG. Pathways of adenine nucleotide catabolism in erythrocytes. *J Clin Invest* 1986;77:824–830.

20. Dixon IMC, Eyolfson DA, Dhalla NS. Sarcolemmal Na^+–Ca^{2+} exchange activity in hearts subjected to hypoxia reoxygenation. *Am J Physiol* 1987;253:H1026–H1034.

21. Mellgren RL. Calcium-dependent proteases: an enzyme system active at cellular membranes. *FASEB J* 1987;1:110–115.

22. Cheung JY, Bonventre JV, Malis CD, Leaf A. Calcium and ischemic injury. *N Engl J Med* 1986;314:1670–1676.

23. Das DK, Engelman RM, Rousou JA, Breyer RH, Otani H, Lemeshow S. Role of membrane phospholipids in myocardial injury induced by ischemia and reperfusion. *Am J Physiol* 1986; 251:H71–H79.

24. Otani H, Prasad MR, Jones RM, Das DK. Mechanism of membrane phospholipid degradation in ischemic-reperfused rat hearts. *Am J Physiol* 1989;257:H252–H258.

25. van der Vusse GJ, van Bilsen M, Reneman RS. Is phospholipid degradation a critical event in ischemia and reperfusion-induced damage? *News Physiol Sci* 1989;4:49–53.

26. Gunn MD, Sen A, Chang A, Willerson JT, Buja LM, Chien KR. Mechanisms of accumulation of arachidonic acid in cultured myocardial cells during ATP depletion. *Am J Physiol* 1985; 249:H1188–H1194.

27. Verkley AJ, Post JA. Physico-chemical properties and organization of lipids in membranes: their possible role in myocardial injury. *Basic Res Cardiol* 1987;82(Suppl 1):85–91.

28. Steenbergen CM, Hill ML, Jenings RB. Cytoskeletal damage during myocardial ischemia: changes in vinculin immunofluorescence staining during total *in vitro* ischemia in canine heart. *Circ Res* 1987;60:476–486.

29. Kako K, Kato M, Matsuoka T, Mustapha A. Depression of membrane-bound Na^+-K^+-ATPase activity induced by free radicals and by ischemia of kidney. *Am J Physiol* 1988; 254:C330–C337.

30. Kleber A. Resting membrane potential, extracellular K^+ activity, and intracellular Na^+ activity during global ischemia in isolated perfused guinea pig hearts. *Circ Res* 1983;52:442–450.

31. Sayeed MM. Ion transport in circulatory and/or septic shock. *Am J Physiol* 1987;252:R809–R821.

32. Chance B, Nioka S, Leigh JS Jr. Metabolic control principles: importance of the steady state reaffirmed and quantified by ^{31}P MRS. In: Bryan-Brown CW, Ayres SM, eds. *Oxygen transport and utilization*. Fullerton, CA: Society for Critical Care Medicine, 1987;215–224.

33. Aprille JR. Regulation of the mitochondrial adenine nucleotide pool size in liver: mechanism and metabolic role. *FASEB J* 1988;2:2547–2556.

34. Dudley GA, Terjung RL. Influence of acidosis on AMP deaminase activity in contracting fast-twitch muscle. *Am J Physiol* 1985;248:C43–C50.

35. Welsh FA. Effect of glucose on recovery of energy metabolism following hypoxia–oligemia in mouse brain: dose-dependence and carbohydrate specificity. *J Cereb Blood Flow Metab* 1983; 3:486–492.

36. Nosek TM, Fender KY, Godt RE. It is diprotonated inorganic phosphate that depresses force in skinned skeletal muscle fibers. *Science* 1987;236:191–193.

37. Gores GJ, Nieminen AL, Fleishman KE, Dawson TL, Herman B, Lemaster JJ. Extracellular acidosis delays onset of cell death in ATP-depleted hepatocytes. *Am J Physiol* 1988;255:C315–C322.

38. Sako ET, Kingsley-Hickman PB, From AH, Foker JE, Ugurbil K. ATP synthesis kinetics and mitochondrial function in the post-ischemic myocardium as studied by ^{31}P NMR. *J Biol Chem* 1988;263:10600–10607.

39. Katz A. G-1, 6-P_2, glycolysis, and energy metabolism during circulatory occlusion in human skeletal muscle. *Am J Physiol* 1988;255:C140–C144.

40. McCord JM. Oxygen-derived free radicals in postischemic tissue injury. *N Engl J Med* 1985;312:159–163.

41. Granger DN. Role of xanthine oxidase and granulocytes in ischemia–reperfusion injury. *Am J Physiol* 1988;255:H1269–H1275.

42. Mallory GK, White PD, Salcedo-Salgar J. The speed of healing of myocardial infarction: a study of the pathologic anatomy in 72 cases. *Am Heart J* 1939;18:647–671.

43. Fishbein MC, MacLean D, Maroko PR. Experimental myocardial infarction in the rat. *Am J Pathol* 1978;90:57–70.

44. Engler RL, Schmid-Schonbein GW, Pavelec RS. Leukocyte capillary plugging in myocardial ischemia and reperfusion in the dog. *Am J Pathol* 1983;111:98–111.

45. Smith III EF, Egan JW, Bugelski PJ, Hillegass LM, Hill DE, Griswold DE. Temporal relation between neutrophil accumulation and myocardial reperfusion injury. *Am J Physiol* 1988;255:H1060–H1068.

46. Grum CM, Ketal LH, Myers CL, Shlafer M. Purine efflux after cardiac ischemia: relevance to allopurinol carioprotection. *Am J Physiol* 1987;252:H368–H373.

47. Eddy LJ, Stewart JR, Jones HP, Engerson TD, McCord JM, Downey JM. Free radical-producing enzyme, xanthine oxidase, is undetectable in human hearts. *Am J Physiol* 1987;253:H709–H711.

48. Grgaard B, Schurer L, Gerdin B, Arfors KE. Delayed hypoperfusion after incomplete forebrain ischemia in the rat. The role of polymorphonuclear leukocytes. *J Cereb Blood Flow Metab* 1989;9:500–505.

49. O'Neill PG, Charlat ML, Michael LH, Roberts R, Bolli R. Influence of neutrophil depletion on myocardial function and flow after reversible ischemia. *Am J Physiol* 1989;256:H341–H351.

50. Tennant R, Wiggers CJ. Effects of coronary occlusion on myocardial contraction. *Am J Physiol* 1935;112:351–361.

51. Neely JR, Grotyohann LW. Role of glycolytic products in damage to ischemic myocardium. *Circ Res* 1984;55:816–824.

52. Hossman KA, Kleihues P. Reversibility of ischemic brain damage. *Arch Neurol* 1973;29:375–382.
53. Nordstrom CH, Rehncrona S, Siesjo BK. Restitution of cerebral energy state, as well as of glycolytic metabolites, citric acid cycle intermediates and associated amino acids after 30 minutes of complete ischemia in rats anesthetized with nitrous oxide or phenobarbital. *J Neurochem* 1978;30:479–486.
54. Rehncrona S, Mela L, Siesjo BK. Recovery of brain mitochondrial function in the rat after complete and incomplete cerebral ischemia. *Stroke* 1979;10:437–446.
55. Gutierrez G, Pohil RJ, Andry JM, Strong R, Narayana P. Bioenergetics of rabbit skeletal muscle during hypoxemia and ischemia. *J Appl Physiol* 1988;65:608–616.
56. McCoy CE. Adenosine triphosphate depletion induces a rise in cytosolic free calcium in canine renal epithelial cells. *J Clin Invest* 1988;82:1326–1332.
57. Chaudry IH, Ohkawa M, Clemens MG. Improved mitochondrial function following ischemia and reflow by ATP-MgCl$_2$. *Am J Physiol* 1984;246:R799–R804.
58. Ohkawa M, Clemens MG, Chaudry IH. Studies on the mechanism of beneficial effects of ATP-MgCl$_2$ following hepatic ischemia. *Am J Physiol* 1983;244:R695–R702.
59. Clemens MG, McDonagh PF, Chaudry IH, Baue AE. Hepatic microcirculatory failure after ischemia and reperfusion: improvement with ATP-MgCl$_2$ treatment. *Am J Physiol* 1985;248:H804–H811.
60. Devous MD, Lewandowski ED. Inosine preserves ATP during ischemia and enhances recovery during reperfusion. *Am J Physiol* 1987;253:H1224–H1233.
61. Ambrosio G, Jacobus WE, Mitchell MC, Litt MR, Becker LC. Effects of ATP precursors on ATP and free ADP content and functional recovery of postischemic hearts. *Am J Physiol* 1989;256:H560–H566.
62. Brown JM. Endotoxin pretreatment increases endogenous myocardial catalase activity and decreases ischemia–reperfusion injury of isolated rat hearts. *Proc Natl Acad Sci USA* 1989;86:2516–2520.
63. Watts JA, Whipple JP, Hatley AA. A low concentration of nisoldipine reduces ischemic heart injury: enhanced reflow and recovery of contractile function without energy preservation during ischemia. *J Mol Cell Cardiol* 1987;19:809–816.
64. van Bilsen M. Effects of pyruvate on post-ischemic myocardial recovery at various workloads. *Pflugers Arch* 1988;413:167–173.
65. Gutterman DD, Chilian WM, Eastham CL, Inou T, White CW, Marcus ML. Failure of pyruvate to salvage myocardium after prolonged ischemia. *Am J Physiol* 1986;250:H114–H120.
66. Drummond JC, Moore SS. The influence of dextrose administration on neurologic outcome after temporary spinal cord ischemia in the rabbit. *Anesthesiology* 1989;70:64–70.
67. Myers R. Lactic acid accumulation as a cause of brain edema and cerebral necrosis resulting from oxygen deprivation. In: Korbin R, Guilleminault C, eds. *Advances in perinatal neurology*. New York: Spectrum, 1979;84–114.
68. Welsh FA, Sims RE, McKee AE. Effect of glucose on recovery of energy metabolism following hypoxia–oligemia in mouse brain: dose-dependence and carbohydrate specificity. *J Cereb Blood Flow Metab* 1983;3:486–492.
69. LeMay DR, Dalecy LG. Insulin administration protects neurologic function in cerebral ischemia in rats. *Stroke* 1988;19:1411–1419.
70. Lundy EF, Kuhn JE, Kwon JM, Zelenock GB, D'Alecy L. Infusion of 5% dextrose increases mortality and morbidity following six minutes of cardiac arrest in resuscitated dogs. *J Crit Care* 1987;2:4–14.

THE LUNG: Scientific Foundations
edited by R.G. Crystal, J.B. West et al.
Raven Press, Ltd., New York © 1991.

CHAPTER 5.5.3.2

Hypoxia and the Brain

Thomas F. Hornbein

While the lung depends upon the brain for the tuning of many aspects of its several functions, the brain depends upon the lung for its fundamental sustenance, the provision of oxygen, and the removal of carbon dioxide. The brain is a demanding organ. While representing only 2–3% of an adult's body weight, it commands about a quarter of the body's resting oxygen consumption, 3–4 ml/100 g/min; moreover, its blood supply of 50–60 ml/100 g/min represents 20% of resting cardiac output. A decrease in the oxygen supplied to the central nervous system, either due to diminution in flow, *ischemia,* or to a deficit of oxygen in the arterial blood, *hypoxia,* will rapidly compromise brain tissue oxygenation and brain function. Hypoxemia resulting from environmental factors, hypoventilation, or impaired gas exchange can cause global central nervous system hypoxia, resulting in consequences ranging from diminished (but reversible) neurobehavioral function to permanent injury or death. My goal in this chapter will be to review the central nervous system's dependence upon oxygen and how a lack of oxygen, in the oft-quoted words of Haldane, "not only stops the machine but wrecks the machinery."

CENTRAL NERVOUS SYSTEM OXYGEN SUPPLY AND DEMAND

Approximately 40% of the central nervous system volume is neuronal mass that possesses a high-energy requirement in order to maintain cell integrity, sustain ionic gradients across cell membranes, and permit the electrical depolarization and neurotransmitter release that underpins central nervous system function. The brain's metabolic needs are met by the consumption of ATP, with the energy required to replenish ATP from ADP being derived aerobically from glucose (1). Glucose is normally the brain's only energy substrate, with 95% being converted to carbon dioxide and water. Minimal reserves of oxygen and glucose are stored within the brain, so that failure of delivery of either will quickly result in energy depletion. Cerebral metabolic rates for oxygen (CMR_{O_2}) and glucose may vary severalfold across different regions of the central nervous system, depending upon such things as neuronal and glial density and neuronal activity; for example, oxygen consumption may differ as much as threefold between white and gray matter.

In addition to the autoregulation that maintains cerebral blood flow approximately constant within a cerebral perfusion pressure (mean arterial pressure minus intracranial venous pressure) range of about 50–150 mmHg, cerebral vessels react to changes in oxygen and carbon dioxide in a manner that minimizes changes in tissue oxygen and carbon dioxide levels in the face of changes in the partial pressure of these gases in arterial blood. Between 20 and 60 mmHg $P_{a}CO_2$, cerebral blood flow increases about 2–3% per mmHg. This reactivity to carbon dioxide is hypothesized to result from the diffusion of carbon dioxide across the blood–brain barrier to alter brain extracellular fluid hydrogen ion concentration. Systemic metabolic acid–base changes of similar magnitude have minimal effect on cerebral blood flow, presumably because of the relative impermeability to H^+ or other ions of brain capillaries with their tight junctions between endothelial cells. Cerebral vascular resistance also decreases appreciably when $P_{a}O_2$ falls below 50–60 mmHg, with cerebral blood flow reaching about twice its normoxic value at 30 mmHg.

Adaptation to chronic hypoxia or sustained changes in carbon dioxide level offsets these acute changes, resulting in a cerebral blood flow that is more akin to the normal state. For example, persons with chronic

T. F. Hornbein: Department of Anesthesiology and Department of Physiology and Biophysics, University of Washington, Seattle, Washington 98195.

obstructive pulmonary disease who are both hypoxic and hypercapnic exhibit near-normal cerebral blood flow. After 24–48 hr of acclimatization to an altitude of 4300 m, cerebral blood flow is at or above the sea-level normal value in spite of the lower $P_{a}CO_2$ (2). These adaptations have been explained as being related to restoration of the brain extracellular fluid pH by rapid regulation of bicarbonate concentration across the blood–brain barrier. Mechanisms underlying adjustment of cerebral vascular caliber in response to changes in perfusion pressure or in oxygen or CO_2 levels focus on the possible role of myogenic responses, effect of autonomic innervation on smooth muscle tone, and modulation by substances such as hydrogen ion, adenosine, prostaglandins, and neuropeptides.

CONSEQUENCES OF OXYGEN LACK

Acute brain hypoxia, either from diminished flow or arterial hypoxemia, yields progressive impairment; outcome depends both on the depth and duration of the hypoxia. Initial compromise of neuronal function is associated with a progressive decrease in electrical activity, although a calibration of loss of consciousness to electrical events has not been well defined in humans. At the point where the electroencephalogram (EEG) passes from a burst–suppression pattern to an isoelectric one, normal levels of ATP and ionic gradients across cell membranes are still preserved. Presumably, at least with brief exposures, the impairment is reversible at this stage upon eliminating the brain hypoxia. In cats and in humans with progressive ischemia the EEG becomes isoelectric at cerebral blood flows between 16 and 18 ml/100 g/min, whereas evoked responses in baboons persist to approximately 15 ml/100 g/min; ionic pump failure does not occur until flows fall below 10 ml/100 g/min (3).

At the concentration of an anesthetic where the EEG becomes isoelectric, CMR_{O_2} is approximately 50% the normal awake value; further increase in anesthetic concentration does not produce additional decrease in CMR_{O_2}. This observation suggests that about half of the brain's oxygen requirement is dedicated to neuronal activity while the other half serves to preserve basal ionic gradients and other housekeeping functions. Not until hypoxia encroaches on this second space do depletion of energy stores, loss of membrane integrity, and the potential for damage occur. Neurons, possibly because of a higher metabolic rate, appear to be more susceptible than glia or vascular cells. Thus, an appropriately titrated dose of hypoxia can cause selective neuronal cell death without producing major changes in the brain macroenvironment. More severe hypoxia will yield additional injury, resulting in loss of endothelial integrity, translocation of water with

generalized brain edema, and increase in intracranial pressure and areas of infarction. Microcirculatory changes resulting from ischemia may account for the absence of blood flow—the *no-reflow phenomenon* originally described by Ames et al. (4)—when a mechanical occlusion to flow is eliminated.

Brain tissue hypoxia is more commonly a consequence of ischemia, either global or focal, than of arterial hypoxemia alone. Most of the research examining the consequences of tissue hypoxia, mechanisms of injury, and ways to prevent or treat injury has involved animal models of complete or partial ischemia. To produce brain injury by arterial hypoxemia alone has proven difficult, because such severe hypoxemia causes cardiovascular depression and hypotension as well (5).

Metabolic Effects

The vulnerability of the brain to oxygen lack is vividly illustrated by the consequences of even a few minutes of the total ischemia associated with cardiac arrest, which can result in permanent impairment of function. With sudden, total ischemia, energy stores are quickly exhausted: In the rat's cerebral cortex, phosphocreatine levels approach zero within the first minute, followed by a similar degree of depletion of ATP in the next 60 sec (6). Mitochondrial ATP production ceases, and anaerobic glycolysis (which also depends on glucose availability) produces too little ATP to sustain either function or cell integrity. Increase in brain lactate concentration tracks closely the fall in ATP, with the extent of lactic acid accumulation being related to glucose availability. Thus, partial ischemia, by continuing to supply glucose, may result in higher tissue lactate concentrations and lower pH than during total circulatory arrest; this results in more severe injury, presumably from the greater tissue acidosis. At about 90 sec, associated with and presumably caused by depletion of energy stores, extracellular fluid ion concentrations show sudden and dramatic changes, representing both pump failure and perhaps alterations in membrane integrity (7); extracellular K^+ concentration precipitously rises to 50–60 mM while extracellular sodium and chloride concentrations decrease to a similar extent; extracellular fluid calcium ion concentration decreases from 1.2 mM toward zero as calcium ions enter cells. These changes are associated with a decrease in the volume of the extracellular space as water follows these osmoles into cells.

The depletion of energy stores and of their ionic and acid–base concomitants are the precursor events related not only to loss of function but also to cell injury. Several hypotheses concerning the mechanism of cell membrane dysfunction and cell death, not necessarily mutually exclusive, have been proposed (7).

Calcium

The rise in free intracellular calcium concentration with energy depletion is thought to result from membrane depolarization opening voltage-sensitive calcium channels and neurotransmitter release opening agonist-operated calcium channels; additionally, with ATP depletion the ability to extrude calcium or to sequester it within sarcoplasmic reticulum is compromised. A surfeit of free calcium ion may activate phospholipase A_2, causing release of free fatty acids that trigger production of prostaglandins, leukotrienes, and free radicals. Proteolysis and lipolysis result, impairing cytoskeletal and cell membrane functions. The greater susceptibility of neurons was thought initially to be due to opening of voltage-sensitive channels, but *in vitro* studies indicate that injury can occur without a rise in intracellular calcium; the rise in intracellular calcium could be a consequence rather than a major cause of injury, or it might contribute selectively to damage of neurons containing a high density of agonist-operated calcium channels gated by excitatory amino acids.

Excitatory Amino Acids

Epilepsy, hypoglycemia, and hypoxia result in an increase in concentration of the excitatory amino acids, glutamate, and aspartate, both by increased release and possibly decreased re-uptake. These neurotransmitters, acting on *N*-methyl-D-aspartate (NMDA) receptors, cause opening of agonist-operated calcium channels as well as sodium and chloride channels via action on kainate and quisqualate receptors. An excess of excitatory amino acids might contribute to neuronal injury by facilitating calcium increase and perhaps also by osmolarity changes secondary to sodium, chloride, and water shifts.

Free Radicals

Reperfusion following partial or complete ischemia provides a potential milieu for formation of free radicals. Hydroxyl (OH·) and superoxide ($·O_2^-$) species produced by the mitochondrial respiratory chain or catalyzed by cyclo-oxygenase and lipoxygenase, as well as radicals resulting from autoxidation of compounds such as catecholamines, are all potential contributors to reperfusion injury when oxygen supply is suddenly restored to an abnormal, energy-depleted environment. The ability to demonstrate the presence of free radicals and to define their contribution to post-

ischemic injury has proven difficult. A mechanism for the conversion of ferric to ferrous ions, with a role for the latter in catalyzing free-radical reactions, has been recently proposed (8). Evidence that free radicals may contribute to injury of vascular cells is better than evidence for similar effects upon neurons and glia.

Acidosis

With partial ischemia a continuous supply of glucose to be metabolized anaerobically would result in a greater intracellular lactic acidosis superimposed upon the tissue hypoxia. Cellular injury may be greater with partial ischemia than with complete ischemia because the effect of this acidosis, possibly acting to inhibit mitochondrial ATP production, may more than offset the enhancement of oxygen delivery. Edema and cell damage can appear after a period of apparently normal reperfusion. Less severe ischemia appears to be associated with a longer latency before edema and seizures occur, anywhere from 1 to 24 hr later. Delayed encephalopathy following cerebral hypoxia from a variety of causes, including cardiac arrest, carbon monoxide poisoning, and inspired hypoxia, is recognized clinically (9). Cognitive, behavioral, and motor impairments are observed. Histologically, demyelination and oligodendroglial destruction predominate over the neuronal loss that is characteristic of acute cerebral hypoxia (10). The reason for the delayed impairment following return to apparently normal function after reperfusion is unclear.

Pathological Changes

The extent of pathological abnormality caused by hypoxia or ischemia depends upon the total dose (i.e., depth and duration). Brierley (5) has pointed out the commonality of pathological changes seen with hypoxia and ischemia, proposing that damage from arterial hypoxemia or anemia is likely not to be pure but, instead, associated with circulatory depression and cerebral hypoperfusion. Thus, the so-called border zone lesions (i.e., the end-arterial regions where perfusion first becomes insufficient) are seen with hypoxia as well as ischemia. With mild injury, the early microscopic findings are of neuronal cell injury: "Dark" neurons are scattered in a multifocal manner through the cortex and basal ganglia; with time after the hypoxic injury, these damaged neurons disappear. With moderate injury, widespread involvement of border zones will be seen scattered through various layers of the cortex, the pyramidal layer of the hippocampus, the neocerebellar cortex, and the brainstem; considerable variability in distribution is generally apparent. With severe hypoxia, petechial hemorrhages are seen scattered throughout the brain, particularly in white matter and the corpus callosum. Slightly less severe hypoxia will cause the ischemic neuronal changes described above as well as causing glial injury, edema, and capillary endothelial changes. Thus with increasing severity of hypoxic or ischemic injury, involvement of glial and endothelial cells in addition to neurons is seen. Brierley (5) has discussed in detail these patterns of ''selective vulnerability'' in such areas as the neocortex, the hippocampus, the basal ganglia, and arterial boundary zones.

Functional Consequences

The effects of acute hypoxia in depressing central nervous system function of humans are described in a venerable literature reviewed recently by Gibson et al. (11). We shall focus on the toxicity of oxygen lack—that is, the residual nervous system impairment after the hypoxia has been relieved. Such changes may occur against the background of the acclimatization to hypoxia that permits the adapted individual to tolerate far lower values of arterial P_{O_2} than are possible acutely (12). Based upon the changes noted in the animal models of central nervous system ischemia that we have reviewed, one is tempted to conclude that arterial hypoxemia in the absence of hypoperfusion should not cause brain injury and residual impairment of function after the hypoxemia has been relieved; that is, lacking an isoelectric EEG or loss of consciousness, subsequent harm ought not to occur. But a study by Dong et al. (13), seeking to identify a threshold for ischemic brain injury, noted histological evidence of neuronal damage in monkeys rendered severely anemic and hypotensive even though an isoelectric EEG and obliteration of the somatosensory evoked potential did not occur.

Assessment of neurobehavioral function in individuals with chronic hypoxemia also suggests that sustained consciousness is not a guarantee against hypoxic injury. Two populations of chronically hypoxic humans have been studied: (i) patients with chronic obstructive pulmonary disease (COPD) and (ii) healthy mountaineers climbing to extremely high altitude.

Observations made during the Nocturnal Oxygen Therapy Trial (NOTT) and the Intermittent Positive Pressure Breathing Trial (IPPBT) sponsored by the National Institutes of Health assessed neurobehavioral function of persons with COPD (14). Together, these two trials afforded evaluation of 302 patients and 99 age- and education-matched controls while also permitting assessment of a chronic hypoxemic state ranging from mild (mean $P_{a_{O_2}}$ = 68 mmHg) to moderate (mean $P_{a_{O_2}}$ = 54 mmHg) to severe (mean $P_{a_{O_2}}$ = 44 mmHg). Although both age and education correlated

with neurobehavioral performance, for our present purposes the relevant observation was the weaker but significant correlation of impairment with severity of hypoxemia. Although verbal I.Q. was not significantly affected, perceptual motor learning and problem solving (Digit Symbol, Trail Making B, Category Test) differed from controls, even in the mildly hypoxemic group. The risk of impairment was estimated to be about 6% with mild, 24% with moderate, and 40% with severe hypoxemia. Changes due to hypoxemia were subtle and did not appear to affect daily function (15).

That the neurobehavioral impairment which correlated with hypoxemia represented something more than acute hypoxic depression is indicated by the effects of nocturnal versus continuous oxygen therapy. Testing was performed while the subjects breathed room air without oxygen supplementation (16). Increase in performance I.Q. and a decrease in average impairment rating were comparable between the two groups after 6 months of oxygen therapy, with the improvement being attributed to practice effects. After 12 months of breathing supplemental oxygen, the continuous oxygen therapy group showed further improvement while the nocturnal oxygen group exhibited a decrement in performance that was attributed to the normal progression of the underlying disease. Also, at 12 months, the mortality of the nocturnal group was 20% as compared with 12% for the continuous oxygen group. These results suggest that the chronic hypoxemia of COPD, which may also be associated with a partially reversible change in the EEG with continuous oxygen therapy (17), results from neuronal injury and not simply hypoxic depression of neural function.

Compatible with the conclusion that hypoxemia too mild to cause major impairment of function may yet produce brain injury if sustained long enough are observations on climbers to extremely high altitudes (conventionally above 8000 m), who have been reported to exhibit neurobehavioral impairment following return to sea level when their performance is compared with that prior to the hypoxic exposure (18). In six subjects participating in a simulated 40-day ascent of Mount Everest in an altitude chamber, arterial P_{O_2} levels achieved a nadir of 27–30 mmHg on the final day of hypoxic exposure; although the duration of hypoxia was brief compared with the COPD population, the severity of the final period of hypoxia was far greater, reaching a level incompatible with survival in the absence of acclimatization. After return to low altitude, these subjects, like actual climbers to extremely high altitudes, exhibited decline in visual and verbal long-term memory, increased errors on an aphasic screening test, and decreased speed of finger tapping with repeated testing. Climbers retested 1 year after an expedition to Mount Everest no longer exhibited memory and aphasic deficits, but finger tapping speed was still impaired. Neurobehavioral abnormalities appeared to be greater in persons who possessed a more vigorous ventilatory response to an acute hypoxic challenge, in spite of the fact that those individuals had a higher arterial oxygen saturation and that persons with a higher hypoxic ventilatory response are reported to perform better while climbing at extremely high altitude. As with the COPD population, changes were subtle, causing no obvious deficits in daily function. On the whole, the abnormalities appeared to be transient, although Regard et al. (19) reported similar deficits in five of eight elite high-altitude mountaineers 2–9 months after the last of repeated sojourns to above 8000 m without the use of supplemental oxygen; three of the five also displayed electroencephalographic abnormalities.

These observations on humans chronically hypoxemic from COPD or from exposure to extremely high altitude imply that central nervous system injury can result from a level of hypoxia that does not cause loss of consciousness; hypoperfusion as a consequence of cerebral vasoconstriction consequent to relative hypocapnia could be a contributing factor, at least in the high-altitude climbers. The lack of movement disorders and extrapyramidal signs in both groups suggests a different distribution of neuronal injury as compared to that seen following cardiac arrest, perhaps describing a pure hypoxemia without ischemia injury. That a fairly functional state is sustained may be because only scattered neurons become sufficiently hypoxic to experience irreversible injury.

PROTECTION OF THE BRAIN FROM HYPOXIA

Behind the question of how hypoxia hurts the brain lurks the hope that understanding may yield ways to protect the central nervous system from the damage wrought by a surfeit of hypoxia. Under certain circumstances, neurons may sustain many minutes without oxygen and still recover apparently normal function (1), thereby presenting a number of opportunities to alter outcome. Protection may take the form of (a) ways to enhance the central nervous system tolerance to a prospective hypoxic event or (b) ways to effect damage control once the hypoxic insult has occurred (3).

Barbiturate Therapy

Decreasing the oxygen needs of the brain may permit it to tolerate better a period of oxygen deprivation. Thiopental produces a dose-related decrease in brain electrical activity (20), electrical silence being associated with a 50% decrease in $CMRo_2$. Thus far barbiturates are the only drugs clearly shown to afford protection. Their efficacy is most apparent in animal models of focal ischemia: Barbiturate administration prior to or early (1–2 hr) after occlusion of the middle cerebral artery decreases the extent of injury if the occlusion is temporary (21) but not if the occlusion is sustained (22); indeed, barbiturates seemed to worsen the outcome with permanent occlusion. Perhaps barbiturates possess actions other than the decrease in $CMRo_2$ that contribute to cerebral protection, such as (a) the capacity to decrease cerebral edema and intracranial pressure or (b) a role as a free-radical scavenger.

Based upon the promise of these studies, the hope was that barbiturate therapy, if it could be implemented soon enough, might also be of value in decreasing the injury too frequently associated with the global ischemia of cardiac arrest (3). A number of animal studies and a multi-institutional clinical trial have concluded that barbiturates are of little or no value when given after cardiac arrest. Their potential use in protecting the brain from anticipated ischemia, such as in certain surgical situations, has not been determined.

The dose-related depression of both brain electrical activity and $CMRo_2$ by isoflurane is like that of barbiturates, suggesting a capacity for similar cerebral protection. Although some controversy exists concerning the relative efficacy of isoflurane versus thiopental (3), a recent study by Newberg Milde et al. (23), where both drugs were titrated to comparable electrical depression and perfusion pressure was controlled, reports comparable efficacy after 5 hr of middle cerebral artery occlusion. These results support the hypothesis that protection may be primarily a consequence of reduction in metabolic requirement.

Other methods to enhance oxygen supply or to decrease demand have been evaluated to a limited extent (3). These include such things as hypercapnic cerebral vasodilation, induced hypertension, and the use of perfluorocarbon (Fluosol DA), which adds modestly to the oxygen-carrying capacity of blood. Demonstrating the efficacy of these approaches is a difficult challenge that has yet to be met. Hypothermia decreases oxygen demand as a function of the extent of cooling and has been well demonstrated to prolong the time that total ischemia is tolerated when the hypothermia is imposed prior to the ischemic event. The efficacy of hypothermia as a treatment modality following hypoxic injury to the brain has not been established. Similarly, lidocaine might provide protection in doses sufficient to suppress neural activity and $CMRo_2$, and lidocaine can also produce additional metabolic depression when superimposed on an EEG already isoelectric from barbiturate administration. The capacity to block sodium channels may provide an additional theoretical basis for protection, but no data demonstrating efficacy for lidocaine yet exist.

Calcium Channel Blockers

Because of their ability to increase flow and to inhibit elevation of intracellular calcium, these slow channel blockers might afford protection. Steen et al. reported better neurological recovery and improved postischemic cerebral blood flow when nimodipine was administered prior to a complete ischemic event (24), but they could not demonstrate benefit when the drug was administered after the ischemic episode even though flow was improved (25). A number of studies have failed to find any benefit of calcium channel blockers for treatment of focal ischemia, either as pretreatment or administered after the occlusion had been effected (3). Because of the apparently beneficial effect of calcium channel blockers on cerebral blood flow, further study of their value in providing brain protection is warranted.

Hyperosmolar Agents

Mannitol is effective in (a) reducing the cerebral edema associated with ischemia, (b) increasing cerebral blood flow, (c) improving blood rheology, and (d) preserving microcirculatory flow in areas of ischemia. Thus, this drug may be of benefit in ameliorating the "no-reflow phenomena" during reperfusion. These theoretical benefits form the basis for its clinical use, although data demonstrating its efficacy are lacking and indeed may be difficult to obtain in the clinical setting, since hyperosmolar agents are rarely used as the sole therapeutic modality.

Other Drugs

Another drug for which efficacy has been suggested but is unproven is naloxone, a pure opioid antagonist. After being shown to be beneficial in the treatment of septic shock, naloxone was evaluated for its effect on both spinal shock and cerebral ischemia; results to date are equivocal. Similarly, phenytoin, butanediol, and γ-hydroxybutyrate have theoretical benefits that are as yet undocumented. Among the critical questions with these and other drugs is the extent to which they may provide protection when given as prophylaxis prior to an ischemic event, as opposed to providing therapeutic benefit when administered after the event.

Corticosteroids may reduce vasogenic edema late in the course of cerebral ischemia, but thus far they have not been shown to be of value in affecting outcome.

Other drugs with theoretical (but as yet unproven) benefit are dimethylsulfoxide, prostacyclin, propanalol, and iron chelators.

CONCLUSION

This brief review is but a sampler of extensive studies of brain hypoxia by many investigators. In compensation, many of the references are reviews that will efficiently extend your explorations of what is known. What is not known is perhaps more intriguing. For example, does continuous oxygen therapy buy more time for better function for the brains of persons hypoxemic with COPD? Will understanding of how hypoxia causes injury to the brain or, conversely, how cells adapt to chronic hypoxia provide wisdom that may lead to better ways to protect the brain from oxygen lack or care for it following hypoxic injury? These are indeed precious questions targeted to our most precious organ.

REFERENCES

1. Siesjö BK. *Brain energy metabolism.* New York: John Wiley & Sons, 1978.
2. Severinghaus JW, Chiodi H, Eger EI II, Brandstater B, Hornbein TF. Cerebral blood flow in man at high altitude. Role of cerebrospinal fluid pH in normalization of flow in chronic hypocapnia. *Circ Res* 1966;19:274–282.
3. Spetzler RF, Nehls DG. Cerebral protection against ischemia. In: Wood JH, ed. *Cerebral blood flow. Physiologic and clinical aspects.* New York: McGraw–Hill, 1987;651–676.
4. Ames A III, Wright RL, Kowada MD, Thurston JM, Majno G. Cerebral ischemia. II. The no-reflow phenomenon. *Am J Pathol* 1968;52:437–453.
5. Brierley JB. In: Blackwood W, Corsellis JAN, eds. *Greenfield's neuropathology.* London: Edward Arnold, 1976;43–85.
6. Nordström CH, Siesjö BK. Effects of phenobarbital in cerebral ischemia. Part I: Cerebral energy metabolism during pronounced incomplete ischemia. *Stroke* 1978;9:327–335.
7. Siesjö BK. Mechanisms of ischemic brain damage. *Crit Care Med* 1988;16:954–963.
8. Krause GS, White BC, Aust SD, Nayini NR, Kumar K. Brain cell death following ischemia and reperfusion: a proposed biochemical sequence. *Crit Care Med* 1988;16:714–726.
9. Plum F, Posner JB, Hain RF. Delayed neurological deterioration after anoxia. *Arch Intern Med* 1962;110:56–63.
10. Bass NH. Pathogenesis of myelin lesions in experimental cyanide encephalopathy. *Neurology* 1968;18:167–177.
11. Gibson GE, Pulsinelli W, Blass JP, Duffy TE. Brain dysfunction in mild to moderate hypoxia. *Am J Med* 1981;70:1247–1254.
12. Schoene RB, Hornbein TF. High altitude adaptation. In: Murray JF, Nadel JA, eds. *Textbook of respiratory medicine.* Philadelphia: WB Saunders, 1988;196–220.
13. Dong WK, Bledsoe SW, Chadwick HS, Shaw CM, Hornbein TF. Electrical correlates of brain injury resulting from severe hypotension and hemodilution in monkeys. *Anesthesiology* 1986;65:617–625.
14. Grant I, Prigatano P, Heaton RK, McSweeny AJ, Wright EC, Adams KM. Progressive neuropsychologic impairment and hypoxemia: relationship in chronic obstructive pulmonary disease. *Arch Gen Psychiatry* 1987;44:999–1006.
15. McSweeney AJ. Quality of life in relation to COPD. In: McSweeney AJ, Grant I, eds. *Chronic obstructive pulmonary disease: a behavioral perspective. Lung biology in health and dis-*

ease vol 36 (Lenfant C, series ed.). New York: Marcel Dekker, 1988;59–85.

16. Heaton RK. Psychological effects of oxygen therapy for COPD. In: McSweeney AJ, Grant I, eds. *Chronic obstructive pulmonary disease: a behavioral perspective. Lung biology in health and disease,* vol 36 (Lenfant C, series ed.). New York: Marcel Dekker, 1988;105–121.

17. Block AJ, Castle JR, Keitt AS. Chronic oxygen therapy treatment of chronic obstructive pulmonary disease at sea level. *Chest* 1974;65:279–288.

18. Hornbein TF, Townes BD, Schoene RB, Sutton JR, Houston CS. The cost to the central nervous system of climbing to extremely high altitude. *N Engl J Med* 1989;321:1714–1719.

19. Regard M, Oelz O, Brugger P, Landis T. Persistent cognitive impairment in climbers after repeated exposure to extreme altitude. *Neurology* 1989;39:210–213.

20. Michenfelder JD. The interdependency of cerebral functional and metabolic effects following massive doses of thiopental in the dog. *Anesthesiology* 1974;41:231–236.

21. Selman WR, Spetzler RF, Roski RA, Roessmann U, Crumrine R, Macko R. Barbiturate coma in focal cerebral ischemia. Relationship of protection to timing of therapy. *J Neurosurg* 1982;56:685–690.

22. Wade JG, Amtorp O, Sorensen SC. No-flow state following cerebral ischemia. *Arch Neurol* 1975;32:381–384.

23. Newberg Milde L, Milde JH, Lanier WL, et al. Comparison of the effects of isoflurane and thiopental on neurologic outcome and neuropathology after temporary focal cerebral ischemia in primates. *Anesthesiology* 1988;69:905–913.

24. Steen PA, Newberg LA, Milde JH, Michenfelder JD. Nimodipine improves cerebral blood flow and neurologic recovery after complete global ischemia in the dog. *J Cereb Blood Flow Metab* 1984;3:38–43.

25. Steen PA, Newberg LA, Milde JH, Michenfelder JD. Cerebral blood flow and neurologic outcome when nimodipine is given after complete cerebral ischemia in the dog. *J Cereb Blood Flow Metab* 1984;4:82–87.

THE LUNG: Scientific Foundations
edited by R.G. Crystal, J.B. West et al.
Raven Press, Ltd., New York © 1991.

CHAPTER 5.5.3.3

Systemic Effects of Hypoxia

Paul T. Schumacker

To support the energetic requirements of their normal metabolic activities, cells must continuously oxidize metabolic substrates. The reducing equivalents that are generated by the oxidation of these substrates are eventually passed to molecular oxygen in the electron transport system of the mitochondrion, and the associated free energy change is conserved in the coupled phosphorylation of ADP to ATP. The rate at which oxygen is consumed in this process is normally limited by the availability of reducing equivalents and of mitochondrial ADP, and these in turn are closely coupled to the rate at which metabolic activity consumes ATP and other high-energy intermediates. Accordingly, the consumption of oxygen by cells normally is coupled tightly to the rate of energy expenditure for biosynthetic, metabolic, contractile, membrane transport, or other particular functions the cell performs, as long as an adequate concentration of oxygen is available to the terminal cytochrome aa3 complex in the mitochondrion. A functional definition of cellular hypoxia is "the condition occurring when convective or diffusive O_2 transport fails to meet this demand and begins to limit the rate of ATP synthesis." When this occurs, a state of supply-limited O_2 uptake occurs, where changes in O_2 uptake parallel adjustments in the O_2 supply. When cellular hypoxia threatens, well-known cellular mechanisms effect a shift in intermediary metabolism toward anaerobic pathways. Recent studies also suggest that cells may respond by augmenting the affinity of the terminal cytochrome aa3 system for oxygen, thereby increasing the ability of the cell to maintain its uptake of oxygen despite a limited supply (1,2). However, the focus of this chapter is to consider the physiological responses of isolated tissues and organ systems to hypoxia.

METABOLIC CONTROL OF LOCAL TISSUE OXYGEN SUPPLY

Classically, limitations in oxygen supply to tissues have been characterized according to the manner in which convective transport is limited. For example: Hypoxic hypoxia generally refers to a lowering of the arterial O_2 tension; anemic hypoxia refers to reductions in hematocrit, hemoglobin concentration, and thus O_2-carrying capacity; and stagnant hypoxia applies to tissue blood-flow limitations. In practice, such pure forms of O_2 supply limitation rarely occur because local or systemic responses to a falling P_{O_2}, hemoglobin concentration, or blood flow can lead to other changes. For example, anemic hypoxia is often accompanied by increases in systemic blood flow.

Local tissue blood flow is normally coupled to the local oxygen availability-to-demand ratio (3), because tissues regulate local flow to maintain oxygen availability and uptake. The metabolic model of microcirculatory control states that microvascular tone is regulated to maintain adequate oxygen availability to the parenchyma (4). As oxygen delivery is reduced (e.g., by lowering the hemoglobin saturation), changes in precapillary sphincter or terminal arteriolar (5) tone lead to an increase in the density of perfused capillaries and a decrease in intercapillary distances. The consequent increase in capillary surface area, decrease in diffusion distance, and increase in capillary transit time will permit a greater arteriovenous extraction of O_2 without causing O_2 supply limitation of metabolism in some regions. If the O_2 demand of the tissue is high, or if the O_2 availability is sufficiently depressed, feedback extends back from the capillary bed to resistance vessels, causing an arteriolar relaxation and a corre-

P. T. Schumacker: Section of Pulmonary and Critical Care Medicine, The University of Chicago, Chicago, Illinois 60637.

sponding increase in local blood flow that opposes existing neurohumoral tone (4,6).

Control of Perfused Capillary Density

The regulation of perfused capillary density is an important mechanism in preventing tissue hypoxia in the face of reduced O_2 supply, and it has been the focus of considerable experimental study. Several excellent reviews have examined this issue and its relevance to specific tissues (6–8). Some of the experimental measurements of perfused capillary density have been carried out using thin muscle or mesenteric preparations, owing to the suitability of these preparations for videomicroscopic assessment of arteriolar diameters and capillary flow velocities. Such thin preparations also facilitate the experimental manipulation of tissue Po_2 by altering the O_2 tension in the superfusate. In this regard, decreasing the O_2 tension in the superfusate elicits an increased diameter of arterioles, an increase in the velocity of flow in perfused capillaries, and a decrease in the mean intercapillary distance (9–11). Similar results are seen in surface vessels of organs when the animal is ventilated with hypoxic gas mixtures (12). Conversely, exposure of the muscle to relatively high oxygen concentrations results in a significant reduction in the number of capillaries receiving blood flow (10). It is likely that these changes in arteriolar tone are influenced by parenchymal interactions, since they are closely linked to the metabolic activity of the tissue (13). However, data also suggest that conducting vessels may respond directly to the intravascular Po_2, and that the site where O_2 is sensed may be the endothelial cell (14).

Other techniques to assess perfused capillary density include (a) measurement of the capillary filtration coefficient (K_f) or (b) the tissue extraction of diffusible and nondiffusible indicators, yielding a permeability–surface-area (PS) product. These methods assume that the measured changes reflect surface area adjustments as opposed to permeability changes. In general, the results from these functional studies are in accord with the conclusions reached using intravital microscopic techniques. For example, using the filtration coefficient method, Granger et al. (15) perfused skeletal muscle with hypoxic blood and found increases in K_f, suggestive of increased capillary recruitment. In pump-perfused small intestine, Granger et al. (16) found that capillary surface area (and thus K_f) increased as blood flow was experimentally reduced, and that Vo_2 was maintained until flow reached a critically low level. Using a diffusible indicator technique in loops of small bowel perfused at constant flow, Shepherd found that ^{86}Rb extraction increased during hypoxic hypoxia, providing evidence that capillary recruitment had occurred (17). When skeletal muscle blood flow was experimentally lowered by norepinephrine infusion, exchange vessels responded by increasing capillary surface area (and thus K_f) (15) to preserve O_2 extraction. Similarly, sympathetic nerve stimulation increased resistance and decreased blood flow; however, perfused capillary density (and thus K_f) increased in response to this stimulation, thereby increasing tissue oxygen extraction ability (18). Collectively, these studies support the general view that local metabolic control of perfused capillary density and red blood cell flow acts to maintain tissue O_2 availability in the face of changing supply. Although local control of blood flow via the myogenic reflex can also influence microvascular tone and capillary density in tissues such as the gut (19), the myogenic response does not appear to interfere with metabolic control when local O_2 delivery is limited (20).

The role of the precapillary sphincter in controlling perfused capillary density in various tissues has been the focus of some discussion. Anatomically, the precapillary sphincter is thought of as a smooth muscle band encircling a capillary at its entrance and being capable of regulating flow. This could function to control flow through capillaries in an on–off manner and could explain the periodic oscillations in capillary perfusion that have been noted in most tissues. Anatomical studies have provided evidence that such sphincters do exist in the viscera, whereas they have failed to locate such a structure in skeketal muscle (5). If precapillary sphincters are absent in muscle, then adjustment of capillary recruitment would presumably have to be controlled by the terminal arteriole; however, this notion conflicts with evidence that resistance and exchange vessels can be controlled independently (15), and that periodic flow in capillaries is not associated with periodic closure of arterioles (21). Recent data suggest that in skeletal muscle the function of regulating capillary flow is carried out by terminal arteriole feeder vessels, and that capillaries are recruited in groups supplied by terminal arterioles arising from these vessels (22). Other data similarly support the notion of recruitment of groups of capillaries, but controlled at the level of the terminal arteriole (23). An alternative suggestion is that changes in tone of resistance vessels act to regulate the hydrostatic pressure across the capillary bed, which, in turn, leads to on–off perfusion resulting from a distribution of slightly different yield shear stresses among capillaries (21). However, if this were true, then on–off flow behavior might be expected among capillaries supplied by the same terminal arteriole, and this is not generally seen (22).

Control of Tissue Blood Flow in Hypoxia

The local tissue blood flow response to hypoxia reflects the integration of the systemic response to hypoxia and the local effects; this response is heavily influenced by the tissue O_2 availability/demand ratio. Using a denervated preparation to separate local from systemic influences in a perfused canine small bowel preparation, Shepherd (17) found that blood flow increased to 146% of control in response to a lowered arterial P_{O_2} (46 torr), while V_{O_2} was nearly maintained. In newborn swine, arterial hypoxemia caused a fall in intestinal blood flow and V_{O_2} that could be prevented by prior gut denervation or alpha-blockade with phentolamine (24). When no attempt was made to limit the neural response to systemic hypoxia, chemoreflex vasoconstriction increased vascular resistance in skeletal muscle in proportion to the severity of the hypoxemia (25). In cremaster muscle, Morff et al. (26) found that local bath hypoxia (P_{O_2} = 4.5 torr) partially inhibited the chemoreflex arteriolar constriction in response to the lowered arterial P_{O_2} ($F_{I_{O_2}}$ = 0.1). Collectively, these results are consistent with a picture of the independent, but coordinated, local control of resistance and exchange vessels acting to preserve tissue O_2 uptake in the face of limited O_2 supply. In response to hypoxia, systemic-chemoreflex-mediated adrenergic vasoconstriction may transiently depress blood flow, but with time, local metabolic vasodilation attentuates this depression (27).

The integration of local and neural control of blood flow also is influenced by the relative level of metabolic activity within the tissue. In skeletal muscle, for example, limitations in O_2 delivery that depress the prevailing tissue and effluent venous P_{O_2} cause a shift in the site of active regulation toward the resistance vessels and intensify the functional hyperemic responses relative to when tissue O_2 availability was unstressed (15). In isolated canine small bowel, vascular autoregulation is more effective when metabolic rate is stimulated by placing transportable solutes into the lumen, as compared to when uptake is minimal (20). In the gut, increases in small intestinal blood flow following a period of hypoxic hypoxia are greater in absorptive than in postabsorptive animals (28). Moreover, the functional hyperemia in the gut during absorption of glucose and bile is limited to the mucosa, whereas muscularis blood flow decreases (29); this further supports the concept of a close coupling between the local level of metabolic activity and metabolic regulation of flow.

However, the integrated tissue response to hypoxia or ischemia may not always be adaptive. For example, in canine myocardium, uneven adrenergic tone in vessels within an ischemic region may lead to heterogeneous perfusion distributions (30). In that study, chronic myocardial denervation or chemical sympathectomy reduced overall O_2 extraction and reduced the number of venules with very low O_2 contents within the ischemic region of the myocardium. Thus, adrenergic tone in resistance vessels may contribute to the heterogeneity of blood flow distribution, apparently to the detriment of tissue oxygen supply.

TISSUE RESPONSES TO HYPOXIA

O_2 Delivery–Uptake Relationships

As the supply of O_2 to a tissue or to the whole body is lowered progressively, O_2 supply dependence occurs at the point where O_2 uptake (V_{O_2}) begins to fall (31). Although some attention has been paid to the average tissue P_{O_2} where this occurs (32), or to the venous O_2 tension at that point (33), the onset of this supply dependence of O_2 uptake most likely signals the point where anoxic loci begin to appear within the tissue. Within such regions, the O_2 concentration available to mitochondria falls below the level needed to adequately oxidize cytochrome aa3. It would seem reasonable to expect that the type of hypoxia imposed should play an important role in determining when this occurs, since differences in the O_2 tension in capillary blood would seem fundamental to the process of diffusion. In this regard, Gutierrez et al. (34) compared progressive hypoxic hypoxia at high and low blood flow rates and found that O_2 uptake by rabbit hindlimb was higher for a similar O_2 delivery when the blood flow was low but capillary P_{O_2} was higher. This suggested that capillary P_{O_2}, rather than convective O_2 transport, limited O_2 uptake. However, when Cain (35) compared progressive anemia and hypoxic hypoxia in a canine model, he found that the point where V_{O_2} began to fall was associated with a single value of oxygen delivery, calculated as the product of cardiac output and arterial O_2 content, regardless of the manner in which delivery was lowered. This critical oxygen delivery was associated with a mixed venous O_2 tension of 17 torr in hypoxic hypoxia versus 45 torr in anemic hypoxia. Subsequent experimental studies have shown that a similar critical oxygen delivery is reached when stagnant hypoxia is used to lower O_2 transport (36). In each case, the point where V_{O_2} became depressed appeared to correlate with the point where lactate accumulation in blood rose steeply (37). Further reductions in O_2 transport below the critical delivery are associated with approximately linear decreases in whole-body oxygen uptake (38). This linear decrease below the critical point is identical with the behavior predicted in a Krogh tissue model when diffusion of O_2 from the capillary surface to the parenchyma limits availability in some tissue regions (39).

Intestine

The metabolic demand of the intestine varies with its metabolic workload, which is increased by the addition of an absorptive load to the lumen. The resting O_2 uptake of the gut is high relative to that of the whole body, and the oxidative work of the mucosa is responsible for a large share of this O_2 uptake. Differential control of mucosal and serosal blood flow has been noted; reactive hyperemic responses occur in the former but not in the latter.

The relationship between O_2 delivery and uptake in the gut appears to parallel the response seen at the systemic level. For example, Kvietys and Granger found that O_2 uptake in isolated canine small bowel was independent of blood flow until flow was reduced below about 40 ml/min per 100 g (40). Using an innervated autoperfused loop of small intestine, Nelson et al. (36) found (a) a range of high O_2 delivery when V_{O_2} was independent of supply and (b) a linear region of O_2-supply-limited uptake when delivery was reduced below a critical level. The O_2 extraction ratio at the critical point was found to be a better index of the efficacy of O_2 utilization than either the critical delivery or critical blood flow, since it is independent of (a) the metabolic rate of the tissue and (b) hemoglobin concentration. In their preparation (36), the critical O_2 extraction ratio in the gut (63%) was not different from that of the whole body (69%), but the gut reached its critical extraction just before the rest of the body did. This behavior is consistent with a somewhat weaker local metabolic vasodilatory competition with central vasoconstrictor tone seen in the gut, as compared with that seen in skeletal muscle (18,41). However, this effect challenges the classical view that gut perfusion is preferentially sacrificed when O_2 supply becomes limited. Mucosal sloughing seen after intestinal ischemia may instead reflect a sensitivity of mucosal cells to hypoxia by virtue of their high metabolic rate.

Skeletal Muscle

Resting muscle exhibits a low metabolic activity, relative to that of other tissues. During progressive stagnant hypoxia, isolated canine resting hindlimb became supply limited at an O_2 extraction of 67% (42), which was not different from the level of 70% seen for the whole body. In exercising skeletal muscle, O_2 extraction increased from under 60% to about 77% during hypoxic hypoxia (43).

During anemic hypoxia, canine hindlimb maintained O_2 uptake by increasing limb blood flow and extracting more of the delivered O_2, at a point where whole-body O_2 uptake was significantly depressed from preanemic levels (44). In contrast, during hypoxic hypoxia ($F_{I}O_2$ = 0.092) there was an early increase in limb resistance and decrease in blood flow, followed by a later fall in limb resistance and augmentation in blood flow (45). This response has been attributed to local metabolic vasodilatation that opposes sympathoadrenergic vasoconstriction, as accumulating tissue metabolites feed back to relax flow-controlling arterioles. The magnitude of this autoregulatory escape is likely related to the limitation of O_2 delivery relative to the metabolic activity in the muscle. Although it has been reported that beta-blockade can prevent this autoregulatory escape (45), this finding does not fit with the notion of local metabolic vasodilatation. On the other hand, alpha-blockade with phenoxybenzamine did prevent the redistribution of blood flow away from the hindlimb during hypoxic hypoxia (46). This also reduced the ability of the whole body to increase O_2 extraction, since the adrenergic redistribution of a limited O_2 supply among organs was impaired. Within the hindlimb, however, inhibition of adrenergic tone had no detrimental effect on the ability to increase O_2 extraction, since this local microvascular adjustment does not require adrenergic mechanisms.

Liver

The liver is a metabolically active organ, with specific O_2 uptake in the range of 5–10 times the body as a whole. In isolated liver, Lutz et al. (47) found that O_2 uptake became supply dependent when blood flow was reduced below a critical level. Samsel et al. (48) studied isolated canine liver that was pump perfused with blood from a normotensive anesthetized support animal. When O_2 supply was reduced by turning down the speed of the pump, a critical O_2 delivery was also found at an O_2 extraction of 68%. In that study, a significant positive slope was noted in the O_2-supply-independent plateau, which suggested that part of the metabolic O_2 demand of the liver may be determined by its blood flow and, hence, the rate of delivery of metabolic substrates. This seems reasonable, considering that the metabolic work of the liver is dominated by biosynthetic, metabolic, and absorptive functions. An alternative explanation is that some O_2 utilization by nonmitochondrial oxidase systems with lower effective O_2 affinities may be decreased as tissue O_2 tension falls.

Kidney

Blood-flow dependence of O_2 uptake above the critical O_2 delivery has also been noted in the kideny (49–51), where O_2 consumption varies almost linearly with blood flow. Because the renal metabolic workload is dominated by the energetic costs for sodium reabsorption, the glomerular filtration rate appears to be the primary determinant of renal O_2 demand. Accordingly, renal O_2 extraction normally remains relatively constant as blood flow is altered. When blood flow is maintained but O_2 delivery is reduced, O_2 uptake can become limited by supply.

Heart

Metabolic workload normally determines O_2 demand; however, when tissue O_2 supply is reduced sufficiently, tissue function becomes compromised. This is clearly demonstrated in the case of the myocardium, where pressure–volume area of the left ventricle normally correlates closely with myocardial V_{O_2} (52). When Walley et al. (53) reduced canine myocardial O_2 delivery with hypoxic hypoxia, pressure–volume area decreased as a result of a fall in blood pressure and a reduction in the end-systolic pressure–volume relationship, since O_2 availability limited myocardial performance. Although the myocardial O_2 extraction ratio increased, this rise was not sufficient to maintain V_{O_2}.

Endocrine Responses

Systemic hypoxia elicits a complex set of endocrine responses that can reflect the type of hypoxia imposed, its duration and severity, and even the species involved. In some cases the response is heavily influenced by the direct effects of hypoxia on the secreting tissue, whereas in other cases it reflects a response to the systemic cardiovascular or endocrine adjustments to the stress of hypoxia.

The release of erythropoietin (EPO) by the kidney in response to hypoxia provides an example of an endocrine response that reflects the direct effect of hypoxia on the tissue. In adult mammals, renal hypoxia leads to the new synthesis and release of EPO, a circulating glycoprotein that binds to erythrocytic progenitor cells in the bone marrow (54) and stimulates proliferation and differentiation. This leads eventually to an increase in the circulating mass of red blood cells, thereby restoring the balance between O_2 supply and demand. The restoration of normoxic conditions in the kidney then reduces EPO release to basal levels in the range of 100–200 pg/ml (55). The primary site of EPO production appears to be in cortical cells of the interstitial spaces adjacent to the proximal tubules (56). Within 1–4 hr of hypoxic exposure, there is an increase in EPO gene transcription (55) and in measured EPO mRNA levels in the kidney (57), indicating enhanced synthesis. The precise mechanism by which the renal

hypoxia is sensed is still not known. Hypoxia, cobalt ions, and nickel ions all stimulate EPO synthesis through a common pathway, and the sensor may involve a heme protein (58), since EPO production at low levels of P_{O_2} is inhibited by carbon monoxide. Although hypoxic, anemic, and stagnant hypoxia of the kidney all appear to stimulate EPO release, anemia appears to be a more potent stimulus than reduced renal blood flow (59). A more complete description of the control, mode of action, biochemistry, and molecular biology of EPO can be found elsewhere (60).

The stress of hypoxia is also a potent stimulus for release of adrenocorticotropic hormone (ACTH). In unanesthetized and unrestrained rats, Raff and Fagin (61) measured a fivefold increase in ACTH and corticosterone within 20 min after exposure to acute isocapnic hypoxia ($F_{I_{O_2}} = 0.07$), whereas normoxic controls showed no increase. In anesthetized dogs, normocapnic hypoxia produced increases in vasopressin, ACTH, and corticosteroids that were related to the severity of the drop in $P_{a_{O_2}}$ (62). Hypercapnic hypoxia augmented this response at all levels of hypoxia, which suggested that the response was mediated by a chemoreceptor reflex. In a subsequent study (63), the response to hypoxia was studied in dogs with chronic carotid body denervation. However, the increases in ACTH during normocapnic hypoxia were attenuated but not ablated after denervation, and the response during hypercapnic hypoxia was not attenuated. In addition, plasma renin activity increases were not attenuated by chemoreceptor denervation, whereas the cardiovascular hemodynamic response was attenuated. Hence, it appears that only part of the ACTH response to hypoxia is mediated by the carotid chemoreceptors. When hypoxia was induced at different rates in anesthesized dogs, the vasopressin, ACTH, and corticosteriod responses were found to depend only on the steady-state level of lowered $P_{a_{O_2}}$ (64). Of note is the observation that the increases in systemic arterial blood pressure tended to lessen the vasopressin, ACTH, and corticosteroid responses to acute hypoxic hypoxia ($P_{a_{O_2}} = 28$ torr).

Other studies have described the effects of hypoxia on plasma renin activity, angiotensin converting enzyme activity, and plasma aldosterone levels (65,66). An antidiuretic hormone (ADH) response to hypoxia ($P_B = 495$ torr) has also been described (67), which may be blocked by cyclo-oxygenase inhibitors (68).

Adrenal Responses

Hypoxia is known to stimulate the adrenal medulla, leading to increased secretion of catecholamines (69). Recently, Nishijima et al. (70) compared the adrenal medullary and cortical responses to hypoxic hypoxia and carbon monoxide hypoxia. Whereas both adrenal medullary and cortical blood flows rose during hypoxic hypoxia, only medullary flow rose with carbon monoxide hypoxia, even though both forms of hypoxia appeared to stimulate medullary and cortical secretory activity.

During whole-body hypoxia, release of catecholamines from the adrenal medulla and from adrenergic nerve endings leads to increased circulating levels (69). Because catecholamines are known to have a calorigenic effect on tissue metabolism (71), their increased levels during hypoxia could heighten O_2 demand, although the effect might not be detected if the reduced O_2 supply had already depressed O_2 uptake. This effect was nicely demonstrated in resting skeletal muscle by Bredle et al. (72), who perfused a canine hindlimb with normoxic blood while the rest of the animal was made hypoxic by ventilation with 9% O_2 in N_2. Within 30–40 min of hypoxia, the limb O_2 uptake was significantly enhanced; an effect that was blocked by the selective beta-2 antagonist ICI 188,551. This is another example of how the systemic sympathoadrenal response to hypoxia appears maladaptive, in the sense that O_2 demand is augmented under conditions of limited O_2 supply.

Collectively, the above regional studies of hypoxia demonstrate that increases in tissue O_2 extraction occur in response to reductions in O_2 delivery or to increases in O_2 demand in skeletal muscle, intestine, liver, and kidney. A similar critical O_2 extraction ratio in the range of 65–75% appears to exist in many tissues. Although further increases in extraction can be achieved, these increases are inadequate to maintain V_{O_2}, which becomes supply limited.

O_2 RELEASE FROM RED BLOOD CELLS AND TISSUE OXYGEN SUPPLY

Classically, the magnitude of the transport resistance to O_2 unloading from red blood cells has been viewed as small, relative to that of the transport resistance encountered in the tissue itself. This was an assumption in Krogh's model (73) of tissue, as well as in many subsequent analyses (74), where capillary blood was treated as a well-mixed solution of hemoglobin. However, recent theoretical analyses of oxygen release from red blood cells passing axisymmetrically through a capillary suggest that the discrete nature of blood contributes significantly to the overall transport resistance to oxygen flow (75–77). When hemoglobin is partially desaturated, the effective diffusion coefficient for O_2 in the red blood cell is greater than that in plasma, because hemoglobin acts to facilitate diffusion. In plasma there is normally no O_2 carrier present to facilitate O_2 transport, so transport is potentially limited

by its lower effective diffusivity. This, combined with the high flux density of O_2 transport in the plasma region immediately surrounding the red blood cell, creates a large partial pressure difference between red blood cell and capillary wall. Stated differently, the high flux density near the red blood cell, combined with the absence of a facilitated carrier in the plasma, can lead to a high transport resistance to unloading and can significantly slow the rate of O_2 release. This effect has been noted previously in stopped-flow studies of red blood cells, where an unstirred plasma layer around the red blood cells can significantly slow the rate of O_2 release (78). This effect leads to a dependence on capillary hematocrit and red blood cell spacing, since the flux of O_2 at the capillary wall can become very small midway between red blood cells. Gayeski et al. (76) have computed the effect of this carrier-free layer on O_2 release rates in exercising muscle, where rapidly frozen spectrophotometric measurements of myoglobin saturation provide a reference measurement of O_2 tension at the capillary boundary (79). During exercise, when capillary transit times may decrease to less than 50 msec, the carrier-free boundary layer is predicted to slow the rate of O_2 release enough that O_2 unloading may become limited. As a result, muscle P_{O_2} falls and the rate of unloading is augmented at a new, lower steady-state tissue O_2 tension.

This carrier-free effect can explain the disparity between the relatively higher venular P_{O_2} and the much lower tissue P_{O_2} values inferred from myoglobin saturation measurements obtained in muscle sections rapidly frozen while exercising near V_{O_2}max (79). If a high transport resistance in the carrier-free plasma layer results in a large partial pressure difference between hemoglobin and capillary boundary, blood in small venules would exhibit a P_{O_2} much higher than pericapillary levels. The model studies suggest that the importance of this effect is highly dependent on the thickness of the carrier-free layer, as well as on the O_2 saturation of the hemoglobin. Obviously, when hemoglobin is nearly fully saturated the effective transport resistance within the erythrocyte rises to become a significant part of the total transport resistance, because hemoglobin-facilitated transport is reduced. Additional work is needed to explore the magnitude of the carrier-free effects on O_2 transport in resting tissues where O_2 fluxes are smaller, in order to resolve conflicts with other experimental results. For example, the analysis of O_2 release from discrete red blood cells (75) would seem to suggest that tissue O_2 uptake should become supply limited earlier during anemic hypoxia than during stagnant hypoxia, due to the shorter transit times and presumably greater red blood cell spacing within the capillary, yet this apparently does not occur (35). Further experimental validation of the theory will be technically difficult in resting muscle, since the myoglobin will likely be fully saturated and thus the measurement of local tissue Po_2 will be problematic. Similar problems are faced in non-myoglobin-containing tissues.

King et al. (43) compared the effects of hypoxic hypoxia and carbon monoxide hypoxia on working muscle O_2 uptake, extraction, and developed tension. Despite similar depressions in blood O_2 content, the developed tension, O_2 uptake, and O_2 extraction ratio were lower in carbon monoxide than in hypoxic hypoxia. These findings might be explained by the binding of CO to cytochromes, or to myoglobin, thereby reducing the facilitation of O_2 diffusion within the muscle cells.

During exercise at Vo_2max, Hogan et al. (80) measured canine gastrocnemius O_2 uptake and isometric tension during graded levels of hypoxic hypoxia. They found a linear decrease in Vo_2max with decreases in venous Po_2 associated with reduced F_1O_2, and they argue that diffusion of O_2 from blood to mitochondria is the factor limiting maximal O_2 uptake. In view of the rapid-freeze measurements made at Vo_2max by Gayeski and Honig (79), it seems reasonable to speculate that the likely location of this diffusion barrier is between the red blood cell interior and the capillary boundary. If this were true, then addition of stroma-free hemoglobin solution to the blood perfusion might significantly enhance Vo_2max at lower levels of arterial Po_2 by reducing the gas transport resistance contributed by the carrier-free zone surrounding the red cells.

SUMMARY

Cellular hypoxia occurs when convective or diffusive O_2 transport fails to meet the tissue demand for O_2 and when the rate of ATP synthesis becomes limited by the O_2 supply. During states of supply-limited O_2 uptake, changes in tissue O_2 uptake parallel adjustments in the O_2 supply. The metabolic model of microcirculatory control states that microvascular tone is regulated to maintain an adequate ratio of oxygen availability to demand in the tissue. When O_2 delivery is reduced, an increase in the density of perfused capillaries leads to an increase in capillary surface area, a decrease in diffusion distances, and an increase in capillary transit times, thereby permitting a greater arteriovenous extraction of O_2 without causing O_2 supply limitation. When the supply-to-demand ratio is further stressed, metabolic feedback dilates resistance vessels, thereby augmenting local blood flow and O_2 transport. The tissue response to hypoxia reflects the integration of systemic and local responses to hypoxia. For example, during hypoxic hypoxia, chemoreceptor reflex adrenergic vasoconstriction initially decreases

muscle blood flow, but autoregulatory escape later restores perfusion as metabolic vasodilatation competes with sympathetic vasoconstrictor effects. As the supply of O_2 to a tissue or to the whole body is lowered progressively, O_2 supply dependence can be detected at the point where O_2 uptake begins to fall. This critical point is associated with a single value of O_2 delivery, regardless of the manner in which delivery was lowered. The relationship between O_2 delivery and uptake in regional tissues parallels the systemic response, and a similar O_2 extraction ratio of 65–75% is achieved at the onset of O_2 supply dependency of the whole body, skeletal muscle, heart, intestine, liver, and kidney. Metabolic workload normally determines O_2 demand; but when tissue O_2 supply is reduced sufficiently, the tissue function becomes compromised. During systemic hypoxia, increased circulating catecholamines can augment tissue O_2 demands, thereby exacerbating the tissue damage in states of limited O_2 supply. Endocrine responses to hypoxia are complex; moreover, they are influenced by the type of hypoxia imposed, its duration, and severity. The response sometimes reflects the direct effects of hypoxia on the endocrine tissue, whereas in other cases it reflects a response to the systemic cardiovascular or endocrine adjustments to the stress of hypoxia.

ACKNOWLEDGMENTS

The author wishes to thank Dr. R. W. Samsel for his helpful comments on the manuscript. This work was supported by NHLBI grants HL-32646 and HL-01682.

REFERENCES

1. Forman NG, Wilson DF. Energetics and stoichiometry of oxidative phosphorylation from NADH to cytochrome c in isolated rat liver mitochondria. *J Biol Chem* 1982;257:12908–12915.
2. Wilson DF, Erecinska M, Drown C, Silver IA. The oxygen dependence of cellular energy metabolism. *Arch Biochem Biophys* 1979;195:485–493.
3. Shepherd AP, Granger HJ, Smith EE, Guyton AC. Local control of tissue oxygen delivery: its contribution to the regulation of cardiac output. *Am J Physiol* 1973;225:747–755.
4. Granger HJ, Goodman AH, Cook BH. Metabolic models of microcirculatory regulation. *Fed Proc* 1975;34:2025–2030.
5. Baez S. Skeletal muscle and gastrointestinal microvascular morphology. In: Kaley G, Altura BM, eds. *Microcirculation*, vol 1. Baltimore, MD: University Park Press, 1977;69–94.
6. Duling BR, Klitzman B. Local control of microvascular function: role in tissue oxygen supply. *Annu Rev Physiol* 1980;42:373–382.
7. Shepherd AP. Local control of intestinal oxygenation and blood flow. *Annu Rev Physiol* 1982;44:13–27.
8. Shepherd AP. Role of capillary recruitment in the regulation of intestinal oxygenation. *Am J Physiol* 1982;242(*Gastrointest Liver Physiol* 5):G435–G441.
9. Morff RJ. Contribution of capillary recruitment to regulation of tissue oxygenation in rat cremaster muscle. *Microvasc Res* 1988;36:150–161.
10. Lindbom L, Tuma RF, Arfors K-E. Influence of oxygen on per-

fused capillary density and capillary red cell velocity in rabbit skeletal muscle. *Microvasc Res* 1980;19:197–208.

11. Lombard JH, Stekiel WJ. Effect of oxygen on arteriolar diameters in the rat mesoappendix. *Microvasc Res* 1985;30:346–349.

12. Ivanov KP, Kalinina MK, Levkovich YI. Microcirculation velocity changes under hypoxia in brain, muscles, liver, and their physiological significance. *Microvasc Res* 1985;30:10–18.

13. Tyml K. Capillary recruitment and heterogeneity of microvascular flow in skeletal muscle before and after contraction. *Microvasc Res* 1986;32:84–98.

14. Pohl U, Busse R, Galle J, Bassenge E. Possible function of endothelial cells as oxygen sensors. In: Acker H, ed. *Oxygen sensing in tissue*. New York: Springer-Verlag, 1988;143–149.

15. Granger HJ, Goodman AH, Granger DN. Role of resistance and exchange vessels in local microvascular control of skeletal muscle oxygenation in the dog. *Circ Res* 1976;38:379–385.

16. Granger DN, Kvietys PR, Perry MA. Role of exchange vessels in the regulation of intestinal oxygenation. *Am J Physiol* 1982;242(*Gastrointest Liver Physiol* 5):G570–G574.

17. Shepherd AP. Intestinal O_2 consumption and ^{86}Rb extraction during arterial hypoxia. *Am J Physiol* 1978;243(*Endocrinol Metab Gastrointest Physiol* 3):E248–251.

18. Cobbold A, Folkow B, Kjellmer I, Mellander S. Nervous and local chemical control of pre-capillary sphincters in skeletal muscle as measured by changes in filtration coefficient. *Acta Physiol Scand* 1963;57:180–192.

19. Johnson PC. Effect of venous pressure on mean capillary pressure and vascular resistance in the intestine. *Circ Res* 1965;16:294–300.

20. Shepherd AP, Riedel GL. Effect of pulse pressure and metabolic rate on intestinal autoregulation. *Am J Physiol* 1982;242(*Heart Circ Physiol* 11):H769–H775.

21. Lindbom L, Arfors K-E. Mechanisms and site of control for variation in the number of perfused capillaries in skeletal muscle. *Int J Microcirc Clin Exp* 1985;4:19–30.

22. Sweeney TE, Sarelius IH. Arteriolar control of capillary cell flow in striated muscle. *Circ Res* 1989;64:112–120.

23. Delashaw JB, Duling BR. A study of the functional elements regulating capillary perfusion in striated muscle. *Microvasc Res* 1988;36:162–171.

24. Nowicki PT, Caniano DA, Szaniszlo K. Effect of intestinal denervation on intestinal vascular response to severe arterial hypoxia in newborn swine. *Am J Physiol* 1987;253(*Gastrointest Liver Physiol* 16):G201–G205.

25. Costin JC, Skinner NS. Effects of systemic hypoxia on vascular resistance in dog skeletal muscle. *Am J Physiol* 1970;218:886–893.

26. Morff RJ, Harris PD, Wiegman DL, Miller FN. Muscle microcirculation: effects of tissue pH, P_{CO_2}, and P_{O_2} during systemic hypoxia. *Am J Physiol* 1981;240(*Heart Circ Physiol* 9):H746–H754.

27. Shepherd AP, Granger HJ. Autoregulatory escape in the gut: a systems analysis. *Gastroenterology* 1973;65:77–91.

28. Szabo JS, Mayfield SR, Oh W, Stonestreet BS. Postprandial gastrointestinal blood flow and oxygen consumption: effects of hypoxemia in neonatal piglets. *Pediatr Res* 1987;21:93–98.

29. Shepherd AP, Riedel GL. Laser-Doppler blood flowmetry of intestinal mucosal hyperemia induced by glucose and bile. *Am J Physiol* 1985;248(*Gastrointest Liver Physiol* 11):G393–G397.

30. Acad B-A, Joselevitz-Goldman J, Scholz PM, Weiss HR. Improved distribution of regional oxygenation in denervated ischemic dog myocardium. *Circ Res* 1988;62:1041–1048.

31. Schumacker TP, Cain SM. The concept of a critical oxygen delivery. *Intensive Care Med* 1987;13:223–229.

32. Tenney SM. A theoretical analysis of the relationship between venous blood and mean tissue oxygen pressures. *Respir Physiol* 1976;20:283–294.

33. Willford DC, Hill EP, White FC, Moores WC. Decreased critical mixed venous oxygen tension and critical oxygen transport during induced hypothermia in pigs. *J Clin Monit* 1986;2:155–168.

34. Gutierrez G, Pohil RJ, Strong R. Effect of flow on O_2 consumption during progressive hypoxemia. *J Appl Physiol* 1988;65:601–607.

35. Cain SM. Oxygen delivery and uptake in dogs during anemic and hypoxic hypoxia. *J Appl Physiol* 1977;42:228–234.

36. Nelson DP, King CE, Dodd SL, Schumacker PT, Cain SM. Systemic and intestinal limits of O_2 extraction in the dog. *J Appl Physiol* 1987;63:387–394.

37. Nelson DP, Beyer C, Samsel RW, Wood LDH, Schumacker PT. Pathological supply dependence of O_2 uptake during bacteremia in dogs. *J Appl Physiol* 1987;63:1487–1492.

38. Samsel RW, Schumacker PT. Determination of the critical oxygen delivery from experimental data: sensitivity to error. *J Appl Physiol* 1988;64:2074–2082.

39. Schumacker PT, Samsel RW. Analysis of oxygen delivery and uptake relationships in the Krogh tissue model. *J Appl Physiol* 1989;67:1234–1244.

40. Kvietys PR, Granger DN. Relation between intestinal blood flow and oxygen uptake. *Am J Physiol* 1982;242(*Gastrointest Liver Physiol* 5):G202–G208.

41. Cobbold A, Folkow B, Lundgren O, Wallentin I. Blood flow, capillary filtration coefficients and regional blood volume responses in the intestine of the cat during stimulation of the hypothalamic 'defence' area. *Acta Physiol Scand* 1964;61:467–475.

42. Samsel RW, Nelson DP, Sanders WM, Wood LDH, Schumacker PT. Effect of endotoxin on systemic and skeletal muscle O_2 extraction. *J Appl Physiol* 1988;65:1377–1382.

43. King CE, Dodd SL, Cain SM. O_2 delivery to contracting muscle during hypoxic hypoxia or CO hypoxia. *J Appl Physiol* 1987;63:726–732.

44. Cain SM, Chappler CK. Oxygen extraction by canine hind limb versus whole dog during anemic hypoxia. *J Appl Physiol* 1978;45:966–970.

45. Cain SM, Chappler CK. Oxygen extraction by canine hindlimb during hypoxic hypoxia. *J Appl Physiol* 1979;46:1023–1028.

46. Cain SM, Chappler CK. O_2 extraction by canine hindlimb during alpha-adrenergic blockade and hypoxic hypoxia. *J Appl Physiol* 1980;48:630–635.

47. Lutz J, Henrich H, Bauereisen E. Oxygen supply and uptake in the liver and intestine. *Pflugers Arch* 1975;360:7–15.

48. Samsel RW, Cherqui D, Pietrabissa A, Sanders WM, Roncella M, Emond JC, Schumacker PT. The limits of oxygen extraction in the isolated canine liver *Physiologist* 1988;31:A147.

49. Gotshall RW, Miles DS, Sexsox WR. Renal oxygen delivery and consumption during progressive hypoxemia in the anesthetized dog. *Proc Soc Exp Biol Med* 1983;174:363–367.

50. Schlichtig R, Kramer DJK, Stein K, Pinsky MR. Renal O_2 consumption is supply-dependent at all levels of renal O_2 delivery during progressive hemorrhage [Abstract]. *Am Rev Respir Dis* 1989;139:A312.

51. Gotshall RW, Miles DW, Sexson WR. Renal oxygen delivery and consumption during progressive hypoxemia in the anesthetized dog. *Proc Soc Exp Biol Med* 1983;174:363–367.

52. Suga H, Hayashi T, Shirahata M, Ninomiya I. Critical evaluation of left ventricular systolic pressure volume area as predictor of oxygen consumption rate. *Am J Physiol* 1981;240:H39–H44.

53. Walley KR, Becker CJ, Hogan RA, Teplinsky K, Wood LDH. Progressive hypoxemia limits left ventricular oxygen consumption and contractility. *Circ Res* 1988;63:849–859.

54. Spivak J. The mechanism of action of erythropoietin. *Int J Cell Cloning* 1986;4:139–166.

55. Schuster SJ, Badiavas EV, Costa-Giomi P, Weinmann R, Erslev AJ, Caro J. Stimulation of erythropoietin gene transcription during hypoxia and cobalt exposure. *Blood* 1989;73:13–16.

56. Koury MJ, Bondurant MC. Localization of erythropoietin synthesizing cells in murine kidneys by *in situ* hybridization. *Blood* 1987;71:524–527.

57. Bauer C, Kurtz A, Eckardt K-U, Tannahill L. Regulation of erythropoietin-binding. *Nephron* 1989;51(Suppl 1):3–10.

58. Goldberg MA, Dunning SP, Bunn HF. Regulation of the erythropoietin gene: evidence that the oxygen sensor is a heme protein. *Science* 1988;242:1412–1415.

59. Pagel H, Jelkmann W, Weiss C. A comparison of the effects of renal artery constriction and anemia on the production of erythropoietin. *Eur J Physiol* 1988;413:62–66.

60. Goldwasser E, Beru N, Smith D. Erythropoietin: the primary regulator of red cell formation. In: Sporn MB, Roberts AB, eds.

Peptide growth factors and their receptors. Handbook of experimental pharmacology. Chap. 18, vol. 95. Berlin, Heidelberg: Springer-Verlag, 1989;747–770.

61. Raff H, Fagin KD. Measurement of hormones and blood gases during hypoxia in conscious cannulated rats. *J Appl Physiol* 1984;56:1426–1430.

62. Raff H, Shinsako J, Keil LC, Dallman MF. Vasopressin, ACTH, and corticosteroids during hypercapnia and graded hypoxia in dogs. *Am J Physiol* 1983;244(*Endocrinol Metab* 7):E453–E458.

63. Raff H, Shinsako J, Dallman MF. Renin and ACTH responses to hypercapnia and hypoxia after chronic carotid chemodenervation. *Am J Physiol* 1984;247:(*Regul Integrative Comp Physiol* 16):R412–R417.

64. Raff H, Shinsako J, Keil LC, Dallman MF. Vasopressin, ACTH, and blood pressure during hypoxia induced at different rates. *Am J Physiol* 1983;245(*Endocrinol Metab* 8):E489–E493.

65. Colice GL, Ramirez G. Effect of hypoxemia on the renin–angiotensin–aldosterone system in humans. *J Appl Physiol* 1985;58:724–730.

66. Milledge JS, Catley DM, Blume FD, West JB. Renin, angiotensin-converting enzyme, and aldosterone in humans on Mount Everest. *J Appl Physiol* 1983;55:1109–1112.

67. Claybaugh JR, Wade CE, Sato AK, Cucinell SA, Lane JC, Maher JT. Antidiuretic hormone responses to eucapnic and hypocapnic hypoxia in humans. *J Appl Physiol* 1982;53:815–823.

68. Walker BR. Inhibition of hypoxia-induced ADH release by meclofenamate in the conscious dog. *J Appl Physiol* 1983;54:1624–1629.

69. Sylvester JT, Scharf SM, Gilbert RD, Fitzgerald RS, Traystman RJ. Hypoxic and CO hypoxia in dogs: hemodynamics, carotid reflexes, and catecholamines. *Am J Physiol* 1979;236(*Heart Circ Physiol* 5):H22–H28.

70. Nishijima MK, Breslow MJ, Raff H, Traystman RJ. Regional adrenal blood flow during hypoxia in anesthetized, ventilated dogs. *Am J Physiol* 1989;256(*Heart Circ Physiol* 25):H94–H100.

71. Blatteis CM, Lutherer LO. Reduction by moderate hypoxia of the calorigenic action of catecholamines in dogs. *J Appl Physiol* 1974;36:337–339.

72. Bredle DL, Chappler CK, Cain SM. Metabolic and circulatory responses of normoxic skeletal muscle to whole-body hypoxia. *J Appl Physiol* 1988;65:2063–2068.

73. Krogh A. The number and distribution of capillaries in muscles with calculations of the oxygen pressure head necessary for supplying the tissue. *J Physiol (Lond)* 1918;52:391–408.

74. Kreuzer F. Oxygen supply to tissues: the Krogh model and its assumptions. *Experientia* 1982;38:1415–1426.

75. Federspiel WJ, Popel AS. A theoretical analysis of the effect of the particulate nature of blood on oxygen release in capillaries. *Microvasc Res* 1986;32:164–189.

76. Gayeski TEJ, Federspiel WJ, Honig CR. A graphical analysis of red cell transit time, carrier-free layer thickness, and intracellular P_{O_2} on blood–tissue O_2 transport. *Adv Exp Med Biol* 1988;222:25–35.

77. Clark A, Federspiel WJ, Clark PAA, Cokelet GR. Oxygen delivery from red cells. *Biophys J* 1985;47:171–181.

78. Huxley VH, Kutchai H. The effect of the red cell membrane and a diffusion boundary layer on the rate of oxygen uptake by human erythrocytes. *J Physiol* 1981;316:75–83.

79. Gayeski TEJ, Honig CR. O_2 gradients from sarcolemma to cell interior in red muscle at maximal V_{O_2}. *Am J Physiol* 1986;251(*Heart Circ Physiol* 20):H789–H799.

80. Hogan MC, Roca J, Wagner PD, West JB. Limitation of maximal O_2 uptake and performance by acute hypoxia in dog muscle *in situ*. *J Appl Physiol* 1988;65:815–821.

THE LUNG: Scientific Foundations
edited by R.G. Crystal, J.B. West et al.
Raven Press, Ltd., New York © 1991.

CHAPTER 5.6.1

Exercise Hyperpnea

Its Characteristics and Control

Hubert V. Forster and Lawrence G. Pan

During exercise, the increase in blood O_2 extraction by the muscles must be replenished, and the CO_2 produced must be eliminated. In addition, during heavy exercise, there is a need to compensate for lactacidosis. Essential to meeting these tasks is an increase in breathing—specifically, an increase in alveolar ventilation, $\dot{V}_A$. In many species, breathing helps regulate temperature during exercise by increasing ventilation of the conducting airways (dead space ventilation, V_D). The increase in pulmonary ventilation ($\dot{V}_E$) required to meet these needs must be achieved efficiently with minimal oxygen consumption ($\dot{V}_{O_2}$) by the respiratory muscles. This chapter, which has as its focus the regulation of breathing in exercise, will discuss (a) the basic "exercise or metabolic stimulus," (b) the stimuli responsible for hyperventilation of exhaustive exercise, (c) thermal-induced exercise hyperpnea, and (d) minimization of the O_2 cost of breathing. The key characteristics of the exercise hyperpnea will be presented first.

CHARACTERIZATION OF BREATHING DURING EXERCISE

Temporal Pattern

The temporal pattern of the breathing response to muscular exercise in humans exhibits three distinct phases

(Fig. 1) (1–12). The first phase is typified by an increase in $\dot{V}_E$ that occurs immediately or within seconds after the onset of exercise. The second phase is the rather slow, gradual increase that occurs over approximately the first 3 min of exercise. During the third phase, breathing is stable in submaximal exercise. During heavy exercise, this steady-state third phase is rarely observed (3,13). Of the total increase in $\dot{V}_E$ from rest, the rise in the second phase is usually slightly larger than the first, and the magnitude of both phases increases as work intensity increases (1,3–5,8,10–12). The decrease in the ventilation once exercise is terminated also has a fast and slow component (1,2,5,7). Mammals other than humans also demonstrate fast and slow breathing responses to exercise (13–18).

Ventilation–Metabolic-Rate Relationship

In humans, $\dot{V}_E$ and $\dot{V}_A$ are curvilinearly related to the increase in metabolic rate during dynamic muscular exercise (Fig. 2) (5,12,19–23). Specifically, between rest and approximately 60–70% of maximal $\dot{V}_{O_2}$, $\dot{V}_E$ and $\dot{V}_A$ increase in a manner nearly proportionate to the increase in $\dot{V}_{O_2}$. But at higher workrates, when lactacidosis is evident, $\dot{V}_E$ and $\dot{V}_A$ increase proportionately more than metabolic rate. The slope of the $\dot{V}_E-\dot{V}_{O_2}$ relationship is influenced by exercise type (24–27), posture (24), muscle mass (20), acid–base status (28,29), levels of oxygenation (20,30–32), and levels of certain hormones or neurotransmitters (33–36). The relationships between $\dot{V}_E$, $\dot{V}_A$, and $\dot{V}_{O_2}$ are less well established for nonhuman mammals, but judging from changes in $P_{a_{CO_2}}$ (presented below), it appears that in most nonhuman species, $\dot{V}_A$ increases during exercise proportionately more than does $\dot{V}_{O_2}$.

H. V. Forster: Department of Physiology, Medical College of Wisconsin and Veterans Administration Medical Center, Milwaukee, Wisconsin 53226.
L. G. Pan: Department of Physiology, Medical College of Wisconsin and Department of Physical Therapy, Marquette University, Milwaukee, Wisconsin 53226.

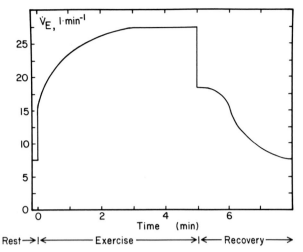

FIG. 1. Schematic representation of the temporal pattern of human pulmonary ventilation ($\dot{V}_E$) during and after exercise at approximately 1.0 liter·min^{-1} oxygen consumption. (Data based on refs. 1, 2, 4–6, 8–10, 37, and 176.)

Tidal Volume (V_T) and Breathing Frequency (f) During Exercise

Usually, both V_T and f increase during exercise (5,21,37). The magnitude of each change is variable and is determined primarily by (a) the impedance of the respiratory system, (b) the role of the respiratory system in temperature regulation, and (c) limb movement frequency and the type of exercise (see section entitled "Minimization of Work of Breathing," below).

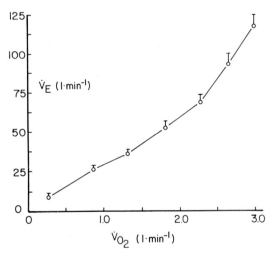

FIG. 2. Relationship of human steady-state pulmonary ventilation ($\dot{V}_E$) and oxygen consumption ($\dot{V}_{O_2}$) during treadmill exercise. Data (mean ± SEM) represent a compilation of several studies in the authors' laboratory ($n = 10$).

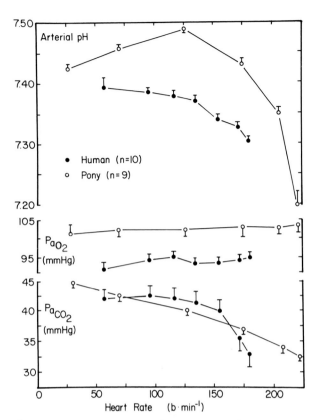

FIG. 3. Relationship of arterial pressure of carbon dioxide (P_aCO_2), arterial pressure of oxygen (P_aO_2), and arterial pH to heart rate in humans (●; $n = 10$) and ponies (○; $n = 9$) during treadmill exercise. Heart rate is utilized as an index of exercise intensity. Data (mean ± SEM) represent a compilation of several studies in the authors' laboratory.

Blood Gases During Exercise

In humans, P_aCO_2 and P_aO_2 change minimally from rest during exercise up to approximately 60–70% of maximal $\dot{V}_{O_2}$ (Fig. 3). In most subjects, there is a transient 1- to 3-mmHg hypocapnia at the onset of exercise; in other subjects, however, P_aCO_2 increases during this transition (38–41). Similarly, during steady-state submaximal exercise, P_aCO_2 differs from rest by at most 1–3 mmHg (5,19,21,22,39,41). However, during heavy exercise coincident with the lactacidosis, P_aCO_2 decreases from rest by as much as 10 mmHg in most humans (Fig. 3) (5,12,19,21,22). Homeostasis of P_aO_2 is nearly maintained during mild, moderate, and heavy exercise (Fig. 3) (5,19,21). Exceptional are superbly conditioned athletes who hyperventilate minimally during heavy exercise; thus, P_aCO_2 remains near resting levels and P_aO_2 is reduced by as much as 30 mmHg below rest (42–45). The relationship of P_aCO_2 to work-rate appears independent of the resting condition. In other words, during such conditions as chronic metabolic acidosis and alkalosis or hormonal changes when P_aCO_2 is altered from normal, exercise results in P_aCO_2 regulation to near the altered resting level (29,36,46). Hypoxia is an exceptional condition in that P_aCO_2 is lower during hypoxic exercise than during hypoxic rest (30,31,36).

In several nonhuman species, P_aCO_2 homeostasis is not maintained during submaximal exercise (Fig. 3) (13–17,27,37,43–53). Ponies (15,48), goats (54), and dogs (47) all decrease P_aCO_2 in rest to work and low to moderate work transitions. Often there is some increase from this nadir in P_aCO_2; however, during steady-state conditions, P_aCO_2 is always below resting levels in a workload-dependent fashion. Most species also hyperventilate during heavy exercise; in ponies, the exercise hypocapnia remains a single function of workrate (53). In contrast to the declining P_aCO_2, P_aO_2 in the steady state of exercise remains near resting levels in most species (17,47,53). Exceptional are horses during heavy exercise. They do not hyperventilate; thus P_aCO_2 is at or above normal and P_aO_2 is below normal (55,56). An alveolar–capillary diffusion limitation is a primary contributor to the hypoxemia (57).

MECHANISM OF BASIC EXERCISE VENTILATORY DRIVE

Few topics in physiology that have been researched to the same extent as has the mechanism of exercise hyperpnea remain as controversial. The controversy centers around the origin of the stimulus that provides for a rapid (Fig. 1) and rather precise adjustment of $\dot{V}_A$ to meet the metabolic demands (Fig. 2) so that P_aO_2 does not decrease and P_aCO_2 does not increase from rest during submaximal exercise (Fig. 3). Most theories that have been advanced fit into one of two categories. One group of theories proposes that the stimulus is "humoral"; that is, exercise causes a change in some blood-borne agent which increases $\dot{V}_A$ through a receptor located outside of the exercising limbs. Other theories propose that the stimulus is "neural"; that is, it originates in the brain or in the exercising muscles and is transmitted to the medullary respiratory centers by either descending or ascending neural pathways. Proponents of each theory provide data which seem to indicate that each (humoral and neural) can totally account for the hyperpnea.

Humoral Theories

Among the first to propose a humoral mechanism for exercise hyperpnea were Geppert and Zuntz in 1888 (58). In 1905 Haldane and Priestley (59), who docu-

mented the important role of P_aCO_2 and P_aO_2 in regulation of breathing, suggested that the increased CO_2 production during exercise could mediate the exercise hyperpnea. However, Douglas and Haldane (60) observed in 1909 that P_aCO_2 did not change sufficiently during exercise to account for the increased breathing. Since then, numerous studies have confirmed the near-constancy of P_aCO_2 during mild and moderate exercise in humans. How then could PCO_2 (or [H$^+$]) mediate the exercise hyperpnea when mean stimulus levels at known chemoreceptors remain nearly constant, or as in most species, when mean PCO_2 and [H$^+$] are below normal?

Changes in PCO_2 could mediate exercise hyperpnea as a result of an increase in sensitivity to CO_2 during exercise. However, an increase has been seen by some (61–63) but not all (7,64,65) investigators who tested this hypothesis. Because the latter group found that the CO_2 response curve is not altered by exercise, they concluded that the "exercise and CO_2 stimuli are additive."

Oscillations of P_aCO_2 about a mean value occur during the breathing cycle (66,67), resulting in swings in carotid chemoreceptor firing (68–70). Despite a near-normal mean P_aCO_2 during exercise, these oscillations increase during exercise (71). It has been shown that changing the oscillatory pattern alters breathing (72), supporting the hypothesis that the increased swings in carotid chemoreceptor discharge could contribute to exercise hyperpnea even though mean P_aCO_2 and the sensitivity to CO_2 are not altered (73–75).

A third theory suggests that the respiratory center functions as an integral controller during exercise (76). A transient hypercapnia at the onset of exercise increases carotid chemoreceptor activity that increases breathing to restore P_aCO_2 to normal. Breathing will stay elevated until there is a transient hypocapnia at the termination of exercise. This theory is not supported by data showing that the predominant P_aCO_2 change at the exercise onset is a slight hypocapnia (39,77).

Results of studies in which carotid chemoreceptor activity has been attenuated or eliminated do not permit conclusive statements regarding the role of these receptors in exercise hyperpnea. Animal studies clearly show that exercise hypocapnia is accentuated following carotid chemoreceptor resection (13–15). Similarly, attenuating chemoreceptor activity by elevating P_aO_2 also accentuates exercise hypocapnia (31). These data suggest the chemoreceptor function in normal animals to dampen and not augment exercise hyperpnea. In normal humans, elevating P_aO_2 slows ventilatory kinetics (78), but during submaximal exercise, high oxygen has minimal effect on $\dot{V}_E$ and P_aCO_2 (5,30,39,79,80). In carotid-chemoreceptor-denervated asthmatic humans, there is a transient hypercapnia during exercise (81). This finding could mean that these receptors provide an important drive to $\dot{V}_A$ during exercise. However, it is conceivable that in these patients the exercise response was hypercapnic prior to carotid denervation as a result of above-normal airway resistance. Alternative conclusions based on all these human and nonhuman data include the following: (a) The carotid chemoreceptors are "fine tuners" of $\dot{V}_A$ during exercise, correcting either an excessive (non-humans) or an insufficient (human asthmatics) $\dot{V}_A$ response, or (b) there are indeed species differences in the role of these chemoreceptors in mediation of exercise hyperpnea.

Other potent chemoreceptors are located within the brainstem. These apparently respond to changes in $[H^+]$ of cerebral interstitial fluid (82–84). The role of these chemoreceptors in control of breathing under any condition is unknown as a result of uncertainties in quantitating stimulus level (82). Nevertheless, it seems unlikely that mean stimulus level increases during exercise, since P_{CO_2} and $[H^+]$ of both arterial blood and cerebrospinal fluid (85) remain near normal or decrease during light and moderate exercise.

Finally, because mixed venous P_{CO_2} in humans increases during exercise (86–88), several investigators have tested the hypothesis that exercise hyperpnea is mediated by chemoreceptors on the venous side of the circulation (89–96) or in the lung (12,23,76,97,98). This theory is based primarily upon data obtained during several different conditions that indicate a high correlation of $\dot{V}_A$ to lung CO_2 delivery and apparent maintenance of arterial isocapnia (12,99–105). To date, however, no chemoreceptors have been documented on the venous side of the circulation (90,92,93,106), nor has a pulmonary CO_2 sensor been identified that could account for exercise hyperpnea (97,98). Moreover, surgical denervation of the lung and heart does not alter P_{aCO_2} during exercise (54,107–110). Accordingly, exercise hyperpnea does not appear to be critically dependent upon venous, cardiac, or lung chemoreceptors.

All of the above humoral theories focus on P_{CO_2} and $[H^+]$ as potential mediators of exercise hyperpnea. Other substances proposed as exercise stimuli include P_{O_2} (80,111), catecholamines (5,112–115), and plasma $[K^+]$ (116–118). There is some evidence that plasma catecholamines (24,119–121) and plasma $[K^+]$ (118, 122) may contribute to exercise hyperpnea, but both the temporal pattern of changes and the magnitude of $\dot{V}_E$ stimulation attributable to these stimuli do not adequately account for hyperpnea during submaximal exercise (12,112,113,118,123). Even though the $\dot{V}_E$ response to hypoxia is increased by exercise (20,32), P_{aO_2} is an unlikely major contributor to exercise hy-

perpnea simply because P_{aO_2} homeostasis is usually maintained over all levels of exercise (Fig. 3).

Neural Theories

Among the first to propose neural mediation of exercise hyperpnea were Krogh and Lindhard in 1913 (9). They believed that the ventilatory response at the onset of exercise was too rapid to be mediated by humoral mechanisms (Fig. 1). They suggested that there might be a signal from the motor cortex to the respiratory center which was proportional to the intensity of motor activity. More recently, Eldridge et al. (124) have proposed that "neural command signals emanating from the hypothalamus are primarily responsible for the proportional driving of locomotion, respiration, and circulatory adjustments during exercise." This is popularly known as the "central command" theory (124–126). It is based on data in decorticate, unanesthetized cats who spontaneously walk or run while being supported on a treadmill. In this preparation, an increase in ventilation precedes locomotion and is proportional to the locomotion. Contrary to this theory, nearly identical $\dot{V}_E$ responses occur to voluntary and electrically induced muscle contractions in humans (127–130), even though there is supposedly no central command when muscles are stimulated electrically.

A second "neural" theory for exercise hyperpnea suggests that the signal originates in the exercising limbs and, through spinal pathways, stimulates the respiratory center appropriately (4,25,93,128,131–137). Major support for this theory was provided by the cross-circulation studies of Kao (93). The abdominal arteries were anastomosed as were the abdominal veins in pairs of anesthetized dogs. Electrically induced muscle contractions of the hind legs were begun in one of the dogs (termed "neural"). $\dot{V}_E$ in this dog increased immediately, whereas in the second (or "humoral") dog, $\dot{V}_E$ did not increase until P_{aCO_2} increased and P_{aO_2} decreased. The $\dot{V}_E$ response in the neural dog was eliminated by ablation of the lateral spinal columns or transection of the spinal cord. Several other studies have also tested this theory using anesthetized preparations, electrical stimulation, and/or cord transection (130,133,137–142). Some, but not all, concluded similarly to Kao (93), who stated: "There is certainly a peripheral neurogenic drive which must be considered as the, or one of the mechanisms of exercise hyperpnea."

Afferents from the respiratory muscles are a third potentially important neural stimulus in exercise hyperpnea (143). Supportive of this concept are data obtained in humans in whom airway resistance is reduced by 50% when switching from a $N_2–O_2$ to a $He–O_2$ inspiratory gas mixture (143). Typically, He–O_2 breathing results in an increase in $\dot{V}_E$ and f and a decrease in $P_{a}CO_2$ (143,144). However, within the first breath of reduced resistance, there is a 20–40% reduction in the amplitude and rate of rise of the diaphragmatic electromyogram (EMG). Accordingly, during normal air breathing, the higher EMG must be due to some reflex sensitive to the resistive load or impedance presented by the lung to the respiratory musculature. The magnitude of this He–O_2 reduction in diaphragmatic activity is workload-dependent (143) and is independent of lung afferents (144). It makes sense, therefore, that a portion of the exercise hyperpnea appears to be due to mechanoreceptor–proprioceptive feedback from the thorax (145).

Neural and Humoral Mediation

It has been proposed that no single factor mediates exercise hyperpnea (146). For example, Dejours (5) and others (see ref. 12) advanced the neurohumoral theory according to which the initial, fast $\dot{V}_E$ response is neurally mediated while the slow rise to a steady-state $\dot{V}_E$ is humorally mediated (Fig. 1). The exact nature of each component was not specified, but it was emphasized that the combined effects of small changes in several blood-borne substances might constitute the humoral stimulus.

Yamamoto (147) proposed what has come to be known as the "occlusion theory." According to this theory, during exercise there are "many sufficient mechanisms, each of which in a given, isolated circumstance explains the whole phenomenon (ventilatory increase). When they act simultaneously, they mask each other." This theory attempts to reconcile the widely differing neural and humoral theories, each of which claims to be capable of explaining the entire exercise hyperpnea.

The neurohumoral and occlusion theories differ primarily on the basis of the background of their origins. Neither proposes stimuli other than those proposed by other theories. Neither of these theories has been adequately tested.

HYPERVENTILATION OF HEAVY EXERCISE

The origin of the hyperventilation of heavy exercise is also controversial. Tradition links this hyperventilation in humans to the onset of anaerobic metabolism (5,12,19,23,148). Arterial acidosis supposedly stimulates carotid chemoreceptors, resulting in hyperventilation and respiratory acid–base compensation. These conclusions are based on correlative data and on evidence that carotid-body-resected asthmatics do not hyperventilate during heavy exercise (23). How-

ever, recent studies have shown a dissociation of hyperventilation from lactacidosis in humans. Hagberg et al. (149) have shown that humans who cannot produce lactic acid (McArdle's syndrome) still hyperventilate during heavy exercise. Others have altered lactic acid production by dietary manipulation and have found a hyperventilation greater than expected from the lactacidosis (150–152). In ponies there is no indication of an "added" ventilatory drive at the onset of lactacidosis, and exercise hypocapnia is a linear function of workrate (53). Finally, surgical resection of the carotid chemoreceptors in ponies accenuates and does not attenuate the hyperventilation (53).

Other factors may contribute to the hyperventilation of heavy exercise. Hyperkalemia (117,118,122) and an increase in plasma catecholamines (5,113,115,123) during heavy exercise potentially could contribute to the hyperventilation through the carotid chemoreceptors. However, the accenuated hyperventilation in carotid-chemoreceptor-resected ponies suggests that substances acting at these receptors are not critical to the hyperventilation (53,118). The increase in body temperature is another potentially important contributor (12,37,111,153,154). Conceivably, the combined effects of many factors may provide the stimulation for the hyperventilation during heavy exercise, or the so-called basic exercise stimulus might elicit hyperventilation during heavy exercise.

CONTRIBUTION OF VENTILATORY SYSTEM TO TEMPERATURE REGULATION

The temporal pattern of breathing during prolonged exercise indicates how breathing may participate in temperature regulation (Fig. 4). In ponies during mild treadmill exercise (1.8 mph, 5% grade, $\dot{V}O_2 = 1.4$ liters·min^{-1}, heart rate = 70 beats·min^{-1}) for 30 min in a neutral temperature environment, breathing frequency increases during the first minute from 6 to 29 breaths and then rises gradually, reaching 76 breaths during the 30th minute (Fig. 4). Between 3 and 30 min, $\dot{V}_E$ similarly increases but $P_{a}CO_2$ and metabolic rate do not change appreciably whereas V_T decreases (authors' laboratory, *unpublished observations*). Accordingly, the progressively increasing $\dot{V}_E$ does not serve pulmonary gas-exchange requirements; it appears to represent only an increase in dead-space ventilation. It thus seems quite likely that tachypneic hyperpnea in this species is fulfilling requirements for temperature regulation to minimize increases in body temperature (Fig. 4). In several other species, breathing similarly provides a major contribution to temperature regulation (155–158).

A time-dependent increase in ventilation also occurs in humans during exercise (24,159). The increase is not

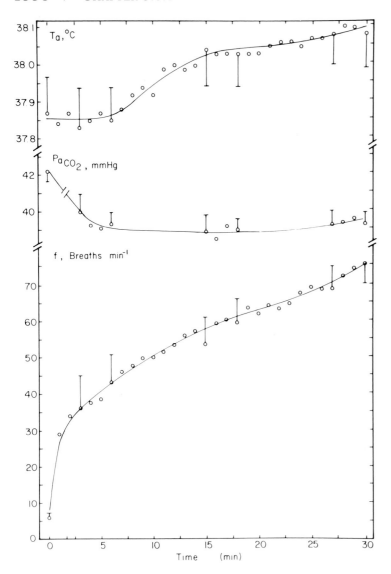

FIG. 4. Temporal pattern of breathing frequency (*f*), arterial pressure of carbon dioxide (P_{aCO_2}), and arterial blood temperature (T_a) during 30 min of treadmill exercise by ponies at 1.8 mph (5% grade) in a neutral temperature environment. These data (mean ± SEM) are from the authors' laboratory (*unpublished observations*).

as great as it is in ponies, and at relatively high work-rates it is associated with progressive hypocapnia. Thus, the greater ventilation results in more than just an increase in dead-space ventilation, suggesting that it might, in addition to temperature regulation, help compensate for increased lactic acid production.

Thermoregulatory changes in breathing are dependent on hypothalamic integration of peripheral and central sensory information (160–162). Changes in skin (155,163,164), airway (156,165), and hypothalamic (157,158) temperatures appear capable of eliciting changes in breathing. During exercise, arterial (Fig. 4), hypothalamic, muscle, and skin temperatures change (65,111,153,154,166–171). These changes might then provide the stimulus for tachypneic hyperpnea. This conclusion is suggested by data on humans showing elimination of a time-dependent hyperventilation during exercise by cooling the skin and maintaining core temperature near constant (159). The change in arterial

and presumably hypothalamic temperature need not be great in some species to elicit a large change in breathing (Fig. 4). Therefore, either the system is highly sensitive to the small changes in hypothalamic temperature, or skin temperature is of major importance. However, in humans it appears that core temperature needs to increase nearly 1°C before the ventilatory drift is evident (12,111,166,171).

MINIMIZATION OF WORK OF BREATHING

The ventilatory control system may operate so as to minimize the force generated by the respiratory muscles or to minimize the O_2 cost of breathing (63,172–174). This cost depends on lung and chest wall compliance and is affected by airway resistance (173–176), but it is also affected by locomotion (161,177,178). Consequently, minimization of total elastic and flow-resistive work during exercise is achieved by (a) appropriate V_T and f responses to exercise, (b) appropriate changes in airway diameter, (c) appropriate recruitment of respiratory muscles, and (d) appropriate inspiratory and expiratory flow profiles.

In humans at low workloads, hyperpnea is accomplished primarily through an increase in V_T (21). Both inspiratory and expiratory reserve volumes are utilized so that the steep, linear portions of the lung and chest wall compliances are utilized. However, compliance begins to decrease as V_T exceeds 65% of V_T; thus, at higher workloads, breathing frequency contributes progressively more to hyperpnea (178). In contrast, with the stiff chest wall and therefore high elastic work in ponies, it is apparently more efficient to increase f at low workloads (16,85). However, there is a limit to the increase in f; thus, when the ventilatory demand is high, V_T becomes increasingly more important in this species.

Because locomotion per se imposes limitations on ventilatory function (161,177,178), breathing is thought to be most efficient when there is a coupling of breath and stride frequency during exercise. In other words, locomotion is associated with cyclic changes that either facilitate or hinder inspiration and expiration. For example, the cyclic "loading" of the respiratory system as the forelimbs strike the ground during a gallop by quadripeds is advantageous for expiration but not for inspiration. Second, the cyclic acceleration and deceleration in the horizontal plane shifts abdominal contents, and thus it is more efficient for inspiration to occur during acceleration when the abdominal contents are moving away from the diaphragm. Finally, both locomotion and respiration involve cycle movements in the ribs, sternum, and associated musculature; thus a coupling or coordination of breath and stride frequency avoids antagonistic actions. This coupling, termed "entrainment," has been observed in several species, including human. In quadripeds, locomotion and breathing are coupled at a constant 1:1 ratio during a gallop (161,177,179). During a trot or walk in these species and during running in humans, the ratio is more variable (17,26,132,176,180–183).

Airway diameter is regulated during exercise, and thus inspiratory and expiratory flow can increase without major changes in airway resistance (184). The large increase in upper airway V_D during exercise is evidence of airway dilation (185). Expiratory flow is also enhanced by elimination of braking (186), which is the active slowing of passive flow early in expiration due to abduction of the laryngeal aperture and sustained contraction of the diaphragm (186,187).

The temporal pattern of inspiratory and expiratory flow is under active regulation (188,189). Theoretically, a rectangular airflow profile is more efficient than a sinusoidal profile (188–191). At rest in humans the profiles tend to be more sinusoidal than rectangular (188,192–195), but during exercise they become more rectangular (188,194). In equines and goats, the airflow profiles are nearly rectangular at rest, during mild and moderate exercise, and during CO_2 inhalation (28,196–198). These profiles are a result of the specific recruitment patterns of the respiratory muscles. For example, the expiratory braking at rest (187) in humans provides for the nearly sinusoidal flow profile. Moreover, the rectangular profiles during exercise are partly due to contraction of expiratory muscles to reduce end-expiratory lung volume (EELV) below the passive functional residual capacity (199,200). There is thus an active and passive component to both inspiration and expiration. Decreasing EELV also enhances the efficiency of breathing by lengthening the diaphragm, which permits generation of increased tension for the same amount of phrenic nerve activation (201).

Essentially, the O_2 cost of breathing during exercise is minimized through appropriate selection of the rate, magnitude, and pattern of activation of inspiratory, expiratory, and airway muscles. Afferents from mechanoreceptors in the chest wall, lung, and possibly the diaphragm are thought to provide crucial information to the respiratory controller for efficient breathing (63,172–174). Changes and/or species differences in respiratory impedance are major determinants of f and V_T. An important role has also been postulated for afferents from the exercising limbs (11,131,161, 180,202). For the same increase in metabolic rate, f increases more when running speed is increased than it does when running incline is increased (17,26, 48,203). Finally, the hypothalamic mechanism appears capable of providing a proportional response in locomotion and breathing without peripheral neural afferents (125–127). The peripheral afferent and central command mechanisms might be of most importance in mediating a so-called "neural" entrainment, but it is likely that lung and chest wall afferents contribute to what can be called a "mechanical" entrainment.

CONCLUSION

The mechanism of the several aspects of exercise hyperpnea remains controversial in part because the phenomenon is difficult to study. Most studies on specific receptors or pathways have been completed under highly unphysiologic conditions. Many of the procedures such as electrical stimulation of muscles and nerves and venous CO_2 loading many not provide a valid simulation of the exercise condition. Many of the clinical models such as spinal-lesioned humans and carotid-chemoreceptor-resected asthmatics may provide misleading data. Denervating a receptor and comparing responses before and after denervation may not provide a valid index of the role of the receptor when intact. Moreover, it is technically difficult to isolate one or more pathways and yet maintain physiologic conditions. These problems are not unique to the studies of exercise hyperpnea, but they seem exaggerated because of the multiplicity of changes that occur during exercise and because of the number of components of this control system.

Not surprisingly then, the conclusion reached regarding exercise hyperpnea mechanisms depends largely upon the assumptions that are made. If it is assumed that denervating a receptor provides a valid index of the normal response, then there seems little doubt that carotid and pulmonary receptors are not critical for exercise hyperpnea. On the other hand, if it is assumed that the response to electrically stimulated muscle contractions in paraplegic humans provides a valid test of the neural theories, then there seems little doubt that the neural pathways are not critical for exercise hyperpnea. If both assumptions are accepted, then the occlusion theory seems most logical. The challenge then is to test these theories under physiologic conditions in chronic animal models.

It seems paramount in future studies that the focus be expanded from most previous studies. The focus has been largely on the human response, that is, the close $\dot{V}_A$ coupling to metabolic rate and near arterial isocapnia during submaximal exercise and the progressive hypocapnia associated with the lactacidosis during heavy exercise. It is now clear though that this pattern is unique to humans; other mammals clearly hyperventilate during submaximal exercise, and lactacidosis does not appear to accentuate the hyperventilation. Of interest are data indicating P_aO_2 homeostasis over all levels of exercise in all but a few exceptional cases. These findings do not necessarily imply that the important aspect of control is P_aO_2 chemoreception; however, it seems unlikely P_{CO_2} is the major regulated variable.

Many factors should be considered in planning future studies. *First*, it seems clear that species differences in the characteristics of exercise hyperpnea provide insights into its mechanism. *Second*, the control system has several tasks, and the specific $\dot{V}_E$ at any time under any condition represents an attempt to "best" meet all the tasks. *Third*, the control system has many components. The close coupling of ventilation and metabolic rate during exercise might represent the combined influence of a very "gross" primary exercise drive with rather precise chemoreceptor "fine tuning" (204). *Fourth*, basic neuronal properties must influence exercise hyperpnea. The phenomenon known as "afterdischarge" (persisting neural activity after cessation of a stimulus) may contribute to the slow components of ventilation during and after ex-

ercise (205). *Fifth*, numerous neuromodulators in the brainstem and spinal cord probably have an important impact on exercise hyperpnea (206). The so-called "interaction of exercise" and other ventilatory stimuli might be mediated by changes in these neuromodulators. In essence, it seems prudent that future studies be planned considering not only what is known about exercise hyperpnea but also what is known about all components of this complex regulatory system.

REFERENCES

1. Asmussen E. Ventilation at transition from rest to exercise. *Acta Physiol Scand* 1973;89:68–78.
2. Beaver WL, Wasserman K. Transients in ventilation at start and end of exercise. *J Appl Physiol* 1968;25:390–399.
3. Casaburi R, Barstow TJ, Robinson T, Wasserman K. Influence of work rate on ventilatory and gas exchange kinetics. *J Appl Physiol* 1989;67:547–555.
4. D'Angelo E, Torelli G. Neural stimuli increasing respiration during different types of exercise. *J Appl Physiol* 1971;30:116–121.
5. Dejours P. Control of respiration in muscular exercise. In: *Handbook of physiology, Section 3: Respiration, vol 1*. Washington, DC: American Physiological Society, 1974;631–648.
6. Diamond LB, Casaburi R, Wasserman K, Whipp BJ. Kinetics of gas exchange and ventilation in transitions from rest or prior exercise. *J Appl Physiol* 1977;43:704–708.
7. Hickman JB, Pryor WW, Page EB, Atwell RJ. Respiratory regulation during exercise in unconditioned subjects. *J Clin Invest* 1951;30:503–516.
8. Jensen JI. Neural ventilatory drive during arm and leg exercise. *Scand J Clin Lab Invest* 1972;29:177–184.
9. Krogh A, Lindhard J. The regulation of respiration and circulation during the initial stages of muscular work. *J Physiol (Lond)* 1913;47:112–136.
10. Pearce DH, Milhorn HT Jr. Dynamic and steady-state respiratory responses to bicycle ergometer exercise. *J Appl Physiol* 1977;42:959–967.
11. Torelli G, Brandi G. Regulation of ventilation at the beginning of muscular exercise. *Int Angew Physiol* 1961;19:134–139.
12. Whipp B. Control of exercise hyperpnea. In: Hornbein TF, ed. *Regulation of breathing*, Part II. New York: Marcel Dekker, 1981;1069–1140.
13. Bisgard G, Forster HV, Messina J, Sarazin RG. Role of the carotid body in hyperpnea of moderate exercise in goats. *J Appl Physiol* 1986;52:1216–1222.
14. Flandrois R, Lacour JF, Eclache JP. Control of respiration in exercising dog: interaction of chemical and physical humoral stimuli. *Respir Physiol* 1974;21:169–181.
15. Pan LG, Forster HV, Bisgard GE, Kaminski RP, Dorsey SM, Busch MA. Hyperventilation in ponies at the onset of and during steady-state exercise. *J Appl Physiol* 1983;54:1394–1402.
16. Powers SK, Beadle RE, Thompson D, Lawler J. Ventilatory and blood gas dynamics at onset and offset of exercise in the pony. *J Appl Physiol* 1987;62:141–148.
17. Smith CA, Mitchell GS, Jameson LC, Musch TI, Dempsey JA. Ventilatory response of goats to treadmill exercise: grade effects. *Respir Physiol* 1983;54:331–341.
18. Szlyk PC, McDonald BW, Pendergast BW, Krasney JH. Control of ventilation during graded exercise in the dog. *Respir Physiol* 1981;46:345–365.
19. Asmussen E. Muscular exercise. In: Fenn WV, Rahn H, eds. *Handbook of physiology, Section 3: Respiration, vol 2*. Washington, DC: American Physiological Society, 1965;939–978.
20. Asmussen E. Exercise and the regulation of ventilation. In: *Physiology of muscular exercise, vol 15*. Washington, DC: American Heart Association, 1967;132–145.
21. Dempsey JA, Rankin J. Physiologic adaptations of gas trans-

port systems to muscular work in health and disease. *Am J Phys Med* 1967;46:582–647.

22. Dempsey JA, Reddan WG, Rankin J, Birnbaum ML, Forster HV, Thoden JS, Grover RF. Effects of acute through life-long hypoxic exposure on exercise pulmonary gas exchange. *Respir Physiol* 1971;13:62–87.

23. Wasserman K, Whipp BJ, Casaburi R, Beaver WL, Brown HV. CO_2 flow to the lungs and ventilatory control. In: Dempsey JA, Reed CE, eds. *Muscular exercise and the lung.* Madison, WI: University of Wisconsin Press, 1977;103–135.

24. Dempsey JA, Gledhill N, Reddan WG, Forster HV, Hanson PG, Claremont AD. Pulmonary adaptation to exercise: effects of exercise type and duration, chronic hypoxia, and physical training. In: Milvey P, ed. *The marathon: physiological, medical epidemiology, and psychological studies. NY Acad Sci* [special edition] 1977;301:243–261.

25. Kay JDS, Petersen ES, Vejby-Christensen H. Breathing in man during steady-state exercise on the bicycle at low pedaling frequencies and during treadmill walking. *J Physiol (Lond)* 1977;272:553–561.

26. McMurray RG, Ahlborn SW. Respiratory reasponses to running and walking at the same metabolic rate. *Respir Physiol* 1982;47:257–265.

27. Szal SE, Schoene RB. Ventilatory response to rowing and cycling in elite oarswomen. *J Appl Physiol* 1989;67:264–269.

28. Forster HV, Brice AG, Lowry TF, Gutting SM. The temporal pattern of inspiratory and expiratory flow in awake goats at rest and during mild exercise. *Proc Int Univ Physiol Sci* 1989;2352.

29. Oren A, Whipp BJ, Wasserman K. Effect of acid–base status on the kinetics of the ventilatory response to moderate exercise. *J Appl Physiol* 1982;52:1013–1017.

30. Dempsey JA, Forster HV, Birnbaum ML, Reddan WG, Thoden J, Grover RF, Rankin J. Control of exercise hyperpnea under varying durations of exposure to moderate hypoxia. *Respir Physiol* 1972;16:213–231.

31. Forster HV, Pan LG, Bisgard GE, Kaminski RP, Dorsey SC, Busch MA. The hyperpnea of exercise at various P_{IO_2} in normal and carotid body denervated ponies. *J Appl Physiol* 1983;54:1387–1393.

32. Weil JV, Byrne-Quinn E, Sodal IE, Kline JS, McCullough, RE, Filley GF. Augmentation of chemosensitivity during mild exercise in normal man. *J Appl Physiol* 1972;33:813–819.

33. Knuttgen HG, Emerson K. Physiological response to pregnancy at rest and during exercise. *J Appl Physiol* 1974;36:546–553.

34. Mitchell GS, Smith CA, Dempsey JA. Changes in the $V_I:V_{CO_2}$ relationship during exercise: role of carotid body. *J Appl Physiol* 1984;57:1894–1900.

35. Pernoll ML, Metcalfe J, Kovach PA, Wachtel R, Dunham M. Ventilation during rest and exercise in pregnancy and postpartum. *Respir Physiol* 1975;25:295–310.

36. Schaefer SL, Mitchell GS. Ventilatory control during exercise with peripheral chemoreceptor stimulation: hypoxia versus domperidone. *J Appl Physiol* 1989;67:2438–2446.

37. Watken RL, Rostosfer HH, Robinson S, Newton JL, Baillie MD. Changes in blood gases and acid–base balance in the exercising dog. *J Appl Physiol* 1962;17:656–660.

38. Barr PO, Beckman M, Bjurstedt H, Brismar J, Hessler CM, Matell G. Time course of blood gas changes provoked by light and moderate exercise in man. *Acta Physiol Scand* 1964;60:1–17.

39. Forster HV, Pan LG, Funahashi A. Temporal pattern of $PaCO_2$ during exercise in humans. *J Appl Physiol* 1986;60:653–660.

40. Oldenburg FA, McCormack DO, Morse JLC, Jones NL. A comparison of exercise responses in stairclimbing and cycling. *J Appl Physiol* 1979;46:510–516.

41. Young IH, Woolcock AJ. Changes in arterial blood gas tension during unsteady-state exercise. *J Appl Physiol* 1978;44:93–96.

42. Dempsey JA, Hanson P, Henderson K. Exercise induced arterial hypoxemia in healthy humans at sea level. *J Physiol (Lond)* 1984;355:161–175.

43. Holmgren A, Linderholm H. Oxygen and carbon dioxide ten-

sion of arterial blood during heavy and exhaustive exercise. *Acta Physiol Scand* 1958;44:203–215.

44. Powers SK, Lawler J, Dempsey JA, Dodd S, Landry G. Effects of incomplete pulmonary gas exchange on V_{O_2}max. *J Appl Physiol* 1989;66:2491–2495.

45. Rowell LB, Taylor HL, Wang Y, Carlson WB. Saturation of arterial blood with oxygen during maximal exercise. *J Appl Physiol* 1984;19:284–286.

46. Forster HV, Klausen K. The effect of chronic metabolic acidose and alkalosis on ventilation during exercise and hypoxia. *Respir Physiol* 1973;17:336–346.

47. Clifford PS, Litzow JT, Coon RL. Arterial hypocapnia during exercise in beagle dogs. *J Appl Physiol* 1986;61:599.

48. Forster HV, Pan LG, Bisgard GE, Flynn C, Dorsey SM, Britton MS. Independence of exercise hypocapnia and limb movement frequency in ponies. *J Appl Physiol* 1984;57:1885–1893.

49. Fregosi RF, Dempsey JA. Arterial blood acid–base regulation during exercise in rats. *J Appl Physiol* 1984;57:396–402.

50. Kiley JP, Kuhlmann WD, Fedde MR. Arterial and mixed venous blood gas tensions in exercising ducks. *Poult Sci* 1980;59:914–917.

51. Kuhlmann WD, Hodgson DS, Fedde MR. Respiratory, cardiovascular and metabolic adjustments to exercise in the hereford calf. *J Appl Physiol* 1985;58:1273–1280.

52. Mitchell GS, Gleason TT, Bennett AF. Ventilation and acid–base balance during activity in lizards. *Am J Physiol* 1981;240:R29–R37.

53. Pan LG, Forster HV, Bisgard GE, Murphy CL, Lowry TF. Independence of exercise hyperpnea and acidosis during high intensity exercise in ponies. *J Appl Physiol* 1986;60:1016–1024.

54. Pan LG, Brice AG, Forster HV, Forster AL, Lowry TF, Murphy CL, Gutting SM, Brown DR. Ventilatory response to treadmill exercise in normal and cardiac denervated goats. *FASEB J* 1989;3:A848.

55. Bayly WM, Grant BD, Breeze RG, Kramer JW. The effects of maximal exercise on acid–base balance and arterial blood gas tensions in thoroughbred horses. In: Snow DH, Persson SG, Rose RJ, eds. *Equine exercise physiology.* Cambridge: Granta Editions, 1983;400–404.

56. Thorston J, Essen-Gustavsson B, Lindholm A, McMicken D, Persson S. Effects of training and detraining on oxygen uptake, cardiac output, blood gas tensions, pH, and lactate concentrations during and after exercise in the horse. In: Snow DH, Persson SG, Rose RJ, eds. *Equine exercise physiology.* Cambridge, UK: Granta Editions, 1983;470–486.

57. Wagner PD, Gillespie JR, Landgren GL, Feddi MR, Jones BW, DeBowes RM, Pieschl RL, Erickson HH. Mechanism of exercise-induced hypoxiemia in horses. *J Appl Physiol* 1989;66:1227–1233.

58. Geppert J, Zuntz N. Ueber die Regulation der Atmung. *Arch Gesamte Physiol* 1888;42:189–245.

59. Haldane JS, Priestley JG. The regulation of the lung-ventilation. *J Physiol (Lond)* 1905;32:225–266.

60. Douglas CG, Haldane JS. The regulation of normal breathing. *J Physiol (Lond)* 1909;38:420–440.

61. Clark JM, Sinclair RD, Lenox JB. Chemical and nonchemical components of ventilation during hypercapnic exercise in man. *J Appl Physiol* 1980;48:1065–1076.

62. Poon C-S, Greene JG. Control of exercise hyperpnea during hypercapnia in humans. *J Appl Physiol* 1985;59:792–797.

63. Poon C-S. Ventilatory control in hypercapnia and exercise: optimization hypothesis. *J Appl Physiol* 1987;62:2447–2459.

64. Asmussen E, Nielsen M. Ventilatory responses to CO_2 during work at normal and at low oxygen tensions. *Acta Physiol Scand* 1957;39:27–35.

65. Cotes JE. The role of body temperature in controlling ventilation during exercise in one normal subject breathing oxygen. *J Physiol (Lond)* 1955;129:554–563.

66. Band DM, Cameron IR, Semple SJG. Oscillations in arterial pH with breathing in the cat. *J Appl Physiol* 1969;26:261–267.

67. Goodman NW, Nail BS, Torrance RW. Oscillations in the discharge of single carotid chemoreceptor fibres of the cat. *Respir Physiol* 1974;20:251–266.

68. Band DM, Willshaw P, Wolff CB. The speed of response of

the carotid body chemoreceptor. In: Paintal AS, ed. *Morphology and mechanisms of chemoreceptors.* New Delhi, India: Navchetan Press, 1976;197–207.

69. Biscoe TJ, Purves MJ. Observations on the rhythmic variation in the cat carotid body chemoreceptor activity which has the same period as respiration. *J Physiol (Lond)* 1967;190:389–412.

70. Black AMS, Torrance RW. Respiratory oscillations in chemoreceptor discharge in control of breathing. *Respir Physiol* 1971;13:221–237.

71. Cross BA, Davey A, Guz A, Katona PG, Maclean M, Murphy K, Semple SJC, Stidwell R. The pH oscillations in arterial blood during exercise: a potential signal for the ventilatory response in the dog. *J Physiol (Lond)* 1982;329:57–73.

72. Black AMS, Goodman NW, Nail BS, Rao PS, Torrance RW. The significance of the timing of chemoreceptor impulses for their effect upon respiration. *Acta Neurobiol Exp* 1973;33:139–147.

73. Grant B, Semple SJG. Mechanisms whereby oscillations in arterial carbon dioxide tension might affect pulmonary ventilation. In: Paintal AS, ed. *Morphology and mechanisms of chemoreceptors.* New Delhi, India: Navchetan Press, 1976;114–121.

74. Saunders KB. Oscillations of arterial CO_2 tension in a respiratory model: some implications for the control of breathing in exercise. *J Theor Biol* 1980;84:163–179.

75. Yamamoto IH, Edwards MW. Homeostasis of CO_2 during intravenous infusion of CO_2. *J Appl Physiol* 1960;15:807–818.

76. Wasserman K, Whipp BJ, Casaburi R, Golden M, Beaver WL. Ventilatory control during exercise in man. *Bull Eur Physiopathol Respir* 1979;15:27–47.

77. Fordyce WE, Bennett FM, Edelman SK, Grodins FG. Evidence for a fast neural mechanism during the early phase of exercise hyperpnea. *Respir Physiol* 1982;48:27–43.

78. Casaburi R, Stremal RW, Whipp BJ, Beaver WL, Wasserman K. Alteration by hyperoxia of ventilatory dynamics during sinusoidal work. *J Appl Physiol* 1980;48:1083–1091.

79. Asmussen E, Nielsen M. Pulmonary ventilation and effect of oxygen breathing in heavy exercise. *Acta Physiol Scand* 1958;43:365–378.

80. Bannister RG, Cunningham DJC. The effects on the respiration and performance during exercise of adding oxygen to the inspired air. *J Physiol (Lond)* 1954;125:118–137.

81. Wasserman K, Whipp BJ, Koyal SN, Cleary MG. Effect of carotid body resection on ventilatory and acid–base control during exercise. *J Appl Physiol* 1975;39:354–358.

82. Bledsoe SW, Hornbein TF. Central chemosensors and the regulation of their chemical environment. In: Hornbein TF, ed. *Regulation of breathing*, Part I. New York: Marcel Dekker, 1981;347–428.

83. Fencl V, Miller TB, Pappenheimer JR. Studies on the respiratory response to disturbances of acid–base balance with deductions concerning the composition of cerebral interstitial fluids. *Am J Physiol* 1966;210:459–472.

84. Pappenheimer JR, Vencl V, Heisey SR, Held D. Role of cerebral fluids in control of respiration as studied in unanesthetized goats. *Am J Physiol* 1965;208:436–450.

85. Bisgard GE, Forster HV, Byrnes B, Stanek K, Klein J, Manohar M. Cerebrospinal fluid acid–base balance during muscular exercise. *J Appl Physiol* 1978;45:94–101.

86. Casaburi R, Daly J, Hansen JE, Effros RM. Abrupt changes in mixed venous blood gas composition. *J Appl Physiol* 1989;67:1106–1112.

87. Edwards RHT, Denison DM, Jones G, Davies CTM, Campbell EJM. Changes in mixed venous gas tensions at start of exercise in man. *J Appl Physiol* 1972;32:165–169.

88. Lindhard J. Ueber das Minutenvolum des Herzens bei Ruhe und bei Muskelarbeit. *Arch Gesamte Physiol* 1915;161:233–283.

89. Armstrong BW, Hurt HH, Blide RW, Workman JM. The humoral regulation of breathing. *Science* 1961;133:1897–1906.

90. Aviado DM, Li TH, Kalow W, Schmidt CF, Turnbull GL, Peskin GW, Hess ME, Weiss AJ. Respiratory and circulatory reflexes from the perfused heart and pulmonary circulation of the dog. *Am J Physiol* 1951;165:261–277.

91. Comroe JH. The location and function of the chemoreceptors of the aorta. *Am J Physiol* 1939;127:176–191.

92. Dejours P, Methoefer JC, Teillac A. Essai de nise en evidence de chemorecepteurs veineux de ventilation. *J Physiol (Paris)* 1955;47:160–163.

93. Kao FF. The peripheral neurogenic drive: an experimental study. In: Dempsey JA, Reed CE, eds. *Muscular exercise and the lung.* Madison, WI: University of Wisconsin Press, 1979;71–85.

94. Lamb TW. Ventilatory responses to intravenous and inspired carbon dioxide in anesthetized cats. *Respir Physiol* 1966;2:99–104.

95. Riley RL. The hyperpnea of exercise. In: Cunningham DJC, Lloyd BB, eds. *The regulation of human respiration.* Oxford: Blackwell, 1963.

96. Zuntz N, Geppert J. Ueber die Natur de normalen Atemreize und den Ort ihrer Wikrung. *Arch Gesamte Physiol* 1986;38:337–338.

97. Green JF, Sheldon MI. Ventilatory changes associated with changes in pulmonary blood flow in dogs. *J Appl Physiol* 1983;54:997–1002.

98. Sheldon JI, Green JF. Evidence for pulmonary CO_2 chemosensitivity: effects on ventilation. *J Appl Physiol* 1982;52:1192–1197.

99. Brown HV, Wasserman K, Whipp BJ. Effect of beta-adrenergic blockade during exercise on ventilation and gas exchange. *J Appl Physiol* 1976;41:886–892.

100. Casaburi R, Whipp BJ, Koyal SN, Wasserman K. Coupling of ventilation to CO_2 production during constant load ergometry with sinusoidally varying pedal rate. *J Appl Physiol* 1978;44:97–103.

101. Jones NL, Haddon RWT. Effect of a meal on cardiopulmonary and metabolic changes during exercise. *Can J Physiol Pharmacol* 1973;51:445–450.

102. Jones WB, Thomas HD, Reeves TJ. Circulatory and ventilatory responses to postprandial exercise. *Am Heart J* 1965;69:668–676.

103. Miyamoto Y, Nakazono Y, Yamakoshi K. Neurogenic factors affecting ventilatory and circulatory responses to static and dynamic exercise in man. *Jpn J Physiol* 1987;37:435–446.

104. Phillipson EA, Bowes G, Townsend ER, Duffin J, Cooper JD. Role of metabolic CO_2 production in ventilatory response to steady-state exercise. *J Clin Invest* 1981;68:768–774.

105. Phillipson EA, Duffin J, Cooper JD. Critical dependence of respiratory rhythmicity on metabolic CO_2 load. *J Appl Physiol* 1981;50:45–54.

106. Cropp GJA, Comroe JH Jr. Role of mixed venous CO_2 in respiratory control. *J Appl Physiol* 1961;16:1029–1033.

107. Banner N, Guz A, Heaton R, Innes JA, Murphy K, Yacoub M. Ventilatory and circulatory responses at the onset of exercise in man following heart or heart–lung transplantation. *J Physiol* 1988;399:437–449.

108. Clifford PS, Litzow JT, von Colditz JH, Coon RL. Effect of chronic pulmonary denervation on ventilatory response to exercise. *J Appl Physiol* 1986;61:603–610.

109. Favier R, Kepenekian G, Desplanches D, Flandrois R. Effects of chronic lung denervation on breathing pattern and respiratory gas exchange during hypoxia, hypercapnia and exercise. *Respir Physiol* 1982;47:107–119.

110. Flynn C, Forster HV, Pan LG, Bisgard GE. Role of hilar nerve afferents in hyperpnea of exercise. *J Appl Physiol* 1985;59:798–806.

111. Dejours P, Teillac A, Girard F, Lacaisse A. Étude du rôle de l'hyperthermie centrale modérée dans la régulation de la ventilation de l'exercice musculaire chez l'homme. *Rev Fr Etudes Clin Biol* 1958;3:755–761.

112. Bannister EW, Griffiths J. Blood levels of adrenergic amines during exercise. *J Appl Physiol* 1972;33:674–676.

113. Euler US von, Hellner S. Excretion of noradrenaline and adrenaline in muscular work. *Acta Physiol Scand* 1952;26:183–191.

114. Flandrois R, Favien R, Pequignot JM. Role of adrenaline in gas exchanges and respiratory control in the dog at rest and exercise. *Respir Physiol* 1977;30:291–303.

115. Gray I, Beetham WP. Changes in plasma concentration of epinephrine and norepinephrine with muscular work. *Proc Soc Exp Biol Med* 1957;96:636–638.

116. Band DM, Linton RAF, Kent R, Kurer FL. The effect of peripheral chemodenervation on the ventilatory response to potassium. *Respir Physiol* 1985;60:217–225.

117. Conway J, Paterson DJ, Petersen ES, Robbins PA. Changes in arterial potassium and ventilation in response to exercise in humans. *J Physiol* 1986;374:26P.

118. Forster HV, Lowry TF, Murphy CL, Pan LG. Role of elevated plasma [K$^+$] and carotid chemoreceptors in hyperpnea of exercise in awake ponies. *J Physiol (Lond)* 1989;417:112p.

119. Coles DR, Duff F, Shepherd WHT, Whelan RF. The effect on respiration of infusions of adrenaline and nonadrenaline into the carotid and vertebral arteries in man. *Br J Pharmacol* 1956;11:346–350.

120. Cunningham DJC, Hey EN, Lloyd BB. The effect of intravenous infusion of noradrenaline on the respiratory response to carbon dioxide. *Q J Exp Physiol* 1958;43:394–399.

121. Whelan RF, Young IM. The effect of adrenaline and noradrenaline infusions on respiration in man. *Br J Pharmacol* 1953;8:98–102.

122. Bascom DA, Clement JD, Cunningham DA, Friedland JS, Paterson DJ, Robbins PA. Changes in arterial plasma potassium [K$^+$] and ventilation (V_E) during exercise in subjects with McArdle's syndrome. *J Physiol* 1989;417:141.

123. Haggendal J, Harley LH, Salten B. Arterial noradrenaline concentration during exercise in relation to the relative work loads. *Scand J Clin Lab Invest* 1970;26:337–342.

124. Eldridge FL, Milhorn DE, Kiley JP, Waldrop TG. Stimulation by central command of locomotion, respiration and circulation during exercise. *Respir Physiol* 1985;59:313–337.

125. DiMarco AF, Romaniuk JR, von Euler C, Yamamoto Y. Immediate changes in ventilation and respiratory pattern associated with onset and cessation of locomotion in the cat. *J Physiol (Lond)* 1983;343:1–16.

126. Waldrop TG, Mullins DC, Millhorn DE. Control of respiration by the hypothalamus and by feedback from contracting muscles in cats. *Respir Physiol* 1986;64:317–328.

127. Adams L, Frankel H, Garlick J, Guz A, Murphy K, Semple SJG. The role of spinal cord transmission in the ventilatory response to exercise in man. *J Physiol* 1984;355:85–97.

128. Asmussen E, Neilsen M, Weith-Pedersen G. Cortical or reflex control of respiration during muscular work? *Acta Physiol Scand* 1943;6:168–175.

129. Brice AG, Forster HV, Pan LG, Funahashi A, Lowry TF, Murphy CL, Hoffman MD. Ventilatory and Paco$_2$ response to voluntary and electrically-induced leg exercise. *J Appl Physiol* 1988;64:218–225.

130. Brice G, Forster HV, Pan L, Funahashi A, Hoffman M, Lowry T, Murphy C. Is the hyperpnea of muscle contractions critically dependent on spinal afferents? *J Appl Physiol* 1988;64:223–226.

131. Agostoni E, D'Angelo E. The effect of limb movements on the regulation of depth and rate of breathing. *Respir Physiol* 1956;27:33–52.

132. Asmussen E, Johansen SH, Jorgensen M, Neilsen M. On the nervous factors controlling respiration and circulation during exercise. *Acta Physiol Scand* 1965;63:343–350.

133. Bennett F. A role for neural pathways in exercise hyperpnea. *J Appl Physiol* 1984;56:1559–1564.

134. Comroe MJ Jr, Schmidt CF. Reflexes from the limbs as a factor in the hyperpnea of muscular exercise. *Am J Physiol* 1943;138:536–547.

135. Dejours, P. La regulation de la ventilation au cours de l'exercise musculaire chez l'homme. *J Physiol (Paris)* 1959;51:163–261.

136. Flandrois R, Lacour JR, Maroquin JI, Charlot J. Limb mechanoreceptors inducing the reflex hyperpnea of exercise. *Respir Physiol* 1967;2:335–343.

137. McCloskey DI, Mitchell JH. Reflex cardiovascular and respiratory responses originating in exercising muscle. *J Physiol (Lond)* 1972;224:173–186.

138. Bessou P, Dejours P, Laporte Y. Action ventilatoire reflexe de fibres afferentes de grand diametre d'origine musculaire chez le chat. *J Physiol (Paris)* 1959;51:400–401.

139. Hornbein TF, Sorensen SC, Parks CR. Role of muscle spindles in lower extremities in breathing during bicycle exercise. *J Appl Physiol* 1969;27:476–479.

140. Lamb TW. Ventilatory responses to hind limb exercise in anesthetized cats and dogs. *Respir Physiol* 1968;6:88–104.

141. Mitchell JH, Reardon WC, McCloskey PI. Reflex effects on circulation and respiration from contracting skeletal muscle. *Am J Physiol* 1977;233:H374–H378.

142. Tibes U, Hemmer B, Boning D. Heart rate and ventilation in relation to venous K$^+$, osmolality, pH, Pco$_2$, Po$_2$, orthophosphate, and lactate at transition from rest to exercise in athletes and non-athletes. *Eur J Appl Physiol* 1977;36:127–140.

143. Hussain SNA, Pardy RL, Dempsey JA. Mechanical impedance as determinant of inspiratory neural drive during exercise in humans. *J Appl Physiol* 1985;59:365–375.

144. Pan LG, Forster HV, Bisgard GE, Lowry TF, Murphy CL. Role of carotic chemoreceptors and pulmonary vagal afferents during helium:O$_2$ breathing in ponies. *J Appl Physiol* 1987;62:1020–1027.

145. Mitchell GS, Douse MA, Foley KT. Receptor interactions in modulating ventilatory activity. *Am J Physiol* 1990;in press.

146. Grodins FS. Analysis of factors concerned in regulation of breathing in exercise. *Physiol Rev* 1950;30:220.

147. Yamamoto WS. Looking at the regulation of ventilation as a signalling process. In: Dempsey JA, Reid CE, eds. *Muscular exercise and the lung*. Madison, WI: University of Wisconsin Press, 1977;137–149.

148. Nielson M, Asmussen E. Humoral and nervous control of breathing in exercise. In: Cunningham DJC, Lloyd BB, eds. *The regulation of human respiration*. Philadelphia: FA Davis, 1963;504–513.

149. Hagberg JM, Coyle EF, Carroll JE, Miller JM, Martin WH, Brooke MH. Exercise hyperventilation in patients with McArdles disease. *J Appl Physiol* 1982;52:991–994.

150. Green HJ, Hughson RL, Orr GW, Ranney DA. Anaerobic threshold, blood lactate and muscle metabolites in progressive exercise. *J Appl Physiol* 1983;54:1032–1038.

151. Hagenhauser GJT, Sutton JR, Jones NL. Effect of glycogen depletion on the ventilatory response to exercise. *J Appl Physiol* 1983;54:470–474.

152. Hughes EF, Turner SC, Brooks GA. Effect of glycogen depletion and pedaling speed on "anaerobic threshold." *J Appl Physiol* 1982;52:1598–1607.

153. Christensen EH. Beitrage zur Physiologie schwerer kopelicher arbeit. II. Die Korpertemperatur wahrend und unmittelbar nach schwerer korperlicher arbeit. *Arbeitsphysiologie* 1931;4:154–174.

154. Henry JD, Bainton CR. Human core temperature increase as a stimulus to breathing during moderate exercise. *Respir Physiol* 1974;21:183–191.

155. Bligh J. The initiation of thermal polypnea in the calf. *J Physiol (Lond)* 1957;136:413–419.

156. Bligh J. The receptors concerned in the thermal stimulus to panting in sheep. *J Physiol (Lond)* 1959;146:142–151.

157. Hales JRS. Changes in respiratory activity and body temperature of the severely heat-stressed ox and sheep. *Comp Biochem Physiol* 1969;31:975–985.

158. Hunter WS, Adams T. Respiratory heat exchange influences on diencephalic temperature in the cat. *J Appl Physiol* 1966;21:873–876.

159. Dempsey JA, Thomson JJ, Alexander SC, Forster HV, Chosy C. Respiratory influences on acid–base status and their effects on O$_2$ transport during prolonged muscular work. In: Howald H, Poortmans JR, eds. *Metabolic adaptation to prolonged physical exercise*. Basel, Switzerland: Birkhauser Verlag, 1975;56–64.

160. Baker MA. Brain cooling in endotherms in heat and exercise. *Annu Rev Physiol* 1982;44:85–96.

161. Bramble DM, Carrier DR. Running and breathing in mammals. *Science* 1983;219:251–256.

162. Lim PK, Grodins FS. Control of thermal panting. *Am J Physiol* 1955;180:445–449.

163. Bligh J. The receptors concerned in the respiratory response to humidity in sheep at high ambient temperature. *J Physiol (Lond)* 1963;168:747–763.

164. Kaminski RP, Forster HV, Bisgard GE, Pan LG, Dorsey SM. Effect of altered ambient temperature on breathing in ponies. *J Appl Physiol* 1985;58(5):1585–1591.

165. McBride B, Whitelaw WA. A physiological stimulus to upper airway receptors in humans. *J Appl Physiol* 1981;51:1189–1197.

166. Barltrop D. The relationship between body temperature and respiration. *J Physiol (Lond)* 1954;125:19P–20P.

167. Buchtal F, Honcke P, Lindhard J. Temperature measurements in human muscles *in situ* at rest and during muscular work. *Acta Physiol Scand* 1944;8:230–258.

168. Lambertsen, CJ. Mechanical and physical aspects of respiration. In: Bard P, ed. *Medical physiology*. St. Louis: CV Mosby, 1961;559.

169. Morgan DP, Kao F, Lim TPK, Grodins FS. Temperature and respiratory responses in exercise. *Am J Physiol* 1955;183:454–458.

170. Nielsen M. Die Regulation der Korpertemperatur bei Muskelarbeit. *Skand Arch Physiol* 1938;79:193–230.

171. Whipp BJ, Wasserman K. Effect of body temperature on the ventilatory response to exercise. *Respir Physiol* 1970;8:354–360.

172. Mead J. Control of respiratory frequency. *J Appl Physiol* 1980;49:528–532.

173. Milic-Emili G, Petit JM. Mechanical efficiency of breathing. *J Appl Physiol* 1960;15:359–362.

174. Otis AB, Fenn WO, Rahn H. Mechanics of breathing in man. *J Appl Physiol* 1950;2:592–607.

175. Margaria R, Milic-Emili G, Petit JM, Cavagna G. Mechanical work of breathing during muscular exercise. *J Appl Physiol* 1960;15:354–358.

176. Thoden JS, Dempsey JA, Reddan WG, Birnbaum ML, Forster HV, Grover RF, Rankin J. Ventilatory work during steady-state response to exercise. *Fed Proc* 1969;28:1316–1320.

177. Attenburrow DP. Time relationship between the respiratory cycle and limb cycle in the horse. *Equine Vet J* 1982;14:69–72.

178. Dempsey JA. Is the lung built for exercise? *Med Sci Sports Exerc* 1986;18:143–155.

179. Hornicke H, Meixner R, Pollmann U. Respiration in exercising horses. In: Snow DH, Persson SG, Rose RJ, eds. *Equine exercise physiology*. Cambridge, UK: Grants Editions, 1982;7–16.

180. Bechbache RR, Duffer J. The entrainment of breathing frequency by exercise rhythm. *J Physiol (Lond)* 1977;272:553–561.

181. Iscoe S. Respiratory and stepping frequencies in conscious exercising cats. *J Appl Physiol* 1981;51:835–839.

182. Jasinskas CL, Wilson BA, Hoare J. Entrainment of breathing rate to movement frequency during work at two intensities. *Respir Physiol* 1980;42:199–209.

183. Kawahara K, Kumagai S, Nakazono Y, Miyamoto Y. Coupling between respiratory and stepping rhythms during locomotion in decerebrate cats. *J Appl Physiol* 1989;67:110–115.

184. Widdicombe JB, Nadel JA. Airway volume, airway resistance, and work and force of breathing: theory. *J Appl Physiol* 1963;18:863–868.

185. Forster HV, Pan LG, Bisgard GE, Flynn C, Hoffer RE. Changes in breathing when switching from nares to tracheostomy breathing in awake ponies. *J Appl Physiol* 1985;59:1214–1221.

186. England SJ, Bartlett D Jr. Changes in respiratory movements of the human vocal cords during hyperpnea. *J Appl Physiol* 1982;52:780–785.

187. Remmers JE, Bartlett D. Reflex control of expiratory airflow and duration. *J Appl Physiol* 1977;42:80–87.

188. LaFortuna CL, Minette AE, Mognoni P. Inspiratory flow pattern in humans. *J Appl Physiol* 1984;57:1111–1119.

189. Yamashiro SM, Grodins FS. Optimal regulation of respiratory airflow. *J Appl Physiol* 1971;30:597–602.

190. Hamalainen RP, Viljanen AA. Modelling the respiratory airflow pattern by optimizing criteria. *Biol Cybern* 1978;29:143–149.

191. Ruttiman VE, Yamamoto WS. Respiratory airflow patterns that satisfy power and force criteria of optimality. *Ann Biomed Eng* 1972;1:146–159.

192. Agostoni EE, Campbell JM, Freedman S. Energetics. In: Campbell EJM, Agostoni E, Newsom Davis J, eds. *The respiratory muscles*. London: Lloyd-Luke, 1970;115–137.

193. Benchetrit G, Shea SA, Pham Dinh T, Bodocco S, Baconnier P, Guz A. Individuality of breathing patterns in adults assessed over time. *Respir Physiol* 1989;75:199–210.

194. Procter DF, Hardy JB. Studies of respiratory airflow. *Bull Johns Hopkins Hosp* 1949;85:253–280.

195. Silverman L, Lee G, Plotkin T, Sawyers LA, Yoncey AR. Airflow measurements on human subjects with and without respiratory resistance at several work rates. *Arch Ind Hyg Occup Med* 1951;3:461–478.

196. Gutting SM, Forster HV, Brice AG, Lowry TF, Pan LG, Murphy CL. Pattern of respiratory muscle activity during exercise in normal and hilar nerve denervated ponies. *FASEB J* 1988;2:5824.

197. Gutting SM, Forster HV, Lowry TF, Pan LG, Forster MA. Effects of hypercapnia on respiratory muscle activity in awake ponies. *FASEB J* 1989;3:3621.

198. Koterba AM, Kosch PC, Beech J, Whitlock T. Breathing strategy of the adult horse (*Equus caballus*) at rest. *J Appl Physiol* 1988;64:337–346.

199. Henke KG, Sharratt M, Pegelow D, Dempsey JA. Regulation of end-expiratory lung volume during exercise. *J Appl Physiol* 1988;64:135–146.

200. Sharratt MT, Henke KG, Aaron EA, Pegelow DF, Dempsey JA. Exercise-induced changes in function residual capacity. *Respir Physiol* 1987;70:313–326.

201. Grimby G, Goldman M, Mead J. Respiratory muscle actions inferred from rib cage and abdominal V-P partitioning. *J Appl Physiol* 1976;41:739–751.

202. Takano N. Effects of pedal rate on respiratory responses to incremental bicycle work. *J Physiol (Lond)* 1988;396:389–397.

203. Hanson P, Claremont A, Dempsey J, Reddan W. Determinants and consequences of ventilatory responses to competitive endurance running. *J Appl Physiol* 1982;52:615–623.

204. Bennett FM, Fordyce WE. Gain of the ventilatory exercise stimulus: definition and meaning. *J Appl Physiol* 1988;65:2011–2017.

205. Eldridge FL. Central neural respiratory stimulatory effect of active respiration. *J Appl Physiol* 1974;37:723–735.

206. Feldman JL, Smith JC. Cellular mechanisms underlying modulation of breathing pattern in mammals. *Ann NY Acad Sci* 1989;563:114–130.

THE LUNG: Scientific Foundations
edited by R.G. Crystal, J.B. West et al.
Raven Press, Ltd., New York © 1991.

CHAPTER 5.6.2.1

Pulmonary Gas Exchange

Paolo Cerretelli and Pietro Enrico di Prampero

The transfer of gases at the pulmonary level is the ultimate manifestation of the metabolic events taking place in the mitochondria and propagating through a cascade of integrated systems. These involve media with highly different physicochemical properties and of remarkable biological relevance. It is therefore understandable that physiologists working in different fields have long been attracted by the study of pulmonary gas exchange.

The present chapter is devoted to a brief discussion of the most relevant aspects of pulmonary gas exchange at steady state (see section entitled "The Steady State") as well as during metabolic transients (see section entitled "The Unsteady State"). The study of the transfer of gases over one breathing cycle (see section entitled "The Breathing Cycle"), showing that the steady state is not so "steady" after all, will bridge the gap between the section on the steady state and the one on the unsteady state. The final section entitled "The O_2 Debt–Deficit" will be devoted to a brief discussion of the O_2 debt–deficit concept.

THE STEADY STATE

Several factors are known to affect gas exchange during exercise in humans. Among these, hyperventilation, hemodynamic variables, hematologic factors, alveolar–end-capillary diffusion disequilibrium, and, particularly, ventilation–perfusion ($\dot{V}_A/\dot{Q}$) mismatch.

A survey of recent data from the literature with regard to alveolar air composition and alveolar–arterial O_2 and CO_2 gradients both at rest and at exercise pro-

vides new information on the role of O_2 diffusion limitation and $\dot{V}_A/\dot{Q}$ inequality in limiting gas exchange.

Arterial O_2 Pressures (P_aO_2)
and Alveolar–Arterial PO_2 Differences ($D_{A-a}O_2$)

From an extensive review of the literature (1), the mean P_aO_2 of moderately active, healthy subjects at rest ($n = 175$) studied by 17 investigators averaged 91.5 ± 4.9 (SD) torr. Submaximum and maximum aerobic exercise did not significantly affect P_aO_2 in these subjects. Hammond et al. (2), studying eight 22-year-old trained subjects ($\dot{V}O_2$max range: 37.4–64.0 ml· kg^{-1}·min^{-1}), found P_aO_2 to drop from 99.1 ± 5.5 (SD) torr at rest down to 90.7 ± 8.2 ($n = 5$) torr at workloads requiring an O_2 consumption of greater than 3.5 liters ·min^{-1}. This trend towards arterial O_2 desaturation with increasing workloads is in agreement with the results of Dempsey et al. (3), who found, in 16 runners capable of achieving and sustaining very high metabolic rates [$\dot{V}O_2$max = 72 ± 2 (SEM) ml·kg^{-1}·min^{-1}] and characterized by an average resting P_aO_2 of 91 ± 0.9 (SEM) torr, a drastic decrease of P_aO_2 to 75 ± 2.3 torr during maximum short-term exercise.

From a survey of the literature (1), the resting alveolar–arterial PO_2 difference ($D_{A-a}O_2$) averages in young healthy untrained male subjects 11.0 ± 3.1 (SD) torr. This value remains essentially unchanged at workloads up to ~40% of $\dot{V}O_2$max (see also ref. 2). A further increase of workload is accompanied by greater values of $D_{A-a}O_2$ up to an average maximum of 24.9 ± 7.2 torr, a value also found by Hammond et al. (2) for loads requiring an O_2 consumption of greater than 3.5 liters·min^{-1} (23.0 ± 8.0). For endurance runners, Dempsey et al. (3) found at $\dot{V}O_2$max an average maximum $D_{A-a}O_2$ of 33 ± 1.8 (SEM) torr. Both athletic condition and training do not seem to greatly affect $D_{A-a}O_2$ at rest or at exercise (3,4).

A widening of $D_{A-a}O_2$ has been found with aging.

P. Cerretelli: Département de Physiologie, Centre Médical Universitaire, 1211 Geneva, Switzerland.
P. E. di Prampero: Istituto di Biologia, Università di Udine, 33100 Udine, Italy.

However, since D_{A-aN_2} in elderly subjects was similar to that in young individuals (5), it was hypothesized that, with aging, the number of lung units with low $\dot{V}_A/\dot{Q}$ ratio remains unchanged. This conclusion is not compatible with the findings obtained by scanning the distribution of radioactive gases in the lung (6). Thus the larger D_{A-aO_2} was attributed to the combined effect of $\dot{V}_A/\dot{Q}$ and $D_L/\dot{Q}$ inequalities (7), a condition compatible with a narrow D_{A-aN_2} (5).

Arterial CO₂ Pressures (P_aCO_2) and Alveolar–Arterial P_{CO_2} Differences (D_{A-aCO_2})

Resting arterial CO₂ partial pressure (P_aCO_2) measured by 14 investigators in 147 subjects (on mouthpiece) averaged 38.2 ± 1.8 (SD) torr (1). In moderately active subjects, P_aCO_2 tends to increase slightly but significantly when raising $\dot{V}O_2$ up to 35% of $\dot{V}O_2$max. In the same subjects, P_aCO_2 decreases with a further increase of workload. Near $\dot{V}O_2$max, P_aCO_2 averages 33.3 ± 3.5 (SD) torr (data from 12 investigators; see ref. 1). The pattern described above applies to nonathletic individuals. However, the trend is similar in athletic subjects. In fact, Dempsey et al. (3) found a drop of P_aCO_2 from 38.9 at rest to 32.5 torr at maximum exercise ($\dot{V}O_2 = 4.81$ liters·min⁻¹) with a further drop to 28.9 torr when breathing 21% O₂ in He, and Hammond et al. (2) observed a reduction from 38.7 ± 2.1 (SD) to 35.2 ± 3.0 torr between rest and a $\dot{V}O_2$ of 3.97 ± 0.29 liters·min⁻¹.

Because of the high diffusivity of CO₂ across the alveolar membrane, the D_{A-aCO_2} should be near zero. However, there are reasons why negative D_{A-aCO_2} could arise [e.g., the relatively slow rate of the chemical reactions involved in the CO₂ transport in blood (see also the section entitled "Lung Diffusing Capacity," below) and the presence of unperfused alveoli (8)]. Moreover, there is experimental evidence that paradoxical negative P_{CO_2} gradients exist between blood and alveolar gas (8). From a survey of the literature, it appears that at rest the D_{A-aCO_2} measured on over 40 subjects is not significantly different from zero, whereas at workloads corresponding to $\dot{V}O_2$ of 1.5–2.5 liters·min⁻¹, the mean CO₂ gradient appears to be slightly negative. Scheid and Piiper (8) consider positive D_{A-aCO_2} the result of artifacts or inadequate measurement techniques.

O₂ Diffusion Limitation

At sea level, O₂ diffusion limitation has generally been considered unlikely even at heavy exercise (10–13), as indicated by the marginal drop of P_aO_2 and small increase of D_{A-aO_2} up to submaximal workloads in healthy untrained individuals.

Wagner (14), however, has demonstrated in mathematical models the importance of the $\bar{P}_{\bar{v}O_2}$ level in achieving P_{O_2} equilibrium between alveolar gas and pulmonary capillary blood. At $\bar{P}_{\bar{v}O_2}$ of 20 torr, P_{AO_2} of 100 torr, and normal diffusing capacity, equilibration would be only 80% complete after 0.3 sec. With increasing capillary volume from 80 to 150–200 ml and cardiac output to 25 liters·min⁻¹, a subject exercising at near $\dot{V}O_2$max ($\bar{P}_{\bar{v}O_2} < 20$ torr) would approach diffusion limitation even with a perfectly homogeneous lung, uniform transit times, and no accumulation of extravascular fluid in the lungs (see ref. 2). Moreover, as $\dot{V}_A/\dot{Q}$ inequality increases during exercise (see next paragraph), maldistribution of diffusive to perfusive conductance (15) may further increase the likelihood of diffusive limitation.

On the above theoretical grounds, Hammond et al. (2) calculated the fraction of the D_{A-aO_2} that at exercise could not be accounted for by measured $\dot{V}_A/\dot{Q}$ inequality. While confirming that trained subjects do not undergo O₂ diffusion limitation at workloads corresponding to $\dot{V}O_2$ of up to 2.5 liters·min⁻¹ (see also ref. 16), these investigators could observe that at $\dot{V}O_2$ of 3.07 and 3.97 liters·min⁻¹ the portion of D_{A-aO_2} unaccounted for was 9.1 and 12.3 torr, respectively. They inferred that, since postpulmonary shunt was negligible and since measured $\dot{V}_A/\dot{Q}$ inequality as well as intrapulmonary shunt could not explain the entire D_{A-aO_2}, this part of the D_{A-aO_2} difference was due to alveolar–end-capillary diffusion limitation developing at heavier workloads. Similarly, even though the various components of the measured D_{A-aO_2} were not assessed, Dempsey et al. (3) hypothesized that the widening of the P_{O_2} gradient found in endurance runners is due, in part, to the development of O₂ diffusion limitation secondary to very short erythrocyte transit times in the lungs. The latter investigators also proved that in their subjects there was no evidence of impaired breathing mechanics (in fact, P_{AO_2} was 108 ± 1.4 torr), a condition, however, that might occur in endurance master athletes (Dempsey, *personal communication*). Wagner et al. (17) recently found that also in the horse most of the exercise-induced hypoxemia is the result of diffusion limitation, which accounts for 76% of the observed D_{A-aO_2} at maximal running speeds of 13–14 m·sec⁻¹.

$\dot{V}_A/\dot{Q}$ Inequality During Exercise

As is well known from radioactive xenon clearance studies, the overall topographical distribution of ventilation and perfusion in the lungs becomes more uniform with exercise (18). On the other hand, recent studies based on the multiple inert gas elimination technique show small increases in $\dot{V}_A/\dot{Q}$ inequality

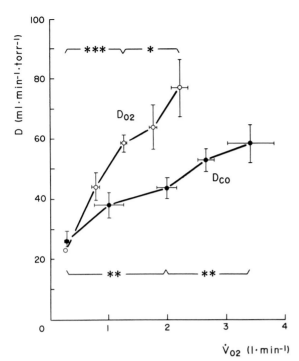

FIG. 1. Mean ($\pm$SD) diffusion capacity for O_2 (D_{O_2}; 44 subjects) and D_{CO} (318 subjects) as a function of $\dot{V}_{O_2}$ by various methods. $*p < 0.05$; $**p < 0.01$; $***p < 0.001$. (Adapted from ref. 1.)

with increasing $\dot{V}_{O_2}$ during exercise in normoxia. Two types of indices of $\dot{V}_A/\dot{Q}$ mismatching in the lungs may be used. One type is calculated from the distributions of the $\dot{V}_A/\dot{Q}$ 50 compartment lung model analysis (19,20), whereas the other is derived directly from retention and excretion of various inert gases (21). These sophisticated analytical approaches show a trend towards inequality of the intraregional $\dot{V}_A/\dot{Q}$ distribution during sea-level exercise that, however, is of borderline statistical significance. The $\dot{V}_A/\dot{Q}$ mismatching is accentuated by hypoxia (21). These results, on the other hand, confirm those of Gledhill et al. (22), who showed that the inspiration of SF_6-enriched air induces a decrease of a preexisting inhomogeneity of $\dot{V}_A/\dot{Q}$ distribution within regions of the lung (intraregional). In contrast, the inhomogeneity between regions, such as that due to the gravitational field, as is well known, is reduced at exercise. The above findings—that is, the improvement of the $\dot{V}_A/\dot{Q}$ distribution between regions and the worsening of the $\dot{V}_A/\dot{Q}$ distribution within given regions of the lung—are only apparently contradictory.

Lung Diffusing Capacity

Mean resting and exercise D_L values for CO ($D_{L_{CO}}$), as assessed by various methods, appear in Fig. 1 (see ref. 1). Despite the large differences among values ob-

tained at rest by various methods, $D_{L_{CO}}$ appears to increase with increasing $\dot{V}_{O_2}$. The same conclusion can be drawn also for $D_{L_{O_2}}$, irrespective of the technique used. The increase in D_L during exercise follows the enlargement of the effective gas–blood contact area, a consequence of the recruitment of vessels unperfused at rest and of increased transmural pressure causing vascular distension and thus also causing increases in capillary blood volume. Additional factors leading to an apparent increase of D_L are (a) the more homogeneous topographical (vertical) distribution of blood perfusion in the lungs during exercise and (b) the reduced negative effect on the estimate of D_L of a given degree of lung inhomogeneity when $\dot{V}_{O_2}$ is above resting (23). Because of the large scatter of the data in Fig. 1, it is impossible to determine whether a plateau for D_L is attained. The existence of a plateau would represent an important indicator for characterizing the maximum capacity of the lungs for diffusive gas exchange across the gas–blood barrier.

Meyer et al. (24) determined rebreathing $D_{L_{CO}}$ and $D_{L_{O_2}}$ from alveolar–mixed-venous equilibration kinetics of $C^{18}O$ and $^{18}O_2$. Relatively high resting D_L values were found ($\sim$50 ml·min^{-1}·torr^{-1}), with only a minor rise of D_L with increasing exercise up to a $\dot{V}_{O_2}$ of $\sim$3 liters·min^{-1}. Whereas the drop of P_{aO_2} found in highly trained athletes at very heavy workloads (3) would be compatible with the leveling off of D_L, the question could be settled only by simultaneous measurements of P_{aO_2}, D_L, and $\dot{Q}$ during maximum exercise, which, to the authors' knowledge, have not been carried out. The ratio of D_L measured with $^{18}O_2$ and $C^{18}O$ by Meyer et al. (24) is, for both rest and exercise, $\sim$1.2 (i.e., close to the ratio of Krogh's diffusion constants K_{O_2}/K_{CO}). This value is compatible with the assumption that diffusion between the gas phase and hemoglobin (Hb) is the main resistive component of the O_2 transfer in the lung as opposed to the rate of reaction with Hb.

Recently, Borland and Higenbottam (25) measured single-breath pulmonary diffusing capacity in humans both at rest and at exercise using nitric oxide (NO). This gas combines with both reduced and oxidized Hb about 1400 times faster than does CO (26). $D_{L_{NO}}$ should therefore represent an index of the diffusing capacity of the alveolar–capillary membrane D_m ("extra erythrocyte" gas transfer). Resting $D_{L_{NO}}$ for three subjects was 160 ± 6.6 ml·min^{-1}·torr^{-1}, as compared with 36.7 ± 2.1 for $D_{L_{CO}}$ (i.e., the former was 4.3 times greater than the latter). At exercise ($\dot{V}_{O_2} = 2.6 \pm 0.1$ liter·min^{-1}), $D_{L_{NO}}$ and $D_{L_{CO}}$ were 209 ($+26\%$ compared to rest) and 58 ($+45\%$) ml·min^{-1}·torr^{-1}, respectively.

Resting $D_{L_{CO_2}}$ values as obtained by the single-breath technique with the stable isotope $^{13}CO_2$ are not significantly different from infinity (27). Measurements carried out by Piiper et al. (28) yielded values of 180 and 300 ml·min^{-1}·torr^{-1} at rest and at exercise (75 W), respectively. From these measurements, the investigators predict at heavy exercise a detectable $P_a CO_2-P_A CO_2$ gradient as a consequence of an equilibration deficit attributable to the relatively slow reaction rates of CO_2 in blood (see refs. 1 and 2), but this has not yet been reported to occur.

THE BREATHING CYCLE

Breath-by-breath (BB) methods allow the assessment of pulmonary gas transfer in the breathing cycle, thus greatly enhancing the temporal resolution of the measurements. They have therefore been fruitfully utilized to investigate the behavior of gas transfer at steady state as well as during the onset and offset of exercise.

Because of the large variability in pulmonary gas stores from one breath to the next, the BB gas transfer measured at the mouth may be considerably different from ''true'' alveolar gas exchange. To overcome this drawback, several groups of investigators have developed computational methods to correct for BB changes in pulmonary stores (29–32), all essentially derived from the original algorithm proposed by Auchincloss et al. (33). This is briefly summarized below.

The alveolar transfer of gas g during breath i (V_i^{galv}) can be calculated provided that the gas transfer at the mouth (V^{gm}) as well as the changes in pulmonary gas stores (ΔV^{gs}) during the same breath are known:

$$V_i^{galv} = V_i^{gm} - \Delta V_i^{gs} \quad [1]$$

The gas transfer at the mouth can be easily obtained by standard respiratory methods:

$$V_i^{gm} = (V_I F_I^g)_i - (V_E F_E^g)_i \quad [2]$$

where F_I^g and F_E^g are the inspiratory and expiratory gas fractions and where V_I and V_E are the corresponding volumes. At variance with V_i^{gm}, the changes of pulmonary gas stores during any given breath (ΔV_i^{gs}) cannot be directly assessed with presently available methods. In an attempt to estimate ΔV_i^{gs}, Auchincloss et al. (33) were the first to express ΔV_i^{gs} as the sum of two terms: (i) variation of alveolar fraction at constant volume and (ii) variation of volume at constant fraction. Whereas the latter term accounts for actual changes in end-expiratory volume, the former term applies whenever any changes in alveolar gas composition have occurred throughout the breath, even without changes in lung volume. If this is so, then

$$\Delta V_i^{gs} = V_{A(i-1)} \cdot (F_{A(i)}^g - F_{A(i-1)}^g) + F_{A(i)}^g \cdot (V_I - V_E)_i \quad [3]$$

where $V_{A(i-1)}$ is the end-expiratory volume at the beginning of breath i and where $F_{A(i)}^g$ and $F_{A(i-1)}^g$ are the

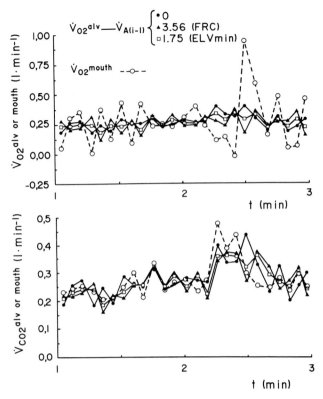

FIG. 2. Breath-by-breath O_2 consumption (*upper curve*) and CO_2 output (*lower curve*) at the mouth and at the alveolar level ($\dot{V}O_2$alv and $\dot{V}CO_2$alv) as a function of time in a sequence of 25 consecutive breaths at rest. $\dot{V}O_2$alv and $\dot{V}CO_2$alv were calculated according to Eq. 5, giving $V_{A(i-1)}$ the indicated values. (Adapted from ref. 35.)

alveolar fractions of gas g at the end and at the beginning of breath i. In turn, the changes of lung volume, ΔV_L, during the *i*th breath ($V_I - V_E)_i$ can be calculated from the nitrogen balance equation, assumed to hold on a BB basis (30,33):

$$\Delta V_{L(i)} = (V_I - V_E)_i = V^{m(i)}N_2 - [(F_{A(i)}N_2 - F_{A(i-1)}N_2 \cdot V_{A(i-1)}]/F_{A(i)}N_2 \quad [4]$$

Thus, as from Eqs. 1, 3, and 4, the complete algorithm for calculating BB alveolar gas exchange turns out to be

$$V_i^{galv} = \pm V_i^{gm} - [V_{A(i-1)} \cdot (F_{A(i)}^g - F_{A(i-1)}^g) + F_{A(i)}^g \cdot \Delta V_{L(i)}] \quad [5]$$

where the plus (+) or minus (−) sign depends on the direction of gas transfer with respect to the alveolar barrier.

In Eq. 5, the only quantity not directly measurable on a BB basis is $V_{A(i-1)}$. Auchincloss et al. (33), as well as others (29,31,32), assumed $V_{A(i-1)}$ to be constant and equal to the subject's functional residual capacity (FRC). Wessel et al. (29,34) proposed that the term containing $V_{A(i-1)}$ be omitted (i.e., they assumed that it was equal to zero) because of the smallness of

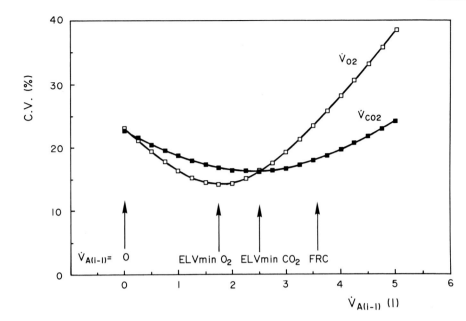

FIG. 3. Variability of $\dot{V}_{O_2}$alv and $\dot{V}_{CO_2}$alv [expressed as coefficient of variation (C.V., %)] as a function of $V_{A(i-1)}$ employed in calculations. Data refer to the same experiment reported in Fig. 2. (Adapted from ref. 35.)

the alveolar fraction differences between subsequent breaths. Swanson (30) introduced the concept of effective lung volume (ELV), to indicate the end-expiratory volume that "effectively" takes part in gas exchange. He also attempted to assign to $V_{A(i-1)}$ a value of ELV constant and equal to that which minimizes BB gas exchange variability throughout any single experiment (see Fig. 3). It goes without saying that such an ELV value can be obtained only by analyzing a series of breaths at steady state.

In a recent study, di Prampero and Lafortuna (35) calculated $\dot{V}_{O_2}$ and $\dot{V}_{CO_2}$ on a BB basis on six subjects at rest over sequences of 100 consecutive breaths both at the mouth and at the alveolar level, according to Eqs. 2 and 5 divided by the breathing period. $\dot{V}_{O_2}$alv and $\dot{V}_{CO_2}$alv were calculated, alternatively assigning to $V_{A(i-1)}$ in Eq. 5 the value of zero, ELVmin [as defined by Swanson (30)], and FRC, estimated from anthropometric data. In three subjects the resting period was followed by 10 min of constant-level (75 W) cycloergometric exercise. The results show that all three nominal values of $V_{A(i-1)}$ adopted for the calculations lead to a reduced BB variability in both $\dot{V}_{O_2}$alv and $\dot{V}_{CO_2}$alv when compared with the corresponding mouth values. The observed reduction of the BB variability of the alveolar gas transfer depends on the fact that $V_{A(i-1)}$ in Eq. 5 multiplies the difference $F^g_{A(i)} - F^g_{A(i-1)} = \Delta F^g_{A(i)}$. The latter, for a given constant alveolar gas exchange, can be positive or negative, depending on the difference in ventilation between subsequent breaths. It follows that $V_{A(i-1)} \cdot F^g_{A(i)}$ becomes a positive or negative term whose amplitude is determined by the nominal value given to $V_{A(i-1)}$. If the value attributed to $V_{A(i-1)}$ is too small (e.g., equals 0), the correction for the

changes in pulmonary stores is also too small. On the contrary, when the value given to $V_{A(i-1)}$ is too large (e.g., FRC or greater), the fluctuations observed at the mouth are overcompensated (see Figs. 2 and 3). Because of the greater solubility and smaller absolute alveolar fractions for CO_2, the effects in the estimate of $\dot{V}_{CO_2}$alv are less marked than for $\dot{V}_{O_2}$alv.

Despite the effects of alveolar gas transfer on BB variability, the nominal value of $V_{A(i-1)}$ employed in the calculations does not affect to any significant extent the average $\dot{V}_{O_2}$ and $\dot{V}_{CO_2}$ calculated over sequences of 100 breaths at rest and during cycloergometric steady-state exercise at 75 W.

In view of the above considerations, it seems legitimate to conclude that the adoption of the nominal values of $V_{A(i-1)}$ proposed in the literature to estimate BB alveolar gas transfer entails arbitrary assumptions.

Finally, experimental and modeling evidence (36,37) has shown that gas mixing—and hence the time course of fractional gas concentration in expired air measured at the mouth—is influenced by respiratory parameters such as tidal volume and ventilation. Thus, for a given alveolar mean fraction, different end-tidal fractions can be achieved, as a function of the respiratory pattern. Conversely, different effective alveolar volumes could match the same end-tidal fraction, depending on the respiratory pattern. Thus the "true values" of $V_{A(i-1)}$ and $F^g_{A(i)}$ do seem to affect each other via the respiratory pattern in a rather complicated manner.

THE UNSTEADY STATE

The kinetics of gas exchange during metabolic transients reflects the integrated responses of (a) the energetic events taking place at the muscle level, (b) the dynamics of the circulatory responses, and (c) the utilization of the gas stores of the body. It is therefore understandable that the study of gas-exchange kinetics in various conditions of work transients has long attracted the interest of physiologists working in different fields.

Because of their good time resolution, BB methods have been widely utilized for assessing the time course of gas-exchange transients. On the basis of the results obtained with these methods, several investigators have developed mathematical models describing in detail the gas-exchange kinetics during work transients (see ref. 1 for review). However, in view of the preceding discussion, the physiologic meaning of these mathematical descriptions seems questionable. Indeed, di Prampero and Lafortuna (35) have shown that the value of $V_{A(i-1)}$ utilized in the calculations (see Eq. 5) can affect by up to three breaths ($\sim$10 sec) the time at which an increase of alveolar $\dot{V}_{O_2}$ is detected upon work onset. Contrary to the delay time, however, the half-time of the alveolar gas-exchange kinetics does not seem to be greatly affected by the value of $V_{A(i-1)}$ used in the calculations. Thus, whereas the $\dot{V}_{O_2}$ kinetics an be considered a reasonable description of the underlying physiologic events, the presence and meaning of initial time delays or cardiodynamic phases should be taken with caution, as being more prone to computational artifacts.

It is therefore unfortunate that the precise assessment of the alveolar gas transients as the onset and offset of exercise will remain elusive as long as the conceptual and practical difficulties concerning the algorithm for BB alveolar gas-exchange measurement is not solved.

THE O$_2$ DEBT–DEFICIT

Even if the precise analysis of the alveolar $\dot{V}_{O_2}$ kinetics at the onset and offset of exercise still remains an unsolved problem, its description seems accurate enough to allow calculating the O$_2$ debt–deficit at the work offset–onset. The present section is devoted to a brief description of the above problem, with the interested reader being referred to the appropriate specific literature (see ref. 1 for review).

During metabolic transients, the actual O$_2$ uptake at any time t ($\dot{V}_t O_2$) lags behind the actual O$_2$ requirement, with this last variable being defined as the $\dot{V}_{O_2}$ that would be attained at steady state for the work intensity prevailing at time t ($\dot{V}_s O_2$).

The O$_2$ debt–deficit is the time integral of the difference between O$_2$ requirement and O$_2$ uptake:

$$O_2 \text{ debt–deficit} = \int (\dot{V}_s O_2 - \dot{V}_t O_2) \, dt \quad [6]$$

The O$_2$ deficit incurred at the onset of exercise has a positive sign, whereas the O$_2$ debt paid after the end of the exercise is negative.

In the case of square-wave aerobic exercise changes, and assuming a monoexponential $\dot{V}_{O_2}$ kinetics, we obtain

$$\dot{V}_s O_2 - \dot{V}_t O_2 = \dot{V}_s O_2 e^{-kt} \quad [7]$$

Hence

$$O_2 \text{ debt–deficit} = \int \dot{V}_s O_2 e^{-kt} \, dt = \dot{V}_s O_2/k \quad [8]$$

Regardless of the detailed shape of the $\dot{V}_{O_2}$ kinetics at work onset, the $\dot{V}_{O_2}$ response can be appropriately described by a "mean" half-time (or time constant). This is defined as the half-time which, given the time course of $\dot{V}_s O_2$ in question and assuming a monoexponential $\dot{V}_{O_2}$ kinetics, would lead to the same O$_2$ debt–deficit as calculated from the empirical function (Eq. 6).

The energy requirement of the working muscles can be assumed to be proportional to $\dot{V}_s O_2$. Hence the O$_2$ deficit is a measure of the energy drawn from sources other than those due to O$_2$ absorption through the upper airways [i.e., phosphocreatine (PC) breakdown, lactate production, and depletion of body O$_2$ stores (see ref. 1)]:

$$O_2 \text{ deficit} = V_{PC O_2} + V_{eLa O_2} + \Delta V_{st O_2} \quad [9]$$

where $V_{PC O_2}$ is the O$_2$ equivalent of the net PC breakdown, $V_{eLa O_2}$ is the net amount of lactate produced before the attainment of the steady state (expressed in O$_2$ equivalents), and $\Delta V_{st O_2}$ is the amount of O$_2$ drawn from the body stores.

At the offset of exercise, PC is resynthesized and $\Delta V_{st O_2}$ rebuilt at the expense of the extra O$_2$ consumed above resting without, however, any significant lactate production. Therefore the O$_2$ debt is the sum of only two of the three terms of Eq. 9:

$$O_2 \text{ debt} = V_{PC O_2} + \Delta V_{st O_2} \quad [10]$$

It appears from Eq. 9 that the O$_2$ deficit—and hence the $\dot{V}_{O_2}$ kinetics at the onset of exercise—depends, other things being equal, on the relative contribution of PC breakdown, early lactate production, and depletion of body O$_2$ stores. Whereas PC breakdown is presumably set by the intrinsic characteristics of the muscle, the latter two terms depend to a large extent on the exercise type and mode, as well as on the training conditions of the subject. Indeed, di Prampero et al. (38) have shown that, for a given square-wave exercise intensity change, the $\dot{V}_{O_2}$ kinetics is faster, and the O$_2$ deficit correspondingly smaller, during stepping than during cycling exercise at high work loads (see Table 1). The slower $\dot{V}_{O_2}$ kinetics and larger O$_2$ deficit in cycling are associated with a larger production of lactate during the transition phase. On the contrary, the $\dot{V}_{O_2}$ kinetics during the recovery following exercise

TABLE 1. *Average "mean" half-times* $t_{1/2}$ *of* $\dot{V}_{O_2}$ *kinetics during square-wave exercise intensity changes from rest to 20% or 40% $\dot{V}_{O_2}$max, from 20% to 40% $\dot{V}_{O_2}$max, and from >25% to 85% $\dot{V}_{O_2}$max during stepping and during cycling[a]*

Condition	Stepping [$t_{1/2}$, sec ($\pm$SD)]	Cycling [$t_{1/2}$, sec ($\pm$SD)]
Rest → 20%	25.4 ($\pm$8.6)	16.1 ($\pm$6.1)
Rest → 40%	31.1 ($\pm$10.1)	29.6 ($\pm$7.9)
20% → 40%	15.6 ($\pm$4.8)	36.0 ($\pm$14.0)
>25% → 85%	35.4 ($\pm$6.3)	49.0 ($\pm$9.6)

[a] Individual "mean" half-times were calculated dividing the measured O_2 deficit by the corresponding $\dot{V}_{O_2}$ amplitude change. (From ref. 38.)

was essentially the same, with the half-times amounting to 20.8 ($\pm$ 5.8) and 22.3 ($\pm$ 6.7) sec in stepping and cycling, respectively.

The above results, together with Eqs. 9 and 10, provide a clue to a comprehensive interpretation of most results obtained by various investigators concerning the $\dot{V}_{O_2}$ kinetics in different experimental situations which so far have led to controversial interpretation. The following examples seem particularly relevant to this discussion (see ref. 38 for details and references): (i) The supine posture, by raising cardiac output and mixed venous blood O_2 content, ultimately leads to an increase of the size of the O_2 stores of the body. Hence the $\dot{V}_{O_2}$ kinetics in the supine posture should be slowed down, as shown experimentally. (ii) Arm exercise is characterized by a greater involvement of glycolytic fibers and, hence, by a larger lactic acid contribution to energy requirement. Thus the $\dot{V}_{O_2}$ kinetics should be slowed down, as experimentally found. (iii) Endurance training, by increasing the fraction of oxidative muscle fibers and improving muscle perfusion, should lead to faster $\dot{V}_{O_2}$ kinetics, as shown experimentally.

Over the last several decades, the extensive literature on the study of gas exchange in the lungs has been mainly concerned with resting humans and/or animals. Steady-state exercise has only occasionally represented a means to stress the cardiopulmonary function in order to enable us to explore the limits and the functional reserve of some of its components. As is well known, most emphasis was put on the following: the mechanics of the ventilatory pump and of the pleural space; the regulation of the airway resistance; the adaptation of the myocardial performance; and, mainly, the characteristics of gas exchange. The patter may undergo remarkable changes when the capillary blood volume is increased, the alveolar–capillary barrier becomes wider and thinner and the distributions of both lung ventilation and perfusion and of their ratio are greatly altered.

Last but not least, the functional condition of un-

steady state has now made its appearance. The results of some preliminary work indicate that this transient or "dynamic" functional phase can be of paramount importance not only for the analysis of anaerobic metabolism but also for the study of gas exchange. In fact, the different time course of the readjustment of its various determinants upon a given metabolic stress may become a useful tool to gain some new insight into their specific role. Together with the study of gas exchange at the tissue level, this seems to represent an interesting development of research in respiratory physiology.

REFERENCES

1. Cerretelli P, di Prampero PE. Gas exchange in exercise. In: Fachi LE, Tenney SM, eds. *Handbook of physiology, Section 3: The respiratory system, vol IV—Gas exchange.* Bethesda, MD: American Physiological Society, 1987;297–339.
2. Hammond MD, Gale GE, Kapitan KS, Ries A, Wagner PD. Pulmonary gas exchange in humans during exercise at sea level. *J Appl Physiol* 1986;60:1590–1598.
3. Dempsey JA, Hanson PG, Henderson KS. Exercise-induced arterial hypoxaemia in healthy human subjects at sea level. *J Physiol* 1984;355:161–175.
4. Hartley LH, Grimby G, Kilbom A, et al. Physical training in sedentary middle-aged and older man. III. Cardiac output and gas exchange at submaximal and maximal exercise. *Scand J Clin Lab Invest* 1969;24:335–344.
5. Bachofen HH, Hobi HJ, Scherrer M. Alveolar–arterial N_2 gradients at rest and during exercise in healthy men of different ages. *J Appl Physiol* 1973;34:137–142.
6. Holland J. Milic-Emili J, Macklem PT, Bates DV. Regional distribution of pulmonary ventilation and perfusion in elderly subjects. *J Clin Invest* 1968;47:81–92.
7. Piiper J. Variations of ventilation and diffusing capacity to perfusion determining the alveolar–arterial O_2 difference: theory. *J Appl Physiol* 1961;16:507–510.
8. Scheid P, Piiper J. Blood/gas equilibrium of carbon dioxide in lungs. A critical review. *Respir Physiol* 1980;39:1–31.
9. Gurtner GH. Can alveolar P_{CO_2} exceed pulmonary end-capillary CO_2? Yes. *J Appl Physiol* 1977;42:323–328.
10. Lilienthal JL Jr, Riley RL, Proemmel DD, Franke RE. An experimental analysis in man of the oxygen pressure gradient from alveolar air to arterial blood during rest and exercise at sea level and at altitude. *Am J Physiol* 1946;147:199–216.
11. Asmussen E, Nielsen M. Alveolo-arterial gas exchange at rest and during work at different O_2 tensions. *Acta Physiol Scand* 1960;50:153–166.
12. Staub NC. Alveolar–arterial oxygen tension gradient due to diffusion. *J Appl Physiol* 1963;18:673–680.
13. West JB, Wagner PD. Predicted gas exchange on the summit of Mt. Everest. *Respir Physiol* 1980;42:1–16.
14. Wagner PD. Influence of mixed venous P_{O_2} on diffusion of O_2 across the pulmonary blood: gas barrier. *Clin Physiol* 1982;2:105–115.
15. Piiper J, Scheid P. Blood-gas equilibrium in lungs. In: West JB, ed. *Pulmonary gas exchange. Ventilation, blood flow, and diffusion,* vol 1. New York: Academic Press, 1980;131–171.
16. Torre-Bueno JR, Wagner PD, Saltzman HA, Gale GE, Moon RE. Diffusion limitation in normal humans during exercise at sea level and simulated altitude. *J Appl Physiol* 1985;58:989–995.
17. Wagner PD, Gillespie JR, Landgren GL, et al. Mechanism of exercise-induced hypoxemia in horses. *J Appl Physiol* 1989;66:1227–1233.
18. Bake B, Bjure J, Widimsky J. The effect of sitting and graded exercise on the distribution of pulmonary blood flow in healthy

subjects studied with the [133]xenon technique. *Scand J Clin Lab Invest* 1968;22:99–106.

19. Wagner PD, Laravuso RB, Uhl RR, West JB. Continuous distributions of ventilation–perfusion ratios in normal subjects breathing air and 100% O_2. *J Clin Invest* 1974;54:54–68.

20. Wagner PD, Saltzman HA, West JB. Measurement of continuous distributions of ventilation–perfusion ratios: theory. *J Appl Physiol* 1974;36:588–599.

21. Gale GE, Torre-Bueno JR, Moon RE, Saltzman RA, Wagner PD. Ventilation–perfusion inequality in normal humans during exercise at sea level and simulated altitude. *J Appl Physiol* 1985;58:978–988.

22. Gledhill N, Froese AB, Buick FJ, Bryan AC. $\dot{V}_A/\dot{Q}$ inhomogeneity and A–a Do_2 in man during exercise: effect of SF_6 breathing. *J Appl Physiol* 1978;45:512–515.

23. Piiper J. Apparent increase of the O_2 diffusing capacity with increased O_2 uptake in inhomogeneous lungs: theory. *Respir Physiol* 1969;6:209–218.

24. Meyer M, Scheid P, Riepl G, Wagner H-J, Piiper J. Pulmonary diffusing capacities for O_2 and CO measured by a rebreathing technique. *J Appl Physiol* 1981;51:1643–1650.

25. Borland CDR, Higenbottam TW. A simultaneous single breath measurement of pulmonary diffusing capacity with nitric oxide and carbon monoxide. *Eur Respir J* 1989;2:56–63.

26. Guenard H, Varene N, Vaida P. Determination of lung capillary blood volume and membrane diffusing capacity in man by the measurements of NO and CO transfer. *Respir Physiol* 1987;70:113–120.

27. Hyde RW, Puy RJM, Raub WF, Forster RE. Rate of disappearance of labelled carbon dioxide from the lungs of humans during breath holding: a method for studying the dynamics of pulmonary CO_2 exchange. *J Clin Invest* 1968;47:1535–1552.

28. Piiper J, Meyer M, Marconi C, Scheid P. Alveolar–capillary equilibration kinetics of [13]CO_2 in human lungs studied by rebreathing. *Respir Physiol* 1980;42:29–41.

29. Wessel HU, Stout RL, Paul MH. Breath-by-breath determination of alveolar gas exchange [Letter to the editor; with a reply by K. Wasserman]. *J Appl Physiol* 1983;54:598–599.

30. Swanson GD. Breath-to-breath considerations for gas exchange kinetics. In: Cerretelli P, Whipp BJ, eds. *Exercise bioenergetics and gas exchange*. Amsterdam: Elsevier/North-Holland, 1980;211–222.

31. Beaver WL, Lamarra N, Wasserman K. Breath-by-breath measurement of true alveolar gas exchange. *J Appl Physiol* 1981; 51:1662–1675.

32. Giezendanner D, Cerretelli P, di Prampero PE. Breath-by-breath alveolar gas exchange. *J Appl Physiol* 1983;55:583–590.

33. Auchincloss JH Jr, Gilbert R, Baule GH. Effect of ventilation on oxygen transfer during early exercise. *J Appl Physiol* 1966;21:810–818.

34. Wessel HU, Stout RL, Bastanier CK, Paul MH. Breath-by-breath variation of FRC: effect on $\dot{V}o_2$ and $\dot{V}co_2$ measured at the mouth. *J Appl Physiol* 1979;46:1122–1126.

35. di Prampero PE, Lafortuna CL. Breath-by-breath estimate of alveolar gas transfer variability in man at rest and during exercise. *J Physiol* 1989;415:459–475.

36. Meyer M, Hook C, Rieke H, Piiper J. Gas mixing in dog lungs studied by single-breath washout of He and SF_6. *J Appl Physiol* 1983;55:1795–1802.

37. Paiva M, Engel LA. Theoretical studies of gas mixing and ventilation distribution in the lung. *Physiol Rev* 1987;67:750–796.

38. di Prampero PE, Mahler PB, Giezendanner D, Cerretelli P. Effects of priming exercise on $\dot{V}o_2$ kinetics and O_2 deficit at the onset of stepping and cycling. *J Appl Physiol* 1989;66:2023–2031.

THE LUNG: *Scientific Foundations*
edited by R.G. Crystal, J.B. West et al.
Raven Press, Ltd., New York © 1991.

CHAPTER 5.6.2.2

Blood-Gas Transport and Acid–Base Regulation

Brian J. Whipp and Karlman Wasserman

The regulation of arterial blood-gas partial pressures (P_aCO_2, P_aO_2) during exercise requires a balance between pulmonary and tissue gas exchange. The regulation of arterial pH requires a balance between the total acid production (chiefly in the form of hydrated CO_2 and organic acids such as lactic, pyruvic, aceto-acetic and β-hydroxybutyric) and utilization, ion translocations between muscle and blood, and the rate of pulmonary CO_2 clearance.

These regulatory processes can be complicated, however, by the competing demands for pulmonary gas exchange under the following circumstances: (a) when O_2 uptake ($\dot{V}O_2$) and CO_2 output ($\dot{V}CO_2$) are markedly different, such as with different substrate utilization patterns or during nonsteady states of altered metabolic rate, and (b) when the CO_2 clearance requirements for maintaining P_aCO_2 differ from that for pH_a regulation. These differences are apparent in the following steady-state relationships:

$$P_{AO_2} = P_{IO_2} \cdot \left[\frac{P_{AN_2}}{P_{IN_2}} \right] - 863 \cdot \frac{\dot{V}O_2}{\dot{V}_A} \quad [1]$$

And as

$$R = \frac{\dot{V}CO_2}{\dot{V}O_2} \quad [2]$$

$$P_{AO_2} = P_{IO_2} \cdot \left[\frac{P_{AN_2}}{P_{IN_2}} \right] - \frac{P_{ACO_2}}{R} \quad [3]$$

$$P_{ACO_2} = 863 \cdot \frac{\dot{V}CO_2}{\dot{V}_A} \quad [4]$$

$$pH_a = pK' + \log \frac{[HCO_3^-]_a}{25.6} \cdot \frac{\dot{V}_A}{\dot{V}CO_2} \quad [5]$$

B. J. Whipp: Department of Physiology, UCLA School of Medicine, Los Angeles, California 90024.

K. Wasserman: Division of Respiratory and Critical Care Physiology and Medicine, Harbor–UCLA Medical Center, Torrance, California 90509.

where: P_{AO_2}, P_{ACO_2}, and P_{AN_2} represent alveolar PO_2, PCO_2, and PN_2, respectively; P_{IO_2} and P_{IN_2} represent inspired PO_2 and PN_2, respectively; $\dot{V}_A$ is alveolar ventilation; pH_a is arterial pH; and $[HCO_3^-]_a$ is the arterial bicarbonate concentration. Consequently, as shown in Eq. 5, arterial pH regulation is inextricably linked to the coupling between ventilation and CO_2 as well as to factors that alter $[HCO_3^-]_a$ (Fig. 1).

As shown in Eqs. 1 and 3, P_{ACO_2} and P_{AO_2} depend upon $\dot{V}CO_2/\dot{V}_A$ and $\dot{V}O_2/\dot{V}_A$, respectively. Because $\dot{V}_A$ has been demonstrated to change in proportion to $\dot{V}CO_2$ as RQ (the average tissue gas-exchange ratio, i.e., $\dot{Q}CO_2/\dot{Q}O_2$) and R (the pulmonary gas-exchange ratio, i.e., $\dot{V}CO_2/\dot{V}O_2$) change, P_{ACO_2} (and hence P_aCO_2) will be regulated; the necessary consequence is that P_{AO_2} (and hence P_aO_2) will decrease as RQ decreases and will increase as RQ increases. These changes are normally of little physiologic significance because, at a P_{ACO_2} of 40 mmHg, P_{AO_2} will only vary by ~10 mmHg as RQ changes with the typical exercise range of ~0.8 to 1.0. When a subject is already hypoxemic (e.g., during a sojourn at high altitude or as a consequence of lung disease), these differences in P_{AO_2} resulting from RQ changes can be more important.

As shown in Eq. 4, P_{ACO_2} can only be regulated at a particular set-point level if $\dot{V}_A$ changes in proportion to $\dot{V}CO_2$. Whether this change in $\dot{V}_A$ is also adequate to maintain P_{AO_2} depends upon the current level of R (Eq. 3); whether it is adequate to maintain pH_a depends upon the current level of $[HCO_3^-]_a$ (Eq. 5).

We shall therefore consider acid–base regulation during exercise within the framework schematized in Fig. 1. We shall also distinguish between two intensity domains: (a) *moderate*, where $[HCO_3^-]_a$ is unchanged because there is no sustained increase in organic acid concentration, and (b) *heavy*, in which $[HCO_3^-]_a$ is reduced as a result of the buffering of the increased concentrations of the organic acids, of which lactic acid is the proportionally dominant component.

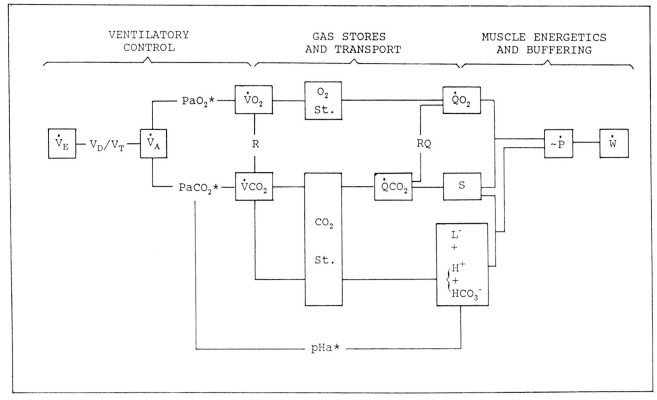

VENTILATORY
CONTROL

GAS STORES
AND TRANSPORT

MUSCLE ENERGETICS
AND BUFFERING

FIG. 1. Schematic representation of physiologic determinants of blood-gas and acid–base regulation. $\dot{W}$ represents the muscular power generation (i.e., work/time); $\sim\dot{P}$ is the high-energy-phosphate utilization rate. Other symbols are standard. The regulated variables are denoted by asterisks.

MODERATE EXERCISE

Steady State

Gas exchange in skeletal muscle during exercise is linked to the mechanisms that furnish the energy for force generation and work. This is provided by the free energy of hydrolysis of the terminal phosphate bond(s) of adenosine triphosphate (ATP). And although the intramuscular concentration of ATP is low ($\sim$5 mM/kg wet wt), its concentration does not change appreciably until near-maximal work rates. For moderate exercise, ATP is regenerated from two distinct, but related, processes.

The first is the decrease in cellular creatine phosphate (CP) concentration, that is,

$$\text{CP} + \text{ADP} \longrightarrow \text{ATP} + \text{C} \qquad [6]$$

This reaction is catalyzed by the enzyme creatine kinase and has an equilibrium constant of $\sim$100. This predicts that the intramuscular ATP concentration will be maintained within 10% of its resting value, even at work rates at which [CP] will have decreased by 90%.

Although this CP reaction does not directly involve O_2 and CO_2 exchange, it serves as a control link (1,2)

to intramitochondrial O_2 uptake ($\dot{Q}O_2$), with the increase in $\dot{Q}O_2$ being proportionally coupled to the decrease in [CP]. In contrast, there appears to be no such direct control link to $\dot{Q}CO_2$; this appears to be dependent upon the $\dot{Q}O_2$ and the metabolic substrate (Fig. 1). Another relevant feature of this creatine kinase reaction is that when CP "donates" its P to ADP, the resulting ATP formation fixes an H^+ ion (3). Consequently, the reaction induces (a) a transient alkalinity when [CP] is decreasing, as in the on-transient of exercise, and (b) an acidity early in recovery as CP is resynthesized. But, as discussed below, the actual intramuscular acid–base changes depend upon other, more dominant mechanisms that occur at the same time.

The second mechanism of ATP regeneration is oxidative phosphorylation. The demands for O_2 utilization depend upon both the ATP turnover rate and the substrate mixture being catabolized. That is, for a given rate of ATP production, both the O_2 cost and the CO_2 yield differ markedly when carbohydrate is the dominant substrate than when lipids are utilized (see Table 1); catabolism of protein is normally quantitatively insignificant. Although from a thermodynamic standpoint, carbohydrate and fatty acid oxidation are

TABLE 1. *Gas-exchange consequences of substrate oxidation*

	RQ	$\dot{V}_{O_2}{}^a$ (liters·min^{-1})	$\dot{V}_{CO_2}$ (liters·min^{-1})	~P:O$_2$	~P:CO$_2$	O$_2$:~P	CO$_2$:~P
Glycogen (G):	1.0	1.0	1.0	6.00	6.00	0.17	0.17
Palmitate (P):	0.7	1.0	0.7	5.65	8.13	0.18	0.12
G/P:	1.43	1.0	1.43	1.06	0.89	0.94	1.42

[a] Values at a particular $\dot{V}_{O_2}$. For a particular work rate or high-energy-phosphate utilization rate, less is needed when glycogen is the substrate than when palmitate is utilized.

virtually equally efficient in conserving free energy in the form of high-energy phosphate (e.g., see ref. 4), carbohydrate may be considered to be more efficient at generating energy compared with fatty acid oxidation when O$_2$ utilization is the frame of reference. But with respect to CO$_2$ production, it is less efficient.

In the steady state of moderate-intensity exercise, therefore, $\dot{V}_A$ normally increases as a linear function of $\dot{V}_{CO_2}$ (5), with a slope of 21.5 at a $P_a\text{CO}_2$ of 40 mmHg; $P_a\text{CO}_2$ is consequently regulated at, or close to, its resting value. Some subjects, however, hyperventilate when they initially breathe through a mouthpiece, and they subsequently return to their regulated level of $P_a\text{CO}_2$ as they exercise; this can be easily misinterpreted as CO$_2$ retention.

Minute ventilation ($\dot{V}_E$) also increases as a linear function of $\dot{V}_{CO_2}$ at this intensity (5–7), but with a slope of approximately 25 and an intercept on the $\dot{V}_E$ axis of about 3 liters/min. This linearity of $\dot{V}_E$ as a function of $\dot{V}_{CO_2}$ (with set-point regulation of $P_a\text{CO}_2$) can only be achieved by the physiologic dead-space fraction of the tidal volume (V_D/V_T) decreasing hyperbolically as work rate is increased (7). Subjects who regulate their $P_a\text{CO}_2$ at lower levels and/or have a high V_D/V_T require appreciably greater increases of $\dot{V}_E$ to effect regulation of $P_a\text{CO}_2$. End-expiratory (end-tidal) $P\text{CO}_2$ ($P_{ET}\text{CO}_2$) should not be used as a direct estimator of $P_a\text{CO}_2$ during exercise, even in normal subjects (6,8,9), since the accelerated rates of alveolar gas exchange (which result from the increased mixed venous $P\text{CO}_2$ and pulmonary blood flow) steepen the alveolar phase of the expired $P\text{CO}_2$ profile. The single-point sample (end-tidal) can therefore exceed the mean level of $P_A\text{CO}_2$ or $P_a\text{CO}_2$ by up to 8 mmHg (8). In normal subjects, however, it is possible to derive both the flow-weighted and the time-averaged $P_{\bar{a}}\text{CO}_2$ as a close estimation of $P_a\text{CO}_2$ during exercise (see ref. 8 for discussion) or to use an empirical equation using V_T and $P_{ET}\text{CO}_2$ derived by Jones et al. (9).

Although both $P_a\text{CO}_2$ and $P_a\text{O}_2$ normally change little in moderate steady-state exercise, the mixed venous concentrations of these gases change appreciably. It has been repeatedly demonstrated that cardiac output ($\dot{Q}$) is linearly related to $\dot{V}_{O_2}$ over a wide range of work rates in normal subjects, but with a positive $\dot{Q}$-inter-

cept of about 5 liters/min and a slope of approximately 5–6; that is,

$$\dot{Q} \text{ (liters/min)} \simeq 5 \times \dot{V}_{O_2} \text{ (liters/min)} + 5 \text{ (liters/min)}$$

or

$$\dot{V}_{O_2} \text{ (liters/min)} \simeq 0.2 \times \dot{Q} \text{ (liters/min)} - 1 \text{ (liter/min)}$$

[7]

This relationship both predicts and accounts for the pattern of change of the mixed venous O$_2$ content ($C_{\bar{v}}O_2$) over this range of work rates; that is,

$$\dot{Q}(C_aO_2 - C_{\bar{v}}O_2) \simeq 0.2\dot{Q} - 1$$

yielding

$$C_aO_2 - C_{\bar{v}}O_2 \simeq 0.2 - \frac{1}{\dot{Q}} \qquad [8]$$

Consequently, the body's arteriovenous difference for O$_2$ increases hyperbolically with increasing work rate, as though to asymptote at the resting arterial O$_2$ content of ~200 ml/liter (although this normally increases slightly during exercise as a result of hemoconcentration). The actual maximum value of $(C_aO_2 - C_{\bar{v}}O_2)$ attained, of course, depends upon the subject's ability to increase $\dot{V}_{O_2}$ and $\dot{Q}$.

It has been reported that the increase in $\dot{Q}$ and the decrease in $C_{\bar{v}}O_2$ ($\Delta C_{\bar{v}}O_2$) tend to offset one another, such that their product (i.e., the vascular O$_2$ flux *into* the lung) is constant during exercise (10). Consequently, $\dot{V}_{O_2}$ must increase in proportion to the vascular O$_2$ flux out of the lung. And because C_aO_2 does not change appreciably at these work rates, the $\dot{V}_{O_2}$ must increase as a direct function of flow *per se* (i.e., $\dot{Q}$).

The amount of "stored O$_2$" used for oxidative phosphorylation during the nonsteady state becomes proportionally reduced as the work rate increases; that is,

Volume of venous blood O$_2$ stores utilized

$$= \Delta C_{\bar{v}}O_2 \cdot V_v \quad [9]$$

where V_v is the effective venous blood volume. By the same reasoning, however, the increase in venous CO$_2$ stores is given by

Volume increase of venous blood CO$_2$ stores

$$= \Delta C_{\bar{v}}\text{CO}_2 \cdot V_v \quad [10]$$

Consequently, the increase in the CO_2 stores only exceeds the decrease in the O_2 stores by the increase in *RQ*.

These steady-state changes explain the amounts of venous blood gas stores that contribute to the apparent deficits in O_2 utilization and CO_2 output at exercise onset; they do not provide information with respect to the patterns of contribution in the nonsteady state.

Nonsteady State

$\dot{Q}O_2$ in skeletal muscle during exercise is controlled by the energy-transferring reactions of the intramuscular "high-energy" phosphate pool (excellent critical analyses of this topic may be found in refs. 1 and 2).

Although there are no direct experimental data showing that the time course of skeletal-muscle $\dot{Q}O_2$ in humans is monoexponential, the pattern of change in [CP] in human muscle (estimated both by ^{31}P nuclear magnetic resonance spectroscopy and by muscle biopsy techniques), along with the coupled exponentiality of the [CP] and $\dot{Q}O_2$ changes in isolated and *in situ* skeletal muscles of other animal species (see refs. 1,2, and 11), makes it highly probable during moderate exercise.

The O_2 concentration in the venous effluent from the contracting muscle ($C_{v(m)}O_2$) will therefore be determined by the ratio of the change in $\dot{Q}O_2$ and the muscle blood flow ($\dot{Q}_m$):

$$C_{v(m)}O_2 = C_aO_2 - (\dot{Q}O_2/\dot{Q}_m) \qquad [11]$$

The increase in $\dot{Q}_m$ will differ only from the increase in the total cardiac output (assumed here to equal the pulmonary blood flow, $\dot{Q}_p$) as a result of (a) the changes in the mean blood flow in the remainder of the body (thought to be small at these work rates) and (b) any changes in the volume of the intervening venous pool. In contrast, the influence of the altered $C_{v(m)}O_2$ on $C_{\bar{v}}O_2$ will be delayed by the transit delay to the pulmonary capillary bed. Consequently, a simple monoexponential increase in $\dot{Q}O_2$ will be transformed into a more complex pattern of change in $\dot{V}O_2$. That is, during the nonsteady-state phase between rest and exercise, there will be an initial gas-exchange phase ("phase 1" or $\phi 1$) which is dominated by changes in $\dot{Q}_p$ and a subsequent phase ("phase 2," or $\phi 2$) in which the altered $C_{v(m)}O_2$ supplements the pulmonary gas exchange.

The notion that pulmonary gas exchange in $\phi 1$ is cardiodynamically mediated is supported by the following findings: (a) There are rapid and proportional increases in both $\dot{Q}_p$ and $\dot{V}O_2$ during $\phi 1$ of exercise in humans (see ref. 12); (b) $\dot{V}O_2$ increases rapidly even when $\dot{V}_E$ is constrained at resting levels at the start of work (13); (c) when the rapid increase of the stroke

volume (SV) is reduced (i.e., either by beginning exercise in the supine posture or from unloaded cycling), the $\phi 1$ increase in $\dot{V}O_2$ is markedly slower (14,15); (d) the surreptitious increase in cardiac output as a result of the paced heart rate in patients with implanted pacemakers at rest and at exercise onset leads to increases in $\dot{V}O_2$ (16); and (e) when the $\phi 1$ increase in $\dot{Q}_p$ is attenuated in certain cardiac and pulmonary diseases, there is also a reduction in the magnitude of the $\phi 1$ $\dot{V}O_2$ response (16–18).

The onset of $\phi 2$ is reflected by: (a) both $\dot{V}O_2$ and $\dot{V}CO_2$ beginning to increase more rapidly (15); (b) the slope of the alveolar PCO_2 and PO_2 profiles steepening, as a result of the increased $P_{\bar{v}}CO_2$ and the decreased $P_{\bar{v}}O_2$; and (c) $P_{ET}CO_2$ increasing and $P_{ET}O_2$ decreasing.

In addition, the $\phi 2$ $\dot{V}O_2$ increases monoexponentially to the steady state with a time constant of response (T) which is relatively independent of work rate (~ 30 sec in normal subjects: see ref. 15 for discussion). $T\dot{V}O_2$ can be appreciably longer under the following circumstances: (a) in patients with cardiorespiratory impairments (16–18); (b) for arm exercise in normal subjects (19), although this is likely to be largely the result of the high relative work rates employed; (c) when hypoxic inspirates are breathed (20); and (d) following beta-adrenergic blockade (21). It is shorter in highly fit or endurance-trained subjects (22).

$\dot{V}CO_2$ also increases monoexponentially during $\phi 2$, but with an appreciably longer time constant, of 50 sec or more (15). Consequently, R begins to *decrease* at the $\phi 1$–$\phi 2$ transition, before increasing until a $\dot{V}CO_2$ steady state is attained. The $\dot{V}CO_2$ kinetics reflect (a) the time course with which CO_2 is produced metabolically and (b) the storage of CO_2 in the exercising tissues (7,23). That is, the difference in $T\dot{V}O_2$ and $T\dot{V}CO_2$ is dominated by storage of CO_2 *within* the muscle. And because the $\phi 2$ $\dot{V}CO_2$ kinetics are as well fit by a simple exponential as are the $\dot{V}O_2$ kinetics, the pattern of cumulative storage in the muscle (V_mCO_2st) will be a sigmoid function of time, reaching a steady-state value of approximately

$$V_mCO_2\text{st} = \Delta\dot{V}_{SS}CO_2 \cdot (T\dot{V}CO_2 - T\dot{V}O_2) \qquad [12]$$

(i.e., ≈ 250 ml for a transition from unloaded cycling to 100 W).

During recovery, the blood-gas stores return to their prior control levels and the extra CO_2 stored in the muscle is discharged; the volume and time course of this discharge are not significantly different from those of the initial storage.

We would therefore predict that altering the tissue CO_2 capacitance should alter $\dot{V}CO_2$ kinetics predictably. This is, in fact, the case. When the prior control phase is light exercise, muscle-tissue PCO_2 will be increased and the slope of the CO_2 dissociation curve will be shallower. This should result in the kinetics of

CO_2 output *from* the working muscle being closer to those of its production rate *within* the muscle. Both $T\dot{V}CO_2$ and $T\dot{V}_E$ are faster under these conditions, although $T\dot{V}O_2$ is not (23). Consequently, the undershoot of R during φ2 is reduced.

The resulting degree of mean alveolar and arterial blood-gas regulation will depend upon the pattern and magnitude of the concomitant ventilatory response. And although the mechanisms of ventilatory control are beyond the scope of this chapter, the characteristics of the control are fundamental to it.

The relative constancy of $P_{ET}CO_2$ and $P_{ET}O_2$ during φ1 suggests that the arterial blood will undergo a slight hyperventilation, reflecting the constant end-tidal value and a steeper expiratory alveolar slope in φ1 (24). Direct sampling of arterial blood has demonstrated that a small, transient φ1 hyperventilation is not uncommon (25,26).

In φ2, $\dot{V}_E$ has been shown to increase monoexponentially, using square-wave, impulse, and sinusoidal exercise (see refs. 12 and 27). Its time constant, however, is *slower* than that of $\dot{V}CO_2$, but only by approximately 10%. This close kinetic coupling means that P_aCO_2 and pH_a will be closely regulated during φ2. The predictably small transient CO_2 retention has, to date, been demonstrated only with averaging of several repetitions of a sinusoidally fluctuating work rate and for ramp-type exercise (7,28). But because $T\dot{V}O_2$ is only 50–60% of $T\dot{V}_E$, a transient hypoxemia in φ2 is predictable (Eq. 1) and has been reported (e.g., see ref. 29). It is also important to recognize that not only are the magnitudes of P_aCO_2 and P_aO_2 change different but so is the time at which the maximum change is attained. This has important implications for the timing of discrete blood samples.

The φ2 $\dot{V}_E$ time constant, both absolutely and relative to that of $\dot{V}CO_2$, changes in proportion to the magnitude of the peripheral chemoreceptor contribution to the hyperpnea (27,30,31). When the peripheral chemoreceptor contribution to $\dot{V}_E$ was varied from ~50% to zero (using inspired O_2 fractions that ranged from 12% to 100%, respectively), $T\dot{V}_E$ changed by fourfold (i.e., from <30 sec to ~2 min). This suggests an important role for the carotid bodies (the predominant ventilatory peripheral chemoreceptors in humans) in modulating φ2 $\dot{V}_E$ dynamics. The speeding of the $\dot{V}_E$ kinetics following a dietary-induced metabolic acidosis (31), along with the fact that $T\dot{V}_E$ was also prolonged following intravenous infusion of dopamine (32), provides further support for this concept. But perhaps the most decisive support for such a concept is provided by observations on subjects who had previously undergone bilateral carotid body resection. In these subjects, the time course of $\dot{V}_E$ was appreciably slower than for control subjects in response to square-wave exercise (33). This suggests that the carotid bodies in

humans play an important role in preventing significant further arterial hypoxemia during nonsteady states of increased metabolic rate in hypoxemic subjects, by tightening the coupling of ventilation to metabolic rate in φ2. And although this has not, to date, been systematically demonstrated with direct arterial blood sampling, the following observation is consistent with the concept: During the φ2 on-transient of exercise, the transient decrease in $P_{ET}O_2$ and the increase in $P_{ET}CO_2$ are markedly greater with hyperoxia and smaller with hypoxia (27,30).

HEAVY EXERCISE

At higher work rates, the control mechanisms that regulate arterial pH and blood-gas tensions are stressed further by the aerobic energy transfer being supplemented by anaerobic–glycolytic processes (i.e., those not utilizing O_2). This leads to a metabolic acidosis, of which the chief metabolic acid is lactic acid. Because lactic acid has an effective dissociation constant (at 25°C) of 1.36×10^{-4}, or a pK' of 3.86, only approximately one molecule per thousand will be in the undissociated form at a muscle cell pH of 6.86; the remainder will be present as lactate ions and hydrogen ions. In fact, the notion that glycolysis produces appreciable quantities of lactic acid which *then* dissociate into lactate and H^+ ions is incorrect; the dissociation is already manifest at the level of pyruvate production (actually from the first triose reaction). The consequent pH changes in the muscle cell and in blood will depend upon both intrinsic buffering mechanisms and H^+ removal.

Although a small transient increase in arterial blood lactate ($[lactate]_a$) can be discerned during the nonsteady-state phase of constant-load moderate exercise, a range of work rates exists during incremental exercise in which $[lactate]_a$ either is unchanged or reflects a small pyruvate-dependent increase (34). As work rate increases further, a demonstrably more rapid rate of increase of $[lactate]_a$ is evident (34) which is well described as a "tear-away" exponential function. The work rate—or, more properly, the $\dot{V}O_2$—at which this occurs may be termed the "lactate threshold." However, not only does $[lactate]_a$ begin to increase at a markedly faster rate at this threshold, but so does the $[lactate]_a/[pyruvate]_a$ ratio (Fig. 2). This threshold is also apparent in muscle [lactate], the muscle [lactate]/[pyruvate] ratio, and a more reduced muscle cellular redox state as evidenced by the (NADH + H^+)/NADH ratio (see refs. 3 and 35 for discussion); that is, the changes in lactate and pyruvate are intimately linked to those of the NAD/NADH redox couple:

$$\frac{[lactate^-]}{[pyruvate^-]} = K_{eq} \cdot \frac{[NADH] \cdot [H^+]}{[NAD^+]} \qquad [13]$$

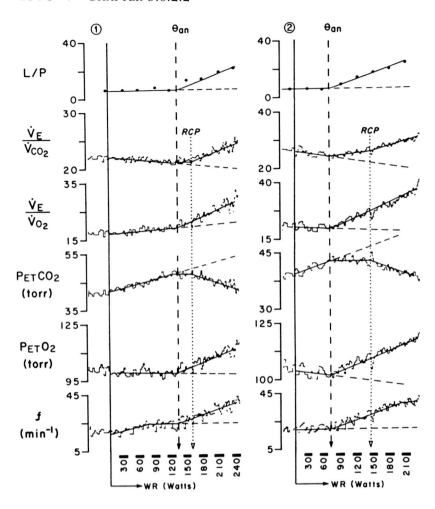

FIG. 2. Breath-by-breath responses of the ventilatory equivalents for CO_2 and O_2 ($\dot{V}_E/\dot{V}_{CO_2}$, $\dot{V}_E/\dot{V}_{O_2}$), end-tidal P_{CO_2} and P_{O_2} ($P_{ET}CO_2$, $P_{ET}O_2$), and breathing frequency (f), together with the blood [lactate]/[pyruvate] ratio (L/P), to a 1-min incremental exercise test to exhaustion. θ_{an} is the anaerobic (or lactate) threshold; RCP indicates the onset of the respiratory compensation for the lactic acidosis. The period of isocapnic buffering (i.e., with $P_{ET}CO_2$ becoming constant between θ_{an} and RCP) is relatively short in subject 1 and much longer in subject 2. (From ref. 28.)

Thus, increases in [H^+] or in [NADH]/[NAD], or in both, will result in an increased [L^-]/[P^-]. Sahlin and co-workers (3,36) have presented data that support the link between lactate production in exercising muscle and a more reduced mitochondrial redox state. Chemical analysis of muscle biopsy samples revealed a decrease in [NADH] at 40% of $\dot{V}_{O_2}$max but showed an increase at 75% and 100%. Furthermore, up to a 4–5 mM/liter increase of [lactate], there appears to be no discernible difference between muscle and blood [lactate] (3,37,38). However, at higher levels, muscle [lactate] exceeds blood [lactate] (3,37), presumably reflecting the saturable lactate-transport kinetics of the muscle sarcolemma and also reflecting the lactate wash-in kinetics into its volume of distribution in the body water.

The induction of a metabolic acidosis prior to exercise results in a reduction of both exercise tolerance and maximum blood [lactate]. Prior bicarbonate loading results in greater values being attained for both. These effects are consistent with the demonstration that lactate efflux from skeletal muscle is slowed by extracellular acidosis but is speeded by extracellular alkalosis.

The bicarbonate system has been demonstrated to

account for 90–95% of the H^+ buffering associated with lactic acidosis, from measurements of arterial blood (6). The remainder reflects intracellular buffering mechanisms. Consequently, the pattern of exercise (6,34) and recovery (38) [HCO_3^-]$_a$ effectively mirrors that of [lactate]$_a$ (Fig. 3).

The resting intramuscular [HCO_3^-] is less than half that of arterial blood, and during exercise the lactate efflux from muscle will be coupled to HCO_3^- influx in addition to cotransport with H^+ ions. The rate of H^+ clearance from exercising muscle has been reported to exceed that of lactate appreciably, at high work rates (e.g., ref. 3). Furthermore, Kowalchuk et al. (38) reported an extensive study of the factors influencing muscle [H^+] during and following high-intensity exercise, and they analyzed their results in accord with Stewart's "strong ion difference" (SID) formulation. Although they questioned the extent to which the [H^+] and [HCO_3^-] changes were consequences of changes in SID resulting from strong-ion translocations (e.g., lactate, K^+, Na^+), they showed that the changes in blood [lactate] and [bicarbonate] were similar; a poor relationship existed for the muscle compartment, however.

The net effect of the buffering reactions is to yield

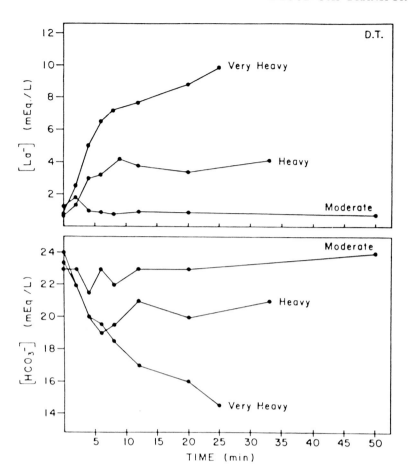

FIG. 3. Responses in blood [lactate] and [bicarbonate] during constant-load moderate, heavy, and very heavy exercise (designated duration: 50 min) in a single subject. Note that the subject could only complete the full 50 min for the moderate test; the final point for the heavy and very heavy tests represents the fatigue point. Note also that the changes in [bicarbonate] mirror those in [lactate]. (From ref. 18.)

an amount of CO_2 (derived from the HCO_3^- component only, however) which is markedly in excess of the equivalent aerobic yield. For example, assuming the net rate of ATP production at a given work rate to be constant, the aerobic ATP yield will be $\simeq 6$ mM ATP/mM CO_2. In contrast, the anaerobic yield from glycolysis will be 6 mM ATP/4 mM lactic acid (i.e., the P:lactate ratio is 1.5); and assuming that 90% of the lactate buffering is accomplished by HCO_3^-, this will produce 3.6 mM CO_2/6 mM ATP (i.e., = [lactate] × HCO_3^- fraction of the buffering, = 4 × 0.9, = 3.6 mM [HCO_3^-] decrease). Subtracting the 1 mM of CO_2 that would have resulted aerobically for the production of 6 mM of ATP, the net increase of CO_2 will therefore be 2.6 mM. The result is a two- to threefold increase in CO_2 production rate from the blood lactate-generating reactions. $\dot{V}_{CO_2}$ therefore increases at an appreciably greater rate than $\dot{V}_{O_2}$ when blood [lactate] is increasing. It should be noted that because the *rate* at which CO_2 is evolved from this reaction is a function not of the *magnitude* of the [HCO_3^-] decrease, but rather of its *rate* of decrease, the $\dot{V}_{CO_2}$ kinetics become more complex in this intensity domain and become highly dependent upon the work-rate forcing regime.

However, as schematized in Table 2, the net gas-exchange consequence of lactic acidosis will be complicated by the fact that the lactate concentration depends upon the relative production and utilization rates, as well as upon the dynamics of the lactate distribution in the body water. It has been demonstrated that lactate can be oxidized to CO_2 and H_2O in muscle and also can be resynthesized to glycogen in liver and skeletal muscle—but presumably not in fibers that are themselves producing lactate. When lactate is produced and immediately oxidized at a local site, the net gas exchange that results will be equivalent to that predicted from its totally aerobic breakdown. This is consistent with the increased lactate turnover rate demonstrated at low work rates. If, however, there is a temporal dissociation between its anaerobic production and its subsequent aerobic utilization, the CO_2 produced (as the H^+ ions are immediately buffered) will have been cleared via ventilation. Hence, the subsequent oxidation will yield a less-than-expected CO_2 production, as HCO_3^- is reformed. If, however, glycogen is being simultaneously synthesized, with restitution of HCO_3^- as shown in Table 2, CO_2 will be fixed, further complicating a simple interpretation of [lactate] changes from current rates of CO_2 evolution. The fact that the increase in [lactate] may be reasonably approximated from the excess CO_2 produced during rapid-incremental exercise presumably reflects the dominance of lactate production over utilization for this particular work-rate forcing.

TABLE 2. *Stoichiometry of lactate metabolism*

Production		Utilization	
Aerobic	Anaerobic[a]	Aerobic	Anaerobic

Production, Aerobic:

$$6O_2 + C_6H_{10}O_5 + H_2O \xrightarrow{37\ ATP} 6CO_2 + 6H_2O$$

Production, Anaerobic[a]:

$$\phi O_2 + C_6H_{10}O_5 + H_2O \xrightarrow{3\ ATP} 2C_3H_5O_3^- + 2H^{+b} + 2HCO_3^- \longrightarrow 2CO_2 + 2H_2O$$

Utilization, Aerobic:

$$6O_2 + 2C_3H_5O_3^- \xrightarrow{34\ ATP} 4CO_2 + 4H_2O + 2HCO_3^-$$

Utilization, Anaerobic:

$$C_6H_{10}O_5 + H_2O + 2HCO_3^- \xrightarrow{3\ ATP} \phi O_2 + 2C_3H_5O_3^- + 2CO_2 + 2H_2O$$

[a] The term "anaerobic" is used in the sense that no (ϕ) O_2 is utilized directly in the reaction.
[b] Note that the H^+ is both "produced" with the lactate and "consumed" in the buffering reactions.

Although these features of cellular and blood buffering have been well described, their control mechanisms remain the topic of considerable debate. The major issue is whether the threshold for lactic acidosis is a manifestation of the onset of tissue anaerobiosis (i.e., local mitochondrial P_{O_2} falling below the critical value for continued O_2 utilization). Resolution of this issue is likely to prove difficult, since regional variations of muscle tissue P_{O_2} are unlikely to be discerned from samples of venous effluent blood, or from spectrophotometric analysis of muscle tissue blocks (even when relatively small). But while convincing evidence of regional anaerobiosis within contracting muscle, and even within a particular muscle fiber, may not be available with current technology [although the work of Connett et al. (39) and Sahlin and co-workers (3,36) comes closest to resolving the issue], there are functionally important inferences for both work performance and acid–base regulation which seem incontrovertible. Exercising-muscle pH does not begin to decrease until ~60% of the muscle's maximum metabolic rate is attained, and thereafter it decreases progressively with further increases in power output, which, for exhausting exercise, can reach a value of 6.5 or less (3). Furthermore, Sahlin and co-workers (see ref. 3 for discussion) have demonstrated that the decrease in muscle pH in humans during exercise is a linear function of the increase of its [lactate] and [pyruvate]. Any of the four accepted mechanisms of tissue hypoxia (i.e., hypoxic, anemic, stagnant, and histotoxic) can decrease the threshold of lactic acidosis and increase [lactate]$_a$ at a particular work rate (see ref. 18 for discussion). The argument that [lactate]$_a$ can be increased by a mechanism such as hyperventilatory alkalosis (as a result of disinhibition of the regulatory glycolytic enzyme phosphofructokinase) seems unlikely to be relevant, since respiratory alkalosis is not a usual consequence of high-intensity exercise.

In this context, a consideration of the $\dot{V}_{O_2}$ kinetics is instructive. It has been demonstrated that the early component of the $\phi 2$ response (i.e., after about 15 sec of exercise) is slowed compared with subthreshold exercise (4), presumably reflecting the O_2 that was not used in the lactate-yielding reactions. But superimposed upon this is a slow component of delayed onset that causes $\dot{V}_{O_2}$ to increase to values greater than those predicted from subthreshold work rates (4). There is, however, a range of suprathreshold work rates at which a steady state may eventually be reached. At even higher work rates, no steady state is attained, and $\dot{V}_{O_2}$ continues to increase until the maximum $\dot{V}_{O_2}$ is attained (40). The highest $\dot{V}_{O_2}$ at which a steady state can be attained appears to coincide with the highest work rate at which blood [lactate] does not continue to rise, and at which pH$_a$ does not continue to fall, during the course of the work (40). In most subjects, this occurs at approximately "halfway" between the lactate threshold and the maximum-attainable $\dot{V}_{O_2}$ (as discerned from a rapid-incremental exercise test) and at a maximum sustainable blood [lactate] of ~5 mEq/liter (although some subjects can sustain a much higher value).

The mechanism of the slower delayed phase, which can lead to an "excess" $\dot{V}_{O_2}$ of more than 1 liter/min, has not been resolved. However, it correlates highly with the magnitude and time course of blood [lactate] increase (40) but correlates poorly with other potential metabolic stimulators such as catecholamine levels, body temperature, and $\dot{V}_E$. Because experimentally increased blood [lactate] in resting animals stimulates $\dot{V}_{O_2}$ and also because physical training proportionally reduces both blood [lactate] and the magnitude of this "excess" $\dot{V}_{O_2}$, the energetics of lactate clearance or the load to—and the proportional utilization of—the mitochondrial hydrogen shuttle mechanisms may be involved; however, Roth et al. (41) were unable to discern any significant difference in the pattern of postexercise $\dot{V}_{O_2}$ when blood [lactate] was elevated to

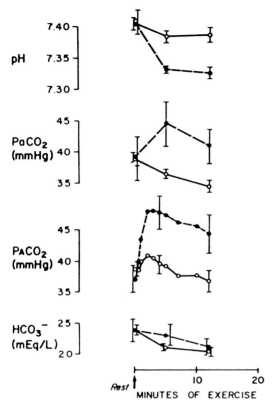

FIG. 4. Average arterial and end-tidal partial pressures ($P_{a}CO_2$, $P_{ET}CO_2$), arterial pH, and [bicarbonate] for control subjects (*solid lines with open symbols*) and carotid-body-resected subjects (*dashed lines with solid symbols*) in response to constant-load exercise above the lactate threshold. (Modified from ref. 33.)

a peak of approximately 5 mM/liter by circulatory occlusion during the work.

In response to lactic acidosis, $\dot{V}_E$ must change in excess of the *total* pulmonary CO_2 load if there is to be respiratory compensation. A dominant mechanism of this hyperventilation appears to be mediated by the carotid bodies in humans (Fig. 3). Consequently, the $\dot{V}_E$ response to high-intensity exercise is markedly attenuated in subjects who have previously had both carotid bodies surgically resected (33) {as a result, they develop a significantly greater acidemia for the same reduction of $[HCO_3^-]_a$ (Fig. 4)}, as well as in subjects breathing high-O_2 gas mixtures (42) (assuming that the high inspired O_2 levels completely attenuated the carotid body responsiveness to H^+). Arterial pH, K^+, circulating catecholamines, osmolarity, and body temperature (but apparently only above a temperature threshold) have all been proposed as potential mediators. However, Rausch (42) has shown recently that (for the same increase in blood [lactate] during sustained constant-load heavy exercise), although the magnitude of the transient pH_a decrement was markedly attenuated in subjects breathing high-O_2 gas mixtures (to suppress carotid chemosensitivity; see refs.

43 and 44), a slow (as well as progressive) compensatory hyperventilation developed. Consequently, although the carotid bodies subserve the major pH regulatory function during acute metabolic acidosis (especially the rapid component), other (presumably central chemoreceptor) mechanisms can also influence acid–base homeostasis.

Furthermore, subjects who do not increase blood [lactate] during exercise, owing to a deficiency of myophosphorylase B (McArdle's syndrome), also hyperventilate at high relative (but low absolute) work rates (45). In contrast to normal subjects, therefore, they develop marked respiratory alkalosis. It is not known, at present, to what extent this hyperventilation results from "unusual" stimulation of muscle type III and IV receptors, or even from hyperkalemic stimulation of the carotid bodies. However, the observation that subjects who do not develop lactic acidosis during exercise can hyperventilate does not rule out the fact that the decrease of pH normally provides an important source of carotid-body-mediated ventilatory drive.

There are interesting temporal characteristics that relate to the development of the respiratory compensation for the metabolic acidosis. In response to incremental exercise of a quasi-steady-state nature (i.e., increment durations of 4 min or longer), as opposed to moderate-intensity exercise, ventilation increases progressively faster relative to work rate and $\dot{V}O_2$ above the lactate threshold. When the work rate is incremented rapidly, a domain of work rates exists within which $\dot{V}_E$ changes at a faster rate than $\dot{V}O_2$ (as was also evident for the longer-duration increments); that is, the ventilatory equivalent for O_2 ($\dot{V}_E/\dot{V}O_2$) and end-tidal P_{O_2} both start to increase immediately above the lactate threshold (Fig. 1). In contrast, however, $\dot{V}_E$ retains its subthreshold proportionality to $\dot{V}CO_2$ more closely over a substantial portion of the suprathreshold work rates, such that there is no decrease in end-tidal P_{CO_2} until a point halfway between the lactate threshold and the maximum-attainable $\dot{V}O_2$ (see Fig. 2). This domain of work, which is evident only when rapidly incrementing work-rate profiles are employed, has been termed the range of "isocapnic buffering" (18,28).

The functional basis for this unusual pattern of response (i.e., hyperventilation relative to O_2 but not to CO_2) is presently uncertain. It has been suggested, however, that the carotid bodies are not immediately responsive to a falling arterial pH, resulting perhaps from an amplitude- or time-related threshold for carotid body excitation.

Although arterial hypocapnia is the common feature of suprathreshold exercise in normal subjects, arterial P_{O_2} at sea level tends to be maintained at or close to resting levels. However, as both the ventilatory equivalent for O_2 ($\dot{V}_E/\dot{V}O_2$) and $P_{ET}O_2$ increase systematically in this work-rate domain (Fig. 2), an important question to be resolved is, Why doesn't P_aO_2 also increase? That is, there is a progressive widening of the alveolar-to-arterial Po_2 gradient ($P_{A-a}O_2$) normally without arterial hypoxemia. However, to date, it has not been demonstrated that this widening of the $P_{A-a}O_2$ begins *precisely* at the lactate threshold.

Clearly, the reduction in $C_{\bar{v}}O_2$ affects $P_{A-a}O_2$ more markedly for any given shunt fraction of the cardiac output ($\dot{Q}_s/\dot{Q}_t$). There is evidence of improved topographical uniformity of $\dot{V}_A$ and $\dot{Q}$ distributions in the lung during exercise; however, evidence from the multiple-inert-gas technique has demonstrated exercise-induced increases in the dispersion of $\dot{V}_A/\dot{Q}$ distribution at high work rates (see ref. 46 for discussion). Gale et al. (47) and Hammond et al. (48), however, could not demonstrate statistically significant changes of either $\dot{V}_A$ or $\dot{Q}$ dispersion for moderate exercise. In contrast, Gledhill et al. (46) did find an increased dispersion of $\dot{V}_A/\dot{Q}$ ratios. Hammond et al. (48) confirmed this increased dispersion at high work rates. They further showed, however, that this dispersion was not sufficient to account for the entire widening of the $P_{A-a}O_2$, and they concluded that there was lack of diffusion equilibrium across the alveolar–capillary membrane at these high work rates. These results supported the contention of Dempsey et al. (49)—who demonstrated arterial hypoxemia at high work rates in some highly fit subjects—that sufficiently high pulmonary blood flows could lead to a pulmonary diffusion "impairment" as a result of some lung regions not having the capacity to recruit adequate pulmonary capillary volume, as capillary flow increased, in order to keep the capillary transit time sufficiently long for diffusion equilibrium of Po_2.

In conclusion, therefore, the acid–base status of the fluid milieux of the contractile units of skeletal muscle can only be maintained during exercise within the relatively narrow range compatible with efficient energy transfer, if there is an integrated system of regulation. This includes the processes governing oxygen delivery to the muscle, intrinsic muscle buffering and ion exchange, CO_2 clearance mechanisms, and ventilatory control. Abnormalities in one or more of these components can therefore result in inappropriate disturbances of acid–base homeostasis and consequent reduction in exercise tolerance.

REFERENCES

1. Mahler M. First-order kinetics of muscle oxygen consumption, and an equivalent proportionality between $\dot{Q}o_2$ and phosphorylcreatine level. *J Gen Physiol* 1985;86:135–165.
2. Krisanda JM, Moreland TS, Kushmerik MJ. ATP supply and demand during exercise. In: Horton ES, Terjung RL, eds. *Exercise, nutrition, and energy metabolism.* New York: Macmillan, 1988;27–44.
3. Hultman E, Sahlin K. Acid–base balance during exercise. In: Hutton RS, Miller DI, eds. *Exercise and sports science reviews,* vol 8. Philadelphia: Franklin Institute Press, 1980;41–128.
4. Whipp BJ. Dynamics of pulmonary gas exchange. *Circulation* 1987;76:VI-18–VI-28.
5. Jones NL. Exercise testing in pulmonary evaluation: rationale, methods, and the normal respiratory response to exercise. *N Engl J Med* 1975;293:541–544.
6. Wasserman K, VanKessel AL, Burton GG. Interaction of physiological mechanisms during exercise. *J Appl Physiol* 1967;22:71–85.
7. Whipp BJ. The control of exercise hyperpnea. In: Hornbein T, ed. *The regulation of breathing.* New York: Marcel Dekker, 1981;1069–1139.
8. Whipp BF, Lamarra N, Ward SA, Davis JA, Wasserman K. Estimating arterial Po_2 from flow-weighted and time-averaged alveolar Pco_2 during exercise. In: Swanson GD, Grodins FS, eds. *Respiratory control: modelling perspective.* New York: Plenum Press, 1990;91–99.
9. Jones NL, Robertson DG, Kane JW. Difference between end-tidal and arterial Pco_2 in exercise. *J Appl Physiol* 1979;47:954–960.
10. Durand J. Circulatory responses to exercise. In: Moret PR, Weber J, Haissly JC, Denolin H, eds. *Lactate: physiologic, methodologic and pathologic approach.* Berlin: Springer-Verlag, 1980;25–34.
11. Meyer RA. A linear model of muscle respiration explains monoexponential phosphocreatine changes. *Am J Physiol* 1988;254:C548–C553.
12. Miyamoto Y. Neural and humoral factors affecting ventilatory response during exercise. *Jpn J Physiol* 1989;39:199–214.
13. Weissman ML, Jones PW, Oren A, Lamarra N, Whipp BJ, Wasserman K. Cardiac output increase and gas exchange at the start of exercise. *J Appl Physiol* 1982;52:236–244.
14. Karlsson H, Lindborg B, Linnarsson D. Time courses of pulmonary gas exchange and heart rate changes in supine exercise. *Acta Physiol Scand* 1975;95:329–340.
15. Whipp BJ, Ward SA, Lamarra N, Davis JA, Wasserman K. Parameters of ventilatory and gas exchange dynamics during exercise. *J Appl Physiol* 1982;52:1506–1513.
16. Casaburi R, Spitzer S, Wasserman K. Effect of altering heart rate on oxygen uptake at exercise onset. *Chest* 1989;95:6–12.
17. Sietsema KE, Cooper DM, Rosove MH, Perloff JK, Child JS, Canobbio MM, Whipp BJ, Wasserman K. Dynamics of oxygen uptake during exercise in adults with cyanotic congenital heart disease. *Circulation* 1986;73:113–114.
18. Wasserman K, Hansen JE, Sue DY, Whipp BJ. *Principles of exercise testing and interpretation.* Philadelphia: Lea & Febiger, 1987.
19. Cerretelli P, Shindell D, Pendergast DP, di Prampero PE, Rennie DW. Oxygen uptake transients at the onset and offset of arm and leg work. *Respir Physiol* 1977;30:81–87.
20. Xing HC, Hughson RL, Northey DR. Investigation of slower kinetics of $\dot{V}O_2$ with hypoxia by frequency domain analysis. *Med Sci Sports Exerc* 1989;21:S20.
21. Hughson RL, Smyth GA. Slower adaptation of Vo_2 to steady state of submaximal exercise with β-blockade. *Eur J Appl Physiol* 1983;52:107–110.
22. Hagberg JM, Hickson RC, Ehsani AA, Holloszy JO. Faster adjustment to and from recovery from submaximal exercise in the trained state. *J Appl Physiol* 1980;48:218–224.
23. Whipp BJ, Ward SA. Physiological determinants of pulmonary gas exchange kinetics during exercise. *Med Sci Sports Exerc* 1990;22:62–71.
24. Ward SA, Lamarra N, Whipp BJ. Gas-exchange inferences for the proportionality of the cardiopulmonary responses during phase 1 of exercise. In: Swanson GD, Grodins FS, eds. *Respiratory control: modelling perspective.* New York: Plenum Press, 1990;137–146.
25. Cochrane GM, Prior JG, Woolf CB. Respiratory arterial pH and Pco_2 oscillations in patients with obstructive airways disease. *Clin Sci* 1981;61:693–702.
26. Forster HV, Pan LG, Funahashi A. Temporal pattern of arterial CO_2 partial pressure during exercise in humans. *J Appl Physiol* 1986;60:653–659.

27. Casaburi R, Whipp BJ, Wasserman K, Stremel RW. Ventilatory control characteristics of the exercise hyperpnea as discerned from dynamic forcing techniques. *Chest* 1978;73S:280S–283S.

28. Whipp BJ, Davis JA, Wasserman K. Ventilatory control of the "isocapnic buffering" region in rapidly-incremental exercise. *Respir Physiol* 1989;76:357–368.

29. Oldenburg FA, McCormack DW, Morse JLC, Jones NL. A comparison of exercise responses in stair-climbing and cycling. *J Appl Physiol* 1979;46:510–516.

30. Griffiths TG, Henson LC, Whipp BJ. Influence of inspired oxygen concentration on the dynamics of the exercise hyperpnea. *J Physiol (Lond)* 1986;380:387–407.

31. Oren A, Whipp BJ, Wasserman K. The effects of acid–base status on the kinetics of ventilatory response to moderate exercise. *J Appl Physiol* 1982;52:1013–1017.

32. Boetger CL, Ward DS. Effect of dopamine on transient ventilatory response to exercise. *J Appl Physiol* 1986;61:2102–2107.

33. Wasserman K, Whipp BJ, Koyal SN, Cleary MG. Effect of carotid body resection of ventilatory and acid–base control during exercise. *J Appl Physiol* 1975;39:354–358.

34. Beaver WL, Wasserman K, Whipp BJ. Bicarbonate buffering of lactic acid generated during exercise. *J Appl Physiol* 1986;60:472–478.

35. Karlsson J. Muscle exercise, energy metabolism and blood lactate. *Adv Cardiol* 1986;35:35–46.

36. Henriksson J, Katz A, Sahlin K. Redox state changes in human skeletal muscle after isometric contraction. *J Physiol (Lond)* 1986;380:441–451.

37. Hirche H, Langohr HD, Wacker U. Lactic acid accumulation in working muscle. In: Keul J, ed. *Limiting factors of physical performance.* Stuttgart: Thieme, 1973;166–171.

38. Kowalchuk JM, Heigenhauser GJF, Lidinger MI, Sutton JR, Jones NL. Factors influencing hydrogen ion concentration in muscle after intense exercise. *J Appl Physiol* 1988;65:2080–2089.

39. Connett RJ, Gayeski TFJ, Honig CR. Lactate accumulation in fully aerobic, working, dog gracilis muscle. *Am J Physiol* 1984;246:H120–H128.

40. Poole DC, Ward SA, Gardner GW, Whipp BJ. Metabolic and respiratory profile on the upper limit for prolonged exercise in man. *Ergonomics* 1988;31:1265–1279.

41. Roth DA, Stanley WC, Brooks GA. Induced lactacidemia does not affect post-exercise O_2 consumption. *J Appl Physiol* 1988;65:1045–1049.

42. Rausch SM. Role of the carotid bodies in the respiratory compensation for metabolic acidosis of exercise in normal humans. *Proc Br Physiol Soc*, Oxford, June 1989;147P.

43. Ward SA, Bellville JW. Peripheral chemoreflex suppression by hyperoxia during moderate exercise in man. In: Whipp BJ, Wiberg DM, eds. *Modelling and control of breathing.* New York: Elsevier, 1983;54–61.

44. Cunningham DJC, MacFarlane DJ. Response of the human arterial chemoreceptors to quick changes in $P_{et}CO_2$, during acute metabolic acidosis. *J Physiol (Lond)* 1985;361:62P.

45. Hagberg JM, Coyle EF, Carroll JE, Miller JM, Martin WH, Brooke MH. Exercise hyperventilation in patients with McArdle's disease. *J Appl Physiol* 1982;52:991–994.

46. Gledhill N, Froese AB, Dempsey JA. Ventilation to perfusion distribution during exercise in health. In: Dempsey JA, Reed CE, eds. *Muscular exercise and the lung.* Madison, WI: University of Wisconsin Press, 1977;325–342.

47. Gale GE, Torre-Bueno J, Moon R, Saltzman H, Wagner PD. V_A/Q inequality in normal man during exercise at sea level and simulated altitude. *J Appl Physiol* 1985;58:978–988.

48. Hammond MD, Gale GE, Kapitan KS, Ries A, Wagner PD. Pulmonary gas exchange in humans during exercise at sea level. *J Appl Physiol* 1986;60:1590–1598.

49. Dempsey JA, Hanson PG, Henderson KS. Exercise-induced arterial hypoxaemia in healthy human subjects at sea level. *J Physiol (Lond)* 1984;355:161–175.

THE LUNG: *Scientific Foundations*
edited by R.G. Crystal, J.B. West et al.
Raven Press, Ltd., New York © 1991.

CHAPTER 5.6.3

Determinants of Maximal Oxygen Uptake

P. D. Wagner, H. Hoppeler, and B. Saltin

DEFINITION OF $\dot{V}_{O_2}$max

Maximum oxygen uptake ($\dot{V}_{O_2}$max) is defined as the rate of oxygen consumption beyond which additional energy demand must be met from anaerobic sources, resulting in an accumulation of lactic acid in working cells and in the plasma (1). $\dot{V}_{O_2}$max is usually elicited during intense activities involving large muscle masses such as running and cycling. Under these conditions, over 90% of the O_2 uptake in the lungs is consumed by skeletal muscle cells (2). However, the catabolic capacity of the myosin ATPase is such that it outstrips by far the capacity of the respiratory system to deliver energy aerobically. Thus, $\dot{V}_{O_2}$max must be determined by the capability to deliver O_2 to muscle mitochondria via the O_2 transport system, rather than by the properties of the muscle's contractile machinery. If we experimentally determine the system's capacity to deliver O_2 we find, for any individual, quite reproducible values for maximal oxygen flow rates, the absolute values of which depend on the specific conditions chosen for measuring $\dot{V}_{O_2}$max. The present chapter describes how the components of the O_2 transport system interact in determining $\dot{V}_{O_2}$max, and it reviews current concepts on the relationships between structure and function.

BALANCE BETWEEN RESPIRATORY STRUCTURES AND FUNCTIONS IN ANIMALS

For the purpose of the current analysis, we consider only the oxygen-transfer-related characteristics of the total respiratory system. In this context, its critical role is to supply oxygen to working cells, ultimately to the terminal substrate oxidases located in the inner mitochondrial membranes of mitochondria. To this end, the respiratory system is organized into a sequence of transfer steps (Fig. 1). In two convective steps (i.e., ventilation and circulation), oxygen flow is determined by the flow rate of a medium (air or blood) multiplied by the specific capacitance of this medium for O_2. In two diffusive steps, oxygen flow is determined by a P_{O_2} difference multiplied by the specific diffusive conductance of the lung and of the muscle tissue gas exchanger, respectively. The rate at which oxygen finally disappears in the mitochondrial oxygen sink is characterized by the number of respiratory complexes multiplied by the rate at which they can operate. Unlike the previous steps, which can be described as relatively simple physical phenomena, this last step seems somewhat more complex, since energy transduction in mitochondria is critically dependent on the specific activity of a large number of enzymes arranged into a metabolic network within the mitochondrial compartments.

At each level, the respiratory system is characterized by a number of structural and functional properties that jointly determine the conditions for oxygen flow. Structural design establishes a topological framework that enables the different compartments to exchange oxygen. Structure can be viewed as a "capacity" for oxygen flow which may be exploited to a variable degree by short-term adjustment of functional variables. The structural design thus sets the upper limits within which functional regulation occurs. However, structural plasticity also exists and is amply demonstrated for many features of the respiratory system in training (3; see also Chapter 5.5.2.6). Structural adaptation requires longer time periods and can be defined as a response of the organism to chronic changes in functional demand.

P. D. Wagner: Department of Medicine, University of California—San Diego, La Jolla, California 92093.
H. Hoppeler: Institute of Anatomy, University of Berne, CH-3000 Berne, Switzerland.
B. Saltin: August Krogh Institute, University of Copenhagen, DK-2100 Copenhagen, Denmark.

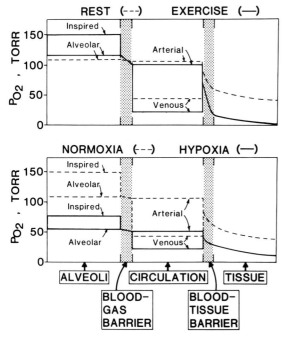

FIG. 1. The P_{O_2} cascade from the environment to the mitochondria. The figure illustrates the sequential movement of O_2 by convective and diffusive processes. Dashed lines reflect the same resting, normoxic conditions in both panels. Solid lines reflect exercise and hypoxia as shown.

It has been hypothesized that animals should be built according to a principle of economic design, whereby morphogenesis during growth and maintenance regulates the size of the structural elements to satisfy, but not to exceed, the functional requirements of the respiratory system (4). This principle of economic design was termed "symmorphosis" and has served as a conceptual framework for an integrated analysis of the respiratory system from lung to skeletal muscle mitochondria. Symmorphosis was experimentally tested by an analysis of how structural and functional variables interact to permit oxygen flow through all compartments of the respiratory system at the limits of functional regulation—at $\dot{V}_{O_2}$max. A first set of experiments on allometric variations (body-mass-related differences in $\dot{V}_{O_2}$max/M_b) provided for a fivefold difference in $\dot{V}_{O_2}$max (5), whereas a second set of experiments on adaptive variations (activity-level-related differences in $\dot{V}_{O_2}$max/M_b) provided for a two- to threefold difference in $\dot{V}_{O_2}$max (6). Taken together, these experiments demonstrate that, with the possible exception of the lungs, there seems to be a close balance between the structural elements along the pathway for oxygen (see ref. 7). That is, the functional limits for oxygen flow at each step are reached at about the same level of oxygen consumption. This implies a match of the structural capacities for oxygen transfer to each other as well as to the oxidative capacity of the working muscle cells (8). The main findings on allometric and adaptive variations can be summarized as follows.

Muscle Oxidative Capacity—Mitochondria

$\dot{V}_{O_2}$max will never exceed the capacity of the final oxygen sink to consume O_2. In adaptive and allometric variations, it is consistently found that higher oxygen consumption rates are achieved only by building more structures (i.e., more mitochondria), and not by changing their specific activity. Mitochondrial oxygen consumption at $\dot{V}_{O_2}$max is found to be constant (3–5 ml O_2/min/ml) for all species except for humans (see below). There is thus essentially a 1:1 match of mitochondrial volume to $\dot{V}_{O_2}$max (Fig. 2). It may be noted that in any one species, more mitochondria may be obtained by increasing the fractional volume of mitochondria in muscles or by increasing lean body mass of the whole animal, or both.

Capillaries in Skeletal Muscle

Higher oxygen flow rates in muscle tissue seem to be mainly achieved by building more capillaries. This reduces the mean diffusion path between capillaries and mitochondria (9), and it increases the capillary wall surface area available for outward diffusion of O_2 from the blood. In adaptive variation, a higher hemoglobin concentration in athletic species also seems to be of advantage for capillary oxygen delivery (10).

Circulatory Transport of Oxygen

In allometric variation, the higher maximal rates of oxygen transport are met entirely by a larger muscle

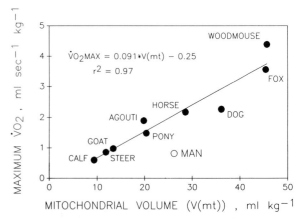

FIG. 2. Relationship between maximum $\dot{V}_{O_2}$ and mitochondrial mass volume across a wide range of mammalian species. Note that man is farthest from the relatively tight linear relationship shown by four-legged mammals, as discussed in the text.

blood flow rate (per kilogram), $\dot{Q}_{max}/M_b$. The larger $\dot{Q}_{max}/M_b$ of the small species is due roughly equally to both higher maximal heart rates (a functional variable) and larger mass-specific stroke volumes (a structural variable). In adaptive variation, there are two mechanisms: (i) a larger $\dot{Q}_{max}/M_b$ of athletic species that is entirely due to a larger stroke volume and (ii) a larger arteriovenous oxygen content difference due to a larger hemoglobin concentration (both structural variables). There may also be greater O_2 extraction in this setting.

Pulmonary Gas Exchanger

If morphometric estimates of diffusing capacity are used to compute the contact time necessary for red blood cells to achieve alveolar–capillary equilibration in the lung, one predicts that even at $\dot{V}_{O_2}$max, such equilibrium is reached before the end of the capillary (11) in all except possibly the smallest species. However, measurements of the degree of alveolar–capillary equilibration made using the multiple inert-gas elimination technique (12–15) clearly show that at $\dot{V}_{O_2}$max, equilibration has not occurred by the end of the capillary. The resolution of these apparently inconsistent conclusions is either that the morphometric estimates of diffusing capacity overestimate actual values [because they are based on full capillary recruitment (16)] or that the assumptions used in computing the available contact time for equilibration are incorrect. In particular, the required assumptions of both $\dot{V}_A/\dot{Q}$ homogeneity and transit time uniformity are obviously not met in reality. On the other hand, estimates of O_2 diffusing capacity in maximally exercising, normal subjects are close to morphometric estimates (15), so that the above assumptions of homogeneity would appear to be the basis for the discrepancy.

STRUCTURE–FUNCTION RELATIONSHIPS UNIQUE TO HUMANS

The basic structural arrangement of skeletal muscles in terms of fiber and capillary geometry appears to be similar between humans and other mammals, with greater differences amongst particular muscle groups than between animals. For example, the hummingbird and pigeon flight muscles are extremely vascular, reflecting adaptation to high O_2 needs (17).

However, Fig. 2 points out a fundamental difference between humans and four-legged mammals. Mitochondrial volume per unit body weight is much higher for humans than for comparably sized nonhuman mammals. Maximum $\dot{V}_{O_2}$/kg on the other hand, is relatively similar. The reasons for this are not clear, but they may well relate to the upright posture and thus unequal

development (and use) of upper versus lower limbs: Because man is dependent on only a part of his muscle mass (i.e., lower limbs predominantly) for $\dot{V}_{O_2}$max, these muscles have adapted so as to possess a higher specific mitochondrial volume. This teleological hypothesis is consistent with the observations of Andersen and Saltin (18) and Rowell et al. (19) that when leg blood flow in humans is *not* limited by cardiac output reaching its maximum value, specific $\dot{V}_{O_2}$ can reach very high levels indeed. Thus, Andersen and Saltin (18) reported values of almost 6 ml sec^{-1} kg^{-1} in such a setting.

CONCEPT OF MULTIPLE DETERMINANTS OF $\dot{V}_{O_2}$max

The above discussion points out that $\dot{V}_{O_2}$max is determined by how much O_2 can be supplied to the muscles, which, in turn, depends on the structural and functional capacities for O_2 transport at each point in the O_2 pathway of Fig. 1. The most important concept to be developed in this chapter is that in any given situation and individual, it is the integrated, interactive effects of each step in the O_2 pathway that set $\dot{V}_{O_2}$max: No single step is "the" limiting one; a change in capacity of *any* one step will alter $\dot{V}_{O_2}$max. As discussed in more detail below, it is clearly evident from the literature that as each step is manipulated experimentally one at a time, $\dot{V}_{O_2}$max is altered predictably. Thus, hypoxia reduces and hyperoxia increases $\dot{V}_{O_2}$max; pulmonary gas exchange inefficiency and impaired cardiac output or hemoglobin concentration reduce $\dot{V}_{O_2}$max, and muscle gas exchange inefficiency also impairs $\dot{V}_{O_2}$max. Showing just how all of these factors interact to set $\dot{V}_{O_2}$max will be a major objective of this chapter.

ROLE OF THE VARIOUS COMPONENTS OF THE OXYGEN DELIVERY SYSTEM IN SETTING $\dot{V}_{O_2}$max

Inspired P_{O_2}

It has been shown repeatedly that reducing inspired P_{O_2} results in a lower $\dot{V}_{O_2}$max. Acute reductions in $P_{I_{O_2}}$ to values as low as 80–90 torr cause $\dot{V}_{O_2}$max to be reduced to some 60–75% of sea-level values (20,21). Further reduction in $P_{I_{O_2}}$ more chronically with increase in altitude produces still greater reductions (22), so that $\dot{V}_{O_2}$max falls to as low as 25% of sea-level values at the $P_{I_{O_2}}$ corresponding to the summit of Mt. Everest, about 43 torr (23). These data are shown in Fig. 3.

Hyperoxia conversely increases $\dot{V}_{O_2}$max (24,25), although the effects are both less dramatic and more

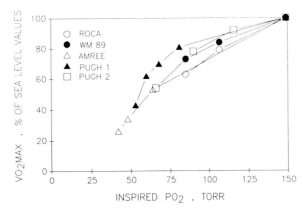

FIG. 3. Reduction in maximum oxygen uptake with increase in altitude, reflected here by inspired P_{O_2}. Five studies are shown; circles indicate acute hypoxia, and triangles and squares indicate chronic hypoxia. $\dot{V}_{O_2}$max is reduced to as much as 25% of sea-level control at the summit of Mt. Everest.

difficult to show because of the flatness of the O_2 dissociation curve above normal sea-level conditions. Thus, some 10–20% increase in $\dot{V}_{O_2}$max is apparent with 100% O_2 breathing and/or hyperbaric O_2 conditions, and Powers et al. (26) recently showed that even elite athletes with $\dot{V}_{O_2}$max as high as 70 ml/kg/min can increase their $\dot{V}_{O_2}$max by breathing O_2-enriched mixtures.

Pulmonary Gas Exchange

The classical view of pulmonary gas exchange is that it is not a factor limiting $\dot{V}_{O_2}$max at sea level but that it is factor at high altitude. More recently, evidence has been produced that demonstrates a small effect even at sea level, especially in elite athletes (26). This effect is due to reduction in arterial P_{O_2} resulting from both ventilation–perfusion mismatching (27,28) and diffusion limitation of O_2 transfer (12–14). However, because of the hyperventilation of exercise and the slope of the O_2 dissociation curve, the degree of arterial desaturation is mild. Thus, even in elite athletes (who show the greatest effect), arterial saturation generally does not fall below 90% (26) from resting values of about 97%. Consequently, maximal O_2 delivery to, and utilization by, muscles is not greatly impaired.

At high altitude, diffusion limitation of O_2 transfer across the blood–gas barrier during heavy exercise considerably reduces arterial oxygenation by as much as 4 ml O_2 per 100 ml blood at altitudes above 5000 m (15). This amounts to a reduction of some 20–25% in arterial O_2 concentration over and above that which would have been caused by reduction in $P_{I_{O_2}}$ alone if the lungs were free from diffusion limitation.

High altitude results in diffusion limitation because

pulmonary O_2 uptake must take place wholly on the steep part of the O_2 dissociation curve. This increases (relative to sea level) the discrepancy between the tissue solubility of O_2 (which governs the rate of diffusion of O_2 through a given area of the blood–gas barrier) and the average slope of the O_2 dissociation curve, which governs the rate at which blood P_{O_2} can rise per milliliter of O_2 reaching the red blood cell. At high altitude, ventilation–perfusion mismatching is of little significance to O_2 exchange in normal humans, however (29).

Hemoglobin Content and the Particulate Nature of Blood

Several studies have shown a strong correlation between $\dot{V}_{O_2}$max and O_2 delivery to muscle as the latter was altered by changing the hemoglobin (Hb) concentration (30–34). Specifically, $\dot{V}_{O_2}$max can be increased by transfusion, and Gledhill concluded that about a liter of blood was required to measurably increase maximum $\dot{V}_{O_2}$ (35).

The real question is whether the dependence of $\dot{V}_{O_2}$max on Hb concentration is due solely to the obvious proportional effect of [Hb] on convective O_2 delivery into the arterial system of the muscle, or whether additional (diffusive) factors are operative. In particular, it is possible that with a reduction in Hb concentration and hence an increase in inter-red blood cell spacing, the instantaneous outward effective diffusing area of the capillary wall is reduced (36,37). The presumption here is that the inter-red blood cell plasma space does not provide a significant route for outward O_2 diffusion because of the very low plasma O_2 solubility. A second potential influence of a reduction in Hb concentration might be a reduction in *total* muscle capillary O_2 off-loading kinetic rates (from red blood cells), not because the off-loading reaction in a given red blood cell is reduced but simply because there are fewer red blood cells per unit of capillary volume.

Recent evidence shows that the effect of Hb concentration on $\dot{V}_{O_2}$max occurs by both convective and diffusive factors. Hogan et al. (38) found that by acutely reducing Hb concentration from 14 to 7 g/100 ml at a constant flow rate, there was a reduction in the effective muscle diffusing capacity of 34%. Whether this was due to increased red blood cell spacing, altered O_2 Hb off-loading kinetics, or perhaps other, as yet undefined factors remains to be determined. However, this observation is consistent with the long-standing observation of Cain (39) that at rest, the critical venous P_{O_2} is much higher in anemia than in hypoxia, explainable by an effect of Hb concentration on muscle O_2 diffusing capacity.

Myocardial Determinants

It has long been known that in normal humans, maximum $\dot{V}O_2$ correlates well with convective O_2 delivery. The latter, the product of blood flow and arterial O_2 concentration, is most dependent on blood flow because in normal subjects, arterial PO_2 and Hb concentration, the determinants of arterial O_2 concentration, are confined to a relatively narrow range. Many studies in both humans and isolated, perfused muscle have shown the correlation between muscle blood flow and $\dot{V}O_2$max (18,19,40–44). Perhaps the closest documentation of this in humans is the work of Andersen and Saltin (18) and Rowell et al. (19) using the functionally isolated knee extensor. They found that $\dot{V}O_2$ and muscle blood flow were tightly correlated over the entire load range to maximum, and that $\dot{V}O_2$max of the exercising leg was maintained in hypoxia as a result of increased blood flow (compensating for the reduced arterial PO_2).

Although this tight correlation has led some others to imply cause and effect [i.e., that $\dot{V}O_2$max was uniquely limited by the cardiovascular system (45)], current thinking would propose a slightly different viewpoint. Thus, in line with the section entitled "Concept of Multiple Determinants of $\dot{V}O_2$max" (see above), cardiac output (or muscle blood flow) is just one of the interacting determinants of $\dot{V}O_2$max. However, it would appear from the above studies that it may be the most important single factor from the quantitative point of view, at least during normoxia.

Finally, it should be pointed out that even during extreme hypoxia equivalent to the summit of Mt. Everest ($P_1O_2 \approx 43$ torr), there is no evidence of impaired myocardial contractility or function per se at $\dot{V}O_2$max. This statement is based on evidence from electrocardiography, echocardiography, and filling-pressure–cardiac-output relationships measured during a simulated ascent of Mt. Everest in 1985 (46). Although maximum cardiac output is reduced under the above conditions (47), this is primarily due to a reduced maximal heart rate, the cause of which is currently unknown.

Peripheral Vascular Determinants

Two interrelated aspects of the skeletal muscle vasculature must be considered here. The first is vascular pressure–flow relationships ("vascular resistance"), and the second is transit time available for O_2 extraction. Mean transit time is given by the ratio of capillary blood volume to muscle blood flow and hence involves both structural (capillary geometry) and functional (flow) components.

It is, of course, well known that at $\dot{V}O_2$max, mean arterial pressure normally rises only slightly whereas cardiac output increases about fourfold, implying an overall reduction in skeletal muscle vasculature resistance as compared to the resting state. However, the work of Andersen and Saltin (18) and Rowell et al. (19) underscores the enormous increase in flow that a functionally isolated muscle (such as the knee extensors) is capable of when it exercises alone, again with essentially normal systemic blood pressures, implying an even greater fall in *local* (exercising) muscle vascular resistance under such conditions. The latter observation then argues clearly that in two-legged exercise at $\dot{V}O_2$max, there must be some degree of vasoconstriction [assuming that all or nearly all capillaries are recruited as thought (48)]. Thus, compared to rest, normal bi-legged exercise could be thought of as causing partial reduction in peripheral vascular tone, but by no means its abolition. Precisely what controls the degree of tone remains unknown. It is felt that the partial reduction in tone not only prevents severe systemic hypertension from occurring, but serves to increase capillary volume and therefore, together with capillary recruitment, buffer red blood cell transit time. In fact, the latter effect is believed by some to be the principal advantage of the above changes (40).

Even so, it would appear that transit time is too short to permit diffusional equilibration of O_2 between red blood cells and mitochondria to occur (40). Certainly, there is a wealth of evidence of incomplete extraction of O_2 from capillary blood (20,40,49,50) at $\dot{V}O_2$max. This has been argued to be mostly, if not completely, on the basis of diffusion limitation—that is, a tissue diffusing capacity too low for the available transit time. The evidence for this conclusion lies in the remarkably consistent proportional relationships found between mean capillary (or muscle venous) PO_2 and $\dot{V}O_2$max itself, concordant with the physical laws of diffusion (20,50). However, other physiological events may contribute to the O_2 present in the muscle venous blood, including (a) heterogeneity of the relationship between $\dot{V}O_2$ and blood flow within the exercising muscle (51), (b) muscle perfusional shunts between arterial and venous blood, and (c) diffusional shunts of O_2 between adjacent arterioles and venules (52). In normal muscle at $\dot{V}O_2$max, these three phenomena are generally considered to be unimportant, although no good methods exist for their quantification.

Oxygen Unloading and Tissue Transport

For O_2 to be transported from the blood to the muscle mitochondria, a number of sequential steps must be executed. First, O_2 must chemically dissociate from Hb in the red blood cell, and then it must diffuse out of the red blood cell through the plasma and through the capillary wall. Diffusion continues outward through the interstitial space and sarcolemma to reach the usually myoglobin-rich interior of the myocyte. Facilitated diffusion of O_2 attached to myoglobin then ensues until O_2 molecules reach their mitochondrial sites of utilization.

Perhaps the key issue here is to ask whether any of these sequential steps is sufficiently slow as to provide a significant impediment to the flow of O_2 to the cytochromes. The presence of considerable amounts of O_2 in the effluent venous blood draining maximally exercising limb muscles (P_{O_2} is commonly 20 torr in femoral venous blood of humans at $\dot{V}_{O_2}max$) would suggest that at one or more of the above sites, there is diffusion limitation of O_2 extraction from the blood. Considerable recent evidence (20,50,53,54) supports this old notion, perhaps first introduced by Krogh (55) at the start of this century. In particular, as would be expected of a diffusion-limited situation, there is a closely proportional relationship between $\dot{V}_{O_2}max$ and calculated mean capillary P_{O_2} as $P_{I_{O_2}}$ is reduced in normal humans (20). Although it is not currently possible to exclude phenomena such as muscle perfusional shunt or perfusion–$\dot{V}_{O_2}$ heterogeneity as additional factors responsible for the incomplete extraction of O_2 at $\dot{V}_{O_2}max$, direct measurement of myocyte myoglobin-associated O_2 saturation indicates very low (1–5 torr) corresponding intracellular P_{O_2} values (56), even while the venous P_{O_2} is some 20 torr.

These data, although perhaps still controversial, imply that the bulk of the resistance to outward flux of O_2 lies between Hb and the myocyte cell wall, a very short physical distance compared to the intercapillary distances within myocyte cytoplasm. However, even if it is correct to narrow down the locations of most resistance to this small component, it still remains to be elucidated what subcomponents are important: chemical dissociation off hemoglobin, subsequent physical diffusion out of the capillary, or the next diffusive step through the interstitial space. Recent data from isolated canine gastrocnemius muscle stimulated to $\dot{V}_{O_2}max$ demonstrate a large effect of Hb concentration (observed by hematocrit reduction) on overall muscle diffusing capacity for O_2 (38). This suggests that inter-red blood cell spacing (36,37) or slowness in the chemical off-loading rates (57), or both, are significant factors, although much more work needs to be done to resolve these questions completely. Such results are consistent with the well-known observation that under resting conditions, anemia results in a considerable elevation of the critical level of P_{O_2} observed in venous blood below which metabolic rate falls (39).

Integrative Analysis of the Determinants of $\dot{V}_{O_2}max$

The foregoing discussion of the individual roles of the many factors important to O_2 supply to mitochondria has prompted a quantitative, integrative analysis of how they might all combine to eventually set $\dot{V}_{O_2}max$ under a particular set of conditions (54,58). While purposefully simple, this analysis does account for current observations on the determinants of $\dot{V}_{O_2}max$ even while ignoring phenomena such as flow–$\dot{V}_{O_2}$ heterogeneity within muscle. It is presented here as a useful conceptual approach, but it is still in the early stages of development. Undoubtedly it will become modified with the acquisition of more data in the future.

The analysis is based simply on two equations accounting for O_2 supply: the equation describing Fick's principle:

$$\dot{V}_{O_2} = \dot{Q}(C_a O_2 - C_v O_2) \qquad [1]$$

and that describing subsequent outward diffusive flux of O_2 according to basic principles of diffusion:

$$\dot{V}_{O_2} = D_{O_2}[P_{\overline{CAP}}O_2 - P_{MITO}O_2] \qquad [2]$$

Here, $\dot{V}_{O_2}$ is O_2 uptake, $\dot{Q}$ is muscle blood flow, D_{O_2} is overall muscle O_2 diffusing capacity (representing all of the steps between Hb and the cytoplasm described above). $C_a O_2$ and $C_v O_2$ are the O_2 concentrations of arterial and effluent venous blood, and $P_{\overline{CAP}}O_2$ and $P_{MITO}O_2$ are, respectively, mean capillary P_{O_2} and mitochondrial P_{O_2}. If (a) $P_{\overline{CAP}}O_2$ and $P_v O_2$ are proportional to one another, as would be the case in a simple diffusion-limited system where P_{O_2} falls essentially exponentially from the arterial to venous end of the capillary, and (b) $P_{MITO}O_2$ is sufficiently close to zero to be neglected compared to $P_{\overline{CAP}}O_2$, which seems to be the case ($P_a O_2 = 100$ torr, $P_v O_2 = 20$ torr, $P_{\overline{CAP}}O_2 \approx 40$ torr, $P_{MITO}O_2 < 1$–5 torr, all at $\dot{V}_{O_2}max$), then Eq. 2 can be rewritten as

$$\dot{V}_{O_2} = D_{O_2} \cdot K \cdot P_v O_2 \qquad [3]$$

where K is the constant relating effluent venous P_{O_2} ($P_v O_2$) to $P_{\overline{CAP}}O_2$.

If $\dot{V}_{O_2}$ is plotted (on the ordinate) against $P_v O_2$ (on the abscissa) for both Eqs. 1 and 3 under conditions of fixed values of $\dot{Q}$, $C_a O_2$, and D_{O_2}, two relationships are apparent as in Fig. 4. Their point of intersection yields $\dot{V}_{O_2}max$ as the highest value of $\dot{V}_{O_2}$ on the line for Eq. 3 still compatible with mass balance (Eq. 1). This simple analysis then shows how each step in the O_2 pathway can alter $\dot{V}_{O_2}max$. Thus, $C_a O_2$ can be altered by changing inspired P_{O_2} or pulmonary gas-exchange efficiency. An increase in $C_a O_2$ will elevate each point on the line for Eq. 1, which will thus intersect that for Eq. 3 at a higher point, indicating how much $\dot{V}_{O_2}max$ will rise for a given rise in $C_a O_2$. In the same way, an increase in muscle blood flow will improve O_2 delivery and elevate the line of Eq. 1, but simultaneously the negative slope of that line becomes greater (see Eq. 1), tending to offset the gain in $\dot{V}_{O_2}max$. This negative effect, intuitively expressed, is the result of reducing

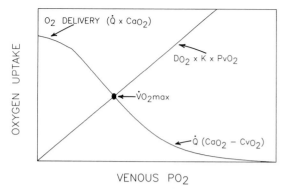

FIG. 4. Integrative analysis of diffusive and convective factors transporting oxygen to muscle. The straight line through the origin reflects Fick's law of diffusion, which linearly relates oxygen uptake to partial pressure gradient. The curved line represents mass balance as expressed by Fick's principle. The intersection of the two relationships gives maximum $\dot{V}_{O_2}$ as explained in the text.

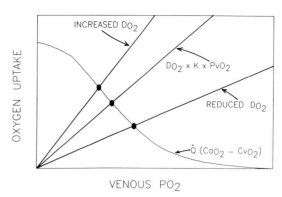

FIG. 6. Potential effects of changes in muscle diffusing capacity at constant convective oxygen delivery. Filled ovals indicate maximum $\dot{V}_{O_2}$ and associated effluent muscle venous P_{O_2} as diffusive capacity is altered up or down.

the transit time (or $D_{O_2}/\dot{Q}$ ratio), thus reducing the amount of O_2 that can diffuse out of the capillaries per red blood cell, all other factors being constant. Alterations of muscle diffusing capacity (e.g., upward by endurance training or downward by disuse atrophy) would alter the slope of the line representing Eq. 3 and thus lead to a correspondingly increased or decreased $\dot{V}_{O_2}$max at the new points of intersection of the two lines. These notions are shown in Figs. 5 and 6.

The power of such analyses, then, is to predict quantitatively from some starting point how the changes in any one or more variables in the O_2 transport pathway combine to alter $\dot{V}_{O_2}$max.

Mitochondrial Oxygen Consumption

Our view of mitochondria as determinants of oxygen flow through the respiratory system remains sketchy.

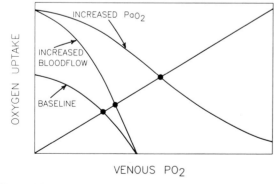

FIG. 5. Effects of increasing convective oxygen delivery to the muscle on maximum $\dot{V}_{O_2}$, compared to baseline conditions. A doubling of oxygen delivery achieved by an increase in P_{O_2} alone produces a greater increment in maximum $\dot{V}_{O_2}$ than does the same increase in oxygen delivery produced by increased muscle blood flow. The reasons are explained in the text.

However, it has been noted above that the rate of global mitochondrial oxygen consumption at $\dot{V}_{O_2}$max is found to be very constant in both allometric and adaptive variation in mammalian species. This notion is somewhat in contrast to findings where $\dot{V}_{O_2}$max was varied with chronic endurance or sprint training as an experimental tool (59–61). Generally speaking, these studies indicate that muscle tissue oxidative capacity is not related to whole-animal $\dot{V}_{O_2}$max and that mitochondrial oxidative capacity is far in excess of the capacity of the respiratory system to deliver oxygen to muscle cells. It remains to be further explored whether and why the ratio of mitochondrial oxygen consumption is lower in muscles of endurance-trained animals as some studies suggest (59). It will be necessary to conduct integrated studies that measure whole-body as well as compartmental oxygen consumptions and possibly even substrate fluxes in a coherent conceptual framework. The question of the maximal rate at which a unit volume of mitochondria can consume oxygen when isolated and optimally supplied with substrate and oxygen has recently been addressed. It was found that mitochondria *in vivo* seem to exploit some 60–80% of their maximal oxygen uptake capacity (62,63). It will indeed be a most important issue to find out whether training is able to change the rate at which mitochondria consume oxygen at $\dot{V}_{O_2}$max in intact animals. The currently available data do not yet allow an answer to this question.

SUMMARY

It appears that $\dot{V}_{O_2}$max, broadly related to mitochondrial volume across a range of species, is, in any individual case, set by O_2 supply rather than by the amount of metabolic machinery in the mitochondria.

In the not-too-distant past it was common to talk in

terms of a "limiting factor" to $\dot{V}O_2$max as if some single step in the O_2 pathway supply was by itself *the rate-limiting component*. The literature shows repeatedly, however, that each and every step in this pathway has the power to alter $\dot{V}O_2$max individually. These diverse observations can conveniently be brought together into a simple integrative analysis of diffusive and convective processes involved in O_2 transport to show just how the steps interact to set $\dot{V}O_2$max in any set of circumstances. Consequently, *all* steps in the O_2 pathway are limiting in that improving their transport capacity will permit a higher $\dot{V}O_2$max up to the point of full exploitation of the biochemical capacity of the mitochondria, a point that has apparently not yet been reached. Finally, however, it must be kept in mind that the processes described in this chapter reflect only $\dot{V}O_2$max—that is, the maximum rate of O_2 utilization. In particular, the relationships between $\dot{V}O_2$max and the closely associated phenomena of physiologically demonstrable muscle fatigue on the one hand, and symptomatic exhaustion on the other, are not clear and remain to be elucidated.

REFERENCES

1. Margaria R. *Biomechanics and energetics of muscular exercise*. Oxford: Clarendon Press, 1976.
2. Mitchell JH, Blomqvist G. Maximal oxygen uptake. *N Engl J Med* 1971;284:1018–1022.
3. Saltin B, Gollnick PD. Skeletal muscle adaptability: significance for metabolism and performance. In: Peach LD, Adrian RH, Geiger SR, eds. *Handbook of physiology, Section 10: Skeletal muscle*. Baltimore: Williams & Wilkins, 1983;555–631.
4. Taylor CR, Weibel ER. Design of the mammalian respiratory system. I. Problem and strategy. *Respir Physiol* 1981;44:1–10.
5. Weibel ER, Taylor CR. Design of the mammalian respiratory system. *Respir Physiol* 1981;44:1–164.
6. Weibel ER, Kayar SR. Matching O_2 delivery to O_2 demand in muscle. I. Adaptive variation. In: Gonzalez NC, Fedde MR, eds. *Oxygen transfer from atmosphere to tissues*. New York: Plenum Press, 1988;159–169.
7. Taylor CR, Karas RH, Weibel ER, Hoppeler H. Matching structures and functions in the respiratory system. In: Wood SC, ed. *Comparative pulmonary physiology*. New York: Marcel Dekker, 1989;27–65.
8. Lindstedt SL, Wells DJ, Jones JR, Hoppeler H, Thronson HA. Limitations to aerobic performance in mammals: interaction of structure and demand. *Int J Sports Med* 1988;9:210–217.
9. Hoppeler H, Kayar SR. Capillarity and oxidative capacity of muscles. *News Physiol Sci* 1988;3:113–116.
10. Conley KE, Kayar SR, Roesler K, Hoppeler H, Weibel ER, Taylor CR. Adaptive variation in the mammalian respiratory system in relation to energetic demand. IV. Capillaries and their relationship to oxidative capacity. *Respir Physiol* 1987;69:47–64.
11. Karas RH, Taylor CR, Jones JJ, Lindstedt SL, Reeves RB, Weibel ER. Adaptive variation in the mammalian respiratory system in relation to energetic demand. VII. Flow of oxygen across the pulmonary gas exchanger. *Respir Physiol* 1987;69:101–115.
12. Torre-Bueno J, Wagner PD, Saltzman HA, Gale GE, Moon RE. Diffusion limitation in normal humans during exercise at sea level and simulated altitude. *J Appl Physiol* 1985;58(3):989–995.
13. Hammond MD, Gale GE, Kapitan KS, Ries A, Wagner PD. Pulmonary gas exchange in humans during exercise at sea level. *J Appl Physiol* 1986;60(5):1590–1598.
14. Wagner PD, Gale GE, Moon RE, Torre-Bueno J, Stolp BW, Saltzman HA. Pulmonary gas exchange in humans exercising at sea level and simulated altitude. *J Appl Physiol* 1986;60(1):260–270.
15. Wagner PD, Sutton JR, Reeves JT, Cymerman A, Groves BM, Malconian MK. Operation Everest II. Pulmonary gas exchange during a simulated ascent of Mt. Everest. *J Appl Physiol* 1988;63(6):2348–2359.
16. Weibel ER, Marques LB, Constantinopol M, Doffey F, Gehr P, Taylor CR. Adaptive variation in the mammalian respiratory system in relation to energetic demand. VI. The pulmonary gas exchanger. *Respir Physiol* 1987;69:81–100.
17. Mathieu-Costello O. Histology of flight: tissue and muscle gas exchange. In: Sutton JR, Coates G, Remmers JE, eds. *Hypoxia: the adaptations*. Toronto: BC Dekker, 1990;12–19.
18. Andersen P, Saltin B. Maximal perfusion of skeletal muscle in man. *J Appl Physiol* 1985;366:233–249.
19. Rowell LB, Saltin B, Kiens B, Christensen NJ. Is peak quadriceps blood flow in humans even higher during exercise with hypoxemia? *Am J Physiol* 1986;251:H1038–H1044.
20. Roca J, Hogan MC, Story D, Bebout DE, et al. Evidence for tissue diffusion limitation of $\dot{V}O_2$max in normal humans. *J Appl Physiol* 1989;67(1):291–299.
21. Bebout DE, Story D, Roca J, et al. Effects of altitude acclimatization on pulmonary gas exchange during exercise. *J Appl Physiol* 1989;67(6):2286–2295.
22. Pugh LGCE, Gill MB, Lahiri S, Milledge JS, Ward MP, West JB. Muscular exercise at great altitudes. *J Appl Physiol* 1964;19(3):431–440.
23. Ward MP, Milledge JS, West JB, eds. *High altitude medicine and physiology*. Philadelphia: University of Pennsylvania Press, 1989.
24. Cerretelli P, Di Prampero PE. Gas exchange in exercise. In: Farhi LE, Tenney SM, eds. *Handbook of physiology, Section 3: The respiratory system, vol IV*. Bethesda, MD: American Physiological Society, 1987;297–339.
25. Welch HG. Hyperoxia and human performance: a brief review. *Med Sci Sports Exerc* 1982;14:253–262.
26. Powers SK, Lawler J, Dempsey JA, Dodd S, Landry G. Effects of incomplete pulmonary gas exchange on $\dot{V}O_2$max. *J Appl Physiol* 1989;66(6):2491–2495.
27. Gledhill N, Froese AB, Dempsey JA. Ventilation to perfusion distribution during exercise in health. In: Dempsey J, Reed CE, eds. *Muscular exercise and the lung*. Madison, WI: University of Wisconsin Press, 1977;325–343.
28. Gale GE, Torre-Bueno J, Moon RE, Saltzman HA, Wagner PD. Ventilation–perfusion inequality in normal humans during exercise at sea level and simulated altitude. *J Appl Physiol* 1985;58(3):978–988.
29. Lilienthal J Jr, Riley RL, Proemmel DD, Franke RE. An experimental analysis in man of the oxygen pressure gradient from alveolar air to arterial blood during rest and exercise at sea level and at altitude. *Am J Physiol* 1946;147:199–216.
30. Buick FJ, Gledhill N, Froese AB, Spriet L, Meyers EC. Effect of induced erythrocythemia on aerobic work capacity. *J Appl Physiol* 1980;48:636–642.
31. Pace N, Lozner EL, Consolazio WV, Pitts GC, Pecora LJ. The increase in hypoxia tolerance of normal men accompanying the polycythemia induced by transfusion of erythrocytes. *Am J Physiol* 1947;148:152–163.
32. Robertson R, Gilcher R, Metz K, et al. Central circulation and work capacity after red blood cell reinfusion under normoxia and hypoxia in women. *Med Sci Sports* 1979;11:98.
33. Spriet LL, Gledhill N, Froese AB, Wilkes DL, Meyers EC. The effect of induced erythrocythemia on central circulation and oxygen transport during maximal exercise. *Med Sci Sports Exerc* 1980;12:122.
34. Williams MH, Wesseldine S, Somma T, Schuster R. The effect of induced erythrocythemia upon 5-mile treadmill run time. *Med Sci Sports Exerc* 1981;13:169–175.
35. Gledhill N. Blood doping and related issues: a brief review. *Med Sci Sports Exerc* 1982;14(3):183–189.
36. Federspiel WJ, Sarelius IH. An examination of the contribution

of red cell spacing to the uniformity of oxygen flux at the capillary walls. *Microvasc Res* 1984;27:273.

37. Federspiel WJ, Popel AS. A theoretical analysis of the effect of the particulate nature of blood on oxygen release in capillaries. *Microvasc Res* 1986;32:164.

38. Hogan MC, Bebout DE, West JB, Wagner PD. Effect of altered Hb concentration on maximal O_2 consumption in canine gastrocnemius *in situ*. *FASEB J* 1990;Pt. II.4(4):5499, A1213.

39. Cain SM. Oxygen delivery and uptake in dogs during anemic and hypoxic hypoxia. *J Appl Physiol* 1977;42(2):228–234.

40. Saltin B. Hemodynamic adaptations to exercise. *Am J Cardiol* 1985;55:42D–47D.

41. Saltin B, Blomqvist G, Mitchell JH, Johnson RL Jr, Wildenthal K, Chapman CB. Response to exercise after bed rest and after training. *Circulation* 1968;38(Suppl 7):1–78.

42. Ekblom B. The effect of physical training on oxygen transport system in man. *Acta Physiol Scand* 1969;328(Suppl):1–45.

43. Blomqvist CG, Saltin B. Cardiovascular adaptations to physical training. *Annu Rev Physiol* 1983;45:169–189.

44. Horstman DH, Gleser M, Delehunt J. Effects of altering O_2 delivery on $\dot{V}O_2$ of isolated working muscle. *Am J Physiol* 1976;230(2):327–334.

45. Barclay JK, Stainsby WN. The role of blood flow in limiting maximal metabolic rate in muscle. *Med Sci Sports* 1975;7(2):116–119.

46. Reeves JT, Groves BM, Sutton JR, et al. Operation Everest II: preservation of cardiac function at extreme altitude. *J Appl Physiol* 1987;63(2):531–539.

47. Pugh LGCE. Cardiac output in muscular exercise at 5,800 m (19,000 ft). *J Appl Physiol* 1964;19(3):441–447.

48. Gray SD, McDonagh PG, Gore RW. Comparison of functional and total capillarity densities in fast and slow muscles of the chicken. *Pflügers Arch* 1983;397:209–213.

49. Pirnay F, Lamy M, Dujardin J, Deroanne R, Petit JM. Analysis of femoral venous blood during maximum muscular exercise. *J Appl Physiol* 1972;33:289–292.

50. Hogan MC, Roca J, Wagner PD, West JB. Limitation of maximal O_2 uptake and performance by acute hypoxia in dog muscle *in situ*. *J Appl Physiol* 1988;65(2):815–821.

51. Duling BR, Damon DH. An examination of the measurement of flow heterogeneity in striated muscle. *Circ Res* 1987;60(1):1–13.

52. Harris PD. Movement of oxygen in skeletal muscle. *News Physiol Sci* 1986;1:147–149.

53. Hogan MC, Roca J, West JB, Wagner PD. Dissociation of maximal O_2 uptake from O_2 delivery in canine gastrocnemius *in situ*. *J Appl Physiol* 1989;66(3):1919–1926.

54. Wagner PD. An integrated view of the determinants of maximum oxygen uptake. In: Gonzalez NC, Fedde MR, eds. *Oxygen transfer from atmosphere to tissues*, vol 227. New York: Plenum Press, 1988;245–256.

55. Krogh A. The number and distribution of capillaries in muscle with calculations of the pressure head necessary for supplying the tissue. *J Physiol (Lond)* 1919;52:409–415.

56. Honig CR, Gayeski TEJ, Federspiel W, Clark A Jr, Clark P. Muscle O_2 gradients from hemoglobin to cytochrome: new concepts, new complexities. *Adv Exp Med Biol* 1984;169:23–38.

57. Gutierrez G. The rate of oxygen release and its effect on capillary O_2 tension: a mathematical analysis. *Respir Physiol* 1986;63:79–97.

58. Wagner PD. The determinants of $\dot{V}O_2max$. In: *Annals of Sports Medicine*, vol 4, Part 4. New York: Oxford University Press, 1988;196–212.

59. Davies KJA, Packer L, Brooks GA. Exercise bioenergetics following sprint training. *Arch Biochem Biophys* 1982;215:260–265.

60. Gollnick PD, Saltin B. Significance of skeletal oxidative enzyme enhancement with endurance training. *Clin Physiol* 1982;66:195–201.

61. Hilty MR, Groth H, Moore RL, Musch TI. Determinants of $\dot{V}O_2max$ in rats after high-intensity sprint training. *J Appl Physiol* 1989;66:195–201.

62. Schwerzmann K, Cruz-Orive LM, Eggmann R, Saenger A, Weibel ER. Molecular architecture of the inner membrane of mitochondria from rat liver: a combined biochemical and stereological study. *J Cell Biol* 1986;102:97–103.

63. Schwerzmann K, Hoppeler H, Kayar SR, Weibel ER. Oxydative capacity of muscle and mitochondria: correlation of physiological, biochemical and morphometric characteristics. *Proc Natl Acad Sci USA* 1988;86:1583–1587.

THE LUNG: *Scientific Foundations*
edited by R.G. Crystal, J.B. West et al.
Raven Press, Ltd., New York © 1991.

CHAPTER 5.6.4

Learning from Comparative Physiology

C. Richard Taylor and Ewald R. Weibel

MODEL AND CONCEPT

The Lung Is an Integrated Part of the Respiratory System

If an ordinary human exercises vigorously (e.g., by running a mile as hard as he or she can), his or her muscles consume about 10 times as much O_2 as at rest in the process of increased energy production by oxidative phosphorylation. A well-trained athlete doing the same may increase his O_2 consumption by up to 20 times, matching his higher power output. In either case, this is accompanied by an increase in cardiac output and heart rate, as well as by an increase in minute ventilation and respiratory frequency: O_2 uptake in the lung and O_2 transport by the circulation of blood must be matched to the O_2 consumption in the mitochondria of the working muscle cells.

What we learn from this is threefold:

1. Respiration is an *integral function* involving the coordinated action of all structures that build the pathway for O_2 from the lung to the respiratory chain enzymes in the mitochondria. The lung cannot be considered in isolation.

2. Respiration is a *regulated process* matched to the instantaneous demands on aerobic metabolism: As ATP consumption increases, O_2 demand is increased proportionately, and this requires appropriate regulation of the various O_2 transport functions.

3. Respiration, or aerobic metabolism, is a *limited function* in the sense that O_2 consumption can rise up to a definable limit, called $\dot{V}_{O_2}max$, beyond which any additional call for energy must be, and is, covered by

anaerobic glycolysis. This limit is a characteristic of the individual, and it is higher in an athlete than in an untrained subject; to a certain extent, it is malleable in that it can be elevated by training.

What Sets the Limit for Aerobic Metabolism Is Not Obvious

In order to approach the question of what sets the limit for aerobic metabolism, we must consider the entire pathway of O_2 from the site of O_2 uptake in the lung to the O_2 sink in the mitochondria. In Fig. 1 this pathway is broken into four steps, and the functional and structural variables that affect the specific transfer function are identified. Under steady-state conditions, the flow rate $\dot{V}_{O_2}$ through each step must be equal to O_2 consumption rate; accordingly, if $\dot{V}_{O_2}max$ is measured under steady-state conditions, such as in endurance exercise, each of the steps experiences the maximal flow rate, or the maximal stress, that is imposed on it by the system.

The obvious question is (a) whether there is a single step in this pathway which sets the limit to $\dot{V}_{O_2}$, with all others maintaining appreciable excess capacity or redundancy, or (b) whether the limits set by the different steps are approximately matched to each other and to the overall limit of the system. We would also like to know whether the limiting factors are primarily structural or functional.

Structural Parameters Are Prime Candidates as Potential Limiting Factors of $\dot{V}_{O_2}max$

Figure 1 shows that structural parameters intervene at all levels of the pathway. For example, the model predicts that the pulmonary diffusing capacity depends on the surface area available for gas exchange between air and blood, that stroke volume is determined by the

---

C. R. Taylor: Museum of Comparative Zoology, Harvard University, Cambridge, Massachusetts 02138.

E. R. Weibel: Department of Anatomy, University of Berne, CH-3000 Berne 9, Switzerland.

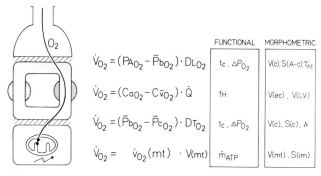

	FUNCTIONAL	MORPHOMETRIC
$\dot{V}_{O_2} = (P_{A_{O_2}} - \bar{P}_{b_{O_2}}) \cdot DL_{O_2}$	t_c, ΔP_{O_2}	$V(c)$, $S(A-c)$, τ_{ht}
$\dot{V}_{O_2} = (C_{a_{O_2}} - C\bar{v}_{O_2}) \cdot \dot{Q}$	f_H	$V(ec)$, $V(LV)$
$\dot{V}_{O_2} = (\bar{P}_{b_{O_2}} - \bar{P}_{c_{O_2}}) \cdot DT_{O_2}$	t_c, ΔP_{O_2}	$V(c)$, $S(c)$, δ
$\dot{V}_{O_2} = \dot{v}_{O_2}(mt) \cdot V(mt)$	$\dot{m}_{ATP}$	$V(mt)$, $S(im)$

FIG. 1. Model of respiratory system identifying, at each level, the functional and morphometric parameters that determine the transfer ratios.

size of the heart ventricles, that the O_2 transport capacity of the blood is determined by the erythrocyte volume, and, finally, that the capacity of cells for oxidative phosphorylation is related to the volume of mitochondria.

Structural parameters cannot be regulated or changed on a short time scale because this requires slow morphogenetic processes, but they can be modified in response to chronically altered functional demand. Thus it is well known that in exercise, cardiac output is regulated by increasing heart frequency up to a certain maximum with stroke volume unchanged; as a consequence of training, however, heart size increases and maximal cardiac output becomes elevated by larger stroke volume at the same maximal frequency [1].

This kind of observation suggests that the limit for $\dot{V}_{O_2}$ may be set primarily by structural parameters.

Good Design Calls for Matched Limits: The Hypothesis of Symmorphosis

The question, therefore, is whether the structural design of the system is such that it allows the limits to $\dot{V}_{O_2}$ of the sequential steps of Fig. 1 to be matched to each other and to the overall limit. In a way, common sense dictates that this should be the case, since it does not make sense for the body to build and maintain, at high cost, structures of a fundamental and vital functional system that it will never use. In order to approach this question, we have proposed the hypothesis of symmorphosis [2], which, in short terms, postulates that the design of all the components making up the system is matched to functional demand, a hypothesis that can be tested.

The test of the hypothesis of symmorphosis can proceed in two ways:

1. We can use structural data to calculate model values for a theoretical functional capacity at each level, and we can test (by experiment) to what extent this capacity is exploited at $\dot{V}_{O_2}$max; this depends on the availability of good theoretical models.

2. In a more pragmatic approach, noting that $\dot{V}_{O_2}$max varies among species and individuals, we can study the variation of structural and functional parameters in relation to the variation in $\dot{V}_{O_2}$max and then try to come to a conclusion with regard to their relative effect on determining $\dot{V}_{O_2}$max.

We shall primarily follow the second approach.

TESTING THE HYPOTHESIS: LEARNING FROM COMPARATIVE PHYSIOLOGY

Variations in $\dot{V}_{O_2}$max Offer Test Cases for the Study of Limiting Factors

The limit of aerobic metabolism in humans ranges from 40 ml O_2 min^{-1} kg^{-1} body mass in an untrained person to about 80 ml O_2 min^{-1} kg^{-1} in a top endurance athlete. Some of this difference is a result of training. More typically, however, systematic training for endurance exercise can increase $\dot{V}_{O_2}$max in an individual by about 1.5-fold [1]. We call this change "induced variation" in $\dot{V}_{O_2}$max.

Larger variations in $\dot{V}_{O_2}$max are observed between mammalian species related to two types of selection pressures:

1. *Allometric variation.* Metabolic requirements are related to body mass (M_b) in such a way that small animals have a higher metabolic rate than large ones; thus, standard $\dot{V}_{O_2}$ is proportional to $M_b^{0.75}$, and $\dot{V}_{O_2}$max $\sim M_b^{0.8}$ [3]. Accordingly, mass-specific $\dot{V}_{O_2}$max/M_b ranges from 48 to 420 ml min^{-1} kg^{-1} [0.8 to 7 ml sec^{-1} kg^{-1}] between a 450-kg cow and a 2-g shrew (Fig. 2), according to $\dot{V}_{O_2}$max/$M_b \sim M_b^{-0.2}$. A useful comparison is to say that, at $\dot{V}_{O_2}$max, a mouse consumes some six times more O_2 than a cow, per unit body mass.

2. *Adaptive variation.* In several size classes, nature has selected species for athletic performance by adaptation to environment and behavioral patterns (Fig. 2). Thus we find that nature's athletes, such as horses, ponies, and dogs, have a $\dot{V}_{O_2}$max that is 2.5 times higher than more normal or sedentary species of similar size, such as steers, calves, and goats [4,5].

A Study of Nature's Experiments Can Reveal Fundamental Design Principles

The combined study of adaptive and allometric variation using the same strategy affords a good set of data

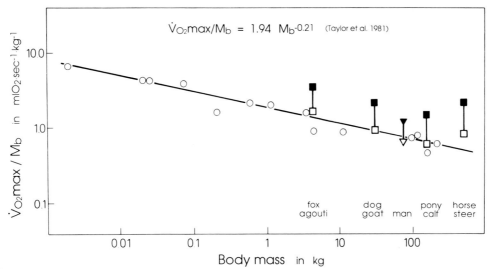

FIG. 2. Mass-specific maximal O_2 consumption as a function of body mass in mammals. Open circles and regression line are for the allometric series ranging from wood mice to elands (3). Squares represent adaptive pairs (4,5); note that the athletic species, as well as human athletes (filled triangle), lie clearly above the allometric range for "normal" $\dot{V}_{O_2}$max.

to test the hypothesis of matched limits or of symmorphosis. The reason is that the causes of variation in $\dot{V}_{O_2}$max are different:

1. In allometric variation the fundamental variable is time: Small animals have a shorter life span; they operate most functions at faster rates (e.g., stride frequency of locomotion, respiratory and heart frequency, etc.), and thus the rate of ATP consumption is higher (6).

2. In adaptive variation, in contrast, time constants are not different between the species pairs, since these have the same body size, and basal or standard metabolic rate is similar; in the athletic species the higher $\dot{V}_{O_2}$max is simply related to their higher work capacity, which involves a larger active muscle mass (7).

The approach will be to go through the respiratory system step by step, beginning at the mitochondria and proceeding to the lung. By comparing the changes in structural and functional variables to the variations in $\dot{V}_{O_2}$max, we will attempt to identify parameters that vary in proportion to $\dot{V}_{O_2}$max, whose ratio to $\dot{V}_{O_2}$max is, accordingly, invariant in both types of variation. We shall specifically be searching for invariant ratios of the type

Design parameter/Functional parameter

where the functional parameter is $\dot{V}_{O_2}$max, the measure of the dominant overall function of the respiratory system.

OXYGEN CONSUMPTION BY THE MITOCHONDRIA: MUSCLES SET THE DEMAND

When humans or animals exercise at their maximal rates of oxygen consumption, the mitochondria located in their skeletal muscles consume more than 90% of the oxygen (8). Therefore, we can concentrate on the design of these particular mitochondria as we begin our search for invariant design parameters in the respiratory system.

First we need to ask, What is the relevant structural parameter of the skeletal mitochondria to relate to the large variations in $\dot{V}_{O_2}$max/M_b with body size and adaptation? The mitochondrion is bounded by a continuous outer membrane and contains a second inner membrane that forms multiple infoldings, the cristae. The oxygen is consumed in the process of oxidative phosphorylation of ATP, and the respiratory chain enzymes that catalyze these reactions are built into the inner membrane. It is estimated that 40% of its surface is made up of these proteins of energy transduction (9). Therefore the surface area of the inner membrane, S(im), appears to be an appropriate structural parameter to relate to $\dot{V}_{O_2}$max; however, in practice it is difficult and time-consuming to measure.

One of the first general findings to emerge from comparative studies is that the area of inner mitochondrial membrane per unit volume of skeletal muscle mitochondria is invariant at 35 $\mu m^2/\mu m^3$ (9,10). It does not depend on whether the mitochondria is in a muscle that is highly aerobic and continuously active (e.g., the diaphragm) or in one that is relatively inactive, or whether it is in a mouse, a horse, a cow, or a human.

It follows from this constant relationship that the volume of mitochondria in the skeletal muscle is a good measure of the quantity of respiratory chain enzymes present (11) and therefore also an appropriate structural parameter to relate to $\dot{V}_{O_2}$max. The maximal rate of oxygen consumption by the mitochondria then can be expressed as the product of V(mt) and a functional parameter:

$$\dot{V}_{O_2}max/M_b = V(mt)/M_b \cdot \dot{v}_{O_2}(mt) \qquad [1]$$

where $\dot{v}_{O_2}(mt)$ is the rate at which each unit volume of mitochondria consumes oxygen.

How do these parameters change as $\dot{V}_{O_2}max/M_b$ is varied with size and adaptation? Since time is the fundamental variable in allometric variation, we would anticipate *a priori* that $\dot{v}_{O_2}(mt)$ would vary directly with $\dot{V}_{O_2}max/M_b$, being six times greater in a mouse than a cow, whereas $V(mt)/M_b$ should be invariant. This would seem to be an eminently reasonable design principle, since the relative volume of the muscle fibers occupied by mitochondria would not increase with demand. This is because the volume of muscle per unit mass, $V(muscle)/M_b$, follows the general allometric rules of organ size and is invariant with body size. On average, skeletal muscles make up about 40–45% of the total body mass (6). If $V(mt)/M_b$ changed with $\dot{V}_{O_2}max/M_b$, the contractile machinery would become progressively more diluted as demand increased; this might pose a serious problem for small animals, in which mitochondria could occupy a significant fraction of the total cell volume.

Contrary to our expectations, small animals have more mitochondria in each gram of their muscles than do large animals. Quantitative measurements of mitochondrial volume in animals spanning a range of body mass from 20 g (wood mice) to 500 kg (horses or steers) reveal that the mitochondrial volume of the skeletal muscles varies nearly directly with $\dot{V}_{O_2}max$ over the entire size range of mammals (12,13), whereas $\dot{v}_{O_2}(mt)$, calculated by dividing $\dot{V}_{O_2}max$ by V(mt), does not change with size (Fig. 3). When compared to the cow, the mouse has six times the volume of mitochondria in its skeletal muscles per M_b, corresponding to the difference in $\dot{V}_{O_2}max$, so that, at $\dot{V}_{O_2}max$, each milliliter of mitochondria in both cow and mouse would consume, on the average, 4–5 ml O_2 min^{-1} (Fig. 3). Thus the 5- to 10-fold difference in $\dot{V}_{O_2}max/M_b$ is matched by corresponding differences in the amount of mitochondrial structure that animals build, whereas the functional parameter, the rate at which each unit of structure consumes oxygen, is the same, irrespective of size.

Why is the fundamental design principle of time con-

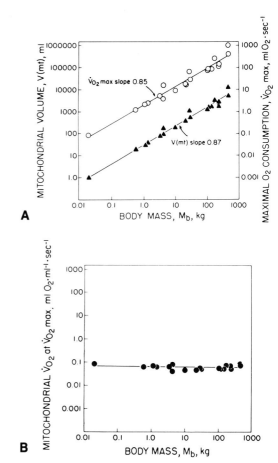

FIG. 3. The $\dot{V}_{O_2}$max and whole-body muscle mitochondrial volume, V(mt), have nearly equal slopes when plotted logarithmically against body mass (**A**), resulting in an invariant mitochondrial O_2 consumption rate at $\dot{V}_{O_2}$max (**B**). (From ref. 19.)

stants varying with size violated with respect to mitochondria? A possible explanation may lie in their origin and their genetics. The enzyme systems of mitochondria and their spatial organization within membranes are very similar to those found in bacteria. So similar, in fact, that it has been suggested that mitochondria evolved from bacteria that were incorporated into the first eukaryotes in an endosymbiotic relationship (14). This is supported by the finding that mitochondria contain their own DNA and ribosomes which are both similar to those of bacteria. If we consider mitochondria simply as endosymbiotic bacteria that respond to increased energy demand by reproducing, then their individual size and composition do not change and there is no reason to expect that the rates of their enzymes will change with O_2 demand.

If we now consider the adaptive pairs, we find that mitochondria have adapted to the 2.5-fold differences in aerobic capacity among animals of the same size in the same way that mitochondria adapted to differences with allometry (11,12). The higher demand is met by simply building more of the same structure. The 2.5 times greater $\dot{V}o_2max/M_b$ of dogs, ponies, and horses compared to that of goats, calves, and steers is matched by a 2.5 times larger volume of mitochondria in their muscles, whereas the average rate at which each milliliter of mitochondria consumes oxygen is the same, namely, 4–5 ml O_2 ml min^{-1} (Table 1).

Overall, this comparative approach has revealed that the rate of maximal O_2 consumption by skeletal muscle mitochondria is invariant at

$$\dot{V}o_2(mt) = 4\text{–}5 \text{ ml } O_2 \text{ ml}^{-1} \text{ min}^{-1}$$

and, accordingly,

$$V(mt)/\dot{V}o_2max = 0.2 \text{ ml}/(ml \ O_2 \ min^{-1}) = \text{Invariant}$$

under all circumstances.

Surprisingly, this invariant parameter also appears to apply reasonably well to the mitochondria of the heart. The oxygen consumption of the left heart has been calculated from measurements of work rate for the adaptive pairs while they exercise at $\dot{V}o_2max$. When this value is divided by the mitochondrial volume, one also obtains approximately 4 ml O_2 ml^{-1} min^{-1} (15).

The invariant 4–5 ml O_2 ml^{-1} min^{-1} is a minimal value for rate of oxygen consumption of the mitochondria, since it assumes that all of the mitochondria are active and consuming oxygen at the same rate. Although this may be a reasonable assumption for the heart where all of the fibers are active, only 30–40% of the muscle fibers are active in the skeletal muscles when animals exercise at $\dot{V}o_2max$ (16). However, it is not as bad as it might seem, since most of the mitochondria are located in these fibers because in heavy endurance exercise it is the oxidative, mitochondria-rich fibers which are active. Recently, it has been found that the respiratory capacity of isolated mitochondria is about 5.8 ml O_2/milliliter of mitochondria when physiologically reasonable substrates such as succinate are used (9). Using this value it appears that animals are able to exploit 60–80% of the *in vitro* oxidative capacity when they exercise at $\dot{V}o_2max$. This indicates that most of the skeletal muscle mitochondria are utilized at $\dot{V}o_2max$ and that they operate at close to their maximal rates. The invariant estimate of $\dot{V}o_2(mt)$ suggests that the same fraction of skeletal muscle mitochondria is utilized in all of the animals.

It should be noted that humans are different (see Chapter 5.6.3.). Because of bipedal locomotion, they normally reach $\dot{V}o_2max$ while performing exercises that do not involve all of their muscles, and average $\dot{V}o_2(mt)$ is only half of what we find in animals. The mitochondria of the muscles that are involved, however, appear to consume oxygen at close to the same

maximal rate that we find in the animal studies (17,18; see also Chapter 5.5.2.1).

We can conclude that there is a good match between structure and function in the design of the respiratory system at the level of the mitochondria with allometric and adaptive variations in $\dot{V}o_2max$. In both cases the differences in maximal rates of oxygen consumption are matched by corresponding differences in the amount of mitochondrial structure, whereas the average rate at which each unit of structure consumes oxygen is invariant.

THE FLOW OF OXYGEN FROM CAPILLARIES TO MITOCHONDRIA

Oxygen diffuses from the capillaries to the mitochondria, and the flow of oxygen at this step can be described as the product of a conductance and a pressure head (Fig. 1):

$$\dot{V}o_2max = DTo_2 \cdot (Pbo_2 - Pco_2) \qquad [2]$$

where Pbo_2 is the mean capillary and Pco_2 is the mean intracellular Po_2. The conductance, DTo_2, extends from the erythrocytes in the capillaries to the mitochondrial oxygen sinks. We do not, as yet, have a model or set of measurements that allows us to formulate the dependence of DTo_2 on functional and structural variables. What can we use as a relevant structural parameter to relate oxygen flow at this step in the respiratory system to the variations in $\dot{V}o_2max$?

In general terms, the maximal conductance must be related to the volume of capillaries in skeletal muscles, V(c), a structural parameter that has been measured. V(c) is directly proportional to the capillary surface area available for diffusion of oxygen out of the blood, since the diameter of capillaries does not change with size or adapatation. V(c) also plays an important role in determining the time available for diffusion as blood transits the capillary network.

Using $V(c)/M_b$ as the structural parameter, we can express the maximal flow of oxygen through this step in the respiratory system in the same way we have considered oxygen consumption by the mitochondria, expressed as the product of $V(c)/M_b$ and a functional parameter, $\dot{V}o_2(c)$, the rate at which oxygen diffuses out of each unit volume of capillaries:

$$\dot{V}o_2max/M_b = [V(c)/M_b] \cdot \dot{V}o_2(c) \qquad [3]$$

We would expect these parameters would change with variations in $\dot{V}o_2max/M_b$ in parallel to the structural and functional parameters of the mitochondria that set the demand. What do we find?

With allometry, small animals have more capillaries in each gram of their muscles than do large animals.

TABLE 1. *Changes of morphometric and physiologic parameters of muscle mitochondria and capillaries, and of heart with adaptive variation of $\dot{V}_{O_2}max$ in three species pairs[a]*

Species pair	Mitochondria			Capillaries			Heart		
	$\dfrac{\dot{V}_{O_2}max}{M_b}$ (ml sec⁻¹ kg⁻¹)	$\dfrac{V(mt)}{M_b}$ (ml kg⁻¹)	$\dfrac{V(mt)}{\dot{V}_{O_2}max}$ (ml ml⁻¹ sec)	$\dfrac{V(c)}{M_b}$ (ml kg⁻¹)	$V_v(ec)$	$\dfrac{V(c) \cdot V_v(ec)}{\dot{V}_{O_2}max}$ (ml ml⁻¹ sec)	f_H (min⁻¹)	$\dfrac{V_s}{M_b}$ (ml kg⁻¹)	$\dfrac{V_s \cdot V_v(ec)}{\dot{V}_{O_2}max/f_H}$ (ml ml⁻¹ sec²)
25–30 kg									
Dog	2.29	40.6	17.7	8.2	0.50	1.79	274	3.17	0.15
Goat	0.95	13.8	14.5	4.5	0.30	1.42	268	2.07	0.144
D/G	2.4*	2.9*	1.2	1.8*	1.68*	1.26	1.02	1.53*	1.04
150 kg									
Pony	1.48	19.5	13.2	5.1	0.42	1.45	215	2.50	0.198
Calf	0.61	9.2	15.1	3.2	0.31	1.63	213	1.78	0.252
P/C	2.4*	2.13*	0.9	1.6*	1.35*	0.89	1.02	1.40*	0.78
450 kg									
Horse	2.23	30.0	13.5	8.3	0.55	2.05	202	3.11	0.228
Steer	0.85	11.6	13.7	5.3	0.40	2.49	216	1.52	0.198
H/S	2.6*	2.6*	1.0	1.6*	1.4*	0.82	0.94	2.1*	1.13

[a] Data from refs. 10–13. Asterisk denotes significant ratio.

When quantitative measurements of capillary volume are made on the same individuals for whom mitochondria volume measurements were made, one finds that average capillary volume/M_b, like mitochondrial volume/M_b, decreases in direct proportion to $\dot{V}O_2max/M_b$ over the size range of 20 g (mice) to 500 kg (horses), whereas the rate of oxygen delivery per milliliter of capillary, $\dot{v}o_2(c)$, is nearly the same over the entire size range of animals (19). Thus we can conclude that

$\dot{V}O_2max/V(c)$ is invariant with size

$$= 15 \text{ ml } O_2 \text{ min}^{-1} \text{ ml}^{-1}$$

This constant value for $\dot{v}o_2(c)$, like that for $\dot{v}o_2(mt)$, is a minimal value which assumes that at $\dot{V}O_2max$, all of the capillaries are utilized and that oxygen diffuses out of all of them at the same rate. Regardless of whether or not this is the case, it clearly indicates that the capillary surface available for diffusion increases directly with the rate of diffusion of oxygen out of the capillaries over the 5- to 10-fold differences in $\dot{V}O_2max/M_b$ with size. Also, we can see the ratio of V (c)/V(mt) must also be invariant (i.e., ~0.3 ml of capillaries for each ml of mitochondria), since both $\dot{V}O_2max/V(mt)$ and $\dot{V}O_2max/V(c)$ are invariant with size (20).

With adaptive variation, we find a different pattern of adjustment of capillaries to oxygen demand (21). Capillary volume/M_b changes by only 1.7-fold with the 2.5-fold difference in $\dot{V}O_2max/M_b$ between the dog–goat, pony–calf, and horse–steer pairs (Table 1). Using Eq. 3, we can calculate that oxygen diffuses out of each milliliter of capillary (each square centimeter of its surface) at 1.5 times the rate in the more aerobic species. Part of the explanation for this higher rate of diffusion lies in a 1.6-fold higher oxygen concentration of the arterial blood entering the capillary and a corresponding 1.6-fold greater extraction of oxygen as the blood transits the capillary bed. This results from a 1.5-fold higher hemoglobin concentration in the blood of the athletic species, which is due to higher hematocrit or erythrocyte concentration, $V_V(ec, blood)$ (Table 1). Multiplying the 1.7-fold greater volume of capillaries by the 1.6-fold greater extraction of oxygen across the capillary provides a 2.7-fold greater oxygen delivery during its transit through the capillary bed.

We can conclude that there is a reasonably good match between structure and function at the level of the capillaries. In the case of allometric variations in $\dot{V}O_2max/M_b$, the higher rates of oxygen consumption are matched by corresponding differences in the amount of capillary structure, whereas the rate at which O_2 diffuses from each square centimeter of capillary surface is invariant in this case. The design of the capillaries at this level is closely matched to that of the mitochondria that consume the oxygen. In adap-

tive variation, capillaries are incompletely matched, but this is compensated by a higher hemoglobin or erythrocyte concentration. For both allometric and adaptive variation, it therefore appears that the mass of hemoglobin in capillaries is matched to the mass of mitochondria; this is achieved by varying capillary volume and hemoglobin concentration. The invariant ratio of structural parameters, therefore, is expressed as

$$V(ec)/V(mt) = M(Hb)/V(mt) \sim 4 \times 10^{-2} \text{ g ml}^{-1}$$

and, consequently, we find that the invariant ratio to $\dot{V}O_2max$ is expressed as

$$\{V(c) \cdot V_V(ec)\}/\dot{V}O_2max = 1.8 \text{ ml}/(\text{ml } o_2 \text{ sec}^{-1})$$

and thus involves two structural variables, namely, capillary volume and erythrocyte concentration in the blood.

CONVECTIVE TRANSPORT OF OXYGEN BY THE CIRCULATION

Oxygen is transported from the capillaries in the lung to the capillaries in the muscle by the circulation. Delivery of oxygen by the circulation depends on the properties of the heart as the pump and on those of the blood as the carrier, and both can be varied to adjust to differences in demand. Oxygen flow at this step can be described as the product of the maximal cardiac output, $\dot{Q}max/M_b$, times the difference in arteriovenous oxygen concentration, $Cao_2 - C\bar{v}o_2$ (Fig. 1):

$$\dot{V}O_2max/M_b = (\dot{Q}max/M_b) \cdot (Cao_2 - C\bar{v}o_2) \quad [4]$$

The relevant structural parameter of the pump is obviously the size of the heart, which determines the amount of blood pumped with each contraction, Vs. The flow of blood at this step is the product of Vs/M_b and a functional parameter, f_H, the maximal frequency of contraction of the pump:

$$\dot{Q}max/M_b = f_H \cdot Vs/M_b \quad [5]$$

$Cao_2 - C\bar{v}o_2$ will depend on a second structural parameter, namely, the amount of hemoglobin or erythrocytes contained in the blood.

In allometric variation we would anticipate that time (i.e., f_H) would vary with size, while the structural parameters, [Hb] and Vs/M_b, would be invariant. What information we have supports this idea. On average, the heart makes up the same fraction of body mass over the size range of mammals from mice to cows, about 0.58% (22); likewise, hemoglobin concentration and oxygen-carrying capacity of the blood do not vary systematically with body size. Mammals spanning a range of body size from bats to horses have, on average, about 13 g of hemoglobin per 100 ml of blood, which can carry 17.5 ml of oxygen (6). The invariant heart size and O_2 capacity of the blood suggest that allometric differences in circulatory transport are brought about entirely by increases in heart frequency. Furthermore, heart frequency at rest varies directly with oxygen consumption (23). This suggests that V_s/M_b and $(Ca_{O_2} - C\bar{v}_{O_2})$ will also be invariant with size at $\dot{V}_{O_2}max$, and a higher f_H will account for all of the variation in $\dot{V}_{O_2}max$. However, measurements of these circulatory parameters at $\dot{V}_{O_2}max$ do not exist for a large enough size range of animals to draw any definitive conclusions.

The structural and functional variations in circulatory transport of oxygen with adaptive variation are very clear-cut. Here the animals follow the general principles of design: f_H is determined by size, and structures vary with O_2 demand (Table 1). Maximal heart frequencies of goats and dogs, ponies and calves, and horses and steers are nearly identical for animals of the same size, despite 1.4- to 2.0-fold differences in $\dot{Q}max/M_b$ and a 2.5-fold difference in $\dot{V}_{O_2}max/M_b$ (5,15). The structural parameters V_s/M_b and hemoglobin concentration account for all of the 2.5-fold difference in oxygen delivery at this step. These studies indicate that these animals are operating at or close to the upper limit of their structural capacity for convective transport of oxygen in the circulatory system at $\dot{V}_{O_2}max$ (4). Available structures (stroke volume and hemoglobin concentration) for both $\dot{Q}max$ and $(Ca_{O_2} - C\bar{v}_{O_2})$ appear fully exploited by the time an animal has increased its oxygen consumption from resting to maximal levels. Thus at this step of O_2 transport in the respiratory system there appears to be a match between maximal rates of O_2 delivery and the structures involved, a finding that is in accord with the predictions of symmorphosis.

The limited information we have therefore suggests that the structural parameters V_s/M_b and $V_v(ec,blood)$ are invariant in allometric variation, but variant in adaptive variation, whereas the functional parameter f_H is invariant in adaptive variation, but variant in allometric variation.

Accordingly, the ratio of design to functional parameters, which is invariant with both allometric and adaptive variation, involves two structural and two functional parameters:

$$\{V_s \cdot V_v(ec,blood)\}/\{\dot{V}_{O_2}max/f_H\} = \text{Invariant}$$

That heart frequency is involved is not surprising, since it must be considered to be a dominant functional parameter when size varies: The heart of a cow cannot beat as fast as that of a mouse.

THE FLOW OF OXYGEN FROM AIR TO BLOOD IN THE LUNG

The transfer of O_2 from the air to the blood in the lung is achieved by diffusion. The O_2 flow rate is determined by the product of the partial pressure difference as driving force and the conductance of the gas exchanger (24), such that (Fig. 1)

$$\dot{V}_{O_2} = DL_{O_2} \cdot (PA_{O_2} - \bar{Pb}_{O_2}) \qquad [6]$$

The partial pressure difference between alveolar air and capillary blood is a functional variable that essentially depends on (a) the ventilation of alveoli through the airways and (b) the perfusion of capillaries by the circulation. In contrast, the diffusion conductance for O_2, the diffusing capacity DL_{O_2}, is largely determined by the following structural parameters (Fig. 1): the alveolar and capillary surface areas [S(A) and S(c)]; the harmonic mean barrier thicknesses of the tissue barrier (τht) and of the plasma layer separating erythrocytes from the endothelium (τhp); and the capillary blood volume [V(c)]. The model used to calculate DL_{O_2} from these morphometric data, as well as its strength and limitations, is discussed in Chapter 4.2.8.

The morphometric parameters entering the calculation of DL_{O_2} are essentially determined by two variables: the lung volume, V(L), and the size or density of the "building blocks" of the gas-exchange units in lung parenchyma. The ultimate building block of the gas exchanger is the alveolar septum, with morphometric characteristics being the fraction of septum occupied by capillaries, the capillary volume per septal (alveolar) surface, V(c)/S(A), and the harmonic mean thickness of the tissue barrier. These septa are built into the acinus as alveolar walls in the form of a three-dimensional maze; accordingly, the alveolar surface density, $S_V(A)$, is a measure of the building-block characteristics of lung parenchyma. This hierarchical design provides several options for varying diffusing capacity. Thus the total alveolar surface area, S(A), is the product of V(L) and the alveolar surface density, $S_V(A)$; furthermore, capillary volume is the product of V(c)/S(A) and S(A). To increase DL_{O_2}, the lung would have to increase, for example, the alveolar surface area, and this can be achieved by either increasing lung volume or increasing the alveolar surface density by packing more alveolar septa into the unit volume of lung parenchyma. Alternatively or additionally, the loading of capillaries onto the septum could be increased.

The first question with respect to design of the gas exchanger is which of these options are used, or whether any of these basic design parameters are invariant with allometric and adaptive variation of $\dot{V}_{O_2}max$.

Let us first consider lung volume. The general notion is that mass-specific lung volume is invariant with body size. At closer inspection we find, however, that VL increases slightly (but significantly) with $M_b^{1.06}$ (25), with the result that VL/M_b varies from 35 ml kg^{-1} in shrews and mice to 60 ml kg^{-1} in dog, man, and cow and can even reach 100 ml kg^{-1} in the horse. In adaptive variation, lung volume is an important variable, being larger in the athletic species (26,27).

Among the building-block characteristics, the parameters that characterize septum structure are invariant in adaptive variation (26,27), but they show a weak allometric variability (25). Thus, capillary loading varies between 0.7 and 1.7 ml m^{-2} from shrew to horse, increasing with $M_b^{0.05}$. The same regression is found for the harmonic mean barrier thickness, which measures 0.27 μm in the shrew and 0.65 μm in the horse. The ratio of tissue to blood in the septum, however, is invariant under all circumstances.

The packing of alveolar septa into lung parenchyma, measured by $S_V(A)$ (which is inversely proportional to alveolar diameter), appears to be invariant in the size range of animals between 1 and 100 kg (28), assuming values of 400–500 cm^{-1}. However, it increases drastically in small mammals, up to 1500 cm^{-1} in the shrews, and it falls to 250 cm^{-1} in large mammals, so that over the entire mammalian size range we find $S_V(A)$ to decrease with $M_b^{-0.11}$. In adaptive variation, $S_V(A)$ is invariant, except in the dog–goat pair (26,27).

As a result of these variations, the combined building-block parameter of the gas-exchange unit, $DLO_2/V(L)$, decreases slightly with $M_b^{-0.07}$ in allometric variation, but it remains invariant in adaptive variation, again with the exception of the dog–goat pair (26,27).

An additional building-block parameter is important, namely, hematocrit or erythrocyte concentration in the blood. As discussed above, this parameter is invariant with allometry, but it is variant in adaptive variation (Table 1).

In conclusion, we find that the fundamental building block, the alveolar septum, is invariant in its composition but that it can vary its thickness (resulting in increased capillary loading and barrier thickness) as well as its packing into the parenchymal air space; this variation occurs with allometry, but not usually in adaptive variation. Mass-specific lung volume is a weak variant with allometry, but it can show important variation in adaptive variation; in a recent study of the pronghorn antelope, whose $\dot{V}O_2$max is twice that of the dog, we found the increase in lung volume (to nearly 5 liters for a 20-kg animal!) to account for most of the adaptive lung change (*unpublished observation*). Quite evidently, all these parameters are subject to a number of constraints. The lung volume is limited by the space available in the chest cavity. The packing of alveolar septa into the air space is limited by the requirements for adequate ventilation, as well as by mechanical constraints related to surface tension. The smaller the alveoli, the greater the surface forces; and the larger the alveoli, the more costly the alveolar ventilation. Mammals may indeed have found an optimum range for the size of these building blocks from which they deviate only in the very small species, and perhaps in the largest but to a lesser extent.

How are these building blocks related to O_2 uptake at $\dot{V}O_2$max? Specifically, is O_2 uptake by the unit capillary volume invariant? We find that it is not. In allometry, $\dot{V}O_2$max/V(c) varies with $M_b^{-0.2}$, ranging from 12 ml O_2 min^{-1} ml^{-1} in large animals to 42 ml O_2 min^{-1} ml^{-1} in small (500 g) animals, and it may go even higher in mice and shrews (25). In adaptive variation, we find that athletic species load about twice as much O_2 onto their blood per unit time, a rate that appears to be about proportional to their higher hematocrit (26,27) (Table 2). Oxygen uptake rate by the pulmonary capillary unit is therefore clearly not invariant, in partial contrast to the muscle capillaries where we have found the discharge rate $\dot{V}O_2$max/V(c) to be invariant with allometric variation, whereas a similar difference was found between the adaptive pairs. It is noteworthy that the rates are similar in lung and muscle capillaries, at least in the nonathletic species; the observed differences can be explained by different transit times.

When we now consider the total pulmonary diffusing capacity, we must note that it is composed of two main components (see Chapter 4.2.8.): (i) the membrane diffusing capacity, DM_{O_2}, which is exclusively determined by structural variables, and (ii) the blood or erythrocyte diffusing capacity, De_{O_2}, which depends on capillary blood volume and hematocrit, two parameters that are also subject to some functional variation.

The hypothesis of symmorphosis predicts that DM_{O_2} and DL_{O_2} should be proportional to $\dot{V}O_2$max. This is not the case. In Fig. 4 we have plotted DL_{O_2} and $\dot{V}O_2$max for the allometric series; we note that mass-specific DL_{O_2} does not change with size, so that the ratio $DL_{O_2}/\dot{V}O_2$max increases with $M_b^{0.2}$. This means that a 300-kg cow has six times as much diffusing capacity available as a 30-g mouse to accomplish O_2 uptake at $\dot{V}O_2$max. What this means is that the driving force for O_2 uptake in the lung is smaller in the cow than in the mouse, but why this occurs is unknown. Various possibilities have been suggested, such as (a) appreciable differences in capillary transit time (29) or (b) differences in the pressure head PA_{O_2} as a result of the fact that the size of acini varies considerably

TABLE 2. Changes of morphometric pulmonary diffusing capacity, mean capillary transit time (tc), and alveolar–capillary P_{O_2} difference at $\dot{V}_{O_2}$max, with adaptive variation of $\dot{V}_{O_2}$max in three species pairs[a]

Species pair	$\dot{V}_{O_2}$max/M_b (ml sec^{-1} kg^{-1})	DL_{O_2}/M_b (ml min^{-1} mmHg^{-1} kg^{-1})	$\dot{V}_{O_2}$max/Vc (ml O_2 sec^{-1} ml^{-1})	tc (sec)	ΔP_{O_2}[b] (mmHg)	DL_{O_2}/$\dot{V}_{O_2}$max (mmHg^{-1})
25–30 kg						
Dog	2.29	7.07	0.54	0.29	22.4	0.052
Goat	0.95	4.78	0.21	0.47	12.5	0.084
D/G	2.4*	1.48*	2.6*	0.62*	1.8*	0.61*
150 kg						
Pony	1.48	4.71	0.47	0.35	21.9	0.053
Calf	0.61	2.99	0.25	0.38	13.7	0.082
P/C	2.4*	1.57*	1.9*	1.04	1.6*	0.65*
450 kg						
Horse	2.23	6.48	0.51	0.40	19.2	0.048
Steer	0.85	3.24	0.31	0.49	15.5	0.064
H/S	2.6*	2.0*	1.6*	0.83	1.24*	0.76*

[a] Data from refs. 26 and 27. Asterisk denotes significant ratio.
[b] From Bohr integration.

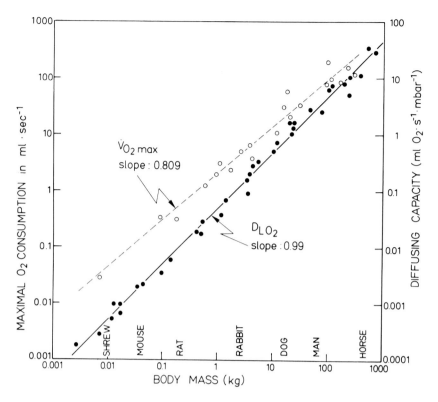

FIG. 4. The allometric slope for morphometric pulmonary diffusing capacity is clearly different from that of $\dot{V}_{O_2}$max. (From ref. 34.)

with body size (30,31), and this could influence alveolar ventilation (32).

In adaptive variation we find that the athletic species have a larger DL_{O_2}/M_b than the nonathletic animals, but this increase is not proportional to the differences in $\dot{V}_{O_2}$max/M_b. Here again, athletic species accomplish their higher O_2 uptake rate by adding to their increased DL_{O_2} an elevated driving force (Table 2). In this instance we were able to show that this is partly due to the fact that the athletic species use a greater fraction of their transit time to accomplish equilibration of the capillary blood with alveolar air, namely about 80%, whereas the sedentary species use only 50%, with the remainder appearing as a redundancy (27,33).

In conclusion, we find that the ratio $DL_{O_2}/\dot{V}_{O_2}$max is not invariant, neither in allometric nor in adaptive variation. To find an invariant ratio we must consider all structural and functional variables, because only the following equation applies:

$$DL_{O_2}/(\dot{V}_{O_2}max/\Delta P_{O_2}) = \text{Invariant}$$

We must therefore conclude that the hypothesis of symmorphosis is not, or only partially, fulfilled with respect to the pulmonary gas exchanger. Functional variables are used to a large extent to modulate the rate of O_2 uptake even at $\dot{V}_{O_2}$max. This is possible because the pulmonary gas exchanger maintains an appreciable level of redundancy or excess capacity (33). One is tempted to speculate that maintaining such re-

dundancy in that part of the respiratory system that forms the interface with the environment may well be a survival strategy, allowing the organism to cope with adverse environmental factors such as hypoxia. It has indeed been shown that goats can maintain their $\dot{V}_{O_2}$max even at high altitude (33), presumably because their gas exchanger is redundant when judged under sea-level conditions.

CONCLUSIONS

In undertaking this integrated study of the respiratory system we have first asked whether O_2 consumption is limited at a single step, with all other steps maintaining excess capacity or redundancy, or whether the conductances at the sequential transfer steps were approximately matched. By comparing allometric and adaptive variation we found that variation in the design parameters and in the functional parameters occurred at every step. The correlations of these variations were variably tight, were strongest with respect to mitochondrial volume, and often involved a combination of several parameters. It therefore appears unlikely that a single step or a single parameter of the pathway is the limiting factor for $\dot{V}_{O_2}$.

We then asked specifically whether the design of the system is such as to allow the limits to $\dot{V}_{O_2}$ at each of the steps to be matched to each other and to the overall limit, namely, the maximal oxygen demand imposed by energy needs. This amounted to testing the hypothesis of symmorphosis. We approached this by searching for structural and functional parameters that remained invariant with allometric and adaptive variation in $\dot{V}O_2$max—on the one hand, parameters that defined structural building blocks of the system; on the other hand, ratios with $\dot{V}O_2$max.

At the level of the mitochondria, the hypothesis of symmorphosis holds in its simplest and tightest form: The mitochondrial building blocks—namely, their inner membrane with the respiratory chain—are invariant in all instances studied, and so is the ratio $V(mt)/\dot{V}O_2$max.

Capillary volume is invariant both with respect to mitochondrial volume and to $\dot{V}O_2$max in allometric variation, but not in adaptive variation. In the latter case we find an important variation in hematocrit. As a result, the ratio of capillary erythrocyte volume to mitochondrial volume, and the ratio $\{V(c)\cdot V_V(ec)\}/\dot{V}O_2$max are invariant. Thus, symmorphosis is fulfilled by the combination of two structural parameters, namely, capillary volume and erythrocyte concentration in the blood.

With respect to O_2 transport by the circulation, none of the structural parameters was found to be invariant with both types of variation. The ratio of stroke volume, as the measure of functional heart size, to $\dot{V}O_2$max was not invariant in either case; the ratio of the erythrocyte volume ejected with each stroke, $Vs(ec)$, to $\dot{V}O_2$max was invariant in adaptive variation only. The simplest invariant ratio was $\{Vs\cdot V_V(ec)\}/\{\dot{V}O_2max/f_H\}$—that is, the ratio of erythrocyte stroke volume to $\dot{V}O_2$max divided by heart frequency. The reason for this is that heart frequency is a very strong and obligatory variable in allometric variation (where time constants are the main variables) and thus is a *dominant* factor in determining design and function of circulation under all circumstances.

The conductance of the pulmonary gas exchanger, its diffusing capacity DL_{O_2}, is determined by a large number of structural variables, some of which, such as hematocrit and capillary volume, may partly be subject to functional regulation. With regard to the structural building-block parameters, we merely found the volumetric composition of the alveolar septum to be invariant in all instances; the other building-block parameters were invariant in adaptive variation but were variant in allometric variation. None of the ratios of $\dot{V}O_2$max to morphometric parameters (single or combined) or to DL_{O_2} was invariant, neither with allometric variation nor with adaptive variation. This refutes the hypothesis of symmorphosis for the pulmonary gas exchanger, although DL_{O_2} did vary consistently in the direction of $\dot{V}O_2$max in adaptive variation, but not to the extent where a match would be achieved. The invariant ratio was $DL_{O_2}/\{\dot{V}O_2max/\Delta P_{O_2}\}$. This may be trivial, but, in analogy to the observation made above that heart frequency is a dominant factor in setting O_2 transport by the blood, we would have to consider whether ΔP_{O_2} could play a similar role in determining O_2 uptake in the lung, since ΔP_{O_2} may well be determined by some strong boundary conditions external to the gas exchanger. On the other hand, we have demonstrated, in the case of adaptive variation, that the pulmonary gas exchanger maintains a certain degree of redundancy which may be variable for reasons yet unknown. The most important consideration, however, is that the lung establishes the interface between the respiratory system and the environment and that the redundancy observed under sea-level conditions disappears in high-altitude hypoxia, where, indeed, the lung can become the limiting factor for O_2 uptake. Redundancy of the pulmonary gas exchanger may be a survival strategy for coping with "dominant" environmental conditions.

REFERENCES

1. Saltin B, Blomqvist B, Mitchell JH, Johnson RL Jr, Wildenthal K, Chapman CB. Response to submaximal and maximal exercise after bed rest and training. *Circulation* 1968(Suppl 7);38:1–78.
2. Taylor CR, Weibel ER. Design of the mammalian respiratory system. I. Problem and strategy. *Respir Physiol* 1981;44:1–10.
3. Taylor CR, Maloiy GMO, Weibel ER, Langman VA, Kamau JMZ, Seeherman MJ, Heglund NC. Design of the mammalian respiratory system. III. Scaling maximum aerobic capacity to body mass: wild and domestic mammals. *Respir Physiol* 1981;44:25–37.
4. Taylor CR, Karas RH, Weibel ER, Hoppeler H. Adaptive variation in the mammalian respiratory system in relation to energetic demand. II. Reaching the limits to oxygen flow. *Respir Physiol* 1987;69:7–26.
5. Jones JH, Longworth KE, Lindholm A, Conley KE, Karas RH, Kayar SR, Taylor CR. Oxygen transport during exercise in large mammals. I. Adaptive variation in oxygen demand. *J Appl Physiol* 1989;67(2):862–870.
6. Schmidt-Nielsen K. *Scaling: Why is animal size so important?* Cambridge, MA: Cambridge University Press, 1984.
7. Weibel ER, Taylor CR, Hoppeler H, Karas RH. Adaptive variation in the mammalian respiratory system in relation to energetic demand. I. Introduction to problem and strategy. *Respir Physiol* 1987;69:1–6.
8. Mitchell JH, Blomqvist G. Maximal oxygen uptake. *N Engl J Med* 1971;284:1018–1022.
9. Schwerzmann K, Hoppeler H, Kayar SR, Weibel ER. Oxidative capacity of muscle and mitochondria: correlation of physiological, biochemical and morphometric characteristics. *Proc Natl Acad Sci USA* 1989;86:1583–1587.
10. Hoppeler H, Mathieu O, Krauer R, Claassen H, Armstrong RB, Weibel ER. Design of the mammalian respiratory system. VI. Distribution of mitochondria and capillaries in various muscles. *Respir Physiol* 1981;44:87–111.
11. Hoppeler H, Kayar SR, Claassen H, Uhlmann E, Karas RH. Adaptive variation in the mammalian respiratory system in relation to energetic demand. III. Skeletal muscles: setting the demand for oxygen. *Respir Physiol* 1987;69:27–46.
12. Mathieu O, Krauer R, Hoppeler H, Gehr P, Lindstedt SL, Alexander RMcN, Taylor CR, Weibel ER. Design of the mammalian respiratory system. VII. Scaling mitochondrial volume in skeletal muscles to body mass. *Respir Physiol* 1981;44:113–128.

13. Hoppeler H, Jones JH, Lindstedt SL, Longworth KE, Taylor CR, Straub R, Lindholm A. Relating maximal oxygen consumption to skeletal muscle mitochondria in horses. In: Gillespie JR, Robinson NE, eds. *Equine physiology II.* Davis, CA: ICEEP, 1987;278–289.

14. Margulis L. *Symbiosis in cell evolution.* San Francisco: Freeman, 1981.

15. Karas RH, Taylor CR, Rösler K, Hoppeler H. Adaptive variation in the mammalian respiratory system in relation to energetic demand. V. Limits to oxygen transport by the circulation. *Respir Physiol* 1987;69:65–79.

16. Armstrong RB, Taylor CR. Relationship between muscle force and muscle area showing glycogen loss during locomotion. *J Exp Biol* 1982;97:411–420.

17. Anderson P, Saltin B. Maximal perfusion of skeletal muscle in man. *J Physiol (Lond)* 1985;366:233–249.

18. Hoppeler H, Lindstedt SL. Malleability of skeletal muscle tissue in overcoming limitation: structural elements. *J Exp Biol* 1985;115:355–364.

19. Taylor CR, Weibel ER, Hoppeler H, Karas RH. Matching structures and functions in the respiratory system: allometric and adaptive variations in energy demand. In: Wood SC, ed. *Comparative pulmonary physiology: current concepts.* New York: Marcel Dekker, 1989;27–65.

20. Hoppeler H, Mathieu O, Weibel ER, Krauer R, Lindstedt SL, Taylor CR. Design of the mammalian respiratory system. VIII. Capillaries in skeletal muscles. *Respir Physiol* 1981;44:129–150.

21. Conley KE, Kayar SR, Rösler K, Hoppeler H, Weibel ER, Taylor CR. Adaptive variation in the mammalian respiratory system in relation to energetic demand. IV. Capillaries and their relationship to oxidative capacity. *Respir Physiol* 1987;69:47–64.

22. Prothero J. Heart weight as a function of body weight in mammals. *Growth* 1979;43:139–150.

23. Stahl WR. Scaling of respiratory variables in mammals. *J Appl Physiol* 1967;22(3):453–460.

24. Bohr C. Ueber die spezifische Tätigkeit der Lungen bei der respiratorischen Gasaufnahme. *Scand Arch Physiol* 1909;22:221.

25. Gehr P, Mwangi DK, Ammann A, Sehovic S, Maloiy GMO, Taylor CR, Weibel ER. Design of the mammalian respiratory system. V. Scaling morphometric pulmonary diffusing capacity to body mass: wild and domestic mammals. *Respir Physiol* 1981;44:61–86.

26. Weibel ER, Marques LB, Constantinopol M, Doffey F, Gehr P, Taylor CR. Adaptive variation in the mammalian respiratory system in relation to energetic demand. VI. The pulmonary gas exchanger. *Respir Physiol* 1987;69:81–100.

27. Constantinopol M, Jones JH, Weibel ER, Taylor CR, Lindholm A, Karas RH. Oxygen transport during exercise in large mammals: oxygen uptake by the pulmonary gas exchanger. *J Appl Physiol* 1989;67(2):871–878.

28. Weibel ER, Gehr P, Cruz-Orive LM, Müller AE, Mwangi DK, Haussener V. Design of the mammalian respiratory system. IV. Morphometric estimation of pulmonary diffusing capacity; critical evaluation of a new sampling method. *Respir Physiol* 1981;44:39–59.

29. Lindstedt SL. Pulmonary transit time and diffusing capacity in mammals. *Am J Physiol* 1984;246:R384–R388.

30. Rodriguez M, Bur S, Favre A, Weibel ER. Pulmonary acinus: geometry and morphometry of the peripheral airway system in rat and rabbit. *Am J Anat* 1987;180:143–155.

31. Haefeli-Bleuer B, Weibel ER. Morphometry of the human pulmonary acinus. *Anat Rec* 1988;220:401–414.

32. Weibel ER, Taylor CR, Gehr P, Hoppeler H, Mathieu O, Maloiy GMO. Design of the mammalian respiratory system. IX. Functional and structural limits for oxygen flow. *Respir Physiol* 1981;44:151–164.

33. Karas RH, Taylor CR, Jones JH, Reeves RB, Weibel ER. Adaptive variation in the mammalian respiratory system in relation to energetic demand. VII. Flow of oxygen across the pulmonary gas exchanger. *Respir Physiol* 1987;69:101–115.

34. Weibel ER. *The pathway for oxygen.* Cambridge, MA: Harvard University Press, 1984.

THE LUNG: *Scientific Foundations*
edited by R.G. Crystal, J.B. West et al.
Raven Press, Ltd., New York © 1991.

CHAPTER 5.7.1

General Physiology of Sleep

Christian Guilleminault and William C. Dement

Sleep influences every physiological process, and it has been shown that each sleep state has not only a unique physiology but a specific pathology as well. Wakefulness, rapid eye movement (REM) sleep, and non-rapid eye movement (NREM) sleep are conventionally defined by brain-wave pattern, muscle tone, and possible oculomotor activity and its type.

Sleep is part of a cyclical phenomenon (1). The sleep/wake rhythm in adults is part of a 24-hr or circadian cycle controlled by an endogenous pacemaker that is active even in an isolated, time-cue-free environment. The nucleus suprachiasmaticus is thought to play a significant role in the maintenance of the mammalian circadian rhythm. At birth, human sleep is not well developed, and its classic index, the 24-hr rhythmic core (in this case, rectal) temperature, is not yet present; it is first noted in a normal full-term infant between 6 and 8 weeks of age (2,3). The sleep/wake cycle and the 24-hr rhythm are therefore progressively established during the first 3 months of life.

INFANT SLEEP (4)

Because the classic states—REM and NREM sleep—cannot be easily identified at birth, sleep has been subdivided into (a) active sleep (AS), which is similar to REM sleep in adults, (b) quiet sleep (QS), and (c) indeterminate sleep (IS) (4). Most of IS and QS are probably NREM sleep, and it is only when a sufficient dendritic sprouting has occurred, near 12 weeks of age, that brain waves are sufficiently characteristic to distinguish between NREM and REM sleep (5–7). Premature and full-term newborn infants exhibit an appreciable lack of concordance between characteristic

electroencephalographic (EEG) patterns, electromyography, eye movements, respiratory patterns, and somatic activity (8). Active (REM) sleep can be recognized by 28 gestational age (GA), but it is only by 36 GA that the sleep of the fetus and the preterm infant begins to assume a more mature character and can be dissociated more easily into AS and QS (8). During the newborn period, infants spend two-thirds of the 24-hr period in sleep; by 6 months of age, they spend only half of their time asleep. The proportion of time spent in AS (REM) during the 24-hr period is gradually reduced from one-third to one-fourth of sleep time. During that period, QS and IS are evolving toward NREM sleep but remain strikingly constant. The reduction in REM sleep is balanced by an increase in wakefulness. This change is associated with a progressive increase in behavioral control of many physiological systems. Simultaneous with the progressive change in state proportion during the 24-hr cycle is a consolidation of each state. Between 6 and 8 weeks of age, sleep becomes more predictable, and by 12 weeks of age, the longest sleep period is distributed between 8 p.m. and 6 a.m. (6). The evolution of the longest wake period is slower but is clearly recognizable in the 3- to 4-month-old infant between 4 and 8 p.m. REM sleep, which at birth is seen at the onset of each sleep period, becomes integrated into the longest sleep period and progresses until it eventually follows NREM sleep. By the time the infant reaches 6 months of age, the so-called sleep onset REM periods, seen at onset of nocturnal sleep and daytime naps, have disappeared, and daytime naps contain disproportionately less REM sleep than exists during nocturnal sleep (5,6). A reorganization of REM sleep during the 24-hr period is occurring. However, it will take nearly 12 months, during which more and more REM sleep is seen at the end of the nocturnal period, to attain the adult pattern.

NREM sleep is considered by most researchers to be scorable as such by the time an infant is 3 months

C. Guilleminault and W. C. Dement: Sleep Disorders Center, Stanford University School of Medicine, Stanford, California 94305.

of age (4). This is related to the development of specific EEG patterns. Although the electroencephalogram is only a poor representation of the underlying neuronal discharges, specific EEG patterns such as sleep spindles, delta waves, and K-complexes indicate that brain activity and the neuronal discharges underwriting physiological behaviors are gradually changing during sleep. Between 2 and 4 months of age, the infant's sleep spindles and K-complexes allow the scoring of stage II NREM sleep (which soon becomes the most important sleep stage) and delta (stages III–IV NREM) sleep. In the 3-month-old infant, delta sleep is already seen, mostly at the beginning of the nocturnal sleep period, after which it decreases significantly by the end of the night. Between 6 and 12 months of age, therefore, the infant exhibits the classic features of sleep stage and state distribution throughout the 24-hr period: (a) nocturnal sleep with a large distribution of delta sleep when sleep commences, along with a large amount of REM sleep toward the end of the nocturnal period; (b) a peak of alertness just before nocturnal sleep; (c) a nap period in the early afternoon (persisting in adulthood as the time of peak daytime drowsiness); and (d) development of clear cycles during nocturnal sleep (4–7).

A cycle is normally defined as a sequence of NREM–REM sleep. The disappearance of the sleep-onset REM period during the first 2 months of age allows calculation of a cycle interval that lasts about 60 min by 6 months of age and that reaches 90 min during early childhood. Very early in life, therefore, the sleep patterns seen in adulthood are established, but the changes that occur during the first weeks of life indicate that adult sleep is the result of a progressive organization that occurs after birth and that is linked to the day/night cycle.

ADULT SLEEP

NREM and REM sleep are seen throughout life, and few changes occur until the onset of old age (9). The cycles persist, with longer REM periods being seen in the early morning hours. The percentage of delta sleep decreases with age. Brief arousals and movement times are much more frequent up to 12 weeks of age and are responsible for the poor sleep efficiency that reappears in old age. Classically, the sleep of a young adult consists of four or five NREM–REM sleep cycles, with sleep onset associated with clear changes in EEG pattern and the appearance of slow eye movements (9). The first cycle is usually shorter than those in the early morning (90 min versus 110 min). The sleeper passes through stage I (light sleep), then stage II and stages III and IV, before reaching REM sleep. The first REM period is short (a mean of 10 min), whereas the early morning REM period can last for 45 min. Delta sleep is prominent during the first two cy-

cles and is not seen in the early morning hours, when stage I and (mostly) stage II represent the NREM sleep that is followed by REM sleep (10).

REM SLEEP

In REM sleep, muscle activity is suppressed or greatly reduced (10–12). This muscle atonia in cats, as well as hypotonia in primates and humans, is related to an active hyperpolarization of spinal-cord motoneurons. The excitability of alpha motoneurons is depressed by a postsynaptic inhibition that is present throughout the entire REM sleep period (12). Although hyperpolarization potentials can be identified throughout REM sleep, these are most prominent during the transition from NREM to REM sleep and whenever intensive clusters of rapid eye movements are present (13). The continuous postural atonia is defined as "tonic" REM sleep, and "phasic" events (such as rapid eye movements or abrupt muscle twitches) occur against this background of tonic, active inhibition. In the cat, these phasic events are associated with neurophysiological events recorded in the pons, the lateral geniculate, and the occipital lobe, as ponto-geniculo-occipital (PGO) waves (12,13). During phasic REM sleep, motor excitations and inhibitions occur, superimposed on the tonic changes of the motor system. The membrane potential of the motoneurons fluctuates rapidly in an apparently random manner. The tonic REM sleep is characterized not only by postural atonia but also by neocortical EEG desynchronization, hippocampal theta waves, brain temperature elevation, and changes in cerebral blood flow. Phasic REM sleep is characterized by twitches of limbs and facial musculature, abrupt autonomic nervous system changes responsible for cardiorespiratory irregularities, and PGO waves.

The anatomical support for REM sleep has been investigated through lesions, stimulation, and the injection of substances (14,15). Bilateral combined mediolateral caudal pontine tegmental lesions induce a loss of muscle atonia. Elimination of REM sleep was seen with combined lesions that also included the nucleus reticularis pontis caudalis. The exact location of the brainstem neurons generating all aspects of REM sleep is still unknown (11–13). However, pharmacologic studies have long suggested an important role for cholinergic muscarinic neurons. Direct injection of the cholinergic agonist carbachol in the pontine tegmentum has been repeatedly shown to elicit a state similar to REM sleep (12,14). Physostigmine injected into a preparation called *cerveau isolé* (15) led to muscle atonia accompanied by rapid eye movement. The dog model of narcolepsy (16), a disease of REM sleep, has been shown to be sensitive to physostigmine, which worsens the abrupt, REM-sleep-like muscle atonia that is, on the other hand, helped by muscarinic antagonists such as atropine. Recently, cholinergic cells in a circuit of interlocking cells and fibers extending from the dorsolateral pons to the ventromedial medulla have been identified and seem to be involved in REM sleep muscle atonia. Also appearing to be involved in REM sleep generation are (a) alpha-1 and alpha-2 adrenergic neurons with pre- and postsynaptic locations and (b) alpha-2 neurons located in the locus ceruleus.

NREM SLEEP

A behavioral quiescent state that occurs periodically is not dependent on the EEG pattern—especially not on delta waves, which are normally used to define sleep. Cats with midbrain transections (high decerebrate proportion) exhibit activity, quiescence, and REM sleep. These states are controlled by brainstem structures below the level of the transection, indicating that behavior signs characteristic of NREM sleep can be seen when the brainstem is sectioned below the intercollicular level (11,13,14). NREM mechanisms have also been linked with forebrain structures (17). Electrical stimulation of the lateral-preoptic–basal-forebrain region induces EEG synchronization and behavioral sleep, as does localized warming or injection of cholinergic substances into this brain region. It thus seems that the neural control of NREM sleep is anatomically diffuse, involving forebrain and brainstem structures (11,13,17).

Although NREM and REM sleep each appear to be linked to specific brain regions, sleep may not be controlled by a specific neuronal network but may, instead, be secondary to the interaction of many neurons in different brain regions.

SLEEP SUBSTANCES (18)

An endogenous basis for sleep has been hypothesized for many years. This suggestion stems from the simple observation that prolonged wakefulness leads to a desire for sleep. Studies of rabbits and goats have also shown that injection of cerebrospinal fluid from sleep-deprived animals has induced sleep. Pappenheimer et al. (19) reported on a factor S that accumulated during wakefulness and led to sleep. Several factors, mostly peptides, have been hypothesized to be responsible for sleep. Factor S has been identified as muramyl peptides, but interleukin I also promotes sleep; moreover, several of the sleep-stimulating peptides have also been shown to stimulate the immune system. However, if certain peptides injected intraventricularly appear to induce sleep, it is unclear whether this is related to a specific effect or whether sleep is secondary to nonspecific changes such as increase in temperature due to the associated activity of the peptides studied.

Borbely and Tobler (20) proposed criteria essential for the identification of a specific sleep substance. The substance must (a) induce and/or maintain physiological sleep, (b) have a dose-related relationship, (c) show no species specificity, (d) be present in the organism, (e) exhibit an endogenous level–state relationship, and (f) be chemically identifiable.

It must be acknowledged that to date no putative sleep peptide fulfills all of the above criteria. Interestingly, most putative sleep factors thus far described are also immunologically active in the sense that they are produced by, or are bound by, leucocytes and/or are implicated in the initiation and/or regulation of the immune response (21). We have mentioned the muramyl peptides and interleukin I, but the list is long and involves the delta-sleep-inducing peptide arginine-vasotocin, vasoactive intestinal peptide, growth-hormone-releasing factor, somatostatin, cholecystokinin, desacetyl alpha-melanocyte-stimulating hormone, corticotropin-like intermediate lobe peptide, neuropeptide Y, alpha-interferon, tumor necrosis factor, lipid A/endotoxin, prostaglandins (PGE_2), veridine, adenosine, and so on (18). Krueger and Karnovsky (21) have emphasized that many regulatory substances are shared by the central nervous system and the immune system and that many of the peptides considered as putative somnogenic agents have clear effects on both sleep and specific aspects of the immune response. Also, infectious disease is associated with an increase in slow-wave (stage III–IV NREM delta) sleep in humans and other mammals. Furthermore, mammalian macrophages process bacterial cell walls that release somnogenic substances such as muramyl peptides, and glia and macrophages both can produce several somnogenic immunoactive substances such as interleukin I, prostaglandin, and alpha-interferon. On the other hand, sleep deprivation and/or the stress associated with it affect certain aspects of the immune response. Krueger and Karnovsky (21) believe that these findings suggest an interaction between sleep and the immune response and that sleep plays a role in the recuperative process. However, even if certain experimental data suggest the participation of such substances in a somnogenic and immunologic response, it is unclear at this time whether, under normal conditions, any of these substances has a physiological role in the control of sleep.

INTERACTION BETWEEN SLEEP AND THE PHYSIOLOGICAL SYSTEM (22)

Endocrine System

We have indicated that sleep/wake is part of the circadian cycle. Many hormones also manifest a circadian variation, often with a peak during the day and a secretory trough during the night (23). The combination of inactivity, sleep, and the nocturnal period has led many initial investigators to ignore the influence of one of these factors in hormonal regulation. However, systematic displacement of the three different variables at various times of the circadian rhythm has allowed investigation of the role of sleep and sleep states in many hormonal secretory patterns. Investigation of release of anterior pituitary hormones has shown that growth hormone secretion is triggered at sleep onset and that sleep fragmentation (and disappearance of delta sleep in children) may greatly reduce its secretion. Prolactin secretion is similarly augmented during sleep, whereas thyroid-stimulating hormone and (to a lesser degree) cortisol are suppressed at sleep onset. Systematic studies have shown that hormones can be subdivided into two groups, depending on the degree of relationship with sleep and sleep states. Growth hormone, prolactin, and luteinizing hormone at puberty, for example, are tightly linked to sleep, whereas cortisol, ACTH, testosterone, and luteinizing hormone in adults are loosely linked to sleep.

Sleep and the Autonomic Nervous System

The interaction between parasympathetic and sympathetic tone during the different sleep states is far from having been entirely explored. As for the endocrine system, there are variations related to inactivity, to the circadian timing, and to sleep and sleep states. Once again, the use of specific protocols with dissociation of each of these three components is necessary to appropriately evaluate the role of sleep states with regard to the autonomic nervous system. The interaction between the autonomic nervous system and sleep was first focused upon during investigation of the cardiovascular system (24). The parasympathetic tone, which is mostly responsible for the modulation of heart rate during sleep, is enhanced during both NREM and tonic REM sleep, whereas the sympathetic tone is reduced. During phasic REM sleep, an inhibition of parasympathetic tone occurs, followed by a phasic inhibition of sympathetic output and simultaneous increase in parasympathetic discharges. These changes occur in rapid succession and have been investigated mostly in cats, using lesion experiments (vagotomy and stellectomy) and pharmacological agonists and antagonists (11,22).

Cardiovascular Physiology

Zanchetti, Mancia, and co-workers (25–28) have performed multiple investigations on cardiovascular regulation during sleep in cats and have applied some of their findings to human investigations. Blood pressure drops during sleep, resulting from the combined effect of circadian timing, supine inactivity, and sleep states. The lowest blood pressure is noted during delta (stage III–IV NREM) sleep. During NREM sleep in cats, there is a change in total peripheral conductance compared with that in wakefulness, with a decrease in cardiac output accompanying a slight reduction in conductance (25). These two contrasting changes prevent blood pressure from showing more than a modest fall. During the tonic phase of REM sleep, there is a drop in cardiac output associated with an increase in total peripheral conductance, leading to a further drop in blood pressure. The vasodilatation is mostly a result of the increase in conductance in mesenteric and renal vascular beds. Local reflexes are responsible for a simultaneous increase in skeletal muscle vesicle resistance, indicating clear regional differences. During phasic REM sleep, blood pressure oscillates and brief rises are noted, both in hypertensive and in normal subjects, with the percentage of change being similar for both groups. Tonic REM sleep hypotension, however, is not seen in humans (25–28).

The coronary circulation in humans is also subject to brief changes in phasic REM sleep pressure. Investigation of the cat has shown that chemoreceptors, and not baroreceptors, are responsible for buffering tonic REM sleep hypotension. Chemoreceptor denervation greatly increases tonic REM sleep hypotension, to the point of impairing cerebral circulation. This action involves chemoreceptor-dependent sinoaortic reflexes. The baroreflexes are also diminished during REM sleep in the cat, but baroreflex control of the heart in humans is monitored during sleep. The reduced renal blood flow noted during phasic REM sleep may play a role in a REM-sleep-related reduction in urine volume. Unlike the changes in mesenteric and renal circulation, the cerebral blood flow is greatly increased during total (tonic and phasic) REM sleep.

Heart rate is greatly influenced by sleep and is reduced during sleep in most animal species and in humans (24). This is an important point, since many (but not all) ventricular arrhythmias are heart-rate-dependent (29,30). Heart rate is lowest during delta sleep, and variability increases during REM sleep—particularly phasic REM sleep, when a short-lasting tachycardia may be followed by a rebound bradycardia following the phasic autonomic nervous system/phasic REM sleep modulation.

The many changes involving the control of (a) ventilation, (b) upper-airway and diaphragmatic muscles, and (c) respiratory accessory muscles will be reviewed in other chapters of this book. But an understanding of the changes in the motor system controls during NREM and REM sleep can help to explain some of the changes, which will be outlined in the other chapters.

THERMOREGULATION AND TEMPERATURE CYCLE (31)

Sleep onset is associated with a fall in rectal temperature and in the temperature of the brain, particularly the hypothalamus, while skin temperature increases with peripheral vasodilatation in the neutrothermic environment, together with increased sweating (32,33). The lowest body temperature is monitored during the early morning hours. During NREM sleep, thermoregulation is maintained, but this involves a lowering of the set-point of control of body temperature. During the transition from wakefulness to sleep, an inactivation of the thermoregulatory mechanisms of cortical control and a release of autonomic controls occur. This transition is associated with instability resulting from the adjustment of the system. When delta sleep occurs, the stability of temperature regulation, dependent on automatic functions, is at its maximum. The hypothalamic thermoregulatory mechanisms control the evolution of the sleep cycle according to the prevailing needs of homeothermic maintenance or sleep (31–33). During NREM sleep, when automatic controls are operating, thermoregulation is dependent on the circadian cycle and inactivity. With the onset of REM sleep, drastic changes occur (31,34). Thermoregulatory responses are greatly abated, and at low ambient temperatures, body temperature decreases. Shivering, thermal vasodilatation, thermal tachypnea (panting), sweating, and overall heat production with oxygen consumption disappear. Neither cooling nor heating of the hypothalamus entrains a thermoregulatory response. The absence of shivering during REM sleep is independent of the REM sleep atonia, as demonstrated by investigation of cats with brainstem lesions that lead to REM sleep without atonia. The inactivation of thermoregulatory mechanisms during REM sleep is the most impressive physiologic change indicative of the nonapplicability of the concept of homeostasis. This is particularly obvious during phasic REM sleep. It is important to note that there is a relationship between (a) outside temperature and (b) sleep and sleep states. High and low temperatures at the limits of acceptability lead to decreased or absent REM sleep (31). There is thus a continuous interaction between thermoregulation (or its absence) and sleep states (31,35). In a neutrothermic environment during an organized day/night, wake/sleep cycle, the 24-hr temperature cycle is linked to the sleep/wake cycle, with the trough of the 24-hr temperature cycle occurring during sleep in the middle of the night. The propensity or likelihood of a subject to present REM sleep onset (i.e., episodes of falling asleep in REM sleep) is maximal close to the trough of the temperature rhythm or during the ascending phase, which would be in the early morning hours. Subjects placed in a time-cue-free environment will have a tendency to move from a sleep/wake cycle based upon a 24-hr day to a genetically based cycle whose population range will be between 23 and 27 hr, with a median around 25 hr. There will thus be a dissociation between the 24-hr temperature rhythm and the sleep/wake cycle that will be monitored. Compared with what is observed in a normal day/night cycle, sleep onset will no longer be seen when the temperature is falling, and the subject may decide to sleep at any point of the temperature rhythm; however, the REM sleep propensity and likelihood of having REM sleep onset will still be linked to the temperature rhythm, with REM sleep still being closely related to temperature minima during the cycle.

METABOLISM AND SLEEP

Metabolic rate and daily amount of sleep are positively correlated across 53 mammalian species (36), as well as in humans, indicating that high energy expenditure during wakefulness is compensated for by increased circadian sleep duration (35).

After 2–3 days of fasting, delta sleep increases in humans and is predominant during the initial 2–3 hr of a normal nocturnal sleep period, when oxygen consumption and body temperature fall precipitously, so that metabolic rates during delta sleep tend to be the lowest of the night. A reduction in oxygen consumption, usually of about 10% but able at times to reach 40%, is noted between relaxed waking and delta sleep. Delta sleep appears to have an energy conservation role, as suggested by increased drive toward delta sleep with elevation in body temperature through a direct thermodynamic influence on metabolic rate. Amount of delta sleep is positively correlated with rectal temperature at delta sleep onset, and mean oxygen consumption is negatively correlated with the magnitude of the decline in rectal and tympanic temperature between sleep onset and end of delta sleep each night. Horne and Shackell (37) also demonstrated that the facilitation of delta sleep by body heating in humans depends on the proximity of heating to sleep onset and that it can be blocked by aspirin. Even during REM sleep (in which, associated with tympanic temperature increase, periodic increases in cerebral metabolism are seen), whole-body energy expenditure remains lower than during wakefulness, indicating that sleep is associated with energy conservation.

CONCLUSIONS

All physiological systems and types of neuronal activity are altered by sleep. Depending on the state of alertness (i.e., wakefulness, NREM sleep, or REM sleep), regulatory processes will exhibit distinct properties.

These clear changes not only will have an impact on the systemic physiology but will be responsible for development of discontinuity of regulation during state transitions, and it will lead to different, state-dependent pathology. Certain deleterious problems will only surface in relation to a specific state, or the latter will be associated with a different risk and different clinical presentations in association with specific organ lesion or dysfunction. During the past 20 years, great attention has been given to (a) the impact of the different states of alertness on the control of ventilation, (b) the interaction between state-dependent changes in motor control and respiratory muscles, and (c) the state-dependent cardiorespiratory pathology. Undoubtedly, many efforts must still be made, and until we have a better understanding of the neuronal reorganization associated with a specific state, we shall not completely apprehend the pathophysiology of many cardiorespiratory events. However, the recognition that exceedingly complex organizational changes occur in the brain with state changes will allow a better understanding of the physiology and pathology of a specific organ such as the lung.

REFERENCES

1. Kleitman N. Sleep and wakefulness, revised edition. Chicago: University of Chicago Press, 1963.
2. Kleitman N, Hoffman H. The establishment of the diurnal temperature cycle. Am J Physiol 1935;119:48–54.
3. Guilleminault C, Gould S, Hayes B, Coons S. Development of temperature rhythm in normal infants. Sleep Res 1987;17:611.
4. Guilleminault C (ed.). Sleep and its disorders in children. New York: Raven Press, 1986.
5. Coons S, Guilleminault C. The development of sleep–wake patterns and non-rapid eye movement sleep stages during the first six months of life in normal infants. Pediatrics 1982;69:793–798.
6. Coons S, Guilleminault C. Development of consolidated sleep and wakeful periods in relation to the day/night cycle in infancy. Dev Med Child Neurol 1984;26:169–176.
7. Hoppenbrouwers T, Hodgman JE, Harper RM, Sterman MB. Temporal distribution of sleep states, somatic activity and autonomic activity during the first half year of life. Sleep 1982;5:131–144.
8. Anders T, Emde R, Parmelee AH (eds.). A manual of standardized terminology, techniques and criteria for scoring states of sleep and wakefulness in newborn infants. Los Angeles: UCLA Brain Information Service/Brain Research Institute, 1971.
9. Rechtschaffen A, Kales A (eds.). A manual of standardized terminology techniques and scoring system for sleep stages of human subjects. Los Angeles: UCLA Brain Information Service/Brain Research Institute, 1968.
10. Lydic R, Biebuyck JL (eds.). Clinical physiology of sleep. Bethesda, MD: American Physiological Society, 1988.
11. Lydic R. Central regulation of sleep and autonomic physiology. In: Lydic R, Biebuyck JL, eds. Clinical physiology of sleep. Bethesda, MD: American Physiological Society, 1988;1–20.
12. Siegel JM. Brain stem mechanisms generating REM sleep. In: Kryger M, Roth R, Dement WC, eds. Principles and practice of sleep medicine. Philadelphia: WB Saunders, 1989;104–120.
13. McGinty DJ, Drucker-Colin R, Morrison A, Parmeggiani PL (eds.). Brain mechanisms of sleep. New York: Raven Press, 1985.
14. Jones BE. Neuroanatomical and neurochemical substrates of mechanisms underlying paradoxical sleep. In: McGinty DJ, Drucker-Colin R, Morrison A, Parmeggiani PL, eds. Brain mechanisms of sleep. New York: Raven Press, 1985;139–156.
15. Jouvet M. Telencephalic and rhombencephalic sleep in the cat. In: Wolstenholme GEE, O'Connor M, eds. The nature of sleep. CIBA Foundation Symposium. London: Churchill, 1961;188–206.
16. Baker TL, Dement WC. Canine narcolepsy–cataplexy syndrome: evidence for an inherited mono-aminergic cholinergic imbalance. In: McGinty DJ, Drucker-Colin R, Morrison A, Parmeggiani PL, eds. Brain mechanisms of sleep. New York: Raven Press, 1985;139–156.
17. McGinty DJ, Sterman MB. Sleep suppression after basal forebrain lesions in the cat. Science 1968;160:1253–1255.
18. Inoue S, Schneider-Helmert D, eds. Sleep peptides: basic and clinical approaches. Berlin: Springer-Verlag, 1988.
19. Pappenheimer JR, Koski G, Fencl V, Karnovsky WL, Krueger JM. Extraction of sleep promoting factor S from cerebrospinal fluid and from brain of sleep deprived animals. J Neurophysiol 1975;38:1299–1311.
20. Borbely AA, Tobler I. The search for an endogenous "sleep substitute." TIPS 1980;1:356–358.
21. Krueger JM, Karnovsky WL. Sleep and the immune response. Ann NY Acad Sci 1987;496:510–516.
22. Orem J, Barnes CD. Physiology in sleep. New York: Academic Press, 1980.
23. Parker DC, Rossman LG, Kripke DF, Hershman JM, Gibson W, Davis C, Wilson K, Pekary E. Endocrine rhythms across sleep–wake cycle in normal young men under basal state conditions. In: Orem J, Barnes CD, eds. Physiology in sleep. New York: Academic Press, 1980;146–180.
24. Baust W, Bohnert B. The regulation of heart rate during sleep. Exp Brain Res 1969;7:169–180.
25. Mancia G, Zanchetti A. Cardiovascular regulation during sleep. In: Orem J, Barnes CD, eds. Physiology in sleep. New York: Academic Press, 1980;1–55.
26. Manilla G, Baccelli G, Adams DB, Zanchetti A. Vasomotor regulation during sleep in the cat. Am J Physiol 1971;220:1086–1093.
27. Baccelli G, Albertini R, Mancia G, Zanchetti A. Control of regional circulation by the sino-aortic reflexes during desynchronized sleep in the cat. Cardiovasc Res 1978;12:523–528.
28. Mancia G, Zanchetti A. Hypothalamic control of autonomic functions. In: Morgans AJ, Panskepp J, eds. Handbook of hypothalamus. New York: Marcel Dekker, 1980;147–222.
29. Winkle RA. The relationship between ventricular ectopic heart rate frequency and heart rate. Circulation 1982;66:439–446.
30. Gillis AM, Guilleminault C, Partinen M, Connolly SJ, Parrish D, Winkle RA. The diurnal variability of ventricular premature depolarizations: influence of heart rate and level of arousal. Sleep 1989:12;391–399.
31. Glotzbach SP, Heller HC. Thermoregulation. In: Kryger M, Roth T, Dement WC, eds. Principles and practice of sleep medicine. Philadelphia: WB Saunders, 1989;300–309.
32. Glotzbach SF, Heller HC. Changes in the thermal characteristics of hypothalamic neurons during sleep and wakefulness. Brain Res 1984;309:17–26.
33. Parmeggiani PL, Cevolani D, Azzaroni A, Ferrari G. Thermosensitivity of anterior hypothalamic–preoptic neurons during the waking–sleep cycle: a study in brain functional states. Brain Res 1987;415:79–89.
34. Palca JW, Walker JM, Berger RJ. Thermoregulation, metabolism and stages of sleep in cold exposed men. J Appl Physiol 1986;61:940–947.
35. Berger RJ, Phillips NH. Regulation of energy metabolism and body temperature during sleep and circadian torpor. In: Lydic R, Biebuyck JL, eds. Clinical physiology of sleep. Bethesda, MD: American Physiological Society, 1988;171–190.
36. Zepelin H, Rechtschaffen A. Mammalian sleep, longevity and energy metabolism. Brain Behav Evol 1976;10:425–470.
37. Horne JA, Shackell BS. Slow wave sleep elevations after body heating: proximity to sleep and effects of aspirin. Sleep 1987;10:383–392.

THE LUNG: Scientific Foundations
edited by R.G. Crystal, J.B. West et al.
Raven Press, Ltd., New York © 1991.

CHAPTER 5.7.2

Effects of Sleep on the Regulation of Breathing and Respiratory Muscle Function

Jerome A. Dempsey, James B. Skatrud, M. Safwan Badr, and Kathe G. Henke

Breathing is governed by a multifaceted control system that ensures not only the precise regulation of alveolar ventilation and arterial blood oxygen acid–base status, but also the production of a mechanically efficient breathing pattern and duty cycle and the coordination of efferent medullary motor output amongst all of the primary and accessory respiratory muscles. Accordingly, in wakefulness, even when the ventilatory control system is severely stressed by the increased requirements for gas exchange demanded by heavy exercise, any significant disruption of the normal breathing pattern is short-lived. Compensations are achieved quickly and are usually near complete in response to mechanical loads, and CO_2 retention and hypoxemia are rarely tolerated and almost always quickly corrected. Furthermore, mechanical impedance to airflow is minimized—even at very high flow rates—because the oral pharyngeal airway is appropriately "stiffened" via tonic and phasic activation of upper-airway abductor muscles so as to protect against any dynamic narrowing of the airway secondary to the development of negative intrathoracic pressure during inspiration.

In this brief review, we will examine the effects of the sleeping state on four critical features of the ventilatory control system, namely: (i) neurophysiologic changes within the central nervous system (CNS); (ii) chemoresponsiveness; (iii) respiratory muscle func-

tion; and (iv) mechanical load compensation. The implications of these fundamental effects to the control of ventilation and the stability of ventilatory pattern during sleep will be examined, with consideration of the nature of the "wakefulness" effect on ventilatory control. We recommend recent extensive reviews on some of these topics (1–4).

NEUROPHYSIOLOGIC EFFECTS OF STATE

In general, three major types of neurophysiologic changes in the CNS with sleep state have potential consequences to the regulation of breathing, namely: (i) withdrawal of the wakefulness stimulus—with major influences in non-rapid eye movement (NREM) sleep; (ii) the state of active inhibition in rapid eye movement (REM) sleep; and (iii) the fluctuating excitatory and inhibitory influences throughout REM sleep. It is likely that the changes in neurophysiologic state of the CNS would have substantial effects on respiratory motor output, given the close proximity of the sleep-state-generating neurons in the reticular activating system to respiratory medullary neurons responsible for ventilatory control. Relatively few, but important, findings in this relationship are available in the chronically instrumented, intact sleeping cat (4,5).

Electrical stimulation of pontine and suprapontine regions can—depending on the area of stimulation—cause either initiation of inspiration (e.g., stimulation of the central nucleus of the amygdala) or inhibition of inspiration (e.g., stimulation of the orbital frontal cortex). Sleep greatly attenuates these effects of stimulation. For example, in NREM sleep, respiration was no longer entrained to stimulation of the central nucleus of the amygdala as it was during wakefulness or

J. A. Dempsey, J. B. Skatrud, M. S. Badr, and K. G. Henke: The John Rankin Laboratory of Pulmonary Medicine, William S. Middleton Memorial Veterans Hospital, Madison, Wisconsin 53705; and Departments of Preventive Medicine and Medicine, University of Wisconsin–Madison, Madison, Wisconsin 53705.

REM sleep, and the average discharge rate of the nucleus was markedly reduced in NREM sleep as opposed to that in wakefulness or REM sleep (5). The spontaneous activity from ventral medullary respiratory modulated neurons decreases markedly in NREM sleep, although the sleep effect is not the same in all medullary neurons. In fact, the sleep effect on neuronal activity was shown to be greatest in those medullary neurons whose activity was *not* tightly linked to phasic respiration as opposed to those which are primarily respiratory in nature (6). Perhaps the activity of the so-called "nonrespiratory" medullary neurons, which is highly state-dependent, is affecting tonic activity to airway abductor muscles (i.e., "accessory" muscles). The sleep effect on medullary respiratory-linked neurons is consistent with the recently demonstrated effect of behavioral or voluntary control of a breath directly on these respiratory medullary neurons (7), as opposed to the traditional view of a separate cortical–spinal neural pathway for the voluntary control of breathing.

In REM sleep, activity of medullary respiratory neurons is sometimes, but not always, correlated with breathing pattern. For example, respiratory-modulated medullary neurons increase their frequency and variability of firing coincident with the variable hyperpnea and tachypnea (but not the apnea) of REM sleep. Also, the atonia of intercostal muscles in REM sleep is not accounted for by reduced central respiratory drive from medullary respiratory areas; instead, active inhibition of these motoneurons probably occurs in REM sleep (4).

Establishing these complex links among neurons concerned primarily with regulation of state and those which are primarily concerned with respiratory rhythm generation may explain the nature of the elusive "wakefulness drive" to breathe (see below).

CHEMORECEPTION

Chemoreceptor feedback is important to the precise control of alveolar ventilation in all physiologic states. During wakefulness, complete chronic denervation of the carotid bodies in mammals reduces V_A only 20–25% at rest or exercise and has no marked effect on breathing pattern (8). Even in the rare, so-called alveolar hypoventilation syndrome in humans, the ventilatory response to CO_2 is completely or almost completely absent, eupneic alveolar ventilation is clearly less, and Pa_{CO_2} is increased, but extreme hypoventilation or apneic episodes do not occur when the subject is awake. In slow-wave sleep the animal with carotid chemoreceptor denervation shows a significantly greater sleep-induced increase in Pa_{CO_2} which means that carotid bodies were important in limiting the sleep-

induced inhibition of ventilation but were not essential to providing "adequate" levels of alveolar ventilation (9). However, when the waking ventilatory response to inhaled CO_2 is absent, then prolonged apnea and marked CO_2 retention occur during sleep (10). The implication here is that while the "wakefulness" stimulus can supplement chemoreceptor stimuli and maintain ventilation, ventilation during slow-wave sleep is critically dependent on metabolic and chemical stimuli. So at least some level of chemoresponsiveness—especially medullary chemoreception—is needed to maintain ventilatory volume and rhythm during sleep. But whether the sleep state actually affects chemoreceptor responsiveness has not been directly tested, and we must depend upon indirect evidence utilizing whole-body ventilatory response tests. This approach has shortcomings.

First, consider NREM sleep effects. According to the conventional method of acutely administering hyperoxic CO_2 or isocapnic hypoxia in NREM sleep, the slope of ventilatory response is reduced by a highly variable amount (i.e., 10–15% below that in wakefulness). There is no fundamental sleep effect on the slope of the basic curvilinear response to hypoxia or the linear response to hypercapnia—at least that portion of the response slope above eupneic levels (11). Combinations of acute hypoxia and hypercapnia (i.e., asphyxia) cause ventilatory stimulation in NREM sleep, but their multiplicative effect is reduced significantly below wakefulness (12).

REM sleep effects on chemoresponsiveness are more complex. There is fairly consistent evidence that hypercapnia and hypoxia have little effect on the irregular and tachypneic pattern of REM sleep (1,10). Also, there are some claims of greatly reduced CO_2 or hypoxic ventilatory response in REM (1,10), but the problem here is that the steady-state response is rarely achieved in REM sleep. Tonic REM sleep is claimed to be identical to slow-wave sleep in terms of ventilatory response, but doubt has been expressed that a significant portion of REM sleep is spent in anything but phasic-type conditions (13). REM influences that may prevent responsiveness to many of these stimuli or inhibitors probably impinge on numerous respiratory sites [including medullary neurons (4) and phrenic spinal motoneurons] and the selective inhibition of some accessory respiratory muscles. Phillipson and Bowes (1) view the reduced response to chemical stimuli in REM sleep as a behavioral system overriding the metabolic control system, and they make interesting analogies to the reduced response of inhaled CO_2 observed in wakefulness during phonation (14).

Limited data suggest that the response to *chronic* ventilatory stimuli during REM and NREM sleep is unchanged from that during wakefulness. This has been shown in normal resting subjects over several days of hypoxic exposure (15) and during chronic progesterone administration and metabolic acidosis secondary to carbonic anhydrase inhibition (16). Chronic hypoventilation in response to sodium bicarbonate-induced metabolic alkalosis was also similar during wakefulness and sleep (3).

It is common to attribute almost any observed change in the ventilatory response to CO_2 or hypoxia in healthy persons to changes in "chemoreceptor sensitivity" of one or more specific chemoreceptors, but this interpretation of these whole-body response tests is unwarranted because the sleeping state exerts other important effects on ventilatory control. These include: (a) sleep-induced increases in airway resistance which reduced ventilatory output for any given motor command (important effects that are discussed in detail below) and (b) sleep-induced increases in cerebral blood flow which would narrow the arterial-to-cerebral venous P_{CO_2} difference and thus reduce cerebral venous effluent P_{CO_2} and presumably medullary chemoreceptor P_{CO_2} and $[H^+]$ at any given systemic P_{CO_2} (17). Thus, one would misinterpret a reduced V_E at any given $P_{ET CO_2}$ because the "actual" stimulus at the medullary chemoreceptor would be lower during sleep. This effect is especially marked in REM sleep, where cerebral blood flow may increase as much as 50–80% greater than wakefulness levels. For the same reason, the so-called isocapnic hypoxic responses would also be uninterpretable in terms of actual chemoreceptor "sensitivity" changes during sleep. In addition to these sleep effects, one cannot discount the possible changes in state of "arousal" during the progressive CO_2 response tests, which would contribute to variability in the response slope in wakefulness.

In contrast to these highly variable effects of sleep on acute and chronic chemoreceptor responses, there is a marked and highly consistent ventilatory inhibition secondary to small reductions in Pa_{CO_2} during NREM sleep. Thus during NREM sleep, as Pa_{CO_2} is gradually reduced via negative- or positive-pressure mechanical ventilation, diaphragmatic electromyogram (EMG) is completely inhibited after a 2 to 4 mmHg reduction in P_{CO_2} (Fig. 1). When Pa_{CO_2} is reduced 3–6 mmHg to the level of normal waking Pa_{CO_2}, and the ventilator abruptly stopped, 5- to 20-sec apneic periods occurred (18,19). As P_{CO_2} is lowered further below this waking set-point (i.e., <40 mmHg Pa_{CO_2}), the duration of post-hyperventilation apnea was prolonged in a linear fashion, reaching 30- to 45-sec apneic periods at −10 mmHg Pa_{CO_2}. Some of the inspiratory muscle inhibition *during* the mechanical ventilation was attributed to a mechanical "unloading" (19), but the posthyperventilation apnea was shown to be due solely to the induced hypocapnia (18,19). These sensitive inhibitory effects of hypocapnia are also produced by active (as well as passive) means as shown by the prolonged ap

neas produced when normoxia is abruptly restored following hypoxic-induced active hyperventilation (18).

We interpret these data to mean that this apneic threshold depends on the overall level of input to respiratory neurons. Thus during wakefulness, reduced input from chemoreceptors, especially central chemoreceptors, clearly inhibits ventilatory drive; however, apnea is prevented over a wide range of respiratory alkalosis because forebrain contributions to inspiratory drive in the awake state are sufficient to "replace" most of the contributions provided by the reduced $[H^+]$. Sleep state—or the loss of wakefulness—removes this extra CNS contribution, thereby unmasking a highly sensitive hypocapnic-induced apneic threshold.

An additional inhibitory influence occurs in NREM sleep because tissue CO_2 production is reduced 10–30%. This will reduce V_A and may also account for some of the increased propensity towards apnea when small reductions in Pa_{CO_2} occur in sleep.

RESPIRATORY MUSCLE FUNCTION

Postural, chest-wall, and upper-airway muscles are all subject, to varying extents, to state-related modulation of their activity. Postural muscle activity is reduced in NREM sleep with little effect on spinal reflex activity, whereas tonic postural activity in REM sleep is completely abolished. Chest-wall respiratory muscles are modified substantially. In NREM sleep, phasic inspiratory muscle EMG activities of both external intercostal and diaphragm muscles are usually increased over wakefulness (20,21). Accessory muscles of respiration may be even more "state-sensitive." For example, scalenus inspiratory muscles (which are commonly phasically active in awake humans) increase their phasic activity in NREM sleep (22) (Fig. 2). Expiratory muscle activity also increases (at least in the deeper stages of NREM sleep), as shown in (a) the internal intercostal muscle activity in the cat (23) and (b) the increased abdominal expiratory muscle activity in humans (21,22). The mechanical consequences of this respiratory muscle recruitment during NREM sleep include an increase in the relative contribution of rib cage versus abdomen to V_T (20), an augmented transdiaphragmatic pressure (21), and evidence in snorers based on gastric pressure changes of chest-wall elastic recoil following active expiration, presumably assisting the initiation of inspiration during NREM sleep (24).

During REM sleep, phasic and tonic intercostal muscle activity is greatly reduced or ceases completely; in the diaphragm, tonic EMG activity is also reduced, but phasic EMG activity continues at an elevated level (20,25). Phasic, and especially tonic, activities of in

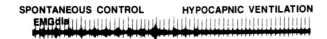

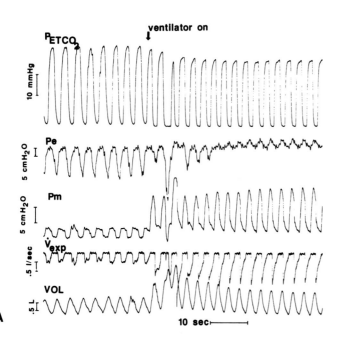

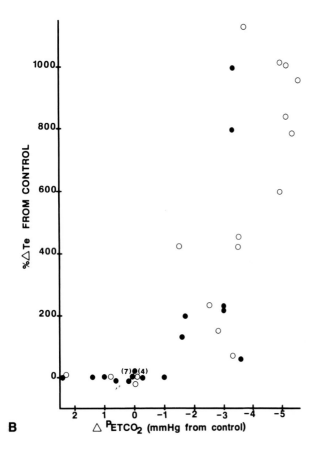

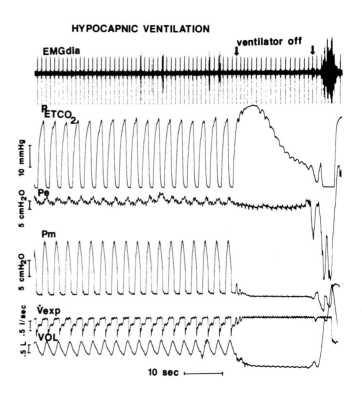

FIG. 1. A: Effects of positive-pressure ventilation and mild hyperventilation on inspiratory muscle effort (esophageal pressure and diaphragmatic EMG). Note the very quick inhibition (within three or four breaths) of inspiratory muscles secondary to the small reductions in P_{ETCO_2}, and also note the mechanical inhibition via positive-pressure ventilation. If P_{ETCO_2} was returned to its normal sleeping level as positive-pressure ventilation continued, inspiratory muscle EMG returned to within 40–60% of the eupneic control values. (From ref. 19.) **B:** Continuation of part A, showing posthyperventilation apnea. This apnea was first detected at 2–3 mmHg below eupneic P_{ETCO_2} (T_E = 2–3 times that of eupnea) and increased linearly so that at 5 torr < normal P_{ETCO_2} posthyperventilation, T_E was 10 times greater than normal T_E. T_E was never prolonged if P_{ETCO_2} was not permitted to fall during the mechanical ventilation period. (From ref. 19.)

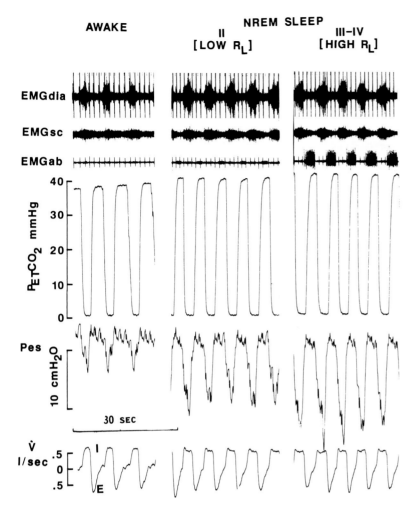

FIG. 2. Effects of NREM sleep on respiratory muscle EMG activity, airway resistance, and P_{ETCO_2} in a healthy subject. Note the augmentation of both diaphragmatic and scalenus inspiratory phasic EMG activity in all stages, and also note the appearance of abdominal muscle EMG activity in deeper (stage III–IV) sleep. Inspiratory resistance increases in all sleep stages. Note that the increased esophageal pressure and truncated inspiratory flow rate, P_{ETCO_2}, increases throughout. (From ref. 22.)

spiratory accessory muscles such as the scalenus and sternocleidomastoids are also markedly reduced in REM sleep (26), possibly causing the reduced functional residual capacity (FRC) commonly seen in REM sleep—at least in patients with obstructive lung disease. Given the marked inhibition of muscle spindle activity in REM, these differences in muscle activities between states may be due to the relative independence of diaphragm recruitment from muscle spindle feedback (27). That the inhibition of intercostal muscle activity is profound in REM sleep is dramatically illustrated by the patient with diaphragmatic paralysis who experiences little ventilatory insufficiency in NREM sleep but is rendered severely hypopneic and hypoxemic upon entering REM sleep and must arouse to resume an adequate breathing pattern (28).

Activity of the accessory respiratory muscles of the upper airway regulating tongue position and pharyngeal and laryngeal caliber is also subject to state-related modulation. In NREM sleep, tonic activity in these muscles, especially the genioglossus, is reduced. During REM sleep, tonic activity is nullified and phasic activity is reduced, often stopping completely for long periods and reappearing with NREM episodes (29).

Thus, the control of ventilatory and accessory respiratory muscles during sleep presents the dilemma that while on the one hand it is important that the diaphragm remains phasically active in all sleep stages, in many cases neither the rib cage nor the oropharyngeal airway is appropriately stiffened in preparation for the negative pressure developed by diaphragmatic contraction. The resultant inefficient (or even completely ineffective) inspiratory effort represents some of the major clinical problems with ventilatory control in sleep.

EFFECT OF SLEEP ON VENTILATORY COMPENSATION FOR MECHANICAL LOADS

The sleeping state imposes a variety of mechanical loads on the ventilatory control system in health and disease. In normal subjects, NREM sleep causes a consistent increase in upper-airway resistance. Snoring represents an extreme form of this complex, sleep-induced mechanical load (Fig. 3). The ability of the control system to respond to these loads is highly selective, depending on the type of load, the sleep state,

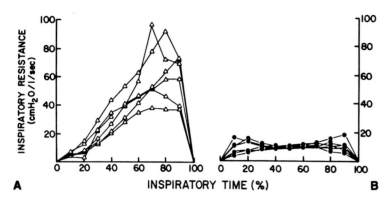

FIG. 3. Variability of resistance in six breaths in a snorer (**A**) versus a nonsnorer (**B**). Note the high resistance and increased within- and between-breath variability in the snorer compared to the nonsnorer. (From ref. 24.)

and the presence of coexistent neuromechanical impairment. Failure to effectively compensate for these spontaneously occurring mechanical loads has adverse effects in terms of CO_2 retention, hypoxemia, and the maintenance of upper-airway patency.

Responses to Mechanical Loads

With load application during wakefulness, both the intensity of the motor output to the respiratory muscles and the inspiratory duration are increased immediately (by the second breath) (30–33), and minute ventilation is preserved. In contrast, during NREM sleep, immediate compensation via increased inspiratory muscle activity is eliminated in sleeping humans (30,31,34) and animals (35,36). Therefore, sleep has a fundamental effect in eliminating the immediate change in intensity of respiratory neural drive in response to mechanical loading.

The effect of mechanical loading during NREM sleep on respiratory cycle timing is more complex and inconsistent. Some human studies with externally applied resistive or elastic loads during sleep have shown a prolongation of T_I (32,33), whereas others have not (30,31,34). Different results are reported when an *internal* resistive load is added or removed. Reduction in the sleep-induced resistance in snorers with either helium or nasal continuous positive airway pressure (CPAP) caused a significant reduction in inspiratory time (21,22). However, a prolongation in inspiratory time in progressing from wakefulness to the higher-resistance NREM sleep state has been reported in some studies (20,37) but not in others (22,24,30). Animal studies have generally shown a prolongation of inspiratory time during resistive loading in sleep (35), but the prolongation of T_I was not sufficient to prevent the fall in tidal volume.

The continued presence of a mechanical load during NREM sleep is associated with progressive augmentation of inspiratory and expiratory muscle activity and a return of minute ventilation toward control levels following the immediate ventilatory depression (Fig. 4) (30–33,35). This restoration of minute ventilation toward unloaded levels is mediated primarily, if not entirely, by chemical stimuli (37,38). Thus, a partial return of minute ventilation toward control levels occurs during NREM sleep, but only at the expense of CO_2 retention and hypoxemia.

Ventilatory compensation during REM sleep has not been well studied in healthy adults. In newborn humans and animals, the response to externally applied mechanical loads is impaired in REM compared to NREM sleep (39–42). This reduced response is related to the reduced activity of intercostal and accessory muscles which places an additional ventilatory demand on the diaphragm. Expiratory muscle activity, which has been shown to be an important component of the ventilatory response to chemical stimuli (43,44), is also likely to be reduced during REM sleep. Therefore, REM sleep interferes with the ventilatory response to chemical stimuli and consequently impairs the most important determinant of ventilatory compensation to sustained loading.

The response to an increased lung volume can be either to restore operating length of the inspiratory muscles back to prehyperinflation levels by activating expiratory muscles or to reflexly augment inspiratory muscle activity in an attempt to preserve minute ventilation. During wakefulness, hyperinflation with either positive pressure applied to the airway or negative pressure applied to the thorax causes both expiratory (45,46) and inspiratory (47,48) muscle activation which restores end-expiratory lung volume to control levels (49) and preserves minute ventilation. During NREM sleep, large increases in end-expiratory lung volume (0.9–1.88 liters) were associated with augmentation of inspiratory muscle activity and preservation of minute ventilation and P_{CO_2} (Fig. 5). In contrast, no augmentation of expiratory muscle activity was noted (50). A similar absence of expiratory muscle recruitment has been reported in humans during anesthesia (51). Respiratory cycle timing was altered by showing a decrease in T_I and an increase in T_E, which had a net effect of slightly decreasing breathing frequency. A confounding effect of an increase in lung

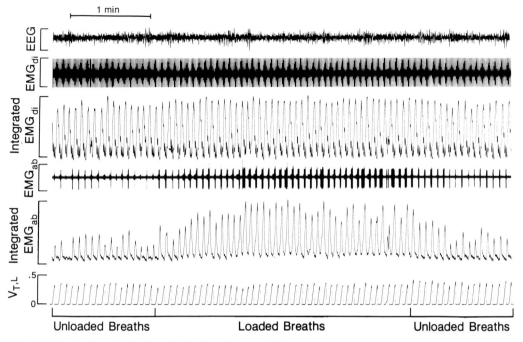

FIG. 4. Effect of sustained resistive loading on tidal volume (V_T), diaphragmatic EMG (EMG_{di}), and expiratory abdominal muscle EMG (EMG_{ab}). Tidal volume decreased immediately upon load application. During sustained loading, EMG_{di} increased slightly whereas EMG_{ab} showed a more pronounced increase. Sleep state remained stable as shown by electroencephalogram (EEG). (From ref. 33.)

volume during NREM sleep is the associated decrease on upper-airway resistance which could have an independent effect on ventilation (52). Thus, the inspiratory muscle response to hyperinflation is preserved during sleep, but the expiratory muscle response is not.

Other examples of significant responses to mechanical loads during sleep are available. The reflex augmentation of upper-airway muscle activity in response to negative pharyngeal pressure is preserved during NREM sleep (53,54). Indirect evidence in humans indicates that decreases in airway resistance during sleep are sensed and responded to, independent of chemical stimuli. When the sleep-induced increase in upper-airway resistance is removed with nasal CPAP, inspiratory and expiratory muscle activity are reduced compared to the high-resistance state even under isocapnic conditions (22). Likewise, unloading of the inspiratory muscles with isocapnic mechanical ventilation during NREM sleep is associated with a reduction in inspiratory and expiratory muscle activity compared to spontaneous breathing levels (19). This indicates that part of the modulation of inspiratory and expiratory muscle activity during steady-state loading or unloading is mediated by neuromechanical reflexes independent of chemical stimuli.

The inhibitory influence of passive mechanical stretch on inspiratory effort also appears to be preserved in the absence of conscious perception. Vagal blockade has a similar effect on breathing pattern during wakefulness and sleep (55). In humans during NREM sleep, isocapnic mechanical ventilation showed an inhibitory effect on inspiratory muscle activity (19). However, the increase in tidal volume during mechanical ventilation was less than 10% in many cases, suggesting that factors other than passive stretch may have mediated the inhibitory effect. Preservation of the Hering–Breuer reflex has been shown in sleeping humans, but only at lung volumes greater than 1–1.5 liters (56). Vagally denervated lung transplant patients have the same breathing pattern during sleep as do vagally intact heart transplant patients (57). Therefore, inhibition of respiratory muscle activity in response to passive mechanical stretch occurs in NREM sleep but probably has a minimal effect in humans in the normal tidal volume range.

Consequences of Mechanical Loading During Sleep

Patients with obstructive or restrictive ventilatory defects are even more susceptible than normals to the adverse effects of sleep because of the added mechanical impairment which is superimposed on an already compromised ventilatory control system. Patients with chronic obstructive pulmonary disease during steady-state NREM sleep show a decrease in

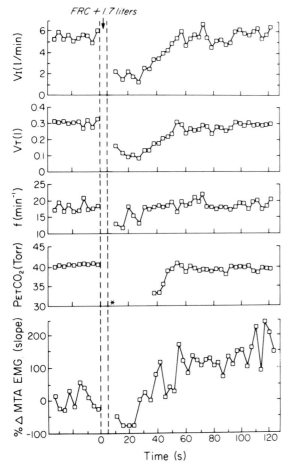

FIG. 5. Breath-by-breath changes in minute ventilation (V$_I$), tidal volume (V$_T$), frequency (f), end-tidal P$_{CO_2}$ (P$_{ETCO_2}$), and slope of the moving time average of surface diaphragmatic electromyogram (MTA EMG) in response to a large sustained hyperinflation induced by a constant negative pressure in a tank ventilator. A P$_{ETCO_2}$ from the first seven breaths could not be precisely measured because of poor waveforms. Note the initial inhibition of ventilatory output. Subsequently, ventilation returns to control levels coincidentally with augmentation of diaphragmatic EMG. (From ref. 49.)

minute ventilation, an increase in Pa$_{CO_2}$ (1–10 mmHg), and a decrease in oxygen saturation (0–10%) compared to wakefulness (58,59). These changes in ventilation and gas exchange are likely to represent an incomplete compensatory response to the increase in upper-airway resistance which normally occurs during sleep.

Episodes of nocturnal asthma provide another example of the effect of a more acute application of an internal resistive load. NREM sleep does not abolish the augmentation of central respiratory drive in response to spontaneously occurring bronchoconstriction (37). Both inspiratory and expiratory muscle EMG activity have been reported to be augmented during nocturnal asthmatic attacks (60). The mechanism of

muscle recruitment is likely to involve both chemical and nonchemical mechanisms (37) and is sufficient to preserve minute ventilation except during periods of REM sleep.

Patients with interstitial lung disease show an increased ventilation and breathing frequency during wakefulness which may be related to perceptual influences (61). In these patients during NREM sleep, ventilation and breathing frequency decreased compared to that during wakefulness. In contrast, normal subjects showed no change in ventilation and an increase in breathing frequency during NREM sleep. One explanation for the elimination of the abnormal breathing pattern during NREM sleep in the patients is that the tachypnea during wakefulness is behaviorally mediated. NREM sleep directly suppresses the cerebral cortex and reduces afferent input to the cortex and could thereby eliminate the behavioral component. This intriguing finding may not be consistent in all types of patients. For example, in patients with chronic obstructive pulmonary disease (COPD) and chronic CO$_2$ retention, their tachypneic pattern of breathing persisted during NREM sleep even when hypoxemia was corrected with supplemental oxygen (59).

In contrast to NREM sleep, REM sleep causes a differential suppression of inspiratory and expiratory muscles which leads to the REM-related episodes of oxygen desaturation commonly observed in patients with lung disease (58,62–64). The intercostal, accessory, and upper-airway muscles show a decrease in activity while the activity of the diaphragm is preserved (25,26,65–67). The inhibitory effect is greater during phasic REM sleep than during tonic REM sleep (25,65–67). The adverse effect of REM sleep in interfering with ventilatory compensation is demonstrated in nocturnal asthma. Inhibition of intercostal muscle activity was associated with inward distortion of the unstable rib cage. Thus, REM-related postsynaptic inhibition (67) is a critical determinant of the elimination of load-compensating mechanisms related to both chemical and neurochemical influences.

The greater inhibition of upper-airway muscle activity during REM compared to NREM sleep causes an increase in upper-airway resistance which increases the mechanical impedance at a time when the control system is least able to compensate for the added load. Adverse effects on ventilation and O$_2$ saturation similar to those observed in patients with COPD have been reported in patients with cystic fibrosis (68), interstitial fibrosis (69), and kyphoscoliosis (70). Thus, the presence of a moderate mechanical load due to lung or chest-wall disease is usually well compensated in NREM sleep because of the preserved response to chemical stimuli. However, during REM sleep, the impairment of inspiratory muscle activity in combination with the disease-related mechanical loads and gas exchange abnormalities can cause severe, sustained episodes of oxygen desaturation.

Patients with neuromuscular disease and CO_2 retention are especially susceptible to hypopnea and oxygen desaturation during sleep (71–74). Load compensation is impaired because of weak muscles and a weak ventilatory response to chemical stimuli, both of which are essential for effective ventilatory compensation. The combination of sleep-induced increase in upper-airway resistance plus weak muscles and reduced ventilatory response to chemical stimuli may account for the episodes of hypoventilation and oxygen desaturation observed in NREM sleep. Further inhibition of respiratory muscles during REM sleep may greatly decrease ventilation. REM-related inhibition of intercostal and accessory muscles is especially important in patients with bilateral diaphragmatic paralysis. These patients develop severe hypoventilation and oxygen desaturation, often requiring nocturnal mechanical ventilation (28).

In summary, the sleeping state places the individual at risk for CO_2 retention and hypoxemia by impairing or eliminating strategies of load compensation which are available during wakefulness. In addition, a sleep-induced increase in upper-airway resistance further compromises alveolar ventilation. The presence of disease states associated with added impedances, weak or inefficient muscles, and/or poor responses to chemical stimuli can lead to severe O_2 desaturation, pulmonary hypertension, cor pumonale, and death. Arousal remains the ultimate response to a sleep-induced load, but the physiologic cost of this response is high in terms of additional morbidity.

WHY IS CO_2 RETAINED IN SLEEP?

This apparently straightforward question is actually fairly complex. The traditional explanation focuses on the true "state effect" of sleep as manifested in the reduced phasic activity of medullary respiratory neurons (4) (see above). However, an important remaining question is, To what extent are these inhibitory effects on some respiratory neurons translated to respiratory muscles and eventually to total ventilatory output in the intact sleeping animal or human? Is this state effect on medullary respiratory neurons directly translatable, or do the other CNS effects of state change (primarily that of increased upper-airway resistance, secondary to reductions in "non- or weak-respiratory" neuronal activity) override this effect and indirectly influence ventilatory output?

First, there is clear evidence of inhibitory effects of

sleep state directly on ventilatory control mechanisms; that is, loss of wakefulness "resets" ventilation and Pa_{CO_2}. This is indicated by sleep-induced hypoventilation in tracheostomized humans, amounting to a 1- to 2-torr increase in Pa_{CO_2} (18,22). Similar data are more plentiful in tracheostomized dogs and cats; however, the waking control values are highly variable, and thus the apparent sleep effects are often uninterpretable (1). Furthermore, in intact humans, when most or all of the sleep-induced increase in airway resistance is removed (see below), some significant level of alveolar hypoventilation does remain. Recently, Rist et al. (75) showed that during wakefulness, when the $P_{ET_{CO_2}}$ was increased to the same level as during NREM sleep, the diaphragmatic EMG activity was elevated above that obtained during sleep. Thus sleep, per se, was apparently producing some depressant effect on respiratory motor output, at least with regard to these respiratory muscles under study.[1] Additional evidence, often used to implicate a direct "state" effect on respiratory motor output, is available from study of the transition from wakefulness to sleep (76,77). A reduction in V_E, an increase in $P_{ET_{CO_2}}$, and an increase in the rib-cage contribution to V_T were often (but not always) shown to precede the initiation of theta activity in the electroencephalogram (denoting onset of stage I) by about 3–10 sec. Many of these data provide only an indirect and incomplete test of state effect on ventilatory control; however, the implications seem clear that a significant effect of loss of wakefulness on medullary output is clearly translatable into a reduced respiratory muscle recruitment and hypoventilation.

There is growing evidence to support a major role for increasing airway resistance as a cause of hypoventilation during sleep. Perhaps the most compelling evidence is the observation in intact humans that the hypoventilation in NREM sleep coexists not with *reduced* respiratory muscle activity but, instead, with *augmented* inspiratory and expiratory muscle activity, as denoted both by EMG recordings in diaphragm, scalenus, intercostal, and abdominal muscles and by mechanical evidence of active expiration, of increased diaphragmatic contraction, and of increased rib-cage contribution to V_T (see section entitled "Respiratory Muscle Function," above). This apparent paradox of

---

[1] There are exceptions to this airway-resistance-dependent increase in respiratory muscle activity in NREM sleep. The internal intercostal muscles in the cat show a NREM state-dependent increase in EMG activity even in the tracheostomized animal (23). In the intact human, the scalenus inspiratory muscle EMG activity rises during NREM sleep (coincident with an increase in airway resistance and $P_{ET_{CO_2}}$) and falls significantly when CPAP normalizes the resistance (to waking levels), but this activity still remains elevated compared to waking levels (22).

the sleeping state holds for all inspiratory muscles in snorers and nonsnorers as resistance increases and Pa_{CO_2} rises through all NREM sleep stages. Abdominal expiratory muscle activation occurs only in the snorer—usually in stage III–IV sleep (22). Furthermore, when this sleep-induced increase in airway resistance is reduced 30–50% via breathing a low-density gas mixture ($He:O_2$) (21), or completely relieved via nasal CPAP (22), V_E rose and Pa_{CO_2} fell to within 1–2 mmHg of that of waking levels, and EMG activity was decreased in inspiratory muscles and completely silenced in abdominal expiratory muscles.[2] Taken together, these data suggest that the state effect of reducing medullary respiratory neuronal activity is not fully realized at the level of respiratory muscles; to the contrary, the secondary effect of an increase in airway resistance intervenes to cause major (further) hypoventilation, CO_2 retention, and feedback stimulation of

respiratory muscle activity. We would also expect these highly state-sensitive and very quick to occur changes in airway resistance (78) to contribute significantly to sudden reductions in ventilation at sleep onset or during any transient changes in sleep state.

THE "WAKEFULNESS" STIMULATION TO VENTILATION

As shown in Fig. 6, wakefulness effects on ventilatory control are more complex than just the suppression of respiratory neuronal activity leading to an increased "set-point" for Pa_{CO_2}. The effects of NREM sleep on tonic and phasic activity of upper-airway muscle secondary to reductions in "nonrespiratory" medullary neuronal activity do contribute significantly to sleep-induced hypoventilation. This effect is potentiated by the loss of immediate compensation to resistive loads during sleep. Presuming that a compensatory response to loading requires "perception" of the added load, suprapontine inhibition in NREM sleep may mediate a loss of vigilance and thus account for this blunted compensatory response. NREM sleep exerts no sig-

---

[2] An alternative explanation of these effects is that the awake subject's cortical perception of the progressive CO_2-induced hyperpnea contributed to the augmentation of inspiratory muscle activity; it is this behaviorally moderated response to stress that is eliminated by NREM sleep.

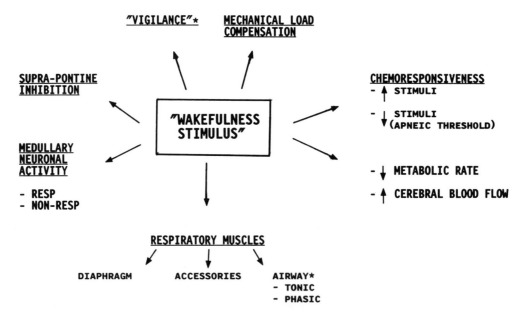

FIG. 6. Removal of the "wakefulness stimulus" in NREM sleep results primarily in (a) the inhibition of higher CNS activity and (b) reduced medullary neuronal activity which is only weakly related to respiration. These fundamental changes manifest themselves in two ways: (i) reduced tonic airway abductor muscle activity causing increased airway resistance; and (ii) removal of "vigilance," and thus perception of the increased resistive load is lost as is the immediate compensation for the load. Thus V_T falls and CO_2 rises: Since chemoreceptor responsiveness to increased stimuli is not appreciably affected by NREM sleep, respiratory motor output is increased to inspiratory and even expiratory accessory muscles. Three important inhibitory influences are also shown: (i) The loss of the "wakefulness stimulus" unmasks a highly sensitive apneic threshold that is responsive to mild hypocapnia; (ii) reduced V_{CO_2}; (iii) increased cerebral blood flow and thus reduced medullary P_{CO_2}; and (iv) reduction in medullary respiratory neuronal activity secondary to removal of wakefulness (higher CNS) stimulus, per se.

nificant effects on chemoresponsiveness, and upper-airway muscles appear to be the only respiratory muscles markedly inhibited via NREM sleep; thus, the respiratory acidosis that occurs secondary to the combination of increased airway resistance and loss of vigilance and load perception provides a strong source of stimulation for primary and accessory muscles of the chest wall and abdomen.

Two other primary effects of sleep state which have a bearing on ventilation (and probably on the ventilatory response to any superimposed stimuli or inhibitors) are (i) the increases in cerebral blood flow (and especially medullary blood flow) as it affects local P_{CO_2} and (ii) the 10–15% reduction in V_{CO_2} in sleep. Finally, the wakefulness influence on ventilatory control is also manifested in the unmasking of a highly sensitive apneic threshold to reduced P_{CO_2} in sleep. This is a prime example of the loss of vigilance in the sleeping control system, which in wakefulness would normally respond quickly and vigorously to cessation of diaphragmatic activity or to apnea. REM sleep clearly represents more than merely the "loss" of these wakefulness influences on ventilatory control; rather, this state involves the acquisition of active and highly selective inhibitions of respiratory motor output and respiratory muscle activity.

SLEEP EFFECT ON VENTILATORY STABILITY

Sleep not only renders the ventilatory control system more susceptible to inhibition but also predisposes it to instability in breathing pattern. This occurrence may be readily demonstrated when healthy persons are exposed during NREM sleep to even moderately hypoxic environments for as little as 10–15 min (79–81) and the effects persist for many days. The susceptibility to hypoxic-induced periodic breathing correlates positively with the magnitude of the waking response to chemoreceptor stimuli—especially to the asphyxic combination of hypoxia and hypercapnia (80). Note the regularly spaced (i.e., every 20–25 sec) cycles of breath clusters followed by apneas. The apneas are almost always of the central type, are 10–15 sec in duration, and occur at the rate of > 150 per hour, so that almost one-half of the NREM sleep time is spent without breathing. Within each breathing cluster, the average V_T and mean inspiratory flow rate are very much larger than those during steady-state nonperiodic breathing, but substantial variability exists and some small tidal volumes (especially toward the end of the cluster) approach dead space volumes and others are as large as one-half the inspiratory lung capacity. Large swings occur in arterial O_2 saturation, and SaO_2 falls out of proportion to the coincident rise in P_{CO_2} during the apneic periods.

What causes periodic breathing? (See Fig. 7.) Two key factors here include: (a) the highly sensitive hypocapnic-induced apneic threshold, which is unmasked in sleep (this initiates hypopneic periods and, eventually, apneas); and (b) the high gain of peripheral chemoreceptors to asphyxic stimuli (which would occur at the termination of an apneic period). This responsiveness is preserved in sleep. In the intact sleeping human, we believe that the powerful combination

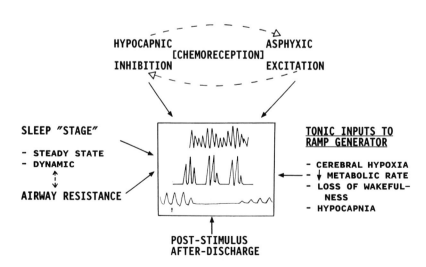

FIG. 7. Three types of unstable breathing are shown here: (i) the waxing-and-waning Cheyne–Stokes pattern; (ii) the periodic, cluster breathing (both of these are observed during NREM sleep in hypoxia); and (iii) the inhibition observed upon abrupt termination of an hypoxic stimulus. We show the chemoreceptor inhibitory–excitatory interaction as a primary underlying mechanism that triggers and perpetuates hypoxia-induced periodic breathing. Other superimposed influences include: (i) dynamic changes in sleep state (which may affect controller gain and/or upper-airway resistance); (ii) changing airway resistance, which will greatly influence ventilatory output at any given motor output; (iii) reduced tonic inputs to the medullary rhythm generator; and (iv) the stabilizing presence or destabilizing absence of afterdischarge of respiratory motor output following sudden withdrawal of the primary stimulus.

[CHEMORECEPTION]

HYPOCAPNIC INHIBITION   ASPHYXIC EXCITATION

SLEEP "STAGE"
- STEADY STATE
- DYNAMIC

AIRWAY RESISTANCE

TONIC INPUTS TO RAMP GENERATOR
- CEREBRAL HYPOXIA
- ↓ METABOLIC RATE
- LOSS OF WAKEFULNESS
- HYPOCAPNIA

POST-STIMULUS AFTER-DISCHARGE

of these chemoreceptor stimuli is essential to the production of instability and periodicity. Nevertheless, a number of additional stabilizers and destabilizing mechanisms also may play an important modulatory role.

1. *Afterdischarge phenomenon: a stabilizer.* Eldridge (82) electrically stimulated the carotid sinus nerves in anesthetized cats, causing phrenic nerve activity to increase. When he suddenly stopped stimulation, phrenic nerve activity returned only very slowly to prestimulus baseline activity. Theoretically, this potentiated "afterdischarge" effect would prevent ventilatory inhibition from occurring, and no periodic breathing would occur. Accordingly, the apnea of hypoxic-induced periodic breathing might then be attributed to the suppression of this afterdischarge by long-standing cerebral hypoxia, as recently suggested by Younes (2). This is an intriguing possibility that needs the clear demonstration of a significant afterdischarge of ventilatory output following a truly physiologic stimulus applied during sleep. We would predict that even very small reductions in P_{CO_2} at the chemoreceptors—especially medullary chemoreceptors—would present a strong inhibition to afterdischarge of inspiratory activity (18), but Eldridge has demonstrated that the afterdischarge to electrical carotid sinus nerve stimulation persists even when the animal's P_{CO_2} is substantially less than his apneic threshold.

2. *The importance of tonic inputs to the respiratory controller.* Generation of the inspiratory "ramp" to permit normal cycling of medullary respiratory neurons requires a critical minimum level of tonic input to the respiratory controller. Several factors might reduce tonic input sufficiently so that periodic breathing simply becomes a "switching" problem (2). Indeed, some have suggested recently that periodicity may simply be an inherent central rhythm exposed by the suppression of "tonic" drives (83). At least four types of important tonic input may be identified.

a. *Hypocapnia,* acting at peripheral and/or medullary chemoreceptors, as described in detail above.

b. *Cerebral hypoxia*—by itself—may act as a tonic depressant of ventilatory drive, at least if hypoxia is of sufficient duration (84).

c. *Reduced metabolic rate* (i.e., V_{CO_2} or V_{O_2}) may also cause destabilization of breathing pattern through reduction in tonic drive, as shown by the central and obstructive apneas observed in the untreated hypothyroid patient during NREM sleep (85). Perhaps the destabilization effects of hypoxia may also be linked to a reduced V_{O_2}. Unfortunately, we have no idea as to receptor site or nervous pathways through which a change in metabolic rate may exert its effect on ventilation or breathing pattern. Periodic breathing, prominent in the hibernating animal, may represent an extreme example of the destabilizing effects of reduced metabolic rate (86).

d. The removal of the *wakefulness drive* to breathe also contributes to a significant reduction in tonic input to the medullary controller. It is unlikely that NREM sleep, per se, is a destabilizer of ventilatory pattern, but it clearly serves a permissive role in the genesis of destabilization via hypocapnia, cerebral hypoxia, or reduced metabolic rate.

3. *Dynamically changing sleep state.* This may be necessary for the perpetuation of periodic breathing by being responsible for the generation of very large breaths at the point that each apneic period was broken. At least a portion of this augmented breath may be the result of the increased gain attributable to the rise in P_{CO_2} from below to above the apneic threshold, combined with the synergistic effect of asphyxic stimuli acting on the carotid body (see above). It is also likely that this apparent increase in gain is attributable to a microarousal immediately prior to, or coincident with, these initiations of the breath. This coincidence may be shown by the simultaneous analysis of the time course of changing ventilatory output versus EEG spectral frequency. Quite often the EEG change precedes the initiation of ventilatory output, especially in very light sleep stages. Much work is needed on this important question, since current analyses suffer from EEG motion artifacts and as yet improperly defined changes in "sleep state." The effect of a true change in state may affect ventilatory response because of a change in controller gain and, perhaps even more importantly, because of a reduction in airway resistance. The most profound effect of state change is observed in REM sleep, where periodic breathing in hypoxia does not occur (79). Perhaps the tonic input to the respiratory controller is so elevated in REM sleep that switching mechanisms are not sufficiently suppressed by hypoxia and/or hypocapnia.

In nonhypoxic states, dynamic changes in sleep state may become powerful destabilizers of ventilatory output. Elderly subjects seem particularly prone to sleep-dependent destabilization of breathing pattern that occurs during stage I–II sleep. This might be related to poorly "consolidated" sleep states in the elderly. Accordingly, Pack et al. (87) used spectral analysis of EEG to demonstrate a coincidence of synchronous oscillations in ventilation and in frequency content of the EEG, a finding that implicates a reduction in the state-dependent input to the ventilatory control system as the primary initiator of apneas during light sleep in these elderly subjects.

4. *Airway impedance*. When airway impedance is elevated in sleep, it may have a significant influence on periodic breathing by preventing instability. A sufficiently high resistance may actually prevent periodic breathing, possibly because the impedance does not permit sufficient hyperventilation and hypocapnia to occur. In snoring subjects, we were only rarely able to produce periodic breathing by administering hypoxia during NREM sleep (78). This effect may also explain why periodic breathing in hypoxic sleep usually occurs in stages lighter than III–IV, since the airway resistance is usually considerably lower in these lighter sleep stages.

ACKNOWLEDGMENTS

We thank Jennifer Thomas for her excellent preparation of the manuscript. Original work reported here was supported by grants from the NHLBI (15469 and HL42242), the Veterans Administration, and the Hazel Mae Mayer Trust. Kathe Henke was a Wisconsin Heart Association pre-doctorate fellow.

REFERENCES

1. Phillipson EA, Bowes G. Control of breathing during sleep. In: Cherniack NS, Widdicombe JG, eds. *Handbook of physiology: the respiratory system.* Bethesda, MD: American Physiological Society, 1986;649–689.
2. Younes M. The physiological basis of central apnea and periodic breathing. In: Simmons DH, ed. *Current pulmonology,* vol 10. Chicago: Year Book Medical Publishers, 1989.
3. Dempsey JA, Skatrud JB. Fundamental effects of sleep state on breathing. In: Simmons DH, ed. *Current pulmonology,* vol 9. Chicago: Year Book Medical Publishers, 1988;267–304.
4. Orem JM. Respiratory neuronal activity in sleep. In: Edelman NH, Santiago TV, eds. *Contemporary issues in pulmonary disease,* vol 5. New York: Churchill Livingstone, 1986;19–44.
5. Frysinger RC, Zhang J, Harper R. Cardiovascular and respiratory relationships with neural discharge in the central nucleus of the amygdala during sleep-waking cycles. *Sleep* 1988;11:317–332.
6. Orem J, Osorio I, Brooks E, Dick T. Activity of respiratory neurons during NREM sleep. *J Neurophysiol* 1985;54:1144–1156.
7. Orem J, Netick A. Voluntary control of breathing in the cat. *Brain Res* 1986;366:238–253.
8. Smith CA, Jameson LC, Mitchell GS, Musch TI, Dempsey JA. Central–peripheral chemoreceptor interaction in the awake CSF-perfused goat. *J Appl Physiol* 1984;56:1541–1544.
9. Guazzi M, Freis ED. Sino-aortic reflexes and arterial pH and Pco_2 in wakefulness and sleep. *Am J Physiol* 1969;217:1623–1627.
10. Sullivan CE, Issa FG, Berthon-Jones M, et al. Patho-physiology of sleep apnea. In: Saunders N, Sullivan C, eds. *Sleep and breathing.* New York: Marcel Dekker, 1984;299–363.
11. Bulow K. Respiration and wakefulness in man. *Acta Physiol Scand [Suppl]* 1963;209.
12. Goethe B, Cherniack N, Williams L. Effect of hypoxia on ventilatory and arousal responses to CO_2 during NREM sleep

with and without flurazepam in young adults. *Sleep* 1986;1:24–37.
13. Orem J. Medullary respiratory neuron activity: relationship to tonic and phasic REM sleep. *J Appl Physiol* 1980;48:54.
14. Phillipson EA, McClean PA, Sullivan CE, et al. Interaction of metabolic and behavioral respiratory control during hypercapnia and speech. *Am Rev Resp Dis* 1978;117:903–909.
15. Berssenbrugge A, Dempsey JA, Skatrud JB. Effects of sleep state on ventilatory acclimatization to chronic hypoxia. *J Appl Physiol* 1984;57:1089–1096.
16. Skatrud J, Dempsey J. Relative effectiveness of acetazolamide versus medroxyprogesterone acetate in correction of chronic CO_2 retention. *Am Rev Resp Dis* 1983;127:405–412.
17. Parisi RA, Neubauer JA. Control of breathing during sleep. In: Edelman NH, Santiago TV, eds. *Breathing disorders of sleep.* New York: Churchill Livingstone, 1986;45–56.
18. Skatrud J, Dempsey J. Interaction of sleep state and chemical stimuli in sustaining rhythmic ventilation. *J Appl Physiol* 1983;55:813–822.
19. Henke KG, Arias A, Skatrud JB, Dempsey JA. Inhibition of inspiratory muscle activity during sleep. *Am Rev Resp Dis* 1988;138:8–15.
20. Tabachnick E, Muller NL, Bryan AC, Levison H. Changes in ventilation and chest wall mechanics during sleep in normal adolescents. *J Appl Physiol: Respir Environ Exerc Physiol* 1981;51:557–567.
21. Skatrud JB, Dempsey JA, Badr S, Begle RL. Effects of high airway impedance on CO_2 retention and respiratory muscle activity during NREM sleep. *J Appl Physiol* 1988;65:1676–1685.
22. Henke KG, Dempsey JA, Kowitz JM, Badr S, Skatrud JB. Effects of sleep-induced increases in upper airway resistance on respiratory muscle activity. *J Appl Physiol* 1989;in press.
23. Dick TE, Parmeggiani PL, Orem J. Intercostal muscle activity during sleep in the cat: an augmentation of expiration. *Respir Physiol* 1982;50:255–265.
24. Skatrud JB, Dempsey JA. Airway resistance and respiratory muscle function in snorers during NREM sleep. *J Appl Physiol* 1985;59:328–335.
25. Tusiewicz K, Moldofsky H, Bryan AC, Bryan MH. Mechanics of the rib cage and diaphragm during sleep. *J Appl Physiol: Respir Environ Exerc Physiol* 1979;43:600–602.
26. Johnson MN, Remmers JE. Accessory muscle activity during sleep in chronic obstructive pulmonary disease. *J Appl Physiol* 1984;57:1011–1017.
27. Corda M, von Euler C, Lennerstrand G. Proprioceptive innervation of the diaphragm. *J Physiol (Lond)* 1965;178:161–177.
28. Skatrud J, Iber C, McHugh W, Rasmussen H, Nichols D. Determinants of hypoventilation during wakefulness and sleep in diaphragmatic paralysis. *Am Rev Resp Dis* 1980;121:587–593.
29. Sauerland EK, Harper RM. The human tongue during sleep: electromyographic activity of the genioglossus muscle. *Exp Neurol* 1976;51:160–170.
30. Iber C, Davies SF, Chapman RC, Mahowald MM. A possible mechanism for mixed apnea in obstructive sleep apnea. *Chest* 1986;89:800–805.
31. Wilson PA, Skatrud JB, Dempsey JA. Effects of slow wave sleep on ventilatory compensation to inspiratory elastic loading. *Respir Physiol* 1984;55:103–120.
32. Wiegand L, Zwillich C, White D. Sleep and the ventilatory response to resistive loading in normal man. *J Appl Physiol* 1988;64:1186–1195.
33. Badr MS, Skatrud JB, Dempsey JA, Begle RL. Effect of mechanical loading on expiratory muscle activity during NREM sleep. *J Appl Physiol* 1989;in press.
34. Hudgel DW, Mulholland M, Hendricks C. Neuromuscular and mechanical responses to inspiratory resistive loading during sleep. *J Appl Physiol* 1987;63:603–608.
35. Bowes B, Kozar LF, Andrey SM, Phillipson EA. Ventilatory responses to inspiratory flow-resistive loads in awake and sleeping dogs. *J Appl Physiol* 1983;54:1550–1557.

36. Santiago TV, Sinha AK, Edelman NH. Respiratory flow-resistive load compensation during sleep. *Am Rev Resp Dis* 1981;123:382–387.

37. Ballard RD, Saathoff MC, Patel DK, Kelly PL, Martin RJ. Effect of sleep on nocturnal bronchoconstriction and ventilatory patterns in asthmatics. *J Appl Physiol* 1989;67:243–239.

38. Bruce EN, Smith JD, Grodins FS. Chemical and reflex drives to breathing during resistance loading in cats. *J Appl Physiol* 1974;37:176–182.

39. Frantz ID III, Adler SM, Abroms IF, Thach BT. Respiratory response to airway occlusion in infants: sleep state and maturation. *J Appl Physiol* 1976;41:634–638.

40. Henderson-Smart DJ, Read DJC. Depression of respiratory muscles and defective responses to nasal obstruction during active sleep in the newborn. *Aust Pediatr J* 1976;12:261–266.

41. Knill R, Andrews W, Bryan AC, Bryan MH. Respiratory load compensation in infants. *J Appl Physiol* 1976;40:357–361.

42. Purcell M. Response in the newborn to raised upper airway resistance. *Arch Dis Child* 1976;51:602–607.

43. Oliven A, Kelsen SG. Effect of hypercapnia and PEEP on expiratory muscle EMG and shortening. *J Appl Physiol* 1989; 66:1408–1413.

44. Smith CA, Ainsworth DM, Henderson KH, Dempsey JA. Differential responses of expiratory muscles to chemical stimuli in awake dogs. *J Appl Physiol* 1989;66:384–391.

45. Campbell EJM, Dickinson CJ, Dinnick OP, Howell JBL. The immediate effects of threshold loads on the breathing of men and dogs. *Clin Sci* 1961;21:309–320.

46. Green M, Mead J, Sears TA. Muscle activity during chest wall restriction and positive pressure breathing in man. *Respir Physiol* 1978;35:283–300.

47. Banzett RB, Inbar GF, Brown R, Goldman M, Rossier A, Mead J. Diaphragm electrical activity during negative lower torso pressure in quadriplegic men. *J Appl Physiol: Respir Environ Exerc Physiol* 1981;51:654–659.

48. Banzett R, Strohl K, Geffroy B, Mead J. Effect of transrespiratory pressure on P_{ETCO_2}–Pa_{CO_2} and ventilatory reflexes in humans. *J Appl Physiol: Respir Environ Exerc Physiol* 1981; 51:660–664.

49. Begle RL, Skatrud JB, Dempsey JA. Ventilatory compensation for changes in functional residual capacity during sleep. *J Appl Physiol* 1987;62:1299–1306.

50. Begle RL, Skatrud JB. Effect of lung volume on expiratory muscle recruitment during wakefulness and NREM sleep. *Am Rev Resp Dis* 1989;139:A82.

51. Derenne J, Whitelaw WA, Couture J, Milic-Emili J. Load compensation during positive pressure breathing in anesthetized man. *Respir Physiol* 1986;65:303–314.

52. Begle RL, Badr S, Skatrud JB, Dempsey JA. Effect of lung inflation on airway resistance during NREM sleep. *Am Rev Resp Dis* 1989; in press.

53. Mathew OP. Upper airway negative-pressure effects on respiratory activity of upper airway muscles. *J Appl Physiol: Respir Environ Exerc Physiol* 1984;56:500–505.

54. Mathew OP, Abu-Osba YK, Thach BT. Influence of upper airway pressure changes on genioglossus muscle respiratory activity. *J Appl Physiol: Respir Environ Exerc Physiol* 1982; 52:438–444.

55. Phillipson EA, Murphy E, Kozar LF. Regulation of respiration in sleeping dogs. *J Appl Physiol* 1976;40:688–693.

56. Hamilton RD, Winning AJ, Horner RL, Guz A. The effect of lung inflation in man during wakefulness and sleep. *Respir Physiol* 1988;73:145–154.

57. Shea SA, Horner RL, Banner NR, McKenzie E, Heaton R, Yacoub MH, Guz A. The effect of human heart-lung transplantation upon breathing at rest and during sleep. *Respir Physiol* 1988;72:131–150.

58. Hudgel DW, Martin RJ, Capehart M, Johnson B, Hill P. Contribution of hypoventilation to sleep oxygen desaturation in chronic obstructive pulmonary disease. *J Appl Physiol* 1983; 55:669–677.

59. Skatrud JB, Dempsey JA, Iber C, Berssenbrugge A. Correction of CO_2 retention during sleep in patients with chronic obstructive pulmonary diseases. *Am Rev Resp Dis* 1981;124:260–268.

60. Issa FG, Sullivan CE. Respiratory muscle activity and thoracoabdominal motion during acute episodes of asthma during sleep. *Am Rev Resp Dis* 1985;132:999–1004.

61. Shea SA, Winning AJ, McKenzie E, Guz A. Does the abnormal pattern of breathing in patients with interstitial lung disease persist in deep, NREM sleep? *Am Rev Resp Dis* 1989;139:653–658.

62. Fletcher EC, Gray BA, Levin DC. Nonapneic mechanisms of arterial oxygen desaturation during rapid-eye-movement sleep. *J Appl Physiol* 1983;54:632–639.

63. Catterall JR, Calverley PMA, MacNee W, Warren PM, Shapiro CM, Douglas NJ, Flenley DC. Mechanism of transient nocturnal hypoxemia in hypoxic chronic bronchitis and emphysema. *J Appl Physiol* 1985;59:1698–1703.

64. Catterall JR, Douglas NJ, Calverley PMA, Shapiro CM, Brezinova V, Brash HM, Flenley DC. Transient hypoxemia during sleep in chronic obstructive pulmonary disease is not a sleep apnea syndrome. *Am Rev Resp Dis* 1983;128:24–29.

65. Duron B. Activité électrique spontanée des muscles intercostaux et du diaphragme chez l'animal chronique. *J Physiol (Paris)* 1982;61:282–289.

66. Parmeggiani PL, Sabattini L. Electromyographic aspects of postural, respiratory and thermoregulatory mechanisms in sleeping cats. *Electroencephalogr Clin Neurophysiol* 1972;33:1–13.

67. Remmers JE. Effects of sleep on control of breathing. *Int Rev Physiol* 1981;23:111–147.

68. Tepper RS, Skatrud JB, Dempsey JA. Ventilation and oxygenation changes during sleep in cystic fibrosis. *Chest* 1983;84:388–393.

69. Perez-Padilla R, West P, Lertzman M, Kryger MH. Breathing during sleep in patients with interstitial lung disease. *Am Rev Resp Dis* 1985;132:224–229.

70. Mezon BL, West P, Israels J, Kryger M. Sleep breathing abnormalities in kyphoscoliosis. *Am Rev Resp Dis* 1980;122:617–622.

71. Naughton J, Block R, Welch M. Central alveolar hypoventilation. *Am Rev Resp Dis* 1971;103:557–565.

72. Farmer WC, Glenn WW, Gee JB. Alveolar hypoventilation syndrome. Studies of ventilatory control in patients selected for diaphragm pacing. *Am J Med* 1978;64:39–49.

73. Bubis MJ, Anthonisen NR. Primary alveolar hypoventilation treated by nocturnal administration of O_2. *Am Rev Resp Dis* 1978;118:947–953.

74. Barlow PB, Bartlett D Jr, Hauri P, et al. Idiopathic hypoventilation syndrome: importance of preventing nocturnal hypoxemia and hypercapnia. *Am Rev Resp Dis* 1980;121:141–145.

75. Rist KE, Daubenspeck JA, McGovern JF. Effects of non-REM sleep upon the respiratory drive and the respiratory pump in humans. *Respir Physiol* 1986;63:241–256.

76. Colrain JM, Trinder J, Fresa G, Wilson GV. Ventilation during sleep onset. *J Appl Physiol* 1987;63:2067–2074.

77. Naifeh KH, Kamiya J. The nature of respiratory changes associated with sleep onset. *Sleep* 1981;4:49–59.

78. Warner G, Skatrud JB, Dempsey JA. Effect of hypoxia-induced periodic breathing on upper airway obstruction during sleep. *J Appl Physiol* 1987;62:2201–2211.

79. Berssenbrugge A, Dempsey JA, Iber C, Skatrud J, Wilson P. Mechanisms of hypoxia-induced periodic breathing during sleep in humans. *J Physiol (Lond)* 1983;343:507–524.

80. Dempsey JA, Skatrud JB. A sleep-induced apneic threshold and its consequences. *Am Rev Resp Dis* 1986;133:1163–1170.

81. Chapman KR, Bruce EN, Gothe B, Cherniack NS. Possible mechanisms of periodic breathing during sleep. *J Appl Physiol* 1988;64:1000–1008.

82. Eldridge FL. Central neural respiratory stimulating effect of active respiration. *J Appl Physiol* 1974;37:723–735.

83. Andrews DC, Johnson P, Symmonds M. Metabolic rate and pe-

riodic breathing in the developing lamb. In: *Proceedings of the Physiological Society—Oxford Meeting*. Oxford, England: 1989;141P.

84. Holtby S, Bereganski D, Anthonisen NR. The effect of 100% O₂ on hypoxic eucapnic ventilation. *J Appl Physiol* 1988; 65:1157–1162.

85. Skatrud JB, Iber C, Ewart R, Thomas G, Rasmussen H,

Schultze B. Disordered breathing during sleep in hypothyroidism. *Am Rev Resp Dis* 1981;124:325–329.

86. Millson WK. Control of arrhythmic breathing in aerial breathers. *Can J Zool* 1988;66:99–108.

87. Pack AI, Cola MF, Goldszmidt A, Silage DA. Coherent oscillations in ventilation and frequency content of the electroencephalogram. *J Appl Physiol* 1989;in press.

THE LUNG: *Scientific Foundations*
edited by R.G. Crystal, J.B. West et al.
Raven Press, Ltd., New York © 1991.

CHAPTER 5.7.3

Upper-Airway Effects on Breathing

Erik van Lunteren

The upper airways are complex structures with multiple functions, some of which are respiratory, and others of which are alimentary, communicative, or olfactory. Their neural regulation provides for proper coordination between breathing, vocalization, mastication, deglutition, and olfaction. Some of the upper-airway structures are derived phylogenetically and embryologically from the gill arches, and hence the respiratory role of the upper airways can be regarded as primary as opposed to secondary.

The upper airways have several different respiratory functions. They serve as the intake for environmental gases, which are subsequently modified with regard to temperature and humidity before entering the lower respiratory tract and the lungs. The resistance of the upper-airway conduit can be altered in several ways and at several sites, and this may participate in the regulation of normal airflow during inspiration and expiration. The impact of the upper airway on breathing during wakefulness and sleep is, to a large extent, mediated via multiple muscles located in and surrounding the upper-airway lumen. In addition, structural factors such as soft tissue of the tongue, adenoids, and pharyngeal adipose tissue, as well as physiological mucosal and submucosal factors including blood flow and secretions, affect airflow; however, these have a slower time course than do neuromuscular factors.

Modulation of airflow during wakefulness and sleep may occur at five general sites of the upper airways. The size of the laryngeal aperture varies dynamically throughout the respiratory cycle, as a result of the inspiratory abduction and the expiratory adduction of the vocal cords. The pharynx undergoes smaller changes in size during normal breathing, yet altera-

tions in pharyngeal size appear to play a major factor in the pathogenesis of the obstructive sleep apnea syndromes. The soft palate regulates the route of airflow between nose and mouth to suit ventilatory demands; in addition, it controls the size of the posterior nasopharynx. The nose contributes the greatest portion of normal resting supraglottic upper-airway resistance, and it is influenced by both neuromuscular and neurovascular factors. Finally, the anterior oral orifice needs to be opened for breathing to switch from the nasal to the oral route; in addition, under some circumstances, narrowing of the oral aperture may be used to regulate airflow during expiration.

Detailed descriptions of upper-airway structure, regulation of upper-airway muscles, and upper-airway effects on breathing during wakefulness and sleep are available in several recent reviews (1–7).

MUSCLES OF THE UPPER AIRWAYS

Anatomy and Mechanical Actions

A heterogeneous group of striated muscles are present in the upper airways (Table 1). These muscles may narrow, dilate, or stiffen the airways, change the route by which airflow traverses the airway, and participate in special respiratory acts such as coughing (2,3,6,7).

The muscles of the larynx consist of an intrinsic and an extrinsic group. The intrinsic muscles of the larynx control the laryngeal inlet and regulate the movements of the vocal cords. The size of the laryngeal inlet is regulated by the oblique arytenoid muscles, which approximate the laryngeal cartilages to one another and draw them forward to the epiglottis. This action serves primarily as a lower-airway defensive function by closing the supraglottic airway during swallowing. The position of the vocal cords is controlled by five other muscles. The posterior cricoarytenoid is the primary muscle that controls laryngeal aperture during resting

E. van Lunteren: Departments of Medicine and Neurosciences, Case Western Reserve University School of Medicine, Cleveland, Ohio 44106.

TABLE 1. *Muscles that alter upper-airway size and configuration*

Intrinsic muscles of the larynx
  Posterior cricoarytenoid
  Thyroarytenoid
  Cricothyroid
  Transverse arytenoid
  Lateral cricoarytenoid
  Oblique arytenoid
Muscles that act directly or indirectly on the hyoid arch
  Geniohyoid
  Sternohyoid
  Thyrohyoid
  Sternothyroid
  Omohyoid
  Mylohyoid
  Stylohyoid
  Digastric
  Hyoglossus
  Genioglossus (some species)
Muscles of the posterolateral pharyngeal wall
  Superior constrictor
  Middle constrictor
  Inferior constrictor
Muscles that act on the tongue
  Intrinsic tongue muscles
    Longitudinal
    Transverse
    Vertical
  Extrinsic tongue muscles
    Genioglossus
    Hyoglossus
    Styloglossus
    Palatoglossus
Muscles that regulate the position of the soft palate
  Levator veli palatini
  Tensor veli palatini
  Musculus uvulae
  Palatopharyngeus
  Palatoglossus
Muscles that control the mandible
  Masseter
  Temporalis
  Lateral pterygoid
  Medial pterygoid
Nasal muscles
  Dilator naris
  Levator alaeque nasi
  Procerus
  Compressor naris

breathing in the adult (8–10); moreover, it acts to abduct the vocal cords by rotating the arytenoid cartilages and therefore moving the vocal cords away from the midline. Movement of the vocal cords towards the midline is accomplished by contraction of the transverse arytenoid, lateral cricoarytenoid, and thyroarytenoid muscles. The former muscle moves the posterior aspects of the arytenoid cartilages together, whereas the latter two muscles displace the vocal processes of the arytenoid cartilages and the vocal cords towards the midline. The adductor laryngeal muscles

appear to participate in breathing especially during early postnatal life, although recent studies suggest that they are active during the respiratory cycle in adults as well (11). Finally, the vocal cords are elongated and tensed by the action of the cricothyroid muscle, which pulls the thyroid cartilages forward and tilts the lamina of the cricoid cartilages backward with the attached arytenoid cartilages. There appears to be great interdependence among the laryngeal muscles with respect to their mechanical actions. For example, the cricothyroid muscle acting alone narrows the laryngeal aperture, but concomitant activation of the posterior cricoarytenoid muscle dilates the larynx to a greater extent than if the posterior cricoarytenoid contracts alone (12). All of the intrinsic muscles of the larynx are supplied by the recurrent laryngeal nerve—with the exception of the cricothyroid muscle, which is supplied by the superior laryngeal nerve.

The extrinsic muscles of the larynx consist of laryngeal elevators (the digastric, stylohyoid, mylohyoid, geniohyoid, stylopharyngeus, salpingopharyngeus, and palatopharyngeus muscles) and laryngeal depressors (the sternothyroid, sternohyoid, and omohyoid muscles). The extrinsic laryngeal muscles are used to change the position of the thyroid cartilage during swallowing, and they act to resist displacement of the larynx during breathing. The latter action is assisted by the elastic recoil of the trachea. The extrinsic laryngeal muscles also have actions on the pharynx, as discussed in greater detail below.

Several groups of muscles may alter the size and configuration of the pharynx. These include the muscles that alter the shape and position of the tongue, muscles located in the anterior and lateral walls of the pharynx which insert on the hyoid bone, and a constrictor group of muscles located mainly laterally and posteriorly. In addition, two other muscle groups may alter pharyngeal size, including those which act on the mandible as well as those which regulate the position of the soft palate.

The muscles of the tongue are classified into two types: intrinsic and extrinsic. Muscles that are totally confined to the tongue comprise the intrinsic group. Their main mechanical roles are to alter the shape of the tongue and to increase the rigidity of the tongue. There are three groups of intrinsic muscles: the longitudinal, transverse, and vertical groups. Despite having no bony attachments, they are able to regulate tongue movements by acting as muscular hydrostats.

Four muscles comprise the extrinsic tongue muscle group. The genioglossus is a fan-shaped muscle located in the midline; some fibers course directly posteriorly from the mandible, whereas other fibers initially course posteriorly and then curve in a more superior and anterior direction towards the top surface and tip of the tongue. The genioglossus is the major muscle that allows the tongue to protrude and, along with the hyoglossus, also depresses the tongue. The tongue is drawn upward and backward by the styloglossus, and the posterior tongue is drawn upward by the palatoglossus. All of the intrinsic and extrinsic tongue muscles (as well as the geniohyoid muscle; see below) are innervated by the hypoglossal nerve, with the exception of the palatoglossus muscle. Studies in which tongue muscles have been electrically stimulated indicate that the genioglossus is responsible for protruding the tongue and, in addition, may also deviate the tip of the tongue ipsolaterally, whereas the intrinsic muscles have actions involved in lateral movements of the tongue. These studies have also pointed out the interrelationships between the mechanical actions of intrinsic and extrinsic tongue muscles contracting alone as compared to contracting simultaneously. Physiological studies have not systematically examined which muscle or muscles of the tongue are most important for altering the size of the posterior phyarnx, although it is quite clear that activity of the genioglossus muscle correlates with increases in pharyngeal airway size (13–15).

A large number of muscles insert on the hyoid arch, a bony structure situated near the junction of the neck with the head. By moving the hyoid arch, these muscles alter the configuration of the pharynx resulting from soft tissue connections between the hyoid arch and the pharyngeal wall. Muscles that insert on the hyoid bone from an inferior direction include the sternohyoid, sternothyroid, and omohyoid. The suprahyoid and infrahyoid muscle groups exert cranial and caudal forces on the hyoid bone, respectively, and, in addition, may move the hyoid anteriorly or posteriorly. Based on studies in which these muscles have been either electrically stimulated or selectively denervated, it is apparent that many of these hyoid muscles, like the genioglossus muscle, have the ability to dilate and/or stabilize the pharynx (13,15–18). Furthermore, there may be some degree of synergy between these muscles when stimulated simultaneously, especially with regard to the combined action of suprahyoid and infrahyoid muscles, which, when acting together, would be expected to produce a vector of forces in an anterior direction on the hyoid bone and, hence, on the anterior pharyngeal wall. Although these muscles act mainly on the lower portions of the pharynx, many of the hyoid muscles produce dilation of the nasopharynx as well.

Three sets of muscles are located on the posterior and lateral walls of the pharynx, and they have a mechanical action of narrowing the pharynx: the superior, middle, and inferior constrictors. They are used primarily during swallowing, although several of these muscles are also spontaneously active in phase with

the respiratory cycle and may help regulate the rate of airflow during expiration.

Muscles that control the position of the jaw may impact on the size of the pharynx in two manners. Protrusion of the jaw moves many of the oral and pharyngeal structures (including the tongue) in an anterior direction, thereby dilating the pharynx. In addition, closure of the mouth produces an anteriorly directed traction on the hyoid arch via its muscular and soft tissue connections with the mandible. Conversely, opening the mouth, and hence relaxation of some of the mandibular muscles, is critical for breathing to traverse the oral route. Muscles that primarily elevate the jaw are the temporalis and the masseter, whereas muscles that primarily protrude the jaw are the medial and lateral pterygoids. Some of these muscles have been shown to be rhythmically active in phase with the respiratory cycle, and their degree of activity appears to correlate with stabilization of the pharyngeal upper airway (19).

The soft palate and uvula are movable tissues suspended from the posterior border of the hard or bony palate and extending downward and backward into the oropharynx. Raising the palate closes the pharyngeal isthmus, thereby promoting oral breathing, whereas moving the palatoglossal arches toward the midline narrows the oral pharyngeal isthmus and favors nasal breathing (20). In addition, movements of the palate towards and away from the posterior nasopharyngeal wall appear to be important determinants of airway obstruction in some subjects with obstructive sleep apnea (21). The five muscles that regulate the position of the soft palate and the palatoglossal arches are the levator veli palatini, tensor veli palatini, musculus uvulae, palatopharyngeus, and palatoglossus. The position of the soft palate appears to be determined by the coordinated activity of groups of antagonistic muscles, especially during speech but probably also during breathing.

The oral aperture is controlled by the mandibular muscles as well as by those muscles which act upon the lips. Multiple dilator muscles radiate out from the lips, allowing fine regional control with regard to dilating the anterior portion of the mouth. Only one muscle acts as a lip sphincter: the orbicularis oris. Its fibers encircle the oral orifice and some are attached to the maxilla, the mandible, and the buccinator muscle.

Several muscles act to dilate or constrict the anterior nasal passages. The dilators in humans include the dilator naris muscle, the levator alaeque nasi muscle, and the procerus muscle. This group of muscles is commonly referred to as the ''alae nasi'' in the respiratory literature. In humans, nasal resistance can be reduced by as much as one-third by voluntary flaring of the external naris. One muscle in the nose acts as a nasal sphincter: the compressor naris.

Activity of muscles in one portion of the upper airway may impact on the luminal diameter of other parts of the upper airway. During inspiration, the amount of subatmospheric pressure generated within the pharynx is determined, to a large extent, by (a) pharyngeal size and compliance and (b) the intensity of the thoracic muscle contraction. However, upstream airway resistance, especially that in the nose, can alter the pressure profiles within the upper airway, so that narrowing at the nose may result in more subatmospheric pressures in the pharynx and increase the tendency of the pharynx to narrow or collapse during inspiration. Other close interrelationships exist among muscles of the pharynx, not only within a given group but also between muscles of the tongue, anterior and posterior pharynx, mandible, and soft palate. It appears that the activity of no single muscle can account for the majority of the changes in pharyngeal resistance that occur during breathing. In addition, the interdependence of muscle action is further complicated by intersubject variability among sleep apnea patients in the site of pharyngeal obstruction (nasopharynx *versus* oropharynx *versus* hypopharynx *versus* combinations of these), which may reflect both neuromuscular and anatomic factors. The neural control of these muscles and their activity in patients with sleep apnea will be discussed subsequently.

Intrinsic Properties of Upper-Airway Muscles

The most extensive information available about the intrinsic properties of upper-airway muscles is for the muscles of the larynx. In general, the laryngeal muscles have physiological and structural properties associated with fast contraction times, yet they are surprisingly resistant to fatigue. The contraction times of the thyroarytenoid, posterior cricoarytenoid, and cricothyroid muscles (22–26) are compared to that of the diaphragm, typical slow limb muscles, and typical fast limb muscles in Fig. 1. From these values it is apparent that contraction times are species-dependent for all of the different muscle groups. The thyroarytenoid and posterior cricoarytenoid are as fast as, if not faster than, many of the fast limb muscles, whereas the cricothyroid muscle is somewhat slower than this although substantially faster than the slow limb muscles. The half-relaxation times of laryngeal muscles tend to be comparable to their contraction times, which is usually the case with the faster striated muscles—in contrast to slower striated muscles, in which half-relaxation times tend to be one to two times as long as contraction times. In the cat, half-relaxation times have been reported to be 41 msec for the cricothyroid muscle, 20–27 msec for the thyroarytenoid muscle, and 29 msec for the posterior cricoarytenoid muscle.

The twitch-to-tetanus ratios of laryngeal muscles are also consistent with their fast physiological profile. In different species, this ratio ranges from 0.10 to 0.16 for the thyroarytenoid muscle and from 0.23 to 0.24 for the cricothyroid muscle. These values contrast with those of the diaphragm, which have much higher twitch-to-tetanus ratios, ranging from approximately 0.36 to 0.37. The low twitch-to-tetanus ratios of the laryngeal muscles allow tension production to be finely regulated. The fast contraction and relaxation times, as well as the low twitch-to-tetanus ratios, are appropriately reflected in the shapes of the force–frequency curves of the laryngeal muscles, which tend to be located to the right of the of many other limb skeletal muscles.

The endurance characteristics of laryngeal muscles

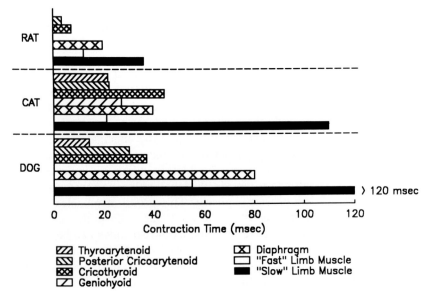

FIG. 1. Isometric contraction times of laryngeal and pharyngeal upper-airway muscles are compared to contraction times of the diaphragm and limb skeletal muscles in three species. Most upper-airway muscles have contraction times on the order of those for fast limb muscles, and they are usually faster than those of the diaphragm. Laryngeal muscle data are from refs. 22–27, pharyngeal muscle data are from ref. 34, and other muscle data are reviewed in ref. 7.

have been assessed in two separate studies. Edstrom et al. (27) found that despite the muscles being fast, the cricothyroid, thyroarytenoid, and lateral cricoarytenoid muscles develop fatigue at a much slower rate than did the tibialis anterior (a typical fast limb muscle); however, their fatigue characteristics were comparable to those of the soleus, a typical slow limb muscle. Hinrichsen and Dulhunty (24) found that the cricothyroid was more resistant to fatigue than was the posterior cricoarytenoid muscle. Both muscles were more resistant to fatigue than would be predicted on the basis of their fast contraction times.

Information is also available regarding the histochemical properties of laryngeal muscles; fiber subtype proportions appear to be both muscle- and species-specific. Edstrom et al. (27) found in cats that the lateral cricoarytenoid and transverse arytenoid muscles were composed of 10% or less slow oxidative fibers, whereas the cricothyroid and posterior cricoarytenoid muscles consisted of approximately 40% slow oxidative fibers. More recently, Teig et al. (28) studied the posterior cricoarytenoid muscles in humans and classified 67% of fibers as slow and 33% as fast. Malmgren and Gacek (29) also assessed human posterior cricoarytenoid muscles; they found 52% of fibers to be slow and 48% of fibers to be fast. Finally, Hinrichsen and Dulhunty (24) found in the rat that the posterior cricoarytenoid had only 3% slow fibers and that the cricothyroid had 16% slow fibers, with the remainder being fast fibers for each muscle. Ultrastructural examination of the posterior cricoarytenoid and cricothyroid muscles by these same investigators revealed (a) well-developed T-tubule systems and sarcoplasmic reticulum, which may be adaptations for very fast contraction times, and (b) high mitochondrial contents, which may be an adaptation that allows good endurance properties.

The histochemical properties of tongue muscles have been examined in two studies. In the cat (30) the extrinsic muscles were found to have fiber subtype proportions of 19–25% slow and 75–81% fast. The intrinsic muscles consisted entirely of fast fibers. In humans (31) the tongue muscles consist of 30–35% slow and 65–70% fast fibers (in this study, no differentiation was made between intrinsic and extrinsic tongue muscles). Of note is that in patients with Down's syndrome, tongue muscles consisted of a lower proportion of slow fibers (approximately 5–20%) and a correspondingly higher proportion of fast fibers, as compared with those in normal subjects. Regarding other muscles that act on the lower pharynx, in the cat the geniohyoid and sternohyoid consist of approximately 14–16% slow fibers, 31–36% fast oxidative glycolytic fibers, and 48–55% fast glycolytic fibers (32). An even greater paucity of slow oxidative fibers has been found in these same muscles in the rat (33). Physiologically,

the geniohyoid muscle of the cat has a relatively fast contraction time (27 msec), a relatively low twitch-to-tetanus ratio, and a force–frequency curve located to the right of the diaphragm. Despite these fast physiological properties, the geniohyoid appears to be quite resistant to fatigue when stimulated at high rates (34). In contrast, the human genioglossus has been reported to be relatively easily fatiguable (35).

The jaw muscles appear to have variable compositions in different species. In humans the lateral pterygoid muscle consists of 70% slow oxidative fibers which account for 81% of the overall fiber cross-sectional area (36). In contrast, in cats the pterygoid muscles consist of 29% slow oxidative fibers, the masseter consists of 10% slow oxidative fibers, and the temporalis consists of 2% slow oxidative fibers (37). In the latter study in the cat, the masseter and temporalis muscles had contraction times of 11–13 msec, with comparable half-relaxation times. In addition, the twitch-to-tetanus ratios were on the order of 0.10 to 0.13, consistent with their fast physiological properties. These muscles tended to reduce their forced output rapidly when stimulated repeatedly.

ACTIVITY OF UPPER-AIRWAY MUSCLES DURING WAKEFULNESS AND SLEEP

Electrical Activity of Upper-Airway Muscles

Many of the upper-airway muscles are electrically active in phase with the respiratory cycle. The extent of activity varies considerably among muscles. Some (e.g., the posterior cricoarytenoid) are consistently active, whereas others are either quiescent or intermittently active during resting breathing and are only recruited as the ventilatory efforts increase. Muscles also differ with respect to the portion of the respiratory cycle during which they are active. Those which dilate the upper airways tend to be active predominantly during inspiration, whereas those which narrow the upper airways tend to be active predominantly during expiration. These muscles are sometimes active exclusively during one phase of the respiratory cycle; more commonly, however, these muscles are predominantly active during one phase, with lower levels of activity during the other phases. Examples of muscles that are active more during inspiration than during expiration include (a) the posterior cricoarytenoid in the larynx, (b) the genioglossus and geniohyoid in the pharynx, and (c) the alae nasi of the nose (8–10,14,17,38–42). Examples of muscles that are active predominantly during expiration include (a) the thyroarytenoid muscle of the larynx and (b) the pharyngeal constrictors (11,39). Despite classification as predominantly inspiratory or expiratory, some muscles may change their predominant phase of activation in response to a variety of chemical or mechanical stimuli.

The timing of the inspiratory onset of upper-muscle activity often differs from that of the diaphragm (41). Many of the upper-airway muscles have been reported to become active up to 50–100 msec prior to the onset of diaphragm activity (this has been called "preactivation"), whereas some muscles may lag behind the diaphragm with regard to inspiratory onset. The exact relationship between the timing of diaphragm and upper-airway muscle inspiratory onset appears to depend on factors such as chemical drive, mechanical afferent input from the upper airways, and the state of arousal. In addition, patients with sleep apnea have been found to have dynamic breath-to-breath alterations in the inspiratory onset of upper-airway muscle activity, which has been postulated to play a role in maintenance of upper-airway patency. To the extent that preactivation of upper-airway muscles occurs, this is felt to dilate (or at least stiffen) the upper airway prior to the onset of inspiratory airflow and, hence, produce an early inspiratory stabilization of upper airways.

The pattern of inspiratory activity, as reflected in the shape of the electromyograms, is typically different for upper-airway muscles than for thoracic inspiratory muscles. In contrast to the progressively incrementing electrical activity of diaphragm inspiratory activity, many of the upper-airway muscles are maximally active during early to mid-inspiration, with a subsequent decrement in activity during the remainder of inspiration (43,44). This pattern is dependent on both vagal and nonvagal mechanisms (see below). The pattern of upper-airway-muscle inspiratory activity resembles, to a certain extent, that of inspiratory airflow. The magnitude of subatmospheric pressures generated in the upper airways during inspiration tends to parallel the instantaneous inspiratory airflow, and hence there appears to be a close matching between the within-breath requirements for pharyngeal stabilization and within-breath activation of upper-airway dilating muscles.

Some of the upper-airway muscles that are active predominantly during inspiration have minimal or no activity during expiration, whereas other muscles may display considerable activity during expiration. Similarly, some muscles that are active predominantly during expiration may display some activity during inspiration as well. Among this latter group of muscles, the thyroarytenoid muscle of the larynx appears to be predominantly active during the early part of expiration (coincident with the postinspiration activity of the diaphragm), whereas other muscles such as the pharyngeal constrictors tend to be active somewhat later during expiration.

Chemical stimuli such as hypercapnia and hypoxia increase the activity of thoracic respiratory muscles and also increase the activity of upper-airway muscles (8,9,17,38,40–42). The CO_2 thresholds of the upper-airway muscles (i.e., the P_{CO_2} at which these muscles become active) tend to be higher than the CO_2 threshold for the diaphragm, and in addition there is considerable variability among upper-airway muscles with regard to the P_{CO_2} at which they become active. For example, the CO_2 threshold of the diaphragm appears to be lower than that of the posterior cricoarytenoid muscle of the larynx, and both are lower than the CO_2 thresholds of most pharyngeal dilating muscles such as the genioglossus and geniohyoid muscles. Once active, the upper-airway muscles increase their activity as the degree of hypercapnia increases. For some upper-airway muscles, the increases in activity in response to hypercapnia are parallel to those of the thoracic respiratory muscles. For other upper-airway muscles, however, there appear to be disproportionate increases in upper-airway muscle activity at high CO_2 levels, resulting in a curvilinear relationship between thoracic and upper-airway muscle activity as CO_2 increases. That is, changes in P_{CO_2} at lower levels of CO_2 are associated with greater increments in diaphragm activity than in upper-airway muscle activity, whereas changes in P_{CO_2} at higher CO_2 levels are associated with relatively greater increments in upper-airway muscle activity.

Hypoxia also influences the activation of upper-airway muscles, with mild to moderate degrees of hypoxia stimulating activity of upper-airway muscles. Again there are muscle-to-muscle and species-to-species differences in both hypoxia thresholds for muscle activation as well as differences in linearity versus alinearity of these responses. With severe or prolonged hypoxia, there is known to be a depressive effect on breathing, and during this time a decrement in upper-airway muscle may occur as well. However, it appears that during the so-called hypoxic depression of breathing, activity of upper-airway muscles may be quite well maintained relative to that of thoracic respiratory muscles. In response to hypoxia and hypercapnia, differences also have been found to occur in the timing over which changes in thoracic versus upper-airway muscle activity occur. Differences in both the magnitude and timing of responses of upper-airway versus chest-wall muscles have been widely implicated in the dynamic fluctuations in upper-airway resistance that may occur during sleep in subjects with obstructive sleep apnea; moreover, these differences may contribute both to the production and relief of upper-airway obstruction.

Receptors located in the lungs, lower airways, and upper airways, and whose afferents are carried via the vagus nerve (including one of its branches, the superior laryngeal nerve), have a profound influence on upper-airway muscle activity. The effect of pulmonary stretch receptors is typically tested by preventing lung inflation during inspiration. During such a maneuver there is an augmentation of upper-airway muscle inspiratory activity which typically exceeds the augmentation of thoracic respiratory muscle activity. Not only does the peak activity of upper-airway muscles increase (Fig. 2), but there also tends to be an especially pronounced increment in activation during late inspiration (43,44). This results in upper-airway muscle activity peaking towards the end of inspiration (when lung inflation is prevented) rather than during early to mid-inspiration (when lung inflation is allowed to occur). This inhibitory influence of lung-volume-related afferent information accounts for much, but not all, of the early peaking pattern of upper-airway muscle electrical activity during inspiration. In contrast to their inhibitory effect on both diaphragm and upper-airway muscle activity during inspiration, it appears that pulmonary stretch receptors may have opposite effects on muscle activity during expiration; that is, their effects inhibit diaphragm activity during expiration but stimulate both laryngeal and pharyngeal dilating muscle activity during early expiration. The effects of pulmonary C-fiber-associated receptors have

been tested by the administration of substances such as capsaicin. During the resulting apnea, the duration of upper-airway muscle quiescence is shorter than that of diaphragm quiescence; furthermore, when breathing resumes, albeit at higher rates and lower tidal volumes, the relative amount of upper-airway muscle activity compared to diaphragm activity is elevated (39).

Receptors in the larynx (and to a lesser extent the pharynx), including pressure, temperature, "drive," and irritant receptors, influence the activity of both upper-airway and thoracic respiratory muscles. Potentially especially relevant to breathing during sleep is the role of pressure receptors (45,46). When subatmospheric pressures are applied to the larynx and pharynx, there is a marked augmentation of activity of upper dilating muscles in the absence of a similar stimulatory effect on thoracic respiratory muscles (Fig. 2). There may be a minor role for pressure (and flow) receptors in augmenting upper-airway muscle activity during the course of normal inspiration. In subjects with obstructive sleep apneas, cyclic subatmospheric pressures are produced in the larynx and pharynx downstream from the site of upper-airway obstruction.

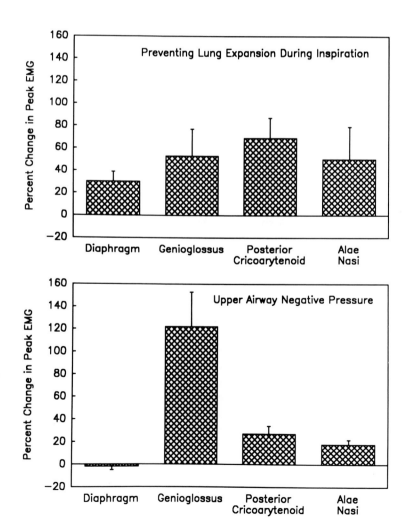

FIG. 2. Effects of respiratory stimuli on electrical activity of the diaphragm and three upper-airway muscles. Values in response to preventing inspiratory lung inflation (**top**) and in response to application of subatmospheric pressures to the upper airways (**bottom**) are depicted as a percent change relative to prestimulus control values. Data are from refs. 44 and 46.

It has been postulated that this reflex may be especially important in restoring upper-airway patency when obstructive apneas occur.

A number of other receptors throughout the body may influence upper-airway muscle activity. These include receptors in the esophagus and other portions of the gastrointestinal tract, in skeletal muscles, and in the cardiovascular system. Afferent inputs from these receptors may not affect all of the respiratory muscles equally; for example, esophageal dilation inhibits crural diaphragm activity but stimulates airway-dilating muscle activity. The exact roles of these reflexes during normal ventilatory homeostasis are unclear, although it should be noted that associations have been described between congestive heart failure and intermittent airway obstruction.

The state of arousal has a strong influence on the respiratory activity of upper-airway muscles (14,21,38, 40,47,48). Most studies have indicated that during both non-rapid eye movement and rapid eye movement sleep there are diminutions of upper-airway dilating muscle activity compared to during wakefulness. The degree to which this occurs varies among the different sleep states, as well as from muscle to muscle. Typically, the reduction of upper-airway muscle activity exceeds the reduction of thoracic respiratory muscle activity. The net effect is an alteration in the relationship between the magnitude of subatmospheric pressures generated in the pharynx due to inspiratory thoracic muscle contraction and stabilization of the upper airways due to contraction of upper dilating muscles. To the extent that the upper airways are destabilized during sleep, and to the extent that anatomic abnormalities are present in the upper airway, the net effect of the relative diminution of upper-airway stabilization may vary from a simple increase in upper-airway resistance to snoring to frank upper-airway obstruction and obstructive sleep apnea (see below).

A wide variety of pharmacological agents affect the activity of upper-airway muscles (reviewed in ref. 4). In general, the direction of the effect on upper-airway muscle activity is similar to that on diaphragm activity and breathing. However, at low doses the upper-airway muscles alone may be affected, and at higher doses the magnitude of the effect on upper-airway muscles may far exceed the magnitude of the effect on thoracic muscle activity. Sites of action of these pharmacological agents are variable, and they include peripheral chemoreceptors, central chemoreceptors, central respiratory neuronal groups, and motoneurons supplying the respiratory muscles. Agents that generally have been found to reduce upper-airway muscle activity include ethanol, benzodiazepines, gamma-aminobutyric acid and related agents, members of the opiate family, and dopamine. Agents that appear to stimulate upper-airway muscle activity include acetylcholine, nicotine, lobeline, sodium cyanide, isoproterenol, protriptyline, and progesterone. For some of these pharmacological agents there are associations between reductions in upper-airway muscle activity and worsening of sleep apnea (ethanol and benzodiazepines), and for other agents there are associations between stimulation of upper-airway muscle activity and alleviation of obstructive sleep apnea (nicotine and protriptyline).

The respiratory control of upper-airway muscles has been examined in greater detail by recording the activity patterns of single motor units of these muscles (49,50). The motor unit, which consists of a motoneuron and the muscle fibers it supplies, is the fundamental entity by which muscle contraction is regulated. For striated muscles it is known that increases in muscle activity are brought about by increasing the frequency of firing of motor units already active, as well as by the recruitment of motor units previously inactive. Conversely, decrements in muscle contraction are produced by slowing the rate of motor unit firing as well as by quiescence of motor units. For nonrespiratory skeletal muscles as well as the diaphragm, during graded contractions there appears to be an orderly recruitment of motor units on the basis of motoneuron size, with smaller motoneurons usually being recruited prior to larger motoneurons. This most likely is due to the intrinsic properties of the motoneurons themselves, although it has been postulated that specific connections between premotoneurons and motoneurons may contribute to this pattern of recruitment. Each motoneuron supplies only a single type of muscle fiber (during adulthood); in general, motor units that contain slower muscle fibers tend to be recruited earlier than motor units that contain faster muscle fibers. For the diaphragm, motor units appear to segregate into early-onset and late-onset subpopulations. A small number of studies have examined the motor-unit behavior of upper-airway dilating muscles. Although these studies generally concur that subpopulations of motor units can be discerned based on their behavior during breathing, studies tend to disagree on the exact classification system for segregating these subpopulations. There do appear to be subpopulations of motor units which are active during inspiration only, as well as others which are more active during inspiration than during expiration. Tonically active motor units have also been described, and some classification schemes have segregated motor units on the basis of exact timing of firing within specific portions of the respiratory cycle. For the diaphragm it appears that a specific motor unit will remain within a subpopulation despite changes in chemical or mechanical stimuli, whereas for some upper-airway motor units it appears that the pattern of firing within specific phases of the respiratory role may change in response to changes in pulmonary stretch receptor or chemoreceptor input. Nonetheless, it does appear that upper-airway muscles use motor-unit strategies to regulate their activity which are similar to strategies used by thoracic respiratory muscles.

Mechanical Consequences of Upper-Airway-Muscle Respiratory Activity

The relationships between upper-airway-muscle electrical activity and the size and configuration of the upper-airway lumen are complex. The upper airways can be dynamically altered at multiple sites, and each segment is unique with regard to the anatomic mechanical arrangement of its muscles. Each part contains multiple muscles, and hence the net effect of muscle contraction on upper-airway size is determined by all of the active muscles. Furthermore, muscles may act on the airway at distal sites. Finally, muscles may act either directly or indirectly on the upper airway. For example, the genioglossus acts directly to move one of the structures which make up the pharyngeal wall (the tongue), whereas the hyoid muscles act on the hyoid arch; moreover, it is only via soft tissue connections between the hyoid arch and the pharyngeal wall that changes in pharyngeal size occur.

Several techniques have been used to assess mechanical effects of spontaneous muscle contraction on the upper airway (8–10,13,15–19,42,51–58). Alterations in the size and configuration of the upper-airway lumen can be visualized directly, usually with fiberoptic or radiographic techniques in conjunction with video cinematography, with subsequent analysis of the recorded images. Airway resistance can be measured either by passing a constant flow through the upper airway or by making use of spontaneous airflow that occurs during the respiratory cycle. Changes in resistance that occur within a breath or in response to respiratory stimuli can be assessed either (a) globally, across the entire upper airway, or (b) regionally, across specific segments of the upper airway. Changes in upper-airway size can be assessed also in terms of their effects on airflow during inspiration and expiration. This technique is most useful when used in conjunction with either electrical recordings of muscle activity or measurements of airway resistance, in order to allow correlation between upper-airway events on the one hand and effects on airflow on the other hand. Changes in the ability of the pharynx to resist collapse have been used to assess both (a) the relaxed mechanics of the upper airway and (b) the effects of muscle activity on upper-airway mechanics. In animal studies using a preparation where the upper airway is isolated from the rest of the respiratory system and sealed, pressure changes and/or changes in upper airway size can be

assessed directly. Finally, mechanical activity of individual muscles has been assessed by directly measuring length changes of the upper-airway muscles using sonomicrometric techniques.

During quiet breathing, the vocal cords move away from the midline during inspiration and return towards the midline during expiration. The latter movement is, in part, accounted for by relaxation of laryngeal abductors, but under some circumstances laryngeal adductors may contribute to the reduction in laryngeal diameter during expiration. These movements of the vocal cords are appropriately reflected in changes in laryngeal resistance, with resistance being lowest during inspiration and highest towards the end of expiration. The reduction in resistance during inspiration augments inspiratory airflow for a given level of thoracic muscle activation, whereas the narrowing of the larynx during expiration acts to retard expiratory airflow. The latter "laryngeal braking" of expiratory airflow acts in conjunction with postinspiratory activity of the diaphragm to maintain the lungs at a higher degree of expansion during a longer portion of expiration than would be predicted based on the passive properites of the lungs and chest wall alone, and it has been postulated to improve the oxygen transfer capacities of the lung. Other portions of the upper airway, including the nose and the pharynx, also undergo cyclic increases in luminal cross-sectional area during inspiration and undergo reductions during expiration. During resting breathing, these changes are substantially less than what is seen in the larynx, however.

Chemical, mechanical, and pharmacological stimuli produce changes in upper-airway size and configuration consistent with their previously described actions on the upper-airway muscles. For example, as the extent of hypercapnia or hypoxia increases, the phasic dilations of the upper airway during inspiration are progressively augmented as well. The relative effects of hypoxia and hypercapnia on upper-airway dimensions during expiration are not always the same at a given level of ventilation, however. For example, some studies have indicated that the early expiratory activity of upper-airway dilating muscles is higher during hypercapnia than during hypoxia; these influences are appropriately reflected in the size and resistance of the larynx and other portions of the upper airway during expiration. Similarly in subjects with asthma, greater expiratory narrowing of both the larynx and the pharynx has been found during induced bronchoconstriction than during resting breathing. This phenomenon appears to be analogous to the pursed-lips breathing that is seen in subjects with severe chronic obstructive pulmonary disease, which also acts to diminish the rate of airflow during expiration.

For the alae nasi there appears to be a close relationship between electromyographic activity and muscle shortening, both during resting breathing and in response to a variety of chemical and mechanical stimuli. In contrast, for the hyoid muscles the relationships between electrical activity and muscle shortening are less predictable (42,58), due to complex interrelationships between the multiple muscles that attach to the hyoid arch, as well as between soft tissue structures (such as the trachea) that are also connected indirectly to the hyoid arch. For the geniohyoid and sternohyoid muscles, changes in muscle length may occur despite the muscles being electrically quiescent; these length changes appear to be due to movements of (a) the chest wall and (b) the muscular and tracheal connections between the chest wall and the upper airway. Furthermore, even when they are electrically active, the hyoid muscles may lengthen, remain the same length, or shorten. The exact pattern of length changes is dependent on the amount of activity of the muscles themselves as well as on the relative forces imparted by adjacent muscles. Even when shortening of the hyoid muscles does not occur, stiffening of these muscles does occur with muscle contraction, and hence the muscles serve to alter the transmission of forces produced through movements of adjacent structures. Despite these complex mechanical behaviors, electrical activity of the hyoid muscles correlates closely with inspiratory increases in upper-airway size. Studies of length changes of other upper-airway muscle groups have not yet been performed, but most likely they will indicate similar complexities of interrelationships among the activity of different muscles.

THE UPPER AIRWAY
AND OBSTRUCTIVE APNEAS DURING SLEEP

Alterations occur in the size and configuration of the upper airways during changes in behavioral state between wakefulness and sleep, as well as among the different sleep states (51–57). Typically, the upper-air-

way lumen is narrower during sleep than during wakefulness and is narrower during stages 3–4 than during stages 1–2 of non-rapid eye movement sleep. When the sleep-associated reductions in upper-airway luminal size are minor, small changes in overall ventilation occur, due in part to the load compensation of motor output to the thoracic respiratory muscles. In some individuals, however, there are large increases in upper-airway resistance associated with sleep and/or the upper airways are structurally narrowed to begin with, so that relatively small changes in upper-airway luminal size produce relatively large changes in resistance. Under these circumstances there may be incomplete closure of the upper airways, resulting in snoring or complete closure of the upper airways and thereby causing obstructive sleep apneas. The most common site at which obstruction occurs is the pharynx, although as discussed below there is considerable heterogeneity of the site of obstruction within this region. Some patients appear to have a laryngeal contribution to airway obstruction during sleep; in addition, alterations in nasal resistance will change the pressures generated within the pharynx during inspiration. Several anatomic and physiological factors contribute to the propensity of the upper airways to obstruct during sleep (Fig. 3).

Structural alterations of the upper airways predispose subjects to develop snoring and/or obstructive apneas during sleep (52,55,57). Examples of focal upper-airway abnormalities include retrognathia, micrognatia, tonsilar hyperplasia, macroglossia, and nasal airway narrowing. In many patients there are no focal abnormalities, but based on cephalometric radiographic, fluoroscopic, computed tomographic, magnetic resonance imaging, and acoustic reflective techniques, it appears that many of these patients have diffuse narrowing of the pharyngeal and oral airway and increased collapsibility of these areas. Much of the reduction in luminal size appears to be secondary to increased submucosal adipose tissue. The role of an-

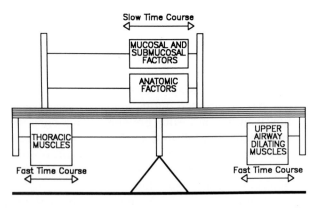

UPPER AIRWAY OBSTRUCTION   UPPER AIRWAY PATENCY

FIG. 3. Schematic of factors that influence the balance of forces leading to patency versus closure of the upper airways. Events with a fast time course include dynamic alterations in upper-airway dilating muscle activity (which promote airway patency) and dynamic alterations in thoracic inspiratory muscle activity (which promote airway closure). Slower alterations (over the course of several minutes to hours, or longer) occur in mucosal and submucosal factors, whereas anatomic factors are relatively stable (or change over weeks to months) in any given individual. The latter two factors predominantly produce narrowing of the upper airways and, hence, predispose to airway closure during periods of reduced upper-airway muscle activity.

atomic changes in predisposition to the obstructive sleep syndrome is further supported by the fact that in a subpopulation of subjects the removal of redundant pharyngeal tissue via uvulopalatopharyngoplasty, or correction of focal abnormalities, can result in the alleviation of sleep apnea. Despite the impressive anatomic evidence of upper-airway narrowing in many subjects with sleep apnea, very few of these subjects have physiological evidence of upper-airway obstruction on pulmonary function testing during wakefulness. Furthermore, during sleep there are differences in propensities for apneas to occur among the different sleep states. Thus it appears that anatomic narrowing of the upper airways plays a permissive role in the pathogenesis of obstructive sleep apnea but that other events with a faster time course explain the periodic production and relief of airway occlusion during sleep.

The site at which the upper airway obstructs during sleep apnea most commonly is the pharynx. However, there is variability in the exact site of closure, with some subjects obstructing the posterior pharynx and/or retropharynx, others the oropharynx, and others the nasopharynx. In addition, the site of obstruction may vary from apnea to apnea in any given patient, and under some circumstances closure of several areas of the pharynx occurs. During obstructive apneas, one or more of the following may occur, based on both endoscopic and fluoroscopic visualization of airway structures: The posterior aspect of the tongue moves further posteriorly; the lateral and posterior pharyngeal walls move toward the middle of the lumen; the mandible and hyoid bone move in a posterior direction; and the soft palate moves toward the posterior wall of the nasopharynx. Typically, progressive narrowing of the upper airway occurs for several breaths prior to frank airway obstruction, resulting in incremental increases in resistance across the upper airway. After several attempted inspiratory efforts against an obstructed airway, patency is then restored as a result of increasing contraction of upper dilating muscles, with either a sudden or gradual relief of the upper-airway obstruction.

Cyclic alterations in the degree of activation of upper-airway muscles are well documented to occur during repetitive obstructive sleep apneas (14,21,51–53,56,57). Reductions in intensity or even the absence of muscle activation leads to and occurs during the apneas, and heightened muscle activity is present during the periods when the upper airways are patent. The role of the genioglossus muscle and the cyclic alterations of pharyngeal luminal diameter has been described extensively, with more recent work examining contributions of other muscles that act on the hyoid bone, mandible, and soft palate in determining upper-airway patency. Current evidence suggests that multiple muscles contribute to this process, with perhaps a few muscles playing a major role and other muscles playing subsidiary roles. Although it is apparent that reductions in upper-airway dilating muscle activity are associated with obstructive apneas, and that increases in upper-airway dilating muscle activity are associated with relief of obstructive apneas, subjects with obstructive apnea may actually have increased overall levels of upper-airway dilating muscle activity than do normals (59). Several explanations may account for the increased level of muscle activation. First, the airway lumen tends to be narrowed to start with, so that a greater amount of muscle activity may be required to maintain a minimal degree of patency. Second, the increase in adipose tissue and/or other soft tissue structures may place an additional load upon the upper-airway muscles, reducing their ability to dilate the pharynx. Finally, alterations in pharyngeal structure may change the resting lengths of the muscles and hence the position on their length-tension relationships, thereby resulting in diminished mechanical output for a given degree of activation.

The role of neuromuscular factors in maintaining airway patency during sleep is further pointed out by the following observations: Pharmacological agents that are known to reduce upper-airway muscle activity are associated with worsening of obstructive apneas; conversely, pharmacologic agents known to increase upper-airway muscle activity appear to have a beneficial effect on upper-airway patency during sleep (60–64). Examples of the former group include ethanol and the benzodiazepines; examples of the latter group include protriptyline and nicotine.

There are several etiologies of the cyclic changes in upper-airway muscle activity that occur during sleep. First, sleep is associated with intrinsic irregularities in breathing pattern, with waxing and waning of the intensity of inspiratory efforts, even apart from any upper-airway influences. The respiratory neural centers that project to thoracic muscles also project to upper-airway muscles via several of the cranial nerves. Any differences between upper-airway muscles and the diaphragm in terms of their responses to these waxing and waning descending respiratory inputs, or any differences in timing of motor responses to these premotor inputs, can result in transient periods where the proper balance between thoracic and upper-airway muscle activity is lost. A second factor is that sleep per se is associated with reductions in the respiratory motor output which appear to be much more pronounced for intercostal and upper-airway muscles than for the diaphragm. Under these circumstances, thoracic respiratory efforts are only minimally reduced, whereas upper-airway dilating efforts are reduced to a greater extent. This may be especially true during rapid eye movement sleep, which is known to be associated with direct inhibition of motoneurons. Finally, there may be a reduced functioning of the load compensation mechanisms of respiratory muscles during sleep as compared to that during wakefulness, so that frank alterations in chemical homeostasis have to occur before the upper-airway muscles are sufficiently activated to reestablish upper-airway patency.

Once upper-airway obstruction occurs, several events contribute to the reestablishment of upper-airway patency. The cessation of effective ventilation leads to hypoxia and hypercapnia. These chemical stimuli, in turn, increase the degree to which upper-airway dilating muscles are activated, which, when sufficiently intense, may be sufficient to reopen the airway at the site of obstruction. A greater increment in upper-airway muscle compared to thoracic muscle force production may result from (a) a curvilinear relationship between thoracic and upper-airway muscles as ventilatory efforts increase and/or (b) alinearities in relationships between increases in muscle activation and resultant effects on thoracic expansion (e.g., for the diaphragm) and upper-airway dilation (e.g., for the genioglossus muscle). A second group of reflexes elicited by upper-airway obstruction are those of mechanoreceptor origin resulting from the absence of lung inflation (pulmonary stretch receptors) or the generation of subatmospheric pressures within the larynx and distal pharynx. Both phenomena would result in a preferential stimulation of upper-airway muscle activity over that of thoracic muscle activity. Finally, obstructive apneas during sleep often lead to frank arousals from sleep to wakefulness, changes in sleep state from rapid eye movement to non-rapid eye movement sleep, changes from a deeper state to a less deep stage within non-rapid eye movement sleep, or small changes in electroencephalographic patterns insufficient to be classified as a full change in sleep stage. Arousals have been well documented to produce sudden increments in upper-airway dilating muscle activity, resulting in a sudden alteration in the balance of forces that determine upper-airway patency. Once airway patency is restored following an obstructive apnea, hypoxia and hypercapnia resolve, lung expansion occurs during inspiration, inspiratory pressures within the laryngeal and pharyneal airways become close to atmospheric, and the electroencephalographic patterns may return to those associated with deeper stages of sleep. These events, in turn, are associated with reductions in upper-airway muscle activity, setting the stage for the subsequent obstructive apnea.

The role of mucosal and submucosal factors in determining nasal airway resistance is well established. The nasal subluminal tissue contains a rich vascular plexus, whose blood vessels are regulated by both neural and humoral factors. Fluctuations in blood volume (and, hence, in nasal resistance) occur normally over a time course of several minutes to hours. Furthermore, the thickness of this tissue is dramatically increased in response to inhaled allergens and infections. Changes in the amount and viscosity of nasal secretions amplify the vascularly mediated alterations in nasal airway resistance. Changes in upstream (nasal) airway resistance alter the pressure profiles produced within the pharynx during inspiration and, hence, can influence the propensity for obstructive apneas to occur during sleep. There has been a recent appreciation for a role of mucosal and submucosal pharyngeal tissues and the nature of pharyngeal secretions in influencing upper-airway patency. Radiographic studies have found that nasopharyngeal tissue of subjects with obstructive sleep apnea has an increased vascular volume compared to that of normals, and histological examination of palatal and retropharyngeal tissue following uvulopalatopharyngoplasty has revealed edematous changes in these tissues in subjects with obstructive sleep apnea. Studies in animal models have indicated that the character of pharyngeal secretions can influence both (a) the magnitude of the subatmospheric intraluminal pressures at which the upper airway both closes and reopens and (b) the difference between closing and opening pressures. The role of alterations in properties of pharyngeal secretions in the pathogenesis of the obstructive sleep in humans awaits further study.

REFERENCES

1. Guilleminault C. Clinical features and evaluation of obstructive sleep apnea. In: Kryger MH, Roth T, Dement WC, eds. *Principles and practice of sleep medicine*. Philadelphia: WB Saunders, 1989;552–559.
2. Mathew OP, Remmers JE. Respiratory function of the upper airway. In: Saunders NA, Sullivan CE, eds. *Sleep and breathing*. New York: Marcel Dekker, 1984;163–200.
3. Remmers JE. Anatomy and physiology of upper airway obstruction. In: Kryger MH, Roth T, Dement WC, eds. *Principles and practice of sleep medicine*. Philadelphia: WB Saunders, 1989;525–537.
4. Robinson RW, Zwillich CW. The effects of drugs on breathing during sleep. In: Kryger MH, Roth T, Dement WC, eds. *Principles and practice of sleep medicine*. Philadelphia: WB Saunders, 1989;501–513.
5. Sullivan CE, Issa FG, Berthon-Jones M, Saunders NA. Pathophysiology of sleep apnea. In: Saunders NA, Sullivan CE, eds. *Sleep and breathing*. New York: Marcel Dekker, 1984;299–364.
6. van Lunteren E, Strohl KP. The muscles of the upper airway. In: Widdicombe JH, ed. *Clinics in chest medicine*, vol 7. Philadelphia: WB Saunders, 1986;171–188.
7. van Lunteren E, Strohl KP. Striated respiratory muscles of the upper airways. In: Mathew OP, Sant'Ambrogio G, eds. *Respiratory function of the upper airway*. New York: Marcel Dekker, 1988;87–124.
8. Bartlett D Jr. Effects of hypercapnia and hypoxia on laryngeal resistance to airflow. *Respir Physiol* 1979;37:293–302.
9. Bartlett D Jr. Effects of vagal afferents on laryngeal responses to hypercapnia and hypoxia. *Respir Physiol* 1980;42:189–198.

10. Brancatisano TP, Dodd DS, Engel LA. Respiratory activity of posterior cricoarytenoid muscle and vocal cords in humans. *J Appl Physiol* 1984;57:1143–1149.

11. Kuna ST, Insalaco G, Woodson GE. Thyroarytenoid muscle activity during wakefulness and sleep in normal adults. *J Appl Physiol* 1988;65:1332–1339.

12. Konrad HR, Rattenborg CC. Combined actions of laryngeal muscles. *Acta Otolaryngol* 1969;67:646–649.

13. Brouillette RT, Thach BT. A neuromuscular mechanism maintaining extrathoracic airway patency. *J Appl Physiol* 1979; 46:772–779.

14. Remmers JE, DeGroot WJ, Sauerland EK, Anch AM. Pathogenesis of upper airway occlusion during sleep. *J Appl Physiol* 1978;44:931–938.

15. Strohl KP, Wolin AD, van Lunteren E, Fouke JM. Assessment of muscle action on upper airway stability in anesthetized dogs. *J Lab Clin Med* 1987;110:221–230.

16. Roberts JL, Reed WR, Thach BT. Pharyngeal airway-stabilizing function of sternohyoid and sternothyroid muscles in the rabbit. *J Appl Physiol* 1984;57:1790–1795.

17. Van de Graaff WB, Gottfried SB, Mitra J, van Lunteren E, Cherniack NS, Strohl KP. Respiratory function of hyoid muscles and hyoid arch. *J Appl Physiol* 1984;57:197–204.

18. van Lunteren E, Haxhiu MA, Cherniack NS. Relation between upper airway volume and hyoid muscle length. *J Appl Physiol* 1987;63:1443–1449.

19. Hollowell DE, Suratt PM. Activation of masseter muscles with inspiratory resistive loading. *J Appl Physiol* 1989;67:270–275.

20. Rodenstein DO, Stanescu DC. The soft palate and breathing. *Am Rev Respir Dis* 1986;134:311–325.

21. Anch AM, Remmers JE, Sauerland EK, deGroot WJ. Oropharyngeal patency during waking and sleep in the Pickwickian syndrome: electromyographic activity of the tensor veli palatini. *Electromyogr Clin Neurophysiol* 1981;21:317–330.

22. Hast MH. Mechanical properties of the cricothyroid muscle. *Laryngoscope* 1966;76:537–548.

23. Hast MH. Mechanical properties of the vocal fold muscle. *Pract Otorhinolaryngol* 1967;29:53–56.

24. Hinrichsen C, Dulhunty A. The contractile properties, histochemistry, ultrastructure and electrophysiology of the cricothyroid and posterior cricoarytenoid muscles in the rat. *J Muscle Res Cell Motil* 1982;3:169–190.

25. Hirose H, Ushijima T, Kobayashi T, Sawashima M. An experimental study of the contraction properties of the laryngeal muscles in the cat. *Ann Otol Rhinol Laryngol* 1969;78:297–306.

26. Martensson A, Skoglund CR. Contraction properties of intrinsic laryngeal muscles. *Acta Physiol Scand* 1964;60:318–336.

27. Edstrom L, Lindquist C, Martensson A. Correlation between functional and histochemical properties of the intrinsic laryngeal muscles in the cat. In: Wyke B, ed. *Ventilatory and phonatory control systems.* London: Oxford University Press, 1974;392–404.

28. Teig E, Dahl HA, Thorkelsen H. Actomyosin ATPase activity of human laryngeal muscles. *Acta Otolaryngol* 1978;85:272–281.

29. Malmgren LT, Gacek RR. Histochemical characteristics of muscle fiber types in the posterior cricoarytenoid muscle. *Ann Otol* 1981;90:423–429.

30. Hellstrand E. Morphological and histochemical properties of tongue muscles in cat. *Acta Physiol Scand* 1980;110:187–198.

31. Yarom R, Sagher U, Havivi Y, Peled IJ, Wexler MR. Myofibers in tongues of Down's syndrome. *J Neurol Sci* 1986;73:279–287.

32. van Lunteren E, Dick TE. Comparison of fiber subtype distribution of pharyngeal dilator muscles and diaphragm in cat [Abstract]. *Soc Neurosci Abstr* 1989;15:1191.

33. Salomone RJ, Dick TE, van Lunteren E. Fiber subtype and capillary distributions of pharyngeal dilator muscles and diaphragm in young and old rats [Abstract]. *Am Rev Respir Dis* 1990;in press.

34. van Lunteren, Salomone RJ, Manubay P, Supinski GS, Dick TE. Comparative contractile and endurance properties of geniohyoid and diaphragm muscles in cats [Abstract]. *Am Rev Respir Dis* 1990:in press.

35. Scardella AT, Co MA, Petrozzino JJ, Krawciw N, Edelman NH, Santiago TV. Strength and endurance characteristics of the normal human genioglossus [Abstract]. *Am Rev Respir Dis* 1989; 139:A449.

36. Eriksson P-O, Eriksson A, Ringqvist M, Thornell L-E. Special histochemical muscle-fibre characteristics of the human lateral pterygoid muscle. *Arch Oral Biol* 1981;26:495–507.

37. Taylor A, Cody FWJ, Bosley MA. Histochemical and mechanical properties of the jaw muscles of the cat. *Exp Neurol* 1973;38:99–109.

38. Haxhiu MA, van Lunteren E, Mitra J, Cherniack NS. Comparison of the response of diaphragm and upper airway dilating muscle activity in sleeping cats. *Respir Physiol* 1987;70:183–193.

39. Haxhiu MA, van Lunteren E, Deal EC, Cherniack NS. Effect of stimulation of pulmonary C fiber receptors on canine respiratory muscles. *J Appl Physiol* 1988;65:1087–1092.

40. Megirian D, Hinrichsen CFL, Sherry JH. Respiratory roles of genioglossus, sternothyroid, and sternohyoid muscles during sleep. *Exp Neurol* 1985;90:118–128.

41. Strohl K, Hensley M, Hallett M, Saunders N, Ingram R Jr. Activation of upper airway muscles before onset of inspiration in normal humans. *J Appl Physiol* 1980;49:638–642.

42. van Lunteren E, Haxhiu MA, Cherniack NS. Mechanical function of hyoid muscles during spontaneous breathing in cats. *J Appl Physiol* 1987;62:582–590.

43. Cohen MI. Phrenic and recurrent laryngeal discharge patterns and the Hering–Breuer reflex. *Am J Physiol* 1975;228:1489–1496.

44. van Lunteren E, Strohl KP, Parker DM, Bruce EN, Van de Graaff WB, Cherniack NS. Phasic volume-related feedback on upper airway muscle activity. *J Appl Physiol* 1984;56:730–736.

45. Mathew OP, Abu-Osba YK, Tach BT. Influence of upper airway pressure changes on genioglossus muscle respiratory activity. *J Appl Physiol* 1982;52:438–444.

46. van Lunteren E, Van de Graaff WM, Parker DM, Mitra J, Haxhiu MA, Strohl KP, Cherniack NS. Nasal and laryngeal reflex responses to negative upper airway pressure. *J Appl Physiol* 1984;56:746–752.

47. Orem J, Lydic R. Upper airway function during sleep and wakefulness: experimental studies on normal and anesthetized cats. *Sleep* 1978;1:49–68.

48. Sauerland ER, Harper RM. The human tongue during sleep: electromyographic activity of the genioglossus muscle. *Exp Neurol* 1976;51:160–170.

49. Mitra J, Cherniack NS. The effects of hypercapnia and hypoxia on single hypoglossal nerve fiber activity. *Respir Physiol* 1983;54:55–66.

50. van Lunteren E, Dick TE. Motor unit regulation of mammalian pharyngeal dilator muscle activity. *J Clin Invest* 1989;84:577–585.

51. Anch AM, Remmers JE, Bunce H III. Supraglottic airway resistance in normal subjects and patients with occlusive sleep apnea. *J Appl Physiol* 1982;53:1158–1163.

52. Haponik EF, Smith PL, Bohlman ME, et al. Computerized tomography in obstructive sleep apnea: correlation of airway size with physiology during sleep and wakefulness. *Am Rev Respir Dis* 1983;127:221–226.

53. Hudgel DW. Variable site of airway narrowing among obstructive sleep apnea patients. *J Appl Physiol* 1986;61:1403–1409.

54. Issa FG, Sullivan CE. Upper airway closing pressure in obstructive sleep apnea. *J Appl Physiol* 1984;57:520–527.

55. Rivlin J, Hoffstein V, Kalbfleisch J, et al. Upper airway morphology in patients with idiopathic obstructive sleep apnea. *Am Rev Respir Dis* 1984;129:355–360.

56. Sanders MH, Moore SE. Inspiratory and expiratory partitioning of airway resistance during sleep in patients with sleep apnea. *Am Rev Respir Dis* 1983;127:554–558.

57. Suratt PM, Dee P, Atkinson RL, Armstrong P, Wilhoit SC. Fluoroscopic and computed tomographic features of the pharyngeal airway in obstructive sleep apnea. *Am Rev Respir Dis* 1983;127:487–492.

58. van Lunteren E, Haxhiu MA, Cherniack NS. Respiratory changes in nasal muscle length. *J Appl Physiol* 1985;59:453–458.

59. Suratt PM, McTier RF, Wilhoit SC. Upper airway muscle activation is augmented in patients with obstructive sleep apnea compared with that in normal subjects. *Am Rev Respir Dis* 1988;137:889–894.

60. Gothe B, Strohl KP, Levin S, Cherniack NS. Nicotine: a different approach to the treatment of obstructive sleep apnea. *Chest* 1985;87:11–17.

61. Haxhiu MA, von Lunteren E, Van de Graaff WG, et al. Action of nicotine on the respiratory activity of the diaphragm and genioglossus muscles and the nerves that innervate them. *Respir Physiol* 1984;57:153–169.

62. Issa FQ, Sullivan CE. Alcohol, snoring and sleep apnea. *J Neurol Neurosurg Psychiatry* 1982;45:353–359.

63. Krol RC, Knuth SL, Bartlett D. Selective reduction of genioglossal muscle activity of alcohol in normal subjects. *Am Rev Respir Dis* 1984;129:247–250.

64. Taasan VC, Block AJ, Boysen PG, Wynne JW. Alcohol increases sleep apnea and oxygen desaturation in asymptomatic men. *Am J Med* 1981;71:240–245.

THE LUNG: Scientific Foundations
edited by R.G. Crystal, J.B. West et al.
Raven Press, Ltd., New York © 1991.

CHAPTER 5.7.4

Gas Exchange During Sleep

David W. Hudgel and Kingman P. Strohl

The physiology of gas exchange changes during sleep. The adaptations occurring in sleep involve pulmonary mechanics, cardiovascular performance, thermoregulation, and organ metabolism (Fig. 1). These normal changes or, alternatively, dysfunctional events in respiratory and cardiovascular performance may result in significant abnormalities in gas exchange and in clinical illness. First, we will discuss the normal function of components of gas exchange during sleep. Next, we will discuss clinical problems of sleep-disordered breathing in which abnormalities in respiratory function and gas exchange during sleep result in morbidity and mortality.

VENTILATION AND CONTROL OF BREATHING DURING SLEEP

In sleep, volitional functions cease or are considerably depressed. Because of this decreased activity, demand for energy is reduced. During non-rapid eye movement (NREM) sleep, respiratory rate and depth are less, resulting in a 6–14% fall in minute ventilation and a 4- to 6-torr increase in arterial CO_2 tension relative to that during wakefulness (1–4). Four factors are primarily responsible for hypoventilation and changes in gas exchange during sleep: an increase in airway resistance, ventilation–perfusion mismatch, a decrease in ventilatory drive, and an altered pattern of breathing.

D. W. Hudgel: Department of Medicine, Case Western Reserve University School of Medicine, Cleveland, Ohio 44106; Division of Pulmonary and Critical Care Medicine, Health Medical Center, Cleveland, Ohio 44109; and Sleep Laboratory, MetroHealth Medical Center, Cleveland, Ohio 44109.

K. P. Strohl: Department of Medicine, Case Western Reserve University School of Medicine, Cleveland, Ohio 44106; and Division of Pulmonary and Critical Care Medicine, University Hospitals of Cleveland, Cleveland, Ohio 44106.

Airway Resistance

In normal, non-snoring individuals, respiratory system resistance rises considerably during NREM sleep. This occurs because of narrowing of the nasopharyngeal airway, since laryngeal and pulmonary airflow resistances do not change (Fig. 2) (4,5). To the degree that upper airway narrowing during sleep does not engage load-compensating mechanisms, minute ventilation will be reduced. Of interest, studies in animals suggest that NREM sleep is accompanied by a fall in airway smooth muscle tone, resulting in mild bronchodilation (3). However, the amount of this bronchodilation is small, and it is not enough to overcome the increase in respiratory system resistance produced by the narrowing of the upper airway.

Ventilation–Perfusion Matching

Changes in lung volume will alter gas exchange by affecting the distribution of ventilation. In normal sleeping subjects, functional residual capacity (FRC) falls slightly (6), presumably as the result of a decrease in postural tone of the chest wall muscles. However, in obese subjects the decrease in lung volume with sleep may be far greater and clinically relevant. In the obese and in patients with asthma or chronic obstructive lung disease, a decrease in lung volume with recumbency alone will result in closure of more gravitationally dependent airways and affect ventilation–perfusion relationships (7).

Ventilatory Drive

A decrease in ventilatory drive activity during sleep may also contribute to the relative hypoventilation observed during sleep (2). Because of the mechanical impediment to breathing produced by an increase in

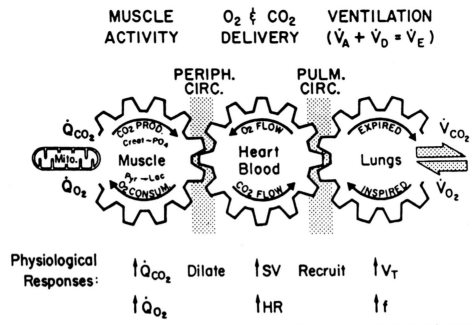

FIG. 1. Scheme depicting the gas transport mechanisms that couple cellular to pulmonary respiration. It represents a functional interdependence of physiologic components of a system of gas exchange. The events during wakefulness can be altered by sleep and the different stages of sleep. Symbols represent various components of ventilation and of oxygen utilization. $\dot{V}_A$ is alveolar ventilation; $\dot{V}_D$ is dead space ventilation; $\dot{V}_E$ is minute ventilation; $\dot{V}_{CO_2}$ is the excretion of CO_2 by the lungs; $\dot{V}_{O_2}$ is the uptake of oxygen by pulmonary respiration; $\dot{Q}_{CO_2}$ is CO_2 production; and $\dot{Q}_{O_2}$ is oxygen consumption. PERIPH. CIRC., peripheral circulation; PULM. CIRC., pulmonary circulation; Mito., mitochondria; Creat $\sim PO_4$, creatine phosphate; Pyr, pyridine; Lac, lactic acid; CO_2 PROD., CO_2 production; O_2 CONSUM., O_2 consumption; SV, stroke volume; HR, heart rate; V_T, tidal volume; f, breathing frequency.

upper-airway resistance, ventilation and the ventilatory responses to chemical stimuli during sleep are not a reliable reflection of central respiratory activity. The occlusion pressure technique for measuring ventilatory responses to chemical stimuli has been used to analyze ventilatory drive status in the presence of a

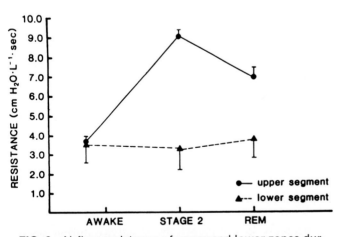

FIG. 2. Airflow resistance of upper and lower zones during sleep in normal humans. During sleep, resistance of larynx and lungs (*lower curve*) does not change whereas resistance above the retroepiglottic space (*upper curve*) increases. (From ref. 5.)

mechanical impediment to breathing. Although this technique is utilized to measure ventilatory drive during sleep (8), its value is questionable because: (a) with the change in lung volume (and, hence, the change in respiratory muscle length) that occurs during sleep, the mechanical output of the diaphragm is different for the same neural input to the muscle; and b) there is no guarantee that neural–muscle coupling is the same during wakefulness as during sleep. In spite of these concerns, this technique may provide more information than ventilation does with regard to respiratory muscle response to stimuli of breathing. White (8) showed no decrease in occlusion pressure responses to hypercapnia during NREM, but he reported a significant decrease during REM sleep. A better variable to gauge ventilatory drive activity would be inspiratory muscle electrical activity. Studies of inspiratory muscle electrical responses to chemical stimuli in sleeping goats showed a decrease in the responses to hypoxia during both NREM and REM sleep (9) and to hypercapnia only during REM sleep (10). During REM sleep, an increase in brain blood flow produces central hypocapnia and alkalosis; both act as respiratory depressants (10). Also, during sleep there is a decreased metabolic rate, which diminishes ventilatory drive activity.

A decrease in respiratory drive usually accompanies a decrease in metabolic rate; however, in REM sleep the metabolic rate can be higher than or equal to that seen in NREM sleep, whereas respiratory drive is significantly lower in REM than in NREM sleep. Therefore, in REM sleep the relationship between metabolism and ventilatory drive does not hold.

Pattern of Breathing

Both respiratory rate and depth are more variable in REM sleep, resulting in fluctuations in arterial blood gases (3,11,12). Periods of hypoventilation resulting in arterial oxygen desaturation to levels approximating 90% will occur in REM sleep (infrequently, however) in healthy subjects. Two respiratory changes in REM sleep may contribute to these periods of hypoventilation and hypoxemia. First, the pattern of breathing may become periodic with phases of shallow, or hypopneic, breathing; and, second, as discussed above, ventilatory drive is reduced. These variables will not affect gas exchange significantly in healthy subjects, but they could result in significant REM-associated hypoxemia in those with preexisting abnormalities in lung mechanics and in ventilation–perfusion disturbances.

Two other factors potentially contribute to hypoxemia during REM sleep in patients with airway disease: heightened airway reactivity and suppressed irritant reflexes. In REM sleep, airway smooth muscle tone varies widely, but the predominant pattern is that of bronchoconstriction (3,7). This could impair ventilation distribution or, subsequently, ventilation–perfusion matching. Also, in REM sleep there is a decreased response to irritating airway stimuli (11). In animal studies, distilled water applied to the larynx or trachea in amounts that cause paroxysmal cough during wakefulness is tolerated in REM sleep without cough or arousal or, even in some instances, without a change in breathing pattern (13). This suppressed defense against noxious stimuli to the respiratory tract in REM sleep could allow for a buildup of intraluminal fluid and airway closure. In individuals with lung disease, gas exchange would be worsened by this mechanism.

METABOLISM DURING SLEEP

It is clear that under normal circumstances the metabolic demands for oxygen are less during sleep than during wakefulness (14–18). However, dispute exists as to whether metabolic rate shows systematic changes across sleep stages. White et al. (14) found a 9% reduction in oxygen consumption that was similar across sleep states for each gender, although metabolic rates

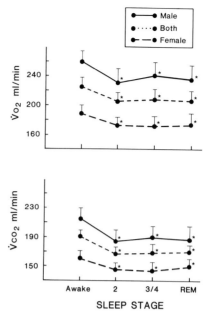

FIG. 3. Effect of various sleep stages on measures of metabolic rate [O₂ consumption (V̇o₂) and CO₂ production (V̇co₂)] demonstrated in male and female subjects. Both V̇o₂ and V̇co₂ were decreased during all stages of sleep compared with wakefulness. The standard error of the mean is shown. *P < 0.05 different from awake. (From ref. 14.)

were higher in men during both wakefulness and sleep (Fig. 3). Haskell et al. (15) found that the drop in oxygen consumption during sleep was altered by ambient temperature changes; both a decrease and increase in ambient temperature from the neutral mean ambient temperature of 29°C resulted in an elevation in metabolic rate. Although there was no difference in the oxygen consumption in NREM and REM sleep at 29°C, changes in ambient temperature resulted in significant differences in oxygen consumption between these two sleep states, with metabolic rate being higher in REM sleep. Interestingly, these investigators found no difference between NREM and REM sleep with respect to rectal temperature, regardless of metabolic rate differences between these sleep stages. This finding implies that there could be differences between NREM and REM sleep with regard to the control of different vascular beds, such that skin vasodilation or constriction may maintain body temperature constant in the face of differing metabolic rates. Brebbia and Altshuler (16) reported differences in oxygen consumption across sleep stages analyzed over the whole night. They found equivalent values for stage 1 and REM sleep. Stage 2 values were lower than values for stage 1 or REM but were higher than stages 3–4. These results persisted even if contiguous 5-min epochs of different sleep stages were analyzed. However, in a recent study by Ryan et al. (17), oxygen consumption was observed to vary more with time than with changes in sleep stage. Oxygen consumption fell gradually over the first 4 hr of sleep and rose gradually over the last 2 hr of sleep. This observation raises the possibility that metabolic changes are more a function of a diurnal rhythm than of sleep stage. Some confounding effects are the result of the aging process. Webb and Hustand (18) studied 20 men between 19 and 63 years of age and found an age effect on nocturnal metabolic rate; as age increased, the fall in metabolic rate with sleep increased. Therefore, age, ambient temperature, time of night, gender, and possibly sleep stage all affect the absolute level and rate of change in metabolism during sleep.

CARDIOVASCULAR FUNCTION DURING SLEEP

Heart rate decreases 10–15% in NREM sleep relative to that in wakefulness (19,20). Snyder et al. (19) found that mean heart rate was increased in REM sleep relative to that in NREM sleep; and, similar to respiration, heart rate is more variable in REM sleep. In NREM sleep there is more parasympathetic nervous system activity relative to sympathetic activity as compared to that in wakefulness; one manifestation is the lower heart rate observed in NREM sleep. However, in REM sleep there is an increase in the sympathetic/parasympathetic activity ratio, resulting in an increased heart rate relative to that in NREM sleep.

In general, changes in blood pressure, cardiac output, and peripheral vascular resistance parallel the changes in heart rate during sleep (19,21,22). Blood pressure may decrease nearly 15% in stages 3 and 4 NREM sleep but may be somewhat higher in REM. The fall in blood pressure in NREM sleep results from a decrease in either cardiac output or peripheral vascular resistance, or in both.

Changes in the peripheral circulation are known to occur in transition from NREM to REM sleep. Blood flow to some organs will increase in REM relative to that in NREM sleep and wakefulness. In REM there are transient surges in brain blood flow (23,24). Skin vasodilation also adjusts body temperature during sleep (25). In addition, studies on NREM sleep in cats have shown an increase in blood flow to the mesentery and kidneys (25,26). During REM sleep a marked vasoconstriction in the skeletal muscle vascular bed was found (25). Whether this decrease in blood flow occurs in respiratory muscles and affects their performance during sleep is unknown.

There are small changes in pulmonary artery pressure during sleep in normal individuals (27). Pulmonary artery pressure is somewhat elevated in heavy snorers without sleep apnea or hypoxemia (27,28). The mechanism of this elevation in pulmonary artery pressure is likely due to swings in thoracic blood volume secondary to greater respiratory excursions in pleural pressure during partial upper airway obstruction (snoring).

BREATH-HOLDING

Pauses in respiration are frequently observed during sleep. Young, healthy subjects may exhibit up to six apneas per hour greater than 10 sec in length, and healthy, elderly subjects often have 10–14 apneas per hour. The events during apnea are in some ways similar to those that occur during breath-holding. Therefore, a review of this physiology is applicable to understanding events that occur during apneas.

Changes in arterial blood-gas tensions during a breath-hold are predominantly dependent on body gas stores. Because the total body oxygen store of 2 liters is considerably less than the CO_2 store of 120 liters (29), oxygen will be depleted rapidly and arterial oxygen tension will fall faster than CO_2 tension rises during a breath-hold. Since a large part of the oxygen in the body is stored in the lungs, one can significantly change the amount of oxygen stored by changing the lung volume at which the breath-hold is initiated. An increase in lung volume in relation to total lung capacity increases oxygen stores, whereas a decrease in lung volume to residual volume diminishes the oxygen store considerably. With the same pulmonary blood flow, lung stores of oxygen will decrease four times as fast when the lung is at residual volume than when it is at total lung capacity (30). Factors that reduce lung volume, such as obesity, and factors that reduce initial alveolar oxygen concentration, such as chronic obstructive lung disease or alveolar hypoventilation (CO_2 retention), will result in more rapid rates of arterial oxygen desaturation during breath-holding (31,32). In fact, as the volume of intrapulmonary oxygen decreases, CO_2 is concentrated in the lung so that late in breath-hold the CO_2 content of alveolar air and arterial blood may actually exceed the CO_2 content of mixed venous blood (33). Motion of the thoracic cage during a breath-hold does not significantly change the rate of desaturation, unless reflex changes in heart rate and circulation time come into play. Exercise will increase peripheral blood flow and utilization of oxygen; therefore, oxygen extraction from the lungs will be increased. During obstructive apnea the vigorous respiratory efforts of obstructive sleep apnea patients markedly enhance oxygen utilization; therefore, reduction in arterial oxygenation can be more rapid than suggested by lung oxygen stores. Thus, even short apneas may result in a considerable hypoxemia, especially in patients with small lungs, with hypoxemia during wakefulness, and with increased skeletal muscle activity during sleep.

CLINICAL DISORDERS

Sleep Apnea

Obstructive sleep apnea (OSA) is characterized by intermittent collapse of the pharyngeal airway during sleep (34–36). Clinically, OSA is characterized by heavy, bedpartner-disturbing snoring and excessive, inappropriate daytime sleepiness (37). With the airway obstruction, arterial oxygen desaturation occurs. This oxygen desaturation and the multiple arousals from sleep result in excessive daytime sleepiness as well as cardiovascular and hematologic complications.

Obstructive sleep apnea syndrome (OSAS) has been recognized for more than 25 years. Two retrospective studies have examined mortality and have come to the conclusion that premature death occurs in the untreated patient population. He et al. (38) found that an untreated group with an initial apnea index of greater than 20 per hour had higher-than-normal mortality rates during the 5 years after the identification of multiple sleep apneas. However, in groups of patients treated with either tracheostomy or nasal continuous positive airway pressure (CPAP), no excess mortality was observed. A retrospective study by Partinen et al. (39) also found an increased mortality rate among patients with more than five apneas per hour who had not been definitively treated for sleep apnea by tracheostomy. The comparison group consisted of patients treated with weight loss alone. Other reports in this population suggest that deaths may be cardiovascular in nature or related to automobile or industrial accidents. Although the available evidence suggests that untreated sleep apnea is associated with excess mortality, the cause-and-effect relationships of mortality to the variables of sleep hypoxia and arousals from sleep have not been clearly defined. Prospective studies are also needed to better determine both (a) the natural history of this disorder and (b) its impact as a co-morbid event.

There is a small group of patients in whom respiratory pauses during sleep are characterized by the absence of respiratory efforts. In these patients it appears that there is a failure of respiratory rhymogenesis. This type of apnea is termed "central" or "diaphragmatic." Patients with recurrent central apneas present with a similar constellation of signs and symptoms as patients with recurrent obstructive apneas and, indeed, patients with central apneas may respond to therapeutic approaches used for obstructive apneas.

Both obstructive and central apnea during sleep may produce varying levels of intermittent hypoxemia. The reduction in tissue oxygen delivery caused by the apnea depends on: lung volume; the degree of venous admixture present; changes in cardiac output during the apnea; changes in cholinergic and/or adrenergic neural activity produced by the apnea; the apnea length; and the sleep stage during which the apnea occurs.

In addition to length of apnea, lung volume and preapneic arterial oxygen tension are the most critical factors determining the extent of hypoxemia (33). Three factors contribute to the reduction in lung volume in OSA: oxygen consumption, obesity, and expiratory lung emptying. The excess work of breathing during an obstructive apnea uses up O_2 that is not completely replaced by the CO_2 produced. Obesity decreases chest wall compliance, leading to a lower initial lung volume. The obstructed upper airway may open during expiration, resulting in expiratory airflow and thus reducing lung volume.

Because of the shape of the hemoglobin–oxygen dissociation curve, there will be a greater rate of decrease in arterial oxygen saturation during an apnea beginning with a P_{aO_2} of less than approximately 60 mmHg than would occur if the P_{aO_2} were higher (Fig. 4). Of course, less hemoglobin oxygen saturation causes a decrease in the oxygen-carrying capacity of blood, thereby decreasing tissue oxygen delivery, unless blood flow and/or oxygen extraction increase in the peripheral vasculature.

Vigorous inspiratory and expiratory efforts against a closed or narrowed upper airway may also influence venous return and cardiac output. Lugaresi et al. (40) demonstrated that the increased negative intrathoracic pressure experienced during an obstructive apnea increased right and left ventricular volume, presumably by increasing both venous return and end-diastolic ventricular volume, or afterload. Therefore, an in-

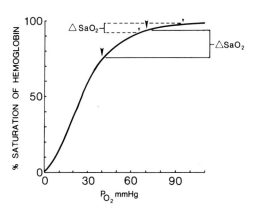

FIG. 4. Oxygen dissociation curve illustrating the impact of an identical change in P_{O_2} on oxygen saturation. The initial starting P_{O_2} before an apnea has a substantial impact on the degree of desaturation observed as a result of an apnea.

crease in wedge pressure and a decrease in cardiac output may occur during obstructive apneas (41,42). During an apnea, relative bradycardia and reduced cardiac output often develop because of increased vagal cholinergic neural output. Along with hemoglobin oxygen desaturation, the result of these changes is less oxygen delivery to the peripheral tissues.

As hypoxia develops, pulmonary and systemic vascular resistances increase (43). It is of interest that patients with dysautonomia syndromes, such as Shy–Drager syndrome, do not have changes in intravascular pressures during hypoxic apneas. An increase in systemic vascular resistance will also contribute to a decrease in tissue oxygen delivery, depending on the site of vascular constriction.

In patients with chronic obstructive lung disease and OSA, Fletcher (30) has demonstrated that the alveolar–arterial oxygen gradient may increase during episodes of arterial oxygen desaturation. The mechanism may relate to acute vasoconstriction in the pulmonary vascular bed or, alternatively, to a fall in lung volume.

As the length of apnea increases and hypoxemia worsens, the inspiratory muscles work harder against the obstruction. Oxygen utilization increases significantly, and peripheral tissue metabolic acidosis may develop. Sleep state affects apnea length and thereby determines the extent of arterial oxygen desaturation. Apnea length increases as much as 50% in REM sleep (33). Therefore, arterial oxygen saturation nadirs following apneas are usually lower in REM sleep than in NREM sleep. The length of the interapnea ventilatory period also affects oxygenation in OSA. If only two or three breaths occur between apneas, the oxygen stores may not be replenished and the mixed venous oxygenation at the beginning of the subsequent apnea may be lower than before the previous apnea. Thus, hypoxemia progressively develops over time.

Myocardial function is important to consider in OSA because of the known association between arrhythmias and apnea (44). During the apnea, when bradycardia is present, myocardial oxygen demand is relatively low. However, during the immediate postapnea period when tachycardia and increases in blood pressure occur, oxygen demand increases. However, oxygen availability is low because of hemoglobin desaturation produced by the previous apnea. Thus, during this phase of the apnea cycle (when myocardium work is increased and oxygen availability is low), myocardial ischemia can occur. Over a period of time, this transient ischemia may increase the risk of arrhythmias and/or myocardial damage.

Some 20% of patients with excessive daytime sleepiness and multiple apneas during sleep will present with hypercapnic respiratory failure (36,45). Many of these individuals will be obese, and usually hypercapnia resolves with successful therapy of sleep-disordered breathing and nocturnal hypoxemia. The observations of Bradley et al. (35) of a correlation between daytime oxygenation and right heart failure suggest that daytime sequela of sleep-disordered breathing, rather than apneas themselves, produce the cardiopulmonary complications of OSA. The mechanism leading to daytime hypoventilation in sleep apnea has not been defined. Clinically, certain overweight patients who hypoventilate improve with weight loss and respiratory stimulants. It may be that certain obese individuals are at risk of developing chronic alveolar hypoventilation due to inadequate respiratory responses to elastic loads (46) or to chemical drive (47). Alternatively, observations that treatment of sleep apnea results is better daytime ventilation suggest that events associated with apnea, such as hypoxia or sleep interruption, impair ventilatory control, resulting (over a period of time) in hypercapnia and hypoxia during wakefulness.

Therapy of patients with obstructive sleep apnea is directed at relieving the hypoxemia. Oxygen administration may clear the hypoxia and its complications, even though it does not prevent the apnea. CPAP applied to the nose, as well as pharmacologic stimulation of upper airway inspiratory dilatory muscle activity, can increase upper airway patency during sleep. Uvulopalatopharyngoplasty surgically increases upper-airway caliber and may resolve the apneas. Use of ventilatory stimulants, such as medroxyprogesterone, often improves hypoventilation. Tracheostomy is needed only if these other therapies fail or are not tolerated. In cases where supplemental oxygen will not improve the oxygenation because of severe hypoventilation, mechanical ventilation is occasionally required. Oftentimes, this may be adequately accomplished through a nasal facemask, obviating the need for tracheostomy.

Upper-Airway Disease

Patients with clinical diseases of the nose, larynx, or pharynx can present with sleep disturbances or with signs and symptoms related to aspiration of secretions. Aspiration may occur in the setting of excessive production of mucus, as exemplified by chronic sinusitis and rhinitis, or in the setting of inadequate neuromuscular tone, caused, for example, by bilateral recurrent laryngeal nerve paralysis. In both instances, frequent arousals from sleep may be associated with cough and/or a choking sensation. During sleep and, in particular, during REM sleep, the cough response is suppressed (13). As a result, greater amounts of secretion are tolerated before a cough ensues. After awakening, this material may precipitate cough paroxysms.

Chronic Obstructive Pulmonary Disease (COPD)

Patients with COPD may present with a variety of complaints related to sleep-disordered breathing. Nocturnal cough can be related to bronchitis. Insomnia may be the consequence of drug therapy, such as aminophylline. Hypoxemia during sleep may occur as a consequence of the mechanical impairment of the airways already present during wakefulness, but the hypoxemia may be exacerbated by the normal changes in gas exchange during sleep (30,33). Cor pulmonale may occur in COPD patients who experience hypoxemia only during sleep. Recognition of these individuals should occur when daytime hypoxemia and hypercapnia are not associated with a severe mechanical defect on pulmonary function testing. Certainly other entities, such as recurrent pulmonary emboli or chest wall muscle weakness, could also produce this presentation. Hypoventilation will occur not only because of sleep apnea but also because of changes in ventilation–perfusion matching and a decrease in respiratory drive, especially during REM sleep. If the problem is sleep apnea, usually there is historical evidence for snoring and restless sleep, and the patient should be treated appropriately for sleep apnea. If apneas are not producing hypoxemia, treatment with supplemental oxygen may not resolve the problem.

Some patients with severe COPD improve their arterial blood gases and lung function after brief periods of time in a negative-pressure chest cuirass ventilator. These changes are associated with improved indices of respiratory muscle strength and endurance. It is thought that these patients may experience respiratory muscle fatigue because of severe impairment of mechanical lung function and that the time in the cuirass serves to rest the muscles of the chest wall. These observations suggest a role for the use of brief periods of ventilatory support, perhaps just during sleep, in the management of patients with COPD.

Asthma

The most common sleep problem associated with asthma is cough. Cough, accompanied by arousals from sleep with cough, may be the presenting complaint of the patient with asthma and increased airway reactivity. Cough may result from changes in airway smooth muscle tone during sleep, as well as from bronchoconstriction during REM sleep (3,7).

A related clinical problem is that of "morning dipping," which refers to the fall in lung function occurring in the early morning hours. Morning dipping has been reported in severe asthmatic attacks and has been held somewhat responsible for deaths from asthma. Morning dipping represents an extreme form of diurnal

variation in lung function present in most patients with airway reactivity. Reports describing morning dipping emphasize that lung function measured some hours later during the day may be normal even though values during the night show moderately severe airway obstruction. The mechanisms for this extreme variation in lung function in asthmatics are not known.

Neuromuscular Disorders

Respiratory disturbances due to obstructive apneas during sleep may occur because upper airway muscles such as the genioglossus are affected by the underlying disease process. Inadequate respiratory activation of upper-airway muscles makes the upper airway vulnerable to collapse during inspiratory efforts by the muscles of the chest wall. Indeed, respiratory failure in the patient with neuromuscular disease may be due to upper airway muscle disease, and its prognostic consequences may be less dire than those due to primary involvement of the chest wall muscles such as the diaphragm.

Disturbances of sleep and respiration during REM sleep in particular may be the first indication of involvement of the respiratory system in the patient with neuromuscular disease. Occasionally, sleep fragmentation and the effects of sleep deprivation dominate the clinical presentation of the patient with neuromuscular disease. After treatment for sleep-disordered breathing, the secondary cardiopulmonary problems improve.

SUMMARY

In healthy subjects there are small decreases in metabolism, blood pressure, cardiac output, peripheral vascular resistance, and ventilation during sleep relative to wakefulness. Some changes are consistent with decreased activity and the lowered metabolic requirements of muscles during NREM sleep. NREM and REM sleep appear to be different physiologic states. In REM sleep, blood flow to certain organs, such as the brain and skin, increases while flow to muscles decreases. Metabolic rate, cardiac output, vascular pressure, and ventilation all become more variable in REM sleep so that, at times, values for these variables are higher than during NREM sleep and comparable to levels during active wakefulness. The mechanisms that explain the variability in physiologic parameters during REM sleep are not known.

There are a number of clinical disorders that are associated with disturbances of ventilation or cardiopulmonary function precipitated or exacerbated by sleep. These clinical syndromes illustrate the impact of sleep and the different stages of sleep on respiratory function of the upper airway, on control of broncho-motor tone, on cardiovascular function, and on lung clearance.

REFERENCES

1. Bulow K. Respiration and wakefulness in man. *Acta Physiol Scand [Suppl]* 1963;209:1–110.
2. Robin ED, Whaley RD, Crump CH, Travia DM. Alveolar gas tensions, pulmonary ventilation, and blood pH during physiologic sleep in normal subjects. *J Clin Invest* 1958;37:981–989.
3. Phillipson EA. Respiratory adaptations in sleep. *Annu Rev Physiol* 1978;40:133–174.
4. Dempsey JA, Skatrud JB. A sleep-induced apneic threshold and its consequences. *Am Rev Respir Dis* 1986;133:1163–1170.
5. Hudgel DW, Martin RJ, Johnson B, Hill P. Mechanics of the respiratory system and breathing pattern during sleep in normal humans. *J Appl Physiol* 1984;56:133–137.
6. Hudgel DW, Devadatta P. Decrease in functional residual capacity during sleep in normal humans. *J Appl Physiol* 1984;57:1319–1322.
7. Ballard RD, Saathoff MC, Patel DK, Kelly PL, Martin RJ. Effect of sleep on nocturnal bronchoconstriction and ventilatory patterns in asthmatics. *J Appl Physiol* 1989;67:243–249.
8. White DP. Occlusion pressure and ventilation during sleep in normal humans. *J Appl Physiol* 1986;61:1279–1287.
9. Parisi RA, Santiago TV, Edelman NH. Genioglossal and diaphragmatic EMG responses to hypoxia during sleep. *Am Rev Respir Dis* 1988;138:610–616.
10. Santiago TV, Neubauer JA, Edelman NH. Correlation between ventilation and brain blood flow during hypoxic sleep. *J Appl Physiol* 1986;60:295–298.
11. Skatrud JB, Dempsey JA. Interaction of sleep state and chemical stimuli in sustaining rhythmic ventilation. *J Appl Physiol* 1983;55:813–822.
12. Gillam PMS. Patterns of respiration in human beings at rest and during sleep. *Bull Physiopathol Respir* 1972;8:1059–1070.
13. Bowes G, Phillipson EA. Arousal responses to respiratory stimuli during sleep. In: Saunders NA, Sullivan CE, eds. *Sleep and breathing*, vol 21 (Lung Biology in Health and Disease Series). New York: Marcel Dekker, 1984;137–161.
14. White DP, Weil JV, Zwillich CW. Metabolic rate and breathing during sleep. *J Appl Physiol* 1985;59:384–391.
15. Haskell EH, Palca JW, Walker JM, Berger RJ, Heller HC. Metabolism and thermoregulation during stages of sleep in humans exposed to heat and cold. *J Appl Physiol* 1981;51:948–954.
16. Brebbia DR, Altshuler KZ. Oxygen consumption rate and electroencephalographic stage of sleep. *Science* 1965;150:1621–1623.
17. Ryan T, Mlynczak S, Erickson T, Paulman SF, Mann GCW. Oxygen consumption during sleep: influence of sleep stage and time of weight. *Sleep* 1989;12:201–210.
18. Webb P, Hustand M. Sleep metabolism and age. *J Appl Physiol* 1975;38:257–262.
19. Snyder F, Hobson JA, Morrison DF, Goldfrank F. Changes in respiration, heart rate, and systolic blood pressure in human sleep. *J Appl Physiol* 1964;19:417–422.
20. Khatri IM, Freis ED. Hemodynamic changes during sleep. *J Appl Physiol* 1967;22:867–873.
21. Zemaityte D. Heart rhythm control during sleep. *Psychophysiol* 1984;21:279.
22. Coccagna G, Mantovani M, Brignani F, Manzini A, Lugaresi E. Arterial pressure changes during spontaneous sleep in man. *Electroencephalogr Clin Neurophysiol* 1971;31:277–281.
23. Reivich M, Isaacs G, Evarts E, Ketty S. The effect of slow wave sleep and REM sleep on regional cerebral blood flow in cats. *J Neurochem* 1968;15:301–306.
24. Parisi RA, Neubauer JA, Frank MM, Santiago TV, Edelman NH. Linkage between brain blood flow and respiratory drive during rapid-eye-movement sleep. *J Appl Physiol* 1988;64:1457–1465.
25. Mancia G, Baccelli G, Adams DB, Zanchetti A. Vasomotor regulation during sleep in the cat. *Am J Physiol* 1971;220:1086–1093.
26. Mancia G, Baccelli G, Zanchetti A. Regulation of renal circulation during behavioral changes in the cat. *Am J Physiol* 1974;227:536–542.
27. Logaresi E, Coccagna G, Girignotta F. Snoring and its clinical implications. In: Guilleminault C, Dement WC, eds. *Sleep apnea syndromes.* New York: Alan R Liss, 1978.
28. Stauffer JL, Davidson WR Jr, Zwillich CW. Echocardiographic and electrocardiographic findings in asymptomatic snoring men. *Am Rev Respir Dis* 1989;139:A113.
29. Cherniack NS, Longobardo GS. Oxygen and carbon dioxide gas stores in the body. *Physiol Rev* 1970;50:196–243.
30. Fletcher EC. Chronic lung disease in patients with sleep apnea. In: Fletcher EC, ed. *Abnormalities of respiration during sleep.* Orlando, FL: Grune & Stratton, 1986;181–202.
31. Findley LJ, Ries AL, Tisie GM. Hypoxemia during apnea in normal subjects: mechanisms and impact of lung volume. *J Appl Physiol* 1983;55:1777–1783.
32. Strohl KP, Altose MD. Oxygen saturation during breath-holding and during apneas in sleep. *Chest* 1984;85:181–186.
33. Shepard JR Jr. Gas exchange and hemodynamics during sleep. *Med Clin North Am* 1985;69:1243–1264.
34. Strohl KP, Cherniack NS, Gothe B. Physiologic basis of therapy for sleep apnea. *Am Rev Respir Dis* 1986;134:791–802.
35. Bradley AJ, Rutherford R, Grossman RF, Lue F, Zamel N, Moldofsky H, Phillipson EA. Role of daytime hypoxemia in the pathogenesis of right heart failure in the obstructive sleep apnea syndrome. *Am Rev Respir Dis* 1985;131:835–839.
36. Sullivan CE, Issa FQ. Obstructive sleep apnea. In: Krygen MH, ed. *Clinics in chest medicine*, vol 6. Philadelphia: WB Saunders, 1985;633–650.
37. Roehrs T, Conway W, Wittig R, Zorick F, Sicklesteel J, Roth T. Sleep–wake complaints in patients with sleep-related respiratory disturbances. *Am Rev Respir Dis* 1985;132:520–523.
38. He J, Kryger MH, Zorick FJ, Conway W, Roth T. Mortality and apnea index in obstructive sleep apnea. *Chest* 1988;94:9–14.
39. Partinen M, Jamieson A, Guilleminault C. Long-term outcome for obstructive sleep apnea syndrome patients. Mortality. *Chest* 1988;94:1200–1204.
40. Lugaresi E, Cirignotta F, Coccagna G, et al. Clinical significance of snoring. In: Saunders NA, Sullivan CE, eds. *Sleep and breathing.* New York: Marcel Dekker, 1984.
41. Buda AJ, Pinky MR, Ingels NB Jr, et al. Effect of intrathoracic pressure on left ventricular performance. *N Engl J Med* 1979;301:453–459.
42. Buda AJ, Schroeder JS, Guilleminault C. Abnormalities of pulmonary artery wedge pressures in sleep-induced apnea. *Int J Cardiol* 1981;1:67–74.
43. Guilleminault C, Motta J, Mihma F, Melvin K. Obstructive sleep apnea and cardiac index. *Chest* 1986;89:331–334.
44. Zwillich C, Devlin T, White D, Douglas N, Weil J, Martin R. Bradycardia during sleep apnea: characteristics and mechanism. *J Clin Invest* 1982;60:1286–1292.
45. Burwell C, Robin E, Whaley R, Bikelman A. Extreme obesity associated with alveolar hypoventilation: a Pickwickian syndrome. *Am J Med* 1956;21:811–818.
46. Lopata M, Onal E. Mass loading, sleep apnea, and the pathogenesis of obesity hypoventilation. *Am Rev Respir Dis* 1982;116:640–645.
47. Gavay SM, Rapoport D, Sorkin B, et al. Regulation of ventilation in the obstructive sleep apnea syndrome. *Am Rev Respir Dis* 1981;124:451–457.
48. Wasserman K, Hansen JE, Sue DY, Whipp BJ. *Principles of exercise testing and interpretation.* Philadelphia: Lee & Febiger, 1987;2.

The Fetal, Perinatal, Postnatal, and Aging Lung

Respiration is a complex process that involves the co-ordination of all the structures involved in gas intake and tissue metabolism. It is controlled and can be adjusted to meet changing environmental and metabolic needs. Neither the lung nor the respiratory system (the respiratory muscles and nervous elements that control them) remains static. The chapters in this section review the dynamic changes in the respiratory system that occur with maturation and aging.

Rapid growth of the lung and the brain occurs in the fetal period. The complexity of dendritic arrangements and of the respiratory arrangements of the medulla, however, simplifies with fetal development. Some neuromodulators increase transiently during the fetal period.

Even though the lung does not subserve a gas-exchanging function in the fetus, breathing movements occur. These movements may affect lung growth. The fetal lung produces and removes large numbers of vasoactive substances.

At birth and in the perinatal period, critical changes occur in lung and thoracic mechanics as the lung is transformed from a fluid-containing to a gas-containing structure. The internal surfactant coat of the lungs is established. Pulmonary vascular resistance declines and extrapulmonary shunts close. These changes depend on the appropriate application of mechanical forces by the infant's respiratory muscles and on the release of appropriate levels of chemical substances. The discontinuous breathing movements of the fetus are changed to a continuous pattern. The chemoreceptors adapt. Peripheral chemoreceptor responses increase, associated with bursts in production (in the medulla) of certain neuromodulators such as the tachykinins.

Each of these steps is crucial, and serious consequences to survival can occur if difficulties arise in these transformations. For example, respiratory failure in the infant can arise from decreased lung surfactant activity. This, in turn, depends on the complex and coordinated production of phospholipids and proteins.

Changes in the respiratory system occur after birth. The tracheobronchial airways become more rigid. Alveolar volume increases more than the volume of the conducting airways. The thorax undergoes great changes, not only in size but in shape. The circular characteristic of the cross-section of the thorax at birth becomes eliptical in the adult. The lungs become more compliant as a result of these changes, the thorax stiffens, and air-trapping is less likely as adulthood is achieved.

With aging, lung function and the ability of the respiratory system to respond to challenges decline. There is a loss of gas-exchanging surface. Lung compliance rises, and the ability to generate large expiratory flows diminishes. As a result, there is a gradual reduction in arterial oxygen partial pressure with advancing age. What is not clear and remains an area of increasing investigation is how much these changes occur as a result of the aging process itself and how much is potentially preventable, arising from exposure to noxious agents in the atmosphere.

While we conventionally believe that breathing is a controlled process, the chapters in this section show that the respiratory system itself (i.e., the structure and function of its components) adjusts continuously in a regulated way to the altered stresses that occur during different stages of life.

The Editors

THE LUNG: Scientific Foundations
edited by R.G. Crystal, J.B. West et al.
Raven Press, Ltd., New York © 1991.

CHAPTER 6.1.1

Fetal Breathing Movements

Richard Harding

Fetal breathing movements (FBMs) may be defined as organized, rhythmical contractions of the respiratory muscles which intermittently reduce intrathoracic pressure during normal intrauterine existence. These movements result from brainstem neural activity, which is relayed principally to skeletal muscles of the thorax and upper respiratory tract. While it is recognized that prenatal breathing movements probably occur in nonmammals and marsupials, the scope of this chapter is restricted to eutherian mammals. A considerable amount of knowledge on FBMs has, of necessity, been obtained in animals, sheep in particular, although with the development of noninvasive monitoring techniques, data on human FBMs have increased greatly in recent years. Together with other biophysical parameters, FBMs are commonly used in the assessment of fetal well-being.

Three forms of respiratory-like movements have been identified in the fetus. The most common, which has been termed "rapid, irregular" breathing movements (1), and which most closely resembles postnatal breathing, involves episodes of rhythmic contractions of the major respiratory muscles, normally of varying frequency and amplitude. In this chapter these are referred to as FBMs. In both fetal sheep (1,2) and humans (3), less frequent, deeper inspiratory efforts also occur. These are particularly common during early human gestation in which they have been termed "hiccups" (4), but little is known of their regulation or function. Under conditions of fetal hypoxia or asphyxia, gasping movements may occur, sometimes as terminal events. These involve intense activation of inspiratory muscles of the thorax and upper airway (5).

The aim of this chapter is to give a concise account of FBMs and their physiological significance. Further details of their neural substrate and regulatory mechanisms can be obtained from more comprehensive reviews (6–9).

MUSCLES INVOLVED IN FETAL BREATHING MOVEMENTS

The diaphragm is the principal thoracic muscle activated during ovine FBMs (10); section of the phrenic nerves greatly reduces or abolishes pressure fluctuations in the trachea (11). During late gestation the intercostal muscles play only a minor role in ovine FBMs (12), although earlier in gestation they are rhythmically active during inspiration (13). The absence of inspiratory intercostal muscle activity during late gestation, coupled with the low compliance of the fetal rib cage, and the small volume changes associated with individual FBMs (1,10,14), presumably account for the inward movement of the rib cage (rib-cage paradox) during the inspiratory phase of FBMs (15,16). During late gestation, pressure fluctuations associated with ovine FBMs are, on average, 3.5–4.0 mmHg below amniotic sac pressure (13). FBMs in the human fetus (34–35 weeks), monitored by ultrasound, cause the anterior chest wall to move inward by 2–5 mm and the anterior abdominal wall to move outward by 3–8 mm (16).

Some of the muscles controlling the dimensions of the upper respiratory tract are rhythmically active during FBMs (17). The principal laryngeal dilator muscle, posterior cricoarytenoid (PCA), contracts increasingly during each inspiratory effort (18). This muscle activity, which rhythmically dilates the glottis, thereby reducing pressure in the upper trachea (when hydraulically isolated from the lower trachea) (19), probably contributes to the tracheal pressure fluctuations associated with FBMs and to the related movements of liquid within the trachea. Activation of the laryngeal dilator muscle (PCA) does not occur in association with the inspiratory phase of isolated deep inspiratory

R. Harding: Department of Physiology, Monash University, Melbourne 3168, Australia.

efforts (2) and probably does not occur during hiccups in the human fetus. In contrast, during asphyxial gasping, inspiratory PCA activation is intense (2). Sustained activity of the major adductor muscle of the larynx (thyroarytenoid) occurs at a low, variable level during fetal apnea (18).

The major muscle of the tongue (genioglossus) is not normally active in phase with ovine FBMs (20) as is the case postnatally in sheep (21). The muscle is, however, active during inspiration in other species after birth (22). Inspiratory activation of the genioglossus muscle can be induced in fetal sheep when FBMs are augmented by cutaneous cold stimulation (23). Similarly, augmented breathing efforts in the postnatal lamb and ewe are associated with inspiratory activation of the genioglossus muscle. The dilator muscles of the nostrils (alae nasi) are also active during many, but not all, inspiratory efforts in the ovine fetus (20,24).

ONTOGENY OF FETAL BREATHING MOVEMENTS

In the exteriorized sheep fetus, infrequent FBMs have been observed following cutaneous stimulation from as early as 40 days (0.28 of term) (1). Spontaneous ovine FBMs, *in utero*, have been detected at 0.34 of gestation (25). Infrequent FBMs (median incidence 2%) can be detected, by ultrasound, in the human fetus as early as 10 weeks (0.25 of term); other body movements can first be detected at 7–8.5 weeks (4). From 10 to 15 weeks of gestation in the human, FBMs and other specific movement patterns increase in frequency and amplitude (4).

Early in ovine gestation (0.3–0.5 of term) there are frequent periods of sustained EMG activity of the diaphragm, usually coincident with activities of other muscles, such as intercostal, abdominal, and external ocular muscles (26,27). Although intrathoracic pressures have not been measured, it is probable that this type of diaphragmatic activity is nonrespiratory, as it persists after cord section at C1 (27) and may be a component of general body movements. With increasing age, the incidence of tonic (nonrespiratory) EMG activity of the diaphragm declines, while that of phasic (respiratory) activity increases (26). During the last third of ovine gestation the frequency of inspiratory efforts during episodes of FBMs is about 0.5–2 Hz (6).

As in the sheep fetus, the incidence of human FBMs (detected as reciprocating movements of the anterior chest and abdominal walls) apparently increases with gestational age, up to 30 weeks. The incidence increases from 2% at 10 weeks, to 6% at 19 weeks (4), 11–13% (depending on time of day) at 22–24 weeks (28), 12–14% at 24–29 weeks (29,30), and to 31% at 30 weeks (31). Between 30 weeks and term (40 weeks)

the daily incidence of FBMs remains at about 31%, with values ranging from 17 to 65% (29,31). The mean frequency of human FBMs at 34–38 weeks was 45–57 breaths/min (16,32), whereas slightly lower rates (42–44 breaths/min) were observed at 24–28 weeks of gestation (30). The incidence of human FBMs, particularly during the second half of gestation, varies with time of day (16,28). Part of this variation is attributable to plasma glucose concentrations, although there is a nocturnal increase in FBM incidence which cannot be attributed to glucose (16). This increase may be due to elevated maternal plasma concentrations of glucocorticoids (33).

RELATIONSHIP BETWEEN FETAL BREATHING MOVEMENTS AND BEHAVIORAL STATES

From the time they first appear, FBMs occur in episodes. As other expressions of fetal neural activity have been studied (e.g., body movements, cortical activity, heart rate variability), it has become apparent that the episodic nature of FBMs is related to activity states of the central nervous system (CNS). During late gestation in sheep (from about 120 days to term), FBMs occur in association with low-voltage electrocortical activity and episodes of rapid eye movements (1). The emergence of high-voltage, slow-wave electrocortical activity coincides with an increase in the duration and incidence of apneic periods (34). This probably results from descending inhibition, as brainstem transection at midcollicular or upper pontine levels does not abolish high-voltage electrocortical activity but dissociates it from periods of fetal apnea (35). Earlier in gestation (95–119 days), before the appearance of high-voltage electrocortical activity, FBMs are associated with episodes of rapid eye movements (13).

In human fetuses, rest–activity cycles have been identified, based on ultrasonically detected eye movements, body movements, and heart-rate variability (36), and have been compared with those present after birth (37). The "rest" or "quiet" phase of the cycle is characterized by the absence of rapid eye movements, low variability of heart rate, and a low incidence of fetal body movements. Although these CNS activity states can be identified at 28 weeks, the incidence of FBMs during periods of increased fetal activity (i.e., rapid eye movements, body movements, and high variability of heart rate) is significantly greater than during "quiet" periods only after 36 weeks (38). It seems likely that periods of reduced motor activity in the human fetus correspond with those of high-voltage electrocortical activity (or slow-wave sleep) in the sheep fetus. Thus, it appears that in both fetal sheep and humans, FBMs, along with other expressions of CNS output, become periodically inhibited with the increasing development of higher levels of the CNS. This state-related inhibition of the central respiratory rhythm must be overridden after birth.

EFFECTS OF FETAL BREATHING MOVEMENTS ON PULMONARY FLUID MOVEMENT

Because FBMs alter pressures within the thorax, it is to be expected that they influence the movement of luminal liquid that is produced by the pulmonary epithelium (39). However, the relationship between FBMs and "airway" fluid movement is not as simple as in the postnatal, air-filled respiratory tract, largely due to physical properties of the liquid and the behavior of the fetal upper airway. The use of electromagnetic flowmeters in sheep (1,10) and ultrasound in humans (40) has shown oscillatory fluid flow related to FBMs. In the ovine fetus, during late gestation, individual FBMs cause small volumes (less than 2 ml) to move to and fro within the trachea, usually with little net volume change (1,10). In contrast, episodes of FBMs may give rise to either a net influx of liquid from the amniotic sac or, more commonly, to a net efflux of liquid from the lungs (14,19).

Little information is available on the relationship between FBMs and "airway" fluid movement during early gestation. Tracheal fluid flow at around 0.6 of term in the ovine fetus shows little variation associated with episodes of FBMs (R. Harding and K. A. Dickson, *unpublished data*). The modulation of tracheal fluid flow during late gestation probably relates to the increased effects of FBMs on luminal pressures (13), the development of increased resistances of the upper respiratory tract (41,42), the increased production and volume of lung liquid (39), and the increased duration of apneic periods (34).

During late ovine gestation (110–145 days), episodes of FBMs, which have an incidence of 40–50%, are normally associated with augmented efflux of pulmonary liquid via the trachea, although episodic influx may occur. That is, the rate of efflux normally exceeds the rate of pulmonary fluid production (14). In contrast, periods of apnea are associated with retardation of tracheal fluid efflux (14) and elevated tracheal pressure (43), due to the increased resistance of the upper respiratory tract to fluid efflux (42). This increase in resistance is largely due to tonic activity in laryngeal adductor muscles and lack of activity in abductor muscles (2,17,18). Retardation of fluid efflux during apnea (below the rate of fluid production) is diminished or abolished by section of the recurrent laryngeal nerves, resulting in a pattern of tracheal fluid flow which is much less modulated by periods of FBMs and apnea (14). In the intact fetus, liquid that has accumulated in the lungs during periods of apnea tends to flow from them during FBM episodes as a result of lowered upper airway resistance. The reduction of this resistance is principally due to (a) an absence of active adduction of the glottis and (b) rhythmic dilation of the glottis due to activity in laryngeal abductor muscles (2,17,18). The driving force for this flow must be a small pressure gradient between the pulmonary lumen and the pharynx or amniotic sac.

The upper airway in the fetus plays a crucial role in the control of pulmonary fluid movement, volume, and composition. If it is functionally removed, by allowing direct continuity between the trachea and amniotic sac, there is a large net movement of amniotic fluid into the lungs during episodes of FBMs (41). In the intact fetus it is unlikely that there is a pool of fluid in the pharynx which is available to be inhaled during FBMs. Attempts to aspirate fluid from the fetal sheep pharynx reveal that it normally contains little fluid (less than 2 ml) and that amniotic fluid cannot normally be sampled from this site (41). This implies (a) that fluid entering the pharynx (via the trachea, nasal cavity, or oral cavity) is rapidly removed, probably by swallowing, and (b) that there is a high resistance to the influx of fluid via the nose or mouth. The presence of a supralaryngeal resistance to the influx of fluid into the trachea is also indicated by the rhythmical reduction of pressures (below amniotic sac pressure) in the upper trachea when it is hydraulically isolated from the lower trachea (19). During some periods of augmented FBMs, amniotic fluid may be drawn into the trachea (19). This presumably occurs owing to either the transient formation of a low-resistance pathway between the larynx and amniotic sac (e.g., by mouth opening) or to the prior accumulation of fluid in the pharynx.

The overall action of the fetal upper respiratory tract appears to be to restrict the entry of amniotic fluid into the lower airways, where it may come into contact with the pulmonary epithelium. Amniotic fluid may interfere with surfactant synthesis (44) and pulmonary function (45), particularly if the fluid is contaminated with meconium (fetal feces) (45,46). The upper airway is also necessary to retard efflux of lung liquid in the absence of FBMs; its functional removal leads to a rapid reduction in lung expansion, accentuated by the compressive effects of uterine motility (41).

INFLUENCE OF HYPOXIA ON FETAL BREATHING MOVEMENTS AND FLUID FLUXES

In the adult, hypoxia is a potent respiratory stimulant, whereas in the fetus it has the effect of depressing breathing movements. Acute reductions in fetal Pa_{O_2}, induced by maternal inhalation of a hypoxic gas mixture, greatly reduce the incidence of FBMs (10,47). In fetal sheep during late gestation, it is necessary to reduce arterial O_2 content by more than 2–2.5 ml/dl to inhibit FBMs (48). It is likely that hypoxia inhibits FBMs via an effect on the CNS, as other motor outputs, including rapid eye movements (47,49,50) and limb movements, are also inhibited (50,51). These responses result in conservation of oxygen in the short term as FBMs are responsible for significant O_2 consumption (52). In healthy fetuses, FBMs are not limited by the low prevailing Po_2. Increasing fetal arterial Po_2, by induction of maternal hyperoxia, has no effect on the incidence of FBMs in sheep (47) or humans (53).

The role of peripheral chemoreceptors in the maintenance of FBMs and their inhibition by acute hypoxia is not clear. It seems likely that aortic chemoreceptors do not play a significant role as vagal section influences neither the incidence of FBMs during normoxia nor the inhibitory effect of acute hypoxia (47). However, there is a continuing controversy as to the role of the carotid bodies in the fetus (54,55). Although they may be active and sensitive to hypoxia during fetal life (56), there is little evidence that they play a significant role in the inhibition of FBMs by hypoxia, although they may affect the rapidity of the response (57).

The inhibitory effect of hypoxia on FBMs can be abolished by transection of the brainstem (35), suggesting that centers in or rostral to the pons are involved. Bilateral electrolytic lesions in the lateral pons, at the level of the trigeminal nuclei, abolish the hypoxic depression of FBMs (58). Evidence in support of such a region activated by hypoxia and with inhibitory effects on breathing has now been presented in the newborn (59). It is possible that this pontine site is also responsible for the inhibition of other motor activities in the fetus during hypoxia. This area may be activated in response to reduced mitochondrial production of ATP, because administration of a mitochondrial ATPase inhibitor (oligomycin B) reduced the incidence of FBMs in sheep (60).

Recently, it has become apparent that, behaviorally, the fetus adapts to chronic hypoxia. Prolonged hypoxia in the sheep fetus, induced either by maternal hypoxia (61) or by restricting uterine blood flow (62,63), initially inhibits FBMs, but after 12–16 hr, the incidence of FBMs (and rapid eye movements) returns to normal. At present, the basis for the adaptation of FBMs to hypoxia is not understood.

Acute hypoxia, depending on its severity, can have a profound effect on tracheal fluid movement. The effect is due partly to the reduced production of lung liquid and partly to the greatly reduced incidence or abolition of FBMs (64). During 4–6 hr of hypoxia the efflux of lung liquid was approximately halved (as was its rate of production), and the influx of liquid via the trachea was virtually abolished; the net effect was a conservation of lung liquid volume. During hypoxia the activity of laryngeal adductor muscles is sustained, or increased, in the absence of FBMs (5); reflex activation of the principal adductor muscle (thyroarytenoid) is increased during periods of low-voltage electrocortical activity, during which there are few FBMs (65). These findings indicate that laryngeal adduction and the resistance of the upper airway are increased during moderate hypoxia or asphyxia, which probably aids in maintaining lung expansion and preventing the entry of amniotic fluid into the lower airways.

Severe gasping, which may be induced by hypoxia or asphyxia, moves only small amounts of fluid in the trachea (less than 2 ml) of the sheep fetus (63). In human fetuses aspiration of amniotic fluid was found to be diminished rather than increased, as might be expected, under conditions of severe distress which culminated in death (66). A study of exteriorized fetal sheep showed that asphyxia, induced by constriction of the umbilical cord, led to the flow of fluid into the lungs but in this study the upper respiratory tract was not in circuit (67), thereby eliminating its valvelike action (41).

Prolonged hypoxia (e.g., 12–24 hr) leads to marked changes in tracheal fluid fluxes which are coincident with the reestablishment of FBMs (63). FBMs during this period result in the net movement of amniotic fluid into the trachea and lungs, probably due to the creation of a low-resistance pathway between the trachea and amniotic sac as a consequence of mouth opening and augmented laryngeal dilation.

CARBON DIOXIDE AND FETAL BREATHING MOVEMENTS

Elevated arterial Pco_2 in the sheep fetus, in the absence of hypoxia, leads to an increase in the amplitude and regularity of FBMs (47,68) and to recruitment of intercostal muscles (69). This stimulation of FBMs occurs only during the behavioral state in which low-voltage electrocortical activity and rapid eye movements are present (70,71). Maternal (and hence fetal) hypercapnia in the human causes an increased incidence of FBMs (72). An inverse relationship between Pco_2 and the incidence of FBMs in the human (73,74) has led to the suggestion that the tonic level of fetal Pco_2 is a primary stimulus for FBMs.

It is likely that the effects of CO_2 are mediated via central chemoreceptors, which are believed to be active from early fetal life (54,75–77). Acidification of blood (78) or CSF (79) increases the incidence of FBMs, whereas reducing the pH of CSF (with bicarbonate) has the opposite effect (79).

NUTRIENT AVAILABILITY

Nutritional state, particularly during late pregnancy, can have a major influence on FBMs. In humans and sheep, fetal hypoglycemia caused by reduced maternal food intake leads to a reduced incidence of FBMs (80). Hypoglycemia induced by insulin administration has a similar effect in fetal sheep (81,82). Administration of glucose following a period of fasting is followed by an increased incidence of FBMs in humans and sheep (80), with the peak incidence occurring 1–2 hr afterward. The incidence of FBMs following oral glucose administered to previously fasted humans was positively correlated with gestational age, there being little effect at 20 weeks (83). An increased incidence of FBMs following glucose administration was first detected at 24 weeks (84). The mechanism whereby circulating glucose concentrations affect FBMs is not clear. Glucose administration is followed by a slight rise in fetal Pa_{CO_2} and a fall in fetal pH (80,82), which could act on central chemoreceptors; the time course of the response to glucose is consistent with this possibility. The effect of glucose administration on fetal movements appears to be specific to breathing movements (85), supporting an action mediated by chemoreceptors.

Hypoglycemia induced by fasting has no effect on blood gas or pH levels, whereas that induced by insulin administration leads to a mild degree of hypoxia (86). Since it is well established that prostaglandin E (PGE) inhibits FBMs (87) and is released into the fetal circulation during hypoglycemia (82), it is possible that it mediates the inhibitory effect of hypoglycemia on FBMs. In contrast, there was no change in PGE concentrations during ovine fetal hyperglycemia, although the incidence of FBMs increased (82). Therefore, it is likely that the effects of hyperglycemia and hypoglycemia on FBMs are mediated by different mechanisms.

EFFECTS OF MATERNAL DRUG INTAKE ON FETAL BREATHING MOVEMENTS

Alcohol

In humans, acute ethanol ingestion during late pregnancy profoundly inhibits FBMs with no effect on other fetal body movements (88,89). Maximum inhibition of FBMs (37–40 weeks gestation) occurred 30 min after ethanol ingestion, when blood levels were greatest (0.33 mg/ml); FBMs remained inhibited for 3 hr, possibly due to alcohol retention in amniotic fluid, although maternal ethanol concentrations rapidly declined (89). Alcohol may cause the fetus to enter slow-wave sleep, although the effects of alcohol on fetal behavioral states have not yet been documented. It is

also possible that alcohol acts via central PGE release (90).

Narcotics and Analgesics

FBMs are inhibited by low doses of many commonly used drugs with sedative, narcotic, or analgesic effects. Maternally administered barbiturates, which readily cross the placenta, profoundly depress or abolish ovine FBMs for long periods (1,10,91). This effect is associated with, and may be due to, a change of fetal behavioral state to one in which FBMs are inhibited (91). The effects of maternally administered diazepam are more equivocal than those of barbiturates. In sheep, diazepam (0.18–0.22 mg/kg) reduced the incidence of FBMs without altering blood gases or pH (92,93), whereas prolonged diazepam administration in sheep led to an increased incidence of FBMs.

Tobacco Smoking

Fetal breathing in humans is inhibited by maternal cigarette smoking (94,95), although this effect is not apparent after maternal glucose ingestion (96). Nicotine administration in pregnant sheep produces a prolonged fetal hypoxia and inhibition of FBMs (97). These effects were prevented by α-adrenergic blockade in the ewe, suggestive of a nicotine-mediated impairment in uterine blood flow. A more recent study, using Doppler ultrasound to assess blood flow velocities, has indicated that maternal cigarette smoking reduces blood flow in the umbilical circulation (98), leading to fetal hypoxia and to inhibition of FBMs.

Opioids

The role of opioids in the regulation of FBMs has received attention recently. Blockade of endogenous opioids, by naloxone, has little effect on the incidence of ovine FBMs (99), although the response to elevated P_{CO_2} is enhanced (100,101). In contrast, exogenous opioids have a complex effect on FBMs and fetal behavior. In fetal sheep, morphine administration is followed, after a substantial delay, by an extended period of vigorous FBMs and desynchronized electrocortical activity (102–104). A similar response, with evidence of fetal arousal, was seen in response to methadone administration (105). At present, the basis for the changes in FBMs and fetal behavior induced by opioids is not understood.

FETAL BREATHING AND LUNG DEVELOPMENT

Observations in human fetuses with congenital abnormalities and experimentation in animals have indicated that FBMs are necessary for normal prenatal lung development (19,106,107). In the human fetus, abnormalities of the innervation or muscles of the thorax, which would be expected to impair FBMs, have been associated with lung hypoplasia (108–110). It is difficult to assess the effects of impaired FBMs per se in these accounts, as the congenital abnormalities associated with lung hypoplasia may also affect thoracic volume (and hence lung expansion). It is well established that available thoracic space and the degree of lung expansion have a potent effect on fetal lung growth (111–113).

Experimentally, attempts have been made to impair or abolish FBMs to determine their influence on fetal lung development. Phrenic nerve section leads to impaired lung growth in fetal sheep (114,115). This procedure, however, leads to atrophy of the diaphragm muscle and probably to its upward displacement, thereby reducing thoracic volume. Section of the cervical spinal cord abolishes the phasic excitation of phrenic motoneurons while leaving intact the phrenic motoneurons themselves and some of their segmental inputs. Therefore, the "tone" of the diaphragm may not be affected. In fetal rabbits this procedure (cord section at C1–C3) led to a reduction in the weight and DNA content of the lungs, which had poorly expanded and thick-walled terminal sacs (116); cord section below the level of phrenic motoneurons (C5–C8) had significant, but less marked, effects on lung growth, suggesting that rhythmic diaphragmatic activation has a stimulatory effect on lung growth. Similar procedures in fetal sheep resulted in reduced pulmonary weights, DNA content, and distensibility (117).

It is possible that high (and low) spinal cord section reduces basal thoracic volume by denervation of intercostal muscles and by reducing segmental inputs to phrenic motoneurons. In none of the experiments described previously (i.e., phrenic or cord section) was the effect on lung expansion or thoracic volume determined. The same concern applies to another study indicative of reduced lung growth and maturation as a result of impaired FBMs. In this study, part of the thoracic wall of fetal sheep was replaced by a silicone rubber membrane, which reduced the measured pressure fluctuations associated with FBMs (118).

It is not clear how FBMs may stimulate lung growth and maturation. Since individual FBMs are essentially isovolumetric, it is unlikely that rhythmical expansion of the whole lung exists as a stimulus to growth. It is possible that lung liquid moves within the lung, with no net change in volume (106) (although no evidence exists for this), or shear forces may be present.

Rather than individual FBMs acting as a stimulus to lung development, it is possible that episodes of FBMs, alternating with periods of apnea, do so through variations in lung liquid volume and hence lung expansion.

These variations result, in part, from the retardation in fluid efflux during apnea (leading to fluid accumulation and lung expansion) and from increased efflux during FBMs (14,119) (leading to a reduction in lung expansion). Superimposed on these variations are increases in lung expansion due to intermittent periods of fluid influx during episodes of augmented FBMs (19,39) and short periods of increased efflux which apparently coincide with fetal body movements. These variations in tracheal flow are likely to lead to changes in lung expansion, as lung liquid production is relatively constant and is not affected by FBM episodes (107,109). Based on measured variations in tracheal fluid flow in fetal sheep, changes in lung expansion have been computed each minute over 4 hr (19). Lung liquid volume varied by 8.4–45.1% (mean 19.6%) of the mean volume, most of the variation occurring during episodes of FBMs.

In conclusion, although definitive evidence is lacking, there is suggestive evidence that FBMs may stimulate lung growth and structural maturation. The mechanisms whereby this stimulatory effect occurs are not clear at present. However, as in several other tissues (19), the growth of lung tissue *in vitro* is stimulated by rhythmical stretch (120).

SUMMARY

Fetal breathing movements are a normal feature of intrauterine life, probably playing a role in the development of the lungs and respiratory muscles. They occur in episodes related to activity states of the fetal central nervous system. The CNS state in which rapid eye movements and desynchronized ECoG are present is permissive to FBMs, and there is evidence of descending inhibition of medullary centers during the quiet sleep, non-REM state. Although individual FBMs are essentially isovolumetric, the flow of liquid in the trachea is influenced by episodes of FBMs, particularly during late gestation. Normally, augmented efflux of lung liquid occurs during these episodes, although net influx of amniotic fluid may occur during bouts of more vigorous FBMs. These fluxes lead to wide variations in fetal lung expansion, although these variations are much greater in the absence of the upper respiratory tract. FBMs are sensitive to variations in maternal and fetal Po_2, Pco_2, and pH. They are not restricted in their incidence or amplitude by the relatively low Po_2 of the fetus; however, further hypoxia (at least acutely) leads to their inhibition. The influence of CO_2 and pH on fetal respiratory drive is similar to that postnatally, indicating that central chemoreceptors are functional in the fetus. Common drugs taken by the mother can have a profound effect on FBMs and associated behavioral states.

REFERENCES

1. Dawes GS, Fox HE, Leduc BM, Liggins GC, Richards RT. Respiratory movements and rapid eye movement sleep in the fetal lamb. *J Physiol* 1972;220:119–143.
2. Harding R. State-related and developmental changes in laryngeal function. *Sleep* 1980;3:307–322.
3. Lewis PJ, Trudinger B. Fetal hiccups. *Lancet* 1977;2:355.
4. De Vries JIP, Visser GHA, Prechtl HFR. Fetal behaviour in early pregnancy. *Eur J Obstet Gynecol Reprod Biol* 1986; 21:271–276.
5. Harding R. Perinatal development of laryngeal function. *J Dev Physiol* 1984;6:249–258.
6. Jansen AH, Chernick V. Development of respiratory control. *Physiol Rev* 1983;63:437–483.
7. Harding R. Fetal breathing. In: Beard RW, Nathanielsz PW, eds. *Fetal physiology and medicine.* New York: Marcel Dekker, 1984;255–286.
8. Bryan AC, Bowes G, Maloney JE. Control of breathing in the fetus and the newborn. In: Fishman AP, Cherniack NS, Widdicombe JG, Geiger SR, eds. *Handbook of physiology,* sec 3, vol 2. Bethesda: American Physiological Society, 1986;621–647.
9. Lagercrantz H, Milerad J, Walker DW. Control of ventilation in the fetus and newborn. In: Crystal RG, West JB, et al, eds. *The lung: scientific foundations,* New York: Raven Press, 1990.
10. Maloney JE, Adamson TM, Brodecky V, Cranage S, Lambert TF, Ritchie BC. Diaphragmatic activity and lung liquid flow in the unanesthetized fetal sheep. *J Appl Physiol* 1975;39:423–428.
11. Fewell JE, Lee CC, Kitterman JA. Effects of phrenic nerve section on the respiratory system of fetal lambs. *J Appl Physiol* 1981;51:293–297.
12. Harding R, Johnson P, McClelland ME, McLeod CN, Whyte PL. Laryngeal function during breathing and swallowing in foetal and newborn lambs. *J Physiol* 1977;272:14P–15P.
13. Clewlow F, Dawes GS, Johnston BM, Walker DW. Changes in breathing, electrocortical and muscle activity in unanesthetized fetal lambs with age. *J Physiol* 1983;341:463–476.
14. Harding R, Sigger JN, Wickham PJD, Bocking AD. The regulation of flow of pulmonary fluid in fetal sheep. *Respir Physiol* 1984;57:47–59.
15. Poore ER, Walker DW. Chest wall movements during fetal breathing in the sheep. *J Physiol* 1980;301:307–315.
16. Patrick J, Fetherston W, Vick H, Voegelin R. Human fetal breathing movements and gross fetal body movements at weeks 34 to 35 of gestation. *Am J Obstet Gynecol* 1978;130:693–699.
17. Harding R. The upper respiratory tract in perinatal life. In: Gluckman PD, Johnston BM, eds. *The development of respiratory function.* Ithaca: Perinatology Press, 1986;332–376.
18. Harding R, Johnson P, McClelland ME. Respiratory function of the larynx in developing sheep and the influence of sleep state. *Respir Physiol* 1980;40:165–179.
19. Harding R, Dickson KA, Hooper SB. Fetal breathing, tracheal fluid movement and lung growth. In: Gluckman PD, Johnston BM, Nathanielsz PW, eds. *Advances in fetal physiology.* Ithaca: Perinatology Press, 1989;153–175.
20. Johnston BM, Gunn TR, Gluckman PD. Genioglossus and alae nasi activity in fetal sheep. *J Dev Physiol* 1986;8:323–331.
21. Harding R, Buttress JA, Caddy DJ, Wood GA. Respiratory and upper airway responses to nasal obstruction in awake lambs and ewes. *Respir Physiol* 1987;68:177–188.
22. Bartlett, D. Upper airway motor system. In: Fishman AP, Cherniack NS, Widdicombe JG, Geiger SR, eds. *Handbook of physiology,* sec 3, vol 2. Bethesda: American Physiological Society, 1986;223–245.
23. Johnston BM, Gunn TR, Gluckman PD. Surface cooling rapidly induces coordinated activity in the upper and lower airway muscles of the fetal lamb *in utero. Pediatr Res* 1988;23:257–261.
24. Jansen AH, Ioffe S, Chernick V. Drug-induced changes in fetal breathing activity and sleep state. *Can J Physiol Pharmacol* 1983;61:315–324.
25. Cooke IRC, Berger PJ. Maturation of respiratory motor activity in the fetal lamb. *Neurosci Lett [Suppl]* 1989;34:573.
26. Ioffe S, Jansen AH, Chernick V. Maturation of spontaneous fetal diaphragmatic activity and fetal response to hypercapnia and hypoxemia. *J Appl Physiol* 1987;62:609–622.
27. Cooke IRC, Berger PJ. The ontogeny of the respiratory pattern generating system of the fetal lamb. *Proc Soc Neurosci* 1988;14:94.
28. De Vries JIP, Visser GHA, Mulder EJH, Prechtl HFR. Diurnal and other variations in fetal movement and heart rate patterns at 20–22 weeks. *Early Hum Dev* 1987;15:333–348.
29. Fox HE, Inglis J, Steinbrecher M. Fetal breathing movements in uncomplicated pregnancies. 1. Relationship to gestational age. *Am J Obstet Gynecol* 1979;134:544.
30. Natale R, Nasello-Paterson C, Connors G. Patterns of fetal breathing activity in the human fetus at 24 to 28 weeks of gestation. *Am J Obstet Gynecol* 1988;158:317–321.
31. Patrick J, Campbell K, Carmichael L, Natale R, Richardson B. Patterns of human fetal breathing during the last 10 weeks of pregnancy. *Obstet Gynecol* 1980;56:24–30.
32. Gennser G, Marsal K. Fetal breathing movements monitored by real-time B-mode ultrasound; basal appearance and response to challenges. *Contrib Gynecol Obstet* 1970;6:66–79.
33. Patrick J, Challis J, Campbell K, Carmichael L, Richardson B, Tevaarwerk G. Effects of synthetic glucocorticoid administration on human fetal breathing movements at 34 to 35 weeks' gestational age. *Am J Obstet Gynecol* 1981;139:324.
34. Bowes G, Adamson TM, Ritchie BC, Dowling M, Wilkinson MH, Maloney JE. Development of patterns of respiratory activity in unanesthetized fetal sheep *in utero. J Appl Physiol* 1981;50:693–700.
35. Dawes GS, Gardner WN, Johnston BM, Walker DW. Breathing in fetal lambs: the effect of brain stem section. *J Physiol* 1983;335:535–553.
36. Nijhuis JG, Prechtl HFR, Martin CB, Bots RSGM. Are there behavioural states in the human fetus? *Early Hum Dev* 1982;6:177–195.
37. Prechtl HFR. The behavioural states of the newborn infant (a review). *Brain Res* 1974;76:185–212.
38. Arduini D, Rizzo G, Giorlandino C. Valensise H, Dell'Acqua S, Romanini C. The development of fetal behavioural states: a longitudinal study. *Prenat Diagn* 1986;6:117–124.
39. Harding R, Fetal lung liquid. In: Brace RA, Ross MG, Robillard JE, eds. *Fetal and neonatal fluid balance.* Ithaca: Perinatology Press, 1989;41–64.
40. Chiba Y, Utsu M, Kanzak T, Hasegawa T. Changes in venous flow and intratracheal flow in fetal breathing movements. *Ultrasound Med Biol* 1985;11:43–49.
41. Harding R, Bocking AD, Sigger JN. Influence of upper respiratory tract on liquid flow to and from fetal lungs. *J Appl Physiol* 1986;61:68–74.
42. Harding R, Bocking AD, Sigger JN. Upper airway resistances in fetal sheep: the influence of breathing activity. *J Appl Physiol* 1986;60:160–165.
43. Vilos GA, Liggins GC. Intrathoracic pressures in fetal sheep. *J Dev Physiol* 1982;4:247–256.
44. Sheldon G, Brazy J, Tuggle B, Crenshaw C, Brumley G. Fetal lamb lung lavage and its effect on lung phosphatidylcholine. *Pediatr Res* 1979;13:599–602.
45. Jose JH, Schreiner RL, Lemons JA, et al. The effect of amniotic fluid aspiration on pulmonary function in the adult and newborn rabbit. *Pediatr Res* 1983;17:976–981.
46. Clarke DA, Nieman GF, Thompson JE, Paskanik AM, Rokhar JE, Bredenbery CE. Surfactant displacement by meconium free fatty acids: an alternative explanation for atelectasis in meconium aspiration syndrome. *J Pediatr* 1987;110:765–770.
47. Boddy K, Dawes GS, Fisher R, Pinter S, Robinson JS. Foetal respiratory movements, electrocortical and cardiovascular responses to hypoxaemia and hypercapnia in sheep. *J Physiol* 1974;243:599–618.
48. Koos BJ, Sameshina H, Power GG. Fetal breathing, sleep state, and cardiovascular responses to graded hypoxia in sheep. *J Appl Physiol* 1987;62:1033–1039.
49. Harding R, Poore ER, Cohen GL. The effect of brief episodes

of diminished uterine blood flow on breathing movements, sleep states and heart rate in fetal sheep. *J Dev Physiol* 1981;3:231–243.

50. Bocking AD, Harding R. Effects of reduced uterine blood flow on electrocortical activity, breathing and skeletal muscle activity in fetal sheep. *Am J Obstet Gynecol* 1986;154:655–662.

51. Natale R, Clewlow F, Dawes GS. Measurement of fetal forelimb movements in the lamb *in utero*. *Am J Obstet Gynecol* 1981;140:545–551.

52. Rurak DW, Gruber NC. Increased oxygen consumption associated with breathing activity in fetal lambs. *J Appl Physiol* 1983;54:701–707.

53. Dornan JC, Ritchie JWK. Fetal breathing movements and maternal hyperoxia in the growth retarded fetus. *Br J Obstet Gynecol* 1983;90:210–213.

54. Walker DW. Peripheral and central chemoreceptors in the fetus and newborn. *Annu Rev Physiol* 1984;46:687–703.

55. Hanson MA. Peripheral chemoreceptor function before and after birth. In: Johnston BM, Gluckman PD, eds. *Respiratory control and lung development in the fetus and newborn*. Ithaca: Perinatology Press, 1986;311–330.

56. Blanco CE, Dawes GS, Hanson MA, McCooke HB. The response to hypoxia of arterial chemoreceptors in fetal sheep and newborn lambs. *J Physiol* 1984;351:25–37.

57. Koos BJ, Sameshina H. Effect of hypoxaemia and hypercapnia on breathing movements and sleep state in sinoaortic denervated fetal sheep. *J Dev Physiol* 1988;10:131–144.

58. Gluckman PD, Johnston BM. Lesions in the upper lateral pons abolish the hypoxic depression of breathing in unanaesthetized fetal lamb *in utero*. *J Physiol* 1987;382:373–383.

59. Martin-Body RL, Johnston BM. Central origin of the hypoxic depression of breathing in the newborn. *Respir Physiol* 1988;71:25–32.

60. Koos BJ, Sameshina H, Power GG. Fetal breathing movement, sleep state and cardiovascular responses to an inhibitor of mitochondrial ATPase in sheep. *J Dev Physiol* 1986;8:67–75.

61. Koos BJ, Kitanaka T, Matsuda K, Gilbert RD, Longo LD. Fetal breathing adaptation to prolonged hypoxaemia in sheep. *J Dev Physiol* 1988;10:161–166.

62. Bocking AD, Gagnon R, Milne KM, White SE. Behavioral activity during prolonged hypoxemia in fetal sheep. *J Appl Physiol* 1988;65:2420–2426.

63. Hooper SB, Harding R. The effect of prolonged hypoxemia on fetal breathing movements and lung liquid volume, secretion and flow. *J Appl Physiol* 1990;in press.

64. Hooper SB, Dickson KA, Harding R. Lung liquid secretion, flow and volume in response to moderate asphyxia in fetal sheep. *J Dev Physiol* 1988;10:473–485.

65. Walker DW, Harding R. Effect of hypoxia on the excitability of two cranial reflexes in unanaesthetized fetal lambs. *J Dev Physiol* 1984;6:387–399.

66. Duenhoelter JH, Pritchard JA. Human fetal respiration. IV. Failure of severe distress to stimulate aspiration of amniotic fluid by the immature human fetus. *Am J Obstet Gynecol* 1978;130:470.

67. Howatt WF, Humphreys PW, Normand ICS, Strang LB. Ventilation of liquid by the fetal lamb during asphyxia. *J Appl Physiol* 1965;20:496–502.

68. Bowes G, Wilkinson MH, Dowling M, Ritchie BC, Brodecky V, Maloney JE. Hypercapnic stimulation of respiratory activity in unanaesthetized fetal sheep *in utero*. *J Appl Physiol* 1981;50:701–708.

69. Dawes GS, Gardner WN, Johnston BM, Walker DW. Effects of hypercapnia on tracheal pressure, diaphragm and intercostal electromyograms in unanaesthetized fetal lambs. *J Physiol* 1982;326:461–474.

70. Jansen AH, Ioffe S, Russell BJ, Chernick V. Influence of sleep state on the response to hypercapnia in fetal lambs. *Respir Physiol* 1982;48:125–142.

71. Rigatto H, Lee D, Davi M, Moore M, Rigatto E, Cates D. Effect of increased arterial CO_2 on fetal breathing and behavior in sheep. *J Appl Physiol* 1988;64:982–987.

72. Ritchie JWK, Lakhani K. Fetal breathing movements in response to maternal inhalation of 5% carbon dioxide. *Am J Obstet Gynecol* 1980;136:386–388.

73. Van Weering HK, Wladimiroff JW, Roodenburg PJ. Effect of changes in maternal blood gases on fetal breathing movements. *Contrib Gynecol Obstet* 1979;6:88–91.

74. Connors G, Hunse C, Carmichael L, Natale R, Richardson B. The role of carbon dioxide in the generation of human fetal breathing movements. *Am J Obstet Gynecol* 1988;158:322–327.

75. Johnston BM, Walker DW. Respiratory responses to changes in oxygen and carbon dioxide in the perinatal period. In: Johnston BM, Gluckman PD, eds. *Respiratory control and lung development in the fetus and newborn*. Ithaca: Perinatology Press, 1986;279–310.

76. Jansen AH. Central chemoreceptor function in the fetus. *Semin Perinatol* 1977;1:323–326.

77. Chernick V, Faridy EE, Pagtakhan RD. Role of peripheral and central chemoreceptors in the initiation of fetal respiration. *J Appl Physiol* 1975;38:407–410.

78. Molteni RA, Melmed MH, Sheldon RE, Jones MD, Meschia G. Induction of fetal breathing by metabolic acidemia and its effect on blood flow to the respiratory muscles. *Am J Obstet Gynecol* 1980;136:609–620.

79. Hohimer AR, Bissonnette JM, Richardson BS, Machida CM. Central chemical regulation of breathing movements in fetal lambs. *Respir Physiol* 1983;52:99–111.

80. Natale R. Maternal plasma glucose concentration and fetal breathing movements: a review. *Semin Perinatol* 1980;4:287–293.

81. Richardson BS, Hohimer AR, Bissonnette JM, Machida CM. Insulin hypoglycemia, cerebral metabolism, and neural function in fetal lambs. *Am J Physiol* 1985;248:R72–R77.

82. Fowden AL, Harding R, Ralph MM, Thorburn GD. Nutritional control of respiratory and other muscular activities in relation to plasma prostaglandin E in the fetal sheep. *J Dev Physiol* 1989;11:253–262.

83. Harper MA, Meis PJ, Rose JC, Swain M, Burns J, Kardon B. Human fetal breathing response to intravenous glucose is directly related to gestational age. *Am J Obstet Gynecol* 1987;157:1403–1405.

84. Nijhuis JG, Jongsma HW, Crijns IJMJ, De Valk IMGM, Van der Velden JWHJ. Effects of maternal glucose ingestion on human fetal breathing movements at weeks 24 and 28 of gestation. *Early Hum Dev* 1986;13:183–188.

85. Bocking AD, Adamson L, Cousin A, et al. Effects of intravenous glucose injections on human fetal breathing movements and gross fetal body movements at 38 to 40 weeks' gestational age. *Am J Obstet Gynecol* 1982;142:606–611.

86. Fowden AL, Harding R, Ralph MM, Thorburn GD. The nutritional regulation of plasma prostaglandin E concentrations in the fetus and pregnant ewe during late gestation. *J Physiol* 1987;394:1–12.

87. Kitterman JA. Arachidonic acid metabolites and control of breathing in the fetus and newborn. *Semin Perinatol* 1987;11:43–52.

88. Fox HE, Steinbrecher M, Pessel D, Inglis J, Medvid L, Angel E. Maternal ethanol ingestion and the occurrence of human fetal breathing movements. *Am J Obstet Gynecol* 1978;132:354–358.

89. McLeod W, Brien J, Loomis C, Carmichael L, Probert C, Patrick J. Effects of maternal ethanol ingestion on fetal breathing movements, gross body movements, and heart rate at 37 to 40 weeks' gestational age. *Am J Obstet Gynecol* 1983;145:251–257.

90. Horrobin DF. A biochemical basis for alcoholism and alcohol-induced damage including the fetal alcohol syndrome and cirrhosis. *Med Hypotheses* 1980;6:929–942.

91. Boddy K, Dawes GS, Fischer RL, Pinter S, Robinson JS. The effects of pentobarbitone and pethidine on foetal breathing movements in sheep. *Br J Pharmacol* 1976;57:311–317.

92. Boddy K. The influence of maternal drug administration on human fetal breathing movements *in utero*. In: Lewis PJ, ed. *Therapeutic problems in pregnancy*. Lancaster. MTP Press, 1977;153–159.

93. Piercy WN, Day MA, Neims AH, Williams RL. Alteration of

ovine fetal respiratory-like activity by diazepam, caffeine, and doxapram. *Am J Obstet Gynecol* 1977;127:43–49.

94. Manning FA, Wyn Pugh E, Boddy K. Effect of cigarette smoking on fetal breathing movements in normal pregnancies. *Br Med J* 1975;1:552.

95. Gennser G, Marsal K, Brantmark B. Maternal smoking and fetal breathing movements. *Am J Obstet Gynecol* 1975;123:861.

96. Thaler I, Goodman JDS, Dawes GS. Effects of maternal cigarette smoking on fetal breathing and fetal movements. *Am J Obstet Gynecol* 1980;138:282–287.

97. Manning F, Walker D, Feyerabend C. The effect of nicotine on fetal breathing movements in conscious pregnant ewes. *Am J Obstet Gynecol* 1978;52:563–568.

98. Morrow RJ, Ritchie JWK, Bull SB. Maternal cigarette smoking: the effects on umbilical and uterine blood flow velocity. *Am J Obstet Gynecol* 1988;159:1069–1071.

99. Adamson SL, Patrick JE, Challis JRG. Effects of naloxone on the breathing, electrocortical, heart rate, glucose and cortisol responses to hypoxia in the sheep fetus. *J Dev Physiol* 1984;6:495–507.

100. Moss IR, Scarpelli EM. CO_2 and naloxone modify sleep/wake state and activate breathing in the acute fetal lamb preparation. *Respir Physiol* 1984;55:325–340.

101. Joseph SA, McMillen IC, Walker DW. Effects of naloxone on breathing movements during hypercapnia in the fetal lamb. *J Appl Physiol* 1987;62:673–678.

102. Sheldon RE, Toubas PL. Morphine stimulates rapid, regular, deep and sustained breathing efforts in fetal lambs. *J Appl Physiol* 1984;57:40–43.

103. Bennet L, Johnston BM, Gluckman PD. The central effects of morphine on fetal breathing movements in the fetal sheep. *J Dev Physiol* 1986;8:297–305.

104. Hasan SU, Lee DS, Gibson DA, et al. Effect of morphine on breathing and behavior in fetal sheep. *J Appl Physiol* 1988;64:2058–2065.

105. Szeto HH. Effects of narcotic drugs on fetal behavioural activity: acute methadone exposure. *Am J Obstet Gynecol* 1983;146:211–216.

106. Liggins GC. Growth of the fetal lung. *J Dev Physiol* 1984;6:237–248.

107. Kitterman JA. Physiological factors in fetal lung growth. *Can J Physiol Pharmacol* 1988;66:1122–1128.

108. Goldstein JD, Reid LM. Pulmonary hypoplasia resulting from phrenic nerve agenesis and diaphragmatic amyoplasia. *J Pediatr* 1980;97:282–287.

109. Page DV, Stocker JT. Anomalies associated with pulmonary hypoplasia. *Am Rev Respir Dis* 1982;125:216–221.

110. Dornan JC, Ritchie JWK, Meban C. Fetal breathing movements and lung maturation in the congenitally abnormal human fetus. *J Dev Physiol* 1984;6:367–375.

111. Alcorn D, Adamson TM, Lambert TF, Maloney JE, Ritchie BC, Robinson PM. Morphological effects of tracheal ligation and drainage in the fetal lamb lung. *J Anat* 1977;123:649–660.

112. Harrison MR, Bressack MA, Chung AM, de Lorimier AA. Correction of congenital diaphragmatic hernia *in utero*. II. Simulated correction permits fetal lung growth with survival at birth. *Surgery* 1980;88:260–268.

113. Moessinger AC, Harding R, Adamson TM, Singh M, Kiu G. Local vs systemic factors at play in fetal lung growth and maturation. *Pediatr Res* 1989;25:56A.

114. Alcorn D, Adamson TM, Maloney JE, Robinson PM. Morphological effects of chronic bilateral phrenectomy or vagotomy in the fetal lamb lung. *J Anat* 1980;130:683–695.

115. Fewell JE, Lee CC, Kitterman JA. Effects of phrenic nerve section on the respiratory system of fetal lambs. *J Appl Physiol* 1981;51:293–297.

116. Wigglesworth JS, Desai R. Effects on lung growth of cervical cord section in the rabbit fetus. *Early Hum Dev* 1979;3:51–65.

117. Liggins GC, Vilos GA, Campos GA, Kitterman JA, Lee CH. The effect of spinal cord transection on lung development in fetal sheep. *J Dev Physiol* 1981;3:267–274.

118. Liggins GC, Vilos GA, Campos GA, Kitterman JA, Lee CH. The effect of bilateral thoracoplasty on lung development in fetal sheep. *J Dev Physiol* 1981;3:275–282.

119. Dickson KA, Maloney JE, Berger PJ. State-related changes in lung liquid secretion and tracheal flow rate in fetal lambs. *J Appl Physiol* 1987;62:34–38.

120. Skinner S, Ashby CA, Low C, et al. The growth of fetal lung structures *in vitro* is stimulated by simulated fetal breathing movements. In: Gluckman PD, Johnston BM, Nathanielsz PW, eds. *Advances in fetal physiology*. Ithaca: Perinatology Press, 1989;153–175.

THE LUNG: Scientific Foundations
edited by R.G. Crystal, J.B. West et al.
Raven Press, Ltd., New York © 1991.

CHAPTER 6.1.2

The First Breath

W. Alan Hodson

The most important single respiratory event of life is the first breath, yet it has been an event particularly elusive to study and therefore lacks our full understanding. The onset of breathing marks the beginning of a remarkable and rapid transition of the respiratory system at birth. How do the lungs, which are fluid-filled and have no prior experience in gas exchange, virtually no pulmonary blood flow, and an erratic system of respiratory control, adjust so rapidly to ventilation and gas exchange? The extraordinary changes in alveolar fluid, mechanical conditions, pulmonary blood flow, and central nervous system control have been well described but are not well understood. Speculations about the mechanisms of the first breath are derived from studies of respiratory control in fetal animals or in newborn human infants during the first several days of life. Successful transition is of utmost importance in preventing hypoxic damage to the infant. Knowledge of physiological events of the first breath is relevant to prevention and treatment of a number of clinical events related to poor respiratory adaptation, including intrapartum asphyxia, hyaline membrane disease, transient tachypnea of the newborn, meconium aspiration, and pneumothorax. Because the first breath is a single event, it has been extraordinarily difficult to study in humans and nearly impossible to study in animals under natural circumstances. Nevertheless, considerable information has been accumulated since Barcroft's pioneering studies of fetal lambs nearly 50 years ago. To quote Barcroft (1): "If I may figure the first breath as a chord struck on an instrument, I may divide a consideration of the subject into some description of the instrument itself, and some investigation of the impact upon it." Indeed, much of the investigation over the past four decades has followed Barcroft's prophetic strategy of describing fetal lung function and the physiological and biochemical changes induced by the first breath.

The first breath must halt the asphyxiating process of disrupted placental O_2 delivery, and therefore its most vital and urgent function is the immediate and effective establishment of gas exchange. This requires the initiation of tidal ventilation, the acquisition of a stable residual gas volume, the removal of fluid from the airways and alveoli, and a marked increase in pulmonary blood flow. The first breath, therefore, is accomplished with unique changes in pulmonary mechanics, cardiopulmonary adjustments, and rapid transalveolar fluid movement.

TRANSITION FROM THE FETAL STATE

Any discussion of transitional physiology at birth requires knowledge of the fetal pulmonary status, including fetal breathing, fetal lung liquid dynamics, and overall lung maturation, which are discussed elsewhere in this book. Fetal breathing (see Chapter 6.1.1) occurs approximately 40% of the time beginning after 20 weeks of gestation. These movements are rapid and shallow and depend on the activity or state of the central nervous system. Fetal breathing movements are characteristically associated with rapid low-voltage electrocortical activity and rapid eye movement (REM) sleep. The on–off phenomenon of fetal breathing movements is intriguing and appears to be unique to the fetus, since this respiratory pattern disappears the instant the first breath is taken. However, anecdotal reports of prolonged apnea occurring during treatment with high-frequency oscillatory ventilation or during extracorporeal membrane oxygenation of newborn infants suggest that postnatal rhythmicity of respiration may be reversible. Recurrent apneic epi-

W. A. Hodson: Pediatric Department, Division of Neonatal and Respiratory Diseases, University of Washington School of Medicine, Seattle, Washington 98195.

sodes of the premature infant may also be a throwback to the fetal state.

The first breath may initiate phasic afferent stimuli from the lungs which are important to the initiation of a type of respiratory rhythmicity quite different from that of the fetus. Although afferent neural activity during fetal breathing has an uncertain role, it appears that fetal breathing is primarily associated with bursts of phrenic nerve and diaphragmatic activity. These fetal respiratory movements decrease with the onset of labor. The utility of fetal breathing movements is unclear, since they are dissimilar to the respiratory pattern following birth. Perhaps diaphragmatic maturation requires conditioning by way of muscular contractions. The stretching of lung tissue with fetal breathing also appears to be an important stimulus to lung growth and differentiation (2). No practice for the first breath seems necessary, however; witness the activity of premature human infants born at 25–26 weeks' gestation who initiate breathing quite well, provided that they are not profoundly asphyxiated during the delivery process.

RESPIRATORY CONTROL MECHANISMS AT BIRTH

Nonspecific Stimuli

A major increase in neural afferent impulses to the central nervous system most likely occurs with the expulsion of the fetus through the narrow birth canal into a new environment of light, sound, air, gravity, and temperature—one that is markedly different from the environment left behind. These afferent impulses do not all converge on the respiratory control centers but probably interact in a complex way to initiate strong efferent respiratory signals. The timing of the first breath may depend on a combination of factors and not simply on stimulation by hypoxic and hypercapnic changes. A number of putative "arousal" stimuli could act synergistically (see Fig. 1). Stimulation from temperature, tactile, proprioceptive, and pain receptors undoubtedly occurs. It is interesting to reflect on the word "gasp," which connotes a sudden reflex inspiration usually in response to fright or pain (3). Perhaps this reflex is a vestigial one related to the first breath? Separation of all of the sensory contributions to the first inspiration is difficult. Individual types of stimuli have been studied in the fetus to determine if they can influence respiration. It has been demonstrated that sciatic nerve stimulation as well as electrical and mechanical stimulation of the skin of the fetal leg produce gasping in the fetal lamb (4–6). The exteriorized fetal lamb has been immersed in a liquid bath and the temperature subsequently varied. Cooling to 10°C results

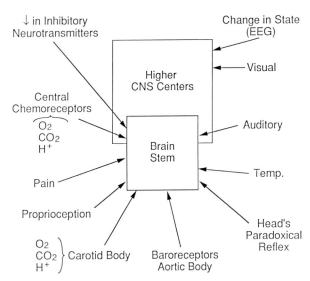

FIG. 1. Putative afferent stimuli influencing the onset of breathing.

in rhythmic breathing, whereas warming to 40°C causes cessation of breathing (7). Merlet et al. (8) produced gasping respirations in partially exteriorized fetal lambs by circulating cold saline around the head.

It is unclear how important these nonspecific stimuli, such as temperature, pain, and proprioception, are to the first breath. They most likely "arouse" a number of central nervous system functions and may increase brain sensitivity to more specific or traditional stimuli.

Peripheral Chemoreceptor Function at Birth

Considerable uncertainty surrounds the exact role and function of the peripheral chemoreceptors at birth. The chemoreceptors are active *in utero* and respond to both hypercapnia and hypoxia (9,10). The fetal carotid body does not appear to be necessary for fetal breathing movements (11). It is clear from studies of fetal sheep that denervation of the carotid body does not prevent or delay the first breath (11–13), not does it prevent or delay the respiratory response to carotid arterial infusions of cyanide or hypoxic and/or hypercapnic blood (14). For several minutes immediately before and after birth, the carotid chemoreceptors are exposed to a wide range of oxygen and carbon dioxide concentrations. Assuming a fetal P_aO_2 of approximately 25 torr, it is of interest to know the vigor with which the carotid chemoreceptors respond to a decrease below this level. The carotid chemoreceptors in the sheep fetus respond to hypoxic stimuli (10,15). Woodrum et al. (9) demonstrated a vigorous response to the infusion of arterial blood with a P_O_2 of 12–15 torr; however, this response was not abolished by carotid sinus denervation. The contribution of cord-clamping to arterial chemoreceptors has been controversial. Fetal chemoreceptor activity increases after cord occlusion (10,16). Biscoe et al. (17,18) demonstrated an increase in carotid sinus nerve activity with cord-clamping; however, if blood gases are kept constant through cross-circulation (19), cord-clamping by itself does not result in breathing. Therefore, the combination of cord-clamping with its attendant ischemia and blood-gas changes may well potentiate carotid chemoreceptor function at birth, but neither event is essential.

The carotid body experiences an abrupt change in Po_2 following the initiation of breathing which is markedly different from that experienced *in utero*. Sympathetic discharge with efferent stimulation of the carotid glomus (20,21) may affect sensitivity to hypoxia; however, studies with sympathetic section do not appear to alter chemoreceptor responses in the fetus (10). It is improbable that adjustments to a new threshold of oxygen/carbon dioxide could occur immediately. Indeed the ventilatory response to a hypoxic stimulus changes over the first several days of life, suggesting the establishment of a new set-point (15,22). Adjustment of the set-point, however, should not affect the response to hypoxia vis-à-vis the first breath, since the fetus has not yet experienced an increase in Po_2. Rather, this readjustment of the chemoreceptors appears to take several days (10,23,24). It is possible that postnatal changes in chemoreceptor sensitivity are a result of central nervous system factors rather than a result of the carotid body itself. Further evidence for the adjustment of the chemoreceptors following birth is obtained from infants with certain abnormal conditions associated with chronic hypoxia [e.g., cyanotic congenital heart disease (25)] and birth at high altitude (26–28). These infants have a blunted ventilatory response to hypoxia. Newborn rats maintained in a chronic hypoxic environment also do not adjust their chemoreceptor sensitivity (29).

The developmental status of the carotid body is of considerable interest even though it is not critical for the first breath. The carotid body has glomus cells at birth and is capable of releasing endogenously produced mediators, including dopamine (30–34). The dopamine concentration of the carotid glomus in the newborn is higher than in the adult and may account for the newborn's decreased sensitivity. The mechanism by which oxygen interacts with glomus cells in the carotid body is complex and poorly understood. Hypoxia appears to modulate potassium conductance in glomus cells through voltage-dependent calcium channels (35). There is virtually no information about the development of Ca^{2+} and K^+ channels in the type I cells of the fetal carotid body. The mechanisms by which chemosensitivity readjusts to postnatal blood gases is out-side the scope of this discussion; however, other changes occurring at the time of birth may include alterations in the microcirculation to the carotid body, the presence of inhibitor substances, decreased receptor sites, decreased accessibility to receptors, or changes in ion channels. All of these aspects need further study.

In conclusion, it appears that the carotid chemoreceptors are not essential for the first breath. There are many other mechanisms at work which act in concert to stimulate the first breath. However, in the abnormal situation, other mechanisms may not function and the peripheral chemoreceptors might therefore act as an important safety factor.

Central Nervous System Factors

Extensive studies on the mechanisms of fetal breathing have attempted to discern the role of the brainstem from that of higher centers (16,36–39). The association between low-voltage REM and fetal breathing movements can be disrupted with rostral section of the brainstem (40,41). Most of the evidence suggests that the suprapontine pathway is necessary for fetal breathing movements. Fetal breathing movements stop during high-voltage electrocortical activity (42,43). The cessation of fetal breathing movements with a modest fall in Po_2 is probably related to higher central nervous system perception and is most likely a response intended for the fetus to conserve oxygen. The mechanisms of this sensing are unclear. Suprapontine section, however, results in a change to near-continuous fetal breathing movements from the usual 40% of the time (41). Following brainstem transection, the response to hypoxia is altered with an increase in fetal breathing movements (40,41). The lateral pontine area of fetal lambs is also involved with the inhibition of breathing during high-voltage electrocortical activity (44). Lateral pontine lesions result in an increased sensitivity to H^+/CO_2 in the fetus. Therefore, there is strong evidence of inhibition of fetal breathing movements from higher centers, which may be important in the transition to postnatal breathing. Clearly this inhibition needs to be altered or stopped if postnatal breathing with regular rhythmicity is to occur. It appears that there are powerful excitatory and inhibitory effects on fetal breathing, brought about by neurotransmitter agonists and antagonists (42); however, if there is a change in these transmitters it is not explained by events surrounding the first breath.

Central Chemoreceptors

If the carotid sinus is denervated in the exteriorized fetal lamb, there is a brisk ventilatory response to a decreased arterial P_{O_2} (25→12 torr) or to an increased P_{CO_2} (~70 torr). Similarly, there is a ventilatory response to the infusion of cyanide into the carotid artery (14). Jansen and Chernick (45) investigated possible sites of central chemoreceptor activity in the fetal lamb. Application of cyanide to the ventral surface of the medulla induced respiratory efforts. Additional studies of the exteriorized fetal lamb led these investigators to propose that histotoxic hypoxia of the medulla initiates respiration by stimulating a site producing gasping rather than stimulating the site responsible for rhythmic breathing (46,47). To test whether the excitation produced from cyanide was due to a secondary increase in the hydrogen ion concentration, they injected acidic mock cerebrospinal fluid (CSF); they concluded that changes in pH on the ventral surface of the medulla did not stimulate respiratory efforts (48). These studies were consistent with earlier observations that low CSF HCO_3^- concentration was not associated with breathing (49). However, with a more prolonged infusion of a solution with a low HCO_3^- concentration into the ventriculocisternal system, there was increased incidence and depth of fetal breathing (39,50). It is interesting to note that hypercapnic infusions in the carotid artery result in gasping ventilation (14). These studies in the unanesthetized fetal lamb suggest that CO_2 changes in the blood may stimulate the central chemoreceptors via H^+ effects at a different central nervous system site than would topical stimulation. Greater chemosensitivity has been shown to result from intravascular stimulation than from medullary surface stimulation (51).

The mechanisms by which hypoxia stimulates vigorous ventilatory effort in the carotid-sinus-denervated fetal lamb are obscure. Hypoxia may depress higher centers that inhibit sustained fetal ventilatory activity, or it may cause the release of a humoral agent necessary for the onset of ventilation at birth or possibly cause a secondary decrease in intracellular pH as a result of anaerobic metabolism. It must be noted that the hypoxic stimulus producing fetal ventilatory activity is greater than that associated with the inhibition of fetal respiratory movements (43). It is also possible that tissue hypoxia following cyanide infusion may mediate a respiratory response via a spinally mediated nonchemoreceptor mechanism (52). The ventilatory responses to hypoxia and hypercapnia in these animals are similar to that seen following cord-clamping and are therefore similar to the first breath. Although it remains speculative, central chemoreceptor response to hypoxia may be the most important stimulus to the vigorous first breath. The exact site of chemosensing in the medulla remains unclear, and the specific neurotransmitters involved are not yet understood (53).

The central chemoreceptors are operative in the fetus, most likely at a different threshold for H^+/CO_2 than after birth. This may be due to inhibitory mechanisms involving the rostral lateral pons (44). Like the peripheral chemoreceptors, the central chemoreceptors may reset after birth. It is unclear whether the mechanism of the first breath is similar to that of the primitive response of autoresuscitation. Such a stimulus seems somewhat harsh if this is an important component of the first breath.

Central chemoreceptor sensitivity may be altered by a variety of neurohumoral substances that change at birth, including neuromodulators and neurotransmitters. Catecholamines, for example, begin to rise during labor, with a marked surge at birth. Hypoxia at birth stimulates an output of catecholamines, adenosine, and opiates; all have a potential to affect respiration. These substances may be more relevant to the understanding of unsuccessful transition following delivery in that they may be more important to inhibition of respiration than to stimulation.

Prostaglandins

Prostaglandins have a considerable influence on respiratory patterns before birth and have been reported to cause apnea in newborn animals. Do they play a role in bringing about the first breath? PGE_2 infused into fetal lambs decreases the frequency of fetal respiratory movements, whereas infusions of a prostaglandin synthase inhibitor (meclofenamate, indomethacin) increase the frequency of breathing (54–61). PGF_2 has a smaller effect than PGE_2, and neither of these is influenced by denervation of peripheral chemoreceptors (55,62). The evidence therefore suggests that tonic inhibition of fetal breathing may be caused by prostaglandins and that this inhibitory function resides in the pons or medulla (63). The rapid reduction in PGE_2 at birth may therefore be important in permitting continuous respiration after birth (64). It seems unlikely, however, that prostaglandins have any role in the first breath in spite of the effects noted on fetal and postnatal breathing.

Other Neuropharmacologic Agents

There has been considerable investigation of (a) the effects of neurotransmitters, neuromodulators, and neuropeptides on the phasic or inhibitory aspects of fetal breathing (65) and (b) the overall effects of opiates on respiratory control (66). This interest has focused primarily on mechanisms of inhibition of fetal breathing and on the modulation of the unique fetal respiratory rhythm. In addition to prostaglandins, serotoninergic and gamma-aminobutyric acid (GABA)-ergic mechanisms have inhibitory effects during high-voltage electrocortical activity. None of the studies has focused on immediate changes at birth. Changes in neuropharmacologic substances at the moment of birth could result from neural input secondary to pain and cooling, along with a decrease in oxygen. Catecholamines, both epinephrine and norepinephrine, increase severalfold at birth; this increase is comparable to that produced by hypoxia (67). Met-enkephalin is also increased with hypoxia in fetal lambs (68). Continuous fetal breathing can be induced by morphine (69–71). This effect follows a period of apnea, and the increase in breathing is associated with a shift from quiet to REM sleep (72). During asphyxia, endogenous opioids are released and depress respiration (73–77). Also, enkephalins are elevated in cord blood at the time of birth (78,79). Naloxone infusion in the fetal lamb does not alter breathing patterns, nor does it alter the depressive response to hypoxia (65); however, Bamford (42) has demonstrated that apomorphine can overcome the inhibition to hypoxia. These findings suggest that endogenous opioids are not important in the regulation of respiration in late gestation and are not important to the mechanisms of the first breath (80). Chernick and co-workers (75,76) have demonstrated a shortening of apnea following asphyxia at birth if naloxone is given. Therefore, endogenous opiates may delay the onset of respiration in the presence of severe asphyxia. Other central neuroactive substances of possible importance to fetal breathing, including thyrotropin-releasing hormone, acetylcholine, substance P, adenosine, and serotonin, have not been related to the onset of breathing, although they have not been specifically studied. Inactivation at birth of some of these neuromodulators may be necessary for the establishment of rhythmic breathing after birth.

Cord-clamping may eliminate humoral inhibitory substances from the mother or from the placenta. Recent studies utilizing a uterine window in fetal lambs suggest that a combination of arousal and an increase in oxygen is required for the maintenance of continuous breathing following birth (81). A rise in P_{O_2} to approximately 100 torr in itself did not induce continuous breathing but required cord occlusion, again suggesting that cord-clamping may decrease circulating respiratory inhibitory substances.

THE MECHANICS OF THE FIRST BREATH

In addition to a remarkable change in the neural control of breathing, quite extraordinary mechanical events occur with the first breath. The gas-exchange area, filled with fetal lung liquid, must be converted to a stable alveolar air–tissue interface with the first breath—no small task! The lung in the fetal state contains liquid that occupies a volume slightly less than the functional residual capacity (FRC). Recent evi-

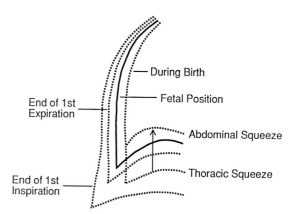

FIG. 2. Hypothetical changes in the position of the thorax and diaphragm before, during, and after the first breath. Note upward movement of the diaphragm (*arrow*) just prior to the first breath.

dence in the fetal lamb suggests that fetal lung liquid absorption begins during labor (82,83) (see Chapter 6.1.3). Therefore, just prior to the first breath the fetal lung fluid may occupy something less than 30% of TLC (Fig. 2). Nevertheless, a relatively large amount of fluid (50–100 ml) must be removed or displaced from the gas-exchange area with the first few breaths.

The First Inspiration

The first inspiration requires a very large negative intrapleural pressure of between 40 and 100 cmH$_2$O (84). Measurements of esophageal pressure before and during the first several breaths in human infants indicate a persistence of high transpulmonary pressures for several breaths (84,85). The high inspiratory pressure is maintained for a mean of 0.58 sec, with a range of 0.29–1.4 sec (86–88). Two general types of inflation patterns have been observed—some requiring high pressure before any volume change occurs, and others with air entry beginning at a lower pressure (Fig. 3). The differences in shape of the pressure–volume loops suggest that in some infants the air entered the lungs only after a 20–40 cmH$_2$O pressure gradient was created (a high opening pressure), whereas in others the pattern would suggest that air might already have entered the lungs. The pressure–volume loops tended to become less square with subsequent breaths. The thoracic recoil following the vaginal squeeze could result in some air entering the lungs prior to the first breath. However, Vyas et al. (89) found a positive esophageal pressure prior to the first breath, making this possibility unlikely. They measured transpulmonary pressures created during the first breath in human infants and determined that esophageal pressure changes averaged −52 cmH$_2$O. During vaginal delivery, the thorax ex-

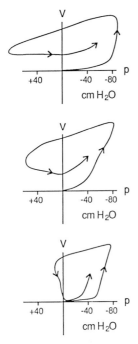

FIG. 3. Schematic representation of the types of pressure–volume changes that may occcur with the first breath. Note differences in opening pressure (*P*). The first expiration requires high positive pressure, and volume (*V*) may return to zero.

periences positive pressures of up to 90 cmH$_2$O from the surrounding birth canal. This external force squeezes some fluid out of the mouth, pharynx, and trachea—perhaps 10–15 ml and sometimes as high as 30 ml (90). The majority of fluid remains behind, however; and with the first inspiration, a small residual air volume is established. The first inspired air, together with the residual alveolar fluid volume, most likely approximates total lung capacity at peak inspiratory pressure.

The relatively large volume of the first breath produced by the high negative pressure appears to be created largely by the diaphragm, since the thorax is not compressed after exit from the vaginal canal and just before the first breath (91). During a vertex delivery, the diaphragm may first be pushed in a caudal direction by the thoracic squeeze and then pushed in a cephalad direction by the abdominal squeeze (Fig. 2). The high position of the diaphragm should be mechanically advantageous for the generation of the high force necessary for the first breath. Evidence for diaphragmatic motion has been observed by x-ray fluoroscopy (92). Other mechanisms that might enhance the first breath have been proposed, including "frog breathing" (93). It was postulated that increased pharyngeal pressure might stimulate Head's paradoxical reflex, which could result in an inspiratory effort. This reflex could also augment the first inspiration. Head's paradoxical

reflex is produced by stimulation of tracheal stretch receptors and is thought to be mediated through the vagus nerve (94).

The high intrapleural pressure is needed to overcome (a) the extremely low compliance of the lung due to its high water content, (b) increased airway resistance due to obstructing airway liquid, (c) the viscous resistance of the fluid-filled airways, and (d) the high surface tension of the air–liquid interface (95). The resistance due to viscosity should change during the course of the first breath; it will be maximal in the trachea at the beginning of inspiration and will decrease as the air–fluid interface moves toward smaller airways. Subsequent breaths should meet with increasingly lower viscous resistance and a higher compliance as fluid moves out of the airways and alveoli. The volume of the first breath should have an effect on the lung compliance of the next breath, which, in turn, should increase the compliance for the next, and so on, as fluid decreases. Compliance measured over the first few breaths was one-fifth to one-third of that measured in older infants (84,96). The glottis may well close at the beginning of inspiration, leading to the creation of higher transpulmonary pressures (97,98). Serial chest radiographs taken at the time of birth indicate moderately good air inflation within 1 sec of the onset of breathing (92).

The total lung capacity of the full-term human infant at birth is estimated to be approximately 85–90 ml/kg, or ~275 ml in an average infant of 3.2 kg. Several investigators have attempted to measure the volume change occurring with the first breath (88,90,99,100). Although a wide range of values (12–67 ml) was found, there is close agreement on the average volume of approximately 40 ml. For an average-sized infant, this is equivalent to 11 ml/kg compared to the average tidal volume of a newborn of 8 ml/kg.

The First Expiration and Establishment of FRC

The volume of the first expiration is considerably less than that inspired, contributing to the establishment of a residual volume. The larger the volume of the first inspiration, the larger the residual volume. This suggests that the recoil pressure at the end of the first inspiration is inversely proportional to the volume (88,89). The first expiration is accomplished with an extremely high positive pressure. Pressures as high as 124 cmH$_2$O have been recorded, with a mean of 71 cmH$_2$O in vaginally delivered infants (85,89). The respiratory pattern over the first few breaths is irregular. The expiratory pressures remain high, and the duration of the first few expirations is extremely variable (see Fig. 4). A range of 0.11 sec to 16 sec was noted for the first expiration in infants born by cesarean section. The

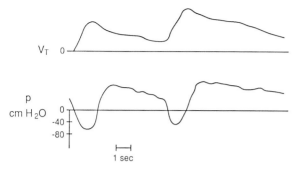

FIG. 4. Volume (*V*) and intrathoracic pressure (*P*) changes occurring during the first two breaths. A large positive pressure occurs during expiration, with the formation of a residual volume. The first several breaths have a prolonged expiratory time.

prolongation and variability implicate an unstable regulation of respiratory rate and depth; perhaps this permissiveness of control is a necessary feature of allowing prolonged expirations with high pressures in order to assist the clearance of lung fluid, the sequential expansion of alveoli, and the lowering of alveolar surface tension. Clearly, the longer the lung is held open, the greater the opportunity for the complex process of forming a surface-active alveolar lining layer. All of these events are critical to the formation of an FRC. The first expiration is longer than subsequent breaths and becomes progressively shorter over the first hour of life, with a mean of 1.86 sec at 30 sec of life and 0.53 sec at 60 min of life (88) (see Fig. 5). How does the infant delay expiration? Adduction of the vocal

cords, resulting in expiratory braking, probably occurs (93,98,101). Vagal afferent traffic carrying pulmonary volume information can activate laryngeal adductor muscles (102). Many full-term infants are noted to have some expiratory grunting during the first minutes of life. Thus glottic narrowing, delayed expiration, and positive pressure should facilitate the progressive increase in the FRC. It is possible that stretch receptors continue to fire throughout expiration, thereby inhibiting or delaying the next inspiration.

FRC Establishment

After the first breath the FRC is only 15% of its eventual size; by 15 min of age it is 40% (88), and by 2 days of age the FRC is approximately 100 ml or 30 ml/kg (103). There is good agreement from a number of studies that residual volume after the first breath is about 15 ml, with considerable variability from 2 to 40 ml (84,88,90,99). There is considerable clinical interest in the effects of cesarean delivery on the first breath. Does the absence of the vaginal squeeze and subsequent thoracic recoil alter the establishment of the FRC and account for the increased respiratory distress experienced by these infants? FRC as well as V_T and V_E are not significantly different after the first breath when cesarean-section infants are compared to those born vaginally (85,88). At 6 hr of age, cesarean-section infants have a lower FRC (104,105); this has been attributed to delayed clearance of lung fluid due to the absence of labor, rather than being attributed to altered mechanical forces at birth (82,83,106).

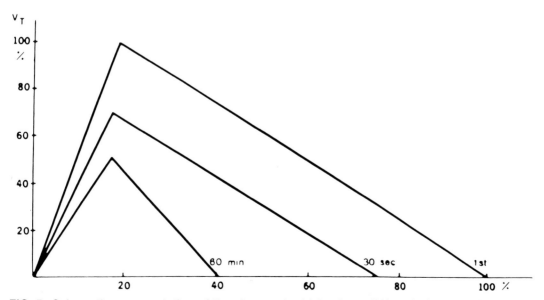

FIG. 5. Schematic representation of the changes in tidal volume (V_T) and of the relationship of inspiratory to expiratory time, for a complete respiratory cycle. The first breath is compared to breaths recorded at 30 sec and 60 min of age. (From ref. 88.)

Air-trapping behind bubbles or foam has been proposed as the mechanism by which air remains in the lung after the first breath (107,108). This interesting hypothesis is supported by stereomicroscopic observations of the first inflation and deflation of near-term fetal rabbit lungs (107,109). Intrapulmonary foam is created by mixing of air and fetal lung liquid that is rich in surfactant. These stable bubbles in small airways may act to maintain the patency of small airways, thereby aiding in the distribution of air distal to the bubble as well as aiding in air-trapping. High expiratory pressures may enhance the production and distribution of bubbles towards the periphery, permitting gas transfer during expiration—perhaps by diffusion of oxygen from within the bubbles (107).

CHANGES IN PULMONARY BLOOD FLOW

So far we have concentrated on changes in respiratory control and the problems of air entry associated with the first breath. Is there sufficient blood flow in the lungs to permit gas exchange with the first breath? A major increase in pulmonary blood flow must occur within minutes of life. The most important function is oxygen extraction from inspired air; however, a secondary function is the removal of fetal lung liquid. Studies in near-term fetal lambs indicate that pulmonary blood flow is less than 10% of cardiac output even though approximately two-thirds of the cardiac output comes from the right ventricle (110,111). Only a small proportion of right ventricular output enters the lungs, as a result of (a) the high pulmonary vascular resistance, (b) the low-resistance flow through the ductus arteriosus, and (c) the low downstream resistance of the umbilical circulation. With the first breath, pulmonary vascular resistance must fall concurrent with a diminution of right to left shunting through the ductus arteriosus.

The mean pulmonary arterial pressure may be as high as 50 torr in the fetus; this is slightly above mean aortic pressure. With the onset of ventilation, pulmonary blood flow will increase from about 50 ml/kg to 400 ml/kg—an approximate eightfold rise (112). It is not known which factors are responsible for the decrease in pulmonary vascular resistance and whether these changes occur after the first breath or after several breaths. Possible mechanisms include the mechanical distension of the lungs and the subsequent increase in P_{O_2}. Ventilation of fetal lungs with a gas, rather than a liquid, without a change in P_{O_2} causes a fall in pulmonary vascular resistance (113,114). This may be due to changes in surface tension which would reduce perivascular tissue pressure (115), although displacement of fetal liquid would more likely increase pressure in the peripheral perivascular spaces. More probably, the mechanical distension might stimulate the release of vasodilator substances.

The mechanical distension of the first breath should therefore have some effect on increasing pulmonary blood flow. The increase in blood flow itself through shear forces may stimulate release of vasodilators from the endothelial cells. As gas exchange improves, the change in $P_{a_{O_2}}$ will also affect pulmonary vascular resistance. An increase in $P_{a_{O_2}}$ has a greater effect on reducing pulmonary vascular resistance than does gaseous ventilation (115–117).

Mediators

There are a number of putative mediators that could account for rapid changes in pulmonary vascular resistance. The low fetal P_{O_2} of < 25 torr may play a role in maintaining pulmonary vasoconstriction in the relatively muscular pulmonary vascular bed. All of the stimuli following the first breath, including mechanical distension, a rise in P_{O_2}, and an increase in blood flow, could act through a common pathway. PGI_2 is a powerful vasodilator produced in the lung. Platelet-activating factor is also a fetal pulmonary vasodilator that is released from a number of cells (118). Bradykinin (117), angiotensin II (119,120), and histamine (121) all have been shown to stimulate PGI_2. The increased pulmonary blood flow results in increased shear forces that could stimulate endothelial cells to produce PGI_2 (122). Much more information is needed on the mechanisms by which these vasoactive mediators are stimulated and released. Suffice it to say, these complex mechanisms are triggered by the first breath.

Other humoral substances such as catecholamines are increased at the time of birth (see above). These could alter pulmonary circulation before the first breath. Beta-adrenergic stimulation decreases pulmonary vascular resistance (113,114), as does acetylcholine infusion (123); however, these effects change postnatally and are probably not important under homeostatic circumstances. It is not known if they are important in the pulmonary circulatory changes associated with the first few breaths.

SUMMARY

The first breath is a seminal respiratory event. Many stimuli appear to interact to trigger it in ways that are incompletely understood. Its vigor and timing are of utmost importance in preventing hypoxic injury to the newborn. The unique aspects of the depth, timing, and pressure of the first breaths, which are somewhat gasping in nature, are in sharp contrast to the preceding pattern of rapid, shallow, and intermittent fetal breathing movements. The first breath is characterized by a large inspiration and an exceedingly long expiration, and it is associated with a high positive intrathoracic pressure. This depends on new muscle functions of the chest wall and diaphragm and also depends on the switch to a new neural control system. The exhaled volume is considerably less than the inhaled volume. As lung liquid is absorbed, a residual volume is established, requiring the rapid formation of a surface-active alveolar lining layer. Blood gases are normalized within an hour of birth (124). A regular, perhaps irreversible, lifelong respiratory pattern is set in place within a few minutes of birth—a remarkable physiological event!

REFERENCES

1. Barcroft J. The onset of respiration at birth. *Lancet* 1942;1:117–120.
2. Alcorn D, Adamson TM, Lambert TF, Maloney JE, Ritchie BC, Robinson PM. Morphological effects of chronic tracheal ligation and drainage in the fetal lamb lung. *J Anat* 1977;123:649–660.
3. Keatinge WR, Nadel JA. Immediate respiratory response to sudden cooling of the skin. *J Appl Physiol* 1965;20:65–69.
4. Scarpelli EM, Condorelli S, Cosmi EV. Cutaneous stimulation and generation of breathing in the fetus. *Pediatr Res* 1977;11:24–28.
5. Condorelli S, Scarpelli E. Somatic-respiratory reflex and onset of regular breathing movements in the lamb fetus *in-utero*. *Pediatr Res* 1975;9:879–894.
6. Chapman RLK, Dawes GS, Rurak DW, Wilds PL. Foetal breathing and nerve stimulation *in-utero*. *J Physiol* 1977;272:13–14.
7. Harned HS, Ferreiro J. Initiation of breathing by cold stimulation: effects of change in ambient temperature on respiratory activity of the full-term fetal lamb. *J Pediatr* 1973;83:663–669.
8. Merlet C, Leanchi J, Rey P, Tchoubroutsky C. Action du refroidissement localisé dans le déclenchement de la respiration chez l'agneau à la noissance. *J Physiol (Paris)* 1967;59:457–458.
9. Woodrum DE, Parer JT, Wennberg RP, Hodson WA. Chemoreceptor response in initiation of breathing in the fetal lamb. *J Appl Physiol* 1972;33(1):120–125.
10. Blanco CE, Dawes GS, Hanson MA, McCooke HB. The response to hypoxia of arterial chemoreceptors in fetal sheep and newborn lambs. *J Physiol* 1984;351:25–37.
11. Jansen AH, Ioffe S, Russel BJ, Chernick V. Effect of carotid chemoreceptor denervation on breathing *in utero* and after birth. *J Appl Physiol* 1981;51:630–633.
12. Harned HS, Griffin CA, Bernyhill WS, MacKinney LG, Sugioka K. Role of carotid chemoreceptors in the initiation of effective breathing of the lamb at term. *Pediatrics* 1967;39:329–336.
13. Chernick V, Faridy EE, Pagtakhan RD. Role of the peripheral and central chemoreceptors in the initiation of fetal respiration. *J Appl Physiol* 1975;38:407–410.
14. Woodrum DE, Standaert TA, Parks CR, Belenky D, Murphy J, Hodson WA. Ventilatory response in the fetal lamb following peripheral chemodenervation. *J Appl Physiol* 1977;42:630–635.
15. Blanco CE, Hanson MA, McCooke HB, Williams BA. Studies of chemoreceptor resetting after hyperoxic ventilation of the fetus *in utero*. In: Ribero JA, Pallot DJ, eds. *Chemoreceptors in respiratory control*. Kent, England: Croom Helm, 1987;369–376.
16. Bystrzycka E, Nail BS, Purves MJ. Central and peripheral neural respiratory activity in the mature sheep foetus and newborn lamb. *Respir Physiol* 1975;25:199–215.
17. Biscoe TJ, Purves MJ, Sampson SR. Types of nervous activity which may be recorded from the carotid sinus nerve in the sheep. *J Physiol* 1969;202:1–23.
18. Biscoe TJ, Purves MJ, Sampson SR. Types of nervous activity which may be recorded from the carotid sinus nerve in the sheep fetus. *J Appl Physiol* 1971;30:382–387.
19. Pagtakhan RD, Faridy EE, Chernick V. Interaction between arterial P_{CO_2} and P_{O_2} in the initiation of respiration of fetal sheep. *J Appl Physiol* 1971;30:382–387.
20. Biscoe TJ, Purves MJ. Cervical sympathetic and chemoreceptor activity before and after the first breath of the newborn lamb. *J Physiol* 1965;181:70P.
21. Jansen AH, Purves MJ, Tan ED. The role of sympathetic nerves in the activation of the carotid body chemoreceptors at birth in the sheep. *J Devel Physiol* 1980;2:305–321.
22. Belenky DA, Standaert TA, Woodrum DE. Maturation of hypoxic ventilatory response of the newborn lamb. *J Appl Physiol* 1979;47:927–930.
23. Hertzberg T, Lagercrantz H. Postnatal sensitivity of the peripheral chemoreceptors in newborn infants. *Arch Dis Child* 1987;62:1238–1241.
24. Cross KW, Warner P. The effect of inhalation of high and low oxygen concentrations on the respiration of the new-born infant. *J Physiol* 1951;114:283–295.
25. Edelman NH, Lahiri S, Braudo L, Cherniack NS, Fishman AP. The blunted ventilatory response to hypoxia in cyanotic congenital heart disease. *N Engl J Med* 1970;202:405–411.
26. Sorensen SC, Severinghaus JW. Respiratory insensitivity to acute hypoxia persisting after correction of tetralogy of Fallot. *J Appl Physiol* 1968;25:221–223.
27. Sorensen SC, Severinghaus JW. Irreversible respiratory insensitivity to acute hypoxia in man born at high altitude. *J Appl Physiol* 1968;25:217–220.
28. Lahiri S, Brody JS, Motoyama EK, Velasquez TM. Regulation of breathing in newborns at high altitude. *J Appl Physiol* 1978;44:673–678.
29. Eden GJ, Hanson MA. Effects of chronic hypoxia on chemoreceptor function in the newborn. In: Ribero JA, Pallot DJ, eds. *Chemoreceptors in respiratory control*. Kent, England: Croom Helm, 1987;369–376.
30. Boyd JD. The development of the human carotid body. *Contrib Embryol Carnegie Inst* 1937;26:1–31.
31. Rogers DC. The development of the rat carotid body. *J Anat* 1965;99:89–101.
32. Hervonen A, Kanerva L, Korkala O, Partanen S. Effects of hypoxia and glucocorticoids on the histochemically demonstrable catecholamines of the newborn rat carotid body. *Acta Physiol Scand* 1972;86:109–114.
33. Mayock DE, Standaert TA, Guthrie RD, Woodrum DE. Dopamine and carotid body function in the newborn lamb. *J Appl Physiol* 1983;54(3):814–820.
34. Korkala O, Hervonen A. Origin and development of the catecholamine-storing cells of the human fetal carotid body. *Histochemie* 1973;37:287–297.
35. Lopez-Barnes J, Lopez-Lopez JR, Urena J, Gonzalez C. Chemotransduction in the carotid body: K^+ current modulated by P_{O_2} in type I chemoreceptor cells. *Science* 1989;241:580–582.
36. Herrington RT, Harnes HS, Ferreiro JI, Griffin CA. The role of the central nervous system in perinatal respiration: studies of chemoregulatory mechanisms in the term lamb. *Pediatrics* 1971;47(5):857–864.
37. Jansen AH, Chernick V. Site of central chemosensitivity in fetal sheep. *J Appl Physiol* 1975;39:1–6.
38. Maloney JE, Adamson TM, Brodecky Y, et al. Modification of respiratory center output in the unanesthetized fetal sheep. *J Appl Physiol* 1975;39:552–558.
39. Bissonnette JM, Hohimer RA, Richardson BS. Ventricular–cisternal cerebrospinal perfusion in unanesthetized fetal lambs. *J Appl Physiol* 1981;50:880–883.
40. Gluckman PD, Johnston BM. Lesions in the upper lateral pons abolish the depression of breathing in unanaesthetized fetal lambs *in-utero*. *J Physiol (Lond)* 1987;382:373–383.
41. Dawes GS, Gardner WN, Johnston BM, Walker DW. Breath-

ing in fetal lambs: the effect of brain stem section. *J Physiol* 1983;335:535–553.

42. Bamford O. Central control mechanisms in fetal breathing. In: Lipshitz J, Maloney J, Nimrod C, Carson G, eds. *Perinatal development of the heart and lung.* Ithaca, NY: Perinatology Press, 1987;233–252.

43. Boddy K, Dawes GS, Fisher K, Pinter S, Robinson JS. Foetal respiratory movements, electrocortical and cardiovascular responses to hypoxemia and hypercapnia in sheep. *J Physiol (Lond)* 1975;39:199–204.

44. Johnston BM, Gluckman PD. Lateral pontine lesions affect central chemosensitivity in unanesthetized fetal lambs. *J Appl Physiol* 1989;67(3):1113–1118.

45. Jansen AH, Chernick V. Respiratory response to central cyanide in fetal sheep after peripheral chemodenervation. *J Appl Physiol* 1974;36:1–5.

46. Jansen AH, Chernick V. Site of central chemosensitivity in fetal sheep. *J Appl Physiol* 1975;39:1–6.

47. Jansen AH, Chernick V. Cardiorespiratory response to central cyanide in fetal sheep. *J Appl Physiol* 1974;37:18–21.

48. Jansen AH, Russel BJ, Chernick V. Respiratory effects of H^+ and dimitrophenol injections into the brain stem subarachnoid space of fetal lambs. *Can J Physiol Pharmacol* 1975;53:733–762.

49. Hodson WA, Fenner A, Brumley G, Chernick V, Avery ME. Cerebrospinal fluid and blood acid base relationships in fetal and neonatal lambs and pregnant ewes. *Respir Physiol* 1968;4:322–332.

50. Hohimer AR, Bissonnette JM, Richardson BS, Machida CM. Central chemical regulation of breathing movements in fetal lambs. *Respir Physiol* 1983;52:99–111.

51. Mitchell RA. Respiratory chemosensitivity in the medulla oblongata. *J Physiol (Lond)* 1969;202:3p–4p.

52. Levine S. Nonperipheral chemoreceptor stimulation of ventilation by cyanide. *J Appl Physiol* 1975;39:199–204.

53. Henderson-Smart DJ, Cohen GL. Chemical control of breathing in early life. *Ann NY Acad Sci* 1988;533:276–288.

54. Kitterman JA, Liggins GC, Ballard PL, Clements JA, Tooley WH. Stimulation of fetal breathing movements in lambs by inhibitors of prostaglandin synthesis. *J Dev Physiol Oxf* 1979;1:453–466.

55. Kitterman JA, Liggins GC, Fewell JE, Tooley WH. Inhibition of breathing movements in fetal sheep by prostaglandins. *J Appl Physiol* 1983;54:687–692.

56. Wallen LD, Murai DT, Clyman RI, Lee CH, Mauray FE, Kitterman JA. Regulation of breathing movements in fetal sheep by prostaglandin E_2. *J Appl Physiol* 1986;60(2):526–531.

57. Kitterman JA. Arachidonic acid metabolites and control of breathing in the fetus and newborn. *Semin Perinatol* 1987; 11:43–52.

58. Wallen LD, Murai DT, Clyman RI, Lee CH, Mauray FE, Kitterman JA. Effects of meclofenamate on breathing movements in fetal sheep before delivery. *J Appl Physiol* 1988;64(2):759–766.

59. Patrick J, Challis JRG, Cross J, Olson DM, Lye SJ, Turliuk R. The relationship between fetal breathing movements and prostaglandin E_2 during ACTH-induced labor in sheep. *J Dev Physiol Oxf* 1987;9:287–293.

60. Hohimer AR, Richardson BS, Bissonnette JM, Machida CM. The effect of indomethacin on breathing movements and cerebral blood flow and metabolism in the fetal sheep. *J Dev Physiol Oxf* 1985;7:217–228.

61. Kitterman JA, Liggins GC, Fewell JE, Tooley WH. Inhibition of breathing movements in fetal sheep by prostaglandins. *J Appl Physiol* 1983;54:687–692.

62. Murai DT, Wallen LD, Chu-Ching HL, Clyman RI, Mauray F, Kitterman JA. Effects of prostaglandins on fetal breathing do not involve peripheral chemoreceptors. *J Appl Physiol* 1987; 62(1):271–277.

63. Koos BJ. Central stimulation of breathing movements in fetal lambs by prostaglandin synthetase inhibitors. *J Physiol* 1985;362:455–466.

64. Challis JRG, Dilley SR, Robinson JS, Thorburn GD. Prosta-

glandins in the circulation of the fetal lamb. *Prostaglandins* 1976;11:1041–1049.

65. Gluckman PD, Bennet L. Neuropharmacology of fetal and neonatal breathing. In: Johnston BM, Gluckman PD, eds. *Respiratory control and lung development in the fetus and newborn.* Ithaca, NY: Perinatology Press, 1986;249–277.

66. Santiago TV, Edelman NH. Opioids and breathing. *J Appl Physiol* 1985;59(6):1675–1685.

67. Lagercrantz H, Bistoletti P. Catecholamine release in the newborn infant at birth. *Pediatr Res* 1973;11:889–893.

68. Martinez AM, Padbury JF, Burnell EE, Thio SL, Hume J. The effects of hypoxia on (methionine) enkephalin peptide and catecholamine release in fetal sheep. *Pediatr Res* 1990;27:52–55.

69. Olsen GD, Hohimer AR, Mathis MD. Cerebral blood flow and metabolism during morphine-induced stimulation of breathing movements in fetal lambs. *Life Sci* 1983;33:751–754.

70. Sheldon RE, Toubas PL. Morphine stimulates rapid, regular, deep and sustained breathing efforts in fetal lambs. *J Appl Physiol* 1984;57(1):40–43.

71. Moss IR, Scarpelli EM. CO_2 and naloxone modify sleep/wake state and activate breathing in the acute fetal lamb preparation. *Respir Physiol* 1984;55:325–340.

72. Hasan SU, Lee DS, Gibson DA, Nowaczyk BJ, Cates DB, Sitar DS, Pinsky C, Rigatto H. Effect of morphine on breathing and behavior in fetal sheep. *J Appl Physiol* 1988;64(5):2058–2065.

73. Grunstein MM, Hazinski TA, Schlueter AM. Respiratory control during hypoxia in newborn rabbits: implied action of endorphins. *J Appl Physiol* 1981;81:122–130.

74. Grunstein MM, Grunstein JS. Maturational effect of enkephalin on respiratory control in newborn rabbits. *J Appl Physiol* 1982;53:1063–1070.

75. Chernick V, Modansky DL, Lawson EE. Naloxone decreases the duration of primary apnea with neonatal asphyxia. *Pediatr Res* 1980;14:357–359.

76. Chernick V, Craig RJ. Naloxone reverses neonatal depression caused by fetal asphyxia. *Science* 1982;216:1252–1253.

77. Jansen AH, Chernick V. Development of respiratory control. *Physiol Rev* 1983;63:437–483.

78. Wardlaw SL, Stark RI, Barc L, Frantz AG. Plasma β-endorphin and β-lipoprotein in the human fetus at delivery: correlation with arterial pH and P_{O_2}. *J Clin Endocrinol Metab* 1979;49:888–891.

79. Moss IR, Conner H, Yee WFH, Iorio P, Scarpelli EM. Human β-endorphin-like immunoreactivity in the perinatal/neonatal period. *J Pediatr* 1982;101:443–446.

80. Long WA, Lawson EE. Developmental aspects of the effect of naloxone on control of breathing in piglets. *Respir Physiol* 1983;51:119–129.

81. Baier RJ, Hasan SU, Cates DB, Hooper DH, Nowaczyk B, Rigatto H. Effect of various concentrations of oxygen and umbilical cord occlusion on fetal breathing and behavior in sheep. *Pediatr Res* 1989;25:301A.

82. Bland RD, Hansen TN, Haberkern CM, Bressack MA, Hazinski TA, Raj JU, Goldberg RG. Lung fluid balance in lambs before and after birth. *J Appl Physiol* 1982;53:992–1004.

83. Bland RD. Lung fluid balance before and after birth. In: Johnston BM, Gluckman PD, eds. *Respiratory control and lung development in the fetus and newborn.* Ithaca, NY: Perinatology Press, 1986;161–205.

84. Karlberg P, Cherry RB, Escardo FE, et al. Respiratory studies in newborn infants. II. Pulmonary ventilation and mechanics of breathing in the first minutes of life, including the onset of respiration. *Acta Paediatr* 1962;51:121–136.

85. Vyas H, Milner AD, Hopkin IE. Intrathoracic pressure and volume changes during the spontaneous onset of respiration in babies born by cesarian section and by vaginal delivery. *J Pediatr* 1981;99:787–791.

86. Milner AD, Saunders RA. Pressure and volume changes during the first breath of human neonates. *Arch Dis Child* 1977;52:918–924.

87. Fawcitt J, Lind J, Wegelius C. The first breath. A preliminary communication describing some methods of investigation of the

first breath of a baby and the results obtained from them. *Acta Pediatr* 1960;49(Suppl 123):5–17.

88. Mortola JP, Fisher JT, Smith JB, Fox GS, Week S, Willis D. Onset of respiration in infants delivered by cesarean section. *J Appl Physiol* 1982;52(3):716–724.

89. Vyas H, Field D, Milner AD, Hopkin IE. Determinants of the first inspiratory volume and functional residual capacity at birth. *Pediatr Pulmonol* 1986;2:189–193.

90. Saunders RA, Milner AD. Pulmonary pressure/volume relationships during the last phase of delivery and the first postnatal breaths in human subjects. *J Pediatr* 1978;93:667–673.

91. Borrel U, Fernström I. The shape of the foetal chest during its passage through the birth canal. A radiographic study. *Acta Obstet Gynecol Scand* 1962;41:213–222.

92. Guebelle F, Karlberg P, Koch G, et al. L'aeration du poumon chez le nouveau-ne. *Biol Neonate* 1959;1:169–210.

93. Bosma JF, Lind J, Gentz N. Motions of the pharynx associated with initial aeration of the lungs of the newborn infant. *Acta Pediatr* 1959;48(Suppl 117):117–122.

94. Cross KW. Head's paradoxical reflex. *Brain* 1961;84:529–534.

95. Agostoni E, Taglietti A, Agostoni AF, et al. Mechanical aspects of the first breath. *J Appl Physiol* 1958;13:344–348.

96. McIlroy MB, Tomlinson ES. The mechanics of breathing in newly born babies. *Thorax* 1955;10:58–61.

97. Harding R, Bocking AD, Sigger JN, Wickham PJD. Laryngeal resistance and lung liquid flow in relation to breathing activity in fetal sheep. In: Jones CT, Nathianielz PW, eds. *Physiological development of fetus and newborn*. New York: Academic Press, 1985;247–251.

98. Harding R. The upper respiratory tract in perinatal life. In: Johnston BM, Gluckman PD, eds. *Reproductive and perinatal medicine. Respiratory control and lung development in the fetus and newborn*, vol III. Ithaca, NY: Perinatology Press, 1986;331–376.

99. Karlberg P. The adaptive changes in the immediate postnatal period, with particular reference to respiration. *J Pediatr* 1960;56:585–604.

100. Karlberg P, Adams FH, Guebelle F, Wallgren G. Alterations of the infant's thorax during vaginal delivery. Physiologic studies. *Acta Obstet Gynecol Scand* 1962;41:223–229.

101. Fisher JT, Mortola JP, Smith JB, Fox GS, Week S. Respiration in newborns: development of the control of breathing. *Am Rev Respir Dis* 1982;125:650–657.

102. Harding R. State-related and developmental changes in laryngeal function. *Sleep* 1980;3:307–322.

103. Polgar G, Weng TR. The functional development of the respiratory system. *Am Rev Respir Dis* 1979;120:625–695.

104. Boon AW, Milner AD, Hopkin IE. Lung volumes and lung mechanics in babies born vaginally and by elective and emergency lower segmental caesarian section. *J Pediatr* 1979;95:1031–1036.

105. Milner AD, Saunders RA, Hopkin IE. Effects of delivery by caesarean section on lung mechanics and lung volume in the human neonate. *Arch Dis Child* 1978;53:545–548.

106. Brown MJ, Olver RE, Ramsden CA, Strang LB, Walters DV. Effects of adrenaline and spontaneous labour on the secretion and absorption of lung liquid in the foetal lamb. *J Physiol (Lond)* 1983;344:137–152.

107. Scarpelli EM. Intrapulmonary foam at birth: an adaptational phenomenon. *Pediatr Res* 1978;12:1070–1076.

108. Grossman G, Robertson B. Lung expansion and the formation of the alveolar lining layer in the full-term newborn rabbit. *Acta Pediatr Scand* 1975;64:7–16.

109. Scarpelli EM. Perinatal lung mechanics and the first breath. *Lung* 1984;162:61–71.

110. Rudolph AM, Heymann MA. Circulatory changes during growth in the fetal lamb. *Circ Res* 1970;26:289–299.

111. Rudolph AM, Heymann MA. The circulation of the fetus *in utero*: methods for studying distribution of blood flow, cardiac output and organ blood flow. *Circ Res* 1967;21:163–184.

112. Rudolph AM. Fetal and neonatal pulmonary circulation. *Ann Rev Physiol* 1979;41:383–395.

113. Cassin S, Dawes GS, Ross BB. Pulmonary blood flow and vascular resistance in immature foetal lambs. *J Physiol (Lond)* 1964;171:80–89.

114. Smith RW, Morris JA, Assali NS. Effects of chemical mediators on the pulmonary and ductus arteriosus circulation in the fetal lamb. *Am J Obstet Gynecol* 1964;89:252–260.

115. Cassin S, Dawes GS, Mott JC, Ross BB, Strang LB. The vascular resistance of the foetal and newly ventilated lung of the lamb. *J Physiol (Lond)* 1964;171:61–79.

116. Assali NS, Kirschbaum TM, Dilts PV Jr. Effects of hyperbaric oxygen on uteroplacental and fetal circulation. *Circ Res* 1968;22:573–588.

117. Heymann MA, Rudolph AM, Nies AS, Melmon KL. Bradykinin production associated with oxygenation of the fetal lamb. *Circ Res* 1969;25:521–534.

118. Accurso F, Abman S, Wilkening RB, Worthen S, Henson PM. Exogenous PAF produces pulmonary vasodilation in the ovine fetus [Abstract]. *Am Rev Respir Dis* 1986;133:11.

119. Dusting AJ. Angiotensin-induced release of a prostacyclin-like substance from the lungs. *J Cardiovasc Pharmacol* 1981;3:197–206.

120. Omini C, Vigano T, Marini A, Pasargiklian R, Fano M, Maselli MA. Angiotensin II: a releaser of PGI_2 from fetal and newborn rabbit lungs. *Prostaglandins* 1983;25:901–910.

121. McIntyre TM, Zimmerman GA, Satoh K, Prescott SM. Cultured endothelial cells synthesize both platelet-activating factor and prostacyclin in response to histamine, bradykinin, and adenosine triphosphate. *J Clin Invest* 1985;76:271–280.

122. Voelkel NF, Chang SW, Pfeffer KD, Worthen SG, McMurtry IF, Henson PM. PAF antagonists: different effects on platelets, neutrophils, guinea pig ileum and PAF-induced vasodilation in isolated rat lung. *Prostaglandins* 1986;32:359–372.

123. Lewis AB, Heymann MA, Rudolph AM. Gestational changes in pulmonary vascular responses in fetal lambs in utero. *Circ Res* 1976;39:536–541.

124. Oliver TK Jr, Demis JA, Bates GD. Serial blood gas tensions and acid–base balance during the first hours of life in human infants. *Acta Paediatr (Stockh)* 1961;50:346–360.

THE LUNG: Scientific Foundations
edited by R.G. Crystal, J.B. West et al.
Raven Press, Ltd., New York © 1991.

CHAPTER 6.1.3

Fetal Lung Liquid and Its Removal Near Birth

Richard D. Bland

Fetal lungs are secretory organs that make breathing-like movements but that serve no respiratory function. They receive less than 10% of the heart's combined ventricular output of blood (1), which, in fetal sheep, supplies sufficient substrate for lung epithelial cells to produce surface-active material and secrete up to 500 ml/day of liquid during the latter part of gestation (2). This liquid flows from terminal respiratory units through conductive airways into the oropharynx, from which it is either swallowed or expelled into the amniotic sac. The balance between production and drainage of luminal liquid has an important effect on lung development before birth: Prolonged outflow obstruction expands the lungs and leads to a decrease in the number of surfactant-producing (type II) cells; continuous and unimpeded removal of luminal liquid decreases lung size, increases apparent tissue density and capillary volume, and stimulates proliferation of type II cells (3).

Rapid removal of liquid from potential air spaces during and soon after birth is a critical event in the timely switch from placental to pulmonary gas exchange. For many years it was thought that mechanical compression of the chest during birth was responsible for squeezing out most of the lung liquid through the mouth, thereby facilitating inflation with air. During the past decade, however, several investigators have presented evidence that the normal transition from liquid to air inflation is considerably more complex than the characteristic oral gush at delivery might suggest. This chapter will review the experimental work that provides the basis for our current understanding of lung liquid clearance near birth, emphasizing the various pathways and mechanisms by which this process occurs.

FORMATION OF LUMINAL LIQUID IN THE FETAL LUNG

In 1923 Fauré-Fremiet and Dragiou (4) reported that the lungs of fetal lambs are filled with liquid, but the source of that liquid was uncertain until 25 years later, when Jost and Policard (5) discovered that ligating the trachea of fetal rabbits caused their lungs to become distended with liquid, implying that the liquid came from within the lungs and was not aspirated from the amniotic sac, as others had suggested (6). Adams et al. (7) showed that the composition of liquid obtained from the trachea of fetal lambs differed considerably from that of plasma and of amniotic liquid sampled from the same animals. These and other investigators found that lung luminal liquid from fetal sheep is rich in chloride, poor in bicarbonate, and almost free of protein (2,7,8) (Table 1). The potassium concentration of luminal liquid is greater than that of plasma and increases toward the end of gestation, when the lung epithelium releases surfactant into potential air spaces (2). A recent report indicates that the composition of lung liquid in fetal dogs is similar to that of fetal lambs, except that the bicarbonate concentration of canine luminal liquid is not significantly different from that of plasma (9).

Figure 1 shows schematically the liquid compartments of the fetal lung: the microcirculation; the interstitium, which is drained by pulmonary lymphatics that empty into the systemic venous system; and potential air spaces. Strang and co-workers (10–13) did extensive studies of water and solute movement across the endothelium and epithelium of the developing lung. They sampled liquid from the trachea, lung lymphatics, and bloodstream of fetal sheep and traced the movement of radiolabeled solutes between the three liquid compartments. These and subsequent studies showed that the pulmonary epithelium forms a tight barrier to macromolecules (12–15), whereas the vascular endo-

R. D. Bland: Department of Pediatrics, Children's Research Center, University of Utah School of Medicine, Salt Lake City, Utah 84132.

TABLE 1. *Composition of lung luminal liquid, lymph, plasma, and amniotic liquid of fetal lambs late in gestation[a]*

Substance	Sodium (mEq/liter)	Potassium (mEq/liter)	Chloride (mEq/liter)	Bicarbonate (mEq/liter)	pH	Total protein (g/dl)
Luminal liquid	150 ± 1	6.3 ± 0.7	157 ± 4	2.8 ± 0.3	6.27 ± 0.01	0.03 ± 0.002
Lung lymph	147 ± 1	4.8 ± 0.5	107 ± 1	25 ± 1	7.31 ± 0.02	3.27 ± 0.41
Plasma	150 ± 1	4.8 ± 0.2	107 ± 1	24 ± 1	7.34 ± 0.04	4.09 ± 0.26
Amniotic liquid	113 ± 7	7.6 ± 0.8	87 ± 5	19 ± 3	7.02 ± 0.09	0.10 ± 0.01

[a] Values are mean ± SEM and are taken from the work of Adamson et al. (8) and Humphreys et al. (10).

thelium has wider openings that allow passage of even large proteins (11,13). Thus, the protein concentration of liquid in the interstitial space, collected as lung lymph, is about 100 times greater than the protein concentration of liquid obtained from the fetal trachea. Despite this large transepithelial protein difference, active transport of chloride ion across the fetal pulmonary epithelium generates an electrical potential difference and causes liquid to flow from the lung microcirculation through the interstitium into potential air spaces (16). As early as mid-gestation, the pulmonary epithelium actively transports chloride in the direction of the lung lumen (14,15). Cassin et al. (17) found that this secretory process can be inhibited by diuretics that block sodium-coupled and potassium-coupled chloride transport. Using a direct micropuncture technique to measure alveolar liquid chloride concentration in lambs before and after birth, Nielson (18) observed that the large chloride gradient between lung luminal liquid and plasma decreases rapidly with the onset of air breathing. The specific site of the fetal "chloride pump" and the forces that regulate the activity of this pump remain unclear.

The volume of liquid in potential air spaces of fetal lambs increases from 4–6 ml/kg body weight at mid-gestation (15) to more than 20 ml/kg near term (10,12,13). The hourly flow rate of tracheal liquid increases from about 2 ml/kg body weight at mid-gestation (15) to about 5 ml/kg at term (2,19,20). This increased production of luminal liquid during development probably reflects an increase in pulmonary microvascular and epithelial surface area that is associated with proliferation and growth of lung capillaries and respiratory units (15,21). The observation that unilateral pulmonary artery occlusion reduces tracheal liquid production in fetal lambs by at least 50% (22) indicates that the pulmonary circulation, rather than the bronchial circulation, is the major source of this liquid. Intravenous infusion of saline solution at a rate sufficient to increase lung microvascular pressure and lung lymph flow in fetal lambs has no effect on the flow of liquid across the pulmonary epithelium (16,23). Thus, transepithelial chloride secretion appears to be the major driving force responsible for the production of luminal liquid in the fetal lung.

In vivo studies, such as those described above, cannot distinguish between distal lung epithelium and airway epithelium with respect to their bioelectric and ion transport properties. At least three groups of investigators have done *in vitro* experiments to help clar-

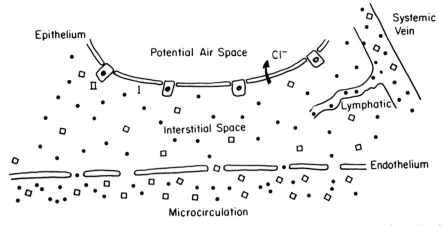

FIG. 1. Schematic diagram of the fluid compartments of the fetal lung, showing the tight epithelial barrier to protein and the more permeable microvascular endothelium which restricts passage of globulins (□) more than it restricts albumin (●). In the mammalian fetus, epithelial chloride secretion provides the driving force for the flow of liquid into the lung lumen. (From ref. 72.)

ify this issue. In studies of excised trachea from fetal and adult sheep, Cotton et al. (24) found that the electrical potential difference across adult airway epithelium was greater (lumen more negative) than it was across fetal epithelium under both open-circuit and short-circuit conditions. Their results indicated that the fetal trachea secretes chloride, whereas the adult trachea absorbs sodium. In studies from another laboratory, however, sodium absorption exceeded chloride secretion in tracheas from both fetal and adult sheep (25). It is unclear why these two laboratories obtained different results using similar techniques and tissues from the same species. Both groups found that isoproterenol stimulated chloride secretion in fetal trachea. Recently, Cotton et al. (9,26) observed chloride secretion, under both open-circuit and short-circuit conditions, in tracheal and bronchial segments taken from fetal dogs. In related studies, Zeitlin et al. (27) measured the bioelectric properties of cultured monolayers of tracheal epithelial cells obtained from fetal and adult rabbits. Their results were consistent with the notion that the fetal airway epithelium secretes chloride. Krochmal et al. (28) demonstrated that cultured cysts of alveolar and tracheal tissue from fetal rats produced luminal liquid that had a higher chloride concentration than that of the external bathing solution. Taken together, these studies provide strong evidence that both proximal and distal portions of the fetal respiratory tract epithelium secrete chloride, which drives liquid toward the lung lumen. Most of this liquid must form in the distal lung, where the total surface area is many times greater than that of the conducting airways.

DECREASE IN LUNG LIQUID BEFORE BIRTH

Several studies have shown that both the rate of liquid formation and the volume within the lumen of the fetal lung normally decrease before birth. Kitterman et al. (20) found that lung liquid secretion in fetal lambs progressively decreases during the 2 days before spontaneous vaginal delivery. Dickson et al. (29) confirmed this observation and showed that the volume of liquid in the lung lumen begins to diminish before the onset of labor in lambs. Brown et al. (30) reported that luminal liquid in fetal sheep may be absorbed rapidly late in labor, a finding that they attributed to a surge in plasma epinephrine concentrations.

In studies performed with fetal rabbits, Bland (31) observed that lung water content was about 25% greater after preterm delivery (28 days gestation) than it was at term (31 days gestation). In related studies, term rabbits that were born either vaginally or by cesarean section following labor had less water in their lungs than did rabbits that were delivered operatively without prior labor (32) (Table 2). Pups that experienced labor also had higher concentrations of protein in their plasma than did pups delivered without labor. Because increased intravascular protein osmotic pressure facilitates absorption of water into the pulmonary circulation, this antenatal increase in plasma protein concentration may contribute to the decrease in fetal lung liquid volume that occurs before birth.

In similar studies done with lambs, the influence of labor on lung water content was even more striking than it was in rabbits (33) (Table 3). Extravascular lung water was 45% less in lambs killed during labor than it was in lambs that had no labor, and there was a further 38% reduction in extravascular lung water measured in lambs that were studied 6 hr after birth. Morphometric analysis of sections of frozen lung obtained from fetal lambs, with and without prior labor, showed that the reduction in lung water content which occurs before birth is the result of a decrease in the volume of liquid in potential air spaces relative to the volume in the interstitium. Collectively, these results indicate that reduced secretion, and perhaps absorption, of luminal liquid before birth leads to about a 15-ml/kg decrease in lung water, leaving a residual volume of approximately 6 ml/kg that must be removed from potential air spaces soon after birth to permit effective pulmonary gas exchange.

It is unknown what causes this reduction in fetal lung liquid secretion before birth, but several studies indi-

TABLE 2. *Effects of gestational age, labor, and type of delivery on lung water content of fetal rabbits*[a]

Gestation days	Number of rabbits	Type of delivery	Labor	Body weight (g)	Plasma protein concentration (g/dl)	Lung water
						Dry lung tissue (g/g)
28 (0.9 term)	16	Operative	−	37 ± 1	3.8 ± 0.1	9.7 ± 0.4
31 (term)	15	Operative	−	51 ± 1[b]	3.9 ± 0.1	8.0 ± 0.4[b]
31 (term)	15	Operative	+	54 ± 3[b]	4.5 ± 0.1[b,c]	6.8 ± 0.2[b,c]
31 (term)	17	Vaginal	+	49 ± 2[b]	4.3 ± 0.1[b,c]	7.1 ± 0.2[b,c]

[a] Values are mean ± SEM and are taken from the work of Bland et al. (31,32).
[b] Significant difference between fetuses born at term and those born prematurely (p < 0.05).
[c] Signficant difference between fetuses born at term following labor and those born without prior labor (p < 0.05).

TABLE 3. *Data from studies of lung water content in fetal and newborn lambs[a]*

Status	Gestation days	Body weight (kg)	Plasma protein concentration (g/dl)	Dry lung weight (g)	Extravascular lung water
					Dry lung tissue (g/g)
Fetuses without labor (n = 10)	138 ± 2	3.3 ± 0.4	3.9 ± 0.1	9.8 ± 1.2	12.3 ± 0.8
Fetuses in labor (n = 9)	139 ± 2	3.3 ± 0.3	4.3 ± 0.1[b]	8.6 ± 0.9	6.8 ± 0.4[b]
Newborns 6 hr after birth (n = 5)	139 ± 3	2.7 ± 0.1	4.7 ± 0.2[b]	8.8 ± 1.3	4.3 ± 0.2[b]

[a] Values are mean ± SEM.
[b] Significantly different from values for fetuses that did not have labor ($p < 0.05$).

cate that hormonal changes, which occur in the fetus just before and during labor, may have an important role in triggering this adaptive process. Several investigators have examined the influence of catecholamines on fetal lung liquid volume. Enhorning et al. (34) showed that injection of β-adrenergic agonists into pregnant rabbits reduced the amount of water in the lungs of their pups. In studies performed with fetal lambs late in gestation, Walters and Olver (35) found that intravenous infusion of epinephrine or isoproterenol, but not norepinephrine, caused reabsorption of liquid from potential air spaces, an effect that β-adrenergic blockade with propranolol prevented. Lawson et al. (36) confirmed the inhibitory effect of epinephrine on secretion of fetal lung liquid and also found that epinephrine increased the concentration of surface-active material in lung liquid. Olver et al. (37) showed that intraluminal administration of amiloride, a sodium transport inhibitor, blocked the effect of epinephrine on fetal lung liquid absorption. This finding suggests that β-adrenergic agonists stimulate sodium uptake by the lung epithelium, which, in turn, drives liquid from the lung lumen into the interstitium, where it can be absorbed into the bloodstream.

Recent studies showed that tracheal instillation of dibuteryl cyclic 3',5'-adenosine monophosphate (db-cAMP) also causes absorption of lung liquid in fetal lambs late in gestation (38,39). The inhibitory effect of both intrapulmonary db-cAMP and intravenous epinephrine on net production of lung luminal liquid increases with advancing gestational age, and both responses are attenuated by prior removal of the thyroid gland (38).

Other hormones that are secreted around the time of birth also may influence net production of lung luminal liquid. Perks and Cassin (40) reported that intravenous infusion of arginine vasopressin reduced lung liquid secretion and in some cases caused reabsorption of liquid from potential air spaces of fetal goats. The magnitude of the response to vasopressin

appears to be less in fetal sheep (41,42). Kitterman (43) reported that intravenous infusion of prostaglandin E₂ reduced tracheal liquid production in fetal lambs. Recent studies indicate that neither β-adrenergic blockade with propranolol nor inhibition of PGE₂ synthesis with meclofenamate prevents the reduction in lung liquid secretion that occurs prior to birth in fetal lambs (44,45). McDonald et al. (46) showed that blockade of β-adrenergic receptors in fetal rabbits does not prevent the normal reduction in lung water that occurs during labor. Thus, the precise role of catecholamines, prostaglandins, and other hormones in regulating lung liquid secretion before, during, and after birth remains to be determined.

POSTNATAL CLEARANCE OF FETAL LUNG LIQUID

Removal of liquid from the lungs continues for several hours after birth. Studies done with fetal and newborn rabbits showed that pulmonary blood volume increases with the onset of breathing, whereas lung water content does not begin to decrease postnatally until the interval between 30 and 60 min after birth (47). When breathing begins, air inflation shifts residual liquid from the lumen into distensible perivascular spaces around large pulmonary blood vessels and bronchi. Accumulation of liquid in these connective tissue spaces, which are distant from sites of respiratory gas exchange, allows time for small blood vessels and lymphatics to remove the displaced liquid with little or no impairment of lung function. In rabbits delivered at term gestation, perivascular cuffs of fluid are of maximal size 30 min after birth, at which time they may store up to 75% of the total amount of extravascular water in the lungs (47); these fluid cuffs normally disappear by 6 hr after birth.

The pattern of lung liquid clearance near birth is similar in lambs (33). As liquid secretion decreases before birth, lung luminal volume also decreases, with a corresponding reduction in the caliber of potential air spaces (Fig. 2A and B). After breathing begins, residual liquid flows into the interstitium and collects around large pulmonary blood vessels and airways (Fig. 2C). These perivascular cuffs progressively decrease in size as aeration of terminal respiratory units improves postnatally (Fig. 2D). Thus, clearance of fetal lung liquid in lambs is complete 6 hr after normal vaginal delivery. The process is slower in preterm lambs (48,49) as well as in preterm rabbits (31).

PATHWAYS FOR REMOVAL OF FETAL LUNG LIQUID

Potential routes for removal of lung luminal liquid at birth include pulmonary lymphatics, the circulation, the pleural space, the mediastinum, and the upper airway. In studies designed to assess the role of lymphatics in removing fetal lung liquid at birth, Humphreys et al. (10) measured pulmonary lymph flow for 1 hr before birth and for 2 hr after the start of mechanical ventilation of lambs delivered by cesarean section. There was a two- to threefold increase in lymph flow after breathing began, and the investigators concluded that pulmonary lymphatics drain about 40% of the liquid contained in potential air spaces of mature lambs before birth. The postnatal increase in lymph flow was less in premature lambs than in lambs delivered at term. These were acute studies performed on anesthetized fetuses immediately following extensive surgery during which the trachea was occluded.

To reexamine the role of lymphatics in removing liquid from the lungs before and after birth, Bland et al. (33) measured vascular pressures, lymph flow, and concentrations of protein in lymph and plasma of five unanesthetized fetal lambs before, during, and after spontaneous vaginal delivery between 132 and 145 days gestation (mean = 139 days). Lymph flow increased postnatally in all five of these lambs, but the increase was transient and small, returning to the prenatal level within 3 hr. The results of these studies suggested that the amount of excess liquid drained postnatally by pulmonary lymphatics accounted for approximately 11% of the residual liquid in the lungs at birth. The concentration of protein in lymph decreased with the onset of ventilation in all five lambs, suggesting that when breathing began, residual liquid in potential air spaces, which contains almost no protein, entered the interstitium and thereby reduced the protein concentration in lymph. With subsequent reabsorption of this liquid into the bloodstream, the concentration of protein in lymph returned to its baseline level. Lymph protein clearance did not change significantly during the course of these studies; this is not surprising, in that liquid from potential air spaces contains less than 0.3 mg protein/ml. These studies, coupled with parallel studies of lung liquid clearance conducted with older newborn lambs, indicate that lung

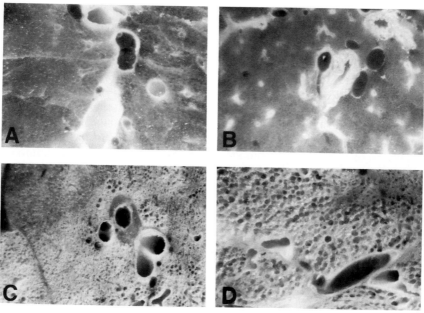

FIG. 2. Sections of rapidly frozen lung taken from lambs that were killed (**A**) without labor (widely patent fluid-filled bronchi), (**B**) during labor (reduced cross-sectional area of bronchi), (**C**) 30 min after birth (perivascular fluid cuffs and fluid in fissure), and (**D**) 6 hr after birth (well aerated, fluid cuffs absent). (From ref. 33.)

lymphatics normally drain only a small fraction of liquid in potential air spaces.

In a sequel to these experiments, Raj and Bland (50) found that left atrial pressure elevation delays, but does not prevent, lung luminal liquid clearance in lambs. More recently, Cummings et al. (51) showed that reduction of plasma protein concentration in newborn lambs also slows the rate at which liquid from potential air spaces is removed from the lungs. These findings provide further evidence that the pulmonary microcirculation absorbs at least some, and perhaps most, of the residual liquid present in potential air spaces at birth. It is also possible that some liquid enters the bloodstream through the mediastinum and pleural space, though studies by Cummings et al. (52) indicate that in normal lambs very little luminal liquid drains by way of the pleural space.

How important is the upper airway as a conduit for draining liquid from the lung lumen at birth? Karlberg et al. (53) measured changes in thoracic pressure and volume in human infants during birth and concluded that chest compression associated with vaginal delivery drives liquid from the lungs into the oropharynx. Other studies, however, indicate that squeezing the thorax during spontaneous birth may not be a critical event in expelling fetal lung liquid. As noted above, animals in labor that are delivered by cesarean section after tracheal ligation have no more water in their lungs than do animals that are born vaginally (32,33). Moreover, studies of lung liquid dynamics in near-term fetal lambs have shown that late in labor, as luminal liquid is absorbed across the epithelium, the upper airway functions as a one-way valve, inhibiting entry of amniotic liquid into the lung lumen and impeding the outward flow of pulmonary liquid into the oropharynx (30). Thus, while the conducting airways may serve as an escape route for lung liquid during delivery without prior labor, they probably play a minor role in liquid clearance during the normal birth process.

There are two components of the process by which liquid in potential air spaces drains from the lungs during and after birth: transepithelial flow into the interstitium, followed by passage of liquid into the bloodstream either directly into the pulmonary circulation or through a network of lymphatics that empty into the systemic venous system. Development of effective respiratory gas exchange and lung volume soon after birth (54) makes it likely that the shift of liquid from air spaces into the interstitium occurs quickly, after which there is slower uptake into the pulmonary circulation or lung lymphatics (33,50). In fetal lambs with an intact placental circulation, absorption of liquid from the lung lumen begins during labor and accelerates immediately after birth (30), perhaps related to a transient increase in hydraulic conductivity of the pulmonary epithelium at the start of air breathing (55).

Studies done with healthy, mature lambs indicate that the transepithelial component of lung liquid clearance takes 2–3 hr and that drainage of liquid from the interstitium into the circulation is complete by 6 hr (33,50).

CHANGES IN LUNG EPITHELIAL CELL ION TRANSPORT AT BIRTH

The stimulus for lung liquid absorption near birth remains unclear, but studies done with living sheep (37,56,57) and with isolated perfused rat lungs (58–60) indicate that active sodium transport across the pulmonary epithelium drives liquid from the lung lumen into the interstitium, with subsequent absorption into the vasculature. Thus, the lung epithelium switches from a predominantly chloride-secreting membrane before birth to a predominantly sodium-absorbing membrane after birth. Consistent with this notion, O'Brodovich et al. (61) recently reported that intraluminal delivery of amiloride, a sodium transport inhibitor, in newborn guinea pigs caused a delay in lung liquid clearance. Likewise, tracheal instillation of amiloride during labor inhibited reabsorption of lung luminal liquid in fetal lambs, whereas β-adrenergic blockade with propranolol did not have this effect (62).

In vitro studies of ion transport and the bioelectric properties of cultured alveolar type II cells harvested from adult rats have provided evidence that the same cells which secrete surfactant into the air spaces also may pump sodium in the opposite direction, thereby generating the driving force for rapid absorption of luminal liquid (63–68). Mason et al. (63) showed that monolayers of cultured rat alveolar type II cells, when mounted in an Ussing-type chamber, maintained a transepithelial electrical potential difference (luminal side negative) which increased in response to β-adrenergic stimulation with terbutaline and which decreased in response to luminal amiloride or abluminal ouabain. Although type II cells occupy only a small portion of the surface area of terminal air spaces, numerous microvilli on the luminal aspect of these cells greatly increase their absorptive surface area (69). It is also possible that sodium pump activity in type I lung epithelial cells might have a role in liquid removal from the air spaces, but studies by Schneeberger and McCarthy (70) showed little or no Na^+, K^+-ATPase on type I cells of adult rat lungs, though it was present on the basolateral surface of type II cells.

To examine the possible link between epithelial cell ion transport and the changes in lung liquid volume that occur during and after birth, Bland and Boyd (71) measured total and ouabain-sensitive rubidium ($^{86}Rb^+$) uptake as an index of Na^+–K^+ exchange and Na^+, K^+-ATPase activity in freshly isolated lung epithelial cells obtained from fetal, newborn, and adult rabbits. Fetal cells took up ^{86}Rb$^+$ (which mimics transmembrane movement of K$^+$) at about 5% of the rate measured for adult cells. Ouabain, a cardiac glycoside that inhibits Na$^+$,K$^+$-ATPase, blocked more than 80% of the ^{86}Rb$^+$ influx with fetal cells and about 50% of the uptake by adult cells. The rate of ^{86}Rb$^+$ entry into cells obtained from newborn pups was three to four times greater than that of fetal cells; ouabain blocked about two-thirds of the ^{86}Rb$^+$ uptake in newborn cells. Amiloride also inhibited ^{86}Rb$^+$ uptake in both adult and newborn cells. These observations support the concept that changes in epithelial cell cation flux may contribute to the shift of lung luminal liquid that occurs around the time of birth.

In related studies, ouabain-sensitive ^{86}Rb$^+$ uptake (an index of sodium pump activity) in cells harvested from fetal rabbits was similar to that from newborn pups that had respiratory distress after premature birth (71). In contrast, there was a threefold or greater increase in ouabain-sensitive ^{86}Rb$^+$ uptake in cells derived from term fetuses that experienced labor. These findings suggest that events associated with labor may stimulate Na$^+$,K$^+$-ATPase activity in lung epithelial cells, possibly contributing to the decrease in lung water that occurs in fetal rabbits during labor (32). The stress of premature birth and subsequent respiratory failure, however, does not increase lung epithelial cell cation flux, an observation that may help to explain the lung fluid retention often associated with premature birth (72). Consistent with these observations, Gowen et al. (73) recently reported a greater electrical potential difference across the nasal mucosa of newborn infants born by cesarean section without prior labor and of infants with respiratory distress from retained fetal lung liquid compared to that of normal infants who experienced labor.

To determine if these developmental changes in epithelial cell cation flux were the result of an increase in the number of sodium pumps or in the activity of these pumps, Chapman et al. (74) recently measured the number of ouabain-binding sites (sodium pumps) and ouabain-sensitive ^{86}Rb$^+$ uptake (to derive a turn-over number) of type II lung epithelial cells obtained from fetal, newborn, and adult rabbits. They measured cell binding of radiolabeled ouabain and cell uptake of ^{86}Rb$^+$ in the presence of 10^{-4} M ouabain, and by Scatchard analysis of ^{3}H-binding they determined a dissociation constant (K_d) and a maximal number of binding sites per cell (U_{max}). Na$^+$,K$^+$-ATPase turnover number was calculated from measurement of ouabain-sensitive ^{86}Rb$^+$ influx and U_{max}. Sodium pump number was the same in fetal and newborn cells, but turn-over number was four times greater in newborn cells than in fetal cells, indicative of increased pump activity after birth (Table 4). Adult cells had almost three times more sodium pumps than did fetal and newborn cells, sufficient to account for the postnatal tripling of ouabain-sensitive ^{86}Rb$^+$ uptake. Turnover number was not significantly different in newborn and adult cells. These findings indicate that sodium pump activity increases at birth, whereas the number of sodium pumps increases after birth.

SUMMARY OF POSTNATAL CLEARANCE OF FETAL LUNG LIQUID

Figure 3 is a schematic diagram of the fluid compartments of the fetal lung and the forces that contribute to liquid clearance. As noted previously, luminal liquid in the fetal lung contains <0.3 mg protein/ml, whereas pulmonary interstitial liquid has a protein concentration of $\sim$30 mg/ml (8,10,33). This transepithelial difference in protein concentration generates an osmotic pressure difference of >10 cmH$_2$O (75), which draws liquid from the lumen into the interstitium, as chloride secretion stops (18). Epithelial sodium pumps and transpulmonary pressure associated with lung inflation also drive liquid from potential air spaces into the interstitium, thereby increasing the protein osmotic pressure difference between plasma and interstitial fluid. Air entry into the lungs not only displaces liquid but also decreases hydraulic pressure in the pulmonary circulation and increases pulmonary blood flow (76), which, in turn, increases lung blood volume and effective vas-

TABLE 4. *Sodium pump number and activity in type II lung epithelial cells derived from fetal, newborn, and adult rabbits[a]*

Status	Number of rabbits	U_{max} (10^3 molecules/cell)	K_m (10^{-7} M)	Ouabain-sensitive ^{86}Rb$^+$ uptake (nmol/10^6 cells/hr)	Turnover number (10^3/min)
Adult	10	166 ± 27[b,c]	2.7 ± 0.4	42 ± 4[b,c]	1.5 ± 0.2[b]
Newborn (litters)	9	64 ± 15	2.7 ± 0.4	16 ± 2[b]	1.6 ± 0.3[b]
Fetus (litters)	7	56 ± 11	5.2 ± 1.3	4 ± 1	0.4 ± 0.1

[a] U_{max}, maximal ouabain binding; K_m, dissociation constant. Data are mean ± SEM.
[b] Significantly different from fetal results ($p < 0.05$).
[c] Significantly different from newborn results ($p < 0.05$).

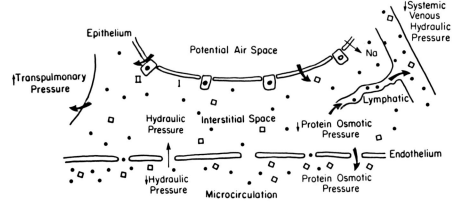

FIG. 3. Schematic diagram of the fluid compartments in the fetal lung, showing the forces that affect fluid clearance near birth. (●) Albumin molecules; (□) globulins. (From ref. 72.)

cular surface area for fluid uptake (77). These circulatory changes facilitate absorption of fluid into the pulmonary vascular bed. About 10% of the luminal liquid leaves the lungs through lymphatics that drain via the thoracic duct into the superior vena cava. With spontaneous breathing, postnatal reduction of intrathoracic pressure decreases systemic venous pressure, which may hasten lymphatic drainage; however, most of the displaced luminal liquid directly enters the pulmonary microcirculation or seeps into the mediastinum with subsequent absorption into the bloodstream.

REFERENCES

1. Rudolph AM, Heymann MA. Circulatory changes during growth in the fetal lamb. *Circ Res* 1970;26:289–299.
2. Mescher EJ, Platzker ACG, Ballard PL, Kitterman JA, Clements JA, Tooley WH. Ontogeny of tracheal fluid, pulmonary surfactant, and plasma corticoids in the fetal lamb. *J Appl Physiol* 1975;39:1017–1021.
3. Alcorn D, Adamson TM, Lambert TF, Maloney JE, Ritchie BC, Robinson PM. Morphological effects of chronic tracheal ligation and drainage in the fetal lamb lung. *J Anat* 1977;123:649–660.
4. Fauré-Fremiet E, Dragiou J. Le développement du poumon foetal chez le mouton. *Arch Anat Microsc* 1923;19:411–424.
5. Jost A, Policard A. Contribution expérimental à l'étude du développement prénatal du poumon chez le lapin. *Arch Anat Microsc* 1948;37:323–332.
6. Addison WHF, How HW. On the prenatal and neonatal lung. *Am J Anat* 1913;15:199–214.
7. Adams FH, Fujiwara T, Rowshan G. The nature and origin of the fluid in the fetal lamb lung. *J Pediatr* 1963;63:881–888.
8. Adamson TM, Boyd RDH, Platt HS, Strang LB. Composition of alveolar liquid in the foetal lamb. *J Physiol* 1969;204:159–168.
9. Cotton CU, Boucher RC, Gatzy JT. Bioelectric properties and ion transport across excised canine fetal and neonatal airways. *J Appl Physiol* 1988;65:2367–2375.
10. Humphreys PW, Normand ICS, Reynolds EOR, Strang LB. Lymph flow and clearance of liquid from the lungs of the lamb at the start of breathing. *J Physiol* 1967;193:1–29.
11. Boyd RDH, Hill JR, Humphreys PW, Normand ICS, Reynolds EOR, Strang LB. Permeability of lung capillaries to macromolecules in foetal and newborn lambs and sheep. *J Physiol* 1969;201:567–588.
12. Normand ICS, Reynolds EOR, Strang LB. Passage of macromolecules between alveolar and interstitial spaces in foetal and newly ventilated lungs of the lamb. *J Physiol* 1970;210:151–164.
13. Normand ICS, Olver RE, Reynolds EOR, Strang LB. Permeability of lung capillaries and alveoli to non-electrolytes in the foetal lamb. *J Physiol* 1971;219:303–330.
14. Schneeberger EE, Walters DV, Olver RE. Development of intercellular junctions in the pulmonary epithelium of the foetal lamb. *J Cell Sci* 1978;32:307–324.
15. Olver RE, Schneeberger EE, Walters DV. Epithelial solute permeability, ion transport and tight junction morphology in the developing lung of the fetal lamb. *J Physiol* 1981;315:395–412.
16. Olver RE, Strang LB. Ion fluxes across the pulmonary epithelium and the secretion of lung liquid in the foetal lamb. *J Physiol* 1974;241:327–357.
17. Cassin S, Gausse G, Perks AM. The effects of bumetamide and furosemide on lung liquid secretion in fetal sheep. *Proc Soc Exp Biol Med* 1986;181:427–431.
18. Nielson DW. Changes in the pulmonary alveolar subphase at birth in term and premature lambs. *Pediatr Res* 1988;23:418–422.
19. Adamson TM, Brodecky V, Lambert TF, Maloney JE, Ritchie BC, Walker AM. Lung liquid production and composition in the "in utero" foetal lamb. *Aust J Exp Biol Med Sci* 1975;53:65–75.
20. Kitterman JA, Ballard PL, Clements JA, Mescher EJ, Tooley WH. Tracheal fluid in fetal lambs: spontaneous decrease prior to birth. *J Appl Physiol* 1979;47:985–989.
21. Schneeberger EE. Plasmalemmal vesicles in pulmonary capillary endothelium of developing fetal lamb lungs. *Microvasc Res* 1983;25:40–55.
22. Shermeta DW, Oesch I. Characteristics of fetal lung fluid production. *J Pediatr Surg* 1981;16:943–946.
23. Carlton DP, Cummings JJ, Bland RD. Increased pulmonary vascular filtration pressure does not affect lung luminal liquid secretion in fetal sheep. *Clin Res* 1989;37:212A.
24. Cotton CU, Lawson EE, Boucher RC, Gatzy JT. Bioelectric properties and ion transport of airways excised from adult and fetal sheep. *J Appl Physiol* 1983;55:1542–1549.
25. Olver RD, Robinson EJ. Sodium and chloride transport by the tracheal epithelium of fetal, newborn and adult sheep. *J Physiol* 1986;375:377–390.
26. Cotton CU, Boucher RC, Gatzy JT. Paths of ion transport across canine fetal tracheal epithelium. *J Appl Physiol* 1988;65:2376–2382.
27. Zeitlin PL, Loughlin GM, Guggino WB. Ion transport in cultured fetal and adult rabbit tracheal epithelia. *Am J Physiol* 1988;254:C691–C698.
28. Krochmal EM, Ballard ST, Yankaskas JR, Boucher RC, Gatzy JT. Volume and ion transport by fetal rat alveolar and tracheal epithelia in submersion culture. *Am J Physiol* 1989;256:F397–F407.
29. Dickson KA, Maloney JE, Berger PJ. Decline in lung liquid volume before labor in fetal lambs. *J Appl Physiol* 1986;61:2266–2272.
30. Brown MJ, Olver RE, Ramsden CA, Strang LB, Walters DV.

Effects of adrenaline and of spontaneous labour on the secretion and absorption of lung liquid in the foetal lamb. *J Physiol* 1983;344:137–152.

31. Bland RD. Dynamics of pulmonary water before and after birth. *Acta Paediatr Scand* 1983;305(Suppl):12–20.

32. Bland RD, Bressack MA, McMillan DD. Labor decreases the lung water content of newborn rabbits. *Am J Obstet Gynecol* 1979;135:364–367.

33. Bland RD, Hansen TN, Haberkern CM, Bressack MA, Hazinski TA, Raj JU, Goldberg RB. Lung fluid balance in lambs before and after birth. *J Appl Physiol* 1982;53:992–1004.

34. Enhorning G, Chamberlain D, Contreras C, Burgoyne R, Robertson B. Isoxsuprine-induced release of pulmonary surfactant in the rabbit fetus. *Am J Obstet Gynecol* 1977;129:197–202.

35. Walters DV, Olver RE. The role of catecholamines in lung liquid absorption at birth. *Pediatr Res* 1978;12:239–242.

36. Lawson EE, Brown ER, Torday JS, Madansky DL, Taeusch HW Jr. The effect of epinephrine on tracheal fluid flow and surfactant efflux in fetal sheep. *Am Rev Respir Dis* 1978; 118:1023–1026.

37. Olver RE, Ramsden CA, Strang LB, Walters DV. The role of amiloride-blockable sodium transport in adrenaline-induced lung liquid reabsorption in the fetal lamb. *J Physiol* 1986;376:321–340.

38. Barker PM, Brown MJ, Ramsden CA, Strang LB, Walters DV. The effect of thyroidectomy in the fetal sheep on lung liquid reabsorption induced by adrenaline or cyclic AMP. *J Physiol* 1988;407:373–383.

39. Walters DV, Ramsden CA, Olver RE. Dibutyryl cyclic AMP induces a gestation-dependent absorption of fetal lung liquid. *J Appl Physiol* 1990;68:2054–2059.

40. Perks AM, Cassin S. The effects of arginine vasopressin and other factors on the production of lung liquid in fetal goats. *Chest* 1982;81(Suppl):63–65.

41. Ross MG, Ervin G, Leake RD, Fu P, Fisher DA. Fetal lung liquid regulation by neuropeptides. *Am J Obstet Gynecol* 1984;150:421–425.

42. Bland RD, Fike CD, Teague WG, Braun D, Keil LC. Vasopressin decreases lung water in fetal lambs. *Pediatr Res* 1985;19:399A.

43. Kitterman JA. Fetal lung development. *J Dev Physiol* 1984;6:67–82.

44. Chapman DL, Carlton DP, Cummings JJ, Poulain FR, Bland RD. Propranolol does not prevent absorption of lung liquid in fetal lambs during labor. *FASEB J* 1990;14:A4111.

45. Wallen LD, Murai DT, Clyman RI, Lee CH, Mauray FE, Ballard PL, Kitterman JA. Meclofenamate does not affect lung development in fetal sheep. *J Dev Physiol* 1989;12:109–115.

46. McDonald JV, Gonzales LW, Ballard PL, Pitha J, Roberts JM. Lung β-adrenoreceptor blockade affects perinatal surfactant release but not lung water. *J Appl Physiol* 1986;60:1727–1733.

47. Bland RD, McMillan DD, Bressack MA, Dong L. Clearance of liquid from lungs of newborn rabbits. *J Appl Physiol* 1980; 49:171–177.

48. Egan EA, Dillon WP, Zorn S. Fetal lung liquid absorption and alveolar epithelial solute permeability in surfactant deficient, breathing fetal lambs. *Pediatr Res* 1984;18:566–570.

49. Bland RD, Carlton DP, Scheerer RG, Cummings JJ, Chapman DL. Lung fluid balance in lambs before and after premature birth. *J Clin Invest* 1989;84:568–576.

50. Raj JU, Bland RD. Lung luminal liquid clearance in newborn lambs. Effect of pulmonary microvascular pressure elevation. *Am Rev Respir Dis* 1986;134:305–310.

51. Cummings JJ, Carlton DP, Poulain FR, Bland RD. Hypoproteinemia slows lung liquid clearance in lambs. *Clin Res* 1990;38:136A.

52. Cummings JJ, Carlton DP, Poulain FR, Bland RD. Lung luminal liquid is not removed via the pleural space in healthy newborn lambs. *Physiologist* 1989;32:202.

53. Karlberg P, Adams FH, Geubelle F, Wallgren G. Alteration of the infant's thorax during vaginal delivery. *Acta Obstet Gynecol Scand* 1962;41:223–229.

54. Milner AC, Saunders RA, Hopkin IE. Effects of delivery by

cesarean section on lung mechanics and lung volume in the human neonate. *Arch Dis Child* 1978;53:545–548.

55. Egan EA, Olver RE, Strang LB. Changes in non-electrolyte permeability of alveoli and the absorption of lung liquid at the start of breathing in the lamb. *J Physiol* 1975;244:161–179.

56. Matthay MA, Landolt CC, Staub NC. Differential liquid and protein clearance from the alveoli of anesthetized sheep. *J Appl Physiol* 1982;53:96–104.

57. Matthay MA, Bertiaume Y, Staub NC. Long-term clearance of liquid and protein from the lungs of unanesthetized sheep. *J Appl Physiol* 1985;59:928–934.

58. Crandall ED, Heming TA, Palombo RL, Goodman BE. Effects of terbutaline on sodium transport in isolated perfused rat lung. *J Appl Physiol* 1986;60:289–294.

59. Basset G, Crone C, Saumon G. Significance of active ion transport in transalveolar water absorption: a study on isolated rat lung. *J Physiol* 1987;384:311–324.

60. Basset G, Crone C, Saumon G. Fluid absorption by rat lung *in situ*: pathways for sodium entry in the luminal membrane of alveolar epithelium. *J Physiol* 1987;384:325–345.

61. O'Brodovich H, Hannam V, Seear M, Mullen JBM. Amiloride impairs lung liquid clearance in newborn guinea pigs. *J Appl Physiol* 1990;68:1758–1762.

62. Chapman DL, Carlton DP, Cummings JJ, Poulain FR, Bland RD. Propranolol does not prevent absorption of lung liquid in fetal lambs during labor. *FASEB J* 1990;in press.

63. Mason RJ, Williams MC, Widdicombe JH, Sanders MJ, Misfeldt DS, Berry LG Jr. Transepithelial transport by pulmonary alveolar type II cells in primary culture. *Proc Natl Acad Sci USA* 1982;79:6033–6037.

64. Goodman BE, Fleischer RS, Crandall ED. Evidence of active Na$^+$ transport by cultured monolayers of pulmonary alveolar epithelial cells. *Am J Physiol* 1983;245:C78–C83.

65. Goodman BE, Brown SES, Crandall ED. Regulation of transport across pulmonary alveolar epithelial cell monolayers. *J Appl Physiol* 1984;57:703–710.

66. Sugahara K, Caldwell JH, Mason RJ. Electrical currents flow out of domes formed by cultured epithelial cells. *J Cell Biol* 1984;99:1541–1544.

67. Cott G, Sugahara K, Mason R. Stimulation of net active ion transport across type II cell monolayers. *Am J Physiol* 1986;250:C222–C227.

68. Cheek JM, Kim KJ, Crandall ED. Tight monolayers of rat alveolar epithelial cells: bioelectric properties and active sodium transport. *Am J Physiol* 1989;256:C688–C693.

69. Weibel ER, Gehr P, Haies D, Gil J, Bachofen M. The cell population of the normal lung. In: Bouhuys A, ed. *Lung cells in disease*. Amsterdam: Elsevier/North-Holland, 1976:3–16.

70. Schneeberger EE, McCarthy KM. Cytochemical localization of Na$^+$-K$^+$-ATPase in rat type II pneumocytes. *J Appl Physiol* 1986;60:1584–1589.

71. Bland RD, Boyd CAR. Cation transport in lung epithelial cells derived from fetal, newborn and adult rabbits. Influence of premature birth, labor and postnatal development. *J Appl Physiol* 1986;62:507–515.

72. Bland RD. Pathogenesis of pulmonary edema after premature birth. *Adv Pediatr* 1987;34:175–222.

73. Gowen CW Jr, Lawson EE, Gingras J, Boucher RC, Gatzy JJ, Knowles MR. Electrical potential difference and ion transport across nasal epithelium of term neonates: correlation with mode of delivery, transient tachypnea of the newborn, and respiratory rate. *J Pediatr* 1988;113:121–127.

74. Chapman DL, Widdicombe JH, Bland RD. Developmental differences in rabbit lung epithelial cell Na$^+$-K$^+$-ATPase. *Am J Physiol* (*Lung Cell Mol Physiol*) 1990;69:in press.

75. Bland RD, Bressack MA. Lung fluid balance in awake newborn lambs with pulmonary edema from rapid intravenous infusion of isotonic saline. *Pediatr Res* 1979;13:1037–1042.

76. Dawes GS, Mott JC, Widdicombe JG, Wyatt DG. Changes in the lungs of the newborn lamb. *J Physiol* 1953;121:141–162.

77. Walker AM, Alcorn DG, Cannata JC, Maloney JE, Ritchie BC. Effect of ventilation on pulmonary blood volume of the fetal lamb. *J Appl Physiol* 1975;39:969–975.

THE LUNG: Scientific Foundations
edited by R.G. Crystal, J.B. West et al.
Raven Press, Ltd., New York © 1991.

CHAPTER 6.1.4

Fetal and Neonatal Pulmonary Circulation

Mary L. Tod and Sidney Cassin

The fetal pulmonary circulation fulfills a unique function: *in utero*, close to term, fetal lungs receive about 8–10% of the combined ventricular output in order to meet the metabolic demands of an actively growing organ, but with the first inspiration of air the pulmonary circulation must accommodate the total cardiac output in order to take over the function of gas exchange. The presence of the large fetal shunts, the foramen ovale and the ductus arteriosus, allows the fetal lung to regulate the amount of blood flow it receives by active vasoconstriction. Before birth the pulmonary vascular resistance is relatively high, but it decreases markedly upon initiation of ventilation of the lungs. The mechanisms by which the fetal pulmonary circulation is regulated and undergoes its transition from a high- to a low-resistance pathway will be the focus of this chapter. Additional information and much of the original source materials can be found in a number of excellent reviews (1–11).

HEMODYNAMIC FEATURES OF THE FETAL AND PERINATAL LUNG

Blood Flow

Although descriptions of the pattern of the fetal circulation were provided by cineangiography almost 50 years ago, these techniques did not allow for quantification of blood flow through the major vessels in the fetal lamb. In 1954, Dawes and co-workers (cited in ref. 6) made the first attempts at quantifying these blood flows based on measurements of O_2 contents in the major blood vessels of the fetal lamb. These investigators were able to calculate that the fetal pulmonary circulation receives approximately 10% of the combined ventricular output by estimating the proportion of mixing which would yield the measured O_2 saturations based on relative flows. Although these measurements were indirect, the estimated blood flows were similar to those measured by other, more direct methods developed more recently. The microsphere technique of measuring organ blood flows has allowed the pulmonary flow to be determined at various gestational ages in the same animal (10). The distribution of combined ventricular output, measured in fetal lambs ranging from 60 to 150 days gestational age, indicates that the lungs receive only 3.5% of the total output at 0.4 term, but the fraction gradually increases to almost 8% at term. In terms of absolute flows, at 60 days the pulmonary blood flow is only 3–5 ml/min, whereas by 150 days it increases to 140 ml/min (10).

This remarkable increase in fetal pulmonary perfusion is presumably related to the growth of the fetal lungs. The lungs increase in weight by 6-fold from midgestation to term (12), and the number of pulmonary vessels increases by more than 10-fold (10). Thus, the tremendous increase in cross-sectional area of the pulmonary vasculature permits pulmonary blood flow to increase throughout gestation. Indeed, in a preliminary report, Morin (13) found that when the increase in perfusion is corrected for the increase in lung weight, pulmonary blood flow remains relatively constant during the latter half of gestation (124 ± 32 ml/100 g/min at 0.6 gestation versus 111 ± 38 ml/100 g/min at term in fetal lambs). Thus, a gradual increase in pulmonary arterial pressure (10), accompanied by a relatively constant flow per unit lung tissue with increasing gestational age, results in fetal pulmonary vascular resistance increasing during the latter portion of gestation (12).

The importance of maintaining a high pulmonary

M. L. Tod: Division of Pulmonary and Critical Care Medicine, Department of Medicine, University of Maryland School of Medicine, Baltimore, Maryland 21201.

S. Cassin: Department of Physiology, University of Florida College of Medicine, Gainesville, Florida 32610.

vascular resistance *in utero* becomes obvious when one considers that the function of gas exchange is performed not by the lungs but instead by the placenta. If fetal lungs were to receive an increased fraction of the right ventricular output, a large arteriovenous shunt would exist between the two sides of the heart, increasing the volume of blood returned to the left ventricle. The major consequence of increased pulmonary perfusion in the fetus would be to increase the workload of the left ventricle. One therefore might expect that elimination of a major fetal extrapulmonary shunt, the ductus arteriosus, would increase pulmonary blood flow. In a recent experiment, fetal lambs were delivered by cesarean section 3–17 days after ductal ligation, and pulmonary pressures and flows were measured (14). This procedure caused newborn lambs to maintain elevated pulmonary arterial pressures and pulmonary vascular resistances when compared with those of nonligated controls. In addition, morphological analysis of the pulmonary vasculature of these lambs which had undergone ligation of the ductus arteriosus *in utero* demonstrated an increase in the medial muscle in the peripheral pulmonary arteries (15), which was similar to that observed in human infants with persistent pulmonary hypertension (11). Recently, partial compression of the ductus arteriosus in fetal lambs, which produced a sustained elevation of pulmonary arterial pressure, was initially accompanied by an increase in pulmonary blood flow; however, despite a constant increase in pulmonary arterial pressure, flow gradually returned to the baseline values (16). These investigators speculated that the fetal lung has regulatory mechanisms which act to maintain a high pulmonary vascular resistance (16). Thus, *in utero*, the pulmonary blood flow is apparently regulated at that level of perfusion which is necessary to meet the metabolic demands of the growing organ.

As early as 1954, evidence of pulmonary O_2 consumption in the fetal lamb was provided by measuring a pulmonary arterial–venous O_2 gradient of 1.6 ml O_2/100 ml blood, a value corresponding to approximately 8% of the total fetal O_2 consumption (6). Subsequently, in elegant studies on anesthetized exteriorized fetal lambs, the O_2 consumption of fetal lungs was reported to be 0.25 ± 0.04 ml/kg·min, or approximately 750 µl of O_2 per minute in a term lamb weighing ~3 kg (6). Recent studies in chronically instrumented fetal lambs (119–141 days of gestation) demonstrated that both O_2 delivery and O_2 consumption increase with increasing gestational age (by 43% and 93%, respectively), with O_2 consumption reaching 952 ± 168 µl/min by late gestation (17), showing excellent agreement with the values reported 20 years earlier (6). Pulmonary arterial and venous glucose and lactate concentrations were also determined in the more recent study (17). In contrast with O_2 consumption, glucose availability and uptake fall significantly with advancing gestation. Lactate is produced by the fetal lung, and the rate of lactate production does not change with age (17).

During the last trimester, the fetal lung is not only undergoing substantial growth but is also maturing with regard to a number of metabolic processes (e.g., production of surfactant). A close relationship between pulmonary perfusion and surfactant production has been proposed (18) whereby hypoperfusion of the fetal lung may lead to inadequate amounts of surfactant at birth and give rise to the respiratory distress syndrome. However, studies in which the left pulmonary artery was ligated, either acutely or chronically, have not demonstrated any alterations in surfactant production or lung morphology (19,20). This suggests that the bronchial blood supply may partially compensate for a lack of pulmonary blood flow before birth, at least within the time frame of these studies. In the normal fetus, bronchial blood flow is estimated to be approximately 14% of pulmonary blood flow (17). The apical lobe of the fetal lung develops surfactant several days earlier than the basilar lobe in lambs; therefore, the distribution of pulmonary perfusion in the fetus was suggested to be directed to those regions of the lung with greater rates of surfactant synthesis and alveolar stability (21). However, when labeled microspheres were injected into the pulmonary circulation of fetal lambs at different gestational ages, the distribution of pulmonary blood flow to the different lobes was similar based on lobar weight (21). From these studies, it appears that pulmonary blood flow in the fetus is uniform, as would be expected based on consideration of the lack of hydrostatic gradients to influence pulmonary vascular pressures in the fluid-filled lung. In contrast, the distribution of blood flow is correlated with the extent of aeration of fetal lungs following initiation of ventilation (22). During the onset of ventilation, there are patchy areas of the lung in which some alveoli appear inflated and others remain collapsed. Those areas with a greater extent of inflation receive a greater proportion of pulmonary blood flow; once a more uniform expansion of the alveoli is achieved, perfusion becomes evenly distributed (22).

In addition to being involved in surfactant production, the fetal lung also produces and removes a large number of vasoactive substances. Many of the compounds that are inactivated by the pulmonary vascular endothelium in the adult are also metabolized by the fetal and neonatal lung; however, the affinity or capacity of the metabolic processes may be different from that observed in the adult. For example, Pitt and Lister (23) evaluated pulmonary angiotensin-converting enzyme activity and serotonin metabolism in newborn lambs at 1 day, 1 week, and 1 month of age, as well as in older sheep at 8–23 weeks of age. Pulmonary removal of serotonin is similar in all age groups; in contrast, there is a gradual increase in metabolism of a substrate for angiotensin-converting enzyme from birth to the older age group. In other studies, pulmonary inactivation of PGE_1 and PGE_2 is significantly less than adult values in fetal and newborn rabbit lungs (24,25), whereas inactivation of norepinephrine is greatest in fetal lungs and least in adult lungs (25). Other investigators reported that pulmonary inactivation of bradykinin is greatest in adult sheep (93%), less in newborn lambs (68%), and least in fetal lambs at term (46%) (10). Bradykinin is not inactivated in the lungs of immature fetal lambs. In addition to developmental differences in pulmonary inactivation of vasoactive compounds, there are differences in production of various vasoactive compounds. Thus, Printz et al. (26) described an age-related increase in lung cyclooxygenase activity in fetal, newborn, and adult sheep. These investigators also reported a developmental increase in fetal lung thromboxane synthase activity, with no developmental change in prostacyclin synthase activity noted (26,27). Furthermore, thromboxane synthesis is especially sensitive to modulation by glutathione in fetal and neonatal lungs (28). Decreases in glutathione levels at the time of birth, as well as variations in response to elevated blood oxygen, may be of significance in the transition from fetus to newborn. The developmental changes in formation as well as inactivation of vasoactive compounds may correlate with the increase in pulmonary perfusion during the last trimester of gestation, since these products may contribute to regulation of fetal pulmonary vascular resistance (see below).

Pressure–Flow Relationships

One approach to studying the hemodynamics of the adult pulmonary circulation has been the analysis of pressure–flow relationships across the lung. These methods have also been adapted to the fetal and neonatal pulmonary circulation as a useful means of assessing changes in pulmonary vascular resistance due to a variety of conditions. Thus, increased pulmonary vascular resistance is measured by an increase in the slope of the pressure–flow curve or by an increase in the zero-flow pressure intercept, or both. In fetal lambs, analysis of instantaneous pressure–flow curves reveals that pulmonary vascular resistance is elevated in mature fetuses as compared with immature fetuses, when expressed in terms of either body weight or lung weight (12,29). However, the pressure intercept at zero flow, extrapolated from the steep portion of the curve, is 33–36 mmHg and is not different at the two gestational ages (29). Using the concept of a Starling resistor to determine the critical pressure of the pulmonary vasculature, results similar to the pressure intercept

from extrapolation are obtained in unventilated fetal goat lungs (1). However, upon ventilation with air, the critical pressure decreases significantly, from 22 mmHg to 13 mmHg (1); in neonatal goats the critical pressure is 11 mmHg and is increased significantly by hypoxia, to 14 mmHg (1). Recently, pressure–flow curves were constructed in intact neonatal piglets by a technique of partially occluding the inferior vena cava to reduce cardiac output (30). These investigators observed a significant increase in the slope of the pressure–flow relationship when the piglets breathed 13% O_2, indicating an increase in resistance in these experiments. Hypoxia has no effect on the extrapolated pressure intercept at zero flow, which is near the origin, suggesting that the neonatal piglet has a minimal critical closing pressure (30). This finding in newborns is strikingly different from that observed in isolated lungs of adult pigs, in which a significant critical pressure exists during normoxia (~15 mmHg) and is increased to ~32 mmHg by hypoxia with no increase in the slope of the pressure–flow curve (31). The differences observed between fetal, neonatal, and adult animals in terms of their pressure–flow relationships may be related to the factors involved in decreasing pulmonary vascular resistance at birth.

Distribution of Pulmonary Vascular Resistance

The distribution of pulmonary vascular resistance across the lung has been used to describe the site of action of vasoactive stimuli; in addition, it can be utilized to describe changes that occur with development of the lungs before and after birth. Several methods have been used to partition the total pulmonary vascular resistance into different regions. One method is based on the behavior of the circulation with respect to elevating outflow pressure, usually called the "Starling resistor technique." This approach defines the lung as consisting of two resistances: one upstream from Starling resistors (or critical pressures) and one downstream (1). Using this method, over 80% of the total pressure drop across the fetal goat lung occurs in vessels located upstream from the critical pressure locus (1). In addition, the effect of ventilating the lungs with a fetal gas mixture that does not change the arterial blood-gas tensions is to reduce the pressure surrounding the vessels that act like Starling resistors, such that the relative distribution remains the same as before ventilation (1). Recently, a different approach based on rapid occlusion of inflow or outflow has been used to partition the pulmonary vascular resistance into resistances across relatively indistensible arterial and venous regions and a relatively compliant middle region, which probably consists of capillaries and small muscular arteries and veins (32). In fetal lambs, the pressure drop across this middle region contributes more than 75% of the total resistance before ventilation; although the middle pressure gradient is significantly decreased after ventilation, it still accounts for approximately 50% of the total resistance (32). The most likely explanation for the differences in distribution of pulmonary vascular resistance in these two studies is the lack of precise anatomical definitions of both (a) the boundaries of the regions determined by occlusion and (b) the location of the vessels that behave as Starling resistors. If the Starling resistor locus were situated within the middle region defined by occlusion, the results are not that dissimilar. The distribution of pulmonary vascular resistance after birth varies as a function of postnatal age in lambs (32), with the total pressure drop across the pulmonary vasculature at a constant flow gradually decreasing from the first day until 2 weeks of age, then increasing slightly at 1 month of age (Fig. 1). The most striking change in the distribution occurs in the middle gradient, which is almost 50% of the total pressure gradient in ventilated fetal lungs (−10 to −15 days) but which is reduced significantly at 0–14 days of age to only 20–25% of the total (32). Finally, at 1 month of age, the pressure drop across the middle region again represents over 40% of the total gradient.

A different approach that partitions pulmonary vascular resistance relies upon anatomical visualization of subpleural vessels with direct micropuncture of 20- to 80-μm arterioles and venules for recording of microvascular pressures. This technique has been used in isolated perfused rabbit lungs at different ages, but a direct comparison of the effect of age was not made in these separate studies (33–35). The results from these studies suggest that there is an age-related change in the distribution of pulmonary vascular resistance in rabbits, with newborns (5–19 days of age) having an arterial–microvascular–venous ratio of 60%–30%–10% (33). By 3–4 weeks of age, the ratio changes slightly to 50%–25%–25% (34). In contrast, in adult rabbit lungs, the ratio of the pressure drops is 33%–60%–7% (35). Taken together, the results of these separate experiments suggest that the major site of resistance shifts from the arteries to the microcirculation as the lung matures.

The reason for these age-related changes in the resistance distribution is not known, but these changes may be due, in part, to anatomical changes that occur in the neonatal pulmonary vasculature (11). In addition, there may be influences by vasoactive substances, especially cyclo-oxygenase products, which may be of relatively greater importance in the younger neonate (36,37). As discussed above, there may also be alterations in the ability to synthesize and/or metabolize a number of other vasoactive compounds during the neonatal period, which could contribute to the changes in the distribution of vascular pressure gradients observed in perinatal lambs. Thus, a number of underlying events may interact to produce the functional pattern of pulmonary vascular resistance changes with developmental age.

EVENTS AT BIRTH

The ability of the fetal pulmonary circulation to rapidly dilate to accept the entire right ventricular output at birth is the centerpiece of the hemodynamic transition that converts the lungs from an organ in parallel with other organs of the systemic circulation to one that is

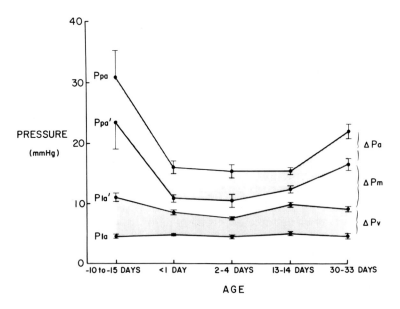

FIG. 1. Average pulmonary vascular pressures as a function of age. Premature lungs (−10 to −15 days) were ventilated, and pulmonary arterial (P_{pa}) and left atrial (P_{la}) pressures were measured at a flow of 100 ml·kg^{-1}·min^{-1} in all age groups. Instantaneous pressures determined from inflow and outflow occlusions are P_{pa}' and P_{la}', respectively. Arterial (ΔP_a), middle (ΔP_m), and venous (ΔP_v) pressure gradients are represented by the differences between the solid lines. (From ref. 32.)

in series between the two ventricles. The factors involved in this remarkable transition have been investigated for almost 40 years; however, they are still not completely understood. Dawes (5,6) has contributed much to our knowledge of the events occurring with the initiation of ventilation by studying the pulmonary circulation of exteriorized fetal lambs. In newborn lambs and goats, pulmonary arterial blood pressure falls almost to adult levels within several hours after birth; in human infants, pulmonary arterial pressure gradually approaches adult values during the first 3 days of life (5). The following major influences on the ventilation-induced decline in pulmonary vascular resistance have been identified: (a) Changing from a fluid-filled to a gas-filled lung results in the establishment of an air–liquid interface in newly inflated alveoli; (b) ventilation with an O_2-containing gas produces greater dilation than does ventilation with a gas that does not alter the fetal arterial O_2 tension; and (c) reducing fetal arterial CO_2 tension causes a further fall in pulmonary vascular resistance (5,6,10).

Expansion of fetal lungs with a gas causes pulmonary vasodilation, even when the gas is nitrogen (6,10). Recently, ventilation of unanesthetized fetal lambs *in utero* with a gas mixture that did not alter fetal arterial O_2 or CO_2 tensions caused a fourfold increase in pulmonary artery blood flow (measured by radioactive microsphere methods) without changing pulmonary arterial pressure (38). These studies confirm earlier experiments in anesthetized fetal lambs and goats (1,6) and suggest that the geometry of the fetal pulmonary vasculature may be altered by the introduction of an air–liquid interface in the alveoli which results in a reduction of perivascular tissue pressure, thus leading to recruitment and/or distention of pulmonary capillaries (10). The significant reduction in the pressure gradient across vessels in the middle region (which contains, but is not limited to, capillaries) with ventilation in fetal lamb lungs also supports the role of surface forces in increasing pulmonary blood flow at birth (32).

Other studies in which fetal lungs were expanded with various liquids reported that fluid expansion, without oxygenation, compresses pulmonary vessels and causes an increase in pulmonary vascular resistance (39). Upon removal of the liquid, pulmonary blood flow returns to the initial level. When an oxygenated fluid is used to expand the fetal lungs, there is a significant decrease in pulmonary vascular resistance; this suggests that mechanical factors of gaseous expansion are not the sole mechanism producing pulmonary vasodilation at birth, and that changes in P_{O_2} and P_{CO_2} exert a local direct effect on pulmonary blood vessels (39). These results are consistent with those in which vasodilation caused by ventilation with nitrogen

or a fetal gas mixture is augmented by the addition of oxygen to the gas mixture (5,6,12,38).

Additional experiments in fetal lambs demonstrated that the P_{O_2} of the blood perfusing the lungs can also influence pulmonary vascular tone (5,6,10,12). Increasing the oxygen tension of the blood perfusing an unventilated fetal lung produces vasodilation, thus providing further evidence for a direct effect of O_2 on pulmonary vessels. However, because the oxygenated blood is obtained from ventilation of the right lung, or from ventilation of a donor lamb, it is not clear whether humoral mediators may have been involved in eliciting the responses in these studies. More recently, during the course of a prolonged exposure of the pregnant ewe to normobaric 100% O_2, which significantly elevates fetal arterial P_{O_2} from 18 to 24 torr, the peak increase in pulmonary blood flow is a function of increasing gestational age (11). However, the increase in fetal pulmonary blood flow noted within the first hour of O_2 administration is not sustained during the second hour of exposure, suggesting that the fetal pulmonary circulation has regulatory mechanisms that may limit the perfusion of the lungs before birth in favor of maintaining blood flow to the systemic circulation (11). Additional observations on the role of oxygenation in unanesthetized fetal lambs have been made by exposing pregnant ewes to hyperbaric oxygen to markedly increase the fetal arterial P_{O_2} without ventilation of fetal lungs (40,41). Increasing the fetal P_{O_2} from 25 to 55 torr results in an 8.8-fold increase in pulmonary blood flow in near-term fetal lambs, which is not prevented by inhibition of prostaglandin synthesis (40,41). In addition, immature fetal lambs (94–101 days gestation) have no change in the fraction of right ventricular output received by the lungs even though the fetal P_{O_2} is increased from 27 to 174 torr, suggesting that some maturational process is involved in the response of the pulmonary circulation to oxygen.

The importance of vasoactive prostaglandins in the transitional pulmonary circulation has been determined by Leffler et al. (36). These studies demonstrated that upon ventilation, fetal lungs release primarily prostacyclin, a potent pulmonary vasodilator, and that the production of prostacyclin by the newly ventilated lungs is an additional factor which contributes to the increase in pulmonary perfusion at birth. The synthesis and release of prostacyclin is related to mechanical ventilation of fetal lungs and is not stimulated by oxygenation alone (42). This suggests that distortion of pulmonary tissues during the establishment of ventilation contributes to the production of prostacyclin and the decrease in pulmonary vascular resistance. The report that the increase in fetal pulmonary blood flow which occurs with hyperbaric oxygenation is not reduced by indomethacin provides additional support for this hypothesis (41).

REGULATION OF FETAL AND PERINATAL PULMONARY CIRCULATION

Mechanical Influences

The relationship between lung volume and pulmonary vascular resistance has been well described for adult lungs using a model in which the lung is comprised of (a) alveolar vessels, which increase resistance as the lung is inflated, and (b) extra-alveolar vessels, which are pulled open by lung inflation and thereby decrease resistance (43). However, the direct effect of lung volume on the pulmonary circulation of the fetus has received little attention. Recently, the effects of increasing and decreasing lung liquid volume in fetal lambs indicate that removal of fetal lung liquid from its initial volume to a minimal volume is accompanied by a doubling of pulmonary vascular conductance and a decrease of the critical closing pressure, estimated from pulmonary pressure–flow curves (44). Expansion of lungs with fluid to twice the initial volume reduces pulmonary vascular conductance to zero and greatly increases the critical closing pressure. Thus, the adult response that is characterized by a U-shaped curve relating vascular resistance to inflation is not observed in fetal lambs, in which pulmonary vascular resistance increases progressively with each level of lung expansion. These results may reflect differences due to the materials used to inflate the lungs (i.e., air versus liquid) or may be related to anatomical differences between fetal and adult pulmonary vessels, with the relatively more muscular fetal pulmonary arteries exhibiting critical closure at higher transmural pressures than observed in adult lungs. As discussed above, ventilation of fetal goat lungs with air significantly decreases the critical pressure from 22 mmHg to 13 mmHg, supporting the first possibility (1). However, papaverine further reduces the critical pressure to 6 mmHg, suggesting that increased vascular smooth muscle tone also contributes to the critical pressure in the perinatal pulmonary circulation (1).

In the neonatal animal, lung inflation by positive-pressure ventilation increases pulmonary vascular resistance, presumably by compressing alveolar vessels. Unilaterally applied positive end-expiratory pressure (PEEP) in intact lambs permits separation of direct effects of airway pressure on the pulmonary circulation of the inflated lung to be compared with the indirect effects of PEEP on overall cardiopulmonary function (45). The contribution of indirect changes in ventricular afterload and cardiac output is small in comparison with the direct effect that increasing PEEP has on

decreasing pulmonary blood flow to the inflated lung (45). These experiments were performed in newborns at 2–3 weeks after birth, at which time the foramen ovale and ductus arteriosus probably were not patent. In other studies using premature ventilated fetal goats, increasing the level of PEEP caused significant right-to-left shunting at extrapulmonary sites in the majority of cases (46). Although pulmonary vascular resistance was not measured, the occurrence of ductal shunting due to increased PEEP with little change in systemic resistance indicates that overinflation of lungs increases pulmonary vascular resistance in these premature animals (46).

High-frequency ventilation, clinically used to improve gas exchange in adults without compromising pulmonary perfusion, is reported to cause an increase in pulmonary arterial pressure and a decrease in pulmonary blood flow in newborn lambs (47,48). Vibratory ventilation in 2- to 4-week-old lambs is associated with (a) decreased P_{aO_2} and cardiac output, (b) elevated pulmonary arterial pressure, and (c) no change in lung lymph flow (47). High-frequency oscillatory ventilation in 4-day-old lambs does not alter gas exchange, measured by the multiple inert gas technique, but significantly increases pulmonary arterial pressure and decreases pulmonary blood flow, both during normoxia and during hypoxia (48). The effect on the pulmonary circulation is to improve ventilation–perfusion matching, as evidenced by an increase in arterial P_{O_2} during normoxic high-frequency ventilation, primarily by altering the distribution of blood flow to the lungs. These studies suggest that newborn lambs may modify pulmonary hemodynamics to achieve better gas exchange, rather than altering the distribution of alveolar ventilation as in adults.

The fetal pulmonary circulation exhibits the ability to autoregulate, or to control the amount of blood flow received. This phenomenon was first described in 1962 by Dawes and Mott (cited in ref. 6), who observed a period of pulmonary ischemia in fetal lambs followed by a period of reactive hyperemia. These observations led Dawes (6) to speculate that local regulation of blood flow to the fetal lung is a protective mechanism which actively limits the amount of perfusion of the developing organ. This hypothesis has been tested recently in intact, unanesthetized fetal lambs in which the existence of mechanisms which act to overcome stimuli that increase pulmonary perfusion in the fetus was described (11,16,49). Diverse stimuli which initially increase pulmonary blood flow include: increased fetal P_{aO_2}; vasodilators such as tolazoline, acetylcholine, histamine, and bradykinin; and partial compression of the ductus ateriosus (11,16,49). With each of these stimuli, pulmonary blood flow is increased for a period of 20–50 min; but despite continued exposure, flow gradually returns to baseline levels. These results support the hypothesis that the fetal pulmonary circulation regulates its perfusion. Preliminary findings suggest that some characteristics of this regulatory mechanism may persist into the immediate neonatal period. Isolated perfused lungs from newborn lambs less than 1 day of age respond to increments in left atrial pressure with significantly greater than one-to-one increases in pulmonary arterial pressure, measured at constant pulmonary blood flow (50). Identical experiments in lambs older than 2–4 days resulted in either the same or smaller pulmonary arterial pressure increase as left atrial pressure was elevated. These results suggest that in younger lambs there is active pulmonary vasoconstriction in response to an increase in transmural pressure, whereas in older lambs there is passive vasodilation in response to the same stimulus (50). These responses are not dependent on production of prostaglandins (16,50). Distention of the main pulmonary artery by balloon inflation in infants results in elevated pulmonary arterial pressure measured distal to the balloon (51), further supporting the hypothesis of autoregulation in the fetus. If similar increases in pulmonary vascular pressures were to occur in the intact newborn, where there is the possibility of patent shunts, the result would be to redirect pulmonary blood flow away from the lungs. This mechanism may be a contributing factor to the development of persistent pulmonary hypertension in the newborn.

Neural Control

Autonomic control of the fetal and neonatal pulmonary circulation has been investigated by use of sympathetic and/or parasympathetic antagonists, transection of neural efferent pathways, stimulation of peripheral ends of cut nerves, and administration of cholinergic and adrenergic agonists (5,6,8,10,52,53). Evidence from those studies in which autonomic input was reduced suggests that the fetal pulmonary vasculature is not tonically controlled by neural reflexes (6,53); however, when stimulated, the fetal pulmonary circulation exhibits significant responses to parasympathetic and adrenergic agents (6,8,52). In particular, the fetal pulmonary circulation vasodilates markedly when acetylcholine is injected, but sectioning the vagus nerve or administering atropine has no effect on baseline pulmonary tone (5,6,8,10,52,53). In addition, some studies suggest that greater responses are observed in mature fetuses than in immature fetuses (8,52); other investigators report that acetylcholine significantly increases pulmonary blood flow in immature fetal lambs at 75–90 days of gestation (5). After the ventilation-induced fall in resistance occurs, either in ventilated mature fetal lambs or in newborns, injections of acetylcholine have minimal impact on the low-re-

sistance pulmonary bed (5,8). Alveolar hypoxia, which elevates baseline tone, permits the vasodilator response to acetylcholine to return (8).

The fetal pulmonary circulation appears to be under some degree of tonic sympathetic influence, since bilateral thoracic sympathectomy results in a slight pulmonary vasodilation (5,6,10). Injection of norepinephrine causes greater pulmonary vasoconstriction with increasing fetal age; direct effects on pulmonary vessels are mediated by alpha-adrenergic mechanisms, whereas indirect effects due to an increase in cardiac output are mediated by beta-receptors (52). Consistent with these observations, norepinephrine has no direct effect on the pulmonary circulation in alpha-blocked newborn lambs during normoxia; however, during hypoxia in these lambs, norepinephrine causes significant vasodilation (8). Neonatal lungs exhibit an increased pulmonary beta-receptor reactivity during hypoxia which resembles the beta-adrenergic response to norepinephrine in immature (0.5–0.6 term) fetal lambs (5,6,29). In summary, it appears that the autonomic system exerts minimal tonic control on the fetal pulmonary circulation but that it can contribute to regulation of pulmonary vascular resistance when stimulated. Additionally, there may be a developmental process involving either the receptors and/or the effector mechanisms.

Oxygen, Carbon Dioxide, and pH

As discussed above, fetal lungs respond to increasing O_2 by vasodilating. Several methods have been used to elevate fetal P_{O_2}, including perfusing an unventilated fetal lung with blood from a donor lung that is ventilated (5,6,10). Although this method causes pulmonary vasodilation to occur, the possible release of vasoactive substances from the ventilated lung is not excluded. Other methods of increasing oxygen in the fetus have demonstrated that oxygen exerts a direct response on the pulmonary vessels and that this response is not mediated by prostaglandins (2,3,5,6,8,10,11,40,41). When the gestational age of the fetus is taken into consideration, the O_2-induced increase in pulmonary perfusion is correlated with increasing gestational age, with no response noted at < 100 days gestation and a threshold occurring between 100 and 115 days (11,40). Neonatal pulmonary vascular responses to hyperoxia are insignificant (54), presumably because they are superimposed on a room-air-dilated vascular bed.

Both fetal and newborn animals display vigorous hypoxic pulmonary vasoconstriction, similar to the response in adult lungs. Although it may be argued that the fetus is normally hypoxic by virtue of a $P_{a}O_2$ of 18–24 torr, and that this is one of the factors which maintains the high pulmonary vascular resistance of the fetus, further vasoconstriction can be demonstrated by reducing fetal O_2 below the normal range of values (5,6,8,10,11). The hypoxic pressor response in the fetus is not due to neural reflexes or catecholamine release; however, the response to decreased O_2 is greater in mature fetuses (5,6,8,10,11). The effect of age on the hypoxic response in the newborn is controversial. Although some investigators report an age-dependent increase in hypoxic pulmonary vasoconstriction (6,32,55,56), others show a decrease with age (57–59) or no effect of age (60). Recently, the age-related increase in hypoxic vasoconstriction in isolated lungs from neonatal lambs was found to be reversed by indomethacin (37). Thus, the discrepancies between the other studies may exist because the young neonate has a greater vasodilator modulation of hypoxic vasoconstriction that diminishes with increasing age. As in the adult, the mechanism(s) by which hypoxic pulmonary vasoconstriction occurs is unknown.

The site of pulmonary vasoconstriction in response to hypoxia is also somewhat controversial. Lung lymph flow increases during hypoxia in unanesthetized newborn lambs but is not affected by hypoxia in adult sheep (61), suggesting an increase in fluid filtration pressure due to pulmonary venous constriction. Other studies support this finding, showing a redistribution of pulmonary blood flow and an increase in small pulmonary wedge pressure during alveolar hypoxia in lambs (62,63). Additional support comes from measurement of microvascular pressures by direct micropuncture of subpleural vessels. Using this anatomical technique, a significant increase in the pressure measured in 20- to 80-μm pulmonary venules is observed with hypoxia (63a). In contrast, with the same technique in isolated neonatal rabbit lungs, only the pulmonary arterial pressure increases during hypoxia, with no change occurring in the microvascular pressures (64). Using a different functional approach of vascular occlusion to partition the pulmonary circulation, other investigators found that hypoxia primarily increases the pressure gradient across the middle region in newborn lambs, with additional increases in the arterial pressure drop as well (32,65). These results are not entirely incompatible with those produced by the micropuncture technique, because the middle region defined by vascular occlusion is probably not limited to microvessels as is the microvascular region determined by micropuncture. Thus, hypoxic constriction of small muscular veins and/or arteries may contribute to the increase in the pressure gradient across the middle region (32,65). In addition, the age-dependent increase in the hypoxic response of the middle region is modified by dilator prostaglandins, such that when the production of prostaglandins is inhibited there is an age-dependent decrease in hypoxic response of the

middle region (65). Additional studies that combine the two techniques to investigate the site of hypoxic pulmonary vasoconstriction in the newborn are needed.

The hypoxic pressor response can be altered by changes in pH and/or P_aCO_2: Acidosis enhances the pressor response, whereas alkalosis blunts this effect (10,66,67). Recently, the attenuation of the hypoxic vasoconstriction by alkalosis was found to result from changes in arterial pH that are independent of changes in P_aCO_2 (68). Thus, both metabolic and respiratory alkalosis produce a decrease in pulmonary vascular resistance that was elevated by hypoxia.

Mediators and Antagonists

Many researchers have investigated vasoactive mediators that could be responsible for maintaining high pulmonary vascular tone in the fetus, just as many have sought to determine the mediator responsible for hypoxic pulmonary vasoconstriction in the adult and newborn. At this time, there does not appear to be a unique substance that is capable of accounting for all the manifestations involved in the regulation of the perinatal pulmonary circulation. Instead, it has become apparent that many substances contribute in various ways to modulating pulmonary vascular responses in the fetus and the newborn, and that the net interaction between these substances eventually results in what we term "regulation of the pulmonary circulation."

Peptides and Biogenic Amines

The perinatal pulmonary circulation is able to respond to a number of endogenous and exogenous neuropeptides and amines. Acetylcholine or histamine infusion produces a profound vasodilation in the fetal lamb, but has little effect on pulmonary vascular resistance after ventilation of the lungs (5,6). Similarly, the normoxic pulmonary circulation of the neonatal lamb is not influenced by acetylcholine; however, during hypoxic vasoconstriction, acetylcholine causes a decrease in pulmonary vascular resistance (69,70). The responses of the fetal and neonatal pulmonary circulation to histamine are similar: Dilation is observed in the fetus and hypoxic newborn, and vasoconstriction is observed in the normoxic newborn (5,6,8,10,70,71). In isolated pulmonary arteries from neonatal and adult dogs, contractile responses to histamine increase with postnatal age, apparently due to the relatively low activity of the H_1-receptor in the newborn (72). There is an enhanced contractile response to histamine in the newborn in the presence of metiamide, an H_2-receptor blocker, suggesting a relatively greater influence of dilator H_2-receptors than of constrictor H_1-receptors in the neonatal period (72). Bradykinin is also a potent pulmonary vasodilator in the fetus, but it has little direct vasodilator effect in the newborn or following ventilation of the fetal lung (8). Although angiotensin II is a potent vasoconstrictor in adult lungs, pulmonary vasodilation was observed in the unanesthetized fetal lamb in response to angiotensin II; however, these investigators suggest that this effect may be mediated by release of dilator prostaglandins (73). Finally, vasoactive intestinal peptide (VIP) is reported to be a powerful pulmonary vasodilator in both normoxic and hypoxic lambs (74). Thus, a variety of endogenous amines and peptides exert vasodilatory effects on the pulmonary circulation in which tone has been elevated, either naturally (as in the fetus) or by hypoxia. The action of catecholamines in the fetal and neonatal pulmonary circulation has been described above.

Eicosanoids

Interest in the role of eicosanoids (a family of products arising from the metabolism of arachidonic acid) in the regulation of the fetal and neonatal pulmonary circulation has remained high for almost 20 years, and several recent reviews provide an excellent summary of much of the earlier research in this area (2,4,7,9). Of particular importance has been the realization that dilator prostaglandins, especially prostacyclin, are involved in the transition from a high-resistance to a low-resistance pulmonary circulation at the time of birth (36). Some areas of current controversy include the identification of the eicosanoid(s) responsible for hypoxic pulmonary vasoconstriction in the neonate, their potential involvement in maintaining high fetal pulmonary vascular resistance, and the use of dilator prostaglandins in the therapy of persistent pulmonary hypertension of the newborn.

Research for the mediators involved in hypoxic pulmonary vasoconstriction suggested that leukotrienes may contribute to the response. For example, leukotrienes C_4 and D_4 were present in the lung lavage fluid of infants with hypoxemia and persistent pulmonary hypertension, but no leukotrienes were found in infants who required ventilatory support but who did not have pulmonary hypertension (2–4,9,11). Subsequent investigations into the effects of leukotrienes on the fetal and neonatal pulmonary circulations have found that LTC_4 and LTD_4 produce pulmonary vasoconstriction (2–4,8,9,11,75); however, part or all of their pressor effect may be mediated by the action of thromboxane A_2 (2–4,9,11,76). Studies using inhibitors of leukotriene synthesis along with antagonists of their receptors yield conflicting results: Some report that hypoxic pulmonary vasoconstriction could be partially or completely reversed (2–4,8,9,11), and others report

no effect on the hypoxic pressor response (2–4,9,11,76). A very interesting study found that the venoconstriction observed in hypoxic lamb lungs could be prevented by inhibitors of thromboxane synthesis or action, but the remaining arterial constriction was reduced only when the effects of lipoxygenase products were removed (77). There is some question as to the specificity of the receptor antagonists and synthesis inhibitors used in many of these studies (75). A recent study using a highly selective receptor antagonist, L 649923, reported complete elimination of pressor responses to LTD_4 in newborn lambs and goats without affecting the pressor response to hypoxia (Fig. 2) (76). This study also demonstrated that the pulmonary vasoconstriction produced by LTD_4 was completely blocked by BW 755C (a dual cyclo-oxygenase and lipoxygenase inhibitor) and by SQ 29548 (a thromboxane receptor antagonist), but the hypoxic pulmonary vasoconstriction was preserved or enhanced in the presence of these inhibitors (Fig. 2) (76).

Similar controversy surrounds the proposition that leukotrienes are responsible for maintaining the high pulmonary vascular resistance of the fetus. There are reports that putative leukotriene synthesis inhibitors and receptor antagonists increase pulmonary blood flow in fetal lambs (2–4,7–9). In contrast, although pulmonary vasodilation was observed in fetal goats when the receptor antagonist FPL 57231 was administered, this compound reduced pressor responses not only to LTD_4 but also to U 46619 (a thromboxane A_2 mimetic) and to phenylephrine (75). This demonstration of a relative lack of specificity of FPL 57231 for the leukotriene receptors weakens the argument for a role for leukotrienes in the regulation of the fetal pulmonary circulation.

A potential goal of the research on the effects of eicosanoids on the perinatal pulmonary circulation is to discover a therapeutic agent that can be used to selectively dilate the pulmonary circulation of infants with persistent pulmonary hypertension. Part of the difficulty involved in treating these neonates is a result of differing etiologies and clinical presentations of a syndrome with significant morbidity and mortality (11). The potency of prostacyclin and PGD_2 in vasodilation of fetal lungs (2,3) has led to clinical trials of these compounds. Thus far these drugs have not proven to be very effective, in part because of the systemic hypotension produced by prostacyclin (78). There was no effect on pulmonary arterial pressure in infants receiving PGD_2 (79); reasons for this ineffectiveness are unknown, but they may be related to species and age differences in the action of PGD_2. Thus, although PGD_2 was originally reported to dilate the pulmonary bed in fetal and hypoxic neonatal lambs (2,3), a recent report in newborn piglets indicates that PGD_2 constricts the pulmonary circulation (80), sug-

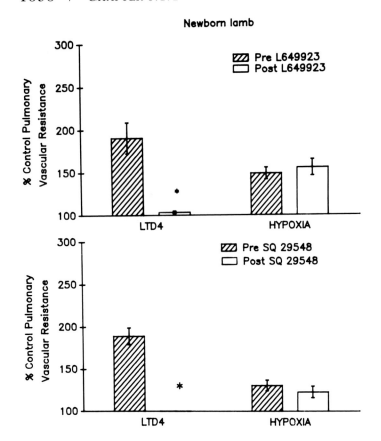

FIG. 2. Effects of a leukotriene D_4 (LTD$_4$) receptor antagonist, L 649923, on pulmonary pressor responses to LTD$_4$ and hypoxia in newborn lambs (**top panel**). Effects of a thromboxane A_2 receptor antagonist, SQ 29548, on pulmonary pressor responses to LTD$_4$ and hypoxia in newborn lambs (**bottom panel**). Asterisks, $p < 0.05$. (From ref. 76.)

gesting that the human infant may respond more like a piglet. Another possibility is that the vasculature of infants with persistent pulmonary hypertension may be unable to respond normally to the vasodilators, perhaps in fact contributing to the original failure to accomplish a normal postnatal transition. One clinical report has suggested that there is an increase in plasma thromboxane levels in patients with persistent pulmonary hypertension (11). Together with the observations that thromboxanes are responsible for the pulmonary hypertension of experimentally induced sepsis in animal models (4,11), it is possible that specific thromboxane synthesis inhibitors or receptor antagonists may prove effective in this disease.

Other Compounds

A potent vasodilator in the adult pulmonary circulation is platelet-activating factor (PAF). Preliminary data indicate that infusion of PAF causes dose-dependent increases in pulmonary blood flow in fetal lambs (8,11). Thus, it is possible that the combined or independent actions of PAF and PGI$_2$ may be responsible for the majority of the postnatal fall in pulmonary vascular resistance (8). Each compound has a number of factors that can elicit its production, and many of these factors are present at the time of birth (8).

With the discovery of endothelium-derived relaxing factor in 1980 by Furchgott and Zawadski (81), there has been growing interest in the interaction of the endothelium and the adjacent vascular smooth muscle. In addition to a relaxing factor produced by the endothelium, a constricting factor has also been described which may be released during hypoxia (11,82). A preliminary report suggests that the bradykinin-induced relaxation of pulmonary arteries is dependent on intact endothelium in older rabbits but that it is independent of the endothelium in younger rabbits (83); however, the ages were not specified in this abstract. The possibility of an age-related change in the role of the endothelium in modulating pulmonary vascular responses warrants investigation.

SUMMARY

Regulation of the perinatal pulmonary circulation involves a complex interaction of anatomical, mechanical, physical, and hormonal factors. Although a number of these factors contribute to the reduction of pulmonary vascular resistance which occurs at birth, a single factor does not appear to be responsible for the high vascular tone which exists in the fetus, the maintenance of low vascular tone in the newborn, or the pulmonary vascular response to hypoxia. Thus, the basic mechanisms of control of the fetal and neonatal pulmonary circulation continue to be actively researched, with the hope of providing a better understanding of, and a rational therapy for, the disorders associated with the failure to achieve a dilated pulmonary vasculature at birth.

REFERENCES

1. Cassin S. The Starling resistor model in the foetal and neonatal pulmonary circulation. In: Comline K, Cross K, Dawes G, Nathanielsz P, eds. *Foetal and neonatal physiology*. London: Cambridge University Press, 1973;112–128.
2. Cassin S. Role of prostaglandins, thromboxanes, and leukotrienes in the control of the pulmonary circulation in the fetus and newborn. *Semin Perinatol* 1987;11:53–63.
3. Cassin S. Mechanisms of control of the perinatal pulmonary circulation. In: Will JA, Dawson CA, Weir EK, Buckner CK, eds. *The pulmonary circulation in health and disease*. Orlando, FL: Academic Press, 1987;469–485.
4. Coceani F, Olley PM. Eicosanoids in the fetal and transitional pulmonary circulation. *Chest* 1988;93:112S–117S.
5. Dawes GS. *Foetal and neonatal physiology*. Chicago: Year Book Medical Publishers, 1968.
6. Dawes GS. Control of the pulmonary circulation in the fetus and newborn. In: Fishman A, Hecht H, eds. *The pulmonary circulation and interstitial space*. Chicago: University of Chicago Press, 1969;293–304.
7. Heymann MA. Postnatal regulation of the pulmonary circulation: a role for lipid mediators. *Am Rev Respir Dis* 1987;136:222–224.
8. Heymann MA, Soifer SJ. Control of fetal and neonatal pulmonary circulation. In: Weir EK, Reeves JT, eds. *Pulmonary vascular physiology and pathophysiology*. New York: Marcel Dekker, 1989;33–50.
9. Kulik TJ, Lock JE. Leukotrienes and the immature pulmonary circulation. *Am Rev Respir Dis* 1987;136:220–222.
10. Rudolph AM, Heymann MA, Lewis AB. Physiology and pharmacology of the pulmonary circulation in the fetus and newborn. In: Hodson W, ed. *Development of the lung*. New York: Marcel Dekker, 1977;497–523.
11. Stenmark KR, Abman SH, Accurso FJ. Etiologic mechanisms in persistent pulmonary hypertension of the newborn. In: Weir EK, Reeves JT, eds. *Pulmonary vascular physiology and pathophysiology*. New York: Marcel Dekker, 1989;335–402.
12. Cassin S, Dawes GS, Mott JC, Ross BB, Strang LB. The vascular resistance of the foetal and newly ventilated lung of the lamb. *J Physiol* 1964;171:61–79.
13. Morin FC III. Pulmonary arterial pressure, blood flow, and resistance in the fetal lamb during advancing gestation [Abstract]. *FASEB J* 1989;3:A979.
14. Morin FC III. Ligating the ductus arteriosus before birth causes persistent pulmonary hypertension in the newborn lamb. *Pediatr Res* 1989;25:245–250.
15. Wild LM, Nickerson PA, Morin FC III. Ligating the ductus arteriosus before birth remodels the pulmonary vasculature of the lamb. *Pediatr Res* 1989;25:251–257.
16. Abman SH, Accurso FJ. Acute effects of partial compression of ductus arteriosus on fetal pulmonary circulation. *Am J Physiol* 1989;257:H626–H634.
17. Simmons RA, Charlton VE. Substrate utilization by the fetal sheep lung during the last trimester. *Pediatr Res* 1988;23:606–611.
18. Chu J, Clements JA, Cotton E, Klaus MH, Sweet AY, Thomas MA, Tooley WH. The pulmonary hypoperfusion syndrome. *Pediatrics* 1965;35:733–742.
19. Adams FH, Nozaki M, Chida N, Salawy AE, Norman A. Effects of hypoxemia, hypercarbia, acidosis, and reduced pulmonary blood flow on the surfactant of fetal lamb lung. *J Pediatr* 1967;71:396–403.
20. Pickard LR, Tepas JJ III, Inon A, Hutchins GM, Shermeta DW, Haller JA Jr. Effect of pulmonary artery ligation on the developing fetal lung. *Am Surg* 1979;45:793–796.
21. Chernick V. Lobar blood flow and maturation of the fetal lamb lung. *Can J Physiol Pharmacol* 1969;47:657–661.
22. Zweizig HZ, Kuhl DE, Katz R, Polgar G. Distribution of pulmonary blood flow in fetal and newborn lambs. *Respir Physiol* 1970;8:160–168.
23. Pitt BR, Lister G. Pulmonary metabolic function in the awake lamb: effect of development and hypoxia. *J Appl Physiol* 1983;55:383–391.
24. Simberg N, Toivonen H, Hartiala J, Bakhle YS. The inactivation of prostaglandin E_2 and 5-hydroxytryptamine in isolated perfused fetal and neonatal rabbit lungs. *Acta Physiol Scand* 1981;113:291–295.
25. Olson EB Jr, Rankin J. Differences in the perinatal development of the isolated rabbit lungs' ability to inactivate vasoactive substances. *Biol Neonate* 1983;44:366–371.
26. Printz MP, Skidgel RA, Friedman WF. Studies of pulmonary prostaglandin biosynthetic and catabolic enzymes as factors in ductus arteriosus patency and closure. Evidence for a shift in products with gestational age. *Pediatr Res* 1984;18:19–24.
27. Skidgel RA, Friedman WF, Printz MP. Prostaglandin biosynthetic activities of isolated fetal lamb ductus arteriosus, other blood vessels, and lung tissue. *Pediatr Res* 1984;18:12–18.
28. Bellan JA, Kerstein MD, Cassin S, Kadowitz PJ, Hyman AL, Rush DS, McNamara DB. Pulmonary thromboxane synthetase activity: a developmental study. *Surg Forum* 1986;37:319–321.
29. Cassin S, Dawes GS, Ross BB. Pulmonary blood flow and vascular resistance in immature foetal lambs. *J Physiol* 1964;171:80–89.
30. Gibson RL, Truog WE, Redding GJ. Hypoxic pulmonary vasoconstriction during and after infusion of Group B Streptococcus in neonatal piglets. Vascular pressure–flow analysis. *Am Rev Respir Dis* 1988;137:774–778.
31. Mitzner W, Sylvester JT. Hypoxic vasoconstriction and fluid filtration in pig lungs. *J Appl Physiol* 1981;51:1065–1071.
32. Tod ML, Sylvester JT. Distribution of pulmonary vascular pressure as a function of perinatal age in lambs. *J Appl Physiol* 1989;66:79–87.
33. Fike CD, Lai-Fook SJ, Bland RD. Microvascular pressures measured by micropuncture in lungs of newborn rabbits. *J Appl Physiol* 1987;63:1070–1075.
34. Raj JU, Chen P. Micropuncture measurement of lung microvascular pressure in profile in 3- to 4-week-old rabbits. *Pediatr Res* 1986;20:1107–1111.
35. Raj JU, Bland RD, Lai-Fook SJ. Microvascular pressures measured by micropipettes in isolated edematous rabbit lungs. *J Appl Physiol* 1986;60:539–545.
36. Leffler CW, Hessler JR, Green RS. The onset of breathing at birth stimulates pulmonary vascular prostacyclin synthesis. *Pediatr Res* 1984;18:938–942.
37. Gordon JB, Tod ML, Wetzel RC, McGeady ML, Adkinson NF Jr, Sylvester JT. Age-dependent effects of indomethacin on hypoxic vasoconstriction in neonatal lamb lungs. *Pediatr Res* 1988;23:580–584.
38. Iwamoto HS, Teitel D, Rudolph AM. Effects of birth-related events on blood flow distribution. *Pediatr Res* 1987;22:634–640.
39. Lauer RM, Evans JA, Aoki H, Kittle CF. Factors controlling pulmonary vascular resistance in fetal lambs. *J Pediatr* 1965;67:568–577.
40. Morin FC III, Egan EA, Ferguson W, Lundgren CEG. Development of pulmonary vascular response to oxygen. *Am J Physiol* 1988;254:H542–H546.
41. Morin FC III, Egan EA, Norfleet WT. Indomethacin does not diminish the pulmonary vascular response of the fetus to increased oxygen tension. *Pediatr Res* 1988;24:696–700.
42. Leffler CW, Hessler JR, Green RS. Mechanism of stimulation of pulmonary prostacyclin synthesis at birth. *Prostaglandins* 1984;28:877–887.
43. Howell JBL, Permutt S, Proctor DF, Riley RL. Effect of inflation of the lung on different parts of the pulmonary vascular bed. *J Appl Physiol* 1961;16:71–76.
44. Walker AM, Ritchie BC, Adamson TM, Maloney JE. Effect of

changing lung liquid volume on the pulmonary circulation of fetal lambs. *J Appl Physiol* 1988;64:61–67.

45. Fuhrman BP, Everitt J, Lock JE. Cardiopulmonary effects of unilateral airway pressure changes in intact infant lambs. *J Appl Physiol* 1984;56:1439–1448.

46. Egan EA, Hessler JR. Positive end expiratory pressure (PEEP) and right to left shunting in immature goats. *Pediatr Res* 1976;10:932–937.

47. Raj JU, Goldberg RB, Bland RD. Vibratory ventilation decreases filtration of fluid in the lungs of newborn lambs. *Circ Res* 1983;53:456–463.

48. Truog WE, Standaert TA. Effect of high-frequency ventilation on gas exchange and pulmonary vascular resistance in lambs. *J Appl Physiol* 1985;59:1104–1109.

49. Accurso FJ, Wilkening RB. Temporal response of the fetal pulmonary circulation to pharmacologic vasodilators. *Proc Soc Exp Biol Med* 1988;187:89–98.

50. Tod ML, Yoshimura K, Pier KG, Rubin LJ. Effect of left atrial pressure (Pla) on neonatal pulmonary pressure gradients [Abstract]. *FASEB J* 1989;3:A372.

51. Baylen BG, Emmanouilides GC, Juratsch CE, Yoshida Y, French WJ, Criley JM. Main pulmonary artery distention: a potential mechanism for acute pulmonary hypertension in the human newborn infant. *J Pediatr* 1980;96:540–544.

52. Nuwayhid B, Brinkman CR III, Su C, Bevan JA, Assali NS. Systemic and pulmonary hemodynamic responses to adrenergic and cholinergic agonists during fetal development. *Biol Neonate* 1975;26:301–317.

53. Nuwayhid B, Brinkman CR III, Su C, Bevan JA, Assali NS. Development of autonomic control of fetal circulation. *Am J Physiol* 1975;228:337–344.

54. Truog WE, Redding GJ, Standaert TA. Effects of hyperoxia on vasoconstriction and $\dot{V}_A/\dot{Q}$ matching in the neonatal lung. *J Appl Physiol* 1987;63:2536–2541.

55. Rendas A, Branthwaite M, Lennox S, Reid L. Response of the pulmonary circulation to acute hypoxia in the growing pig. *J Appl Physiol* 1982;52:811–814.

56. Fike CD, Hansen TN. Hypoxic vasoconstriction increases with postnatal age in lungs from newborn rabbits. *Circ Res* 1987;60:297–303.

57. Reeves JT, Leathers JE. Circulatory changes following birth of the calf and the effect of hypoxia. *Circ Res* 1964;15:343–354.

58. Sidi D, Kuipers JRG, Teitel D, Heymann MA, Rudolph AM. Developmental changes in oxygenation and circulatory responses to hypoxemia in lambs. *Am J Physiol* 1983;245:H674–H682.

59. Custer JR, Hales CA. Influence of alveolar oxygen on pulmonary vasoconstriction in newborn lambs versus sheep. *Am Rev Respir Dis* 1985;132:326–331.

60. Redding GJ, McMurtry I, Reeves JT. Effects of meclofenamate on pulmonary vascular resistance correlate with postnatal age in young piglets. *Pediatr Res* 1984;18:579–583.

61. Bland RD, Bressack MA, Haberkern CM, Hansen TN. Lung fluid balance in hypoxic, awake newborn lambs and mature sheep. *Biol Neonate* 1980;38:221–228.

62. Hansen TN, Le Blanc AL, Gest AL. Hypoxia and angiotensin II infusion redistribute lung blood flow in lambs. *J Appl Physiol* 1985;58:812–818.

63. Hazinski TA, Kennedy KA. Alveolar hypoxia increases small pulmonary wedge pressure in awake young lambs. *Pediatr Res* 1987;22:679–682.

63a. Raj JU, Chen P. Micropuncture measurement of microvascular pressures in isolated lamb lungs during hypoxia. *Cir Res* 1986;59:398–404.

64. Fike CD, Lai-Fook SJ, Bland RD. Microvascular pressures during hypoxia in isolated lungs of newborn rabbits. *J Appl Physiol* 1988;65:283–287.

65. Gordon JB, Hortop J, Hakim TS. Developmental effects of hypoxia and indomethacin on distribution of vascular resistances in lamb lungs. *Pediatr Res* 1989;26:325–329.

66. Johnson GH, Kirschbaum TH, Brinkman CR III, Assali NS. Effects of acid, base, and hypertonicity on fetal and neonatal cardiovascular hemodynamics. *Am J Physiol* 1971;220:1798–1807.

67. Johnson CH, Brinkman CR III, Assali NS. Response of the hypoxic fetal and neonatal lamb to administration of base solution. *Am J Obstet Gynecol* 1972;114:914–922.

68. Lyrene RK, Welch KA, Godoy G, Philips JB III. Alkalosis attenuates hypoxic pulmonary vasoconstriction in neonatal lambs. *Pediatr Res* 1985;19:1268–1271.

69. Shepard FM, Blankenship W, Stahlman M. Cardiovascular response of the neonatal lamb to acetylcholine. *Am J Physiol* 1967;213:895–898.

70. Lock JE, Hamilton F, Olley PM, Coceani F. The effect of alveolar hypoxia on pulmonary vascular responsiveness in the conscious newborn lamb. *Can J Physiol Pharmacol* 1980;58:153–159.

71. Woods JR Jr, Brinkman CR III, Assali NS. Fetal and neonatal cardiopulmonary response to histamine. *Obstet Gynecol* 1976;48:195–202.

72. Newman JH, Souhrada JF, Reeves JT, Arroyave CM, Grover RF. Postnatal changes in response of canine neonatal pulmonary arteries to histamine. *Am J Physiol* 1979;237:H76–H82.

73. Iwamoto HS, Rudolph AM. Effects of angiotensin II on the blood flow and its distribution in fetal lambs. *Circ Res* 1981;48:183–189.

74. Kulik TJ, Johnson DE, Elde RP, Lock JE. Pulmonary vascular effects of vasoactive intestinal peptide in conscious newborn lambs. *Am J Physiol* 1984;246:H716–H719.

75. Gause GE, Baker R, Cassin S. Specificity of FPL 57231 for leukotriene D_4 receptors in fetal pulmonary circulation. *Am J Physiol* 1988;254:H120–H125.

76. Cassin S, Gause G, Davis T, ter Riet M, Baker R. Do inhibitors of lipoxygenase and cyclooxygenase block neonatal hypoxic pulmonary vasoconstriction? *J Appl Physiol* 1989;66:1779–1784.

77. Raj JU, Chen P. Role of eicosanoids in hypoxic vasoconstriction in isolated lamb lungs. *Am J Physiol* 1987;253:H626–H633.

78. Kaapa P, Koivisto M, Ylikorkala O, Kouvalainen K. Prostacyclin in the treatment of neonatal pulmonary hypertension. *J Pediatr* 1985;107:951–953.

79. Soifer SJ, Clyman RI, Heymann MA. Effects of prostaglandin D_2 on pulmonary arterial pressure and oxygenation in newborn infants with persistent pulmonary hypertension. *J Pediatr* 1988;112:774–777.

80. Coe JY, Olley PM, Hamilton F, Vanhelder T, Coceani F. A method to study pulmonary vascular response in the conscious newborn piglet. *Can J Physiol Pharmacol* 1987;65:785–790.

81. Furchgott RF, Zawadski JV. The obligatory role of endothelial cells in the relaxation of arterial smooth muscle by acetylcholine. *Nature* 1980;288:373–376.

82. Holden WE, McCall E. Hypoxia-induced contractions of porcine pulmonary artery strips depend on intact endothelium. *Exp Lung Res* 1984;7:101–112.

83. Diamantis W, Chand N, Mahoney TP, Sofia RD. Mechanism of bradykinin (BK)-induced relaxation of rabbit pulmonary arteries (PA) [Abstract]. *Pharmacologist* 1986;28:187.

THE LUNG: *Scientific Foundations*
edited by R.G. Crystal, J.B. West et al.
Raven Press, Ltd., New York © 1991.

CHAPTER 6.1.5

Fetal Gas Exchange

Lawrence D. Longo

Development of the embryo, fetus, and newborn infant demands appropriate respiratory exchange of oxygen and carbon dioxide. During intrauterine life the placenta serves as the lung for the fetus; however, in addition it fulfills the functions of many organs essential to extrauterine existence.

With birth, physiologically one of the most tumultuous events of life, the responsibility for respiratory function shifts from the placenta to the newborn lung, which, within a matter of seconds, must change from a relatively passive structure with fluid-filled airways to an active member with relatively full functional capacity.

RESPIRATORY GAS EXCHANGE IN THE PLACENTA

The placenta serves to couple substrate delivery to the fetus by the mother, in parallel with other vascular beds. It supplies about 8 ml O_2 per minute per kilogram fetal mass (about twice that of an adult per-weight basis, e.g., 24 ml/min for a 3-kg term fetus), and because fetal blood O_2 stores are only sufficient for 1–2 min, this must be continuous on a moment-to-moment basis. Table 1 gives normal values of blood gases and pH in maternal and fetal placental exchange vessels.

Factors Affecting Placental Oxygen Transfer

Placental O_2 exchange is altered by varying the properties of maternal or fetal blood, such as O_2 capacity or affinity, or by variations in maternal or fetal placental blood flow. Respiratory gas transfer is also dependent upon the spatial configuration of the blood

vessels (countercurrent blood flow being more efficient than concurrent) and upon the diffusion characteristics of the placental membranes (1,2). Table 2 lists some of these factors and their components. Many of the variables that affect placental gas exchange are interdependent, thus complicating the design and interpretation of experiments. Although ideally the exchange process should be studied by sampling inflowing and end-capillary blood within a single exchange unit, this is experimentally impossible. Uterine and umbilical venous outflows, rather than representing blood from a single exchange unit, consist of blood from numerous compartments with differing O_2 and CO_2 tensions and contents. This probably results from a combination of nonuniform distribution of maternal and fetal placental blood flows, nonuniform distribution of diffusing capacity to blood flows, vascular shunts, and so on. An additional problem for one investigating placental exchange dynamics is that experimental change of a given variable to stress the system results in physiological compensations that mask the effect of a given change. Thus, details of the relative roles of the various factors must be inferred from manipulation of the maternal and fetal arterial inputs and mixed venous outputs.

Placental Diffusing Capacity

As in the lung, the quantity of O_2 crossing the placenta is a function of the so-called "diffusing capacity" and the partial pressure gradient. The diffusion characteristics of the placental membrane may be described by Fick's first law:

$$\frac{dQ}{dt} = \frac{AD\Delta C}{\Delta X} \qquad [1]$$

where dQ/dt is the quantity of a given substance (e.g., O_2) crossing the placental membrane per unit time, A

L. D. Longo: Department of Physiology, Loma Linda University, Loma Linda, California 92350.

is the exchange area, D is the diffusion constant (cm^2/sec), ΔC is the concentration difference (by volume) across the membrane, and ΔX is the diffusion distance.

The placental membrane is a complex structure: Its thickness and permeability vary with location. At a given locus, however, the permeability, diffusibility, and thickness may be treated as constants and combined into a single term that expresses the membrane diffusion characteristics:

$$\frac{dQ}{dt} = \frac{1}{P_z} = D_p \qquad [2]$$

where D_p is the placental diffusing capacity in milliliters per minute per torr partial pressure difference for gas z. For respiratory gases, the Bunsen solubility coefficient (α) and the partial pressure difference (ΔP) are used rather than the concentration difference (ΔC) in derivations from Fick's law. Thus placental diffusing capacity is commonly expressed as

$$D_p = \frac{\dot{V}}{\bar{P}_m - \bar{P}_f} \qquad [3]$$

where $\dot{V}$ is the quantity of respiratory gas exchanging across the placental membrane per unit time, and $\bar{P}_m - \bar{P}_f$ is the mean partial pressure difference between maternal and fetal placental exchange vessels (3).

Ideally, one would like to study O_2 or CO_2 exchange using those gases; as noted above, this is not practical for several reasons. First, significant amounts of the total O_2 exchanging are consumed by the placenta, probably close to one-third at term (4). Second, uterine and umbilical mixed venous blood samples must be used

TABLE 1. *Normal values of O_2, CO_2, and pH in human maternal and fetal blood*

Variable	Maternal uterine		Fetal umbilical	
	Artery	Vein	Vein	Artery
P_{O_2} (torr)	95	38	30	22
HbO_2 (% saturation)	98	72	75	50
O_2 content (ml/dl)	16.4	11.8	16.2	10.9
O_2 content (mM)	7.3	5.3	7.2	4.5
Hb (g/dl)	12.0	12.0	16.0	16.0
O_2 capacity (ml/dl)	16.4	16.4	21.9	21.9
O_2 capacity (mM)	7.3	7.3	9.8	9.8
P_{CO_2} (torr)	32	40	43	48
CO_2 content (mM)	19.6	21.8	25.2	26.3
HCO_3	18.8	20.7	24.0	25.0
pH	7.42	7.35	7.38	7.34

[a] P_{O_2} and P_{CO_2} are partial pressures of O_2 and CO_2, respectively; Hb stands for hemoglobin.

TABLE 2. *Principal fators affecting placental oxygen transfer*

Variable	Associated components
Placental diffusing capacity	Membrane diffusing capacity (area, thickness, O_2 solubility, diffusivity of tissues); capillary blood volume; diffusing capacity of blood (O_2 capacity, hemoglobin reaction rates, concentration of reduced hemoglobin)
Maternal arterial P_{O_2}	Inspired P_{O_2}; alveolar ventilation; mixed venous P_{O_2}; pulmonary blood flow; pulmonary diffusing capacity
Fetal arterial P_{O_2}	Umbilical venous P_{O_2}; fetal O_2 consumption; peripheral blood flow; maternal arterial P_{O_2}; maternal placental hemoglobin flow; placental diffusing capacity
Maternal placental hemoglobin flow rate	Arterial pressure; placental resistance to blood flow; venous pressure; O_2 capacity of blood
Fetal placental hemoglobin flow rate	Umbilical arterial blood pressure; umbilical venous blood pressure (or maternal vascular pressure under conditions of sluice flow); placental resistance to blood flow; blood O_2 capacity
Spatial relation of maternal to fetal flow	—
Amount of CO_2 exchange	—

for the calculations, which, as noted above, represent a mixture of blood from compartments with differing ratios of maternal-to-fetal blood flow (5,6), and probably differing ratios of diffusing capacity for blood flows (7). Thus, under almost all circumstances, O_2 exchange is limited by blood flow rather than by diffusion; moreover, as in the lung, a metabolically inert gas whose exchange is limited by diffusion (and which combines with hemoglobin) is used.

Carbon monoxide in low concentrations has been shown to be the most practical gas for studies of transplacental diffusion. The placental diffusing capacity for carbon monoxide (D_pCO) can be calculated by use of the Haldane relation:

$$\frac{[HbCO]}{[HbO_2]} = \frac{P_{CO} \cdot M}{P_{O_2}} \qquad [4]$$

where [HbCO] is the carboxyhemoglobin concentration, [HbO$_2$] is the oxyhemoglobin saturation, Pco is the CO partial pressure (in torr), and M is the relative affinity of hemoglobin for CO and O$_2$.

Placental CO diffusing capacity equals about 0.5 ml/min/torr/kg fetal weight in several species (sheep, dog, macaque monkeys) (3,8); however, in the rabbit and guinea pig it is severalfold greater (9,10). Such studies suggest that the mean maternal–fetal partial pressure difference for O$_2$ equals only about 6 torr, a value similar to that of the pulmonary alveolar–capillary Po$_2$ difference (3). In turn, this suggests that the placenta does not constitute a significant barrier to respiratory gas diffusion, and that placental O$_2$ exchange is limited by blood flow rather than by diffusion (3).

During the course of gestation, the placental mass and exchange area increase to meet the demands of the developing conceptus. Nonetheless, during the last trimester while fetal mass increases severalfold (from 1000 to 3500 g) and placental mass doubles so that the ratio of placental to fetal mass is halved (from 0.22 to 0.14), $D_p$co calculated in terms of fetal weight remains constant (8,11). During prolonged antenatal hypoxia in guinea pigs with the mother breathing 12% O$_2$ from day 15 to 62 gestation (term = 64 days), $D_p$co increased ~63% (10). These changes are associated with an increase in placental vascular volume and a decrease in diffusion distance, which suggests the dependence of $D_p$co on placental structure (12). In contrast to the increase in $D_p$co in long-term hypoxemia, in pregnant guinea pigs that exercised from 15 to 60 min per day throughout gestation there was an approximately 34% decrease in $D_p$co, with the decrease being proportional to exercise duration (10,13). Again, under these circumstances there was an inverse relation between exercise duration and both $D_p$co and the maternal and fetal placental exchange area (14).

Unfortunately, no reliable measurements of $D_p$co in humans are available. The value would be predicted to decrease in conditions in which the placental membranes are thickened (e.g., diabetes mellitus, syphillis, edema), in association with intrauterine growth retardation, and in association with decreased blood volume or hemoglobin concentrations in the placental exchange vessels. However, none of these clinical associations have been established.

Maternal and Fetal O$_2$ Partial Pressures

Both theoretical and experimental studies suggest that placental O$_2$ exchange is particularly sensitive to changes in maternal or fetal arterial O$_2$ tensions. Decreases in maternal arterial Po$_2$ to ~70 torr appear to have little effect on placental O$_2$ exchange and fetal oxygenation, since this would decrease [HbO$_2$] only

~5%. Above ~70 torr the oxyhemoglobin saturation curve is relatively flat and oxyhemoglobin remains saturated. However, a decrease in maternal arterial Po$_2$ below this value results in decreased amounts of O$_2$ crossing to the fetus (15). Contrariwise, raising maternal arterial Po$_2$ to ~600 torr by breathing 100% O$_2$ will slightly increase the amount of O$_2$ in maternal blood and will increase fetal umbilical venous O$_2$ tension by 3–5 torr. Although probably of little value under normal circumstances, such an increase in fetal blood O$_2$ tension may be of great benefit in instances of fetal hypoxemia.

Fetal arterial O$_2$ tensions also influence placental O$_2$ exchange, with the amount of such exchange varying inversely with the umbilical arterial Po$_2$ value (1). Of course, fetal arterial Po$_2$ is in turn a function of transplacental O$_2$ exchange, umbilical venous Po$_2$, and the rate of fetal O$_2$ consumption.

Umbilical venous O$_2$ tension is normally 10–15 torr less than that of the uterine venous blood (Table 1) (2). The blood-gas values shown in Table 1 are based on studies in chronically catheterized sheep and monkeys, as well as being based on recent human data obtained by puncture of the umbilical cord under ultrasonic guidance (cordocentesis). Nonetheless, many of the data presented and discussed are derived from studies in experimental laboratory animals. A number of factors could theoretically affect placental O$_2$ exchange and could account for the O$_2$ tension difference between uterine and umbilical venous blood. Such factors include (a) the geometric relation of fetal vessels to maternal blood in the exchange area, (b) placental shunts in which uterine or umbilical arterial blood enters the venous circulation without traversing the exchange areas, and (c) nonuniform or uneven distribution of maternal and fetal blood flow in localized regions of the placenta. Such maternal–fetal perfusion inequalities could act as an effective shunt and could account for the uterine–umbilical O$_2$ tension difference (6,16).

Maternal and Fetal Blood O$_2$ Affinity and Capacity

Hemoglobin in maternal blood contributes considerably to placental O$_2$ transfer. The reduced form of hemoglobin binds with O$_2$ to form oxyhemoglobin. Because this binding is reversible, hemoglobin can unload O$_2$ to diffuse across the placenta as the O$_2$ partial pressure decreases. The ability of hemoglobin to bind oxygen depends not only upon the Po$_2$ but also upon the hemoglobin–O$_2$ affinity, as indicated by the sigmoid-shaped oxyhemoglobin saturation curve.

The P_{50} describes the O$_2$ partial pressure required to half-saturate hemoglobin. Under standard conditions (pH = 7.40, Pco$_2$ = 40 torr, 37°C) the P_{50} for normal adult human blood, including that of the pregnant mother, is 26.5 torr (Fig. 1). The curve is shifted to the right (i.e., lowered O_2 affinity) in association with increased concentrations of CO_2, hydrogen ion (H^+), 2,3-diphosphoglycerate (2,3-DPG), adenosine triphosphate, and/or chloride ion. In many species, but not all, the fetal oxyhemoglobin saturation curve is shifted to the left as compared to that of maternal blood. The P_{50} for fetal blood near term is about 20 torr (Fig. 1). Under physiologic conditions *in vivo* the maternal curve is shifted to the left (pH = 7.42, P_{CO_2} = 34 torr) while that of the fetus is shifted to the right (pH = 7.35, P_{CO_2} = 45 torr, T = 37.5°C), so that they are, in fact, almost superimposed (Fig. 1).

Blood oxygen capacity is the maximum amount of O_2 that can reversibly bind with hemoglobin. With a hemoglobin concentration of 14 g/dl the nonpregnant woman has a blood O_2 capacity of ~19 g/dl ([Hb] $\times$ 1.36). During the course of gestation a physiologic hemodilution occurs: Plasma volume increases ~50% while erythrocyte mass increases ~25% (17). Thus, near term the maternal hemoglobin concentration decreases to ~11.5 g/dl, with an O_2 capacity of 15.6 g/dl (18). In humans, fetal hemoglobin concentration increases from 8.5 g/dl at 10 weeks' gestation to a mean value of 16.5 g/dl at term (19). Thus, during the last third of gestation the fetal blood O_2 capacity exceeds that of the mother.

As noted above, *in vivo* the maternal and fetal O_2 saturation curves are probably superimposed. Figure 2 shows maternal and fetal blood O_2 content as a function of O_2 partial pressure. This illustrates that a normal fetal umbilical venous P_{O_2} of only ~28 torr is associated with an O_2 content of 15.5 ml/dl, a value as great as the maternal O_2 content of 15.4 ml/dl. Thus, despite the fetal hemoglobin being only ~75% saturated compared to ~98% in the adult, its greater hemoglobin concentration allows for a higher O_2 content. The maternal and fetal blood oxyhemoglobin saturations have important implications for placental O_2 transfer. An increase of either maternal or fetal O_2 capacity will promote placental O_2 exchange (1,20). Other factors remaining constant, the larger the sum of maternal and fetal blood O_2 capacity, the greater the O_2 exchange before equilibration of P_{O_2} values in these bloodstreams is reached.

Bohr and Haldane Effects

As maternal and fetal blood course through placental exchange vessels, H^+ and CO_2 diffuse from fetal blood across the placenta so that maternal blood becomes more acidotic and hypercarbic, shifting the oxyhemoglobin saturation curve to the right and thereby increasing the O_2 available for transfer. At the same time, the fetal curve is shifted to the left, thereby promoting O_2 uptake by the fetal erythrocytes. Theoretical studies suggest that this mechanism, the so-called "Bohr effect," accounts for ~8% of placental O_2 exchange (21).

As a consequence of this exchange process, deox-

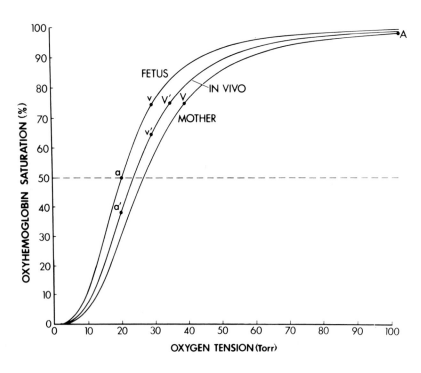

FIG. 1. HbO$_2$ saturation curves for human maternal and near-term fetal blood. Maternal and fetal HbO$_2$ affinities (P_{50}) are 26.5 and 20 torr, respectively. *A* and *V,* maternal arterial and venous values, respectively, under standard conditions; *a* and *v,* umbilical arterial and venous values, respectively; *V', a',* and *v',* probable *in vivo* maternal venous, umbilical arterial, and umbilical venous values, respectively.

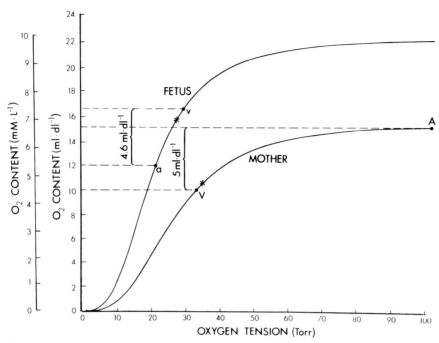

FIG. 2. Blood O_2 content as a function of P_fO_2 for maternal hemoglobin (12 g/dl) and P_{50} (26.5 torr) and for near-term fetal hemoglobin (16.5 g/dl) and P_{50} (20 torr). *Asterisks,* mean maternal and fetal PO_2; *A* and *V,* maternal arterial and venous values; *a* and *v,* umbilical arterial and venous values.

yhemoglobin concentration increases in the maternal placental blood, while decreasing in that of the fetus. Because deoxyhemoglobin binds CO_2 to a greater extent than oxyhemoglobin, CO_2 exchange from fetal to maternal blood is augmented. In fact, this so-called "Haldane effect" is calculated to account for ~46% of placental CO_2 exchange (21).

Maternal and Fetal Placental Blood Flow

To a great extent, placental O_2 and CO_2 exchange depend upon the rates of uterine and umbilical blood flows. During the course of gestation, uteroplacental blood flow increases from very little to 700–1000 ml/min at term (22,23); 80–90% of this flow supplies the placenta and is thus available for O_2 and nutrient transfer to the fetus. In the human, maternal blood from uterine spiral arteries enters the intervillous space and is diverted toward the placental villi. After bathing fetal vessels contained in the villi, uterine blood spreads laterally into the uterine venous sinuses. Experiments in the monkey (24), sheep (25), and other species indicate that placental O_2 exchange varies as a function of uterine blood flow.

The role of uterine blood flow on placental O_2 exchange and fetal oxygenation has obvious clinical im-

plications. For example, uteroplacental blood flow is reduced during the uterine contractions of labor, and this is associated with transient decreases in O_2 transfer to the fetus (2). In addition, blood flow may be decreased in women with vascular disease or hypertensive disorders of pregnancy. Fetal O_2 transfer is highly dependent upon the rate of uterine blood flow (1,26,27).

As with uteroplacental blood flow, the importance of umbilical flow on placental O_2 exchange is difficult to assess because of compensatory changes in other factors that affect such flow. In an effort to minimize this problem, Power and Jenkins (15) perfused *in situ* an isolated cotyledon of the sheep placenta with blood of known O_2 tension, O_2 content, and O_2 flow rate. Thus, these investigators demonstrated the dependence of venous outflow O_2 tension and the rate of O_2 transfer of fetal cotyledonary blood flow. Outflow O_2 tension varied inversely with the cotyledonary flow rate, whereas the O_2 exchange rate increased with increased blood flow (15).

In most vascular beds, blood flow is proportional to the hydrostatic pressure difference between arterial and venous vessels. However, in the placenta, because of the close association between maternal and fetal circulations, evidence suggests that increases in maternal placental blood volume may impinge upon fetal vessels in placental villi, thereby increasing the resistance of umbilical flow (28). Under such conditions, fetal placental blood flow would be proportional to the fetal inflow pressure minus the surrounding maternal placental blood pressure. Such a "sluice" or "waterfall" relation, in which the surrounding pressure affects vascular resistance, has been described in the lung. In addition, evidence suggests that such a mechanism may also operate so that increases in fetal placental blood volume affect maternal placental flow (29,30). In a pregnant woman near term, in the supine position the gravid uterus may compress the inferior vena cava, impeding uterine venous outflow and causing intervillous space pressure to rise. Thus, fetal placental vessels would be compressed, thereby increasing the vascular resistance and decreasing the umbilical flow. Of course, fetal placental flow would

be restored once fetal arterial pressure increased sufficiently.

Maternal and Fetal Placental Oxygen Flow

Oxygen delivery to an organ equals the product of blood flow and blood O_2 content. In many respects, although not all, a given decrease in hemoglobin concentration has an effect similar to that of decreasing blood flow on O_2 delivery and exchange. In the maternal circulation, decreases in hemoglobin concentration may be compensated for by increases in uteroplacental blood flow. Figure 3 depicts how changes in uteroplacental blood flow and O_2 flow affect placental O_2 exchange.

For the fetus, similar principles apply (Fig. 4). How-

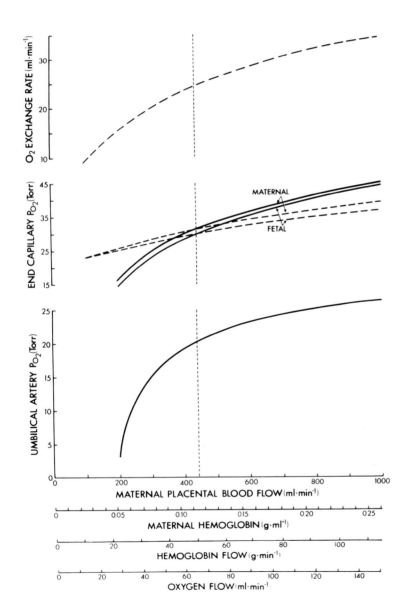

FIG. 3. Calculated effects of changes in maternal placental blood flow, in maternal hemoglobin, in hemoglobin flow, and in O_2 flow on transient maternal and fetal placental end-capillary Po_2 values and Vo_2 (*dashed lines*) and on steady-state end-capillary Po_2 values and fetal arterial Po_2 (*solid lines*).

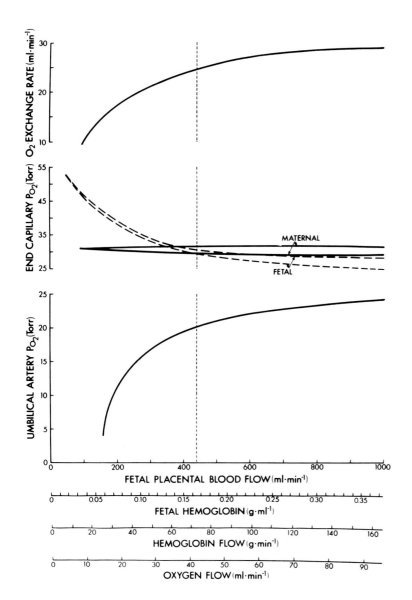

FIG. 4. Calculated effects of changes in fetal placental blood flow, in fetal hemoglobin, in hemoglobin flow, and in O_2 flow on transient maternal and fetal placental end-capillary P_{O_2} values and $\dot{V}_{O_2}$ (*dashed lines*) and on steady-state end-capillary P_{O_2} values and fetal arterial P_{O_2} (*solid lines*).

ever, the fetus has a limited ability to increase its already relatively high cardiac output, and thus its uteroplacental blood flow. Under some conditions of fetal hypoxia (31) or asphyxia (32), hemoglobin concentration increases, presumably as a result of water movement from the vascular to the extravascular compartment.

RESPIRATORY GAS EXCHANGE IN THE NEWBORN LUNG

An understanding of the events associated with the transition from respiratory gas exchange by the placenta to air breathing by the newborn requires a knowledge of lung development, the associated synthesis of pulmonary surfactant, the phenomenon of breathing movements by the fetus, the events associated with the first breath, and the establishment of breathing in the newborn infant. Because several of these topics are covered elsewhere, they will be considered only briefly here.

Prenatal Lung Development and Fetal Breathing

In humans, lung development may be considered in four stages: (i) the early embryonic period of the first 5 weeks, during which time the lung primordium undergoes epithelial proliferation and lobar buds appear; (ii) the glandular or pseudoglandular period extending to the 17th week, during which time bronchial segmentation, cartilage formation, and bronchial artery development occur; (iii) the canalicular period, from about the 13th to 25th weeks, during which time the primitive gas-exchange units, the respiratory bron-

TABLE 3. *Measurements on the newborn and adult human lung*

Variable	Newborn	Adult
Body weight (kg)	3.5	70
Surface area (m²)	0.21	1.90
Lung weight (g)	50	800
Tracheal diameter (mm)	8	18
Bronchiole diameter (mm)	0.1	0.2
Number of airways ($\times 10^6$)	1.5	14.0
Alveolar diameter (m)	50–100	200–300
Alveolar surface area (m²)	4	80
Number of alveoli ($\times 10^6$)	24	296
Total lung capacity (ml/kg)	63	82
Inspiratory capacity (ml/kg)	33	52
Vital capacity (ml/kg)	35	66
Functional residual capacity (ml/kg)	30	34
Dead space (ml/kg)	2.2	2.2
Tidal volume (ml/kg)	6	7
Closing volume (ml/kg)	12	7
Respiratory rate at rest	40	20
Alveolar ventilation (ml/kg·min)	100–150	60
Oxygen consumption at rest (ml/kg·min)	6	3
Compliance, total (liters/cmH₂O·liters lung volume)	0.03	0.03
Compliance, chest wall (liters/cmH₂O·liters lung volume)	0.26	0.06
Compliance, lung tissue (liters/cmH₂O·liters lung volume)	0.055	0.06
O₂ cost (% of O₂ consumption)	6	2

[a] Adapted from refs. 54–56.

chioles, emerge; and (iv) the terminal air sac period, beginning at the 24th week, with development of alveolar ducts or saccules and some alveoli. During this latter period (the so-called "viable stage"), the epithelium in terminal air spaces flattens and the type II cells or granular pneumocytes appear. Postnatally, the alveoli increase in both number and size (Table 3). For instance, at birth there are only about 20×10^6 alveoli, as contrasted with about 300×10^6 in the adult.

The near-term fetal lung is fluid-filled, containing ~20 ml/kg, which is about equivalent to functional residual capacity (33). Lung volume is a function of this fluid volume. During the third trimester of gestation, this lung fluid flows via the trachea into the pharynx, where most is expelled into the amniotic fluid and some is swallowed. From studies in chronically catheterized near-term fetal animals, the rate of such fluid flow averages 17 ± 2 ml/hr and the rate increases in association with low-voltage, high-frequency, rapid-eye-movement-like electroencephalographic (EEG) activity (34). Rather than representing an ultrafiltrate of fetal plasma, this lung fluid is actively secreted, and in comparison to plasma its pH is 6.43, its [HCO₃⁻] is 2.8 mEq, and its protein is 27 mg/dl (35). At the time of normal vaginal delivery, roughly one-third of this fluid is squeezed out of the mouth and nose, one-third

is absorbed by the pulmonary lymphatics, and the balance is absorbed by the capillaries (36).

As noted above, beginning at about the 24th week of gestation the type II alveolar epithelial cells appear. These pneumocytes contain an abundance of large lamellar inclusions rich in acid phosphatase. They also contain surfactant, a lipoprotein complex, the principal lipid of which is 2-phosphatidylcholine, or lecithin. By the 32nd week of gestation, phosphatidylglycerol and lecithin concentrations rise, whereas those of phosphatidylinositol and sphingomyelin decrease. The developmental pattern of these lipids constitutes a lung "profile" from which strong inferences regarding the degree of fetal maturation can be made (37). The surface-tension-lowering properties of pulmonary surfactant help in establishing the air–liquid interface and stabilize expiratory lung volume (functional residual capacity), which is important for establishing the lung as a functional organ postnatally.

The occurrence of respiratory-like activity by the fetus has been recognized since the late 19th century. Only in recent years, however, has it become appreciated that such fetal "breathing" is a normal phenomenon. In near-term humans and sheep it is episodic (occurring 40–50% of the time) and is influenced by a number of factors (38). In the sheep, but not in humans, it is associated with rapid eye movements and low-voltage, high-frequency EEG activity; this species difference probably occurs because of a less mature central nervous system in the term human fetus. The regulation of fetal "breathing," as well as its role in the preparation for extrauterine existence, has received considerable attention.

Pulmonary Circulation and the Changes at Birth

During the course of fetal development, the pulmonary vascular tree grows in concert with the ventilatory apparatus and the rest of the lung. In the near-term sheep fetus the cardiac output (combined right and left ventricles) equals about 500 ml/min/kg, with the right ventricle contributing ~60% (39–41). The lungs receive about 3–4% of right ventricular output, with the balance being shunted through the ductus arteriosus (39). Maintenance of the relatively high pulmonary vascular resistance is thought to be due to (a) relatively low arterial O₂ tension and (b) vasoconstrictors such as the leukotrienes C₄ and D₄, which are arachidonic acid metabolites synthesized through the lipoxygenase pathway.

At birth a number of events occur almost simultaneously. The umbilical circulation ceases rather abruptly, systemic arterial pressure rises, and with lung expansion the pressure in the pulmonary bed falls. For a varying period the central circulation is in a state of transition with continued patency of both the foramen ovale and ductus arteriosus. Over a period of hours to days (depending on maturity at birth and the state of health) these two shunts gradually decrease. Foramen ovale closure results largely from hydrostatic pressure changes; this is because with umbilical circulating arrest, less blood returns to the right side of the heart while at the same time relatively more returns to the left atrium via the pulmonary veins. The mechanism of closure of the ductus arteriosus is more complex. Considerable evidence indicates that *in utero* ductus patency is maintained, at least in part, by the vasodilatory prostaglandins PGE_2 and PGI_2, which are cyclo-oxygenase-mediated products of arachidonic metabolism (42,43). With birth, there appears to be a shift in the balance of the vasodilatory–vasoconstrictor eicosanoids; furthermore in conjunction with increased O_2 tensions, a change in the balance of endothelium-derived constricting versus relaxing factors, and other phenomena, the ductus arteriosus gradually closes.

Respiration at Birth

For the pulmonologist, birth may be considered the process wherein the lung liquid is replaced by air as the fetus emerges as a newborn infant. The success of this transition is essential for fulfillment of one's potential as a person. The inspiratory gasp shortly following birth is believed to result from the combination of (a) the sudden release of pressure on the squeezed head and chest, (b) tactile stimuli, (c) exposure to a cooler environment, and (d) the partial asphyxia associated with a decrease in arterial P_{O_2} and increase in P_{CO_2} which stimulate central and peripheral chemoreceptors. Following the first few gasps, respiration becomes regular and rhythmic. With increased neuronal traffic the respiratory center assumes a greater role in regulation, the carotid body becomes sensitive to O_2 tensions less than 60 torr, and central chemoreceptors respond to increased P_{CO_2} values (44). Lung inflation and deflation become influenced by the Hering–Breuer reflex, and the regulation of respiration in the infant is essentially the same as that of the adult.

Factors Affecting Pulmonary O_2 and CO_2 Exchange

Because the factors that affect O_2 and CO_2 exchange in the newborn lung are essentially those of the adult, we will consider chiefly those instances in which they differ.

Rather than being a replica in miniature of the adult lung, the lung of the newborn differs in many regards (Table 3). Because of the newborn's relatively greater mass of highly metabolizing organs such as brain, and also because of its relatively smaller mass of more slowly metabolizing bone and fat, the basal O_2 consumption rate of the newborn equals 6–8 ml/min/kg (i.e., twice that of an adult on a per-kilogram basis); moreover, the newborn can increase its rate of O_2 consumption to 12–15 ml/min/kg when crying. With a pulmonary compliance about equal to that of an adult, the basal O_2 cost of breathing in a healthy infant in a warm environment is about 1.8 ml O_2 per liter of ventilation (45)—that is, about 6% of total O_2 consumption, as compared with 2% in the adult under comparable circumstances. This difference is mostly attributed to the almost twofold greater alveolar ventilation (Table 3) and the unsteady character of breathing in the newborn. Following the first minute or two of respiration, alveolar ventilation is relatively well distributed in the newborn as compared with the adult (46), probably because gravitational forces are less. For the same reason, the variation in blood flow to different parts of the lung, with respect to their height relative to the heart (47), is probably less in the newborn. This may be particularly so when pulmonary arterial pressure is high shortly after birth.

From a mechanical standpoint, pulmonary function of the newborn differs little from that of the adult. Nonetheless, the newborn's chest wall is relatively unstable, resulting in mechanical differences. For instance, the newborn infant's chest wall compliance is relatively great and its functional residual capacity is low (Table 3). With its normal relatively low tidal volume (near the airway closing volume), the infant compensates with tachypnea. With relative thoracic wall instability, the infant engages in diaphragmatic and/or paradoxical respiration. Thus, under these circumstances any disease that decreases lung compliance can result in chest wall collapse.

Important differences between newborns and adults exist with regard to ventilatory regulation. In response to hypoxia, hyperpnea in both the mature (48) and premature (49) newborn is sustained for only a few minutes, unlike that in the adult. This hyperpnea varies with environmental temperature, being abolished in a cold environment. By 3 days of age, hypoxia-induced hyperpnea is maintained (50). The cause of this biphasic response in the newborn may result from metabolic and endocrine differences, but this is not established.

Newborn respiratory responses to CO_2 and combined hypercapnea and hypoxia are similar to those of the adult (50). Exposure to a cold environment stimulates newborn breathing (51), presumably because of augmented sensory input. In general, pulmonary reflexes are well developed in both mature and premature infants. For instance, Hering–Breuer inflation-deflation reflex is present in the newborn (52). The sensory mechanisms responsible for coughing or transient apnea on presentation of a noxious stimulus to the airways are also functional.

Asphyxia, analgesics, and anesthetics greatly impair pulmonary competence in the newborn. For instance, even light anesthesia decreases O_2 consumption during cold exposure. Small doses of analgesics reduce ventilatory response to CO_2. Progressive hypoxemia leads to deterioration with abrupt respiratory arrest. Comparison with the adult is difficult in these regards. On the one hand, the newborn can withstand stresses that might prove fatal to the adult. On the other hand, the newborn is extremely fragile and vulnerable to these stresses.

COMPARISON OF GAS EXCHANGE IN THE PLACENTA AND LUNG

Sir Joseph Barcroft first explored the question of how respiratory gas exchange in the placenta compares with that of the lung, estimating that the lung is "... perhaps twenty times as efficient or more"(53). Of course, the outcome of such a comparison will vary depending upon the function being compared. Table 4 presents comparative values for several measures of placental and infant pulmonary respiratory gas exchange and blood flow.

Despite the similar weights of these organs, 10- to 20-fold more O_2 is exchanged per minute in the lungs than in the term placenta, in rough accord with the mass of organism supplied. Although in the lungs O_2 consumption by parenchymal tissue is an insignificant fraction of the total quantity exchanged, at term 20–50% or more of the O_2 derived from maternal blood is consumed by placental tissue before it reaches the fetus (4). In both organs, O_2 and CO_2 exchange mutually enhance one another; moreover, the placenta shows double Bohr and Haldane effects because these reactions occur in both maternal and fetal blood.

Both organs receive a generous blood supply. However, in the placenta 20–36% of flow functionally bypasses gas-exchange sites, a fraction much larger than that in the lung. Although some of the placental shunt may be anatomical, probably most is physiologic, analogous to the nonuniform ventilation–perfusion distribution in the lung. Both organs have flow characterized by a sluice or waterfall phenomenon. Although the pulmonary circulation displays active and precise

TABLE 4. *Comparisons of blood flow and gas exchange in placenta and lungs*[a]

Variable	Placenta	Lungs
CO diffusing capacity (ml/min·torr)	1.81	25
CO diffusing capacity (ml/min·torr·kg body wt)	0.60	0.42
CO diffusing capacity (ml/min·torr·kg organ wt)	3.6	42
O_2 diffusing capacity (liters/min·torr)	2.3	30
Mean alveolar–pulmonary capillary P_{O_2} difference (torr)		8
Mean maternal–fetal placental P_{O_2} difference (torr)	8	
O_2 transfer rate (ml/min)	24	300
O_2 transfer per unit blood flow (ml/min)	6	54
Tissue O_2 consumption and CO_2 production	Significant	Insignificant
Interaction of O_2 and CO_2	Double Bohr and double Haldane effects	Bohr and Haldane effects
Fixed acid transfer	Significant	Insignificant
Blood flow (% of cardiac output)	45	100
Distribution	Uneven maternal flow/fetal flow	Uneven ventilation/blood flow
Shunt (%)	20	2
Type of flow	Sluice (maternal vascular pressure surrounding fetal capillaries)	Sluice (alveolar pressure surrounding pulmonary capillaries)
Regulation	Unknown	Active and precise

[a] From ref. 2.

regulation, the regulation of maternal and fetal placental blood flows remains poorly understood.

Another question concerns the relative efficiency of placental O_2 exchange. A large exchange surface with a small barrier (as expressed by the D_p) is advantageous for substrate exchange. In addition, both a uniform distribution of maternal-to-fetal placental flow and a countercurrent flow pattern optimize exchange. Placental "efficiency" may be considered from several points of view—for example, the magnitude of the degree of arterialization of umbilical venous blood, the maternal–fetal venous P_{CO_2} and P_{CO_2} differences, the umbilical arterial–venous P_{O_2} difference, and the percentage of O_2 extracted from maternal arterial blood. Until relatively recently, the placenta was believed to be optimally designed to facilitate respiratory gas exchange. We now appreciate, however, that the vascular architecture is not arranged most efficiently, that O_2 consumption and CO_2 production occur in the regions of gas transfer, and that inhomogeneities of several types introduce further inefficiency. Although it was previously thought that the membranes separating maternal and fetal blood were a significant barrier to diffusion, we now realize that these tissues constitute only a minor resistance to exchange.

Formerly, the placenta was considered as a glorified sieve separating the fetus from the mother. It now is understood to perform complex metabolic syntheses in the interplay of hormones between the two organisms and to serve other metabolic and immunologic functions as vital as respiratory gas exchange. Finally, it is designed for rapid growth during a relatively brief lifespan. In view of the diversity of placental morphologic types and vascular arrangements in the various mammalian species, it is evident that a wide divergence of architecture is compatible with similar physiologic functions. None of this new information denies the fact that the respiratory function of the placenta is of critical importance for optimal fetal development. It does, however, suggest that the respiratory function may be a subsidiary consideration in the design of the placenta.

ACKNOWLEDGMENTS

I thank Brenda Kreutzer for helping to prepare this manuscript. This work was supported by USPHS grant HD-03807.

REFERENCES

1. Longo LD, Hill EP, Power GG. Theoretical analysis of factors affecting placental O_2 transfer. *Am J Physiol* 1972;22:730–739.
2. Longo LD. Respiratory gas exchange in the placenta. In: Fishman AP, Farhi LE, Tenney SM, eds. *Handbook of physiology, Section 3: The respiratory system, vol IV—Gas exchange.* Washington, DC: American Physiological Society, 1987;351–401.
3. Longo LD, Power GG, Forster RE II. Respiratory function of the placenta as determined with carbon monoxide in sheep and dogs. *J Clin Invest* 1967;46:812–828.
4. Meschia G, Battaglia FC, Hay WW Jr, et al. Utilization of substrates by the ovine placenta *in vivo. Fed Proc* 1980;39:245–249.
5. Longo LD, Power GG. Analysis of P_{O_2} and P_{CO_2} differences between maternal and fetal blood in the placenta. *J Appl Physiol* 1969;26:48–55.
6. Power GG, Longo LD, Wagner HN Jr, et al. Uneven distribution of maternal and fetal placental blood flow, as demonstrated using macroaggregates, and its response to hypoxia. *J Clin Invest* 1967;46:2053–2063.
7. Power GG, Hill EP, Longo LD. Analysis of uneven distribution of diffusing capacity and blood flow in the placenta. *Am J Physiol* 1972;222:740–746.
8. Bissonnette JM, Longo LD, Novy MJ, et al. Placental diffusing capacity and its relation to fetal growth. *J Dev Physiol* 1979;1:351–359.
9. Bissonnette JM, Wickham WK. Placental diffusing capacity for carbon monoxide in unanesthetized guinea pigs. *Respir Physiol* 1977;31:161–168.
10. Gilbert RD, Cummings LA, Jachau MR, et al. Placental diffusing capacity and fetal development in exercising or hypoxic guinea pigs. *J Appl Physiol* 1979;46:828–834.
11. Longo LD, Ching K. Placental diffusing capacity for carbon monoxide and oxygen in unanesthetized sheep. *J Appl Physiol* 1977;43:885–893.
12. Bacon BJ, Gilbert RD, Kaufmann P, et al. Placental anatomy and diffusing capacity in guinea pigs following long-term maternal hypoxia. *Placenta* 1984;5:465–488.
13. Nelson PS, Gilbert RD, Longo LD. Fetal growth and placental diffusing capacity in guinea pigs following long-term maternal exercise. *J Dev Physiol* 1983;5:1–10.
14. Smith AD, Gilbert RD, Lammers RJ, et al. Placental exchange area in guinea pigs following long-term maternal exercise: a stereological analysis. *J Dev Physiol.* 1983;5:11–21.
15. Power GG, Jenkins F. Factors affecting O_2 transfer in the sheep and rabbit placenta perfused *in situ. Am J Physiol* 1975; 229:1147–1153.
16. Power GG, Dale PS, Nelson PS. Distribution of maternal and fetal blood flow within cotyledons of the sheep placenta. *Am J Physiol* 1981;241:H486–H496.
17. Longo LD, Hardesty JS. Maternal blood volume: measurement, hypothesis of control, and clinical considerations. *Rev Perinat Med* 1984;5:35–59.
18. Pritchard JA, Hunt CF. A comparison of the hematologic responses following the routine prenatal administration of intramuscular and oral iron. *Surg Gynecol Obstet* 1958;106:516–518.
19. Oski TA. Hematological problems. In: Avery GB, ed. *Neonatology. Pathophysiology and management of the newborn.* Philadelphia: JB Lippincott, 1975;379–422.
20. Bartels H. *Prenatal respiration.* Amsterdam: North-Holland, 1970.
21. Hill EP, Power GG, Longo LD. A mathematical model of carbon dioxide transfer in the placenta and its interaction with oxygen. *Am J Physiol* 1973;224:283–299.
22. Assali NS, Douglas RA Jr, Baird WW, et al. Measurements of uterine blood flow and uterine metabolism. IV. Results in normal pregnancy. *Am J Obstet Gynecol* 1953;66:248–253.
23. Metcalfe J, Romney SL, Ramsey LH, et al. Estimation of uterine blood flow in normal human pregnancy at term. *J Clin Invest* 1955;34:1632–1638.
24. Parer JT, de Lannoy CW, Hoversland AS, et al. Effect of decreased uterine blood flow on uterine oxygen consumption in pregnant macaques. *Am J Obstet Gynecol* 1968;100:813–820.
25. Fuller EO, Manning MW, Nutter DO, et al. A perfused uterine preparation for the study of uterine and fetal physiology. In: Longo LD, Reneau DD, eds. *Fetal and newborn cardiovascular physiology, vol 2: Fetal and newborn circulation.* New York: Garland Press, 1978;421–435.
26. Clapp JF III. The relationship between blood flow and oxygen

uptake in the uterine and umbilical circulations. *Am J Obstet Gynecol* 1978;132:410–413.

27. Dawes GS, Mott JC. Changes in O₂ distribution and consumption in foetal lambs with variations in umbilical blood flow. *J Physiol (Lond)* 1964;170:524–540.

28. Power GG, Longo LD. Sluice flow in placenta: maternal vascular pressure effects on fetal circulation. *Am J Physiol* 1973;225:1490–1496.

29. Cottle MKW, Van Petten GR, Van Muyden P. Depression of uterine blood flow in response to cord compression in sheep. *Can J Physiol Pharmacol* 1982;60:825–829.

30. Hasaart THM, De Haan J. Depression of uterine blood flow during total umbilical cord occlusion in sheep. *Eur J Obstet Gynecol Reprod Biol* 1985;19:125–131.

31. Born GVR, Dawes GS, Mott JC. Oxygen lack and autonomic nervous control of the foetal circulation in the lamb. *J Physiol (Lond)* 1956;134:149–166.

32. Adamsons K, Beard RW, Myers RE. Comparison of the composition of arterial, venous, and capillary blood of the fetal monkey during labor. *Am J Obstet Gynecol* 1970;107:435–440.

33. Avery ME, Cook CD. Volume–pressure relationships of lungs and thorax in fetal, newborn, and adult goats. *J Appl Physiol* 1961;16:1034–1038.

34. Dickson KA, Maloney JE, Berger PJ. State-related changes in lung liquid secretion and tracheal flow rate in fetal lambs. *J Appl Physiol* 1987;62:34–38.

35. Adamson TM, Boyd RDH, Platt HS, et al. Composition of alveolar liquid in the foetal lamb. *J Physiol (Lond)* 1969;204:159–168.

36. Humphreys PW, Normand ICS, Reynolds EOR, et al. Pulmonary lymph flow and the uptake of liquid from lungs of the lamb at the start of breathing. *J Physiol (Lond)* 1967;193:1–29.

37. Kulovich MV, Hallman MB, Gluck L. The lung profile. I. Normal pregnancy. *Am J Obstet Gynecol* 1979;135:57–63.

38. Koos BJ. Central stimulation of breathing movements in fetal lambs by prostaglandin synthetase inhibitors. *J Physiol (Lond)* 1985;362:455–466.

39. Anderson DV, Bissonnette JM, Faber JJ, et al. Central shunt flows and pressures in the mature fetal lamb. *Am J Physiol* 1981;241:H60–H66.

40. Gilbert RD. Control of fetal cardiac output during changes in blood volume. *Am J Physiol* 1980;238:H80–H86.

41. Rudolph AM, Heymann MA. Circulatory changes during growth in the fetal lamb. *Circ Res* 1970;26:289–299.

42. Cassin S, Winikor I, Tod M, et al. Effects of prostacyclin on the fetal pulmonary circulation. *Pediatr Pharmacol* 1981;1:197–207.

43. Tripp ME, Heymann MA, Rudolph AM. Prostaglandin E₁ and pulmonary vascular resistance in neonatal lambs. *Pediatr Res* 1977;11:401.

44. Blanco CE, Dawes GS, Hanson MA, et al. The response to hypoxia of arterial chemoreceptors in fetal sheep and new-born lambs. *J Physiol (Lond)* 1984;351:25–37.

45. Thibeault DW, Clutario B, Auld PAM. The oxygen cost of breathing in the premature infant. *Pediatrics* 1966;37:954–959.

46. Nelson NM. Neonatal pulmonary function. *Pediatr Clin North Am* 1966;13:769–799.

47. West JB. *Ventilation/blood flow and gas exchange.* Oxford: Blackwell Scientific Publications, 1965.

48. Cross KW, Warner P. The effect of inhalation of high and low oxygen concentrations in the respiration of the newborn infant. *J Physiol (Lond)* 1951;114:238–295.

49. Cross KW, Oppé TE. The effect of inhalation of high and low concentrations of oxygen on the respiration of the premature infant. *J Physiol (Lond)* 1952;177:38–55.

50. Brady JP, Ceruti E. Chemoreceptor reflexes in the new-born infant: effects of varying degrees of hypoxia on heart rate and ventilation in a warm environment. *J Physiol* 1966;184:631–645.

51. Ceruti E. Chemoreceptor reflexes in the newborn infant: effect of cooling on the response to hypoxia. *Pediatrics* 1966;37:556–564.

52. Cross KW, Klaus M, Tooley WH, et al. The response of the new-born baby to inflation of the lungs. *J Physiol (Lond)* 1960;151:661–665.

53. Barcroft J. *The respiratory function of the blood. Part II. Haemoglobin.* Cambridge, England: Cambridge University Press, 1928;52.

54. Avery GB, ed. *Neonatology. Pathophysiology and management of the newborn,* 2nd ed. Philadelphia: JB Lippincott, 1981;158–159.

55. Dawes GS. *Foetal and neonatal physiology. A comparative study of the changes at birth.* Chicago, Year Book Publishers, 1968;185.

56. Smith CA, Nelson NM. *The physiology of the newborn infant,* 4th ed. Springfield, IL: Charles C Thomas, 1976;207.

THE LUNG: Scientific Foundations
edited by R.G. Crystal, J.B. West et al.
Raven Press, Ltd., New York © 1991.

CHAPTER 6.1.6

Control of Ventilation in the Neonate

Hugo Lagercrantz, Josef Milerad, and David Walker

Fetal breathing movements are episodic and are frequently interrupted by apnea which is related to high-voltage electrocortical activity. Although fetal breathing movements are influenced by CO_2, metabolic rate, and nutritional supply, fetal respiratory activity is more governed by behavioral and sleep states than by metabolism. After birth, breathing movements become continuous and are strongly affected by the carbon dioxide chemostat both in the term (1–3) and the prematurely born (4) infant. This transition of respiratory control could be due to increased firing activity in the rhythm-generating neurons in the medulla, increased respiratory drive inputs, disappearance of fetal inhibitory influences of breathing, or a combination of these mechanisms. Before these possibilities can be discussed we have to consider whether there are any major structural changes of the bulbopontine neurons controlling respiration or whether the relative importance of the various drive mechanisms changes during development until the mature pattern is established.

DEVELOPMENT OF NEURONAL NETWORK CONTROLLING RESPIRATION

In the newborn the brainstem is relatively more mature than the more rostral brain structures. Neuronal pathways and neurotransmitter systems develop in a caudocranial direction. The neurons constituting the bulbopontine respiratory control system are probably formed during the proliferative phase at an early fetal stage—in the human, between the 10th and 20th gestational week. However, the differentiation of central

respiratory neurons, accompanied by the formation of the respiratory neuronal network, probably also occurs to a large extent during the neonatal period (5,6).

There is a redundancy of neurons during early fetal life, and about half of the neurons disappear by programmed cell death (7,8). There is also an overgrowth of dendrites, dendritic spines, and synapses, which become more structured during the neonatal period (9).

The development of the dendritic arrangement in respiratory-related areas in the medulla in 5- to 60-day-old mice has been investigated by using Golgi electron microscopy and immunohistochemistry, combined with retrograde labeling with gold/fluorescent microspheres injected into phrenic motor neurons. Axons and dendrites were then reconstructed by three-dimensional computer-assisted contour analysis, and the spatial integration of respiratory groups could then be mapped (1,5). Most of the labeled phrenic motor neurons (61%) were found to terminate in the contralateral nucleus tractus solitarius (nTS), with the remaining ones terminating in equal numbers in the nucleus ambiguus and the reticular formation. By further use of these tools, the neuronal network controlling respiration in the neonate can be elucidated in further details.

In contrast to our knowledge of the neuronal network controlling respiration in adult mammals (10), much less is known about the structural organization of the central respiratory neurons in the human infant. The organization of the dendritic pathways and the formation of synapses are probably not complete at term and are consequently even less complete in the preterm infant. Neuronal immaturity has therefore been postulated to be the major cause of respiratory irregularity, often interrupted by short apnea, in the neonate (11,12). It has been estimated that to elicit an action potential in an intercostal motoneuron, the motoneuron has to receive excitatory inputs from at least 200 synapses from other nerves (11,13).

H. Lagercrantz and J. Milerad: Department of Pediatrics and the Nobel Institute for Neurophysiology, Karolinska Institute, S-104 01 Stockholm, Sweden.

D. Walker: Department of Physiology, Monash University, Melbourne, Victoriam Australia 3168.

The assumption that the immaturity of connectivity is involved in the genesis of apnea of prematurity is corroborated by the finding that there is a correlation between increased latency of brain auditory responses and the frequency of apnea in preterm infants (12). The latency of the brainstem auditory response is assumed to be related to the neuronal conductivity. Because the auditory pathways are localized closely to the central respiratory neurons, it can be assumed that there might be a parallelism between the maturation of the auditory pathways and the development of the stability of breathing.

CHEMICAL NEUROANATOMY

The neurotransmitters and neuromodulators controlling central respiratory activity are scarcely known in the adult (see Chapters 5.4.1–5.4.7) and even less so in the neonate. However, there are some neuromodulators that are transiently expressed in high concentrations during ontogeny, and this raises interesting questions as to their involvement in respiratory control in the fetus and the neonate (14).

Excitatory amino acids such as glutamate and aspartate increase the firing rate in respiratory neurons in the adult (15,16). The glutaminergic concentration is transiently very high in the human fetal brain, but it is lower in the brain of the newborn than in that of the adult (17). Aspartate has been found to occur in lower concentrations in the infant than in the adult (18). Inhibitory amino acids such as gamma-aminobutyric acid (GABA) and taurine seem to be expressed at an earlier stage than excitatory ones such as glutamate and aspartate (19).

Classical neurotransmitters such as serotonin and noradrenaline appear early during ontogeny (14). Noradrenergic neurons originating from the locus coeruleus sprout into the fetal rat cortex and brainstem, so that noradrenaline is transiently the dominating neurotransmitter in the brain (20). By increasing the postsynaptic noradrenaline concentration in the brain with tricyclic antidepressive and catecholamine-releasing drugs, continuous breathing can be triggered in the fetal sheep (21).

Some neuropeptides (e.g., somatostatin) are expressed in fairly high concentrations during early development and then disappear (22). Because somatostatin is a very potent respiratory inhibitory agent (23,24), somatostatin neurons might contribute to the inhibition of fetal breathing. However, since there is no specific somatostatin antagonist available, we do not know whether there is a tonic somatostatin inhibition.

Endogenous opioids have been suggested to suppress breathing tonically both in the fetus and the new-born, since naloxone was found to stimulate breathing at least in the exteriorized fetus (25,26). Also, naloxone was found to increase the fetal breathing response to CO_2 in sheep (27). Furthermore, met-enkephalin has been found in higher concentrations in respiratory nuclei in the brainstem in newborn rabbit pups as compared with older ones (28). However, there is some controversy as to whether endogenous opioids are really involved in the inhibition of eupneic breathing in the fetus and the neonate (29). In fetal sheep it was found that intracerebroventricular infusion of beta-endorphin did not change breathing movements (30).

Substance P is the most abundant neuropeptide in the nTS and has been suggested to be involved in the mediation of the hypoxic drive at both a peripheral and a central level (31). Substance P immunofluorescence-like activity is low in the carotid chemoreceptors of the newborn kitten but is more abundant after 2 weeks (32).

Each central respiratory neuron probably receives thousands of synapses that release many different kinds of neurotransmitters. Interneurons with endorphins, somatostatin, and other neuropeptides might modulate the effect of the more classical neurotransmitters. There are also nonsynaptic neuromodulators such as adenosine and prostaglandins, which have effects at a pre- or a postsynaptic level (Fig. 1).

There might be some dominance of inhibitory neuroactive agents terminating at the respiratory neurons before birth, possibly related to the lower fetal P_{O_2} (19). After birth there is both an immediate and a more long-term reorganization of the synapses with regard to neurotransmitter content, as reported by recent experiments in newborn rabbits (33).

Analysis of mRNA for substance P somatostatin and cholecystokinin by the Northern blot technique showed substantial increases of these neuropeptides in respiratory-related brain structures of the rabbit pup during the first 2 days of life as compared to the fetus (33). This pattern differed significantly from the expression of these neuropeptides in the striatum, which was used as the hybridizing control. This "switch on" of neuropeptides could be associated with birth and is possibly related to the postnatal increase in P_aO_2.

RESPIRATORY DRIVE MECHANISMS

Respiratory Rhythmic Generation

The exact locus where the respiratory rhythm is generated in the adult mammal is not known (10), in spite of a number of neurophysiological studies (34). By the use of a brainstem–spinal-cord preparation, respiratory-rhythm-generating neurons were detected in new-

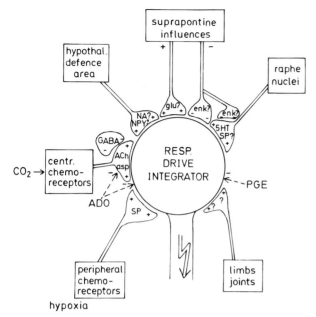

hypoxia

FIG. 1. Putative neurotransmitter and neuromodulators involved in the respiratory driving and inhibitory mechanisms, which, to a large extent, converge onto the nucleus paragigantocellularis lateralis and go from there to the dorsal and ventral respiratory groups in the medulla, where the central respiratory pattern is generated. Each neuron probably receives thousands of synapses. The neuropeptides occur in specific neurons, probably often coexisting with classical neurotransmitters. Neuromodulators such as adenosine (ADO) and prostaglandins (PGE) are formed more ubiquitously during, for example, hypoxia. Key: glu, glutamic acid; asp, aspartic acid; ACh, acetylcholine; NA, noradrenaline; 5-HT, 5-hydroxytryptamine or serotonin; enk, enkephalin; SP, substance P; NPY, neuropeptide Y.

born rat pups (0–5 days) (34,35). Spontaneously firing units were found in the rostral ventrolateral medulla; these appeared in bursts with the same rhythmic frequency as the nervous activity recorded from the C4 ventral root, which was shown to be related to respiration. The firing activity was found to precede inspiratory activity. The region seemed to correspond to the nucleus reticularis rostroventrolateralis (RVL) in the adult rat, which has been found to contain adrenaline neurons and which has been assumed to act as a tonic vasomotor center (36). After electrolytic lesion of this region, the respiratory rhythmic activity disappeared. Vagal afferent activity was not found to affect this respiratory rhythm generation.

The different types of respiratory-related neurons that may be present in the brainstem of newborn animals are not known in detail. However, some idea of the developmental changes that must occur can be assessed from the changes in respiratory pattern and timing. Inspiratory time increases with development in many species, from values of less than 100 msec to typical adult values of greater than 400 msec, depend-

ing on the species being examined (37–39). Spike discharge rate of phrenic and laryngeal motor neurons is low in the immature newborn kitten (40) and opossum (41). These observations suggest that there may be changes in the medulla which increase the internal connectivity of neurons and which allow greater local self-excitation of the inspiratory neuronal pool.

Medullary expiratory neurons have been shown to be tonically active in apneic and anesthetized fetal sheep (42). However, in lightly anesthetized air-breathing opossums, few expiratory neurons were found to be active at normal lung volumes, but there was increased activity when breathing was loaded by increasing the airway pressure by approximately 3 cmH$_2$O (43). Abdominal expiratory activity was not recruited in the smallest newborn opossum, but it occurred during loaded breathing in the 4th to 5th postnatal week (43). Firing rates of expiratory neurons increased with developmental age, as found previously for inspiratory neurons. These observations suggest that there is considerable postnatal development of the expiratory neuronal network in the brainstem, which occurs after the development of the inspiratory network. However, the expiratory responses prompted by lung inflation may be dependent on the development of afferent fibers in the lung.

Other observations indicate that mechanoreceptor activity in the lung is important in the maintenance of normal ventilation in the newborn—as shown by the disruption of breathing pattern in lambs after removal of end-expired pressure, accompanied by a sixfold increase of expiratory duration after vagotomy, in unanesthetized newborn rat pups (44). Vagotomy also increased inspiratory time (as expected) in these rat pups, but there was a fall in ventilation in pups <11 days old, whereas there was no change in adult rats (44). Thus, vagal afferent input from the very immature lung appears to provide a critical feedback to the brainstem maintaining normal breathing rhythm and tidal volume, although the mechanism by which expiratory time is modified is not clear. The number and diameter of myelinated vagal fibers increase after birth in several species (45,46), but the changes in the smaller-fiber populations in the lung have not been described.

Suprapontine Drives

Breathing is controlled by autonomic and voluntary mechanisms (Fig. 2). In the awake adult the forebrain drive overrides the metabolic or autonomic control of breathing (10). Respiration during wakefulness is therefore fairly irregular and can easily be modulated by sensory inputs. This is probably also true for the infant, although the periods of wakefulness are shorter.

The newborn term infant spends about 50% of the

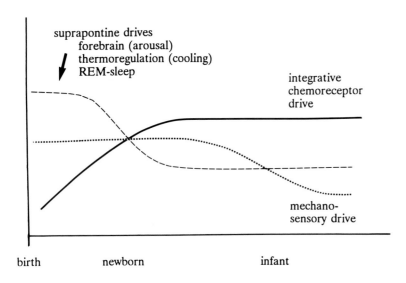

suprapontine drives
forebrain (arousal)
thermoregulation (cooling)
REM-sleep

integrative
chemoreceptor
drive

mechano-
sensory drive

birth   newborn   infant

FIG. 2. Schematic representation of the relative importance of different respiratory drive mechanisms after birth. Cooling of the skin and the increased arousal induced by labor and delivery are important for initiation of breathing at birth. Mechanosensory information constitutes a major drive to sustain regular and efficient breathing during the first few weeks of life. The importance of the peripheral chemoreceptor drive, as well as of the integration and modulation of various respiratory and nonrespiratory stimuli, increases after the newborn period. [Figure based on an original concept of P. Johnson, Oxford University (1984).]

time in active sleep corresponding to rapid eye movement (REM) sleep. Preterm infants do so even more, although the sleep states are not so well organized. The increased neuronal activity in the brainstem reticular system during REM sleep seems to have a profound effect on respiration. This activity is the main drive of fetal respiratory movements (see Chapter 6.1.1) and is probably also of importance to sustain breathing in the infant. If a preterm baby is hyperventilating slightly during artificial ventilation, spontaneous breathing ceases during quiet sleep (non-REM sleep) but is sustained during REM sleep in spite of low P_{CO_2} (47).

However, breathing during REM sleep is, to some extent, less efficient. As a result of a decrease in the intercostal muscle tone there are periods of paradoxical respiration with chest and abdominal excursions out of phase (48). The percentage of inward rib cage motion decreases over the first few months of life (49). The stability of upper airways is lower in REM sleep (see below), and the cyclic fluctuations in the depth and rate of breathing are often in phase during active sleep. The simultaneous decrease in respiratory rate and tidal volume may lead to periods of hypoventilation (50).

A diurnal rhythm in breathing is present before birth in the human and sheep. This might be a true circadian rhythm (i.e., of suprachiasmatic origin), since it persists after removal of diurnal variation of plasma nutrients such as glucose (51) as well as after removal of the maternal (and fetal) nocturnal rise of plasma melatonin (52). However, the time of the rise and fall in incidence of fetal breathing movements during the day and night is altered after maternal pinealectomy, indicating that maternal melatonin may provide the fetal brain with information about the time of day. These observations have importance for the understanding of the response of infants to the day/night cycle. Circa-

dian variation of plasma prolactin and temperature are present from birth in lambs and in the human neonate.

Hypothalamic input to the central respiratory neurons is probably also important for the infant. Fetal lambs show a panting response to increased core temperature (53,54), and tachypnea has been reported in the human fetus during maternal fever. These observations suggest that hypothalamic mechanisms which increase ventilation are developed before birth. Also, fetal lambs respond to surface cooling by onset of shivering accompanied by a switch of pattern from discontinuous to continuous breathing (55), demonstrating the prenatal development of temperature-sensitive mechanisms in the brain.

Karlberg (56) found that the breathing of newborn babies delivered by cesarean section became shallower and sometimes ceased when they were immersed in warm water, but their breathing started again immediately when they were removed from the bath. This confirms the importance of skin temperature receptors in providing a potent drive to breathing in the perinatal period (see below), although it is not clear whether the absolute skin temperature, the skin-to-core temperature difference, and the sensation of surface cooling or warming (i.e., rate of change of temperature) are each important in respiratory effects. It has been noted that the incidence of apnea in premature infants is greater during increases of incubator air temperature, indicating (a) a dynamic sensitivity by the infant to ambient temperatures and (b) a risk of inadvertent, transient increases of temperature to the newborn (57). It has also been suggested that hyperthermia may permit reflex laryngeal closure in the newborn, because high body temperatures were associated with decreased threshold and latency for reflex contraction of the laryngeal adductor reflex in newborn dogs (58).

The effects of changing ambient temperature are,

however, complex; these changes alter the metabolic rate, which is a major stimulus for breathing during the neonatal period, and is probably also of importance to sustain breathing in the infant.

Feeding regimens and glucose availability are now well-established factors influencing breathing movements in the human and sheep fetus. Other nutrients such as amino acids, along with the hormonal changes that follow ingestion and digestion, may also affect breathing either directly or via their influence on sleep and wakefulness. For instance, the sleeping pattern of 2- to 3-day-old infants can be modified by alteration of the amino acid composition of the diet (59), indicating that there is active and competitive uptake of amino acids into the brain, which may influence neurotransmitter turnover (60).

Central Chemoreceptor Drive Mechanisms

When inhaling CO_2, newborn infants seem to increase breathing to about the same extent as adults do (2), although their response curve is shifted to the left as a result of lower resting P_aCO_2 levels in the newborn period. Compared to that of the adult, the ventilatory response of the neonate to CO_2 is more greatly influenced by factors other than the excitability of central and peripheral chemoreceptors.

Behavioral State

In one study, lower CO_2 sensitivity was found in REM sleep than in quiet sleep (61), although other investigators could not confirm this difference (3,62).

Temperature

The CO_2 threshold for initiating breathing movements from apnea is higher in the fetus than in the newborn (63). Cooling results in a shift of the CO_2 response curve to the left, also resulting in an increase in the slope (i.e., sensitivity). This effect is rapid, suggesting that skin receptors mediate the response initially (63), but the subsequent decrease of the core temperature probably results in (a) stimulation of central thermoreceptors and (b) increased nonspecific activity in brainstem reticular neurons. It is noteworthy that cooling altered the behavioral state in the fetal lamb to an aroused (i.e., awake-like) state, an effect that would also augment the ventilatory drive (55,63). The interaction of temperature with blood gases at birth indicates that cooling (a) overrides the mildly inhibitory effects of hypoxia and (b) counteracts any absence of ventilatory drive due to hypocapnia, if it were to be present. This indicates the potency of

temperature as a determinant of the onset of breathing at birth.

P_{O_2} Level

Whereas hypoxia potentiates the CO_2 response in the adult, it has the opposite effect in the infant (4,64). This is probably due to the depressive effect of hypoxia on breathing control in the infant (see below).

Pulmonary Mechanics

The chest-wall distortion during active sleep has been found to decrease or disappear during CO_2 inhalation (62,65). Some of the recorded increase in ventilation may thus be attributed to a more efficient breathing pattern rather than being attributed to an increased ventilatory drive.

Another confounding factor is that arterial CO_2 tension usually remains unchanged during inhalation of low concentrations of CO_2. It therefore appears that the CO_2 response may, in part, be mediated by stimulation of airway receptors (66). These receptors have been assumed to be identical to the sensory nerve endings of the slowly adapting pulmonary stretch receptor (67).

The rebreathing method used in many adult studies to test central chemoreceptor responsiveness is not easily used with infants. The sleep epochs of infants are short, and a change of behavioral state may occur before steady state is reached. Most investigators have therefore used steady-state methods giving 2% and 4% CO_2. The usefulness of this method is also limited to arousals and change of sleep state (3). In addition, recordings of breathing volumes in infants are difficult because application of a face mask affects the normal control of breathing (68).

To what extent CO_2 sensitivity changes during development has not been finally resolved. Some of the studies are summarized in Table 1. The CO_2 responsiveness has been found to increase with postnatal age in preterm monkeys (69) and in preterm (70), but not in term (2,3), infants. The ventilatory response to CO_2 has also been found to increase with gestational age (70). Significantly lower CO_2 sensitivity has been found in preterm infants with recurrent apnea (64,71). Godfrey (72) tried to explain the notion of an increase of CO_2-response slope with age with changes in the dynamics of breathing during the first few months of life. His conclusions were not supported by Rigatto (64), who reinvestigated CO_2 responsiveness, trying to avoid the mechanical problem by recording a diaphragm electromyogram (EMG). By using this approach, he still found a lower CO_2 response in preterm, as compared to term, infants. An increase in response

TABLE 1. *Effects of REM sleep (REM), gestational age (GA), and postnatal age (PA) on CO$_2$ sensitivity[a]*

Subjects	CO$_2$ test	Method	GA	PA	REM	Reference
Term infants	Rebr	Pneumotachometer	—	↔	—	2
Term infants	2% SS	Barometric chamber	—	↔	—	3
Term infants	Rebr	Pm 0.1	—	↑	—	73
Preterm infants	2% and 4% SS	Pneumotachometer	↑	↑	—	70
Preterm and term infants	Rebr	Diaphragm EMG	↑	↑	↔	64
Preterm and term infants	3% SS	Pneumotachometer	↑	—	↔	62

[a] SS, steady state; Rebr, rebreathing; ↑, increase in sensitivity; ↔, no change in sensitivity; —, effects not analyzed; Pm 0.1, pressure fall during 0.1 sec airway occlusion.

to CO$_2$, measured as respiratory drive (by the Pm 0.1 method) in relation to postnatal age, has been reported by Taeusch et al. (73).

Peripheral Chemoreceptor Drive

Until recently, the peripheral chemoreceptors were thought to be silent in the fetus and then activated shortly after birth (74). In fact, they were suggested to be responsible for the switch from episodic fetal breathing to continuous breathing after birth (75). However, this idea was rejected when it was found that, at birth, carotid-denervated fetal sheep did not start to breathe later than sham-operated ones (76).

Furthermore, recent studies have demonstrated that the peripheral chemoreceptors are tonically active before birth in the lamb fetus (77). When the P_{O_2} level was further decreased either by occluding the umbilical cord or by giving a hypoxic gas mixture to the ewe, a similar stimulus–response curve, relating firing rate to $P_{a}O_2$, was observed in the fetus as in the adult. The fetal response curve was, however, located far to the left. If these studies performed in exteriorized and anesthetized fetal sheep are valid also for the fetus in the normal state, we can conclude that the threshold for the sensitivity to hypoxia is lower in the fetus than in the adult.

After birth, the peripheral chemoreceptors reset to a higher P_{O_2} level. This resetting occurs subsequently during the first week in the lamb (77). Similar adaptation has been seen in the neonatal rat (78). These results have been confirmed in newborn infants where hyperoxia was used to produce physiological chemodenervation (79,80). Hence it appears that tonic chemoreceptor activity during normoxia does not become effective until a few days after birth.

Thus the tonic input from peripheral chemoreceptors during normoxia does not seem to be of major importance to sustain breathing in newborn mammals. However, the relative importance of the peripheral chemoreceptor drive as measured in terms of an immediate rise in ventilation in response to mild hypoxia seems to increase progressively during the first few weeks of life (82). At about 10 days it may contribute to almost 50% of the ventilatory drive in the lamb (83) and also in the rat (78). Fetal sheep that were chemodenervated before birth survived the newborn period without any problems, but they died suddenly after a few weeks (83). The importance of the peripheral chemoreceptor drive also seems to increase as the human baby matures (80). However, when evaluating the effects of the chemodenervation experiments, it has to be borne in mind that chemoreceptive structures at other peripheral sites may take over the role of carotid bodies following their denervation (84).

The mechanism for this resetting of the peripheral chemoreceptor reflex has not yet been elucidated. However, recent studies indicate that dopamine might be involved (79). Dopamine modulates peripheral chemoreceptor activity in the adult. In the newborn, relatively high levels of dopamine in the carotid chemoreceptor tissue are present during the first few hours after birth. The turnover of dopamine is also high immediately after delivery. Subsequently the dopamine concentration increased whereas turnover decreased, suggesting that very little dopamine was being released. These changes in dopamine turnover occur during the same period of time as the appearance of the peripheral chemoreflex (Fig. 3).

The role of CO$_2$ for stimulation of the peripheral chemoreceptors is less clear. Sudden changes of CO$_2$ seem to affect ventilation significantly, whereas the tonic drive of CO$_2$ via the peripheral chemoreceptors is weak. The peripheral chemoreceptor response to CO$_2$ has been tested by giving a single bolus of a gas mixture with high CO$_2$ content to babies; the immediate response has been assumed not to be affected by the central chemoreceptor response. In this way a progressive rise of the peripheral CO$_2$ response was demonstrated to occur during the first 3 months of life (11).

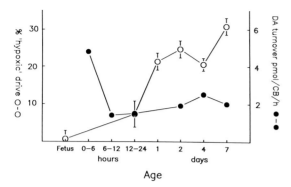

FIG. 3. Peripheral chemosensitivity was tested by giving extra oxygen to nonanesthetized rat pups. Respiration was monitored by plethysmography, and the relative decrease during O_2 exposure was used as an index of peripheral chemoreceptor activity. The test was carried out in near-term pups delivered by cesarean section and in vaginally born rats on the day of birth. The vaginally born group was then tested repeatedly over the first week of life. From 1 day of age and thereafter, ventilation decreased significantly, suggesting an increase in chemoreceptor activity with increasing age. Dopamine turnover in the carotid bodies was measured after inhibition of synthesis with alpha-methyl-*p*-tyrosine. Note the relatively high turnover rate of dopamine immediately after birth, and also note the marked decrease in turnover rates only a few hours later. These results suggest that dopamine might be involved in the resetting of the carotid bodies after birth. (From ref. 79.)

INHIBITORY MECHANISMS

Suprapontine Inhibition

Fetal breathing is partially suppressed (see Chapter 6.1.1) from a suprapontine level. This was first pointed out in the 1930s by Sir Joseph Barcroft, who observed continuous breathing in sheep fetus after transecting the fetal brain above the pontine level. Later studies in the adult cat showed also that in the adult there is some cortical inhibition of breathing (85).

More recent studies in the fetal sheep have shown that midcollicular decerebration results in continuous breathing activity dissociated from the behavioral state (86). The most striking effect was that the hypoxic inhibition of fetal breathing was removed by the transection (see below).

Whether decerebration increases normal breathing in the neonate has not been shown, although it effectively removes the depressive phase of the hypoxic response (87). But we have to postulate that there must be some kind of cortical inhibition of breathing also in the infant like in the fetus and the adult. It is possible that this suprapontine inhibition is, to some extent, related to the development of babbling and speech, when autonomic breathing is less convenient. It is tempting to draw some parallel with the cortical

suppression of neonatal reflexes which starts from about 2 months of age.

Hypoxic Inhibition

The ventilatory response to hypoxia in the infant is characterized by an initial increase and then a decrease—that is, a biphasic response. The response of the newborn thus appears to be an intermediate between the fetal and the adult pattern. A number of studies have been devoted to investigate the mechanism behind this biphasic response. The decerebration studies (87,88) exclude the possibility that there is some kind of medullary depression behind the inhibition of breathing, as first believed (89). Furthermore, it is not due to failure of peripheral chemoreceptor function (81). Depression of intercostal muscles and/or diaphragm also seems to be unlikely (90).

Recent research has been focused on the possibility that hypoxia activates neurochemical mechanisms that affect breathing. The possible role of various neurochemical substances causing ventilatory depression was based on findings that specific antagonists could block the so-called "hypoxic depression." The most widely studied neurotransmitters/modulators in this respect have been endorphins, GABA, adenosine, and dopamine (91,92).

The role of endorphins mediating the depressive phase of the biphasic ventilatory response in the infant has been based on the findings that naloxone could block the ventilatory depression in the rabbit pup (93,94), the piglet (91), and even the human baby (95). Furthermore, enkephalin analogues were found to markedly depress breathing in the neonate (92). However, relatively high concentrations (milligrams) of naloxone were needed to prevent the hypoxic ventilatory depression. This dose of naloxone increases the plasma catecholamine levels (96), which could eliminate the hypoxic inhibition of breathing (93).

GABA and its analogues have been found to inhibit breathing in fetal sheep (97). Although GABA is a potent inhibitor of respiration, it does not seem to be involved in the hypoxic depression of breathing, since the GABA antagonist could not block the hypoxic respiratory depression in the fetal sheep (98).

Adenosine is another neuromodulator of interest with regard to the hypoxic depression of the neonate (99). Adenosine is released from many tissues during hypoxia, as a result of the increased turnover of ATP. Adenosine has a well-known central action in depressing respiration, although it can stimulate breathing via the peripheral chemoreceptors (100,101).The role of adenosine causing ventilatory depression in the newborn is suggested by the finding of increased levels of hypoxanthine—the main metabolite of adenosine in plasma and extracellular fluid during asphyxia in the newborn (102,103). Furthermore, the hypoxic depression could partially be blocked with theophylline and enhanced with dipyridamole, which increases the endogenous levels of adenosine.

The depressive phase of breathing caused by hypoxia could also be blocked with specific dopamine D1-receptor antagonists in rabbit pups, suggesting that also dopamine is involved (104). Using a microdialysis technique, dopamine was found to be released in increased concentrations during hypoxia in the nTS region of the adult rabbit brain. This dopamine release did not occur after carotid body denervation, suggesting that the respiratory depression effect may be partially mediated via the peripheral chemoreceptors (105).

PATTERN FORMATION

Pulmonary Reflexes

Receptors situated in the tracheobronchial tree and within lung parenchyma do not play a very important regulatory role during quiet air breathing in adult mammals. However, in the newborn and preterm infant, they have significant effects in maintaining lung volume and promoting inflation.

The classical Hering–Breuer inflation reflex (i.e., termination of inspiration in response to lung distension) has been found to be more active in the newborn, particularly in the preterm baby (11). This has been most commonly investigated by measuring the prolongation of inspiratory time after end-expiratory airway occlusion. In one study, the stretch receptor activity was found to increase between the 32nd and 38th weeks of gestation, reaching a peak at the 38th week and then declining thereafter towards term (106). It is suggested that the functional significance of the Hering–Breuer reflex is to maintain adequate lung volumes (107). According to this hypothesis, the high respiratory rate due to shortened inspiration prevents emptying of the lung below the resting residual capacity. This is corroborated by the finding that lung volume is reduced during REM sleep, which is a period when the Hering–Breuer reflex is less effective (108).

The Hering–Breuer reflex also facilitates active expiration, particularly at increased distending pressures. The clinical applications of this phenomenon may commonly be observed in babies receiving ventilatory support. Active expiration during assisted ventilation ("fighting the ventilator") can lead to pneumothorax in ventilated preterm infants (109). Another common clinical application of this reflex is observed during respiratory stimulation by low distending air-way pressures such as those used in continuous positive airway pressure (CPAP) treatment (110).

A rapid and forceful inspiration may, in some instances, fail to produce a reflex inhibition of inspiration and instead augment inspiration. This phenomenon, known as "Head's paradoxical inflation reflex," is normally only encountered during the newborn period. This response is probably mediated by the irritant receptors situated in the mucosa of the major airways (11)—that is, a mechanism analogous to augmented breaths in the adult (111). The increased activity of this reflex following respiratory pauses is assumed to promote reinflation of the lungs when they tend to collapse.

Other C-fiber receptors in the bronchial and alveolar walls are stimulated by several lung conditions, including congestion and edema. Some of their respiratory actions include apnea followed by rapid shallow breathing, bronchoconstriction, and laryngeal constriction. Our knowledge of the activity of C-fiber receptors in newborns is scarce (112). It has been speculated that apneic spells associated with patent ductus arteriosus in preterm infants may be associated with C-fiber receptor activation.

Sighs are more common in infants than in adults (113). This may seem paradoxical, since irritant receptor activity related to airway defense mechanisms such as cough and bronchial constriction do not seem to be fully developed in infants, particularly not before the 35th week of gestation (114). Stimulation of carinal mucosa produces slowing of respiration, but not cough, in preterm infants (114). The adult response (i.e., coughing, hyperventilation, and arousal) appears in infants who are closer to conceptual term age. These age-dependent differences in response may be due to receptor or central immaturity or to incomplete myelinization of small vagal afferents in the younger infants (46,115).

Control of Upper-Airway Patency

The smaller size of the airways in infants makes them more susceptible to collapse during increased negative airway pressures. For example, while a negative nasal pressure of around 13 cmH$_2$O is needed to induce upper-airway collapse in the sleeping adult (116), the airways of a healthy infant start to close already at a negative pressure of about 4 cmH$_2$O (117).

Nevertheless, in spite of a number of factors that may decrease the airway stability (particularly during active sleep), clinically significant airway obstructions are not frequent among healthy infants, indicating the existence of efficient defense mechanisms (118).

Airway Control During Quiet Breathing

During the newborn period the anatomical relation between the tongue soft palate and the posterior pharyngeal wall favors nasal breathing; this breathing route also offers the lowest airway resistance (119, 120).

A coordination between upper-airway, chest-wall, and diaphragm muscles is well developed in the term newborn (121,122). During inspiration there is a sequential activation of the alae nasi (120), the genioglossus, and the vocal cord abductors before the diaphragm contracts. The ability to synchronize the air-pumping and upper-airway activities is related to gestational age, and the high incidence of respiratory dysrhythmias seen in preterm babies may partly be related to lack of coordination (12,123).

The timing of these events is partly related to sensory information from the nasopharyngeal pathway. When this input is abolished either by diverting tidal airflow or by topical anesthesia of the nasopharyngeal membranes, the normal pattern is lost and a tonic contraction of the pharynx occurs. In species such as rabbits, the airway constriction is particularly intense and may lead to asphyxia and even death (124). Whether this mechanism is of clinical importance in the human infant remains to be elucidated.

The upper laryngeal mucosa also contains receptors sensitive to mechanical, as well as to chemical and thermal, stimuli. The excitation of laryngeal chemoreceptors with liquid induces apnea and airway constriction as a protective reflex against aspiration of foreign matter (125). The reflex response is particularly intense in newborn animals and infants (126). In addition to the changes in ventilation, the laryngeal chemostimulation induces cardiovascular effects such as bradycardia, peripheral vasoconstriction and blood-flow redistribution (125). The apneic and bradycardic components are powerfully reinforced by hypoxia, a finding of potential significance with regard to life-threatening apnea of infancy and the sudden infant death syndrome (SIDS) (127).

Effect of Behavioral State

During active sleep the airway stability is compromised as a result of several factors. Loss of skeletal muscle tone in the tongue and pharyngeal muscles affects the patency of larynx during active sleep. Reduction in laryngeal expiratory activity (128) decreases lung volume and pulmonary stretch receptor activity (129). A decrease in lung mechanoreceptor feedback is associated with a lower activity in the upper airways (130).

Cyclic fluctuation in the depth and rate of breathing may be in phase during active sleep; that is, a decrease in rate may be synchronous with a decrease in tidal volume (48), possibly sometimes leading to chest-wall collapse (128). Such a decrease in ventilation also reduces airway patency, since the dilating activity of the genioglossus and the posterior cricoarytenoid parallels the central inspiratory drive (129,130). A cessation of breathing movements may thus induce airway closure in infants (131).

Sudden changes in upper-airway resistance such as nasal occlusion will significantly increase the muscular activity of the tongue, leading to dilatation of the pharyngeal pathway (117,132). In relative terms, this increase is more pronounced and comes earlier than the increase in inspiratory diaphragmatic activity. This may partly explain why airway patency is usually maintained during induced obstructive episodes (131).

These defense mechanisms are particularly apparent when there is an increase in ventilatory drive (and, consequently, augmented phasic activity) in pulmonary stretch receptors. When breathing is stimulated by application of a face mask, an airway occlusion generating negative pressures of around 30 cmH_2O may still not collapse the airways (133).

Arousal in response to airway stimulation also seems to be increased during active sleep (11). The ability to arouse is further facilitated by the increase in systemic blood pressure during this sleep state (134).

It is of clinical interest that several of the escape mechanisms mentioned above are suppressed by sleep deprivation. Even a short period of forced wakefulness leads to a significant increase of obstructive events during active sleep (135).

Effect of Hypoxia and Hypercapnia

The inspiratory activity of the upper airway is not uniformly increased by chemosensory stimulation. The CO_2 threshold seems to be higher for the genioglossus than for the alae nasi and the diaphragm (136), which may affect the airway patency during hypercapnia. Whether this is related to differential output from the central chemosensory area or attributable to stimulation of airway CO_2 receptors is not clear.

Some studies in animals may suggest that hypoxic stimulation has a greater influence on tongue activity than does hypercapnic stimulation (137). The significance of these observations has not been confirmed in human infants.

CONCLUSIONS

The control of breathing is switched from discontinuous and metabolically less-dependent fetal breathing movements to continuous metabolically related breathing at birth. This transition is only instantaneous. Cooling of the infant seems to be important in stimulating breathing initially and in triggering the increased CO_2 sensitivity. Thermoreceptor-mediated respiratory drive might be very important during the first few days of life. Mechanoreceptor influences on breathing also seem to be important at an early stage. Peripheral chemoreceptor drive is reset from Po_2 to the extrauterine Po_2 a few days after birth; in the infant, this drive becomes important after the newborn period.

REFERENCES

1. Chernick V, Warshaw JB, Kiley JP. Development neurobiology of respiratory control. *Am Rev Respir Dis* 1989;139:1295–1301.
2. Avery ME, Chernick V, Dutton RE, Permutt S. Ventilatory response to inspired CO_2 in infants and adults. *J Appl Physiol* 1963;18:895–903.
3. Haddad GC, Leistner HL, Epstein MAF, Grodin WK, Mellins RB. O_2 induced changes in ventilation and ventilatory pattern in normal sleeping infants. *J Appl Physiol* 1980;48:684–688.
4. Rigatto H, Torre V de la, Cates D. Effects of CO_2 on the ventilatory responses to CO_2 in preterm infants. *J Appl Physiol* 1975;39:896–899.
5. Quattrochi JJ, Madison R, Kljavin IJ, Marsala J, Kosik KS. Integrative structural correlates of central respiratory rhythmicity: a new hypothesis. In: von Euler C, Lagercrantz H, eds. *Neurobiology of the control of breathing.* New York: Raven Press, 1986;231–241.
6. Cameron WE, Averill DB, Berger AJ. Evidence for differential inputs to phrenic motoneurons based on dendritic morphology. In: Bianchi AL, Denavit-Saubi M, eds. *Neurogenesis of central respiratory rhythm.* London: MTP Press, 1985;230–233.
7. Conradi S, Ronnevi L-O. Ultrastructure and synaptology of the initial axon segment of cat spinal moto-neuron during early post-natal development. *J Neurocytol* 1977;6:195–210.
8. Cowan WM. The development of the brain. *Sci Am* 1979; 241(3):106–117.
9. Purpura DP. Development of pathobiology of cortical neurons in immature human brain. In: Gluck L, ed. *Intrauterine asphyxia and the developing fetal brain.* Chicago: Year Book Medical, 1977;349–373.
10. von Euler C. Brain stem mechanisms for generation and control of breathing pattern. In: Fishman AP, Cherniack NS, Widdicombe JG, eds. *Handbook of physiology.* Baltimore: Williams & Wilkins, 1986;1–67.
11. Bryan AC, Bowes G, Maloney JE. Control of breathing in the fetus and the newborn. In: Fishman AP, Cherniack NS, Widdicombe JG, eds. *Handbook of physiology.* Baltimore: Williams & Wilkins, 1986;621–647.
12. Henderson-Smart DJ, Pettigrew AG, Campbell DJ. Clinical apnea and brain-stem neural function in preterm infants. *N Engl J Med* 1983;308:353–357.
13. Sears TA. The respiratory motor neurone and apneusis. *Fed Proc* 1977;36:2412.
14. Lagercrantz H. Neuromodulators and respiratory control during development. *TINS* 1987;10:368–372.
15. Foutz AS, Champagnat J, Denavit-Saubié M. *N*-Methyl-D-aspartate (NMDA) receptors control respiratory off-switch in cat. *Neurosci Lett* 1988;87:221–226.
16. Brew S, Castro D de, Sinclair JD. Studies of glutamate as the transmitter of respiratory stimulation in hypoxia. *Isac Warsawa* Warsaw: Intern. Society for Arterial Chemocephon, 1989;9:10.
17. Barks JD, Silverstein FS, Sims K, Greenamyre JT, Johnston MV. Glutamate recognition sites in human fetal brain. *Neurosci Lett* 1988;84:131–136.
18. Man EH, Fisher GH, Payan IL, Cadilla-Perezrios R, Garcia NM, Chemburkar R, Arends G, et al. D-Aspartate in human brain. *J Neurochem* 1987;48:510–515.
19. Lagercrantz H. Neurochemical modulation of fetal behaviour and excitation at birth. In: von Euler C, Forssberg H, Lagercrantz H, eds. *Neurobiology of early infant behaviour.* Stockholm: Stockholm Press, 1989;19–29.
20. Walker DW, Joseph SA. Chemical and non-chemical control of fetal breathing. In: Gluckman PD, Johnston BM, eds. *The Liggins symposium. Fetal and neonatal medicine.* New York: Perinatology Press, 1989.
21. Felten D, Hallman H, Jonsson G. Evidence for a neurotropic role of noradrenaline neurons for the postnatal development of rat cerebral cortex. *J Neurocytol* 1982;11:119–135.
22. Cavanagh ME, Parnavelas JG. Development of somatostatin immunoreactive neurons in the rat occipital cortex: a combined immunocytochemical-autoradiographic study. *J Comp Neurol* 1988;268:1–12.
23. Härfstrand A, Fuxe K, Kalia M, Agnati F. Somatostatin induced apnoea; prevention by central and peripheral administration of the opiate receptor blocking agent naloxone. *Acta Physiol Scand* 1985;125:91–95.
24. Yamamoto Y, Runold M, Pantaleo T, Lagercrantz H. Somatostatin in the control of respiration. *Acta Physiol Scand* 1988; 134:529–533.
25. Hazinski TA, Grunstein MM, Schlueter MA, Tooley WH. Effect of naloxone on ventilation in newborn rabbits. *J Appl Physiol* 1981;50:713–717.
26. Moss IR, Denavit-Saubie M, Eldridge FL, Gillis RA, Herkenham M, Lahiri S. Neuromodulators and transmitters in respiratory control. *Fed Proc* 1986;45:2133–2147.
27. Joseph SA, McMillen IC, Walker DW. Effects of naloxone on breathing movements and plasma beta-endorphin concentrations during hypercapnia in the fetal lamb. *J Appl Physiol* 1987;62:673.
28. Gingras-Leatherman JL, McNamara MC, Hong JS, Lawson EE. Development of methionine-enkephalin in microdissected areas of the rabbit brain. *Brain Res* 1985;336:73–80.
29. Gluckman PD, Bennet L. Neuropharmacology of fetal and neonatal breathing. In: Johnston BM, Gluckman PD, eds. *Respiratory control and lung development in the fetus and newborn. The scientific basis of clinical practice. Reproductive and perinatal medicine.* Ithaca, New York: Perinatology Press, 1986; 249–277.
30. McMillen IC, Walker DW. Effect of beta-endorphin on fetal breathing movements in sheep. *J Appl Physiol* 1986;6:1005.
31. Prabhakar NR, Runold M, Yamamoto Y, Lagercrantz H, von Euler C. Effect of substance P antagonists on the hypoxia-induced carotid chemoreceptor activity. *Acta Physiol Scand* 1984;121:301–303.
32. Scheibner T, Read DJC, Sullivan CE. Substance P immunoreactivity in the developing kitten carotid body. *Brain Res* 1988;453:72–78.
33. Lagercrantz H, Persson H, Srinivasen M, Yamamoto Y. The developmental expression of some neuropeptide genes in respiration-related areas of the rabbit brain. *J Physiol* 1989;417:25.
34. Speck DF, Feldman JL. The effects of microstimulation and microlesions in the ventral and dorsal respiratory groups in medulla of cat. *J Neurosci* 1982;2:744–757.
35. Onimaru H, Homma I. Respiratory rhythm generator neurons in medulla of brainstem-spinal cord preparation from newborn rat. *Brain Res* 1987;403:380–384.
36. Ross CA, Ruggiero DA, Joh TH, Park DH, Reis DJ. Rostral ventrolateral medulla: selective projections to the thoracic autonomic cell column from the region containing Cl adrenaline neurons. *J Comp Neurol* 1984;228:168–185.
37. Clewlow F, Dawes GS, Johnston BM, Walker DW. Changes in breathing, electrocortical and muscle activity in the mature sheep foetus and newborn lamb. *Respir Physiol* 1975;25:199–215.
38. England SJ, Kent G, Strogryn HAF. Laryngeal muscle and diaphragmatic muscle activities in conscious rat pups. *Respir Physiol* 1985;60:95–108.

39. Parot SM, Bonora M, Gautier H, Marlot D. Developmental changes in ventilation and breathing pattern in unanaesthetized kittens. *Respir Physiol* 1984;58:253–262.

40. Suthers GK, Henderson-Smart DJ, Read DJC. Postnatal changes in the rat of high frequency bursts of inspiratory activity in cats and dogs. *Brain Res* 1977;132:537–540.

41. Farber JP. Medullary inspiratory activity during opossum development. *Am J Physiol* 1988;254:R578–R584.

42. Bystrzycka W. Nail BS, Purves MJ. Central and peripheral neural respiratory activity in the mature sheep foetus and newborn lamb. *Respir Physiol* 1975;25:199–215.

43. Farber JP. Expiratory motor responses in the suckling opossum. *J Appl Physiol* 1983;54:919–925.

44. Fedorko L, Kelly EN, England SJ. Importance of vagal afferents in determining ventilation in newborn rats. *J Appl Physiol* 1988;65:1033–1039.

45. Marlot B, Duron B. Postnatal development of vagal control of breathing in the kitten. *J Physiol* 1979;75:891–900.

46. Schwieler GH. Respiratory regulation during postnatal development in cats and rabbits and some of its morphological substrate. *Acta Physiol Scand [Suppl]* 1968;304:49–63.

47. Curzi-Dascalova L, Lebrun F, Korn G. Respiratory frequency according to sleep states and age in normal premature infants: a comparison with full term infants. *Pediatr Res* 1983;17:152–156.

48. Hathorn MKS. The depth and rate of breathing in newborn infants in different sleep states. *J Physiol (Lond)* 1974;243:101–113.

49. Gaultier C, Praud JP, Canet E, Delaperche MF, D'Allest AM. Paradoxical inward rib cage motion during rapid eye movement sleep in infants and young children. *J Dev Physiol* 1987;9:391–397.

50. Hathorn MKS. Analysis of periodic changes in ventilation in newborn infants. *J Physiol* 1978;285:85–99.

51. Calka J, McMillen IC, Walker DW. Effect of feeding regime on the diurnal variation of breathing movements in the late gestation fetal sheep. *J Appl Physiol* 1989;68:in press.

52. McMillen IC, Nowak R, Walker DW, Young IR. Maternal pinealectomy alters the daily pattern of fetal breathing in sheep. *J Appl Physiol* 1990;258:R284–R287.

53. Walker DW, Davies AN. Effects of hyperthermia on fetal breathing movements. *J Dev Physiol* 1986;8:485–497.

54. Walker DW. Effects of increased core temperature on fetal breathing movements and electrocortical activity in fetal sheep. *J Dev Physiol* 1988;10:513–523.

55. Gluckman PD, Gunn TR, Johnston BM. The effect of cooling on breathing and shivering in unanesthetized fetal lambs *in utero*. *J Physiol* 1983;343:495–506.

56. Karlberg P, Wennergren G. Respiratory control during onset of breathing. *Cardiovasc Respiratory Physiol Fetus Neonate* 1986;133:131–144.

57. Perlstein P, Edwards H, Sutherland J. Apnea in premature infants and incubator-air temperature changes. *N Engl J Med* 1970;282:461.

58. Haraguchi S, Fung RO, Sasaki CT. Effect of hyperthermia on the laryngeal closure reflex. Implications in the sudden infant death syndrome. *Ann Otol Rhinol Laryngol* 1983;92–94.

59. Yogman MW, Zeisel SH. Diet and sleep patterns in newborn infants. *N Engl J Med* 1983;309:1147–1149.

60. Wurtman RJ. Nutrients that modify brain function. *Sci Am* 1982;246:50–59.

61. Bryan AC, Bryan MH. Control of respiration in the newborn. *Clin Perinatol* 1978;5:269–281.

62. Davi M, Sankaran K, Maccallium M, Cates D, Rigatto H. Effect of sleep state on chest distortion and on the ventilatory response to CO_2 in neonates. *Pediatr Res* 1979;13:982–986.

63. Moss IR, Mautone AJ, Scarpelli EM. Effect of temperature on regulation of breathing and sleep/wake state in fetal lambs. *J Appl Physiol* 1983;54:536–543.

64. Rigatto H. Control of ventilation in the newborn. *Annu Rev Physiol* 1984;46:661–674.

65. Andersson D, Gennser G, Johnson P. The effect of carbon dioxide inhalation on phase characteristics of breathing movements in healthy newborn infants. *J Dev Physiol* 1986;8:147–157.

66. Johnson P. Evidence for lower airway chemoreceptors in newborn lambs. *Pediatr Res* 1976;10:462.

67. Sant'Ambrogio G, Miserocchi G, Mortola J. Transient responses of pulmonary stretch receptors in the dog to inhalation of carbon dioxide. *Respir Physiol* 1974;22:191–197.

68. Fleming PJ, Levine MR, Goncalves A. Changes in respiratory pattern resulting from the use of facemask to record respiration in newborn infants. *Pediatr Res* 1982;16:1031–1034.

69. Guthrie RD, Standeart TA, Hodson WA, Woodrum DE. Sleep and maturation of eucapnic ventilation and CO_2 sensitivity in the premature primate. *J Appl Physiol* 1980;48:347–354.

70. Rigatto H, Brady JP, Torre VR del. Chemoreceptor reflexes in preterm infants. I. The effect of gestational age on the ventilatory response to inhalation of 100% and 15% oxygen. II. The effect of gestational and postnatal age on the ventilatory response to inhaled CO_2. *Pediatrics* 1975;55:604–620.

71. Gerhardt T, Bancalari E. Apnea of prematurity. I. Lung function and regulation of breathing. *Pediatrics* 1984;74:58–62.

72. Godfrey S. Growth and development of the respiratory system: functional development. In: Davis JA, Dobbing J, eds. *Scientific foundations of paediatrics*, 2nd ed. London: Heinemann, 1981;432–450.

73. Taeusch HW Jr, Carson S, Frantz ID III, Milic-Emili J. Respiratory regulation after elastic loading and CO_2 rebreathing in normal term infants. *Pediatrics* 1976;88:102–111.

74. Biscoe TJ, Purves MJ, Sampson SR. Types of nervous activity which may be recorded from the carotid sinus nerve in the sheep fetus. *J Physiol (Lond)* 1969;202:1–23.

75. Purves MJ. The effects of hypoxia in the new-born lamb before and after denervation of the carotid chemoreceptors. *J Physiol* 1966;185:60–77.

76. Jansen AH, Ioffe S, Rusell BJ, Chernick V. Effect of carotid chemoreceptor denervation on breathing *in utero* before and after birth. *J Appl Physiol* 1981;5i:630–633.

77. Blanco CE, Dawes GS, Hanson MA, McCooke HB. The response to hypoxia of arterial chemoreceptors in fetal sheep and newborn lambs. *J Physiol* 1984;351:25–37.

78. Hertzberg T, Hellström S, Lagercrantz H, Pequignot JM. Resetting of arterial chemoreceptors and carotid body catecholamines in the newborn rat. *J Physiol* 1990; in press.

79. Girard F, Lacaisse A, Dejours P. Le stimulus O_2 ventilatoire à la période neonatale chez l'homme. *J Physiol (Paris)* 1960;52:108–109.

80. Hertzberg T, Lagercrantz H. Postnatal sensitivity of the peripheral chemoreceptors in newborn infants. *Arch Dis Child* 1987;62:1238–1241.

81. Blanco CE, Hanson MA, Johnson P, Rigatto H. Breathing pattern of kittens during hypoxia. *J Appl Physiol* 1984;56:12–17.

82. Bonora M, Marlot D, Gautier H, Duron B. Effects of hypoxia on ventilation during postnatal development in conscious kittens. *J Appl Physiol* 1984;56:1464–1471.

83. Bureau MA, Begin R. Postnatal maturation of the response to O_2 in awake newborn lambs. *J Appl Physiol* 1982;52:428–433.

84. Sinclair JD. Respiratory drive in hypoxia: carotid body and other mechanisms compared. *NIPS* 1987;2:57–60.

85. Tenney SM, Ou LC. Ventilatory response of decorticate and decerebrate cats to hypoxia and CO_2. *Respir Physiol* 1977;29:81.

86. Dawes GS, Gardner WN, Johnston BM, Walker DW. Breathing in fetal lambs: the effect of brain stem and mid-brain transection. *J Physiol* 1983;335:535–553.

87. Martin-Boddy RL, Johnston BM. Central origin of the hypoxic depression of breathing in the newborn. *Respir Physiol* 1988;71:25–32.

88. Dawes GS, Fox HE, Leduc BM, Liggins GC, Johnston BM, Walker DW. Breathing patterns in lambs after midbrain transection. *J Physiol* 1980;308:20P.

89. Cross KS, Oppe TW. The effect of inhalation of high and low concentrations of oxygen on the respiration of the premature infant. *J Physiol* 1952;117:38–55.

90. Haddad GG, Mellins RB. Hypoxia and respiratory control in early life. *Annu Rev Physiol* 1984;46:629–643.

91. Moss IR, Runold M, Dahlin I, Fredholm BB, Nyberg F, Lagercrantz H. Respiratory and neuroendocrine responses of piglets to hypoxia during postnatal development. *Acta Physiol Scand* 1987;131:533–541.

92. Moss IR, Luman JG. Neurochemicals and respiratory control during development. *J Appl Physiol* 1989;67:1–13.

93. Srinivasan M, Yamamoto Y, Lagercrantz H. Ventilatory effects of naloxone via the sympathoadrenal system in the neonate. *Neurosci Lett* 1988;90:159–164.

94. Grunstein MM, Hazinski TA, Schlueter MA. Respiratory control during hypoxia in newborn rabbits: implied action of endorphins. *J Appl Physiol* 1981;51:122–130.

95. Boeck C de, Reempts R van, Rigatto H, Chernick V. Naloxone reduces decrease in ventilation induced by hypoxia in newborn infants. *J Appl Physiol* 1984;56:1507–1511.

96. Padbury JF, Agata Y, Polk DH, Wang DL, Callegari CC. Neonatal adaptation: naloxone increases the catecholamine surge at birth. *Pediatr Res* 1987;21:590.

97. Hedner T, Iversen K, Lundborg P. GABA concentrations in the cerebrospinal fluid of newborn infants. *Early Hum Dev* 1982;7:53–58.

98. Johnston BM, Gluckman PD. GABA-mediated inhibition of breathing in the late gestation sheep fetus. *J Dev Physiol* 1983;5:353–360.

99. Runold M, Lagercrantz H, Fredholm B. Ventilatory effect of an adenosine analogue in unaesthetized rabbits during development. *J Appl Physiol* 1986;61:255–259.

100. McQueen DS, Mir AK. Changes in carotid body amine levels and effects of dopamine on respiration in rats treated neonatally with capsaicin. *Br J Pharmacol* 1984;83:909–918.

101. Runold M, Lagercrantz H, Prabhakar NR, Fredholm BB. Role of adenosine in hypoxic ventilatory depression. *J Appl Physiol* 1989;67:541–546.

102. Saugstad O. Hypoxanthine as a measurement of hypoxia. *Pediatr Res* 1975;9:158–161.

103. Irestedt L, Dahlin I, Hertzberg T, Sollevi A, Lagercrantz H. Adenosine concentration in umbilical cord blood of newborn infants after vaginal delivery and cesarean section. *Pediatr Res* 1989;26:106–108.

104. Srinivasan M, Lagercrantz H, Yamamoto Y. A possible dopaminergic pathway mediating hypoxic depression in neonatal rabbits. *J Appl Physiol* 1989;67:1271–1276.

105. Goiny M, Lagercrantz H, Srinivasan M, Ungerstedt U, Yamamoto Y. Hypoxia-mediated *in vivo* release of dopamine in the nucleus tractus solitarii of the rabbit. *J Appl Physiol* 1989;submitted for publication.

106. Bodegård G, Schwieler G, Skoglund S, Zetterström R. Control of breathing in newborn babies. *Acta Paediatr Scand* 1969;58:567–571.

107. Olinsky AM, Bryan H, Bryan AC. Influence of lung inflation on respiratory control in neonates. *J Appl Physiol* 1974;36:426–429.

108. Henderson-Smart DJ, Read DJC. Reduced lung volume during behavioural active sleep in the newborn. *J Appl Physiol* 1979;46:1081–1085.

109. Greenough A, Wood S, Morley CJ, Davies JA. Pancuronium prevents pneumothoraces in ventilated premature babies who actively expire against positive pressure ventilation. *Lancet* 1984;i:1–4.

110. Martin RJ, Nearman HS, Katona PG, Klaus MH. The effect of a low continuous positive airway pressure on the reflex control of ventilation of the preterm infant. *J Pediatr* 1977;90:976–981.

111. Sant'Ambrogio G. Information arising from the tracheobronchial tree of mammals. *Physiol Rev* 1982;62:531–569.

112. Trippenbach T. Development of aspects of respiratory reflexes. In: von Euler C, Lagercrantz H, eds. *Neurobiology of the control breathing.* New York: Raven Press, 1986;283–290.

113. Fleming PJ, Goncalves AL, Levine MR, Woolard S. The development of stability of respiration in human infant: changes in ventilatory responses to spontaneous sighs. *J Physiol (Lond)* 1984;347:1–16.

114. Fleming PA, Bryan AC, Bryan MH. Functional immaturity of pulmonary irritant receptors and apnea in newborn preterm. *Pediatrics* 1978;61:515–518.

115. Sachis RN, Armstrong DL, Becker LE, Bryan AC. The vagus nerve and sudden infant death syndrome, a morphometric study. *J Pediatr* 1981;98:278–280.

116. Schwartz AR, Smith PL, Wise RA, Gold AR, Permutt S. Induction of upper airway occlusion in sleeping individuals with subatmospheric nasal pressure. *J Appl Physiol* 1988;64:535–542.

117. Roberts JL, Reed WR, Mathew OP, Menon AA, Thach BT. Assessment of pharyngeal airway stability in normal and micrognathic infants. *J Appl Physiol* 1985;58:290–299.

118. Guilleminault CH, Araigno R, Korobkin R. Mixed and obstructive sleep apnea in near miss for sudden infant death syndrome. *Pediatrics* 1979;64:882.

119. Mortola JP, Fisher JT. Mouth and nose resistance in newborn kittens and puppies. *J Appl Physiol* 1981;51:641–645.

120. Carlo WA, Martin RJ, Bruce EN, Strohl KP, Fanaroff AA. Alae nasi activation (nasal flaring) decreases nasal resistance in preterm infants. *Pediatrics* 1983;71:383.

121. Roberts JL, Reed WR, Mathew OP, Thach BT. Control of respiratory activity of the genioglossus muscle in micrognathic infants. *J Appl Physiol* 1986;61:1523–1533.

122. Kosch PC, Hutchison AA, Wozniak JA, Carlo WA, Stark AA. Posterior cricoarytenoid and diaphragm activities during tidal breathing in neonates. *J Appl Physiol* 1988;64:1969–1978.

123. Milner AD, Boon AW, Saunders RA, Hopkins IE. Upper airway obstructions and apnoea in preterm babies. *Arch Dis Child* 1980;55:22–25.

124. Abu-Osba YK, Mathew OP, Thach BT. An animal model for airway sensory deprivation producing obstructive apnea with postmortem findings of sudden infant death syndrome. *Pediatrics* 1981;68:796–801.

125. Daly M de Burgh, Angell-James JE, Elsner R. Role of carotid body chemoreceptors and their reflex interactions in bradycardia and cardiac arrest. *Lancet* 1979;I:764–767.

126. Harding R, Johnson P, McClelland ME. Liquid sensitive laryngeal receptors in the developing sheep, cat, and monkey. *J Physiol* 1978;277:409–422.

127. Wennergren G, Hertzberg T, Milerad J, Bjure J, Lagercrantz H. Hypoxia reinforces laryngeal reflex bradycardia in infants. *Acta Paediatr Scand* 1989;78:11–17.

128. Harding R, Johnson P, McClelland ME. Respiratory function of the larynx in the developing sheep and the influence of sleep state. *Respir Physiol* 1980;40:165–179.

129. Barlett D, Remmers JE, Gauthier H. Laryngeal regulation of respiratory airflow. *Respir Physiol* 1973;18:194–204.

130. Lunteren E van, Graaf WB van der, Parker DM, Strohl KP, Mitra J, Salamone J, Cherniack NS. Activities of the upper airway muscles during augmented breaths. *Respir Physiol* 1983;53:87–89.

131. Milner AD, Saunders RA, Hopkins IE. Apnoea induced by airflow obstructions. *Arch Dis Child* 1977;52:379–382.

132. Carlo WA, Miller MJ, Martin RJ. Differential response of respiratory muscles to airway occlusion in infants. *J Appl Physiol* 1985;59:847–852.

133. Cohen GL, Henderson-Smart DJ. Upper airway stability and apnea during nasal occlusion in newborn infants. *J Appl Physiol* 1986;60:1517–1521.

134. Fewell JE, Johnson P. Acute increases in blood pressure cause arousal from sleep in lambs. *Brain Res* 1984;311:259–265.

135. Canet E, Gaultier C, D'Allest A-M, Dehan M. Effects of sleep deprivation on respiratory events during sleep in healthy infants. *J Appl Physiol* 1989;66:1158–1163.

136. Carlo WA, Martin RJ, Abboud EF, Bruce EN, Strohl KP. Effect of sleep state and hypercapnia on alae nasi and diaphragm EMG in preterm infants. *J Appl Physiol* 1983;54:1590–1596.

137. Brouillette RT, Thach BT. Control of genioglossus muscle inspiratory activity. *J Appl Physiol* 1980;49:801–808.

THE LUNG: Scientific Foundations
edited by R.G. Crystal, J.B. West et al.
Raven Press, Ltd., New York © 1991.

CHAPTER 6.1.7

Pulmonary Surfactant and Respiratory Distress Syndrome in the Premature Infant

Jeffrey A. Whitsett

Respiratory failure is caused by decreased surfactant activity in the lungs of prematurely born infants. Efforts to improve the diagnosis and treatment of respiratory distress syndrome (RDS) have resulted in a more complete understanding of the various molecules required for reduction of surface tension in the alveolus of the lung. The complexity of the alveolar surfactant system has increased with the identification of macromolecules and their aggregate forms that constitute pulmonary surfactant. The controlled synthesis, secretion, and catabolism of the lipids and proteins that comprise the active surfactant complex are critical to the reduction of surface tension in the alveolus. In the present work, we will consider factors involved in reduction of surface tension from the perspective of the pathogenesis and treatment of RDS in premature infants. The concepts derived from the study of surfactant in the developing lung will hopefully be applicable to respiratory failure accompanying surfactant deficiency or surfactant dysfunction in older patients such as those with adult respiratory distress syndrome (ARDS).

INTERFACIAL FORCES AT THE ALVEOLAR SURFACE

Distinct phase boundaries at the alveolar surface create significant collapsing forces relating primarily to the unequal forces generated by water molecules at the air–liquid–tissue interfaces. These forces were first

recognized by the observed differences in the filling pressures of air-filled as compared to liquid-filled lungs (1). Avery and Mead (2) demonstrated decreased surface active material in lung lavage from premature infants with RDS compared to that from infants dying from other causes. The surface active material from mature lungs was identified as consisting primarily of phospholipids, leading to the concept that the phospholipids in the alveolar space created a monolayer at the air-liquid interface capable of reducing collapsing surface forces (3). The monolayer, in effect, creates a phase boundary capable of generating extremely low surface tension. Lack of surfactant material in the normal lung (e.g., after removal by lavage) results in a rapid loss of compliance and residual lung volume leading to hypoxia and hypercarbia. The physiologic abnormalities of the surfactant-deficient lung can be resolved by repletion of surfactant material in the alveolar space; recovery of normal pressure–volume relationships is a rapid, physical phenomenon, occurring as readily in the intact as in the excised lung. Surfactant replacement is now widely used for prevention and treatment of RDS in premature infants.

COMPOSITION AND STRUCTURAL FEATURES OF PULMONARY SURFACTANT

Pulmonary surfactant is obtained by lung lavage with isotonic solutions and is further purified by centrifugation (4). A variety of physical forms can be separated on the basis of their distinct buoyant densities (5). The most surfactant active material sediments at low gravitation forces and consists primarily of large macromolecular aggregates (called "tubular myelin") and large multilamellated structures. Smaller vesicular material containing abundant quantities of phospholipid

J. A. Whitsett: Division of Pulmonary Biology, Children's Hospital Research Foundation, Children's Hospital Medical Center, Cincinnati, Ohio 45267; and Division of Neonatology, Department of Pediatrics, University of Cincinnati College of Medicine, Cincinnati, Ohio 45267.

is also present in lung lavage; however, this material is much less surface active than tubular-myelin-rich fractions (5). Surfactant aggregates exist in a state of dynamic flux. The various macromolecular forms are likely generated by changes in protein and phospholipid composition, as well as by mechanical forces produced during the respiratory cycle.

Pulmonary surfactant is synthesized by specialized cells termed "type II epithelial cells." After secretion, the larger lamellar forms unravel to form tubular myelin. This process is likely facilitated by the presence of high extracellular Ca^{2+} and by the incorporation of surfactant proteins into the phospholipids. Tubular myelin consists of highly organized protein lipid complexes that consist of parallel square tubes of 40–60 nm/face (Fig. 1). This material is relatively enriched in surfactant proteins (5). Tubular myelin and/or the large lamellar forms of surfactant are likely to provide the alveolar pool of phospholipid from which the surfactant monolayer is formed. Lighter surfactant fractions are somewhat depleted of surfactant proteins and are considerably less surface active. The lighter, vesicular forms appear later, after secretion of lamellar forms and generation of tubular myelin; several studies support the concept that the smaller, lighter vesicles represent catabolic products derived primarily from tubular myelin or from the surface monolayer. Re-uptake of phospholipid occurs at high rates. There is considerable *in vivo* and *in vitro* evidence that pulmonary surfactant lipids are re-utilized and metabolized by type II epithelial cells (Fig. 2).

Surfactant Phospholipids

Phospholipids represent the most abundant molecules comprising pulmonary surfactant (approximately 85–90%) (for review, see ref. 6). Protein, glycolipid, and neutral lipids contribute to most of the remaining fraction. The phospholipids in surfactant are enriched in disaturated phosphatidylcholine (DSPC), and the acyl chains are predominantly disaturated palmitoyl groups (DPPC) (Fig. 3). The head groups of the surfactant phospholipids are comprised primarily of choline, glycerol, and lesser amounts of serine, inositol, and ethanolamine. These highly charged regions of the molecule interact strongly at the aqueous phase and are closely associated with each other by strong charge-dependent interactions of the head groups. The acyl chains are highly hydrophobic and are excluded

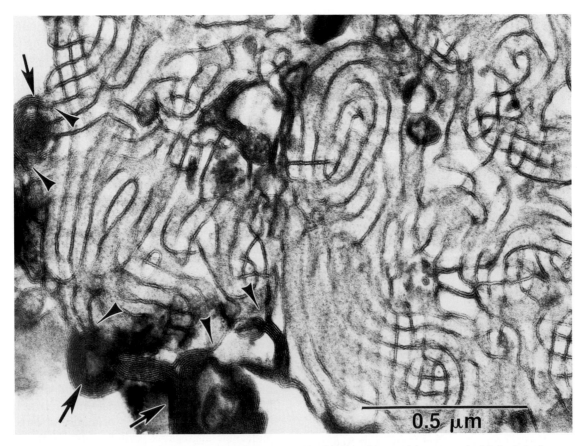

FIG. 1. Phospholipid membrane of secreted lamellar bodies (*arrows*) is converted into tubular myelin in the alveolar lumen. ×100,000. (Courtesy of S. Wert.)

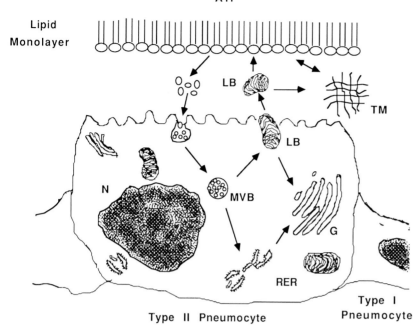

Air

Lipid
Monolayer

FIG. 2. Life cycle of pulmonary surfactant. Phospholipids are synthesized in the rough endoplasmic reticulum (RER) and are stored in large inclusions, refered to as "lamellar bodies" (LB). Lamellar bodies are exocytosed into the alveolar lumen. Interactions of the phospholipids with calcium and surfactant protein result in the formation of tubular myelin (TM). The monolayer is likely formed by movement of lipids from the lamellar and tubular myelin aggregates. Smaller vesicles are generated from the monolayer and are taken up by the type II cells, likely entering multivesicular bodies (MVB) and are either catabolized or directly neutrilized. N, nucleus; G, Golgi bodies.

Type II Pneumocyte

Type I Pneumocyte

from the aqueous phase. The density of packing depends primarily upon the structures of the acyl chains (saturated molecules being more densely packed because of the lack of kinks in their acyl chains). This packing is also likely to be influenced by the relative composition of the lipids or by the presence of proteins that may insert, or be strongly associated with, either acyl chains or head groups. Interactions among phospholipids and proteins are, in turn, highly dependent upon temperature. DPPC is capable of packing densely at an air–liquid interface and is ideally suited for the reduction of surface tension. Monolayers derived from phosphatidylcholine (PC) generate low surface tensions, similar to those of pulmonary surfactants. The precise roles of the various phospholipids [e.g., phosphatidylglycerol (PG) and phosphatidylinositol (PI)] are unclear at present, although they represent 10–15% of the surfactant phospholipids. The acidic phospholipid, PG, is detected in surfactant phospholipid from most vertebrates studied. However, surfactant deficient in PG is highly functional (7). Acidic phospholipids appear to be capable of strong charge-dependent interactions with calcium and may be associated with surfactant proteins and therefore may play an important role in surfactant organization or homeostasis.

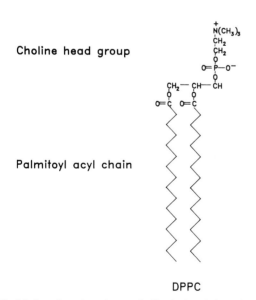

Choline head group

Palmitoyl acyl chain

DPPC

FIG. 3. Molecular structure of dipalmitoylphosphatidylcholine (DPPC). The charged head group consists of choline that interacts with the aqueous environment and the choline groups of neighboring DPPC molecules. The acyl chain, consisting of 16 carbons, is hydrophobic and interacts with neighboring acyl chains to form membranes, monolayers, vesicles, and other organized aggregate forms.

**Unique Physical Properties
of Pulmonary Surfactant**

Surfactant-like phospholipids alone are capable of generating a monolayer with low surface tension at the air–liquid interface but do not have the complete biophysical properties of native surfactant. The difference lies primarily in (a) the rapidity with which the phospholipid molecules can absorb to the surface and (b) their stability after compression and decompression during the respiratory cycle. At physiologic temperatures (i.e., below their phase transition temperature), most phospholipids are in a gel or crystalline state and are not freely mobile from aggregate or vesicular forms. Thus, the ability of pure phospholipids to move from large aggregated forms (such as tubular myelin) to a monolayer would be limited. Moreover, during compression, there is likely purification of the phospholipids by "squeeze out." The abundance of DPPC in the monolayer would be enriched by this process. Less biophysically stable molecules, both phospholipids and proteins, are likely to be excluded from the surface of the monolayer by compression and decompression. The mechanisms controlling the movement of lipids from the lamellated or tubular myelin forms to the monolayer and ultimately to the smaller catabolic remnants have not been elucidated. However, there is increasing evidence that the surfactant-associated proteins may enhance the biophysical activity of surfactant phospholipids.

Surfactant Proteins

Because phospholipids comprise the largest fraction of pulmonary surfactant, the focus of surfactant research was initially prioritized toward the elucidation of the structure, function, and the regulation of synthesis and catabolism of phospholipids in the developing lung. Initial clinical trials with exogenous surfactant replacement therapy for respiratory distress utilizing phospholipids alone were relatively unsuccessful (8,9), leading to an increased interest in the nature of the other components in surfactant. Since organic solvent extracts of pulmonary surfactant which were relatively devoid of proteins were highly surface active and provided an exogenous surfactant with properties and efficacy similar to that of whole surfactant, research attention was initially focused primarily on the phospholipids rather than on the small amounts of associated proteins (10,11). The unique properties of some of the surfactant proteins made the elucidation of their structure and function even more elusive.

Hundreds of proteins can be detected in pulmonary surfactant by sensitive silver stain analysis of the pulmonary lavage. Many of these are serum proteins, including albumin and immunoglobulins, whereas the surfactant proteins are lung-specific. At present, four distinct surfactant-associated proteins have been isolated from pulmonary surfactant. All are secretory products of the type II epithelial cells. The four proteins are now termed surfactant proteins A, B, C, and D (Table 1). The role of these proteins in surfactant structure, function, and metabolism is an active area of research interest and has been subject to several recent reviews (12–14).

TABLE 1. *Surfactant proteins*

Surfactant protein	Characteristics	Monomeric size (kDa)	Glycosylation
SP-A	Collagenous and lectin domains	28–36	+
SP-B	Hydrophobic	8	−
SP-C	Hydrophobic	3.8	−
SP-D	Collagenous domain	43	+

Surfactant Protein A (SP-A)

SP-A, the most abundant surfactant-phospholipid-associated protein (15), is a 28- to 36-kDa glycoprotein that forms larger sulfhydryl-dependent oligomers in the alveolus. The entire structure was deduced from cDNAs encoding the protein (see Fig. 4). SP-A is encoded by approximately 4.5 kilobases of genomic DNA located on the long arm of human chromosome 10 (16,17). This locus consists of five exons, some of which encode discrete protein domains. The amino-terminal portion of the SP-A is approximately 10 kDa and contains a large collagenous domain with Gly-X-Y-Gly repeats rich in hydroxyproline. Intermolecular disulfide linkages form dimers, trimers, and larger oligomers.

Electron-microscopic studies demonstrated the presence of octadecamers arranged as a "bunch of flowers," with the adjacent stems being formed by the close association of the collagenous, NH_2-terminal domains of the SP-A molecules (18). The precise role of SP-A has not been clarified; however, a number of *in vitro* experiments provide strong inferences regarding its potential functions. SP-A binds aggregates and phospholipids in a calcium-dependent manner, and intermolecular interactions of SP-A and phospholipids are critical to the formation of tubular myelin (19,20). SP-A, when mixed with phospholipid, SP-B, and calcium, generated tubular myelin forms *in vitro* (21). The carboxy-terminus of the SP-A molecule is homologous to mammalian lectins such as mannose-binding proteins. SP-A binds carbohydrates in a calcium-dependent manner and thus is, itself, a mammalian lectin (22). The presence of collagenous, lipid-binding, and lectin-like domains supports the premise that SP-A may interact with cell surfaces or other cell-associated molecules. SP-A binding sites and receptor-mediated endocytosis of SP-A have recently been demonstrated in type II epithelial cells (23,24), and binding sites were also observed in alveolar macrophages. *In vitro*, SP-A enhances the uptake of phospholipids and inhibits the secretion of phospholipids by type II epithelial cells, supporting its role in recycling and regulation of

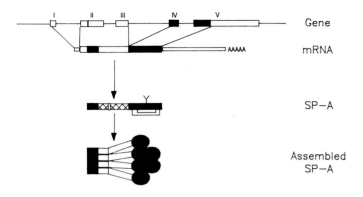

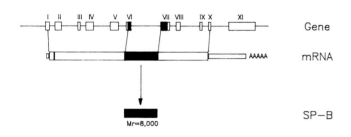

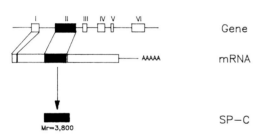

FIG. 4. Gene, mRNA, and protein structure of SP-A, SP-B, and SP-C. Each of the proteins is encoded by distinct genetic loci located on different human chromosomes (10, 2, and 8, respectively). After transcription, the introns are spliced from the mRNA, which is comprised of translated and both 3′ and 5′ nontranslated regions terminating in a polyadenylated 3′ region. The exons are represented by Roman numerals. The mRNAs are translated to form precurser proteins. SP-A and SP-B are glycosylated (Y) and are proteolytically processed. The active SP-C polypeptide is formed by proteolysis but is not glycosylated. Assembled SP-A consists of hexamers (shown) and octadecamers formed by interactions in the collagenous domain (open); the globular, lectin-like regions (filled spheres) comprise the carboxyterminus which is formed by sulfhydryl bonds between Cys residues (buackets) within each SPA molecule.

secretion of surfactant phospholipids (25–27). A variety of immune functions have been ascribed to whole surfactant, and some of these may be related to SP-A. Recent studies support the role of the SP-A in host defense. For example, SP-A, the C1q component of

complement, enhances phagocytic activity of alveolar macrophages (28). Although surfactants prepared with synthetic lipids and SP-A are not highly active (29), SP-A enhances the biophysical activity of phospholipid mixtures containing the two, more hydrophobic, lower-molecular-weight proteins SP-B and SP-C (30,31). Thus, considerable *in vitro* evidence supports the importance of SP-A in host defense surfactant homeostasis and function; its role *in vivo* remains to be discerned with more clarity.

Hydrophobic Surfactant Proteins

The presence of hydrophobic proteins in surfactant was demonstrated by Phizackerley et al. (32) and Suzuki (33). Their precise identity and structures were not clarified until relatively recently. Two low-molecular-weight proteins are relatively insoluble in aqueous environments and are strongly associated with surfactant phospholipids. Both proteins are soluble in mixtures of chloroform/methanol and in other nonpolar solvents. The proteins were isolated from organic solvent extracts of lung surfactants and are termed SP-B and SP-C (14). These proteins confer important biophysical properties to surfactant phospholipids and are present in surfactant extracts used for surfactant replacement therapy (34,35).

SP-B

SP-B is an approximately 87-kDa polypeptide encoded by a single human gene located on chromosome 2. The SP-B gene is located within approximately 10 kilobases of DNA and is comprised of 11 exons and 10 introns (36) from which the SP-B mRNA (approximately 2 kilobases) is transcribed (see Fig. 4) (37,38). The SP-B peptide is highly hydrophobic but contains a number of positively charged amino acids. SP-B forms sulfhydryl-dependent oligomers in alveolar lavage, where it is tightly associated with surfactant phospholipids. The SP-B peptide is translated as a preproprotein that is proteolytically processed by removal of a hydrophobic leader sequence. Further proteolytic processing is required to generate the carboxy and amino terminus of the active 79-amino-acid peptide found in the airway (39). The active SP-B peptide has been detected in phospholipid-rich inclusions in the type II epithelial cell and in association with phospholipids in pulmonary surfactant (40,41). Although the function of SP-B is not known with precision, SP-B confers dramatic surfactant-like activity to synthetic phospholipid mixtures and aids in the formation of tubular myelin (21,42). The mechanisms by which relatively small amounts (less than 1% by weight) of the SP-B polypeptide dramatically alter the rate of spreading and adsorption of phospholipid molecules have not been discerned. Native and synthetic SP-B peptides enhance the uptake of phospholipids by type II epithelial cells *in vitro* (43). Thus, SP-B may also play a role in the recycling of surfactant in the alveolus. The secretory and catabolic pathways controlling SP-B content in the airway have not been clarified at present.

SP-C

Human SP-C is a 3.7-kDa polypeptide encoded by a single gene located on chromosome 8 (44,45). The human SP-C gene spans approximately 3.5 kilobases of contiguous DNA comprised of six exons and five introns (Fig. 4). The active peptide, consisting of 35–36 amino acids, is derived by the proteolytic processing of a 22-kDa precursor translated from a 0.9-kilobase mRNA (46,47), and SP-C is selectively expressed in lung and is synthesized by purified type II epithelial cells *in vitro* (48). SP-C is an extraordinarily hydrophobic peptide containing a domain rich in valine which is likely inserted into the membrane. Like SP-B, SP-C enhances surfactant properties of phospholipid vesicles, enhancing both the rate of their absorption and the rate of spreading (34,49,50). The SP-C peptide enhances the uptake of phospholipid vesicles by type II epithelial cells *in vitro* and therefore may also play a role in the movement of lipids between various aggregate forms in the alveolus and in surfactant recycling (43).

SP-D

SP-D was identified in rat surfactant by its migration during electrophoresis and by its sensitivity to collagenase (51). SP-D is a 43-kDa glycoprotein which migrates in sodium dodecyl sulfate/polyacrylamide gel electrophoresis and which, like SP-A, has a large collagen-like domain. SP-D is synthesized by type II cells. The abundance of SP-D in alveolar surfactant is considerably less than SP-A, and its biological functions have not been discerned at present.

SURFACTANT PRODUCTION AND DIFFERENTIATION OF THE TYPE II CELLS

The lungs of premature infants have not had sufficient time for the differentiation of the distal airway epithelial cells required for synthesis and secretion of pulmonary surfactant. During prenatal development, "immaturity" of any of the components critical to the production of an adequate quantity and quality of pulmonary surfactant may contribute to the pathogenesis

of respiratory distress. Because surfactant is not required in intrauterine life, the genetic and synthetic apparatus controlling surfactant production has not been fully developed in the premature infant with RDS. It is surprising, however, that many infants, even those who are extremely premature (24–25 weeks gestation), do not have RDS and appear to have a highly functional surfactant system. Surfactant is produced by type II epithelial cells in the distal respiratory epithelium. These cells are derived by differentiation of precursors in the fetal lung (pre-type II cells). In the human lung, type II cells are generally recognizable by approximately 22–24 weeks of gestation. Morphologic differentiation of the fetal precursor cells is associated with the appearance of lamellar osmiophilic inclusions, glycogen depletion, and the appearance of surfactant proteins such as SP-A and SP-B. With advancing gestation, epithelial cells of the distal airway become more cuboidal and a distinct microvillous membrane is observed at the apical pole of the cells. The biosynthetic pathways critical to the production of surfactant are also not fully active in the immature lung. The expression of genes controlling surfactant phospholipid and surfactant protein production appear to be closely linked to the mature type II cell phenotype.

REGULATION OF EXPRESSION OF SURFACTANT PROTEINS AND LIPIDS

The synthesis of the phospholipid and protein components of surfactant increases dramatically prior to birth. Control of phospholipid synthesis and of the enzymes involved in phospholipid synthesis has been studied intensively during the last decade; these advances have recently been reviewed (6,52–54). The numbers of lamellar bodies in the differentiating respiratory epithelial cells increase in late gestation. The differentiated type II cells are rich in the surfactant phospholipids DSPC and PG. Synthesis of surfactant phospholipid is increased by a number of hormones, including glucocorticoids, thyroid hormones, epidermal growth factor (EGF), and cyclic adenosine monophosphate (cAMP). These hormones also enhance the morphologic differentiation of fetal pre-type II cells. In contrast, surfactant phospholipid synthesis is inhibited by testosterone and insulin; both male infants and infants of diabetic mothers are at higher risk for RDS (for review, see refs. 52–54). The study of the molecular events controlling surfactant phospholipid biosynthesis has been complicated by the inability to purify and characterize these proteins from the developing lung. The genes encoding many of the critical enzymes have not been isolated. Characterization of the regulation of genes encoding cytidylyltransferase, choline phosphotransferase, fatty acid synthase, and others might provide a more complete understanding of the potential gene regulation and the post-translational modifications of enzymes that control the increase in phospholipid synthesis in the respiratory cells of the developing lung. There is strong evidence that glucocorticoids enhance enzymes important in phospholipid biosynthesis, including fatty acid synthase, choline phosphotransferase, lysolecithin acetyltransferase, glycerol phosphate phosphatidyltransferase, phosphatidylglycerol phosphatase, choline phosphate cytidylyltransferase, and phosphatidate phosphatase in the developing lung (52,54). Maternal administration of glucocorticoids enhances pulmonary maturation in the newborn lamb and is now used to decrease the risk of RDS in premature infants (55,56).

REGULATION OF SURFACTANT PROTEIN SYNTHESIS

Surfactants A, B, and C are not expressed in high levels in fetal lung until late in gestation. Expression of the surfactant protein genes also accompanies the morphologic differentiation of type II epithelial cells and corresponds, in time, to the increase in surfactant lipid biosynthesis observed in animal models and in human fetal lung tissue during explant culture (for recent review, see refs. 12 and 57). Surfactant protein genes are expressed in a highly cell-selective manner, and the abundance of the mRNAs encoding them increases in late gestation. It is increasingly apparent that surfactant protein genes are subject to rigorous humoral and cell-specific controls. The distal respiratory epithelium of the fetal lung undergoes dramatic differentiation in the perinatal period to form type II epithelial cells that express surfactant proteins and lipids. The pre-type II cells line the developing distal airway and provide the stem cells from which type II and type I epithelial cells are generated. Type II epithelial cells also serve as progenitor cells after injury, restoring the alveolar epithelium after lung damage. There is close linkage between the surfactant protein expression and type II epithelial cell phenotype. Surfactant protein expression is also subject to numerous humoral influences. Although the developmental appearance and regulation of surfactant proteins are somewhat similar, they are also subjected to unique regulatory influences. SP-A gene expression is enhanced by cAMP and EGF and is inhibited by insulin and transforming growth factor beta (TGF-β). Both stimulatory and inhibitory effects of glucocorticoid on SP-A gene expression have been observed in fetal lung explant culture (58–61). Glucocorticoids directly stimulate SP-B and SP-C expression in vitro in human fetal lung explant cultures and in a pulmonary adenocarcinoma cell line (62,63). SP-A, SP-B, and SP-C expression increase concomitantly

TABLE 2. Factors regulating surfactant phospholipid secretion from type II cells in vitro[a]

Stimulatory	Inhibitory
Phorbol esters	SP-A
ATP, adenosine	Colchicine
Prostaglandins, leukotrienes	Compound 48/80
Catecholamines	Plant lectins
Ionomycin, A23187	
Cytochalasins	

[a] ATP, adenosine triphosphate; SP-A, surfactant protein A.

during perinatal development in the fetal rat lung (64). Several studies support the concept that SP-A expression is influenced after injury or inflammation. For example, SP-A content and mRNA are increased markedly by exposure of adult rats to 85% oxygen (65). Silicosis stimulates SP-A content in the rat lung (66).

Regulation of gene expression, occurring at both transcriptional and post-transcriptional levels, mediates the developmental and hormonal production of surfactant. Although the synthesis of the phospholipids and proteins of surfactant occurs concomitantly during development, it is also clear that each can be modulated independently to control the relative abundance of surfactant components in the alveolus.

SECRETORY MECHANISMS

The regulated storage and secretion of surfactant by type II cells is likely to be critical for successful perinatal adaptation at birth. Secretion of pulmonary surfactant occurs by an exocytotic mechanism into the alveolar lumen and is influenced by a number of humoral and mechanical stimuli (for review, see refs. 52, 53, and 67). in the adult animal, ventilation, mediated in part by β-adrenergic mechanisms, is a potent stimulus for surfactant secretion and may also mediate the enhanced phospholipid secretion observed during parturition. Surfactant phospholipid secretion has been extensively studied in vitro utilizing primary cultures of adult type II epithelial cells (for review, see refs. 67 and 68). Catecholamines, phorbol esters, and a variety of other pharmacologic agents enhance phospholipid secretion from type II cells (see Table 2). Activation of either cAMP-dependent protein kinase or protein kinase C increases phospholipid secretion by type II cells. Inhibitory factors influencing surfactant secretion have also been identified (Table 2). Most importantly, SP-A is a potent inhibitor of both kinase C and cAMP-mediated phospholipid secretion in vitro (26,27). Thus, SP-A may provide an important counterregulatory signal controlling surfactant homeostasis, both increasing phospholipid re-uptake and inhibiting its secretion.

The identity of proteins and receptors mediating the secretion and re-uptake of surfactant by type II cells has not been ascertained. The cell-surface receptors and proteins involved in receptor signaling and secretion coupling are likely to be critical to surfactant homeostasis in the developing lung. Nevertheless, the ontogenic regulation of the cellular components controlling surfactant secretion is likely to play a role in the pathogenesis of RDS in premature infants.

KINETICS OF SURFACTANT SYNTHESIS AND SECRETION

The life cycle of surfactant has become increasingly complex. An important feature of the biosynthesis and secretion of pulmonary surfactant is the relatively long time period required for its production and entry into the alveolus (for review, see ref. 69). Isotopic labeling of phospholipids in the adult sheep lung reaches maximal specific activity in the airway 24 hr after labeling. This relatively long time period is even more prolonged in the newborn animal, with surfactant reaching maximal labeling after 50 hr. The slow time course for the production and secretion of surfactant may be critical to the generation of an adequate alveolar pool of surfactant at birth or in restoring extracellular surfactant pools once they are depleted after lung injury.

SURFACTANT RECYCLING

The relative sizes and turnover rates of the intracellular pools of surfactant may also be critical factors in perinatal lung function. The recycling of lung surfactant has been recently reviewed (67,69). Comparison of the extracellular pools of surfactant with that expected to be required for the generation of monolayer suggests that extracellular surfactant phospholipid is not present in great excess. Thus, secretion re-uptake and recycling of surfactant is likely to be required for maintenance of lung function. Surfactant lipid is present in kinetically distinct intracellular pools—one in the lamellar body, another in more proximal components of the biosynthetic pathway, and a third in the alveolus. The presence of relatively large, nonlamellar body intracellular pools in the adult lung suggests that the capacity to generate the surfactant pools by biosynthesis or by recycling may be limited in the developing lung. For example, immediately following birth, lamellar body numbers increase even as the alveolar (extracellular) pool is rapidly increasing, suggesting the potential importance of this large prelamellar body phospholipid pool.

The re-uptake, re-utilization, and catabolism of surfactant are important processes in the life cycle of pulmonary surfactant. Surfactant is not lost by uptake via alveolar microphage or via the trachea. Exogenous surfactant is taken up by the lung at high rates, and the uptake process is not readily saturable. Approximately 90% of labeled surfactant is lost from the air space after the administration of exogenous surfactant in the adult rabbit after 24 hr (69). Both recycling and catabolism of pulmonary surfactant have been observed in vivo and in vitro. There is evidence that surfactant phospholipid is both directly re-utilized or is catabolized and (then re-utilized) for biosynthesis of new surfactant by type II epithelial cells (67). In vitro, β-adrenergic agents enhance the uptake and metabolism of phospholipids in the perfused rat lung (70). This clearance process is much slower in the newborn animal: Only 50% is lost from the alveolar space after administration of exogenous surfactant after 24 hr. Thus, phospholipid surfactant is recycled more slowly in the newborn than in the adult lung (69).

PERINATAL GENERATION OF AGGREGATE FORMS OF PULMONARY SURFACTANT

There is little extracellular surfactant prior to birth. The life cycle of the aggregate forms of surfactant can be readily appreciated by observing the time of appearance of the various forms after birth (71). The abundance of dense, tubular-myelin-rich fractions is highest prior to birth, and the lighter, vesicular forms, while lacking immediately following birth, appear with increasing abundance within hours of ventilation, reaching adult proportions several hours after birth. Pulse labeling of the surfactant phospholipids in the mouse lung demonstrates (a) the early labeling in very dense fractions and (b) subsequent time-dependent appearance of label in lighter, vesicular forms (72). The secretory and catabolic cycle appears to be generated rapidly following birth. Surfactant phospholipids are secreted as the relatively dense phospholipid material that interacts with calcium and surfactant proteins, SP-A and SP-B, to form tubular myelin. Smaller, vesicular forms of surfactant are relatively lacking in SP-A, are less surface active, and may represent catabolic products derived from the monolayer.

SURFACTANT FUNCTION AFTER INJURY

Severe epithelial cell injury is detected immediately after mechanical ventilation of the immature, surfactant-deficient lung. The injury is prominent in the distal respiratory tract, particularly in respiratory bronchioli (73). Both mechanical and oxidant injury may lead to increased capillary leakage of fluid and proteins during mechanical ventilation and oxygen exposure in the premature lung. Protein leakage from the capillary to the alveolar space may lead to disruption of the surfactant complex with loss of surface activity related to the effects of albumin, fibrinogen, and other proteins (52). The surface activity of the alveolar material from premature lambs with respiratory failure is distinctly inferior to that of natural surfactant but can be improved by repeated washing. A serum-surfactant-inhibiting protein of approximately 110 kDa has been described (74,75). Development of surfactant preparations that maintain their surface properties in the presence of severe alveolar capillary leak may therefore be critical to therapy after lung injury has been established. Because surfactant may also decrease alveolar capillary leakage, early treatment of surfactant deficiency may be an important consideration in clinical care of premature infants at risk for hyaline membrane disease.

EXOGENOUS SURFACTANT THERAPY

The advances in our understanding of surfactant structure and function have led to the use of exogenous surfactant replacement for treatment and prevention of RDS in premature infants. There has now been nearly a decade of experience with surfactant replacement since the first successful clinical trials of Fujiwara et al. (11). Widespread use of surfactant replacement has occurred in Japan, Europe, and the United States, and numerous controlled clinical trials support its efficacy for prevention and treatment of established RDS (for review, see refs. 69 and 76). A variety of preparations, some containing surfactant proteins and some with preparations lacking protein (77,78), have been used successfully with marked reduction of morbidity and mortality from RDS. Improvements in our clinical use of surfactant preparations for treatment of neonatal RDS are expected in the coming years, and extension of surfactant replacement to other pulmonary disorders with decreased surfactant is highly likely, especially for patients with ARDS.

SUMMARY

Knowledge gained from the analysis of the ontogenic appearance of the proteins and lipids critical to lung function in the newborn has important implications for therapy of adult disorders characterized by lung injury, surfactant deficiency, or dysfunction. The identification of the roles played by the individual components of this remarkably complex system will be required for rational treatment of disorders characterized by surfactant deficiency. It is clear that surfactant homeostasis is maintained by complex humoral, mechanical, and cellular factors that keep the alveolus from collapse. It is a dynamic system with large pools and rapid flux rates among intracellular and extracellular pools.

Therapeutic strategies based on the knowledge of gene regulation, biochemistry, and physiology of the surfactant system will likely lead to exciting new therapies for treatment of pulmonary disorders in the future.

REFERENCES

1. VanNeergaard K. Neue Auffassunder uber einen Grundbegriff der Atemmechanik. Die Retraktionskraft der Lunge abhangig von der Oberflacshens pannung in der Alveolar. 2. *Gesamte Exp Med* 66:373–394.
2. Avery ME, Mead J. Surface properties in relation to atelectasis and hyaline membrane disease. *Am J Dis Child* 1959;97:517–523.
3. Pattle RE. Properties, function and origin of the alveolar lining layer. *Nature* 1955;175:1125–1126.
4. King RJ, Clements JA. Surface active materials from dog lung. II. Composition and physiological correlations. *Am J Physiol* 1972;223:715–726.
5. Wright JR, Benson BJ, Williams MC, Goerke J, Clements JA. Protein composition of rabbit alveolar surfactant subfractions. *Biochim Biophys Acta* 1984;791:320–332.
6. Harwood JL. Lung surfactant. *Prog Lipid Res* 1987;26:211–256.
7. Beppu OS, Clements JA, Goerke J. Phosphatidylglycerol-deficient lung surfactant has normal properties. *J Appl Physiol* 1983;55:496–502.
8. Chu J, Clements JA, Cotten EK, Klaus MH, Sweet AY, Tooley WH. Neonatal pulmonary ischemia, Part I: clinical physiological studies. *Pediatrics* 1967;40:709–782.
9. Robillard E, Alarie Y, Dagenais-Perusse P, Baril E, Guilbeault A. Microaerosol administration of synthetic β-γ-diplamitoyl-L-α-lecithin in the respiratory distress syndrome: a preliminary report. *Can Med Assoc J* 1964;90:55–57.
10. Adams FH, Enhorning G. Surface properties of lung extracts. I. A dynamic alveolar model. *Acta Physiol Scand* 1966;68:23–27.
11. Fujiwara T, Maeta H, Chida S, Morita T, Watabe Y, Abe T. Artificial surfactant therapy in hyaline membrane disease. *Lancet* 1980;55–59.
12. Weaver TE. Pulmonary surfactant-associated proteins. *Gen Pharmacol* 1988;19:361–368.
13. Hawgood S. Pulmonary surfactant apoproteins: a review of protein and genomic structure. *Am J Physiol (Lung Cell Mol Physiol)* 1989;1:13–22.
14. Possmayer F. A proposed nomenclature for pulmonary surfactant-associated proteins. *Am Rev Respir Dis* 1988;138:990–998.
15. King RJ, Klass DJ, Gikas EG, Clements JA. Isolation of apoproteins from canine surface active material. *Am J Physiol* 1973;224:788–795.
16. White RT, Damm D, Miller J, et al. Isolation and characterization of the human pulmonary surfactant apoprotein gene. *Nature* 1985;317:361–363.
17. Bruns G, Stroh H, Veldman GM, Latt SA, Floros J. The 35 kd pulmonary surfactant-associated protein is encoded on chromosome 10. *Hum Genet* 1987;76:58–62.
18. Voss T, Eistetter H, Schafer KP. Macromolecular organization of natural and recombinant lung surfactant protein SP 28-36. *J Mol Biol* 1988;201:219–227.
19. King RJ, Carmichael MC, Horowitz PM. Reassembly of lipid–protein complexes of pulmonary surfactant. Proposed mechanism of interaction. *J Biol Chem* 1983;258:10672–10680.
20. King RJ, MacBeth MC. Interaction of the lipid and protein components of pulmonary surfactant. Role of phosphatidylglycerol and calcium. *Biochim Biophys Acta* 1981;647:159–168.
21. Suzuki Y, Fujita Y, Kogishi K. Reconstitution of tubular myelin from synthetic lipids and proteins associated with pig pulmonary surfactant. *Am Rev Respir Dis* 1989;140:75–81.
22. Haagsman HP, Hawgood S, Sargeant T, et al. The major lung surfactant protein, SP 28-36, is a calcium-dependent, carbohydrate-binding protein. *J Biol Chem* 1987;262:13877–13880.
23. Ryan RM, Morris RE, Rice WR, Ciraolo G, Whitsett JA. Bind-

ing and uptake of pulmonary surfactant protein (SP-A) by pulmonary type II epithelial cells. *J Histochem Cytochem* 1989; 37:429–440.

24. Kuroki Y, Mason RJ, Voelker DR. Alveolar type II cells expressing a high affinity receptor for pulmonary surfactant protein A. *Proc Natl Acad Sci USA* 1988;85:5566–5570.

25. Wright JR, Wager RE, Hawgood S, Dobbs L, Clements JA. Surfactant apoprotein Mr = 26–36,000 enhances uptake of liposomes by type II cells. *J Biol Chem* 1987;262:2888–2894.

26. Rice WR, Ross GF, Singleton FM, Dingle S, Whitsett JA. Surfactant-associated protein inhibits phospholipid secretion from type II cells. *J Appl Physiol* 1987;63:692–698.

27. Dobbs LG, Wright JR, Hawgood S, Gonzales R, Venstrom K, Nellenbogen J. Pulmonary surfactant and its components inhibit secretion of phosphatidylcholine from cultured rat alveolar type II cells. *Proc Natl Acad Sci USA* 1987;84:1010–1014.

28. Tenner AJ, Robinson SL, Borchelt J, Wright JR. Human pulmonary surfactant protein (SP-A), a protein structurally homologous to C1Q, can enhance Fcr-mediated and Cr1-mediated phagocytosis. *J Biol Chem* 1989;264:13923–13928.

29. Ross GF, Notter RH, Meuth J, Whitsett JA. Phospholipid binding and biophysical activity of pulmonary surfactant-associated protein (SAP) 35 and its non-collagenous COOH-terminal domains. *J Biol Chem* 1986;261:14283–14291.

30. Hawgood S, Benson BJ, Schilling J, Damm D, Clements JA, White RT. Nucleotide and amino acid sequences of pulmonary surfactant protein SP 18 and evidence for cooperation between SP 18 and SP 28-36 in surfactant lipid adsorption. *Proc Natl Acad Sci USA* 1987;84:66–70.

31. Chung J, Show-Hwa Y, Whitsett JA, Harding PGR, Possmayer F. Effect of surfactant-associated protein-A (SP-A) on the activity of lipid extract surfactant. *Biochim Biophys Acta* 1989; 1002:348–358.

32. Phizackerley PJR, Town M-H, Newman GE. Hydrophobic proteins of lamellated osmiophilic bodies isolated from pig lung. *Biochem J* 1979;183:731–736.

33. Suzuki Y. Effects of protein, cholesterol and phosphatidylglycerol on surface activity of lipid-protein complex reconstituted from pig pulmonary surfactant. *J Lipid Res* 1982;23:62–69.

34. Whitsett JA, Ohning BL, Ross GF, et al. Hydrophobic surfactant-associated protein in whole lung surfactant and its importance for biophysical activity in lung surfactant extracts used for replacement therapy. *Pediatr Res* 1986;20:460–467.

35. Taeusch HW, Keough KMW, Williams M, et al. Characterization of bovine surfactant for infants with respiratory distress syndrome. *Pediatrics* 1986;77:572–581.

36. Pilot-Matias TJ, Kister SE, Fox JL, Kropp K, Glasser SW, Whitsett JA. Structure and organization of the gene encoding human pulmonary surfactant phospholipid SP-B. *DNA* 1989; 8:75–86.

37. Glasser SW, Korfhagen TR, Weaver TE, Pilot-Matias T, Fox JL, Whitsett JA. cDNA and deduced amino acid sequence of human pulmonary surfactant-associated proteolipid SPL(Phe). *Proc Natl Acad Sci USA* 1987;84:4007–4011.

38. Jacobs KA, Phelps DS, Steinbrink R, et al. Isolation of a cDNA clone encoding a high molecular weight precursor to a 6-kDa pulmonary surfactant-associated protein. *J Biol Chem* 1987; 262:9808–9811.

39. Curstedt T, Johansson J, Barros-Soderling B, et al. Low molecular mass surfactant protein type I. *Eur J Biochem* 1988; 172:521–525.

40. Suzuki Y, Kogishi K, Fujita Y, Kina T, Nishikawa S. A monoclonal antibody to the 15,000 dalton protein associated with porcine pulmonary surfactant. *Exp Lung Res* 1986;11:61–73.

41. Weaver TE, Sarin VK, Sawtell N, Hull WM, Whitsett JA. Identification of surfactant proteolipid SP-B in human surfactant and fetal lung. *J Appl Physiol* 1988;65:982–987.

42. Revak SD, Merritt TA, Degryse E, et al. Use of human surfactant low molecular weight apoproteins in the reconstitution of surfactant biologic activity. *J Clin Invest* 1988;81:826–833.

43. Rice WR, Sarin VK, Fox JL, Baatz J, Wert S, Whitsett JA. Surfactant peptides stimulate uptake of phosphatidylcholine by isolated cells. *Biochim Biophys Acta* 1989;1006:237–245.

44. Johansson J, Curstedt T, Robertson B, Jornvall H. Size and structure of the hydrophobic low molecular weight surfactant-associated polypeptide. *Biochemistry* 1988;27:3544–3547.

45. Glasser SW, Korfhagen TR, Perme CM, Pilot-Matias TJ, Kister SE, Whitsett JA. Two genes encoding human pulmonary surfactant proteolipid SP-C. *J Biol Chem* 1988;263:10326–10331.

46. Glasser SW, Korfhagen TR, Weaver TE, et al. cDNA, deduced polypeptide structure and chromosomal assignment of human pulmonary surfactant proteolipid: SPL(pVal). *J Biol Chem* 1988;263:9–12.

47. Warr RG, Hawgood S, Buckley DI, et al. Low molecular weight human pulmonary surfactant protein (SP5): isolation, characterization and cDNA and amino acid sequences. *Proc Natl Acad Sci USA* 1987;84:7915–7919.

48. Liley HG, White RT, Warr RG, Benson BJ, Hawgood S, Ballard PL. Regulation of messenger RNAs for the hydrophobic surfactant proteins in human lung. *J Clin Invest* 1989;83:1191–1197.

49. Takahashi A, Fujiwara T. Proteolipid in bovine lung surfactant: its role in surfactant function. *Biochem Biophys Res Commun* 1986;135:527–532.

50. Notter RH, Shapiro DL, Ohning B, Whitsett JA. Biophysical activity of synthetic phospholipids combined with purified lung surfactant 6,000 dalton apoprotein. *Chem Phys Lipids* 1987; 44:1–17.

51. Persson A, Rust K, Chang D, Moxley M, Longmore W, Crouch E. CP4: a pneumocyte-derived collagenous surfactant-associated protein. *Biochemistry* 1988;27:8576–8585.

52. VanGolde LMG, Batenburg JJ, Robertson B. The pulmonary surfactant system: biochemical aspects and functional significance. *Physiol Reviews* 1988;68:374–455.

53. Post M, VanGolde LMG. Metabolic and developmental aspects of the pulmonary surfactant system. *Biochim Biophys Acta* 1988;947:259–286.

54. Rooney SA. Lung surfactant. *Environ Health Perspect* 1984;55:205–226.

55. Liggins GC. Premature delivery of foetal lamb infused with glucocorticoids. *J Endocrinol* 1969;45:515–523.

56. Liggins GC, Howie RN. A controlled trial of antepartum glucocorticoid treatment for treatment and prevention of the respiratory distress syndrome in premature infants. *Pediatrics* 1972; 50:515–525.

57. Ballard PL. Hormonal regulation of pulmonary surfactant. *Endocr Rev* 1989;10:165–181.

58. Whitsett JA, Pilot T, Clark JC, Weaver TE. Induction of surfactant protein in fetal lung. *J Biol Chem* 1987;262:5256–5261.

59. Ballard PL, Hawgood S, Liley H, et al. Regulation of pulmonary surfactant apoprotein SP 28-36 gene in fetal human lung. *Proc Natl Acad Sci USA* 1986;83:9527–9531.

60. Whitsett JA, Weaver TE, Lieberman MA, Clark JC, Daugherty C. Differential effects of epidermal growth factor and transforming growth factor-β on synthesis of Mr = 35,000 surfactant-associated protein in fetal lung. *J Biol Chem* 1987;262:7908–7913.

61. Mendelson CR, Chen C, Boggaram V, Zacharias C, Snyder JM. Regulation of the synthesis of the major surfactant apoprotein in fetal rabbit lung tissue. *J Biol Chem* 1986;261:9938–9943.

62. Whitsett JA, Weaver TE, Clark JC, et al. Glucocorticoid enhances surfactant proteolipid Phe and pVal synthesis and RNA in fetal lung. *J Biol Chem* 1987;262:15618–15623.

63. O'Reilly MA, Gazdar AF, Clark JC, et al. Glucocorticoids regulate surfactant protein synthesis in a pulmonary adenocarcinoma cell line. *Am J Physiol* 1989;257:L385–L392.

64. Schellhase DE, Emrie PA, Fisher JH, Shannon JM. Ontogeny of surfactant apoproteins in the rat. *Pediatr Res* 1989;26:167–174.

65. Nogee LM, Wispé JR, Clark JC, Whitsett JA. Increased synthesis and mRNA of surfactant protein A in oxygen-exposed rats. *Am J Respir Cell Mol Biol* 1989;1:119–125.

66. Kawada H, Horiuchi T, Shannon JM, Kuroki Y, Voelker DR, Mason RJ. Alveolar type II cells, surfactant protein A (SP-A) and the phospholipid components of surfactant in acute silicosis in the rat. *Am Rev Respir Dis* 1989;140:460–470.

67. Wright JR, Clements JA. Metabolism and turnover of lung sur-factant. *Am Rev Respir Dis* 1987;135:426–444.
68. Mason RJ. Surfactant synthesis, secretion, and function in al-veoli and small airways. *Respiration* 1987;51(Suppl 1):3–9.
69. Jobe A, Ikegami M. Surfactant for the treatment of respiratory distress syndrome. *Am Rev Respir Dis* 1987;136:1256–1275.
70. Fisher AB, Dodia C, Chander A. Secretagogues for surfactant increase lung uptake of alveolar phospholipids. *Am J Physiol (Lung Cell Mol Physiol)* 1989;257:L248–L252.
71. Bruni R, Baritussio A, Quaglino D, Gabelli C, Benevento M, Ronchetti IP. Postnatal transformations of alveolar surfactant in the rabbit: changes in pool size, pool morphology and isoforms of the 32–38 kDa apoprotein. *Biochim Biophys Acta* 1988; 958:255–267.
72. Gross NJ, Narine KR. Surfactant subtypes in mice: character-ization and quantification. *J Appl Physiol* 1989;66:342–349.
73. Nilsson R, Grossman G, Robertson B. Lung surfactant and the pathogenesis of neonatal bronchiolar lesions induced by artificial ventilation. *Pediatr Res* 1978;12:249–255.
74. Jobe A, Ikegami M, Jacobs H, Jones S, Conaway D. Permea-bility of premature lamb lungs to protein and the effect of sur-factant on that permeability. *J Appl Physiol* 1983;55:169–176.
75. Ikegami M, Jobe A, Berry D. A protein that inhibits surfactant in respiratory distress syndrome. *Biol Neonate* 1986;50:121–129.
76. Whitsett JA, Weaver TE. Pulmonary surfactant proteins: im-plications for surfactant replacement therapy. In: Shapiro DL, Notter RH, eds. *Surfactant replacement therapy*. New York: Alan R Liss, 1989;71–89.
77. Durand DJ, Clyman RI, Heymann MA, et al. Effect of a protein-free synthetic surfactant on survival and pulmonary function in preterm lambs. *J Pediatr* 1985;107:775–780.
78. Morley CJ, Miller N, Bangham AD, Davis JA. Dry artificial lung surfactant and its effect on very premature babies. *Lancet* 1981; 6468–6470.

THE LUNG: *Scientific Foundations*
edited by R.G. Crystal, J.B. West et al.
Raven Press, Ltd., New York © 1991.

CHAPTER 6.2.1

Physiology of Postnatal Growth

Jacopo P. Mortola

METABOLIC AND VENTILATORY RATES

The newborn mammal, not dissimilarly from the adult, can be looked at as a biochemical machinery transforming chemical energy via a number of complex metabolic processes. Anaerobic pathways of energy supply do not represent a durable and effective alternative to aerobic energy production. Gas exchange via the skin may have some practical importance only for CO_2 elimination in the smallest newborn mammals, like some marsupials that are born at a very early stage of development (1). Therefore, in newborns as in adults, the whole metabolic process can be simplified into a chemical reaction, of which oxygen (O_2) is one of the reagents and carbon dioxide (CO_2) one of the products, with lung ventilation ($\dot{V}E$) representing the pathway common to both O_2 and CO_2 exchange. Hence, a close relationship between $\dot{V}E$ and the metabolic requirement of the organism [conveniently expressed by the rates of O_2 use ($\dot{V}O_2$) and of CO_2 elimination ($\dot{V}CO_2$)] should be expected. This is indeed the case. *Among newborns of different species* $\dot{V}E$ and $\dot{V}O_2$ (per unit of animal's weight, i.e., specific $\dot{V}E$ and $\dot{V}O_2$) change in close proportion, the values of the smallest newborns being higher than those of newborns of larger species. *Within the same species*, with growth, specific $\dot{V}E$ and $\dot{V}O_2$ gradually decline in parallel; the result is that blood gases, after the early postnatal period, remain almost unchanged throughout life.

At least in part, the differences in metabolic and ventilatory rates with age reflect the unescapable fact that newborns are smaller than adults. In fact, geometrical considerations indicate that the smaller the animal the larger its body surface-to-volume ratio, hence the higher the ratio between the primary source of heat

dissipation (body surface) and heat production (body mass). But because many newborns have metabolic rates that are higher than those of similiar size adults of different species (2), the high specific $\dot{V}O_2$ and $\dot{V}CO_2$ of the newborn mammal also reflect less effective thermoinsulation and thermoregulatory mechanisms.

The developmental and interspecies differences in specific $\dot{V}E$ are almost exclusively determined by differences in breathing frequency, while specific VT is approximately constant, around 8–10 ml/kg, independent of species size and almost unaffected by age. Breathing rate is usually much higher in the newborn than in the adult (e.g., about three to four times higher in the resting human infant than in the adult human), although the magnitude of the age difference depends on the species, being usually less pronounced in the smallest mammals (3,4).

NEONATAL BREATHING PATTERN

The scanty information available on the evolution of the breathing pattern in the neonatal period is almost exclusively from studies in the human infant (5–8), and it can be summarized in the following manner. The first breath after birth is usually deep and slow, almost twice the VT of the resting infant at a few days. The first expiration is less than the first inspiration, and the difference in air volume reflects the beginning in the establishment of the functional residual capacity (FRC) (Fig. 1). This is the result of purely mechanical factors, which include the tensioactive properties of surfactants and the viscous characteristics of the neonatal lung tissue. After several breaths at relatively low rate, for the next few hours respiration becomes rapid (averaging 70–90 breaths/min at 90 min after birth), often shallow and extremely irregular (Fig. 1). Short apneas alternate with bursts of tachypnea, and expiratory flows are often interrupted for periods of variable duration by complete laryngeal closure, with lung

J. P. Mortola: Department of Physiology, McGill University, Montreal, Quebec H3G 1Y6, Canada.

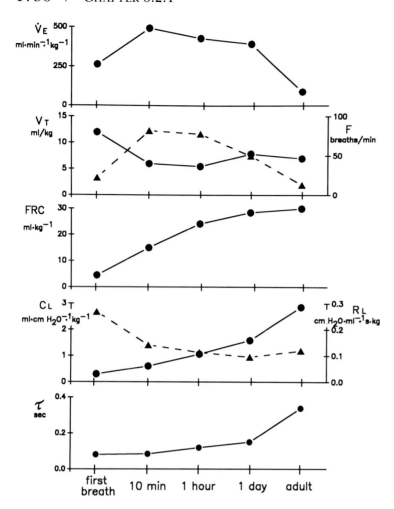

FIG. 1. Values of some respiratory variables in humans during the early phases after birth and adulthood (data from refs. 2 and 9). C_L, lung compliance; F, breathing frequency (*dashed line*); FRC, functional residual capacity; R_L, total pulmonary resistance (*dashed line*); τ, lung time constant; $\dot{V}_E$, expired volume per minute; V_T, tidal volume.

volume maintained above FRC (8,10,11). This rapid, irregular breathing, common to all normal infants, irrespective of their mode of delivery or type of maternal anesthesia, and also observed in some newborn mammals in their early postnatal phases (12,13), usually disappears within the first day. However, it could persist much longer in infants with delay in lung fluid clearance and associated low lung compliance.

It is difficult to sort out to what extent the characteristics of the neonatal breathing pattern are the consequence of the rapidly changing phenomena occurring in the respiratory system during the early postnatal period or reflect a programmed routine with specific physiological aims. The notion that pulmonary fluid absorption in the newborn requires several hours (2,14) supports the view that the rapid breathing of the first hours is reflex in nature; in fact, stimulation of a group of pulmonary unmyelinated fibers by an increase in interstitial pressure is known to determine rapid and shallow breathing. From an energetics viewpoint, the fast and shallow pattern minimizes the higher external work of breathing determined by the low lung compliance.

The laryngeal occlusions during the first hours are the most apparent manifestation of the phenomenon of expiratory adduction of the vocal folds, which is physiological in adult mammals and also pronounced in the first days after birth ("grunting"). Since during the laryngeal occlusion above FRC the inspiratory muscles are relaxed (13,15), airway pressure rises; therefore, laryngeal closure (and, to a minor extent, grunting) may contribute to the absorption of the pulmonary fluid. In addition, the braking of expiration effectively prolongs the time constant of the respiratory system, raising the FRC above the passive resting volume of the respiratory system (Vr) (16–18). Laryngeal closures and braking are observed not only in infants but also in many newborn mammals during the first hours postnatally. The inputs from pulmonary vagal receptors seem to be important in the laryngeal control of expiratory flow, although the full details of the mechanisms involved are not clear. Bypassing of the vocal folds in clinical or experimental conditions (tracheostomy) decreases the newborn's lung compliance and promotes respiratory problems. In intubated infants, this is avoided by the common practice of adding an end-expiratory positive pressure, which, by mechanically substituting the larynx, keeps lung volume and compliance elevated.

STRUCTURE AND FUNCTION

The overall design of the respiratory system in the neonatal and young mammal is as in the adult. However, some characteristics of its structural constituents need to be mentioned, because they are the basis of age-related differences in the mechanical behavior of the respiratory pump and in some aspects of respiratory control.

Upper Airways

In the human infant the laryngeal block is located higher, with respect to its projection on the vertebral column, than in the adult (19). The oropharyngeal region is therefore relatively narrower than in the adult, and the easier apposition of the posterior portion of the tongue with the soft palate facilitates the separation of the oral cavity from the nasopharyngeal pathway. This is important for the generation of the negative mouth pressures required for sucking, a fundamental function for all newborn mammals which can effectively occur without interference with the breathing act.

Infants, as most newborn mammals, are often considered to be obligatory nose breathers (20). In reality, breathing through the mouth can and does occur, although nose breathing is easier in infants, because of the incomplete formation of the turbinate nasal bones; switching to mouth breathing when nasal resistance is increased may be delayed or difficult particularly in prematures (21). The nose-breathing attitude does not seem to have a mechanical basis, since mouth resistance is not higher than in adults; rather, it may represent a behavioral phenomenon, possibly related to incomplete development of the neural circuitry that coordinates breathing with the nonrespiratory functions of the upper airways (20).

In adult mammals afferents from the laryngeal area have been extensively studied. Most receptors are sensitive to changes in laryngeal pressure, while a lower percentage is specifically responding to activity of upper airway muscles or to changes in upper airway airflow and temperature. In newborn dogs qualitatively similar populations of receptors have been found, although there would seem to be a lower concentration of airflow (or cold) sensitive receptors. In addition, the receptor activity at any given laryngeal pressure is much attenuated (22). Despite these differences, the reflex ventilatory response to pressure and flow stimuli in the newborn is much more pronounced than in the adult. For example, experimentally applied steady flows through the upper airways can substantially decrease ventilation in kittens and puppies, with minimal or no effects in adult cats and dogs (23).

Chemosensitive free endings responding to water and, particularly, to changes in the ionic composition and pH of their microenvironment have been described in both newborns and adults (24,25). These receptors are considered responsible for the reflex responses to instillation of liquid in the larynx, with apnea, bradycardia, and hypotension, which, as the reflex responses to physical stimuli, are much more dramatic in the newborn than in the adult. They have been the object of considerable attention because of the possible implication in the pathophysiology of the sudden infant death syndrome.

The much stronger reflex responses to upper airway stimuli in newborns than in adults, and the observation that comparable stimulation of laryngeal afferents induces apnea only in the newborn, are some of the data supporting the concept that the central processing of the upper airway inputs is not the same throughout postnatal life but is undergoing important maturational changes.

Cough, a defense mechanism against stimuli in the upper and lower airways, has a low incidence in the first days after birth and it gradually develops postnatally, the maturation of the response to laryngeal stimuli possibly preceding that to stimulation of the lower airways (Fig. 2). While one may expect that cough is suppressed in the fetus, in whom all the airways are liquid filled, its low incidence in the newborn period is puzzling. Ventilatory inhibition and apnea may be regarded as appropriate protective responses to upper airway disturbances, but, if not associated with an effective expulsive act, they could become a risky defense strategy.

Lung and Lower Airways

At birth, the development of the lower respiratory tract is far from complete (26,27). The most peripheral airways are absent or only partly formed, and only a fraction of the adult population of alveoli is present. In fact, in some of the smallest species, no true alveoli are recognized at birth, and saccule septation and alveolar formation can begin after a few days. One may therefore expect that in the newborn the volume of the conducting airways, relative to that of the gas exchange area, is larger than in the adult; indeed, the relationship between compliance (mostly reflecting the volume of the peripheral airspaces) and resistance (mostly determined by the size of the large conducting airways) changes with age, as discussed later. In ad-

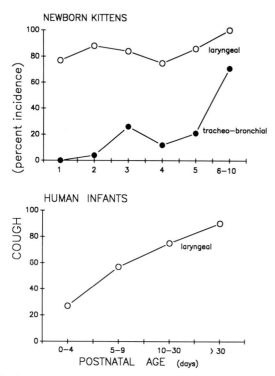

FIG. 2. Percent incidence of the cough reflex in anesthetized kittens and full-term infants during the first days of life. (Modified from ref. 20.)

dition, one may expect that the mechanical function of the lung and airways may differ from later developmental stages. Trachea and lower airways are highly compliant in both term and premature newborns (28), which, coupled to the low lung recoil mostly resulting from the low elastin and collagen pulmonary content, is the structural basis for the susceptibility of the newborn's tracheobronchial tree to dynamic airway compression. Air trapping and uneven air distribution become a less likely event with postnatal growth, which sees a gradual increase in lung recoil, stiffening of the airways, and the rise in the FRC (2).

Pulmonary Afferents and Reflexes

Recordings from the pulmonary afferents of the peripheral cut end of the vagi nerves have indicated the presence in newborns, as in adults, of two major populations of airway receptors, the slowly adapting receptors (SARs) and the rapidly adapting receptors (RARs). The former are chiefly involved in the regulation of the breathing pattern; the latter are thought to be part of pulmonary defense mechanisms, including periodic sighs for airway reexpansion and cough.

In newborns, however, the percentage of RARs is substantially less than in the adult, possibly contributing to the above mentioned low incidence of cough in the neonatal period. In addition, in the newborn the

SARs are less active, at similar transpulmonary pressures, and very few fire spontaneously at end-expiration (22). These differences may reflect incomplete structural maturation of the neurons and their axons (in particular, partial myelination) as well as differences in airway tension. In fact, at any given transpulmonary pressure P, the local tension, $T = P \times r$, is the appropriate stimulus of these receptors; because the radius of curvature r of the airways is much smaller in the newborn, T is also expected to be smaller.

The apnea following lung inflation (Hering–Breuer reflex), which represents the pulmonary vagal reflex contributing to the regulation of the depth and frequency of breathing, is often reported to be stronger in the newborn than in the adult, at least for comparable, body weight normalized, lung volume changes. This would be at odds with the finding of lower SAR activity in the newborn and would call attention to important age-related differences in the central integration of these pulmonary inputs. However, an opposite conclusion can be reached with respect to the strength of the Hering–Breuer reflex when transpulmonary pressure, rather than lung volume, is used as the reference parameter in the comparison between ages, therefore taking into account the lower lung compliance of the newborn and the proper stimulus of the airway receptors (29).

Thorax

The major change readily apparent in the infant's thorax during growth is the progressive modification in shape. From an almost circular profile at birth, the cross section of the thorax becomes more elliptical, with the lateral diameter exceeding the anterior–posterior dimension. In addition, the angle of attachment of the ribs to the vertebral column, close to 90°, gradually increases with age. The pull due to the hydrostatic force generated by the abdominal content in the vertical posture is the most likely explanation for these changes, probably combined with the increased muscle mass and the progressive mineralization of the soft thoracic structures. Functionally, this results in a progressive stiffening of the chest wall (defined physiologically, rather than anatomically, comprising any structure outside the lung that moves during passive changes in lung volume), which contributes to the increase in Vr and to greater chest stability against changes in pleural pressure. In addition, the change in rib orientation and the progressive increase in the area of the lower rib cage facing the abdomen (apposition area) gradually increase the expanding inflationary action of the abdominal pressure on the rib cage during contraction of the diaphragm in inspiration.

Respiratory Muscles

The mass of diaphragm and intercostal muscles (per unit of body weight) does not appreciably differ between newborns and adults. The concentration of type 1 slow-twitch, high-oxidative "fatigue-resistant" fibers was found to be low in the muscles of premature infants (30), but other studies in different species indicated that the newborn's respiratory muscles are well equipped for fast oxidative requirements (31–33).

No information is available on the developmental aspects of the mechanical properties of the respiratory muscles (force–length and force–velocity relationships) and their individual contribution to lung expansion (ventilatory action). What is known is that the inspiratory (negative) pleural pressures can be extremely high, up to 70 cmH$_2$O during the first breath at birth (2,5,6), and maximal inspiratory and expiratory pressures in children are very close to the adult values (34). These results can be explained by reminding ourselves that pressure is equal to the ratio between force and area; the former is proportional to the cross section of the muscle, the latter to the area over which the muscle force is applied, which, in first approximation, is the thorax surface. Because during growth respiratory muscle mass increases in proportion to body mass, muscle cross section and thorax surface area are expected to increase uniformly, yielding age-independent values of maximal inspiratory muscle pressure. Departures from this prediction could reflect the above mentioned developmental differences in the geometry of the chest wall, notable among which is the increase in curvature of the diaphragm dome with growth.

MECHANICAL BEHAVIOR OF THE VENTILATORY PUMP

In the newborn, static lung compliance (C$_L$) tends to be smaller, per unit of lung weight, than in the adult and increases progressively with age (2,35). The low C$_L$ of the early postnatal period is probably more because of the smaller volume of the airspaces than because of differences in pulmonary tissue distensibility. During spontaneous breathing, dynamic C$_L$ in the newborn can be even lower than the static value, partly because of the relatively high breathing rate and asynchronous behavior of peripheral lung units, and mostly because of the viscous properties of the newborn lung, which are much more marked than in the adult (36). With growth, as C$_L$ increases, resistance (R$_L$) decreases, the former reflecting the progressive expansion of the lung peripheral airways, and the latter the increase in the cross section of the larger airways. However, as one may expect from the notion that the peripheral airways and alveoli are far more incomplete

at birth than the larger airways are, the postnatal increase in C$_L$ exceeds the decrease in R$_L$. Because the product of compliance and resistance has the physical dimension of time, and indeed C$_L$ × R$_L$ represents the time constant of the lung (τ), it follows that τ increases from birth to adulthood (Fig. 1). It is of interest that as τ increases breathing frequency decreases with growth in what may seem a perfect matching between the metabolic and ventilatory requirements of the organism and the mechanical behavior of its respiratory pump.

Because in newborns the outward recoil of the chest is very small and chest wall compliance (Cw) is high, it follows that the Cw/C$_L$ ratio is high in both static and dynamic conditions, a characteristic that represents the fundamental aspect of neonatal respiratory mechanics (2). The little outward pull of the chest on the lung implies that (a) the passive resting volume of the respiratory system (Vr), per unit of lung weight, is small and (b) the recoil pressure of the lung at Vr is less negative (usually about half) than the adult value (37,38). This has several functional implications, two of which are briefly examined.

Control of Functional Residual Capacity

A low Vr could mean small O$_2$ reserve, large oscillations in blood gases with each breathing cycle, and possibly closure of some airways with ventilation distribution inequalities and higher inspiratory work. All the above is avoided in the infant by dynamically maintaining the end-expiratory level (FRC) above Vr via mechanisms that prolong the expiratory time constant of the respiratory system (39). They include the postinspiratory activity of the inspiratory muscles and the expiratory adduction of the vocal cords. The final result is that human infants breathe with an FRC − Vr difference of about 10–15 ml, or about 3 ml/kg; in other words, through the control of the duration of expiration and of the magnitude of expiratory flow, the end-expiratory level is kept above the value that one would expect on the basis of the passive characteristics of the infant's respiratory system. The advantages of an increased mean lung volume (and FRC) are obvious and were mentioned previously. One possible disadvantage is the extra cost related to the contraction of the inspiratory muscles without inspiratory flow during the very early phase of inspiration (since airway pressure must decrease below the recoil pressure of the respiratory system at FRC before inspiratory airflow can occur). This and other potential problems may explain why in the smallest newborn mammalian species, which have very high metabolic and ventilatory requirements, the dynamic elevation of the FRC is present only in the first hours after birth (when it is probably crucial for lung expansion and fluid reabsorption), while afterward it is abandoned.

Chest Wall Distortion

In the mammalian respiratory system, the main pressure generator, the diaphragm, faces both the lungs and the inner side of the thorax. Therefore, the mechanical design is such that whenever the diaphragm contracts and lowers the pleural pressure not only do the lungs tend to inflate but the rib cage also tends to cave inward. A clear example of the mere action of the diaphragm on the chest wall is offered by patients with no activity of the intercostal muscles (tetraplegic patients) [40]. The fact that rib cage paradoxical inward motion in inspiration occurs only occasionally in healthy term infants and very rarely in normal adults implies that extradiaphragmatic muscles are offsetting the distorting action of the diaphragm. In other words, outward motion of the chest during inspiration in a way that may seem similar to that occurring during artificial ventilation (in which the rib cage is expanded by the increase in pleural pressure) should not be interpreted as absence of distortion (where distortion is defined as a different configuration of the chest wall from the configuration assumed under passive condition *at the same lung volume*), but rather as compensation of distortion [41]. The two concepts are totally different when examined from the viewpoint of the energetics of breathing.

In newborns, the high C_W/C_L ratio, coupled to other structural characteristics of the thorax mentioned above and the incomplete proprioceptive control of the intercostal muscles [42], favors chest distortion; this can become very apparent in the form of inward paradoxical motion of the thorax during inspiration, particularly in premature infants and during REM sleep.

RESPONSE TO HYPOXIA: ADAPTATION AND ACCLIMATIZATION

When faced by acute hypoxia the human infant increases $\dot{V}_E$ only transiently; in a few minutes $\dot{V}_E$ can be back to the normoxic value or even below it [43]. This pattern, often labeled *biphasic ventilatory response*, has attracted much attention because it would seem to indicate that the newborn is deprived of one of the basic mechanisms of acclimatization to the decrease in O_2 availability. After the immediate increase, the drop in $\dot{V}_E$ (which, to a minor extent and over a longer period of time, occurs also in the adult) is due entirely to a decrease in V_T, while breathing rate remains elevated. Measurements of chemoreceptor activity, in anesthetized animals, did not show signs of adaptation, nor could the phenomenon be explained as

the result of an increase in the mechanical impedance of the ventilatory pump or fatigue of the respiratory muscles. In newborn infants [44] as in newborns of many other species born relatively immature [4,45], the metabolic rate drops in hypoxia rather rapidly, to such an extent that the $\dot{V}_E/\dot{V}_{O_2}$ ratio is increased even in those cases in which the absolute value of $\dot{V}_E$ during hypoxia is below the normoxic value. As a result, the decline in $\dot{V}_E$ does not yield an increase in Pa_{CO_2}: on the contrary, Pa_{CO_2} decreases, indicating that the newborn is hyperventilating during hypoxia relative to its new low metabolic requirements [45]. The hypoxic newborn mammal is therefore combining strategies of acclimatization (among which is the increase in $\dot{V}_E$) and of adaptation, with a drop in metabolic rate reminiscent of the hypoxic response of lower vertebrates and of mammalian hibernation. The disadvantage of this double strategy is that, by lowering metabolic rate, body growth is impaired, and some organs are affected more than others. Indeed, some of the structural changes of chronic neonatal hypoxia can persist well beyond the removal of the hypoxic stimulus. On the other hand, the obvious advantage of adaptation is that tissue P_{O_2} is not as low as it would be with the only acclimatization. The end result is that the newborn mammal, by renouncing the homeothermic privilege and reducing O_2 needs, can survive hypoxia much better than the adult.

The mechanisms that allow the hypometabolic response of the newborn mammal against hypoxia are not known. It is therefore presently impossible to say whether the declining phase of $\dot{V}_E$ during the response to hypoxia is the direct consequence of the drop in metabolic rate or is a parallel phenomenon determined by as yet obscure O_2-mediated responses in the central nervous system [46].

REFERENCES

1. Baudinette RV, Runciman SIC, Frappell PF, Gannon BJ. Development of the marsupial cardiorespiratory system. In: Tyndale-Biscoe CH, Janssens PA, eds. *The developing marsupial. Models for biomedical research.* Berlin, Springer-Verlag, 1988;132–147.
2. Mortola JP. Dynamics of breathing in newborn mammals. *Physiol Rev* 1987;67:187–243.
3. Mortola JP, Noworaj A. Breathing pattern and growth: comparative aspects. *J Comp Physiol B* 1985;155:171–176.
4. Mortola JP, Rezzonico R, Lanthier C. Ventilation and oxygen consumption during acute hypoxia in newborn mammals: a comparative analysis. *Respir Physiol* 1989;78:31–43.
5. Karlberg P, Cherry RB, Escardo FE, Koch G. Respiratory studies in newborn infants. II. Pulmonary ventilation and mechanics of breathing in the first minutes of life, including the onset of respiration. *Acta Paediatr* 1962;51:121–136.
6. Saunders RA, Milner AD. Pulmonary pressure/volume relationships during the last phase of delivery and the first postnatal breaths in human subjects. *J Pediatr* 1978;93:667–673.
7. Mortola JP, Fisher JT, Smith JB, Fox GS, Weeks S, Willis D. Onset of respiration in infants delivered by cesarean section. *J Appl Physiol* 1982;52:716–734.

8. Fisher JT, Mortola JP, Smith JB, Fox GS, Weeks S. Respiration in newborns. Development of the control of breathing. *Am Rev Respir Dis* 1982;125:650–657.
9. Polgar G, Weng TR. The functional development of the respiratory system. From the period of gestation to adulthood. *Am Rev Respir Dis* 1979;120:625–695.
10. Milner AD, Saunders RA, Hopkin IE. Effects of delivery by caesarean section on lung mechanics and lung volumes in the human neonate. *Arch Dis Child* 1978;53:545–548.
11. Radvanyi-Bouvet MF, Monset-Couchard M, Morel-Kahn F, Vilente G, Dreyfus-Brisac C. Expiratory patterns during sleep in normal full-term and premature neonates. *Biol Neonate* 1982;41:74–84.
12. Farber JP. Laryngeal effects and respiration in the suckling opossum. *Respir Physiol* 1978;35:189–201.
13. Mortola JP. Breathing pattern in newborns. *J Appl Physiol* 1984;56:1533–1540.
14. Humphreys PW, Normand ICS, Reynolds EOR, Strang LB. Pulmonary lymph flow and the uptake of liquid from the lungs of the lamb at the start of breathing. *J Physiol (Lond)* 1967;193:1–29.
15. Harrison VC, Heese HdeV, Klein M. The significance of grunting in hyaline membrane disease. *Pediatrics* 1968;41:549–559.
16. Mortola JP, Fisher JT, Smith B, Fox G, Weeks S. Dynamics of breathing in infants. *J Appl Physiol* 1982;52:1209–1215.
17. Mortola JP, Milic-Emili J, Noworaj A, Smith B, Fox G, Weeks S. Muscle pressure and flow during expiration in infants. *Am Rev Respir Dis* 1984;129:49–53.
18. Kosch PC, Stark AR. Dynamic maintenance of end-expiratory lung volume in full-term infants. *J Appl Physiol* 1984;57:1126–1133.
19. Bosma JF. Functional anatomy of the upper airway during development. In: Mathew OP, Sant'Ambrogio G, eds. *Respiratory function of the upper airway*. New York: Marcel Dekker, 1988;47–86.
20. Mortola JP, Fisher JT. Upper airway reflexes in newborns. In: Mathew OP, Sant'Ambrogio G, eds. *Respiratory function of the upper airway*. New York: Marcel Dekker, 1988;303–357.
21. Rodenstein DO, Perlmutter N, Stanescu DC. Infants are not obligatory nasal breathers. *Am Rev Respir Dis* 1985;131:343–347.
22. Fisher JT, Sant'Ambrogio G. Airway and lung receptors and their reflex effects in the newborn. *Pediatr Pulmonol* 1985;1:112–126.
23. Al-Shway SF, Mortola JP. Respiratory effects of airflow through the upper airways in newborn kittens and puppies. *J Appl Physiol* 1982;53:805–814.
24. Storey AT, Johnson P. Laryngeal water receptors initiating apnea in the lamb. *Exp Neurol* 1975;47:42–55.
25. Boggs DF, Bartlett D Jr. Chemical specificity of a laryngeal apneic reflex in puppies. *J Appl Physiol* 1982;53:455–462.
26. Burri PH. Develoment and growth of the human lung. In: Fishman AP, Fisher AB, eds. *Handbook of physiology. The respiratory system*, vol 1. Bethesda: American Physiological Society, 1985;1–46.
27. Brody JS, Thurlbeck WM. Development, growth, and aging of the lung. In: Macklem PT, Mead J, eds. *Handbook of physiology. The respiratory system*, vol 3, part 1. Bethesda: American Physiological Society, 1986;355–386.
28. Croteau JR, Cook CD. Volume–pressure and length–tension measurements in human tracheal and bronchial segments. *J Appl Physiol* 1962;16:170–172.
29. Gaultier C, Mortola JP. Hering–Breuer inflation reflex in young and adult mammals. *Can J Physiol Pharmacol* 1981;59:1017–1021.
30. Keens TG, Bryan AC, Levison H, Ianuzzo CD. Developmental pattern of muscle fiber types in human ventilatory muscles. *J Appl Physiol* 1978;44:909–913.
31. Lieberman DA, Maxwell LC, Faulkner JA. Adaptation of guinea pig diaphragm muscle to aging and endurance training. *Am J Physiol* 1972;222:556–560.
32. Maxwell LC, McCarter RJM, Kuehl TJ, Robotham JL. Development of histochemical and functional properties of baboon respiratory muscles. *J Appl Physiol* 1983;54:551–561.
33. Tamaki N. Effect of growth on muscle capillarity and fiber type composition in rat diaphragm. *Eur J Appl Physiol* 1985;54:24–29.
34. Gaultier C, Zinman R. Maximal static pressures in healthy children. *Respir Physiol* 1983;51:45–61.
35. Cook CD, Helliesen PJ, Agathon S. Relation between mechanics of respiration, lung size and body size from birth to young adulthood. *J Appl Physiol* 1958;13:349–352.
36. Sullivan KJ, Mortola JP. Age related changes in the rate of stress relaxation within the rat respiratory system. *Respir Physiol* 1987;67:295–309.
37. Fisher JT, Mortola JP. Statics of the respiratory system in newborn mammals. *Respir Physiol* 1980;41:155–172.
38. Frappell PB, Mortola JP. Respiratory mechanics in small newborn mammals. *Respir Physiol* 1989;76:25–36.
39. Mortola JP. Establishment of the end-expiratory level (FRC) in newborn mammals. In: Walters DV, Strang LB, Geubelle F, eds. *Physiology of the fetal and neonatal lung*. Lancaster: MTP Press Limited, 1987;129–136.
40. Mortola JP, Sant'Ambrogio G. Motion of the rib cage and the abdomen in tetraplegic patients. *Clin Sci Mol Med* 1978;54:25–32.
41. Mortola JP, Saetta M, Fox G, Smith G, Weeks S. Mechanical aspects of chest wall distortion. *J Appl Physiol* 1985;59:295–304.
42. Trippenbach T. Chest wall reflexes in newborns. *Bull Eur Physiopathol Respir* 1985;21:115–122.
43. Jansen AH, Chernick V. Development of respiratory control. *Physiol Rev* 1983;63:437–483.
44. Cross KW, Tizard JPM, Trythall DAH. The gaseous metabolism of the newborn infant breathing 15% oxygen. *Acta Paediatr* 1958;47:217–237.
45. Mortola JP, Rezzonico R. Metabolic and ventilatory rates in newborn kittens during acute hypoxia. *Respir Physiol* 1988;73:55–68.
46. Moss IR, Inman JG. Neurochemicals and respiratory control during development. *J Appl Physiol* 1989;67:1–13.

THE LUNG: Scientific Foundations
edited by R.G. Crystal, J.B. West et al.
Raven Press, Ltd., New York © 1991.

CHAPTER 6.3.1

Morphology of the Aging Lung

William M. Thurlbeck

That morphologic changes occur in the lung with age is incontrovertible. However, the issue of whether these are due to aging or associated with aging is not often addressed. One only has to read the older literature concerning the physiologic changes in the lung with age to recognize an obvious problem, not recognized at the time: The subjects studied were thought to be healthy, but smokers were included. This problem now exists concerning the morphologic changes described in aged lungs in humans. Smokers have never been rigorously excluded, and completely credible information in unlikely to be obtained from retrospective review of the clinical records of patients whose lungs are obtained at autopsy. More subtle problems also exist, and perhaps the best analogy is wrinkles due to aging. Wrinkles are associated with aging, and many would consider them to be caused by aging. A little reflection suggests that this idea is not entirely true. The severity of wrinkling is widely different between subjects, and those heavily exposed to sunshine have more wrinkling. In any given person, wrinkling varies topographically: It is most severe in areas most exposed to the sun (the face), less severe in areas exposed to a lesser degree (arms), and may be absent in regions hardly ever exposed (buttocks). Wrinkling is thus best thought of as representing a normal process, which is exaggerated and hastened in nearly all people by sunlight. The lung may be similar. The great majority of people are exposed to environmental pollutants throughout life, and the degree of exposure varies widely. It is also true that the human lungs that have been studied in autopsies have come from major urban centers. The situation may not be very different in experimental animals: In most instances, they breathe the same air as we do, and partial filtering may not remove significant noxious agents. Perhaps the ideal animals in which to study normal aging are those that were raised in totally sterile conditions and that breathed completely filtered air. The constraints, of course, are the assumptions that different types of animals age in the same way and that strains of the same species do the same.

That aging affects all organ systems is unargued. Thus, evidence that a particular structural or functional change is due to aging requires that the change must be universal. This statement must be modified, since there has to be a normal biological variation. The confounding factor is disease, which may mimic aging but which, by definition, is separate. This chapter will first consider structural aging in the human lung. Paradoxically, it is difficult to understand because of our detailed knowledge of disease and of the most relevant human condition, emphysema. This chapter will then consider aging in animals where reasonably precise morphologic data are available and where the circumstances are easier to control.

AGING OF THE HUMAN LUNG

Until the 1950s it was thought that emphysema was a normal accompaniment of aging, so-called senile emphysema. The detailed morphologic changes of the human lung were first described in the 1960s. The lung changes in shape with age, and this was described by Anderson and Anderson (1) using paper-mounted whole lung (Gough–Wentworth) sections of inflated lung. They noted that up to age 60 years there was an increase in both anteroposterior diameter and lung height, but the anteroposterior diameter increased more. After age 60 years, only the anteroposterior diameter increased. The net effect is one of "rounding" of the shape of the lung in these midsagittal sections, and they found that the "index of rounding" (anter-

W. M. Thurlbeck: Department of Pathology, Faculty of Medicine, University of British Columbia, Vancouver, British Columbia V6T 1W5, Canada.

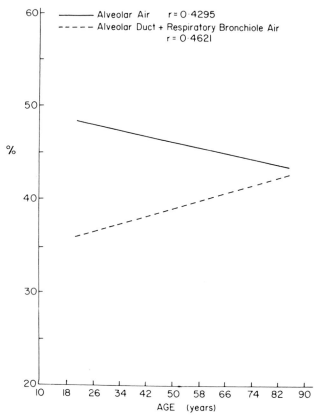

FIG. 1. Regression lines for the proportion of alveolar air and alveolar duct air versus age. Alveolar air diminishes significantly, and alveolar duct air increases significantly. (From ref. 37.).

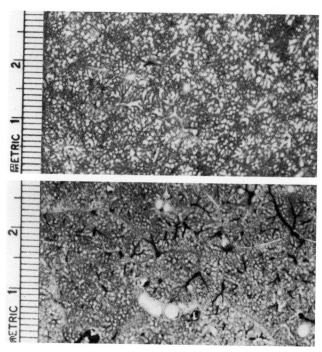

FIG. 3. A paper-mounted whole lung section from an 85-year-old woman (**top**) shows enlarged air spaces when compared to that of a 45-year-old woman (**bottom**). [From refs. 37 (**bottom**) and 38 (**top**).]

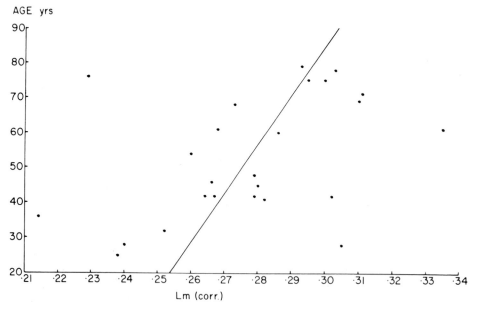

FIG. 2. The average interalveolar wall distance, Lm (corr.), increases with age. (From ref. 3.)

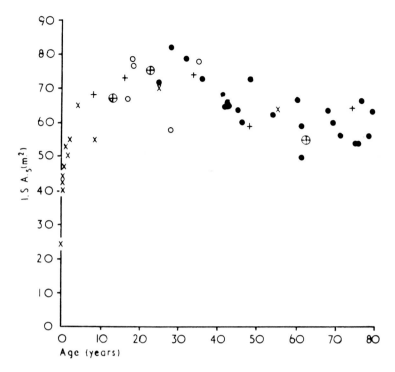

FIG. 4. When alveolar surface area is normalized to a standard volume of 5 liters, an initial increase is seen with growth, but there is a steady decrease after age 20–30 years. Data calculated from published data: ×, from refs. 39 and 40; ○, from ref. 41; +, from ref. 9; ●, from ref. 3; ⊕, from ref. 42. (From ref. 43.)

oposterior diameter/lung height) increased with age. Ryan et al. (2) measured the inner and outer diameters of alveolar ducts and respiratory bronchioles in a 26-year-old man and an 82-year-old man. They found that the inner diameter, representing the distance between mouths of alveoli, increased markedly and that alveoli flattened. They coined the term "ductectasia" for the changes and found that there was a steady increase in its frequency after age 40 years. A study of a fairly large number of nonemphysematous lungs (3) indicated that alveolar air decreased with age and that the proportion of alveolar duct and respiratory bronchiolar air (the air in the "core" of these structures internal to the mouths of alveoli) increased (Fig. 1). It should be noted that the correlation was of low order but was statistically significant. The net effect of the change in the internal geometry of the gas-exchanging parenchyma results in an increase of the average distance between alveolar walls (3,4). This distance—the mean linear intercept (MLI or Lm)—increases with age (Fig. 2). MLI is primarily a function of the size of both alveolar ducts and alveoli, and its increase is consistent with the above. The surface-to-volume ratio, which, in the method used, is directly reciprocally related to the MLI, decreases with age. Using the paper-mounted whole-lung-section technique, several investigators (5–8) noted that with increasing age the smallest visible air space increased with age, so that these spaces could be visualized at increasing distance from the observer (Fig. 3). Because of the thickness of paper-mounted whole lung sections (0.3–0.5 mm), alveoli are not vis-

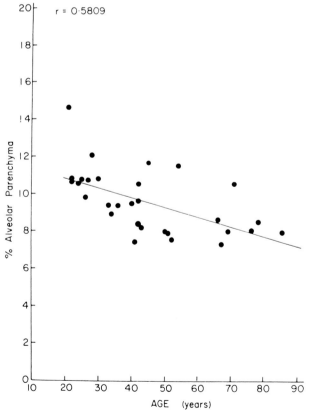

FIG. 5. The proportion of the lung formed by alveolar walls (parenchyma) shows a gradual decrease with age. (From ref. 37.)

ualized and the smallest air spaces are alveolar ducts and sacs.

Using microscopic sections, Weibel (9) provided the first quantitative data. He found that the proportion of lung formed by alveolar ducts increased. The effect is loss of gas-exchanging surface area; the results collated from various studies, normalized to a lung volume of 5 liters, are shown in Fig. 4. This shows that the changes start between 20 and 30 years of age.

The proportion of alveolar parenchyma decreases with age; this is substantial, with a loss of approximately 30% (Fig. 5). The nature of this loss is uncertain. The number of alveoli per unit volume decreases with age (*unpublished data*). Since maximum lung volume does not increase with age (10), this implies that there may be loss of alveoli. Another change with age that has been described is an increase in the number and/or size of the pores of Kohn (11,12). In other organs there is a loss in capillary number with age, and this may also occur in the lung. The average amount of emphysema increases in nonsmokers (13), and this is greater in men than in women and occurs in the latter decades of life (Fig. 6). The emphysema is mainly panacinar in type and is usually found in the lower zones of the lungs, especially close to the pleura. Whether this is a normal process or represents disease is debatable, but this author considers it an exaggeration of the aging changes described above. It may also contribute to the loss of alveolar parenchyma.

An early subjective description of elastic tissue indicated that the thickness of elastic fibers decreases with age (7), but a more recent study showed no change in the number of elastic fibers (14). Electron microscopically, no alteration in collagen or elastin was seen (15). Biochemical studies have shown no change in parenchymal elastin content, but there was an increase in pleural elastin and a decrease in airway and vascular elastin (16,17). The amino acid composition of elastin changes with age, with the amounts of polar amino acids being increased (17). Most authors have found that collagen content of the lung remains constant (16). With age, soluble collagen decreases and insoluble collagen increases (18,19). Collagen also becomes more stable, more resistant to thermal and chemical denaturation, and less susceptible to collagenase digestion (20). These changes are due to increased numbers of molecular collagen cross-links with fewer reducible links being available (21).

CHANGES IN ANIMALS

There are a number of studies of aging laboratory animals (22–30) but not as many as there should be, per-

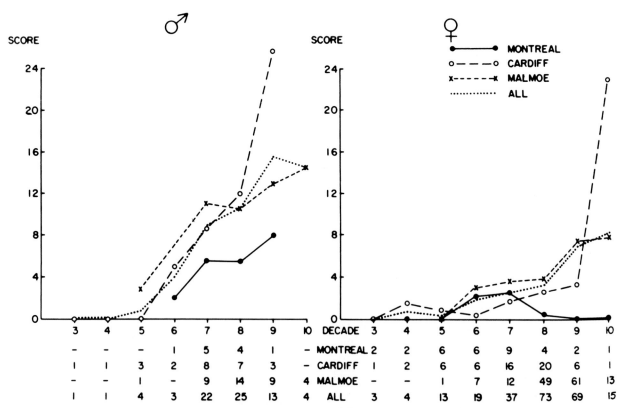

FIG. 6. The average severity of emphysema in nonsmokers in three cities, along with the mean of the three cities (ALL). There is a gradual increase with age and a higher average emphysema score in males compared to females. (From ref. 44.)

haps because of the high maintenance cost. The increase in MLI has been shown in rabbits (27), dogs (24,25), mice (28), hamsters (26), and Sprague–Dawley rats (23). However, one study of BALB/cNNia mice did not demonstrate age-related changes (30). These animals were raised and maintained in sterile conditions, and they breathed highly filtered air in a rural animal facility. The authors raised the notion that age-related changes in humans and other animals might be due to environmental factors. Another series of experiments on virally induced bronchiolitis (Sendai virus) showed subsequent disordered alveolar formation (31). The morphometric changes are also similar to those found in aging, and it may be that childhood infections result in age-related changes. This is unlikely, however, since the changes observed in humans affect almost all subjects.

Pores of Kohn have been more thoroughly studied in animals. Older reports indicated that pores of Kohn were absent in young mammals and numerous in older animals (32,33). In mice, another report showed that there was a rapid increase in the number of pores of Kohn in early life and no significant increase thereafter (29). In dogs, the number of pores were found to increase until 1 year of age, but there was no further increase (22). A quantitative scanning electron-microscopic study of the sterile, environmentally protected mice showed that the proportion of alveolar wall consisting of pores increased rapidly between 2 and 6 months of age, with no increase occurring after this (30). The size of the pores was unchanged.

In mice, total elastic fiber length was unchanged, although biochemically the elastin content was reduced (28). This suggested either that the elastic fibers were thinned or that some were lost and the remainder were stretched. Pinkerton et al. (34) performed a quantitative light- and electron-microscopic study in specific pathogen-free rats. They found that alveolar and capillary surface area did not decrease between 5 and 26 months of age. The ratio of type II alveolar cells to type I alveolar cells decreased, and the total interstitial matrix volume (noncellular connective tissue compared to the alveolar wall) increased 39% in males and 89% in females. The significance of these findings is hard to interpret, and the difference between these animals and humans is unexplained. These have also been supported in rats and hamsters (35,36), in which biochemical measurements have shown an increase. In mice, however, the amount of collagen remained unchanged (28). There was no change in the distribution of parenchymal versus airway collagen. Age-related change in collagen type has not been studied.

CONCLUSIONS

In summary, I have briefly considered the morphologic changes in the lungs of humans and laboratory animals

that occur with age. The point was made that it is difficult to separate changes that occur *with* age from changes that occur *because* of age. Relatively few studies have considered changes in nonsmoking humans, and even these studies would not satisfy rigorous epidemiologic scrutiny, since the smoking history has been obtained retrospectively from patients' records. In both humans and laboratory animals, environmental factors may produce changes. In humans, the shape of the entire lung changes because it increases more in the anteroposterior diameter. In humans and animals, there is a decrease in alveolar air and an increase in alveolar duct air (defined here as the core of air central to the openings of alveoli in alveolar ducts and sacs). As a consequence, there is loss of the surface-to-volume ratio of the gas-exchanging part of the lung. Observations that are not yet fully resolved include (a) loss of gas-exchanging parenchyma, which may be due to loss of alveoli, and (b) mild localized panacinar emphysema in nonsmoking older humans. The exact status of collagen, elastin, and pores of Kohn in both laboratory animals and humans is not completely certain. Further studies might include (a) examination of the lungs of documented nonsmokers living a lifetime in a rural environment, such as certain religious orders, and (b) examination of wild animals in remote, nonurban areas.

ACKNOWLEDGMENT

The author's laboratory is supported by grant MT-7124 from the Medical Research Council of Canada.

REFERENCES

1 Anderson WF, Anderson AE Jr, Hernandez JA, Foraker AG. Topography of aging and emphysematous lungs. *Am Rev Respir Dis* 1964;90:411–423.
2. Ryan SF, Vincent TN, Mitchell RS, Filey GF, Dart G. Ductectasia: an asymptomatic pulmonary change related to age. *Med Thorac* 1965;22:181–187.
3. Thurlbeck WM. The internal surface area of non-emphysematous lungs. *Am Rev Respir Dis* 1967;95:765–773.
4. Hasleton PS. The internal surface area of the adult human lung. *J Anat* 1972;112:391–400.
5. Heard BE. A pathological study of emphysema of the lungs with chronic bronchitis. *Thorax* 1958;13:136–149.
6. Heppleston AG, Leopold JG. Chronic pulmonary emphysema: anatomy and pathogenesis. *Am J Med* 1961;31:279–291.
7. Wright RR. Elastic tissue of normal and emphysematous lungs—tridimensional histologic study. *Am J Pathol* 1961;39:355–367.
8. Thurlbeck WM. The incidence of pulmonary emphysema. *Am Rev Respir Dis* 1963;87:206–215.
9. Weibel ER. *Morphometry of the human lung.* Heidelberg: Springer-Verlag, 1963.
10. Thurlbeck WM. Postmortem lung volumes. *Thorax* 1979; 34:735–739.
11. Macklin CC. Alveolar pores and their significance in the human lung. *Arch Pathol* 1936;21:202–226.
12. Pump KK. Emphysema and its relation to age. *Am Rev Respir Dis* 1976;114:5–13.
13. Thurlbeck WM, Ryder RC, Sternby N. A comparison of the

severity of emphysema in necropsy populations in three different countries. *Am Rev Respir Dis* 1974;109:239–248.

14. Niewoehner DE, Kleinerman J. Morphometric study of elastic fibers in normal and emphysematous human lungs. *Am Rev Respir Dis* 1977;115:15–21.

15. Adamson JS. An electron microscopic comparison of the connective tissue from the lungs of young and elderly subjects. *Am Rev Respir Dis* 1968;98:399–406.

16. Pierce JA, Hocott JB. Studies on the collagen and elastin content of the human lung. *J Clin Invest* 1960;39:8–14.

17. John R, Thomas J. Chemical composition of elastins isolated from aortas and pulmonary tissues of humans of different ages. *Biochem J* 1972;127:261–269.

18. Rickert WS, Forbes WF. Changes in collagen with age. VI. Age and smoking related changes in human lung connective tissue. *Exp Gerontol* 1976;11:89–101.

19. Prockop DJ, Kivirikko KI, Tuderman L, Guzman N. The biosynthesis of collagen and its disorders. *N Engl J Med* 1979; 301:77–85.

20. Vidik A. Connective tissue—possible implications of the temporal changes for the aging process. *Mech Ageing Dev* 1979; 9:267–285.

21. Bailey AJ, Robins SP, Balian G. Biological significance of the intermolecular crosslinks of collagen. *Nature* 1974;251:105–109.

22. Martin HB. The effect of aging on the alveolar pores of Kohn in the dog. *Am Rev Respir Dis* 1963;88:773–778.

23. Johanson WG Jr, Pierce AK. Lung structure and function with age in normal rats and rats with papain emphysema. *J Clin Invest* 1973;52:2921–2927.

24. Robinson NE, Gillespie JR. Morphologic features of the lungs of aging beagle dogs. *Am Rev Respir Dis* 1973;108:1192–1199.

25. Hyde DM, Robinson NE, Gillespie JR, Tyler WS. Morphometry of the distal air spaces in lungs of aging dogs. *J Appl Physiol* 1977;43:86–91.

26. Snider GL, Sherter CB. A one-year study of the evolution of elastase-induced emphysema in hamsters. *J Appl Physiol* 1977;43:721–729.

27. Boatman ES, Arce P, Luchtel D, Pump KK, Martin CJ. Pulmonary function, morphology and morphometrics. In: Bowden DM, ed. *Aging in nonhuman primates.* New York: Van Nostrand Reinhold, 1979;292–313.

28. Ranga V, Kleinerman J, Ip MPC, Sorensen J. Age-related changes in elastic fibers and elastin of lung. *Am Rev Respir Dis* 1979;119:369–381.

29. Ranga V, Kleinerman J. Interalveolar pores in mouse lungs. Regional distributions and alterations with age. *Am Rev Respir Dis* 1980;122:477–481.

30. Kawakami M, Paul JL, Thurlbeck WM. The effect of age on lung structure in male BALB/cNNia inbred mice. *Am J Anat* 1984;170:1–21.

31. Castleman WL, Sorkness RL, Lemanske RF, Grasee G, Suyemoto MM. Neonatal viral bronchiolitis and pneumonia induces bronchiolar hypoplasia and alveolar dysplasia in rats. *Lab Invest* 1988;59:387–396.

32. Loosli CG. Intralveolar communications in normal and pathologic mammalian lungs: review of the literature. *Arch Pathol* 1937;24:743–776.

33. Macklem PT. Airway obstruction and collateral ventilation. *Physiol Rev* 1971;51:368–436.

34. Pinkerton KE, Barry BE, O'Neil JJ, Raub JA, Pratt PC, Crapo JD. Morphologic changes in the lung during the lifespan of Fischer 344 rats. *Am J Anat* 1982;164:155–174.

35. Juricova M, Deyl Z. Aging processes in collagens from different tissues of rats. *Adv Exp Med Biol* 1975;53:351–357.

36. Goldstein M. The response of the aging hamster lung to elastase injury. *Am Rev Respir Dis* 1982;125:295–298.

37. Thurlbeck WM. Chronic airflow obstruction in lung disease. In: Bennington JL, ed. *Major problems in pathology,* vol 5. Philadelphia: WB Saunders, 1976.

38. Thurlbeck WM, Dunnill MS, Hartung W, Heard BE, Heppleston AG, Ryder RC. A comparison of three methods of measuring emphysema. *Hum Pathol* 1970;1:215–226.

39. Dunnill MS. Postnatal growth of the lung. *Thorax* 1962;17:329–333.

40. Dunnill MS. Evaluation of a simple method of sampling the lung for quantitative histological analysis. *Thorax* 1964;19:443–448.

41. Duguid JB, Young A, Cauna D, Lambert MW. The internal surface area of the lung in emphysema. *J Pathol Bacteriol* 1964; 88:405–421.

42. Hicken P, Brewer D, Heath D. The relation between the weight of the right ventricle of the heart and the internal surface area and number of alveoli in the human lung and emphysema. *J Pathol Bact* 1966;92:529–546.

43. Thurlbeck WM. Internal surface area and other measurements of emphysema. *Thorax* 1967;22:483–496.

44. Thurlbeck WM, Ryder RC, Sternby N. A comparative study of the severity of emphysema in necropsy populations in three different countries. *Am Rev Respir Dis* 1974;109:239–248.

THE LUNG: Scientific Foundations
edited by R.G. Crystal, J.B. West et al.
Raven Press, Ltd., New York © 1991.

CHAPTER 6.3.2

Physiology of the Aging Lung

Ronald J. Knudson

As one grows older, a variety of exogenous factors to which the lung is exposed, often coupled with innate host susceptibility, may result in injury or disease adversely affecting lung function. Myriad factors, such as environmental or industrial exposures, the disturbed microenvironment associated with smoking, altered immune mechanisms, weakened defense mechanisms, or the injurious effects of past disease which may occur as early as childhood, may, if not actually causing disease, nevertheless adversely affect lung function. Inasmuch as the effects of many of these factors may be cumulative, they may become manifest only later in life.

It is a relatively rare individual who, as he ages, maintains lung function unaffected by life's earlier experiences. Though such individuals make up a relatively small cohort of any randomly selected population, it is from studies of such individuals that investigators have attempted to describe the subtle changes that are the normal effects of aging alone. Most such studies are cross-sectional and make the perhaps incorrect assumption that a description of the differences between age groups accurately reflects the changes that actually occur over time. There are relatively few longitudinal studies that follow a population of subjects over a substantial period of time, and most of these have been limited to spirometric testing. It is possible, therefore, that the descriptions of aging presented here may need to be changed as data accumulate in future years.

It is important to recognize the relatively subtle changes that are normal to the aging process in order to distinguish them from the changes that are caused by lung disease. The changes that occur as a consequence of aging are similar to, but less pronounced than, the changes that are observed in disease and in emphysema in particular. Indeed, Bates and Christie (1) stated that "emphysema is a gross exaggeration of what happens to the lung with advancing years." One should not infer, however, that emphysema is part of the normal aging process.

Inasmuch as growth and development are the subjects of another chapter, this review will focus primarily on changes that accrue once maturation has been achieved. Those are interrelated changes and are discussed in the following sequence:

Loss of lung elastic recoil
Increase in closing volume
Changes in subdivisions of lung volume
Decrease in maximum expiratory flows
Decrease in diffusing capacity (transfer factor) of the lung
Decrease in arterial oxygen tension
Changes in response to stimuli

LUNG ELASTIC RECOIL

The relationship of lung volume to distending pressure describes the elastic characteristic of the lung. A reasonable approximation of the static deflation pressure–volume (P–V) curve of the lung can be derived *in vivo* by using an esophageal balloon to measure static transpulmonary pressure [$P_{st}(L)$] during stepwise deflation from total lung capacity (TLC). The position of the curve relative to the pressure axis is highly dependent upon technique of measuring pressure. Perhaps as a result, the changes in curve position with age were assessed with conflicting results. One study suggested no change in recoil with age (2), whereas others reported a parallel shift toward lower distending pressures (3). Other studies examined changes in compliance. Lung compliance, measured as the slope of the

R. J. Knudson: Department of Internal Medicine, Division of Respiratory Sciences, University of Arizona College of Medicine, Tucson, Arizona 85724.

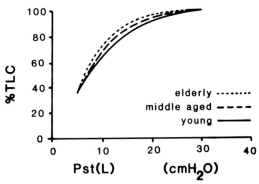

FIG. 1. Changes in the static deflation pressure–volume curve with age. To compensate for size, lung volume is expressed as percent of TLC. Age groups are defined as follows: young = 25–35 years of age; middle-aged = 36–64 years; elderly = 65–75 years. (Redrawn from ref. 12.)

P–V curve over the tidal volume range above functional residual capacity (FRC), describes a segment of the curve but is influenced by FRC itself, which may change with age. Many studies reported no change in compliance with age (2,4–6), whereas others found that compliance was increased in older subjects (7,8).

As techniques improved and more data became available, it became apparent that loss of lung elastic recoil is a normal consequence of aging (4,6–12). The studies by Turner et al. (11) and Knudson et al. (12) have shown that, with aging, the loss of recoil is greater at higher lung volumes than at lower ones and that it becomes insignificant below 50% TLC; these studies have also shown that there is a change in curve shape

rather than a simple parallel shift of the P–V curve, as shown in Fig. 1.

Because curve position can be a function of measurement technique and because compliance describes only a segment of the curve treated as a linear function, mathematical descriptors of curve shape were developed. In recent years, an exponential expression has been widely adopted which provides a numerical expression for curve shape (13–15). For pressure and volume data points between FRC and TLC, an iterative least-mean-square regression can be derived to fit the exponential equation:

$$V = V_{max} - Ae^{-kP}$$

where V and P are volume and pressure, respectively, V_{max} is the volume extrapolated to infinite pressure, and A is the difference between V_{max} and volume (V_0) extrapolated to $P = 0$. The constant k (in units of cm H_2O^{-1}) is a descriptor of curve shape. As k increases, the curve becomes more curvilinear and concave relative to the pressure axis. This is illustrated in Fig. 2. The change in shape of the P–V curve with age, which is a consequence of greater loss of recoil at higher lung volumes, is reflected by an increase in k (13,14,16). The relationship of k to age is highly significant and is expressed in the following regression equation (16), where age is expressed in years:

$$k = (0.000672 \times age) + 0.10656$$

In normal subjects, the natural log of k (ln k), rather than k itself, shows a Gaussian distribution (16) and has proven to be a reproducible measurement in serial testing (17). The equivalent age regression for ln k is as follows (16):

$$\ln k = (0.00406 \times age) - 2.19812$$

These changes in the lung's mechanical properties with aging appear to be correlated with structural changes described in the preceding chapter 6.3.1. The shape constant k has been found to be linearly related to measured mean linear intercept (L_m), the morphometric index of size of terminal air spaces (18,19). The disruption of lung architecture, along with the consequent enlargement of terminal air spaces characteristic of emphysema, is well recognized. Values of k above the normal range have been reported in several studies of patients with this disease (13,18,20). In a study of three different animal species in which no disease process was involved, L_m explained 86% of the variance in k between and within species, and k was clearly related to air-space size (19). Thus the increase of k with advancing age may be a reflection of the age-related increase in interalveolar wall distance, or L_m, with advancing age. The underlying mechanisms involving collagen, elastin, collagen–elastin fiber interactions, and biochemical changes with aging which ex-

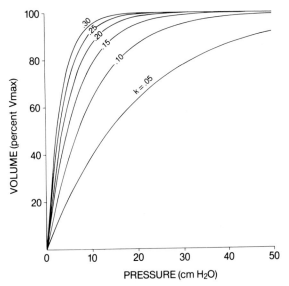

FIG. 2. Pressure–volume curves showing the relationship of the exponential shape constant k to curve shape for values of k from 0.05 to 0.30. Volume is expressed as percent of V_{max}, with $V_0 = 0\%$. (From ref. 16.)

plain both the mechanical and morphological changes observed are the subject of another chapter but remain areas for future investigation.

CLOSING VOLUME

When a normal adult fully expires and the lung approaches residual volume, airways supplying dependent regions close and those regions cease to contribute to volume expired (21,22). This nonuniform behavior of the lung, which is otherwise assumed to have uniform mechanical properties, has been attributed to the gravity-dependent gradient of pleural, and hence transpulmonary, pressure (23,24) (see Chapter 5.1.2.6). In a field of gravity, transpulmonary pressure diminishes with distance from the apex down the lung. The site of airway closure appears to be at the level of terminal bronchioles (25), airways that depend on lung recoil for their external support. Consequently, airways in the dependent regions are first to close.

The volume at which these airways begin to close, the closing volume (26), has been shown to increase with advancing age (22,26,27). In very young people, the closing volume may be equal to residual volume and may remain below FRC in young adulthood. However, as the closing volume increases with age, it can exceed FRC and encroach on the tidal volume range. The alternate closing and opening of small airways when breathing at different frequencies has been suggested as the explanation for the increase in frequency dependence of dynamic compliance observed in the elderly (28,29).

Several phenomena contribute to the increase in closing volume with advancing age. The loss of lung recoil with advancing age would allow the small airways, which depend on lung recoil for their patency, to close at higher lung volumes. There is also evidence that the transpulmonary pressure at which these airways close, the closing pressure, is greater in the elderly than in younger subjects (26). If, as suggested (12), the intrapulmonary airways themselves lose recoil with advancing age, they may tend to close more readily. There are morphologic data from study of lungs from men who died of nonrespiratory causes showing that, after 30 years of age, there is a significant decrease in the diameter of membranous bronchioles with advancing age (30). It would seem likely, therefore, that such airways, already smaller in the elderly, would close more readily during expiration. The increase in closing volume, as we shall see (*vide infra*), affects gas exchange in the elderly.

LUNG VOLUMES

In a healthy normal individual, TLC is closely correlated with a function of height. Once full growth and maturation have been achieved, TLC remains essentially constant throughout adult life. With age, the chest wall becomes less compliant (6). At the same time, the lung loses elastic recoil. It appears that any limitation to expansion of a stiff chest wall at TLC in the elderly is offset by the increase in lung compliance, resulting in little change in TLC. Loss of stature and diminished inspiratory muscle strength with age may contribute to the small decrease in TLC observed in the elderly. The subdivisions of lung volumes are affected by age, however.

FRC is determined by the balance of lung and chest wall elastic forces at resting end-tidal expiration. As the lung becomes more compliant and the chest wall less compliant with age (6), FRC increases with advancing age (11) in the normal healthy adult. As FRC increases, the transpulmonary pressures at FRC appear to remain unchanged (4); several studies have reported no age-related change in lung compliance in the tidal volume range above FRC (2,4–6).

Residual volume (RV) is determined primarily by the balance between (a) the outward recoil of the chest wall at low lung volumes and (b) the maximal force that expiratory muscles are able to generate (31). Reflex contraction of the diaphragm at the end of maximum expiration opposes expiratory forces generated by muscles of the abdominal wall and limits further expiration at RV (32). A slightly lower lung volume can be reached if expiratory forces are artificially augmented at RV (31). Other factors contribute to the determination of RV as one ages. Expiratory flow becomes flow-limited at very low lung volumes, and continued effort is required to achieve RV. Artificial augmentation of expiratory forces will not result in further volume decrease in the elderly (31). Residual volume is also increased as small airways close at higher lung volume in the elderly and as the lung units served by those airways cease to contribute to the expirate, as described in the preceding section.

The consequence of the increase in RV with age is, of course, a decrease in vital capacity. The time course of these changes is a matter of some interest. Because vital capacity is the easiest to measure and is the most commonly employed test of lung function, plentiful date regarding this subdivision of lung volume are available for examination and analysis. From a merging of cross-sectional and longitudinal observations, a temporal description has begun to emerge encompassing phases of growth, maturation, and subsequent decline in lung function reflected by changes in vital capacity (33,34). This description, inferred from these studies, is approximated in Fig. 3 and may be summarized as follows. In early life, the increase in vital capacity parallels somatic growth including the adolescent growth spurt, though rate of lung maturation appears to lag slightly behind height, reaching peak

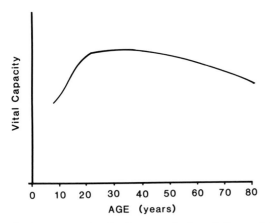

FIG. 3. An approximate temporal description of the changes of vital capacity (unscaled) over a lifetime. The evolution of the FEV$_1$ over time follows a similar pattern.

growth velocity almost a year after the most rapid rate of increase in height. Full lung growth appears to be achieved at about age 18 years in females and 19 years in males. For the next two decades, vital capacity remains at a virtual plateau. In reality, the process of maturation appears to continue in a subtle fashion, gradually merging with an equally subtle phase of decrease in vital capacity. The rate of decline accelerates with age and becomes readily apparent only after about 40 years of age. Thereafter, vital capacity continues to decrease at a rate that increases with time, with the annual decline becoming greater as one ages.

This description of change with advancing age differs from that derived from most cross-sectional studies. Even the largest cross-sectional studies are limited by the nature of such studies and the quantity of data representing the various age groups. In most cases, data have been fitted to best-fit linear regressions, which appear to show a constant rate of decline in function after about 20 years of age. Such linear regressions are commonly used to determine "normal values" in most laboratories. It is becoming apparent,

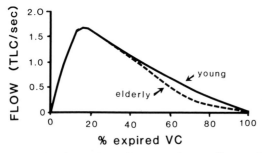

FIG. 4. Comparison of maximum expiratory flow–volume curves of young (aged 25–35 years) and elderly (aged 65–75 years) subjects. To compensate for size, flow is expressed as TLC/sec and volume is expressed as percent expired VC. (Redrawn from ref. 12.)

however, that such models do not adequately describe biological reality.

It is reasonable to assume that vital capacity is an appropriate surrogate for TLC in the first several decades of life. We can assume, therefore, that the increase in TLC, accompanied by the plateau in function, through the fourth decade of life parallels that of vital capacity. Thereafter, it is the increase in RV (and not the change in TLC) which results in the decline in vital capacity in later life.

MAXIMUM EXPIRATORY FLOW

The most common test of ventilatory function involves the forced vital capacity (FVC) maneuver from which measurements of expiratory flow can be derived. The maximum expiratory flow–volume (MEFV) curve is the graphical expression of the relationship between maximum expiratory flow ($\dot{V}_{max}$) and expired volume during the FVC maneuver. There is a modest decrease in $\dot{V}_{max}$ with advancing age. This is illustrated in Fig. 4 where $\dot{V}_{max}$ is expressed as TLC/sec to compensate for lung size. In studies of healthy adults, it appears that the decrease in $\dot{V}_{max}$ with aging becomes statistically significant only over the terminal 30–40% of the expired FVC, whereas $\dot{V}_{max}$ is well preserved at high lung volumes (12,35). Consequently, the MEFV curve exhibits a change in shape with increasing convexity in the direction of the volume axis (12,35,36).

The equal pressure point theory of flow limitation proposed by Mead et al. (35) has been used to explain the age-associated changes in $\dot{V}_{max}$. According to this concept, maximum expiratory flow at any given lung volume is determined by the relationship $\dot{V}_{max} = P_{st}(L)/R_{us}$, where $P_{st}(L)$ is the lung recoil at that volume, derived from the static deflation P–V curve, and R_{us} is the resistance of airways upstream of points at which lateral airway pressure is equal to pleural pressure, the equal pressure points (EPP). Decrease in $P_{st}(L)$ with aging would, in part, contribute to a decrease in $\dot{V}_{max}$. Moreover, the intraparenchymal airways upstream of the EPP depend on lung recoil for their external support and might narrow with loss of lung recoil, contributing to an increase in R_{us}.

This simple explanation, however, is not sufficient to explain a seeming paradox in the age-associated changes in lung recoil and maximum expiratory flow. The loss of lung recoil, we have seen, is greatest at high lung volumes and becomes insignificant at low lung volumes, whereas $\dot{V}_{max}$ is well preserved at high lung volumes. Thus $\dot{V}_{max}$ is well preserved at high lung volumes in the face of loss of recoil. Conversely, $\dot{V}_{max}$ decreases at low lung volumes, where the loss of recoil is least significant.

It seems likely that the resting length of all elastic

structures, airways as well as lung parenchyma, increases with age. Thus, though lung recoil provides external support for intrapulmonary airways, the airways may also lose recoil at a rate at least commensurate with the loss of lung parenchymal recoil. Consequently, the resting cross-section of airways may remain unchanged or even increase with age as $P_{st}(L)$ decreases, allowing $\dot{V}_{max}$ to be preserved at high lung volumes. In support of this is the observation that upstream segment conductance (G_{us}, the reciprocal of R_{us}) has been shown to increase with age at high lung volumes (35,37). The length of the upstream segment also affects its resistance. From *in vivo* studies of young adults (38), it was determined that EPP are located at the level of lobar or segmental bronchi at high lung volumes and then migrate toward alveoli after approximately 75% of the vital capacity has been expired. Subsequent studies of excised lungs obtained at autopsy revealed that in the elderly the EPP migrate toward alveoli at higher lung volumes (39), suggesting that the shorter upstream segment in older subjects may contribute to the higher G_{us}.

At low lung volumes, where the decrease in $\dot{V}_{max}$ with aging is most apparent, there is minimal age-related loss of lung recoil (11,12,35). The EPP have migrated toward alveoli, and the resistance of peripheral airways is the major determinant of $\dot{V}_{max}$ at low lung volumes. A high correlation between mean bronchiole diameter and pulmonary conductance has been confirmed (30). This study, based on lungs obtained at autopsy of men who died of nonrespiratory causes, also revealed that, after 30 years of age, there was a significant progressive decrease in the mean diameter of membranous bronchioles with advancing age though no change in dimensions of segmental bronchi was observed (30). This provides a morphological basis for the decrease in $\dot{V}_{max}$. In addition, as described earlier, the closing volume increases with advancing age. This contributes to the reduction in $\dot{V}_{max}$ near the end of the FVC maneuver as terminal airways close at progressively higher lung volumes in the elderly and as the lung units served by those airways cease to contribute to expiratory flow.

How aging affects the several factors influencing wave speed flow can, in the absence of data, only be postulated. The wave speed theory of flow limitation is described in detail in another chapter (see Chapter 5.1.2.4) but can be summarized here as follows. Maximum expiratory flow, or flow at wave speed, is determined when the local flow velocity at some critical point in the airways, the "choke point," equals tube wave speed (40–45). Flow at wave speed ($\dot{V}_{ws}$) can be expressed by the equation

$$\dot{V}_{ws} = \left(\frac{1}{\rho}\right)^{0.5} \left(\frac{dP_{tm}}{dA}\right)^{0.5} A^{1.5}$$

where ρ = gas density, A is the cross-sectional area of the airway at the choke point under flow-limiting conditions, and dA is the change in cross-sectional area at the choke point for a given change in airway transmural pressure, dP_{tm}. Thus dP_{tm}/dA is an expression of airway elasticity.

If maximum expiratory flow, or $\dot{V}_{ws}$, remains well preserved at high lung volumes in the elderly, it follows that the choke point does not change in location or at least that $(dP_{tm}/dA)^{0.5} A^{1.5}$ does not change appreciably. However, the decrease of $\dot{V}_{ws}$ at low lung volumes associated with aging suggests that, compared to young subjects, in the elderly the choke point at lower lung volumes is in a different location, where the area A is smaller and/or the airway is more compliant so that dP_{tm}/dA is smaller. Unfortunately, we lack direct measurements of the pertinent variables and information about the influence of age on these variables. Thus, this brief summary of age-associated changes in flow based on wave speed theory must be considered speculative.

Because measurement of the forced expiratory volume in the first second (FEV_1) of the FVC maneuver is reproducible and easy to make, it has been the measurement of expiratory flow most often used in clinical evaluation and epidemiological studies. It represents the average flow over that initial second of forced expiration. Inasmuch as the normal healthy person can expire in excess of 80% of the FVC in the first second (47), the FEV_1 includes flows near the terminal portion of the MEFV curve; the decreases in $\dot{V}_{max}$ with aging will also affect this measurement.

Data obtained from testing populations of healthy subjects of a wide range of ages have been used to derive regression equations that yield "normal values" for each sex. Most of these equations for adults are of a linear form and include (a) a height coefficient to account for body size and (b) an age coefficient to describe the decrease in FEV_1 with aging. Such equations assume a linear decline in FEV_1 with time, and the age coefficient is in units of liters/year of age. The age coefficients that appear in 14 reference equations for white males (47–60) published over 25 years from 1961 to 1986 range from −0.023 to −0.033, with a mean of −0.028 (46). If the decline in FEV_1 is indeed linear and the age coefficient is a reasonable estimate of the annual rate of change, one would conclude that the FEV_1 in men systematically falls at the rate of approximately 28 ml/year after about 25 years of age.

These regression equations are based on cross-sectional analysis of data obtained in a single survey of a population of healthy subjects of various ages. The estimate of the linear decline in FEV_1 is based on the assumption that the younger individuals will, in time, come to resemble the older subjects. In fact, from a merging of cross-sectional and longitudinal observa-

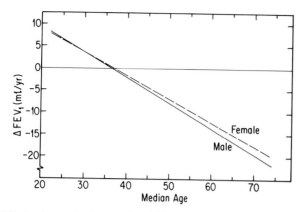

FIG. 5. Annual change in FEV₁ (expressed in milliliters per year), plotted against mean age (expressed in years). (Modified from ref. 61 and taken from ref. 46.)

tion, it appears that the temporal sequence of changes in FEV₁ closely parallels the sequence described for vital capacity (*vide supra*) (33,34). Once full lung growth has been attained, FEV₁ may continue to increase almost imperceptibly and then, equally imperceptibly, begin to decline, after which the rate of decline accelerates with advancing age.

From longitudinal analysis of data obtained by sequential testing of healthy adult nonsmokers followed over approximately 10 years, Burrows et al. (61) determined the annual change in FEV₁ (ΔFEV₁, expressed in milliliters per year) for each subject by linear regression. The results are shown in Fig. 5, where mean ΔFEV₁ is plotted against median age for subjects tested. The results differ from those obtained in cross-sectional studies from which prediction equations are derived. Real decline does not commence until well into the fourth decade of life, but changes are quite subtle even into the fifth decade. Once FEV₁ becomes negative, the annual rate of decline accelerates with age and does not approach the 28 ml/year anticipated by prediction equations until a very advanced age.

The rate of decline has also been shown to be proportional to body size (61–63) and ΔFEV₁, best expressed by an equation that includes a function of height (H^2 or H^3) as well as age. Because FEV₁ is proportional to height, the decline in FEV₁ with age is proportional to FEV₁ itself: The taller person with a large FEV₁ will exhibit a more rapid decline in FEV₁ over time than his shorter counterpart. If the rate of decline in FEV₁ is proportional to age × H^2, the decline in the younger adult is relatively small, is determined by size, and accelerates with age, as data seem to show.

Longitudinal studies follow a given population sample over a specified length of time. Cross-sectional studies, on the other hand, include different age cohorts, each of which has been exposed to environmental and social conditions unique to its life span;

moreover, these studies assume, in the analysis, that the young cohorts will nevertheless come to resemble the older cohorts. Older subjects are also, by definition, survivors. It is important to recognize that the cross-sectional studies that have been used to derive the commonly used reference equations include this cohort effect. Though these equations are often called "prediction equations," they may not actually predict the changes that occur as one ages.

DIFFUSING CAPACITY

The most readily applicable measurement of the transfer of gas from the gaseous phase in the terminal lung units to the blood–liquid phase in the pulmonary capillaries is the carbon monoxide (CO) diffusing capacity (D_L), or transfer factor, of the lung, a test that takes advantage of the high affinity of CO for hemoglobin. This is the subject of another chapter (see Chapter 5.3.3). The D_L, expressed in units of ml/min/mmHg pressure difference, is dependent on lung volume and can also be expressed as specific diffusing capacity, or D_L per liter alveolar volume (D_L/V_A). The normal evolution of the D_L with time in healthy subjects has been demonstrated in many studies, and the resulting regression equations (64–72) include age coefficients to express the decrease in D_L and D_L/V_A with advancing age in the adult. Figure 6 shows plots of such regression equations from several recent studies (69–72) and illustrates the age-related decrease in this measurement of lung function.

To explain the decline in diffusing capacity with aging, the several phenomena that can affect the measurement may be considered. These are: (a) distribution of the inspired test gas, (b) flow and distribution of blood within the lung, (c) the available gas-exchanging surface, and (d) the resistance to transfer of gas molecules from the gas phase to attachment to the hemoglobin molecule (46).

The single-breath carbon monoxide diffusing capacity test requires inspiration of a vital capacity of the test gas. Because of the gravity-dependent gradient of transpulmonary pressure, the inspired gas is not homogeneously distributed (21,22) and an increase in this nonhomogeneity with age could contribute to a decrease in D_L. This does not appear to be the case, however. In healthy subjects, the alveolar volume, V_A, measured from the single-breath D_L test does not differ significantly from TLC measured by a multiple-breath equilibration technique regardless of age, suggesting that any increase in nonhomogeneity of gas distribution with age is negligible (73). Moreover, radioactive xenon studies have demonstrated that the gas distribution of an inspired vital capacity is similar in elderly and young subjects (26). Thus increased nonhomo-

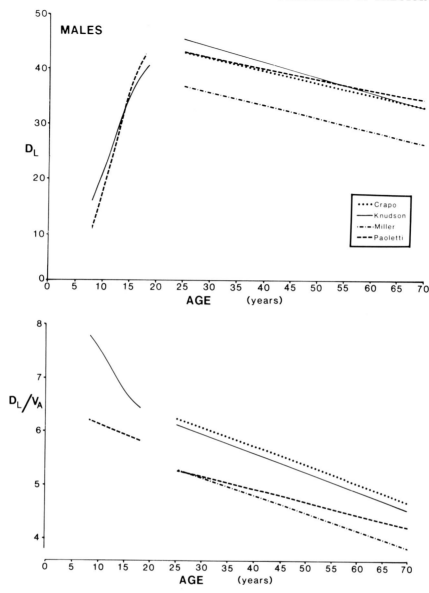

FIG. 6. Plots of regression equations of Crapo and Morris (69), Miller et al. (70), Paoletti et al. (71), and Knudson et al. (72) for D_L **(upper panel)** and D_L/V_A **(lower panel)**, showing relationship of these measurements to age. (From ref. 72.)

geneity of gas distribution cannot explain the decrease in D_L with age.

The total diffusion resistance, $1/D_L$, has been considered to be the sum of two resistances in parallel (100):

$$\frac{1}{D_L} = \frac{1}{D_M} + \frac{1}{\phi V_c}$$

where V_c is the pulmonary capillary blood volume, ϕ is the reaction rate of combination of CO in ml/min/mmHg CO tension per milliliter of blood, and D_M is the membrane diffusing capacity. If cardiac output decreased with age, perfusion (and hence V_c) could be diminished, resulting in a decrease in D_L. In healthy adults, however, cardiac output at rest has not been

found to decrease with age (74). There have been few studies on the effect of age on V_c. One such study on subjects under 60 years of age failed to find a change in V_c with age (75), whereas another study of nonsmoking subjects aged 18–78 years revealed some decrease in V_c only in the very few subjects over 70 years of age (73). Thus, evidence for a change in V_c with age is scanty; if there is a decrease, it may be a very late phenomenon and cannot explain the progressive decrease in D_L throughout adult life. There is also scanty evidence of an age effect on diffusion/perfusion or D_L/V_A inhomogeneities, although there are age-related changes in ventilation/perfusion distribution during quiet breathing. One study (26) demonstrated an increase in perfusion to upper lung zones in elderly subjects compared to young subjects, but perfusion of dependent zones was similar. Changes in perfusion (or changes in perfusion distribution) appear to explain little, if any, of the observed decrease in diffusing capacity with age.

The membrane component, D_M, includes the permeability of the alveolar–capillary membrane, the total gas-exchanging surface or membrane available, and any other factors that affect the movement of gas molecules from gas to blood phase. A decrease of D_M with age has been demonstrated (73,75). There is no evidence for any age-related change in the permeability of the membrane across which gas exchange actually occurs. The morphological changes described in Chapter 6.3.1, however, could affect D_M. If there was a decrease in internal surface area available for gas exchange, this would result in a decrease in D_M, and hence in D_L, with age. One must also postulate that the alveolar–capillary surface area, which is the pertinent area for gas exchange, also decreases with age. One study, however, did not report a change in capillary density with age while confirming the increase in air-space diameter (76).

The observed increase in air-space size, reflected by the increase in mean linear intercept (L_m) with age, may introduce another phenomenon contributing to decrease in D_M. With the marked increase in total cross-sectional area of air passages within the terminal lung unit, convective movement of inspired gas becomes less effective than gaseous diffusion as the primary mechanism for moving gas molecules. At the level of the pulmonary acinus, therefore, the distance to be traversed by gaseous diffusion becomes a gas-phase resistance to CO uptake. The age-associated increase in size of air spaces and of distance to be traversed increases this gas-phase component of resistance (77–79) which is included in the measurement of D_M, observed to decrease with age.

There are several observations that support the concept of the morphological changes (described in Chapter 6.3.1) of the aging lung introducing a gas-phase diffusion barrier. As noted in a previous section (*vide supra*), the shape constant, k, from exponential analysis of the $P–V$ curves shows a high correlation with L_m. A significant inverse correlation has been demonstrated between k and D_L/V_A (80,81), which suggests that increasing L_m is associated with decrease in D_L/V_A. Moreover, k and L_m have been shown to increase with age while D_L/V_A decreases, and all of these measurements are independent of lung size. In the absence of direct measurements, assessing the magnitude of the gas-phase diffusion barrier has proven difficult but has been the subject of investigation (78,79,82,83). It has been estimated that it may represent from 20% to 40% of the total resistance to oxygen uptake from gas in the alveolar space (79).

The structural and morphologic changes in the lung associated with aging which affect the membrane component, D_M, appear sufficient to explain the observed decrease in D_L, whereas there is little evidence of changes in perfusion or distribution of inspired gas with age.

ARTERIAL OXYGEN TENSION

Blood gases and ventilation/perfusion relationships are the subject of a separate chapter (see Chapter 5.3.4). Arterial blood pH and carbon dioxide tension are maintained within narrow limits throughout adult life by homeostatic mechanisms. An increase in resting minute ventilation with advancing age helps to maintain carbon dioxide tension in this normal range (84,85). As a consequence of the several phenomena of aging described above, however, there is a gradual decrease in arterial oxygen tension (Pa_{O_2}) with advancing age (86–89). For adults over 20 years of age, residing at sea level, the change in Pa_{O_2} with age can be described by the following regression equation (87):

$$Pa_{O_2} = 100.1 - 0.323A$$

where A is age in years.

The morphological changes that are responsible for the decrease in D_L with age also, of course, affect oxygen transfer. The decrease in Pa_{O_2} with age, however, is primarily the result of an increase in ventilation/perfusion mismatching (86,88,90). As previously noted, there is evidence of an increase in perfusion to superior regions of the lung in the elderly (26), regions that receive less ventilation. Perfusion to dependent regions, however, is unchanged. Closure of terminal airways is a phenomenon observed in dependent regions of the lung. As previously described, the closing volume encroaches upon, and can exceed, FRC in older persons, and airway closure may therefore be present during tidal breathing. As units close, dependent regions of the lung receive less ventilation while perfusion is maintained. With advancing age, these factors combine to produce ever-increasing inequality in ventilation/perfusion relationships, contributing to a decrease in Pa_{O_2} and increasing alveolar–arterial oxygen gradient (88,90,91) observed in the elderly.

RESPONSES TO STIMULI

In addition to structural and physiological phenomena of aging which directly involve the lung, there are other changes worth brief mention which affect respiration. With aging, there appears to be a decrease in ventilatory response to hypoxia and hypercapnia. The anticipated increase in heart rate in response to hypoxia, but not to hypercapnia, is also less in the elderly (92).

The diminished ventilatory response to stimuli in the elderly was considered to be too great to be accounted for by changes in the mechanical properties of the respiratory system, suggesting that aging may attenuate chemoreceptor function.

It has long been recognized that maximal aerobic performance, assessed by measurement of peak oxygen consumption in response to vigorous exercise, decreases with age (93). The role of the respiratory and cardiovascular systems in this phenomenon has been the subject of several studies (94–100). In summary, the ventilatory or gas-exchanging capabilities of the aging respiratory system are not limiting factors to maximal oxygen consumption. The cardiovascular system is also well maintained, and cardiac output can respond appropriately to exercise stress in healthy elderly people (74). Lifestyles of the elderly may lead to some loss of fitness and to a decrease in muscle mass (101). This phenomenon and other local phenomena, such as decrease in mitochondrial density (102) at the level of the exercising muscle itself, appear to be primarily responsible for the decline in aerobic work capacity with advancing age.

REFERENCES

1. Bates DV, Christie RV. Effects of ageing on respiratory function in man. In: Wolstenholme EW, Cameron MF, eds. *Ciba Foundation Colloquia on Ageing. General aspects*, vol I. Boston: Little, Brown, 1955;58.
2. Permutt S, Martin HB. Static pressure–volume characteristics of lung in normal males. *J Appl Physiol* 1960;15:819–825.
3. Pride NB. Pulmonary distensibility in age and disease. *Bull Physiol Pathol Respir* 1974;10:103–108.
4. Frank NR, Mead J, Ferris BG Jr. The mechanical behavior of the lungs in healthy elderly persons. *J Clin Invest* 1957;36:1680–1687.
5. Butler J, White HC, Arnott WM. The pulmonary compliance in normal subjects. *Clin Sci* 1957;16:709–729.
6. Mittman C, Edelman NH, Norris AH, et al. Relationship between chest wall and pulmonary compliance and age. *J Appl Physiol* 1965;20:1211–1216.
7. Pierce JA, Ebert RV. The elastic properties of the lungs in the aged. *J Lab Clin* 1958;51:68–71.
8. Cohn JE, Donoso HD. Mechanical properties of lung in normal men over 60 years old. *J Clin Invest* 1963;42:1406–1410.
9. Bode FR, Dosman J, Martin RR, et al. Age and sex differences in lung elasticity, and in closing capacity in non-smokers. *J Appl Physiol* 1976;41:129–135.
10. Gibson GJ, Pride NB, O'Cain C, et al. Sex and age differences in pulmonary mechanics in normal smoking subjects. *J Appl Physiol* 1976;41:20–25.
11. Turner JM, Mead J, Wohl ME. Elasticity of human lungs in relation to age. *J Appl Physiol* 1968;25:664–671.
12. Knudson RJ, Clark DF, Kennedy TC, et al. Effect of aging alone on mechanical properties of the normal adult human lung. *J Appl Physiol* 1977;43:1054–1062.
13. Gibson GJ, Pride NB, Davis J, et al. Exponential description of the static pressure-volume curve of normal and diseased lungs. *Am Rev Respir Dis* 1970;120:799–811.
14. Colebatch HJH, Greaves IA, Ng CKY. Exponential analysis of elastic recoil and aging in healthy males and females. *J Appl Physiol* 1979;47:638–691.
15. Colebatch HJH, Ng CKY, Nikov N. Use of an exponential function for elastic recoil. *J Appl Physiol* 1979;46:387–393.
16. Knudson RJ, Kaltenborn WT. Evaluation of lung elastic recoil by exponential curve analysis. *Respir Physiol* 1981;46:29–42.
17. McCuaig KE, Vessal S, Cappin K, et al. Variability in measurements of pressure–volume curves in normal subjects. *Am Rev Respir Dis* 1985;131:656–658.
18. Greaves IA, Colebatch HJH. Elastic behavior and structure of normal and emphysematous lungs post mortem. *Am Rev Respir Dis* 1980;121:127–136.
19. Haber PS, Colebatch HJH, Ng CKY, et al. Alveolar size as a determinant of pulmonary distensibility in mammalian lungs. *J Appl Physiol* 1983;54:837–845.
20. Pare PD, Brooks LA, Bates J, et al. Exponential analysis of the lung pressure–volume curve as a predictor of pulmonary emphysema. *Am Rev Respir Dis* 1982;126:54–61.
21. Milic-Emili J, Henderson JAM, Dolovich MB, et al. Regional distribution of inspired gas in the lung. *J Appl Physiol* 1966;21:749–759.
22. Dollfuss RE, Milic-Emili J, Bates DV. Regional ventilation of the lungs, studied with boluses of xenon. *Respir Phys* 1967;2:234–246.
23. Turner JM. Distribution of lung surface pressure as a function of posture in dogs. *Physiologist* 1962;5:223.
24. Hoppin FG Jr, Green ID, Mead J. Distribution of pleural surface pressure in dogs. *J Appl Physiol* 1969;27:863–873.
25. Hughes JM. Site of airway closure in dog lungs. *Bull Physiopathol Respir* 1970;6:877–879.
26. Holland J, Milic-Emili J, Macklem PT, et al. Regional distribution of pulmonary ventilation and perfusion in elderly subjects. *J Clin Invest* 1968;47:81–92.
27. Anthonisen NR, Danson J, Robertson PC, et al. Airway closure as a function of age. *Respir Physiol* 1970;8:58–65.
28. Begin R, Renzetti AD Jr, Bigler AH, et al. Flow and age dependence of airway closure and dynamic compliance. *J Appl Physiol* 1975;38:199–207.
29. Cohn JE, Donoso HD. Mechanical properties of lung in normal men over 60 years old. *J Clin Invest* 1963;42:1406–1410.
30. Niewoehner DE, Klienerman J. Morphologic basis of pulmonary resistance in the human lung and effects of aging. *J Appl Physiol* 1974;36:412–418.
31. Leith DE, Mead J. Mechanisms determining residual volume of the lungs in normal subjects. *J Appl Physiol* 1967;23:221–227.
32. Agostoni E, Torri G. Diaphragm contraction as a limiting factor to maximum expiration. *J Appl Physiol* 1962;17:427–428.
33. Tager IB, Segal MR, Speizer FE, Weiss ST. The natural history of forced expiratory volumes; effect of cigarette smoking and respiratory symptoms. *Am Rev Respir Dis* 1988;138:837–849.
34. Sherrill DL, Camilli A, Lebowitz MD. On the temporal relationships between lung function and somatic growth. *Am Rev Respir Dis* 1989;140:638–644.
35. Mead J, Turner JM, Macklem PT, et al. Significance of the relationship between lung recoil and maximum expiratory flow. *J Appl Physiol* 1967;22:95–108.
36. Green M, Mead J, Hoppin F, et al. Analysis of the forced expiratory maneuver. *Chest* 1973;63:33S–35S.
37. Yernault JC, De Troyer A, Rodenstein D. Sex and age differences in intrathoracic airways mechanics in normal man. *J Appl Physiol* 1979;46:556–564.
38. Macklem PT, Wilson NJ. Measurement of intrabronchial pressure in man. *J Appl Physiol* 1965;20:653–663.
39. Silvers GW, Maisel JC, Petty TL, et al. Flow limitation during forced expiration in excised human lungs. *J Appl Physiol* 1974;36:737–744.
40. Dawson SV, Elliott EA. Wave-speed limitation on expiratory flow—a unifying concept. *J Appl Physiol* 1977;43:498–515.
41. Elliott EA, Dawson SV. Test of wave-speed theory of flow limitation in elastic tubes. *J Appl Physiol* 1977;43:516–522.
42. Dawson SV, Elliott EA. Use of the choke point in the prediction of flow limitation in elastic tubes. *Fed Proc* 1980;39:2765–2770.
43. Mead J. Expiratory flow limitation: a physiologist's point of view. *Fed Proc* 1980;39:2771–2775.
44. Shapiro AH. Steady flow in collapsible tubes. *J Biomech Eng* 1977;99:126–147.

45. Griffiths DJ. Negative-resistance effects in flow through collapsible tubes. *Med Biol Eng* 1975;13:785–802.

46. Knudson RJ. Aging of the respiratory system. *Curr Pulmonol* 1989;10:1–24.

47. Knudson RJ, Lebowitz MD, Holberg CJ, et al. Changes in the normal maximal expiratory flow–volume curve with growth and aging. *Am Rev Respir Dis* 1983;127:725–734.

48. Kory RC, Callahan R, Boren HG, et al. The Veterans Administration–Army cooperative study of pulmonary function. I. Clinical spirometry in normal men. *Am J Med* 1961;30:243–258.

49. Berglund E, Birath G, Bjure J, et al. Spirometric studies of normal subjects. I. Forced expirograms in subjects between 7 and 70 years of age. *Acta Med Scand* 1963;173:185–192.

50. Ferris BG Jr, Anderson DO, Zickmantel R. Prediction values for screening tests of pulmonary function. *Am Rev Respir Dis* 1965;91:252–261.

51. Cotes JE. Average normal values for the forced expiratory volume in white Caucasian males. *Br Med J* 1966;1:1016–1018.

52. Dickman ML, Schmidt CD, Gardner RM, et al. On-line computerized spirometry in 738 normal adults. *Am Rev Respir Dis* 1969;100:780–790.

53. Morris JF, Koski A, Johnson LC. Spirometric standards for healthy nonsmoking adults. *Am Rev Respir Dis* 1971;103:57–67.

54. Cherniack RM, Raber MB. Normal standards for ventilatory function using an automated wedge spirometer. *Am Rev Respir Dis* 1972;106:38–46.

55. Schmidt CD, Dickman ML, Gardner RM, et al. Spirometric standards for healthy elderly men and women. *Am Rev Respir Dis* 1973;108:933–943.

56. Higgins MW, Keller JB. Seven measures of ventilatory lung function. Population values and a comparison of their ability to discriminate between persons with and without chronic respiratory symptoms and disease, Tecumseh, Michigan. *Am Rev Respir Dis* 1973;108:258–272.

57. Knudson RJ, Slatin RC, Lebowitz MD, et al. The maximal expiratory flow volume curve. Normal standards, variability and effects of age. *Am Rev Respir Dis* 1976;113:587–600.

58. Crapo RO, Morris AH, Gardner RM. Reference spirometric values using techniques and equipment that meet ATS recommendations. *Am Rev Respir Dis* 1981;123:659–664.

59. Paoletti P, Pistelli G, Fazzi P, et al. Reference values for vital capacity and flow–volume curves from a general population study. *Bull Eur Physiopathol Respir* 1986;22:451–459.

60. Miller A, Thornton JC, Warshaw R, et al. Mean and instantaneous expiratory flows, FVC and FEV_1: prediction equations from a probability sample of Michigan, a large industrial state. *Bull Eur Physiopathol Respir* 1986;22:589–597.

61. Burrows B, Lebowitz MD, Camilli AE, et al. Longitudinal changes in forced expiratory volume in one second in adults; methodological considerations and findings in healthy nonsmokers. *Am Rev Respir Dis* 1986;133:974–980.

62. Cole TJ. The influence of height on the decline in ventilatory function. *Int J Epidemiol* 1974;3:145–152.

63. Van der Lende R, Kok TJ, Peset R, et al. Decreases in VC and FEV_1 with time: indicators for effects of smoking and air pollution. *Bull Eur Physiopathol Respir* 1981;17:775–792.

64. Burrows B, Kasik JE, Niden AH, et al. Clinical usefulness of the single-breath pulmonary diffusing capacity test. *Am Rev Respir Dis* 1961;84:789–806.

65. Van Ganse WF, Ferris BG, Cotes JE. Cigarette smoking and pulmonary diffusing capacity (transfer factor). *Am Rev Respir Dis* 1972;195:30–40.

66. Gaensler EA, Smith AA. Attachment for automated single breath diffusing capacity measurement. *Chest* 1973;63:136–145.

67. Bates DV, Macklem PT, Christie RV. *Respiratory function in disease.* Philadelphia: WB Saunders 1971.

68. Teculescu DB, Stanescu DC. Lung diffusing capacity: normal value in male smokers and nonsmokers using the breath-holding technique. *Scand J Respir Dis* 1970;51:137–149.

69. Crapo RO, Morris AH. Standardized single breath normal values for carbon monoxide diffusing capacity. *Am Rev Respir Dis* 1981;123:185–189.

70. Miller A, Thornton JC, Warshaw R, et al. Single breath diffusing capacity in a representative sample of the population of Michigan, a large industrial state. *Am Rev Respir Dis* 1983;127:270–277.

71. Paoletti P, Viegi G, Pistelli G, et al. Reference equations for the single-breath diffusing capacity a cross-sectional analysis and effects of body size and age. *Am Rev Respir Dis* 1985;132:806–813.

72. Knudson RJ, Kaltenborn WT, Knudson DE, et al. The single breath carbon monoxide diffusing capacity: reference equations derived from a healthy non-smoking population and effects of hematocrit. *Am Rev Respir Dis* 1987;135:805–811.

73. Georges R, Saumon G, Loiseau A. The relationship of age to pulmonary membrane conductance and capillary blood volume. *Am Rev Respir Dis* 1978;117:1069–1078.

74. Rodeheffer RJ, Gerstenblith G, Becker LC, et al. Exercise cardiac output is maintained with advancing age in healthy human subjects: cardiac dilation and increased stroke volume compensate for a diminished heart rate. *Circulation* 1984;69:203–213.

75. Hamer NAJ. The effect of age on the components of the pulmonary diffusing capacity. *Clin Sci* 1962;23:85–93.

76. Butler C, Kleinerman J. Capillary density: alveolar diameter, a morphometric approach to ventilation and perfusion. *Am Rev Respir Dis* 1970;102:886–894.

77. Gomez DM. A physicomathematical study of lung function in normal subjects and in patients with obstructive pulmonary disease. *Med Thorac* 1965;22:275–294.

78. Rahn H, Paganelli CV. The role of gas-phase diffusion at altitude. In: Loeppley JA, Riedesel ML, eds. *Oxygen transport to human tissues.* New York: Elsevier/North-Holland, 1982;213–221.

79. Scheid P, Piiper J. Intrapulmonary gas mixing and stratification. In: West JB, ed. *Pulmonary gas exchange, vol I: Ventilation, blood flow, and diffusion.* New York: Academic Press, 1980;87–130.

80. Knudson RJ, Bloom JW, Knudson DE, et al. Subclinical effects of smoking: physiologic comparison of healthy middle-aged smokers and nonsmokers and interrelationships of lung function measurements. *Chest* 1984;86:20–29.

81. Habib MP, Klink ME, Knudson DE, et al. Physiologic characteristics of subjects exhibiting accelerated deterioration of ventilatory function. *Am Rev Respir Dis* 1987;136:638–645.

82. Engel LA. Gas mixing within the acinus of the lung. *J Appl Physiol: Respir Environ Exercise Physiol* 1983;54:609–618.

83. Engel LA, Paiva M. *Gas mixing and distribution in the lung.* New York: Marcel Dekker, 1985.

84. Tenney SM, Miller RM. Dead space ventilation in old age. *J Appl Physiol* 1956;9:321–327.

85. Lefrak SS, Campbell EJ. Structure and function of the aging respiratory system. In: Gracey DR, ed. *Pulmonary disease in the adult.* Chicago: Year Book Medical Publishers, 1981;12–51.

86. Sorbini CA, Grassi V, Solinas E, et al. Arterial oxygen tension in relation to age in healthy subjects. *Respiration* 1968;25:3–13.

87. Murray JF. *The normal lung.* Philadelphia: WB Saunders, 1976.

88. Raine JM, Bishop JM. A–a difference in O_2 tension and physiologic dead space in normal man. *J Appl Physiol* 1963;18:284–288.

89. Mellemgaard K. The alveolar–arterial oxygen difference: its size and components in normal man. *Acta Physiol Scand* 1966;67:10–20.

90. Muiesan G, Sorbini CA, Grassi V. Respiratory function in the aged. *Bull Physiopathol Respir* 1971;7:973–1009.

91. Kanber GJ, King FW, Eshchar YR, et al. The alveolar–arterial oxygen gradient in young and elderly men during air and oxygen breathing. *Am Rev Respir Dis* 1968;97:376–381.

92. Kronenberg RS, Drage CW. Attenuation of the ventilatory and heart rate responses to hypoxia and hypercapnia with aging in normal men. *J Clin Invest* 1973;52:1812–1819.

93. Robinson S. Experimental studies of physical fitness in relation to age. *Arbeitphysiologic* 1938;10:251–323.

94. Julius S, Amery A, Whitlock LS, et al. Influence of age on the hemodynamic response to exercise. *Circulation* 1967;36:222–232.

95. Hossack KF, Bruce RA. Maximal cardiac function in sedentary normal men and women: comparison of age-related changes. *J Appl Physiol* 1982;53:799–804.

96. Astrand I. Aerobic work capacity in men and women with special reference to age. *Acta Physiol Scand* 1960;169:169–192.

97. Astrand PO, Rodahl K. *Textbook of work physiology*. New York: McGraw-Hill, 1977; 318–325.

98. Higginbotham MB, Morris KG, Williams RS, et al. Physiologic basis for the age-related decline in aerobic work capacity. *Am J Cardiol* 1986;57:1374–1379.

99. Kanstrup I-L, Ekblom B. Influence of age and physical activity on central hemodynamics and lung function in active adults. *J Appl Physiol* 1978;45:709–717.

100. Lakatta EG, Mitchell JH, Pomerance A, et al. Human aging: changes in structure and function. *J Am Coll Cardiol* 1987;10:42A–47A.

101. Fleg JL, Lakatta EG. Role of muscle loss in the age-associated reduction in $V_{O_2}max$. *J Appl Physiol* 1988;63:1147–1151.

102. Orlander J, Kiessling K-H, Larson L, Karlsson J, Aniasson A. Skeletal muscle metabolism and ultrastructure in relation to age in sedentary man. *Acta Physiol Scand* 1978;104:249–261.

THE LUNG: Scientific Foundations
edited by R.G. Crystal, J.B. West et al.
Raven Press, Ltd., New York © 1991.

SECTION 7

Lung Injury, Defense, and Repair

Section 7 covers the fundamental mechanisms involved in lung injury, the various aspects of lung defense, and repair mechanisms. As in other sections of the book, individual chapters reflect different approaches ranging from physiology to molecular biology but, taken together, provide an integrated picture of the complex processes involved in lung injury and repair, which are relevant to normal lung function and to many lung diseases.

The first subsection is devoted to proteases and antiproteases. There have been enormous advances in our understanding of lung proteases and how their activity is controlled by antiproteases. The balance between protease and antiprotease activity is critical and fundamental to our understanding of emphysema. Advances in molecular biology have provided important new insights into regulation of antiproteases and have led to new therapeutic options using genetically engineered antiproteases; in the future, these advances will lead to gene therapy for α_1-antitrypsin deficiency.

The second subsection deals with oxidants and antioxidants. The different types of reactive oxygen species, their source, and the mechanism by which they induce cellular injury are discussed in detail. Reactive oxygen species are increasingly recognized to be important in a number of inflammatory lung diseases, and, as with proteases, the balance between oxidants and antioxidants is of critical importance. Intracellular antioxidant defenses are now much better understood, and the development of antioxidants as therapeutic agents is also discussed. The prospect of developing far more effective antioxidants will undoubtedly lead to a greater interest in the role of reactive oxygen species in lung diseases beyond emphysema.

The respiratory epithelium is exposed to many inhaled gases and particles and has involved sophisticated defense systems. The third, fourth, and fifth subsections deal with particulates and infectious agents.

The principles of particle deposition in the respiratory tract are discussed in some detail, since they are fundamental to our understanding of the site of deposition of inhaled particles in the respiratory tract and are relevant to understanding the principles of aerosol therapy. Mucociliary clearance is an important defense mechanism in the airways from the larynx to terminal bronchioles, and we now have a much greater understanding of the factors which alter clearance. This information should be related to the chapters in subsection 3.1, which deal with (a) the structure and function of ciliated epithelial cells and (b) the synthesis, propulsion, and rheology of airway mucus. Cough is an important defense mechanism in larger airways, and the different factors that are involved in cough control are discussed. Macrophages are the predominant defense mechanism in the alveoli, and the multiple responses of these phagocytic cells are becoming increasingly complex. It is clear that macrophages may show very different patterns of response with different stimuli, and this may be an important determinant in the way in which diseases may develop. Many minerals are inhaled and may lead to different patterns of lung injury. The cellular basis of these responses is discussed. The different mechanisms of the lung also include various immune mechanisms that are particularly important in defending against infections. Immunodeficiency predisposes to chronic lung infection and highlights the critical role of lung immune defense mechanisms. Immune mechanisms may also lead to lung injury such as granuloma formation and immune-complex-related lung injury, which are discussed in detail.

The sixth subsection deals with environmental contaminants. This is a highly topical area of research, and we are exposed to an increasing number of contaminants in the atmosphere as a result of industrialization. The multiple environmental contaminants are discussed, and cigarette smoking is given special consideration. The ways in which cigarette smoking leads to lung injury are still debated, and multiple interactive factors seem likely.

The seventh subsection considers other mechanisms of lung injury and discusses injury from inflammatory cells (particularly neutrophils and eosinophils), which play an important pathogenetic role in many airway and parenchymal diseases. An increasing number of drugs are implicated in lung injury, and many different patterns of pathologic responses to drugs have now been recognized, although the particular mechanisms involved are often far from understood. Adult respiratory distress syndrome represents a type of gross lung injury with many different causes, but common underlying mechanisms, such as neutrophil-dependent endothelial cell injury and the role of cytokines, are now providing clues toward a greater understanding of the syndrome.

The eighth subsection discusses lung fibrosis, which is essentially a reaction to lung injury and is part of the normal repair process in the lung. The role of mesenchymal cells and their regulation is discussed, giving insights into the mechanisms of fibrosis in various chronic fibrosing lung conditions. Animal models have thrown light on the mechanisms involved in lung fibrosis, and molecular approaches are increasingly being used to understand the regulation of matrix protein production.

In the ninth subsection, the role of genetic factors in susceptibility to lung injury is discussed. It is clear that many lung diseases in which injury is important have a genetic basis, while most emphasis has been placed on α_1-antitrypsin deficiency, it is becoming increasingly clear that genetic factors also apply to many other lung diseases. This may be due to defects in epithelial cells, disordered mucosal immunity, or defects in lung function.

Section 7 thus covers a wide range of topics relating to lung injury and defense which are relevant to virtually all lung diseases and are fundamental to the function of the normal lung. The chapters, written from several different perspectives, provide an up-to-date overview and should be read in conjunction with the earlier sections of the book dealing with structure and formation of the various epithelial cell elements involved in lung defense.

The Editors

THE LUNG: Scientific Foundations
edited by R.G. Crystal, J.B. West et al.
Raven Press, Ltd., New York © 1991.

CHAPTER 7.1.1

Proteases

Richard C. Hubbard, Mark L. Brantly, and Ronald G. Crystal

"Proteases" are proteins that function as enzymes and that have the capacity to degrade proteins by hydrolyzing peptide bonds (1–3). Other terms used to describe this class of enzymes include "proteinases" and "peptidases," to separate enzymes that cleave proteins (the "proteinases") from those that act to cleave oligopeptide substrates (the "peptidases") (see ref. 1 for a review of this nomenclature). In modern usage, the proteases are divided into "exopeptidases" (proteases whose function is restricted to N- or C-terminal peptide linkages) and "endopeptidases" (proteases not so restricted). The proteases are further subdivided on the basis of critical components of the catalytic mechanisms they use to cleave the peptide bonds, including: serine, cysteine, aspartic, metallo, and unclassified (1–3). Beyond this mechanistic categorization, proteases vary in their substrate specificity, defined by primary, secondary, and tertiary structures of their targets. Some proteases are highly specific and will attack only one type or class of proteins, whereas others have a broad range of potential targets.

In the lung, some proteases function within cells while others are released by cells into the local milieu. In the latter category, a variety of proteases are capable of modifying the extracellular matrix components and/or the cells of the lung parenchyma. Extracellular proteases also play a central role in the lung by modifying proteins that participate in the complement system, in coagulation, and in other protein cascade systems (see Chapters 3.2.3 and 3.4.4). In this chapter we will focus on extracellular proteases relevant to the structure of the normal lung, as well as on those relevant to the derangements of the lung parenchyma in a broad variety of acute and chronic lung disorders. In general, these proteases are endopeptidases; they function in the pH and ionic conditions of the extracellular milieu of the lung, and their catalytic function depends on serine or metallo-type processes. For a general description of how such proteases evolved and how they function, several reviews are available (1–3). We will limit the discussion to human "proteases." With regard to proteases relevant to the lung of experimental animals, the overall concepts for the human proteases are generally applicable, but there are sufficient differences such that the reader should consult the literature specific to each species.

ANTIPROTEASES VERSUS NATURAL SUBSTRATES

By necessity, proteases capable of attacking extracellular components of the lung parenchyma must be controlled. In the lung, as elsewhere, this is provided by antiproteases, proteins that inhibit proteases, usually by interacting with the catalytic site of the protease. The known extracellular lung antiproteases relevant to the proteases discussed in this chapter are α_1-antitrypsin, secretory leukoprotease inhibitor (SLPI), α_1-antichymotrypsin, α_2-macroglobulin, and tissue inhibitor of metalloprotease (TIMP). For a full discussion of these antiproteases, see Chapter 7.1.2.

In general, antiproteases function as such because the concentration–time kinetics of their interaction with the protease is more favorable than that of the protease with tissue components. If the protease concentration in the local milieu overwhelms the local antiprotease screen, the result is degradation of one or more protein components of the lung parenchyma. Furthermore, while interaction with an antiprotease generally provides permanent inhibition of the protease (depending on the protease and the antiprotease, as well as on the concentration of each), once a protease interacts with and cleaves a natural substrate,

R. C. Hubbard, M. L. Brantly, R. G. Crystal: Pulmonary Branch, National Heart, Lung and Blood Institute, National Institutes of Health, Bethesda, Maryland 20892.

the protease is usually free to continue to destroy other tissue components.

The evidence that a variety of proteases are capable of functioning to cleave normal lung parenchymal components comes from several sources, including instillation of the proteases into the airways of experimental animals, *in vitro* addition of protease to explants of lung tissue or cultures of lung parenchymal cells, and *in vitro* studies with purified lung components, particularly components of the extracellular matrix.

SOURCES OF EXTRACELLULAR PROTEASES RELEVANT TO LUNG PARENCHYMAL COMPONENTS

Because of the abundance of antiproteases in plasma (4), proteases released outside of the lung likely never reach the lung; therefore, the only sources of proteases relevant to destruction of lung parenchymal components are derived from inflammatory cells within the lung (or possibly originating in pulmonary capillaries) and from lung parenchymal cells. Without question, the major sources of proteases potentially injurious to the lung are inflammatory cells, particularly the neutrophil (Table 1). Other inflammatory cells capable of releasing proteases within the lung are alveolar macrophages, T-lymphocytes, eosinophils, basophils, and mast cells. There is also evidence that cells which comprise the lung parenchyma, such as fibroblasts, can

release proteases. In general, parenchymal cell-derived extracellular proteases are thought to function in normal growth and development and in normal extracellular protein turnover, whereas inflammatory cell-derived extracellular proteases are a major source of lung parenchymal derangement in lung disease.

NEUTROPHIL PROTEASES

Because of the prominent role of the neutrophil in releasing proteases into the extracellular environment in inflammatory reactions, neutrophils have been referred to as the "secretory organs of inflammation" (5) (see Chapter 3.4.7 for a more detailed description of neutrophil function). At least six proteases that function extracellularly have been identified in human neutrophils, including neutrophil elastase, cathepsin G, collagenase, gelatinase, proteinase-3, and plasminogen activator (1,6–9). Except for plasminogen activator, all are stored within cytoplasmic granules in the intact neutrophil and are disgorged extracellularly, or intracellularly into phagolysosomes as part of the neutrophil's response to various stimuli (6–11). The proteases are stored within neutrophils in one of three types of granules: azurophilic (primary), specific (secondary), and tertiary (C-particle). Azurophilic granules—so named because they contain myeloperoxidase, which imparts a bluish color to the granules when the cell is stained with the common Wright–Giemsa stain—con-

TABLE 1. *Characteristics of proteases relevant to the lung[a]*

Protease	Category[b]	Molecular mass[c] (kDa)	Cell source	Substrate[d]
Neutrophil elastase	Serine	29	Neutrophil, basophil, mast cell	Elastin, type I–IV collagen, fibronectin, laminin, proteoglycans
Cathepsin G	Serine	30	Neutrophil	Fibronectin, proteoglycans, elastin, type IV collagen
Collagenase	Metalloprotease	75, 57	Neutrophil, fibroblast, macrophage	Type I, III–V, and VII collagen; gelatin; fibronectin
Gelatinase	Metalloprotease	225, 94, 30	Neutrophil, fibroblast, macrophage	Laminin, elastin, fibronectin, gelatin, Type V and VII collagen
Proteinase-3	Serine	27	Neutrophil	Type I and III collagen
Plasminogen activator	Serine	54	Neutrophil, macrophage	Elastin
Cathepsin D	Aspartic	42	Monocyte, neutrophil, fibroblast, macrophage	Proteoglycans, type IV collagen, fibronectin
Cathepsin L	Cystiene	25	Macrophage	Type IV collagen, fibronectin
Cathepsin B	Cystiene	29	Macrophage	Elastin
Granzymes 1–6[e]	Serine	60–70	T cell	Cellular matrix

[a] Only proteases listed are those known to be from humans.
[b] Classification of proteases by active-site catalytic mechanisms.
[c] Molecular mass observed in nonreducing conditions.
[d] Substrates listed are restricted to extracellular matrix components.
[e] Several human granzymes have been reported, but the biological function of only granzyme 1 has been evaluated.

tain neutrophil elastase, cathepsins B, D and G, and proteinase-3. Collagenase is contained within specific granules, whereas gelatinase is contained within the tertiary and specific granules. All of these proteases are stored in an inactive form. It is likely that the granule form protects the neutrophil from self-destruction by its own proteases, thus enabling the neutrophil to serve as a transport "mule" capable of delivering and discharging its potent burden of proteases directly to an inflammatory locus.

The stored neutrophil proteases are released from their respective granules in different ways depending on the manner in which the cell responds to various stimuli (Fig. 1). For example, intracellular degranulation occurs following phagocytosis by opsonized bacteria, in a process that includes fusion of storage granules with portions of plasmalemma that form the phagocytic vacuoles (8–10). This process is not perfect, however, and invariably there is exocytosis of granule proteases into the extracellular milieu. With some stimuli, such as phorbol esters, lipopolysaccharides, and N-formyl-methionyl-leucyl-phenylalanine (FMLP), there is direct exocytosis of protease granules (8–11). Furthermore, the direct extracellular release of the contents of azurophilic and specific granules appears to be under separate control (10). For example, the proteases contained within the azurophilic granules are those which are used principally for extracellular

release as part of inflammatory responses, a process that also includes the respiratory burst and myeloperoxidase-mediated oxidant production (8). In contrast, migration of neutrophils, through filters in vitro and through tissues in vivo in response to chemotactic stimuli, results in preferential discharge of specific granules (10,11). Relevant to this process, some neutrophil plasma-membrane receptors, including the FMLP receptor and the complement receptor CR3 (which binds the C3b fragment C3bi), exist in a preformed pool on the specific granule membrane. In this reaction, C3b-directed neutrophil chemotaxis through tissues is probably aided by C3b, inducing specific release of collagenase and thus likely helping neutrophil movement through tissues.

In addition to "leak" associated with phagocytosis and direct exocytosis, granule proteases can reach the extracellular milieu following neutrophil damage and death. The neutrophil is a short-lived cell with a lifespan of 1–2 days within the circulation and 1–2 days after leaving the circulation (12). It is likely that many neutrophils die within the lung, as a result of either (a) normal senescence or (b) inflammation within pulmonary capillaries or in the parenchyma. In these circumstances, disruption of the cell results in the indiscriminate release of all cellular enzymes, potentially leading to uncontrolled proteolysis. Another mechanism that can result in nonselective liberation of gran-

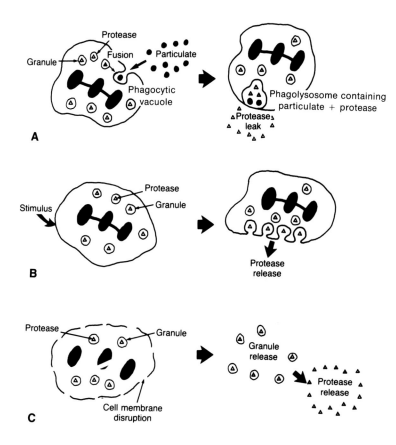

FIG. 1. Mechanisms by which neutrophils release proteases into the extracellular milieu. **A:** "Leaky phagocytosis." Proteases are released from neutrophils during the process of phagocytosis of particulates (such as bacteria). As the cell engulfs the particulate into a phagocytic vacuole, there is fusion of the vacuole with cytoplasmic granules containing proteases. The process of degranulation into the forming phagolysosome is associated with some "leak" of proteases outside of the cell. **B:** Inflammation. Proteases are released extracellularly at the surface of the neutrophil in response to an inflammatory stimulus. **C:** Cell death. Neutrophil autolysis leads to release of cytoplasmic granules containing proteases into the extracellular space.

ule enzymes is the toxic accumulation of soluble agents within lysosomes (e.g., material leached from silica) following endocytosis, resulting in rupture of lysosomes from within, leading to cytolysis.

Neutrophil Elastase

Neutrophil elastase, NE (EC 3.4.21.37), is the major protease contained within the azurophilic granules of neutrophils (6–9,13). NE is also the most potent of the neutrophil proteases with respect to its broad substrate specificity and kinetics of proteolysis. In this regard, NE plays a major role in the pathogenesis of a variety of human lung disorders (see below and Chapters 7.2.1, 7.2.4, 7.5.2, 7.7.1, 7.7.3.1, 7.9.1, 7.9.2, and 8.2.2). Because of the central importance of this protease in the lung, NE will be used as a prototype protease to demonstrate the general structure and expression of a protease gene and the structure and function of the protease itself.

NE is coded for by a single-copy, 4-kb gene on chromosome 11 at q14, including five exons and four introns (14). The exon structure predicts a primary translation product of 267 amino acid residues, including a 29-residue N-terminal precursor containing (a) a 27-residue "pre" signal peptide followed by a "pro$_n$" dipeptide and (b) a 20-residue C-terminal peptide. Following synthesis, the inactive precursor molecular form is trimmed, glycoslyated with complex carbohydrates, transported to the Golgi, and ultimately carried to the azurophilic granules. Although NE is carried by neutrophils within their granules, mature neutrophils do not synthesize neutrophil elastase (15). *In situ* hybridization studies have demonstrated that the NE gene is first detectable within blast cells and maximally expressed during the promyelocyte stage (15,16). Thereafter, neutrophil elastase mRNA levels decline such that they are undetectable by the stage of the neutrophil metamyelocyte. This suggests that the NE gene is activated in promyelocytes, myelocytes, and metamyelocytes but is shut down prior to the departure of the mature neutrophil from the bone marrow. NE mRNA transcripts appear in marrow differentiation in a relatively similar fashion as transcripts of myeloperoxidase, an enzyme also found in azurophilic granules.

While it is clear that NE gene expression is tightly controlled, the mechanisms underlying this control are not well understood. Analysis of the 5′ flanking region of the NE gene demonstrates consensus promoter elements, including a CAAT box, a TATA box, and a GC box (14). This region also contains a number of internal repeats, including a 317-bp sequence containing six tandem repeats of 53 or 52 bp that are nearly identical. NE gene expression and myelocytic differentiation can be induced in HL-60 promyelocytic leukemia cells by exposure to dimethylsulfoxide, with the rate of NE gene transcription increasing 1.9-fold and NE transcript number increasing 2.5-fold over 5 days (15,17). In contrast, exposure to phorbol esters leads to a marked reduction in the rate of NE gene transcription and in the number of NE mRNA transcripts, accompanied by induction toward monocytic differentiation. Thus, NE gene expression is intimately linked to neutrophil differentiation, and it is restricted to immature neutrophil precursors.

The mature neutrophil elastase protein is a single-chain, 220-amino-acid glycoprotein with four intramolecular disulfide bonds linking eight half-cystine residues (16,18,19). The carbohydrate side chains account for about 20% of the molecular weight, and differences in the content of the carbohydrates due to variable glycosylation likely account for the isozyme character of elastase seen on gel electrophoresis (19,20). NE is a very basic protein; because of its high content of arginine residues, it has an isoelectric point of 9.4.

The catalytic site of NE includes the triad His[41]–Asp[88]–Ser[173] (21). This triad (also called the "charge-relay system") functions by transfer of electrons from the carboxyl group of Asp[88] to the oxygen of Ser[173], which then becomes a powerful nucleophile able to attack the carbonyl carbon atom of the peptide bond of the substrate (Fig. 2). This catalytic triad is highly conserved among all serine proteases. The other important component of the active center of NE is the substrate binding site, which is responsible for the substrate specificity of neutrophil elastase (21). Studies using synthetic substrates have demonstrated that the binding site specifically prefers substrates containing nonbulky amino acids, especially Val and Ala (13,20,21).

NE derives its name from its ability to cleave the peptide bonds of elastin, a rubber-like macromolecule that gives the lung elastic recoil and that is resistant to most proteases (22). NE will also cleave many other proteins that contain appropriate surface-exposed amino acid sequences. In the context of the extracellular matrices of the lung, other proteins cleaved by NE include collagen (types I–IV), fibronectin, laminin, and cartilage proteoglycans (1,20,22–24). In addition, NE can cleave coagulation factors (fibrinogen and Factors V, VII, XII, and XIII), plasminogen, IgG and IgM, complement factors C3 and C5, *Escherichia coli* cell walls, and gp120, the coat protein of the human immunodeficiency virus (7,20,25). It may also cleave other proteases found within neutrophil granules, including the latent form of gelatinase (6).

Neutrophils contain approximately 1 pg of NE per cell, although several studies have indicated that the NE content per neutrophil varies among individuals

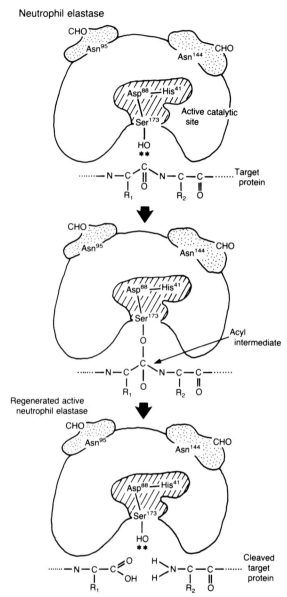

Neutrophil elastase

Regenerated active
neutrophil elastase

FIG. 2. Protease attack of a protein. As an example, shown is the mechanism by which neutrophil elastase (NE) cleaves a typical target protein. **Top:** The NE molecule is globular and is comprised of two complex carbohydrate (CHO) side chains attached to Asn^{95} and Asn^{144}. The catalytic site of the NE molecule is in an indentation of the molecule and is composed of the triad His^{41}–Asp^{88}–Ser^{173}, in which the γ-oxygen of serine becomes a powerful nucleophile able to attack a suitably located carbonyl group on the target substrate. The bond to be cleaved must fit into the active site pocket of the NE, held there by change interactions mediated by the residues forming the pocket. The peptide bond under attack is between two amino acid residues identified by their side chains R_1 and R_2. NE preferentially attacks peptide bonds adjacent to small side chains such as found on Val or Ala residues. **Middle:** An acyl–enzyme intermediate molecule is formed between serine and the carbonyl group on the target protein. **Bottom:** The acyl–enzyme complex is hydrolyzed with subsequent regeneration of active NE and cleavage of the protein.

over approximately a 2.5-fold range (26). This may be relevant to the "individual susceptibility" of individuals to emphysema. For example, individuals with the hereditary disorder α1-antitrypsin deficiency who have higher NE levels per neutrophil appear to have more severe emphysema than those with less NE per cell, despite their similar levels of plasma α1-antitrypsin (27) (see Chapter 7.9.1).

There are many lines of evidence that NE plays a major role in a variety of lung disorders. Perhaps the most important is the observation that intrapulmonary instillation of NE can produce emphysema (28,29). Furthermore, NE has been identified in association with elastin and connective tissue fibers in emphysematous lung tissue resulting from intratracheal injection into normal animals (29,30). Lungs in animal models of NE-induced emphysema show reduction in elastin content, whereas repeated pulmonary sequestration of neutrophils by endotoxin causes elastolysis (29–31). Acute pulmonary injury, such as that associated with hemorrhagic shock, hyperoxia, or microembolic lung injury, is characterized by (a) an increased concentration of neutrophils in lung and (b) increased concentrations of NE and neutrophils in bronchoalveolar lavage fluid (32–34).

Cathepsin G

Cathepsin G (EC 3.4.21.20) is the other neutral protease contained within the primary (azurophilic) neutrophil granule (6,7,13,35). It is a so-called "chymotrypsin-like" enzyme, because it is sensitive to inhibitors of chymotrypsin and also because it hydrolyzes the same synthetic substrates as does bovine chymotrypsin A (35). The cathepsin G gene has been localized to chromosome 14 at q11.2, near the α/δ T-cell receptor locus (36). The structure of the cathepsin G gene is very similar to that of NE (14,36). It spans 2.7 kb of genomic DNA and is composed of five exons and four introns. Southern blot analysis has shown that, unlike the NE gene, which seems to be unique, there are several other cathepsin-G-like genes in the human genome, which could represent pseudogenes or highly related genes (36).

Cathepsin G is an approximately 30-kDa glycoprotein with four distinct forms visible on gel electrophoresis (35). The mature protein contains three disulfide bonds, is glycoslyated at only one site (Asn^{51}), and has an isoelectric point near 13.0. Like NE, it has a catalytic triad His^{57}–Asp^{120}–Ser^{195}. The amino acid sequence has a 37% homology with NE. Mature neutrophils contain approximately 1–2 pg of cathepsin G per cell (6).

Cathepsin G can cleave a number of proteins of pulmonary matrix, including collagen types I and III, fibronectin, and laminin (1,6,35,37). It can also destroy histones, fibrinogen, and hemoglobin (6). However, the role of cathepsin G in extracellular matrix degradation is unclear. Despite the equal amounts of neutrophil elastase and cathepsin G in azurophilic granules, much less cathepsin G is released from neutrophils following stimulation (6,11). Cathepsin G can activate gelatinase and collagenase from their intracellular latent forms, has bactericidal activity, and appears to potentiate the degradation of elastin by elastase (although this is controversial) (6,35,38,39). It has been suggested that its principal role is to function as an intracellular protease active within phagosomes, rather than to degrade extracellular proteins (6).

Collagenase

Neutrophil collagenase (EC 3.4.24.7) is a member of the vertebrate collagenase gene family, composed of at least four closely related metalloproteases, including collagenase, stromolysin, stromolysin-2, and putative metalloprotease ("PUMP-1") (40–43). In neutrophils, collagenase is contained within the secondary (specific) granules as an inactive proenzyme which can be activated extracellularly by NE, cathepsin G, plasmin, and possibly other proteases (43–45). It is likely, but not conclusively proven, that neutrophil collagenase is identical to fibroblast collagenase, an enzyme coded by a 10-exon, 9-intron, 2.0-kb segment on chromosome 11 at q21–22.1 (41).

Neutrophils secrete two forms of collagenase: a 75-kDa protein and a 57-kDa protein (42). Another form, a 22-kDa molecule, has been observed, representing a degradation product of the 57-kDa molecule (42). Neutrophil collagenase degrades both type I and type III collagen but is characterized by its ability to cleave type I collagen at a 15-fold greater rate than it cleaves type III collagen (43–45). In contrast, collagenase from macrophages, eosinophils, and fibroblasts are equally active against type I and type III collagen. In contrast to NE and cathepsin G, neutrophil collagenase is a metalloprotease; that is, it utilizes a heavy metal (Zn^{2+}) at its catalytic site (42,44–46). Interestingly, collagenase is inhibited by gold compounds, which interact with a heavy-metal-binding site on the collagenase molecule to cause noncompetitive enzyme inhibition (46). This may, in part, explain the positive effects of gold therapy in rheumatoid arthritis, in which collagenase released by inflammatory cells plays a significant role in joint destruction.

Gelatinase

Gelatinase is a metalloprotease contained within both secondary and tertiary granules (C-particles) of neu-

trophils (6,47,48). It is classified as a member of the collagenase family of proteases because of its ability to degrade type IV collagen, but it also degrades fibronectin, gelatin (denatured type I collagen), and collagens type V and VII (6,45,47,48). Gelatinase consists of three proteins (225, 130, and 92 kDa) under nonreducing conditions but consists of a single protein (92 kDa) under reducing conditions (47). Stored as an inactive proenzyme, it appears to be secreted by the neutrophil in response to such stimuli as FMLP (47). Gelatinase is activated by NE and possibly by other neutrophil serine proteases. Unlike other metalloproteases, gelatinase is not efficiently activated by trypsin, plasmin, or cathepsin G. The role of gelatinase in the lung is not understood.

Proteinase-3

Proteinase-3 is an incompletely defined serine protease contained within azurophilic granules (49). Its molecular weight (approximately 27 kDa) is similar to that of NE and cathepsin G. On acrylamide gel electrophoresis, it appears as three isozymes. Proteinase-3 is active at neutral pH. Like NE, it is capable of degrading elastin, but its preferred site of proteolytic attack appears to be different from that of NE (49). Although capable of inducing emphysematous changes when instilled intratracheally in the hamster, its role in the human lung is unknown.

Plasminogen Activator

Plasminogen activator (EC 3.4.21.31) is unique among neutrophil neutral proteinases in that it is not stored in latent form within granules but is an active protease bound to the cell membrane (6,50). Furthermore, its activity in neutrophils can be modulated (50). The major function of plasminogen activator is to cleave plasminogen to release the active protease plasmin. With regard to extracellular lung components, plasmin can degrade fibronectin and laminin and can activate latent collagenase (50). The role of plasminogen activator in the lung in health and disease is not defined.

Other Proteases

Neutrophils also contain proteases that require a low pH for optimal function, including cathepsin B and cathepsin D (6,51,52). Because they function only in acid conditions, with regard to tissue damage they likely function only within the neutrophil to help digest phagocytosed tissue components.

ALVEOLAR MACROPHAGE PROTEASES

Alveolar macrophages, the resident phagocytic cells of the alveolar epithelial surface, are capable of elaborating a vast array of inflammatory mediators (see Chapter 3.4.5), including proteases capable of degrading proteins of the extracellular matrix. However, the degree to which alveolar macrophages contribute *in vivo* to lung matrix protein degradation is much less well defined than for neutrophils, and it is unclear whether the proteolytic activities which have been detected in macrophages in culture are relevant to the lung in health and disease. Alveolar macrophages contain neutral proteases capable of degrading extracellular proteins; they also contain a broad array of lysosomal acid proteases, including the cathepsins B, D, and L, which are active within the acid milieu of phagolysosomes but which are rapidly inactivated at neutral pH.

Macrophage Elastases

Long the subject of debate, it is now established that human alveolar macrophages secrete proteases capable of degrading elastin (53). However, there has been considerable difficulty in identifying and characterizing the proteases responsible for macrophage elastinolytic activity, due to the fact that alveolar macrophages have a surface receptor that readily binds and internalizes free NE (54). Moreover, monocytes, the precursor cell for alveolar macrophages, contain small amounts of elastase, but there is no evidence that they actually synthesize the enzyme (15,55). Given these factors, a large degree of uncertainty has surrounded the identity of true alveolar macrophage "elastase," and it is likely that the elastinolytic activity of alveolar macrophages is due to at least three identified proteases, and possibly a fourth.

Cathepsin B (EC 3.4.22.1), cathepsin L (EC 3.4.22.15), cathepsin D (EC 3.4.23.5), plasminogen activator, and an as-yet-unidentified metalloprotease are all capable of release by alveolar macrophages and have the capacity to cleave elastin (51,53,56–58). Cathepsins B and L are cysteine proteases (i.e., the thiol group of amino acid cysteine plays a central role at the active site), whereas cathepsin D is an aspartic protease (i.e., the carboxyl groups of aspartic acid are essential for the active site). All three cathepsins are acid hydrolases, and therefore by themselves they likely do not play a significant role in degrading extracellular elastin, due to their low degree of activity of the neutral pH of the extracellular milieu (51,52). Furthermore, the cathepsins are predominantly lysosomal proteases; thus, while they may be secreted extracellularly, their role is more likely to degrade phagocytosed macromolecules.

Plasminogen Activator

Macrophage plasminogen activator is a 67-kDa serine protease which has a wide spectrum of substrates, including elastin, fibronectin, laminin, and other extracellular glycoproteins (57–59). Macrophage plasminogen activator is antigenically similar to urokinase and is membrane-bound. In the presence of plasminogen, macrophage plasminogen activator is thought to enhance elastin degradation by removing elastin-associated glycoproteins, thus uncovering elastin fiber (57). Plasminogen activator seems to work in concert with other macrophage proteases to degrade matrix proteins, possibly by helping the macrophage to create an acidic microenvironment at contact points with macrophages, thus allowing acid proteases to function (57–59).

Macrophage Metalloproteases

Alveolar macrophages produce a number of metalloproteases which can degrade extracellular matrix proteins. Three distinct collagenases, with maximal activity against type III, type IV, and type V collagen, have been identified and are antigenically identical to their neutrophil and skin fibroblast counterparts (60–62). Alveolar macrophages also release stromolysin, a 47-kDa protease that is active against both collagen and elastin (53). Finally, a protease has been identified in supernates of cultured alveolar macrophages which degrades elastin in the presence of both serine and cysteine protease inhibitors but which is inhibited by the tissue inhibitor of metalloproteinase. This enzyme is distinct from other macrophage metalloproteases, and it is necessary for the macrophage to directly contact elastin in order to degrade it with this enzyme (53).

LYMPHOCYTE PROTEASES

Cytotoxic T-lymphocytes contain cytoplasmic granules that have been implicated in the cytotoxic mechanism of cell-mediated cytolysis (63–67). Murine studies have shown that these granules contain a pore-forming protein (perforin), cytolysin, proteoglycan, and a family of serine proteases (64–67). The latter have been named *granzymes,* of which at least three and as many as six types in humans have been identified (64–67). Analysis by gel filtration shows that granzymes have a molecular weight ranging between 60 and 70 kDa but that under reducing conditions their molecular weight is approximately 30 kDa, suggesting that in their native form they exist as dimers. Their native substrates are not definitively known, but elastin and fibronectin can be cleaved by granzyme 1 (67). It appears that granzymes mediate cytotoxicity by working in concert with perforin and cytolysin to form pores in target cell membranes, causing DNA release and breakdown (64–66).

EOSINOPHIL PROTEASES

Eosinophils contain a collagenase which equally degrade types I and III collagen (68). This enzyme is probably identical to the metalloprotein collagenase of macrophages but is distinguishable from neutrophil collagenase, which cleaves type I collagen at a much greater rate than it cleaves type III. Cathepsin G and gelatinase have also been described in eosinophils (69). In contrast to neutrophils, eosinophil granules do not contain proteases in significant quantity. Instead, they contain a group of basic proteins which are the major part of the antiparasitic armamentarium of eosinophils (see Chapter 7.4.9). It is doubtful that, by themselves, any of these eosinophil enzymes play a major role in degrading elastin or other matrix proteins, but they may play a role in a multienzyme inflammatory reaction with neutrophil or other cellular proteases (68,69).

BASOPHIL AND MAST CELL PROTEASES

Elastase

Basophils and mast cells contain an enzyme which has properties similar to that of NE (70,71). On a per-cell basis, it is estimated that levels of elastase are 3–20% that of neutrophils. Elastase has been identified within these cells by an antineutrophil elastase antibody and by both immunofluorescence and immunogold techniques. It is as yet unclear whether mast cells and basophils contain elastase as a result of biosynthesis by precursor forms, or as a result of uptake of neutrophil elastase released by neutrophils.

Chymase

Chymase (EC 3.4.21.39) is a 30-kDa chymotrypsin-like serine protease (72). With optimal proteolytic activity at pH 7.5–9.5, it is capable of function within the extracellular milieu. Although the substrate specificity of human chymase is not clearly established, it is structurally very similar to that of rat mast cell chymase, which can degrade collagen, fibronectin, and proteoglycans (72).

PARENCHYMAL CELL PROTEASES

Fibroblasts

Fibroblasts, the predominant cell type within lung interstitial tissues, are capable of synthesizing both collagenases and gelatinase (41,45,73,74). Like macrophages, fibroblasts secrete collagenases with differing activities against collagen subtypes, with type III, type IV, and type V collagenases being produced by fibroblasts. Fibroblast interstitial collagenase (collagenase type III) is synthesized in pre-proenzyme form, and the secretion products consist of a minor glycosylated form (57 kDa) and a major unmodified peptide (52 kDa) (73).

EVIDENCE OF A ROLE FOR PROTEASES IN THE LUNG

It is very likely, but not proven, that a variety of the proteases discussed above play an important role in the lung during normal growth and development as well as in the normal turnover of parenchymal components. In contrast, the evidence is overwhelming that proteases play a central role in the connective tissue destruction that characterizes a number of lung diseases, including α_1-antitrypsin deficiency (see Chapter 7.9.1), smoking-related emphysema (75–77), cystic fibrosis (Chapter 7.9.2), bronchiectasis (78), bronchitis (78), and the adult respiratory distress syndrome (Chapter 7.7.3.1). An important concept for each of these disorders is that there is an imbalance between proteases and protease inhibitors in the lung, such that proteases are able to attack and degrade extracellular matrix proteins uninhibited by the normal concentration of antiproteases (79). The result is damage, which is generally a slow, inexorable process that culminates in sufficient lung function abnormalities to cause impairment of the ability of the lung to exchange gas in a normal fashion. Direct evidence of enhanced extracellular matrix destruction in some of these disorders is the finding of elevated levels of degradation products of lung connective tissue in the serum and urine of affected individuals (77). Furthermore, in emphysema, there is a quantitative relationship between the distribution of NE in contact with alveolar interstitial elastin fibers and the local presence of emphysematous changes in the lung (80).

Emphysema associated with cigarette smoking is a condition associated with an excess of proteases in the lung and an acquired deficiency of antiproteases (75–77). The protease burden in cigarette smokers' lungs is chronically increased due to a number of factors, including (a) a chronic macrophage and neutrophil alveolitis resulting from the deposition of particulates inhaled in cigarette smoke, thereby inducing alveolar macrophage release of chemotactic factors, and (b) the neutrophil chemotactic effects of nicotine and elastin degradation fragments (81–83). These same cells, in addition to increasing the protease burden in the lung, drastically reduce the effective antiprotease screen by releasing greatly exaggerated amounts of oxidants, including O_2^{-}, H_2O_2, hydroxyl radical, and $HOCl^{-}$. These oxidants, along with the inhaled oxidants present in cigarette smoke, oxidize and inactivate α_1-antitrypsin, rendering it ineffective as an inhibitor of NE (84–87). Consistent with this knowledge, oxidized α_1-antitrypsin has been found in bronchoalveolar lavage fluid of smokers; moreover, the α_1-antitrypsin in the lungs of cigarette smokers has a significantly reduced rate of association for NE compared to that of nonsmokers (88,89).

In bronchitis, bronchiectasis, and cystic fibrosis, a similar condition exists except that the major tissue derangement occurs to a greater degree in airways than in the lower respiratory tract (78,90). In these conditions, the presence of increased amounts of mucus is associated with (a) acute and chronic bacterial colonization and (b) neutrophil-dominated airway inflammation (78,90,91). The neutrophils release their proteases and oxidants, leading to a regional protease-antiprotease imbalance within the affected airway, ultimately resulting in protease-mediated destruction of the bronchial wall. For example, bronchoalveolar lavage fluid analysis in cystic fibrosis demonstrates normal to high levels of α_1-antitrypsin, but even higher levels of active NE, due to the fact that the α_1-antitrypsin has been oxidized and/or proteolytically cleaved by neutrophil proteases (92,93).

In many individuals with the adult respiratory distress syndrome, bronchoalveolar lavage fluid contains oxidized and cleaved forms of α_1-antitrypsin and free NE, along with cleaved complement proteins and clotting factors, all evidence that the antiprotease screen has been overwhelmed (94,95). The tremendous oxidant and inflammatory cell burdens represent an extreme form of stress upon the pulmonary antiprotease and antioxidant defenses, such that the degree and time course of lung damage are far more acute than in emphysema due to α_1-antitrypsin deficiency, cigarette smoking, bronchiectasis, or cystic fibrosis.

REFERENCES

1. Barrett AJ. An introduction to proteases. In: Barrett AJ, Salvesen G, eds. *Protease inhibitors.* New York: Elsevier, 1986;1–22.
2. Barrett AJ. *Proteases in mammalian cells and tissues.* New York: Elsevier/North-Holland, 1977.
3. Barrett AJ, McDonald JK. *Mammalian proteases.* New York: Academic Press, 1986.
4. Travis J, Salvesen GS. Human plasma proteinase inhibitors. *Annu Rev Biochem* 1983;52:655–709.
5. Weissmann G, Zurier RB, Hoffstein S. Leukocytes as secretory organs of inflammation. *Agents Actions* 1973;3:270–279.
6. Senior RM, Campbell EJ. Neutral proteinases from human inflammatory cells. *Clinics Lab Med* 1983;3:645–666.
7. Havemann K, Janoff A. *Neutral proteases of human polymorphonuclear leukocytes.* Baltimore: Urban & Schwarzenberg, 1978.
8. Falloon J, Gallin JI. Neutrophil granules in health and disease. *J Allergy Clin Immunol* 1986;77:653–662.
9. Wright DG. Human neutrophil degranulation. *Methods Enzymol* 1988;162:538–551.
10. Baggiolini M, Dewald B. Exocytosis by neutrophils. In: *Regulation of leukocyte function.* New York: Plenum Press, 1984;221–246.
11. Goldstein IM. Neutrophil degranulation. In: *Regulation of leukocyte function.* New York: Plenum Press, 1984;189–219.
12. Golde DW. Neutrophil kinetics. In: Williams WJ, Beutler EW, Erslev AJ, Lichtman MA, eds. *Hematology,* 4th ed. New York: McGraw-Hill, 1990;734–753.
13. Travis J. Structure, function, and control of neutrophil proteinases. *Am J Med* 1988;84:37–43.
14. Takahashi H, Nukiwa T, Yoshimura K, Quick CD, States DJ, Homles MD, Whang-Peng J, Knutsen T, Crystal RG. Structure of the human neutrophil elastase gene. *J Biol Chem* 1988;263:14739–14747.
15. Takahashi H, Nukiwa T, Basset P, Crystal RG. Myelomonocytic cell lineage expression of the neutrophil elastase gene. *J Biol Chem* 1988;263:2543–2547.
16. Fouret P, DuBois RM, Bernaudin J, Takahashi H, Ferrans VJ, Crystal RG. Expression of the neutrophil elastase gene during human bone marrow cell differentiation. *J Exp Med* 1989;169:833–845.
17. Yoshimura K, Crystal RG. Transcriptional and posttranscriptional modulation of human neutrophil elastase gene expression. *Am Rev Respir Dis* 1990;141:A353.
18. Barrett AJ. Leukocyte elastase. *Methods Enzymol* 1981;80:581–588.
19. Sinha S, Watorek W, Karr S, Giles J, Bode W, Travis J. Primary structure of human neutrophil elastase. *Proc Natl Acad Sci USA* 1987;84:2228–2232.
20. Bieth JG. Elastases: catalytic and biological properties. In: Mecham R, ed. *Regulation of matrix accumulation.* New York: Academic Press, 1986;217–320.
21. Bode W, Meyer E, Powers JC. Human leukocyte and porcine pancreatic elastase: x-ray crystal structures, mechanism, substrate specificity, and mechanism-based inhibitors. *Biochemistry* 1989;28:1951–1962.
22. Janoff A, Scherer J. Mediators of inflammation in leukocyte lysosomes. IX. Elastinolytic activity in granules of human polymorphonuclear leukocytes. *J Exp Med* 1968;128:1137–1155.
23. Janoff A. Elastase in tissue injury. *Annu Rev Med* 1985;36:207–216.
24. Gadek JE, Fells GA, Wright DG, Crystal RG. Human neutrophil elastase functions as a type III collagen "collagenase." *Biochem Biophys Res Commun* 1980;95:1815–1822.
25. States DJ, Fells GA, Crystal RG. Susceptibility of the HIV envelope protein to attack by neutrophil elastase. *Clin Res* 1989;37:482A.
26. Galdston M, Janoff A, Davis AL. Familial variation of leukocyte lysosomal protease and serum α1-antitrypsin as determinants in chronic obstructive pulmonary disease. *Am Rev Respir Dis* 1973;107:718–725.
27. Hubbard R, McElvaney N, Crystal RG. Amount of neutrophil elastase carried by neutrophils may modulate the extent of emphysema in α1-antitrypsin deficiency. *Am Rev Respir Dis* 1990;141:A682.
28. Gross P, Pfitzer EA, Tolker E, Babyak MA, Kaschak M. Experimental emphysema. *Arch Environ Health* 1965;11:50–58.
29. Karlinsky J, Snider GL. Animal models of emphysema. *Am Rev Respir Dis* 1978;117:1109–1133.
30. Kuhn C, Yu S, Chraplyvy M, Linder H, Senior RM. The in-

duction of emphysema with elastase. *Lab Invest* 1976;34:372–380.

31. Guenther CA, Coalson JJ, Jacques J. Emphysema associated with intravascular leukocyte sequestration. *Am Rev Respir Dis* 1981;123:79–84.

32. Spragg RG, Cochrane CG. Human neutrophil elastase and acute lung injury. In: Zapol WM, Fakke KJ, eds. *Acute respiratory failure.* New York: Marcel Dekker, 1982;379–405.

33. Crapo JD, Barry B, Foscue H, Shelburne J. Structural and biochemical changes in rat lungs occurring during exposure to lethal and adaptive doses of oxygen. *Am Rev Respir Dis* 1980;122:123–143.

34. Flick MR, Perel A, Staub NC. Leukocytes are required for increased lung microvascular permeability after microembolization in sheep. *Circ Res* 1981;48:344–351.

35. Barrett AJ. Cathepsin G. *Methods Enzymol* 1981;80:561–565.

36. Hohn PA, Popescu NC, Hanson RD, Salvesen G, Ley TJ. Genomic organization and chromosomal localization of the human cathepsin G gene. *J Biol Chem* 1989;264:13412–13419.

37. Capodici C, Berg RA. Cathepsin G degrades denatured collagen. *Inflammation* 1989;13:137–145.

38. Capodici C, Muthukumaran G, Amoruso MA, Berg RA. Activation of neutrophil collagenase by cathepsin G. *Inflammation* 1989;13:245–258.

39. Reilly CF, Fukunaga Y, Powers JC, Travis J. Effect of neutrophil cathepsin G on elastin degradation by neutrophil elastase. *Hoppe-Seyler's Physiol Chem* 1984;365:1131–1135.

40. Muller D, Quantin B, Gesnel M, Millon-Collard R, Abecassis J, Breathnach R. The collagenase gene family in humans consists of at least four members. *Biochem J* 1988;253:187–192.

41. Collier IE, Smith J, Kronberger A, Bauer EA, Wilheim SM, Eisen AZ, Goldberg GI. The structure of the human skin fibroblast collagenase gene. *J Biol Chem* 1988;263:10711–10713.

42. Hasty KA, Hibbs MS, Kang AH, Mainardi CL. Secreted forms of human neutrophil collagenase. *J Biol Chem* 1986;261:5645–5650.

43. Horwitz AL, Hance AJ, Crystal RG. Granulocyte collagenase: selective digestion of type 1 relative to type III collagen. *Proc Natl Acad Sci USA* 1977;74:897–901.

44. MaCartney HW, Tschesche H. Latent and active human polymorphonuclear leukocyte collagenases isolation, purification and characterisation. *Eur J Biochem* 1982;121:70–78.

45. Harris ED Jr, Welgus HG, Krane SM. Regulation of the mammalian collagenases. *Collagen Rel Res* 1984;4:493–512.

46. Mallya SK, Van Wart HE. Mechanism of inhibition of human neutrophil collagenase by gold(I) chrysotherapeutic compounds. *J Biol Chem* 1989;264:1594–1601.

47. Hibbs MS, Bainton DF. Human neutrophil gelatinase is a component of specific granules. *J Clin Invest* 1989;84:1395–1402.

48. Murphy G, Hembry RM, McGarrity AM, Reynolds JJ, Henderson B. Gelatinase (type IV collagenase) immunolocalization in cells and tissues: use of an antiserum to rabbit bone gelatinase that identifies high and low M_r forms. *J Cell Sci* 1989;92:487–495.

49. Kao RC, Wehner NG, Skubitz KM, Gray BH, Hoidal JR. Proteinase 3: a distinct human polymorphonuclear leukocyte proteinase that produces emphysema in hamsters. *J Clin Invest* 1988;82:1963–1973.

50. Granelli-Piperno A, Vassalli J, Reich E. Secretion of plasminogen activator by human polymorphonuclear leukocytes. *J Exp Med* 1977;146:1693–1706.

51. Barrett AJ, Kirschke H. Cathepsin B, cathepsin H, and cathepsin L. *Methods Enzymol* 1980;80:535–565.

52. Clausbruch UCV, Tschesche H. Cathepsin D from human leukocytes. *Biol Chem Hoppe-Seyler* 1988;369:683–691.

53. Senior RM, Connolly NL, Cury JD, Welgus HG, Campbell EJ. Elastin degradation by human alveolar macrophages. *Am Rev Respir Dis* 1989;139:1251–1256.

54. Campbell EJ, White RR, Senior RM, Rodriquez RJ, Kuhn C. Receptor-mediated binding and internalization of leukocyte elastase by alveolar macrophages in vitro. *J Clin Invest* 1979;64:824–833.

55. Welgus HG, Connolly NL, Senior RM. 12-*O*-Tetradecanoyl-phorbol-13-acetate-differentiated U937 cells express a macro-

phage-like profile in neutral proteinases. *J Clin Invest* 1986;77:1675–1681.

56. Burnett D, Crocker J, Stockley RA. Cathepsin B-like cysteine proteinase activity in sputum and immunohistologic identification of cathepsin B in alveolar macrophages. *Am Rev Respir Dis* 1983;128:915–919.

57. Chapman HA, Reilly JJ, Kobzik L. Role of plasminogen activator in degradation of extracellular matrix protein by live human alveolar macrophages. *Am Rev Respir Dis* 1988;137:412–419.

58. Reilly JJ, Chapman HA. Association between alveolar macrophage plasminogen activator activity and indices of lung function in young cigarette smokers. *Am Rev Respir Dis* 1988;138:1422–1428.

59. Chapman HA, Stone OL. Characterization of a macrophage-derived plasminogen-activator inhibitor. *Biochem J* 1985;230:109–116.

60. Welgus HG, Campbell EJ, Bar-Shavit Z, Senior RM, Teitelbaum SL. Human alveolar macrophages produce a fibroblast-like collagenase and collagenase inhibitor. *J Clin Invest* 1985;76:219–224.

61. Garbisa S, Ballin M, Daga-Gordina D, et al. Transient expression of type IV collagenolytic metalloproteinase by human mononuclear phagocytes. *J Biol Chem* 1986;261:2369–2375.

62. Hibbs M, Hoidal JR, Kang AH. Expression of a metalloproteinase that degrades native type V collagen and denatured collagens by cultured human alveolar macrophages. *J Clin Invest* 1987;80:1644–1650.

63. Hameed A, Lowrey DM, Lichtenheld M, Podack ER. Characterization of three serine esterases isolated from human IL-2 activated killer cells. *J Immunol* 1988;141:3143–3147.

64. Pasternack MS, Eisen HN. A novel serine esterase expressed by cytotoxic T lymphocytes. *Nature* 1985;314:743–745.

65. Pasternack MS, Verret CR, Liu MA, Eisen HN. Serine esterase in cytolytic T lymphocytes. *Nature* 1986;322:740–743.

66. Masson D, Tschopp J. A family of serine esterases in lytic granules of cytolytic T lymphocytes. *Cell* 1987;49:679–685. .

67. Hayes MP, Berrebi GA, Henkart PA. Induction of target cell DNA release by the cytotoxic T lymphocyte granule protease granzyme A. *J Exp Med* 1989;170:933–946.

68. Davis WB, Fells GA, Sun X, Gadek JE, Venet A, Crystal RG. Eosinophil-mediated injury to lung parenchymal cells and interstitial matrix. *J Clin Invest* 1984;74:269–278.

69. Gleich GJ, Adolphson CR. The eosinophilic leukocyte: structure and function. *Adv Immunol* 1986;39:177–253.

70. Meier HL, Heck LW, Schulman ES, MacGlashan DW Jr. Purified human mast cells and basophils release human elastase and cathepsin G by an IgE-mediated mechanism. *Int Arch Allergy Appl Immunol* 1985;77:179–183.

71. Meier HL, Schulman ES, Heck LW, MacGlashan D, Newball HH, Kaplan AP. Release of elastase from purified human lung mast cells and basophils identification as a Hageman factor cleaving enzyme. *Inflammation* 1989;13:295–308.

72. Wintroub BU, Kaempfer CE, Schechter NM, Proud D. A human lung mast cell chymotrypsin-like enzyme. *J Clin Invest* 1986;77:196–201.

73. Wilhelm SM, Collier IE, Marmer BL, Eisen AZ, Grant GA, Goldberg GI. SV40-transformed human lung fibroblasts secrete a 92-kDA type IV collagenase which is identical to that secreted by normal human macrophages. *J Biol Chem* 1989;264:17213–17221.

74. Mauch C, Adelmann-Grill B, Hatamochi A, Krieg T. Collagenase gene expression in fibroblasts is regulated by a three-dimensional contact with collagen. *FEBS Lett* 1989;250:301–305.

75. Gadek JE, Fells GA, Crystal RG. Cigarette smoking induces functional antiprotease deficiency in the lower respiratory tract of humans. *Science* 1979;206:1315–1316.

76. Janoff A, Carp H, Lee DK, Drew RT. Cigarette smoke inhalation. *Science* 1979;206:1313–1314.

77. Janoff A. Elastases and emphysema. *Am Rev Respir Dis* 1985;132:417–433.

78. Stockley RA. Proteolytic enzymes, their inhibitors and lung diseases. *Clin Sci* 1983;64:119–126.

79. Gadek JE, Fells GA, Zimmerman RL, Rennard SI, Crystal RG.

Antielastases of the human alveolar structures. *J Clin Invest* 1981;68:889–898.

80. Damiano VV, Tsang A, Kucich U, Abrams WR, Rosenbloom J, Kimbel P, Fallahnejad M, Weinbaum G. Immunolocalization of elastase in human emphysematous lungs. *J Clin Invest* 1986;78:482–493.

81. Hunninghake GW, Crystal RG. Cigarette smoking and lung destruction—accumulation of neutrophils in the lungs of cigarette smokers. *Am Rev Respir Dis* 1983;128:833–838.

82. Totti N, McCusker RT, Campbell EJ, Griffin GL, Senior RM. Nicotine is chemotactic for neutrophils and enhances neutrophil responsiveness to chemotactic peptides. *Science* 1984;223:169–171.

83. Senior RM, Griffin GL, Mecham RP. Chemotactic activity of elastin derived peptides. *J Clin Invest* 1980;66:859–862.

84. Ossanna PJ, Test ST, Matheson NR, Regiani S, Weiss SJ. Oxidative regulation of neutrophil elastase-alpha-1-proteinase inhibitor interactions. *J Clin Invest* 1986;77:1939–1951.

85. Zaslow MC, Clark RA, Stone PJ, Calore JD, Snider GL, Franzblau C. *Am Rev Respir Dis* 1983;434–439.

86. Padrines M, Schneider-Pozzer M, Bieth JG. Inhibition of neutrophil elastase by alpha-1-proteinase inhibitor oxidized by activated neutrophils. *Am Rev Respir Dis* 1989;139:783–790.

87. Hubbard RC, Ogushi F, Fells GA, Cantin AM, Jallat S, Courtney M, Crystal RG. Oxidants spontaneously released by alveolar macrophages of cigarette smokers can inactivate the active site of α1-antitrypsin, rendering it ineffective as an inhibitor of neutrophil elastase. *J Clin Invest* 1987;80:1289–1295.

88. Fells GA, Ogushi F, Hubbard RC, Crystal RG. α1-antitrypsin in the lower respiratory tract of cigarette smokers has a decreased association rate constant for neutrophil elastase. *Am Rev Respir Dis* 1987;135:A291.

89. Carp H, Miller F, Hoidal JR, Janoff A. Potential mechanism of emphysema: α1-proteinase inhibitor recovered from lungs of cigarette smokers contains oxidized methionine and has decreased elastase inhibitory capacity. *Proc Natl Acad Sci USA* 1982;79:2041–2045.

90. Wood R, Boat T, Doershuk CF. Cystic fibrosis. *Am Rev Respir Dis* 1976;113:833–878.

91. Goldstein W, Doring G. Lysosomal enzymes from polymorphonuclear leukocytes and proteinase inhibitors in patients with cystic fibrosis. *Am Rev Respir Dis* 1986;134:49–56.

92. Suter S, Schaad UB, Roux L, Nydegger UE, Waldvogel FA. Granulocyte neutral proteases and Pseudomonas elastase as possible causes of airway damage in patients with cystic fibrosis. *J Infect Dis* 1984;149:523–531.

93. McElvaney N, Hubbard RC, Fells G, Chernick M, Kaplan D, Crystal RG. Aerosolization of α1-antitrypsin to establish a functional anti-neutrophil elastase defense of the respiratory epithelia in cystic fibrosis. *Clin Res* 1990;38:485A.

94. Cochrane CG, Spragg R, Revak SD. Pathogenesis of the adult respiratory distress syndrome—evidence of oxidant activity in bronchoalveolar lavage fluid. *J Clin Invest* 1983;71:754–761.

95. Lee CT, Fein AM, Lippmann M, Holtzman H, Kimbel P, Weinbaum G. Elastolytic activity in pulmonary lavage fluid from patients with adult respiratory-distress syndrome. *N Engl J Med* 1981;304:192–196.

THE LUNG: Scientific Foundations
edited by R.G. Crystal, J.B. West et al.
Raven Press, Ltd., New York © 1991.

CHAPTER 7.1.2

Antiproteases

Richard C. Hubbard and Ronald G. Crystal

Antiproteases are molecules that combine with proteases in a fashion that prevents the protease from acting on its natural substrates (1–3). In this context, an antiprotease is distinguished from natural protein substrates by virtue of the time and concentration kinetics of its interaction with the protease; that is, the antiprotease is sufficiently "attractive" to the protease that the protease prefers interacting with the antiprotease rather than with the natural substrate. Furthermore, given the appropriate relative concentrations, a competent antiprotease interacts with the protease in a fashion that prevents the protease from subsequently interacting with other molecules (1–4).

In this chapter we will limit the discussion to extracellular antiproteases that normally protect the human lung from proteases capable of attacking components of the extracellular matrix [see Chapter 7.1.1 for a discussion of the relevant proteases; Chapters 3.3.1–3.3.6 for details concerning matrix components; Chapters 3.4.1, 3.4.5, 3.4.7, 3.4.9–3.4.11 for the information concerning inflammatory cells that are the sources of the proteases; and Chapters 7.1.3 and 7.9.1 for the consequences (to the lung) of unopposed proteases]. For a discussion of antiproteases that modulate intracellular protease function, see ref. 5; for a discussion of extracellular antiproteases that modulate the complement, coagulation, and other regulatory pathways (e.g., antithrombin III, α_2-antiplasmin, C1 inhibitor), the reader is referred to general texts on these subjects (1,2).

The extracellular antiproteases that serve to protect the lung are all proteins and include α_1-antitrypsin (α_1AT), secretory leukoprotease inhibitor (SLPI), α_1 antichymotrypsin (α_1ACT), tissue inhibitor of metalloproteases (TIMP), and α_2-macroglobulin (α_2M). Although we will detail all of these extracellular antiproteases, we will place most emphasis on α_1AT and SLPI, the major antiproteases in the lung.

HOW ANTIPROTEASES FUNCTION

Since, by definition, the function of a protease is to destroy proteins, the concept of a protein as an inhibitor of a protease appears paradoxical. However, the protein antiproteases are able to function as such by virtue of their ability to tightly bind to the protease, usually in the region surrounding its active catalytic site. Subsequent to this tight interaction, the protein antiproteases generally function in one of two ways: (i) The protease cleaves a peptide bond at the reactive site of the antiprotease in a fashion similar to that of its normal proteolytic activity, but the cleavage is sufficiently slow and the protease–antiprotease binding sufficiently tight that the result is inhibition of the protease; or (ii) the protease is "trapped" within the antiprotease. The mechanisms of protease inhibition have been studied in detail, and several excellent reviews are available on this subject (1,6).

In regard to antiprotease defense of the lung, it is important to consider the kinetics of the inhibition process. In this context, antiproteases are classified as irreversible or reversible inhibitors, although this distinction is sometimes blurred (1,7). The two can usually be distinguished by diluting the concentration of the protease–antiprotease complex; if the two proteins do not come apart, the inhibition is said to be irreversible. The major antiproteases in the lung (α_1AT and SLPI) are reversible inhibitors; however, since they are very slowly reversible, they act as "pseudo-irreversible inhibitors" (1,3,7,8).

The concept of the kinetics of protease inhibition relates to both time of inhibition and the concentration of antiprotease (relevant to the protease) required for

R. C. Hubbard and R. G. Crystal: Pulmonary Branch, National Heart, Lung and Blood Institute, National Institutes of Health, Bethesda, Maryland 20892.

inhibition (7–9). Except for α_2M (see below), all of the pulmonary-relevant antiproteases inhibit proteases on a molecule for molecule basis; that is, one antiprotease molecule interacts with only one protease molecule. For the reversible inhibitors, the time–concentration kinetics are expressed in two ways: (i) equilibrium constant (i.e., the molarity at which 50% of the protease and antiprotease molecules will form a complex) and (ii) association rate constant (a measure of the rate at which the complex is formed, a parameter commonly used when the association of the two molecules is far in excess of dissociation, a common occurrence with the major pulmonary antiproteases) (1,7–9).

None of the pulmonary protein antiproteases are protease-specific; they all inhibit more than one protease. However, most are protease class-specific; that is, one antiprotease inhibits the class of serine proteases, whereas another inhibits the class of metalloproteases (see Chapter 7.1.1). For example, α_1AT and SLPI inhibit serine proteases, whereas TIMP inhibits metalloproteases (1–4,8–11).

An often overlooked aspect of the function of antiproteases is the translation of these *in vitro* concepts of protease inhibition to actual *in vivo* potency. In general, *in vivo* potency depends upon two factors: (i) the rate at which inhibition takes place and (ii) the stability of the protease–antiprotease complex (7,9). Since the major pulmonary antiproteases exhibit such high association rate constants and low dissociation rate constants (and thus act essentially as pseudo-irreversible inhibitors), the *in vivo* potency can be defined in terms of two critical parameters: (i) the association rate constant and (ii) the concentration of the inhibitor in the lung. This concept has been quantified by Bieth (7) in terms of a parameter referred to as "the delay time of inhibition": delay time of *in vivo* inhibition = 5/(*in vitro* measured association rate constant × *in vivo* inhibitor concentration). For example, if the inhibition of neutrophil elastase (NE) by α_1AT were to occur *in vitro* with an association rate constant of approximately 10^7 M^{-1} sec^{-1} assuming an *in vivo* concentration of functional α_1AT in normal lower respiratory tract epithelial lining fluid (ELF) of 2.5 μM, the delay time of *in vivo* inhibition would be 0.2 sec; that is, in the milieu of ELF *in vivo*, it would take about 0.2 sec for α_1AT to inhibit an equal amount of NE. In contrast, since the concentration of active SLPI in lower respiratory tract ELF is only about 0.6 μM, even though the association rate constant of SLPI for NE is about the same as that of α_1AT, the *in vivo* delay time for NE inhibition is five-fold greater than that of α_1AT. Thus, under normal conditions, SLPI contributes much less to lower respiratory tract anti-NE protection than does α_1AT.

This concept of *in vivo* potency is very important in conceptualizing the development of artificial antiproteases for therapeutic use in augmenting pulmonary antiprotease protection. For efficient protection, the obvious goal is to have the *in vivo* delay time as low as possible. However, if the artificial antiprotease is a reversible inhibitor, it is estimated that 1000-fold greater concentrations of the inhibitor may be needed to achieve the same *in vivo* delay time exhibited by the normal protein antiproteases (7).

α_1-ANTITRYPSIN

α_1-Antitrypsin (α_1AT) is a 52-kDa serine protease inhibitor produced primarily by liver hepatocytes (3,12). Although α_1AT is a broad-spectrum inhibitor of serine proteases (see Chapter 7.1.1), its major role is to inhibit neutrophil elastase (3,8,13). α_1AT is the most abundant extracellular antiprotease in the lung and provides greater than 90% of the anti-NE protection of the lower respiratory tract (14,15).

Gene Structure

α_1AT is coded for by a single 12.2-kb gene on chromosome 14 at q31-32.3 and consists of seven exons and six introns (Fig. 1) (16,17). Analysis of DNA sequences 12 kb 3' to exon V of the α_1AT gene demonstrates a gene with similar characteristics, referred to as the "α_1AT-like gene" (18). Although controversial, the α_1AT-like gene is probably a pseudogene; that is, it is nonfunctional and likely evolved by duplication of the true α_1AT gene.

The first three exons of the α_1AT gene (I_A, I_B, and I_C) code for untranslated regions of α_1AT mRNA, with different lengths of 5' untranslated region partially dependent on cell type (see below). The structural information for the α_1AT protein is coded for by the last four exons (II, III, IV, and V). The coding sequence for the α_1AT protein starts with a sequence for a 24-amino-acid hydrophobic signal peptide that forms the N-terminal portion of the α_1AT as it is translated; the signal peptide is removed in the rough endoplasmic reticulum (RER), leaving the mature 394-amino-acid molecule (16,17,19,20). The active-site Met^{358} (see below) is coded for by sequences residing in exon V.

Cell Expression

By far, the major site of α_1AT gene expression is the hepatocyte (3,12,21). Other human cells that synthesize α_1AT include mononuclear phagocytes and neutrophils. There is indirect evidence that megakaryocytes, islet cells, and intestinal epithelial cells also express the α_1AT gene (22–24). Despite this apparent

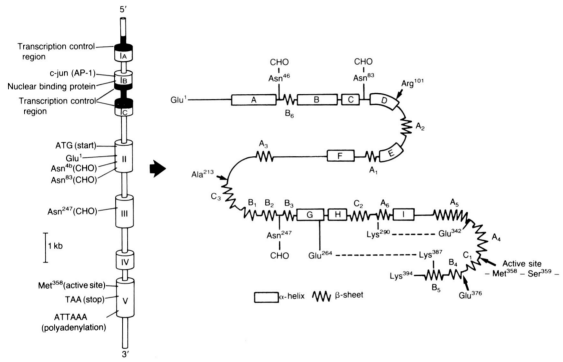

FIG. 1. Structure of the normal α₁-antitrypsin (α₁AT) gene and protein. **Left:** Schematic representation of the α₁AT gene. The gene is 12.2 kb in length and is composed of three noncoding exons (I$_A$, I$_B$, and I$_C$), four coding exons (II, III, IV, and V), and six introns. The cis-acting consensus controlling regions are located in exons I$_A$, I$_B$, and I$_C$ and flanking regions, as indicated. Exon I$_B$ contains a region capable of binding at least two different hepatocyte nuclear proteins, and it also contains sequences capable of binding the *c-jun* protein (AP-1). The start codon (ATG) is in exon II, followed by residues coding for a 24-residue signal peptide. The sequences for the mature 394-residue protein begin in exon II (Glu^1) and end in exon V at the stop signal (TAA). Carbohydrate attachment sites (Asn^{46}, Asn^{83}, and Asn^{247}) and the location for the codon for the active site (Met^{358}) are indicated. The stop codon (TAA) and the polyadenylation signal (ATTAAA) are in exon V. **Right:** Linear form of the normal α₁AT protein, demonstrating the 394-residue single chain containing three asparaginyl-linked complex carbohydrate side chains (CHO) at residues 46, 83, and 247. The tertiary structure of the molecule is a result of the nine α-helices (A–I) and three β-pleated sheets: sheet A (strands A$_1$–A$_6$), sheet B (strands B$_1$–B$_6$), and sheet C (strands C$_1$–C$_3$). Two internal salt bridges (Glu^{342}--Lys^{290} and Glu^{264}--Lys^{387}) help stabilize the molecule and play an important role in the pathogenesis of common deficiency states. Shown are the residues at positions 101, 213, and 376 for the common M1(Ala^{213})allele. Residues at these alleles define the differences among the four common normal α₁AT alleles (see Table 1). The active inhibitory site at Met^{358}–Ser^{359} is located in a loop protruding from the molecule (see Fig. 2 and ref. 36 for details).

broad expression of the α_1AT gene, all available evidence suggests that lung levels of α_1AT are modulated by plasma α_1AT levels, which, in turn, are modulated by hepatocytes, with other cells contributing very little (12,17,19).

Transcription of the α_1AT gene is controlled by sequences 5' to the middle of exon I_C and 5' to exon I_A (16,21,25). The region 5' to exon I_C is used primarily by hepatocytes, but it is also used by activated mononuclear phagocytes (21,25,26). Within the 5' portion of I_C are consensus promoter elements; 5' to this, in exon I_B, there are two regions capable of binding the nuclear protein AP-1 (the product of the *c-jun* proto-oncogene) (27–29). The region between I_B and I_C contains sequences recognized by liver-specific trans-activating nuclear proteins. There are also consensus promoter elements 5' to exon I_A, but these controlling elements seem to modulate constitutive transcription in both mononuclear phagocytes and hepatocytes (26).

Modulation of α_1AT Expression

Normal α_1AT serum levels are 20–53 μM. The levels are increased in trauma, pregnancy, hemorrhage, and neoplasia (12,30), but the mechanisms responsible for the up-regulation of the α_1AT gene *in vivo* are unknown. In cell culture, α_1AT mRNA levels are increased by phorbol esters and interleukin 6 (interferon β_2), but not by interleukin 1 or tumor necrosis factor (31). *In vivo* administration of typhoid vaccine or estrogens increases α_1AT serum levels in normal humans, but *in vivo* administration of lipopolysaccharide has no effect, despite its marked effect on increasing other serum "acute-phase reactants" (*unpublished observations*).

Protein Structure and Function

The mature α_1AT molecule is a 52-kDa glycoprotein comprised of a single chain of 394 amino acids with three carbohydrate side chains N-linked to amino acids Asn^{46}, Asn^{83}, and Asn^{247} of the polypeptide chain (20,32) (Fig. 1). The side chains are composed of *N*-acetylglucosamine, mannose, galactose, and sialic acid, arranged as a common-core sequence with two or three "antennae" coming off to form "biantennary" or "triantennary" configurations (3,32,33).

Isoelectric focusing analyses of serum of normal individuals homozygous for the same α_1AT allele demonstrate two major and three minor forms of α_1AT focusing in the range of 4.1 to 4.8 (34,35). The two major forms differ only by the carbohydrates; one has three biantennary side chains, whereas the other has two biantennary chains (Asn^{46}, Asn^{247}) and one triantennary chain (Asn^{83}). One minor form has one bian-

tennary and two triantennary chains. The other two minor bands have the same carbohydrate side chains as the two major bands, but the protein is missing five N-terminal residues. The post-translational processes responsible for use of these differences are unknown.

Crystallographic analysis of the mature protein reveals a globular structure 6.7 nm by 3.2 nm with the three carbohydrates on the external side of one end of the molecule (36). The internal structure is highly ordered with 30% in the form of α-helices and 40% in β-pleated sheets (Fig. 1). Two intramolecular salt bridges (Glu^{342}--Lys^{290} and Glu^{264}--Lys^{387}) help maintain the three-dimensional structure and play an important role in the pathogenesis of common α_1AT deficiency states (see Chapter 7.9.1).

The major function of α_1AT is to inhibit neutrophil elastase (NE), a powerful protease capable of cleaving a wide spectrum of extracellular matrix proteins (see Chapter 7.1.1). *In vitro*, α_1AT is capable of inhibiting a variety of other human serine proteases, including trypsin, chymotrypsin, cathepsin G, plasmin, thrombin, tissue kallikrein, factor X_a, and plasminogen; however, it inhibits these far less effectively than it inhibits NE (9). The active inhibitory site of α_1AT is centered at Met^{358}–Ser^{359}, part of a highly stressed external loop protruding from the molecule (36). When the Met^{358}–Ser^{359} bond is cleaved, the stress is released and the two residues are separated widely. It is the conformation of the active-site loop that gives the exquisite sensitivity of α_1AT for NE. Presented on this stressed loop, the Met^{358}–Ser^{359} is highly attractive to the active-site pocket of NE (Fig. 2). A tight, noncovalent interaction occurs between the inhibitor and the NE reactive-site pocket, and the NE is prevented from functioning. Under normal conditions, the interaction between the two molecules is a suicide interaction for both, with the unmodified (but inhibited) NE remaining attached to the α_1AT. In most instances the α_1AT remains intact. However, the NE can cleave the Met^{358}–Ser^{359} bond of the α_1AT; if this occurs under normal conditions, the NE remains bound to the N-terminal portion of α_1AT ending with Met^{358}, and the 36-amino-acid C-terminal peptide (Ser^{359}–Lys^{394}) is released (37). Interestingly, this cleaved C-terminal fragment of α_1AT is chemotactic for neutrophils, further increasing the local burden of NE (37).

The association rate constant for complex formation (K_a) of α_1AT and NE is extremely rapid, approximately 10^7 M^{-1} sec^{-1} (9) (Table 1). The K_a of α_1AT for NE is higher than the K_a of α_1AT for any of the other serine proteases, consistent with the principal function of α_1AT as the major physiologic inhibitor of NE (9). The rate of dissociation of NE from α_1AT is negligible. When α_1AT is exposed to oxidants (electrophilic molecules, including physiologic radicals such as O_2^-, H_2O_2, OH$\cdot$, and HOCl$^-$ (see Chapter

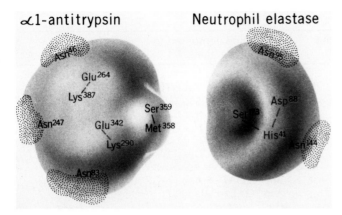

FIG. 2. Interaction between α_1-antitrypsin (α_1AT) and neutrophil elastase (NE). The α_1AT molecule is globular in shape, with its active inhibitory site (Met[358]–Ser[359]) protruding from the opposite end of the molecule from the carbohydrate side chains at asparaginyl residues 46, 83, and 247. The NE enzyme is also globular and is glycosylated at Asn[95] and Asn[144]. The active site of NE is centered in a pocket that contains the catalytic triad Ser[173]--His[41]--Asp[88]. When NE attacks a protein substrate like elastin, a portion of this protein is locked into this pocket, triggering the transfer of an electron within the catalytic triad and converting the Ser[173] into a reactive nucleophile that attacks and cleaves a peptide bond of the target. The cleaved protein is released, allowing NE to attack again (see Chapter 7.7.1). In contrast, when NE interacts with α_1AT, the Met[358]–Ser[359] of α_1AT fits into the active-site pocket of NE and the catalytic triad is activated, but the interaction is such that the α_1AT–NE complex remains intact, resulting in inhibition of the NE.

7.2.1), its interaction with NE changes dramatically, due to the effect of the oxidants on sensitive amino acids of the α_1AT molecule (38–40). Included among these residues is the Met[358] at the active site; when Met[358] is oxidized, the K_a of α_1AT for NE decreases by approximately 2000-fold, and the rate of dissociation increases (9,38). NE is able to cleave oxidized α_1AT at the Met[358]–Ser[359] active site; the cleaved ox-

idized α_1AT cannot maintain its interaction with NE, permitting the NE to be released, and cannot function again as an active antiprotease.

Recombinant forms of α_1AT produced in *Escherichia coli* or yeast have no carbohydrate side chains, but they inhibit NE with a K_a similar to that of the natural molecule (41–43). Several recombinant variants of the α_1AT have been synthesized that differ from normal α_1AT by changes in active-site residues (41–44). Interestingly, substitution of the Met[358] by Val, Ala, or Leu confers to the α_1AT molecule the ability to resist oxidation (see Chapter 7.9.1 for details).

Different Normal α_1AT Alleles

The α_1AT gene is pleomorphic, with approximately 75 normal alleles known (12,17,19,25) (for alleles associated with α_1AT deficiency or dysfunction, see Chapter 7.9.1). By definition, a normal allele codes for an α_1AT protein that is synthesized in normal amounts and functions in a normal fashion. Most data regarding α_1AT polymorphisms are from the Caucasian populations of European descent. Among this group there are four common normal α_1AT alleles: M1(Ala[213]), M1(Val[213]), M3, and M2 (Table 2) (12,17,19,25). M1(Ala[213]) is believed to be the "oldest" human α_1AT allele (see below). The M1(Val[213]), M3, and M2 alleles differ from the M1(Ala[213]) by single bases, respectively, resulting in single amino acid substitutions. Most other normal alleles are rare.

Evolution of the α_1AT Gene

Comparison of the α_1AT gene sequence to that of other serine protein inhibitors has led to the concept of the

TABLE 1. *Major antiproteases relevant to the lung[a]*

Antiprotease	Molecular weight (kDa)	Form[b]	Amino acids[c]	Disulfide bonds	Number of carbohydrate side chains	Antiprotease spectrum relevant to the lung extracellular matrix	Concentration in normal plasma (μM)	Concentration in ELF (μM)
α_1-Antitrypsin	52	1	394	No	3	NE, cathepsin G	20–53	2–6
SLPI	12	1	107	Yes	0	NE, cathepsin G, chymase	0.004–0.007	1–1.2
α_1-Antichymotrypsin	68	1	408	Yes	Yes[d]	Cathepsin G	6–8	0.5–1
TIMP	29	1	184	Yes	Yes[d]	Collagenases, stromolysins, PUMP-1	0.03	ND
α_2-Macroglobulin	720	4	1451	Yes	8	All classes of proteases	2.5–5	0.01

[a] Abbreviations: SLPI, secretory leukoprotease inhibitor; TIMP, tissue inhibitor of metalloproteinases; NE, neutrophil elastase; ELF, epithelial lining fluid; ND, not determined; PUMP-1, putative metalloproteinase 1.
[b] Number of polypeptide chains in intact molecule.
[c] Number of amino acids in each polypeptide chain.
[d] Glysosylated, but number of carbohydrate chains not known.

TABLE 2. *Normal α₁-antitrypsin alleles*

Category[a]	Allele	Base allele[b]	Mutation site (exon)	Sequence compared to base allele	Allelic frequency[c]
Common	M1(Ala^{213})	—	—	—	0.20–0.23
	M1(Val^{213})	M1(Ala^{213})	III	Ala^{213} G<u>C</u>G → Val G<u>T</u>G	0.44–0.49
	M3	M1(Val^{213})	V	Glu^{376} GAA → Asp GA<u>C</u>	0.10–0.11
	M2	M3	II	Arg^{101} CG<u>T</u> → His CA<u>T</u>	0.14–0.19
Rare	M4	M1(Val^{213})[d]	II	Arg^{101} CG<u>T</u> → His CA<u>T</u>	0.01–0.05
	B$_{alhambra}$	Unknown	Unknown	Lys → Asp	Rare
	F	M1(Val^{213})	III	Arg^{223} <u>C</u>GT → Cys <u>T</u>GT	Rare
	P$_{saint albans}$	M1(Val^{213})	V	Asp^{341} GA<u>C</u> → Asn A<u>A</u>C	Rare
			III	Asp^{256} GA<u>T</u> → Asp GA<u>C</u>	
	V$_{munich}$	M1(Val^{213})	II	Asp^2 GA<u>T</u> → Ala G<u>C</u>T	Rare
	X	M1(Val^{213})	III	Glu^{204} → Lys	Rare
	X$_{christchurch}$	Unknown	V	Glu^{363} → Lys	Rare
	Other[e]	?	?	?	?

[a] Common = allelic frequency ≥ 10%; rare = allelic frequency < 10%.
[b] "Base allele" is the common normal allele from which the mutation developed.
[c] Allelic frequency based on U.S. Caucasian population.
[d] Assumed.
[e] Other rare normal alleles include: B, B$_{saskatoon}$, C, D, E, E$_{cincinnatti}$, E$_{franklin}$, E$_{lemberg}$, E$_{matsue}$, E$_{tokyo}$, G, G$_{cler}$, J$_{houyao}$, L, L$_{beijing}$, M$_{chapel hill}$, M$_{salla}$, M5$_{germany}$, N, N$_{adelaide}$, N$_{grossoeure}$, N$_{hampton}$, N$_{letrait}$, N$_{agato}$, N$_{yerville}$, P$_{budapest}$, P$_{castoria}$, P$_{clifton}$, P$_{kyoto}$, P$_{oki}$, P$_{saint louis}$, P$_{weishi}$, R, T, V, W$_{finneytown}$, W$_{salerno}$, X$_{alban}$, X$_{hagi}$, X$_{fengcheng}$, Y$_{brighton}$, Y$_{toronto}$, and Z$_{pratt}$; the sequence of these alleles is unknown.

"serpins" (*serine proteinase inhibitors*), molecules that evolved from an ancestral serine protease inhibitor and that consequently have common tertiary structures, functional domains, and reactive centers (45). Among this list are molecules with very different inhibitory profiles, including α₁-antichymotrypsin (an inhibitor of cathepsin G), antithrombin III (thrombin), C1 inhibitor (C1s component of complement, kallikrein), α₂-antiplasmin (plasmin), heparin cofactor II (thrombin), protein C inhibitor (activated protein C), plasminogen activator inhibitor (plasminogen activator), and angiotensinogen (no known substrate). All are single-chain glycoproteins with a molecular weight of 40–60 kDa, and all are suicide inhibitors that form one-to-one complexes with their target proteases. All have Glu--Lys internal salt bridges, an interesting observation in the context that the mutations causing the two most common α₁-At deficiency alleles (Z and S) both involve Glu--Lys salt bridges (see Chapter 7.9.1) (12,25). In the genes coding for the serine proteases, the number and position of the introns are rigidly conserved, suggesting an ancestral gene that may have duplicated relatively late in evolution; in contrast, the number and position of the introns among the serpin genes vary significantly, suggesting early duplication before divergence (45,46). The concept of early duplication of the serpins before divergence is also consistent with the observation of an α₁AT-like gene 12 kb 3' to the α₁AT gene (18).

Evaluation of all known sequences of α₁AT genes has led to the concept that the M1(Ala^{213}) gene is the "oldest" human gene (see below) (12). In this regard,

the baboon, gorilla, and chimpanzee α₁AT genes and the human M1(Ala^{213}) gene have GCG (Ala) coding for residue 213, whereas for all other known normal α₁AT genes, this codon is CTG (Val). Furthermore, comparison of sequences of the human α₁AT genes with those of the primates has revealed that the coding exons of the human M1(Ala^{213}) gene differ from those of the chimpanzee by only 11 bases (causing only two amino acid changes), from those of the gorilla by 20 bases (eight amino acid changes), and from those of the baboon by 64 bases (30 amino acid changes) (T. Nukiwa and R. Crystal, *unpublished observations*). In contrast, all of the other sequenced human α₁AT genes differ from those of the chimpanzee by more bases (and amino acid changes) than does the M1(Ala^{213}) gene.

SECRETORY LEUKOPROTEASE INHIBITOR

The secretory leukoprotease inhibitor (SLPI; also referred to as "bronchial mucous inhibitor," "mucous proteinase inhibitor," "human seminal inhibitor," and "antileukoprotease") is a 12-kDa, nonglycosylated serine antiprotease produced by mucosal cells, including those in the large and small airways (10,47,48). In the lung, the major role of SLPI is to protect the upper respiratory tract from NE (10,49–53).

Gene Structure

SLPI is coded for by a single gene which has not yet been assigned to a chromosome. The gene consists of four exons and three introns and spans approximately 2.6 kb (Fig. 3) (10,54–56). Exon III contains sequences for the active inhibitory site. The region 5' to the gene contains consensus TAAAT and CAAT promoter sequences within 95 bp of the transcription initiation site.

Cells Producing SLPI

SLPI is synthesized and secreted by mucosal cells widely dispersed throughout the upper and lower respiratory tract (47,48). In the central airways, immunohistologic studies demonstrate SLPI in serous and goblet cells of the submucosal glands as well as in surface epithelium of the bronchial mucosa. In the distal airways, SLPI is present in nonciliated (Clara) epithelial cells.

The mechanisms of control of the SLPI gene are not known. *In vitro*, SLPI is produced by the H24 squamous cell line (57). SLPI mRNA transcripts in these cells are approximately 0.9 kb. The putative primary

translation product is a 132-amino-acid protein, containing a 25-residue N-terminal signal peptide which is cleaved prior to secretion of the final SLPI protein.

Protein Structure and Function

SLPI is a 107-residue, nonglycosylated single chain with eight intramolecular disulfide links (Fig. 3) (10,58). Crystallographic analysis demonstrates that the tertiary structure has a boomerang shape and is composed of two similar domains of approximately the same size (an N-terminal region covered by residues 1–54, along with a C-terminal region containing residues 55–107) (58). The polypeptide segments of each domain are interconnected by four disulfide bridges. Overall, the two domains have a similar structure. The active site for protease inhibition is contained within the C-terminal domain, at Leu^{72}–Met^{73}. The corresponding residues in the N-terminal domain (Arg^{20}–Tyr^{21}) were hypothesized to be specific for inhibition

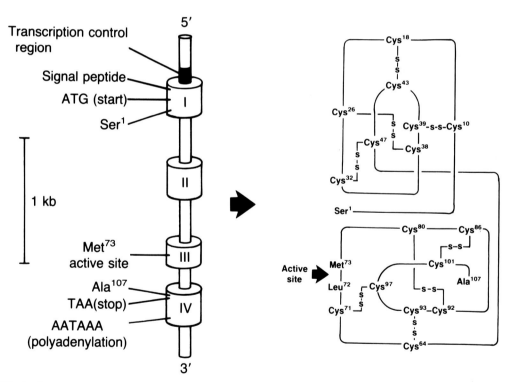

FIG. 3. The secretory leukoprotease inhibitor (SLPI) gene and protein. **Left:** The SLPI gene is 2.4 kb in length and consists of four exons and three introns. A cis-acting transcriptional control region is located 5' to exon I. Sequences for the 25-residue signal peptide, the start codon (ATG), and the first amino acid of the mature protein (Ser^1) are located in exon I. Exon III includes sequences for the active-site Met^{73}. Exon IV codes for a single amino acid (the C-terminal Ala^{107}), the stop codon (TAA), and the polyadenylation signal (AATAAA). **Right:** The SLPI protein is a single-chain, nonglycosylated polypeptide extending from Ser^1 to Ala^{107}. The three-dimensional structure has a boomerang shape and includes two domains. Each domain contains four disulfide bonds (—S—S—) located between Cys residues as indicated. The protease inhibitory site is located at Leu^{72}–Met^{73} (*arrow*). The inner loop of each domain forms β-sheet structures, while the remainder of each domain is arranged in spiral chains (see ref. 58 for details).

of trypsin (10,55), but it is now recognized that all proteases interact only with the Leu^{72}–Met^{73} site in the C-terminal domain (58).

SLPI inhibits a variety of serine proteases, including NE, cathepsin G, trypsin, chymotrypsin, and mast cell chymase, forming a one-to-one complex with each enzyme (8,10,59). The rate of association is highest with neutrophil elastase, with an association rate constant of 10^7 M^{-1} sec^{-1} (8). This high K_a value, together with a very low rate of dissociation of SLPI–NE complexes, makes SLPI an excellent physiologic inhibitor of NE. Furthermore, SLPI is acid-stable, which may enable it to remain functional in the decreased pH in the vicinity of activated neutrophils (59). SLPI has a pI greater than 9, very similar to that of NE (pI 10.8), and thus may localize and bind to tissue sites favored by NE, such as elastin. In the lung, the concentration of SLPI is highest on the epithelial surfaces (see below). Some SLPI is found in serum, but at low concentrations (4–7 nM) (49,50).

α₁-ANTICHYMOTRYPSIN

α_1-Antichymotrypsin (α_1ACT), a 68-kDa glycosylated serine antiprotease, is present in the lung, although its role in defending the lung is not clear. It is capable of inhibiting a variety of serine proteases released by inflammatory cells, but its likely physiologic function is to inhibit the neutrophil serine protease cathepsin G (1–3,60).

Gene Structure and Expression

α_1ACT is a member of the serpin family, and the gene shares many similarities with α_1AT, including its genomic structure (45,61,62). The exon sequence has a 56% homology with α_1AT, the protein sequence has a 45% homology, and the active sites are in similar locations. The α_1ACT gene occupies 12 kb of chromosome 14 in the same general region as α_1AT (61,63). The gene contains five exons and four introns. Exon II contains the translation initiation codon. The active site (Leu^{358}–Ser^{359}) is in exon V. The exon structure predicts a 22- or 25-residue signal peptide; the exact size is unclear due to the presence of two closely spaced in-phase translation initiation codons. The signal peptide is cleaved during intracellular processing, leaving the mature 408-residue molecule. The α_1ACT gene is expressed in hepatocytes and, experimentally, in a human histiocytic cell line (64). α_1ACT is an acute-phase reactant; its serum concentration rises rapidly in a variety of conditions, including surgery, burn injuries, inflammatory bowel disease, and some types of cancer. Normal serum α_1ACT levels range from 6 to 8 μM (2,3).

Protein Structure and Function

The mature α_1ACT protein functions as a serine antiprotease in the same manner as does α_1AT, forming one-to-one complexes with a target protease (1–3). Its rate of association is highest for cathepsin G, with a K_a of 5×10^7 M^{-1} sec^{-1} (8). It also inhibits chymotrypsin and mast cell chymase, but it has no inhibitory activity against NE or trypsin (3,8).

Recombinant α_1ACT produced in E. coli is nonglycosylated, but it is similar to normal human α_1ACT in its antiprotease spectrum (65). Interestingly, recombinant α_1ACT with a Leu^{358}→Met substitution (i.e., conferring an active site similar to α_1AT) still does not inhibit NE.

TISSUE INHIBITORS OF METALLOPROTEINASES

As the name suggests, the tissue inhibitors of metalloproteinases (TIMP) is specific inhibitor of the "metallo" class of proteases such as collagenase (11,66–69). TIMP is a 29-kDa single-chain glycoprotein produced by several cells, including fibroblasts and mononuclear phagocytes. Although little is known about TIMP in lung, it theoretically could play an important role in protecting the matrix from a variety of metalloproteases, including interstitial collagenase (type I collagenase), neutrophil collagenase, type IV collagenases (gelatinase), the stromolysins, and putative metalloproteinase 1 (PUMP-1) (see Chapter 7.7.1).

Gene Structure and Expression

The genoamic structure and chromosomal location of TIMP are not known. Recently a similar gene (TIMP-2) has been described, suggesting that TIMP belongs to a multigene family (11,70). The cDNA sequence predicts a 23-residue leader sequence followed by a 184-residue polypeptide containing two attachment sites for complex carbohydrate side chains (71). The expression of the gene is up-regulated in cultured fibroblasts by phorbol esters and interleukin 1 (67).

Protein Structure and Function

The TIMP molecule contains six intramolecular disulfide links. It forms a one-to-one complex with its target protease (11). Little is known about the TIMP–protease interaction, although it is believed to be less effective than α_2-Macroglobulin (α_2M) as an inhibitor of interstitial collagenase (11,69).

α₁-MACROGLOBULIN

α₂Macroglobulin (α₂M) is a 720-kDa glycoprotein that functions as a "universal" antiprotease, capable of inhibiting the majority of proteases from all four catalytic classes (see Chapter 7.1.1) (1–3,72). Although present in small amounts in the lung (see below), its broad spectrum and its ability to form tight complexes with proteases suggest that it may play a role in protecting pulmonary tissues, at least in the localized areas where α₂M is produced.

Gene Structure and Expression

The α₂M gene is located on the short arm of chromosome 12 at p12.3-13.3 (72–75). Sequence homologies suggest that α₂M belongs to a gene family that includes the complement factors of C3, C4, and C5 (see Chapter 3.4.6) (3,72). The genomic structure of the human α₂M gene is not known. The sequence of the α₂M cDNA predicts that the primary translation product includes a 23-amino-acid N-terminal hydrophobic signal peptide followed by a mature 1451-residue polypeptide used to form the actual α₂M molecule. The α₂M gene is expressed in a variety of cell types, such as hepatocytes, fibroblasts, and mononuclear phagocytes (including aveolar macrophages) (72). Normal serum levels range from 2.5 to 5 μM. Although human α₂M is an acute-phase reactant in many mammalian species, its levels do not increase with trauma or other forms of stress (72,76). In experimental animals, the acute-phase process is modulated in hepatocytes by a combination of transcriptional and post-transcriptional processes (76).

Protein Structure and Function

The mature 720-kDa α₂M molecule is built from four 1451-residue polypeptide chains (72,77–80). Each chain contains 22 cysteine residues; 20 are involved in intrachain disulfide bonds, and two are used in interchain disulfide bonds that link two chains into a covalently bonded dimer of 180 kDa. The dimers form the basic subunit of the molecule, with two subunits joining in a noncovalent fashion to form the final molecule. α₂M is highly glycosylated, with each polypeptide chain containing eight asparaginyl-linked oligosaccharide side chains. Each of the two subunits of the final α₂M molecule contains a specific region, referred to as the "bait region," which is attractive to proteases and highly susceptible to proteolytic cleavage. When the protease interacts with α₂M, it cleaves the bait region, yielding two polypeptides (85 and 95 kDa) that remain linked. Cleavage of the peptide bond within the bait region causes the molecule to undergo a rapid con-

formational change which physically entraps the protease molecule within the bulk of the α₁M molecule, resulting in sterically induced inhibition of the protease. The resulting complex is very stable; once bound, a protease cannot be displaced. Because there are two bait regions per molecule (one for each subunit), two protease molecules can be inhibited by one α₂M molecule. The K_a of α₂M for each proteases differs, with a value of 4×10^7 M^{-1} sec^{-1} for NE and 3.1×10^6 M^{-1} sec^{-1} for cathepsin G.

In addition to the trapping mechanism described above, there is evidence that α₂M can link covalently with nucleophilic groups on proteases (3,72,81). Using such a mechanism, α₂M can interact with proteins such as platelet-derived growth factor and transforming growth factor-β, preventing these molecules from functioning in a normal fashion (72) (see Chapters 2.8, 2.9, 3.4.5, and 7.8.1).

Receptors for α₂M–protease complexes have been identified on hepatocytes, fibroblasts, and mononuclear phagocytes (72). These likely serve to "clear" α₂M–protease complexes.

OTHER ANTIPROTEASES

Other antiproteases with possible relevance to the pulmonary extracellular matrix include the plasma antiproteases α-cysteine proteinase inhibitor and inter-α-trypsin inhibitor. α₂-Cysteine protease inhibitor is a 57-kDa protein with high inhibitory activity against cathepsins H and L, significantly higher than that against cathepsin B (2–4). This antiprotease does not inhibit NE. Inter-α-trypsin inhibitor is a 180-kDa inhibitor of serine proteases, including trypsin, chymotrypsin, and plasmin (2–4). It does not inhibit NE or cathepsin G; *in vitro*, NE cleaves inter-α-trypsin inhibitor.

ROLES OF ANTIPROTEASES IN PROTECTING THE LUNG

The definitive example of the critical importance of antiproteases in the lung is provided by α₁AT deficiency, a hereditary disorder associated with emphysema caused by unopposed destruction of the alveolar walls by NE (see Chapter 7.9.1). For the other antiproteases, the evidence is indirect, as detailed below.

Locations and Levels

The locations and amounts of the antiproteases in the lung are dictated by where they are synthesized and their physical properties (Table 1). Most available information relates to α₁AT and SLPI.

For the antiproteases derived primarily from plasma

(e.g., α_1AT), the concentrations in various lung compartments are dictated by the plasma concentration and the molecular mass. Most data in humans come from bronchoalveolar-lavage-derived estimates of epithelial lining fluid (ELF) levels (14,82–86). Concentrations of the 50- to 70-kDa proteins (e.g., α_1AT) in ELF are approximately 10% that in plasma, whereas concentrations of the 80- to 230-kDa proteins in ELF are 5–10% that in plasma. Very large proteins, such as α_2M (720-kDa), are present in ELF in very low concentrations. Of the plasma protease inhibitors less than 70-kDa in size, only α_1AT and α_1ACT have high enough concentrations in plasma that their levels in ELF are of potential physiologic significance. For example, α_1AT diffuses across the capillary endothelium into the lung interstitium, and across epithelium to the epithelial surface. Consequently, the α_1AT within the lung in different anatomic spaces (e.g., interstitial versus epithelial) is not compartmentalized differently between the upper and lower respiratory tracts. This has been verified by bronchoalveolar lavage studies demonstrating that ELF levels of α_1AT in large airways are equal to those in the alveoli (87). Levels of α_1AT in lung interstitium are between the alveolar and plasma levels. Normally, proteins that diffuse from the plasma into the interstitium are removed via interstitial fluid flowing into the pulmonary lymphatics, with only a fraction passing across the epithelium. For α_1AT it has been estimated that interstitial levels are 50–70% of the plasma levels (88). Since the normal range of plasma α_1AT is between 20 and 53 μM, the alveolar interstitial level is approximately 10–40 μM.

In contrast to the predominantly liver-produced α_1AT, almost all of the SLPI and TIMP in the lung are produced by cells normally present within the lung. SLPI is produced locally within large-airway serous cells of submucosal glands, as well as by Clara cells in the small airways, but not by cell types in the alveoli (47,48). Consequently, concentrations of SLPI are highest on the epithelial surface in upper airways; they are lower in alveolar regions, and likely lower in lung interstitium as well (52,53). TIMP is produced within the lung by fibroblasts and alveolar macrophages. Although regional levels of TIMP within the lung are not known, it is likely that TIMP concentrations are highest around locations of alveolar macrophages and fibroblasts (11).

Although α_2M is a plasma antiprotease, its large molecular mass precludes significant diffusion across the alveolar wall from plasma (14,82–86). It is produced by fibroblasts and, to a small extent, by alveolar macrophages; and thus, like SLPI and TIMP, it is likely present near these cells. However, the mass of this protein is such that it likely does not diffuse a significant distance from its site of production, forming a "moat" of antiprotease protection around the synthe-

TABLE 3. *Kinetics of inhibition of neutrophil elastase by antiproteases normally present in the lung*

Antiprotease	Association rate constant (M^{-1} sec^{-1})	In vivo inhibition time (sec)[a]
α_1-Antitrypsin	10^7	0.08–0.25
Secretory leukoprotease inhibitor	10^7	0.45–0.50
α_1-Antichymotrypsin	0	—
Tissue inhibitor of metalloproteases	0	—
α_2-Macroglobulin	4×10^7	6

[a] "*In vivo* inhibition" time refers to the estimated time it would take an antiprotease (at levels found in lung epithelial lining fluids) to inhibit 97% of the activity of an equal concentration of protease (7).

sizing cell. The lack of diffusion of α_2M is reflected in the low concentrations (0.01 μM) in normal ELF (14,84).

Protection Against NE

Direct assessment of ELF in normal individuals has shown that α_1AT is the principal inhibitor of NE, contributing approximately 90% of the total anti-NE capacity (14,15). The remainder of ELF NE inhibition is caused by SPLI and, to a very limited degree, by α_2M. The ELF at α_1AT level in normal individuals ranges between 2 and 5 μM. Normally, greater than 90% of ELF α_1AT is functionally capable of inhibiting NE (89).

SLPI is present in significant amounts on the epithelial surface, predominantly in larger airways, with a level over 10-fold higher than in the alveoli (53). Compared to α_1AT, SLPI levels are nearly twofold higher in the airways, but the α_1AT concentration is over threefold higher than SLPI in the alveoli. Inexplicably, the SLPI present on the lung epithelial surface is largely inactive, with only one-third functionally capable of inhibiting NE (53). Thus, despite generally comparable overall levels of SLPI and α_1AT on the lung epithelial surface, SLPI contributes far less to the anti-NE protection than does α_1AT, except perhaps in the large airways, where SLPI concentrations are highest.

Put in the context of the kinetics of inhibition of NE, for the concentrations of functional inhibition present, α_1AT is clearly the major defense against this protease (Table 3). In this regard, the "*in vivo* inhibition time" of α_1AT for NE is two- to fivefold faster than that for SLPI. On a molecule-for-molecule basis, α_2M is even more effective than α_1AT as an NE inhibitor, but the concentrations in the lung are so low that it plays little, if any, significant role in defending against this protease.

Protection Against Other Proteases

The hierarchy of lung antiprotease defense against proteases other than NE is less well understood. α_1AT, SLPI, α_1ACT, and α_2M all inhibit cathepsin G, with α_1ACT the most effective (8,10,72). It is assumed, but not proven, that TIMP forms the major defense against metalloproteases, but the levels and function of TIMP in the normal human lung are unknown.

Protease–Antiprotease Balance in the Lung

There are several roles for antiproteases protecting the extracellular matrix from proteolytic attack. First, the extracellular matrix of the normal lung is a dynamic structure, with new components being synthesized constantly, necessitating the removal of similar components. Presumably there is an array of proteases that subserve this function (e.g., fibroblast interstitial collagenase), and the antiproteases likely serve to dampen the potential for damage. Second, within the normal lung there are inflammatory cells (such as alveolar marcophages and neutrophils) that have the capacity to release proteases with the potential for damaging the extracellular matrix. All available evidence suggests that there is excess antiprotease protection that serves as a defensive barrier against adverse proteolytic attack from the normal, low-burden inflammatory-cell-derived proteases. This is particularly true for the defenses against NE. Finally, the lung is a common place for acute and chronic inflammatory processes, events that are associated by varying burdens of different types of proteases. In some situations, the antiprotease screen is effective, but it is often overwhelmed, permitting unopposed proteolytic attack. In this regard, the intensity, location, and specificity of the protease burden determines the extent, site, and kind of damage to the extracellular matrix. Furthermore, just as there are various mechanisms by which the protease burden can be increased, there are a variety of processes that can leave the lung "deficient" in antiprotease protection. The most dramatic example of this is the hereditary deficiency of α_1AT, but there are a number of other acquired processes that attack the structure and/or function of the antiproteases, resulting in an equivalent antiprotease deficiency state (see Chapter 7.9.1 for details).

REFERENCES

1. Barrett AJ. An introduction to proteases. In: Barrett AJ, Salvesen G, eds. *Protease inhibitors.* New York: Elsevier, 1986; 1–22.
2. Sottrup-Jensen L. In: Putnam FW, ed. *The plasma proteins,* 2nd ed. Orlando FL: Academic Press, 1987;191–291.
3. Travis J, Salvesen GS. Human plasma proteinase inhibitors. *Annu Rev Biochem* 1983;52:655–709.
4. Laskowski M, Kato I. Protein inhibitors of proteinases. *Annu Rev Biochem* 1980;49:593–626.
5. Barrett AJ, ed. *Proteinases in mammalian cells and tissues.* Amsterdam: Elsevier, 1977.
6. Knight CG. The characterization of enzyme inhibition. In: Barrett AJ, Salvesen G, eds. *Protease inhibitors.* New York: Elsevier, 1986;23–51.
7. Bieth JG. *In vivo* significance of kinetic constants of protein proteinase inhibitors. *Chem Med* 1984;32:387–397.
8. Beatty K, Bieth J, Travis J. Kinetics of association of serine proteinases with native and oxidized α-1-proteinase inhibitor and α-1-antichymotrypsin. *J Biol Chem* 1980;255:3931–3934.
9. Smith CE, Johnson DA. Human bronchial leucocyte proteinase inhibitor. *Biochem J* 1985;225:463–472.
10. Thompson RC, Ohlsson K. Isolation, properties, and complete amino acid sequence of human secretory leukocyte protease inhibitor, a potent inhibitor of leukocyte elastase. *Proc Natl Acad Sci USA* 1986;83:6692–6696.
11. Matrisian LM. Metalloproteinases and their inhibitors in matrix remodeling. *Trends Genet* 1990;6:121–125.
12. Crystal RG. The α1-antitrypsin gene and its deficiency states. *Trends Genetics* 1989;5:411–417.
13. Bieth JG. Elastases: catalytic and biologic properties. In: Mecham R, ed. *Regulation of matrix accumulation.* New York: Academic Press, 1986;217–320.
14. Gadek JE, Fells GA, Zimmerman RL, Rennard SI, Crystal RG. Antielastases of the human alveolar structures—implications for the protease–antiprotease theory of emphysema. *J Clin Invest* 1981;68:889–898.
15. Wewers MD, Casolaro MA, Crystal RG. Comparison of alpha-1-antitrypsin levels and antineutrophil elastase capacity of blood and lung in a patient with the alpha-1-antitrypsin phenotype null–null before and during alpha-1-antitrypsin augmentation therapy. *Am Rev Respir Dis* 1987;135:539–543.
16. Long GL, Chandra T, Woo SLC, Davie EW, Kurachi K. Complete sequence of the cDNA for human α1-antitrypsin and the gene for the S-variant. *Biochemistry* 1984;23:4828–4837.
17. Brantly M, Nukiwa T, Crystal RG. Molecular basis of alpha-1-antitrypsin deficiency. *Am J Med* 1988;84:13–31.
18. Hofker MH, Nelen M, Klasen EC, Nukiwa T, Curiel D, Crystal RG, Frants RR. Cloning and characterization of an α1-antitrypsin like gene 12 kb downstream of the genuine α1-antitrypsin gene. *Biochem Biophys Res Commun* 1988;155:634–642.
19. Crystal RG, Brantly ML, Hubbard RC, Curiel DT, States DJ, Holmes MD. The alpha 1-antitrypsin gene and its mutations. *Chest* 1989;95:196–208.
20. Carrell RW, Jeppsson J-O, Laurell C-B, et al. Structure and variation of human α1-antitrypsin. *Nature* 1982;298:329–334.
21. Perlino E, Cortese R, Ciliberto G. The human α₁-antitrypsin gene is transcribed from two different promoters in macrophages and hepatocytes. *EMBO J* 1987;6:2767–2771.
22. Kelsey GD, Povey S, Bygrave AE, Lovell-Badge RH. Species- and tissue-specific expression of human alpha 1-antitrypsin in transgenic mice. *Genes Dev* 1987;1:161–171.
23. Ruther U, Tripodi M, Cortese R, Wagner EF. The human alpha 1-antitrypsin gene is efficiently expressed from two tissue-specific promoters in transgenic mice. *Nucleic Acids Res* 1987; 15:7519–7529.
24. Carlson JA, Rogers BB, Sifers RN, Hawkins HK, Finegold MJ, Woo SLC. Multiple tissues express alpha 1-antitrypsin in transgenic mice and man. *J Clin Invest* 1988;82:26–36.
25. Crystal RG. α1-Antitrypsin deficiency, emphysema and liver disease: genetic basis and strategies for therapy. *J Clin Invest* 1990;85:1343–1352.
26. Trapnell BC, Nagaoka I, Chytil A, Crystal RG. Surface activation-induced upregulation of α1-antitrypsin gene expression in mononuclear phagocytes is associated with selective 5' noncoding exon usage. *Clin Res* 1989;37(2):482A.
27. Courtois G, Morgan JG, Campbell LA, Fourel G, Crabtree GR.

Interaction of a liver-specific nuclear factor with the fibrinogen and α1-antitrypsin promoters. *Science* 1987;240:688–692.

28. Li Y, Shen R-F, Tsai SY, Woo SLC. Multiple hepatic *trans-*acting factors are required for *in vitro* transcription of the human alpha 1-antitrypsin gene. *Mol Cell Biol* 1988;8:4362–4369.

29. Monaci P, Nicosia A, Cortese R. Two different liver-specific factors stimulate *in vitro* transcription from the human α1-antitrypsin promoter. *Embo J* 1988;7:2075–2078.

30. Hubbard RC, Crystal RG. Alpha-1-antitrypsin augmentation therapy for alpha-1-antitrypsin deficiency. *Am J Med* 1988;84:52–62.

31. Perlmutter DH, May LT, Sehgal PB. Interferon β2/interleukin 6 modulates synthesis of α1-antitrypsin in human mononuclear phagocytes and in human hepatoma cells. *J Clin Invest* 1989;84:144–148.

32. Mega T, Lujan E, Yoshida A. Studies on the oligosaccharide chains of human α1-protease inhibitor. II. Structure of oligosaccharides. *J Biol Chem* 1980;255:4057–4061.

33. Carrell RW, Jeppsson J-O, Vaughan L, Brennan SO, Owen MC, Boswell DR. Human α1-antitrypsin: carbohydrate attachment and sequence homology. *FEBS Lett* 1981;135:301–303.

34. Gadek JE, Crystal RG. α1-Antitrypsin deficiency. In: Stanbury JB, Wyngaarden JB, Frederickson DC, Goldstein JL, Brown MS, eds. *Metabolic basis of inherited disease.* New York: McGraw–Hill, 1982;1450–1467.

35. Cox DW, Johnson AM, Fagerhol MK. Report of nomenclature meeting for α1-antitrypsin: INSERM, Rouen Bois-Guillaume. *Hum Genet* 1980;53:429–433.

36. Loebermann H, Tokuoka R, Deisenhofer J, Huber R. Human α1-proteinase inhibitor: crystal structure analysis of two crystal modifications, molecular model and preliminary analysis of the implications for function. *J Mol Biol* 1984;177:531–556.

37. Banda MJ, Rice AG, Griffin GL, Senior RM. The inhibitory complex of human α1-proteinase inhibitor and human leukocyte elastase is a neutrophil chemoattractant. *J Exp Med* 1988;167:1608–1615.

38. Johnson D, Travis J. The oxidative inactivation of human α-1-proteinase inhibitor—further evidence for methionine at the reactive center. *J Biol Chem* 1979;254:4022–4026.

39. Carp H, Janoff A. Potential mediator of inflammation—phagocyte-derived oxidants suppress the elastase-inhibitory capacity of alpha1-proteinase inhibitor *in vitro. J Clin Invest* 1980;66:987–995.

40. Hubbard RC, Ogushi F, Fells GA, Cantin AM, Jallat S, Courtney M, Crystal RG. Oxidants spontaneously released by alveolar macrophages of cigarette smokers can inactivate the active site of α1-antitrypsin, rendering it ineffective as an inhibitor of neutrophil elastase. *J Clin Invest* 1987;80:1289–1295.

41. Courtney M, Buchwalder A, Tessier L-H, et al. High-level production of biologically active human α1-antitrypsin in *Escherichia coli. Proc Natl Acad Sci USA* 1984;81:669–673.

42. Rosenberg S, Barr PJ, Najarian RC, Hallewell RA. Synthesis in yeast of a functional oxidation-resistant mutant of human α1-antitrypsin. *Nature* 1984;312:77–80.

43. Travis J, Owen M, George P, Carrell R, Rosenberg S, Hallewell RA, Barr PJ. Isolation and properties of recombinant DNA produced variants of human α1-proteinase inhibitor. *J Biol Chem* 1985;260:4384–4389.

44. Jallat S, Carvallo D, Tessier LH, Roecklin D, Roitsch C, Ogushi F, Crystal RG, Courtney M. Altered specificities of genetically engineered α1 antitrypsin variants. *Protein Eng* 1986;1:29–35.

45. Carrell RW, Boswell DR. Serpins: the superfamily of plasma serine proteinase inhibitors. In: Barrett AJ, Salvesen G, eds. *Protease inhibitors.* New York: Elsevier, 1986;403–419.

46. Nukiwa T, Satoh K, Brantly ML, Ogushi F, Fells GA, Courtney M, Crystal RG. Identification of a second mutation in the protein-coding sequence of the Z type alpha 1-antitrypsin gene. *J Biol Chem* 1986;261:15989–15994.

47. Mooren H, Kramps JA, Franken C, Meijer C, Dijkman JA. Localisation of a low-molecular-weight bronchial protease inhibitor in the peripheral human lung. *Thorax* 1983;38:180–183.

48. Franken C, Meijer CJLM, Dijkman JH. Tissue distribution of antileukoprotease and lysozyme in humans. *J Histochem Cytochem* 1989;37:493–498.

49. Fryksmark U, Prellner T, Tegner H, Ohlsson K. Studies on the role of antileukoprotease in respiratory tract diseases. *Eur J Respir Dis* 1984;65:201–209.

50. Kramps JA, Franken C, Dijkman JH. ELISA for quantitative measurement of low-molecular-weight bronchial protease inhibitor in human sputum. *Am Rev Repir Dis* 1984;129:959–963.

51. Hutchison DCS. The role of proteases and antiproteases in bronchial secretions. *Eur J Respir Dis* 1987;71:78–85.

52. Kramps JA, Franken C, Dijkman JH. Quantity of anti-leucoprotease relative to α1-proteinase inhibitor in peripheral airspaces of the human lung. *Clin Sci* 1988;75:351–353.

53. Vogelmeier C, Hubbard R, Geiger R, Fritz H, Crystal RG. Secretory leukoprotease inhibitor levels in normal upper and lower respiratory tract epithelial lining fluid of normals. *Am Rev Respir Dis* 1990;141(4):A47.

54. Stetler G, Brewer MT, Thompson RC. Isolation and sequence of a human gene encoding a potent inhibitor of leukocyte proteases. *Nucleic Acids Res* 1986;14:7883–7896.

55. Ohlsson K, Rosengren M. In: Mittman C, ed. *Pulmonary emphysema and proteolysis.* Orlando, FL: Academic Press, 1987;307–322.

56. Heinzel R, Appelhans H, Gassen G, Seemuller U, Machleidt W, Fritz H, Steffens G. Molecular cloning and expression of cDNA for human antileukoprotease from cervix uterus. *Eur J Biochem* 1986;160:61–67.

57. Appelhans B, Ender B, Sachse G, Nikiforou T, Appelhans H, Ebert W. Secretion of antileukoprotease from a human lung tumor cell line. *FEBS Lett* 1987;224:14–18.

58. Grutter MG, Fendrich G, Huber R, Bode W. The 2.5 Å X-ray crystal structure of the acid-stable proteinase inhibitor from human mucous secretions analysed in its complex with bovine α-chymotrypsin. *EMBO J* 1988;7:345–351.

59. Fritz H. Human mucous proteinase inhibitor (human mpi). *Biol Chem Hoppe Seyler* 1988;369(Suppl):79–82.

60. Berman G, Afford SC, Burnett D, Stockley RA. α1-Antichymotrypsin in lung secretions is not an effective proteinase inhibitor. *J Biol Chem* 1986;261:14095–14099.

61. Chandra T, Stackhouse R, Kidd VJ, Robson KJH, Woo SLC. Sequence homology between human α1-antichymotrypsin, α1-antitrypsin, and antithrombin III. *Biochem* 1983;22:5055–5061.

62. Bao J-J, Sifers RN, Kidd VJ, Ledley FD, Woo SLC. Molecular evolution of serpins: homologous structure of the human α1-antichymotrypsin and α1-antitrypsin genes. *Biochemistry* 1987;26:7755–7759.

63. Rabin M, Watson M, Kidd V, Woo SLC, Breg WR, Ruddle FH. Regional location of α1-antichymotrypsin and α1-antitrypsin genes on human chromosome 14. *Somatic Cell Mol Genet* 1986;12:209–214.

64. Berman G, Burnett D, Woo SLC, Stockley RA. Production of alpha 1-antichymotrypsin by the J 111 cell line. *Biol Chem Hoppe Seyler* 1988;369:23–26.

65. Rubin H, Wang ZM, Nickbarg EB, et al. Cloning, expression, purification, and biological activity of recombinant native and variant human α1-antichymotrypsins. *J Biol Chem* 1990;265:1199–1207.

66. Welgus HG, Stricklin GP. Human skin fibroblast collagenase inhibitor—comparative studies in human connective tissues, serum, and amniotic fluid. *J Biol Chem* 1983;258:12259–12264.

67. Murphy G, Reynolds JJ, Werb Z. Biosynthesis of tissue inhibitor of metalloproteinases by human fibroblasts in culture—stimulation by 12-O-tetradecanoylphorbol 13-acetate and interleukin 1 in parallel with collagenase. *J Biol Chem* 1985;260:3079–3083.

68. Welgus HG, Campbell EJ, Bar-Shavit Z, Senior RM, Teitelbaum SL. Human alveolar macrophages produce a fibroblast-like collagenase and collagenase inhibitor. *J Clin Invest* 1985;76:219–224.

69. Albin RJ, Senior RM, Welgus HG, Connolly NL, Campbell EJ. Human alveolar macrophages secrete an inhibitor of metalloproteinase elastase. *Am Rev Respir Dis* 1987;135:1281–1285.

70. Goldberg GI, Marmer BL, Grant GA, Eisen AZ, Wilheim S, He C. Human 72-kilodalton type IV collagenase forms a complex with a tissue inhibitor of metalloproteases designated TIMP-2. *Proc Natl Acad Sci USA* 1989;86:8207–8211.

71. Carmichael DF, Sommer A, Thompson RC, Anderson DC,

Smith CG, Welgus HG, Stricklin GP. Primary structure and cDNA cloning of human fibroblast collagenase inhibitor. *Proc Natl Acad Sci USA* 1986;83:2407–2411.

72. Sottrup-Jensen L. α-Macroglobulins: structure, shape, and mechanism of proteinase complex formation. *J Biol Chem* 1989; 264:11539–11542.

73. Bell GI, Rall LB, Sanchez-Pescador R, Merryweather JP, Scott J, Eddy RL, Shows TB. Human α₂-macroglobulin gene is located on chromosome 12. *Somatic Cell Mol Genet* 1985;11:285–289.

74. Fukushima Y, Bell GI, Shows TB. The polymorphic human α₂-macroglobulin gene (A2M) is located in chromosome region 12p12.3-p13.3. *Cytogenet Cell Genet* 1988;48:58–59.

75. Kan C-C, Solomon E, Belt KT, Chain AC, Hiorns LR, Fey G. Nucleotide sequence of cDNA encoding human α₂-macroglobulin and assignment of the chromosomal locus. *Proc Natl Acad Sci USA* 1985;82:2282–2286.

76. Gehring MR, Shiels BR, Northemann W, de Bruijn MHL, Kan C-C, Chain AC, Noonan DJ, Fey GH. Sequence of rat liver α₂-macroglobulin and acute phase control of its messenger RNA. *J Biol Chem* 1987;262:446–454.

77. Sottrup-Jensen L, Lonblad PB, Jones CM, Stepanik TM. Primary structure of human α₂-macroglobulin. II. Primary structure of eight CNBr fragments located in the NH₂-terminal half of α₂-macroglobulin, accounting for 603 amino acid residues. *J Biol Chem* 1984;259:8304–8309.

78. Stepanik TM, Sottrup-Jensen L. Primary structure of human α₂-macroglobulin. III. Primary structure of three large disulfide-bridged CNBr fragments, located in the COOH-terminal part of α₂-macroglobulin and accounting for 301 residues. *J Biol Chem* 1984;259:8310–8312.

79. Sottrup-Jensen L, Stepanik TM, Kristensen T, et al. Primary structure of human α₂-macroglobulin. V. The complete structure. *J Biol Chem* 1984;259:8318–8327.

80. Jensen PEH, Sottrup-Jensen L. Primary structure of human α₂-macroglobulin. Complete disulfide bridge assignment and lo-calization of two interchain bridges in the dimeric proteinase binding unit. *J Biol Chem* 1986;261:15863–15869.

81. Feldman SR, Salvatore VP. A three-dimensional model of a unique proteinase inhibitor: α₂-macroglobulin. *Semin Thromb Hemost* 1986;12:223–225.

82. Hubbard RC, Casolaro MA, Mitchell M, Sellers SE, Arabia F, Matthay MA, Crystal RG. Fate of aerosolized recombinant DNA-produced α₁-antitrypsin: Use of the epithelial surface of the lower respiratory tract to administer proteins of therapeutic importance. *Proc Natl Acad Sci USA* 1989;86:680–684.

83. Reynolds HY, Fulmer JD, Kazmierowski JA, Roberts WC, Frank MM, Crystal RG. Analysis of cellular and protein content of broncho-alveolar lavage fluid from patients with idiopathic pulmonary fibrosis and chronic hypersensitivity pneumonitis. *J Clin Invest* 1977;59:165–175.

84. Bell DY, Haseman JA, Spock A, McLennan G, Hook GER. Plasma proteins of the bronchoalveolar surface of the lungs of smokers and nonsmokers. *Am Rev Respir Dis* 1981;124:72–79.

85. Warr GA, Martin RR, Sharp PM, Rossen RD. Normal human bronchial immunoglobulins and proteins—effects of cigarette smoking. *Am Rev Respir Dis* 1977;116:25–30.

86. Delacroix DL, Marchandise FX, Francis C, Sibille Y. Alpha-2-macroglobulin, monomeric and polymeric immunoglobulin A, and immunoglobulin M in bronchoalveolar lavage. *Am Rev Respir Dis* 1985;132:829–835.

87. Rennard SI, Ghafouri M, Thompson AB, et al. Fractional processing of sequential bronchoalveolar lavage to separate bronchial and alveolar samples. *Am Rev Respir Dis* 1990;141:208–217.

88. Hubbard RC, Crystal RG. Strategies for therapy of α₁-antitrypsin deficiency by the aerosol route. *Eur J Resp Dis* 1990;in press.

89. Ogushi F, Fells GA, Hubbard RC, Straus SD, Crystal RG. Z-type α₁-antitrypsin is less competent than M1-type α₁-antitrypsin as an inhibitor of neutrophil elastase. *J Clin Invest* 1987; 80:1366–1374.

THE LUNG: Scientific Foundations
edited by R.G. Crystal, J.B. West et al.
Raven Press, Ltd., New York © 1991.

CHAPTER 7.1.3

Consequences of Proteolytic Injury

Edgar C. Lucey, Phillip J. Stone, and Gordon L. Snider

Inflammatory reactions are highly complex, redundant processes. Cells of the inflammatory system, particularly neutrophils and mononuclear phagocytes, are capable of elaborating oxidants, cationic proteins, and proteases into the extracellular milieu, all of which have the potential to injure normal tissue. Normal tissues, rather than the invading microbe or the inhaled agent, may bear the brunt of the attack, and the injury of normal tissues may then result in persistence of the inflammatory response (1). This chapter will focus on the role of proteases in injuring lung parenchymal connective tissue and altering the phenotypic expression of bronchial epithelial cells. Although fibroblasts, eosinophils, mast cells, platelets, and bacteria are also potential sources of proteases in the lungs (see Chapter 7.1.1), the emphasis will be on proteases originating in neutrophils and macrophages.

NEUTROPHILS

The neutrophil enzymes with the most potential for tissue injury are (a) the neutral serine proteases, elastase and cathepsin G, which are stored in the azurophilic granules, and (b) two metalloproteases, collagenase and gelatinase, found in the specific granules and tertiary granules, respectively. These enzymes all have the potential for attacking key elements of the extracellular matrix of the lungs, namely, collagen, elastin, and proteoglycans. Neutrophil elastase is misnamed, since it is a protease which has broad specificity and which also has the potential for cleaving a variety of proteins and for attacking intact cells. It has recently

been reported that human neutrophil granules also contain another serine protease, designated proteinase 3 (2). Its ability to degrade elastin at pH 6.5 is slightly greater than that of human neutrophil elastase, but it is less active than neutrophil elastase at pH 7.4 or 8.9.

Specific granules contain receptors for the *Escherichia coli* chemoattractant, f-Met-Leu-Phe (3); these granules fuse with the plasma membrane as they approach the inflammatory site and can release their contents into the extracellular milieu. In contrast, azurophilic granules fuse with phagosomes and do not, in general, release their contents extracellularly (4,5), although there can be "leakage" of granule contents into the extracellular space, especially if the phagocytosed particle is large (6). In the event that elastase or cathepsin G does enter the extracellular milieu, as certainly happens after cell death, an elaborate defense exists to protect against tissue injury (see Chapter 7.1.2 for a discussion of the antiproteases screen of the lung).

A portion of the circulating neutrophils passing through the lungs adhere transiently to the capillary endothelium, forming the marginated pool of cells in the pulmonary vascular bed (see Chapter 3.4.8). Neutrophils are normally sparse in the alveolar space, but they can migrate from the capillaries into the alveolar space in great numbers in response to concentration gradients of chemotactic substances. Neutrophils can release their granule proteases while marginated in the capillary, while migrating through the thin or thick portion of the alveolar walls, or after gaining access to the alveolar space. Neutrophils can exclude α_1-antitrypsin from penetrating into zones of contact with opsonized surfaces (7), and stimulated adherent neutrophils can degrade surface-bound substrates *in vitro* even in the presence of high concentrations of protease inhibitors (8,9).

E. C. Lucey and G.L. Snider: Pulmonary Section, Boston D.V.A. Medical Center, Boston, Massachusetts 02130.

P. J. Stone: Department of Biochemistry, Boston University School of Medicine, Boston, Massachusetts 02118.

MACROPHAGES

Macrophages are resident in the lung, but their numbers increase greatly in many chronic lung diseases. They are concentrated in the centriacinar lung zones of smokers, and there has been much question as to the role they play in the degradation of matrix proteins, especially elastin, in the genesis of smoker's emphysema (10). Lysosomes within macrophages contain a variety of hydrolytic enzymes such as acid phosphatase and cathepsins. Macrophages secrete a group of metalloproteases, including collagenases, gelatinases, stromelysin, and an as yet poorly characterized metalloelastase (11). Macrophages may also be carriers of other proteases. Cultured macrophages demonstrate receptor-mediated ingestion of neutrophil elastase and can subsequently secrete a portion of the elastase in active form into the medium (12–14).

EFFECT OF PROTEASES ON EXPERIMENTAL ANIMALS

Information on the role of proteases as agents capable of injuring tissues has come from studies using purified and partially purified enzymes in experimental animal studies, in tissue culture systems, and in *in vitro* studies using natural or synthetic substrates. More direct evidence for the role of proteases in causation of human disease has come from studies of lung tissues and fluids in human diseases.

Exogenous Proteases

Papain and Pancreatic Elastase

The concept that proteases instilled into the lung could cause emphysema in experimental animals evolved from the serendipitous observation by Gross et al. (15) that intratracheal administration of papain to rats causes a condition resembling human emphysema.

Pathology

The inhalation of an aerosol or intratracheal instillation of papain or pancreatic elastase into hamsters or rats results (within a few hours) in hemorrhage, destruction of alveolar walls, and a mild inflammatory cell influx. The edema, hemorrhage, and inflammation disappear, and the alveolar enlargement with destruction that is characteristic of emphysema is fully evident (Fig. 1). Enzymes without elastolytic properties, such as pancreatic trypsin or bacterial collagenase, cause acute lung injury along with inflammatory cell infiltration,

but the lungs heal completely after the injury; emphysema is not induced (16).

Ultrastructural studies of lung tissue soon after the administration of pancreatic elastase to hamsters show some injury to a variety of cells (17,18), but most alveoli continue to be lined by an uninterrupted layer of epithelium (19,20). Pancreatic elastase passes into the interstitium via pinocytotic vesicles of type I cells. Degradation of elastic fibers begins within 15 min of the instillation of the elastase and progresses rapidly with evidence of rupture of alveolar walls and air-space enlargement (21). By 4 days, synthesis of new elastic fibers has begun, with the appearance of small clumps of microfibrils in close association with interstitial cells, fibroblasts, and smooth muscle cells. There is a limited amount of proliferation of alveolar type II cells. Small elastic fibers seen in the late stages of repair may indicate structural abnormalities in newly synthesized elastic fibers (19,20).

Despite preservation of alveolar type I cells, heparan sulfate proteoglycans are markedly decreased in the epithelial basal lamina 2 hr after pancreatic elastase treatment, as shown ultrastructurally with ruthenium red staining of anionic sites. Similar but less extensive changes are observed in the capillary basal lamina. Regeneration of the anionic sites is complete by 10 days (22).

Pancreatic elastase treatment of hamsters cause increased alveolar epithelial permeability for [^{14}C]sucrose and ^{125}I-bovine serum albumin by 3 hr after treatment, but this permeability is back to normal at 5 days (23). Widespread mitotic activity is also induced by pancreatic elastase treatment of hamster lungs; the peak labeling index is seen in nonciliated, nongranulated bronchial cells at 24 hr, in type II alveolar cells at 2 days, and in endothelial cells at 4 days (24).

Thirty days after pancreatic elastase treatment of hamsters, twice as many cells and a higher percentage of neutrophils are recovered in bronchoalveolar lavage fluid than in saline-treated control animals (25,26). At 24 hr, but not at 4 weeks, a heat-stable chemoattractant for neutrophils is found in the BAL supernatant.

Biochemistry

Twenty-four hours after treatment with pancreatic elastase, the total elastin content of hamster lungs is reduced to about one-third of normal. There is minimal reduction of lung collagen. A rapid burst of new connective tissue synthesis restores the lung content of both of these proteins to values slightly above normal within several weeks (27–32).

In vitro radiolabeling with [^{14}C]proline shows increased amounts of both collagen and elastin in the

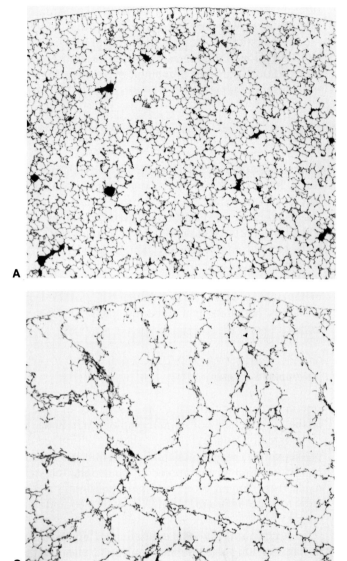

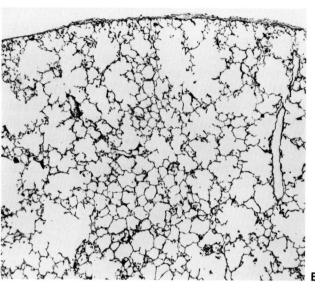

FIG. 1. Photomicrographs of hamster lungs, untreated (**A**) and 3 days after the intratracheal instillation of 300 μg of human neutrophil elastase (**B**) or of 300 μg of porcine pancreatic elastase (**C**). For each panel, the pleurae are at the top margin. The lungs were lavaged with saline prior to fixation to aid in the measurement of air-space size by removing blood cells. The mean linear intercept (MLI) of the untreated animal is 55 μm. The neutrophil elastase treatment caused distortion and mild enlargement of air spaces (MLI = 65 μm). The pancreatic elastase treatment produced severe distortion and enlargement of air spaces (MLI = 83 μm). Hematoxylin–eosin stain, magnification ×30.

lungs 14 and 20 days after instillation of papain to rats (33). There are increases in specific as well as total radioactivity of both proteins during the first 6 days, indicating that biosynthesis is occurring. Studies (34) have also shown parallel increases of lysyl oxidase activity and *in vivo* incorporation of [^{14}C]lysine into desmosine and isodesmosine, which peak about 1 week after elastase treatment. Incorporation of [^{14}C]proline into collagen hydroxyproline was elevated above control in pancreatic elastase-treated hamster lungs over the period of 21–360 days after treatment (35); total lung collagen levels rose by the same amount in both control and elastase-treated lungs over the 1-year period.

Thus, in addition to showing elastin damage and repair, these studies and the organ culture studies (35) discussed below confirm that alteration and the laying down of new collagen are a part of pancreatic elastase-induced emphysema. However, the proportion of total lung collagen turned over must be very small, since sensitive radiolabeling methods must be used to show it, and ultrastructural studies have not demonstrated its site.

The lungs of hamsters treated with pancreatic elastase 3–4 weeks previously contain more glycosaminoglycans than do lungs of saline-treated control animals (36). The increase is limited to the dermatan sulfate subtype. Incorporation of [^{14}C]glucosamine into glycosaminoglycans was greatest in hamster lung explants over the period of 1–5 days after treatment with pancreatic elastase, returning to normal by 21 days (35). The amount of heparan sulfate remains low in relation to the amounts of collagen and elastin in the explants from elastase-treated as compared with control lungs (35). Thus, it appears that lung injury from pancreatic elastase treatment results in an activation of metabolism of all connective tissue elements, but with a change in the balance of lung connective tissue components. These findings likely reflect an imperfection of the repair process as compared with normal fetal pulmonary organogenesis and postnatal growth.

Total lung lipids, triglycerides, total and esterified cholesterol, and total phospholipid of rats treated intratracheally with papain are increased, whereas diglycerides are decreased (37). In rabbits rendered emphysematous with pancreatic elastase, phospholipid content (and therefore total lung lipid content) is decreased. The decrease in phospholipid is due to decreased lecithin and lysolecithin fractions (38).

Degradation Products of Elastin

The degradation of elastin produces peptides that are found in the serum and excreted in the urine. Two amino acids, desmosine and isodesmosine, found in cross-links are unique to elastin. A 1978 study (39) established the basis for measurement of desmosines in the urine as an indicator of elastin degradation. Desmosine and isodesmosine were recoverable from the urine of hamsters after the intratracheal injection of pancreatic elastase; only trace quantities were detected in the feces. Dietary elastin does not confound the results, because radiolabeled desmosine given by gastric intubation fails to reveal radiolabeled desmosines in the urine (40). In contrast, desmosines injected intraperitoneally are recovered in the urine.

A sensitive radioimmunoassay has been used to monitor the excretion of desmosine in the urine after the treatment of male sheep with pancreatic elastase (41). Most of the elevation in urinary desmosine excretion occurred in the first 48 hr after elastase administration. The increase in desmosine excretion was positively correlated with the dose of the enzyme and with the anatomic and physiologic estimates of severity of emphysema.

A study using a hemagglutination–inhibition assay showed that immunoreactive elastin-derived peptides could be detected in serum of dogs for a period of 12 days after the administration of a single 25- or 50-mg dose of pancreatic elastase and for at least 40 days after a 100-mg dose (42). This latter finding likely reflects a combination of proteolytic destruction of elastin and its repair.

Effects on Respiratory Function

The functional abnormalities of animals with experimental emphysema are similar to those seen with the human disease (16). Briefly, the lungs show increased compliance, functional residual capacity, residual volume, and total lung capacity. There is airflow limita-

tion and decreased diffusing capacity. The breathing pattern is slower and deeper than normal. Arterial blood gas studies show hypoxemia usually without CO_2 retention. Pulmonary hypertension and cor pulmonale, only partially prevented by oxygen therapy, have been documented.

Effects on Nonrespiratory Functions of the Lung

There is evidence that angiotensin conversion is reduced in papain-treated dogs, due to the hypoxia (43). There was no effect on 5-hydroxytryptamine uptake by pancreatic elastase-treated hamster lungs (44). Thirty days after pancreatic elastase treatment, hamsters cleared endotracheally administered inocula of *Staphylococcus aureus* in saline as rapidly as did control hamsters (45). But after infection with *S. aureus* in mucus (as a virulence enhancing factor), emphysematous hamsters had impaired clearance and decreased survival.

Neutrophil Enzymes

The neutrophil is thought to be the source of elastase in the pathogenesis of human emphysema. First, homogenates of leukocytes were shown to produce emphysema in experimental animals (46–48). Soon after, highly purified preparations of neutrophil elastase, made from human blood and purulent sputum, were shown to produce emphysema in dogs (49) and hamsters (50,51).

Destruction of alveolar epithelium is much greater in hamster lung after human neutrophil elastase than after pancreatic elastase administration (19), but the severity of the emphysema is less than that produced by pancreatic elastase. Like pancreatic elastase and papain, human neutrophil elastase treatment causes decreased elastin content (50), increased air-space size (Fig. 1), and increased lung volumes (49–51). The emphysema persists indefinitely but without progression (52). Increasing the dose of neutrophil elastase in order to produce more severe emphysema results in death of the animals from pulmonary hemorrhage (50,51).

It is not fully known why the emphysema induced by human neutrophil elastase is less severe than that induced by pancreatic elastase. Increased bleeding into the lung resulting in inactivation of human neutrophil elastase by α_1-antitrypsin has been suggested (50). However, the half-life in the lung of instilled enzymatically active human neutrophil elastase is similar to that of pancreatic elastase (53). Various elastases have well-described differences in substrate preference (49,54). Such differences, along with differing accessibility of the enzymes to elastic fibers in the alveolar walls, could cause the differing severity of induced emphysema.

Using two purification schemes and testing every fraction for its emphysema-inducing potency, one group found that only the elastase-containing fractions of dog neutrophil granule homogenates were capable of inducing experimental emphysema (55). A study with human neutrophils found two separate fractions with emphysema-inducing properties. One contained the well-characterized human neutrophil elastase; the other, containing proteinase 3, induced more severe emphysema in hamsters than did human neutrophil elastase (2).

Human neutrophil cathepsin G, an enzyme as plentiful in the neutrophil as elastase but with only weak elastolytic activity, does not cause emphysema when given intratracheally to hamsters and does not potentiate the emphysema induced in hamsters by human neutrophil elastase (56).

Macrophage Enzymes

Macrophages are the predominant cell in the respiratory bronchiolitis of smokers, and there has been much interest in this cell as a source of neutrophil chemotactic factor and as a possible source of elastase for the production of emphysema. It has not been considered as seriously as neutrophil elastase because the macrophage elastase is not stored in the cell but rather is produced constitutively. Even so, mild emphysema was produced in dogs by treating them with aerosolized homogenates of alveolar macrophages (46). Although there has been extensive *in vitro* study of the possible role of the macrophage in tissue injury, there are no definitive studies in animal models with this cell or its products.

Nonelastolytic Proteases

As already noted, instillation of nonelastolytic enzymes into the lungs results in acute lung injury, but after the acute injury has resolved there is no emphysema.

A small but significant increase in total lung capacity is seen in hamsters treated with bacterial collagenase (57,58), an enzyme specific for collagen but different from all human collagenases. This is of interest, however, because the lung is relatively deficient in anti-collagenase activity (59).

The administration of trypsin or chymotrypsin to hamsters 24 hr after pancreatic elastase treatment produces more severe emphysema than does elastase alone (60). Elastin degradation after 1 week was similar in all groups, but elastin resynthesis was impaired in the elastase–trypsin and elastase–chymotrypsin

groups. The effect might be due to destruction of the microfibrillar components of the elastic fiber by the trypsin and chymotrypsin, thus removing the template requisite for resynthesis of pulmonary elastic fibers (see Chapter 3.3.3). These observations raise the possibility of cooperative effects between elastolytic and nonelastolytic enzymes in the pathogenesis of emphysema.

Effects on the Airway Epithelium

Secretory cell metaplasia (SCM) is defined as the development of secretory granules in nongranulated secretory epithelial cells, accompanied by an increase in the number of granules in granulated secretory cells. SCM is induced in the hamster by a single intratracheal instillation of a serine protease, which must be enzymatically active but which need not have elastolytic activity (61). The lesion is also induced by hydrogen ions (62).

Secretory granule discharge occurs within 2 hr of neutrophil elastase instillation, followed by (a) restoration of granule density to normal by day 3, (b) development of SCM by day 8, and (c) progression of the lesion to day 21 (63,64) (Fig. 2). The phenotypic expression of the cell is permanently changed, since the lesion persists indefinitely (52). Enzyme-induced SCM is prevented by prior treatment with antiproteases such as α_1-antitrypsin (65) or recombinant secretory leukocyte protease inhibitor (66), but not by administration of the anti-inflammatory agent flurbiprofen. This observation raises the possibility that the *in vivo* function of secretory leukocyte protease inhibitor, which is secreted by human bronchial glands and airways secretory cells, is to protect the epithelium from inflammatory cell and bacterial proteases. SCM is not induced in trachea or bronchioles (67), suggesting that airway regional differences in the susceptibility to induction of SCM should shed light on the pathogenesis of SCM. Enzyme-induced secretory granule discharge is not sufficient to cause SCM, since granule discharge does occur in the trachea, followed by restoration to normal granule density (67).

Neutrophil elastase treatment causes changes in lectin-binding sites on the luminal surface of Clara cells (68), which may be related to the signal that induces SCM.

Human neutrophil elastase as well as bacterial elastases has been shown to impair mucociliary clearance (69–71). The effect on ciliated cells as well as the effect on secretory cells may be caused by enzymatic cleavage of the attachments of the cells to the basement membrane and neighboring cells. In this regard, it is known that some proteases can initiate cell division and permit cells to escape from contact inhibition in

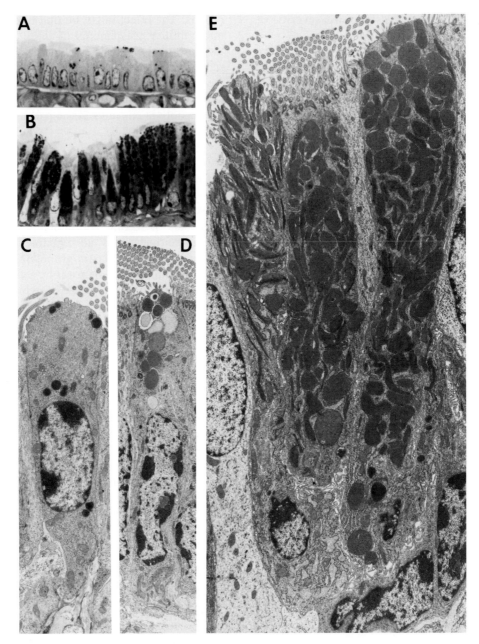

FIG. 2. Effect of neutrophil elastase on the airways of the hamster. Shown are photomicrographs and electron micrographs of plastic-embedded sections from the main left intrapulmonary bronchi of hamsters. **A, C,** and **D:** Hamster treated intratracheally with normal saline solution. Panels **B** and **E:** Hamster treated 16 days previously with 350 μg of human neutrophil elastase. In the photomicrograph of the saline-treated control animal (**A**), only a few secretory cells with dark granules are seen; secretory cells with no visible granules are also present. In the elastase-treated animal (**B**), most secretory cells are stuffed with large numbers of granules, with a resultant increase in the height of the bronchial epithelium (toluidine blue stain). Transmission electron micrographs of a Clara cell (**C**) and a mucus cell (note heterogeneity of granules) (**D**) from a saline-treated control hamster are shown for comparison with three secretory cells from an elastase-treated hamster (**E**). Note the large, dense, sometimes elongated granules that fill the apical cytoplasm and greatly enlarge the cells of the elastase-treated animal. (From ref. 135.)

cell culture, and that in higher concentrations these proteases can lift and separate epithelial cells off their basement membrane.

Eliciting Neutrophils to the Lungs

Intravenous administration of endotoxin causes intravascular pulmonary leukocyte sequestration. Mild emphysema arose after 10 weekly intravenous injections of endotoxin in rhesus monkeys (72) or after 50 intravenous injections over 17 weeks in dogs (73). Combining D-galactosamine treatment of rats (which decreases α_1-antitrypsin levels) with repeated injections of endotoxin resulted in emphysema after 10 weeks (74); treatment with endotoxin alone produced milder changes. In these experiments, it is postulated that the emphysema is induced by release of enzymes from sequestered leukocytes.

Other Models of Proteolytic Injury

A number of laboratories have observed air-space enlargement with exposure of rats (75–77), hamsters (78–80), mice (81), rabbits (82), and dogs (83) to NO_2. Hamsters exposed to 30 ppm NO_2 showed decreased lung elastin and collagen content 4 and 10 days (respectively) after starting exposure. The collagen content returned to control levels by day 14 of exposure. Total elastin did not return to control levels until after NO_2 exposure stopped (84). During exposure, neutrophils accumulated rapidly in the lungs, and there was evidence suggesting that the neutrophils released elastase during their migration through the lung interstitium (76).

Exposure of rats to hyperoxia can lead to air-space enlargement (85). There is evidence of collagen degradation (86). Exposure of lung tissue slices to hyperoxia with and without added protease inhibitors suggests that collagen degradation is mediated by proteases (87). In neonatal guinea pigs exposed to hyperoxia (88) there was increased elastolytic activity in the lung epithelial lining fluid recovered by lavage.

EFFECTS OF PROTEASES ON TISSUE AND ORGAN CULTURE

Connective Tissue Matrix

Human macrophages do not elaborate a measurable amount of metalloelastase into culture medium, but they are capable of degrading elastin when cultured on elastin-rich [^{3}H]lysine-labeled extracellular matrices deposited by rat smooth muscle cells (89) or when cultured in direct contact with radiolabeled elastin (11).

The elastin degradation was inhibited by the tissue inhibitor of metalloproteases, but it was inhibited minimally or not at all by inhibitors of cysteine proteases or by the serine protease inhibitor, eglin-c. Cooperative interaction was shown between a neutral protease (plasminogen activator) and an elastolytic acid protease (thought to be cathepsin L) (89). The plasminogen activator may enhance elastin degradation by removing glycoproteins covering the elastic fibers.

Purification of collagen and elastin removes the proteoglycan ground substance in which these protein fibers reside in the native state; the microfibrillar component of the elastic fiber is also removed during preparation of purified elastin. Removal of the proteoglycans by plasmin or trypsin treatment of rat heart muscle cell cultures enhanced susceptibility of elastin in the system to degradation by mouse macrophage metalloelastase (90). The elastin component of neonatal rat aorta smooth muscle cell cultures is 10-fold less susceptible to solubilization by human neutrophil elastase than is the corresponding purified elastin substrate (91).

Neutrophil elastase is capable of degrading the core protein of proteoglycans in an elastin-rich culture system (92). Neutrophil cathepsin G and the neutrophil myeloperoxidase–halide–oxidant system play minor roles in degrading proteoglycans. Degradation of proteoglycans in the alveolar basement membrane may affect solute exchange (92).

In a study of protease-damaged elastin in neonatal rat aortic smooth muscle cell cultures, repair was operationally defined as restoration of resistance to elastin solubilization by hot alkali (93). Immediately after pancreatic elastase treatment, only 6% (relative to control) of the elastin was resistant to hot alkali. Four weeks later, resistance to hot alkali had increased by 90%. Repair was found to require relatively little new tropoelastin incorporation into the cell layer, suggesting a salvage repair mechanism. Frayed elastic fibers which were seen immediately after treatment were replaced or remodeled within 2 weeks by continuous bands of elastin that resembled those in control cultures.

Airway Epithelium

In a primary culture of hamster tracheal epithelial cells (94), as well as in tracheal explants (95,96), it was found that neutrophil elastase, acting as a protease, released mucins bound to the secretory cell apical surface. Much of the released mucin was also degraded by the elastase. Studies of cultured bovine airway glandular serous cells (97) showed that both neutrophil elastase and cathepsin G stimulate secretion of chondroitin sulfate proteoglycan and also degrade the proteoglycan.

EVIDENCE OF PROTEASE INVOLVEMENT IN HUMAN PATHOLOGY

Investigators have sought evidence for direct involvement of proteases in human pathology in several ways. They have (a) measured protease activity in circulating neutrophils or alveolar macrophages, (b) used immunologic methods to measure small amounts of protease bound to antiproteases in blood, (c) measured protease activity in epithelial lining fluid recovered by lavage, (d) measured degradation products of collagen and elastin in blood and urine, and (e) used immunohistologic methods to demonstrate the presence of proteases in lung tissue in relation to their substrates. The last-mentioned method is the only one that provides direct evidence of the presence of extracellular proteases in the lung tissue. The other methods are all indirect, and there is no way of knowing how well they reflect the microenvironments of the lungs. Attempts have been made to give relevance to these studies by relating these measurements to an index of disease severity, such as lung function measurements or comparing a diseased population with a suitable control population.

Emphysema

Laurell and Ericksson (98) first noticed an association between a deficiency in the plasma protein, α_1-antitrypsin, and the occurrence of early onset emphysema. There has been little question that the emphysema is caused by insufficient protease inhibitor to balance the effects of elastase(s) (see Chapter 7.9.1 for details).

Some investigators have reported an association between blood leukocyte elastase concentration and airflow obstruction, in homozygous or heterozygous α_1-antitrypsin deficiency (99–102), whereas others have not (103,104); the same controversy surrounds persons with normal serum levels of α_1-antitrypsin, with some reports supporting the concept (103,104) and others not (105).

Minute amounts of pancreatic elastase have been demonstrated in normal human serum, in the preactivated proelastase form or bound to α_2-macroglobulin. It has been suggested that these complexes might be taken up by monocytes before they migrate into the lungs, where free elastase could then be released (106). Elevated levels of several pancreatic enzymes in the circulation of cigarette smokers have also been reported (107). But the blood seems unlikely as a portal of entry of proteases into the lungs, since a large amount of pancreatic elastase administered to hamsters intravenously does not produce emphysema (108). Furthermore, although serum immunoreactive leukocyte elastase concentration in chronic obstruc-

tive bronchitis was found to be double that in age-matched controls, patients with other active lung diseases have similarly increased leukocyte elastase concentrations in serum (109). Elastase-like esterase activity in lavage fluid has been reported to be lower in smokers than in nonsmokers (110,111). Much of this activity appears to be due to a metalloprotease (111).

Investigators have not found elevated levels of desmosine in the urine of smokers with chronic obstructive pulmonary disease (COPD) when compared with those of normal smokers or nonsmokers (112,113). Urinary desmosines were similar in normals, in individuals with the Z homozygous form of α_1-antitrypsin deficiency with emphysema, and in subjects with interstitial lung diseases; furthermore, this marker was not elevated in children with α_1-antitrypsin deficiency (114). Studies with an enzyme-linked immunoassay for elastin fragments (115) have shown that patients with COPD have elevated plasma elastin peptide levels compared with levels in normal nonsmokers; normal smokers had intermediate values, but the three groups overlapped.

Controversy surrounds a report that provides direct evidence of the protease–antiprotease hypothesis of emphysema in smokers. One group (116) has shown immuno-ultrastructurally that neutrophil elastase is bound to elastic fibers in the lungs of smokers and that the amount of elastase is proportional to the amount of emphysema that is present. Another group reports inability to reproduce these findings (117).

In summary, pathologic studies (118) unequivocally show that elastic fiber fraying and rupture occur in human emphysema. There is powerful indirect evidence from *in vitro* and experimental studies that elastases of neutrophil origin play a role. To a far lesser extent, macrophage elastases have been implicated. However, there is no clear, direct evidence of the precise mechanism by which the elastic fibers are damaged in emphysema.

Adult Respiratory Distress Syndrome

The adult respiratory distress syndrome (ARDS) is an acute interstitial pulmonary disease of diverse etiology. Although there is powerful evidence that neutrophils contribute importantly to the injury of the lungs in this condition, the place of proteolytic injury is not clear (119). Elevated elastolytic activity was found in association with reduced levels of functional α_1-antitrypsin in lavage fluid of about half the patients with ARDS (120,121). In other studies (122,123), although elastase was detected immunologically, elastolytic activity was not detected in lavage fluid; neutrophil collagenase and myeloperoxidase were readily detected (123,124). Macrophages in the lavage fluid of ARDS patients elaborate a peptide that releases neutrophil enzymes (125).

Bronchiectasis and Cystic Fibrosis

In infected bronchiectasis and cystic fibrosis, the airways are the site of severe suppuration with large numbers of neutrophils. In cystic fibrosis the predominant organisms are, most frequently, *Pseudomonas aeruginosa* and *Pseudomonas cepacia,* organisms which can elaborate elastase and other proteases. Destructive changes in the airways, and to a much lesser extent in the lung parenchyma, are features of both disorders. Elastolytic activity has been demonstrated in the secretions of patients with both cystic fibrosis and bronchiectasis (126–130). Elastase levels are higher in purulent than in mucoid sputum (127), and in both disorders there is more impairment of lung function with higher elastase levels (128). Neutrophils recovered in lavage fluid of cystic fibrosis patients have marked down-regulation of CR1, the C3b receptor; they also have decreased ability to kill *P. aeruginosa.* This down-regulation appears to be due to exposure to neutrophil elastase activity (131).

Interstitial Fibrosis

An increased number of cells, often with an increased proportion of neutrophils, are found in lavage fluid of persons with idiopathic pulmonary fibrosis (IPF) and other forms of interstitial fibrosis. In these disorders, active neutrophil collagenase and myeloperoxidase are elevated as is immunologically determined elastase; although elastase activity is not usually detected (132,133). While these enzymes may contribute to lung injury, the exact significance of finding these enzymes in lavage fluid is not clear.

The neutrophil products, collagenase and myeloperoxidase, have also been found in lavage fluid of adult patients with bronchiolitis (134). Elastase has also been demonstrated in the lavage fluid of patients with pneumonia (121), a condition usually followed by complete healing of the lungs.

CONCLUSION

Depending on the circumstances and location, large amounts of proteases are present in the cells and fluids of the body. Antiproteases of diverse nature are also present to control the many and critically important functions of these agents. There is little doubt that proteases confer important survival value in pulmonary disease states. For example, neutrophils and their proteases play a key role in exteriorizing noxious micro-

organisms by contributing to lung abscess formation with tissue liquefaction and external drainage of the resultant purulent material. Proteases also contribute to solubilizing inflammatory products that have served their purpose and that need to be cleared from the lungs. The enzymes may also serve to remove inappropriately laid-down matrix proteins during the process of lung repair. However, there are many lung diseases where the body's proteases may contribute to further injury of lung tissue as well as serving a useful purpose.

Evidence of a role for proteases in the pathogenesis of human lung diseases is most powerful for emphysema. However, except in severe α_1-antitrypsin deficiency, the evidence is, for the most part, indirect; also, the precise mechanism by which protease–antiprotease imbalance gives rise to emphysema is unknown. Although proteases have been demonstrated in secretions and lavage fluid of interstitial fibrosis, their pathogenetic role remains uncertain. There is good evidence that proteases play an important role in airway epithelial secretory cell metaplasia, which is a feature of many chronic lung diseases. There is also good evidence that proteases result in bronchial wall injury in infected bronchiectasis and cystic fibrosis. However, it is unclear why the enormous increase in elastase burden of the lungs in these two diseases does not give rise to overt emphysema.

REFERENCES

1. Henson PM, Johnston RB. Tissue injury in inflammation: oxidants, proteinases, and cationic proteins. *J Clin Invest* 1987;79:669–674.
2. Kao RC, Wehner NG, Skubitz KM, Gray BH, Hoidal JR. Proteinase 3: a distinct human polymorphonuclear leukocyte proteinase that produces emphysema in hamsters. *J Clin Invest* 1988;82:1963–1973.
3. Fletcher MP, Gallin JI. Human neutrophils contain an intracellular pool of putative receptors for the chemoattractant *N*-formyl-methionyl-leucyl-phenylalanine. *Blood* 1983;62:792–799.
4. Malech HL, Gallin JI. Neutrophils in human diseases. *N Engl J Med* 1987;317:687–694.
5. Gallin JI. Neutrophil specific granules in health and disease. *Clin Res* 1984;32:320–328.
6. Weissman G, Zurier RB, Spieler PJ, Goldstein IM. Mechanisms of lysosomal enzyme release from leukocytes exposed to immune complexes and other particles. *J Exp Med* 1971;134:149s–165s.
7. Campbell EJ, Campbell MA. Pericellular proteolysis by neutrophils in the presence of proteinase inhibitors: effects of substrate opsonization. *J Cell Biol* 1988;106:667–676.
8. Campbell EJ, Senior RM, McDonald JA, Cox DL. Proteolysis by neutrophils: relative importance of cell-substrate contact and oxidative inactivation of proteinase inhibitors *in vitro. J Lab Invest* 1982;70:845–852.
9. Weiss SJ, Regiani S. Neutrophils degrade subendothelial matrices in the presence of alpha-1-proteinase inhibitor: cooperative use of lysosomal proteinases and oxygen metabolites. *J Clin Invest* 1984;73:1297–1303.
10. Janoff A. Elastase and emphysema. Current assessment of the

protease-antiprotease hypothesis. *Am Rev Respir Dis* 1985;132:417–433.

11. Senior RM, Connolly NL, Cury JD, Welgus HG, Campbell EJ. Elastin degradation by human alveolar macrophages: a prominent role of metalloproteinase activity. *Am Rev Respir Dis* 1989;139:1251–1256.

12. Campbell EJ. Human leukocyte elastase, cathepsin G, and lactoferrin: family of neutrophil granule glycoproteins that bind to an alveolar macrophage receptor. *Proc Natl Acad Sci USA* 1982;79:6941–6945.

13. McGowan SE, Arbeit RD, Stone PJ, Snider GL. A comparison of the binding and fate of internalized neutrophil elastase in human monocytes and alveolar macrophages. *Am Rev Respir Dis* 1983;128:688–694.

14. White R, Janoff A, Gordon R, Campbell E. Evidence for *in vivo* internalization of human leukocyte elastase by alveolar macrophages. *Am Rev Respir Dis* 1982;125:779–781.

15. Gross P, Babyak MA, Tolker E, Kaschak M. Enzymatically produced pulmonary emphysema: a preliminary report. *J Occup Med* 1964;6:481–484.

16. Snider GL, Lucey EC, Stone PJ. Animal models of emphysema. *Am Rev Respir Dis* 1986;133:149–169.

17. Kuhn C, Tavassoli F. The scanning election microscopy of elastase-induced emphysema: a comparison with emphysema in man. *Lab Invest* 1976;34:2–9.

18. Yu SY, Sun CN, Still MF. Ultrastructural changes of elastic tissue in hamster lung during elastase-emphysema. *Adv Exp Med Biol* 1977;79:39–56.

19. Kuhn C, Slodkowska J, Smith T, Starcher B. The tissue response to exogenous elastase. *Bull Eur Physiopathol Respir* 1980;16(Suppl):127–139.

20. Morris SM, Stone PJ, Snider GL, Albright JT, Franzblau C. Ultrastructural changes in hamster lung four hours to twenty-four days after exposure to elastase. *Anat Rec* 1981;201:523–535.

21. Morris SM, Kagan HM, Stone PJ, Snider GL, Albright JT. Ultrastructural changes in hamster lung 15 minutes to 3 hours after exposure to elastase. *Anat Rec* 1986;215:134–143.

22. Vaccaro CA, Wu Z, Hinds A, Snider GL. Altered basement membrane proteoglycans in pancreatic elastase-induced emphysema. *Am Rev Respir Dis* 1985;131:A387.

23. Schmid RP, Wangensteen D, Hoidal J, Gosnell B, Niewoehner D. Effects of elastase and cigarette smoke on alveolar epithelial permeability. *J Appl Physiol* 1985;59:96–100.

24. Weinberg KS, Hayes JA. Elastase-induced emphysema: asynchronous bronchial, alveolar and endothelial cell proliferation during the acute response to injury. *J Pathol* 1982;136:253–264.

25. Vered M, Dearing R, Janoff A. A new elastase inhibitor from *Streptococcus pneumoniae* protects against acute lung injury induced by neutrophil granules. *Am Rev Respir Dis* 1985;131:131–133.

26. Verghese A, Franzus B, Stout R. Characterization of bronchoalveolar lavage cells and macrophage-derived chemoattractant activity in pancreatic elastase-induced emphysema in hamsters. *Exp Lung Res* 1988;14:797–810.

27. Karlinsky JB, Snider GL. Animal models of emphysema. *Am Rev Respir Dis* 1978;117:1109–1113.

28. Yu SY, Keller NR, Yoshida A. Biosynthesis of insoluble elastin in hamster lungs during elastase-emphysema. *Pro Soc Exp Biol Med* 1978;157:369–373.

29. Yu SY, Keller NR. Synthesis of lung collagen in hamsters with elastase-induced emphysema. *Exp Mol Pathol* 1978;29:37–43.

30. Fonzi L, Lungarella G. Correlation between biochemical and morphological repair in rabbit lungs after elastase injury. *Lung* 1980;158:165–171.

31. Valentine R, Rucker RB, Chrisp CE, Fisher GL. Morphological and biochemical features of elastase-induced emphysema in strain A/J mice. *Toxicol Appl Pharmacol* 1983;68:451–461.

32. Osman M, Keller S, Cerreta JM, Leuenberger P, Mandl I, Turino GM. Effect of papain-induced emphysema on canine pulmonary elastin. *Proc Soc Exp Biol Med* 1980;164:471–477.

33. Kobrle V, Hurych J, Holusa R. Changes in pulmonary connective tissue after a single intratracheal instillation of papain in the rat. *Am Rev Respir Dis* 1982;125:239–243.

34. Osman M, Kaldany RR, Cantor JO, Turino GM, Mandl I. Stimulation of lung lysyl oxidase activity in hamsters with elastase-induced emphysema. *Am Rev Respir Dis* 1985;131:169–170.

35. Karlinsky JB, Fredette J, Davidovits G, Catanese A, Snider R, Faris B, Snider GL, Franzblau C. The balance of lung connective tissue elements in elastase-induced emphysema. *J Lab Clin Med* 1983;102:151–162.

36. Karlinsky JB. Glycosaminoglycans in emphysema and fibrotic hamster lungs. *Am Rev Respir Dis* 1982;125:85–88.

37. Singh WG, Charles AK, Venkitasubramanian TA. Lung lipids in experimental emphysema. *Indian Biochem Biophys* 1980;17:61–66.

38. Rosario E, Gonzalez-Santos P. Rabbit lung lipids in experimental fibrosis and emphysema: lipolytic activity and content and distribution of lipids. *Eur J Clin Invest* 1983;13:237–242.

39. Goldstein RA, Starcher BC. Urinary excretion of elastin peptides containing desmosine after intratracheal injection of elastase in hamsters. *J Clin Invest* 1978;61:1286–1290.

40. Starcher BC, Goldstein RA. Studies on the absorption of desmosine and isodesmosine. *J Lab Clin Med* 1979;94:848–852.

41. Janoff A, Chanana AD, Joel DD, Susskind H, Laurent P, Yu SY, Dearing R. Evaluation of the urinary desmosine radioimmunoassay as a monitor of lung injury after endobronchial elastase instillation in sheep. *Am Rev Respir Dis* 1983;128:545–551.

42. Kucich U, Christner P, Weinbaum G, Rosenbloom J. Immunologic identification of elastin-derived peptides in the serums of dogs with experimental emphysema. *Am Rev Respir Dis* 1980;122:461–465.

43. Stalcup SA, Leuenberger PJ, Lipset JS, Osman MM, Cerreta JM, Mellin RB, Turino GM. Impaired angiotension conversion and bradykinin clearance in experimental canine pulmonary emphysema. *J Clin Invest* 1981;67:201–209.

44. Ryerson G, Block ER, Harris JO, Cannon JK. 5-hydroxytryptamine uptake by lungs of hamsters with pulmonary emphysema. *Exp Lung Res* 1981;2:241–248.

45. Verghese A, Catanese A, Arbeit RD. *Staphylococcus aureus* pneumonia in hamsters with elastase-induced emphysema—the virulence enhancing activity of mucin. *Proc Soc Exp Biol Med* 1988;188:1–6.

46. Mass B, Ikeda T, Meranze DR, Weinbaum G, Kimbel P. Induction of experimental emphysema. Cellular and species specificity. *Am Rev Respir Dis* 1972;106:384–391.

47. Fonzi L, Lungarella G. Elastolytic activity in rabbit leukocyte extracts. Effects of the whole leukocyte homogenate on the rabbit lung. *Exp Molec Pathol* 1979;31:486–491.

48. Tarjan E, Tolnay P, Appel J, Peto L, Dienes Z. Experimental pulmonary emphysema: its induction in rats by leuko-elastase extracted from purulent sputum. *Acta Med Acad Sci Hung* 1980;37:217–223.

49. Janoff A, Sloan B, Weinbaum G, Damiano V, Sandhaus RA, Elias J, Kimbel P. Experimental emphysema induced with purified human neutrophil elastase: tissue localization of the instilled protease. *Am Rev Respir Dis* 1977;115:461–478.

50. Senior RM, Tegner H, Kuhn C, Ohlsson K, Starcher BC, Pierce JA. The induction of pulmonary emphysema with human leukocyte elastase. *Am Rev Respir Dis* 1977;116:469–475.

51. Snider GL, Lucey EC, Christensen TG, Stone PJ, Calore JD, Catanese A, Franzblau C. Emphysema and bronchial secretory cell metaplasia induced in hamsters by human neutrophil products. *Am Rev Respir Dis* 1984;129:155–160.

52. Lucey EC, Stone PJ, Christensen TG, Breuer R, Snider GL. An 18-month study of the effects on hamster lungs of intratracheally administered human neutrophil elastase. *Exp Lung Res* 1988;14:671–686.

53. Stone PJ, Lucey EC, Calore JD, McMahon MP, Snider GL, Franzblau C. Defenses of the hamster lung against human neutrophil and porcine pancreatic elastase. *Respiration* 1988;54:1–15.

54. Senior RM, Bielefeld DR, Starcher BC. Comparison of the elastolytic effects of human leukocyte elastase and porcine pancreatic elastase. *Biochem Biophys Res Commun* 1976;72:1327–1334.

55. Sloan B, Abrams WR, Meranze DR, Kimbel P, Weinbaum G.

Emphysema induced *in vitro* and *in vivo* in dogs by a purified elastase from homologous leukocytes. *Am Rev Respir Dis* 1981;124:295–301.

56. Lucey EC, Stone PJ, Breuer R, Christensen TG, Calore JD, Catanese A, Franzblau C, Snider GL. Effect of combined human neutrophil cathepsin G and elastase on induction of secretory cell metaplasia and emphysema in hamsters, with *in vitro* observations on elastolysis by these emzymes. *Am Rev Respir Dis* 1985;132:362–366.

57. Snider GL, Sherter CB, Koo KW, Karlinsky JB, Hayes JA, Franzblau C. Respiratory mechanics in hamsters following treatment with endotracheal elastase or collagenase. *J Appl Physiol* 1977;42:206–215.

58. Karlinsky JB, Snider GL, Franzblau C, Stone PJ, Hoppin FG. *In vitro* effects of elastase and collagenase on mechanical properties of hamster lungs. *Am Rev Respir Dis* 1976;113:769–777.

59. Gadek JE, Fells GE, Zimmerman RL, Crystal RG. The normal lower respiratory tract is relatively deficient in anti-collagenase activity. *Am Rev Respir Dis* 1981;123:224.

60. Osman M, Keller S, Hosannah Y, Cantor JO, Turino GM, Mandl I. Impairment of elastin resynthesis in the lungs of hamsters with experimental emphysema induced by sequential administration of elastase and trypsin. *J Lab Clin Med* 1985;105:254–258.

61. Breuer R, Lucey EC, Stone PJ, Christensen TG, Snider GL. Proteolytic activity of human neutrophil elastase and porcine pancreatic trypsin causes bronchial secretory cell metaplasia in hamsters. *Exp Lung Res* 1985;9:167–175.

62. Christensen TG, Lucey EC, Breuer R, Snider GL. Acid-induced secretory cell metaplasia in hamster bronchi. *Environ Res* 1988;45:78–90.

63. Breuer R, Christensen TG, Lucey EC, Stone PJ, Snider GL. An ultrastructural morphometric analysis of elastase-treated hamster bronchi shows discharge followed by progressive accumulation of secretory granules. *Am Rev Respir Dis* 1987;136:698–703.

64. Christensen TG, Breuer R, Hornstra LJ, Lucey EC, Stone PJ, Snider GL. An ultrastructural study of the response of hamster bronchial epithelium to human neutrophil elastase. *Exp Lung Res* 1987;13:279–297.

65. Stone PJ, Lucey EC, Snider GL. Induction and exacerbation of emphysema in hamsters with human neutrophil elastase inactivated reversibly by a peptide boronic acid. *Am Rev Respir Dis* 1990;141:47–52.

66. Lucey EC, Stone PJ, Ciccolella DE, Breuer R, Christensen TG, Thompson RC, Snider GL. Recombinant human leukocyte protease inhibitor ameliorates human neutrophil elastase-induced emphysema and secretory cell metaplasia in the hamster. *J Lab Clin Med* 1990;115:224–232.

67. Christensen TG, Breuer R, Lucey EC, Stone PJ, Snider GL. Regional difference in airway epithelial response to neutrophil elastase: tracheal secretory cells discharge and recover in hamsters that develop bronchial secretory cell metaplasia. *Exp Lung Res* 1989;15:943–959.

68. Christensen TG, Breuer R, Lucey EC, Hornstra LJ, Stone P, Snider GL. Lectin cytochemistry of hamster tracheobronchial epithelium: regional differences in surface glycoconjugates and in the secretory cell response to neutrophil elastase. *Am J Respir Cell Mol Biol* 1990;in press.

69. Tegner H, Ohlsson K, Toremalm NG, von Meckleburg C. Effect of human leukocyte enzymes on tracheal mucosa and its mucociliary activity. *Rhinology* 1979;17:199–206.

70. Sykes DA, Wilson R, Greenstone M, Currie DC, Steinfort C, Cole PJ. Deleterious effects of purulent sputum sol on human ciliary function *in vitro*: at least two factors identified. *Thorax* 1987;42:256–261.

71. Smallman LA, Hill SL, Stockley RA. Reduction of ciliary beat frequency *in vitro* by sputum from patients with bronchiectasis: a serine proteinase effect. *Thorax* 1984;39:663–667.

72. Wittels EH, Coalson JJ, Welch MH, Geunter CA. Pulmonary intravascular leukocyte sequestration: a potential mechanism of lung injury. *Am Rev Respir Dis* 1974;109:502–509.

73. Guenter CA, Coalson JJ, Jacques J. Emphysema associated with intravascular leukocyte sequestration: comparison with papain-induced emphysema. *Am Rev Respir Dis* 1981;123:79–84.

74. Blackwood RA, Moret J, Mandl I, Turino GM. Emphysema induced by intravenously administered endotoxin in an alpha$_1$-antitrypsin-deficient rat model. *Am Rev Respir Dis* 1984;130:231–236.

75. Freeman G, Crane SC, Stephens RJ, Furiosi NJ. Pathogenesis of the nitrogen dioxide-induced lesion in the rat lung: a review and presentation of new observations. *Am Rev Respir Dis* 1968;98:429–443.

76. Glasgow JE, Pietra GG, Abrams WR, Blank J, Oppenheim DM, Weinbaum G. Neutrophil recruitment and degranulation during induction of emphysema in the rat by nitrogen dioxide. *Am Rev Respir Dis* 1987;135:1129–1136.

77. Blank J, Glasgow JE, Pietra GG, Burdette L, Weinbaum G. Nitrogen-dioxide-induced emphysema in rats: lack of worsening by beta-aminopropionitrile treatment. *Am Rev Respir Dis* 1988;137:376–379.

78. Lam C, Kattan M, Collins A, Kleinerman J. Long-term sequelae of bronchiolitis induced by nitrogen dioxide in hamsters. *Am Rev Respir Dis* 1983;128:1020–1023.

79. Kleinerman J, Ip MPC, Gordon RE. The reaction of the respiratory tract to chronic NO$_2$ exposure. In: Scarpelli DG, Craighead JE, Kaufman N, eds. *The pathologist and the environment.* Baltimore: Williams & Wilkins, 1985;200–210.

80. Lafuma C, Harf A, Lange F, Bozzi L, Poncy JL, Bignon J. Effect of low-level NO$_2$ chronic exposure on elastase-induced emphysema. *Environ Res* 1987;43:75–84.

81. Blair WH, Henry MC, Ehrlich R. Chronic toxicity of nitrogen dioxide: effect on histopathology of lung tissue. *Arch Environ Health* 1969;18:186–192.

82. Haydon GB, Davidson JT, Lillington GA. Nitrogen dioxide-induced emphysema in rabbits. *Am Rev Respir Dis* 1967;95:797–805.

83. Hyde D, Orthoeffer J, Dungworth D, Tyler W, Carter R, Lum H. Morphometric and morphologic evaluation of pulmonary lesions in beagle dogs chronically exposed to high ambient levels of air pollutants. *Lab Invest* 1978;38:455–469.

84. Kleinerman J, Ip MPC. Effect of nitrogen dioxide on elastin and collagen contents of lung. *Arch Environ Health* 1979;34:228–232.

85. Riley DJ, Berg RA, Edelman NH, Prockop DJ. Prevention of collagen deposition following pulmonary oxygen toxicity in the rat by *cis*-4-hydroxy-1-proline. *J Clin Invest* 1980;65:643–651.

86. Riley DJ, Kramer MJ, Kerr JS, Chae CU, Yu SY, Berg RA. Damage and repair of lung connective tissue in rats exposed to toxic levels of oxygen. *Am Rev Respir Dis* 1987;135:441–447.

87. Kerr JS, Chae CU, Nagase H, Berg RA, Riley DJ. Degradation of collagen in lung tissue slices exposed to hyperoxia. *Am Rev Respir Dis* 1987;135:1334–1339.

88. Merritt TA. Oxygen exposure in the newborn guinea pig lung lavage cell populations, chemotactic and elastase response: a possible relationship to neonatal bronchopulmonary dysplasia. *Pediatr Res* 1982;16:798–805.

89. Chapman HA, Reilly JJ, Kobzik L. Role of plasminogen activator in degradation of extracellular matrix protein by live human alveolar macrophages. *Am Rev Respir Dis* 1988;137:412–419.

90. Werb Z, Banda MJ, Jones PA. Degradation of connective tissue matrices by macrophages. I. Proteolysis of elastin, glycoproteins, and collagen by proteinases isolated from macrophages. *J Exp Med* 1980;152:1340–1357.

91. Stone PJ, McMahon MP, Morris SM, Calore JD, Franzblau C. Elastin in a neonatal rat smooth muscle cell culture has greatly decreased susceptibility to proteolysis by human neutrophil elastase. An *in vitro* model of elastolytic injury. *In Vitro Cell Dev Biol* 1987;23:663–676.

92. McGowan SE. Mechanisms of extracellular matrix proteoglycan degradation by human neutrophils. *Am J Respir Cell Mol Biol* 1990;2:271–279.

93. Stone PJ, Morris SM, Martin BM, McMahon MP, Faris B, Franzblau C. Repair of protease-damaged elastin in neonatal

rat aortic smooth muscle cell cultures. *J Clin Invest* 1988;82:1644–1654.

94. Kim KC, Wasano K, Niles RM, Schuster JE, Stone PJ, Brody JS. Human neutrophil elastase releases cell surface mucins from primary cultures of hamster tracheal epithelial cells. *Proc Natl Acad Sci USA* 1987;84:9304–9308.

95. Niles R, Christensen TG, Breuer R, Stone PJ, Snider GL. Serine proteases stimulate mucous glycoprotein release from hamster tracheal ring organ culture. *J Lab Clin Med* 1986;108:489–497.

96. Breuer R, Christensen TG, Niles RM, Stone PJ, Snider GL. Human neutrophil elastase causes glycoconjugate release from the epithelial cell surface of hamster trachea in organ culture. *Am Rev Respir Dis* 1989;139:779–782.

97. Sommerhoff CP, Nadel JA, Basbaum CB, Caughey GH. Neutrophil elastase and cathepsin G stimulate secretion from cultured bovine airway gland serous cells. *J Clin Invest* 1990;85:682–689.

98. Laurell CB, Ericksson S. The electrophoretic alpha-1-globulin pattern of serum in alpha-1-antitrypsin deficiency. *Scand J Clin Lab Invest* 1963;15:132–140.

99. Galdston M, Melnick EL, Goldring RM, Levytska V, Curasi CA, Davis AL. Interactions of neutrophil elastase, serum trypsin inhibitory activity, and smoking history as risk factors for chronic obstructive pulmonary disease in patients with MM, MZ, and ZZ phenotypes for alpha$_1$-antitrypsin. *Am Rev Respir Dis* 1977;116:837–846.

100. Kidokoro Y, Kravis TC, Moser KM, Taylor JC, Crawford IP. Relationship of leukocyte elastase concentration to severity of emphysema in homozygous alpha$_1$-antitrypsin-deficient persons. *Am Rev Respir Dis* 1977;115:793–803.

101. Abboud RT, Rushton JM, Grzybowski S. Interrelationships between neutrophil elastase, serum alpha$_1$-antitrypsin, lung function and chest radiography in patients with chronic airflow obstruction. *Am Rev Respir Dis* 1979;120:31–40.

102. Lam S, Abboud RT, Chan-Yeung M, Rushton JM. Neutrophil elastase and pulmonary function in subjects with intermediate alpha$_1$-antitrypsin deficiency (MZ phenotype). *Am Rev Respir Dis* 1979;119:941–951.

103. Rodriguez JR, Seal JE, Radin A, Lin JS, Mandl I, Turino GM. Neutrophil lysosomal elastase activity in normal subjects and in patients with chronic obstructive pulmonary disease. *Am Rev Respir Dis* 1979;119:409–417.

104. Kramps JA, Bakker W, Dijkman JH. A matched-pair study of the leukocyte elastase-like activity in normal persons and in emphysematous patients with and without alpha-1-antitrypsin deficiency. *Am Rev Respir Dis* 1980;121:253.

105. Binder R, Stone PJ, Calore JD, Dunn DM, Snider GL, Franzblau C, Valeri CR. Serum antielastase and neutrophil elastase levels in PiM phenotype cigarette smokers with airflow obstruction. *Respiration* 1985;47:267–277.

106. Geokas MC, Brodrick JW, Johnson JH, Largman C. Pancreatic elastase in human serum: determination by radioimmunoassay. *J Biol Chem* 1977;252:61–67.

107. Balldin G, Borgstrom A, Eddeland A, Genell S, Hagberg L, Ohlsson K. Elevated serum levels of pancreatic secretory proteins in cigarette smokers after secretin stimulation. *J Clin Invest* 1980;66:159–162.

108. Ip MPC, Kleinerman J, Sorensen J. The effect of elastase on pulmonary elastin and collagen: comparison of intravenous and intratracheal exposure. *Exp Lung Res* 1980;1:181–189.

109. Stockley RA, Ohlsson K. Serum studies of leucocyte elastase in acute and chronic lung diseases. *Thorax* 1982;37:114–117.

110. Janoff A, Raju L, Dearing R. Levels of elastase activity in bronchoalveolar lavage fluids of healthy smokers and nonsmokers. *Am Rev Respir Dis* 1983;127:540–544.

111. Niederman MS, Fritts LL, Merrill WW, Fick RB, Matthay RA, Reynolds HY, Gee JBL. Demonstration of a free elastolytic metalloenzyme in human lung lavage fluid and its relationship to alpha$_1$-antiprotease. *Am Rev Respir Dis* 1984;129:943–947.

112. Davies SF, Offord KP, Brown MG, Campe H, Niewoehner D. Urine desmosine is unrelated to cigarette smoking or to spirometric function. *Am Rev Respir Dis* 1983;128:473–475.

113. Harel S, Janoff A, Yu SY, Hurewitz A, Bergofsky EH. Desmosine radioimmunoassay for measuring elastin degradation *in vitro*. *Am Rev Respir Dis* 1980;122:769–773.

114. Pelham F, Wewers M, Crystal R, Buist AS, Janoff A. Urinary excretion of desmosine (elastase cross-links) in subjects with PiZZ alpha-1-antitrypsin deficiency, a phenotype associated with hereditary predisposition to pulmonary emphysema. *Am Rev Respir Dis* 1985;132:821–823.

115. Kucich U, Christner P, Lippmann M, Kimbel P, Williams G, Rosenbloom J, Weinbaum G. Utilization of a peroxidase antiperoxidase complex in an enzyme-linked immunosorbent assay of elastin-derived peptides in human plasma. *Am Rev Respir Dis* 1985;131:709–713.

116. Damiano VV, Tsang A, Kucich U, Abrams WR, Rosenbloom J, Kimbel P, Fallahnejad M, Weinbaum G. Immunolocalization of elastase in human emphysematous lungs. *J Clin Invest* 1986;78:482–493.

117. Fox B, Bull TB, Guz A, Harris E, Tetley TD. Is neutrophil elastase associated with elastic tissue in emphysema? *J Clin Pathol* 1988;41:435–440.

118. Wright RR. Elastic tissue of normal and emphysematous lungs: a tridimensional histological study. *Am J Pathol* 1961;39:355–363.

119. Tate RM, Repine JE. Neutrophils and the adult respiratory distress syndrome. *Am Rev Respir Dis* 1983;128:552–559.

120. Lee CT, Fein AM, Lippmann M, Holtzman H, Kimbel P, Weinbaum G. Elastolytic activity in pulmonary lavage fluid from patients with adult respiratory-distress syndrome. *N Engl J Med* 1981;304:192–196.

121. Cochrane CG, Spragg RG, Revak SD, Cohn AB, McGuire WW. The presence of neutrophil elastase and evidence of oxidation activity in bronchoalveolar lavage fluid of patients with adult respiratory distress syndrome. *Am Rev Respir Dis* 1983;127:S25–S27.

122. Idell S, Kucich U, Fein A, Kueppers F, James HL, Walsh PN, Weinbaum G, Colman RW, Cohen AB. Neutrophil elastase-releasing factors in bronchoalveolar lavage from patients with adult respiratory distress syndrome. *Am Rev Respir Dis* 1985;132:1098–1105.

123. Weiland JE, Davis WB, Holter JF, Mohammed JR, Dorinsky PM, Gadek JE. Lung neutrophils in the adult respiratory distress syndrome: clinical and pathophysiologic significance. *Am Rev Respir Dis* 1986;133:218–225.

124. Christner P, Fein A, Goldberg S, Lippmann M, Abrams W, Weinbaum G. Collagenase in the lower respiratory tract of patients with adult respiratory distress syndrome. *Am Rev Respir Dis* 1985;131:690–695.

125. Cohen AB, MacArthur C, Idell S, Maunder R, Martin T, Dinarello CA, Griffith D, Mclarty J. A peptide from alveolar macrophages that releases neutrophil enzymes into the lungs in patients with the adult respiratory distress syndrome. *Am Rev Respir Dis* 1988;137:1151–1158.

126. Stockley RA. Proteolytic enzymes, their inhibitors and lung diseases. *Clin Sci* 1983;64:119–126.

127. Stockley RA, Hill SL, Morrison HM, Starkie CM. Elastolytic activity of sputum and its relation to purulence and to lung function in patients with bronchiectasis. *Thorax* 1984;39:408–413.

128. Bruce MC, Poncz L, Klinger JD, Stern RC, Tomashefski JF, Dearborn DG. Biochemical and pathologic evidence for proteolytic destruction of lung connective tissue in cystic fibrosis. *Am Rev Respir Dis* 1985;132:529–535.

129. Tournier JM, Jacquot J, Puchelle E, Bieth JG. Evidence that *Pseudomonas aeruginosa* elastase does not inactivate the bronchial inhibitor in the presence of leukocyte elastase. *Am Rev Respir Dis* 1985;132:524–528.

130. Suter S, Schaad UB, Tegner H, Ohlsson K, Desgrandchamps D, Waldvogel FA. Levels of free granulocyte elastase in bronchial secretions from patients with cystic fibrosis: effect of antimicrobial treatment against *Pseudomonas aeruginosa*. *J Infest Dis* 1986;153:902–909.

131. Berger M, Sorensen RU, Tosi MF, Dearborn DG, Doring G. Complement receptor expression on neutrophils at an inflam-

matory site, the *Pseudomonas*-infected lung in cystic fibrosis. *J Clin Invest* 1989;84:1304–1313.

132. Gadek JE, Kelman JA, Fells G, Weinberger SE, Horwitz AL, Reynolds HY, Fulmer JD, Crystal RG. Collagenase in the lower respiratory tract of patients with idiopathic pulmonary fibrosis. *N Engl J Med* 1979;301:737–742.

133. Garcia JGN, James HL, Zinkgraf S, Perlman MB, Keogh BA. Lower respiratory tract abnormalities in rheumatoid interstial

lung disease: potential role of neutrophils in lung injury. *Am Rev Respir Dis* 1987;136:811–817.

134. Kindt GC, Weiland JE, Davis WB, Gadek JE, Dorinsky PM. Bronchiolitis in adults: a reversible cause of airway obstruction with airway neutrophils and neutrophil products. *Am Rev Respir Dis* 1989;140:483–492.

135. Snider GL. Protease–antiprotease imbalance in the pathogenesis of emphysema and chronic bronchial injury: a potential target for drug development. *Drug Dev Res* 1987;10:235–253.

THE LUNG: Scientific Foundations
edited by R.G. Crystal, J.B. West et al.
Raven Press, Ltd., New York © 1991.

CHAPTER 7.2.1

Oxidants:

Types, Sources, and Mechanisms of Injury

Ingrid U. Schraufstätter and Charles G. Cochrane

SOURCE AND TYPE OF OXIDANTS INVOLVED IN PULMONARY PATHOLOGY

Involvement of oxygen radicals has been associated with a number of pulmonary diseases (Table 1). The source of oxidants varies considerably for each specific case:

Stimulated leukocytes [both polymorphonuclear leukocytes (PMNs) and macrophages] are the primary source of oxidants in adult respiratory distress syndrome (ARDS) and presumably other inflammatory diseases. In addition, both PMNs and macrophages are secondarily attracted to the lungs, where they undergo their respiratory burst following oxidative damage by many other agents. In addition to leukocytic cells, endothelial cells themselves are capable of O_2^- formation under certain conditions. The NADPH oxidase/cytochrome$_{b554}$ system in the plasma membrane of stimulated PMNs forms O_2^- (1). The local concentrations of oxidants formed by PMNs can be extremely high: 2×10^6 PMNs stimulated with 10^{-8} M f-Met-Leu-Phe produce 10 nmoles O_2^- within 1 min in a volume of 1–2 μl. In the absence of O_2^- degrading pathways, this would be a local concentration of 5–10 mM. O_2^- itself is not indiscriminately reactive, although it selectively damages a limited number of targets (e.g., catalase) (2). Its protonated form, $HO_2 \cdot$ (pK_a = 4.8), can, however, directly attack polyunsaturated fatty acids (3), similar to $\cdot OH$. O_2^- quickly dismutates to H_2O_2. For extracellular O_2^-, this reaction is no-

nenzymatic and is presumably supported by the acidic pH in the proximity of stimulated PMNs. In the presence of transition metal the extremely toxic $\cdot OH$ radical can be formed in a Fenton-type reaction:

$$Fe^{2+} + H_2O_2 \rightarrow Fe^{3+} + \cdot OH + OH^-$$

Fe^{3+} can be rereduced by O_2^- or other reducing agents (e.g., ascorbate, glutathione):

$$Fe^{3+} + O_2^- \rightarrow Fe^{2+} + O_2$$

Since H_2O_2 easily diffuses through cell membranes (4), $\cdot OH$ formation may occur extra- or intracellularly. Because of its extremely high reactivity, $\cdot OH$ will always cause site-directed damage at the site of its formation.

Myeloperoxidase, abundantly present in PMNs and released during the respiratory burst, converts H_2O_2 into HOCl (5), a very reactive oxidant which can further react to form more long-lived chloramines.

Hyperoxia leads to intracellular O_2^- formation by electron-slip of mitochondrial (6) as well as "microsomal" respiratory chains. O_2^- is degraded to H_2O_2 by cellular superoxide dismutase (SOD). This reaction is essentially diffusion-limited. H_2O_2 itself is further degraded to H_2O. However, a certain percentage of O_2^- and H_2O_2 escape the cellular defense mechanisms under the conditions of increased formation during hyperoxia.

Asbestos contains high concentrations of iron [2.7–28%, depending on the particular type (7)]. In the presence of O_2, O_2^- can be formed directly:

$$(Asbestos)-Fe^{2+} + O_2 \rightarrow (Asbestos)-Fe^{3+} + O_2^-$$

In the presence of H_2O_2, it can be formed indirectly:

$$(Asbestos)-Fe^{3+}$$

$$+ H_2O_2 \rightarrow (Asbestos)-Fe^{2+} + O_2^- + 2H^+$$

I. U. Schraufstätter and C. G. Cochrane: Division of Vascular Biology and Inflammation, Department of Immunology Research, Scripps Clinic, La Jolla, California 92037.

TABLE 1. *Examples of pulmonary diseases in which oxygen radicals are thought to be involved*[a]

Condition	Source of oxidant
ARDS	Stimulated PMNs
Hyperoxia	O_2^- formation from electron transport chains
Asbestosis	Fe^{2+}, stimulated macrophages
Paraquat toxicity	Redox cycling
Bleomycin toxicity	Formation of O_2^-/$\cdot OH$ from Fe^{2+}–bleomycin complex
Cigarette smoking	H_2O_2, NO, peroxyl compounds, quinones, stimulated PMNs, and macrophages
Ionizing radiation	$\cdot OH$ formation by ionization

[a] ARDS, adult respiratory distress syndrome; PMNs, polymorphonuclear leukocytes.

Consequent formation of $\cdot OH$ has been shown using electron spin resonance spectroscopy and the spin trap dimethylpyroline-*N*-oxide (DMPO) (7,8). In addition, frustrated phagocytosis of asbestos fibers by macrophages will lead to activation of their respiratory burst.

The herbicide paraquat (PQ^{2+}), which accumulates in lung epithelium, causes oxidant formation as a result of redox cycling (9):

$$NADPH \rightarrow NADP \qquad PQ^{2+} \leftarrow PQ^+ \qquad O_2^- \leftarrow O_2$$

The reduction of PQ^{2+} by NADPH (the reduced form of nicotinamide-adenine dinucleotide phosphate, NADP) is dependent on cytochrome P_{450} reductase present in the endoplasmic reticulum (ER). A mitochondrial enzyme chain can also reduce PQ^{2+}.

Bleomycin leads to similar redox cycling except that it is strictly Fe-dependent (10). Because bleomycin binds avidly to DNA, much of the site-directed $\cdot OH$ formation will lead to DNA damage.

Cigarette smoke contains a multitude of oxidizing compounds, some of which are listed in Table 1. In addition, cigarette smoking attracts macrophages into the lungs. The effects of cigarette smoking on lung pathology are described in more detail in Chapter 7.6.3.

Finally, ionizing radiation directly produces $\cdot OH$ without the necessity for transition metal.

With the exception of cigarette smoke and ionizing radiation, all other oxidant-producing mechanisms begin with the formation of O_2^-. The rate, concentration, and site of formation (e.g., plasma membrane, nucleus, mitochondria, ER) of O_2^- vary considerably, however, which may cause damage of different targets.

EVIDENCE FOR OXIDANT INVOLVEMENT *IN VIVO*

As described above, oxidants are assumed to contribute to pulmonary injury under various conditions. Evidence for oxidative processes—determined as inactivation of α_1-antitrypsin inhibitor (α_1-AT) due to methionine sulfoxide formation of its active site—has been found in lavage fluids of patients with ARDS (11) or other inflammatory pulmonary diseases as well as in cigarette smokers (12). Because α_1-AT inhibits neutrophil elastase present in the same lavage fluids, part of the oxidant-induced injury may be due to secondary, proteolytic damage caused by this enzyme (see Chapters 7.7.1, 7.7.2, and 7.9.1). Generally, oxidants and proteases may enhance each other's damaging effects. Oxidants formed in the lung cause attraction of protease-containing neutrophils. Leukocytic proenzymes (e.g., collagenase) are activated by oxidative processes (13), and oxidatively modified proteins are preferred targets of certain proteases (14).

In experimental animals it was found that oxidant-producing enzymes [xanthine oxidase + hypoxanthine (15) or glucose oxidase (16)] cause increased vascular permeability, anoxia, and attraction of neutrophils. Hence, oxidants by themselves are capable of producing pulmonary injury. Various PMN-stimulating agents [formylated peptides; phorbol myristate acetate (PMA); cobra venom factor, which activates complement] have been found to cause pulmonary edema in various laboratory animals (rats, rabbits, sheep, rhesus monkeys) (16–19). The pathology could be prevented by neutrophil depletion, and it could be greatly attenuated by antioxidants such as catalase (16) and the iron chelator deferoxamine (17). In isolated, perfused lungs, PMA-stimulated neutrophils cause increased vascular permeability, whereas stimulated neutrophils of a patient with chronic granulomatous disease, which do not generate oxidants, failed to show this effect (20).

The biochemical pathways involved in oxidant-induced pathology are poorly understood *in vivo*. A primary reason for this is the lack of knowledge of the molecular targets that are affected by various oxidants. The situation is complicated by two facts: (i) Quantitative determination of short-lived oxidants *in vivo* is almost impossible, although there are methods of qualitatively detecting their presence [e.g., by the use of electron spin resonancy in the presence of spin traps (21), by H_2O_2-dependent inactivation of catalase in the presence of aminotriazole (16), or by glutathione oxidation]. (ii) Various oxidants (e.g., H_2O_2, $\cdot OH$, HOCl) affect cells in very different ways, thus invalidating the notion of a unified scheme for oxidative injury.

BIOCHEMICAL PATHWAYS AFFECTED BY OXIDANTS *IN VITRO*

Effect of Neutrophil-Derived Oxidants on Cell Viability

When target cells were exposed to stimulated neutrophils or macrophages, cell lysis occurred over a period of several hours. The oxidant species causing cell death in most cases was H_2O_2, which induced cell lysis in various tumor cell lines (22), endothelial cells (23), and fibroblasts (24). Cell lysis could be prevented by addition of catalase but not by addition of SOD, OH, or HOCl scavengers. When comparing the susceptibility of various tumor cells to H_2O_2-induced cell lysis, a correlation between cellular glutathione (GSH) and the flux of H_2O_2 causing 50% lysis was observed (25).

In certain cell types, other oxidants were, however, found to cause cell death: Cell lysis in mouse tumor cells was dependent on myeloperoxidase activity (26) and was prevented by scavengers of HOCl such as methionine. The reason for the different behavior of these cells is not known, but certain cells appear to be unusually sensitive to lysis by HOCl-derived chloramines (27). Cells normally killed as a result of myeloperoxidase activity could be lysed via an H_2O_2-dependent pathway if myeloperoxidase-deficient neutrophils were used, although the time required for cell lysis was prolonged.

Cell lysis in erythrocytes could be prevented by extracellular SOD, but this does not necessarily indicate that O_2^- caused cell lysis directly (28): O_2^- can be transported through an anion channel (29)—the most abundant protein of red cell membranes with 10^6 copies/cell. It is conceivable that O_2^- was taken up by erythrocytes prior to dismutation. O_2^- uptake by the anion transporter, which is present in considerably lower concentrations in other cell types, presumably cannot compete in these cell types with extracellular dismutation of O_2^-.

Assessment of cell viability gives only limited information. It is an insensitive and late event of cell damage and does not elucidate the pathways of cell injury. For this reason, pathways of oxidative injury were followed in more detail using selected oxidants.

Pathways of Cellular Damage Caused by H_2O_2

Concentrations of H_2O_2 of 20–120 μM—well within the range produced by stimulated PMNs—caused formation of DNA strand breaks in various target cells (30–32). These strand breaks were observed within seconds after the addition of oxidant, and they could be prevented by the addition of catalase or cell-permeable Fe-chelators (phenanthroline, deferrithiocine, and prolonged incubation with deferoxamine) (31). H_2O_2-induced deoxyribonucleic acid (DNA) strand breaks in isolated DNA were Fe-dependent and inhibitable by ·OH scavengers (8,30). ·OH radical formation could be directly detected with the spin trap DMPO (32), and finally DNA base hydroxylations, a definite footprint of ·OH formation, could be detected in isolated DNA exposed to H_2O_2 + Fe^{2+}/ethylenediaminetetraacetic

TABLE 2. Susceptibility to H_2O_2-induced DNA strand breaks in different cell types[a]

Cell	D_{50} (μM H_2O_2)	Catalase content (ng/10^6 cells)	$t_{1/2}$ H_2O_2 (min)
Macrophage	170	850	0.8
PMN	94	503	2.5
GM1380	58	213	5.5
P388D1	35	20	14.0
Lymphocyte	20	4	24.0
Macrophage + 12 mM AT	13.5	<2	120.0

[a] D_{50} represents the concentration of H_2O_2 that led to unwinding in alkali of 50% of the DNA. The cells used were rabbit alveolar macrophages, human neutrophils, GM1380 human embryo lung fibroblasts, the murine leukocytic tumor cell line P388D1, and human peripheral lymphocytes. AT (aminotriazole) inhibits catalase activity. (From ref. 31.)

acid (EDTA) or stimulated PMNs (33). It is therefore clear that ·OH or a transition-metal–H_2O_2 complex with the reactivity of ·OH was ultimately responsible for damage in isolated DNA and presumably also in whole cells. Susceptibility to H_2O_2-induced DNA strand breaks in different cell types was inversely correlated with H_2O_2 degrading capacity, at this concentration of H_2O_2 primarily a function of catalase content (Table 2).

Formation of DNA strand breaks by various agents leads to activation of poly-adenosine diphosphate (ADP)-ribose polymerase (34), a nuclear enzyme hydrolyzing nicotinamide-adenine dinucleotide (NAD) into ADP-ribose and nicotinamide. ADP-ribose is joined into polymers that are covalently attached to various nuclear proteins (e.g., histones and the poly-ADP-ribose polymerase itself) (35). Following H_2O_2-induced DNA strand breakage, an increase in the concentration of poly-ADP-ribose polymer is observed (36,37). Because the turnover of this polymer is very high (on the order of 1 min), the most striking effect of the activation of poly-ADP-ribose polymerase is severe depletion of cellular NAD levels (36). Whereas nicotinamide can be quantitatively recovered in the extracellular fluid, ADP-ribose disappears into the adenine nucleotide pool. The fall in NAD results in loss of adenosine triphosphate (ATP) (36,38). Although the mechanism involved is poorly understood, ATP depletion with low concentrations of H_2O_2 (50–200 μM) appears to be a direct consequence of loss of NAD and can be prevented in the presence of inhibitors of poly-ADP-ribose polymerase (39). At higher concentrations of H_2O_2, ATP synthesis is directly affected, resulting in inhibition of both glycolysis and mitochondrial respiration (40). Inhibition of glycolysis is due to inactivation of glyceraldehyde-3-phosphate dehydrogenase (GAPDH) (40) and can be accounted for by a combined effect of altered cellular NAD/NADH ratios and direct inhibition of the enzyme (40). GAPDH is the only enzyme of the glycolytic pathway that is inhibited, and the inactivation does not depend on $\cdot OH$ as an intermediate. Enzyme inhibition appears to be due to disulfide formation between Cys^{149} and the spatially related Cys^{153} in a short alpha-helix of the molecule.

DNA strand break formation (41), activation of poly-ADP-ribose polymerase (36), and ATP depletion (42) have all been observed in target cells exposed to PMA-stimulated PMNs.

At slightly higher concentrations of H_2O_2 (43) or in the presence of redox cycling drugs (44), an increase of intracellular Ca^{2+} is observed, primarily due to release from intracellular stores, but is eventually followed by influx of Ca^{2+} from the extracellular medium. The increase of free Ca^{2+} is prevented by inhibitors of poly-ADP-ribose polymerase, although the connection between these two phenomena is not yet understood. Increase of free intracellular Ca^{2+} activates a number of potentially harmful enzymes (Ca^{2+}-dependent proteases, endonuclease, and phospholipase A_2). Finally, cytoskeletal derangement and bleb formation are shortly followed by cell lysis. Lipid peroxidation is only observed if Fe^{2+} is added extracellularly. Under these conditions, polyunsaturated fatty acid—primarily phosphatidylcholine and phosphatidylethanolamine—are oxidized. Concomitantly, aldehydes are generated, the major ones being malonaldehyde, hexanal, and 4-hydroxynonenal. These aldehydes are detected in their free form as well as in their bound form (the latter presumably being bound to the free amino and thiol groups of membrane lipids and proteins). Protein-bound aldehydes can secondarily inactivate plasma membrane proteins such as Na^+,K^+-ATPase.

Figure 1 summarizes the effect of a bolus of H_2O_2 on target cells.

Long-Term Effects of H_2O_2

Low doses of H_2O_2 (50–150 μM) cause DNA strand breaks but do not result in cell death. These strand breaks are repaired within 2–4 hr, and although cell replication is delayed, it will occur eventually. Hence, there is the risk of misrepair of DNA and of H_2O_2-induced somatic mutations: Strand breaks may, for example, cause chromosome rearrangements, and base hydroxylation may result in point mutations: Not only did 8-hydroxydeoxyguanosine (the major base hydroxylation formed by $\cdot OH$) mismatch with thymidine, but adjacent pyrimidines were also misread (45). Further point mutations caused by oxidants involved substitution of deoxyadenosine for thymidine opposite a template deoxyadenosine (46), and, finally, oxidants

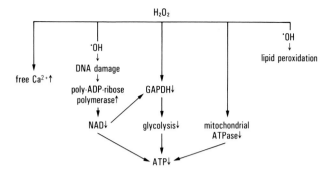

FIG. 1. Cellular targets of H_2O_2. Lipid peroxidation is dependent on the presence of extracellular iron or copper. None of the other pathways needs extracellular transition metal, but they occur intracellularly following diffusion of the H_2O_2 into the cell. The source of transition metal for site-directed $\cdot OH$ formation under these conditions is the cell itself.

caused abnormal cytosine methylation of the c-*abl* oncogene (47). Background levels of DNA base hydroxylations can even be found during normal cellular metabolism (48), but the concentrations increased following oxidative stress (48).

When C3H10T1/2 cells were exposed to either PMA-stimulated PMNs or xanthine oxidase/hypoxanthine, transformed foci were formed that could be prevented in the presence of antioxidants (49). When injected into nude mice, these cells caused tumors (50). H_2O_2 thus has the potential of being a mutagen and carcinogen. In addition, H_2O_2 is capable of initiating lipid peroxidation in the presence of metal ions, and a number of these products (fatty acid hydroperoxides, aldehydes, and cholesterol hydroperoxides) are themselves mutagens.

Thus, formation of oxidants may explain the association of chronic inflammation with carcinogenesis, observed in disorders such as ulcerative colitis, tuberculosis, asbestosis, and may be a contributing factor in carcinogenesis due to cigarette smoking.

Role of Transition Metal in Oxidative Injury

Most of the H_2O_2-induced damage is dependent on the formation of $\cdot OH$ radical in the presence of transition metal, primarily iron. Yet, free iron is too low to be detected in normal plasma (<1–2 μM), and protein-bound iron does not support $\cdot OH$ formation in the surrounding medium. A small, mobile iron pool (e.g., chelated to ATP and citrate) may exist intracellularly, and it is possible that DNA damage is caused by traces of iron bound to DNA. Iron contained in asbestos is able to support $\cdot OH$ formation directly.

In addition, iron can be released from various proteins during oxidative or inflammatory processes: H_2O_2 can cause iron release from hemoglobin (51), and this released iron is then responsible for ·OH formation and, for example, lipid peroxidation. Similarly, Fe^{3+} can be released from the ferritin molecule (the major cellular iron storage protein) by O_2^-, and this has been shown to occur in the presence of stimulated macrophages (52). Fe^{2+} bound to transferrin, the plasma transporter protein for iron, easily detaches from transferrin once the pH falls below 6, a pH that can be reached in the microenvironment of activated phagocytes (53). While evidence for the presence of reactive iron in an area of oxidative injury is still mostly indirect (hypothesized from the beneficial effect of iron chelators), these iron-released pathways may well be operating *in vivo*. The location of reactive iron will determine primary sites of ·OH-induced damage: Iron released from transferrin may thus initiate lipid peroxidation of plasma membranes, whereas iron bound to DNA will cause DNA damage in the presence of H_2O_2.

Effects of Hyperoxia

While it is known that hyperoxia leads to increased intracellular O_2^- production, only limited data are available on the biochemical mechanisms involved in cytotoxicity. Hyperoxia is clearly genotoxic, and it results in inhibition of DNA synthesis (54) partially due to inhibition of thymidine kinase (55), formation of chromosomal aberrations (56), and mutations (56). RNA synthesis is particularly sensitive to hyperoxia (57). DNA strand break formation and NAD depletion were barely detectable, which may, however, simply reflect that DNA repair and NAD resynthesis proceeded at a rate similar to that of the level of damage induced by prolonged exposure to a low concentration of oxidant. Differences in the toxic effects of a bolus of H_2O_2 versus prolonged low-level oxidative stress during hyperoxia may, at least partially, be due to the different rates of H_2O_2 formation: At high concentrations of H_2O_2, its reaction rate with catalase is diffusion-limited; at low concentrations the low affinity of catalase makes it a poor defense system, and H_2O_2 consumption by the glutathione cycle becomes the major detoxifying route. Oxidation of glutathione and consequent oxidation of NADPH can be severe during hyperoxic injury, but this is only of minor importance when a bolus of H_2O_2 is added. Depletion of reduced glutathione (oxidized glutathione can be transported out of cells) may be deleterious to cells (sustaining lipid peroxidation and allowing oxidation of protein sulfhydryls) and may contribute to the injury observed during hyperoxia.

Effect of Redox Cycling Agents

Because redox cycling agents cause intracellular formation of O_2^-, it would be expected that their mechanism of toxicity should be similar to that of hyperoxia. Keeping in mind that the concentrations of oxidants formed by the doses of these agents normally used during *in vitro* experiments are considerably higher than those achieved during hyperoxia, this hypothesis appears to be generally supported by experimental evidence.

Paraquat leads to oxidation of glutathione, loss of oxidized glutathione from the cell, oxidation of cellular NADPH, and formation of lipid peroxides (9). These changes have also been observed in lung tissue of rats that had received paraquat subcutaneously (58). Glutathione oxidation is followed by protein sulfhydryl oxidation and release of Ca^{2+} from cellular stores. Mitochondrial Ca^{2+} is released when oxidized intramitochondrial NAD(P) is hydrolyzed to nicotinamide and ADP-ribose (59). Inactivation of Ca^{2+}-ATPases of the plasma membrane and the ER can be reversed by disulfide reducing agents such as glutathione or dithiothreitol (60) and thus appears to be caused by sulfhydryl oxidation. ATP depletion has not been studied in detail in this system. The final pathology of increased free Ca^{2+}, plasma membrane blebbing, and cell lysis appears to be similar to that observed with a bolus of H_2O_2. Redox cycling agents have also been found to cause DNA damage, and they are mutagenic in the Ames test (61).

Cytotoxic Effects of HOCl and Chloramines

HOCl formed by neutrophilic myeloperoxidase in the presence of H_2O_2 is a very potent microbicidal agent. Its microbicidal activity appears to be due to inactivation of various membrane proteins: Bacterial respiration is inhibited—in particular, succinate oxidase activity (62). At the same time, various transporter systems are affected (e.g., β-galactosidase) (63). HOCl is very reactive, especially with various protein moieties (e.g., amino groups, sulfhydryls, methionines, tyrosines) (64,65). *In vivo*, inactivation of α_1-AT due to methionine sulfoxide formation of its active site (11) is thought to be mediated by HOCl. Because of its high reactivity, HOCl is likely to react with whatever protein moieties it encounters first, presumably plasma and plasma membrane proteins. In protein-free medium it is extremely toxic to target cells, where it inactivates various sulfhydryl-dependent transporter systems (glucose transporter, various amino acid transporters, Na^+,K^+-ATPase) and, generally speaking, causes a poorly defined "leakiness" to small molecules, resulting in cell swelling and eventually cell lysis. No specific pathway involved in cell lysis has been determined, and cell death appears to result from the combined effect on various independent targets. Table 3 shows a comparison between cellular targets

TABLE 3. *Comparison between cellular targets of H_2O_2 and $HOCl^a$*

	H_2O_2	HOCl
Degradation:	Degraded enzymatically (catalase, GSH cycle)	Degraded by reactions with amino acids, proteins, etc.
Location of targets:	Diffuses freely into cells; site-directed damage due to metal-dependent ·OH formation	Reacts with closest target
Cell death:	Lysis after several hours (threshold dose: 250–300 μM)	Lysis within 1 hr (threshold dose: 25–35 μM)
Sulfhydryl oxidation		
Total —SH:	No general —SH oxidation at millimolar concentrations; very specific targets (e.g., GAPDH)	50% oxidation at 100 μM; multiple molecular targets
Extracellular —SH:	25% oxidation at 700 μM H_2O_2; no functional consequences	50% oxidation at 12 μM; dysfunction of —SH-dependent plasma membrane proteins
ATP depletion:	Caused by inactivation of GADPH and by inhibition of mitochondrial ADP-phosphorylation; preceding cell death by hours	Caused by inactivation of GADPH, inhibition of mitochondrial ADP-phosphorylation, and inhibition of cell transport; barely preceding cell death
DNA:	DNA strand breaks at <100 μM; base hydroxylations; activation of poly-ADPRP, causing severe NAD depletion	No DNA strand breaks at 200 μM; base oxidation products unknown; NAD loss at time of cell lysis

^{a} Molarities refer to results obtained in P388D1 cells.

of H_2O_2 and HOCl, clearly depicting distinct sites of oxidative damage by the two oxidants. Effects of HOCl at low concentrations are closely simulated by the poorly cell-permeable sulfhydryl reagent para-chloromercuriphenylsulfonate, and since HOCl causes oxidation of plasma membrane sulfhydryls, these are the likely site of initial attack. In the presence of free amino acids, HOCl readily forms chloramines, which are toxic by themselves (64) but not as reactive as HOCl. Chloramines thus can diffuse over longer distances before they react with a target and are able to reach intracellular sites. Different chloramines show differences in toxic potential: Addition of taurine (for example) to HOCl, leading to taurinemonochloramine formation, will protect from HOCl-induced injury, whereas NH_2Cl (formed by HOCl in the presence of ammonia) is toxic by itself and affects targets similar to those of HOCl, leading to sulfhydryl depletion and inhibition of glutamine uptake (27). The toxic effect of both compounds can, however, be differentiated in certain systems: Using erythrocytes, HOCl is cytolytic at one-tenth the concentration of NH_2Cl, but NH_2Cl oxidizes intracellular hemoglobin prior to cell lysis (66). Because concentrations of protein versus amino acid cannot be estimated at the site of adherence of a stimulated neutrophil to a target cell, it is not clear which chlorinating compounds are responsible for oxidative damage *in vivo*. Indeed, both HOCl and chloramines appear considerably less toxic in the *in vivo* situation (67) than would be anticipated from their *in vitro* behavior. One may even speculate that myelo-

peroxidase converts a reasonable microbicidal agent (H_2O_2) into an outstanding one (HOCl) and at the same time diverts the genotoxic H_2O_2 into HOCl, which is too reactive to reach nuclear sites of intact cells. Future experimentation will have to define the role of myeloperoxidase-derived oxidants in tissue damage.

Although there has been considerable progress in recent years in the definition of cellular targets of oxidants *in vitro*, and although it is clear that oxidants are involved in edema formation *in vivo* and are probably contributing to the development of fibrosis, the connections between biochemistry and pathology are still poorly understood and await future investigation. Interactions between oxidants, proteases, lipid metabolites, and cytokines are expected and need to be determined in order to understand the complex scenario.

REFERENCES

1. Babior BM, Kipnes RS, Curnutte JT. Biological defense mechanisms: the production by leukocytes of superoxide, a potential bactericidal agent. *J Clin Invest* 1973;52:741.
2. Fridovitch I. Biological effects of the superoxide radical. *Arch Biochem Biophys* 1986;247:1.
3. Bielski BHJ, Arudi RL, Sutherland MW. A study of the reactivity of perhydroxyl radical/superoxide ion with unsaturated fatty acids. *J Biol Chem* 1973;258:4759.
4. Chance B, Sies H, Boveris E. Hydroperoxide metabolism in mammalian organs. *Physiol Rev* 1979;59:527.
5. Klebanoff SJ. Oxygen metabolism and the toxic properties of phagocytes. *Ann Intern Med* 1980;93:480.
6. Freeman BA, Crapo JD. Hyperoxia increases oxygen radical production in rat lungs and lung mitochondria. *J Biol Chem* 1981;256:10986.

7. Weitzman SA, Gracefa P. Asbestos catalyzes hydroxyl and superoxide radical generation from hydrogen peroxide. *Arch Biochem Biophys* 1983;228:373.

8. Jackson J, Schraufstatter IU, Hyslop PA, Vosbeck K, Sauerheber R, Weitzman SA, Cochrane CG. Role of oxidants in DNA damage: hydroxyl radical mediates the synergistic DNA damaging effects of asbestos and cigarette smoke. *J Clin Invest* 1987;80:1090.

9. Sandy MS, Moldeus P, Ross D, Smith MT. Role of redox cycling and lipid peroxidation in biperidyl herbicide cytotoxicity. *Biochem Pharmacol* 1986;35:3095.

10. Giloni L, Takeshita M, Johnson F, Iden C, Grollman AP. Bleomycin-induced strand-scission of DNA. *J Biol Chem* 1981; 256:8608.

11. Cochrane CG, Spragg RG, Revak SD. Pathogenesis of the adult respiratory distress syndrome. *J Clin Invest* 1983;71:754.

12. Gadek JE, Fells GA, Crystal RG. Cigarette smoking induces antiprotease deficiency in the lower respiratory tract of humans. *Science* 1979;206:1315.

13. Weiss SJ. Tissue destruction by neutrophils. *N Engl J Med* 1989;32:365.

14. Davies JAK, Goldberg AL. Oxygen radicals stimulate intracellular proteolysis and lipid peroxidation by independent mechanisms. *J Biol Chem* 1987;262:8220.

15. Johnson KJ, Fantone JC, Kaplan J, Ward PA. *In vivo* damage of rat lungs by oxygen metabolites. *J Clin Invest* 1981;67:983.

16. Schraufstatter IU, Revak SD, Cochrane CG. Proteases and oxidants in pulmonary inflammatory injury. *J Clin Invest* 1984; 73:1175.

17. Ward PA, Till GO, Kunkel R, Beachamp C. Evidence for the role of hydroxyl radical in complement and neutrophil dependent tissue injury. *J Clin Invest* 1983;72:789.

18. Heflin C, Brigham K. Prevention by granulocyte depletion of increased vascular permeability of sheep lung following endotoxemia. *J Clin Invest* 1981;68:1253.

19. Revak SD, Rice CL, Schraufstatter IU, Halsey WA, Bohl BP, Clancy RM, Cochrane CG. Experimental pulmonary inflammatory injury in the monkey. *J Clin Invest* 1985;76:1182.

20. Shasby DM, Vanbenthuysen KM, Tate RM, Shasby SS, McMurtry I, Repine JE. Granulocytes mediate acute edematous lung injury in rabbits and in isolated perfused rabbit lungs perfused with phorbol myristate acetate: Role of oxygen radicals. *Am Rev Respir Dis* 1982;125:443.

21. Zweier JL, Flaherty JT, Weisfeldt ML. Direct measurement of free radical generation following reperfusion of ischemic myocardium. *Proc Natl Acad Sci USA* 1987;84:1404.

22. Nathan CF, Arrick BA, Brukner LH, Cohn ZA. Extracellular cytolysis by activated macrophages and granulocytes: hydrogen peroxide as a mediator of cytotoxicity. *J Exp Med* 1979;149:100.

23. Weiss SJ, Young J, LoBuglio AF, Slivka A, Nimeh NF. Role of hydrogen peroxide in neutrophil-mediated destruction of cultured endothelial cells. *J Clin Invest* 1981;68:714.

24. Simon RH, Scoggin CH, Patterson D. Hydrogen peroxide causes the total injury to human fibroblasts exposed to oxygen radicals. *J Biol Chem* 1981;256:7181.

25. Nathan CF, Arrick BA, Murray HW, DeSantis NM, Cohn ZA. Tumor cell anti-oxidant defenses: inhibition of the glutathione redox-cycle enhances macrophage-mediated cytolysis. *J Exp Med* 1980;153:766.

26. Clark RA, Klebanoff SJ. Neutrophil-mediated tumor cell cytotoxicity: Role of the peroxidase system. *J Exp Med* 1975; 141:1442.

27. Learn DB, Thomas EL. Inhibition of tumor cell glutamine uptake by isolated neutrophils. *J Clin Invest* 1988;82:789.

28. Weiss SJ, LoBuglio AF. Biology of disease: phagocyte-generated oxygen metabolites and cellular injury. *Lab Invest* 1982;47:5.

29. Lynch RE, Fridovich I. Effects of superoxide on the erythrocyte membrane. *J Biol Chem* 1978;253:1838.

30. Brawn K, Fridovich I. DNA strand scission by enzymatically generated oxygen radicals. *Arch Biochem Biophys* 1980;206:414.

31. Schraufstatter IU, Hyslop PA, Jackson JH, Cochrane CG. Oxidant-induced DNA damage of target cells. *J Clin Invest* 1988;82:1040.

32. Bradley MO, Erickson LC. Comparison of the effects of hydrogen peroxide and x-ray irradiation on toxicity, mutation, and DNA damage/repair in mammalian cells (V-79). *Biochim Biophys Acta* 1981;654:135.

33. Jackson JH, Gajewski E, Schraufstatter IU, Hyslop PA, Fuciarelli AF, Dizdaroglu M, Cochrane CG. Damage to the bases in DNA induced by stimulated neutrophils. *J Clin Invest* 1989;84:1644.

34. Skidmore CJ, Davies MI, Goodwin PM, Halldorsson H, Lewis PJ, Shall S, Zia'ee AA. The involvement of poly-ADP-ribose-polymerase in the degradation of NAD caused by gamma-irradiation and *N*-methyl-*N*-nitrosourea. *Eur J Biochem* 1979; 101:135.

35. Ueda K. ADP-ribosylation. *Annu Rev Biochem* 1985;54:73.

36. Schraufstatter IU, Hinshaw DB, Hyslop PA, Spragg RG, Cochrane CG. Oxidant injury of cells: DNA strand breaks activate poly-ADP-ribose polymerase and lead to depletion of NAD. *J Clin Invest* 1986;77:1312.

37. Carson DA, Seto S, Wasson DB. Lymphocyte dysfunction after DNA damage by toxic oxygen species: a model of immunodeficiency. *J Exp Med* 1986;163:746.

38. Sims JL, Berger SL, Berger NA. Poly-ADP-ribose polymerase inhibitors preserve NAD and ATP levels in DNA-damaged cells: mechanism of stimulation of unscheduled DNA synthesis. *Biochemistry* 1983;22:5188.

39. Schraufstatter IU, Hyslop PA, Hinshaw DB, Spragg RG, Sklar LA, Cochrane CG. Hydrogen peroxide-induced injury of cells and its prevention by inhibitors of poly-ADP-ribose polymerase. *Proc Natl Acad Sci USA* 1986;83:498.

40. Hyslop PA, Hinshaw DB, Halsey WA, Schraufstatter IU, Sauerheber RD, Spragg RG, Jackson JH, Cochrane CG. Mechanisms of oxidant-mediated cell injury: the glycolytic and mitochondrial pathways of ADP-phosphorylation are major intracellular targets inactivated by hydrogen peroxide. *J Biol Chem* 1988; 263:1665.

41. Birnboim HC. DNA strand breakage in human leukocytes exposed to a tumor promotor, phorbol myristate acetate. *Science* 1982;215:1247.

42. Spragg RG, Hinshaw DB, Hyslop PA, Schraufstatter IU, Cochrane CG. Alterations in ATP and energy charge in endothelial and P388D1 cells after oxidant injury. *J Clin Invest* 1985;76:1471.

43. Hyslop PA, Hinshaw DB, Schraufstatter IU, Sklar LA, Spragg RG, Cochrane CG. Intracellular calcium homeostasis during H_2O_2 injury to cultured P388D1 cells. *J Cell Physiol* 1986; 129:356.

44. Jewel SA, Bellomo G, Thor H, Orrenius S, Smith MT. Bleb formation in hepatocytes during drug metabolism is caused by disturbances in thiol and calcium homeostasis. *Science* 1982;217:1257.

45. Kuchino Y, Mori F, Kasai H, Inoue H, Iwai S, Miura K, Ohtsuka E, Nishimura S. Misreading of DNA templates containing 8-hydroxydeoxyguanosine at the modified base and at adjacent residues. *Nature* 1987;327:77.

46. Loeb L, James EA, Waltersdorph AM, Klebanoff SJ. Mutagenesis by the autoxidation of iron with isolated DNA. *Proc Natl Acad Sci USA* 1988;85:3918.

47. Weitzman SA, Lee RM, Ouellette AJ. Alterations in c-abl gene methylation in cells transformed by phagocyte-generated oxidants. *Biochem Biophys Res Commun* 1989;158:24.

48. Richter C, Park JW, Ames BN. Normal oxidative damage to mitochondrial and nuclear DNA is extensive. *Proc Natl Acad Sci USA* 1988;85:6465.

49. Zimmermann R, Cerutti P. Active oxygen acts as a promotor of transformation in mouse embryo C3H/10T1/2 fibroblasts. *Proc Natl Acad Sci USA* 1984;81:2085.

50. Weitzman S, Weitberg AB, Clark EP, Stossel TP. Phagocytes as carcinogens: malignant transformation produced by human neutrophils. *Science* 1985;227:1231.

51. Gutteridge JMC. Iron promotion of Fenton reaction and lipid peroxidation can be released from haemoglobin by peroxides. *FEBS Lett* 1986;201:291.

52. Biemond P, van Eijk HG, Swask AJG, Koster JF. Iron mobilization from ferritin by superoxide derived from stimulated leukocytes. *J Clin Invest* 1984;73:1576.

53. Halliwell B, Gutteridge JMC, Blake D. Metal ions and oxygen radical reactions in human inflammatory joint disease. *Philos Trans R Soc Lond* 1985;311:659.

54. Drew RM, Painter RB, Feinendegen LE. Oxygen inhibition of nucleic acid synthesis in HeLa S3 cells. *Exp Cell Res* 1964;36:297.

55. Junod AF, Clement A, Jornot L, Petersen H. Differential effects of hyperoxia and hydrogen peroxide on thymidine kinase and adenosine kinase activities of cultured endothelial cells. *Biochim Biophys Acta* 1985;847:20.

56. Sturrock JE, Nunn JF. Chromosomal damage and mutations after exposure of Chinese hamster cells to high concentrations of oxygen. *Mutat Res* 1978;57:27.

57. Wittner M, Rosenbaum RM. Inhibition and reversal of intranuclear RNA synthesis in cultured mammalian cells. *J Appl Physiol* 1972;33:820.

58. Keeling PL, Smith LS. Relevance of NADPH depletion and mixed disulfide formation in rat lung to the mechanism of cell damage following paraquat administration. *Biochem Pharmacol* 1982;31:3243.

59. Richter C, Frei B. Ca^{2+} release from mitochondria induced by prooxidants. *Free Rad Biol Med* 1988;4:365.

60. Moore M, Thor H, Moore G, Nelson S, Moldeus P, Orrenius S. The toxicity of acetaminophen and *N*-acetyl-*p*-benzoquinone in isolated hepatocytes is associated with thiol depletion and increased cytosolic Ca^{2+}. *J Biol Chem* 1985;260:13035.

61. Moody CS, Hassan HN. Mutagenicity of oxygen radicals. *Proc Natl Acad Sci USA* 1982;79:2853.

62. Rosen H, Rakita RM, Waltersdorph AM, Klebanoff SJ. Myeloperoxidase-mediated damage to the succinate oxidase system of *Escherichia coli*. *J Biol Chem* 1987;242:15004.

63. Albrich JM, Gilbaugh JH, Callahan KB, Hurst JK. Effects of the putative neutrophil-generated toxin, hypochlorous acid, on membrane permeability and transport systems of *Escherichia coli*. *J Clin Invest* 1986;78:177.

64. Grisham MB, Jefferson MM, Melton DF, Thomas EL. Chlorination of endogenous amines by isolated neutrophils. *J Biol Chem* 1984;259:10404.

65. Fliss H, Weissbach H, Brot N. Oxidation of methionine residues in proteins of activated human neutrophils. *Proc Natl Acad Sci USA* 1983;80:7160.

66. Grisham MB, Jefferson MM, Thomas EL. Role of monochloramine in the oxidation of erythrocyte hemoglobin by stimulated neutrophils. *J Biol Chem* 1984;259:6766.

67. Weiss SJ. Tissue destruction by neutrophils. *N Engl J Med* 1989;320:365.

THE LUNG: Scientific Foundations
edited by R.G. Crystal, J.B. West et al.
Raven Press, Ltd., New York © 1991.

CHAPTER 7.2.2

Antioxidants and the Lung

John E. Heffner and John E. Repine

THE LUNG IS EXPOSED TO MANY OXIDANTS

Oxidants appear to play important roles in the lung in both health and disease (1,2). Under normal circumstances, generation of oxidants by phagocytic cells (alveolar macrophages, monocytes, and neutrophils) residing in the lung probably occurs daily and is essential for effective host-defense against invading microorganisms. The latter premise is indirectly but well supported by the frequent, often life-threatening infections of patients with chronic granulomatous disease (CGD)—a condition in which neutrophils and microphages fail to generate O_2 metabolites and correspondingly do not kill bacteria well *in vitro* (3,4) (see Chapter 7.4.2). It is also likely that O_2 metabolites serve as key mediators in a variety of biologically relevant control processes which are not well defined at the present time.

Considerable evidence also links oxidants to the development of a number of human lung diseases (see Chapters 7.2.1, 7.2.4, 7.3.5, 7.7.1, 7.7.2, 7.9.1, and 8.2.2). Oxidants can be generated by endogenous mechanisms involving phagocytes, xanthine oxidase, cytochrome P450 oxidases, mitochondria, and arachidonic acid metabolism. Lung oxidants can also be increased from exogenous sources, such as inspiration of polluted air and cigarette smoke. Pathologic processes accounting for increased production of oxidants internally include inflammation, ischemia–reperfusion (hypoxia–reoxygenation) insults, inhalation of toxic gases or inert particles, and intake of certain delete-

J. E. Heffner: Medical Intensive Care Unit, Department of Medicine, St. Joseph's Hospital and Medical Center, Phoenix, Arizona 85013.

J. E. Repine: Department of Medicine, Webb Waring Lung Institute, University of Colorado Health Sciences Center, Denver, Colorado 80262.

rious drugs. Indeed, it is probable that oxidants contribute to tissue injury in inflammatory phases of the adult respiratory distress syndrome (ARDS), in xenobiotic exposure (e.g., bleomycin, paraquat, and nitrofurantoin), in inorganic dust inhalation (fibrosis, silicosis), in toxic gas inhalation (e.g., hyperoxia, ozone, NO_2), in ischemia–reperfusion disorders (transplantation, pulmonary embolism), and in emphysema (directly and indirectly via inactivation of antiproteases). These contributions of oxidants to beneficial and detrimental lung processes are described in detail in other chapters (see above list) and in prior reviews (5–21).

ANTIOXIDANT DEFENSES: SOME GENERAL CONCEPTS

Some general concepts have emerged regarding the action of antioxidants which relate to the varied and highly reactive nature of toxic oxygen metabolite species.

First, there is a *specificity* in the scavenging ability of various antioxidants. Nearly every cell contains a number of enzymatic scavengers, including superoxide dismutase (SOD), catalase, and glutathione redox systems which degrade specific oxidants in specific ways (Fig. 1). For example, SOD converts superoxide anion (O_2^-) to hydrogen peroxide (H_2O_2), whereas catalase preferentially degrades H_2O_2.

Second, there is often a selective *localization* within cells of each antioxidant. For example, manganese-rich SOD is localized near mitochondrial structures, whereas SOD rich in copper–zinc is primarily localized in cytoplasmic areas. The significance of this localization is not fully appreciated.

Third, antioxidant levels and activities are not stable. Antioxidant enzymes can be inactivated by oxidants. SOD is susceptible to inactivation by H_2O_2, and O_2^-, can inactivate catalase. Moreover, appropriate stimulation, such as sublethal exposure to oxidants,

1. *Superoxide dismutase (SOD)*

   a. Manganese SOD:mitochondrial
   b. Copper–Zinc SOD:cytosol/nuclear

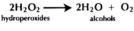

$$2O_2^- + 2H^+ \longrightarrow H_2O_2 + O_2$$

superoxide anion → hydrogen peroxide

2. *Catalase*

$$2H_2O_2 \longrightarrow 2H_2O + O_2$$

hydrogen peroxide → water

3. *Glutathione redox cycle*

$$2H_2O_2 \longrightarrow 2H_2O + O_2$$

hydroperoxides → alcohols

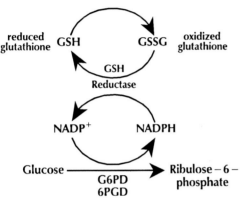

FIG. 1. Lung intracellular antioxidant enzyme systems. The three major systems—superoxide dismutase, catalase, and the glutathione redox cycle—are shown (see text for details).

can increase antioxidants through genetic and other mechanisms.

Fourth, a large number of extracellular antioxidants exist whose relative importance is unclear (see Chapter 7.2.3). These include ceruloplasmin, extracellular SOD, lactoferrin, β-carotene, bilirubin, albumin, and other molecules. The importance of these extracellular antioxidants is unknown, but they appear to be necessary for maintaining oxidant–antioxidant balance, especially along blood endothelial barriers. In addition, blood cells contain antioxidants and can travel to, as well as augment, lung antioxidants. It has recently been observed that antioxidants in erythrocytes, leukocytes, and platelets can decrease oxidants *in vitro* and can also decrease oxidant-mediated injury to bystanding tissues. The latter raises the intriguing possibility that antioxidants can be selectively increased locally during inflammation, hemorrhage, or transudation of fluid into lung parenchymal and even alveolar spaces.

Fifth, the ability to increase antioxidants by pharmacologic methods has not been satisfactory. Primarily, it is difficult to keep high concentrations of highly efficient antioxidant enzymes in the circulation. At-

tempts at increasing antioxidant enzyme half-life by polyethylene glycol conjugation or liposome have improved antioxidant activity but have inherent limitations. Thus, on the one hand, the large size of antioxidant enzymes has limited the accessibility of these large effective antioxidant enzymes to key locations. On the other hand, the effectiveness of small permeant chemical scavengers has been limited by their lack of efficiency in degrading O_2 metabolite species. These molecules are metabolized by reaction with oxidants, and thus it is very difficult to maintain sufficient concentrations of these agents.

DIRECT ANTIOXIDANT MECHANISMS: ANTIOXIDANT ENZYME SYSTEMS (FIG. 1)

Catalase, SOD, and the enzymes of the glutathione redox cycle are primary intracellular antioxidant defense mechanisms. These antioxidant enzymes eliminate O_2 radicals and hydroperoxides that may subsequently oxidize crucial cellular structures. These antioxidant enzyme systems also inhibit free-radical chain reactions by decreasing radicals which initiate the process.

Catalase is one of the antioxidant enzymes which has appreciable reductive activity for H_2O_2 and other small methyl or ethyl hydroperoxides but which does not metabolize large-molecule peroxides, such as lipid peroxide products of lipid peroxidation. Catalase is located primarily in peroxisomes, which contain many of the enzymes that generate H_2O_2 in aerobic cells (22).

The *glutathione redox cycle* is a central mechanism for reduction of intracellular hydroperoxides. This mechanism complements catalase as a reducing system for H_2O_2, but it most likely exceeds catalase in its capacity to eliminate additional toxic hydroperoxides (23). Glutathione metabolism also degrades large-molecule lipid peroxides (formed through free-radical action on polyunsaturated lipid membranes) and products of lipoxygenase-catalyzed reactions. The key enzyme in the glutathione redox cycle responsible for reduction of hydroperoxides is glutathione peroxidase (GSH-Px). Nonstressed cells maintain a high intracellular GSH/GSSG ratio (GSH stands for reduced glutathione; GSSG stands for oxidized glutathione) to ensure availability of GSH and thereby promote active reduction of hydroperoxides through the glutathione redox cycle. Cells maintain a high GSH/GSSG ratio in two ways. First, in contrast to GSH, GSSG can be transported out of the cell. Transmembrane transport systems occur in liver and heart cells and undoubtedly occur in the lung (24). Second, GSSG is converted to GSH by GSH reductase, which catalyzes reduction of other low-molecular-weight disulfides but not mixed disulfides (25). The capacity to recycle GSH makes the

GSH redox cycle a pivotal antioxidant defense mechanism for cells and prevents the depletion of cellular thiols. Regeneration of GSH requires nicotinamide-adenine dinucleotide phosphate (NADP)-reducing equivalents that are supplied through glucose-6-phosphate dehydrogenase (G6PD) activity in the hexose monophosphate shunt. Cellular distribution of GSH-Px is tightly bound to GSH reductase. Both enzymes exist predominantly in the cytosol; however, mitochondria also have some GSH redox activity, and a GSH-Px exists in human plasma (26). The GSH redox cycle may be the more important antioxidant peroxidase in mammalian species. Studies of human inborn errors of metabolism confirm that the importance of catalase deficiency is secondary to that of the defects in GSH redox function in removing H_2O_2 produced in rats (27). The importance of the GSH redox cycle relative to that of catalase for the reduction of H_2O_2 may be a consequence of several factors. First, catalase activity is largely confined to peroxisomes, whereas enzymes of the GSH redox cycle are distributed throughout the cytosol, allowing greater availability and a higher likelihood of contact with oxidants. Second, the substrate concentration that produces half-maximal velocity is lower for GSH-Px than for catalase (28). This suggests that GSH-Px is the preferential pathway for the degradation of low concentrations of H_2O_2 present in intact cells. Although catalase has a low affinity for H_2O_2, it has a higher capacity for hydroperoxide metabolism. Accordingly, catalase appears to be more important when rates of H_2O_2 generation are increased to levels where a greater enzyme rate constant becomes necessary.

G6PD and *6-phosphogluconate dehydrogenase* are significant antioxidant enzymes, because they catalyze reactions that supply NADPH (the reduced form of NADP) for completion of the redox cycle regeneration of GSH (29). This postulate is most convincingly supported by the observation that cells deficient in G6PD activity are sensitive to oxidant injury. More specifically, erythrocytes from patients with G6PD deficiency are easily lysed by oxidants (30). This metabolic pathway also serves as an antioxidant system in other cell lines, and G6PD is increased in rat liver cells under oxidative stress. The antioxidant capacity of the generated NADPH is limited to the GSH redox cycle.

SOD is an enzyme which uses superoxide anion (O_2^-) as a substrate (31,32). SOD has variable effectiveness in protecting against oxidant damage. For example, in some systems SOD enhances lipid peroxidation, whereas in others it limits membrane injury. These opposing effects may be determined by local concentrations of free iron and catalase. The concentration of SOD may be a key determinant. In the presence of excess iron, SOD can increase OH· formation and tissue injury by generating H_2O_2, which then reacts with Fe^{3+} in the Haber–Weiss reaction. If tissue iron is compartmentalized and unavailable for reaction, catalase or peroxidases can reduce H_2O_2 generated by SOD to nontoxic products. In this latter condition, SOD would have protective antioxidant effects by eliminating O_2^- that would otherwise reduce Fe^{3+} to Fe^{2+} and thereby promote OH· formation (33). In conditions wherein catalase activity is insufficient to metabolize generated H_2O_2, SOD may increase oxidant tissue injury (34).

Taken *en toto*, SOD, catalase, and GSH peroxidase are highly complementary enzyme systems that optimally combine to limit oxidant stress (35). These antioxidants also protect each other from oxidant inactivation. For example, H_2O_2 can inactivate SOD, and O_2^- can inhibit catalase and peroxidase function (36).

Nonenzymatic Antioxidants

Vitamin E is a lipid-soluble antioxidant which limits oxidant-induced membrane injury in human tissue (37). By virtue of its hydrophobicity, vitamin E partitions into lipid membranes, thereby being positioned optimally for maximal antioxidant effectiveness. Vitamin E is a particularly effective antioxidant which converts O_2^-, OH·, and lipid peroxyl radicals to less reactive O_2 metabolites. Although present in extracellular fluids, the antioxidant activity of vitamin E is localized predominantly in the cell membrane.

Beta-carotene is a metabolic precursor to vitamin A. It accumulates in high concentrations in the membranes of certain tissues. Furthermore, it can scavenge O_2^- and react directly with peroxyl-free radicals, thereby serving as an additional lipid soluble antioxidant (38).

Vitamin C is widely available in both extracellular and intracellular spaces in most biologic systems where it can participate in redox reactions. Vitamin C can directly scavenge O_2^- and OH·, forming a semidehydroascorbate-free radical that is subsequently reduced by GSH to generate dehydroascorbate and GS; it can also neutralize several oxidants present in the blood of smokers (39). Vitamin C is usually not considered a major antioxidant, because it also has additional pro-oxidant properties. Vitamin C is probably the only cellular reducing agent (other than O_2^-) capable of converting Fe^{3+} to Fe^{2+}, which can then react with H_2O_2 to form OH· by Haber–Weiss-type mechanisms.

Uric acid, formed by the catabolism of purines, may have antioxidant properties (40). Urate primarily scavenges (a) OH· formed by the reaction of peroxides with hemoglobin and (b) peroxyl radicals from lipid peroxidation. Additionally, uric acid prevents the oxidation of vitamin C and binds transition metal in forms that will not stimulate free-radical reactions.

Taurine is an amino acid which is distributed in both extracellular and intracellular spaces. Taurine accumulates to high intracellular concentrations, particularly in cells normally associated with high rates of oxygen radical generation or in cells rich in membranes (41). In addition to its established role in xenobiotic conjugation reactions, taurine may also protect against reactive oxygen radicals, because it reacts directly with such species as hypochlorous acid (HOCl) to form less reactive species.

Albumin is an additional antioxidant that can bind copper tightly and iron weakly to its surface (27,42). Other noncrucial molecules, such as mucus, may also provide protection.

INDIRECT ANTIOXIDANT MECHANISMS

The potential for assault by endogenous and exogenous oxidants mandates that all cells use many different antioxidant strategies, including some indirect approaches to prevent or limit oxidant injury (43). Some of these indirect mechanisms provide antioxidant protection by preventing formation of free radicals, preventing conversion of oxidants to more toxic species, and/or effectively repairing molecular defects resulting from oxidants.

Reduction of Oxidant Formation

Decreasing excess oxidant formation is a first step in improving cell survival. Considerable oxygen radical formation occurs during normal cellular oxidative phosphorylation. Within mitochondria, the majority of oxygen metabolized in the respiratory chain is reduced to water without significant formation of free radicals. However, conditions such as hyperoxia can result in enhanced oxygen radical formation from the mitochondrial electron-transport chain. Minimizing substrate and stimuli which increase O_2 radical production is a reasonable strategy for antioxidant defense. O_2 metabolite production by phagocytes can also be reduced by decreasing the number of cells or by preventing their adherence to key structures. The latter capitalizes on the short half-lives of oxygen species which require their generation in close apposition to the target. Inhibition of O_2 metabolite generating NADPH oxidase activation in phagocyte membranes also provides a way of decreasing O_2 metabolite formation. Reduction of O_2 metabolites by xanthine oxidase can also be accomplished by allopurinol or tungsten treatment. Reduction of O_2 metabolite generation has intrinsic advantages over attempts to scavenge O_2 metabolites, which can never be totally complete.

Removal of Factors Which Enhance Oxidant Toxicity

Certain substances convert less toxic O_2 metabolite species to more toxic O_2 metabolite species. Transitional metal ions, most notably iron, play a major role in the generation of more toxic oxygen species in facilitating Haber–Weiss chemical reaction (27,44). The intense reactivity and cytotoxicity of OH· found by reaction of O_2^- and H_2O_2 with Fe^{2+} suggests that prevention of OH· formation through limitation of transitional metal availability is an important cell defense process. The extracellular space is a particularly important arena for control of transition metal OH· generation. Substrates for the Haber–Weiss reaction, O_2^- and H_2O_2, are present through release from phagocytic cells, and a relative lack of extracellular antioxidant enzyme systems exists to eliminate these species.

The availability of free extracellular iron to react with O_2^- and H_2O_2 is avoided through several mechanisms. Hemoglobin is stored and protected within erythrocytes that are rich in antioxidant defense mechanisms (45). The majority of remaining extracellular iron is bound avidly (in the form of ferric ion) to transferrin and lactoferrin, which are iron-binding glycoproteins that transport iron in the circulation (46). The transferrin- or lactoferrin-bound iron is unavailable for participation in the Haber–Weiss reaction. Lactoferrin has a greater affinity for iron than does transferrin at low pH and is also only partially loaded at basal conditions. Ceruloplasmin, a plasma glycoprotein acute-phase reactant, is an important extracellular antioxidant that functions coordinately with transferrin to promote iron binding and prevention of metal-catalyzed, free-radical reactions; it also prevents the nonenzymatic generation of O_2^-, scavenges O_2^- and H_2O_2, and suppresses the oxidative inactivation of proteases by products of the leukocyte myeloperoxidase system. Lastly, ceruloplasmin binds copper, preventing its participation in H_2O_2-forming reactions.

Cellular iron is unavailable for participation in free-radical reactions because it is bound to ferritin. Iron-catalyzed reactions may be limited by the presence of human plasma of transferrin in concentrations in excess of that required for iron transport. This unexplained excess may support tissue and alveolar transferrin concentrations in regions of alveolitis to allow rapid binding of free iron released from macrophages in smokers (47). Additionally, release of lactoferrin from phagocytes may be a biologic protective mechanism for removing extracellular iron produced through cellular inflammation.

Repair of Oxidant Injury

Molecular repair has been investigated thoroughly in the effects of ionizing radiation on nucleic acid injury and carcinogenesis (48). Injury occurs by radical attack (on the pyrimidine) of deoxyribose sugar-phosphate bonds, causing liberation of free bases from the nucleotide. In chemical systems of free-radical injury of endothelial cells, H_2O_2 combined with intracellular iron causes DNA single-strand breakage (49). Minor-to-moderate damage is repaired by activation of a nuclear enzyme (namely, protein ADP ribosyl transferase) that causes excision–repair to occur. Severe damage, however, causes protein ADP ribosyl transferase to greatly deplete cellular NAD^+ levels and initiate cytotoxicity. The latter function of the enzyme may be an attempt to sacrifice the individual cell with a damaged genome in favor of preservation of the whole organism.

ANTIOXIDANT RESPONSES OF THE LUNG

Interest in increasing endogenous antioxidant enzyme activity was pioneered by the striking observation that rats exposed to a sublethal concentration of oxygen were protected from the lethality of subsequent exposure to normobaric hyperoxia (50)—a protective effect which correlated with increased intracellular SOD, catalase, G6PD, and GSH-Px activity. The potential protective role of the induced antioxidant enzymes was also suggested when a similar type of protection against hyperoxia was observed in neonatal rats. Young rats can rapidly induce antioxidant enzymes after exposure to sublethal partial pressures of oxygen which fail to induce enzymes (and fail to confer tolerance to hyperoxia) in older rats (51). The capacity of pulmonary antioxidant enzymes to increase in rat lung cells may be an adaptive mechanism of the fetus in preparation for exposure to oxygen after birth. Indeed, lung SOD, GSH-Px, catalase, and G6PD activities increase in fetal lungs toward term. In contrast, adult animals may lose this adaptive ability. For unexplained reasons, adult rats do not increase SOD activities after oxygen exposure.

It is uncertain whether observations suggesting a role for intracellular antioxidants in the protection against hyperoxia can be applied to other species other than the rat. Mice, guinea pigs, and hamsters reveal little or no induction of SOD after exposure to sublethal hyperoxia, and tolerance to lethal concentrations of hyperoxia does not occur. In addition, a patient with partial monosomy 21 has recently been studied who had an apparent increased sensitivity to pulmonary oxygen toxicity (52). Because the gene for CuZnSOD is on chromosome 21, contained in the missing genome segment, the patient's SOD activity in blood samples was decreased. Catalase activity was normal. After an inadvertent 4.5-hr exposure to 100% inspired oxygen, the patient developed pulmonary respiratory failure which was attributed to oxygen toxicity. This single case report suggests the importance (in humans) of intracellular SOD in the protection against hyperoxic lung injury.

The role of intracellular antioxidant enzymes has also been investigated in studies of endotoxin-induced tolerance to hyperoxia. Endotoxin pretreatment decreases lethality in adult rats exposed to normobaric hyperoxia; SOD, catalase, and GSH-Px activities increase and correlate with survival (53). Lung antioxidant enzyme activities increase, but the contribution of the increased antioxidant enzymes to improved survival is uncertain. In addition, endotoxin prevents hyperoxic injury to cultured endothelial cells in the absence of SOD induction. Furthermore, serum from endotoxin-treated rats protects recipient rats against hyperoxic lung injury without altering lung SOD activity. Antecedent tissue necrosis factor/cachectin (TNF/C) and interleukin-1 (IL-1) treatment also protected rats from hyperoxia. Interestingly, induction of lung antioxidant enzymes had not occurred after 52 hr of hyperoxia exposure—a time which was just before control (54). In later investigations, however, it was noted that lung G6PD, SOD, GSH-Px, GSH reductase, and catalase levels were increased after 72 hr of hyperoxia in rats treated with TNF/C and IL-1—again a time when all control rats had already died. Only GSH reductase and G6PD activities were slightly increased earlier after 4 or 16 hr of exposure. These studies suggest that TNF/C and IL-1 infusion may mediate lung protection from hyperoxia, possibly through antioxidant enzyme induction and/or possibly via other mechanisms such as recruitment to the lung of more resistant cell lines. Other investigators have demonstrated induction of mitochondrial MnSOD in cultured cells exposed to TNF/C and to IL-1 (55).

Alterations in the GSH redox cycle may contribute to defense against oxidants generated in the extracellular space. Inhibition of lung GSH reductase activity after infusion of 1,3-bis(2-chloroethyl)-1-nitrosourea (BCNU) augments antioxidant responses. Inhibition of lung G6PD activity, the supportive system supplying reducing equivalents to the GSH redox cycle, caused lung edema after infusion of a previously sublethal dose of xanthine oxidase. These findings were supported by cell culture studies, with endothelial and epithelial cells demonstrating potentiation of H_2O_2 toxicity with inhibition of various enzymes in the GSH redox cycle (56).

Airway Localization of Antioxidant Activity

The alveolar space can recruit additional antioxidant activity from the epithelial lining fluid. Alveolar fluid contains large amounts of GSH, in concentrations exceeding plasma concentrations by 100 times or more (57). Over 90% of the GSH exists in the reduced form in sufficient concentrations to protect against H_2O_2 generated by stimulated alveolar macrophages. The source of alveolar GSH is uncertain but is suspected to be the epithelial cell. Catalase is also found in large quantities in the epithelial lining fluid. Additional antioxidants contained in the alveolar space in low concentrations include ceruloplasmin, transferrin, ascorbate, vitamin E, ferritin, other serum protein, and small molecules such as bilirubin and methionine. These compounds help broaden the spectrum of antioxidant protection of the lower respiratory tract.

Pulmonary Recruitment of Cells with Antioxidant Potential

Erythrocytes are rich in antioxidant systems that include SOD, catalase, and components of the GSH redox cycle (58). Additionally, erythrocyte membranes contain an anion channel through which O_2^- can enter the cell, thereby becoming available for dismutation by erythrocyte SOD. H_2O_2 is also freely diffusible across erythrocyte membranes. Erythrocytes decrease the toxicity of an O_2^-/H_2O_2 generating system on the lysis of murine leukemia cells *in vitro* (59). Furthermore, erythrocytes from patients with a smoking history contain more GSH and catalase than do those from nonsmokers, presumably because the erythrocytes of smokers are constantly exposed to oxidative stress and undergo induction of protein synthesis (60). These antioxidant-enhanced erythrocytes protect endothelial cells in culture from H_2O_2 more effectively than do those from nonsmokers. Whether certain smokers who resist vascular injury from smoking do so because they have the ability to increase antioxidants in their erythrocytes and other cells is unknown. When infused into the isolated perfused rabbit lung, erythrocytes attenuated lung edema formation caused by addition of xanthine oxidase into the otherwise cell-free perfusate (58). The mechanism of protection depended on erythrocyte catalase. In addition, isolated rabbit lungs exposed to ischemia undergo less edema formation and decreased malonaldehyde (a product of lipid peroxidation) release in the presence of erythrocytes (61). Ischemic, isolated hearts incurred less injury and exhibited decreased tissue H_2O_2 concentrations when reperfused with erythrocytes; protection also occurred after the addition of glutaraldehyde-fixed erythrocytes, which do not release SOD or catalase after treatment with H_2O_2 (62). Insufflation of erythrocytes into the airways of rabbits protected lung function from injury after a subsequent exposure to hyperoxia (63). Most of these studies have identified erythrocyte catalase as the most active reductant in

protecting the lung, although a role for erythrocyte GSH redox cycle also appears likely.

Platelets also contain catalase and components of the GSH redox cycle; they are equal to erythrocytes with regard to intracellular GSH content, and they are several times more active in terms of GSH-Px function. The antioxidant potential of platelets is supported by the finding that gel-filtered platelets consume extracellular H_2O_2 in the range of zero to 400 μM at an exponential rate *in vitro*. Furthermore, incubation of platelets *in vitro* with xanthine oxidase is associated with marked stimulation of their hexose monophosphate shunt pathway that results in the metabolism of generated H_2O_2 through the GSH redox cycle. Platelets decreased oxidant-induced lung injury in isolated perfused rabbit lungs. Infusion of washed human platelets reduced oxidant-mediated lung edema generated by the coinfusion of xanthine oxidase. Because lung protection was blocked by inhibition of platelet GSH redox cycle enzymes but not by inhibition of catalase, platelet protection appeared to depend on reduction of H_2O_2 by GSH-dependent mechanisms (64). Platelets also decreased ischemia–reperfusion injury in the isolated rabbit lungs—a finding which further emphasizes the ability of intravascular antioxidants to scavenge intracellularly generated oxygen metabolites (65). These observations, suggesting a role for platelets in attenuating oxidant-induced injury, are supported by findings *in vivo* in rats that lung toxicity from α-naphthylthiourea is potentiated in the absence of circulating platelets. This impression is supported by studies in the isolated perfused rabbit lung demonstrating that human platelets depleted of G6PD augment oxidant lung injury, whereas control platelets prevent it (66).

Phagocytes might contribute to antioxidant defense mechanisms. Phagocytes (alveolar macrophages, monocytes, and neutrophils) contain considerable antioxidants and lower H_2O_2 concentration *in vitro* (67).

ANTIOXIDANT PHARMACOLOGY: TREATMENT WITH ANTIOXIDANT ENZYMES (FIG. 2)

The use of SOD and catalase as a treatment to decrease oxidant-induced lung injury has produced variable results. Infusion of catalase decreased pulmonary edema generated by air emboli, immune-complex alveolitis, alveolar damage after airway instillation of phorbol myristate acetate (PMA), and diffuse pulmonary microvascular injury after systemic activation of complement. Exogenous SOD treatment decreased lung edema in sheep after infusion of microemboli and prolonged survival in rats exposed to hyperoxia when SOD was infused continuously in the peritoneal space.

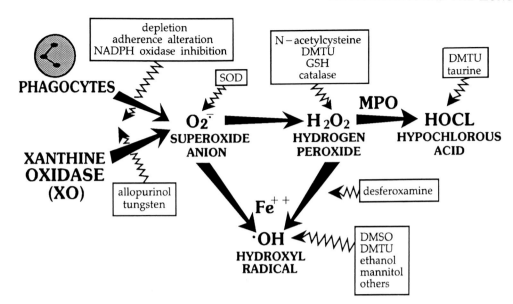

FIG. 2. Common experimental strategies regarding oxidants in the lung. Two sources of oxidants are phagocytes and xanthine oxidase. In boxes are indicated the specific antioxidants that inhibit specific oxidants or that inhibit conversion from one oxidant to another (see text for details and abbreviations). Abbreviations not found in text: DMSO, dimethyl sulfoxide; MPO, monoamine peroxidase.

However, increasing plasma levels of SOD did not decrease lung toxicity after neonatal hyperoxic exposure in the rat. SOD also did not decrease injury to cultured endothelial cells after incubation with stimulated neutrophils or glucose oxidase. The effectiveness of SOD and catalase may be limited by their large molecular mass (which prevents intracellular transport) or by their charge (which prevents their adherence to targets). At the present time, major benefits of exogenous catalase and SOD may be considered to involve elimination of extracellular oxidants that either directly alter membrane permeability or serve as neutrophil chemotactic factors.

Liposome encapsulation has been used to improve the intracellular uptake of SOD and catalase. Liposome-encapsulated SOD increased intracellular SOD concentrations to 6–12 times normal values in cultured aortic endothelial cells (68). Furthermore, liposomal antioxidant enzymes injected into intact animals or instilled into the airway prolong survival after exposure to hyperoxia. Effectiveness of liposomes in animals may require that they not become engulfed by phagocytes (69); in these models, phagocytes may need to be removed by, or at least be preoccupied with, latex beads. Conjugation of antioxidant enzymes with polyethylene glycol (PEG) decreases pulmonary oxygen toxicity in rats (70) and reduces alveolar capillary membrane permeability after the infusion of endotoxin in pigs (71).

The antioxidant activities of PEG-conjugated antioxidants may relate to the enhanced survival and OH· scavenging ability of protein-bound PEG (70). PEG-conjugated antioxidants also have the ability to interact with membrane surfaces in ways that may enhance their effectiveness (72).

Exogenous GSH treatment improved the antioxidant capacity of lung cells. Survival time was prolonged in rodents exposed to hyperoxia following supplementation with exogenous GSH (73). Additionally, cultured rat type II alveolar cells were more resistant to paraquat-induced injury in the presence of added extracellular GSH. Limitation of cellular GSH uptake with transport-blocking agents prevented protection by exogenous GSH in hyperoxic or paraquat-induced injury, indicating that transmembrane GSH transport is occurring.

Supplementation with Nonenzymatic Antioxidants

Vitamin E only protects vitamin E-deficient animals from oxidant-mediated damage. Studies clearly indicate that rodents with preexisting vitamin E deficiency have increased oxidant injury after exposure to hyperoxia, endotoxin, or ozone (74) and that the degree of injury can be attenuated with repletion of vitamin E (75). However, normal animals receive little benefit from additional pharmacologic supplementation with vitamin E. Despite the fact that some studies show protection from lung injury and decreased lipid peroxidation in rodents, there is little beneficial effect of supplemental vitamin E in antioxidant-replete animals after exposure to oxidant challenge.

N-*acetylcysteine* treatment has decreased oxidant injury in several models of lung damage. Smoke instilled in the airways of isolated rat lungs caused a rapid and dose-dependent depletion of total lung GSH which was attenuated when N-acetylcysteine was added to the perfusate (76). This antioxidant effect was mediated through accelerated GSH biosynthesis rather than through direct antioxidant mechanisms. The latter hypothesis was advanced because buthionine sulfoximine, a GSH synthesis inhibitor, blocked the protective effect. Infusing N-acetylcysteine into cannulated sheep reduced lung lymph clearance after endotoxin infusion (77).

Dimethylthiourea (DMTU) is a low-molecular-weight scavenger of OH·, H_2O_2, and HOCl (78,79). DMTU has a long biologic half-life and distributes well across cell membranes because of its small size. DMTU decreases (a) oxidant-induced injury in hyperoxic toxicity to alveolar macrophages *in vitro*, (b) neutrophil and oxygen metabolite-mediated edema in isolated perfused lungs, and (c) lung injury in intact rats exposed to hyperoxia, PMA, or thiourea. DMTU has furthered research into the development of a small, permeant, inexpensive scavenger capable of producing a marker of antioxidant activity, thereby detecting oxidant-mediated mechanisms in pulmonary disease.

FUTURE POSSIBILITIES

Genetic control and induction of antioxidants by altering their synthesis at fundamental levels holds great promise for understanding and controlling oxidant-mediated processes. Increases in antioxidants that occur in rats exposed to hyperoxia, hypoxia, cytokines, or endotoxin are most likely mediated by genetic control mechanisms (80). The system involves pretranslational synthesis of the enzyme under normal gestational and postgestational conditions; pretranslational changes occur in neonatal rats, and post-translational changes occur in adult rats exposed to hyperoxia. Furthermore, fibroblast cell clones generated by recombinant gene technology that overproduce human CuZnSOD are relatively resistant to injury caused by hypoxia (81). It is also intriguing that cytokine products from endotoxin treatment can also induce antioxidant enzymes. Induction of MnSOD mRNA was found after treatment with TNF-β, IL-1a, and IL-1B, but not after treatment with other cytokines. TNF-α induces MnSOD mRNA in a variety of cell lines and in various organs of mice *in vivo*.

It has become increasingly clear that free radicals contribute in varying degrees to the pathogenesis of several pulmonary conditions. It has also become equally clear that the lung depends on a delicate balance between oxidant and antioxidant systems to maintain normal cellular function. Much remains to be learned about intracellular and extracellular antioxidants in the lung, and also about their function, in health and disease.

REFERENCES

1. Weiss SJ. Oxygen, ischemia, inflammation. *Acta Physiol Scand* 1986;548:9–37.
2. Halliwell B, Grootveld M. The measurement of free radical reactions in humans. Some thoughts for future experimentation. *FEBS Lett* 1987;213:9–14.
3. Holmes B, Page AR, Good RA. Studies of the metabolic activity of leukocytes from patients with a genetic abnormality of phagocytic function. *J Clin Invest* 1967;46:1422–1428.
4. Hoidal JR, Fox RB, Repine JE. Defective oxidative metabolic reponses *in vitro* of alveolar macrophages in chronic granulomatous disease. *Am Rev Respir Dis* 1979;120:613–618.
5. Harlan JM, Killen PD, Harker LA, Striker GE. Neutrophil-mediated endothelial injury *in vitro*. *J Clin Invest* 1981;68:1394–1403.
6. Shasby DM, Vanbenthuysen KM, Tate RM, Shasby SS, McMurtry I, Repine JE. Granulocytes mediate acute edematous lung injury in rabbits and in isolated rabbit lungs perfused with phorbol myristate acetate: role of oxygen radicals. *Am Rev Respir Dis* 1982;125:443–447.
7. Varani J, Fligiel SEG, Till GO, Kunkel RG, Ryan US, Ward PA. Pulmonary endothelial cell killing by human neutrophils: possible involvement by hydroxyl radical. *Lab Invest* 1986;53:656–663.
8. Test ST, Lampert MB, Ossanna PJ, Thoene JG, Weiss SJ. Generation of nitrogen–chlorine oxidants by human phagocytes. *J Clin Invest* 1984;74:1342–1349.
9. Baldwin SR, Grum CM, Boxer LA, Simon RH, Ketai LH, Devall LJ. Oxidant activity in expired breath of patients with adult respiratory distress syndrome. *Lancet* 1986;1:11–13.
10. Cochrane CG, Spragg R, Reval SD. Pathogenesis of the adult respiratory distress syndrome: evidence of oxidant activity in bronchoalveolar lavage fluid. *J Clin Invest* 1983;71:754–758.
11. Brigham KL, Meyrick B, Berry LC Jr, Repine JE. Antioxidants protect cultured bovine lung endothelial cells from injury by endotoxin. *J Appl Physiol* 1987;63:840–850.
12. Smith LL. The response of the lung to foreign compounds that produce free radicals. *Annu Rev Physiol* 1986;48:681–692.
13. Smith P, Heath D. Paraquat. *CRC Crit Rev Toxicol* 1976;4:411–445.
14. Snider GL, Hayes JA, Korthy AL. Chronic interstitial pulmonary fibrosis produced in hamsters by endotracheal bleomycin. *Am Rev Respir Dis* 1978;177:1099–1108.
15. Martin WJ. Nitrofurantoin. Potential direct and indirect mechanisms of lung injury. *Chest* 1983;83(Suppl):51S–52S.
16. Mossman BT. Alteration of superoxide dismutase activity in tracheal epithelial cells by asbestos and inhibition of cytotoxicity by antioxidants. *Lab Invest* 1986;54:204–212.
17. DeLucia AJ, Hoque PM, Mustafa MG, Cross CE. Ozone interaction with rabbit lung. I. Effect of sulfhydryls and sulfhydryl-containing enzyme activities. *J Lab Clin Med* 1972;80:559–566.
18. Pryor WA, Dooley MM, Church DR. The mechanisms of the inactivation of human alpha-1-proteinase inhibitor by gas-phase cigarette smoke. *Adv Free Radical Biol Med* 1986;2:161–188.
19. Hoidal JR, Fox RB, Le Marbe PH, Perri R, Repine JE. Altered oxidative metabolic responses *in vitro* of alveolar macrophages from asymptomatic cigarette smokers. *Am Rev Respir Dis* 1981;123:85–89.
20. Carp H, Miller F, Hoidal JR, Janoff A. Potential mechanism of emphysema: alpha-1-proteinase inhibitor recovered from lungs of cigarette smokers contains oxidized methionine and has decreased elastase inhibiting activity. *Proc Natl Acad Sci USA* 1982;79:2041–2045.
21. Turrens JF, Freeman BA, Crapo JD. Hyperoxia increases H_2O_2

release by lung mitochondria microsomes. *Arch Biochem Biophys* 1982;217:411–421.

22. Chance B, Sies H, Boveris A. Hydroperoxide metabolism in mammalian organs. *Physiol Rev* 1979;59:527–605.
23. Ross D, Norbeck K, Moldeus P. The generation and subsequent fate of glutathionyl radicals in biological systems. *J Biol Chem* 1985;260:155028–155032.
24. Sies H, Akerboom TPM. Glutathione disulfide (GSSG) efflux from cells and tissues. *Methods Enzymol* 1984;105:445–451.
25. Nishiki K, Jamieson D, Oshino N, Chance B. Oxygen toxicity in the perfused rat liver and lung under hyperbaric conditions. *Biochem J* 1976;160:343–355.
26. Maddepati KR, Gasparski C, Marnett LJ. Characterization of the hydroperoxide-reducing activity of human plasma. *Arch Biochem Biophys* 1987;254:9–17.
27. Halliwell B, Gutteridge JMC. Oxygen free radicals and iron in relation to biology and medicine: some problems and concepts. *Arch Biochem Biophys* 1986;246:501–514.
28. Jones DP, Eklow L, Thor H, Orrenius S. Metabolism of hydrogen peroxide in isolated hepatocytes: relative contributions of catalase and glutathione peroxidase in decomposition of endogenously generated H_2O_2. *Arch Biochem Biophys* 1981;210:505–516.
29. Jacob HS, Jandl JH. Effects of sulfhydryl inhibition on red blood cells. II. Glutathione in the regulation of the hexose monophosphate pathway. *J Biol Chem* 1966;241:4243–4250.
30. Cohen G, Hochstien P. Glucose-6-phosphate dehydrogenase and detoxification of hydrogen epoxide in human erythrocytes. *Science* 1961;134:1756–1757.
31. Fridovich I, Freeman B. Antioxidant defenses in the lung. *Annu Rev Physiol* 1986;48:693–702.
32. McCord JM, Fridovich I. Superoxide dismutase: an enzymic function for erythrocuprein (hemocuprein). *J Biol Chem* 1969;244:6049–6055.
33. Fridovich IA. The biology of oxygen radicals. *Science.* 1978;201:875–880.
34. Scott MD, Meshnick SR, Eaton JW. Superoxide dismutase-rich bacteria: paradoxical increase in oxidant activity. *J Biol Chem* 1987;262:3640–3645.
35. Heffner JA, Repine JE. State of the art—pulmonary strategies of antioxident defense. *Am Rev Respir Dis* 1989;140:531–534.
36. Kono Y, Fridovich I. Superoxide radical inhibits catalase. *J Biol Chem* 1982;257:5751–5754.
37. Burton GW, Ingold KU. Autooxidation of biological molecules. 1. The antioxidant activity of vitamin E and related chain-breaking phenolic antioxidants *in vitro*. *J Am Chem Soc* 1981;103:6472–6477.
38. Foote CS, Denny RW. Chemistry of singlet oxygen VII. Quenching by beta-carotene. *J Am Chem Soc* 1968;90:6233–6235.
39. Anderson R, Theron AJ, Ras GJ. Ascorbic acid neutralizes reactive oxidants released by hyperactive phagocytes from cigarette smokers. *Lung* 1988;166:149–159.
40. Ames BN, Cathcart R, Schwiers E, Hochstein P. Uric acid provides an antioxidant defense in humans against oxidant- and radical-caused aging and cancer: a hypothesis. *Proc Natl Acad Sci USA* 1981;78:6858–6862.
41. Wright CE, Tallen HH, Lin YY. Taurine: biological update. *Annu Rev Biochem* 1986;55:427–453.
42. Brown JM, Beehler CJ, Berger EM, Grosso MA, Whitman GJ, Terada LS, Leff JA, Harken AH, Repine JE. Albumin decreases hydrogen peroxide and reperfusion injury in isolated rat hearts. *Inflammation* 1989;13:583–589.
43. Sies H. Antioxidant activity in cells and organs. *Am Rev Respir Dis* 1987;136:478–480.
44. Halliwell B, Gutteridge JMC. The importance of free radicals and catalytic metal ions in human diseases. *Mol Aspects Med* 1985;8:89–193.
45. Gutteridge JMC. Ion promoters of the Fenton reaction and lipid peroxidation can be released from haemoglobin by peroxides. *FEBS Lett* 1986;201:291–295.
46. Gutteridge JMC. Antioxidant properties of the proteins caeruloplasmin, albumin and transferrin. A study of their activity in serum and synovial fluid from patients with rheumatoid arthritis. *Biochim Biophys Acta* 1986;869:119–127.
47. Pacht ER, Davis WB. Role of transferrin and ceruloplasmin in antioxidant activity of lung epithelial lining fluid. *J Appl Physiol* 1988;64:2092–2099.
48. Berger NA. Poly(ADP-ribose) in the cellular responses of DNA damage. *Radiat Res* 1985;101:4–15.
49. Schraufstatter IR, Hinshaw DB, Hyslop PA, Spragg RG, Cochrane CG. Oxidant injury of cells. *J Clin Invest* 1986;77:1312–1320.
50. Crapo JD, Tierney DF. Superoxide dismutase and pulmonary oxygen toxicity. *Am J Physiol* 1974;226:1401–1407.
51. Frank L, Bucher JR, Roberts RJ. Oxygen toxicity in neonatal and adult animals of various species. *J Appl Physiol* 1978;45:699–704.
52. Ackerman AD, Fackler JC, Tuck-Muller CM, Tarpey MM, Freeman BA, Rogers MC. Partial monosomy 21, diminished activity of superoxide dismutase, and pulmonary oxygen toxicity. *N Engl J Med* 1990;318:1666–1669.
53. Frank L, Yam J, Roberts RJ. The role of endotoxin in protection of adult rats from oxygen-induced lung toxicity. *J Clin Invest* 1978;61:269–275.
54. White CW, Ghezzi P, Dinarello CA, Caldwell SA, McMurtry IF, Repine JE. Recombinant tumor necrosis factor/cachectin and interleukin 1 pretreatment decreases lung oxidized glutathione accumulation, lung injury, and mortality in rats exposed to hyperoxia. *J Clin Invest* 1987;79:1868–1873.
55. Wong GHW, Goeddel DV. Induction of manganous superoxide dismutase by tumor necrosis factor: possible protective mechanism. *Science* 1988;242:941–949.
56. Suttorp N, Seeger W, Schmidt F, Simon LM, Neuhof H, Roka L. Importance of the glutathione cycle in the defense of lung tissue against a peroxide attack. *Eur J Respir Dis [Suppl]* 1983;126:473.
57. Cantin AM, North SL, Hubbard RC, Crystal RG. Normal alveolar epithelial lining fluid contains high levels of glutathione. *J Appl Physiol* 1987;163:152–157.
58. Toth KM, Clifford DP, Berger EM, White CW, Repine JE. Intact human erythrocytes prevent hydrogen peroxide-mediated damage to isolated perfused rat lungs and cultured bovine pulmonary artery endothelial cells. *J Clin Invest* 1984;74:292–295.
59. Agar NS, Sadradeh SMH, Hallaway PE, Eaton JW. Erythrocyte catalase. A somatic oxidant defense. *J Clin Invest* 1986;77:319–321.
60. Toth KM, Berger EM, Beehler CJ, Repine JE. Erythrocytes from cigarette smokers contain more glutathione and catalase and protect endothelial cells from hydrogen peroxide better than do erythrocytes from nonsmokers. *Am Rev Respir Dis* 1986;134:281–284.
61. Mann J, Hoidal JR, Rao NV, McCusker KT, Kennegy TP. Erythrocytes protect the ischemic lung from oxidant injury during reperfusion [Abstract]. *Am Rev Respir Dis* 1988;137:396.
62. Brown JM, Grosso MA, Terada LS, Repine JE. Erythrocytes decrease myocardial hydrogen peroxide levels and reperfusion injury. *Am J Physiol* 1989;256:H584–H588.
63. Van Asbeck BS, Hoidal J, Vercellotti GM, Schwartz BA, Moldow CF, Jacob HS. Protection against lethal hyperoxia by tracheal insufflation of erythrocytes: role of red cell glutathione. *Science* 1985;227:756–759.
64. Heffner JE, Katz S, Haushka PV, Cook J. Human platelets attenuate oxidant lung injury in isolated rabbit lungs. *J Appl Physiol* 1988;65:1258–1266.
65. Zamora CA, Baron DA, Heffner JE. Human platelets attenuate lung edema induced by ischemia-reperfusion [Abstract]. *Clin Res* 1989;37:26A.
66. Heffner JE, Cook JA, Halushka PV. Platelets modulate edema formation in isolated rabbit lungs. *J Clin Invest* 1989;84:757–764.
67. Berger EM, Beehler CJ, Harada RN, Repine JE. Phagocytic cells as scavengers of hydrogen peroxide (H_2O_2) [Abstract]. *Clin Res* 1987;35:170A.
68. Turrens JF, Crapo JD, Freeman BA. Protection against oxygen toxicity by intravenous injection of liposome-entrapped catalase and superoxide dismutase. *J Clin Invest* 1984;73:87–95.

69. McDonald RJ, Berger EM, White CW, White JG, Freeman BA, Repine JE. Effect of superoxide dismutase encapsulated in liposomes or conjugated with polyethylene glycol on neutrophil bactericidal activity *in vitro* and bacterial clearance *in vivo*. *Am Rev Respir Dis* 1985;131:633–637.

70. White CW, Jackson JH, Abuchowski A, Berger EM, Freeman BW, Repine JE. Polyethylene glycol-attached antioxidant enzymes decrease pulmonary oxygen toxicity in rats. *J Appl Physiol* 1989;66:584–590.

71. Olson NC, Grizzle MK, Anderson DL. Effect of polyethylene glycol-superoxide dismutase and catalase on endotoxemia in pigs. *J Appl Physiol* 1987;63:1526–1532.

72. Beckman JS, Minor RL, White CW, Repine JE, Rosen GM, Freeman BA. Superoxide dismutase and catalase conjugated to polyethylene glycol increase endothelial enzyme activity and oxidant resistance. *J Biol Chem* 1988;283:1–9.

73. Gerschman R, Gilbert DL, Caccamise D. Effects of various substances on survival times of mice exposed to different high oxygen tensions. *Am J Physiol* 1958;192:563–571.

74. Dillard CJ, Litov RE, Savin WM, Dumelin EE, Tappel AL. Effects of exercise, vitamin E and ozone on pulmonary function and lipid peroxidation. *J Appl Physiol* 1978;45:927–932.

75. Yoshikawa T, Furukawa Y, Murakami M, Watanabe K, Kondo M. Effect of vitamin E on endotoxin-induced disseminated intravascular coagulation in rats. *Thromb Haemost* 1982;48:235–237.

76. Moldeus P, Berggren M, Grafstrom R. *N*-Acetylcysteine protection against the toxicity of cigarette smoke and cigarette smoke condensates in various tissues and cells *in vivo*. *Eur J Respir Dis* 1985;66(Suppl 139):123–129.

77. Bernard GR, Lucht WD, Niedermeyer ME, Snapper JR, Ogletree ML, Brigham KL. Effect of *N*-acetylcysteine on the pulmonary response to endotoxin in the awake sheep and upon *in vitro* granulocyte function. *J Clin Invest* 1984;73:1772–1784.

78. Fox RB. Prevention of granulocyte-mediated oxidant lung injury in rats by a hydroxyl radical scavenger, dimethylthiourea. *J Clin Invest* 1984;74:1456–1564.

79. Fox RB, Harada RN, Tate RM, Repine JE. Prevention of thiourea-induced pulmonary edema by hydroxyl radical scavengers. *J Appl Physiol* 1983;55:1456–1459.

80. Hass MA, Igbal J, Clerich LB, Frank L, Massaro D. Rat lung Cu,Zn superoxide dismutase latin and sequence of a full length DNA and studies of enzyme induction. *J Clin Invest* 1989;83:1241–1246.

81. White CW, Shanley PF, Rosandich ME, Repine JE. Overexpression of superoxide dismutase (SOD) protects against cell death due to severe hypoxia [Abstract]. *Clin Res* 1989;37:579A.

THE LUNG: Scientific Foundations
edited by R.G. Crystal, J.B. West et al.
Raven Press, Ltd., New York © 1991.

CHAPTER 7.2.3

Extracellular Antioxidant Defenses

W. Bruce Davis and Eric R. Pacht

Most research examining lung antioxidant defenses has focused on intracellular antioxidants. There is increasing evidence that extracellular substances also provide antioxidant protection. Lung extracellular fluid compartments include airway secretions, interstitial fluid, lymph, pleural fluid, and alveolar epithelial lining fluid (ELF). Most of these compartments have not been studied with respect to antioxidant defenses. By far the best-studied extracellular compartment is ELF, since this thin layer of fluid is readily accessible by bronchoalveolar lavage (BAL). This chapter will review the current evidence that ELF provides antioxidant protection for the alveolar epithelium, the region of the lung in closest proximity to the high oxygen concentrations and other oxidants in ambient air. Examples are provided which show that the protection afforded by ELF under baseline conditions is altered in response to acute and chronic oxidant stress. Several antioxidants have been identified in ELF (Table 1). This list is probably incomplete, and other antioxidants will doubtless be identified in future investigations.

SERUM PROTEINS

Several of the individual serum proteins, including albumin, ceruloplasmin, and transferrin, have specific antioxidant functions (see below). In addition, serum proteins en masse may have antioxidant protective effects by virtue of their presence in large amounts (7–8 g/dl). This concept holds that serum proteins act as "sacrificial" antioxidants, reacting with a variety of reactive oxygen species, thereby sparing host cells and tissues (1). One of the best examples of this type of

W. B. Davis and E. R. Pacht: Division of Pulmonary and Critical Care, Department of Internal Medicine, The Ohio State University, Columbus, Ohio 43210.

TABLE 1. *Epithelial lining fluid (ELF) antioxidants*

Serum proteins
Total protein
Albumin
Ceruloplasmin
Transferrin
Lactoferrin
Superoxide dismutase
Catalase
Glutathione
Vitamin E
Vitamin C
Others

reaction is the oxidation of serum proteins by hypochlorous acid (2,3). The hypochlorous acid is scavenged, leading to oxidation of both critical and noncritical residues in the component proteins. An example of critical injury is the oxidation of the active-site methionine in the serum protein α_1-antitrypsin (2). Noncritical oxidation presumably occurs in the other methionine residues of α_1-antitrypsin, as well as in other proteins not yet studied. Continuing antioxidant protection can be provided as these damaged proteins are replaced by newly synthesized proteins.

Serum proteins are easily detectable in human BAL, and their concentration in ELF has been estimated at 7 mg/ml, or 10% of serum levels (4,5). The presence of such high amounts of protein is surprising, since the alveolar epithelium is considered relatively impermeable to serum proteins (6). Thus, serum proteins must gain access to the alveolar space either by the small, but finite, epithelial transport or by other mechanisms. There is some evidence that the normal alveolar epithelium has size-selective sieving properties with respect to serum proteins (5,7). Except for transferrin, serum proteins of less than 200,000 daltons are distributed equally between serum and BAL; that is, each component protein in this size range comprises the same percentage of BAL total protein and serum total protein. Large-molecular-weight proteins such as α_2-macroglobulin (820,000 daltons) and immunoglobulin M (900,000 daltons) are largely excluded from the alveolar space.

Conditions of acute lung injury are associated with marked increases in alveolar fluid total protein. This has been shown in adult respiratory distress syndrome (ARDS) patients in both tracheal aspirate (8,9) and BAL (5) studies. These techniques have used total protein concentrations to separate patients with high-permeability pulmonary edema (e.g., ARDS) from patients with cardiac edema. There is some evidence that the normal size-selectivity of the alveolar epithelium is lost in ARDS such that both large and small serum proteins flood the alveolar space (5). There is also evidence that the large increases in epithelial lining fluid proteins provide increased antioxidant activity (10).

ALBUMIN

Albumin, molecular weight 68,000, is the principal protein constituent in normal BAL fluid. Its concentration in human ELF has been estimated at 3.5 mg/ml, approximately 50% of ELF total protein (4,5). Since albumin also comprises about 50% of serum total protein, the proportion of albumin is equal in serum and ELF.

Since albumin is present in ELF in such high concentrations, albumin probably functions as a nonspecific "sacrificial" antioxidant, as previously discussed. In addition, albumin has more specific antioxidant functions (reviewed in ref. 1). Albumin binds iron and copper, thus preventing lipid peroxidation. Albumin inhibits hydroxyl (OH·) production and inhibits hypochlorous acid-mediated oxidation of α_1-antitrypsin (3). Other antioxidant properties include inhibition of neutrophil chemiluminescence, scavenging of peroxy radicals, and binding of bilirubin, an inhibitor of lipid peroxidation.

Similar to total protein, ELF concentrations of albumin increase in acute lung injury (5). For example, BAL albumin concentration was 548 µg/ml in ARDS patients compared to 36 µg/ml in normal volunteers (5).

CERULOPLASMIN

Ceruloplasmin is an α_2-globulin protein with a molecular weight of 124,000. Each molecule contains six to eight copper atoms and is present in normal human serum at approximately 140–400 µg/ml. It is produced in the liver and is considered an acute-phase reactant. Ceruloplasmin is a potent antioxidant and, along with transferrin, accounts for greater than 90% of serum's antioxidant activity in assays of lipid peroxidation. Lipid peroxidation is believed to be initiated by, or dependent on, trace amounts of metals, particularly iron (11,12). Thus, ceruloplasmin is believed to inhibit lipid peroxidation by its ferroxidase activity, which oxidizes iron from the reduced (ferrous, Fe^{2+}) form to the oxidized (ferric, Fe^{3+}) form. Once ceruloplasmin has oxidized iron to the Fe^{3+} state, ferric ions can be tightly bound to transferrin and used for storage of iron. Although ceruloplasmin's ferroxidase activity is its principal antioxidant mechanism, several other antioxidant functions have been described. These include inhibition of copper-catalyzed lipid peroxidation (13), suppression of oxidative inactivation of α_1-antitrypsin (14,15), inhibition of neutrophil myeloperoxidase (15), and dismutation of superoxide (16).

Alterations in ceruloplasmin ferroxidase appear to explain a deficit in the antioxidant activity of serum from cigarette smokers. Smoker serum contains approximately 15% more antigenic ceruloplasmin than does nonsmoker serum (14,17,18). Paradoxically, smoker serum has 7–12% less antioxidant activity than does nonsmoker serum (14,17,18). This paradox may be explained by an acquired biochemical defect in ceruloplasmin ferroxidase activity in smokers (18). The mechanism for this defect is unknown, although oxidants are known to destroy the functional properties of ceruloplasmin (19).

Ceruloplasmin is present in normal human BAL fluid. One BAL study estimated the ELF concentration at 25 µg/ml, or approximately 0.20 µM (20). This concentration of ceruloplasmin was sufficient to inhibit in vitro lipid peroxidation (20). ELF ceruloplasmin concentration increases in conditions of altered epithelial permeability (5,10). This appears to occur as a generalized increase in protein permeability, which may have a net protective effect. The functional activity of ELF ceruloplasmin under conditions of increased oxidant stress has not been studied.

TRANSFERRIN

Transferrin is a beta-globulin protein with a molecular weight of 77,000. The concentration of transferrin in normal human serum is 2–4 mg/ml. Like ceruloplasmin, transferrin is synthesized in the liver and is an acute-phase reactant. Each molecule of transferrin is capable of binding two ferric iron molecules. Saturation of iron receptor sites destroys transferrin's antioxidant properties (12). Since transferrin is only 30–35% saturated in vivo, it has the ability to bind free iron and prevent hydroxyl (OH·) formation and lipid peroxidation (12). Thus, ceruloplasmin, via its ferroxidase activity, and transferrin, via its iron binding properties, inhibit iron-catalyzed lipid peroxidation. A separate, but important, biologic function of transferrin is its ability to inhibit bacterial growth by binding iron (21,22).

Transferrin is easily detectable in normal human BAL fluid (5,7,20). ELF concentration was 324 μg/ml (4.2 μM) in one study (20). There is evidence that transferrin may be selectively accumulated in ELF. This is based on distribution coefficient data in which the transferrin/total protein ratio in BAL fluid was higher than this ratio in serum (5,7). Selective accumulation might be explained by an unknown transport mechanism, by charge, or by local production by alveolar leukocytes. There is also evidence that transferrin is the principal component of ELF responsible for its antioxidant activity (20). ELF from normal humans inhibits *in vitro* lipid peroxidation (Fig. 1). Pretreatment of ELF with Fe^{3+} saturates the transferrin and destroys approximately 90% of ELF antioxidant activity (20). Although ceruloplasmin is also present in ELF, several experimental observations suggest that transferrin is the more important ELF antioxidant (20). ELF concentrations of transferrin increase in conditions of acute lung injury, including oxygen toxicity (23) and ARDS (5,10). ARDS ELF was shown to be more protective than normal ELF as an inhibitor of lipid peroxidation (10). An important role for transferrin was suggested by iron-loading experiments (10).

LACTOFERRIN

Lactoferrin is an 80,000-dalton protein found in exocrine secretions and in the specific granule of neutrophils (12,24). It is produced by various epithelial cells, including bronchial epithelial cells (25). Lactoferrin and transferrin are immunologically distinct. How-

ever, similar to transferrin, lactoferrin's biologic activity is directly related to its ability to bind extracellular iron and prevent lipid peroxidation. In addition to its antioxidant properties, lactoferrin is antibacterial, probably because it decreases the iron available for bacterial growth (21,22). Lactoferrin also facilitates leukocyte adherence (26) and blocks complement activation by the classical pathway (27).

Lactoferrin is present in normal human BAL fluid at a concentration of approximately 0.5 μg/ml (28). There is some evidence that lactoferrin is more "bronchial" than "alveolar," since lavage concentrations of lactoferrin decrease with successive lavage aliquots (28). This finding is consistent with the known production of lactoferrin by bronchial glandular acini (25). Lactoferrin can be detected in sputum, and there is evidence that concentrations of lactoferrin increase in inflammatory airway diseases. For example, BAL lactoferrin levels are increased in chronic bronchitis patients compared to normal volunteers (28). In addition, BAL levels of lactoferrin increased dramatically following induction of pneumonia in mice (22). Although lactoferrin released by recruited neutrophils could account for some of these increases, current evidence favors increased local production of lactoferrin in disease states (28). BAL lactoferrin has not been studied with respect to its iron saturation, antioxidant activity, or other functional properties.

SUPEROXIDE DISMUTASE

Superoxide dismutase (SOD) is usually regarded as an intracellular antioxidant enzyme. Extracellular fluids contain very low concentrations of the two prin-

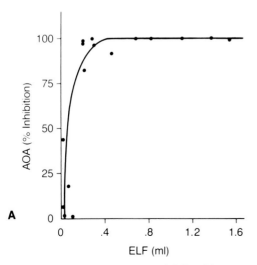
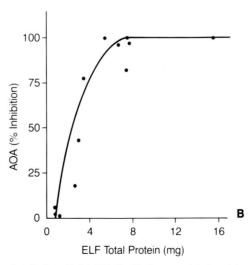

FIG. 1. Antioxidant activity (AOA) of human epithelial lining fluid (ELF). ELF was obtained by bronchoalveolar lavage. Increasing ELF volumes **(A)** and ELF total protein **(B)** were incubated in an assay of lipid peroxidation. ELF inhibited lipid peroxidation, as shown by its AOA. (From ref. 20.)

cipal forms of SOD, namely, copper–zinc (Cu–Zn) SOD and manganese (Mn) SOD. The low levels may represent background leakage of enzyme from cells. For example, serum Cu–Zn SOD content was 11.2 µg/liter in one report (29). Levels of these SOD enzymes in ELF or BAL fluid are not known.

A third form of the enzyme (extracellular SOD) appears to be the principal SOD in extracellular fluids (29,30). This enzyme was discovered by Marklund et al. (29,30), who found that Cu–Zn SOD accounted for only a small fraction of total SOD activity of extracellular fluids. Characterization of extracellular SOD shows that it is distinct from the other SOD enzymes in terms of amino acid composition, antigenic properties, electrophoresis, and behavior during protein separation (30). Extracellular SOD is a 135,000-dalton glycoprotein composed of four equal noncovalently bound subunits. The enzyme contains four copper atoms, which probably accounts for its enzymatic activity. It also contains four zinc atoms. The enzyme is cyanide-sensitive and catalyzes a first-order dismutation of superoxide anion. It is hydrophobic and has an affinity for heparin, a finding that may explain its binding to endothelial cell surfaces (30). It has been detected in all human extracellular fluids investigated, including plasma, serum, synovial fluid, ascites, and cerebrospinal fluid. It has also been detected in several human tissues, including lung, and in human cell lines (30). Thus, extracellular SOD is presumably present in normal human ELF, although this has not been studied.

CATALASE

Catalase is present in most cells, including lung parenchymal cells. Catalase is the principal intracellular mechanism for removal of H_2O_2, along with myeloperoxidase and the glutathione system. The importance of catalase as an intracellular antioxidant has been demonstrated in multiple tissues, including lung (31). The concentration of catalase in extracellular fluids is low and probably represents background leakage from cellular sources. Unlike SOD, no specific extracellular catalase has been identified.

Normal human ELF catalase was found to be 154 units/mg albumin in one study (32). Levels increased nearly threefold in idiopathic pulmonary fibrosis patients (32). The presence of catalase in an extracellular fluid is roughly analogous to the addition of exogenous catalase in various experimental conditions. Under *in vitro* conditions, catalase is highly effective in scavenging H_2O_2, in preventing formation of OH· and MPO products, and in preventing oxidant-mediated cytotoxicity (31). The importance of extracellular catalase in biologic fluids will await the demonstration that it

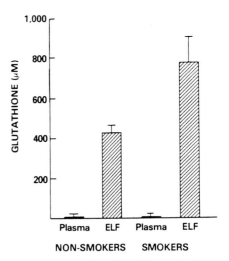

FIG. 2. Plasma and epithelial lining fluid (ELF) glutathione levels in smokers and nonsmokers. ELF glutathione levels are much higher than plasma levels. (From ref. 35.)

can serve as an antioxidant *in vivo*. In this context, one study (32) has shown that normal human ELF containing catalase can inhibit H_2O_2- and myeloperoxidase-mediated lung cell injury in *in vitro* cytotoxicity experiments.

GLUTATHIONE

Glutathione (GSH) is a sulfhydryl-containing tripeptide that is present in all cells in millimolar concentrations. GSH, both alone and in concert with GSH peroxidase and GSH reductase, is one of the most important intracellular antioxidant defenses. Antioxidant functions include the removal of H_2O_2, lipid peroxides, and myeloperoxidase products (31). GSH provides protection against lipid peroxidation in tissues, including lung (31), and is also important in metabolism of various drugs and toxins (33). Proof of the importance of GSH as an intracellular antioxidant has been provided by studies using various pharmacologic agents to deplete intracellular stores of GSH (34).

There is increasing evidence that GSH is an important epithelial lining fluid antioxidant. The concentration of GSH in plasma is low (~3 µM) (Fig. 2). The low plasma concentration is probably explained by the action of the cell-surface enzyme γ-glutamyl transpeptidase, which is especially active in kidney and which functions to remove extracellular GSH from plasma (35). In contrast to plasma, GSH levels in normal human ELF were 429 µM, approximately 140-fold higher than plasma levels (35). These GSH concentrations were protective in cytotoxicity experiments using relevant concentrations of H_2O_2 (35). Possibilities for why ELF GSH is so elevated include local production by alveolar cells and/or decreased clearance of GSH from the alveolar space. The latter could be the result of low levels of lung γ-glutamyl transpeptidase or decreased epithelial permeability favoring local accumulation (35). In addition to being present in high concentrations, GSH is present almost entirely (>96%) in its reduced form (35). The mechanism by which ELF GSH is maintained in reduced form, even in a tissue exposed to high oxidant burden, is unclear. This contrasts with the known production of oxidized GSH (i.e., GSSG) in certain models of lung injury (36).

GSH concentrations in ELF have also been studied in various inflammatory lung diseases. GSH levels in young asymptomatic cigarette smokers were 80% higher than in nonsmokers (Fig. 2), and the GSH was also maintained in reduced form. The increased GSH was interpreted as an adaptive response to chronic oxidant stress. BAL glutathione levels also increased in the lungs as well as in BAL fluid of rats exposed to 80% oxygen for 5 days (37). In contrast, ELF GSH in idiopathic pulmonary fibrosis (IPF) patients was only 25% of normal levels (38). The mechanism for the deficiency is unexplained, but low GSH levels may contribute to the marked epithelial injury characteristic of IPF.

The importance of GSH as an antioxidant has suggested therapeutic strategies to increase lung tissue levels of GSH. One approach is the intravenous infusion of N-acetylcysteine. This approach has been utilized successfully in sheep (39) and is currently being studied in ARDS patients (40). This approach depends on the uptake of N-acetylcysteine by lung cells, leading to net synthesis of GSH. It is not known whether this therapeutic strategy would increase ELF GSH levels. Another approach is inhalation of GSH. Recent work suggests the feasibility of this route in humans.

VITAMIN E

Vitamin E (α-tocopherol) is a naturally occurring lipid antioxidant. It is lipid soluble and is principally located in cell membranes. Vitamin E reduces O_2^-, OH·, singlet oxygen, and lipid peroxy radicals, thereby preventing lipid peroxidation in cells (31). Numerous animal models have demonstrated the importance of vitamin E in oxidant lung injury. Antioxidant protection in these systems is directly related to the cellular content of vitamin E.

Vitamin E is also present in extracellular fluids, where it is carried bound to circulating lipids. Serum concentrations of vitamin E are 8–12 μg/ml in normal humans (Fig. 3). Serum vitamin E is probably the source of vitamin E for tissues and other extracellular fluids, and it presumably is in a dynamic equilibrium with these various compartments. Vitamin E is also

present in normal human BAL fluid and was measured at 20.7 ng/ml in one study (41) (Fig. 3). Assuming 100-fold dilution by instilled saline, normal human ELF would be expected to contain about 2 μg/ml, a level about 10–20% that of serum. BAL fluid levels are directly related to lung tissue levels (41). Both serum and BAL levels can be augmented by supplementation with high-dose oral vitamin E (41).

Since the main function of vitamin E is to protect membrane lipids, it is not clear how vitamin E might function as an antioxidant in extracellular fluids. Perhaps it protects circulating lipids such as lipoproteins or surfactant. Alternatively, extracellular vitamin E might provide antioxidant protection at the interface between cells and extracellular fluid. Regardless of how it functions as an extracellular antioxidant, it has been clearly shown that human BAL fluid contains the oxidative metabolite, vitamin E quinone (41). Also, BAL from cigarette smokers contains significantly lower levels of vitamin E than does nonsmoker fluid. This deficiency has been attributed to increased oxidation of vitamin E in smokers and/or increased uptake by lung parenchymal cells and alveolar macrophages (41).

VITAMIN C

Vitamin C (ascorbate) is an antioxidant that can also function as a pro-oxidant at certain concentrations. Vitamin C is water soluble and is found in most cells and in extracellular fluids. Normal serum concentration is about 50 μM (42). As an antioxidant, vitamin C reduces and regenerates oxidized vitamin E and lipid peroxides (31). It scavenges neutrophil oxidants released extracellularly (43). Vitamin C has enhanced uptake into alveolar macrophages and type II cells (44). The existence of a specific ascorbic acid transport system in these two cell types may explain their resistance to oxidant injury. Finally, vitamin C is protective in some animal models of oxidant lung injury (45).

There is some evidence that vitamin C functions as an extracellular antioxidant in the lung. In one study, 30% of the ascorbic acid in rat lung slices was removed by washing the slices in buffer for 2 min. The authors concluded that this 30% of ascorbic acid represented the amount present in the epithelial lining fluid (46). The ascorbic acid was not bound to protein, and its concentration was estimated at 3.5 mg/ml. Another BAL study in rats estimated the alveolar fluid concentration at 1.1 mg/ml (47). Since the concentration in rat serum is only 14 μg/ml, the high ascorbate level suggests that it is selectively accumulated in alveolar fluid. One study showed that alveolar fluid ascorbic acid was measurable even in vitamin C-deficient animals with very low lung tissue levels (48).

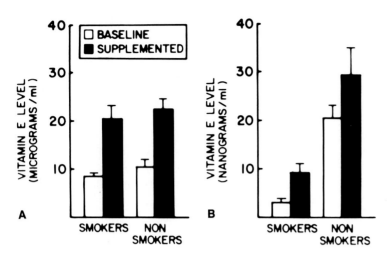

FIG. 3. Serum **(A)** and bronchoalveolar lavage (BAL) fluid **(B)** levels of vitamin E were measured on a baseline diet (*unfilled bars*) and following 3 week high-dose supplementation with vitamin E (*filled bars*). Serum levels were the same in smokers and nonsmokers. In contrast, cigarette-smoker BAL fluid had low levels of vitamin E. (From ref. 41.)

Two experimental observations support an antioxidant role for vitamin C in ELF. First, cigarette-smoker alveolar macrophages accumulate more ascorbic acid and dehydroascorbate (the oxidized metabolite) than do nonsmoker macrophages. A faster rate of accumulation was noted for smoker cells from both humans and hamsters (42). Following internalization by alveolar macrophages, dehydroascorbate was reduced to ascorbic acid. The authors speculated that vitamin C functions as an ELF antioxidant *in vivo*. Oxidized vitamin C (dehydroascorbate) is then taken up by alveolar macrophages, reduced to vitamin C, and recycled to the alveolar fluid, where it can again be used for antioxidant protection (42). The second observation is that extracellular vitamin C (0.025 mM) can inhibit the extracellular release of oxidants by human neutrophils (43). This concentration is below the estimated level of vitamin C in rat epithelial lining fluid (6.3 mM).

OTHERS

Any biologic molecule can potentially serve as an electron acceptor and thus has the potential for antioxidant function. An example of this type of antioxidant may be surfactant. Surfactant and other associated lipids in ELF may be protective, since oxidized lipid products have been recovered in BAL fluid from animals with acute lung injury (49).

SUMMARY

This chapter has reviewed the evidence that extracellular antioxidants in ELF provide antioxidant protection for the alveolar epithelium. This is a relatively new concept derived from BAL studies in which various antioxidants have been identified and quantitated (Table 1). Many of these antioxidants are altered in acute and chronic diseases. In addition, ELF concentrations of several of the components have antioxidant activity in *in vitro* experiments. However, there is currently no direct experimental proof that ELF or ELF components provide *in vivo* antioxidant protection. Future studies in animals and in humans should be designed to show which ELF components are critical for antioxidant protection.

ACKNOWLEDGMENT

W. Bruce Davis is the recipient of an American Lung Association Career Investigator Award.

REFERENCES

1. Halliwell B. Albumin—an important extracellular antioxidant? *Biochem Pharmacol* 1988;37:569–571.
2. Weiss SJ. Tissue destruction by neutrophils. *N Engl J Med* 1989;320:365–376.
3. Wasil M, Halliwell B, Hutchison DCS, Baum H. The antioxidant action of human extracellular fluids. *Biochem J* 1987;243:219–223.
4. Rennard SI, Gasset G, Lecossier D, O'Donnell KM, Pinkston P, Martin PG, Crystal RG. Estimation of the volume of epithelial lining fluid recovered by lavage using urea as marker of dilution. *J Appl Physiol* 1986;60:532–538.
5. Holter JF, Weiland JE, Pacht ER, Gadek JE, Davis WB. Protein permeability in ARDS: loss of size selectivity of the alveolar epithelium. *J Clin Invest* 1986;78:1513–1522.
6. Taylor AE, Gaar KA. Estimation of equivalent pore radii of pulmonary capillary and alveolar membranes. *Am J Physiol* 1970;218:1133–1140.
7. Bell DY, Haseman JA, Spock A, McLennan G, Hook GER. Plasma proteins of the bronchoalveolar surface of the lungs of smokers and nonsmokers. *Am Rev Respir Dis* 1981;124:72–79.
8. Fein A, Grossman RF, Jones JG, Overland E, Pitts L, Murray JF, Staub NC. The value of edema fluid protein measurement in patients with pulmonary edema. *Am J Med* 1979;67:32–38.
9. Sprung CL, Rackow EC, Fein IA, Jacob AI, Isikoff SK. The spectrum of pulmonary edema: differentiation of cardiogenic, intermediate, and noncardiogenic forms of pulmonary edema. *Am Rev Respir Dis* 1981;124:718–722.
10. Lykens ML, Davis WB, Pacht ER. Increase in alveolar epithelial lining fluid antioxidant activity in ARDS. *Clin Res* 1988;36:508A.

11. Stocks J, Gutteridge JMC, Sharp RJ, Dormandy TL. Assay using brain homogenate for measuring the antioxidant activity of biological fluids. *Clin Sci Mol Med* 1974;47:215–222.

12. Halliwell B, Gutteridge JMC. Oxygen free radicals and iron in relation to biology and medicine: some problems and concepts. *Arch Biochem Biophys* 1986;246:501–514.

13. Gutteridge JMC, Richmond R, Halliwell B. Oxygen free radicals and lipid peroxidation: inhibition by the protein caeruloplasmin. *FEBS Lett* 1980;112:269–272.

14. Galdston M, Levytska V, Schwartz M, Magnusson B. Ceruloplasmin: increased serum concentration and impaired antioxidant activity in cigarette smokers and ability to prevent suppression of elastase inhibitory capacity of alpha-1-proteinase inhibitor. *Am Rev Respir Dis* 1984;129:258–263.

15. Taylor JC, Oey L. Ceruloplasmin: plasma inhibitor of the oxidative inactivation of alpha-1-protease inhibitor. *Am Rev Respir Dis* 1982;126:476–482.

16. Goldstein IM, Kaplan HB, Edelson HS, Weissman G. Ceruloplasmin: a scavenger of superoxide anion radicals. *J Biol Chem* 1979;254:4040–4045.

17. Galdston M, Feldman JG, Levytska V, Magnusson B. Antioxidant activity of serum ceruloplasmin and transferrin available iron-binding capacity in smokers and nonsmokers. *Am Rev Respir Dis* 1987;135:783–787.

18. Pacht ER, Davis WB. Decreased ceruloplasmin ferroxidase activity in cigarette smokers. *J Lab Clin Med* 1988;111:661–668.

19. Winyard P, Lunec J, Brailsford S, Blake D. Action of free radical generating systems upon the biological and immunological properties of ceruloplasmin. *Int J Biochem* 1984;16:1273–1278.

20. Pacht ER, Davis WB. Role of transferrin and ceruloplasmin in antioxidant activity of lung epithelial lining fluid. *J Appl Physiol* 1988;64:2092–2099.

21. Bullen JJ, Rogers HJ, Leigh L. Iron-binding proteins in milk and resistance to *Escherichia coli* infection in infants. *Br Med J* 1972;1:69–75.

22. LaForce FM, Boose DS, Ellison RT III. Effect of aerosolized *Escherichia coli* and *Staphylococcus aureus* on iron and iron-binding proteins in lung lavage fluid. *J Infect Dis* 1986;154:959–965.

23. Davis WB, Rennard SI, Bitterman PB, Crystal RG. Pulmonary oxygen toxicity: early reversible changes in human alveolar structures induced by hyperoxia. *N Engl J Med* 1983;309:878–883.

24. Ward PA, Till GO, Kunkel R, Beauchamp C. Evidence for role of hydroxyl radical in complement and neutrophil-dependent tissue injury. *J Clin Invest* 1983;72:789–801.

25. Masson PL, Heremans JF, Prignot JJ, Wauters G. Immunohistochemical localization and bacteriostatic properties of an iron-binding protein from bronchial glands. *Thorax* 1977;21:538–544.

26. Oseas R, Yang HH, Baehner RL, Boxer LA. Lactoferrin: a promoter of polymorphonuclear leukocyte adhesiveness. *Blood* 1981;57:939–945.

27. Kijlstra A, Jeurissen HM. Modulation of classical C3 convertase of complement by tear lactoferrin. *Immunology* 1982;47:263–270.

28. Thompson AB, Bohling T, Payvandi F, Rennard SI. Lower respiratory tract lactoferrin and lysozyme arise primarily in the airways and are elevated in association with chronic bronchitis. *J Lab Clin Med* 1990;115:148–158.

29. Marklund SL, Holme E, Hellner L. Superoxide dismutase in extracellular fluids. *Clin Chim Acta* 1982;126:41–51.

30. Marklund SL. Extracellular superoxide dismutase in human tissues and human cell lines. *J Clin Invest* 1984;74:1398–1403.

31. Freeman BA, Crapo JD. Free radicals and tissue injury. *Lab Invest* 1982;47:412–426.

32. Cantin AM, North SL, Fells GA, Hubbard RC, Crystal RG. Oxidant-mediated epithelial cell injury in idiopathic pulmonary fibrosis. *J Clin Invest* 1987;79:1665–1673.

33. Dawson JR, Vahakangas K, Jernstrom B, Moldeus P. Glutathione conjugation by isolated lung cells and the isolated, perfused lung. Effect of extracellular glutathione. *Eur J Biochem* 1984;138:439–443.

34. Arrick BA, Nathan CF, Griffin OW, Cohn ZA. Glutathione depletion sensitizes tumor cells to oxidative cytolysis. *J Biol Chem* 1982;257:1231–1237.

35. Cantin AM, North SL, Hubbard RC, Crystal RG. Normal alveolar epithelial lining fluid contains high levels of glutathione. *J Appl Physiol* 1987;63:152–157.

36. Jenkinson SG, Marcum RF, Pickard JS, Orzechowski Z, Lawrence RA, Jordan JM. Glutathione disulfide formation occurring during hypoxia and reoxygenation of rat lung. *J Lab Clin Med* 1988;112:471–480.

37. Jenkinson SG, Black RD, Lawrence RA. Glutathione concentrations in rat lung bronchoalveolar lavage fluid: effects of hyperoxia. *J Lab Clin Med* 1988;112:345–351.

38. Cantin AM, Hubbard RC, Crystal RG. Glutathione deficiency in the epithelial lining fluid of the lower respiratory tract in idiopathic pulmonary fibrosis. *Am Rev Respir Dis* 1989;139:370–372.

39. Bernard GR, Lucht WD, Niedermeyer ME, Snapper JR, Ogletree ML, Brigham KL. Effect of *N*-acetylcysteine on the pulmonary response to endotoxin in the awake sheep and upon *in vitro* granulocyte function. *J Clin Invest* 1984;73:1772–1784.

40. Bernard GR, Swindell BB, Meredith MJ, Carroll FE, Higgins SB. Glutathione (GSH) repletion by *N*-acetylcysteine (NAC) in patients with the adult respiratory distress syndrome (ARDS). *Am Rev Respir Dis* 1989;139:A221.

41. Pacht ER, Kaseki H, Mohammed JR, Cornwell DG, Davis WB. Deficiency of vitamin E in the alveolar fluid of cigarette smokers. *J Clin Invest* 1986;77:789–796.

42. McGowan SE, Parenti CM, Hoidal JR, Niewoehner DE. Ascorbic acid content and accumulation by alveolar macrophages from cigarette smokers and nonsmokers. *J Lab Clin Med* 1984;104:127–134.

43. Anderson R, Theron AJ, Ras GJ. Regulation by the antioxidants ascorbate, cysteine, and dapsone of the increased extracellular and intracellular generation of reactive oxidants by activated phagocytes from cigarette smokers. *Am Rev Respir Dis* 1987;135:1027–1032.

44. Castranova V, Wright JR, Colby HD, Miles PR. Ascorbate uptake by isolated rat alveolar macrophages and type II cells. *J Appl Physiol* 1983;54:208–214.

45. Matzen RN. Effect of vitamin C and hydrocortisone on the pulmonary edema produced by ozone in mice. *J Appl Physiol* 1957;11:105–109.

46. Willis RJ, Kratzing CC. Ascorbic acid in rat lung. *Biochem Biophys Res Commun* 1974;59:1250–1253.

47. Snyder A, Skoza L, Kikkawa Y. Comparative removal of ascorbic acid and other airway substances by sequential bronchoalveolar lavages. *Lung* 1983;161:111–121.

48. Willis RJ, Kratzing CC. Extracellular ascorbic acid in lung. *Biochim Biophys Acta* 1976;444:108–117.

49. Roehm JN, Hadley JG, Menzel DB. Antioxidants vs lung disease. *Arch Intern Med* 1971;128:88–93.

THE LUNG: Scientific Foundations
edited by R.G. Crystal, J.B. West et al.
Raven Press, Ltd., New York © 1991.

CHAPTER 7.2.4

Consequences of Oxidant Injury

Jeffrey S. Warren, Kent J. Johnson, and Peter A. Ward

GENERAL EFFECTS OF OXIDANTS ON LUNG MORPHOLOGY AND FUNCTION

Much of the morphological and functional data cogent to oxidant-mediated pulmonary disease in humans has come from clinical studies of acutely ill patients and from examination of lung tissue obtained by biopsy or postmortem examination. Perhaps the least equivocal example of oxidant-mediated lung injury in humans is the diffuse alveolar damage associated with iatrogenic hyperoxia. Although molecular oxygen (O_2) is required (at approximately 0.2 atm) to maintain aerobic oxidative metabolism in humans, higher concentrations have deleterious effects. Because oxygen is toxic at high concentrations and also because high concentrations of oxygen are frequently required to support patients in respiratory failure, considerable attention has been directed towards understanding the mechanisms by which oxygen and its metabolites injure cells and tissues. At oxygen concentrations exceeding an F_iO_2 of 0.5 (at 1.0 atm), the likelihood of developing pulmonary oxygen toxicity is accelerated (1,2). Examination of lung tissue from humans and experimental animals has provided insight into the pathogenesis of hyperoxic lung injury. Based on morphologic analyses, the principal sites of oxygen-induced lung injury appear to be type I alveolar pneumocytes and pulmonary capillary endothelial cells. The earliest alterations that can be discerned ultrastructurally include endothelial cell swelling (hydropic degeneration), cytoplasmic bleb formation, and the disruption of intercellular tight junctions. Slightly later, there are detachment and necrosis of type I pneumocytes accompanied by the formation of hyaline membranes.

These alterations are variously accompanied by type II pneumocyte hyperplasia, intra-alveolar fibrosis, and, in some cases, the development of interstitial fibrosis (3). This constellation of morphologic alterations constitutes the familiar picture of the adult respiratory distress syndrome (ARDS). It is now clear that, in addition to oxygen toxicity, a variety of pulmonary insults can trigger similar or identical morphologic alterations. Biochemical analyses of bronchoalveolar lavage fluids obtained from patients undergoing hyperoxic lung injury have provided evidence, albeit indirect in humans, that oxygen metabolites (and proteases) are important mediators of hyperoxic lung injury. The hypothesis that oxygen metabolites are toxic in this setting is supported by the retrieval of elevated concentrations of lipid peroxidation products and oxidatively inactivated proteins (e.g., α_1-antitrypsin) in lung lavage fluid (2). These clinical data are supported by experimental studies of hyperoxic lung injury in animals. For instance, hyperoxia leads to augmented intrapulmonary production of superoxide anions and hydrogen peroxide in rats (4). Conversely, systemic treatment of rats with pharmacologic doses of antioxidant compounds such as superoxide dismutase, vitamin C, and low-molecular-weight sulfhydryl-reducing agents results in significant resistance to the adverse effects of supranormal oxygen concentrations (4–6). Similarly, physiological or pharmacological augmentation of endogenous antioxidant enzyme systems such as superoxide dismutase, catalase, and glutathione peroxidase also results in resistance to the deleterious effects of hyperoxia (7–12).

Oxygen radicals and their metabolites also appear to be principal mediators of inflammatory and immunologic lung injury. In these settings, host cells convert molecular oxygen into a series of metabolites that can alter cell function and damage biomolecules. An array of experimental systems have been devised to examine lung injury mediated by endogenously generated ox-

J. S. Warren, K. J. Johnson, and P. A. Ward: Department of Pathology, University of Michigan Medical School, Ann Arbor, Michigan 48109.

ygen metabolites. *In vivo* oxidant-mediated lung injury models display the gamut of morphological and functional aberrations. Animal studies have provided quantitative morphological and functional data that have helped clarify the role of oxidants in the pathogenesis of lung injury. Among the most extensively investigated lung injury models are: cobra venom factor (CVF)-induced alveolar endothelial injury; a rat model of systemic complement activation resulting in neutrophil-mediated endothelial disruption; IgG and IgA immune complex alveolitis; rat models of neutrophil-mediated and monocyte–macrophage-mediated alveolitis, respectively; and bleomycin-induced pulmonary fibrosis in a variety of animal models.

In the mid-1970s, Craddock et al. (13) proposed that acute lung injury which sometimes occurs in burn, trauma, or hemodialysis patients is the result of activation of plasma mediator systems and sequestration of neutrophils within pulmonary alveolar capillaries. Subsequent studies suggested that intravascular complement activation leads to endothelial cell lysis by C5a-activated neutrophils (14,15). Neutrophil-dependent acute lung injury develops rapidly (30 min) following intravenous bolus infusion of CVF into rats

(16). CVF infusion results in systemic complement activation, appearance of C5a in the serum, and intrapulmonary neutrophil sequestration. Antioxidant intervention studies suggest that the hydroxyl radical (HO·) may be the principal oxidant mediator of CVF-induced lung injury (17). Morphologically, CVF-induced lung injury is characterized by intra-alveolar edema and hemorrhage, destruction of endothelial cells, and the appearance of intracellular gaps between pulmonary capillary endothelial cells (Fig. 1). In this model, as well as in others, lung injury has been quantitated by morphometric analysis, by increases in lung weight, and by measuring the leakage of ^{125}I-labeled serum proteins from the vascular space into the pulmonary parenchyma. This model serves as a paradigm for acute lung injury in which the endothelium is the primary target of phagocyte-mediated injury.

Acute IgG immune complex-mediated alveolitis, like CVF-induced injury, is neutrophil-, complement-, and oxygen metabolite-mediated (18,19). Despite these similarities, it has become clear that mediators derived from alveolar macrophages are also important in the pathogenesis of immune complex-induced injury (20) (see Chapter 7.5.2). In this respect, immune complex

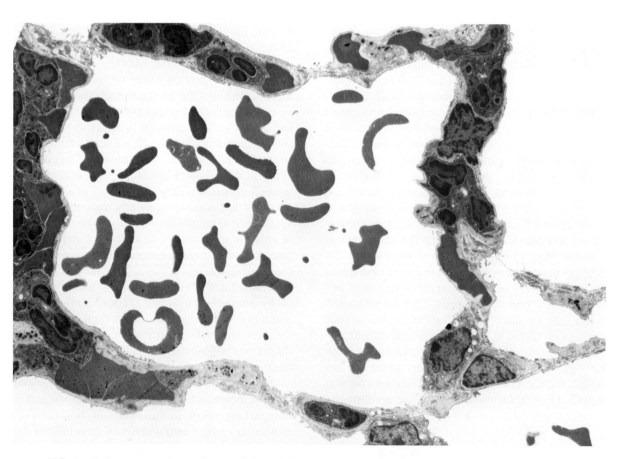

FIG. 1. Cobra venom factor-induced lung injury. There are aggregates of intravascular neutrophils accompanied by endothelial cell damage and intra-alveolar hemorrhage. ×2900.

injury seems to evolve from both the vascular and air-space compartments of the lung. In IgG immune complex injury, an intense neutrophilic alveolitis is attended by endothelial and alveolar epithelial cell destruction, hemorrhage, and edema. Amorphous, electron-dense deposits of immune complexes can be seen within phagocytes that have been recruited into sites of inflammation (Fig. 2). The extent of lung damage can also be quantitated by measuring increases in lung weight or by measuring the leakage of radiolabeled colloid into the pulmonary parenchyma.

The relevance of IgA immune complex lung injury to human lung disease is controversial, even though there are a variety of extrapulmonary human diseases in which IgA complexes seem pivotal. Despite this caveat, IgA immune complex lung injury in the rat is an interesting model because it is complement-dependent and oxygen metabolite-mediated but does not require the participation of neutrophils (21,22). This observation is reflected in the morphologic evidence of extensive alveolar damage accompanied by increased numbers of pulmonary macrophages (Fig. 3).

Interstitial pulmonary fibrosis is a frequent sequel to a diverse group of lung injuries associated with oxygen-derived free radicals and their metabolites. Included among these diseases are chronic hyperoxic lung injury, radiation pneumonitis, paraquat toxicity, collagen-vascular diseases, and a variety of drug-induced pulmonary lesions (23–28). Bleomycin, which includes a mixture of glycopeptides derived from *Streptomyces verticillus*, is a potent chemotherapeutic agent known to induce pulmonary fibrosis in patients (27). Several investigators have developed and characterized animal models of pulmonary fibrosis in which bleomycin is instilled into the animals' lungs via a tracheostomy (29–32) (Fig. 4). Pulmonary fibrosis develops over a period of several weeks and is associated with a marked intrapulmonary increase in collagen synthesis. Antioxidant interventions and direct measurements of endogenous antioxidant enzyme activities have revealed that the role of oxidants varies depending upon the stage of development of the injury (33). This lung injury model has provided insights into the pathogenesis of oxidant-mediated chronic fibrosing lung disease and is beginning to yield new information relevant to the regulation of growth control and connective tissue synthesis (34). Lung injury is quantitated by morphological analysis, measurement of net in-

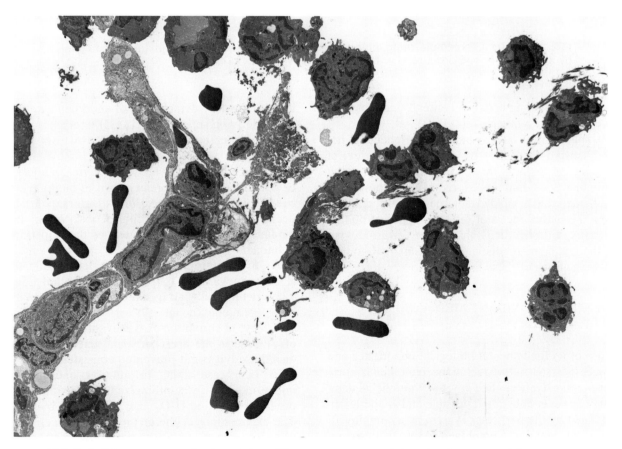

FIG. 2. IgG immune complex lung injury. There are numerous intra-alveolar neutrophils accompanied by intra-alveolar hemorrhage. Several neutrophils contain electron-dense immune deposits. ×2575.

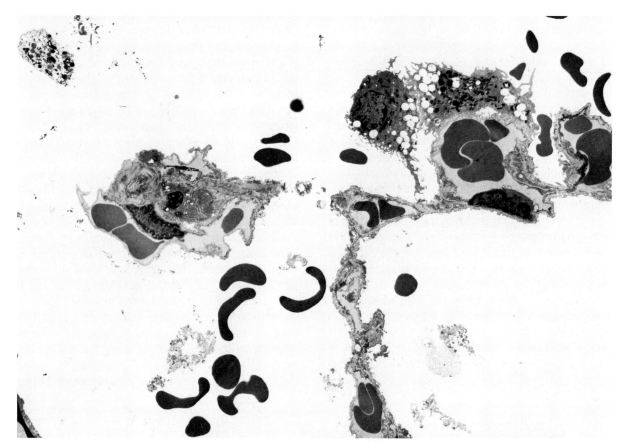

FIG. 3. IgA immune complex lung injury. There are several alveolar macrophages accompanied by intra-alveolar hemorrhage. No neutrophils are evident. ×2575.

creases in whole-lung collagen content, and measurement of collagen synthesis rates.

This spectrum of *in vivo* lung injury models is not comprehensive but serves to illustrate the variety of morphological patterns that can develop as the result of pulmonary oxidant exposure. More importantly, these models have yielded a large body of data regarding the pathogenesis of different types of pulmonary injury. Current focus has shifted toward delineating the endogenous regulatory systems that control the pathogeneses of these diseases.

EVIDENCE FOR OXIDANT-MEDIATED CELLULAR INJURY

Because of its fundamental biological importance and advances in tissue culture technique, endothelial injury has been intensively studied *in vitro*. Endothelial damage may be reversible or irreversible and is operationally defined by the particular *in vitro* assay employed. In the most commonly employed cytotoxicity assay, endothelial cells are labeled with chromium-51, which is released into the culture supernatant when cell lysis or leakage occurs. In other systems, cell injury has been defined by detachment of endothelial cells from the underlying support matrix (35), morphologic alterations, or decreased rates of cell growth in replating assays (36).

The capacity for activated phagocytes to injure (lyse or detach) endothelial cells grown in monolayers has been reported by numerous investigators over the past decade. Subsequent to the clinical observation that hemodialysis patients can sometimes develop transient pulmonary dysfunction secondary to complement activation and intrapulmonary neutrophil sequestration (13,14), Sacks et al. (15) demonstrated that C5a-activated neutrophils can lyse monolayers of human umbilical vein endothelial cells.

Release of chromium-51 is prevented by the addition of catalase in the presence or absence of superoxide dismutase but is not prevented consistently by superoxide dismutase alone. In addition, endothelial cell injury induced by xanthine/xanthine oxidase (which produces O_2^- and H_2O_2) can be blocked by catalase. The explanation for the inconsistent protective effect of superoxide dismutase is not known with certainty but may be attributable to its capacity to catalyze the formation of H_2O_2 and O_2^- or by the ability of O_2^- to function as a reducing agent, thereby favoring the

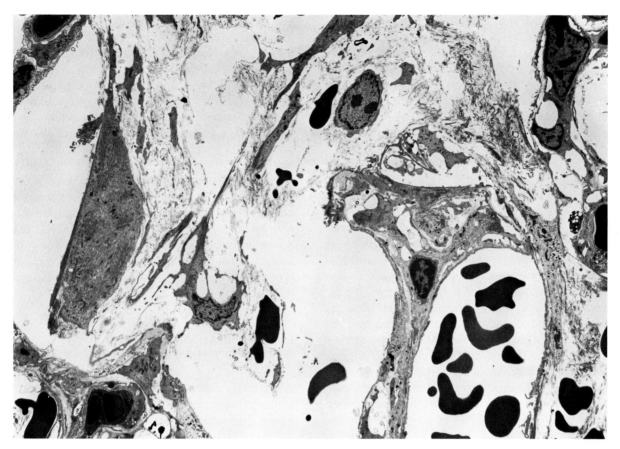

FIG. 4. Bleomycin-induced pulmonary fibrosis. This (early) lesion is characterized by rare inflammatory cells and some hemorrhage. There is an increased amount of interstitial collagen. ×2775.

iron-catalyzed Fenton reaction. Addition of purified myeloperoxidase or lysozyme to endothelial cell cultures does not increase the release of chromium-51 compared to that of controls. This observation suggests that these granular constituents are not critical in neutrophil-triggered endothelial injury.

Weiss et al. (37) have demonstrated that phorbol myristate acetate (PMA)-stimulated human neutrophils can lyse umbilical vein endothelial cells. The inability of PMA-activated chronic granulomatous disease (CGD) neutrophils (genetically incapable of oxidant burst) to cause endothelial cell lysis has provided further evidence that oxygen metabolites are important in phagocyte-mediated endothelial injury. These investigators have also shown that hypohalous acid scavengers and myeloperoxidase inhibitors (azide and cyanide) do not block neutrophil-triggered endothelial cell lysis when the neutrophils are activated with PMA.

The role of toxic oxygen products in the killing of endothelial cells by neutrophils is predicated partly on the strong correlation between endothelial cell killing and the effectiveness of neutrophils activated by agonists that preferentially trigger oxidant release rather

than maximum degranulation. Varani et al. (38) have suggested that $HO^{\cdot}$ is the principal oxygen-derived mediator of endothelial cell injury. Also, a battery of hydroxyl radical scavengers (D-mannitol and N,N-dimethylthiourea) and iron chelators (deferoxamine but not iron-saturated deferoxamine) have been shown to prevent neutrophil-mediated endothelial lysis. This observation not only supports the conclusion that $HO^{\cdot}$ is important but also supports the hypothesis that iron is required for cell killing. The requirement for iron is consistent with the hypothesis that $HO^{\cdot}$ formed by the Fenton reaction is a relevant pathogenetic mechanism in oxidant-mediated tissue injury (see Chapter 7.2.1). Recent studies by Gannon et al. (36) suggest that the endothelial cells themselves are the chief source of iron in neutrophil-mediated endothelial lysis.

It should be noted that there are also *in vitro* data which suggest that neutrophil-mediated endothelial injury can occur by nonoxidant-mediated mechanisms. Harlan et al. (35) have demonstrated that addition of zymosan-activated neutrophils to endothelial monolayers causes endothelial cell detachment without lysis (chromium-51 release). Interestingly, direct addition of reagent H_2O_2 to endothelial cell monolayers induces cell lysis, whereas the addition of CGD neutrophils causes detachment but not lysis. Either catalase or superoxide dismutase blocks endothelial lysis but does not block detachment. Endothelial cell detachment can also be induced by the addition of neutrophil lysates and by purified granular constituents. Because endothelial cell detachment can be inhibited by neutral protease inhibitors, it has been suggested that this process is mediated by neutrophil elastase-like enzymes.

In studies using monolayers of human microvascular endothelial cells (from omental fat), Smedly et al. (39) have provided additional evidence that nonoxidant pathways of neutrophil-mediated endothelial injury may be important. Pretreatment of neutrophils with lipopolysaccharide, followed by activation with either C5a or synthetic formyl peptides, results in endothelial injury that occurs in a temporal pattern similar to that induced by direct addition of purified neutrophil elastase to endothelial cells. Both neutrophil-mediated and elastase-mediated endothelial injury can be blocked with synthetic elastase inhibitors. Although the studies by Harlan et al. (35) and Smedley et al. (39) suggest that nonoxidant mechanisms are important, they do not necessarily exclude oxidant-mediated injury mechanisms. For instance, C5a and PMA, the agonists used by Sacks et al. (15) and Weiss et al. (37), are potent agonists for neutrophil oxidant production. However, these agonists are also weak neutrophil granule secretagogues. There is also emerging evidence that endothelial cells derived from different vascular beds may differ in their patterns of susceptibility to oxidant and nonoxidant mechanisms of injury. The endothelial cells employed by Sacks et al. (15), Weiss et al. (37), and Harlan et al. (35) were obtained from human umbilical veins. The endothelial cells utilized by Smedly et al. (39) were obtained from omental capillaries. The availability of ultrapure recombinant enzymes, chemically defined oxidant-generating systems, and absolutely specific enzyme and oxidant antagonists, along with greater availability of endothelial cells from different anatomic sites, will help clarify these issues.

Although great attention has been directed towards elucidating pathways of endothelial cell injury, concomitant studies utilizing nonendothelial target cells have also provided important insights into mechanisms of oxidant-mediated (and nonoxidant-mediated) cell injury. For instance, Klebanoff and Clark (40) and Clark and co-workers (41,42) have shown that myeloperoxidase-dependent oxidants (hypohalous acids) can lyse red blood cells and some types of tumor cells. Baehner et al. (43) have shown that neutrophil function can be altered through a mechanism involving autooxidation, and Simon et al. (44) have shown that cultured human fibroblasts can be killed by hydrogen peroxide exposure. Perhaps more cogent to the effects of oxidants on lung function and integrity are studies by

Cantin et al. (45). These investigators have shown that lung inflammatory cells obtained from patients with idiopathic pulmonary fibrosis spontaneously release exaggerated amounts of O_2^- and H_2O_2 compared to normal unstimulated cells. In addition, epithelial lining fluid obtained from idiopathic pulmonary fibrosis patients contains above-normal concentrations of myeloperoxidase. Compared to cytotoxicity of alveolar epithelial cells by lung inflammatory cells or lining fluid alone, incubation of inflammatory cells plus epithelial lining fluid results in a synergistic increase in *in vitro* cytotoxicity of alveolar epithelial cells maintained in culture. In this system, cellular injury can be blocked with methionine, a scavenger of O_2^- and $HO^{\cdot}$ and also a myeloperoxidase pathway scavenger. These observations serve to emphasize the wide spectrum of cell types and oxidants that appear to be operative in cell injury processes.

BIOCHEMICAL MECHANISMS OF OXIDANT-MEDIATED CELLULAR INJURY

A plethora of mechanisms have been invoked to explain the molecular bases of oxidant-mediated cellular injury. For instance, several investigators have temporally linked oxidant-mediated tissue injury with rises in tissue and plasma lipid peroxidation products (46,47). In the CVF-induced acute lung injury model described by Till et al. (16), as well as in a closely related acute lung injury that is triggered by thermal skin injury (48), systemic complement activation leads to neutrophil-mediated lung damage followed rapidly by the appearance of conjugated dienes, lipid hydroperoxides, and N,N'-iminopropenes (Schiff bases) in lung homogenates and plasma (49). Pretreatment of these rats with antioxidants or iron chelators reduces the extent of lung injury (as determined by determination of lung permeability indices) and suppresses the appearance of lipid peroxidation products. Presumably, these lipid-derived compounds arise from oxidant-damaged cytoplasmic and organelle membranes. Although various alterations in membrane-associated function and a variety of peroxidation products have been described, interpretation of these data is difficult because of the technical difficulties with many of the assays for lipid peroxidation products, instability of many of the oxidant product of lipids, and uncertainty as to whether the appearance of lipid peroxidation products reflects direct cell injury or an epiphenomenon.

Other potentially important mechanisms of oxidant-mediated cell injury have also been implicated (50). Protein polymerization can result secondary to the incorporation of lipid peroxide-derived oxidation products or as the result of direct reaction of proteins with oxygen radicals (51,52). Sulfoxide formation from sulfhydryl groups, disulfide cross-linking of proteins, and structural alteration of cells following cross-linkage of cytoskeletal proteins have all been linked to oxidant-mediated processes (53). Direct oxidant-mediated structural cell damage can easily be envisioned as a consequence of these reactions.

There are several well-characterized examples of cytotoxicity resulting from oxidant-mediated alteration of normal intracellular metabolism. Drapier and Hibbs (54) have shown that activated murine macrophages can damage tumor cells through a mechanism in which oxidants inactivate cis-aconitase. Schraufstatter et al. (55,56) have shown that hydrogen peroxide can induce target cell lysis through activation of poly-adenosine diphosphate (ADP)-ribose polymerase, a nuclear enzyme associated with deoxyribonucleic acid (DNA) damage and repair. Activation of poly-ADP-ribose polymerase with high concentrations of H_2O_2 leads to target cell lysis following intracellular depletion of nicotinamide-adenine dinucleotide (NAD) and adenosine triphosphate (ATP). Depletion of NAD (and ATP) induced by H_2O_2 is prevented by addition of 3-aminobenzamide or theophylline, inhibitors of poly-ADP-ribose polymerase. In addition, H_2O_2 induces DNA strand breaks, an event known to be associated with activation of poly-ADP-ribose polymerase. These investigators have shown that DNA strand breaks can be produced in rabbit pulmonary endothelial cells with relatively lower concentrations of H_2O_2 than required to cause strand breaks in rabbit alveolar macrophages or human monocytes. They have postulated that this difference in susceptibility could be explained by the differing concentrations of protective antioxidant enzymes present in these different cell types. Recently, Hyslop et al. (57) have shown that exposure of P388D1 cells (murine leukocytic tumor) to micromolar concentrations of H_2O_2 results in inactivation of glycolysis at the glyceraldehyde-3-phosphate dehydrogenase step. Three different mechanisms of inactivation appear to play a role: direct inactivation of the intracellular enzyme, reduction of the intracellular concentrations and redox potentials of its nicotinamide cofactors, and a cytosolic pH shift. Exposure of P388D1 cells to higher concentrations of H_2O_2 (300–800 μM) impairs mitochondrial contribution of ATP to the intracellular ATP pool.

Finally, Phan et al. (58) have recently defined a mechanism through which products of activated neutrophils can accelerate the conversion of xanthine dehydrogenase to xanthine oxidase in endothelial cells maintained in monolayers. Xanthine oxidase, as well as its formation from xanthine dehydrogenase, has received considerable attention in the context of ischemia–reperfusion-associated tissue injury (59). It appears that intracellular xanthine dehydrogenase is cleaved into xanthine oxidase through a calpain-dependent proteolytic mechanism triggered by ischemia (59). Xanthine oxidase catalyzes the formation of O_2^- and uric acid from xanthine and hypoxanthine. For this process to be relevant to the process of cell injury, it must also be assumed that substrate (xanthine, hypoxanthine) for xanthine oxidase becomes available as a result of cell exposure to H_2O_2. Studies by Phan et al. (58) suggest that neutrophils may not only directly injure endothelial cells but may also induce endothelial cells to hasten their own destruction by producing oxidants.

OXIDANT-MEDIATED DAMAGE OF MATRIX MOLECULES

Oxygen radicals and metabolites may amplify cell and tissue injury through a variety of indirect mechanisms. The effects of oxidants on extracellular matrix material have not been extensively examined, but there are several examples of interactions that have relevance to tissue injury. Superoxide anions cause the depolymerization of hyaluronate, a glucosaminoglycan that is the chief constituent of synovial fluid (60). Depolymerized hyaluronate is susceptible to digestion by β-N-acetyl-glucosaminidase. The tertiary structure of hyaluronate can be altered by singlet oxygen. The conformational change in hyaluronic acid results in decreased viscosity of hyaluronic-acid-containing solutions. Similarly, cartilage and collagen proteoglycans can also be damaged by O_2^- and its metabolites (61). Fligiel et al. (62) have shown that hydrogen peroxide can alter glomerular basement membranes and purified target proteins such as hemoglobin and fibronectin, rendering them more susceptible to subsequent proteolysis by lysosomal proteases. This change in the proteins induced by exposure to H_2O_2 is not associated with any detectable change in molecular weight (either up or down). These examples illustrate potential mechanisms of oxidant-mediated tissue injury that are independent of cellular injury per se. They also illustrate the importance of interplay among different mediator systems in the pathogenesis of tissue injury.

OXIDANT MODULATION OF INFLAMMATORY MEDIATOR SYSTEMS

There is increasing recognition that the pathophysiology of tissue injury is greatly influenced by interactions that occur among various soluble mediator systems. Two of the earliest demonstrated examples of such mediator interactions were described in the late 1970s. Carp and Janoff (63) demonstrated that neutrophil-derived oxidants can inactivate serum elastase inhibitor. Matheson et al. (64) demonstrated that neutrophil peroxidase can give rise to oxidants that inactivate α_1-antitrypsin. Inactivation of proteins that normally counter the effects of proinflammatory proteases may compromise host defense systems, thereby amplifying inflammatory tissue injury.

It has been postulated that a chemotactic lipid is derived from oxygen-radical-induced modification of arachidonic acid (65). Superoxide anion has been implicated, since the generation of this chemotactic activity in plasma can be blocked with superoxide dismutase. The precise biochemical identity of this chemotactic factor has not been elucidated. Shingu and Nobunaga (66) have shown that exposure of C5 to an oxygen-radical-generating system (xanthine/xanthine oxidase) results in the formation of a chemotactic peptide that has the same molecular weight and functional profile as C5a. More recently, Vogt et al. (67) have demonstrated that H_2O_2 can cause conformational changes in the alpha chain of purified C5, enabling it to initiate the assembly of C5b-9 (membrane attack complex), as demonstrated by the appearance of an activity that causes "reactive lysis" of erythrocytes. In this pathway, C5 cleavage does not occur. Addition of H_2O_2 to whole plasma or serum also results in complement activation, including the cleavage of C5 into C5a. These observations serve to emphasize the multiplicity of amplification mechanisms that may play roles in acute inflammation.

There is increasing evidence for proinflammatory interactions between oxygen metabolites and lysosomal proteases. Exposure of isolated macrophages to leukocytic proteases results in amplified O_2^- responses following cell activation with various soluble stimuli (68). Similarly, exposure of ex vivo perfused rabbit lungs to limiting concentrations of either leukocytic lysosomal extracts or a cell-free O_2^--generating system (xanthine/xanthine oxidase) results in minimal lung injury. In contrast, when these materials are perfused simultaneously, there is significant lung injury, indicating a synergistic proinflammatory interaction (69). Weiss et al. (70) have recently shown that physiological concentrations of hypohalous acid (derived from H_2O_2 and myeloperoxidase) will activate latent collagenase after its release from specific granules of human neutrophils. These investigators have also shown that latent gelatinase can be activated through a similar mechanism (71). Friedl et al. (72) have recently shown that histamine and several of its metabolites, including methylhistamine, imidazole-4-acetic acid, and methylimidazole-4-acetic acid, can increase the catalytic activity of xanthine oxidase in rat plasma and rat pulmonary artery endothelial cells. This observation may explain the therapeutic efficacy of xanthine oxidase inhibitors, histamine receptor antagonists, and cromolyn in the reduction of xanthine oxidase-dependent, neutrophil-independent skin edema that occurs secondary to thermal skin trauma. The many interactions among inflammatory mediator systems serve to reemphasize the complexity of oxidant-mediated tissue injury. It will be a continuing challenge to identify the relevant phlogistic pathways in clinical states and to devise therapeutic strategies to exploit this information.

ACKNOWLEDGMENTS

The authors would like to thank Kimberly Drake and Jennifer Fricke for manuscript preparation; they would also like to thank Robin Kunkel for preparation of transmission electron micrographs. This work was supported, in part, by National Institutes of Health grants HL-40526, HL-34635, and HL-31963.

REFERENCES

1. Mustafa MG, Tierney DF. Biochemical and metabolic changes in the lung with oxygen, ozone, and nitrogen dioxide toxicity. *Am Rev Respir Dis* 1978;118:1061–1090.
2. Fisher AB. Oxygen therapy: side effects and toxicity. *Am Rev Respir Dis* 1980;112:61–69.
3. Adamson IYR, Bowden DH, Wyatt JP. Oxygen poisoning in mice, ultrastructural and surfactant studies during exposure and recovery. *Arch Pathol Lab Med* 1970;90:463–472.
4. Freeman BA, Crapo JD. Hyperoxia increases oxygen radical production in rat lungs and lung mitochondria. *J Biol Chem* 1981;256:10986–10992.
5. Crapo JD, McCord JM. Oxygen-induced changes in pulmonary superoxide dismutase assayed by antibody titrations. *Am J Physiol* 1976;231:1196–1203.
6. Forman HJ, York JL, Fisher AB. Mechanism for the potentiation of oxygen toxicity of disulfiram. *J Pharmacol Exp Ther* 1980;212:452–455.
7. Crapo JD, Barry BE, Foscue HA, et al. Structural and biochemical changes in rat lungs occurring during exposures to lethal and adaptive doses of oxygen. *Am Rev Respir Dis* 1980;122:123–136.
8. Forman HJ, Fisher AB. Antioxidant enzymes of rat granular pneumocytes: constitutive level effect of hyperoxia. *Lab Invest* 1981;45:1–6.
9. Steinberg H, Greenwald RA, Moak SA, et al. The effect of oxygen adaption on oxyradical injury to pulmonary endothelium. *Am Rev Respir Dis* 1983;128:94–97.
10. Frank L, Summerville J, Massaro D. Protection from oxygen toxicity with endotoxin: role of the endogenous antioxidant enzymes of the lung. *J Clin Invest* 1980;65:1104–1110.
11. Freeman BA, Young SL, Crapo JD. Liposome-mediated augmentation of superoxide dismutase in endothelial cells prevents oxygen injury. *J Biol Chem* 1983;258:12534–12542.
12. Turrens JF, Crapo JD, Freeman BA. Protection against oxygen toxicity by intravenous injection of liposome-entrapped catalase and superoxide dismutase. *J Clin Invest* 1984;73:87–95.
13. Craddock PR, Fehr J, Brigham KL, Kronenberg RS, Jacob HS. Complement and leukocyte mediated pulmonary dysfunction in hemodialysis. *N Engl J Med* 1977;196:769–775.
14. Craddock PR, Fehr J, Brigham KL, Kronenberg RS, Jacob HS. Pulmonary vascular leukostasis resulting from complement activation by dialyzer cellophane membranes. *J Clin Invest* 1977;59:879–889.
15. Sacks T, Moldow CF, Craddock PR, Bowers TK, Jacob HS. Oxygen radical mediated endothelial cell damage by complement-stimulated granulocytes: an *in vitro* model of immune vascular damage. *J Clin Invest* 1978;61:1161–1167.

16. Till GO, Johnson KJ, Kunkel R, Ward PA. Intravascular activation of complement and acute lung injury. Dependency on neutrophils and toxic oxygen metabolites. *J Clin Invest* 1982;69:1126–1132.

17. Ward PA, Till GO, Kunkel R, Beauchamp C. Evidence for role of hydroxyl radical in complement and neutrophil-dependent tissue injury. *J Clin Invest* 1983;72:789–801.

18. Johnson KJ, Ward PA. Acute immunologic pulmonary alveolitis. *J Clin Invest* 1974;54:349–356.

19. Johnson KJ, Ward PA. Role of oxygen metabolites in immune complex injury of lung. *J Immunol* 1981;126:1365–1369.

20. Warren JS, Yabroff KR, Remick DG, Kunkel SL, Chensue SW, Kunkel RG, Johnson KJ, Ward PA. Tumor necrosis factor participates in the pathogenesis of acute immune complex alveolitis in the rat. *J Clin Invest* 1989;84:1873–1882.

21. Johnson KJ, Wilson BS, Till GO, Ward PA. Acute lung injury in rat caused by immunoglobulin A immune complexes. *J Clin Invest* 1984;74:358–366.

22. Johnson KJ, Ward PA, Kunkel RG, Wilson BS. Mediation of IgA induced lung injury in the rat. Role of macrophages and reactive oxygen products. *Lab Invest* 1986;54:499–508.

23. Chvapil M, Peng YM. Oxygen and lung fibrosis. *Arch Environ Health* 1975;30:528–532.

24. Gross NJ. Pulmonary effects of radiation therapy. *Ann Intern Med* 1977;86:81–92.

25. Autor AP, Schmitt SL. Pulmonary fibrosis and paraquat toxicity. In: Autor AP, ed., *Biochemical mechanisms of paraquat toxicity*. London: Academic Press, 1977;175–186.

26. Hunninghake GW, Fauci AS. Pulmonary involvement in the collagen vascular diseases. *Am Rev Respir Dis* 1978;119:471–503.

27. Weiss RB, Muggia FM. Update on cytotoxic drug-induced pulmonary disease. *Am J Med* 1980;68:259–266.

28. Johnson KJ, Fantone JC, Kaplan J, Ward PA. *In vivo* damage of rat lungs by oxygen metabolites. *J Clin Invest* 1981;67:983–993.

29. Thrall RS, McCormick JR, Jack RM, McReynolds RA, Ward PA. Bleomycin-induced pulmonary fibrosis in the rat. *Am J Pathol* 1979;95:117–127.

30. Phan SH, Thrall RS, Ward PA. Bleomycin-induced pulmonary fibrosis in rats: biochemical demonstration of increased rate of collagen synthesis. *Am Rev Respir Dis* 1980;121:501–506.

31. Adamson IYR, Bowden DH. The pathogenesis of bleomycin-induced pulmonary fibrosis in mice. *Am J Pathol* 1974;77:185.

32. Fleischman RW, Barker JR, Thompson GR, Schaeppi UH, Illevski VR, Cooney DA, Davis RD. Bleomycin-induced interstitial pneumonia in dogs. *Thorax* 1971;26:675.

33. Fantone JC, Phan SH. Oxygen metabolite detoxifying enzyme levels in bleomycin-induced fibrotic lungs. *Free Rad Biol Med* 1988;4:399–402.

34. Fantone JC, Ward PA. Oxygen-derived radicals and their metabolites: relationship to tissue injury. In: *Current concepts*. Kalamazoo, MI: Upjohn Company, 1985;51–59.

35. Harlan JM, Killen PD, Harker LA, Striker GE, Wright DG. Neutrophil-mediated endothelial injury *in vitro*: mechanisms of cell detachment. *J Clin Invest* 1981;68:1394–1401.

36. Gannon DE, Varani J, Phan SH, et al. Source of iron in neutrophil-mediated killing of endothelial cells. *Lab Invest* 1987;57:37–44.

37. Weiss SJ, Young J, LoBuglio AF, Slivka A, Nimeh NF. Role of hydrogen peroxide in neutrophil-mediated destruction of cultured endothelial cells. *J Clin Invest* 1981;68:714–721.

38. Varani J, Fligiel SEG, Till GO, Kunkel RG, Ryan US, Ward PA. Pulmonary endothelial cell killing by human neutrophils. Possible involvement of hydroxyl radical. *Lab Invest* 1985;53:665–674.

39. Smedly LA, Tonnesen MG, Sanhaus RA, Haslett C, Gutherie LA, Johnston RB, Henson PM, Worthen GS. Neutrophil-mediated injury to endothelial cells. Enhancement by endotoxin and essential role of neutrophil elastase. *J Clin Invest* 1986;77:1233–1239.

40. Klebanoff SJ, Clark RA. Hemolysis and iodination of erythrocyte components by a myeloperoxidase-mediated system. *Blood* 1975;45:699–707.

41. Clark RA, Klebanoff SJ. Neutrophil-mediated tumor cell cytotoxicity: role of the peroxidase system. *J Exp Med* 1975; 141:1442–1447.

42. Clark RA, Klebanoff SJ, Einstein AB, Fefer A. Peroxidase-H_2O_2–halide system: cytotoxic effect on mammalian tumor cells. *Blood* 1975;45:161–170.

43. Baehner RL, Boxer LA, Allen JM, Davis J. Autooxidation as a basis for altered function by polymorphonuclear leukocytes. *Blood* 1977;50:327–335.

44. Simon RH, Scoggin CH, Patterson D. Hydrogen peroxide causes the fatal injury to human fibroblasts exposed to oxygen radicals. *J Biol Chem* 1981;256:7181–7186.

45. Cantin AM, North SL, Fells GA, Hubbard RC, Crystal RG. Oxidant-mediated epithelial cell injury in idiopathic pulmonary fibrosis. *J Clin Invest* 1987;79:1665–1673.

46. Fletcher BL, Dillard CJ, Tappel AL. Measurement of fluorescent lipid peroxidation products in biological systems and tissues. *Anal Biochem* 1973;52:1–9.

47. Riley CA, Cohen G, Lieberman M. Ethane evolution: a new index of lipid peroxidation. *Science* 1974;183:208–210.

48. Till GO, Beauchamp C, Menapace D, Tourtellotte W, Kunkel R, Johnson KJ, Ward PA. Oxygen radical dependent lung damage following thermal injury of rat skin. *J Trauma* 1983;23:269–277.

49. Till GO, Hatherill JR, Tourtellotte WW, Lutz MJ, Ward PA. Lipid peroxidation and acute lung injury after thermal trauma to skin. Evidence for a role for hydroxyl radical. *Am J Pathol* 1985;119:376–384.

50. Freeman BA, Crapo JD. Free radicals and tissue injury. In: Rubin E, Damjanov I, eds. *Advances in the biology of disease*, vol 1, 1st ed. Baltimore, MD: Williams & Wilkins, 1984;26–40.

51. Roubul WT, Tappel AL. Polymerization of protein induced by free radical lipid peroxidation. *Arch Biochem Biophys* 1966; 173:150–155.

52. Roubul WT, Tappel AL. Damage to protein, enzymes and amino acids by peroxidizing lipids. *Arch Biochem Biophys* 1966;113:5–8.

53. Fantone JC, Ward PA. Role of oxygen-derived free radicals and metabolites in leukocyte-dependent inflammatory reactions. *Am J Pathol* 1982;107:395–418.

54. Drapier JC, Hibbs JB. Murine cytotoxic activated macrophages inhibit aconitase in tumor cells. Inhibition involves the iron–sulfur prosthetic group and is reversible. *J Clin Invest* 1986; 78:790–797.

55. Schraufstatter IU, Hinshaw DB, Hyslop PA, Spragg RG, Cochrane CG. Oxidant injury of cells, DNA strand-breaks activate polyadenosine diphosphate-ribose polymerase and lead to depletion of nicotinamide adenine dinucleotide. *J Clin Invest* 1986;77:1312–1320.

56. Schraufstatter IU, Hyslop PA, Jackson J, Cochrane CG. Induction of DNA strand breaks by H_2O_2 and PMA. *Fed Proc* 1986;45(3):451.

57. Hyslop PA, Hinshaw DB, Halsey WA, Schraufstatter IU, Sauerhaber RD, Spragg RG, Jackson JH, Cochrane CG. Mechanisms of oxidant-mediated cell injury. The glycolytic and mitochondrial pathways of ADP phosphorylation are major intercellular targets inactivated by hydrogen peroxide. *J Biol Chem* 1988; 263:1665–1675.

58. Phan SH, Gannon DE, Varani J, Ryan US, Ward PA. Xanthine oxidase activity in rat pulmonary artery endothelial cells and its alteration by activated neutrophils. *Am J Pathol* 1989;134:1201–1211.

59. McCord JM. Oxygen-derived radicals: a link between reperfusion injury and inflammation. *Fed Proc* 1987;46:2402–2406.

60. Greenwald RA, Moy WW. Effects of oxygen-derived free radicals on hyaluronic acid. *Arthritis Rheum* 1980;23:455–463.

61. Greenwald RA, Moy WW. Inhibition of collagen gelatin by action of superoxide radical. *Arthritis Rheum* 1979;22:251–259.

62. Fligiel SEG, Lee EC, McCoy JP, Johnson KJ, Varani J. Protein degradation following treatment with hydrogen peroxide. *Am J Pathol* 1984;115:418–425.

63. Carp H, Janoff A. In vitro suppression of serum elastase inhibitory capacity by reactive oxygen species generated by phagocytosing polymorphonuclear leukocytes. *J Clin Invest* 1979; 63:793–797.

64. Matheson NR, Wong DS, Travis J. Enzymatic inactivation of human alpha-1-proteinase inhibitor by neutrophil peroxidase. *Biochem Biophys Res Commun* 1989;88:402–409.

65. Perez HD, Weksler BB, Goldstein JM. Generation of a chemotactic lipid from arachidonic acid by exposure to a superoxide generating system. *Inflammation* 1980;4:313–328.

66. Shingu M, Nobunaga M. Chemotactic activity generated in human serum from the fifth component of complement by hydrogen peroxide. *Am J Pathol* 1984;117:201–206.

67. Vogt W, Zabern I von, Hesse D, Notte R, Haller Y. Generation of an activated form of human C5 (C5b-like) by oxygen radicals. *Immunol Lett* 1987;14:209–215.

68. Speer CP, Pabst MJ, Hedegaard HB, Rest RF, Johnston RB, Jr. Enhanced release of oxygen metabolites by monocyte-derived macrophages exposed to proteolytic enzymes: activity of neutrophil elastase and cathepsin G. *J Immunol* 1984;133:2151–2156.

69. Fox RB, Merrigan MJ. Synergism of oxygen radicals and elastase in the pathogenesis of acute permeability pulmonary edema. *Am Rev Respir Dis* 1986;133:A153.

70. Weiss JS, Peppin G, Ortiz H, Ragsdale C, Test SI. Oxidative autoactivation of latent collagenase by human neutrophils. *Science* 1985;227:747–749.

71. Peppin GJ, Weiss SJ. Activation of the endogenous metalloproteinase, gelatinase, by triggered human neutrophils. *Proc Natl Acad Sci USA* 1986;83:4322–4326.

72. Friedl HP, Till GO, Trentz O, Ward PA. Roles of histamine, complement and xanthine oxidase in thermal injury of skin. *Am J Pathol* 1989;135:203–218.

THE LUNG: *Scientific Foundations*
edited by R.G. Crystal, J.B. West et al.
Raven Press, Ltd., New York © 1991.

CHAPTER 7.3.1

Particle Deposition

David C. F. Muir

Lister (1) observed in 1868 that air entering the pleural cavity from the lung did not cause infection. He suggested that inhaled air was filtered of germs by the air passages, one of whose functions was to arrest inhaled particles of dust. Tyndall (2), an eminent Victorian physicist, examined exhaled air with the aid of a bright beam of light and found that deep lung air was absolutely free from suspended matter. Owens (3) extended these experiments and showed that airborne dust was, in fact, present in the deep lung air following a deep inhalation but that particles did not reach the alveoli during quiet breathing.

These authors clearly developed the idea that the bronchial tree has a most important physiological function as a filter that prevents much inhaled dust from reaching the alveoli. Findeisen (4), a meteorologist, was the first to apply information about the dynamics of airborne particles in order to predict their total and regional deposition in the lung. He used anatomical data available at the time to calculate flow rates in each generation of airways as a function of minute ventilation and combined this with the factors that were known to cause particle deposition in branching tubes. He treated the airways as a series of filters during both inhalation and exhalation. Three deposition mechanisms were identified.

1. *Gravitational settlement.* Each particle settles with a uniform speed that is proportional to its density and square of its diameter.

2. *Inertial impaction.* When airstreams change direction or velocity, the inertia of the entrained particles causes them to maintain their original direction for a distance that depends on the particle density and square of its diameter.

3. *Diffusion.* Airborne particles acquire a random motion as a result of bombardment by the surrounding gas molecules. Diffusivity is inversely proportional to particle diameter but is insensitive to its density. Correction factors are required when the size of the particle is less than that of the mean free path of the air molecules ($\sim$0.5 μm).

These mechanisms determine the probability that an inhaled particle will touch the surface of the respiratory tract where it is held by surface tension and other forces. Such a particle is considered to be deposited or filtered from the airstream. Each behaves as an independent unit, and deposition does not depend on the numerical concentration.

An aerosol (being defined as a volume of gas containing suspended solid or liquid particles) is drawn into the bronchial tree during inspiration, to a depth that depends on the tidal volume and at a rate that depends on the frequency of breathing. The approach used by Findeisen (4) and by subsequent authors was to calculate the transit time of a particle in each airway and to estimate its deposition probability according to (a) the dimensions of that airway and (b) the diffusivity and sedimentation velocity of the particle. The latter are functions of residence time within each airway. As far as inertial impaction is concerned, it is necessary to calculate the rate of airflow at each bifurcation and, making assumptions about the branching angle, to estimate the probability that a particle will touch the airway in the proximity of the bifurcation. It follows that the probability of a particle being deposited in a given airway as a result of gravity or diffusion increases as the rate of airflow at the mouth slows or during breath-holding. Conversely, the impaction probability increases with more rapid airflow.

In general terms, large particles are trapped in the nose and upper airways as a result of inertial impaction. Smaller particles are deposited mainly by gravitational settlement in the deeper lung, whereas the

D. C. F. Muir: Occupational Health Program, McMaster University, Hamilton, Ontario L8N 3Z5, Canada.

very smallest particles, which have a high coefficient of diffusion, are completely filtered out in the nose or upper airways during inhalation. Between these extremes of size, particles are able to penetrate the protective filter of the bronchial tree and reach the alveoli. Particles of approximately 0.5-μm diameter have such a low settling velocity and diffusivity that they penetrate to the alveoli during inhalation, but most remain airborne and appear at the mouth during the subsequent exhalation. As a result, their total deposition in the respiratory tract during breathing is minimal and does not normally exceed about 15%. Particles larger and smaller than 0.5 μm penetrate beyond the terminal bronchioles during inhalation and may be deposited in the alveoli. Only those larger than 0.5 μm contribute a sufficient mass to be of general importance in human health. The range of these particles that deposit in the alveoli is between 1 and 5 μm and probably reaches a maximum between 2 and 3 μm. Particles smaller than 0.5 μm are also thought to have a peak value for alveolar deposition, but, as noted above, their mass is exceedingly small.

Following Findeisen's original calculations (4), improved anatomical models (5–7) and deposition formulae (8–10) have been used to predict particle behavior in the lung (11,12). The irregular branching pattern of the bronchial tree is a formidable barrier to the theoretician, and impaction calculations are very sensitive to assumptions about the branching angle of the smaller airways. Moreover, it is known that the pattern of airflow at bifurcations is complex (13) and is probably asymmetrical during inhalation and exhalation. Another source of asymmetry during the breathing cycle is attributable to the fact that air decelerates during its passage from large to small airways but accelerates during exhalation. There is uncertainty about the effect of laminar flow patterns in the small airways on deposition probabilities. As a result of velocity gradients normal to the airway diameter in fully developed laminar viscous flow, it is probable that a unit of tidal air enters the smallest lung units along the central axis and is surrounded by a sheath of clean air derived from the air originally in the lung at the start of inhalation. This effect has been discussed by Davies (14) and needs further study.

Total deposition of particles in the lung has been reported by many authors using optical or mechanical systems for measuring particle concentration at the mouth or nose during breathing (15–19). Only limited data are available in the case of very fine aerosols because of the technical difficulties of producing and measuring the concentrations of these particles (20,21).

Deposition experiments are generally carried out using apparatus provided with a mouthpiece. Most re-

cently, it has been recognized that only a fraction of the ambient dust can enter the nose and mouth during inhalation (22). This is termed the *breathable* or *inhalable* fraction, and the concept is important in determining the uptake of toxic particles by the body. In applying deposition calculations to the problem of ambient aerosols it is important to allow for possible changes in particle size as a result of evaporation or hygroscopic growth (23). Electrostatic charge can be relevant in some industrial situations or in aerosol therapy. In experimental apparatus it is important to neutralize electrostatic charges, since these can have significant effects on particle deposition (24,25). Concentrations must be corrected for instrumental dead space and for any changes in moisture content in exhaled air.

Regional deposition cannot be measured directly in human subjects. Inferences about regional deposition have been made by examining the distribution of particles in exhaled air (8,11,15,26). Deposition on the ciliated airways is now most generally measured by using radioactively labeled aerosols and by assuming that the fraction cleared within the first 24 hr corresponds closely with that deposited on the ciliated airways (27), or by extrapolation from long-term retention curves (28). The two approaches produce similar, but not identical, results; in both methods the assumption is made that insoluble particles deposited on the ciliated airways are cleared rapidly and do not enter the mucosa. Regional deposition in models of the human nose and upper airways has been measured in a number of elegant experiments (29,30). Turbulent deposition at the bifurcation of the major airways results in high local concentrations in these regions. This may be an important factor in the pathogenesis of malignant disease of the bronchus resulting from inhaled carcinogens (31).

Lister would no doubt have been intrigued by one property of the upper airway filter. As the frequency of breathing increases during exercise, the time available for particle sedimentation is reduced; however, the probability of impaction is increased, and the physiological efficiency of the system is maintained. More information is needed about the change from nose to mouth breathing and about the filtration efficiency of each in order to determine how exercise relates to protection of the lungs.

An overview of total and regional deposition as a function of particle size is shown in Fig. 1. This figure has been widely used since its publication some years ago. A committee is currently reviewing the recent deposition data, and a new curve should be available shortly. It is emphasized that the deposition values shown in Fig. 1 refer to the fate of particles after they have entered the nose or mouth. No account is taken

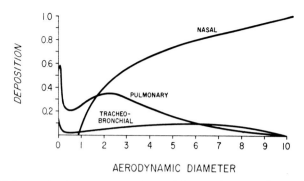

FIG. 1. Regional deposition of inhaled aerosols as a function of particle size (expressed in microns). Nose breathing was observed at 15 respirations per minute and at a 750-cm³ tidal volume. The pulmonary compartment refers to deposition beyond the terminal bronchiole. (From ref. 49.)

of that fraction of ambient dust which fails to enter the oral or nasal orifices.

The effects of dust exposure in industry depend on the site of deposition as well as on the toxicity of the particles. Interest has been focused on (a) nasal cancer caused by the deposition of wood dust or compounds of nickel in the nose, (b) lung cancer caused by deposition of a number of carcinogens on the bronchial tree, and (c) pneumoconiosis caused by deposition and accumulation of dust in the alveoli. Industrial sampling apparatus usually cannot separate out this alveolar fraction of the airborne dust. As a surrogate it is usual to estimate the airborne hazard when alveolar dust is important by using respirable dust samplers. The respirable fraction is defined as that fraction of airborne particles entering the mouth or nose which are able to penetrate beyond the terminal bronchi during inhalation.

In industry it is uncommon to find particles of uniform density or of regular shape, and it is convenient to describe the behavior of such particles in terms of their aerodynamic diameter, defined as that size of unit density sphere which has the same settling velocity as the particle in question and which therefore has the same intrapulmonary deposition pattern. In the case of aerosols containing a range of particle sizes, the aerodynamic mass median diameter (AMMD) is the most appropriate parameter for describing the intrapulmonary deposition of the whole cloud. Half the total particulate mass consists of particles whose size is below the AMMD, and the other half of the mass consists of particles that are larger than the stated size. This is an important concept in experimental work when regional dose is being studied, especially in the case of therapeutic aerosols.

TURBULENCE IN THE AIRWAYS, AND THE EXCHANGE OF AEROSOLS BETWEEN TIDAL AIR AND LUNG AIR

Owens (3) suggested that there was only slight mechanical mixing at the points of contact between inhaled air and lung air during breathing. Altshuler et al. (32) were able to measure the amount of this mechanical mixing and found that it was about 15% of the tidal volume. Possible mechanisms include (a) turbulent mixing in the upper airways and (b) various forms of nonreversible flow in the small airways. The amount of mixing may determine the minimum deposition value in a given subject rather than particle size. In addition, Heyder et al. (19) could find little effect of particle size on deposition for the case of particles ranging from 0.2 to 1 μm in diameter. They suggested that the deposition of particles of this size was determined by mechanical mixing of air volumes during breathing rather than by the intrinsic mobility of the particles. The limitation of particle exchange between tidal air and lung air contrasts strongly with the very rapid equilibration of gas molecules during breathing, which is caused by the very high diffusion coefficient of gas molecules. Davies (14) considered that mechanical mixing could occur only in the upper airways and that the Reynolds number in the depths of the lung was far too low to permit any form of mechanical mixing. However, on the basis of their experimental work, Taulbee et al. (33) felt that mixing of a mechanical nature occurred at all levels of the bronchial tree. Even though turbulent mixing may not occur in the smaller airways, it seems to the present reviewer that airflow between alveoli or asymmetrical airflow at airway bifurcations may contribute a nonreversible component that appears to an observer at the mouth, as if mechanical mixing of air had occurred at all levels of the bronchial tree during breathing.

The degree of turbulence in the larger airways is of practical importance in determining the risk of lung cancer caused by the inhalation of radon progeny. The unattached fraction of radon progeny has a particle size of about 0.001 μm in diameter and is deposited as a result of diffusion. The flux of particles to the surface of the trachea is much greater in turbulent flow than in laminar flow. This was determined experimentally by Cohen (30) and is a key factor in calculating the radiation dose to the lower bronchial tree.

VARIABILITY BETWEEN SUBJECTS, AND THE EFFECT OF LUNG VOLUME

Significant differences in deposition pattern between subjects has been reported (14,34). The reasons for this are uncertain, but Davies (14) considered one source of variability to be failure to standardize for lung volume. Two groups (14,35) have shown that intrapulmonary deposition for aerosols of about 0.5 μm diameter is inversely proportional to functional residual capacity (FRC). However, Muir and Cena (36) could detect no effect when using particles of about 0.01 μm in diameter. The reasons for the sensitivity of particle deposition to FRC in the case of 0.5-μm-diameter aerosols are uncertain. Evidently, the airways are larger when lung volume increases, and this not only increases the mean distance between the particles and the wall of the airway but also affects the development of turbulent airflow. Interestingly, Davies (14) observed no difference in the distribution of aerosol in exhaled air in relation to changes in FRC and considered that this excluded any change in the mechanical mixing of air volumes during breathing. The distribution of inhaled air to regions of the upright lung has been shown to change with lung volume, and this might be a factor affecting particle deposition. In experiments to study the effect of tidal volume on deposition, it is probable that the midthoracic volume should be held constant, since this is the normal physiological response to increasing tidal volume during exercise (37).

THE DEVELOPING LUNG

Children are susceptible to biological aerosols, may be sensitive to radon progeny, and are commonly treated with therapeutic aerosols. Calculations of particle deposition in the infant and child lung indicate a relatively greater deposition efficiency in the upper airway compared to the adult lung (38,39). In combination with the high metabolic activity of children, this may cause a significantly greater deposition of particles per unit surface area of airway compared to that of the adult and must be evaluated when estimating relative risks.

THE EFFECT OF ABNORMAL LUNG ANATOMY OR AIRFLOW: USE OF AEROSOLS FOR DIAGNOSTIC PURPOSES

The fractional deposition of inhaled particles of approximately 1.0 μm in diameter was found to be increased as a result of obstructive airways disease (40). The effect of abnormal airflow or of narrowed airways on regional deposition is likely to be complex. For particles of 0.2–1 μm in diameter, which, as noted by Heyder et al. (19), are deposited in proportion to the mechanical mixing of air, it is probable that there is enhanced alveolar deposition. For somewhat larger particles, which have a significant impaction probability, Sanchis et al. (41) found that there was increased

central or upper airway deposition and that there was restricted access of these particles to the alveoli. They suggested that this might reduce the probability that workers with obstructive airways disease would develop pneumoconiosis, but no epidemiological evidence for this has been found (42). The proximal deposition of particles was proposed as a possible test of disease of the small airways (43), and this has been confirmed by Emmett et al. (44).

The proximal deposition of particles in the presence of abnormal airflow is a determinant of subsequent clearance patterns and must be considered when interpreting experimental data.

The possibility of using aerosols to detect abnormal patterns of airflow was proposed by Altshuler et al. (32). Muir (45) showed that the distribution of aerosols in exhaled air was abnormal in the presence of airflow obstruction and that this effect was most easily shown by the use of a bolus of inhaled particles. However, there does not appear to be any fundamental difference in the information that is obtained about airflow in the lung whether a single inhalation or a bolus is used. The bolus technique is convenient, and Altshuler et al. (32) have suggested that this can be expressed in nondimensional units as the ratio between the height and the half-width of the exhaled bolus (32). It appears to be a very sensitive method of detecting abnormal airflow (46).

Palmes (47) has shown that the deposition of particles during breathholding can be used for estimating the size of the intrapulmonary air spaces. It may provide a method of detecting emphysema during life, although there are likely to be difficulties resulting from the limited access of particles to dilated air spaces.

These exciting techniques provide most interesting possibilities. The methodologies have been worked out, and the next steps must include epidemiological surveys.

ELONGATED PARTICLES

Fibrous or elongated particles such as asbestos are intercepted at the bifurcation of airways if their length is a significant fraction of the airway diameter. They have a settling velocity equivalent to that of a sphere having a diameter approximately one-third that of the fiber (48). In laminar flow they have an irregular or tumbling motion, and their intrapulmonary deposition pattern is complex. The curled shape of chrysotile fibers probably causes them to be deposited at a higher level in the respiratory tract than the needle-like fibers of amosite or crocidolite, and this may be a factor in the relative toxicity of these different varieties of asbestos.

REFERENCES

1. Lister J. An address on the antiseptic system of treatment in surgery. *Br Med J* 1868;2:53–56.
2. Tyndall J. On dust and disease. *Proc R Inst* 1870;6:1–14.
3. Owens JS. Dust in expired air. *Trans Med Soc Lond* 1923;45:79–90.
4. Findeisen W. Uber das Absetzen Kleiner, in der Luft suspendierten Teilchen in der menschlichen Lunge bei der atmung. *Pflugers Arch Ges Physiol* 1935;236:367–379.
5. Weibel ER. *Morphometry of the human lung.* Berlin: Springer-Verlag, 1963.
6. Horsefield K, Dart G, Olsen DE, et al. Models of the human bronchial tree. *J Appl Physiol* 1971;31:207–217.
7. Yeh HC, Schum GM. Models of human lung airways and their application to inhaled particle deposition. *Bull Math Biol* 1980;42:461–480.
8. Landahl HD. On the removal of airborne droplets by the human respiratory tract. I. The lung. *Bull Math Biophys* 1950;12:43–56.
9. Yeh HC, Phalen RF, Raabe OG. Factors in influencing the deposition of inhaled particles. *Environ Health Perspect* 1976;15:147–156.
10. Martin D, Jacobi W. Diffusion deposition of small-sized particles in the bronchial tree. *Health Phys* 1972;23:23–29.
11. Landahl HD. Particle removal by the respiratory system. *Bull Math Biophys* 1963;25:29–39.
12. Beeckmans JM. The deposition of aerosols in the respiratory tract. I. Mathematical analysis and comparison with experimental data. *Can J Physiol Pharmacol* 1965;43:157–172.
13. Olsen DE, Sudlow MF, Horsfield K, Filley GF. Convective patterns of flow during inspiration. *Arch Int Med* 1973;131:51–57.
14. Davies CN. Breathing of half-micron aerosols. *J Appl Physiol* 1972;32:601–611.
15. Brown JH, Cook KM, Ney FG, Hatch T. Influence of particle size upon the retention of particulate matter in the human lung. *Am J Public Health* 1950;40:450–458.
16. Altshuler B, Yarmus L, Palmes ED, Nelson N. Aerosol deposition in the human respiratory tract. *AMA Arch Ind Health* 1957;15:293–303.
17. Muir DCF, Davies CN. The deposition of 0.5 micron diameter aerosol in the lungs of man. *Ann Occup Hyg* 1967;10:161–174.
18. Davies CN, Heder J, Subba Rammu MC. Breathing of half-micron aerosols. *J Appl Physiol* 1972;591–600.
19. Heyder J, Gebhart J, Heigver G, et al. Experimental studies of the total deposition of aerosol particles in the human respiratory tract. *J Aerosol Sci* 1973;4:191–208.
20. Muir DCF, Cena K. Deposition of ultrafine aerosols in the human respiratory tract. *Aerosol Sci Technol* 1987;6:183–190.
21. Schiller DHF, Gebhart J, Heyder J, et al. Deposition of monodisperse insoluble aerosol particles in the 0.05 to 0.2 μm size range within the human respiratory tract. *Ann Occup Hyg* 1988;32(Suppl 1):41–49.
22. Ogden TL, Birkett JL. The human head as a dust sampler. In: Walton WH, ed. *Inhaled paricles IV.* Oxford: Pergamon Press, 1975;93–105.
23. Morrow PE. Factors determining hygroscopic aerosol deposition in airways. *Physiol Rev* 1986;60:330–376.
24. Melandri C, Prodi V, Tarron G, et al. On the deposition of unipolarly charged particles in the human respiratory tract. In: Walton WH, ed. *Inhaled particles IV.* Oxford: Pergamon Press, 1977;193–201.
25. Chan TL, Yu CP. Charge effects on particle deposition in the human tracheobronchial tree. In: Walton WH, ed. *Inhaled particles V.* Oxford: Pergamon Press, 1982;26:65–75.
26. Altshuler B, Palmes ED, Nelson N. Regional aerosol deposition in the human respiratory tract. In: Davies CN, ed. *Inhaled particles II.* Oxford: Pergamon Press, 1965;323–337.
27. Chan TL, Lippman M. Experimental measurements and empirical modelling of the regional deposition of inhaled particles in humans. *Am Ind Hyg Assoc J* 1980;41:399–409.
28. Stahlhofen W, Gebhart J, Heyder J. Biological variability of regional deposition of aerosol particles in the human respiratory tract. *Am Ind Hyg Assoc J* 1981;42:348–352.
29. Schlesinger RB, Lippmann M. Particle deposition in casts of the human upper tracheobronchial tree. *Am Ind Hyg Assoc J* 1972;33:237–251.
30. Cohen BS. Deposition of ultrafine particles in the human tracheobronchial tree. In: *Radon and its decay products.* Washington, DC: American Chemical Society, 1987;475–486.
31. Schlesinger RB, Lippmann M. Selective particle deposition and bronchogenic carcinoma. *Environ Res* 1978;15:424–431.
32. Altshuler B, Palmes ED, Yarmus L, Nelson N. Intrapulmonary mixing of gases studied with aerosols. *J Appl Physiol* 1959;14:321–327.
33. Taulbee DB, Yu CP, Heyder J. Aerosol transport in the human lung from analysis of single breaths. *J Appl Physiol* 1978;44:803–812.
34. Heyder J, Gebhardt J, Stahlhofen W, Stuck B. Biological variability of particle deposition in the human respiratory tract during controlled and spontaneous mouth breathing. *Ann Occup Hyg* 1982;26:137–147.
35. Tarroni G, Melandri C, Prodi V, et al. An indication on the biological variability of aerosol total deposition in humans. *Am Ind Hyg Assoc J* 1980;41:826–831.
36. Muir DCF, Cena K. To be published.
37. Lind L, Hesser CM. Breathing pattern and lung volumes during exercise. *Acta Physiol Scand* 1984;120:123–129.
38. Hislop A, Muir DCF, Jacobsen M, et al. Postnatal growth and function of the pre-acinar airways. *Thorax* 1972;27:265–274.
39. Phalen RF, Oldham MJ, Kleinman MT, et al. Tracheobronchial deposition predictions for infants, children and adolescents. *Ann Occup Hyg* 1988;32(Suppl I):11–21.
40. Love RG, Muir DCF. Aerosol deposition and airway obstruction. *Am Rev Respir Dis* 1976;114:891–897.
41. Sanchis J, Dolovitch M, Chalmers R, et al. Regional distribution and lung clearance mechanisms in smokers and non-smokers. In: Walton WH, ed. *Inhaled particles III.* Old Woking: Unwin, 1971;183–188.
42. Muir DCF, Burns J, Jacobsen M, Walton WH. Pneumoconiosis and chronic bronchitis. *Br Med J* 1977;2:424–427.
43. Dolovitch MB, Sanchis J, Rossman C, et al. Aerosol penetrance: a sensitive index of peripheral airways obstruction. *J Appl Physiol* 1976;40:468–471.
44. Emmett PC, Love RG, Hannan WJ, et al. The relationship between the pulmonary distribution of inhaled fine aerosols and tests of small airway function. *Bull Environ Physiopathol Respir* 1984;20:325–332.
45. Muir DCF. The effect of airways obstruction on the single breath aerosol curve. In: Bouhuys A, ed. *Airway dynamics.* Spingfield, IL: Charles C Thomas, 1970;319–325.
46. McCawley M, Lippmann M. Development of an aerosol dispersion test to detect early changes in lung function. *Am Ind Hyg Assoc J* 1988;49:357–366.
47. Palmes ED. Measurement of pulmonary air-spaces using aerosols. *Arch Int Med* 1973;131:76–79.
48. Timbrell V. The inhalation of fibrous dusts. *Ann NY Acad Sci* 1965;132:255–273.
49. Deposition and Retention Models for Internal Dosimetry of the Human Respiratory Tract. International Commission on Radiological Protection. *Health Phys* 1969;12:173–207.

THE LUNG: *Scientific Foundations*
edited by R.G. Crystal, J.B. West et al.
Raven Press, Ltd., New York © 1991.

CHAPTER 7.3.2

Mucociliary Clearance

Stewart W. Clarke and Demetri Pavia

Mucociliary clearance in the air passages of the nose and trachea was first described comprehensively in 1835 by Sharpey (1). Subsequently, observations on mucociliary motion were made over many decades, culminating in the seminal paper by Lucas and Douglas in 1934 (2); these investigators suggested that the mucus is propelled by the tips of the cilia, which themselves move in a low-viscosity layer beneath the mucus—a concept which is still held, though modified, today. With the advent of electron microscopy, the morphology of the cilia has been explored, together with its dynamic characteristics; studies were initially performed in lower species but were subsequently performed in mammalian respiratory membranes, including those of humans (3).

The purpose of this chapter is to review mucociliary clearance in its entirety (principally in humans) and to discuss its relationship to disease where relevant. Subjects relevant to mucociliary clearance can also be found in Chapters 3.1.2 (structure and function of cilia), 3.1.3 (synthesis and composition of mucus), 3.3.1 (particle deposition), and 7.4.1 (integrated defense).

The air we breathe is loaded with particulate matter which may include microorganisms, pollutants, and allergens, all of which may injure the lung in a variety of ways if not cleared rapidly. It is often stated that the alveolar capillary surface area of the lung is about equivalent to that of a tennis court onto which flows a daily volume of air (and particles) sufficient to fill an average swimming pool (4). Hence the opportunity for damage to the lung is potentially enormous, although it is mitigated by the excellence of the defense mech-

anisms—chief of which is mucociliary clearance (5). The other mechanisms such as cough (6) and bronchoalveolar clearance (7) act as reserve and additional mechanisms, respectively.

It should be emphasized that many, if not most, lung diseases are caused by inhaled particles: Most cases of pneumonia and pulmonary tuberculosis are caused by microorganisms; extrinsic bronchial asthma and allergic alveolitis (e.g., bird-fancier's lung) are caused by inhaled allergens; silicosis, pneumoconiosis, and asbestosis are caused by inhaled dusts; and chronic bronchitis and carcinoma of the lung are caused by inhaled cigarette smoke. This list could be enlarged considerably.

TRACHEOBRONCHIAL DEPOSITION

Particle deposition within the tracheobronchial tree and lung (see above) is an important aspect to consider (8,9). In general, large particles (>10 μm) will be filtered out of the inhaled airstream by the aerodynamic filters of the nose (nasal vibria and mucociliary clearance), nasopharynx (and oropharynx), and larynx. Soluble gases may be dissolved in the nose. The change in cross-sectional areas within these sites, coupled with the change in direction of the airflow as it passes through the nose and beyond, is highly efficient in depositing the larger particles by inertial impaction followed by swallowing (mainly) or expectoration (occasionally)—at least in healthy individuals. Thus it is only the smaller particles which penetrate into the lung, and the smaller they become the deeper the penetration (Fig. 1). However, particles below 1 μm in diameter may act like a nonrespiratory gas and not be deposited at all. Particles of approximately 3 μm in diameter are deposited in the alveoli, whereas those of approximately 5–8 μm in diameter are deposited in the tracheobronchial tree.

S. W. Clarke: Department of Thoracic Medicine, The Royal Free Hospital and School of Medicine, Hampstead, London NW3 2QG, England.

D. Pavia: Medical Division, Boehringer Ingelheim (UK), Ltd., Bracknell, Berkshire RG12 4YS, England.

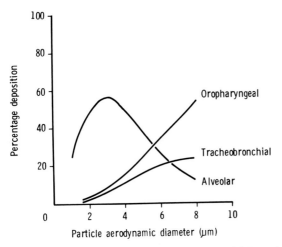

FIG. 1. Percentage of alveolar, tracheobronchial, and oropharyngeal deposition for various size of inhaled aerosols.

NASAL CLEARANCE

Mucociliary clearance starts in the nose, where ciliated mucosa is seen at the anterior aspect of the nasal septum and turbinates lining the nasal cavities and ending in the nasopharynx where there is transition from columnar ciliated to squamous epithelium.

Clearance of secretions in the nose is chiefly by mucociliary action sweeping the mucus backwards at about 6 mm min^{-1}, either to be swallowed imperceptibly or to be cleared from the throat. Mucus in the anterior nose may be blown away voluntarily or by sneezing (two-phase flow) (10) or may be wiped away.

Mucociliary Escalator

Anatomy (3)

From below the larynx, the tracheobronchial tree is lined by pseudostratified ciliated columnar epithelium with frequent goblet cells and submucosal glands which contribute to the "mucus blanket" overlying the mucosal surface. This extends to embrace lobar, segmental, and subsegmental bronchi, bronchioles, and ultimately the terminal bronchioles, which divide into three generations of respiratory bronchioles about 0.5 mm in diameter where additionally there are some Clara cells, the mucosa changing from having a thick submucosal layer to having nonciliated low cuboidal epithelium thereafter. This region is about the 16th generation of airways designated by Weibel (11) and reflects a watershed in clearance at this level, where mucociliary activity peters out and where bronchoalveolar clearance involving surfactant and alveolar macrophages takes over (see below).

Cilia (3)

The engine which drives mucus cephalad is constituted by the cilia (Fig. 2). The ciliated cells have on their mucosal surface about 200 cilia per cell (density 6–8 μm^{-2}) and are also characterized by their long cytoplasmic projections and numerous microvilli. Their length is about 6 μm in large airways and 5 μm in small ones. The shaft is formed of longitudinal fibers having a very characteristic structure with nine outer and two central microtubules. The outer ones each have one complete and one incomplete microtubule attached laterally and combining to form a doublet. They are composed of tubulin, a contractile protein. Dynein arms connect the adjacent doublets [dynein consists of adenosinetriphosphatase (ATPase) protein, the major protein component of the axoneme], deriving energy from adenosine triphosphate (ATP) distributed along the length of the cilium and providing the motive force for cilial beating. The cilial tip has a crown which consists of three to seven short claws (each claw is 25–35 nm long) and which probably grips the mucus blanket and helps propulsion. The ciliary basal body has a foot,

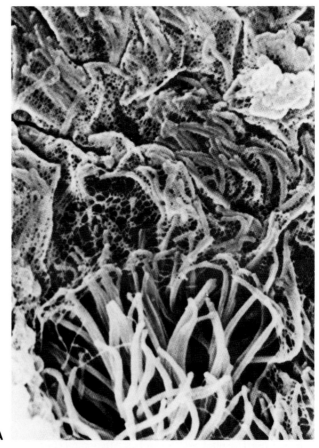

A

FIG. 2. A: Scanning electron micrograph of human bronchial epithelium showing cilia and flakes of mucus. (×6666.) **FIG. 2. *Continues.***

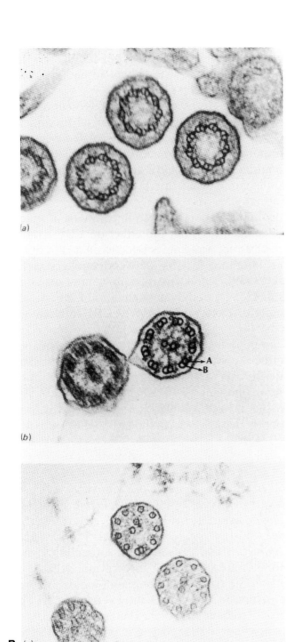

FIG. 2. *Continued.* **B:** Transmission electron micrographs of cross-sections of cilia showing the normal microtubular arrangement at the base (a), mid-shaft (b), and tip (c), (×100,000.)

short striated rootlets, attached cytoplasmic microtubules providing anchorage, and common orientation with adjacent cilia.

Ciliary Beat. During the ciliary beat cycle there is an effective stroke and a recovery stroke. In the effective stroke, the cilia are fully extended perpendicular to the cell surface and sweep the mucus cephalad. In the recovery stroke, the cilia are bent and flexed near the cell surface and take twice as long as for the active stroke (29 versus 15 msec^{-1}, with a maximal cilial tip speed of 1000 μm sec^{-1}). The outer nine microtubule doublets of the ciliary axoneme actively slide

forwards and backwards against one another when propelled by molecular bridges of dynein utilizing energy from ATP to produce cyclical shape changes, the basis of the active sliding movements along the whole length of the cilium, controlling the shape at any stage in the beat cycle. The radial spokes probably provide resistance to sliding and promote bending.

Recent animal and human studies have both indicated that calcium and cyclic adenosine monophosphate (cAMP) are important for ciliary movement (3,12) and the regulation of ciliary beat frequency (CBF). Cyclic AMP activates protein kinase A (PKA), which, in turn, phosphorylates a number of larger proteins using enzyme-bound ATP as the phosphate donor.

Groups of cilia beat spontaneously with metachronal waves in a coordinated fashion independent of nervous control with viscochemical coupling to the overlying mucus blanket. Cilia probably work best in a viscoelastic medium such as coiled macromolecular networks, which provide the consistency and integrity required for transport. The presence of fluid helps to organize coordinated beating, thereby ensuring metachronal waves; the original description of Lucas and Douglas (2) probably still holds true. They reported investigations of nasal epithelia in monkeys and found that particles were usually transported on a layer of mucus, leading them to propose the hypothesis of two distinct fluid layers: (i) an upper fibrous layer of mucus just penetrated by the cilia (the gel layer or epiphase) and (ii) a watery sublayer in which most ciliary movement takes place (the sol layer or hypophase).

Whereas it was often believed that the mucus blanket was uniformly 5–10 μm thick, present evidence suggests that mucus may normally be present in smaller amounts (droplets) on resting epithelia in smaller airways originating around inhaled particles. In larger airways these droplets may aggregate into flakes (10–70 μm in diameter) or plaques rather than forming a blanket. The 10 ml of mucus estimated to be generated daily by a healthy adult human represents a layer of mucus 10 μm thick propelled continuously up the trachea at about 0.2 mm sec^{-1}.

The dimensional length scales are important with respect to mucociliary interaction: Molecular length scales are related to the biochemical structure of mucus; larger scales are associated with the cilial tip (0.1–1 μm); even larger scales are related to cilial length, cell size, ciliary wavelength, and coherence of mucus plaque (5–50 μm); and macroscopic scales are related to the length of an airway (5–10 mm) (3).

Factors Affecting Ciliary Function. CBF is normally 12–14 beats per second, and mucus transport rate is usually 100 μm sec^{-1}. Temperature increase leads to a monotonic rise in CBF of threefold between 20°C and 40°C (13). A decrease in relative humidity of the local airflow leads to a sharp decrease in CBF, particularly at high temperatures (40°C). Mechanical stimulation increases local CBF (14) by way of calcium (Ca^{2+}) influx. Adjacent cells also respond after a brief delay possibly caused by diffusible intracellular messenger (12).

Ionizing radiation both reduces (15) and increases (16,17) ciliary activity, when given in high and low dosage, respectively (18). Hyperosmolality (19) decreases CBF; human nasal cilia are most active in iso-osmotic saline (NaCl 9 g liter^{-1}), with falls in ciliary activity above and below that point in concentrations ranging from 5 to 12 g liter^{-1} (80–200 mmol liter^{-1}) (20). An increase in viscosity in the medium retards ciliary activity, and the optimum pH in human bronchial cells is 7.0–9.0 (20).

As mentioned above, calcium appears to play an important role: Changes in intracellular Ca^{2+} modulate ciliary activity (21) augmented by calmodulin (22) and Ca^{2+} ionophore (12). Potassium also affects ciliary activity (23).

Mediators of ciliary function. Histamine's effects are indeterminate, and on occasion it causes ciliary incoordination (23); likewise for serotonin. Prostaglandins, with the exception of prostaglandin $F_{2\alpha}$ ($PGF_{2\alpha}$), generally increase CBF (24). Leukotrienes [LT; formerly known as "slowly reacting substances of anaphylaxis" (SRS-A)] LTC_4 and LTD_4 produce dose-dependent increases in CBF in sheep, the latter acting indirectly via activation of cyclo-oxygenase (25). Neuropeptide substance P (SP) is another agent involved in inflammatory reactions. Capsaicin causes the release of SP-like immunoreactivity from central and peripheral sensory nerve endings, and its administration has been shown to result in cilia stimulation (26,27) attributable to multiple neurally mediated pathways, one of which may be peptidergic and two of which may involve the release of prostaglandins. Bradykinin is a mediator released in the airway during an allergic challenge, and it increases CBF in animals (28). This increase was inhibited by both hexamethonium and indomethacin, suggesting that neural and cyclo-oxygenase pathways were involved. Finally, antigen challenge in allergic sheep produced (a) a modest increase in CBF (29), though paradoxically, and (b) a reduction in tracheal mucus velocity (TMV). Norepinephrine is inhibitory, whereas epinephrine is excitatory. Lidocaine may be ciliostatic *in vitro* but may have no effect *in vivo*. Codeine, but not morphine, is inhibitory (30).

Beta agonists and antagonists. It is worth noting that there have been many reports confirming that beta agonists increase mucociliary clearance (as well as being bronchodilators) in healthy subjects as well as in patients with chronic obstructive pulmonary disease (COPD) and cystic fibrosis (31). Similarly, in many studies an increase in CBF has been found (32,33), with a decrease after the use of beta-adrenergic blocking drugs (beta blockers) (34).

Cholinergic drugs increase mucus secretion from both glands and CBF, effects blocked by anticholinergics (32,33). Local steroids cause a decrease in CBF (35), though this is not necessarily clinically relevant.

Xanthines increase CBF and mucociliary clearance in humans (36), and this is probably therapeutically important.

Alcohol ingestion leads to impairment of mucociliary clearance (37), but the effect on CBF is not uniform. Cigarette smoking is toxic to cilia (38), but there is no difference in CBF between smokers and non-smokers (39). Sulfur dioxide and ozone cause depression in TMV but oddly enough not in CBF, at least in sheep (40). Lysozyme improves CBF in human nasal mucosa (41).

Cilio-inhibitory factors. Cilio-inhibitory factors are described in serum and in leukocytes, particularly in cystic fibrosis (42). However, *in vitro* CBF in cystic fibrosis is normal (43). A similar ciliostatic factor has been found from asthmatics (44); perhaps it is major basic protein (MBP) from the eosinophils (see Chapter 3.4.9) (45).

Local bacterial infection and purulent secretions can delay CBF and mucociliary clearance (47). Bacteria involved include *Hemophilus influenzae* (48), *Pseudomonas aeruginosa* (48), *Mycoplasma pneumoniae*, *Staphylococcus aureus* (49), and *Streptococcus pneumoniae* (50).

Mucolytics and expectorants. Mucolytics and expectorants are often used to help mucociliary clearance and the traditional potassium iodide and ammonium chloride are both cilio-excitatory. The drug ambroxol (related to bromhexine) is similar (51). Compounds with free sulfhydryl groups such as acetyl cysteine and S-carboxymethylcysteine are probably able to split the disulfide bonds of the lung glycoproteins of mucus and thus reduce its viscosity. At lower concentrations they may stimulate CBF, but at high concentrations they may actively retard it (52). However, no effect on ciliary activity was found in patients with cystic fibrosis or primary ciliary dyskinesia after 3 months of treatment with N-acetyl cysteine (53).

Finally, cilia not only can transport secretions against gravity, but also can carry weights of up to 10 g cm^{-2} without slowing (54), can survive freezing for up to a month with a return to normal beating on rewarming (55), and can continue beating for some hours after death.

Experimental work on ciliary function has been done in a wide variety of primitive organisms as well as in mammals (including rats, guinea pigs, cats, dogs, ferrets, sheep, and humans), and this has to be considered when assessing results. The same applies to lung mucociliary clearance; however, the number of species tested is fewer, and most of the work has been performed in humans.

Methods for Measuring Ciliary Function (56). Nasal cilia are readily obtained, preferably by brush biopsy via a nasal speculum rather than by forceps. Tracheobronchial cilia are usually sampled through a fiberoptic bronchoscope, which is more invasive but is of low risk. There is little or no difference between cilia at the two sites, and the nasal origin is preferable. The specimen needs careful and rapid immersion in tissue culture medium and requires stability of temperature (37°C). Cilial movement can be seen at high magnification under the microscope, and a motility index can be devised from looking at a graticule slide and classifying a given number of graticule squares as containing either motile or immotile cilia. The ratio of motile squares to the number counted is termed the "motility index."

CBF, which is usually measured by a photometric technique, ranges between 12 and 14 beats per second in normal human subjects; it slows down with reduced temperature, speeding up with beta agonists. In some patients with the disorder formerly termed "immotile cilia syndrome" (54), further work has shown impaired motility but by no means complete stasis. Hence the term "primary ciliary dyskinesia" has been coined. An example of this is seen in Kartagener's syndrome with situs inversus, bronchiectasis and sinusitis.

Under high ($\times 30,000$) magnification, the morphological characteristics of the cilia can be clearly seen. Abnormalities such as microtubular anomalies (with less than the $9 + 2$ arrangement), compound cilia, loss of dynein arms, and radial spokes can be assessed by standardized techniques which avoid sampling errors.

In vivo studies of cilial motion are often performed on the nasal mucosa. The most popular is the saccharin test, in which a particle of saccharine is placed in the inferior nasal turbinate and timed until the characteristic sweet taste is noted in the pharynx, with the normal time being 30 min. Its usefulness and reproducibility have been closely defined. Other methods have utilized droplets of dye (for visual measurement), a radiolabeled resin particle, or radiographic contrast medium (57).

Surface Mucosa (58)

In addition to the easily distinguishable columnar ciliated cells, the ciliated epithelial surface contains seven other types of cell. These are glandular, goblet, serous, and Clara; the latter two contain secretory granules producing watery secretions in smaller airways, with the added capacity to transform into goblet cells. The brush cell has a border of microvilli (2 μm in length) and a possible absorptive function. Intermediate cells lie between the others.

Submucosal glands are numerous throughout the cartilaginous airways, whereas goblet cells become progressively sparser in the finer bronchioles. The submucosal glands are branching tubular structures with serous cells at their distal ends and mucus cells proximally, with the main ducts being ciliated.

Secretory granules (1–2 μm) appear near the cell apices of both goblet cells and glandular mucus cells and contain acid glycoprotein; some cells contain secretory carbohydrate, particularly sialic acid. The volume of submucosal glands is about 40 times that of goblet cells in humans. The tracheal epithelium has about one goblet cell per five ciliated cells, the apices of which form a virtually continuous surface cover. In the smaller airways, however, brush and intermediate cells increase. The submucosal gland orifices (diameter 50 μm) and airway branches interrupt the mucosal surface continuity.

Mucus

Mucus and secretions (59), formed within Golgi-derived vesicles of goblet and mucus gland cells, are released by exocytosis in the form of 1- to 2-μm drops of concentrated glycoprotein which rapidly swell by absorption of water from serous fluid. By so doing, their volume increases by a factor of several hundred-fold over about 3 sec or so. These droplets are drawn out into strands, small flakes, or larger plaques, by cilial action. This may serve to maintain the depth of periciliary "sol" by pumping fluid from one region to another and through chloride secretion and sodium absorption, across the epithelium (60). Should the periciliary layer become too deep, then contact between cilia and mucus will fail until excess fluid is removed by the cilia. The converse may happen with too little fluid. The flow of periciliary fluid in the terminal airways may draw surfactant and macrophages onto the mucociliary escalator, aided by compression and expansion on the surface tension of surfactant during breathing (61). Surplus fluid is probably subsequently absorbed by brush cells.

Tracheobronchial mucus—a mixture of secretions from the surface epithelium, submucosal glands, and tissue fluid transudate (62)—is comprised of water (95%), glycoproteins (2–3%), proteoglycans (0.1–0.5%), lipids (0.3–0.5%), other proteins, and occasionally DNA (from white cells); about 6 mg ml^{-1} is secreted daily in health, with a threefold increase in chronic bronchitis or asthma and a 10-fold increase in cystic fibrosis. The main structure of the viscoelastic hydrophilic gel is formed by glycoproteins and proteoglycans, with lipid making up about 30% of the non-aqueous secretion. Three other proteins protect against microorganisms, secretory IGA, lactoferrin, and lysozyme aided by oligosaccharides.

The glycoproteins are of prime importance in giving mucus its characteristic elasticity; the lengthy glycoprotein molecules are probably intertwined or entangled, with their coils held together by weak noncovalent bonds or cross-linked into a three-dimensional network by intra- or intermolecular disulfide bonds. Whatever, mucus gradually dissolves in water, in keeping with noncovalent bonding.

The more forceful the cilia beat, the more easily it is moved. The mucus is seen by the cilia as an elastic structure which is able to store energy and which is then able to convert this energy into motion. This aspect is probably more important than viscosity, though that must be kept within reasonable limits. Mucus also exhibits spinnability or thread-forming properties, which may also affect mucociliary transport (63).

Tracheal submucosal glands are supplied by cholinergic efferent nerves from the vagus nerve; stimulation of these nerves causes secretion, blocked by atropine. Adrenergic nerves may also regulate submucosal gland function, but to a lesser degree. Nonadrenergic noncholinergic nerves may also regulate gland secretion; vasointestinal peptides (VIP) and SP are possible modulators together with other neuropeptides.

In conclusion, the rheological characteristics of sputum seem well fitted to act in tandem with cilia to produce an energy-efficient coupling mechanism which has power in reserve.

AIRFLOW AND MUCUS INTERACTION

Two-phase air–liquid flow whereby energy is transferred from the airstream to the liquid mucus layer (the liquid mucus layer has higher flows and airway narrowing, favoring expiratory clearance) is a possible mechanism helping mucociliary clearance (64). However, significant interaction only occurs at higher flow rates and with turbulent flow regimens (such as may occur during hyperventilation or on exercise), and certainly it occurs with coughing (65). During quiet tidal breathing, airflow only reaches a linear velocity of 10 m sec^{-1} in the narrowest part of the nose, where there may be interaction (interaction occurs during sneezing); it falls to 1 m sec^{-1} in the trachea and to 10 mm sec^{-1} in the respiratory bronchioles, with both figures being far too low for significant interaction. However, at higher rates (10–25 m sec^{-1}), annular flow will occur; at >25 m sec^{-1} there will be mist flow with production of small aerosol droplets (66), particularly with thicker mucus layers (67).

Estimation of flow and shear rates in the lung is dif-ficult, owing to (a) the branching airway geometry, (b) the changing dimensions during phasic flow, and (c) high Reynolds numbers—usually 2000 for the transition from laminar (or streamline) to turbulent flow with short airway lengths (between branches) insufficient to smooth flow even during normal breathing.

The effect of airflow on mucus transport has been summarized as follows: On inspiration there is a thin boundary layer on the inner wall of the bifurcation; this consists of primary and secondary flow patterns tending to shift mucus to the outer wall, though with overall little effect at the usual low flows. On expiration there are thin boundary layers around the walls, indicating higher shear rates and possible two-phase flow conditions for positive mucus transport. Experiments support an increase in viscous dissipation by 20–30% on expiration, commensurate with a net positive mucus clearance. This is supported by cough clearance, which of course is much greater.

MUCOCILIARY AND TERMINAL AIRWAY CLEARANCE

In the bronchoalveolar region, terminal airway clearance interfaces with the peripheral limit of mucociliary clearance proper. This interface is rather poorly defined and is of great interest, since up to 50% of inhaled particles 2–5 μm in diameter may be deposited in this region depending on the mode of breathing (68). Alveolar clearance (69) is either *nonabsorptive*, whereby particles are transported from alveoli to cilial airways by surfactant and then cleared by mucociliary clearance (this involves a very small proportion of particles), or *absorptive* by (a) direct penetration into epithelial cells with subsequent cell death and transport of debris to the mucociliary escalator or the interstitial space, (b) transport through the epithelial wall by transcellular and paracellular pathways, (c) phagocytosis and destruction within the phagocytic system, or (d) transport to lymphatics.

Transcellular Transport

Macromolecules of different size and composition may be handled by (a) endocytosis, (b) lysozyme digestion involving alveolar type 1 cells, and (c) passage to the interstitial space. Paracellular transport involves the passage of hydrophilic substances through the intracellular tight junction by passive diffusion. The permeability (or leakiness) of the epithelial barrier, as measured by diethylenetriaminepentaacetic acid (DTPA) is increased in several conditions (e.g., with smoking, infections, and interstitial lung diseases) (70).

Phagocytosis by alveolar macrophages is the fate of the majority of deeply inhaled particles; some are cleared by mucociliary transport directly, whereas some migrate through the alveolar wall into the interstitial space and lymphatics (71).

Alveolar clearance is slow: An initial *fast* phase lasts about 24 hr, an *intermediate* phase lasts from 3 to 20 days, and a *slow* phase may go on for 100 days or more (72).

Measurement of Lung Mucociliary Clearance in Humans

The objective measurement of mucus transport in the human lung can be achieved primarily in two ways (73). The first way involves the measurement of the actual linear flow of the mucus, and the second way involves the rate of removal of inhaled, deposited particles (usually radioaerosols) in the lungs; the resulting value is an index of mucus flow efficiency.

Measurement of Mucus Velocity

The measurement of mucus velocity involves timing the movement of marker(s), over a given distance. This measurement is invariably undertaken in the trachea, an anatomically well-defined airway; measurement of the velocity of mucus has also been reported for the main bronchi. With the technology currently available, the measurement of mucus flow from more distal airways is complicated by the degree of invasiveness of the method and/or by the amount of overlap of the airways when these are seen in a two-dimensional display.

At present, there are three popular techniques which are used for measuring mucus velocity:

1. *The cinefiberscopic technique* (74) involves the insufflation of Teflon disks through the fiberoptic bronchoscope onto the tracheal mucosa in a circumferential distribution (Fig. 3). These Teflon marker disks are filmed and timed over a given distance to obtain TMV; usually the mean of measurements is determined by performing the technique on approximately 10–20 disks.

2. *The roentgenographic technique* is a modification of the cinefiberscopic method but is somewhat less invasive (75); the Teflon disks are made radio-opaque by coating with bismuth trioxide (Fig. 4). The disks are blown through the bronchoscope (located at the vocal cords) into the trachea, and their movement is recorded with a fluoroscope plus image intensifier, TV monitor, and videotape. A number of x-rays are taken at 1-min intervals, and the average distance traveled by several disks during the procedure gives an average measurement of TMV.

3. *The radioaerosol boli method* (76) for measuring

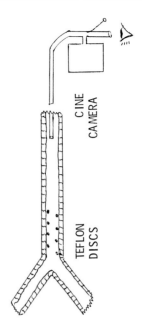

FIG. 3. Schematic diagram of the cinefiberscopic technique for measuring tracheal mucus velocity.

TMV is noninvasive and involves inhaling radioaerosol at a fast rate from near total lung capacity, thereby ensuring predominantly local concentrated deposition in the large, proximal airways. The marker boli are recorded by a gamma camera linked to a computer during transport up the trachea. The TMV is determined from the distance moved in a given time (Fig. 5).

The degree of invasiveness of a technique appears to be related to the measurement of TMV (77). The mean ± SD TMV quoted for healthy nonsmokers using the cinefiberscopic, roentgenographic, and radioaerosol boli techniques are 2.15 ± 0.55 cm min^{-1} (78), 1.14 ± 0.38 cm min^{-1} (75), and 0.44 ± 0.13 cm min^{-1} (76), respectively.

Tracheobronchial Clearance

The second method which assesses lung mucociliary clearance efficiency involves the use of inhaled ra-

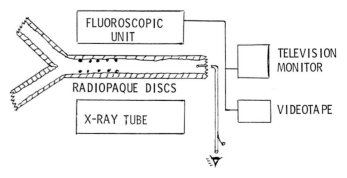

FIG. 4. Schematic diagram of the roentgenographic technique for measuring tracheal mucus velocity.

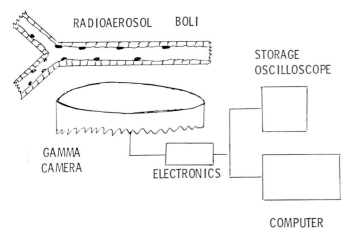

FIG. 5. Schematic diagram of the radioaerosol boli technique for measuring tracheal mucus velocity.

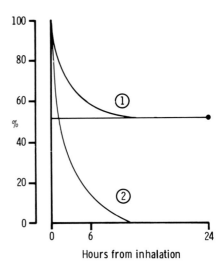

Hours from inhalation

FIG. 6. Schematic illustration of whole (1) and tracheobronchial (2) retention curves for a normal subject. Subtracting whole-lung retention at 24 hr gives tracheobronchial retention.

dioaerosol and was first reported in 1955 (79). This technique involves the inhalation of an aerosol firmly labeled with a gamma-emitting radionuclide such as technetium-99m (physical half-life: 6 hr). The aerosol particles must be insoluble in the lungs. Several types of materials have been used for measuring lung mucociliary clearance: Teflon, polystyrene, albumin microspheres, erythrocytes, iron oxide, and resin (80). Measurement of the radiation originating from the subject's chest immediately after inhalation gives a measure of the amount of radioaerosol which has been initially deposited within the lungs. Serial counting after inhalation shows a decrease in lung radioactivity due to (a) biological clearance and (b) physical decay of the radionuclide. It is an easy matter to correct for the contribution of radionuclide decay by knowing the physical half-life of the radionuclide.

The instrument of choice for measuring the amount of deposited radioaerosol cleared from the lungs is a large-field-of-view gamma-camera linked to a computer. Such an instrument not only provides information regarding radioaerosol retention, but also permits a measure of the distribution within the lungs, thus enabling regional clearance measurements to be made (81). Whole-lung retention can also be achieved with a simpler detection system such as the use of suitably collimated (wide-angle field-of-view) scintillation counter(s) located over the chest.

Plotting initial lung burden (%) against time after inhalation results in a whole-lung clearance curve of the deposited radioaerosol. This clearance curve generally consists of two phases: (i) a fast phase (several hours in duration) due to mucociliary clearance and (in disease) cough and (ii) a slow phase due to alveolar clearance (Fig. 6). Clearance of particles from the nonciliated alveolar regions of the lungs is a slow process, with a biological half-life on the order of several months. In practice, the amount of radioaerosol

present in the lungs after 24 hr is taken to represent the proportion of the radioaerosol deposited beyond the reach of the mucus (i.e., in the alveolated regions) (82,83). By subtracting this estimate of alveolar deposition from the whole-lung clearance curve, a 24-hr trancheobronchial clearance curve can be obtained (36,84). In health, all other things being equal, the amount of radioaerosol that has been cleared first must have been initially deposited near the top of the lungs (i.e., trachea), and the amount coming up last must have originated from the distal ciliated airways (i.e., terminal bronchioles).

The initial site of deposition of radioaerosol within the lungs is directly related to its subsequent clearance rate (85). Factors that govern the deposition into the lungs of inhaled aerosols are the physical properties of the aerosol particles, the mode of inhalation, and the patency of the airways (86). It is imperative that a measure be made of the initial topographical distribution of deposited radioaerosol before a comparison of lung mucociliary clearance is undertaken between or within subjects. The gamma-camera yields such a measure in the form of the penetration index (87). Alternatively, the estimate of alveolar deposition yields the percentage of radioaerosol that is deposited on the ciliated airways (i.e., initial deposition minus alveolar deposition) and has been cleared via the mucociliary escalator.

PHYSIOLOGICAL ASPECTS OF MUCOCILIARY CLEARANCE

Circadian rhythm does not appear to affect mucociliary function. In a randomized fashion, healthy subjects had their mucociliary clearance measured identically on two occasions, starting at midday and at midnight. No difference in clearance was observed between the two assessments (88).

Sleep retardation in lung mucociliary clearance has been reported both in healthy subjects and in asthmatics (88,89). This impairment may result in undue retention of inhaled industrial pollutants in shift workers and may well be of importance in patients with COPD, further compromising their already depressed mucociliary clearance.

Posture does not seem to play a role in the function of mucociliary clearance in health. Clearance was unaltered irrespective of whether the subject was standing, was in the supine position (88,89), or was in the 25° head-down position (90). Of course, in patients with excessive secretions, posture appears to play a major role in the rate of clearance of their lung secretions (91).

Studies have failed to show any difference between the two sexes; with age, however, clearance slows (92,93).

Exercise such as performing routine duties within a hospital (over a 6-hr period), as opposed to relaxation, does not appear to have any effect on lung mucociliary clearance (88). However, brisk exercise such as pedaling for half an hour on a bicycle ergometer, as opposed to quiet breathing, resulted in an enhancement of lung mucociliary transport (94). Eucapnic hyperventilation also resulted in an increased lung mucociliary clearance, although to only 50% of that achieved during exercise. This increase in mucus transport was attributed to either (a) a mechanical effect of increased lung movement or (b) an effect of the autonomic nervous system producing stimulation of airway glands and/or CBF by increased circulating catecholamines.

ENVIRONMENTAL POLLUTANTS

1. *Tobacco smoking.* Tobacco smoking results in the replacement of ciliated cells by goblet cells. Cigarette smoke is also ciliotoxic (38). Studies on the long-term effects of tobacco smoking in asymptomatic smokers have, on the whole, demonstrated a reduced tracheobronchial clearance. Giving up smoking has been shown, in asymptomatic smokers, to return this impaired mucociliary transport to normality within 2–3 months of giving up the habit (95). However, mucociliary clearance in patients with chronic bronchitis who had given up cigarette smoking for more than 1 year was found to be no different than that in current cigarette smokers (96). Studies of the acute effects of cigarette smoking on lung mucociliary clearance have produced conflicting results (5).

2. *Sulfuric acid.* One-hour exposures of healthy subjects to 0.5 μM sulfuric acid (H_2SO_4) mist at 100 and 1000 μg/m^3 concentrations have been reported to produce transient alterations of tracheobronchial clearance in a dose-dependent manner. The reduction in tracheobronchial clearance as a result of doubling the length of exposure to H_2SO_4 mist was as great as or greater than an order of magnitude increase in the concentration of H_2SO_4 (97).

3. *Urban factor.* The effect of living in an urban environment on lung mucociliary clearance was investigated in nonsmoking, monozygotic twins: One of each pair lived in a rural district, whereas the other lived in a city. On average, lung mucociliary clearance was found to be similar in the two pairs of twins (98).

4. *Sulfur dioxide.* SO_2 is a major constituent of urban pollution and has been shown to impair nasal mucociliary clearance. A 3-hr exposure of healthy subjects to 5 ppm of SO_2 has been shown not to affect lung mucociliary clearance other than causing a transient speeding up of clearance after 1 hr of exposure (99).

5. *Ozone.* Exposure of conscious sheep for 2 hr to ozone at a concentration of 0.5 ppm was found not to alter tracheal mucus velocity, although it gave rise to airway hyperreactivity (100).

6. *Formaldehyde.* Both domestic and occupational exposure to formaldehyde were common. Nasal mucociliary clearance was significantly delayed and the sense of smell was significantly reduced in a group of subjects exposed to formaldehyde as compared to an unexposed group of subjects. The effects were correlated with the duration and degree of exposure (101).

7. *Miscellaneous.* Low nickel concentrations result in a reduction of CBF (102), and chromate has a more severe effect (103). Woodworker's dust exposure slows nasal mucociliary clearance severely (104), and failure of this clearance mechanism may play a role in the nasal adenocarcinomas reported in woodworkers.

8. *Hair spray.* Hair spray was found to depress tracheal mucus transport for over 1 hr (105).

EFFECTS OF PHARMACOLOGICAL AGENTS ON LUNG MUCOCILIARY CLEARANCE

Drugs That Enhance Lung Mucociliary Clearance

1. *Mucolytics and expectorants.* Mucolytics and expectorants are used frequently, though with little scientific justification (106). By measuring lung mucociliary clearance (107), limited evidence of enhancement of clearance has been demonstrated following the administration of bromhexine, guaiphenesin, hypertonic saline, sodium 2-mercaptoethane sulfonate, and tap

water (108) to patients with chronic bronchitis or healthy subjects.

2. *Bronchodilators.* Theophyllines and beta agonists are standard bronchodilators. Both groups have an additional effect—namely, enhancement of lung mucociliary clearance (36,109–111). This arises because of ciliostimulation and/or alterations in the mucus production and its physicochemical characteristics. The amount of topical β_2 agonist required to achieve bronchodilatation is small and enhances mucociliary clearance only when given in larger doses (i.e., doses 2.5-fold larger than that recommended for bronchodilatation) (112).

Although anticholinergic drugs (e.g., scopolamine, atropine) reduce mucociliary clearance in humans when given orally or subcutaneously (113,114), the topical administration of the synthetic anticholinergic bronchodilators ipratropium bromide and oxitropium bromide have no such effect (115,116).

3. *Sodium cromoglycate.* Sodium cromoglycate, used prophylactically in asthma, has no effect on mucociliary clearance in healthy subjects but improves, by one-third, the depressed TMV of asymptomatic asthmatics (117).

4. *Corticosteroids.* Because of the possibility that aerosolized steroids may play a role in the increased incidence of chest infections, a study was undertaken in patients with COPD. However, no difference in lung mucociliary clearance was found in a group of subjects who received beclomethasone dipropionate compared to those who received placebo (118).

The administration of oral corticosteroids (prednisolone 15–30 mg daily) in stable asthmatics resulted in improvement of peripheral lung mucociliary clearance (119). This may reduce mucus plugging in small airways.

Drugs That Impair Lung Mucociliary Clearance

1. *Beta blockers.* In vitro animal experiments have shown that low concentrations of propranolol (0.1 μM) block the cilioexcitatory effect of beta agonists. On the other hand, similar concentrations of propranolol (in the absence of beta agonists) have been shown to have no effect on ciliary activity (120). High concentrations of propranolol (100 μM) result in a slowing of ciliary activity, possibly due to the local anesthetic properties of the drug. The administration of propranolol, atenolol, and pindolol has been reported to retard lung mucociliary clearance in healthy subjects (121), chronic bronchitics (122), and patients with coronary heart disease (123).

2. *Aspirin.* Acetylsalicylic acid is claimed to inhibit prostaglandin (PG) synthesis. *In vitro* studies have

shown that exogenous PGs increase bronchial fluid secretion, and PGE_1 and PGE_2 have been reported to be ciliostimulators. Sodium salicylate, on the other hand, has been shown to decrease the output of serous and mucous cells of human bronchial epithelium. Gerrity et al. (124) studied the effect of a single dose of aspirin (16 mg/kg body weight) on lung mucociliary clearance in healthy subjects. This upper range of a single dose of the drug (e.g., for antipyretic purposes) resulted in a small retardation of lung mucociliary clearance.

3. *Oxygen therapy.* The possibility of pulmonary oxygen toxicity on lung mucociliary clearance has been investigated by several groups. Animal experiments have shown that 100% O_2 results in a marked impairment of tracheal mucus flow in cats. Healthy subjects, after breathing 90–95% O_2 for 6 hr, showed evidence of tracheitis. However, within 3 hr of commencement of breathing O_2, tracheal mucus transport was depressed (125). Administration of a β_2 agonist restored the depressed mucus flow rate to control levels.

4. *Narcotics and sedatives.* Opiates appear to depress mucociliary clearance, with a few exceptions (126). Narcotics such as codeine, normethadone, and morphine have been reported to reduce the ciliary activity of the oyster gill. Animal experiments have shown (a) depression of CBF in a dose-dependent fashion (127) and (b) impairment of tracheobronchial clearance (128). In healthy subjects a single dose of 10 mg of temazepam, a benzodiazepine, slowed down lung mucociliary clearance (129).

Anesthetics

1. *Local anesthetics.* The effects of local anesthetics on ciliary activity have been studied *in vitro* using ferret tracheal rings (130). Mepivacaine was found to be the least toxic, with no effect on ciliary activity at 1.0% concentration; bupivacaine was found to be the most toxic, with irreversible damage to the respiratory epithelium at a concentration of 0.13%. Lidocaine, procaine, and chloroprocaine also depressed ciliary activity temporarily (131). At a pH of 7, local anesthetics arrested ciliary activity; however, lowering the pH made these drugs less ciliotoxic.

2. *General anesthetics.* Anesthetics such as halothane, thiopental, pentobarbital, and diethyl ether have been reported, from animal experiments and in humans, to depress lung mucociliary transport temporarily for several hours (132–135). In humans this is a direct effect of the anesthetic rather than being a result of nervous regulation (136).

EFFECTS OF DISEASE
ON LUNG MUCOCILIARY CLEARANCE

Diseases That Do Not Appear
to Impair Mucociliary Transport

Patients with emphysema due to α_1-antitrypsin deficiency but with no associated chronic bronchitis have unaltered mucociliary function of the proximal airways (137). The same was also found to be true for patients with asbestosis (85).

Since rheumatoid disease is a multisystem disorder, its potential involvement in the function of this host defense mechanism was investigated in a group of patients with this disease (138). The mucociliary clearance of the patients, who were on nonsteroidal anti-inflammatory drugs, was found to be similar to that of a control group.

The drying of secretions in the eyes, nose, and mouth of patients with Sjögren's syndrome led Fairfax et al. (139) to examine whether this phenomenon also extended into the lungs and thereby adversely affected the clearance of lung secretions. Mucociliary clear-ance was, however, found to be within the normal range.

Diseases That Affect Mucociliary Transport

In chronic bronchitis the reduction in ciliated cells in favor of goblet cells, together with the associated increase in secretions with abnormal physicochemical properties, results in a grossly impaired mucociliary transport (Fig. 7). The degree of impairment is not related to any of the pulmonary function indices. Cough, the backup clearance mechanism for mucus, plays a major compensating role (140).

Asymptomatic nonsmokers with ragweed asthma, when challenged with ragweed extract, had their TMV reduced by some 25% from baseline value, with return to baseline within 2 hr (141). This finding indicated that slowly reacting substance of anaphylaxis (SRS-A), liberated during airway anaphylaxis, impairs mucociliary clearance.

Stable asthmatics have been reported to have tracheal and main bronchus mucus velocities that are one-half and one-third, respectively, of those for healthy

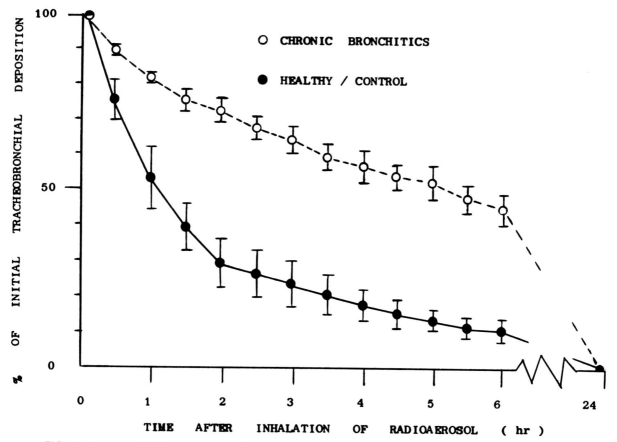

FIG. 7. Mean ± SEM tracheobronchial retention curves for a group of chronic bronchitics with mucoid sputum (*n* = 9) and a group of healthy/control subjects (*n* = 9).

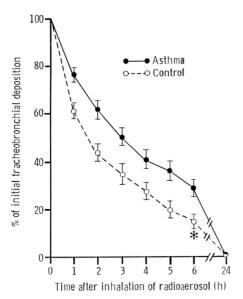

FIG. 8. Mean ± SEM tracheobronchial retention curves for a group of stable mild asthmatics and a group of healthy/control subjects (*p < 0.01).

subjects (142). The overall lung mucociliary clearance efficiency has also been reported to be statistically significantly reduced (Fig. 8) for stable asthmatics as compared to healthy, nonsmoking subjects (143). Furthermore, asthmatics who were in complete remission and who required no medication whatsoever for a period of 1–6 months prior to the study were found to have an impaired lung mucociliary clearance (144). These observations raise the question as to whether asthma ever remits completely.

Bateman et al. (145) demonstrated that the impairment of lung mucociliary clearance observed in a group of asthmatics who were hospitalized because of an acute exacerbation of their disease did not improve 2–4 months later, despite improvements in symptoms and pulmonary function.

The abnormal mucociliary transport in bronchiectatics, originally reported by Lourenco et al. (146), has been confirmed of late (147,148). The degree of mucociliary transport impairment in bronchiectatics is similar to that seen in chronic bronchitics.

Impaired clearance has been reported in patients infected with influenza A virus within days of the onset of symptoms, with recovery 2–3 months later (149,150). Impaired mucociliary clearance accompanies *Mycoplasma pneumoniae*, in keeping with the damage caused to the ciliated epithelium (151). In this instance, however, there is evidence suggesting suboptimal mucociliary transport 1 year after the onset of the symptoms. As early as 1965 Wagner et al. (152) reported, in patients with tuberculosis, evidence of areas in the lung with decreased ciliary activity resulting in local pooling of tracer radioactive particles.

Immunoglobulin deficiency may well be accompanied by impaired mucociliary function (153; see also Chapter 7.4.2).

Patients with bronchial carcinomas have been shown to have a reduced or absent mucociliary clearance from the proximal airways (154). Mucociliary clearance of the bronchial tree post-lobectomy has been found to be intact, although prolonged; however, it has been found to improve with time, reverting to normal values 5–12 months post-surgery (155).

Patients with cystic fibrosis (156), Young's syndrome (157), and primary ciliary dyskinesia (including Kartagener's syndrome) (158) have, on the whole, been shown to have an impaired mucociliary clearance (see Chapter 7.9.3).

REFERENCES

1. Sharpey W. Cilia. In: Todd RB, ed. *Cyclopaedia of anatomy and physiology.* London: Longman, Brown, Longmans and Roberts, 1835;606–638.
2. Lucas AM, Douglas MJ. Principals underlying ciliary activity in the respiratory tract. IIA. Comparison of nasal clearance in man, monkey and other mammals. *Arch Otolaryngol* 1934;20:518–541.
3. Sleigh MA, Blake JR, Liron N. The propulsion of mucus by cilia. *Am Rev Respir Dis* 1988;137:726–741.
4. Green GM, Jakab GJ, Low RB, Davis GS. Defence mechanisms of the respiratory membrane. *Am Rev Respir Dis* 1977;115:479–514.
5. Pavia D. Lung mucociliary clearance. In: Clarke SW, Pavia D, eds. *Aerosols and the lung.* London: Butterworth, 1984;127–155.
6. Leith DE. Cough. In: Proctor DF, Reid LM, eds. *Respiratory defence mechanisms,* Part II. New York: Marcel Dekker, 1977;545–592.
7. Jones JG. Clearance of inhaled particles from the alveoli. In: Clarke SW, Pavia D, eds. *Aerosols and the lung.* London: Butterworth, 1984;170–196.
8. Proctor DJ. The upper airways. I. Nasal physiology and defence of the lungs. *Am Rev Respir Dis* 1977;115:97–129.
9. Proctor DF. The upper airways. II. The larynx and trachea. *Am Rev Respir Dis* 1977;115:315–342.
10. Clarke SW. Role of two-phase flow in bronchial clearance. *Bull Eur Physiopathol Respir* 1973;9:359–372.
11. Weibel ER. *Morphometry of the human lung.* Berlin: Springer, 1963.
12. Sanderson MJ, Dirksen ER. Mechanosensitive and beta-adrenergic control of the ciliary beat frequency of mammalian respiratory tract cells in culture. *Am Rev Respir Dis* 1989;139:432–440.
13. Konietzko N, Nakhosteen JA, Mizera W, Kasparek R, Hesse H. Ciliary beat frequency of biopsy samples taken from normal persons and patients with various lung diseases. *Chest* 1981;80(Suppl):855–857.
14. Toremalm NG, Mercke V, Reimer A. The mucociliary activity of the upper respiratory tract. *Rhinology* 1975;13:113–120.
15. Fuziwara K, Hakansson CH, Toremalm NG. Influence of ionizing radiation on the ciliary cell activity in the respiratory tract. *Acta Radiol (Ther)* 1972;11:513–520.
16. Baldetorp B. Comparison between the immediate effects of photon and electron radiation on the ciliary activity of the trachea of the rabbit. An *in-vitro* investigation. *Acta Radiol (Oncol)* 1985;24:279–284.
17. Baldetorp B, Huberman D, Hakansson CH, Toremalm NG. Effects of ionizing radiation on the activity of the ciliated epithelium of the trachea. *Acta Radiol (Ther)* 1976;15:225–232.

18. Albertsson M. Dose–response studies of single dose ionizing radtion on the ciliated epithelium of the trachea of the rabbit. A physiologic and ultrastructural investigation. *Acta Radiol (Oncol)* 1985;24:433–443.
19. Van de Donk HJM, Zuidema J, Merkhus FWHM. The influence of the pH and osmotic pressure upon tracheal ciliary beat frequency as determined with a new photo-electric registration device. *Rhinology* 1980;18:93–104.
20. Luk CK, Dulfano MJ. Effect of pH, viscosity and ionic-strength changes on ciliary beating frequency of human bronchial explants. *Clin Sci* 1983;64:449–451.
21. Girard PG, Kennedy JR. Calcium regulation of ciliary activity in rabbit tracheal epithelial explants and outgrowth. *Eur J Cell Biol* 1986;40:203–209.
22. Verdugo P, Raess BV, Villalon M. The role of calmodulin in the regulation of ciliary movement in mammalian epithelial cilia. *J Submicroscop Cytol* 1983;15:95.
23. Mellville GN, Iravani J. Factors affecting ciliary beat frequency in the intrapulmonary airways of rats. *Can J Physiol Pharmacol* 1975;53:1122–1128.
24. Wanner A, Maurer D, Abraham WM, Szepfalusi Z, Sielczak M. Effects of chemical mediators of anaphylaxis on ciliary function. *J Allergy Clin Immunol* 1983;72:663–667.
25. Wanner A, Sielczak M, Mella JF, Abraham WM. Ciliary responsiveness in allergic and nonallergic airways. *J Appl Physiol* 1986;60:1967–1971.
26. Lindberg S, Mercke U. Capsaicin stimulates mucociliary activity by releasing substance P and acetylcholine. *Eur J Respir Dis* 1986;68:96–106.
27. Yeates DB, Wong LB, Miller IF. Capsaicin stimulation of ciliary beat is mediated by both neural and humoral mechanisms. *Eur Respir J* 1988;1(Suppl 1):114S.
28. Yeates DB, Wong LB, Miller IF. Stimulation of tracheal ciliary beat frequency by bradykinin. *Eur Respir J* 1988;1(Suppl 1):114S.
29. Maurer DR, Sieleczak M, Oliver W Jr, Abraham WM, Wanner A. Role of ciliary motility in acute allergic mucociliary dysfunction. *J Appl Physiol Respir Environ Exercise Physiol* 1982;52:1018–1023.
30. Iravani J, Melville GN. Mucociliary function in the respiratory tract as influenced by physicochemical factors. *Pharmacol Ther (B)* 1976;2:471–492.
31. Wanner A. Alteration of tracheal mucociliary transport in airway disease. Effect of pharmacologic agents. *Chest* 1981;80(Suppl):867–870.
32. Wong LB, Miller IF, Yeates DB. Stimulation of ciliary beat frequency by autonomic agonists: *in-vivo*. *J Appl Physiol* 1988;65:971–981.
33. Wong LB, Miller IF, Yeates DB. Regulation of ciliary beat frequency by autonomic mechanisms: *in-vitro*. *J Appl Physiol* 1988;65:1895–1901.
34. Van de Donk HJM, Merkhus FWHM. Decrease in ciliary beat frequency due to intranasal administration of propranolol. *J Pharm Sci* 1982;71:595–596.
35. Stafanger G. *In-vitro* effect of beclomethasone dipropionate and flunisolide on the mobility of human nasal cilia. *Allergy* 1987;42:507–511.
36. Sutton PP, Pavia D, Bateman JRM, Clarke SW. The effect of oral aminophylline on lung clearance in man. *Chest* 1981;80(Suppl):889–892.
37. Venizelos DC, Gerrity TR, Yeates DB. Response of human mucociliary clearance to acute alcohol administration. *Arch Environ Health* 1981;36:194–201.
38. Kensler GJ, Battista SP. Components of cigarette smoke with ciliary depressant activity. *N Engl J Med* 1963;269:1161–1166.
39. Stanley PJ, Wilson R, Greenstone MA, MacWilliam L, Cole PJ. Effect of cigarette smoking on nasal mucociliary clearance and ciliary beat frequency. *Thorax* 1986;41:519–523.
40. Abraham WM, Sielczak MW, Delehunt JC, Marchette B, Wanner B. Impairment of tracheal mucociliary clearance but not ciliary beat frequency by a combination of low level ozone and sulfur dioxide in sheep. *Eur J Respir Dis* 1986;68:114–120.
41. Hisamatsu KI, Yamauchi Y, Uchida M, Murakaimi Y. Pro- motive effect of lysozyme on the ciliary activity of the human nasal mucosa. *Acta Otolaryngol (Stockh)* 1986;101:290–294.
42. Spock A, Heick HMC, Cress H, Logan WS. Abnormal serum factor in patients with cystic fibrosis of the pancreas. *Pediatr Res* 1967;1:173–177.
43. Rossman CM, Lee RMKW, Forrest JB, Newhouse MT. Nasal ciliary ultrastructure and function in patients with primary ciliary dyskinesia compared with that in normal subjects and in subjects with various respiratory diseases. *Am Rev Respir Dis* 1984;129:161–167.
44. Dulfano MJ, Luk CK. Sputum and ciliary inhibition in asthma. *Thorax* 1982;37:341–347.
45. Hastie AT, Loegering DA, Gleich GJ, Kueppers F. The effect of purified human eosinophil major protein on mammalian ciliary activity. *Am Rev Respir Dis* 1987;135:848–853.
46. Wilson R. Secondary ciliary dysfunction. *Clin Sci* 1988;75:113–120.
47. Johnson AP, Inzana TJ. Loss of ciliary activity in organ cultures of rat trachea treated with lipo-oligosaccharide isolated from *Haemophilus influenzae*. *J Med Microbiol* 1986;22:265–268.
48. Wilson R, Pitt T, Taylor G, et al. Pyocyanin and 1-hydroxy-phenazine produced by *Pseudomonas aeruginosa* inhibit the beating of human respiratory cilia *in-vitro*. *J Clin Invest* 1987;79:221–229.
49. Wilson R, Roberts D, Cole P. Effect of bacterial products on human ciliary function *in-vitro*. *Thorax* 1985;40:124–131.
50. Steinfort C, Wilson R, Sykes D, Cole PJ. Effect of *Streptococcus pneumoniae* on human ciliary function *in-vitro*. *Thorax* 1986;41:253.
51. Disse BG, Ziegler HW. Pharmacodynamic mechanism and therapeutic activity of ambroxol in animal experiments. *Respiration* 1987;51(Suppl 1):15–22.
52. Iravani J, Melville GN, Horstmann G. *N*-acetylcysteine and mucociliary activity in mammalian airways. *Arzneimittelforschung* 1978;28:250–254.
53. Stafanger G, Bisgaard H, Pedersen M, Morkussel E, Koch C. Effect of *N*-acetylcysteine on the human nasal ciliary activity *in-vitro*. *Eur J Respir Dis* 1987;70:157–162.
54. Maxwell SS. The effect of salt solutions on ciliary activity. *Am J Physiol* 1905;13:154–170.
55. Di Benedetto G, Gill J, Lopez-Vidriero MT, Clarke SW. The effect of cryopreservation on ciliary beat frequency of human respiratory epithelium. *Cryobiology* 1989;26:328–332.
56. Rutman A, Dewar A, MacKay I, Cole PJ. Primary ciliary dyskinesia; cytological and clinical features. *Q J Med* 1988;67:405.
57. Puchelle E, Aug F, Pham QT, Bertrand A. Comparison of three methods for measuring nasal mucociliary clearance in man. *Acta Otolaryngol* 1981;91:297–303.
58. Jeffery PK, Reid LM. The respiratory mucus membrane. In: Brain JD, Proctor DF, Reid LM, eds. *Respiratory defence mechanisms, Part I.* New York: Marcel Dekker, 1977;193–245.
59. Jeffery PK. The origins of secretions in the lower respiratory tract. *Eur J Respir Dis* 1987;71(Suppl 153):34–42.
60. Welsh MJ, Liedtke CM. Chloride and potassium channels in cystic fibrosis airway epithelia. *Nature* 1986;322:467–470.
61. Litt M. Physiocochemical determinants of mucociliary flow. *Chest* 1989;80S:846–849.
62. Lopez-Vidriero MT. Lung secretions. In: Clarke SW, Pavia D, eds. *Aerosols and the lung.* London: Butterworth, 1984;19–48.
63. Puchelle E, Zahm JM, Duvivier C. Spinability of bronchial mucus. Relationship with viscoelasticity and mucous transport properties. *Biorheology* 1983;20:239–249.
64. Kim CS, Iglesias AJ, Sackner MA. Mucus clearance by two-phase gas–liquid flow mechanism: asymmetric periodic flow model. *J Appl Physiol* 1987;62:959–971.
65. Jones JG, Clarke SW. Dynamics of cough. *Br J Anaesth* 1970;42:280–285.
66. Leith DE. Cough. *Phys Ther* 1968;48:439–447.
67. Scherer PW. Mucus transport by cough. *Chest* 1981;80(Suppl):830–833.
68. Agnew JE. Physical properties and mechanisms of deposition

of aerosols. In: Clarke SW, Pavia D, eds. *Aerosols and the lung.* London: Butterworth, 1984;49–70.

69. Morrow PE. Alveolar clearance of aerosols. *Arch Intern Med* 1973;131:101–108.

70. Jones JG, Minty BD, Lawler P, Hulands G, Crawley JCW, Veall N. Increased alveolar epithelial permeability in cigarette smokers. *Lancet* 1980;i:66–68.

71. Lauweryns JM, Baert JH. Alveolar clearance and the role of the pulmonary lymphatics. *Am Rev Respir Dis* 1977;115:625–683.

72. Bailey MR, Fry FA, James AC. Long-term retention of particles in the human respiratory tract. *J Aerosol Sci* 1985;16:295–305.

73. Pavia D, Sutton PP, Agnew JE, Lopez-Vidriero MT, Newman SP, Clarke SW. Measurement of bronchial mucociliary clearance. *Eur J Respir Dis* 1983;64(Suppl 127):41–56.

74. Sackner MA, Rosen MJ, Wanner A. Estimation of tracheal mucous velocity by bronchofiberscopy. *J Appl Physiol* 1973;34:495–499.

75. Friedman M, Stott FD, Poole DO, et al. A new roentgenographic method for estimating mucous velocity in airways. *Am Rev Respir Dis* 1977;115:67–72.

76. Yeates DB, Aspin N, Levison H, Jones MT, Bryan AC. Mucociliary tracheal transport rates in man. *J Appl Physiol* 1975;39:487–495.

77. Clarke SW, Pavia D. Comparison of techniques for measuring tracheal mucous velocities *in-vivo* in man. In: Nakhosteen JA, Maassen W, eds. *Bronchology: research, diagnostic and therapeutic aspects.* Hague: Martinus Nijhoff, 1981;469–472.

78. Santa Cruz R, Landa J, Hirsch J, Sackner MA. Tracheal mucous velocity in normal man and patients with obstructive lung disease; effects of terbutaline. *Am Rev Respir Dis* 1974; 109:458–463.

79. Albert RE, Arnett LC. Clearance of radioactivity dust from the lung. *Arch Environ Health* 1955;12:99–106.

80. Newman SP. Production of radioaerosols. In: Clarke SW, Pavia D, eds. *Aerosols and the lung.* London: Butterworth, 1984; 71–79.

81. Agnew JE, Bateman JRM, Pavia D, Clarke SW. A model for assessing bronchial mucus transport. *J Nucl Med* 1984;24:170–176.

82. Camner P, Philipson K. Human alveolar deposition of 4 mcg Teflon particles. *Arch Environ Health* 1978;36:181–185.

83. Agnew JE, Bateman JRM, Watts M, Paramananda V, Pavia D, Clarke SW. The importance of aerosol penetration for lung mucociliary clearance studies. *Chest* 1981;80(Suppl):843–846.

84. Foster WM, Langenback E, Bergofsky EH. Measurement of tracheal and bronchial mucus velocities in man: relation to lung clearance. *J Appl Physiol Respir Environ Exercise Physiol* 1980;48:965–971.

85. Thomson ML, Short MD. Mucociliary function in health chronic obstructive airway disease and asbestosis. *J Appl Physiol* 1969;26:535–539.

86. Pavia D, Thomson ML, Clarke SW, Shannon HS. Effect of lung function and mode of inhalation on penetration of aerosol into the human lung. *Thorax* 1977;32:194–197.

87. Agnew JE, Pavia D, Clarke SW. Airways penetration of inhaled radioaerosol: an index to small airways function? *Eur J Respir Dis* 1981;62:239–255.

88. Pavia D. Mucociliary clearance at night—effect of physical activity, posture, and circadian rhythm. In: Barnes PJ, Levy J, eds. *Nocturnal asthma.* Royal Society of Medicine International Congress Symposium Series, vol 73. London: 1984;29–38.

89. Pavia D, Agnew JE, Clarke SW. Physiological, pathological and drug-induced alterations in the tracheobronchial mucociliary clearance. In: Isles AF, von Wichert P, eds. *Sustained release theophylline and nocturnal asthma.* Amsterdam: Excerpta Medica, 1985;44–59.

90. Wong JW, Keens TG, Wannamaker EM, et al. Effects of gravity on tracheal mucus transport rates in normal subjects and in patients with cystic fibrosis. *Paediatrics* 1977;60:146–152.

91. Sutton PP, Parker R, Webber BA, et al. Assessment of the forced expiration technique, postural drainage and directed coughing in chest physiotherapy. *Eur J Respir Dis* 1983;64:62–68.

92. Goodman RM, Yergin BM, Landa JF, Golinvaux MH, Sackner MA. Relationship of smoking history and pulmonary function tests to tracheal mucus velocity in non-smokers, young smokers, ex-smokers, and patients with chronic bronchitis. *Am Rev Respir Dis* 1978;117:205–214.

93. Puchelle E, Zahm JM, Bertrand A. Influence of age on bronchial mucociliary transport. *Scand J Respir Dis* 1979;60:307–313.

94. Wolff RF, Dolovich MB, Obminski G, Newhouse MT. The effects of exercise and eucapnic hyperventilation on bronchial clearance in man. *J Appl Physiol* 1977;43:46–50.

95. Camner P, Philipson K, Arvidsson T. Withdrawal of cigarette smoking. A study on tracheobronchial clearance. *Arch Environ Health* 1973;26:90–92.

96. Agnew JE, Little P, Pavia D, Clarke SW. Mucus clearance from the airways in chronic bronchitis—smokers and ex-smokers. *Bull Eur Physiopathol Respir* 1982;18:473–484.

97. Spektor DM, Yen BM, Lippmann M. Effect of concentration and cumulative exposure of inhaled sulphuric acid on tracheobronchial particle clearance in healthy humans. *Environ Health Perspect* 1989;79:167–172.

98. Camner P, Philipson K. Urban factor and tracheobronchial clearance. *Arch Environ Health* 1973;27:81–84.

99. Wolff RK. Effects of airborne pollutants on mucociliary clearance. *Environ Health Perspect* 1986;66:223–237.

100. Abraham WM, Januszkiewicz AJ, Mingle M, Welker M, Wanzer A, Sackner MA. The sensitivity of bronchoprovocation and tracheal mucous velocity in detecting airway irritation after ozone exposure in conscious sheep. *Am Rev Respir Dis* 1979;119(No. 4, Part 2):198.

101. Holmstrom M, Wilhelmsson B. Respiratory symptoms and pathophysiological effects of occupational exposure to formaldehyde and wood dust. *Scand J Work Environ Health* 1988;14:306–311.

102. Adalis D, Gardner D, Miller F. Cytotoxic effects of nickel on ciliated epithelium. *Am Rev Respir Dis* 1978;118:347–353.

103. Mass MJ, Lane BP. Effect of chromates on ciliated cells of rat tracheal epithelium. *Arch Environ Health* 1976;31:96.

104. Black A, Evans J, Hadfield E, Macbeth R, Morgan A, Walsh M. Impairment of nasal mucociliary clearance in woodworkers in the furniture industry. *Br J Ind Med* 1974;31:10–17.

105. Friedman M, Dougherty R, Nelson S, White R, Sackner M, Wanner A. Acute effects of an aerosol hair spray on tracheal mucociliary transport. *Am Rev Respir Dis* 1977;116:281–286.

106. Richardson PS, Phipps RJ. The anatomy, physiology, pharmacology and pathology of tracheobronchial mucus secretion and the use of expectorant drugs in human subjects. *Pharmacol Ther (B)* 1978;3:441–479.

107. Clarke SW, Thomson ML, Pavia D. Effect of mucolytic and expectorant drugs on tracheobronchial clearance in chronic bronchitis. *Eur J Respir Dis* 1980;61(Suppl 110):179–191.

108. Foster WM, Bergofsky EH, Bohning DE, Lippmann M, Albert RE. Effect of adrenergic agents and their mode of action on mucociliary clearance in man. *J Appl Physiol* 1976;41:146–152.

109. Weich DJ, Viljoen H, Sweetlove MA, et al. Investigation into the effect of fenoterol on mucociliary clearance in patients with chronic bronchitis. *Eur J Nucl Med* 1988;14:533–537.

110. Matthys H, Daikeler G, Krauss B, Vastag E. Action of tulobuterol and fenoterol on the mucociliary clearance. *Respiration* 1987;51:105–112.

111. Yeates DB, Spektor DM, Pitt BR. Effect of orally administered orciprenaline on tracheobronchial mucociliary clearance. *Eur J Respir Dis* 1986;69:100–108.

112. Pavia D, Agnew JE, Lopez-Vidriero MT, Newman SP, Clarke SW. The effect of metered dose aerosols on the viscoelastic properties and clearance of bronchial secretions. In: Epstein, SW, ed. *Metered dose inhalers.* Mississauga: Astra, 1984;38–48.

113. Pavia D, Thomson ML. Inhibition of mucociliary clearance from the human lung by hyoscine. *Lancet* 1971;i:449–450.

114. Annis P, Landa J, Lichtiger MC. Effects of atropine on velocity

of tracheal mucus in anesthetized patients. *Anesthesiology* 1976;44:74–77.

115. Wanner A. Effect of ipratropium bromide on airway mucociliary function. *Am J Med* 1986;81:23–27.

116. Taylor RG, Pavia D, Agnew JE, et al. Effect of four weeks' high dose ipratropium bromide treatment on lung mucociliary clearance. *Thorax* 1986;41:295–300.

117. Mezey RJ, Cohn MA, Fernandez RJ, Janszkiewicz AJ, Wanner A. Mucociliary transport in allergic patients with antigen-induced bronchospasm. *Am Rev Respir Dis* 1978;118:677–684.

118. Fazio F, Lafortuna CL. Beclomethasone dipropionate does not affect mucociliary clearance in patients with chronic obstructive lung disease. *Respiration* 1986;50:62–65.

119. Agnew JE, Bateman JRM, Pavia D, Clarke SW. Peripheral airways mucus clearance in stable asthma is improved by oral corticosteroid therapy. *Bull Eur Physiopathol Respir* 1984; 20:295–301.

120. Verdugo P, Johnson NT, Tam PY. β-Adrenergic stimulation of respiratory ciliary activity. *J Appl Physiol* 1980;48:868–871.

121. Pavia D, Bateman JRM, Lennard-Jones AM, Agnew JE, Clarke SW. Effect of selective and non-selective beta blockade on pulmonary function and tracheobronchial mucociliary clearance in healthy subjects. *Thorax* 1986;41:301–305.

122. Matthys H, Vastag E, Daikeler G, Kohler D. The influence of aminophylline and pindolol on the mucociliary clearance in patients with chronic bronchitis. *Br J Clin Pract [Suppl]* 1983;23:82–86.

123. Dorow P, Weiss T, Felix R, Schmutzler H, Schiess W. Influence of propranolol, metoprolol and pindolol on mucociliary clearance in patients with coronary heart disease. *Respiration* 1984;45:286–290.

124. Gerrity TR, Cotromanes E, Garrard CS, Yeates DB, Lourenco RV. The effect of aspirin on lung mucociliary clearance. *N Engl J Med* 1983;308:139–141.

125. Sackner MA, Landa J, Hirsch J, Zapata A. Pulmonary effects of oxygen breathing. A 6-hour study in normal man. *Ann Intern Med* 1975;82:40–43.

126. Nomura S. Influence of narcotics on ciliary movement of gill of oyster. *Proc Soc Exp Biol Med* 1928;25:252.

127. Iravani J, Melville GN. Wirkung von pharmaka und milicuanderungen auf die flimmertatig keit der atemwege. *Respiration* 1975;32:157.

128. Dongen KV, Leusink H. The action of opium-alkaloids and expectorants on the ciliary movements in the air passages. *Arch Int Pharmacodyn Ther* 1953;93:261.

129. Spiteri MA, Pavia D, Lopez-Vidriero MT, Agnew JE, Clarke SW. Is tracheobronchial clearance affected by temazepam? *Thorax* 1986;41:727.

130. Manawadu BR, Mostow SR, Laforce FM. Local anesthetics and tracheal ring ciliary activity. *Anesth Analg* 1978;57:448–452.

131. van de Donk HJM, van Egmond ALM, van den Heuvel AGM, Zuidema J, Merkus FWHM. The effects of drugs on ciliary motility. III. Local anaesthetics and anti-allergic drugs. *Int J Pharmacol* 1982;12:77–85.

132. Forbes AR. Halothane depresses mucociliary flow in the trachea. *Anesthesisology* 1976;45:59–63.

133. Forbes AR, Gamu G. Mucociliary clearance in the canine lung during and after general anesthesia. *Anesthesiology* 50:26–29.

134. Patrick G, Stirling C. Measurement of mucociliary clearance from the trachea of conscious and anesthetized rats. *J Appl Physiol* 1977;42:451–455.

135. Lichtiger M, Landa JF, Hirsch JA. Velocity of tracheal mucus in anesthetized women undergoing gynecologic surgery. *Anesthesiology* 1975;42:753–756.

136. Cavaliere F, Carducci P, Schiavello R, et al. Halothane induced mucociliary depression: some data about a direct inhibition *in vivo*. *Riv Ital Otorinolaryngol Audiol Foniatr* 1985;5:105–107.

137. Moseberg B, Philipson K, Camner P. Tracheobronchial clearance in patients with emphysema associated with alpha₁-antitrypsin deficiency. *Scand J Respir Dis* 1978;59:1–7.

138. Sutton BP, Kadir N, Pavia D, Sheahan NF, Clarke SW. Lung mucociliary clearance in rheumatoid disease. *Ann Rheum Dis* 1982;41:49–51.

139. Fairfax AJ, Haslam PL, Pavia D, et al. Mucociliary clearance in Sjögren's syndrome. *Thorax* 1981;36:226–227.

140. Puchelle E, Zahm JM, Girard F, et al. Mucociliary transport *in-vivo* and *in-vitro*. Relations to sputum properties in chronic bronchitis. *Eur J Respir Dis* 1980;61:254–264.

141. Ahmed T, Greenblatt DW, Birch S, Marchette B, Wanner A. Abnormal mucociliary transport in allergic patients with antigen-induced bronchospasm: role of slow reacting substance of anaphylaxis. *Am Rev Respir Dis* 1981;124:110–114.

142. Foster WM, Langenback EG, Bergofsky EH. Lung mucociliary function in man: interdependence of bronchial and tracheal mucus transport velocities with lung clearance in bronchial asthma and healthy subjects. *Ann Occup Hyg* 1982;26:227–244.

143. Bateman JRM, Pavia D, Sheahan NF, Agnew JE, Clarke SW. Impaired tracheobronchial clearance in patients with mild stable asthma. *Thorax* 1983;38:463–467.

144. Pavia D, Bateman JRM, Sheahan NF, Agnew JE, Clarke SW. Tracheobronchial mucociliary clearance in asthma: impairment during remission. *Thorax* 1985;40:171–175.

145. Bateman JRM, Newman SP, Sheahan NF, Pavia D, Clarke SW. Tracheobronchial clearance during recovery from acute severe asthma. *Thorax* 1983;38:220.

146. Lourenco RV, Loddenkemper R, Carton RW. Pattern of distribution and clearance of aerosols in patients with bronchiectasis. *Am Rev Respir Dis* 1972;106:857–866.

147. Currie DC, Pavia D, Agnew JE, et al. Impaired tracheobronchial clearance in bronchiectasis. *Thorax* 1987;42:126–130.

148. Camner P, Strandberg K, Philipson K. Mucociliary clearance in relation to clinical features in patients with bronchiectasis. *Eur J Respir Dis* 1986;68:267–278.

149. Camner P, Stradberg K, Philipson K. Increased mucociliary transport by cholinergic stimulation. *Arch Environ Health* 1974;29:220–224.

150. Garrard CS, Levandowski RA, Gerrity TR, Yeates DB, Klein E. The effects of acute respiratory virus infection upon tracheal mucus transport. *Arch Environ Health* 1985;40:344–345.

151. Jarstrand C, Camner P, Philipson K. *Mycoplasma pneumoniae* and tracheobronchial clearance. *Am Rev Respir Dis* 1974; 110:415–419.

152. Wagner HN, Jr., Lopez-Majano V, Langen JK. Clearance of particulate matter from the tracheobronchial tree in patients with tuberculosis. *Nature* 1965;205:252–254.

153. Mossberg B, Bjorkander J, Afzelius BA, Camner P. Mucociliary clearance in patients with immunoglobulin deficiency. *Eur J Respir Dis* 1982;63:570–578.

154. Matthys H, Vastag E, Köhler D, Daikeler G, Fischer J. Mucociliary clearance in patients with chronic bronchitis and bronchial carcinoma. *Respiration* 1983;44:329–337.

155. Kosuda S, Kubo A, Sanmiya T, et al. Assessment of mucociliary clearance in patients with tracheobronchoplasty using radioaerosol. *J Nucl Med* 1986;27:1397–1402.

156. Kollberg H, Mossberg B, Afzelius BA, Philipson K, Camner P. Cystic fibrosis compared with the immotile-cilia syndrome. *Scand J Respir Dis* 1978;59:297–306.

157. Pavia D, Agnew JE, Bateman JRM, et al. Lung mucociliary clearance in patients with Young's syndrome. *Chest* 1981; 80(Suppl):892–895.

158. Rossman CM, Forrest JB, Lee RMKW, Newhouse AF, Newhouse MT. The dyskinetic cilia syndrome. Abnormal ciliary motility in association with abnormal ciliary ultrastructure. *Chest* 1981;80(Suppl):860–864.

THE LUNG: Scientific Foundations
edited by R.G. Crystal, J.B. West et al.
Raven Press, Ltd., New York © 1991.

CHAPTER 7.3.3

Cough

R. W. Fuller

Cough has two important physiological roles: It acts as a final pathway of mucociliary clearance, and it serves as part of the defense mechanism of the airways against inhaled particles and noxious substances. Cough is therefore a desirable response of the airways under physiological and some pathological circumstances. Cough is a symptom of many respiratory diseases, mostly as a consequence of excess mucus production (Table 1). However, in some diseases, especially viral respiratory infections, cough occurs without obvious mucus clearance or need to protect the airways. This nonproductive cough can be significantly distressing for the patients by causing social embarrassment and loss of sleep. In order to target therapeutic interventions so that they will reduce unwanted cough, it is important to understand why physiological cough occurs and what is abnormal in nonproductive pathological cough. This chapter will discuss these factors and the currently available antitussive medication.

SENSORY INPUT
INTO THE COUGH REFLEX

The anatomical type of the sensory nerves involved in the human cough reflex is unknown. Histology has revealed unmyelinated nerve endings, some containing neuropeptides, in or below the airway epithelium (1). It is not, however, known whether these connect to myelinated nerves before entering to the central nervous system or whether the nerves remain unmyelinated.

The anatomical site of the cough-sensitive nerves extends from the larynx to the division of the segmental bronchi (2,3), and there is no good evidence for more peripheral cough receptors in the human lung.

Animal studies suggest that there may be a number of possible nerve fibers involved in the cough reflex (1). The fiber involved in human cough is unknown; however, comparing the physiology and pharmacology of human cough with information from animal studies may make it possible to infer the type of nerve(s) involved. Of the possibilities, the myelinated irritant receptor (3) and the unmyelinated C fibers found in the territory of the bronchial artery circulation (4) seem to be the most promising candidates. The slowly adapting stretch receptors (5), when stimulated, do not cause cough but may have a modulatory role (5). The C fibers accessible by the pulmonary artery (6) are not in the correct anatomical position to be responsible for human cough, although parenteral dosing with both lobiline (7) and capsaicin (8) causes cough in humans. These observations were not detailed enough to firmly establish the site of the tussive nerves.

The information from animal studies is confusing because there are marked differences between the response of different species, and few studies have been performed to compare directly both cough response to inhaled tussive agents and their effect on nerves monitored by single-fiber recording. Even mechanical stimulation appears not to activate only myelinated irritant receptors, since C fibers in the dog can also be activated by touch (1). Other stimuli also cause cough and stimulate a number of different fiber types (e.g., prostaglandins, bradykinin, sulfur dioxide), and low chloride solutions stimulate both myelinated and unmyelinated fibers (1). Capsaicin—which at low doses is a relatively selective unmyelinated nerve stimulus (4) and tussive in humans (9), despite stimulating C fibers and (at high concentration) myelinated fibers in the dog (1)—causes no coughing. However, in the cat it is tussive (10), apparently through C-fiber stimulation in the larynx (11). Stimulation of C fibers lower in the respira-

R. W. Fuller: Department of Clinical Pharmacology, Royal Postgraduate Medical School, London W12 ONN, England.

TABLE 1. *Various causes of cough*

Mechanical	Inflammatory mediators/irritants	Extrathoracic	Abnormal cough reflex	Central
Acute/chronic bronchitis	Asthma	Postnasal drip	Viral infections	Psycogenic
Pneumonia	Viral infections	Esophageal reflux	Asthma	
Bronchiectasis	Pollutants	Middle ear disease	Interstitial lung disease	
Cystic fibrosis	Interstitial lung disease		Idiopathic dry cough	
Asthma	Angiotensin converting enzyme inhibitors		Angiotensin converting enzyme inhibitors	
Tumor				
Granuloma				
Blood				
Edema				
Foreign body				

tory tract in the cat, however, inhibits the cough reflex (12). It is therefore difficult to resolve the sensory route and tussive signals from studies promoting cough. The use of inhibitors such as local anesthetics and opiates in humans should be more helpful, because in animal studies their use has shown differential effects of local anesthetics between mechanical (myelinated) (13) and chemical (unmyelinated) (13) stimuli. Likewise, the effect of peripheral-acting opiates (14), which are likely to suppress the action of C fibers more than that of myelinated fibers, have also suggested a role for C fibers in cough.

It is therefore difficult to determine which sensory fibers are inputting into the human cough reflex, because we lack specific stimuli or inhibitors for the different types of fiber. There is, however, good evidence to suggest that the tussive fiber(s) differs from those which cause reflex airway narrowing, and it most likely that more than one fiber type will be involved in coughing, depending upon the stimulus or the pathological condition.

CENTRAL NERVOUS SYSTEM RELAY FOR THE COUGH REFLEX

The site of the central relay (cough center) in humans is unknown. The best-studied species is the cat, where the site for the center has been identified in the medulla oblongata in an area adjacent to the trigeminal tract and nucleus (15). Evidence is also available that some "centrally" acting antitussives such as opiates have their effect at this site (16).

Transmitters involved in transmitting the relay in humans are likewise unknown. In the cat, both serotonergic (17) and catecholinergic nerves (18) are probably involved. The former are inhibitory and appear to mediate the effect of opiate antitussives (19); and the latter, which inhibit respiration in a manner similar to that of serotonin, may also be inhibitory to the cough

reflex. The transmitter that facilitates the cough reflex is, however, unknown. Other potential inhibitory transmitters are those of the gamma-aminobutyric acid (GABA) series, because the benzodiazepine (clonazepam) has been shown to inhibit the cough reflex in the cat (15).

THE MECHANICS OF COUGH

Although the nerves that initiate the cough and the central relay mechanism are still largely unknown, in humans the effect of coordinated activation of the efferent pathway is well established (20). There are four important phases to cough which are designed to create maximum airflow in the upper airway. This flow is required in order to cause the sheer force necessary to separate mucus from the airway walls, to cause its expulsion. The phases are as follows:

1. *Inspiration.* This occurs depending on the part of the respiratory cycle at which cough is initiated to achieve optimum thoracic gas volume to allow the most efficient use of the expiratory muscles.

2. *Compression.* Activation of the rib cage and abdominal musculature at a time that the glottis is closed rapidly leads to high intrathoracic pressures. Coincident with the compression phase, there is narrowing of the bronchi by active bronchoconstriction which will increase the sheer force at the airway wall.

3. *Expression.* When the glottis is open, high airflows are achieved which generate the high sheer forces in the airway wall. These forces are increased by collapsing of the airways following the explosive decompression caused by the glottic opening.

4. *Relaxation.* At the end of the cough, there is a fall in intrathoracic pressure associated with relaxation of the expiratory muscles and transient bronchodilatation.

THE HUMAN COUGH REFLEX

In humans, cough can be provoked by a large number of irritants, given either by inhalation or by intravenous injection; this gives some insight into the mechanism of the human cough reflex. These tussive agents can be classified into a number of different groups (Table 2). Most of these agents (e.g., citric acid) cause cough that is rapidly tachyphylactic, requiring subject selection in order to perform physiological and pharmacological studies. Others, such as capsaicin (9) and nicotine (21), are more robust, causing coughing in most people which is reproducible. The capsaicin cough challenge has therefore been used to evaluate the sensitivity of the cough reflex in patients with cough (22) and to assess the effectiveness of antitussives in normal volunteers (23). So far, no patterns have evolved which give clear insight into the type of nerve or sensory receptor involved in cough. Most studies, however, suggest that the larynx is the major site of cough receptors, although experiments with laryngectomized patients and bronchoscopy do indicate that cough receptors are present at least at the main corini.

THE COUGH REFLEX IN PATIENTS WITH COUGH

Recent studies have been performed in patients with cough to establish whether it is associated with a normal or abnormal sensitivity of the cough reflex.

Patients with Productive Cough

Our studies in patients with productive cough have shown that in most cases the sensitivity of the cough reflex is normal. Figure 1 shows the cough response in patients with chronic obstructive airways diseases and bronchiectasis. These patients with stable productive cough have a normal cough reflex. This finding of a normal cough reflex in patients with productive cough is predictable, since the coughing is presumably due to the mechanical stimulation of the cough reflex to initiate clearance of the mucus, although with inflammatory exacerbations of the illness it is likely that the cough reflex may well be abnormal, making the coughing worse.

Patients with Dry Nonproductive Cough

In a group of patients with a complaint of nonproductive cough due to various etiologies, there was an abnormal increase in the sensitivity of the cough reflex (Fig. 2). This was seen in 109 of 121 patients, and in a few of these patients the test has been repeated and the abnormality remains for at least a 4-week follow-up period. No difference can be seen between the patient groups with respect to their cough reflex sensitivity. Some patients with a history of postnasal drip, however, have only a moderate increase in the sensitivity to their cough reflex, and it is therefore not clear whether this is the cause of the cough or the postnasal drip itself.

Mechanism of the Abnormal Cough Reflex

Epithelial Damage

The increase in the cough reflex has been observed in patients with acute upper respiratory infections, suggesting that perhaps viral epithelial damage may explain the increase (24). Most of these patients in the present study who have had bronchoscopy had normal epithelium.

Asthma

Another explanation is the bronchoconstriction or asthmatic airway hyperreactivity, because this has also been observed following a respiratory tract infection (25) and because cough is a frequent symptom

TABLE 2. *Tussive agents in humans*

Inflammatory mediators	Chemical irritants	Osmotic/low Cl$^-$ solutions	Mechanical
Histamine	Capsaicin	Distilled water	Bronchoconstriction
Bradykinin	Nicotine	Hypertonic saline	Instrumentation
Prostaglandin E$_2$	Metabisulfite	Urea solutions	Lactose
Prostaglandin F$_{2\alpha}$	Sulfur dioxide	Sugar solutions	Aerosols
	Cs gas		Dust
	Lobiline		
	Citric acid		
	Acetic acid		
	Acetylcholine		

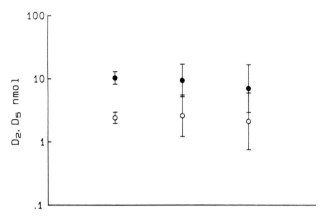

FIG. 1. Dose of capsaicin causing two or five (or more) coughs [D_2 (○) and D_5 (●)] in normal people ($n = 74$) (*left*), in patients with productive cough due to chronic obstructive airways disease ($n = 7$) (*middle*), and in patients with bronchiectasis lung disease ($n = 7$) (*right*).

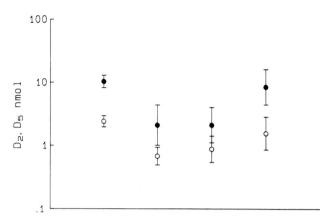

FIG. 2. Dose of capsaicin causing two or five (or more) coughs [D_2 (○) and D_5 (●)] in normal people ($n = 74$) (*left*), in patients with nonproductive cough with unknown diagnosis ($n = 42$) (*second from left*), patients with postviral cough ($n = 7$) (*third from left*), and in patients with postnasal drip ($n = 14$) (*right*).

of asthma. In our patients we have observed an abnormally sensitive cough reflex in asthmatics with cough. However, other asthmatics without cough had a normal cough reflex (Fig. 3) in the presence of the characteristic abnormal bronchoconstrictor response to an inhaled spasmogen, namely, histamine. Likewise, we have performed histamine challenge in the lung in a number of patients with an abnormal cough reflex and found that the majority are normal. It appears that asthma and an abnormal cough reflex can occur together; however, the presence of one does not necessarily mean that the other is also present. This has important implications in the therapy of nonproductive cough.

Angiotensin Converting Enzyme Inhibitor Cough

Recently, cough has been reported as a side effect of therapy with angiotensin converting enzyme inhibitors. It occurs with all known agents and is therefore

not an idiosyncratic reaction to one of them. Retrospective analysis suggests that the cough may be dose-dependent and more frequent if diuretics are also used. They also suggest an increased incidence in females and nonsmokers. Prospective studies, however, are awaited to clarify this picture. The cough is associated with an abnormal increase in the cough reflex (22) (Fig. 4), which only occurs in patients developing the cough and is not a universal finding (26). The change in the cough reflex is reversible as is the cough. The reason for the cough is not yet known. However, the most likely mechanisms involve an increase in bradykinin resulting from inhibition of its metabolism. Bradykinin is indeed a tussive agent (27), although an increased response to inhaled bradykinin has not been demonstrated in asthmatics treated with ramipril (28). Bradykinin itself, unlike prostaglandin E_2 (Fig. 5), did not

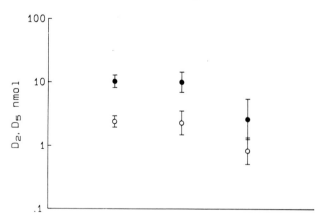

FIG. 3. Dose of capsaicin causing two or five (or more) coughs [D_2 (○) and D_5 (●)] in normal people ($n = 74$) (*left*), in asthmatics without cough ($n = 16$) (*middle*), and in asthmatics with cough ($n = 24$) (*right*).

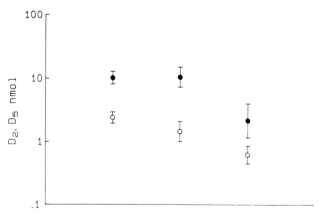

FIG. 4. Dose of capsaicin causing two or five (or more) coughs [D_2 (○) and D_5 (●)] in nomal people ($n = 74$) (*left*), in patients taking angiotensin converting enzyme inhibitors without cough ($n = 37$) (*middle* panel), and in patients taking angiotensin converting enzyme inhibitors with cough ($n = 27$) (*right*).

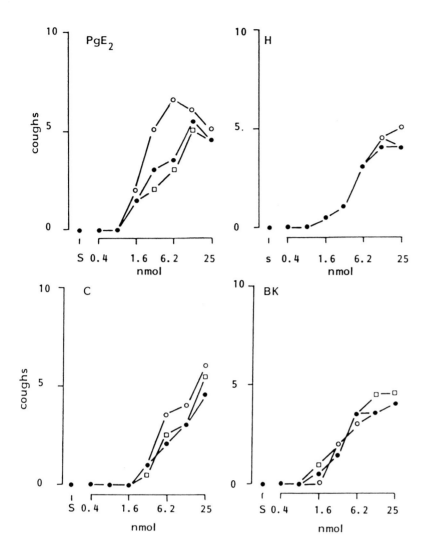

FIG. 5. Median number of coughs before (●), 5 min after (○), and 30 min after (□) treatment with prostaglandin E_2 (**upper left-hand panel**), histamine (**upper right-hand panel**), citric acid (**lower left-hand panel**), and bradykinin (**lower right-hand panel**) (*n* = 6).

increase the sensitivity of the cough reflex (29). In favor of a role for prostaglandins is the observation that sulindac (30) is able to reduce both the cough symptoms and abnormal cough reflex in patients with angiotensin converting enzyme inhibitor cough but not in those with cough due to other causes. It appears likely that in those 5–10% of patients who complain of cough there is an increase in tissue bradykinin levels leading to a secondary increase in prostaglandins which leads to the heightened response of the cough reflex and to the symptoms of cough.

Reduced Cough Response

Some patients have a reduced cough that may increase the risk of respiratory infection. Indeed we have shown that a reduced cough reflex is present in some patients with stroke in whom the efferent pathway was intact. Others have shown that patients post-operation have a similar reduction in the cough response, the mechanism for which is still obscure.

PHARMACOLOGY OF COUGH

The frequency of cough as a symptom has led to a prolonged search for a tolerable, safe, and effective therapy. It should, however, be stated that this goal has not yet been achieved. The drugs evaluated to date fall into two categories: those with a predominantly central action and those with a predominantly peripheral action.

Opiates

As a result of being the longest known antitussive agents, opiates have been extensively studied and reviewed (31). There is clear evidence that high doses of opiates usually administered parenterally are effectiv in reducing the sensitivity of the cough reflex (23). Doses such as those achieved by oral administration of codeine (23) or dextromethorphan (32) have been shown to only cause marginal reduction in the sensitivity of the cough reflex. Despite possible peripheral actions (14), this has not been demonstrated in humans, where the predominant site for opiates appears to be in the central nervous system. Unless a truly peripheral antitussive effect of opiates exists, it may well be impossible to produce effective opiate antitussives that are free of the other central nervous system side effects.

Other Centrally Acting Drugs

There are a number of transmitter systems involved in the relay of cough in the central nervous system, and therefore drugs that inhibit or activate these receptors may be antitussive. Indeed there are reports of antitussive effects of nonspecific antihistamines that are sedative. These effects may be due to inhibition of histamine receptors or to inhibition of serotonin or acetylcholine receptors. In animal studies the benzodiazepine clonazepam is antitussive, and such effects in humans require evaluation (15). Recently the effect of the serotonin receptor antagonist BRL 43694A, which is a potent antiemetic agent, was assessed and found not to alter the cough reflex in normals, suggesting that the receptors are not involved in the normal cough reflex (33). Clearly this is an area of great potential for the development of novel antitussive drugs.

Demulcents

Cough remedies containing syrups are the most widely used by the general public (24). There is anecdotal and objective evidence for their effectiveness at suppressing cough (34). However, the effect is relatively short-lived (less than 10 min). The mechanism of their effect is obscure and may relate to coating of cough receptors in the pharynx, although there is little evidence for these receptors in humans. More likely explanations are that the demulcents stimulate inhibitory reflexes, such as those found in the cat (12), or that the act of swallowing itself may be antitussive. This is an interesting area, since it could be very useful to develop long-acting demulcent-like drugs that may be safe antitussives.

Local Anesthetics

A sufficient dose of local anesthesia will inhibit the sensory input into the cough reflex; this can be achieved during bronchoscopy when the drug is administered by direct vision. Local anesthetics are available as oral lozenges or spray marketed for the treatment of sore throat. None of these treatments is designed to deliver the drugs to the respiratory tract. Nevertheless, if a phenol-containing spray that has local anesthetic (35) properties is given using a tongue depressor, then it does reduce the sensitivity to the cough reflex in normal volunteers. Nebulized lidocaine has also proven to be inhibitory on the cough reflex at a dose that does not reduce reflex bronchoconstriction (36). However, dyclonine given in the same study was ineffective. This implies that local anesthetics have to penetrate the mucosa to inhibit the reflex; this property may differ between drugs. In the nose the effect of lidocaine is enhanced by coadministration with a vasoconstrictor (37). This approach has not been used in the treatment of cough. The development of an effective means of administering local anesthetics in the upper airways would prove to be a valuable treatment of nonproductive cough.

Anti-Inflammatory/Antiallergic Agents

The cough associated with asthma is effectively reduced by inhaled steroids and cromoglycate. In the absence of asthma, the effectiveness of these agents is less clear. There are only anecdotal reports of the effectiveness of inhaled steroids in cough. Cromoglycate and nedocromil sodium have, however, been shown to inhibit cough stimulated in normal volunteers by some, but not all, stimuli (38). These intriguing observations require full study in patients with cough to evaluate their role as antitussives.

Bronchodilators

Inhaled β_2 agonists, like inhaled steroids, are antitussive in asthmatics (39). In normal volunteers there is some evidence for reduction of the cough reflex by both β_2 agonists and anticholinergic bronchodilators (40). These agents, like inhaled steroids, have not yet been evaluated in patients with cough but no asthma.

Expectorants/Mucolytics

In patients with productive cough, such drugs are favored above placebo by patients, although there is little objective evidence for their effect on mucociliary clearance. Patients with dry cough often complain of a feeling that they have mucus in the airways which they fail to clear. With this in mind, they are often treated with expectorants. If the cause for the cough is an increase in the sensitivity of the cough reflex, then it is likely that if a drug is effective in increasing mucus production, it will make the coughing worse rather than better. Few expectorants have been evaluated in patients with dry cough; and when an evaluation has been performed, little benefit was recorded.

CONCLUSION

Cough is undoubtedly the "Cinderella" of respiratory symptoms. Most people will suffer with cough from time to time, whether due to excess mucus production or to an increase in the sensitivity to the cough reflex. Treatment of the symptom remains difficult. If there is an underlying treatable disease, such as bacterial respiratory infection or asthma, then successful treatment will be achieved. However, in the majority this will not be possible. If the disease is short-lived and self-limiting, the use of sedative doses of opiates is justifiable. If the symptom is prolonged, the only options are to treat with demulcents and local anesthetics, which at best only provide temporary relief. The need for safe, tolerable, and effective antitussives is obvious.

REFERENCES

1. Karlsson J-A, Sant'Ambrogio G, Widdicombe J. Afferent neural pathways in cough and reflex bronchoconstriction. *J Appl Physiol* 1988;65:1007–1023.
2. Larsell O, Gurget GE. The effects of mechanical and chemical stimulation of the tracheo-bronchial mucous membrane. *Am J Physiol* 1924;70:311–321.
3. Widdicombe JG. Respiratory reflexes from the trachea and bronchiole of the cat. *J Physiol (Lond)* 1954;123:55–70.
4. Coleridge HM, Coleridge JCG, Roberts AM. Rapid shallow breathing evoked by selective stimulation of bronchial C-fibers in dogs. *J Physiol (Lond)* 1983;340:415–433.
5. Coleridge HM, Coleridge JCG. Reflexes evoked from tracheobronchial tree and lungs. In: Cherniack NS, Widdicombe JG, eds. *Handbook of physiology, Section 3: The respiratory system, vol 2—Control of breathing, Part 1.* Bethesda, MD: American Physiological Society, 1986;395–429.
6. Coleridge HM, Coleridge JCG, Luck JC. Pulmonary afferent fibers of small diameter stimulated by capsaicin and by hyperinflation of the lungs. *J Physiol (Lond)* 1965;179:248–262.
7. Jain SK, Subramanian S, Julka DB, Guz A. Search for evidence of lung chemoreflexes in man: study of respiratory and circulatory effects of phenyldiguanide and lobeline. *Clin Sci* 1972;42:163–177.
8. Winning AJ, Hamilton RD, Shea SA, Guz A. Respiratory and cardiovascular effects of central and peripheral intravenous injections of capsaicin in man: evidence for pulmonary chemosensitivity. *Clin Sci* 1986;71:519–526.
9. Collier JG, Fuller RW. Capsaicin inhalation in man and the effects of sodium cromoglycate. *Br J Pharmacol* 1984;81:113–117.
10. Adcock JJ, Smith TW, Widdicombe JG. Role of the vagus nerves in bronchoconstriction induced by inhaled histamine and capsaicin in normal and hyperreactive airways: irritant versus C-fibre receptors. *Eur Respir J* 1989;2:287s.
11. Adcock JJ, Smith TW. Inhibitory effects of the opioid peptide BW 443C on smaller diameter sensory nerve activity in the vagus. *Br J Pharmacol* 1987;92:596P.
12. Tatar M, Webber SE, Widdicombe JG. Lung C-fibre receptor activation and defensive reflexes in anaesthetized cats. *J Physiol (Lond)* 1988;402:411–420.
13. Karlsson J-A. Airway anaesthesia and the cough reflex. *Bull Eur Physiopathol Respir* 1987;23(Suppl 10):29s–36s.
14. Adcock JJ, Schneider C, Smith TW. Effects of codeine, morphine and a novel opioid pentapeptide BW 443C on cough nociception and ventilation in the unanaesthetised guinea-pig. *Br J Pharmacol* 1988;93:93–101.
15. Chou DT, Wang SC. Studies on the localization of central cough mechanism; site of action of antitussive drugs. *J Pharmacol Exp Ther* 1975;194:499–505.
16. Chakravarty NK, Matallana A, Jensen R, Borison HL. Central effects of antitussive drugs on cough and respiration. *J Pharmacol Exp Ther* 1956;117:127–135.
17. Kamei J, Hosokawa T, Yanaura S, Hukuhara T. Involvement of central serotonergic mechanisms in the cough reflex. *Jpn J Pharmacol* 1986;42:531–538.
18. Bolme P, Corrodi H, Fuxe K, Hokfelt T, Lidbrink P, Goldstein M. Possible involvement of central adrenaline neurons in vasomotor and respiratory control. Studies with clonidine and its interactions with piperoxane and yohimbine. *Eur J Pharmacol* 1974;28:89–94.
19. Kamei J, Hosokawa T, Yanaura S, Hukuhara T. Effects of methysergide on the cough reflex. *Jpn J Pharmacol* 1986;42:450–452.
20. Leith DE, Butler JP, Sneddon SL, Brain JD. Cough. In: *Handbook of physiology, Section 3: Respiration, vol 2—Mechanisms of breathing, Part 1.* Bethesda, MD: American Physiological Society 1986;315–336.
21. Hansson L, Karlsson J-A, Choudry N, Fuller R. Human airway reflexes: effects of inhaled nicotine. *Thorax* 1988;43:836P.
22. Fuller RW, Choudry NB. Increased cough reflex associated with angiotensin converting enzyme inhibitor cough. *Br Med J* 1987;295:1025–1026.
23. Fuller RW, Karlsson J-A, Choudry NB, Pride NB. Effect of inhaled and systemic opiates on responses to inhaled capsaicin in humans. *J Appl Physiol* 1988;65:1125–1130.
24. Higenbottam T. Cough induced by changes of ionic composition of airway liquid. *Bull Eur Physiopathol Respir* 1984;20:553–562.
25. Empey DW, Laitinen LA, Jacobs L, Gold WM, Nadel JA. Mechanisms of bronchial hyperreactivity in normal subjects after upper respiratory tract infection. *Am Rev Respir Dis* 1976;113:131–139.
26. McEwan JR, Choudry N, Street R, Fuller RW. Change in cough reflex after treatment with enalapril and ramipril. *Br Med J* 1989;299:13–16.
27. Fuller RW, Dixon CMS, Cuss FMC, Barnes PJ. Bradykinin-induced bronchoconstriction in humans. *Am Rev Respir Dis* 1987;135:176–180.
28. Dixon CMS, Fuller RW, Barnes PJ. The effect of angiotensin converting enzyme inhibition, ramipril on bronchial responses to inhaled histamine and bradykinin in asthmatic subjects. *Br J Pharmacol* 1987;23:91–93.
29. Choudry NB, Fuller RW, Pride NB. Sensitivity of the human cough reflex: effect of inflammatory mediators prostaglandin E₂, bradykinin and histamine. *Am Rev Respir Dis* 1989;140:137–141.
30. Fuller RW, McEwan JR, Choudry NB. The abnormal cough reflex: role of prostaglandins. *Am Rev Respir Dis* 1989;139:A586.
31. Eddy NB, Friebel H, Hohn K, Halback H. Codeine and its alternatives for pain and cough relief. *Bull WHO* 1969;40:639–719.
32. Fuller RW, Haase G, Choudry NB. The effects of dextromethorphan cough syrup on capsaicin-induced cough in normal volunteers. *Am Rev Respir Dis* 1989;139:A11.
33. Choudry NB, McEwan J, Lavender E, Williams A, Fuller RW. The effect of BRL 43694A (Granisetron) on capsaicin induced cough in man. *Br J Pharmacol* 1990;in press.
34. Packman EW, London SJ. The utility of artificially induced cough as a clinical model for evaluating the antitussive effects of aromatics delivered by inunction. *Eur J Respir Dis* 1980;110:101–109.
35. Choudry NB, Fuller RW. Effect of 1.4% phenol spray on the cough reflex in healthy volunteers. *Eur Respir J* 2:390s.
36. Choudry NB, Fuller RW, Anderson N, Karlsson J-A. The antitussive properties of inhaled local anaesthetics. *Thorax* 1989;44:355P.
37. Stjarne P, Lundblad L, Lundberg JM, Anggard A. Capsaicin and nicotine-sensitive afferent neurones and nasal secretion in healthy human volunteers and in patients with vasomotor rhinitis. *Br J Pharmacol* 1989;96:693–701.
38. Hansson L, Choudry NB, Fuller RW, Pride NB. Effect of nedocromil sodium on the airway response to inhaled capsaicin in normal subjects. *Thorax* 1988;43:935–936.
39. Ellul-Micallef R. Effect of terbutaline sulphate in chronic "allergic" cough. *Br Med J* 1983;287:940–943.
40. Poundsford JC, Birch MJ, Saunders KB. Effect of bronchodilators on the cough response to inhaled citric acid in normal and asthmatic subjects. *Thorax* 1985;40:662–667.

THE LUNG: Scientific Foundations
edited by R.G. Crystal, J.B. West et al.
Raven Press, Ltd., New York © 1991.

CHAPTER 7.3.4

Mineral Analysis of the Lung Parenchyma

Andrew Churg

The traditional method of evaluating the pathogenesis of mineral-dust-induced disease in humans has been to rely largely on gross and microscopic pathologic studies of lung tissue. Little information has been published about the lung dust burden in the morphologically normal lung, and although there are numerous studies on lung mineral content in workers with specific types of dust exposure, these have usually been based on methods that produce gravimetric estimates of the amount of dust of a specific type present.

Experimental studies in animals have made it clear that mineral-dust-related parameters such as particle size, number, and shape play an extremely important role in the pathogenesis of disease. Because of the small size of most inhaled dust particles, the light microscope is unsuited for their evaluation, and the inability to accurately identify mineral dusts with an ordinary electron microscope has prevented examination of the importance of these various parameters in human tissue.

With the invention of the analytical electron microscope, it has become possible to examine on a particle-to-particle and site-to-site basis the exact numbers, types, and sizes of mineral particles in any area of the lung, as well as to evaluate the influence of these parameters on disease patterns. Because these techniques are extremely slow and expensive to perform, relatively few systematic studies have been carried out. Furthermore, this type of analysis is essentially a research technique with few standards and considerable variation in results from laboratory to laboratory (see below). Nonetheless, sufficient data have been accumulated for two broad groups—namely, the general population without occupational mineral dust ex-

posure, and workers with occupational asbestos exposure—to allow some conclusions to be drawn about dust-related parameters and their relation to disease in persons with these types of exposures. Numerous individual reports of analysis of the lung content of other types of dust exist in the literature; references to these studies can be found in refs. 1 and 2.

METHODS

A large variety of analytic techniques are potentially available to evaluate the mineral dust content of lung tissue (see Table 1.5 in ref. 1 for a detailed listing of the methods and their applications). So-called macroanalytic techniques in which a bulk (at some scale) analysis is performed can provide quantitative estimates of the amount of a particular element or of a very specific mineral species. Examples are (a) the use of atomic absorption spectroscopy to determine lung beryllium content and (b) x-ray diffraction to determine the amount of a specific polymorph of silica which may be present. These techniques are limited in their application because of (a) the relatively small amount of dust present in many lungs, (b) the inability of most of the techniques to separate combinations of minerals with any accuracy, and (c) the requirement that the lung tissue be destroyed in order to perform the analysis, thus often obliterating information about local conditions.

Microanalytic techniques are those that allow a particle-by-particle analysis. The most commonly used procedure, and the one that will be the basis of the information presented here, is energy-dispersive x-ray spectroscopy, often referred to as EDAX analysis. The principle underlying this type of analysis is straightforward: When specimens are bombarded by the electron beam in an electron microscope, each atom in the specimen gives off secondary x-rays with characteristic energies. By positioning a suitable detector near

A. Churg: Department of Pathology and University Hospital, University of British Columbia, Vancouver, B.C. V6T 2B5, Canada.

the specimen, it is possible to count and determine the energy of each incoming x-ray photon. The usual device consists of a specially doped silicon dioxide crystal maintained at liquid nitrogen temperature, connected via suitable electronics to amplifiers and a small computer that displays the number of photons of a given energy as peaks that can be assigned to individual elements. Thus a very accurate quantitative microchemical analysis of the specimen can be performed.

In general, a microchemical analysis alone is insufficient for specific identification of a mineral particle. It is also necessary to know something about the morphology, and it is often necessary to know the crystalline structure as determined by electron diffraction. For example, a crystalline particle that produces only a silicon peak is most likely silicon dioxide (quartz or one of its polymorphs), whereas a noncrystalline, fibrous-appearing fragment that produces only a silicon peak is probably a piece of man-made mineral fiber. In the case of asbestos fibers, the combination of morphology, chemistry, and, when necessary, diffraction analysis is sufficient to unequivocally identify virtually all asbestos fibers (see below). For other minerals, identification is often less exact; however, sufficiently broad categories can be created to provide the desired information.

There is considerable variability from laboratory to laboratory in both the instruments used and the methods of specimen preparation, all of which markedly influence the results obtained. The term "analytical electron microscope" as used in this chapter refers to either a scanning, transmission, or scanning/transmission electron microscope equipped with an EDAX spectrometer. Because the resolution of scanning microscopes is considerably lower than that of transmission microscopes, use of a scanning scope may produce quite different qualitative and quantitative results if small particles are the structures of interest. For example, it is much easier to detect chrysotile fibers (which are very fine, measuring down to below 100 Å in diameter) with a transmission scope than with a scanning scope.

Furthermore, the choice of specimen and the method of specimen preparation greatly affect the results. It is possible to identify mineral particles in tissue sections cut for light or electron microscopy (3), but the volume of such specimens is extremely small; as a rule, few particles are found, even when the dust burden is very large. Extrapolation of results from such sections back to the common denominator of particles per gram of lung requires multiplying by a very large number (since the tissue volume is very small), and thus errors resulting from random variations in tissue concentration can be extremely large. This problem is not trivial: Several studies have shown that there are marked variations from site to site within the lung in asbestos fiber concentration over very small areas (4–6). In addition, because tissue sections often cut through a particle, it is difficult to obtain accurate particle sizing. This is especially true of mineral fibers. The one advantage of tissue sections is that it is possible to localize particles to specific lesions.

Because of the difficulties inherent in the use of sections, most investigators have chosen to use larger pieces of tissue along with a digestion procedure that removes the organic component, thus effectively concentrating the mineral particles. By picking specific sites within the lung or specific lesions, a good correlation of mineralogic parameters and pathologic reactions can be obtained in this way.

The choice of agent for removing the organic portion of the lung varies from laboratory to laboratory: Activated oxygen generated in a plasma asher, sodium hypochlorite (laundry bleach), and sodium hydroxide have all been used, and each of these agents has its advantages and disadvantages (see ref. 2 for a review). In our laboratory we use bleach digestion because it does not affect mineral chemistry and does not lead to fiber fragmentation.

After the organic tissue is destroyed, the mineral particles are collected on membrane filters (most laboratories use either Millipore or Nuclepore filters) with a pore size that is small enough to retain the particles of interest. If the specimen is to be examined in a scanning microscope, then in general a membrane filter with a smooth surface is preferable; this filter can be carbon-coated and directly examined. For transmission electron microscopy the particles must be transferred to plastic/carbon-coated electron-microscope grids. The standard method is the so-called Jaffe washer technique: Pieces of the membrane filter are placed particle side down on the coated electron-microscope grids, and the grid/filter assembly is set on top of a sponge that rests in a dish of solvent such as chloroform or acetone. Capillary action draws the solvent onto the grid and slowly dissolves the filter, leaving the mineral particles on top of the carbon/plastic coating. More details of the methods are available in refs. 1 and 2.

The specimen then can be examined in the analytical electron microscope. If a scanning scope is used, a set area is examined; in general, in a transmission scope a set number of grid squares are evaluated. The operator counts, identifies, and measures all of the particles encountered. Because the weight of tissue that was dissolved to make the preparation and the area of the membrane filter examined are known, it is possible to calculate the concentration of particles of specific types per gram of lung in the original lung sample. More details of the techniques can be found in refs. 1 and 2.

These techniques are simple in principle but tedious to perform accurately in practice. As noted above, there are marked variations in the results from laboratory to laboratory. The problem appears to be more severe when attempting to count asbestos fibers than when counting nonfibrous particles. A recent report (7) makes this point explicitly clear: Seven different experienced laboratories examined the same specimens; although all of the laboratories reported the "high specimens" as high and the "low specimens" as low, the absolute value of the particle counts showed marked discrepancies from laboratory to laboratory. Whether these differences relate to preparation methods, counting methods, or totally idiosyncratic factors such as the skill of the operator remains unclear; a further trial is in progress to clarify the situation.

This problem has an important practical consequence: Great care must be taken in comparing results from laboratory to laboratory, and more useful information is often obtained by making comparisons within sets of data generated by a particular laboratory from one type of disease to another.

MINERAL PARTICLES
IN THE GENERAL POPULATION

Particles in the Lung Parenchyma

Few studies have provided detailed information on mineral particles in the general population. Four such studies are summarized in Tables 1 and 2. It is of interest that all four found roughly an order-of-magnitude difference in concentration between the individuals with the highest and lowest particle burden, but, as noted above, the absolute values reported are discrepant, with Paoletti et al. (8) finding approximately one-tenth the mean number of particles when compared to the data of Churg and Wiggs (9), Stettler et al. (10), and Kalliomaki et al. (11).

The potential sources of these discrepancies are worth noting. The subjects are unmatched in terms of age, sex, and smoking history among the four studies; in fact, three of the studies include both smokers and nonsmokers. Moreover, all four studies employed different preparatory techniques and counted different classes and sizes of particles; for example, Churg and Wiggs (9) specifically excluded particles that might be of endogenous origin, whereas approximately 20% of the particles reported by Stettler et al. (10) fell into this category. Whether the closeness of the numbers can therefore even be viewed as real rather than as good luck is a matter of conjecture. Nonetheless, it is clear from all four studies that, simply in terms of concentration, the particulate burden of the normal lung is numerically substantial.

Table 2 shows the breakdown of the types of minerals found in the reports of Stettler et al. (10), Churg and Wiggs (9), and Kalliomaki et al. (11), with the data translated into the categories used by Stettler et al. (10). The results in the three studies are strikingly similar, and, provided that mineral identification is accurate, this type of breakdown is much less subject to preparation variations and other idiosyncratic factors than are concentration data. These data are also fairly similar to those reported by Paoletti et al. (8), who found 54% of the particles to be silicates and 46% to be oxides and sulfates, assuming that they are including silicon dioxide in the latter category. These studies suggest that overall, silicates, largely aluminum silicates, constitute the largest single group of minerals, followed by silicon dioxide (quartz), with smaller amounts of metal oxides and a variety of other types of particles.

These minerals are a good match to those reported in air samples from a variety of areas (12–14); the one exception is that lead particles have been found with a high frequency in the fine particle fraction of air (14) but were extremely rare in our experience in these lungs, suggesting that the lead must rapidly dissolve. Paoletti et al. (8) note that their analysis of particles in the ambient air yields a ratio of silicates to oxides/sulfates which is fairly similar to that seen in the lung. Kalliomaki et al. (11) point out that the minerals found in the lungs that they examined are very similar to the

TABLE 1. *Exogenous mineral particle concentration in the general population (all values $\times\ 10^6$ per gram dry lung)[a]*

Report	Subjects	Mean	Median	Range
Churg and Wiggs (9)	S/M	470	340	180–1090
Kalliomaki et al. (11)	S/NS/M[b]	970[c]		
Paoletti et al. (8)	S/NS/M/F[b]	25–50[d]		10–280
Stettler et al. (10)[e]	S/NS/M/F[b]	570	480	110–1610

[a] S, smokers; NS, nonsmokers; M, males; F, females.
[b] Includes some workers with occupational dust exposure.
[c] Average for smokers and nonsmokers.
[d] My estimate from their Table 1.
[e] Includes some particles that may be of endogenous origin.

TABLE 2. *Parenchymal exogenous mineral species in the general population (value as percent of total)*

Mineral	Churg and Wiggs (9)	Kalliomaki et al. (11)[a]	Stettler et al. (10)
Talc	7	4	3
Aluminum silicates[b]	53	59	38
Silica[c]	20	11	17
Aluminum[d]	4	1	1
Titanium[e]	6	6	12

[a] Cigarette smokers only.
[b] Including kaolin, micas, and feldspar.
[c] Particles analyzing as silicon only, presumably silica (quartz).
[d] Particles analyzing as aluminum only, presumably alumina.
[e] Particles analyzing as titanium only, presumably rutile (TiO_2).

mineral making up Finnish bedrock. It appears likely that the typical burden seen in the urban dweller is derived from atmospheric particles, and most of these are derived, in turn, from rock and soil weathering.

Less information is available about the distribution and sizes of particles in the normal lung. Overall, both Stettler et al. (10) and Churg and Wiggs (9) found that the mean case-to-case particle size was 0.4–0.7 μm. Churg and Wiggs were unable to find any concentration differences in random samples of peripheral upper and lower and central upper and lower lobes; however, they did find that the particles in the upper lobe were slightly but significantly larger than those in the lower lobe. The striking thing in both these studies was the small variation from case to case in mean particle size, implying that the lung retains a very selected fraction of dust from the atmosphere.

Experimentally, cigarette smoking has been shown to slow clearance of inert test particles in humans (15,16). Attempts to determine the effects of smoking on long-term particle concentration by analytical electron microscopy have yielded contradictory results: Vallyathan and Hahn (17) analyzed the concentration of aluminum and silicon and found that it correlated with the amount of smoking. Paoletti et al. (8) suggested that, at any age, particle concentration was greater in smokers than in nonsmokers. Churg and Wiggs (9) found a positive correlation between pack-years of smoking and particle concentration in the upper, but not the lower, lobe. On the other hand, Stettler et al. (10) failed to find any differences between smokers and nonsmokers, and Kalliomaki et al. (11) found that although the particle concentrations were not different between smokers and nonsmokers, smokers had smaller particles than did nonsmokers. At this

point the effects of smoke on long-term particle retention are unclear.

Particles in the Airway Mucosa

Little attention has been paid to mineral particles in airway mucosa. Using a modification of the technique employed for the parenchyma, Churg and Stevens (18) examined the particle concentration in airway mucosa carefully dissected free of surrounding tissue. In a series of lungs from smokers, they found that the particle concentration in the very large airways overall averaged about one-third of that in the parenchyma, a substantial number. A higher ratio of bronchial mucosal to parenchyma particle concentration was noted in a later study of 11 lungs from lifetime nonsmokers (19). In the latter study a distinct correlation of airway generation and particle concentration was noted: Per gram of dry tissue, the main-stem bronchus had considerably fewer particles than did the upper or lower bronchi, and the latter airways had somewhat fewer particles than did the segmental bronchi. Particle concentration showed a positive correlation with increasing distance from the carina and decreasing airway diameter, and particle size also increased as airway diameter decreased (Fig. 1). These patterns were remarkably constant from patient to patient.

A somewhat surprising finding in both these studies was the observation that the types of particles found in the airways were quantitatively different from those found in the parenchyma (Table 3). Silica in particular was concentrated in the airways, whereas silicates such as kaolinite and mica appeared in increasing concentrations as airway diameter narrowed; these silicates constituted an even greater proportion of total particles in the parenchyma (19).

These observations suggest that in the larger airways of the structurally normal nonsmoker lung, airway diameter, airway generation, and path length are the major influences on long-term bronchial particle concentration and size. The patterns of concentration and size are similar from individual to individual, and the concentration patterns (generation by generation) resemble those seen acutely in experimental subjects given inert dusts (20).

What conclusions can be drawn from these studies? The most striking is that, given a fairly low burden of dust, the lung maintains particle concentration, size, and distribution within a remarkably narrow range. The fact that the distribution of dust in the airways after a lifetime resembles that seen in acute experimental studies implies that initial particle deposition patterns are translated into chronic particle burden patterns, probably by translocation of a fraction of the

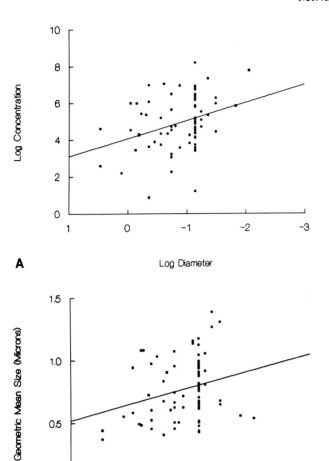

A

Log Concentration

Log Diameter

B

Geometric Mean Size (Microns)

Log Diameter

FIG. 1. Log particle concentration (**A**) and geometric mean particle size (**B**) versus log airway diameter. Note that airway diameter *decreases* along the x-axis in both graphs. (From ref. 19.)

TABLE 3. *Types of particles in airway versus those in parenchyma (as mean percent of total particles)[a]*

Mineral type	Parenchyma	Airway mucosa
Talc	3.4	5.1
Kaolin	17.7	5.4
Mica	23.1	4.3
Feldspar	8.2	7.2
Silica	32.1	66.9
Rutile	4.8	7.2
Miscellaneous	7.2	3.6

[a] From ref. 18.

particles through the airway epithelium into the wall where they lodge permanently (21).

Correlation with Disease

In a general sense, the particle burden in the "normal" lung is tolerated without the appearance of disease. Smoking probably perturbs both particle concentration and distribution, but its exact effects are uncertain. Oddly enough, there is no information on the fraction of particles in the lung which are derived from cigarette smoke, in part because of lack of detailed information about the minerals found in smoke. Recent reports of the types of minerals found in the smoke itself (22) may make it feasible to determine the types and locations of such particles in the human lung. The particulate fraction of cigarette smoke elicits an inflammatory response in the lung in both animals and humans, and this process is probably related to the development of emphysema and small-airway disease (23,24); however, no studies have specifically addressed the relationship between obstructive lung disease and particle burden and/or distribution in humans.

More suggestive data exist for the relationship between mineral particles, derived from smoke and/or air, and lung cancer. In some epidemiologic studies there are correlations between lung cancer rates and concentrations of particulate air pollutants (25–27), and air pollution may be the factor accounting for differences in lung cancer rates previously seen between urban and rural areas (25). Experimentally it has been shown that intratracheal installation of carcinogens such as benzo[a]pyrene along with noncarcinogenic (inert) mineral particles such as iron oxide will greatly increase the number of lung tumors over those found with administration of the carcinogen alone (28). The same effect can be seen if a crude particulate fraction isolated from air is used instead of a pure mineral dust; moreover, since cigarette smoke contains both chemical carcinogens and mineral particles that may adsorb carcinogens from the smoke or from the air, smoke may behave in a similar fashion (29–31). Biochemical studies indicate that this process relates to increases in uptake of carcinogens when bound to particles, as well as relating to redirection of carcinogen metabolism (29–31). In addition, small atmospheric (and presumably also smoke) particles concentrate toxic trace elements by adsorption (32), and particles in smoke may also adsorb radioactive particles (33). Explicit models for the mechanism of particle-enhanced carcinogen transport have been developed by Gerde and Scholandere (34).

Of particular interest is the work of Schlesinger and Lippmann (35). Using a hollow cast of the bronchial tree, they examined the deposition of inert particles and showed that there was a good correlation between the number of particles deposited in various lobar bronchi and the relative incidence of lung cancer in the same lobes. Correlative data in this regard were obtained by Churg and Stevens using human lungs with or without lung cancer (18). These investigators found that bronchial particle concentrations in the mucosa of upper- or lower-lobe bronchi leading to lobes containing lung cancers were significantly higher than in lobes without tumors. No such difference was found for the particle concentration in the lobar parenchyma. These data imply that the distribution of particles within the bronchial mucosa is important in the genesis of carcinoma, and they further raise the possibility that lung structural factors particular to each individual—for example, airway size, which is a major determinant of the deposition of particles (36)—play an important role in this process.

DISEASE CAUSED BY ASBESTOS

The chronic inhalation of asbestos is associated with a variety of changes in the lung, including benign pleural changes (plaques, fibrosis, effusion, and rounded atelectasis), malignant pleural disease (mesothelioma, also occurring in the peritoneum), and parenchymal lung disease (asbestosis, carcinoma). The relationship between asbestos exposure and disease is an area in which there are numerous and extensive epidemiologic studies, as well as sufficiently detailed characterizations of the asbestos minerals (37) to permit very exact identification by analytical electron microscopy. As a result, asbestos-related disease has been a particularly fruitful area for illuminating the relationship between mineral fiber parameters and pathologic reactions.

Asbestos is a general term for a variety of naturally fibrous silicate minerals that have the common properties of high tensile strength, high heat resistance, and relatively high chemical resistance. At present, six types of asbestos are recognized (Table 4). Of these minerals, only chrysotile, amosite, and crocidolite have had any extensive commercial exploitation; tremolite, actinolite, and anthophyllite are largely encountered as contaminants of other minerals. In particular,

TABLE 4. *Types of asbestos*

Chrysotile
Amphiboles
    Amosite
    Crocidolite
    Tremolite
    Actinolite
    Anthophyllite

tremolite and actinolite are found to be contaminants of talc and of chrysotile asbestos ore. Historically, chrysotile has constituted more than 90% of the asbestos used, and at present it constitutes virtually all of the imports into most countries.

Mineralogically, the asbestos minerals can be separated into two groups: Chrysotile comprises one; and amosite, crocidolite, tremolite, actinolite, and anthophyllite comprise the other. The latter five types of fiber are all members of the much larger mineral group known as "amphiboles." This classification is based on physical and chemical properties, but it is of considerable biologic importance. Analytic studies indicate quite clearly that chrysotile, compared to amphiboles, does not accumulate very readily in either human or experimental animal lungs. The reason(s) for this phenomenon is unclear. It has been claimed that the long curly fibers of chrysotile impact high in the bronchial tree and do not penetrate very far into the lung (38), but actual analyses show that the shorter fibers of chrysotile certainly reach the periphery of the lung (39). It has also been claimed that chrysotile fibers dissolve in lung fluid by magnesium leaching (40,41), but studies of both human and animal lungs have failed to find evidence of such leaching in the face of considerable chrysotile loss (42,43). More recent data suggest that chrysotile fibers fragment into very short and narrow pieces which are easily removed by macrophages (43).

In contrast, the amphiboles are chemically stable in the lung even after decades of residence and do not appear to fragment to any great degree. Furthermore, it has been proposed that their straight shape causes them to be carried in the airstream farther into the periphery of the lung than is chrysotile (38). In the lung, the much greater durability of amphibole compared to chrysotile fibers may be the reason why amphiboles are much more carcinogenic in terms of mesothelioma induction in man than are chrysotile fibers (see below).

Asbestos Bodies and Fibers

A great deal of information is available about the forms of asbestos found in lung. The majority of fibers in every lung appear as the bare mineral—that is, the form inhaled. In general, such bare fibers are too small to be reliably identified or even seen in light-microscopic sections of lung, nor can they be distinguished by light microscopy from the non-asbestos fibers found to a greater or lesser extent in every lung.

A variable portion of asbestos fibers in lung acquire an iron protein coat that renders them visible in the light microscope. These are referred to as "asbestos bodies." They appear as linear golden yellow structures in which the coating is variably knobbed and segmented; the underlying transparent, colorless, and usually straight fiber is often visible. The coating appears to be acquired in the phagosomes of macrophages that have engulfed the fibers (1).

Asbestos bodies were first reported early in the 20th century in asbestos workers (reviewed in ref. 1), where they were thought to be specific markers of asbestosis. It was soon realized that they could be found in the lungs of any worker who had asbestos exposure, and thus the name was changed from the original "asbestosis body" to the current "asbestos body" (illustrations of the various forms of asbestos body can be found in refs. 1 and 44).

Because they are readily visible in the light microscope, even in routinely stained sections (and even better in sections stained to demonstrate iron where the stain highlights the coat) asbestos bodies are useful markers of asbestos exposure. They can also be extracted from the lung by the same types of digestion methods used for extracting other mineral particles, and they can be counted either on membrane filters or in a counting chamber. Roggli and Pratt (45) have shown that when there is fairly substantial occupational exposure to amphibole asbestos, a good correlation exists between carefully performed counts of bodies in iron-stained tissue sections and the number of bodies determined by digestion techniques. Thus a relatively crude semiquantitative estimate of asbestos content can be obtained by counting bodies in light-microscopic sections; the drawback to this procedure is that tissue sections are, overall, relatively insensitive detectors of asbestos bodies. The more numerous asbestos fibers, which are invisible by light microscopy, provide a considerably better estimate of asbestos exposure.

Asbestos Burden in Persons with Environmental Asbestos Exposure

In the early 1960s, Thomson et al. (46) reported the startling observation that, if a suitable concentration technique was applied, it was possible to find asbestos bodies in about 25% of the general autopsy population of Cape Town. This was an extremely surprising finding at the time, because it had been previously believed that asbestos bodies were only found in persons with occupational asbestos exposure. The observations of Thomson et al. (46) have been confirmed by numerous subsequent studies, and it is generally agreed that asbestos bodies can be found in the lungs of virtually everyone in the population if suitable techniques are applied (1).

The obvious corollary to this observation was the idea that everyone in the population had a "background" asbestos exposure. However, this notion was challenged by Gross et al. (47,48), who demonstrated that, in experimental animals, instillation of non-asbestos fibers such as fiberglass or fibrous aluminum silicate resulted in the formation of structures morphologically identical to asbestos bodies. They coined the term "ferruginous bodies" as a name for any iron-coated mineral fiber, and they further concluded that, in the general population, ferruginous bodies were not formed on asbestos fibers.

The ideas of Gross et al. (47,48) were refuted by Churg and Green (reviewed in ref. 1), who extracted asbestos bodies from the lungs of persons in the general population without historical asbestos exposure, and who showed that all structures with the appearance described above did in fact contain asbestos. An interesting finding in these studies was that virtually all such bodies were formed on amphiboles, although corollary studies on uncoated fibers indicated that the majority of uncoated fibers in the lungs of such persons were chrysotile (see below). The reason for this phenomenon is not entirely clear, since chrysotile forms asbestos bodies readily in those with occupational chrysotile exposure (49–51); however, since asbestos body formation appears to require a fairly long fiber (49,50) and since most of the chrysotile found in the lungs of the general population is in the form of very short fibers (52), it is possible that the proper underlying fiber structure for asbestos body formation is not present. It is also possible that, because of the fragility of asbestos fibers, asbestos bodies which do form readily fragment into structures that are not recognizable as asbestos bodies, and that it is only in those with very substantial chrysotile exposure that enough morphologically typical asbestos bodies remain for practical recognition.

The ideas of Gross et al. (47,48) concerning the formation of ferruginous bodies are not entirely wrong: Bodies with cores of minerals other than asbestos can indeed be found in human lung. However, the same types of analytic procedures have indicated that such bodies are always morphologically distinguishable from true asbestos bodies at the light-microscopic level. For example, bodies with black cores may have particles of carbon, iron, rutile, or coal fly ash (mullite) as their nucleating agent. Sheet silicate minerals such as talc and mica form bodies in which the cores are plate-like and have a pale yellow color. Illustrations of these various ferruginous bodies can be found in ref. 1. The importance of such bodies is that, since they are readily observed in the light microscope, they may provide important clues to the nature of dust exposure in a given individual, but it is crucial that they not be confused with true asbestos bodies.

As noted, asbestos bodies constitute a minority of the total asbestos burden in the lung. From electron-microscopic studies it has been found that the ratio of fibers to bodies is quite variable; in the general population it may be as high as 10,000 fibers to one body, whereas in those with heavy occupational exposure to amphiboles the ratio may be as low as 5–10 to 1 (1,53). Moreover, there appear to be marked variations in the ability of different individuals to form asbestos bodies, and some persons form relatively few bodies even in the presence of relatively high amphibole loads (54). Thus the use of asbestos body counts to indicate total lung asbestos burden suffers from severe limitations, and there are even rare cases of asbestosis (diffuse interstitial fibrosis) in which a very high fiber burden has been demonstrated by analytical electron microscopy, but in which asbestos bodies could not be found in tissue sections (a combination of diffuse fibrosis and asbestos bodies in tissue sections is the traditional pathological requirement for the diagnosis of asbestosis) (1,44).

It should not be inferred from the above that counting asbestos bodies is useless; on the contrary, the technique is quick, economical, and does not require any equipment more specialized than an ordinary light microscope. Also, if one is dealing with individuals with substantial occupational amphibole exposure, there are clear correlations of asbestos body counts and disease patterns (see below and see also ref. 1 for a listing of quantitative studies of asbestos bodies in various diseases).

As implied above, the observation that asbestos bodies could be found in the lungs of virtually everyone in the population led to the realization that, at least in urban areas, there is extensive atmospheric contamination by asbestos. This idea has been proved by direct demonstration of fibers in the air (55,56). The amphibole fibers amosite and crocidolite are certainly derived from commercial product that has gained access to the atmosphere, and this is true of some of the chrysotile; however, there are extensive outcrops of asbestiform rock in North America, particularly in the west, and natural rock weathering is undoubtedly a source of some of the background levels of chrysotile asbestos.

The relative proportions of fibers found in the lungs of the general population vary considerably, depending on the technique used for counting. In my experience (1), which is derived from examining the lungs of the general populations of San Francisco and Vancouver, and counting all fibers longer than 0.5 μm, the vast majority of the fibers are short pieces of chrysotile. The most common amphibole is tremolite, likely a contaminant of the chrysotile. Amosite and crocidolite are present in very small amounts, if they can be demonstrated at all (Table 5). However, if one counts only long fibers—for example, fibers longer than 5 μm, as reported by Case et al. (57) for a series of accident victims from across Canada (Table 5)—then a much

TABLE 5. *Concentration of abestos fibers per gram dry lung in the general population*

Report/fiber	Mean	Median	95th Percentile
Churg and Wiggs (52) (fibers >0.5 μm)[a]			
Chrysotile	300,000	200,000	1,100,000
Tremolite	400,000	200,000	1,200,000
Amosite/crocidolite	1,000	0	10,000
Case et al. (57) (fibers >5 μm)[b]			
Chrysotile	62,000		
Tremolite	14,000		
Amosite/crocidolite	10,000		

[a] General hospital autopsy population.
[b] Accident victims aged 61 or greater.

greater relative fraction of amosite and crocidolite are found because these fibers do not readily fragment into short lengths. To the extent that long fibers are likely more dangerous than short fibers in the induction of disease, particularly mesothelioma (58–60), one can argue for counting only long fibers as the most important measure of disease potential; however, doing so may lose information about subtle differences in fiber size in different populations (e.g., see Table 6), differences that may relate to the presence or absence of disease.

The asbestos burden carried by members of the general population is numerically substantial. In my laboratory, levels of up to about 1,000,000 fibers of chrysotile, 1,000,000 fibers of tremolite, and 10,000 fibers of amosite plus crocidolite per gram of dry lung may be found (Table 5). The practical consequence of this observation is that the mere qualitative demonstration of the presence of asbestos in the lung is of no diagnostic, investigational, or epidemiologic use. Quantitative levels are required, and any laboratory supplying such levels must also supply the values seen in their background population. This requirement is commonly overlooked.

There are few data on the effects of age or place of residence on asbestos fiber counts in the general population. Data derived largely from counting asbestos bodies suggest that rural dwellers carry lower burdens than do urban dwellers (1,56,61,62), but the problems of comparing results from laboratory to laboratory make it difficult to know exactly how large these differences might be. Case et al. (57) have suggested that there is a trend toward increasing concentration of asbestos bodies, as well as a lesser trend toward increasing concentration of asbestos fibers with age, but we were unable to demonstrate any age-related increase in asbestos bodies in members of the population of Chicago (63). However, we did find that smokers ap-

TABLE 6. *Geometric mean fiber length/aspect ratios in various populations (fiber lengths in microns)[a]*

Population	Chrysotile	Tremolite	Amosite and crocidolite
General population Vancouver, B.C.	1.3/24	1.6/7	
Residents of Thetford Mines, Quebec	2.4/80	2.2/11	
Chrysotile miners, Thetford Mines	2.7/70	2.2/11	
Shipyard workers, insulators, and others exposed to chrysotile and amphiboles	2.5/60	2.5/10	3.9/22 (Amosite) 2.3/33 (Crocidolite)

[a] Data were taken from refs. 52 and 69.

peared to have greater numbers of bodies in their lungs than did non-smokers (63).

Within the last few years the issue of the possible health effects of environmental exposure to asbestos has reached public consciousness, and it has led to both litigation and regulatory-agency-sponsored efforts to remove asbestos from public buildings. Whether any risk exists from such exposures is a subject of considerable debate (55,64,65), in large part because it is impossible to directly demonstrate effects of the extremely low fiber levels found in air in asbestos-containing buildings [the one study which has actually looked at workers in asbestos insulated buildings (66) failed to find any effects compared to a control group], levels that are orders of magnitude below the exposure of occupational groups. Thus a great deal of energy has been expended on mathematical extrapolations from high to low exposure levels, extrapolations that are of questionable scientific validity (64).

Some useful light has been shed on this question by analytical studies of the lungs of individuals living in the chrysotile mining townships of eastern Quebec. Because of the presence of chrysotile/tremolite-bearing rock and soil, mine tailings, and open pit mines, individuals living in these areas are exposed for a lifetime to atmospheric levels of chrysotile and tremolite several hundred times greater than found in the air of most cities in North America (67,68). This relatively high environmental exposure results in measurably increased asbestos body and asbestos fiber burdens in the lungs of those who have lived in or downwind from the mining townships even if they have never worked in the asbestos industry; persons residing in the town of Thetford Mines, for example, carry chrysotile and tremolite burdens of approximately 5–10 times higher than do residents of Vancouver (56,69,70), and a similar result has been shown for the town of Asbestos (56,70); the burden is directly proportional to time lived in the area (56). In addition, the fibers found in the lungs of such persons are considerably longer than fibers seen in the general population of urban areas (52,56,69), a potentially important observation because of the likely enhanced pathogenicity of long fibers (58–60) (see below).

Despite the clear demonstration that persons resi-

dent in these areas carry much higher fiber burdens and considerably longer fibers than do dwellers in urban areas of North America, epidemiologic studies thus far have failed to show an increase in the incidence of either mesothelioma or lung cancer in individuals resident in the townships who have never worked in the asbestos industry (reviewed in refs. 64 and 69). These observations suggest that the lung can tolerate chrysotile and tremolite burdens considerably greater than that ordinarily found in the general population of North American cities without the development of asbestos-related disease. Conversely, these observations imply that the much lower levels of asbestos to which the usual North American urban dweller is environmentally exposed are certainly not going to produce any type of asbestos-related disease.

Populations with Occupational Exposure to Amphiboles

Evaluation of the relationship of asbestos lung burden and disease in occupationally exposed populations is complicated by two factors. The first is that the majority of persons with historic asbestos exposure have been exposed to both amphibole and chrysotile asbestos; thus, sorting out the different effects of the different fiber types is difficult. It is possible to find a few selected populations with exposure to chrysotile (which in North America contains a variable proportion of tremolite)—for example, the chrysotile mining populations of Quebec. However, in North America it is extremely difficult (with a few rare exceptions such as the amosite plant in Tyler, Texas) to find populations with pure amphibole exposure.

An additional difficulty arises from the fact, noted above, that chrysotile fails to accumulate in lung to any great extent. Some possible explanations for this phenomenon have been proposed above, but the practical consequence is that, even in populations with known substantial exposure to both chrysotile and amphiboles, electron-microscopic analysis performed years after the exposure may reveal only elevated levels of amphibole, or greatly elevated levels of amphiboles with minimally elevated levels of chrysotile and tremolite (52,71–73). To a certain extent, tremolite, which in most contexts appears to be associated with chrysotile, may serve as a partial marker for chrysotile exposure, since it, like other amphiboles, is preferentially accumulated in the lung. Indeed in the lungs of Quebec chrysotile miners and millers from Thetford Mines, tremolite is usually present in much higher concentrations than is chrysotile (39,52,74). However, when the chrysotile ore is processed into a form suitable for use in secondary products, some amount of tremolite appears to be removed (52,75–77). The variability of the amount of tremolite relative to chrysotile found in groups such as insulators suggests that in fact different products contain quite different amounts of tremolite (52,75). Even analysis of tremolite burden may provide a poor guide to chrysotile exposure levels. Thus, as a rule, electron-microscopic analysis will greatly underestimate chrysotile exposure in occupationally exposed populations.

A further problem with analysis of lung burden is that, virtually by definition, such analyses are performed at only one point in time, but the burden present at that time must obviously be the result of some balance between deposition and clearance. Unfortunately, little information is available about clearance patterns in humans, and in most studies it has not been possible to match patients exactly for amount and time pattern of exposure.

Reference 1 presents tables with detailed listings of the amounts of amphibole fibers found in populations with asbestos exposure and various asbestos-related diseases. Because of the lack of populations in North America with pure amphibole (amosite or crocidolite) exposure and because the lungs of most populations with mixed exposure contain relatively little chrysotile, I have chosen to treat these various reports as if the workers were exposed only to amphibole in order to conceptualize the relationship between residual fiber burden and the type of asbestos disease present. In the instance of mesothelioma (see below), this is probably a reasonable approximation, but for diseases such as asbestosis, and probably for benign pleural changes as well, the contribution of chrysotile, which is undoubtedly quite important, is ignored.

The distillation of a large number of individual reports suggests that for the amphiboles, chronic exposures to mean fiber concentrations of approximately one order of magnitude above the general population are associated with pleural plaques, exposures of an additional order of magnitude are associated with an increased risk for pleural mesothelioma, and exposures of approximately two additional orders of magnitude are associated with an increased risk for asbestosis. Despite the problems caused by the marked variation in absolute numbers of fibers found from laboratory to laboratory (see above), this pattern is read-

ily apparent when data from different types of diseases are generated by any one laboratory, and this is true whether one counts asbestos bodies (53,62,78,79), uncoated fibers by light microscopy [which in populations with sufficient amphibole exposure are virtually all amphiboles (53,80)], or uncoated fibers by electron microscopy (1,53,62,73,78,79,81–83). Asbestosis appears at much higher lung burdens than does pleural mesothelioma, and mesothelioma appears at higher lung burdens than do benign pleural changes such as plaques. Finally, and most importantly, asbestos disease appears at lung burdens some two to three orders of magnitude greater than that found in the general population.

Several diseases have not been included in the schema because few data are available for these conditions. If one accepts the proposition that asbestos-related lung carcinoma only appear in the presence of asbestosis (84), then the associated burden for lung carcinoma is at the high end of the asbestosis scale (85). Peritoneal mesotheliomas, of which relatively few have been analyzed, appear at higher fiber burdens than do pleural mesothelioma (85), a finding not surprising if one considers the epidemiologic evidence that peritoneal mesothelioma requires fairly substantial occupational exposure for its genesis (86). It is important to point out that some persons with mesothelioma have no history of asbestos exposure; moreover, analysis of lung content fails to show increases over background, a finding that supports the proposition that some proportion of mesotheliomas are unrelated to asbestos exposure (87). An additional finding, noted in a variety of studies, is that if one grades asbestosis pathologically to evaluate the severity of fibrosis, the higher fibrosis grades consistently have higher asbestos counts than do the lower fibrosis grades (53,73,80).

Several broad conclusions emerge from this schema: (a) Despite the fairly wide variation in fiber counts for any given disease, disease appears at a much higher amphibole burden than is found in members of the general population; (b) there is a dose relationship between fiber burden and type of disease present; (c) the pleura is much more sensitive to amphibole exposure than is the parenchyma, and this observation is true of both benign changes and malignant pleural disease; (d) asbestosis is only seen with very high lung burdens, and the grade of asbestosis (i.e., the amount of scarring) is proportional to the asbestos burden.

Populations with Occupational Exposure to Chrysotile

As noted above, there are few populations with even putative exposure to chrysotile alone, and one of the important discoveries made by analytical electron microscopy has been the extent to which many such populations have had occult exposure to amosite and crocidolite (75,76,85). Given the apparent marked differences in the mesothelial carcinogenicity of chrysotile compared to that of amphiboles (see below), such occult exposures are extremely important confounders of attempts to determine dose responses for mesothelioma and have led to the use of inappropriate populations for predictions of asbestos-related disease. For example, Peto (88) has made a variety of projections of potential asbestos disease at different possible chrysotile exposure standards, but Wagner et al. (85) have shown by analysis of lung mineral content that the workers at the factory used for these projections, namely the "chrysotile" textile plant at Rochdale, in fact had widespread exposure to crocidolite.

This problem notwithstanding, one can, using data from industries in which chrysotile was at least the predominant fiber utilized, as well as using data from the chrysotile mining and milling industry, look at reports from various laboratories and construct the same type of scheme for fiber burden versus disease as was just done for amphiboles (39,52,56,69,75–77,89,90). There are quite marked differences in the relationship between fiber burden and disease when comparing chrysotile-exposed to amphibole-exposed populations. In this regard, the general population in mining townships have a chronic exposure to mean fiber concentrations of approximately two orders of magnitude above that of the chrysotile/tremolite general population of urban areas, and neither is at risk for asbestos-related disorders. Exposure to concentrations one order of magnitude higher than that of the mining townships is associated with pleural plaques. It requires at least two additional orders of magnitude of exposure to present a risk for the development of early morphologic changes in the lung, such as the development of airway changes. Another order of magnitude of exposure to chrysotile/tremolite is required to present an increased risk for asbestosis and mesothelioma.

It is apparent from this summary that for chrysotile/tremolite, disease appears at considerably greater lung burdens than are seen in the general population of urban areas in North America, and for that matter greater than the general populations of the mining townships. Indeed, it is remarkable how much chrysotile and tremolite can be tolerated, even in the lungs of miners and millers with long years of exposure, without the appearance of disease; for example, in a series of miners and millers who had no demonstrable asbestos-related disease, the mean chrysotile burden was 20,000,000 fibers and the mean tremolite burden was 50,000,000 fibers per gram dry lung (90; compare Table 5).

The second conclusion of considerable importance is that, as opposed to exposure to amphiboles such as amosite and crocidolite, in which mesothelioma appears at much lower burdens than does asbestosis, in those with chrysotile/tremolite exposure both mesothelioma and asbestosis appear at about the same burden, and this is an extraordinarily high one.

A third conclusion is that, as is true for amphibole-induced asbestosis, there is also a gradient between chrysotile/tremolite fiber burden and the grade of asbestosis, an observation that has been made in both textile workers (76) and chrysotile miners and millers (91). It is interesting that in the latter study a considerably stronger correlation was found for tremolite fiber concentration and grade of fibrosis in local areas of lung than for chrysotile fiber concentration and grade of fibrosis. Whether this indicates that, on a one-to-one basis, tremolite fibers are really more fibrogenic than chrysotile fibers, or whether this problem illustrates the difficulty of using mineral analysis to examine the very small residual fiber burden of chrysotile, is unclear.

As has been indicated above, there is considerable interest in the question of whether some fiber types are more pathogenic than others in regard to the induction of asbestos disease. Epidemiologic studies present this case quite clearly in regard to mesothelioma, for which experimental animal studies have suggested that chrysotile is a very much weaker mesothelial carcinogen than is amosite or crocidolite (86). This question can also be approached by examining the relative burdens of chrysotile (with accompanying tremolite) or amphibole (amosite and crocidolite) in the lungs of workers with any particular disease. As noted above, it appears that vastly greater burdens of chrysotile plus tremolite than of amosite or crocidolite can be tolerated without the appearance of disease, and, conversely, for any given disease, the associated burden of chrysotile plus tremolite appears to be markedly greater than the burden of amosite and crocidolite (e.g., see Table 7). One can take this one step further and note our good fortune that chrysotile, and not amosite or crocidolite, was the major asbestos fiber of historic use. If the numbers of fibers of chrysotile/tremolite routinely found in the general population of North America had, instead, been fibers of amosite/crocidolite, undoubtedly there would have been a mesothelioma epidemic of vast proportion.

The limitations of these types of analyses caused by the failure of chrysotile accumulation should not be ignored. For example, McDonald et al. (92) have recently compared the fiber burden in a series of mesothelioma cases and controls from across Canada, and they claimed that because the distribution of chrysotile fibers in the test series was similar to that in the control series, chrysotile explained very few, if any, mesothelioma cases. However, as has been shown for workers with very substantial historic chrysotile exposure such as shipyard workers and insulators (52), the re-

TABLE 7. *Median concentrations of chrysotile/tremolite or amosite/crocidolite in a series of age- and exposure period-matched workers with mining or shipyard/insulating exposure[a]*

Workers and disease	Concentration of chrysotile/tremolite ($\times 10^6$ fibers per gram dry lung)	Concentration of amosite/crocidolite ($\times 10^6$ fibers per gram dry lung)
Chrysotile miners and millers		
With asbestosis	110	—
With mesothelioma	290	—
Shipyard workers/insulators		
With asbestosis	—	26
With mesothelioma	—	0.7

[a] From ref. 98.

sidual chrysotile burden years after the exposure can be no different from that of the general population. Thus the approach used by McDonald et al. (92) might miss an effect simply because the fiber of interest is no longer present in concentrations related to those of the actual exposure.

EFFECTS OF INTRAPULMONARY FIBER DISTRIBUTION AND SIZE

Most studies that have examined the fiber content of the lung have only considered the question of fiber concentration, and although this variable is both epidemiologically and analytically clearly a major determinant of disease, there is no doubt that both fiber distribution within the lung and fiber size play a role as well.

The importance of fiber distribution is emphasized by the anatomic distribution of certain asbestos-related diseases. For example, asbestosis is always more severe in the lower lobes and in the periphery of the lower lobes, an effect that has never been explained. Pinkerton et al. (93) have shown that, in the rat, fiber burden as well as interstitial fibrosis was greatest in the portions of parenchyma served by short airways with few branches. These observations may indicate that the distribution of fibrosis in human lung reflects the underlying lung airway structure. It appears logical also to assume that the development of both benign pleural changes and malignant pleural disease is related to the number, types, and fiber sizes of fibers that reach the pleura, but little information is available about this question.

As noted above, evaluation of the distribution of fibers within the lung is complicated by the fact that there may be as much as 10-fold differences in fiber concentration between adjacent sites located 1 cm apart under the pleura (6). Morgan and Holmes (4,5) have performed very careful studies in which the whole periphery of the lungs of a small number of workers was examined. Using light microscopy they were unable to find any consistent upper-versus-lower lobe distributions, although they did conclude that in some workers, specific sites in the periphery of the lung, especially the lobar tips, appear to accumulate higher fiber burdens. It has also been suggested that fiber distribution varies within the lung by fiber type. For example, Sebastien et al. (94), examining the lungs of a series of workers with both amphibole and chrysotile exposure, found that chrysotile was always present in the pleura, whereas amphibole often could not be detected. However, we have been unable to find any consistent differences in the distribution of tremolite compared to that of chrysotile within the lung in chrysotile miners and millers (39,90).

A recent observation from our laboratory suggests that fiber distribution must be looked at in a very detailed fashion that relates to the underlying anatomic structures. Examining the numbers and sizes of fibers in a series of carefully defined portions of the peripheral and central upper and lower lobes, we found that in cases of amphibole-associated mesothelioma there was accumulation of long amphibole fibers in the peripheral upper lobe and in the central lower lobe (95). The peripheral upper-lobe fibers were longer than those in the central upper lobe, thereby contradicting theoretic predictions of deposition patterns that would have the longest fibers depositing in the most central locations (38); this also implies either that there is selective redistribution of fibers in some segments of the lung after initial deposition or that, in a fashion analogous to the experimental data of Pinkerton et al. (93), factors such as airway length produce marked inhomogeneities in the intrapulmonary distribution of fibers. The exact relationship between fiber distribution and disease remains to be clarified.

There are a great deal of experimental animal data which indicate that fiber size is important in the pathogenesis of disease; in general, on a one-to-one basis, long fibers appear to be more fibrogenic, and long, high-aspect (length to width) ratio fibers are more dangerous in regard to the production of mesotheliomas than are short- or low-aspect ratio fibers (58–60,96,97), but few data exist on the relationship between fiber size and disease patterns in humans. As shown in Table 6, the chrysotile and tremolite fibers seen in the lungs of the general population are, on average, extremely short, whereas in those with occupational chrysotile exposure the fibers are much longer. In addition, the average length of amosite and crocidolite in the lungs of both members of the general population and those with occupational exposure areas is considerably longer than the average length of tremolite or chrysotile (50,52,69). The differences between chrysotile and amphiboles in this regard undoubtedly reflect fiber durability as explained previously, and, to the extent that long fibers are necessary for the induction of mesothelioma, these differences may serve as a partial explanation for the greater incidence of mesothelioma in those with amphibole, as compared with chrysotile, exposure.

CONCLUSION

The invention of the analytical electron microscope has allowed detailed systematic study of the mineral content of human lung. In members of the general population without occupational dust exposure, such studies reveal that both the parenchyma and the airway mucosa carry substantial mineral particle burdens. There is a surprisingly reproducible pattern of particle distribution within the bronchial tree and parenchyma from person to person. The types of particles seen in the lungs of the general population are similar to those found in urban air, but there are differences between large airways and parenchyma, with the former concentrating silica and the latter concentrating silicates. In the large airways, particle concentration and particle size increase as airway diameter decreases. The long-term distribution of particles in the large airways is similar to that seen in acute experimental studies in humans. When particle burden is relatively low, the lung appears to maintain particle concentration, size, and distribution within fairly narrow limits. Little information is available concerning particle burden and the effects of smoking or disease, but there does appear to be a correlation between particle burden in the large airways and lung cancer.

A large body of information is available concerning the types and concentrations of asbestos fibers within the lung, particularly in those with occupational exposure. The lung appears to be a much better detector of amphibole asbestos than most direct analytic methods, and lung analysis is a particularly sensitive way of determining cumulative exposure to amphiboles; however, chrysotile does not accumulate in lung to anywhere near the same extent. Everyone in the population is exposed to asbestos from air contamination,

but for both chrysotile and amphibole (amosite/crocidolite) asbestos, disease appears at much higher fiber concentrations than are seen in the general population. In general, the lung can tolerate much greater burdens of chrysotile than of amphiboles without the development of disease. There is a dose relationship between fiber burden and type of disease present. Asbestosis is only seen with very high lung burdens, and the grade of asbestosis (i.e., the amount of scarring) is proportional to the asbestos burden. For workers with amphibole exposure, the pleura appears to be much more sensitive than the parenchyma, and this observation is true of both benign pleural changes and malignant pleural disease; however, for workers with chrysotile exposure, malignant pleural disease (mesothelioma) is seen only with extraordinarily high lung burdens. The effects of fiber size and distribution in humans are unclear thus far, although they likely play a role in the genesis of disease.

ACKNOWLEDGMENTS

This work has been supported by grants from the National Cancer Institute of Canada and the Medical Research Council of Canada.

REFERENCES

1. Churg A, Green FHY. *Pathology of occupational lung disease.* New York: Igaku-Shoin, 1988.
2. Ingram P, Shelburne JD, Roggli VL, eds. *Microprobe analysis in medicine.* New York: Hemisphere Press, 1989.
3. Pickett JP, Ingram P, Shelburne JD. Identification of inorganic particles in a single histologic section using both light microscopy and x-ray microprobe analysis. *J Histotechnol* 1980;3:155–158.
4. Morgan A, Holmes A. Distribution and characteristics of amphibole asbestos fibers, measured with the light microscope, in the left lung of an insulation worker. *Br J Indust Med* 1983;40:45–50.
5. Morgan A, Holmes A. The distribution and characteristics of asbestos fibers in the lungs of Finnish anthophyllite mine-workers. *Environ Res* 1984;33:62–75.
6. Churg A, Wood P. Observations on the distribution of asbestos fibers in human lungs. *Environ Res* 1983;31:374–380.
7. Gylseth B, Churg A, Davis JMG, et al. Analysis of asbestos fibers and asbestos bodies in human lung tissue samples. An international laboratory trial. *Scand J Work Environ Health* 1985;11:107–110.
8. Paoletti L, Eibenschutz L, Cassano AM, et al. Mineral fibres and dust in lungs of subjects living in an urban environment. In: Bignon J, Peto J, Saracci R, eds. *Non-occupational exposure to mineral fibres.* Lyon: IARC, 1989;354–360.
9. Churg A, Wiggs B. Types, numbers, sizes, and distribution of mineral particles in the lungs of urban male cigarette smokers. *Environ Res* 1987;42:121–129.
10. Stettler LE, Growth DH, Platek SF, Burg JR. Particulate concentrations in urban lungs. In: Ingram P, Shelburne JD, Roggli VL, eds. *Microprobe analysis in medicine.* New York: Hemisphere Press, 1989;133–146.
11. Kalliomaki PL, Taikina-aho O, Paakko P, et al. Smoking and the pulmonary mineral particle burden. In: Bignon J, Peto J,

Saracci R, eds. *Non-occupational exposure to mineral fibres.* Lyon: IARC, 1989;323–329.

12. Berry JP, Galle P. Chemical and crystallographic microanalysis of fine particles in the urban atmosphere. *Environ Res* 1980;12:150–164.

13. Windon H, Griffin J, Goldberg ED. Talc in atmospheric dusts. *Environ Sci Technol* 1967;1:923–926.

14. Corn M. Aerosols and the primary air pollutants—nonviable particles. In: Stern AC, ed. *Air pollution,* 3rd ed, vol 1. New York: Academic Press, 1976;77–168.

15. Cohen D, Arai SF, Brain JD. Smoking impairs long-term clearance from the lung. *Science* 1979;204:514–516.

16. Bohning DE, Atkins HL, Cohn SH. Long-term particle clearance in man: normal and impaired. *Ann Occup Hyg* 1982;26:259–271.

17. Vallyathan V, Hahn LH. Cigarette smoking and inorganic dust in human lungs. *Arch Environ Health* 1985;40:69–73.

18. Churg A, Stevens B. Association of lung cancer and airway particle concentration. *Environ Res* 1988;45:58–63.

19. Churg A, Stevens B. Exogenous mineral particles in the human bronchial mucosa and lung parenchyma. I. Nonsmokers in the general population. *Exptl Lung Res*; in press.

20. Lippmann M, Yeates DB, Albert RE. Deposition, retention, and clearance of inhaled particles. *Br J Indust Med* 1980;37:337–362.

21. Gore DJ, Patrick G. A quantitative study of the penetration of insoluble particles into the tissue of the conducting airways. *Ann Occup Hyg* 1982;26:149–161.

22. Langer AM, Nolan RP, Bowes DR, Shirey SB. Inorganic particles found in cigarette tobacco, cigarette ash, and cigarette smoke. In: Wehner AP, Felton D, eds. *Biological interactions of inhaled mineral fibers and cigarette smoke.* Columbus, OH: Batelle Press, 1989;421–440.

23. Abrams WR, Kucich U, Kimbel P, Glass M, Weinbaum G. Acute cigarette smoke exposure in dogs: the inflammatory response. *Exptl Lung Res* 1988;14:459–475.

24. Hunninghake GW, Gadek JE, Kawanami O, Ferrans VJ, Crystal RG. Inflammatory and immune processes in the human lung in health and disease; evaluation by bronchoalveolar lavage. *Am J Pathol* 1979;97(1):149–198.

25. Doll R. Atmospheric pollution and lung cancer. *Environ Health Perspect* 1978;22:23–31.

26. Vena JE. Air pollution as a risk factor in lung cancer. *Am J Epidemiol* 1982;116:42–56.

27. Hitosugi M. Epidemiological study of lung cancer with special reference ot the effect of air pollution and smoking habit. *Inst Public Health Bull (Jpn)* 1968;17:237–256.

28. Safiotti U, Montesano R, Sellakumar AR, Cetis F, Kaufman DG. Respiratory tract carcinogenesis in hamsters induced by benzo(*a*)pyrene and ferric oxide. *Cancer Res* 1972;32:1073–1081.

29. Stenback F, Rowland J, Sellakumar A. Carcinogenicity of benzo(*a*)pyrene and dusts in the hamster lung. *Oncology* 1976;33:29–34.

30. Lubawy WC, Isaac RS. Acute tobacco smoke exposure alters the profile of metabolites produced by benzo(*a*)pyrene by the isolated perfused rabbit lung. *Toxicology* 1980;18:37–47.

31. Warshawsky D, Bingham E, Niemeier RW. Influence of airborne particulate on the metabolism of benzo(*a*)pyrene in the isolated perfused lung. *J Toxicol Environ Health* 1983;11:503–517.

32. Natusch DFS, Wallace JR, Evans CA. Toxic trace elements: preferential concentration in respirable particles. *Science* 1974;183:202–204.

33. Martell EA. Radiation at bronchial bifurcations of smokers from indoor exposure to radon progeny. *Proc Natl Acad Sci USA* 1983;80:1285–1289.

34. Gerde P, Scholandere P. A model for the influence of inhaled mineral fibers on the pulmonary uptake of polycyclic aromatic hydrocarbons (PAH) from cigarette smoke. In: Wehner AP, Felton D, eds. *Biological interactions of inhaled mineral fibers and cigarette smoke.* Columbus, OH: Batelle Press, 1989;97–120.

35. Schlesinger RB, Lippmann M. Selective particle deposition and bronchogenic carcinoma. *Environ Res* 1978;15:424–431.

36. Yu CP, Nicolaides P, Soong TT. Effect of random airway sizes on aerosol deposition. *Am Indust Hyg Assoc J* 1979;40:999–1005.

37. Champress PE, Cliff G, Lorimer GW. The identification of asbestos. *J Microsc* 1976;108:231–249.

38. Timbrell V. The inhalation of fibrous dusts. *Ann NY Acad Sci* 1965;132:255–273.

39. Churg A, Wiggs B, DiPaoli L, Kempe B, Stevens B. Lung asbestos content in chrysotile workers with mesothelioma. *Am Rev Respir Dis* 1984;130:1042–1045.

40. Jaurand MC, Gaudichet A, Halpern S, Bignon J. *In vitro* biodegradation of chrysotile fibres by alveolar macrophages and mesothelial cells in culture: comparison with a pH effect. *Br J Indust Med* 1984;41:389–395.

41. Morgan A, Davies P, Wagner JC, Berry G, Holmes A. The biological effects of magnesium-leached chrysotile asbestos. *Br J Exp Pathol* 1977;58:465–473.

42. Churg A, DePaoli L. Clearance of chrysotile from human lung. *Exptl Lung Res* 1988;14:567–574.

43. Churg A, Wright JL, Gilks B, DePaoli L. Rapid short term clearance of chrysotile compared to amosite asbestos in the guinea pig. *Am Rev Respir Dis* 1989;139:885–890.

44. Craighead J, Abraham J, Churg A, et al. Pathology standards for the diagnosis of asbestos-related diseases. *Arch Pathol Lab Med* 1982;106:541–597.

45. Roggli VL, Pratt PC. Numbers of asbestos bodies in iron-stained tissue sections in relation to asbestos body counts in lung tissue digests. *Hum Pathol* 1983;106:544–596.

46. Thomson JG, Kaschula ROC, MacDonald RR. Asbestos as a modern urban hazard. *S Afr Med J* 1983;37:77–81.

47. Gross P, Cralley LJ, DeTreveille RTP. "Asbestos" bodies: their nonspecificity. *Am Indust Hyg Assoc J* 1967;28:541–542.

48. Gross P, deTreveille RTP, Haller MN. Pulmonary ferruginous bodies in city dwellers. A study of their central fiber. *Arch Environ Health* 1969;19:186–188.

49. Pooley FD. Asbestos bodies: their formation, composition, and character. *Environ Res* 1972;5:363–379.

50. Pooley FD. Electron microscope characteristics of inhaled chrysotile asbestos fibre. *Br J Indust Med* 1972;29:146–153.

51. Holden J, Churg A. Asbestos bodies and the diagnosis of asbestosis in chrysotile workers. *Environ Res* 1986;39:232–236.

52. Churg A, Wiggs B. Fiber size and number in users of processed chrysotile ore, chrysotile miners, and members of the general population. *Am J Indust Med* 1986;9:143–152.

53. Ashcroft T, Heppleston AG. The optical and electron microscope determination of pulmonary asbestos fibre concentrations and its relation to the human pathological reaction. *J Clin Pathol* 1973;26:224–234.

54. Dodson R, Williams MG, O'Sullivan MF, et al. A comparison of the ferruginous body and uncoated fiber content in the lungs of former asbestos workers. *Am Rev Respir Dis* 1985;132:143–147.

55. *Report of the Royal Commission on Matters of Health and Safety Arising from the Use of Asbestos in Ontario.* Queen's Printer for Ontario, 1984.

56. Case BW, Sebastien P. Fibre levels in lung and correlation with air samples. In: Bignon J, Peto J, Saracci R, eds. *Non-occupational exposure to mineral fibres.* Lyon: IARC, 1989;207–219.

57. Case BW, Sebastien P, McDonald JC. Lung fiber analysis in accident victims: a biological assessment of general environmental exposure. *Arch Environ Health* 1988;43:178–179.

58. Davis JMG, Addision J, Bolton RE, Donaldson K, Jones AD, Smith T. The pathogenicity of long versus short fibre samples of amosite asbestos administered to rats by inhalation and intraperitoneal injection. *Br J Exp Pathol* 1986;67:415–430.

59. Stanton MF, Layard M, Tegeris A, et al. Relation of particle dimension to carcinogenicity in amphibole asbestos and other fibrous minerals. *JNCI* 1981;67:965–975.

60. Wagner JC, Chamberlin M, Brown RC, et al. Biological effects of tremolite. *Br J Cancer* 1982;45:352–360.

61. Dodson RF, Greenberg SD, Williams, MG, et al. Asbestos content in lungs of occupationally and nonoccupationally exposed individuals. *JAMA* 1984;252:68–71.

62. Roggli VL. Human disease consequences of fiber exposures—

a review of human lung pathology and fiber burden data. *Environ Health Perspect* 1990; in press.

63. Churg A, Warnock ML. Correlation of quantitative asbestos body counts and occupation in an urban population. *Arch Pathol Lab Med* 1977;101:629–634.

64. McDonald JC. Health implications of environmental exposure to asbestos. *Environ Health Perspect* 1985;62:328–329.

65. Hughes JM, Weill H. Asbestos exposure—quantitative assessment of risk. *Am Rev Respir Dis* 1986;133:5–13.

66. Cordier S, Lazar P, Brochard P, Bignon J, Ameille J, Proteau J. Epidemiologic investigation of respiratory effects related to environmental exposure to asbestos inside buildings. *Arch Environ Health* 1987;42:303–309.

67. Sebastien P, Plourde M, Robb R, et al. *Ambient air asbestos survey in Quebec mining towns. Part 2—Main study.* Environment Canada Report 5/AP/RQ-2E, 1986.

68. Siemiatycki J. Health effects on the general population (mortality in the general population in asbestos mining areas). *Proceedings of the World Symposium on Asbestos, Montreal, 1982.* Montreal: The Asbestos Institute, 1982;347–348.

69. Churg A. Lung asbestos content in long-term residents of a chrysotile mining town. *Am Rev Respir Dis* 1986;134:125–127.

70. Case BW, Sebastien P. Environmental and occupational exposures to chrysotile asbestos: a comparative microanalytic study. *Arch Environ Health* 1987;42:85–191.

71. Jones JSP, Roberts GH, Pooley FD, et al. The pathology and mineral content of lungs in cases of mesothelioma in the United Kingdom in 1976. In: Wagner JC, ed. *Biological effects of mineral fibres.* Lyon: IARC, 1980;187–200.

72. McDonald AD, McDonald JC, Pooley FD. Mineral fiber content of lung in mesothelial tumors in North America. *Ann Occup Hyg* 1982;26:417–422.

73. Wagner JC, Newhouse ML, Corrin B, Rossiter CER, Griffiths DM. Correlation between fibre content of the lung and disease in East London asbestos factory workers. *Br J Indust Med* 1988;45:305–308.

74. Rowlands N, Gibbs GW, McDonald AD. Asbestos fibers in the lungs of chrysotile miners and millers. A preliminary report. *Ann Occup Hyg* 1982;26:411–415.

75. Churg A. Chrysotile, tremolite, and malignant mesothelioma in man. *Chest* 1988;93:621–628.

76. Green FHY, Harley R, Vallyathan V, Dement J, Pooley F, Althouse R. Pulmonary fibrosis and asbestos exposure in chrysotile asbestos textile workers: preliminary results. *Accomplishments Oncol* 1986;1:59–68.

77. Pooley FD, Mitha R. Fiber types, concentrations, and characteristics found in lung tissues of chrysotile-exposed cases and controls. *Accomplishments Oncol* 1986;1:1–11.

78. Roggli VL. Pathology of human asbestosis: a critical review. In: Fenoglio-Preiser CM, ed. *Advances in pathology,* vol 2. New York: Yearbook Publishers, 1989;28–49.

79. Roggli VL. Scanning electron microscopic analysis of mineral fibers in human lungs. In: Ingram P, Shelburne JD, Roggli VL, eds. *Microprobe analysis in medicine.* New York: Hemisphere Press, 1989;97–110.

80. Whitwell F, Scott J, Grimshaw M. Relationship between occupations and asbestos-fibre conent of the lungs in patients with pleural mesothelioma, lung cancer, and other disease. *Thorax* 1977;32:377–386.

81. Churg A, Wiggs B. Fiber size and number in amphibole asbestos-associated mesothelioma. *Am J Pathol* 1984;115:437–452.

82. Roggli VL, McGavran MH, Subach J, et al. Pulmonary asbestos body counts and electron probe analysis of asbestos body cores in patients with mesothelioma. *Cancer* 1982;50:2423–2432.

83. Roggli VL, Pratt PC, Brody AR. Asbestos content of lung tissue in asbestos associated disease: a study of 110 cases. *Br J Indust Med* 1986;43:18–29.

84. Hughes J, Weill H. Asbestos related cancer in relation to x-ray evidence of pulmonary fibrosis. *Am Rev Respir Dis* 1989;137(Pt 2):A214.

85. Wagner JC, Berry G, Pooley FD. Mesotheliomas and asbestos type in asbestos textile workers: a study of lung contents. *Br Med J* 1982;285:603–606.

86. Berry G. Chrysotile and mesothelioma. *Accomplishments Oncol* 1986;1:123–131.

87. Gibbs AR, Jones JSP, Pooley FD, Griffiths DM, Wagner JC. Non-occupational malignant mesothelioma. In: Bignon J, Peto J, Saracci R, eds. *Non-occupational exposure to mineral fibres.* Lyon: IARC, 1989;219–228.

88. Peto J. The hygiene standard for chrysotile asbestos. *Lancet* 1978;1:484–488.

89. McConnochie K, Simonato L, Mavrides P, Chrisofides P, Pooley FD, Wagner JC. Mesothelioma in Cyprus: the role of tremolite. *Thorax* 1987;42:342–347.

90. Churg A. Asbestos fibre content of the lungs of chrysotile miners with and without asbestos airways disease. *Am Rev Respir Dis* 1983;127:470–473.

91. Churg A, Wright JL, DePaoli L, Wiggs B. Mineralogic correlates of fibrosis in chrysotile miners and millers. *Am Rev Respir Dis* 1989;139:891–896.

92. McDonald JC, Armstrong B, Case B, Doell D, McCaughey WTE, McDonald AD, Sebastien P. Mesothelioma and asbestos fiber type. Evidence from lung tissue analysis. *Cancer* 1989;63:1544–1547.

93. Pinkerton KE, Plopper CG, Mercer RR, et al. Airway branching patterns influence asbestos fiber location and the extent of tissue injury in the pulmonary parenchyma. *Lab Invest* 1986;55:688–695.

94. Sebastien P, Janson Z, Gaudichet A, et al. Asbestos retention in human respiratory tissues. Comparative measurements in lung parenchyma and in parietal pleura. In: Wagner JC, ed. *Biological effects of mineral fibers.* Lyon: IARC, 1980;237–246.

95. Churg A, Wiggs B. Accumulation of long asbestos in the peripheral upper lobe of patients with mesothelioma. *Am J Indust Med* 1987;9:143–152.

96. Adamson IYR, Bowden DH. Response of mouse lung to crocidolite asbestos. I. Minimal fibrotic reaction to short fibres. *J Pathol* 1987;152:99–107.

97. Adamson IYR, Bowden DH. Response of mouse lung to crocidolite asbestos. II. Pulmonary fibrosis after long fibres. *J Pathol* 1987;152:109–117.

98. Churg A, Wright JL. Fibre content of lung in amphibole- and chrysotile-induced mesothelioma. Implications for environmental exposure. In: Bignon J, Peto J, Saracci R, eds. *Non-occupational exposure to mineral fibres.* Lyon: IARC, 1989;314–318.

THE LUNG: Scientific Foundations
edited by R.G. Crystal, J.B. West et al.
Raven Press, Ltd., New York © 1991.

CHAPTER 7.3.5

Consequences of Chronic Inorganic Dust Exposure

William N. Rom and Ronald G. Crystal

Chronic exposure to high concentrations of airborne inorganic dusts can result in a form of interstitial lung disease referred to as a "pneumoconiosis" (1–9). Like other interstitial lung disorders, the pneumoconioses are chronic fibrotic disorders confined to the lower respiratory tract, primarily the alveolar walls (10–14). The three major classes of inorganic dusts that can cause interstitial lung disease are asbestos (the cause of "asbestosis"), silica ("silicosis"), and coal workers' "pneumoconiosis" (CWP) (1–9,11). In this chapter, we will use these three disorders as naturally occurring "models" to examine the mechanisms by which inherently innocuous materials—in this case, inorganic dusts—can cause human disease by subverting normal biologic processes to damage and scar normal tissues. We will focus only on the biologic processes that lead to interstitial lung disease. Details concerning the physical aspects of these dusts can be found in references 1–3 and 5–9. An overview of the clinical presentations of the interstitial lung disorders caused by inorganic dusts can be found in general tests and reviews (1–14).

Inorganic dusts are normal components of the ambient air, as a result of natural erosion and industrial use. Despite this, and despite the presence of inorganic dusts in the normal human lung (see Chapter 7.3.4), the pneumoconioses are not diseases of the general population but are, instead, confined to individuals chronically exposed to high concentrations of these dusts in the occupational setting. In this regard, it is clear from controlled epidemiologic studies that exposures to inorganic dusts must be high and for a long period of time for the exposure to pose a risk to the individual to develop interstitial lung disease (1–9,15). The reasons why nonoccupational exposures are not associated with disease are linked to many factors, dominated by the concepts of host defense and individual susceptibility.

With regard to host defense, the lung has many mechanisms to prevent dusts from reaching the alveoli. Further, if inorganic dusts do deposit on the alveolar surface, additional defenses include (a) removing dusts from the alveolar air spaces and the interstitium, (b) rendering dusts within the lung "impotent," and (c) repairing damage resulting from inflammatory processes, thereby preventing interstitial lung disease. An overview of some of these processes is presented below; for further details concerning lung defense see Chapters 3.1.2 (structure and function of cilia), 3.1.3 (synthesis and composition of mucus), 3.4.5 (alveolar macrophages), 7.1.2 (antiproteases), 7.2.2 and 7.2.3 (antioxidants), 7.3.1 (particle deposition), 7.3.2 (mucociliary clearance), 7.4.1 (integrated defense), and 7.6.2 (biologic consequences of environmental contaminants).

With regard to individual susceptibility, epidemiologic studies have demonstrated wide variations in the response of different individuals to similar exposures. The reasons for this variation are not known. It is generally assumed that the mechanisms underlying individual susceptibility are complex and rooted in the multitude of processes modulating host defense. Individual susceptibility is also undoubtly linked to genetic factors, although these also remain undefined at this time.

In the context of these considerations, in order to describe the biologic processes underlying the devel-

W. N. Rom: Division of Pulmonary and Critical Care Medicine, NYU Medical Center, New York, New York 10016.

R. G. Crystal: Pulmonary Branch, National Heart, Lung and Blood Institute, National Institutes of Health, Bethesda, Maryland 20892.

opment of the pneumoconioses, we will take as a starting point that the individuals (or experimental animals) being discussed are "susceptible," and that the burden of inorganic dusts to which they have been exposed has overwhelmed the pulmonary host defenses; that is, for the purposes of discussion of the processes that cause disease, we will assume that disease will occur.

SOURCES OF CHRONIC PARTICULATE EXPOSURE IN THE WORKPLACE

The source of exposure for the pneumoconioses is mostly >20-year workplace exposure (1–9,15). The predominant exposures to asbestos are associated with the construction trades. Most cases of asbestosis occur in three groups: insulators, sheet-metal workers, and boilermakers. Other trades with potentially significant exposures include plumbers, engineers, plasterers, carpenters, general laborers, and electricians. Factory workers exposed to asbestos include those involved in the manufacture of textiles, gaskets and friction products, roofing materials, wallboard, and asbestos–cement pipes. Shipyard workers are exposed in confined spaces, and "rip-out" of insulation materials from older ships presents an exposure situation.

Silica exposure occurs in underground mines and attendant crushing operations, in foundries where sand is used in making molds, in refractories making bricks, pottery, or enamel such as for bathroom accessories, sand-blasting pipes, steel structures, or buildings, in glass-making, and in the production or use of silica flour materials. Calcined diatomaceous earth contains a high percentage of crystalline silica and is used to produce dental materials. Granite quarry workers have some exposure, but the incidence of silicosis among this population is very low as a result of stringent dust controls.

CWP occurs in coal miners working in underground mines—with greatest risk for those working at the face, including continuous miner–operators, drillers, shuttle-car operators, and roof bolters. The latter are also exposed to silica (as are underground railroad operators) when sand is applied to the tracks for traction. Long-wall operations produce the greatest amount of dust. Anthracite miners have increased exposures due to the narrowness and tilting of the seams exposing the workers to intervening hard rock. Surface workers have minimal dust exposure, although surface drillers are exposed to silica-containing hard rock and may have sufficient exposures to develop silicosis.

DEPOSITION, RETENTION, AND CLEARANCE OF INORGANIC DUSTS

For inorganic dusts to cause interstitial lung disease, the dusts have to reach the lower respiratory tract. The anatomy of the lung conspires to prevent this (see Chapter 7.3.1). Particles deposit in the tracheobronchial tree by gravitational sedimentation, impaction, Brownian diffusion, and interception. Sedimentation and impaction are the most important deposition mechanisms for particles larger than 1 μm (16,17). In large airways, deep-breathing enhances sedimentation whereas rapid, shallow breathing increases impaction. Impaction concentrates particles at the bifurcations of airways. Deposition of particles through Brownian diffusion becomes significant for particles with aerodynamic diameters less than 1 μm. Deposition by diffusion tends to be uniform; it is greatest in the alveoli, where velocities are very low, giving particles time to diffuse to the surrounding surfaces. Fibers align themselves with air streamlines, effectively resisting impaction and sedimentation until the periphery of the lung, where air turbulence may flip them end-for-end, resulting in interception in the walls of the gas-exchange structures. There is greater alveolar deposition with mouth breathing, approaching 50% for 3-μm particles, whereas nose breathing results in alveolar deposition of 25% for 2.5-μm particles and falls to zero for 8-μm particles. Cigarette smoking and bronchitis produce proximal shift in the deposition pattern (18).

If the particles bypass the defenses established by virtue of the lung anatomy and impact on the airway epithelial surface, they are generally cleared by the "mucociliary escalator," a mechanism by which ciliated epithelial cells propel the fluid lining the airways toward the pharynx (see Chapter 7.3.2). The fluid lining the airways includes mucins produced by submucosal glands and goblet cells (Chapter 3.1.3). Combining with water, electrolytes, and a variety of molecules diffusing from plasma and secreted from epithelial cells, the fluid lining the airways separates into two phases under the continuous beating of cilia: a low-viscosity sol underlying a discontinuous viscoelastic gel phase in which the long-chain mucopolysaccharide molecules are concentrated. The submucosal glands are under the influence of the autonomic nervous system and can be influenced by drugs (e.g., isoproterenol increases secretion, atropine decreases secretion) and irritants (cigarette smoke increases secretion). Metabolites (acetaldehyde, a metabolite of ethanol) inhibit ciliary function. Mucociliary clearance varies among individuals, ranging from 2 to 20 hr (16).

Particles that reach the alveolar epithelial surface are cleared mostly by alveolar macrophages that phagocytize the particle, and subsequently move upward on the epithelial surface (see Chapter 3.4.5). Alveolar epithelial clearance has two phases: a fast phase averaging about 3 weeks and a slow phase lasting approximately 1 year (16). Thus, many particles reaching the alveolar epithelial surface are retained for some time, particularly particles that are ≤1 μm. Particles not cleared by movement upward on the epithelial surface may be cleared by direct penetration into the interstitium and then by the lymphatics.

There are differences in the function of these defense systems depending on the clinical state of the individual, on the specific exposure, and on environmental factors. For example, individuals with chronic obstructive lung disease may lose the fast phase and have a prolonged slow phase of clearance (16). In the pneumoconioses, coal miners with advanced disease retain more quartz than do those without disease or with mild disease, despite similar exposure patterns (19). In humans with chronic exposure to asbestos, there is a greater asbestos burden among those with airway abnormalities than among those with normal airways, and there are far more fibers in lung tissue in those individuals who develop asbestosis (20,21) (see Chapter 7.3.4). In rats, asbestos fibers tend to locate in longer airways and in areas of tissue injury (22). Interestingly, exposure of rats to ozone for 6 weeks followed by asbestos results in decreased clearance of the fibers (23). With regard to specific types of asbestos fibers, intratracheal inoculation of a mixture of fiber types (chrysotile and amosite) demonstrates (in guinea pigs) a differential clearance of fiber types, with chrysotile clearing faster (24). In rats exposed to chrysotile, amosite, or crocidolite, there was less retention of chrysotile than of amphiboles, and the clearance of the amphiboles appeared to be dose-related (25). In rats, about 25% of respirable fibers deposit in the lungs, and there is a tendency for longer fibers of both chrysotile and amphibole to be retained within lung tissue, whereas longitudinal splitting with progressive decrease in mean fiber diameter occurs primarily with chrysotile (26).

THE TWILIGHT ZONE: THE TRANSITION FROM DEFENSE TO DISEASE

In conceptualizing the pathogenesis of the pneumoconioses, two general facts are evident: (i) The lung has many mechanisms by which it is protected from inhaled inorganic particulates, and (ii) in some circumstances, given a sufficient burden, the chronic inhalation of particulates results in interstitial lung disease. From all available evidence, the pathogenesis of the interstitial disease involves normal biologic processes, albeit exaggerated. The fundamental concept is similar to that for all interstitial lung diseases: The damage and subsequent scarring are caused by chronic inflammation in the lung parenchyma (10–14). In the context of the pneumoconioses, the inorganic particulates in the lung initiate a chronic inflammatory process in which the inflammatory cells are activated, thereby releasing mediators that damage the architecture and

promote the accumulation of mesenchymal cells and their connective tissue products (see below).

What is not well understood is what modulates the transition whereby the host defense systems fail to protect against inhaled particulates and whereby normal biologic processes are subverted to injure the lung and promote the development of fibrosis (Fig. 1). At least part of the transition must be associated with the failure of the host defense system to keep up with the chronic burden of particulates impinging on the alveolar epithelial surface. Consistent with this concept is the quantitative evidence that individuals with chronic inorganic dust exposure who develop interstitial lung disease have far more particulates in the lung parenchyma than do normal individuals or individuals with exposure but who do not develop disease (see Chapter 7.3.4).

Accumulation of particulates is only part of the story, however, since the inorganic dusts themselves cause little damage. The damage and the ensuing fibrosis are caused by the inflammation initiated by the accumulated particulates. Termed the "alveolitis" because of its location in the alveolar structures, the inflammation of asbestosis, silicosis, and CWP is dominated by alveolar macrophages, with some lymphocytes and relatively few neutrophils and eosinophils (see ref. 27 for a general review). Thus, the alveolar macrophage plays not only a central role in the clearance of inorganic particulates, but also a central role in the pathogenesis of the interstitial disorders caused by these dusts. It is that transition (i.e., from the alveolar macrophage as the defender to the alveolar macrophage as the offender) that is not understood and remains as the "twilight zone" in understanding the pathogenesis of the pneumoconioses (see Chapter 3.4.5 for a discussion of the alveolar macrophage as a "two-edged-sword" in defending the normal lung).

From what is known, it appears that the alveolar macrophages are responding in a normal fashion to activation stimuli. Thus, the "transition" from defense to disease may simply be a matter of numbers: If the host defense systems are sufficiently overwhelmed by chronic exposure to sufficient amounts of inorganic particulates, if sufficient numbers of alveolar macrophages are activated, and if the normal repair processes cannot keep up with the ensuing damage, the consequences are inevitable—that is, disease.

ROLE OF ALVEOLAR MACROPHAGES IN THE PATHOGENESIS OF THE PNEUMOCONIOSES

Evidence that alveolar macrophages play a central role in the pathogenesis of the pneumoconioses comes from *in vitro* studies with alveolar macrophages recovered

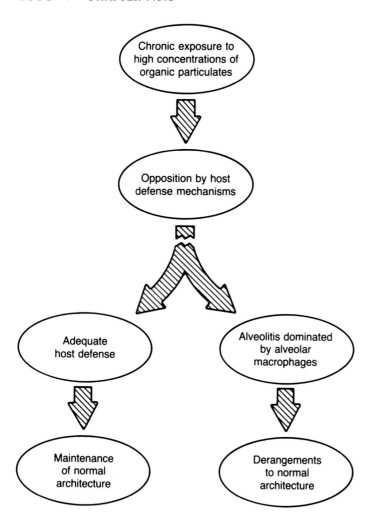

FIG. 1. Consequences of chronic exposure to high concentrations of inorganic particulates. In most circumstances, the host defense systems are adequate to deal with the chronic particulate burden and thus the normal architecture is maintained. In some individuals, however, for reasons that are not completely understood, the host defense system is overwhelmed, and an alveolitis dominated by alveolar macrophages develops, leading to derangements of the normal architecture.

from normal experimental animals and humans, *in vivo* exposures of experimental animals to inorganic particulates, and evaluation of alveolar macrophages of individuals exposed to airborne inorganic dusts in occupational settings.

Phagocytosis of Inorganic Particulates

Alveolar macrophages are capable of ingesting inorganic particulates in a nonspecific manner without the aid of specific ligands (see Chapters 3.4.5 and 3.4.6). *In vitro*, alveolar macrophages from humans and experimental animals readily ingest asbestos, silica, and coal particles (see ref. 28 for review). Morphologic evaluation of alveolar macrophages of experimental animals exposed to inorganic dusts demonstrates the presence of intracellular particulates, suggesting that this process occurs *in vivo* (Fig. 2) (29–43). For example, in rats inhaling silica, two-thirds of the alveolar macrophages contained silica 24 hr following exposure (44). In rats exposed to asbestos, the fibers preferentially deposited at alveolar duct bifurcations, the same

locations where alveolar macrophages are observed to accumulate (43). In rats, asbestos fibers penetrate type I alveolar epithelial cells and are phagocytosed by interstitial macrophages. Up to 3 months following exposure, practically all of the macrophages contain fibers, mostly uncoated, but by 12 months most of the fibers were located in the interstitium (45). In experimental animals, the initial macrophage response to particulate deposition in the alveoli includes a mobilization of phagocytic cells to preferential sites of deposition, an increase in the number of these cells, and an activation process concomitant with phagocytosis. For example, in rats, there was an 88% increase in the number of alveolar macrophages 3 months after chrysotile exposure (42).

Humans exposed to inorganic dusts in occupational settings have increased numbers of alveolar macrophages in the lung. Furthermore, they show evidence of intracellular dusts in alveolar macrophages recovered by bronchoalveolar lavage or in those evaluated in biopsy or autopsy specimens (see ref. 28 for review). The mechanisms responsible for the increased numbers of macrophages in the alveoli in response to

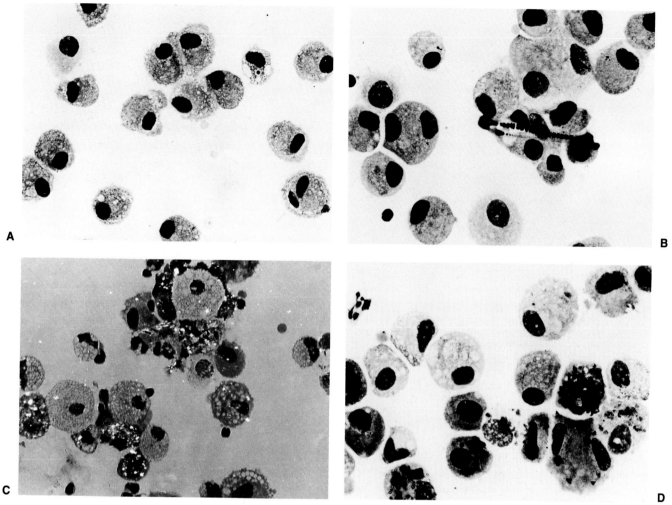

FIG. 2. *In vivo* phagocytosis of particulates by alveolar macrophages of individuals with chronic exposure to inorganic dusts. **A:** Alveolar macrophages from a normal individual. **B:** Alveolar macrophages of an individual with chronic exposure to asbestos demonstrating a group of macrophages surrounding two asbestos bodies (dark-staining, long, beaded structures with clubbed ends). **C:** Polarized light evaluation of alveolar macrophages of an individual with chronic silica exposure showing intracytoplasmic birefringent particles. **D:** Alveolar macrophages from a coal worker demonstrating variously shaped intracytoplasmic particles. All specimens were from nonsmokers. All panels are cytocentrifuge preparations stained with Wright–Giemsa stain, ×400. (From ref. 28.)

particulates are not fully understood, but they likely result from a combination of recruitment of blood monocytes and an increased rate of replication of macrophages *in situ* (46). Morphologic evaluation of these alveolar macrophages demonstrated particulates mostly within phagolysosomes, and occasionally free in the cytoplasm (28) (Figs. 2 and 3). For some inorganic particulates, such as asbestos, there is modification of the fibers within the alveolar macrophage. For example, chrysotile breaks down into smaller fragments (see Chapter 7.3.4). Large asbestos fibers may be coated to form "asbestos bodies" (1,5,8,9,30). The

process of asbestos body formation within alveolar macrophages has been observed in *in vivo* studies in hamsters. Within 2 weeks after exposure, small collections of iron are noted adjacent to phagocytosed asbestos fibers (47). The addition of glycoproteins to these particles leads to the typical beaded appearance of asbestos bodies with clubbed ends.

Activation of Alveolar Macrophages

In the process of phagocytosis of inorganic particulates *in vitro*, alveolar macrophages become activated (see

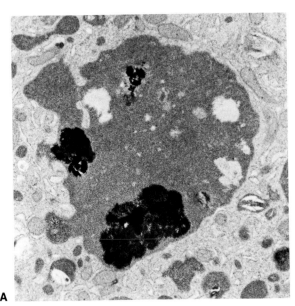 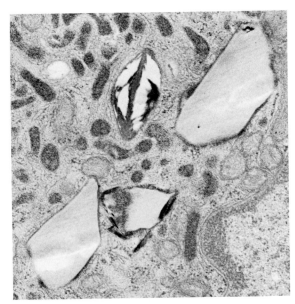

FIG. 3. Inorganic particulates in phagolysosomes of alveolar macrophages of individuals with chronic exposure to inorganic dusts. **A:** Electron-dense, irregularly shaped particles in phagolysosomes of alveolar macrophages of an individual exposed to asbestos (transmission electron micrograph, ×17,000). **B:** Rectangular particles within phagolysosomes of an alveolar macrophage of a coal miner. Transmission electron micrograph, ×30,000. The individuals were nonsmokers. (From ref. 28.)

refs. 2,5–8,15, and 27–31 for review). Two lines of evidence suggest that this process occurs in the lung in association with chronic exposure to high concentrations of airborne particulates. First, in addition to their content of particles, alveolar macrophages from dust-exposed experimental animals and humans show morphologic evidence of activation (Figs. 4–7) (28). Second, alveolar macrophages recovered from the lungs of dust-exposed animals and humans spontaneously release an array of mediators typically produced by activated alveolar macrophages.

With regard to the morphologic evidence, alveolar macrophages of dust-exposed individuals have a higher frequency of multinucleation: Many macrophages contain two to four nuclei, and occasional giant cells contain as many as 20 (Fig. 4). Furthermore, alveolar macrophages display rough surfaces with prominent filopodia, blebs, and rufflings and have increased numbers of intracytoplasmic organelles (Figs. 5–7). Studies of alveolar macrophages of experimental animals exposed to inorganic dusts also show morphologic evidence of activation (28,31,32,34,48,49).

With regard to the release of mediators, evaluation of alveolar macrophages from individuals chronically exposed to airborne inorganic dusts in industrial settings and from experimental animal exposures demonstrates the exaggerated release of mediators capable of injuring the lung parenchyma and promoting the growth of mesenchymal cells.

Mediators That Can Cause Injury

Alveolar macrophages recovered from nonsmoking individuals exposed to airborne asbestos, silica, or coal are releasing two- to threefold more oxygen radicals than are normal macrophages, including superoxide anion and hydrogen peroxide (27). This observation is important because the lung parenchyma, particularly the epithelium and endothelium, are susceptible to injury by these radicals (8,15,50; see Chapters 7.2.1 and 7.2.4). Furthermore, alveolar macrophages recovered from a sheep model of asbestosis and from individuals with asbestosis release plasminogen activator, a protease that converts plasminogen to plasmin, and may play a role in injury to the parenchyma and in the development of intra-alveolar fibrosis on a fibrin substrate (51; see Chapters 3.3.4 and 7.1.1).

Mediators That Promote Mesenchymal Cell Growth

In addition to injuring the parenchyma, alveolar macrophages are capable of promoting the development of fibrosis by releasing polypeptide growth factors that stimulate mesenchymal cells to proliferate. In humans, these mediators include platelet-derived growth factor (PDGF) (W. Rom and R. Crystal, *unpublished observations*; 52,53), fibronectin (28,54), and the alveolar macrophage form of insulin-like growth factor 1 (28,55,56; see Chapters 2.9, 3.4.5, and 7.8.1 for details

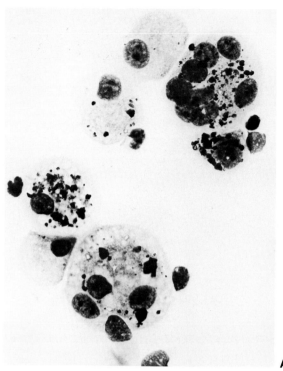

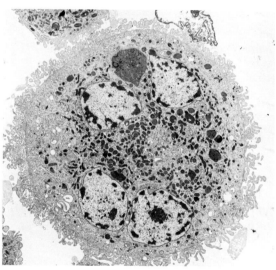

FIG. 4. Examples of multinucleated alveolar macrophages in individuals with chronic exposure to inorganic dusts. **A:** Multinucleated alveolar macrophages from a coal miner. Two of the macrophages have four or more nuclei and numerous intracytoplasmic particles. Wright–Giesma stain, ×630. **B:** Multinucleated alveolar macrophage from an asbestos-exposed individual. The cell is large (20 μm), has four nuclei, and has an increase in lysosomes and phagolysosomes compared to those in normal alveolar macrophages. Transmission electron micrograph, ×4400. The individuals were nonsmokers. (From ref. 28.)

concerning these mediators). Consistent with these observations, immunohistologic staining of lung specimens of individuals with asbestosis, silicosis, and CWP demonstrates intense staining for fibronectin in regions of fibrosis (57). Fibronectin levels in epithelial lining fluid are increased in individuals with these disorders (58,59). The evidence from experimental animals is consistent with the human data, but the mediators are not as well defined. For example, alveolar macrophages lavaged from rats or sheep following asbestos installation spontaneously release growth factors for fibroblasts as early as 1 week after exposure and persisting for many months thereafter (32). It is likely that at least some of these mediators are the same as those observed in humans, since fibronectin is increased in epithelial lining fluid in asbestos-exposed sheep and a PDGF-like molecule is released by rat alveolar macrophages exposed to asbestos (59,60).

Other Mediators

In vitro incubation of inorganic particulates with alveolar macrophages demonstrates that in the process of phagocytizing these materials, the alveolar macrophages are activated to release a variety of molecules associated with activated macrophages (see Chapter 3.4.5). It is not known whether this occurs with *in vivo* exposures. However, in view of the broad armamentarium of mediators available to the alveolar macrophage, as well as the general nonspecificity of the phagocytic process in activating macrophages, it is likely that a variety of mediators are being chronically released by alveolar macrophages of individuals with a high burden of particulates in the lung parenchyma.

Is the Alveolar Macrophage Solely Responsible for the Injury and Fibrosis?

The paradigm of phagocytosis of particulates activating the alveolar macrophage to release mediators that cause injury and fibrosis is logical, and there is little doubt that this dominates the pathogenesis of the pneumoconioses. However, there are observations to suggest it does not explain all aspects of the pathogenesis of these disorders. First, chronic exposure of individuals to dusts of tin, silver, iron, or barium is associated with (a) localized accumulations of alveolar macrophages around the particulates, and (b) although there are rounded opacities on the chest x-ray, there is no significant decrement in lung function despite the fact that alveolar macrophages phagocytize these materials (2); that is, the process of phagocytosis per se may not be sufficient to activate the alveolar macrophage in such a manner as to release the full range of mediators necessary to cause injury and mesenchymal cell pro-

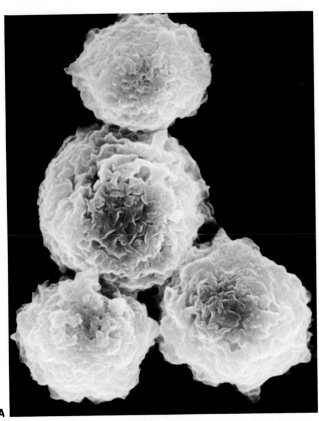 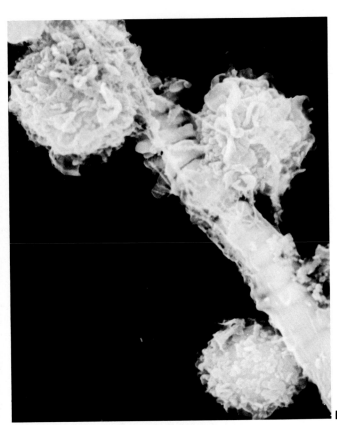

FIG. 5. Scanning electron micrographs showing the difference in surface features of normal alveolar macrophages compared to those of alveolar macrophages activated by attempting to phagocytize an asbestos fiber. **A:** Macrophage from a normal, unexposed individual demonstrates an undulating, smooth surface. ×3000. **B:** Alveolar macrophages of an asbestos-exposed individual attempting to encircle a beaded, long asbestos body. The macrophages have put out long, thin, thread-like filopodia, and the macrophage surfaces show ruffling and blebs. ×3000. The individuals were nonsmokers. (From ref. 28.)

liferation sufficient to cause disease. Second, alveolar macrophages of individuals exposed to inorganic dusts such as asbestos, silican, and coal release exaggerated amounts of fibronectin, a glycoprotein believed to play an important role in the remodeling of the lung parenchyma in the interstitial lung disorders (27,54; see Chapter 3.3.4). However, *in vitro* exposure of human alveolar macrophages to inorganic dusts fails to increase fibronectin release, suggesting that additional mechanisms may be involved (W. Rom, S. Rennard, P. Bitterman, and R. Crystal, *unpublished observations*). Finally, the patterns of injury and fibrosis among the common pneumoconioses are different. Whereas asbestosis shows a pattern typical for interstitial lung disease such as idiopathic pulmonary fibrosis, silicosis tends to be associated with a nodular process; CWP is often a mixture of interstitial lung disease and destructive lung disease (1–14). While some of these differences are likely associated with differences in patterns of deposition of the particulates within the parenchyma and may be modified by ad-

ditional exposures such as cigarette smoking, it is possible that other inflammatory cells participating in the alveolitis play different roles in association with different exposures.

Neutrophils

Some bronchoalveolar lavage studies of inorganic dust-exposed individuals have demonstrated an increase in the number of neutrophils compared to that in normals (27,61–63). In part, this may be due to the inclusion of cigarette smokers in some study groups, but it is also observed (to a small degree) in nonsmoking individuals with asbestosis, silicosis, or CWP (27). An increase in neutrophils has been noted in French, British, and Australian asbestos workers (61,62,64). In Spanish asbestos cement workers, most of whom had a history of smoking, many with asbestosis had a significant increase in neutrophils (63). Since the activated alveolar macrophage is capable of

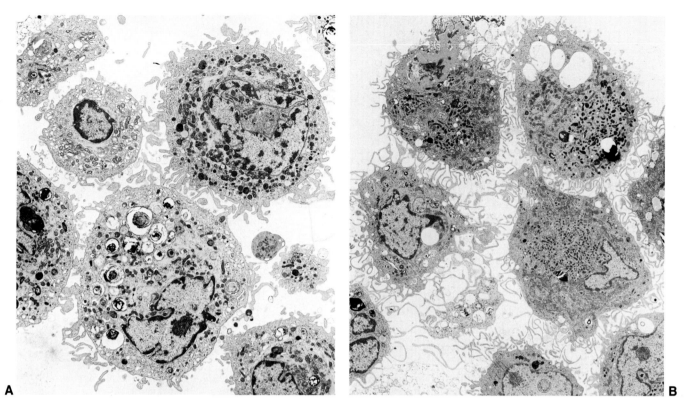

A   B

FIG. 6. Comparison of surface features of alveolar macrophages of a normal individual to those of an individual with chronic silica exposure. **A:** Alveolar macrophage of a normal, unexposed individual showing pseudopodia and few filopodia. **B:** Alveolar macrophage of a silica-exposed individual showing marked filopodia. Both panels are from nonsmokers; both are transmission electron micrographs, ×4000. The individuals were nonsmokers. (From ref. 28.)

releasing chemotactic factors for neutrophils (see Chapters 2.10 and 3.4.5), it is likely that the process of phagocytosis of inorganic dusts is associated with the release of such mediators (65,66). Consistent with this, alveolar macrophages from individuals with asbestosis are releasing increased amounts of leukotriene B4, a chemoattractant for neutrophils (66). While the role of neutrophils in the pathogenesis of the pneumoconioses is unknown, their presence in low (but increased) numbers in the lung parenchyma in association with chronic particulate exposure suggests that neutrophils may modulate at least some of the injury that is observed (see Chapters 3.4.7 and 7.7.1).

Lymphocytes

There is no evidence that the pneumoconioses are immune-mediated disorders; nevertheless, immune-related processes are observed in association with these disorders. For example, up to 20% of individuals with the pneumoconioses have increased serum levels of immunoglobulins, antinuclear antibodies, or immune complexes (1,9,67,68). Furthermore, increased amounts of lymphocytes and lymphocyte products are occasionally observed in the lung of humans and experimental animals exposed to inorganic dusts (27,69–73). For example, bronchoalveolar lavage studies demonstrate that some individuals with asbestos exposure have increased numbers of lymphocytes in epithelial lining fluid (27,69,70,73). In general, there appears to be no skewing in the relative proportions of the major lymphocyte subtypes observed (69,70). Lavage studies of granite workers with silica exposure but without silicosis revealed increased lymphocytes and immunoglobulins in epithelial lining fluid (71). A rat silicosis model demonstrated an increase in the numbers of lymphocytes in lavage fluid, with a predominance of helper T-lymphocytes (72). Mixed dust pneumoconioses with coal mine dust exposure revealed an increase in suppressor/cytotoxic T-cells (70). In asbestos-exposed individuals with increased lymphocytes in lavage fluid, increased amounts of interferon-γ were released by the cells recovered by bronchoalveolar lavage (73). Other animal models of asbestos exposure have documented apparent B-cell hyperactivity and increases in serum immunoglobulins (74). It is difficult to put these observations together in a cohesive pic-

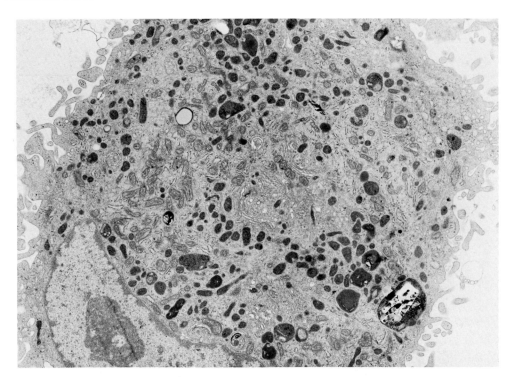

FIG. 7. Demonstration of the striking increase in intracytoplasmic organelles observed in alveolar macrophages of individuals with chronic particulate exposure. Shown is a transmission electron micrograph of an alveolar macrophage of a nonsmoking coal miner demonstrating an increase in the numbers of lysosomes, mitochondria, and components of endoplasmic reticulum compared to those of a normal alveolar macrophage. ×9300. (From ref. 28.)

ture, but at least for now they are considered to be epiphenomena not directly related to the pathogenesis of the pneumoconioses.

DEFENSE AND REPAIR IN RESPONSE TO INFLAMMATORY MEDIATORS

The fact that the alveolar macrophages (and possibly other inflammatory cells) are activated by particulates and releasing mediators with the capacity to injure the lung parenchyma does not necessarily mean that injury is inevitable, since the lower respiratory tract is protected by defensive molecules, particularly antioxidants and antiproteases (see Chapters 7.1.2, 7.2.2, and 7.2.3). Similarly, the presence of an increased burden of polypeptide growth factors is not always followed by proliferation of mesenchymal cells and fibrosis, since there are inhibitory molecules [such as prostaglandin E (PGE)] that suppress the response of mesenchymal cells to exogenous growth signals (see Chapters 3.4.5 and 7.8.1). Furthermore, even if there is injury to the parenchyma, the remaining parenchymal cells in the local milieu have the capacity to renew themselves and thus repair the injury. An increase in the amounts of mesenchymal cells and their collagenous products can also be balanced, at least in part,

by proteolytic enzymes such as collagenases (see Chapter 7.1.1). These concepts of defense and repair, while not completely defined with regard to the response of the lung to chronic particulate exposure, likely play an important role in the differential response of individuals to the same exposure.

CHRONICITY, RATE OF PROGRESSION, AND THERAPY

Knowledge of the pathogenesis of the pneumoconioses helps to explain why the majority of cases are chronic but relatively mild and only slowly progressive. Furthermore, it helps to explain why these disorders are not treated with conventional anti-inflammatory drugs, yet it opens the possibility of new approaches to therapy.

Chronicity

Since the inflammation is initiated by the burden of particulates in the lung if the particulates are not cleared, it follows that the lung must contend with a population of activated macrophages as the macrophages encounter and phagocytize the dusts. In this regard, typical cases of asbestosis, silicosis, and CWP are chronic, with an alveolar macrophage-dominated alveolitis that is rarely suppressed spontaneously.

Rate of Progression

Although occasional cases of the pneumoconioses are observed that have a relatively rapid course, progression is slow for the vast majority of patients seen today; in some individuals the clinical disorder stabilizes, despite the continued alveolitis. This observation is consistent with the knowledge that the alveolitis of the pneumoconioses is alveolar macrophage-dominated. Although the alveolar macrophage has many mediators available to it, overall the activated alveolar macrophage is far less damaging to the lung parenchyma than is the neutrophil (see Chapters 3.4.5, 3.4.7, and 7.7.1). Thus, in contrast to a disease such as idiopathic pulmonary fibrosis, in which neutrophils are an important part of the alveolitis and progression is relatively rapid, the pneumoconioses are much slower; that is, an alveolar macrophage-dominated alveolitis causes less damage to the parenchyma than does an alveolitis that includes a significant proportion of neutrophils (1–14).

Therapy

Conventionally, the fibrotic forms of interstitial lung disease are treated with glucocorticoids (10–14). Although there has never been a controlled trial to evaluate anti-inflammatory drugs in the pneumoconioses, these disorders are generally regarded to be untreatable, despite the fact that the derangement of the pulmonary architecture results from chronic inflammation. With an understanding of the pathogenesis of these disorders as inflammation initiated by the burden of particulates in the lower respiratory tract, it is unlikely that the anti-inflammatory drugs available today (such as glucocorticoids) would be capable of suppressing the activation of the alveolar macrophages if the burden remains chronic. However, it may be possible to protect against the mediators released by the activated macrophages. In this regard, local administration of antioxidants may provide a protective screen against damage mediated by the activated alveolar macrophage (75). With regard to the fibrosis, recent studies have demonstrated that it is possible to augment PGE levels in lower respiratory tract epithelial lining fluid by aerosolization of PGE; that is, it may be possible to capitalize on the antiproliferative capacity of this molecule to prevent mesenchymal cells from responding to alveolar-macrophage-released growth signals (76).

REFERENCES

1. Selikoff IJ, Lee DHK. *Asbestos and disease*. New York: Academic Press, 1978.
2. Morgan WKC, Seaton A. *Occupational lung disease*, 2nd ed. Philadelphia: WB Saunders, 1984.
3. Selikoff IJ, Key MM, Lee DHK. Coal workers' pneumoconiosis. *Ann NY Acad Sci* 1972;200:1–855.
4. Selikoff IJ, Hammond EC, eds. Health hazards of asbestos exposure. *Ann NY Acad Sci* 1979;330:1–811.
5. Rom WN. Asbestos and related fibers. In: Rom WN, ed. *Environmental and occupational medicine*. Boston: Little, Brown & Co., 1983;157–182.
6. Jones RN. Silicosis. In: Rom WN, ed. *Environmental and occupational medicine*. Boston: Little, Brown & Co., 1983;197–206.
7. Merchant JA, Reger RB. Coalworkers' respiratory disease. In: Rom WN, ed. *Environmental and occupational medicine*. Boston: Little, Brown & Co., 1983.
8. Mossman BT, Gee JBL. Asbestos-related diseases. *N Engl J Med* 1989;320:1721–1730.
9. Parkes WR. *Occupational lung disorders*. London: Butterworth, 1982.
10. Crystal RG, Gadek JE, Ferrans VJ, Fulmer JD, Line BR, Hunninghake GW. Interstitial lung disease: current concepts of pathogenesis, staging, and therapy. *Am J Med* 1981;70:542–568.
11. Davis WB, Crystal RG. Chronic interstitial lung disease. In: Simmons D, ed. *Current pulmonology*, vol V. New York: Wiley, 1984;347–473.
12. Crystal RG, Bitterman PB, Rennard SI, Hance A, Keogh BA. Interstitial lung disease of unknown cause: disorders characterized by chronic inflammation of the lower respiratory tract. *N Engl J Med* 1984;310:154–166, 235–244.
13. Crystal RG. Interstitial lung disorders. In: Braunwald G, Isselbacher KJ, Petersdorf RG, Wilson JD, Martin JB, Fauci AS, eds. *Harrison's principles of internal medicine*, 11th ed. McGraw–Hill, 1987;1095–1102.
14. Crystal RG. Interstitial lung disease. In: Wyngaarden JB, Smith LH Jr, eds. *Cecil textbook of medicine*, 18th ed. Philadelphia, WB Saunders, 1988;421–435.
15. Mossman BT, Bignon J, Corn M, Seaton A, Gee JBL. Asbestos: scientific developments and implications for public policy. *Science* 1990;247:294–301.
16. Bohning DE. Particle deposition and pulmonary defense mechanisms. In: Rom WN, ed. *Environmental and occupational medicine*. Boston: Little, Brown & Co., 1983;85–98.
17. Brain JD, Valberg PA. Deposition of aerosol in the respiratory tract. *Am Rev Respir Dis* 1979;120:1325–1366.
18. Lippman M, Yeates DB, Albert RE. Deposition, retention, and clearance of inhaled particles. *Br J Indust Med* 1980;37:337–362.
19. Davis JMG, Ottery J, LeRonx A. The effect of quartz and other non-coal dusts in coalworkers' pneumoconiosis. Part II: Lung autopsy study. In: Walton WH, ed. *Inhaled particles. IV*. Oxford: Pergamon Press, 1977;691–702.
20. Churg A. Asbestos fiber content of the lungs in patients with and without asbestos airways disease. *Am Rev Respir Dis* 1983;127:470–473.
21. Churg A. Fiber counting and analysis in the diagnosis of asbestos-related disease. *Hum Pathol* 1982;13:381–392.
22. Pinkerton KE, Plopper CG, Mercer RR, et al. Airway branching patterns influence asbestos fiber location and the extent of tissue injury in the pulmonary parenchyma. *Lab Invest* 1986;55:688–695.
23. Pinkerton KE, Brody AR, Miller FJ, Crapo JD. Exposure to low levels of ozone results in enhanced pulmonary retention of inhaled asbestos fibers. *Am Rev Respir Dis* 1989;140:1075–1081.
24. Churg A, Wright JL, Gilks B, Depaoli L. Rapid short-term clearance of chrysotile compared with amosite asbestos in the guinea pig. *Am Rev Respir Dis* 1989;139:885–890.
25. Middleton AP, Beckett ST, Davis JMG. A study of the short-term retention and clearance of inhaled asbestos by rats, using UICC standard reference samples. In: Walton WH, ed. *Inhaled particles. IV*. Oxford: Pergamon Press, 1977;247–258.
26. Roggli VL, George MH, Brody AR. Clearance and dimensional changes of crocidolite asbestos fibers isolated from lungs of rats following short-term exposure. *Environ Res* 1987;42:94–105.
27. Rom WN, Bitterman PB, Rennard SI, Cantin A, Crystal RG.

Characterization of the lower respiratory tract inflammation of nonsmoking individuals with interstitial lung disease associated with chronic inhalation of inorganic dusts. *Am Rev Respir Dis* 1987;136:1429–1434.

28. Takemura T, Rom WN, Ferrans VJ, Crystal RG. Morphological characterization of alveolar macrophages from individuals with occupational exposure to inorganic particles. *Am Rev Respir Dis* 1989;140:1674–1685.

29. Ziskind M, Jones RN, Weill H. Silicosis. *Am Rev Respir Dis* 1976;113:643–665.

30. Craighead JE, Mossman BT. The pathogenesis of asbestos-associated diseases. *N Engl J Med* 1982;306:1446–1455.

31. Miller K. The effects of asbestos on macrophages. *CRC Crit Rev Toxicol* 1978;5:319–354.

32. Lemaire I, Rola-Pleszczynski M, Begin R. Asbestos exposure enhances this release of fibroblast growth factor by sheep alveolar macrophages. *J Reticuloendothel Soc* 1983;33:275–285.

33. Tetley TD, Hext PM, Richards RJ, McDermott M. Chrysotile-induced asbestosis: changes in the free cell population, pulmonary surfactant and whole lung tissue of rats. *Br J Exp Pathol* 1976;57:505–514.

34. Miller K, Kagan E. The *in vivo* effects of quartz on alveolar macrophage membrane topography and on the characteristics of the intrapulmonary cell population. *J Reticuloendothel Soc* 1977;21:307–316.

35. Dodson RF, Williams MG Jr, Hurst GA. Early response of free airway cells to "Amosite"; a correlated study using electron microscopy and energy dispersive X-ray analysis. *Lung* 1980;157:143–154.

36. Kagan E, Oghiso Y, Hartmann D-P. The effects of chrysotile and crocidolite asbestos on the lower respiratory tract: analysis of bronchoalveolar lavage constituents. *Environ Res* 1983;32:382–397.

37. Lemaire I. Characterization of the bronchoalveolar cellular response in experimental asbestosis. Different reactions depending on the fibrogenic potential. *Am Rev Respir Dis* 1985;131:144–149.

38. Schoenberger CI, Hunninghake GW, Kawanami O, Ferrans VJ, Crystal RG. Role of alveolar macrophages in asbestos: modulation of neutrophil migration to the lung following acute asbestos exposure. *Thorax* 1982;37:803–809.

39. Begin R, Rola-Pleszczynski M, Masse S, Lemaire I, Sirois P, Boctor M, Nadeau D, Bureau MA. Asbestos-induced lung injury in the sheep model: the initial alveolitis. *Environ Res* 1983;30:195–210.

40. Bozelka BE, Sestini P, Gaumer HR, Hammad Y, Heather CJ, Salvaggio JE. A murine model of asbestosis. *Am J Pathol* 1983;112:326–337.

41. Dauber JH, Rossman MD, Pietra GG, Jimenez SA, Daniele RP. Experimental silicosis. Morphologic and biochemical abnormalities produced by intratracheal instillation of quartz into guinea pig lungs. *Am J Pathol* 1980;101:595–612.

42. Barry BE, Wong KC, Brody AR, Crapo JD. Reaction of rat lungs to inhaled chrysotile asbestos following acute and subchronic exposures. *Exp Lung Res* 1983;5:1–22.

43. Brody AR, Hill LH, Adkins B Jr, O'Connor RW. Chrysotile asbestos inhalation in rats: deposition pattern and reaction of alveolar epithelium and pulmonary macrophages. *Am Rev Respir Dis* 1981;123:670–679.

44. Brody AR, Roe MW, Evans JN, Davis GS. Deposition and translocation of inhaled silica in rats. *Lab Invest* 1982;47:533–541.

45. Pinkerton KE, Pratt PC, Brody AR, Crapo JD. Fiber localization and its relationship to lung reaction in rats after chronic inhalation of chrysotile asbestos. *Am J Pathol* 1984;117:484–498.

46. Spurzem JR, Saltini C, Rom W, Winchester RJ, Crystal RG. Mechanisms of macrophage accumulation in the lungs of asbestos-exposed subjects. *Am Rev Respir Dis* 1987;136:276–280.

47. Suzuki Y, Churg J. Structure and development of the asbestos body. *Am J Pathol* 1969;55:79–107.

48. Miller K. Alterations in the surface-related phenomena of al-veolar macrophages following inhalation of crocidolite asbestos and quartz dusts: an overview. *Environ Res* 1979;20:162–182.

49. Davis GS, Hemenway DR, Evans JN, Lapenas DJ, Brody AR. Alveolar macrophage stimulation and population changes in silica-exposed rats. *Chest* 1981;80(Suppl):8S–10S.

50. Jackson JH, Schraufstatter IU, Hyslop PA, et al. Role of oxidants in DNA damage. Hydroxyl radical mediates the synergistic DNA damaging effects of asbestos and cigarette smoke. *J Clin Invest* 1987;80:1090–1095.

51. Cantin A, Allard C, Bégin R. Increased alveolar plasminogen activator in early asbestosis. *Am Dis* 1989;139:604–609.

52. Mornex J-F, Martinet Y, Yamauchi K, Bitterman P, Grotendorst GR, Chytil-Weir A, Martin GR, Crystal RG. Spontaneous expression of the c-sis gene and release of a platelet-derived growth factor-like molecule by human alveolar macrophages. *J Clin Invest* 1986;78:61–66.

53. Martinet Y, Rom WN, Grotendorst GR, Martin GR, Crystal RG. Exaggerated spontaneous release of a platelet-derived growth factor by alveolar macrophages from patients with idiopathic pulmonary fibrosis. *N Engl J Med* 1987;317(4):202–209.

54. Rennard SI, Hunninghake GW, Bitterman PB, Crystal RG. Production of fibronectin by the human alveolar macrophage: mechanism for the recruitment of fibroblasts to sites of tissue injury in interstitial lung diseases. *Proc Natl Acad Sci USA* 1981;78:7147–7151.

55. Bitterman PB, Adelberg S, Crystal RG. Mechanisms of pulmonary fibrosis: spontaneous release of the alveolar macrophage derived growth factor in the interstitial lung disorders. *J Clin Invest* 1983;72:1801–1813.

56. Rom WN, Basset P, Fells GA, Nukiwa T, Crystal RG. Alveolar macrophages release an insulin-like growth factor I-type molecule. *J Clin Invest* 1988;82:1685–1693.

57. Wagner JC, Burns J, Munday DE, McGee JOD. Presence of fibronectin in pneumoconiotic lesions. *Thorax* 1982;37:54–56.

58. Rennard SI, Crystal RG. Fibronectin in human bronchopulmonary lavage fluid: elevation of patients with interstitial lung disease. *J Clin Invest* 1982;69:113–122.

59. Bégin R, Martel M, Desmarais Y, Drapeau G, Boileau R, Rola-Pleszczynski M, Massé S. Fibronectin and procollagen 3 levels in bronchoalveolar lavage of asbestos-exposed human subjects and sheep. *Chest* 1986;89:237–243.

60. Bauman MD, Jetten AM, Brody AR. Biologic and biochemical characterization of a macrophage-derived growth factor for rat lung fibroblasts. *Chest* 1987;91(Suppl):15–16.

61. Jaurand MC, Gaudichet A, Atassi K, Sébastien P, Bignon J. Relationship between the number of asbestos fibres and the cellular and enzymatic content of bronchoalveolar fluid in asbestos exposed subjects. *Bull Eur Physiopathol Respir* 1980;16:595–606.

62. Hayes AA, Rose AH, Musk AW, Robinson WS. Neutrophil chemotactic factor release and neutrophil alveolitis in asbestos-exposed individuals. *Chest* 1988;94:521–525.

63. Xaubet A, Rodriguez-Roisin R, Bombi JA, Marin A, Roca J, Agusti-Vidal A. Correlation of bronchoalveolar lavage and clinical and functional findings in asbestosis. *Am Rev Respir Dis* 1986;133:848–854.

64. Gellert AR, Langford JA, Winter RJD, Uthayakumar S, Sinha G, Rudd RM. Asbestosis: assessment by bronchoalveolar lavage and measurement of pulmonary epithelial permeability. *Thorax* 1985;508–514.

65. Schoenberger CI, Hunninghake GW, Kawanami O, Ferrans VJ, Crystal RG. Role of alveolar macrophages in asbestosis: modulation of neutrophil migration to the lung after acute asbestos exposure. *Thorax* 1982;37:803–809.

66. Garcia JGN, Griffith DE, Cohen AB, Callahan KS. Alveolar macrophages from patients with asbestos exposure release increased levels of leukotriene B$_4$. *Am Rev Respir Dis* 1989;139:1494–1501.

67. Lange A, Nineham L, Garncarek D, Smolik R. Circulating immune complexes and antiglobulins (IgG and IgM) in asbestosis-induced lung fibrosis. *Environ Res* 1983;31:287–295.

68. Zone JJ, Rom WN. Circulating immune complexes in asbestos workers. *Environ Res* 1985;37:383–389.

69. Wallace JM, Oishi JS, Barbers RG, Batra P, Aberle DR. Bronchoalveolar lavage cell and lymphocyte phenotype profiles in healthy asbestos-exposed shipyard workers. *Am Rev Respir Dis* 1989;139:33–38.
70. Costabel U, Bross KJ, Huck E, Guzman J, Matthys H. Lung and blood lymphocyte subsets in asbestosis and in mixed dust pneumoconiosis. *Chest* 1987;91:110–112.
71. Christman JW, Emerson RJ, Graham WGB, Davis GS. Mineral dust and cell recovery from the bronchoalveolar lavage of healthy Vermont granite workers. *Am Rev Respir Dis* 1985;132:393–399.
72. Struhar D, Harbeck RJ, Mason RJ. Lymphocyte populations in lung tissue, bronchoalveolar lavage fluid, and peripheral blood in rats at various times during the development of silicosis. *Am Rev Respir Dis* 1989;139:28–32.
73. Robinson BWS, Rose AH, Hayes A, Musk AW. Increased pulmonary gamma interferon production in asbestosis. *Am Rev Respir Dis* 1988;138:278–283.
74. Bozelka BE, Sestini P, Gaumer HR, Hammad Y, Heather CJ, Salvaggio JE. A murine model of asbestosis. *Am J Pathol* 1983;112:326–337.
75. Borok Z, Buhl R, Grimes G, Bokser A, Hubbard R, Czerski D, Cantin AM, Crystal RG. Glutathione aerosol therapy to augment the alveolar epithelial antioxidant screen in idiopathic pulmonary fibrosis. *Am Rev Respir Dis* 1990;141:A320.
76. Borok Z, Gillissen A, Buhl R, Hoyt RF, Hubbard RC, Crystal RG. Augmentation of functional prostaglandin E levels on the respiratory epithelial surface by aerosol administration. *Clin Res* 1990;38:485A.

THE LUNG: Scientific Foundations
edited by R.G. Crystal, J.B. West et al.
Raven Press, Ltd., New York © 1991.

CHAPTER 7.4.1

Integrated Host Defense Against Infections

Herbert Y. Reynolds

Infection involving some portion of the respiratory tract is one of the most frequent afflictions that humans have to endure. Although serious infection such as pneumonia is rare for the normal host, milder or nuisance kinds of viral rhinitis or tracheobronchitis and bacterial bronchitis can strike healthy people during epidemics or unpredictably at any time. The morbidity and associated economic impact of mild respiratory infections are enormous. When people with bronchitis from smoking-related chronic lung disease, pneumonia, and deficiencies in lung host defenses and immunity that predispose to sinopulmonary infection are added, the importance of lung infection is considerable in relation to all pulmonary health problems (1). Nosocomial pneumonia will occur in about 5% of hospitalized patients and may affect 25% of patients in specialized intensive care units (2). Pneumonia continues to be a leading cause of death (1).

From a different perspective, it is surprising that respiratory infections are not more of a problem, given the vast array of microbes and multiple strains within each species, the burden of them in ambient air, and the huge number of bacteria contained in naso-oropharyngeal secretions that can be aspirated into the lower airways, even in normals during sleep (3). An effective host defense apparatus (4–11) is able to remove or to contain microbes that alight in the respiratory tract, and the opportunity for infection to develop does not occur. However, this defense system can be overwhelmed by a new, never before encountered microbe by the host, by a particularly virulent strain, or by a large inoculum, as could occur with direct aero-

solization of bacteria into the airways from contaminated ventilatory equipment (12). This is now an exceptional circumstance. Under usual conditions of exposure, human airways below the level of the major bronchi are relatively sterile (13–15) and contain only a small number of culturable bacteria, as found in protected bush catheter specimens taken from normals (16).

An overview of the host defenses spaced along the respiratory tract is given in Fig. 1 (17). As mentioned, microbes enter the airways if they are aerosolized in inhaled ambient air or aspirated with naso-oropharyngeal secretions, which can contain large numbers of organisms (up to 10^8 per milliliter of saliva). Bacteria may reach alveolar tissue if carried in pulmonary artery blood as in septicemia, or they may be introduced directly from an external source as with penetrating trauma or thoracic surgery; these latter two routes will not be discussed. As inhaled air is humidified in the upper respiratory tract, particulates and microbes are enveloped in moisture and assume dimensional and aerodynamic characteristics that determine how deeply they are carried with the airstream into the airways and where they impact or land. Macroscopic particulates are filtered out in the nose and mouth, whereas small ones (<2–3 μm in diameter) can travel to the alveolar surface. Thus, bacteria of this critical size can potentially inoculate the alveoli and cause pneumonia.

Opposing this influx of bacteria and the other noxious contaminates in inhaled air is the defense system. In the upper tract, where the density of microbes is greatest, largely mechanical barriers and reflex mechanisms operate (sneezing, coughing, and ciliary action of epithelial cells in the mucosa). Local secretory immunoglobulin A (S-IgA) antibody might prevent a virus or bacterial species from attaching to the epithelial sur-

H. Y. Reynolds: Department of Medicine, The Milton S. Hershey Medical Center, The Pennsylvania State University, Hershey, Pennsylvania 17033.

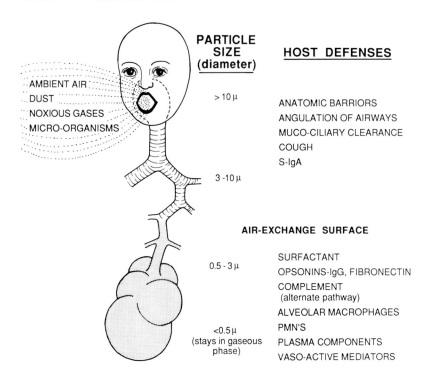

PARTICLE SIZE (diameter)

> 10 μ

3 - 10 μ

0.5 - 3 μ

<0.5 μ (stays in gaseous phase)

HOST DEFENSES

ANATOMIC BARRIORS
ANGULATION OF AIRWAYS
MUCO-CILIARY CLEARANCE
COUGH
S-IgA

AIR-EXCHANGE SURFACE

SURFACTANT
OPSONINS-IgG, FIBRONECTIN
COMPLEMENT
(alternate pathway)
ALVEOLAR MACROPHAGES
PMN'S
PLASMA COMPONENTS
VASO-ACTIVE MEDIATORS

AMBIENT AIR
DUST
NOXIOUS GASES
MICRO-ORGANISMS

FIG. 1. Host defenses spaced along the airways. Ambient air, along with its impurities, is filtered in the naso-oropharynx and in the conducting airways, where large particulates and most microbes are blocked out (glottis) or impacted against the mucosa and are removed by sneezing, coughing, and mucociliary clearance. Aspirated secretions are handled in a similar manner. A few smaller particles and bacteria may escape clearance and reach the alveolar ducts and acini, thereby posing a threat to the air-exchange surface. As air velocity and flow have ceased at this level in the airways, other defense mechanisms are required to cleanse the alveolar surface. These consist of opsonins, immune and nonimmune components, phagocytic cells (especially macrophages), and various components of systemic immunity which can enter the alveoli if inflammation occurs to alter permeability of the air–blood interface. S-IgA, secretory immunoglobulin A; IgG, immunoglobulin G; PMNS, polymorphonuclear leukocytes. (From ref. 17.)

face. Diversion of the laminar airflow in the larger bronchi at dichotomous branching points may deflect particles carried in the airstream against the mucosal surface. At such points of impaction and around an orifice to a bronchial division, lymphoid structures in the mucosa, termed *bronchial-associated lymphoid tissue* (BALT), can capture airborne particles and microbes. Clearance may be accomplished by phagocytic cells in the lymphoepithelium that covers BALT, and immune reactions may be initiated (as will be discussed later). A caveat to consider is that well-defined BALT structures in canines, subhuman primates, and humans are lacking, or at least they are not as obvious as in fowl, rabbits, and rodents, and hence they may be of relatively less importance in airway host defense in higher species.

Final arborizations of the conducting airways merge into the respiratory bronchioles, from which the alveolar ducts and alveoli extend to create the air-exchange surface. The respiratory bronchioles represent, therefore, a transitional zone that also has a role in host defense.

The air-exchange surface in aggregate represents an alveolar surface area that is estimated to be about the area of a tennis court or about 150 m² (18). Because it is possible for very small particles and microbes in inhaled air to reach this surface (the size has to range from 0.5 to less than 3 μm), appropriate components of host defense are needed to deal with them. Because the flow velocity of air molecules virtually ceases when the large cross-sectional area of the alveolar units or acini (18) is reached, particulates will no longer force-

fully strike the surface, as may have occurred in the branching bronchi and bronchioles. However, the dynamic expansion and closure of the alveoli with respiration may compress and force particulates against the alveolar walls so that they become enmeshed in the alveolar lining film. A number of immune and nonimmune substances are contained within the surfactant-rich lipoprotein film that can function as opsonins to coat particulates (surfactant itself, fibronectin fragments, immunoglobulins, and certain complement factors) and condition them for phagocytosis by the scavenger alveolar macrophages that exist just beneath or within the alveolar film and by other inflammatory cells, particularly polymorphonuclear neutrophils, that may be on the alveolar surface. With irritation, plasma components leak in, or locally produced mediators (such as histamine) can be present (19). All may be part of the host defense effort.

With this general overview of host defense components spaced along the airways and in the alveoli, a more in-depth review will be given of the interaction between microbes and respective immune and cellular factors that try to eliminate them.

COLONIZATION AND ENTRY OF MICROBES INTO THE AIRWAYS

The naso-oropharyngeal surface has a complex microbial flora (20) of aerobic and anaerobic bacteria that symbiotically exist in normals without untoward effects and for, as yet, an unknown purpose. Certainly, microorganisms on the nasal mucosa do not seem to have a role in a process like digestion that requires microbes in the terminal small bowel and colon for proper function. Common isolates in cultures of the nose and throat include *Neisseria* species (sp.), *Branhamella catarrhalis*, *Staphylococcus* sp., and a variety of *Streptococcus* sp. In many people with chronic obstructive airways disease, *Streptococcus pneumoniae* and *Hemophilus* sp. or fungi and protozoa can be recovered. Quantitatively, anaerobic bacteria around the teeth and gums are most numerous, possibly reaching 10^8 microorganisms per milliliter of oral secretions, and comprise many varied species but usually not *Bacteroides fragilis*. However, the prevalence of aerobic gram-negative bacilli such as Enterobacteriaceae and *Pseudomonas* sp. in the nasopharynx is low and may be isolated from about 15% of the area swab cultures taken from normals (21). Viruses are also not routinely found. It is likely that some mixture of the normally colonizing bacteria are aspirated into the airways during sleep, even in normal people (3), but are effectively cleared by ciliary action in the tracheobronchial tree or with coughing. Whether microorganisms consistently inhabit the more distal bronchi and small airways is uncertain. Various reports have considered this portion of the respiratory tract beyond the trachea and major bronchi to be sterile; more likely, very low colony numbers can exist in normals (16). Normal airways effectively keep the counts low—in contrast to areas of bronchiectasis and excessive mucus accumulation, where low-grade microbial infection occurs readily.

The interaction, however, between microbes and the airway mucosa and the host defenses inherent to it is dynamic (22,23) and features many different strategies by microbes to gain a foothold on the mucosa, as opposed to a rather limited repertoire of responses available to the host. These microbial attachments are illustrated in Fig. 2.

Respiratory infection may always develop if a new species is introduced into the community and the host (as happens with antigenic shifts in influenza viruses) or if a particularly virulent strain occurs. Also, a very large infecting dose or inoculum, as can be delivered by direct aerosol from contaminated ventilatory equipment (reviewed in ref. 26), has a better chance of causing illness, perhaps by overwhelming host defenses. Otherwise, respiratory infection may occur only if some part of the host defense apparatus is inoperant to allow the entering microbe a significant survival advantage. In this respect, all infecting microbes that succeed might be opportunistic ones that exploit two situations in the host: (i) a void of susceptible organisms in the wake of broad spectrum antibiotic therapy or (ii) malfunction of selective host defenses that alters the complexion of the colonizing flora. Particular examples of infection will be used that involve the conducting airways and the alveolar spaces.

CONDUCTING AIRWAYS

In Fig. 3, a segment of the bronchial airways illustrates the variety of defense mechanisms that deal with microbes that attempt to colonize the mucosa or alight on the surface (11). The airway surface has three layers, which, from the bottom outward, include the lamina propria or submucosa, the basement membrane,

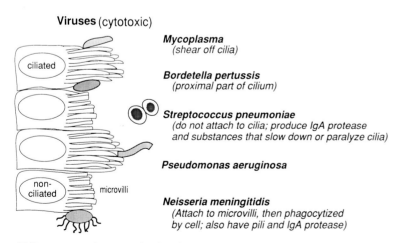

Viruses (cytotoxic)

ciliated

non-ciliated   microvilli

Mycoplasma
(shear off cilia)

Bordetella pertussis
(proximal part of cilium)

Streptococcus pneumoniae
(do not attach to cilia; produce IgA protease
and substances that slow down or paralyze cilia)

Pseudomonas aeruginosa

Neisseria meningitidis
(Attach to microvilli, then phagocytized
by cell; also have pili and IgA protease)

FIG. 2. The respiratory epithelium of the conducting airways consists principally of ciliated cells that are interspersed with goblet cells, ducts leading from bronchial glands, and some absorptive cells that have microvilli instead of cilia. For the interaction with microbes, the ciliated and microvillous cells are most involved. Viruses have the property of invading the cell to integrate into the nuclear apparatus for replication, eventually causing cytotoxicity and death of the epithelial cell. A variety of bacteria attack the cellular appendages. *Mycoplasma pneumoniae* bind to receptors on cilia and can shear them off, whereas *Bordetella pertussis* do the same thing but attack at a more proximal location on the cilium. Adherence of *Pseudomonas aeruginosa* to human epithelial cell cilia (24) may require metabolic changes first in a chronically ill host that affect mucosal cells and facilitate colonization (25). In contrast, certain *Neisseria* sp. attach to the microvilli of these absorptive cells. Bacteria usually have several weapons to overcome the host defenses in the area, i.e., ciliary motion and secretory immunoglobulin A (S-IgA). Pili and adhesion substances on bacteria increase their attachment sites, proteolytic enzymes can selectively degrade S-IgA$_1$, or cilotoxic factors can slow or paralyze ciliary motion, perhaps allowing attachment to occur more readily. *Streptococcus pneumoniae*, *Hemophilus influenzae*, *Neisseria meningitidis*, and some gram-negative baccili such as *Pseudomonas aeruginosa* can secrete IgA proteases.

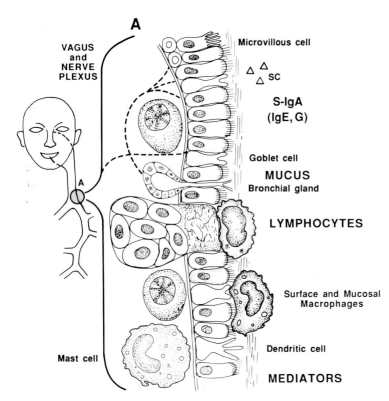

FIG. 3. A portion of the conducting airway surface is enlarged (A) and depicts the mucosa and its submucosal structures. The pseudostratified ciliated epithelium has a covering layer of mucus (produced by goblet cells and bronchial glands) and fluid that contains various proteins, including immunoglobulins and secretory component (SC). A few surface cells may be present, such as lymphocytes (from bronchial-associated lymphoid aggregates) and macrophages. Among the epithelial cells are absorptive microvillous cells and dendritic cells whose cellular processes do not reach to the mucosal surface. In addition, the epithelial cells can produce arachidonic acid metabolites that influence mucosal swelling and permeability. In the submucosa below the basement membrane, plasma cells and mast cells reside that secrete local immunoglobulins (such as IgA) and mediators (such as histamine). Joining all of these glandular and cellular networks together are nerves, perhaps exerting their control through neuropeptides, and by adrenergic and cholinergic nerve fibers. A rich vascular supply exists also. S-IgA, secretory immunoglobulin A; IGE,G, immunoglobulins E and G. (Adapted from ref. 11.)

and a pseudostratified columnar epithelium. In the submucosa, the basal portion of bronchial glands and plasma cells reside, whereas autonomic nerves traverse and become afferent and efferent fibers in the mucosa (27). Tissue mast cells are also located here. The basement membrane is relatively permeable and will allow access to intercellular channels between the epithelial cells. The outermost epithelial cells have movable cilia and form tight junctions between the apical edges. In addition, numerous goblet cells are interspersed, as well as serous cells with absorptive microvillous structures. In areas closer to the respiratory bronchioles, dendritic cells are found with multiple cytoplasmic processes that do not quite reach up to the surface. At points of airway bifurcation and around the opening of bronchial branches, a specialized lymphoepithelium, devoid of ciliated cells, overlies the nodules of lymphoid tissue referred to as BALT. On the luminal surface, a semiliquid or gel mixture consists of (a) mucus, produced from goblet cells and bronchial glands, (b) immunoglobulins, especially IgA but trace amounts of others, (c) cells, including surface macrophages and lymphocytes, (d) local mediators such as histamine and possibly neuropeptides (28), and (e) foreign debris and microbial antigens. Rapid ciliary movement (29,30) sweeps this mucous mixture up the airways. Several structures and substances in this portion of the airways are important in determining host susceptibility to infection and will be presented in more detail.

Immunoglobulins

In the upper respiratory tract, the content of immunoglobulins in external secretions from the nasal mucosa and the parotid and salivary glands, as well as in related secretions (from lacrimal glands and in earwax), accounts for approximately 10% of the protein content. IgA constitutes the largest amount (31); IgG is minimal (about 1%); and IgE is in trace amounts unless allergic rhinitis or atopy is present. In proceeding down the trachea and into the major bronchi, the relative proportions of IgA to IgG still pertain. In the smaller bronchi, it is likely that IgG begins to increase and assume more importance in host defense. This is an assumption, because direct measurements are difficult in this portion of the airways, but selective deficiencies in certain IgG subclasses (namely, IgG$_2$ and/or IgG$_4$) are associated with bronchiectasis. In the alveolar spaces, as sampled in bronchoalveolar lavage (BAL) fluid, the concentrations of IgG and IgA have reversed and IgG seems to be the predominant immunoglobulin (32). This gradual change-over of the IgA and IgG concentrations was also documented to occur in the canine airways (33).

Because IgA is present in greatest amount in upper airway secretions, it is presumably the most important for host defense. Just how it participates in this still remains as something of an enigma (34). IgA in external secretions is predominantly polymeric in form (about 80%): The so-called secretory IgA (S-IgA) consists of two monomers of IgA, each composed of two linked alpha and light chains which are held together by a joining chain and by another glycoprotein produced by serous and epithelial cells, called *secretory component* (SC) (34,35). Thus, S-IgA is the product of two cell types: (i) plasma cells, located in the submucosa of the respiratory tract in this case (36), and (ii) cells in the epithelial lining. Complexing of the SC to the IgA dimer is required for final absorption and transport of IgA through the bronchial glands and epithelial cells, as well as for its extrusion onto the airway luminal surface. This is a remarkable biologic journey that requires an adequate supply of free or unbound SC (37–39). Two subclasses of IgA exist; these are determined by the structure of the heavy chains, known as $alpha_1$ and $alpha_2$ (34). In bronchial secretions, about two-thirds of IgA is of the $alpha_1$ type (IgA_1) and about one-third is $alpha_2$ (IgA_2) (40). External secretions generally have slightly more IgA_2 than found in serum (mean of 33% in bronchial secretions versus 18% in serum, for example).

With respect to S-IgA and its interactions with microbes in the airways, four situations seem evident. First, IgA is the class of immunoglobulins that is produced by the body in greatest amounts, estimated to be grams per day (41), especially in the bile and gastrointestinal tract. Because IgA is a significant component in airway secretions that bathe the mucosal surface, it contributes to the barrier function that helps protect the surface from penetration of noxious substances. Tight cellular junctions (42) and the constant ciliary cleaning are also of great importance in this function.

Second, IgA has demonstrable antibody activity against a variety of microorganisms that can colonize or infect the airways. For example, specific IgA antibody in nasopharyngeal secretions and saliva from patients with pertussis could be detected against *Bordetella pertussis* toxin and filamentous hemagglutinin antigen (HA) with enzyme-linked immunosorbent assays (43). Following experimental secondary infection with influenza A virus in human volunteers, nasal wash fluid contained IgA HA antibodies (44). Although both IgA_1 and IgA_2 antibodies could be detected, IgA_1 accounted for most of the rise in antibody titers in nasal wash after infection. Development of respiratory IgA antibody has been reviewed extensively (34,45). Certainly, this is a major biologic function of this immunoglobulin class, especially on external mucosal surfaces (46).

However, it has proved difficult to find optimal strategies to predictably induce sustained IgA antibody production in the nasopharynx or lower airways in humans after primary immunization. Unfortunately, a polio-like viral vaccine that so effectively induces protective IgA in the gastrointestinal tract does not have a similar effect in the respiratory tract. Because IgA is found on many mucosal surfaces throughout the body and is produced by external secretory glands (parotid, lacrimal, salivary, and breast) and visceral organs (such as the gallbladder), IgA is part of an intricate network of humoral immunity which may be quite different from its intravascular role (46). This interlocking function of mucosal surfaces permits specific immunization of one part and development of local IgA immunity, especially in the gastrointestine; furthermore, a redistribution of the antibody response occurs by homing of primed lymphocytes and plasma cells to other distant sites, particularly to breast tissue in lactating females. It should be possible to exploit these relationships to induce IgA antibody in the respiratory tract. However, as yet, various orally administered bacterial antigens and viral agents stimulate relatively low antibody titers in saliva, tears, and nasal secretions (reviewed in ref. 47), so this approach has not been used as preventive therapy for infections.

Third, the principal amount of S-IgA belongs to the $alpha_1$ heavy chain type, and should natural antibody be produced, it is likely to be IgA_1 (44). The predicament for the host in its confrontation with certain microbes that may be attempting to colonize the airways (Fig. 2) is that IgA_1 is vulnerable to specific bacterial proteases. As mentioned, some of the most common bacteria causing respiratory infections are the ones capable of producing these proteases. Selective advantage might be gained by the host if IgA_2 antibody could be increased preferentially as a substitute.

Fourth, mechanisms by which IgA antibody might participate in additional facets of host immunity against microbes need further exploration in light of new studies that are changing existing concepts about its function. For example, IgA fixes complement poorly, and it is not as effective as IgG as an opsonin for bacterial uptake by phagocytes such as alveolar macrophages (48), perhaps due to the paucity of IgA receptors on them (49). However, experimental use of IgA antibody in assays that do not dissociate the different biologic activities of the IgA subclasses may mask individual effects. When human IgA_1 antibody, obtained from volunteers vaccinated with a tetravalent meningococcal polysaccharide vaccine, was used, classical complement pathway-mediated killing of Group C *Neisseria meningitidis* occurred (50); heretofore, the blocking effect of IgA antibody was thought to be more important. Recent receptor analysis of human alveolar macrophages has disclosed the presence of IgA receptors that will bind either IgA_1 or IgA_2 (51). Cytophilic antibody on these cells is IgA_1 entirely.

Iron Binding Proteins That Inhibit Bacterial Growth

For microorganisms to successfully colonize mucosal surfaces or to live within a host, a mechanism to obtain iron must be found, as this essential ingredient for survival, including for bacteria, is kept sequestered within cells or firmly complexed to transport proteins (52). In plasma, transferrin has this function but lactoferrin is the transport molecule in mucosal secretions. To compete for iron, microbes have developed their own chelators, generally known as *siderophores*.

Because these iron transport proteins are present in airway mucosal secretions and in alveolar lining fluid, they may be host factors in the regulation of bacterial growth. Several reports have identified transferrin (a 90,000-Da protein) in normal BAL fluid (32,53). Transferrin was present in concentrated BAL fluids in amounts that, on average, were 40% more than in matched serum; values were not different for smokers and nonsmokers (53). It was suggested that local secretion of this protein might occur in the alveoli, possibly by lymphocytes and macrophages. In contrast, lactoferrin may not be identified consistently in BAL unless inflammation with polymorphonuclear leukocytes (PMNs) is present. In BAL fluid from normal mice, values for transferrin are about 8 μg/ml and for lactoferrin about 3 μg/ml (54). Iron in the lavage fluid is about 80 ng/ml.

Along the airways, lactoferrin can be found. When the initial BAL fluid aliquot is analyzed separately, since the first sample contains more airway proteins than do subsequent ones, lactoferrin concentrations are much greater than in the remainder of the pooled lavage (11.8 μg/ml versus 0.7 μg/ml) from normals (55).

If these iron transport proteins—lactoferrin predominantly along the airways and transferrin in the alveolar spaces (56)—effectively complex any free iron in mucosal secretions and alveolar lining fluid, then bacterial growth might be suppressed if this nutrient is not readily available. Moreover, human lactoferrin has been shown to have antimicrobial activity against certain bacteria such as *Streptococcus mutans, S. pneumoniae, Escherichia coli,* and *Legionella pneumophila* (57,58). Thus, the availability of iron-binding proteins in the airways could affect the containment of bacteria and be an important nonimmune component of host defense.

Surface Phagocytosis and Antigen Processing Cells

Along the conductive airways (Fig. 3), several opportunities exist for microbes or aerosolized antigens and particles to be captured and eliminated, or to be processed for subsequent use in immune responses. The overall importance of surface phagocytosis in the lungs is uncertain and may be dependent upon the species of animal. Two components, bronchial-associated lymphoid tissue (BALT) and phagocytic cells of the dendritic and macrophage types, are involved.

The respiratory tract contains a considerable amount of lymphoid tissue which is in various forms (59) such as (a) lymph nodes positioned in the mediastinum and hilar areas of the lungs, (b) tonsils and adenoids in the naso-oropharynx, (c) submucosal aggregates spaced along the airways at branching points, and (d) detachable or free lymphoid cells on the alveolar surface. Considerable attention has been given to BALT in rodents, rabbits, and fowl. BALT structures are relatively similar to Peyer's patches in the small intestine (60,61). Similar lymphoid structures in the airways of dogs, primates, and humans (62–64) are not nearly so prominent and possibly are of less significance in airway host defense. Nevertheless, the strategic location of BALT at branching points of the airways suggests that these structures are part of the afferent pathway for local immunity. The structures may intercept any particulates deflected from the airstream, because their specialized covering, which is devoid of ciliated cells and goblet cells, seems suitable for capturing and retaining substances that alight (it is considered to be a sticky surface) (65). Antigen uptake and processing by stimulated (with lipopolysaccharide) dendritic cells and macrophages within BALT may initiate an antibody response (66). BALT is considered to be part of a more extensive common mucosal lymphoid network (67). A feature of this network is that immunization could occur at a remote site (such as in the gastrointestine), and through the redistribution of lymphocytes or plasma cells to other mucosal surfaces, antibodies could be provided there (68). In studies on the IgA system, references were made to this phenomenon (34,47).

It is probable that microbes or organic antigens are processed at other points along the airways by phagocytic cells that are on the mucosal surface or adjacent to it. A few macrophages may reside on the mucociliary surface, since they are retrieved with bronchial lavage (69). They represent either cells that are leaving the alveolar surface to be expelled from the lungs, because they are effete or senescent cells, or ones that are patrolling the airways. Little is known of their function, which might not be of great importance because their number is small. In contrast, dendritic cells are dispersed throughout the columnar epithelium of large and small bronchi (70,71) and represent approximately 1% of all the epithelial cells in human tissue (71). Their cytoplasmic extensions do not quite reach to the bronchial lumen. They are different from macrophages, yet they retain phagocytic capacity and are efficient as antigen presenting cells (72). These cells have potent accessory cell function when mixed with lymphocytes and would seem to be important in initiating immune responses. Dendritic cells also exist in alveolar septa, and the interstitium and their function can be distinguished from alveolar macrophages (73,74). Their strong assessory function is in contrast to the overall suppressive effects attributed to alveolar macrophages (75).

AIR-EXCHANGE AREA: ALVEOLAR UNITS

The conducting airways end at the level of the respiratory bronchioles, where significant anatomic changes develop as airflow velocity ceases and as molecular diffusion carries air into the alveoli, culminating in gas exchange across the epithelial–endothelial layers of the air–blood interface. The large increase in cross-sectional area of the alveolar acini causes this reduction in airflow velocity. In this transitional area of the respiratory bronchioles, host defense mechanisms radically change because those in the upper airways are no longer operant (e.g., mucociliary clearance, coughing, lesser amounts of S-IgA). Here the lymphatic channels originate, which provides the alveolar surface with access to draining lymph nodes in the lung hila and permits egress of phagocytic cells, such as macrophages, from the lung. As the secretory cells and glands of the conducting airways are eliminated with the transition to a single-layer epithelial surface in the alveoli, greater dependence can be envisioned for intravascular humoral components to diffuse into the alveolar lining fluid and for phagocytic cells to emigrate from the interstitial and capillary areas.

The upper respiratory defenses are superbly efficient in removing microbes and particulates that can potentially reach the air-exchange surface via aerodynamic filtration mechanisms; however, very small particulates, between 0.5 and 3 μm in diameter, may elude these mechanisms, and a few can reach the alveoli (Fig. 1). The above dimensions include the size of many bacteria. The other direct route of microbes to the alveolar units is through the pulmonary artery blood flow, where the filtering effect of capillaries can capture them on the endothelial surface and where inflammatory reactions can develop.

Components of Host Defense in the Alveolar Spaces

Because other chapters include details about various alveolar cells (macrophages, Chapter 3.4.5; lymphocytes, Chapter 3.4.1; neutrophils, Chapter 3.4.7) and immunologic components (complement, Chapter 3.4.4), a brief review only will be given about the major immune and nonimmune opsonins and interacting cell types found in normal humans (Fig. 4). A detailed analysis of cellular and noncellular elements can be found in other reviews (32,53,58,76).

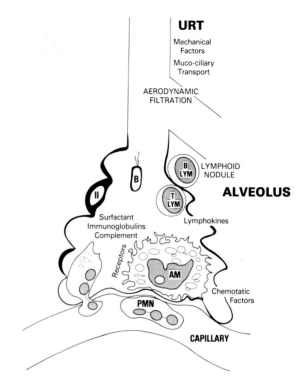

FIG. 4. Clearance of bacteria (B) that escape the upper respiratory tract (URT) and reach the alveolus (represented by enlargement of one) is complex. A bacterium deposited in an alveolus may encounter surfactant (secreted by type II epithelial cells) and/or immunoglobulins (antibodies) and complement proteins which condition it for phagocytosis by a resident alveolar macrophage (AM). Antibody with specific opsonizing potential can facilitate attachment of the bacterium to the AM surface membrane through Fc gamma cell receptors. Other mechanisms can be used to enhance killing and clearance of the microbe. First, the AM can liberate chemotactic factors that attract nearby polymorphonuclear phagocytes (PMN), marginated in a lung capillary adjacent to the alveolus, and thus initiate an inflammatory response. Second, the bacterium may trigger immune lymphocytes (T LYM) to release effector substances (lymphokines or polypeptide mediators) that can activate or stimulate AM phagocytic and bactericidal capacity. (From ref. 100.)

Noncellular Components in Epithelial Lining Fluid (as Sampled by Bronchoalveolar Lavage)

Several components in normal BAL fluid have the capability of coating, in a nonspecific manner, certain bacteria that will enhance phagocytic uptake by alveolar macrophages, thus qualifying as nonimmune opsonins. Strains of staphylococci and rough mutant strains of certain gram-negative bacilli such as *E. coli* are coated with surfactant (77,78). Large fragments of fibronectin seem to facilitate the uptake of bacteria by macrophages *in vitro* (79). Because fibronectin is a prominent component of the epithelial lining fluid (ELF) and can be secreted by alveolar macrophages (80), it is reasonable to believe it has opsonic activity in the lungs. Other acute-phase reactants such as C-reactive protein (81) might have a similar role; however, it is not a component of normal BAL fluid (53).

Immunoglobulins that develop specific antibody activity following antigenic exposure are the principal immune opsonins. Because of its large size, IgM is only present in trace amounts in normal ELF (32). Since IgA, especially S-IgA, does not have an obvious similar secretory mechanism to deliver it into the ELF, as is found in the airways, IgA that is present in ELF may, in fact, be washed from more proximal airway mucosal surfaces during lavage (76), or conceivably an "aspiration" mechanism might carry it into the alveoli. Most serum IgA is in monomeric form, but about 90% of IgA in lavage fluid is in dimeric or polymeric form that has J-chain and SC attached (32). It is uncertain whether monomeric units could be assembled in the alveoli. However, free secretory component can be detected in BAL fluid (39). As mentioned, the role of IgA antibody in the alveoli milieu needs to be reevaluated in view of recent experimental work, although IgA is not likely to be a potent form of opsonizing antibody.

IgG, which constitutes about 5% of the total protein content of normal BAL fluid (32), seems to be the predominant immunoglobulin in the alveoli and also seems to be the most clearly identified with opsonic activity. IgG, which is a heterogeneous population of four heavy-chain subclasses, has individual functional characteristics (82,83) and also has a pattern of distribution in BAL fluid that closely resembles that in serum. In BAL fluid of nonsmokers, IgG_1 and IgG_2 are present in greatest concentrations (65% and 28%, respectively), whereas IgG_3 and IgG_4 together account for less than 10% (1.8% and 5.2%, respectively) (82); virtually the same percentages were measured in the serum of these subjects. IgG_4, however, is found in slightly greater amount in BAL fluid than in serum. In addition, the normal cigarette smokers studied had less IgG_2 in serum and BAL lavage than did the nonsmokers (13% versus 28% in BAL fluid). In terms of host defense, IgG_1 and IgG_3 are considered to be important antibodies because, of the four IgG subclasses, only these two antibodies fix complement. IgG_2 is the repository of type-specific antibody against polysaccharide antigens from important respiratory pathogens such as *Streptococcus pneumoniae* and *Hemophilus influenzae* (84). Antibody against techoic acid from *Staphylococcus aureus* and against lipopolysaccharide from *Pseudomonas aeruginosa* (85) is IgG_2. IgG_4, although seemingly a minor component, can have several effects: to act as a reaginic antibody in allergic disease; to be increased in hypersensitivity pneumonitis (86,87); or, if absent, to predispose to sinopulmonary infections and bronchiectasis (88).

Potentially, complement components can interact with microbes in several ways. Activation of an entire complement pathway in the presence of a microbe could result in its lysis and killing. Partial activation can generate an intermediate component C_3b, which has opsonic activity and promotes receptor-mediated phagocytosis by PMNs and macrophages, or can create C_5a, which has phlogistic properties because of its chemoattractant effect for PMNs. Whether any or all of these functions operate in the normal alveolar space is uncertain. Experimental ablation of the systemic complement system will impair somewhat the lung's clearance of certain encapsulated bacteria (89). In humans, properidin factor B is present in normal BAL fluid (90), and components C_4 and C_6 are proportionally lower than in serum (ratios of hemolytic titer per albumin concentration determined in serum and concentrated BAL fluid) (32). C_{1q} was not detected (32). Taken together, it is possible that complement activity can be generated locally in the airways, but via the alternative pathway. In such chronic diseases as idiopathic pulmonary fibrosis and hypersensitivity pneumonitis, no evidence of complement abnormalities was found (91).

Cells in the Alveolar Spaces

With BAL of 100–300 ml of normal nonsmokers, the recovery of lung cells is approximately 15 million cells having a cell viability of greater than 90%; a minimal number of red cells (about 5%) and ciliated epithelial cells (about 1%, depending on how much coughing occurred during the lavage) are present. The cellular profile is at least 85% alveolar macrophages, about 10% lymphocytes, 1–3% PMNs, and the remaining percentage being eosinophils and mast cells (32). A few platelets may be found. Alveolar macrophages appear in different sizes and have been shown to represent a heterogeneous population of cells with varying functional characteristics (32,92,93). Alveolar macrophages develop from monocyte precursor cells and require a period of maturation and differentiation which occurs in the interstitial compartment of the lung. Whether multiple cell replications occur is uncertain but likely. Once these cells are on the alveolar surface, a very low degree of replication may occur (about 1%) (94); this process is found to be higher in interstitial diseases, where the macrophage population is expanded and more active (95). Among the lymphocytes, most are T-cells (about 70%), of which the majority are of the T-helper/inducer (T_H) subset of T-cells and a smaller percentage (about 30%) are T-suppressor/cytotoxic (T_S) cells (96); the resulting T_H/T_S ratio is about 1.5, which is similar to that found for normal peripheral blood T-lymphocytes. Among the T-helper cells, about 7% of cells are HLA-DR antigen positive and secrete much of the interleukin-2 (97). The killer lymphocytes seem to be nonactivated in the normal lung (98). For the non-T-cell lymphocytes, a mixture of plasma cells and B-lymphocytes constitutes these, some of which seem to contain surface immunoglobulins that can be released (99). About 5% of the lung lymphocyte population are untypable and may represent "null" cells.

Integrated Host Responses in the Alveolar Space

Some of the options with which the host can respond to microbes that reach the alveoli surface are shown in Fig. 4 (100). In this case, a bacterium that has eluded the aerodynamic defenses in the upper airways and has not landed on the mucociliary apparatus nor been snared elsewhere along the conducting airways may enter the air-exchange area. The host must remove it or risk that the bacterium can initiate infection and create inflammation that would seriously alter capillary and epithelial permeability and jeopardize gas exchange in the area. At least four interactions are possible which could be utilized sequentially to build an escalating response if necessary to eliminate the invading microbe. What dictates this hierarchy of responsiveness is unknown. However, some sensing device must recognize characteristics of the microbe that are unique [i.e., inoculum size, special virulence, or resistance properties (enzyme adaptation to resist antibiotics may not be possible to anticipate for the host)] and must know the inventory of the host's armentarium (i.e., availability of specific antibody and, importantly, what deficits exist in current host defenses that will need compensation). Whether this "intelligence" resides with macrophages and lymphocytes or relies on some other mediator messenger system is an unanswered, intriguing question.

The bacterium (Fig. 4) entering the alveolus is likely to first be thrust up against, or to bump into, the alveolar wall, at which time it will become enmeshed in the ELF. It could become coated with the various non-immune opsonins and with specific IgG antibody, if appropriate humoral immunity exists. At this point, two things could occur. The antibody creates an antigen–antibody reaction that activates a complement sequence resulting in bacterial lysis. Of greater probability is that a mixture of opsonins sticks on the bacterium and facilitates its ingestion by an alveolar macrophage. This would be especially true of encapsulated bacteria such as *Streptococcus pneumoniae*. The macrophage is a mobile scavenger that can patrol several alveoli and effectively ingest debris. It has a longevity of months to possibly several years and can have numerous phagocytic encounters, thus being a reusable phagocyte. Experimentally, when a bacterial

inoculum is aerosolized or instilled onto the alveolar surface, bacteria remain free for only a short time (30 min or so) before they are internalized within a macrophage (101,102).

Once the bacterium is within the macrophage, at least two things could happen. The macrophage's bactericidal mechanisms could proceed to kill and destroy the microbe; these mechanisms will not be reviewed here. Or, the microbe could prove to be difficult to destroy, and the macrophage would need to be activated to complete the mission (103). This interaction is complex and involves T-lymphocytes and a variety of cells. Mediators such as interleukin 2, gamma-interferon, and migration inhibitory factor are among the more important ones involved. A predictable group of obligatory intracellular microbes are generally difficult for tissue macrophages in the reticuloendothelial system to contain, and in the lung a number of these are especially important (100). These microbes include: *Mycobacterium tuberculosis, Pneumocystis carinii, Legionella* sp., cytomegalovirus, certain fungi, and human immunodeficiency virus (104). Once the macrophage can become activated or can acquire cellular immunity, it can control the intracellular multiplication of the microbe at least and contain it. This has been shown for *Legionella pneumophila* (105). In addition, the activated macrophage and the lymphocyte team of cells can participate in granuloma formation, which is required to contain some organisms, namely, the tubercle and fungi.

Finally, if local mechanisms and macrophage killing do not suffice to destroy the bacterium and its offspring, the host can recruit additional phagocytes such as PMNs and create an inflammatory response (106). This is predicated on the availability of PMNs, which are stored in the lung capillaries as part of the marginated intravascular pool. Commonly in the immunocompromised patient with bone marrow insufficiency, granulocytopenia is present and the inflammatory reaction is suboptimal, which predisposes the lung, as well as other organs, to infection with aerobic gram-negative bacilli and certain fungi. Under ordinary circumstances, the inflammatory reaction gives access to the resources of systemic immunity and broadens considerably the kind of attack the host can mount towards microbes. For example, the wholesale change in alveolar permeability that occurs with inflammation will allow the large antibody molecules of IgM and IgA to enter; also, more complement components could gain access. Control of both the inflammatory reaction from the air side and active recruitment of PMNs likely resides with the alveolar macrophage. Among the vast array of cytokine mediators this cell type can secrete (107), especially when activated, are several that exert chemoattractant effects on PMNs (108,109). Another possibility is that complement activation in the airway can generate C_5a, which is a potent chemotaxin. Once an influx of PMNs has occurred into the alveoli and these cells begin to release their proteolytic enzymes, other systems such as the coagulation and kinin pathways can generate chemotaxins and help perpetuate the inflammatory reaction. This results in pneumonitis, which is the ultimate response to infection that the lung defenses can mount and represents the culmination of the various intermediate steps described.

In summary, local alveolar host defenses may suffice to handle certain microbes easily, but ever-increasingly potent backup mechanisms exist that can be employed should one fail or become overwhelmed. As examples, nonimmune opsonins can facilitate microbial uptake by phagocytes, but IgG antibody directed against encapsulated bacteria may be more effective. However, to develop antibody requires natural exposure or immunization. For special organisms that alveolar macrophages (AMs) cannot contain and kill (despite specific opsonins that promote ingestion), cellular activation or acquisition of cell-mediated immunity (CMI) is required. Various mediators produced by T-lymphocytes accomplish this. As mentioned, AM require CMI to contain *Legionella* sp., mycobacteria, and certain fungi, but killing and elimination of the microbe from the cell may not occur, so an ongoing process of containment is required that involves granuloma formation. In contrast, respiratory infections in acquired immunodeficiency syndrome (AIDS) patients reflect an inadequate CMI response in which the T-helper lymphocyte machinery is deficient or is overbalanced by T-suppressor cell proliferation in the lung (110–114) that may prevent proper AM stimulation. *Pneumocystis carinii*, fungi, mycobacteria, and even common bacterial pathogens cause infection in this situation. Thus, in AIDS or in patients receiving immunosuppressive chemotherapy, the backup mechanisms—CMI and granuloma formation—are impaired. The ultimate mechanism that is available is the inflammatory response which provides intensive phagocytic help and draws in elements of systemic immunity, creating pneumonitis. Yet, in the compromised host who may have bone marrow failure and inadequate reserves of PMNs, inflammation may not be effective and opportunistic bacterial infections, particularly with aerobic gram-negative bacilli and fungi, occur. With this failure of the inflammatory reaction, the host is in grave danger from septicemia and nosocomial pneumonia. Thus, what is envisioned to be an orderly sequence of alveolar mechanisms that, in stepwise increments, can lead up to pneumonitis may be crippled at several points by either host deficiencies or specific microbes that allow respiratory infections to develop. However, creation of better therapies in the future to

intervene at these points will bolster or restore host defenses and improve success against infection.

REFERENCES

1. Lenfant C. Lung disease. In: Fishman AP, Gail D, Peavy H, Thom TJ, eds. *Magnitude of the problem*, vol 3. NIH publication 84-2358. Washington, DC: National Heart, Lung and Blood Institute, US Department of Health and Human Services, 1982;7–30.
2. Reynolds HY. Prevention and future control of hospital-associated infections commonly caused by gram-negative bacteria. *Prev Med* 1974;3:507–514.
3. Huxley EJ, Viroslav J, Gray WR, Pierce AK. Pharyngeal aspiration in normal adults and patients with depressed consciousness. *Am J Med* 1978;64:564–568.
4. Green GM. In defense of the lung: the J. Burns Amberson Lecture. *Am Rev Respir Dis* 1970;102:691–703.
5. Newhouse M, Sanchis J, Bienenstock J. Lung defense mechanisms. *N Engl J Med* 1976;295:990–997, 1045–1051.
6. Cohen AB, Gold WM. Defense mechanisms of the lungs. *Annu Rev Physiol* 1975;37:325–350.
7. Green GM, Jakab GJ, Low RB, Davis GS. Defense mechanisms of the respiratory membrane. *Am Rev Respir Dis* 1977;115:479–514.
8. Kazmierowski JA, Aduan RP, Reynolds HY. Pulmonary host defenses: coordinated interaction of mechanical, cellular and humoral immune systems of the lung. *Bull Eur Physiopathol Respir* 1977;13:103–116.
9. Brain JD, Proctor DF, Reid LM, eds. *Respiratory defense mechanisms*. New York: Marcel Dekker, 1977.
10. Reynolds HY. Lung host defense: a status report. *Chest* 1979;75:239S–242S.
11. Reynolds HY. Pulmonary host defense—state of the art. *Chest* 1989;95:223S–230S.
12. Pierce AK, Sanford JP, Thomas GD, Leonard JS. Long term evaluation of decontamination of inhalation-therapy equipment and the occurrence of necrotizing pneumonia. *N Engl J Med* 1970;282:528–531.
13. Lees AW, McNaught W. Bacteriology of the lower respiratory tract secretions, sputum, and upper respiratory tract secretions in "normals" and chronic bronchitis. *Lancet* 1959;2:1112–1125.
14. Laurenzi GA, Potter RT, Kass EH. Bacteriologic flora of the lower respiratory tract. *N Engl J Med* 1961;265:1273–1278.
15. Potter RT, Rotman F, Fernandez F, McNeil TM. The bacteriology for the lower respiratory tract: bronchoscopic study of 100 clinical cases. *Am Rev Respir Dis* 1968;97:1051.
16. Halperin SA, Suratt PM, Gwaltney JM, Groschel DHM, Hendley JO, Eggleston PA. Bacterial cultures from the lower respiratory tract in normal volunteers with and without experimental rhinovirus infection using a plugged double catheter system. *Am Rev Respir Dis* 1982;125:678–680.
17. Reynolds HY. Host defense impairments that may lead to respiratory infections. *Clin Chest Med* 1987;8:339–358.
18. Weibel ER, Taylor CR. Design and structure of the human lung. In: Fishman AP, ed. *Pulmonary diseases and disorders*, 2nd ed. New York: McGraw-Hill, 1988;11–60.
19. Rankin JA, Kaliner M, Reynolds HY. Histamine levels in bronchoalveolar lavage from patients with asthma, sarcoidosis and idiopathic pulmonary fibrosis. *J Allergy Clin Immunol* 1987;79:371–377.
20. Mackowiak PA. The normal microbial flora. *N Engl J Med* 1982;307:83–93.
21. Rosenthal S, Tager I. Prevalence of gram negative rods in the normal pharyngeal flora. *Ann Intern Med* 1975;83:355–357.
22. Cassell G, ed. *Microbial surfaces: determinants of virulence and host responsiveness. Rev Infect Dis* 1988;10:S273–S456 [special edition].
23. Reynolds HY. Bacterial adherence to respiratory tract mu-

cosa—a dynamic interaction leading to colonization. *Semin Respir Med* 1987;2:8–19.

24. Franklin AL, Todd T, Gurman G, Black D, Mankinen-Irvin PM, Irvin RT. Adherence of *Pseudomonas aeruginosa* to cilia of human tracheal epithelial cells. *Infect Immunol* 1987; 55:1523–1525.

25. Neiderman MS, Merrill WW, Ferranti RD, Pagano KM, Palmer LB, Reynolds HY. Nutritional status and bacterial binding in the lower respiratory tract in patients with chronic tracheostomy. *Ann Intern Med* 1984;100:795–800.

26. Craven DE, Connolly MG, Lichtenberg DA, Primeau PH, McCabe WR. Contamination of mechanical ventilators with tubing changes every 24 to 48 hours. *N Engl J Med* 1982; 306:1505–1509.

27. Barnes PJ. Neural control of human airways in health and disease. *Am Rev Respir Dis* 1986;134:1289–1314.

28. Barnes PJ. Airway neuropeptides: roles in fine tuning and in disease. *News Physiol Sci* 1989;4:116–120.

29. Rutland W, Griffin M, Cole PJ. Human ciliary beat frequency in epithelium from intrathoracic and extrathoracic airways. *Am Rev Respir Dis* 1982;125:100–105.

30. Wong LB, Miller IF, Yeates DB. Stimulation of ciliary beat frequency by autonomic agonists: in vivo. *J Appl Physiol* 1988;65:971–981.

31. Merrill WW, Hyun H, Strober W, Rankin J, Fick RB, Reynolds HY. Correlations between respiratory tract proteins obtained from upper (nasal) and lower (bronchial lavage) sites. *Am Rev Respir Dis* 1982;125:268A.

32. Reynolds HY, Newball HH. Analysis of proteins and respiratory cells obtained from human lungs by bronchial lavage. *J Lab Clin Med* 1974;84:559–573.

33. Kaltreider HB, Chan MKL. The class specific immunoglobulin composition of fluids obtained from various levels of the canine respiratory tract. *J Immunol* 1976;116:428–429.

34. Mestecky J, McGhee JR. Immunoglobulin A: molecular and cellular interactions involved in IgA biosynthesis and immune response. *Adv Immunol* 1987;40:153–245.

35. Thompson RE, Reynolds HY, Waxdal MJ. Structural composition of canine secretory component and immunoglobulin A. *Biochemistry* 1975;142:2853–2860.

36. Burnett D, Crocker J, Stockley RA. Cells containing IgA subclasses in bronchi of subjects with and without chronic obstructive lung disease. *J Clin Pathol* 1987;40:1217–1220.

37. Goodman MR, Link DW, Brown WR, Nakane PK. Ultrastructure evidence of transport of secretory IgA across bronchial epithelium. *Am Rev Respir Dis* 1981;123:115–119.

38. Strober W, Krakauer R, Kleavemen HL, Reynolds HY, Nelson DL. Secretory component deficiency: a unique disorder of the IgA immune system. *N Engl J Med* 1976;294:351–366.

39. Merrill WW, Goodenberg D, Strober W, Matthay RA, Naegel GP, Reynolds HY. Free secretory component and other proteins in human lung lavage. *Am Rev Respir Dis* 1980;122:156–161.

40. Delacroix DL, Dive C, Rambaud JC, Vaerman JP. IgA subclasses in various secretions and in serum. *Immunology* 1982;47:383–385.

41. Jonard PP, Rambaud JC, Dive C, Vaerman JP, Galian A, Delacroix DL. Secretion of immunoglobulins and plasma proteins from the jejunal mucosa—transport rate and origin of polymeric immunoglobulin A. *J Clin Invest* 1984;74:525–535.

42. Marada JL. Loosening tight junctions—lessons from the intestine. *J Clin Invest* 1989;83:1089–1094.

43. Granström G, Askelöf P, Granström M. Specific immunoglobulin A to *Bordetella pertussis* antigens in mucosal secretions for rapid diagnosis of whooping cough. *J Clin Microbiol* 1988;26:869–874.

44. Brown TA, Murphy BR, Radl J, Haaijman JJ, Mestecky J. Subclass distribution and molecular form of immunoglobulin A hemagglutinin antibodies in sera and nasal secretions after experimental secondary infection with influenza A virus in humans. *J Clin Microbiol* 1985;22:259–264.

45. Reynolds HY, Merrill WW. Lung immunology: humoral and cellular immune responsiveness of the respiratory tract. *Curr Pulmonol* 1981;3:381–422.

46. Conley ME, Delacroix DL. Intravascular and mucosal immunoglobulin A: two separate but related systems of immune defense. *Ann Intern Med* 1987;106:892–899.

47. Bergmann KC, Waldman RH. Stimulation of secretory antibody following oral administration of antigen. *Rev Infect Dis* 1988;10:939–950.

48. Reynolds HY, Kazmierowski JA, Newball HH. Specificity of opsonic antibodies to enhance phagocytosis of *Pseudomonas aeruginosa* by human alveolar macrophages. *J Clin Invest* 1975;56:376–385.

49. Reynolds HY, Atkinson JP, Newball HH, Frank MM. Receptors for immunoglobulin and complement on human alveolar macrophages. *J Immunol* 1975;114:1813–1819.

50. Jarvis GA, Griffiss JM. Human IgA1 initiates complement-mediated killing of *Neisseria meningitidis*. *J Immunol* 1989; 143:1703–1709.

51. Sibille Y, Chafelain B, Staquet P, Merrill WW, Delacroix DL, Vaerman JP. Surface IgA and Fc-alpha receptors on human alveolar macrophages from normals and patients with sarcoidosis. *Am Rev Respir Dis* 1986;139:292–297.

52. Finkelstein RA, Sciortino CV, McIntosh MA. Role of iron in microbe–host interactions. *Rev Infect Dis* 1983;5:S759–S777.

53. Bell DY, Haseman JA, Spock A, McLennan G, Hook GER. Plasma proteins of the broncho alveolar surface of the lungs of smokers and non-smokers. *Am Rev Respir Dis* 1981;124:72–79.

54. LaForce FM, Boose DS, Ellison RT. Effect of aerosolized *Escherichia coli* and *Staphylococcus aureus* on iron and iron-binding proteins in lung lavage fluid. *J Infect Dis* 1986;154:959–965.

55. Thompson AB, Bohling T, Payvandi F, Rennard SI. Lower respiratory tract lactoferrin and lysozyme arise primarily in the airways and are elevated in association with chronic bronchitis. *J Lab Clin Med* 1990;115:148–150.

56. Reynolds HY, Chretien J. Respiratory tract fluids: analysis of content and contemporary use in understanding lung diseases. *DM* 1984;30;1–103.

57. Arnold RR, Brewer M, Gauthier JJ. Bactericidal activity of human lactoferrin: sensitivity of a variety of microorganisms. *Infect Immun* 1980;28:893–898.

58. Bortner CA, Miller RD, Arnold RR. Bactericidal effect of lactoferrin on *Legionella pneumophila*. *Infect Immun* 1986; 51:373–377.

59. Kaltreider HB. Initiation of immune responses in the lower respiratory tract with red cell antigens. In: Kirkpatrick CH, Reynolds HY, eds. *Immunologic and infectious reactions in the lung*. New York: Marcel Dekker, 1976;73–100.

60. Bienenstock J. Bronchus-associated lymphoid tissue. In: Bienenstock J, ed. *Immunology of lungs and upper respiratory tract*. New York: McGraw-Hill, 1984;96–118.

61. Bienenstock J, Befus D. Gut and bronchus associated lymphoid tissue. *Am J Anat* 1984;170:437–445.

62. Brownstein DG, Rebar AH, Bice DE, Muggenburg BA, Hill JO. Immunology of the lower respiratory tract: serial morphologic changes in the lungs and tracheobronchial lymph nodes of dogs after intrapulmonary immunization with sheep erythrocytes. *Am J Pathol* 1980;98:499–514.

63. Moritz ED, Naegel GP, Smith GJW, Reynolds HY. Bronchus associated lymphoid tissue in a sub-human primate model of cell mediated immunity. *Am Rev Respir Dis* 1984;129:A7.

64. Clancy RL, Pucci AA, Jelihovsky T, Bye P. Immunologic "memory" for microbial antigens in lymphocytes obtained from human bronchus mucosa. *Am Rev Respir Dis* 1978; 117:513–518.

65. Racz P, Tenner-Racz K, Myrvik QN, Fainter LK. Functional architecture of bronchial associated lymphoid tissue and lymphoepithelium in pulmonary cell-mediated reactions in the rabbit. *J Reticuloendothel Soc* 1977;22:59–83.

66. Van der Brugge-Gamelkoorn GJ, Van de Ende MB, Sminia T. Non-lymphoid cells of bronchus-associated lymphoid tissue of the rat in situ and in suspension—with special reference to interdigitating and follicular dendritic cells. *Cell Tissue Res* 1985;239:117–182.

67. Mestecky J. The common mucosal immune system and current

strategies for induction of immune responses in external secretions. *J Clin Immunol* 1987;7:265–276.

68. Weisz-Carrington P, Grimes SR Jr, Lamm ME. Gut-associated lymphoid tissue as source of an IgA immune response in respiratory tissues after oral immunization and intrabronchial challenge. *Cellular Immunology* 1987;106:132–138.

69. Fick RB, Richerson HB, Zavala DC, Hunninghake GW. Bronchoalveolar lavage in allergic asthmatics. *Am Rev Respir Dis* 1987;135:1204–1209.

70. Sertl K, Takemura T, Tschachler E, Ferrans VJ, Kaliner MA, Shevach EM. Dendritic cells with antigen-presenting capability reside in airway epithelium, lung parenchyma, and visceral pleura. *J Exp Med* 1986;163:436–451.

71. Holt PG, Schon-Hegrad MA, Oliver J. MHC class II antigen-bearing dendritic cells in pulmonary tissues of the rat. *J Exp Med* 1988;167:262–274.

72. VanVoorhis WC, Witmer MD, Steinman RM. The phenotype of dendritic cells and macrophages. *Fed Proc* 1983;42:3114–3118.

73. Weissler JC, Lyon CR, Lipscomb MF, Toews GB. Human pulmonary macrophages. Functional comparison of cells obtained from whole lung and by bronchoalveolar lavage. *Am Rev Respir Dis* 1986;133:473–477.

74. Nicod LP, Lipscomb MF, Weissler JC, Lyons CR, Albertson J, Towes GB. Mononuclear cells in human lung parenchyma—characterization of a potent accessory cell not obtained by bronchoalveolar lavage. *Am Rev Respir Dis* 1987;136:818–823.

75. Kaltreider HB. Alveolar macrophages—enhancers or suppressors of pulmonary immune reactivity? *Chest* 1982;82:261–262.

76. Reynolds HY. Bronchoalveolar lavage—state of the art. *Am Rev Respir Dis* 1987;135:250–263.

77. O'Neill SJ, Lesperance E, Klass DJ. Human lung lavage surfactant enhances staphylococcal phagocytosis by alveolar macrophages. *Am Rev Respir Dis* 1984;130:1177–1179.

78. Coonrod JD. The role of extracellular bactericidal factors in pulmonary host defenses. *Semin Respir Infect* 1986;1:118–129.

79. Czop JK, McGowan SE, Center DM. Opsonin-independent phagocytosis by human alveolar macrophages: augmentation by human plasma fibronectin. *Am Rev Respir Dis* 1982;125:607–609.

80. Rennard SI, Hunninghake GW, Bitterman PB, Crystal RG. Production of fibronectin by the human alveolar macrophage: a mechanism for the recuitment of fibroblasts to sites of tissue injury in the interstitial lung diseases. *Proc Natl Acad Sci USA* 1981;78:7147–7151.

81. Mold C, Rogers CP, Kaplan RL, Gewurz H. Binding of human C-reactive protein to bacteria. *Infect Immun* 1982;38:392–395.

82. Merrill WW, Naegel GP, Olchowski JJ, Reynolds HY. Immunoglobulin G subclass proteins in serum and lavage fluid of normal subjects: quantitation and comparison with immunoglobulins A and E. *Am Rev Respir Dis* 1985;131:584–591.

83. Reynolds HY. Immunoglobulin G and its function in the human respiratory tract. *Mayo Clinic Proc* 1988;63:161–174.

84. Siber GR, Schur PH, Aisenberg AC, Weitzman SA, Schiffman G. IgG₂ concentrations and the antibody response to bacterial polysaccharide antigens. *N Engl J Med* 1980;303:178–182.

85. Fick RB, Olchowski J, Squier SU, Merrill WW, Reynolds HY. Immunoglobulin-G subclasses in cystic fibrosis: IgG₂ response to Pseudomonas lipopolysaccharide. *Am Rev Respir Dis* 1986;133:418–420.

86. Patterson R, Wang JLK, Fink JN, Calvanico NJ, Roberts M. IgA and IgG antibody activities of serum and bronchoalveolar fluid from symptomatic and asymptomatic pigeon breeders. *Am Rev Respir Dis* 1979;120:1113–1118.

87. Calvanico NJ, Ambegaonkar SP, Schlueter DP, Fink JN. Immunoglobulin levels in bronchoalveolar lavage fluid from pigeon breeders. *J Lab Clin Med* 1980;96:129–140.

88. Beck CS, Heiner DC. Selective immunoglobulin G₄ deficiency and recurrent infections of the respiratory tract. *Am Rev Respir Dis* 1981;124:94–96.

89. Gross GM, Rehm SR, Pierce AK. The effect of complement depletion on lung clearance of bacteria. *J Clin Invest* 1978;62:373–378.

90. Robertson J, Caldwell JR, Castle JR, Waldman RH. Evidence for the presence of components of the alternate (properdin) pathway of complement activation in respiratory secretions. *J Immunol* 1976;117:900–903.

91. Reynolds HY, Fulmer JD, Kazmierowski JA, Roberts WC, Frank MM, Crystal RG. Analysis of cellular and protein components of bronchoalveolar lavage fluid from patients with idiopathic pulmonary fibrosis and hypersensitivity pneumonitis. *J Clin Invest* 1977;59:165–177.

92. Hance AF, Douches S, Winchester RJ, Ferrans VJ, Crystal RG. Characterization of mononuclear phagocytic subpopulation in the human lung by using monoclonal antibodies. *J Immunol* 1985;134:284–292.

93. Sandron D, Reynolds HY, Laval AM, Venet A, Israel-Biet D, Chretien J. Human alveolar subpopulations isolated on discontinuous albumin gradients—cytological and functional heterogeneity. *Eur J Respir Dis* 1986;68:177–185.

94. Golde DW, Byers LA, Finley TN. Proliferative capacity of human alveolar macrophage. *Nature* 1974;247:373–375.

95. Bitterman PB, Saltzman LE, Adelberg S, Ferrans VJ, Crystal RG. Alveolar macrophage replication—one mechanism for the expansion of the mononuclear phagocyte population in the chronically inflammed lung. *J Clin Invest* 1984;74:460–469.

96. Hunninghake GW, Crystal RG. Pulmonary sarcoidoses: a disorder mediated by excess helper T-lymphocyte activity at sites of disease activity. *N Engl J Med* 1981;305:429–434.

97. Saltini C, Spurzem JR, Lee JJ, Pinkston P, Crystal RG. Spontaneous release of interleukin 2 by lung T lymphocytes in active pulmonary sarcoidosis is primarily from the Leu + DR + T cell subset. *J Clin Invest* 1988;77:1962–1970.

98. Robinson BWS, Pinkston P, Crystal RG. Natural killer cells are present in the normal human lung but are functionally impotent. *J Clin Invest* 1984;74:942–950.

99. Rankin JA, Naegel GP, Schrader CE, Matthay RA, Reynolds HY. Airspace immunoglobulin production and levels in bronchoalveolar lavage fluid of normals and patients with sarcoidosis. *Am Rev Respir Dis* 1983;127:442–448.

100. Reynolds HY. Respiratory infections may reflect deficiencies in host defense mechanisms. *DM* 1985;31:1–98.

101. Green GM, Kass EH. The role of the alveolar macrophage in the clearance of bacteria from the lung. *J Exp Med* 1964;119:167–175.

102. Jackson AE, Southern PM, Pierce AK, Fallis BD, Sanford JP. Pulmonary clearance of gram negative bacilli. *J Lab Clin Med* 1967;69:833–841.

103. Murray HW. Interferon-gamma, the activated macrophage, and host defense against microbial challenge. *Ann Intern Med* 1988;108:595–608.

104. Salahuddin SZ, Rose RM, Groopman JE, Markham PD, Gallo RC. Human T lymphotropic virus type III infection of human alveolar macrophages. *Blood* 1986;68:281–284.

105. Nash TW, Libby DM, Horwitz MA. IFN-gamma activated human alveolar macrophages inhibit the intracellular multiplication of *Legionella pneumophila*. *J Immunol* 1988;140:3978–3981.

106. Reynolds HY. Lung inflammation: normal host defense or a complication of some diseases. *Annu Rev Med* 1987;38:295–323.

107. Nathan CF. Secretory products of macrophages. *J Clin Invest* 1987;79:319–326.

108. Sibille Y, Naegel GP, Merrill WW, Young KR, Reynolds HY. Neutrophil chemotactic activity produced by normal and activated human lung cells. *J Lab Clin Med* 1987;110:624–633.

109. Martin TR, Raghu G, Merritt TL, Henderson WR Jr. Relative contribution of leukotriene B₄ to the neutrophil chemotactic activity by the resident human alveolar macrophage. *J Clin Invest* 1987;80:1114–1124.

110. Rankin JA, Collman R, Daniele RP. Acquired immune deficiency syndrome and the lung. *Chest* 1988;94:155–164.

111. Wallace JM, Barbers RG, Oishi J, Prince H. Cellular and T-lymphocyte subpopulation profiles in bronchoalveolar lavage fluid from patients with acquired immunodeficiency syndrome and pneumonitis. *Am Rev Respir Dis* 1984;130:786–790.

112. Venet A, Clavel F, Israel-Biet D, Rouzioux C, Dennewald G,

Stern M, Vittecoq D, Régnier B, Cayrol E, Chrétien J. Lung in acquired immune deficiency syndrome: infectious and immunological status assessed by bronchoalveolar lavage. *Bull Eur Physiopathol Respir* 1985;21:535–543.

113. Young KR, Rankin JA, Naegel GP, Paul ES, Reynolds HY. Bronchoalveolar lavage cells and proteins in patients with the acquired immunodeficiency syndrome—an immunologic analysis. *Ann Intern Med* 1985;103:522–533.

114. Agostini C, Poletti V, Zambello R, et al. Phenotypical and functional analysis of bronchoalveolar lavage lymphocytes in patients with HIV infection. *Am Rev Respir Dis* 1988;138:1609–1615.

THE LUNG: Scientific Foundations
edited by R.G. Crystal, J.B. West et al.
Raven Press, Ltd., New York © 1991.

CHAPTER 7.4.2

Deficiency in Host Defense

Kenneth J. Holroyd and Ronald G. Crystal

To perform its function as the organ for gas exchange, the lung by necessity is exposed to microorganisms that may be present in air and blood. To appropriately deal with these organisms, the lung has a complex host defense system to immobilize, suppress, destroy, and remove infectious agents (see Chapters 2.10, 3.1.2, 3.1.3, 3.4.1–3.4.8, 7.3.1, 7.3.2, and 7.4.1). Although the major components of pulmonary host defense are conveniently categorized into discrete "systems" such as antibody (B-cell)-mediated, T-cell-mediated, phagocytic, mucociliary clearance, and complement, there are multiple complex interactions among these components as they help defend the organ.

One approach to help understand the relative importance of each of these systems is to evaluate the "immunodeficiency" disorders, a group of hereditary and acquired diseases, many of which have pulmonary manifestations (Table 1). In this regard, we will focus on three human immunodeficiency diseases where pulmonary manifestations are relatively important: chronic granulomatous disease (CGD), infection with the human immunodeficiency virus (HIV), and immunoglobulin (Ig) A deficiency. Each of these disorders serves as a model to understand the importance of different components of lung host defense: CGD as a model for understanding phagocytic cell defenses; infection with HIV as an example of a disorder that affects multiple components of the host defense, including cell-mediated immunity, antibody-mediated immunity, and phagocytic cells, eventually leading to the acquired immune deficiency syndrome (AIDS); and IgA deficiency as a model to evaluate the contribution of epithelial antibody defenses. For details concerning the insights gained in pulmonary defense regarding the other components of the host defense system, the reader is referred to the above-mentioned chapters and to recent reviews (1–3).

CHRONIC GRANULOMATOUS DISEASE

Chronic granulomatous disease is a heritable, usually fatal, disease characterized by phagocytic cells with absent or severely deficient ability to respond to activation signals to generate a "respiratory burst"— that is, the production of superoxide anion (O_2^-) and other reactive oxygen species (4,5). It serves as a remarkable example of the critical importance of phagocytes (mononuclear phagocytes and neutrophils) in pulmonary antimicrobial host defense. Clinically, the disease results in recurrent, severe bacterial and fungal infections typically involving the skin, soft tissues, lymph nodes, liver, spleen, and respiratory tract (6). CGD, which is an uncommon disorder, has been used to define the mechanisms by which phagocytic cells generate O_2^-, a process that is central to the role of phagocytes in host defense. Recently, biochemical and molecular genetic techniques have led to an understanding of (a) the components of phagocytic cells that generate O_2^- and (b) the gene abnormalities that cause CGD. The definition of specific defects in the condition has led to a better understanding of the normal functioning of this important host defense system and to new treatment strategies for the disorder.

Clinical Manifestations

CGD is characterized by recurrent infections, suppurative granulomas, and infiltration of viscera with pigmented, lipid-laden macrophages (6,7). The disorder is usually diagnosed before 1 year of age. The disease may be inherited in an X-linked fashion (65%) or on an autosomal recessive basis (35%) (5,7). In addition,

K. J. Holroyd and R. G. Crystal: Pulmonary Branch, National Heart, Lung and Blood Institute, National Institutes of Health, Bethesda, Maryland 20892.

TABLE 1. *Disorders of host defense with prominent pulmonary manifestations*[a]

Category	Disorder
Phagocytic dysfunction	Chronic granulomatous disease
	Glucose 6-phosphate dehydrogenase deficiency
	Chédiak–Higashi syndrome
Cellular (T-cell) deficiency	Human immunodeficiency virus (HIV) infection[b]
	Congenital thymic aplasia
	Nucleoside phosphorylase deficiency
Antibody (B-cell) deficiency	Selective IgA deficiency
	Selective deficiency of IgG subclasses
	Hyper-IgM immunodeficiency
	Common variable immunodeficiency
	Infantile X-linked hypogammaglobulinemia
	Thymoma-associated immunodeficiency
	Kappa light-chain deficiencies
	Hyper-IgE syndrome
Combined (B- and T-cell) deficiency	Ataxia–telangiectasia syndrome
	Adenosine deaminase deficiency
	Wiskott–Aldrich syndrome
	Classical severe combined immunodeficiency
Mucociliary transport defect	Immotile cilia syndromes
	Kartagener's syndrome
Complement deficiency	C3 deficiency

[a] Three of these disorders (CGD, HIV infection, and IgA deficiency) are used in this chapter as examples of disorders of pulmonary host defense; for a review of the general group of disorders see ref. 98.

[b] While HIV infection causes a major deficiency of the cellular immune system, it is also associated with abnormalities in phagocyte and B-cell function (see text).

a kindred with probable autosomal dominant inheritance has been described (8). Patients with the autosomal recessive form may have less severe symptoms and onset later in life (9). Carriers of X-linked CGD do not have increased susceptibility to infection, but they have been observed to have an increased frequency of discoid lupus erythematosus and aphthous stomatitis (10).

Infections may occur in any organ, but sites normally exposed to or colonized by fungi or bacteria present the greatest risk. Thus, involvement of the respiratory tract is frequent, with infections of the lower respiratory tract being the most common cause of death (6). Usually, the lung infections are caused by *Staphylococcus aureus,* enteric bacteria, or aspergillus species. The pneumonias may be accompanied by hilar adenopathy, but abscess formation is uncommon (11).

Repeated infections may lead to chronic lung disease with granulomatous inflammation and pulmonary fibrosis (12). The granulomas include multinucleated giant cells, macrophages, lymphocytes, and plasma cells (6). The macrophages often contain pigmented lipid material, the genesis of which is not understood, although it is likely that both the granuloma formation and lipid inclusions are related in some manner to the incomplete degradation of phagocytosed material.

Biochemistry of the Respiratory Burst

When phagocytes engulf bacteria or other particulate material, a marked change in cellular metabolism occurs, during which cellular utilization of oxygen increases rapidly, leading to large amounts of O_2^{-}, hydrogen peroxide (H_2O_2), hydroxyl radical (OH^-), and possibly singlet oxygen release by these cells into their phagolysosomes and, to a lesser extent, into the extracellular milieu (13). Because myeloperoxidase is also released into phagocytic vacuoles in neutrophils, the respiratory burst is accompanied by the conversion of H_2O_2 to the very toxic hypohalide radical. This reaction, known as the "respiratory burst," begins 30–60 sec after contact with the phagocytic cellular membrane is made by the microorganism (7,13). During this delay, the signal transduction steps take place that lead to activation of the respiratory burst oxidase, referred to as "NADPH oxidase" because of its use of reduced nicotinamide-adenine dinucleotide phosphate (NADPH). The generation of these highly reactive oxygen species plays a central role in the ability of phagocytes to kill microorganisms (14). Interestingly, the organisms that most commonly cause infections in CGD contain catalase, an antioxidant enzyme that neutralizes H_2O_2 (15); that is, in the context of an impotent respiratory burst, the catalase-containing organisms have an even further advantage over the host defense system.

Many stimuli activate the respiratory burst *in vitro,* including the following: phorbol esters; calcium ionophores; plant lectins; inert particles; peptides (synthetic, bacteria-derived, and complement-derived); fluoride ion; immune complexes; products of arachidonic acid metabolism; phospholipase C; analogues of inositol and diacylglycerol; antineutrophil antibodies; detergents; cytochalasin E; platelet-activating factor; leukotriene B$_4$; and platelet-derived growth factor (7,16–18). At least two pathways of activation are thought to exist. One is associated with binding to G-protein-associated cellular receptors, such as the receptors for the chemotactic peptide N-formyl-methionyl-leucyl-phenylalanine (f-Met-Leu-Phe) (19). Alternatively, phorbol esters are thought to directly activate protein kinase C, leading to phosphorylation of

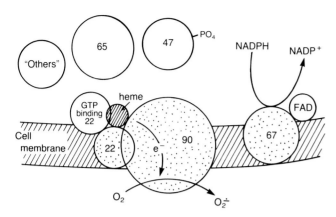

FIG. 1. Components of the NADPH oxidase system used by phagocytes to generate oxidants. As a unit, the NADPH oxidase system transfers an electron (e^-) from reduced nicotinamide-adenine dinucleotide phosphate (NADPH) to oxygen, causing the formation of superoxide anion (O_2^-) and oxidized adenine dinucleotide phosphate ($NADP^+$), which is subsequently regenerated. Components of NADPH oxidase include 90- and 22-kDa heme-associated membrane-bound proteins, a 22-kDa GTP-binding protein, a 67-kDa membrane protein able to bind NADPH and flavin adenine dinucleotide (FAD), a phosphorylated (PO_4) 47-kDa and a 66-kDa cytoplasmic protein, and possibly "other" proteins. Mutations of the genes coding for various components of the NADPH oxidase result in chronic granulomatous disease and its associated deficiency in the phagocytic arm of the host defense system.

multiple proteins, including phosphorylation of components of NADPH oxidase (19).

The generation of O_2^- is mediated by the NADPH oxidase, using NADPH as an electron donor in the one-electron reduction of O_2 to produce O_2^- (Fig. 1) (20,21). Although the structure of NADPH oxidase is not completely understood, the general structure has been determined by protein purification methods and the identification of several genes involved in CGD.

NADPH oxidase is a multicomponent enzyme complex, part of which is located in the plasma membrane. Cell fractionation experiments have shown that the dormant oxidase is located in the plasma membrane and that it requires a cytosolic component for activation (21). Attempts to purify the membrane complex of proteins responsible have not been unequivocally successful; this is because of the instability of the complex (particularly with regard to salts), making separations difficult on most chromatographic media, and because of its inactivity without stimulation (22).

The plasma membrane components include a 90-kDa glycosylated subunit and a 22-kDa nonglycosylated subunit. Together, the two subunits are tightly associated and contain a heme group, likely bound to the 22-kDa subunit (8,23,24). The 90-kDa and 22-kDa subunits and heme act as a unit to form the terminal component of the NADPH oxidase, since it directly

reduces O_2 to O_2^-. This membrane-bound unit of the NADPH oxidase system is referred to as cytochrome b_{-245} (the midpoint potential of the cytochrome is -245 mV) or cytochrome b_{558} (it absorbs at 558 nm). Another membrane component is a 67-kDa protein, likely a flavoprotein, requiring flavin adenine dinucleotide (FAD) to function (25,26). This protein can bind NADPH, and it probably acts to convert intracellular NADPH to $NADP^+$ (8,25). Quinn et al. (27) reported that a 22-kDa GTP-binding protein with characteristics of a ras oncogene product was isolated with the 22-kDa cytochrome b_{-245} subunit (27). In addition to the membrane components, there are at least two, and probably three or more, cytoplasmic subunit components (28). One, a 47-kDa protein, is phosphorylated following stimuli which activate the respiratory burst. The second is a 65-kDa protein of unknown function which migrates from the cytosol to the plasma and phagolysosomal membranes following NADPH oxidase activation. Other cytoplasmic components of the complex have been suggested but have not been definitively identified (29).

Hereditary Forms of CGD

The identification of the gene responsible for the sex-linked form of CGD was a major breakthrough in understanding how the NADPH oxidase system works and also in understanding its relationship to CGD and host defense in general. The strategy used was a novel approach that capitalized on the identification of an individual missing a portion of the X chromosome. The observation that some CGD patients have an increased frequency of the blood antigen Xg, and that some have an absence of the Kell-related antigen Kx (30), led to assignment of the defective gene to the short arm of the X chromosome (Xp). Then, in the context that the cell line HL-60 was known to contain the respiratory burst oxidase, a subtraction library was made using (a) cDNA from the HL-60 cell line and (b) RNA from an individual with a deletion of Xp (31,32). The remaining cDNA, now enriched for respiratory burst-related transcripts from the Xp, was hybridized to a collection of genomic bacteriophage clones from Xp. Two bacteriophage clones were reactive; using this portion of the bacteriophage clones as a probe, a 4.5-kb mRNA was isolated (by Northern blot analysis) from HL-60 cells and from other phagocytic cells (31,32). Other cell types did not contain this mRNA species. The importance to X-linked CGD was demonstrated by its absence in three of the first four of such patients who were examined. This mRNA was subsequently shown to be the 90-kDa subunit of cytochrome b_{-245} (33,34).

In the vast majority of X-linked CGD patients examined to date, the 90-kDa subunit is absent on Western blot analysis of neutrophils (8). The defects in the gene are heterogeneous; only a minority result from gene deletions large enough to be detected by conventional Southern blot analysis (32). The remaining X-linked patients show a variety of functional defects of the NADPH oxidase, reflecting a variety of mutations in the CGD gene that are as yet undefined (8,32).

The concept of autosomal recessive CGD having a different molecular defect than the X-linked form became evident from *in vitro* studies in which the respiratory burst was reconstructed by fusing phagocytes (or components of phagocytes) from individuals with CGD with different inheritance of the disease. Hybrid monocytes, created by *in vitro* fusion of cells from X-linked and autosomal recessive CGD patients, demonstrated normal respiratory burst activity as evidenced by reduction of the dye nitroblue tetrazolium (NBT) (35). Similarly, respiratory burst activity generated in a cell-free system including subcellular fractions of disrupted cells showed that whereas most X-linked CGD patients had defective activity of their membrane fraction, most autosomal recessive patients had defective activity in their cytosolic fraction (28,29,36,37). One subgroup of individuals with the autosomal recessive form of CGD are missing the 47-kDa cytoplasmic component of the NADPH oxidase system. The function of this protein is not clear; however, it has been found that this protein translocates from the cytoplasm into the membranes upon activation of the NADPH oxidase (38). Interestingly, this translocation does not occur in X-linked CGD, suggesting that the membrane binding of the 47-kDa protein is likely to cytochrome b_{-245} or to an associated molecule (32). A deficiency of the 65-kDa cytoplasmic protein has been found in a few individuals with the autosomal recessive form of CGD (28). The molecular defects for the remainder of the autosomal recessive form of CGD are unknown.

Modulation of the NADPH Oxidase System with Interferon-γ

The understanding of the NADPH oxidase system at the molecular and biochemical levels, and of its relevance to CGD, has led to the development of a specific therapy for this disorder with interferon-γ (IFN-γ), a cytokine that normally plays a major role in phagocyte activation. When normal mononuclear phagocytes, including alveolar macrophages, are exposed to IFN-γ *in vitro,* there is an enhancement of the respiratory burst, with increased production of O_2^- and more efficient killing of microorganisms (39). With regard to the components of the NADPH oxidase system, when monocytes, neutrophils, the promonocytic cell lines THP-1 and U937, or alveolar macrophages are cul-

tured in the presence of IFN-γ, the level of the mRNA transcripts for the 90-kDa subunit of cytochrome b_{-245} is increased (40,41). It is not clear how this occurs in the THP-1 cells, but it likely is through transcriptional regulation. Tumor necrosis factor was observed to have a similar effect on mRNA levels. Cytochrome b_{-245} protein levels are also increased in cells incubated in IFN-γ. IFN-γ has no effect on the mRNA level of the 22-kDa cytochrome b_{-245} subunit, but it does cause an increase in the level of the 47-kDa cytoplasmic phosphorylated protein (8).

Depending on the subgroup, similar effects are observed when IFN-γ is added to phagocytic cells of CGD patients *in vitro*. Most autosomal recessive patients whose cells contained cytochrome b_{-245} showed an increase in oxidase activity from undetectable levels to approximately 15% of normal (8,32). In contrast, most X-linked individuals whose cells are cytochrome b_{-245}-deficient showed no response, though some showed a partial response. Some individuals with abnormalities in other components of the NADPH oxidase also show a response. Furthermore, subcutaneous administration of IFN-γ to patients with CGD showed changes in NADPH oxidase activity in neutrophils and monocytes that mimic the *in vitro* responses (32). Importantly, the changes in oxidase activity reflected improvements in *in vitro* bacterial killing, with marked improvement in NADPH oxidase activity to approximately 10% of normal. The *in vivo* effects of IFN-γ on autosomal recessive patients are thought to result, at least in part, from improved interaction between the NADPH-binding molecule and the cytochrome b_{-245}, conceivably by the increased synthesis of the 47-kDa phosphoprotein. In X-linked patients, IFN-γ responders are thought to have an increase in partially functional cytochrome b_{-245}; nonresponders likely have large gene deletions. It is quite likely, however, that IFN-γ induces other components of the NADPH oxidase system and that it possibly enhances nonoxidative mechanisms of bacterial killing.

Based on these concepts, a multi-institutional clinical trial of chronic IFN-γ treatment of CGD was initiated, and results demonstrated a marked decrease in the numbers and severity of infections in treated individuals (42). With regard to the lung, direct administration of IFN-γ to the lower respiratory tract by aerosol has been shown to be safe and capable of directly activating alveolar macrophages (43). Although this strategy has not been tried in CGD, it may offer some advantage for prevention of pulmonary infection. Gene therapy with hematopoietic stem cells containing the normal gene is a potential approach to future therapy.

HUMAN IMMUNODEFICIENCY VIRUS INFECTION

The human immunodeficiency virus (HIV) is the etiologic agent of the acquired immunodeficiency syndrome (AIDS), a disorder characterized by (a) low numbers of CD4$^+$ T-lymphocytes in blood, (b) opportunistic infections, and (c) unusual neoplasms, including Kaposi's sarcoma (44). Infection of the lower respiratory tract is the most common presentation of AIDS, and it is the leading cause of morbidity and mortality in this disease. HIV infection occurs principally through sexual contact, the use of infected syringes for intravenous drug abuse, and the administration of infected blood products. In this context, with the knowledge that HIV principally infects cells of the immune system, it serves as an example of the importance of components of the host defense system in protecting the lung.

Pneumocystis carinii is the most frequent cause of pneumonia, with *Mycobacterium avium-intracellulare, Mycobacterium tuberculosis,* cytomegalovirus, and a variety of other organisms being less frequent (45). The spectrum of pulmonary infections associated with AIDS varies depending on geographic location and consequent exposure to specific pathogens. For example, *Mycobacterium tuberculosis* infection is more common in African than in North American

AIDS patients. The kind of infections in AIDS patients may eventually provide clues to the specific nature of the immunodeficiency in AIDS and might help to understand the relationship of different components of the host defense system in protecting the lung. For example, the nature of an immune defect that greatly increases the risk of pneumocystis infection over all other infections is unknown, as is the nature of an immune defect that allows infection with *Mycobacterium avium-intracellulare* to increase greatly but that allows infection with other atypical mycobacteria to increase only slightly.

Structure of HIV

HIV is an RNA retrovirus; that is, it is composed of nucleic acid in the RNA form, and it carries the enzyme reverse transcriptase that allows the virus to make DNA from viral RNA once inside the cell (46) (Fig. 2). A central cone-shaped core contains the RNA, reverse transcriptase, and the p7 and p9 structural proteins associated with the viral RNA. The cone-shaped core is composed of the structural protein p24, which is surrounded by a circular coat of p17 protein. A membrane bilayer, derived from the cell from which the virus has bud, surrounds the p17 layer. Through the membrane bilayer sticks the glycoprotein gp41, at-

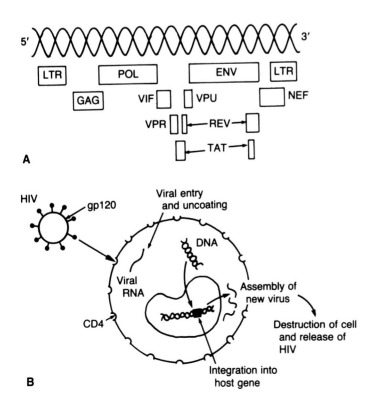

FIG. 2. Structure and function of the human immunodeficiency virus (HIV). **A:** Structure of the HIV provirus. Shown is the double-stranded DNA form of HIV that inserts into the genome. The overall length is 9.7 kb. The structural genes of HIV, along with their function, include: LTR (5' and 3' long terminal repeats; insertion and transcription); gag (core proteins); pol (enzymes); env (envelope proteins); tat (positive regulator); rev (differential regulator); vif (infectivity factor); vpr (positive regulator?); vpu (packaging factor); and nef (negative regulator). See text for details. **B:** Consequences of infection of CD4$^+$ T cells by HIV. The gp120 coat protein of HIV binds to the CD4 protein on the surface of the T cell, permitting viral entry and uncoating. The viral RNA is converted into double-stranded DNA by the reverse transcriptase carried by the virus. The virus integrates into the host genome and directs the synthesis of new virus, destroying the host T cell and releasing new infectious HIV.

tached to which is the knob-shaped glycoprotein gp120 on the surface of the virus.

The 9.7-kb HIV genome contains the standard retroviral env (coding for gp41 and gp120), gag (coding for the structural proteins noted above), and pol (coding for reverse transcriptase and the associated RNase H and protease) genes, as well as the 5' and 3' long terminal repeat (LTR) containing viral integration and regulatory sequences. Most of the other HIV genes are used for regulation. The tat gene codes for a viral trans-activating factor that up-regulates viral replication (47). The rev gene product alters the splicing pattern of viral RNA, resulting in greater production of gag and env gene products than of regulatory gene products (48). Vif (viral infectivity factor) enhances the infectivity of HIV by an unknown mechanism (49). Expression of the nef gene likely down-regulates viral replication, though this point is controversial (50,51). Vpu protein is involved in proper viral maturation and release from cells (52). Vpr may be an additional enhancer of viral replication (53).

Cellular Infection and Viral Life Cycle

HIV can infect two major components of the host defense system, CD4$^+$ helper/inducer T-lymphocytes and mononuclear phagocytes. Infection begins by the binding of viral gp120 to the cell-surface CD4 molecule (54), a glycoprotein present in large numbers on the surface of the CD4$^+$ T cell and, to a far lesser extent, on the surface of mononuclear phagocytes. The virus then fuses with the cellular membrane, most likely with the assistance of gp41, and enters the cytoplasm (55). Viral uncoating of the core RNA and reverse transcriptase ensues, and viral RNA is transcribed into DNA and then integrated into the cellular genome. This integrated DNA form of the virus is known as the *provirus*. Evidence suggests that usually only one copy of the provirus incorporates into the genome of the host cell (56). A pathway of viral entry that may be important for mononuclear phagocytes is the one that occurs via the immunoglobulin G Fc receptor. In this scenario, antibody formed in response to HIV infection binds to the virus, the complex of antibody and HIV is bound by the Fc receptor, and the virus is able to enter the cell (57). Cell-to-cell spread of the virus is also postulated (58).

In the blood, the principal infected cell during asymptomatic HIV infection and in AIDS seems to be the CD4$^+$ lymphocyte, though some individuals have evidence of HIV infection of monocytes, as assessed by polymerase chain reaction of purified cell populations (59,60). It is possible that monocytes sometimes are the first cell population infected (61), since the virus can be isolated (in some individuals) from puri-fied monocytes but not from purified T cells. However, other observers have cast doubts about this circumstance being a frequent occurrence (62). In the lung, it is known that alveolar macrophages are infectable by HIV *in vitro* (63), and virus has been isolated from bronchoalveolar lavage samples (64). Viral RNA has been demonstrated in lung inflammatory cells by *in situ* hybridization, but the percentage of positive cells is only 0.0002% (65). There is no direct information regarding which lung inflammatory cells are infected, although it is likely that both lung CD4$^+$ T cells and alveolar macrophages are targets for the virus. Although the *in situ* hybridization data suggest that the extent of infection is not great, this methodology is relatively insensitive, because it cannot evaluate cells in which HIV is integrated into the host genome but which express RNA at low levels or which remain in a latent state with no RNA transcription.

Increased replication of proviral DNA in T cells is caused by activation of the T cells, such as by antigen or mitogen. Activation of the T cell causes cellular factors such as NFkB to bind to the viral LTR and activate tat gene transcription (66). Tat proteins may act as a viral-produced cell-to-cell "hormone" to increase replication, since tat is taken up by lymphocytes and macrophage cell lines *in vitro*, causing activation of viral replication (67). Cytokines such as tumor necrosis factor may influence similar pathways in both T cells and mononuclear phagocytes, and they can modify viral replication *in vitro* (68,69). Following transcription of viral sequences, assembly of virions is associated with viral budding in T cells until the rate of viral replication becomes so high that the cell lyses. In mononuclear phagocytes, virions may be retained in large numbers in the cytoplasm (70).

Early Immune Dysfunction Following HIV Infection

There is clear evidence that asymptomatic HIV-seropositive individuals have dysfunction of various components of the host defense system prior to the actual development of opportunistic infections and AIDS. Lymphoid hyperplasia, B-cell activation with hypergammaglobulinemia, and autoantibody formation are common (71). T cells respond poorly to soluble recall antigens such as tetanus toxoid, although their proliferation in response to mitogens is usually unaltered (72). B cells are less able to respond to antigens or mitogens. There is some evidence that blood monocytes may have decreased ability to present antigens to T cells, as well as decreased ability to act as accessory cells for T-cell activation (73).

The mechanism of these abnormalities is not known. One of the remaining questions regarding HIV infection is, How does the low viral burden of HIV, measured by polymerase chain reaction DNA analysis (56,59,60) or by quantitative culture of blood mononuclear cells (74), average only one cell in 500–5000 cells and yet clearly influence the remaining immune cells? It has been suggested that a soluble mediator(s) influenced or produced by infected cells may adversely affect immune function in these individuals, or that suppressor lymphocytes may develop in response to viral antigens. One example of such a mediator includes tumor necrosis factor (TNF), known to be produced by virus-infected mononuclear phagocytes and shown in vitro to influence other immune cells (68). Another example is the systemic deficiency of the tripeptide glutathione (GSH) observed in plasma and lung epithelial lining fluid of asymptomatic HIV-seropositive individuals (75). Although the pathogenesis of the systemic GSH deficiency in HIV-seropositive individuals is unknown, GSH appears to be necessary for optimal T-cell and B-cell function; that is, a GSH-deficient state in concert with other HIV-induced abnormalities may help expand the immunodeficiency consequences of HIV infection.

Progression to AIDS

The average time from HIV infection to progression to AIDS is 10 years, with shorter periods for infants, the elderly, and transfusion-related AIDS (76). Over this period of time, there is a gradual evolution of the virus in each individual. In this regard, a genetic heterogeneity of HIV isolates exists in each individual (77), and sequential isolates in an individual show increased ability to replicate and cause cytopathicity as AIDS approaches (78). The virus can also lose its ability to respond to negative regulatory signals such as the nef protein (79). Viral replication increases during progression to AIDS, as assessed by quantitative cultures and increasing plasma levels of viral antigens (80). Furthermore, the ability of CD8[+] T cells to inhibit viral replication decreases shortly before the decline in the blood CD4[+] T-cell count; this may be due to declining CD4[+] T-cell function in giving help for cytotoxic responses, or it may be a function of the evolution of the virus.

As AIDS approaches there is a progressive and often rather precipitous decline in CD4[+] T-lymphocyte count (81). "Memory" T cells primed to respond to recall antigens seem to be preferentially depleted. Compared to asymptomatic HIV-seropositive individuals, AIDS patients have a higher blood burden of virus, with an average of about one in 100 CD4[+] T cells infected; this may gradually cause significant T-cell depletion through viral replication, thereby causing cell lysis (59). Immune destruction of T cells that

have taken up, processed, and presented gp120 as an antigen is another possible mechanism of T-cell loss (82).

Responses of the Lung to HIV Infection

Bronchoalveolar lavage studies have demonstrated that a CD8[+] T-cell alveolitis exists in many asymptomatic individuals with HIV infection (83). At least some of these lymphocytes are able to participate in cytotoxic responses against autologous alveolar macrophages and other cells expressing HIV antigens such as p17 in a class I histocompatibility locus-restricted manner (84,85).

Consistent with these lavage findings, morphologic studies have demonstrated a lymphocyte interstitial pneumonitis in up to 40% of individuals with blood CD4[+] T-cell counts of less than 200 (86,87). Biopsy specimens show lymphoid interstitial infiltrates or lymphoid aggregates, usually in a perivascular or peribronchial location. There can be an associated cough and low-grade fever. This pneumonitis is independent of identifiable lung infection other than HIV, although it is conceivable that it results from a pathogen such as cytomegalovirus. Lymphoid interstitial pneumonitis, characterized by infiltration of the lung with a mixture of lymphocytes, plasma cells, and immunoblasts, is more common in children infected with HIV (88). Again, the relationship of this pathology to the HIV is unknown; however, in this syndrome the highest level of viral RNA is detected by in situ hybridization (0.1% positive cells), and the highest level of HIV p24 antigen is detected in bronchoalveolar lavage (64,65)—consistent with the concept that the virus may play a direct role.

Augmentation of Pulmonary Host Defense in HIV Infection

The primary therapeutic strategy in HIV infection is to suppress viral replication throughout the body with drugs such as azidothymidine (AZT) (89). With regard to augmenting pulmonary host defense, delivery of pentamidine by aerosol has resulted in a marked reduction in the incidence of pulmonary infection by Pneumocystis carinii. Other lung-specific strategies being considered to augment pulmonary host defense include aerosol delivery of IFN-γ and GSH (43,90).

IMMUNOGLOBULIN A DEFICIENCY

Selective immunoglobulin A (IgA) deficiency is defined by very low levels of serum IgA (<5 mg/dl; normal 61–330 mg/dl) in the presence of normal or increased serum IgG and IgM levels (91). The serum deficiency of IgA in these individuals is reflected in a deficiency of IgA on their mucosal surfaces, including the upper respiratory tract, where IgA is normally the major immunoglobulin isotype (see Chapters 3.4.3, 7.4.1). IgA deficiency is the most common primary immunodeficiency, occurring in about one in 600 individuals of European ancestry, although it is less common in Japanese and blacks. Its occurrence is usually sporadic, but instances of familial IgA deficiency have been reported with both autosomal dominant and recessive inheritance (92,93), with rare reports of abnormalities of chromosome 18 (93). In addition, IgA deficiency has been associated with congenital infection with rubella, as well as with administration of the drug phenytoin (94,95).

Despite the fact that IgA is the most common immunoglobulin on the mucosal surface of the upper respiratory tract, its role in pulmonary host defense is unclear, as evidenced by the fact that most individuals with IgA deficiency are asymptomatic (96,97). However, some IgA-deficient individuals have an increased number of respiratory tract infections, including bronchitis and pneumonia, with upper respiratory infection being more common than infection of the lower respiratory tract. Streptococcus and hemophilus species are the most common organisms. The infections usually are less severe than in panhypoglobulinemic patients, and chronic pulmonary disease with bronchiectasis is unusual (98).

Structure and Function of IgA

IgA exists predominantly as a monomer in the serum, but it exists mostly as a polymer (usually dimers) on mucosal surfaces (99,100). Dimeric IgA is found on the respiratory tract epithelial surface combined with two glycoproteins, a 15.6-kDa joining (J) chain and a 70-kDa secretory component (SC) (Fig. 3). The IgA is synthesized by B cells in the bronchial wall along with J chain, forming an IgA-dimer–J-chain complex. The SC is synthesized by the epithelial cells, and it sits on the basolateral membrane of these cells to help transport the IgA across the epithelial cell into the bronchial lumen as an IgA-dimer–J–SC complex. In addition to helping the IgA bind to secretory component, the J chain increases IgA's avidity for antigen but decreases its susceptibility to proteolytic attack. Secretory IgA is thus unique among immunoglobulins, because its components are synthesized by two different cell types and also because it exists in its natural milieu in combination with two other proteins.

Experimental manipulation of amounts of IgA on mucosal surfaces has shown a clear protective effect of increasing amounts of IgA on organisms that affect mucosa or that gain systemic entry through the mucosa. Although a number of theories have been advanced, the mechanism of the protective effect of IgA on mucosal surfaces is not well understood. IgA-mediated activation of the alternative complement pathway has been demonstrated (101), but it is not likely

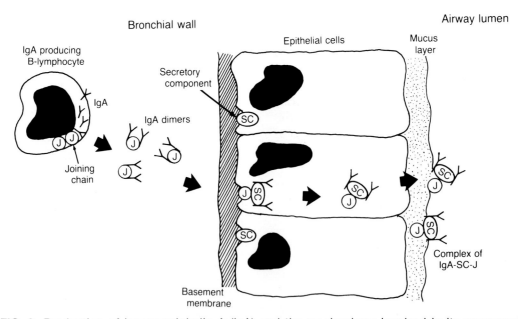

FIG. 3. Production of immunoglobulin A (IgA) and the mechanisms involved in its movement onto the respiratory epithelial surface. IgA produced by B-lymphocytes in the bronchial wall is secreted into the interstitium along with the joining chain (J), forming an IgA-dimer–J complex. This is picked up by the secretory component (SC) on the basolateral surface of epithelial cells, transported through the epithelial cell, and secreted onto the mucosal complex of the airway lumen as an IgA dimer–SC–J complex.

important on the respiratory epithelial surface, where concentrations of complement are very low. Direct killing of type 8 pneumococci was demonstrated by the first IgA monoclonal antibody of known specificity, obtained by immortalizing B cells from a patient immunized with Pneumovax vaccine (102); however, other examples of this phenomenon have not been demonstrated. Neutrophils, monocytes, and lymphocytes have surface receptors for IgA, and cellular cytotoxicity to bacteria in the presence of IgA has been demonstrated using human cells for pseudomonas, salmonella, and staphylococcal species (103–106). The most likely role for IgA is to bind to bacteria, particularly to bacterial structures that bind to cellular receptors—thereby preventing attachment and colonization of mucosal surfaces, and enhancing clearance by the epithelial cilia (107). IgA is also important in protecting the respiratory epithelium from viruses, although the mechanisms involved are not well understood (108,109).

Pathogenesis of IgA Deficiency

Almost all individuals with IgA deficiency have apparently normal IgA genes, and they also have B cells that bear IgA on their surface. However, these B cells also express IgM, as is normally the case in newborns but not in immunologically mature individuals. These B cells fail to undergo plasma cell differentiation, leading to IgA deficiency (110,111). Although T-cell development appears normal in these individuals, it is conceivable that suppressor T cells exist for IgA plasma cell development; such T cells have been demonstrated to exist in a few IgA-deficient individuals, although their importance in creating the deficiency is unknown (112,113). Anti-IgA antibodies have been found in a few individuals (114–116). An increase in class I histocompatibility locus B8 has been associated with IgA deficiency (117,118), but HLA identical twins may be discordant for IgA deficiency (98). Thus, the pathophysiology of IgA deficiency remains unknown.

The reasons for the clinical spectrum of IgA-deficient individuals from normal to increased susceptibility to infection are also unclear. An individual with an IgA level of less than 5 mg/dl is more likely to have infections than an individual with a level that is more than 2 standard deviations below normal but above 5 mg/dl (119). However, even the severely deficient may be asymptomatic. About 15% of IgA-deficient individuals are also IgG2, IgG3, and/or IgG4 subclass-deficient, and some reports have suggested that this group is more predisposed to infection (i.e., those susceptible may have immunoglobulin deficiencies) (120,121), although this association has not been confirmed (122). Some individuals can compensate for IgA deficiency

by increasing the number of IgM plasma cells and antibody on the mucosal surface, where they are normally rare (123,124).

Therapy of IgA Deficiency

Most individuals with IgA deficiency do not require therapy. In symptomatic patients, vigorous antibiotic therapy is employed; for individuals with frequent infections, prophylactic antibiotics are used. Intravenous immunoglobulin therapy is rarely needed, and with this therapy there is a potential risk of anti-IgA antibody formation with subsequent anaphylaxis upon reexposure (96).

IMPLICATIONS FOR UNDERSTANDING PULMONARY HOST DEFENSE

Comparison of the clinical manifestations of CGD, HIV infection, and IgA deficiency shows a remarkable disparity in the types and severity of abnormalities in pulmonary host defense. In contrast to CGD, where impairment of the ability of phagocytes to generate oxidants is associated with an inability of the pulmonary host defense system to clear organisms such as staphylococcus, enteric bacteria, or aspergillus, the CD4+ T cell and mononuclear phagocyte infection of HIV causes a very different problem for the lung, primarily with unusual organisms such as pneumocystis, mycobacteria and cytomegalovirus. Despite the differences in CGD and HIV infection, and the differences in types of resulting pulmonary infections, both are fatal disorders; that is, the impairments in pulmonary host defenses rendered by loss of normal phagocytic oxidant production or the loss of T cells (and other abnormalities in HIV) lead to the obvious conclusion that these functions are critical to pulmonary host defense, or that there is a lack of mechanisms to compensate for their loss. In contrast, IgA deficiency causes only a relatively mild problem, and only in a proportion of affected individuals, suggesting that its role in respiratory host defense is minor and that there are sufficient overlapping systems to compensate for its loss.

REFERENCES

1. Afzelius BA, Mossberg B. Immotile-cilia syndrome (primary ciliary dykinesia) including Kartagener syndrome. In: Scriver CR, Beaudet AL, Sly WS, Valle D, eds. *The metabolic basis of inherited disease.* New York: McGraw–Hill, 1989;2739–2750.
2. Glass DN, Fearon DT, Austen KF. Inherited abnormalities of the complement system. In: Stanbury JB, Wyngaarden JB, Fredrickson DS, Goldstein JL, Brown MS, eds. *The metabolic*

basis of inherited disease. New York: McGraw–Hill, 1983; 1934–1955.

3. Holmes ER, Whaley W. Complement and related clinical disorders. *Blood Rev* 1989;3:120–129.

4. Tauber AI, Borregaard N, Simons E, Wright J. Chronic granulomatous disease: a syndrome of phagocyte oxidase deficiencies. *Medicine* 1983;62:286–309.

5. Curnutte JT, ed. Phagocytic defects II: abnormalities of the respiratory burst. *Hematol/Oncol Clin North Am* 1988;2:1–336.

6. Johnston RB, Newman SL. Chronic granulomatous disease. *Pediatr Clin North Am* 1977;24: 365–376.

7. Forehand JR, Nauseef WM, Johnston RB. Inherited disorders of phagocyte killing. In: Scriver CR, Beaudet AL, Sly WS, Valle D, eds. *The metabolic basis of inherited disease.* New York: McGraw–Hill, 1989;2779–2801.

8. Gallin JI, Malech HL. Update on chronic granulomatous diseases of childhood. *JAMA* 1990;263:1533–1537.

9. Weening WS, Adriaansz LH, Weemaes CMR, Lutter R, Roos D. Clinical differences in chronic granulomatous disease in patients with cytochrome b-negative or cytochrome b-positive neutrophils. *J Pediatr* 1985;107:102–104.

10. Schaller J. Illness resembling lupus erythematosus in mothers of boys with chronic granulomatous disease. *Ann Intern Med* 1972:747–750.

11. Wolfson JJ, Quie PG, Laxdal SD, Good RA. Roentgenologic manifestations in children with a genetic defect of polymorphonuclear leukocyte function. *Radiology* 1968;91:37–48.

12. Dilworth JA, Mandell GL. Adults with chronic granulomatous disease of "childhood." *Ann Intern Med* 1977;63:233–243.

13. Klebanoff SJ. Phagocytic cells: products of oxygen metabolism. In: Gallin JI, Goldstein IM, Snyderman R, eds. *Inflammation.* New York: Raven Press, 1988;391–444.

14. Johnston RB, Keele BB, Misra HP, et al. The role of superoxide anion generation in phagocytic bactericidal activity. *J Clin Invest* 1975;55:1357–1372.

15. Mandell GL, Hook EW. Leukocyte bactericidal activity in chronic granulomatous disease: correlation of bactrial hydrogen peroxide production and susceptibility to intracellular killing. *J Bacteriol* 1969;100:531–532.

16. Curnutte JT, Babior BM. Chronic granulomatous disease. *Adv Hum Genet* 1987;10:229–297.

17. Tzeng DY, Deuel TF, Huang JS, Senior RM, Boxer LA, Baehner RL. Platelet-derived growth factor promotes polymorphonuclear leukocyte activation. *Blood* 1984;64:1123–1128.

18. Ingraham LM, Coates TD, Allen JM, Higgins CP, Baehner RL, Boxer LA. Metabolic, membrane, and functional responses of human polymorphonuclear leukocytes to platelet-activating factor. *Blood* 1982;59:1259–1266.

19. Andrews PC, Babior BM. Phosphorylation of cytosolic proteins by resting and activated human neutrophils. *Blood* 1984;64:883–890.

20. Clark RA, Leidal KG, Pearson DW, Nauseef WM. NADPH oxidase of human neutrophils. *J Biol Chem* 1987;262:4065–4074.

21. Curnutte JT, Kuver R, Scott PJ. Activation of neutrophil NADPH oxidase in a cell free system. *J Biol Chem* 1987;262:5563–5569.

22. Segal AW. The electron transport chain of the microbicidal oxidase of phagocytic cells and its involvement in the molecular pathology of chronic granulomatous disease. *J Clin Invest* 1989;83:1785–1793.

23. Parkos CA, Allen RA, Cochrane CG, Jesaitis AJ. Purified cytochrome b from human granulocyte plasma membrane is comprised of two polypeptides with relative molecular weights of 91,000 and 22,000. *J Clin Invest* 1987;80:732–742.

24. Nugent JHA, Gratzer W, Segal AW. Identification of the haembinding subunit of cytochrome b_{-245}. *Biochem J* 1989;264:921–924.

25. Gabig TG, Lefker BA. Deficient flavoprotein component of the NADPH-dependent O_{2-} generation oxidase in the neutrophils from three male patients with chronic granulomatous disease. *J Clin Invest* 1984;73:701–705.

26. Cross AR, Jones OTG. The association of FAD with the cytochrome b_{-245} of human neutrophils. *Biochem J* 1982; 208:759–763.

27. Quinn MT, Parkos CA, Walker L, Orkin SH, Dinauer MC, Jesaitis AJ. Association of a ras-related protein with cytochrome b of human neutrophils. *Nature* 1989;342:198–200.

28. Volpp BD, Nauseef WM, Clark RA. Two cytosolic neutrophil oxidase components absent in autosomal chronic granulomatous disease. *Science* 1988;242:1295–1297.

29. Curnutte JT, Scott PJ, Mayo LA. Cytosolic components of the respiratory burst oxidase: resolution of four components, two of which are missing in complementing types of chronic granulomatous disease. *Proc Natl Acad Sci USA* 1989;86:825–829.

30. Marsh WL, Uretsky SC, Douglas SD. Antigens of the Kell blood group system on neutrophils and monocytes: their relation to chronic granulomatous disease. *J Pediat* 1975; 87:1117–1120.

31. Royer-Pokora B, Kunkel LM, Monaco AP, et al. Cloning the gene for an inherited human disorder—chronic granulomatous disease—on the basis of its chromosomal location. *Nature* 1986;322:32–38.

32. Orkin SH. Molecular genetics of chronic granulomatous disease. *Annu Rev Immunol* 1989;7:277–307.

33. Teahan C, Rowe P, Parker P, Totty N, Segal AW. The X-linked chronic granulomatous disease gene codes for the β-chain of cytochrome b_{-245} *Nature* 1987;327:720–721.

34. Dinauer MC, Orkin SH, Brown R, Jesaitis AJ, Parkos CA. The glycoprotein encoded by the X-linked chronic granulomatous disease locus is a component of the neutrophil cytochrome b complex. *Nature* 1987;327:717–720.

35. Hamers MN, De Boer M, Meerhof LJ, Weening RS, Roos D. Complementation in monocyte hybrids revealing genetic heterogeneity in chronic granulomatous disease. *Nature* 1984; 307:553–555.

36. Nunoi H, Rotrosen D, Gallin JI, Malech HL. Two forms of autosomal chronic granulomatous disease lack distinct neutrophil cytosol factors. *Science* 1988;242:1298–1301.

37. Lomax KJ, Leto TL, Nunoi H, Gallin JI, Malech HL. Recombinant 47-kilodalton cytosol factor restores NADPH oxidase in chronic granulomatous disease. *Science* 1989;245:409–412.

38. Clark RA, Volpp BD, Leidal KG, Nauseef WM. Two cytosolic components of the human neutrophil respiratory burst oxidase translocate to the plasma membrane during cell activation. *J Clin Invest* 1990;85:714–721.

39. Murray HW. Interferon-gamma, the activated macrophage, and host defense against microbial challenge. *Ann Intern Med* 1988;108:595–608.

40. Newberger PE, Ezekowitz RAB, Whitney C, Wright J, Orkin SH. Induction of phagocyte cytochrome b heavy chain gene expression by interferon γ. *Proc Natl Acad Sci USA* 1988; 85:5215–5219.

41. Jaffe HA, Buhl R, Borok Z, Trapnell B, Crystal RG. Activated alveolar macrophages express increased levels of cytochrome b-245 heavy chain mRNA transcripts correlating with enhanced capacity to release oxidants. *Clin Res* 1989;37:477A.

42. International collaborative study group to assess rIFN-γ in CGD. Clinical efficacy of recombinant human interferon gamma (rIFN-γ) in chronic granulomatous disease (CGD). *Clin Res* 1990;38:465A.

43. Jaffe HA, Buhl R, Mastrangeli A, et al. Organ specific cytokine therapy: upregulation of interferon-γ specific genes in alveolar macrophages by aerosolization of recombinant interferon-γ to the human lung. *Clin Res* 1990;38:405A.

44. Levy JA, ed. *AIDS: pathogenesis and treatment.* New York: Marcel Dekker, 1989.

45. Rankin JA, Collman R, Daniele RP. Acquired immune deficiency syndrome and the lung. *Chest* 1988;94:155–164.

46. Haseltine WA, Wong-Staal F. The molecular biology of the AIDS virus. *Sci Am* 1988;Oct:52–63.

47. Muessing MA, Smith DH, Capon DJ. Regulation of mRNA accumulation by a human immunodeficiency virus trans-activator protein. *Cell* 1987;48:691–701.

48. Malim MH, Hauber J, Le S-Y, Maizel JV, Cullen BR. The HIV-1 rev trans-activator acts through a structured target sequence

to activate nuclear export of unspliced viral mRNA. *Nature* 1989;338:254–257.

49. Fisher AG, Ensoli B, Ivanoff L, et al. The sor gene of HIV-1 is required for efficient virus transmission *in vitro. Science* 1987;237:888–893.

50. Ahmad N, Venkatesan S. Nef protein of HIV-1 is a transcriptional repressor of HIV-1 LTR. *Science* 1988;241:1481–1485.

51. Kim S, Ikeuchi K, Byrn R, Groopman J, Baltimore D. Lack of a negative influence on viral growth by the nef gene of human immunodeficiency virus type 1. *Proc Natl Acad Sci USA* 1989;86:9544–9548.

52. Klimkait T, Strebel K, Hoggan MD, Martin MA, Orenstein JM. The human immunodeficiency virus type 1-specific protein vpu is required for efficient virus maturation and release. *J Virol* 1990;64:621–629.

53. Cohen EA, Terwilliger EF, Jalinoos Y, Proulx J, Sodroshi JG, Haseltine WA. Identification of HIV-1 vpr product and function. *J AIDS* 1990;3:115–122.

54. Sattenau QJ, Weiss RA. The CD4 antigen: physiological ligand and HIV receptor. *Cell* 1988;52:631–633.

55. Gallaher WR. Detection of a fusion peptide sequence in the transmembrane protein of human immunodeficiency virus. *Cell* 1987;50:327–328.

56. Simmonds P, Balfe P, Peutherer JF, Ludlam CA, Bishop JO, Brown AJL. Human immunodeficiency virus-infected individuals contain provirus in small numbers of peripheral mononuclear cells and at low copy numbers. *J Virol* 1990;64:864–872.

57. Takeda A, Tuazon CU, Ennis FA. Antibody-enhanced infection by HIV-1 via Fc receptor-mediated entry. *Science* 1988;242:580–583.

58. Fauci AS. The human immunodeficiency virus: infectivity and mechanisms of pathogenesis. *Science* 1988;239:617–622.

59. Schnittman SM, Psallidopolous MC, Lane HC, et al. The reservoir for HIV-1 in human peripheral blood is a T cell that maintains expression of CD4. *Science* 1989;245:305–308.

60. Psallidopolous MC, Schnittman SM, Thompson LM, et al. Integrated proviral human immunodeficiency virus type 1 is present in CD4+ peripheral blood lymphocytes in healthy seropositive individuals. *J Virol* 1989;63:4626–4631.

61. Popovic M, Gartner S. Isolation of HIV-1 from monocytes but not T lymphocytes. *Lancet* 1987;ii:916.

62. McElrath MJ, Pruett JE, Cohn ZA. Mononuclear phagocytes of blood and bone marrow: comparative roles as viral reservoirs in human immunodeficiency virus type 1 infections. *Proc Natl Acad Sci USA* 1989;86:675–679.

63. Salahuddin SZ, Rose RM, Groopman JE, Markham PD, Gallo RC. Human T lymphocyte virus III infection of human alveolar macrophages. *Blood* 1986;68:281–284.

64. Linneman CC, Baughman RP, Frame PT, Floyd R. Recovery of human immunodeficiency virus and detection of p24 antigen in bronchoalveolar lavage fluid from adult patients with AIDS. *Chest* 1989;96:64–67.

65. Chayt KJ, Harper ME, Marselle LM, et al. Detection of HTLV-III RNA in lungs of patients with AIDS and pulmonary involvement. *JAMA* 1986;256:2356–2359.

66. Nabel G, Baltimore D. An inducible transcription factor activates expression of human immunodeficiency virus in T cells. *Nature* 1987;326:711–713.

67. Frankel AD, Pabo CO. Cellular uptake of the tat protein from human immunodeficiency virus. *Cell* 1988;55:1189–1193.

68. Folks TM, Justement J, Kinter A, Dinarello CA, Fauci AS. Cytokine induced expression of HIV-1 in a chronically infected promonocyte cell line. *Science* 1987;238:800–802.

69. Koyanagi Y, O'Brien WA, Zhao JQ, Golde DW, Gasson JC, Chen ISY. Cytokines alter production of HIV-1 from primary mononuclear phagocytes. *Science* 1988;241:1673–1675.

70. Orenstein JM, Meltzer MS, Phipps T, Gendelman HE. Cytoplasmic assembly and accumulation of human immunodeficiency virus types 1 and 2 in recombinant human colony-stimulating factor-1 treated human monocytes: an ultrastructural study. *J Virol* 1988;62:2578–2586.

71. Edelman AS, Zolla-Pazner S. AIDS: a syndrome of immune dysregulation, dysfunction, and deficiency. *FASEB J* 1989;3:22–30.

72. Lane HC, Depper JM, Greene WC, Whalen G, Waldmann TA, Fauci AS. Qualitative analysis of immune function in patients with the acquired immunodeficiency syndrome. *N Engl J Med* 1985;313:79–84.

73. Chantal Petit AJ, Tersmette M, Terpstra FG, et al. Decreased accessory cell function by human monocytic cells after infection with HIV. *J Immunol* 1988;140:1485–1489.

74. Ho DD, Moudgil T, Alam M. Quantitation of human immunodeficiency virus type 1 in the blood of infected persons. *N Engl J Med* 1989;321:1621–1625.

75. Buhl R, Jaffe HA, Holroyd KJ, et al. Systemic glutathione deficiency in symptom-free HIV-seropositive individuals. *Lancet* 1989;ii:1294–1298.

76. Bacchetti P, Moss AR. Incubation period of AIDS in San Francisco. *Nature* 1989;338:251–253.

77. Fisher AG, Ensoli B, Looney D, et al. Biologically diverse molecular variants within a single HIV-1 isolate. *Nature* 1988;334:444–447.

78. Tersmette M, Lange JMA, deGoede REY, et al. Association between biological properties of human immunodeficiency virus variants and risk for AIDS and AIDS mortality. *Lancet* 1989;i:983–985.

79. Cheng-Mayer C, Iannello P, Shaw K, Luciw PA, Levy JA. Differential effects of nef on HIV replication: implications for viral pathogenesis in the host. *Science* 1989;246:1629–1632.

80. Redfield RS, Burke DS. HIV infection: the clinical picture. *Sci Am* 1988;Oct:90–98.

81. Polk BF, Fox R, Brookmeyer R, et al. Predictors of the acquired immunodeficiency syndrome developing in a cohort of seropositive homosexual men. *N Engl J Med* 1987;316:61–66.

82. Siliciano RF, Lawton T, Knall C, et al. Analysis of host–virus interactions in AIDS with anti-gp120 T cell clones: effect of HIV sequence variation and a mechanism for CD4+ cell depletion. *Cell* 1988;54:561–575.

83. Guillon J-M, Autran B, Denis M, et al. Human immunodeficiency virus-related lymphocytic alveolitis. *Chest* 1988;94:1264–1270.

84. Plata F, Autran B, Martins LP, et al. AIDS-virus specific cytotoxic T lymphocytes in lung disorders. *Nature* 1987;328:348–351.

85. Autran B, Mayaud CM, Raphael M, et al. Evidence for a cytotoxic T-lymphocyte alveolitis in human immunodeficiency virus-infected patients. *AIDS* 1988;2:179–183.

86. Suffredini AF, Ognibene FP, Lack EE, et al. Nonspecific interstitial pneumonitis: a common cause of pulmonary disease in the acquired immunodeficiency syndrome. *Ann Intern Med* 1987;107:7–13.

87. Ognibene FP, Masur H, Rogers P, et al. Nonspecific interstitial pneumonitis without evidence of *Pneumocystis carinii* in asymptomatic patients infected with human immunodeficiency virus (HIV). *Ann Intern Med* 1988;109:874–879.

88. White DA, Matthay RA. Noninfectious pulmonary complications of infection with the human immunodeficiency virus. *Am Rev Respir Dis* 1989;140:1763–1787.

89. Polsky B. Antiviral chemotherapy for infection with human immunodeficiency virus. *Rev Infect Dis* 1989;11:S1648–1663.

90. Buhl R, Holroyd KJ, Borok Z, et al. Reversal of the glutathione deficiency in the lower respiratory tract of HIV-seropositive individuals by glutathione aerosol therapy. *Clin Res* 1990;in press.

91. Amman AJ, Hong R. Selective IgA deficiency: presentation of 30 cases and a review of the literature. *Medicine* 1971;60:223–236.

92. Wilton AN, Cobain TJ, Dawkins RL. Family studies of IgA deficiency. *Immunogenetics* 1985;21:333–342.

93. Grundbacher FJ. Genetic aspects of selective immunoglobulin A deficiency. *J Med Genet* 1972;9:344–347.

94. Soothill JF, Hayes K, Dudgeon JA. The immunoglobulins in congenital rubella. *Lancet* 1966;i:1385–1388.

95. Gilhus NE, Aarli JA, Thorsby E. HLA antigens in epileptic patients with drug-induced immunodeficiency. *J Immunopharmacol* 1982;4:517–520.

96. Hanson LA, Bjorkander J, Carlsson B, Robertson D, Soderstrom T. The heterogeneity of IgA deficiency. *J Clin Immunol* 1988;8:159–162.

97. Morgan G, Levinsky RJ. Clinical significance of IgA deficiency. *Arch Dis Child* 1988;63:579–581.

98. Cooper MD, Butler JL. Primary immunodeficiency diseases. In: Paul WE, ed. *Fundamental immunology.* New York: Raven Press, 1989;1033–1057.

99. Childers NK, Bruce MG, McGhee JR. Molecular mechanisms of immunoglobulin A defense. *Annu Rev Microbiol* 1989; 43:503–536.

100. Conley ME, Delacroix DL. Intravascular and mucosal immunoglobulin A: two separate but related systems of immune defense? *Ann Intern Med* 1987;106:892–899.

101. Hiemstra PS, Gorter A, Stuurman ME, Leendert AVE, Daha MR. Activation of the alternative pathway of complement by human serum IgA. *Eur J Immunol* 1987;17:321–326.

102. Steinitz M, Tamir S, Ferne M, Goldfarb A. A protective human monoclonal IgA antibody produced *in vitro*: anti-pneumococcal antibody engendered by Epstein-Barr virus-immortalized cell line. *Eur J Immunol* 1986;16:187–193.

103. Monteiro RC, Kubagawa H, Cooper MD. Cellular distribution, regulation, and biochemical nature of an Fcα receptor in humans. *J Exp Med* 1990;171:597–613.

104. Gorter A, Hiemstra PS, Leijh PCJ, et al. IgA- and secretory IgA-opsonized *S. aureus* induce a respiratory burst and phagocytosis by polymorphonuclear leucocytes. *Immunology* 1987;61:303–309.

105. Tagliabue A, Villa L, de Magistris MT, et al. IgA-driven T cell-mediated anti-bacterial immunity in man after live oral Ty 21a vaccine. *J Immunol* 1986;137:1504–1510.

106. Tagliabue A, Villa L, Boraschi D, et al. Natural anti-bacterial activity against *Salmonella typhi* by human T4+ lymphocytes armed with IgA antibodies. *J Immunol* 1985;135:4178–4182.

107. Stokes CR, Soothill JF, Turner MW. Immune exclusion is a function of IgA. *Nature* 1975;255:745–746.

108. Taylor HP, Dimmock NJ. Mechanism of neutralization of influenza virus by secretory IgA is different from that of monomeric IgA or IgG. *J Exp Med* 1985;161:198–209.

109. Possee RD, Schild GC, Dimmock NJ. Studies on the mechanism of neutralization of influenza virus by antibody: evidence that neutralizing antibody (anti-haemagglutinin) inactivates influenza virus *in vivo* by inhibiting virion transcriptase activity. *J Gen Virol* 1982;58:373–386.

110. Levitt D, Cooper MD. Immunoregulatory defects in a family with selective IgA deficiency. *J Pediatr* 1981;98:52–58.

111. Conley ME, Cooper MD. Immature IgA B cells in IgA-deficient patients. *N Engl J Med* 1981;305:495–497.

112. Schwartz SA. Heavy chain-specific suppression of immunoglobulin synthesis and secretion by lymphocytes from patients with selective IgA deficiency. *J Immunol* 1980;124:2034–2041.

113. Atwater JS, Tomas TB. Suppressor cells and IgA deficiency. *Clin Immunol Immunopathol* 1978;9:379–384.

114. Mellander L, Bjorkander J, Carlsson B, Hanson LA. Secretory antibodies in IgA-deficient and immunosuppressed individuals. *J Clin Immunol* 1986;6:284–291.

115. Vyas GN, Holmdahl L, Perkins HA, Fudenberg HH. Serologic specificity of human anti-IgA and its significance in transfusion. *Blood* 1969;34:573–581.

116. van Loghem E. Familial occurrence of isolated IgA deficiency associated with antibodies to IgA. *Eur J Immunol* 1974;4:57–60.

117. Hammarstrom I, Smith CIE. HLA-A, B, C and DR antigens in immunoglobulin A deficiency. *Tissue Antigens* 1983;21:75–79.

118. Hammarstrom I, Axelson U, Bjorkander J, Hanson LA, Moller E, Smith CIE. HLA antigens in selective IgA deficiency. *Tissue Antigens* 1984;24:35–39.

119. Plebani A, Ugazio AG, Monafo V, Burgio GR. Clinical heterogeneity and reversibility of selective immunoglobulin A deficiency in 80 children. *Lancet* 1986;i:829–831.

120. Bjorkander J, Bake B, Oxelius V-A, Hansson LA. Impaired lung function in patients with IgA deficiency and low levels of IgG2 or IgG3. *N Engl J Med* 1985;313:720–724.

121. Beard LJ, Ferrante A, Oxelius V-A, Maxwell GM. IgG subclass deficiency in children with IgA deficiency presenting with recurrent or severe respiratory infections. *Pediatr Res* 1986; 20:937–942.

122. Plebani A, Ugazio AG, Monafo V. Selective IgA deficiency: an update. *Curr Probl Dermatol* 1989;18:66–78.

123. Brandtzaeg P, Fjellanger I, Gjeruldsen ST. Immunoglobulin M: synthesis and selective secretion in patients with immunoglobulin A deficiency. *Science* 1968;160:789–791.

124. Plebani A, Mira E, Mevio E, et al. IgM and IgD concentrations in the serum and secretions of children with selective IgA deficiency. *Clin Exp Immunol* 1983;53:689–696.

THE LUNG: Scientific Foundations
edited by R.G. Crystal, J.B. West et al.
Raven Press, Ltd., New York © 1991.

CHAPTER 7.5.1

Granulomatous Processes

Roland M. du Bois, Kenneth J. Holroyd, Cesare Saltini,
and Ronald G. Crystal

As the organ of gas exchange, the lung is chronically exposed to the ambient air and the entire cardiac output and is therefore exposed to a broad array of contaminants, including infectious agents, inorganic particulates, and foreign antigens. When the contaminant is not easily degraded and/or slowly released, the inflammatory/immune system within the lung sometimes resorts to a host defense strategy referred to as "granuloma formation," a process characterized by the accumulation of cells of the mononuclear phagocyte system into relatively discrete structures (1–3). For pulmonary granulomas, these mononuclear phagocytes include (to varying degrees depending on the age of the granuloma and the inciting agent): freshly recruited blood monocytes; alveolar macrophages; and two forms of differentiated macrophages, epithelioid cells and giant cells (4). Most pulmonary granulomas also contain lymphocytes. Some contain Langerhans' cells, whereas others include neutrophils and/or eosinophils (5–7).

Although granuloma formation is not unique to the lung, the mechanism of granuloma formation likely evolved as a form of host defense, and thus the lung is a common site for granulomas. Pulmonary granulomas may become troublesome for two reasons. First, the sheer volume of inflammatory cells may distort the interstitial architecture, thereby interfering with the normal process of gas exchange. Second, the inflammatory process may cause tissue damage and fibrosis, which can result in permanent dysfunction and significant morbidity (8–10).

There are various approaches to the classification of granulomas (1,3,11). Some are based on mechanisms ("nonimmune" and "immune" granulomas) or the relative rate of turnover of the composite cells ("high turnover" versus "low turnover"). Clinical approaches to classification are usually based on morphology of the granuloma ("epithelioid," "caseating" or "necrotic," or "Langerhans' cell"), location ("vascular" or "bronchocentric"), or the overall clinical syndrome ("Churg–Strauss granulomatosis"). In the context that the most common forms of pulmonary granulomatous disorders are mediated by specific immune processes, this chapter will take a mechanistic approach to discussing granulomas and will focus on "immune granulomas." Foundations for this discussion can be found in the chapters on lung lymphocytes (3.4.1), alveolar macrophages (3.4.5), the normal immune response (3.4.5), accessory cell–lymphocyte interactions (3.4.2), consequences of chronic particulate exposure (7.3.5), and integrated defense (7.4.1). For details concerning other forms of granuloma, several reviews are available (5–7,11–13).

GENERAL CONCEPTS
OF IMMUNE GRANULOMAS

"Immune" granulomas are complex structures resulting from specific cell-mediated immune mechanisms. The general paradigm of immune granuloma formation suggests a specific, T-cell-mediated response to an antigenic agent that has been processed by macrophages and presented to antigen-specific T-lymphocytes. The T-cells, in turn, direct the accumulation and differ-

R. M. du Bois: Interstitial Disease Unit, National Heart and Lung Institute, London SW3 6LR, England.

K. J. Holroyd and R. G. Crystal: Pulmonary Branch, National Heart, Lung and Blood Institute, Bethesda, Maryland 20892.

C. Saltini: Pulmonary Branch, National Heart, Lung and Blood Institute, Bethesda, Maryland 20892; and Institute for Tuberculosis and Pulmonary Diseases, University of Modena, Modena, Italy 41100.

entiation of mononuclear phagocytes in the local milieu (8,9,14).

Immune granulomas are often referred to as "epithelioid cell granulomas" because the dominant cell is the "epithelioid cell," a differentiated form of the mononuclear phagocyte (15,16). There is a central core of large (20–40 μm), polygonal epithelioid cells containing abundant cytoplasm and pale-staining nuclei surrounded by a mantle of lymphocytes and mature tissue macrophages. Some immune granulomas contain giant cells, which are derivatives of mononuclear phagocytes with multiple nuclei (16). Interspersed among the epithelioid and giant cells are small numbers of CD4+ helper–inducer T-lymphocytes. The mantle of cells surrounding the epithelioid cells consists mainly of T-cells (some with the CD4+ phenotype and some with the CD8+ suppressor–cytotoxic cell phenotype) and mature macrophages (17–19). Early fibrotic changes may be seen at the periphery of the granuloma, including fibroblasts and collagen (20).

Electron microscopic studies demonstrate that most epithelioid cells have the characteristics of a secretory cell: abundant rough endoplasmic reticulum (RER), a developed Golgi complex and prominent nucleoli, and a plasma membrane forming an interdigitating boundary which interacts with other inflammatory cells (15,21). Some epithelioid cells have less RER but more vesicles; these cells likely represent a more advanced stage of epithelioid cell evolution (21). The origins of the epithelioid cell are clearly established as being of the mononuclear–phagocyte series and thus are derived from blood monocytes. Similarly, giant cells are mononuclear phagocyte-derived (22,23), developing when two or more macrophages fuse.

Models of Granuloma Formation

A variety of strategies have been used to define the character, dynamics, and mechanisms of function of immune granulomas. Although many are not lung-specific, all available evidence suggests that the processes observed are directly relevant to immune granuloma in the lung. Among the most useful of these strategies are variants of the murine *Schistosoma* model, in which schistosomes, its eggs, or inert beads coated with egg antigens are utilized to investigate immune effector function (24–27). Leprosy has been widely used as a clinical model of immune granuloma formation, particularly cutaneous leprosy (19,28). The best-studied pulmonary human "models" of immune granuloma include the clinical disorders sarcoidosis, chronic beryllium disease, tuberculosis, and hypersensitivity pneumonitis (see refs. 10 and 29–31 for a general clinical review of these disorders). One particularly useful strategy to understand human granu-

loma formation relevant to the lung is use of the Kveim–Siltzbach reagent, a suspension of human sarcoid spleen extracted with saline (32). When administered by intradermal injection to patients with early sarcoidosis, localized granulomas develop in 4–6 weeks in 70–80% of cases, whereas no granulomas are observed in normal individuals or in other granulomatous disorders (32,33). Granulomas resembling those obtained with Kveim–Siltzbach reagent have been obtained in individuals with sarcoidosis by intradermal administration of autologous lung cells obtained by bronchoalveolar lavage (34).

Kinetics of Granuloma Formation

Cells of the mononuclear phagocyte family are the first cells to arrive at a site of a developing granuloma (33,35,36) (Fig. 1). In the lung, at least some of these cells are alveolar macrophages, with the remainder being monocytes newly arrived from the circulation. Over several days, the mononuclear phagocytes mature into epithelioid cells and giant cells. Simultaneously, lymphocytes infiltrate into the aggregates of maturing mononuclear phagocytes. The majority of these lymphocytes are CD4+ helper–inducer T-cells. As the granuloma matures, it becomes compact, with the aggregated mononuclear phagocytes and interspersed CD4+ T-cells surrounded by a rim of lymphocytes, consisting mostly of CD4+ T-cells but also containing CD8+ suppressor–cytotoxic T-cells.

Quantitative estimates of the cellular composition of human pulmonary granulomas are imprecise, even with the utilization of monoclonal antibodies to improve cell identification. In pulmonary sarcoidosis, a typical lung biopsy demonstrates granulomas containing 15–60% lymphocytes and 40–85% mononuclear phagocytes (37,38). Studies of the spatial arrangement of T-cell subsets in lymph nodes from patients with sarcoidosis have demonstrated that the ratio of CD4+ to CD8+ T-cells in the central region of the granuloma is 3–20:1, but significantly lower at the periphery of the granuloma (18,37,39). Approximately 50% of the mononuclear phagocytes are epithelioid cells, with the remainder being other forms of mononuclear phagocytes. Giant cells are usually less than 5%.

Granulomas are dynamic structures: Freshly recruited monocytes are continually entering, with mature epithelioid cells either leaving or dying. There is some proliferation of mononuclear phagocytes in granulomas, but the majority of new cells are freshly recruited (40,41). Granulomas may resolve or become fibrosed, usually by proliferation of fibroblasts in the periphery, moving inward in a centripetal fashion, resulting in a small scar.

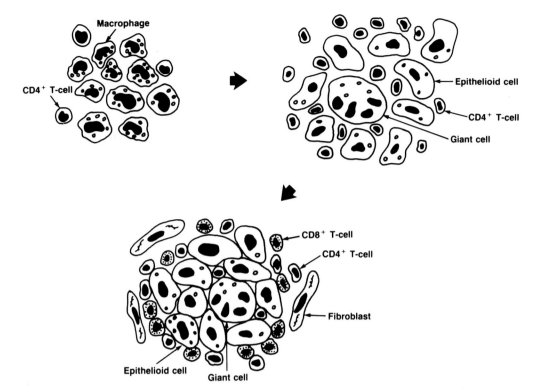

FIG. 1. The evolution of a mature immune granuloma. Shown are three stages of granuloma formation in response to a slowly degradable stimulus inducing an antigen-specific cellular immune process. **Top left:** Macrophages accumulate during the early stages. **Top right:** Coincident with an influx of CD4$^+$ helper–inducer T-cells, macrophages differentiate into epithelioid cells and giant cells. **Bottom:** In the more mature granulomas, the epithelioid and giant cells have aggregated into a compact structure. CD4$^+$ T-cells remain in close association with the central core of epithelioid cells. CD4$^+$ T-cells and CD8$^+$ suppressor–cytotoxic T-cells are observed in the area around the granuloma together with fibroblasts.

Initiation of Immune Granuloma Formation

Pulmonary immune granulomas may be initiated by infectious agents, inorganic agents, and organic particulates; the factor common to all is their low biodegradability and/or persistence, often within macrophages (Table 1) (13). The known responsible agents all act as antigens. Some, such as *Mycobacteria* species or *Thermophylic actinomycetes*, are very complex antigens, whereas others such as beryllium likely act as haptens (29,42).

All models of immune granuloma consistently demonstrate that the first step in granuloma formation is the attempt by tissue macrophages to ingest the inciting agent. For example, following the intradermal administration of the Kveim-Siltzbach reagent, the first cells to appear are mononuclear phagocytes that loosely accumulate in the local milieu (33,35,36). Within the lung, the initial cell to encounter the stimulus is the alveolar macrophage, which ingests the foreign material. Depending on the nature and quantity of the material, it either is totally degraded, is slowly degraded, or persists unchanged within the macro-

phage (43). Substances which are antigenic are internalized and processed within the antigen-presenting cell and coexpressed on its surface together with the class II major histocompatibility complex (MHC) molecules. These class II MHC molecules are necessary for antigen presentation to CD4$^+$ T-cells and are therefore necessary for the subsequent development of a cell-mediated immune response (44–48) (Fig. 2). For a T-cell-mediated response to develop, the antigenic material must be expressed on the surface of the cell as small peptide fragments (49,50). The antigenic epitopes that drive T-cell responses are "hidden" in the tertiary structure of the native molecule and are "exposed" by processing. This is in contrast to epitopes that drive B-cell responses, which are usually on the external regions of the intact protein (50).

Cellular Mechanisms of Granuloma Development

The ingestion and processing of antigen by the macrophage are followed by two processes in parallel: (i) differentiation of the macrophage into epithelioid cells

TABLE 1. *Human lung disorders characterized by granulomas*

Category	Disorder	Cells accompanying mononuclear phagocyte[a]	Dominant site of granulomas	Likely mechanism characterizing granuloma formation
Known	Foreign body[b]	None	Alveoli	Nonimmune
	Infections[c]	Lymphocyte	Alveoli	Immune
	Chronic beryllium disease	Lymphocyte	Alveoli	Immune
	Hypersensitivity pneumonitis	Lymphocyte	Alveoli	Immune
Unknown	Sarcoidosis	Lymphocyte	Alveoli, airway	Immune
	Wegener's granulomatosis	Neutrophil	Vascular, airways	Unknown
	Churg–Strauss syndrome	Eosinophil	Vascular	Unknown
	Lymphomatoid granulomatosis	Lymphocyte	Vascular	Unknown
	Bronchocentric granulomatosis	Lymphocyte, neutrophil, eosinophil	Airways	Unknown
	Langerhans' cell granulomatosis[d]	Langerhans' cell	Terminal bronchioles	Unknown

[a] Cell type usually present in addition to cells of the mononuclear phagocyte series.
[b] Relatively unusual to present as a clinically relevant problem except for rare cases such as talc inhalation or following intravenous drug use; most are alveolar based except for intravenous drug use.
[c] Common agents include myobacteria, fungi, protozoa, viruses, bacteria, and worms.
[d] Also referred to as "histiocytosis X" or "eosinophilic granuloma."

and (ii) the influx of CD4$^+$ T-cells (33). Since epithelioid cells may also exhibit surface class II MHC molecules (33,37), it is possible that both alveolar macrophages and epithelioid cells are involved in presenting the responsible antigens to specific T-cells.

The T-cell plays a central role in the early development of the immune granuloma, as evidenced by poor immune granuloma development in athymic nude mice (51–53). As in the initiation of all cell-mediated immune reactions, the CD4$^+$ T-cell recognizes the antigen presented by the macrophage in the context of the class II molecules. In addition to the direct macrophage to T-cell contact, the ensuing development of the granuloma is augmented by release of cytokines by the macrophages. The importance of at least two cytokines, interleukin 1 (IL-1) and tumor necrosis factor alpha (TNF-α), has been implicated in granuloma formation by studies utilizing an agarose bead model of granuloma formation in mice (see Chapter 2.8 for details concerning these molecules). When uncoated agarose beads are instilled into the trachea of mice, there is a minimal cellular tissue response. In contrast, beads coated with IL-1 or TNF-α produce a vigorous granulomatous response (54,55). Furthermore, aqueous extracts of granulomas produced *in vivo* by antigen-coated beads in sensitized BALB/c mice contain abundant IL-1 (56). Other macrophage mediators implicated in granuloma formation include arachidonic acid metabolites, which may play a regulatory role by their effects on class II molecule expression. Prostaglandin E down-regulates class II molecule expression on macrophages comprising granulomas, whereas prostaglandin F$_{2\alpha}$ up-regulates the expression of these molecules (57,58).

Antigen presentation, in association with secondary cytokine signals, stimulates T-cells to proliferate and to release a number of lymphokines that activate macrophages and lymphocytes and that provide the building blocks from which granulomas are formed (8,9,59). The defined lymphokines of most relevance to the generation of granulomas are interleukin 2 (IL-2, the T-cell growth factor) and interferon gamma (IFN-γ, a potent activator of macrophages). Consistent with this concept, monocytes and alveolar macrophages can be stimulated *in vitro* by IFN-γ to increase the expression of class II surface antigens, Fc receptors, IL-2 receptors, and transferrin receptors. Furthermore, under appropriate circumstances, mononuclear phagocytes will form giant cells under the influence of IFN-γ. Also implicated are lymphokines that are not fully characterized, such as monocyte chemotactic factor (a mediator that attracts monocytes), migration inhibitory factor (an inhibitor of the migration of macrophages), and macrophage-activating factor [molecule(s) that activates macrophages] (23,60–64). The relative contributions of other lymphokines to granuloma formation are not known.

The general model of the development of immune granulomas suggests that following presentation of the antigen, the activated CD4$^+$ T-cell releases a number of cytokines which drive the accumulation of antigen-specific T-cells in the local milieu. Presumably working in concert, IFN-γ, monocyte chemotactic factor, macrophage migration inhibitory factor, and macrophage-activating factor act to recruit mononuclear phagocytes. The recruited mononuclear phagocytes are then immobilized at the site of the ongoing reaction, and they are subsequently activated to mature

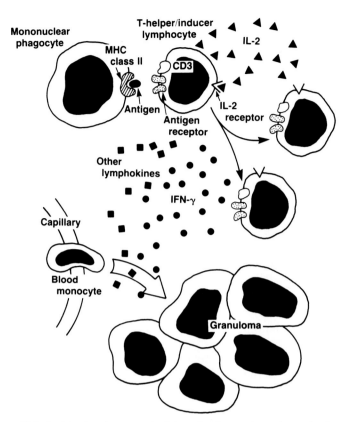

FIG. 2. Mechanisms underlying the formation of a typical immune granuloma. Antigen is presented to an antigen-specific CD4$^+$ helper–inducer T-cell by a mononuclear phagocyte in association with a class II major histocompatibility complex (MHC) molecule. The MHC–antigen complex on the mononuclear phagocyte is recognized by the antigen-specific T-cell antigen receptor (TCR). Signal transduction occurs through CD3 (a TCR-associated surface complex of glycoproteins), down-regulation, and the activation of a number of genes, including the interleukin-2 (IL-2) receptor and the lymphokines IL-2 and interferon-γ (IFN-γ). Together, these and other less well defined lymphokines amplify the immune effector cell response by recruiting more T-lymphocytes and mononuclear phagocytes to the site of inflammation where they aggregate, are activated, and differentiate, forming a granuloma.

and differentiate into epithelioid and giant cells by the same cytokines.

Further details of the cell–cell interactions and mediators involved in granuloma formation have come from the study of murine models of granuloma formation in response to *Schistosoma mansoni* antigens. These models show that granuloma formation and its modulation are under the control of a complex system of distinct T-cell subsets and secretory factors.

In humans, infection with the *Schistosoma mansoni* trematode results in liver granulomas and fibrosis (65). In the latter stages of the disease, there are pulmonary granulomas and fibrosis. *Schistosoma mansoni* infects the human host through the skin, develops into mature

organisms during transit through the lung, and is deposited in the mesenteric venules where eggs are produced. The eggs travel to the liver and, eventually, to the lung; subsequently, granulomas develop around the eggs. In experimental models of this disease, advantage is taken of the knowledge that it is the soluble egg antigen which is responsible for evoking the cell-mediated immune response (65). When pulmonary granulomas are produced in mice by the intravenous injection of *Schistoma mansoni* eggs, the granulomatous response peaks 8 weeks after injection. A decrease or "dampening" of the granulomatous inflammation then follows during more chronic infection (66).

The T-cells responsible for the initiation and maintenance of this granulomatous response bear the murine markers Lyt1$^+$, L3T4$^+$, and Ia$^-$, equivalent to human CD4$^+$ T-cells (67,68). Confirmation that the immunological response is T-cell-mediated is provided by the observations that: (a) adaptive hypersensitivity can be transferred by lymphocytes but not by antibody; (b) the response can be prevented by the administration of antilymphocyte and antithymocyte antibodies; (c) only poorly formed granulomas can be obtained in athymic mice; and (d) there is an association between granuloma formation and T-cell lymphokine production (65). As examples of the last point, T-cells obtained from acute-phase granulomas, as well as T-cell clones derived from spleens of animals at the peak of the granulomatous response, produce IL-2 and migration inhibitory factor following *in vitro* stimulation with specific soluble egg antigen (69,70).

To study the mechanisms responsible for the dampening of the granulomatous response to *S. mansoni* infection, various experimental models have been developed, including: (a) infection of animals with *S. mansoni*; (b) the *in vivo* production of synchronous pulmonary granulomas by intravenous administration of *S. mansoni* eggs; (c) *in vitro* models of granuloma formation in which immune effector cells interact with *S. mansoni* eggs or beads coated with soluble egg antigen; and (d) transferring lymphocytes from chronically infected animals to newly infected animals and observing the consequences to the granulomatous response (65,68,71–74). These models have illustrated that, in addition to the T-helper cell population which initiates and develops the granuloma, immune granulomas contain two populations of suppressor cells that dampen the granulomatous response: suppressor–inducer T-cells (murine T-cell markers Lyt1$^+$ and Ia$^+$) and suppressor–effector T-cells (murine T-cell markers Lyt2$^+$ and Ia$^+$) (70,75–78). These cells function by direct cell–cell contact as well as by releasing soluble mediators that transmit suppressor signals between cell subsets. In regard to soluble mediators, in murine *Schistosoma mansoni* infection there is a suppressor–inducer factor that stimulates T-cells to release a suppressor–effector mediator, which, in turn, suppresses granuloma formation (78–82). Consequent to these processes, there is an impaired capacity of the cells comprising the granuloma to produce lymphokines such as migration inhibitory factor (75,78,83), accompanied by a general suppression of macrophage function (84,85). These processes occur without a decrease of expression of MHC molecules on macrophages comprising the granulomas (86). In addition, the ratio of T-cells within the granulomas bearing the murine equivalent of the CD4$^+$ phenotype to the CD8$^+$ phenotype shifts from 2–3:1 to 1:1 as the lesions are modulated from the vigorous granulomatous process to the more chronic lesion (70).

HOST MODULATION OF GRANULOMA FORMATION

The variation in extent of the granulomatous response of different individuals to a common agent known to incite granuloma formation has led to the concept that there are genetic and/or acquired host factors which modulate granuloma formation.

In the context that immune granulomas are intimately linked to CD4$^+$ T-cell responses, it is not surprising that class II MHC molecules play a critical role in evoking the granulomatous response. In this regard, although non-MHC-linked genetic factors are also involved, evidence from animal models has shown that animals with certain MHC genotypes respond with a high density of granulomas, whereas others have a mild response to the same granulomagenic stimulus (87,88).

One human example of the range of granulomatous response of different individuals to a common stimulus is the different clinical manifestations of infection with *Mycobacterium leprae,* the causative agent of leprosy. In some individuals, the disease manifests by an intense immunologic granulomatous response (tuberculoid leprosy), whereas in others there is a less developed immunological response (lepromatous leprosy) (19,28,89,90). In tuberculoid leprosy, histological examination of the lesions reveals well-formed epithelioid cell granulomas and very few bacilli; that is, the host has successfully dealt with the infection by confining it to a localized area. The relationship of CD4$^+$ to CD8$^+$ T-lymphocytes within and around the granulomas is similar to the pattern of increased numbers of CD4$^+$ T-cells observed in other immune granulomas (91,92). In contrast, the appearance of lepromatous leprosy suggests a defective host response. The lesions are characterized by a collection of macrophages, rare epithelioid cells, an abundance of organisms, and a paucity of T-cells. Furthermore, of the T-cells present, there is a preponderance of CD8$^+$ T-

cells within the relatively scant inflammatory exudate (91,92). In this regard, quantitative assessment demonstrates that the ratio of CD4$^+$ to CD8$^+$ T-cells in tuberculoid lesions is in the range of 1.2–5:1, compared to 0.2–1:1 in lepromatous lesions (93). Thus, it appears that individuals who develop tuberculoid leprosy in response to *M. leprae* are able to mount a clearly developed cellular immune response, at least to the *M. leprae* group of antigens. In contrast, individuals who develop lepromatous leprosy appear to be unable to mount an immune granulomatous response to the same antigenic challenge. The reasons for the striking differences in responses of different individuals to *M. leprae* are not clear. Some can be explained on the basis of MHC differences (89,94). However, there is also evidence that the apparent immunologic impotent state of lepromatous leprosy is, in part, a consequence of local control mechanisms which are capable of being up-regulated by appropriate signals (19,95). For example, if lepromatous leprosy lesions are injected with IFN-γ, the immune response is up-regulated, as evidenced by the accumulation of monocytes and lymphocytes in the lesion (96).

HUMAN PULMONARY IMMUNE GRANULOMAS

Several human lung disorders of known and unknown etiology are characterized by the presence of granulomas in the alveolar, bronchial, and/or vascular walls (Table 1). The pathogenesis of three of these disorders—sarcoidosis, chronic beryllium disease, and hypersensitivity pneumonitis—has been carefully studied in humans. Each one is based on immune processes; for each, a general picture has emerged of the mechanisms of immune granuloma formation.

Sarcoidosis

Sarcoidosis is a chronic, multiorgan disorder of unknown etiology characterized in affected organs by an accumulation of T-lymphocytes and mononuclear phagocytes, noncaseating epithelioid cell granulomas, and derangements of normal tissue architecture (8–10). All parts of the body can be involved, but the lung is the organ most frequently affected. The disease can present in an acute or subacute form and is often self-limited, but in many other cases it is chronic, with variable disease activity over many years. Sarcoidosis is found worldwide, although it has predilections for certain areas (United States, Europe, Japan) and races (blacks in the United States, whites in northern Europe) (10,97).

Although the etiology of sarcoidosis is unknown, the available evidence suggests that it is caused by specific antigens driving cell-mediated immune processes associated with granuloma formation. The earliest stages of pulmonary sarcoidosis are characterized by the accumulation of mononuclear phagocytes and CD4$^+$ T-lymphocytes. The initial mononuclear cell alveolitis precedes the development of granulomas (98), consistent with the data from experimental models of immune granulomas and from studies of the evolution of dermal responses to Kveim–Siltzbach reagent and to a "Kveim–Siltzbach"-type preparation from autologous lung cells in individuals with sarcoidosis. Sarcoid granulomas are "classic" immune granulomas—that is, compact structures composed of a discrete aggregate of mononuclear phagocytes (macrophages, epithelioid cells, giant cells) and scattered CD4$^+$ T-cells, surrounded by a rim of CD4$^+$ and CD8$^+$ T-cells (18,19,37). Analyses of lung epithelial lining fluid recovered by bronchoalveolar lavage from sarcoid patients have demonstrated a severalfold increase in the numbers of T-cells and mononuclear phagocytes compared to that of normal individuals (99). Several studies have demonstrated that the cells recovered by lavage are representative of those within the tissues (37,38).

Lymphocytes

Because the etiology of sarcoidosis is unknown, the major evidence that the granulomas are immune-based comes from analysis of the lymphocyte populations by lavage and in tissue samples. Although sarcoidosis is a systemic disorder, the lymphocyte populations are strikingly compartmentalized. At sites of disease activity such as the lung, there is a marked expansion in lymphocyte numbers, whereas in the blood there is a lymphopenia (100). Consistent with the concept of compartmentalization, the lung lymphocytes are dominated by CD4$^+$ T-cells, with the ratio of CD4$^+$ to CD8$^+$ populations within the lung being 3–10:1. In comparison, the CD4$^+$-to-CD8$^+$ ratio in normal lung is 2:1, approximately 1–1.5:1 in sarcoid blood, and 1.5–2:1 in normal blood (100). The T-cells within the lung are proliferating spontaneously at an exaggerated rate and show evidence of activation (101). Lung T-cells of individuals with active sarcoidosis are spontaneously producing lymphokines, including IL-2, IFN-γ, monocyte chemotactic factor, and migration inhibitory factor (101–104), mediators involved in the recruitment or activation of lymphocytes and mononuclear phagocytes into the local microenvironment. In addition to the secretory function of the lung T-cells, the T-cells express the surface markers of activation, including high-affinity IL-2 receptors (IL-2R), HLA-DR class II MHC molecules, and the VLA-1 marker of late activation (105–107). In contrast to lung, blood T-cells in active pulmonary sarcoidosis appear relatively quiescent, with no evidence of lymphokine re-

lease (108). However, although some blood T-cells do express activation markers such as IL-2R and class II MHC molecules, these cells likely represent T-cells which are activated in tissues such as the lung and which have migrated to blood (108,109).

There is also evidence of B-cell activation in pulmonary sarcoidosis. Levels of immunoglobulins in blood and lung are often elevated (89,110,111), and immune complexes are found in both blood and epithelial lining fluid of some patients (8,110). The available evidence suggests the immunoglobulin-secreting B-cells are likely in the lung parenchyma, not on the pulmonary epithelial surface (112,113). Furthermore, B-cell activation appears to be a nonspecific polyclonal activation of these cells by T-helper cells in the local milieu (110,114). Interestingly, anti-T-lymphocyte antibodies are observed in sarcoidosis in blood and lung (115). They are predominantly IgM and mostly directed toward CD8$^+$ T-cells. No functional role has been identified for these antibodies.

Mononuclear Phagocytes

There is evidence from a variety of sources that the mononuclear phagocytes participating in the granulomas in sarcoidosis are recruited both from blood and from local proliferation and are activated. These observations are consistent with the status of mononuclear phagocytes participating in experimental immune granulomas (40,41,116,117). In this regard, studies of lung macrophages using monoclonal antibodies have demonstrated that the cells bear the phenotype of young, recently recruited monocytes (41,118). The pulmonary mononuclear phagocyte population in sarcoidosis is also proliferating at a rate that is two to three times normal (41). Consistent with the concept that lung mononuclear phagocytes are activated, the surface density of all categories of class II MHC molecules is increased on these cells (116,117). Because lung T-cells in sarcoidosis are releasing IFN-γ, and because IFN-γ augments class II MHC molecule surface density on alveolar macrophages, it is likely that the T-cells are participating, at least in part, in the lung macrophage activation process.

It is possible that macrophage cytokines are involved in the development of sarcoid granulomas, although the evidence for this is not unequivocal. Evaluation of the release of IL-1 by alveolar macrophages from individuals with sarcoidosis has led to conflicting reports: Some studies show no increase, whereas others show an increase, compared with controls (118–121). However, evaluation of IL-1 mRNA transcript numbers in sarcoid macrophages shows no difference from controls, and the *in vitro* responses of control and sarcoidosis monocytes and macrophages to lipopolysaccharide are similar, suggesting that there is no difference in the regulation of IL-1 production in sarcoidosis (121,122).

Alveolar macrophage secretion of TNF-α has been evaluated in patients with sarcoidosis in comparison with normals, and no difference was observed (123). However, when normal macrophages are cultured in the presence of IL-2, increased amounts of TNF-α mRNA transcripts are found (124). Because lung CD4+ MHC class II+ T-cells are releasing IL-2 in sarcoidosis (125), it is possible that CD4+ T-cells are activating genes such as that for TNF-α in lung macrophages in this disease.

Antigen Presentation

In a T-cell-mediated immune response such as sarcoidosis, antigens must be processed and presented by antigen-presenting cells to T-cells. In sarcoidosis, there is evidence that alveolar macrophages have a greater capacity to present antigen than do normal macrophages. In this regard, alveolar macrophages from patients with sarcoidosis, in comparison to those from normal individuals, are capable of increased presentation of nonrelevant antigen, such as tetanus toxoid, to lymphocytes (126,127). In addition, accessory molecules, such as the macrophage adhesion molecules [intercellular adhesion molecule 1 (ICAM-1), lymphocyte function-associated antigen 3 (LFA-3); see Chapter 3.4.1], probably also play a role during antigen presentation in the cell-surface-triggered events leading to lymphocyte activation (128,129). In this context, sarcoid lung lymphocytes express an increased surface density of the CD2 (the sheep erythrocyte receptor) molecule, the natural receptor for LFA-3, believed to be an important accessory receptor in T-cell activation (130).

Further evidence that lung macrophages are presenting antigens to T-cells in sarcoidosis comes from analysis of the numbers of surface antigen receptors on lung T-cells. Recognition of antigen–class II complexes by specific T-cell antigen receptors (TCRs) is an absolute prerequisite for an antigen to be capable of driving a T-cell response. One consequence of T-cell antigen receptor triggering is the down-regulation of surface TCR molecules and the up-regulation of TCR mRNA transcript numbers (131,132). If TCR triggering occurs in sarcoidosis, it would be expected that T-cells from active disease sites would exhibit the appropriate surface and mRNA changes. This is the case compared to blood T-cells; sarcoid lung T-lymphocytes exhibit a decrease in density of surface TCR molecules, and they express increased numbers of TCR β-chain mRNA transcripts (133).

Etiology

Although the process initiating and perpetuating the granulomatous response in sarcoid is unknown, there is increasing evidence that, just as in experimental models of immune granulomas, the disease is caused by several agents acting as specific antigens to drive the T-cell-mediated granulomatous process. This evidence comes from analysis of T-cell antigen receptor usage in sarcoidosis.

As described in detail in Chapter 3.4.1, the enormous diversity of T-cells for specific antigens is created by rearrangement of germline variable (V), diversity (D), junctional (J), and constant (C) region elements of the two types (αβ and γδ) of T-cell antigen receptors. Theoretically, analysis of the relative usage of these elements in T-cell antigen receptors should yield evidence as to whether the T-cells accumulate in a random polyclonal fashion (as might be expected if there was a failure of control of cytokine release), in a monoclonal fashion (e.g., as in a malignancy such as the human T-cell leukemia/lymphoma virus 1), or in relatively biased fashion, with exaggerated use of specific TCR elements [as would be expected if sarcoidosis resulted from persistent, specific antigen(s), in association with enhanced antigen presentation/T-cell triggering].

The evidence from analysis of TCRs in sarcoidosis points to the persistent antigen hypothesis. For example, in one subgroup of patients there is an exaggerated usage of the Vβ8 element of the αβ TCR (134). In this subgroup there is compartmentalization of Vβ8+ CD4+ T-cells to the lung (the site of the granulomas) and Vβ8+ CD8+ T-cells to the blood; that is, the CD8+ suppressor–cytotoxic T-cells likely have been stimulated by the same antigen but are not localizing to the site of the disease.

Further evidence of exaggerated TCR usage in sarcoidosis comes from analysis of T-cells bearing the γδ TCR. Theoretically, the γδ TCR is of particular relevance to sarcoidosis because at least some γδ+ T-cells in normal individuals respond to *Mycobacterium tuberculosis*, an agent known to evoke a granulomatous response (135,136). In normal individuals, less than 10% of blood and lung T-cells use this TCR, but in a subgroup of individuals with sarcoidosis there is a marked expansion in the numbers of γδ T-cells—particularly in blood, but also in lung (137). Furthermore, in some individuals a large proportion of these T-cells use the same γ chains and the same δ chains, leading to the conclusion that they were amplified as a result of a specific, persistent antigenic stimulus (138).

Together, these data are compatible with the concept that sarcoidosis is caused by persistent, specific antigens (exogenous and/or self) that induce a cell-mediated immune response; that is, the disease is not due to the nonspecific accumulation of T-cells at disease sites, nor is it a neoplastic-like disorder caused by the clonal expansion of one cell. In accord with this concept, it is commonly observed that sarcoidosis resolves spontaneously (139). Why this occurs is unknown, but one possibility is that the macrophage–T-cell processes remove the antigen, or that exposure to an inciting external stimulus has been removed. Furthermore, the diversity of the biases in TCR usage may reflect more than one etiology of sarcoidosis, where the different antigens induce a similar type of response, but with T-cells of different specificities.

Chronic Beryllium Disease

Inhalation of low levels of beryllium dusts or salts over months to years is associated with a chronic interstitial pulmonary granulomatous disorder indistinguishable from sarcoidosis (140–142). The concept that the granulomas of chronic beryllium disease are T-cell-mediated immune granulomas is supported by the observations that: (a) beryllium (i.e., the antigen) persists in the lung for long periods (143); (b) large numbers of T-cells and noncaseating granulomas are present in the lung (142); (c) in response to beryllium salts, lung and blood T-cells proliferate and release lymphokines (144,145); and (d) intradermal administration of beryllium salts induces a local granulomatous response in these individuals (146).

In chronic beryllium disease, as in sarcoidosis, the lung T-cell population is predominantly of the CD4$^+$ phenotype (145,147). These CD4$^+$ T-cells—as compared to blood T-cells from the same individual, or compared to T-cells from normals—exhibit increased proliferation in response to beryllium (145,147). As in sarcoidosis, the T-cells are activated, expressing HLA class II molecules and IL-2R and releasing IL-2 (147,148). Furthermore, the beryllium-induced lung T-cell proliferation is class II-restricted. Analysis of T-cell lines and T-cell clones of individuals with this disease confirmed that the beryllium-induced response is antigen-specific and that all of the responder cells are CD4$^+$ T-cells (147).

Thus, from the information available, it appears that chronic beryllium disease is a classic example of an immune granuloma host response. Why an element like beryllium should do this is not clear, but two not mutually exclusive hypotheses could explain it. First, it is likely that most disease is caused by dusts of beryllium metal or salts, so that the particulate forms a nidus around which macrophages ingest, allowing the beryllium to be slowly released. Second, soluble beryllium salts interact with proteins, such that the beryllium becomes an immunogenic hapten in the context of the protein.

Hypersensitivity Pneumonitis

Hypersensitivity pneumonitis, also called "extrinsic allergic alveolitis," is a granulomatous interstitial lung disorder caused by organic dusts from living sources (149). Examples of the common causes of hypersensitivity pneumonitis include thermophilic organisms of the *Micropolyspora* and *Thermoactinomyces* groups, as well as those derived from avian proteins (150). The most common exposure situations involve farmers working with moldy hay, individuals exposed to organisms growing in humidifiers and air conditioners, and bird breeders. Chronic exposure to these organic dusts results, in some individuals, in a lymphocyte–macrophage alveolitis, accompanied by loosely formed granulomas in the alveolar interstitium. For details concerning the clinical presentation and the many causes of hypersensitivity pneumonitis, see refs. 149–152.

Although hypersensitivity pneumonitis is believed to be an example of a human immune granulomatous host response, the granulomatous chronic inflammation of hypersensitivity pneumonitis differs from that of sarcoidosis in a number of ways. First, the agent is known and affected individuals have specific precipitating antibodies in blood and lung directed against the agent (149). Second, the hypersensitivity pneumonitis usually resolves spontaneously on removal from the antigenic exposure (152). Third, histological examination of the lung in hypersensitivity pneumonitis shows that the granulomas are less compact, are defined less clearly in terms of cell–cell interrelationships, and are associated with a significantly more diffuse interstitial mononuclear cell infiltrate than is observed in sarcoidosis (149,153). Fourth, the immunologic mechanisms which give rise to the inflammation are not purely T-cell-mediated, and data suggest that a number of other immunological events may be involved (see below). Finally, hypersensitivity pneumonitis is restricted to the lung, whereas sarcoidosis is a systemic, albeit compartmentalized, disorder.

Pathogenesis

A number of animal models have shown that chronic antigen inhalation in a sensitized animal can induce a clinical picture similar to that observed in hypersensitivity pneumonitis, involving (a) specific antibody production to the inhaled antigen and (b) the pulmonary histological appearances of human hypersensitivity pneumonitis (154–159). In a typical example, footpad injections of ovalbumin in Freund's complete adjuvant were used to sensitize guinea pigs (157). The animals were then challenged by intratracheal injections of ovalbumin, resulting in a pulmonary histologic appearance of hypersensitivity pneumonitis. In another model, repeated intratracheal inoculations of *Micropolyspora faeni* to the rabbit produce similar lesions (158). In these models, initially there is neutrophil inflammation in the lung, followed by an influx of lymphocytes and macrophages. In humans, a similar early neutrophil influx into the lung is observed following inhalational antigen challenge of a sensitized patient (160). Over several days the pattern of cellular infiltrate changes from polymorphonuclear to mononuclear, and after 10 days the morphology has returned almost to normal. The percentage of T-cells in the lung increases by 24 hr after challenge. Furthermore, at least in experimental animals, these T-cells are specifically sensitized to the inciting antigen (157).

The inflammatory processes underlying the early neutrophil infiltration are not clear, but there is evidence suggesting that it results from the formation of immune complexes in the lung. In this regard, locally formed immune complex may activate alveolar macrophages, causing the generation of neutrophil chemoattractants (161–163) (see Chapter 3.4.5). A role for complement has been proposed but has not been proven. Studies in humans have also demonstrated an increase in mast cell numbers in the early phase of the disease, suggesting that mast cell degranulation plays a role in the early inflammation (164,165). Consistent with this concept, elevated levels of histamine are observed in epithelial lining fluid (161).

The fundamental role of the T-cell in the pathological process is demonstrated by studies in experimental animals, showing that immune responsiveness can be transferred to nonsensitized animals by T-lymphocytes from sensitized animals (166). In humans, the chronic form of hypersensitivity pneumonitis is associated with a T-lymphocytic alveolitis, with percentages of T-cells in lavage fluid often as high as 70–80% (167). The increase in T-cell numbers is due to an expansion of both the $CD4^+$ and $CD8^+$ subsets, but preferentially the $CD8^+$ T-cell subset. In this regard, the ratio of lung $CD4^+$ to $CD8^+$ cells is reduced from the 2:1 of normals to nearer 1:1 in this disease (168,169). Lymphocytes in the lung of individuals with hypersensitivity pneumonitis are activated, as evidenced by (a) the increased number of T-cells expressing class II molecules (170), (b) lung T-cells secreting lymphokines such as migration inhibitory factor in response to specific antigens (171), and (c) lung T-cells proliferating in response to the specific causative antigen (171). However, the mechanisms whereby hypersensitivity pneumonitis evolves from a process believed to be immune complex-mediated (in the acute stages) into a more chronic granulomatous inflammatory state are unclear.

THERAPY FOR PULMONARY IMMUNE GRANULOMATOUS DISORDERS

The conventional strategy for therapy of immune granulomas of the lung is to remove the individual from the causative agent (if known) and to suppress the T-cell component of the disorder with glucocorticoids (8,149,152). This approach has varying success, depending on the specific disease and on the amount of derangement of the lung parenchyma.

For sarcoidosis, the etiology is unknown, so the only available therapeutic strategy is to suppress the mechanisms of granuloma function. For individuals with an active $CD4^+$ T-cell alveolitis, glucocorticoids are effective. However, when there is sufficient derangement of the parenchyma, other inflammatory processes are likely ongoing, limiting the effectiveness of this therapy. Attempts at more specific therapy with cyclosporin A, an inhibitor of T-cell activation thought to act at the level of lymphokine mRNA production, have not been successful (172). One reason for this discordance may be the lack of drug penetration into tissue. Alternatively, it may result from an inhibitory effect of cyclosporin A on suppressor cells (similar to the effect of cyclosporin A seen in the *Schistosoma mansoni* model) (173), or from the lack of sensitivity of $CD4^+$ T-cells involved in granuloma formation to cyclosporin A (174).

For chronic beryllium disease, it is possible to remove the individual from future inhalation exposure, but unfortunately the beryllium remains in the lung (i.e., a persistent, undegradable stimulus, chronically involving a granulomatous host response).

For hypersensitivity pneumonitis, removal from inhalation of the organic antigens is helpful, but as with sarcoidosis, if sufficient derangement of the lung parenchyma has occurred, intervention with glucocorticoids is not sufficient, and progression is common.

REFERENCES

1. Boros DL. Granulomatous inflammations. *Prog Allergy* 1978;24:183–267.
2. Adams DO. The granulomatous inflammatory response. A review. *Am J Pathol* 1976;84:164–191.
3. Spector WG. The granulomatous inflammatory exudate. *Int Rev Exp Pathol* 1969;8:1–55.
4. Spector WG. Epithelioid cells, giant cells, and sarcoidosis. *Ann NY Acad Sci* 1976;778:3–6.
5. Liebow AA. Pulmonary angiitis and granulomatosis. *Am Rev Respir Dis* 1973;108:1–18.
6. Fauci AS, Haynes BF, Katz P. The spectrum of vasculitis: clinical, pathologic, immunologic and therapeutic considerations. *Ann Intern Med* 1978;89:660–676.
7. Basset F, Corrin B, Spencer H, et al. Pulmonary histiocytosis X. *Am Rev Respir Dis* 1978;118:811–820.
8. Crystal RG, Bitterman PB, Rennard SI, Hance AJ, Keogh BA. Interstitial lung diseases of unknown cause: disorders char-

acterized by chronic inflammation of the lower respiratory tract. *N Engl J Med* 1984;310:154–165, 235–244.

9. Thomas PD, Hunninghake GW. Current concepts of the pathogenesis of sarcoidosis. *Am Rev Respir Dis* 1987;135:747–760.

10. Mitchell DN, Scadding JG. Sarcoidosis. *Am Rev Respir Dis* 1974;110:774–802.

11. Jung-Legg Y, Legg MA. Pulmonary granulomas. In: Ioachim HL, ed. *Pathology of granulomas.* New York: Raven Press, 1983;223–256.

12. Warren KS. A functional classification of granulomatous inflammation. *Ann NY Acad Sci* 1976;778:7–18.

13. Boros DL. Experimental granulomatosis. *Clin Dermatol* 1986;4:10–21.

14. Daniele RP, Dauber JH, Rossman MD. Immunologic abnormalities in sarcoidosis. *Ann Intern Med* 1980;92:406–416.

15. Soler P, Basset F, Bernaudin JF, Chretien J. Morphology and distribution of the cells of a sarcoid granuloma: ultrastructural study of serial sections. *Ann NY Acad Sci* 1976;718:147–160.

16. Mitchell DN, Scadding JG, Heard BE, Hinson KFW. Sarcoidosis: histopathological definition and clinical diagnosis. *J Clin Pathol* 1977;30:395–408.

17. van Maarsseven AC, Mullink H, Alons CL, Stam J. Distribution of T-lymphocyte subsets in different portions of sarcoid granulomas: immunohistologic analysis with monoclonal antibodies. *Hum Pathol* 1986;17:493–500.

18. Mishra BB, Poulter LW, Janossy G, James GJ. The distribution of lymphoid and macrophage like cell subsets of sarcoid and Kveim granulomata: possible mechanism of negative PPD reaction in sarcoidosis. *Clin Exp Immunol* 1983;54:705–715.

19. Narayanan RB. Immunopathology of leprosy granulomas—current status: a review. *Lepr Rev* 1988;59:75–82.

20. Scadding JG, Mitchell DN. *Sarcoidosis,* 2nd ed. London: Chapman & Hall, 1985.

21. Jones-Williams W, Erasmus DA, James EMV, Davies T. The fine structure of sarcoid and tuberculosis granulomas. *Postgrad Med J* 1970;46:496–500.

22. Postlethwaite AE, Jackson BK, Beachey EH, Kang AH. Formation of multinucleated giant cells from human monocyte precursors. *J Exp Med* 1982;155:168–178.

23. Nagasawa H, Miyaura C, Abe E, Suda T, Horiguchi M, Suda T. Fusion and activation of human alveolar macrophages induced by recombinant interferon-γ and their suppression by dexamethasone. *Am Rev Respir Dis* 1987;136:916–921.

24. Boros DL. Immunoregulation of granuloma formation in murine *Schistosomiasis mansoni. Ann NY Acad Sci* 1986;465:313–323.

25. Boros DL. Immunoregulatory mechanisms active in the suppression of the schistosome egg granuloma. In: Yoshida T, Torisu M, eds. *Basic mechanisms of granulomatous inflammation.* New York: Elsevier, 1989;143–157.

26. Perrin PJ, Phillips SM. The molecular basis of receptor mediated regulation of granulomatous hypersensitivity. In: Yoshida T, Torisu M, eds. *Basic mechanisms of granulomatous inflammation.* New York: Elsevier, 1989;185–202.

27. Chensue SW, Kunkel SL. Monokine production and orchestration in hypersensitivity (*Schistosoma mansoni* egg) and foreign body-type granuloma formation. In: Yoshida T, Torisu M, eds. *Basic mechanisms of granulomatous inflammation.* New York: Elsevier 1989;221–236.

28. Kaplan G, Cohn ZA. The immunobiology of leprosy. *Int Rev Exp Pathol* 1986;28:45–78.

29. Kriebel D, Brain JD, Sprince NL, Kazemi H. The pulmonary toxicity of beryllium. *Am Rev Respir Dis* 1988;137:464–473.

30. Fink JN. Hypersensitivity pneumonitis. *Chest* 1979;75:270–276.

31. Daniel TM, Oxtoby MJ, Pinto E, Moreno S. The immune spectrum in patients with pulmonary tuberculosis. *Am Rev Respir Dis* 1981;123:556–559.

32. Teirstein AS, Brown LK. The Kveim–Siltzbach test in 1987. In: Grassi C, Rizzato G, Pozzi E, eds. *Sarcoidosis and other granulomatous disorders.* New York: Elsevier, 1988;7–18.

33. Munro CS, Mitchell DN. The Kveim response: still useful, still a puzzle. *Thorax* 1987;42:321–331.

34. Holter JF, Kataria YP, Park HK. Cutaneous granulomata in response to injection with autologous bronchoalveolar lavage cell preparations in sarcoidosis patients. In: Grassi C, Rizzato G, Pozzi E, eds. *Sarcoidosis and other granulomatous disorders.* Amsterdam: Elsevier, 1988;139–142.

35. Mishra BB, Poulter LW, Janossy G, Sherlock S, James DG. The Kveim–Siltzbach granuloma. A model for sarcoid granuloma formation. *Ann NY Acad Sci* 1976;278:164–175.

36. Munro CS, Mitchell DN, Poulter LW, Cole PJ. Early cellular responses to intradermal injection of Kveim suspension in normal subjects and those with sarcoidosis. *J Clin Pathol* 1986;39:176–182.

37. Campbell DA, Poulter LW, du Bois RM. Immunocompetent cells in bronchoalveolar lavage reflect the cell populations in transbronchial biopsies in pulmonary sarcoidosis. *Am Rev Respir Dis* 1985;132:1300–1306.

38. Semenzato G, Chilosi M, Ossi E, et al. Bronchoalveolar lavage and lung histology. Comparative analysis of inflammatory and immunocompetent cells in patients with sarcoidosis and hypersensitivity pneumonitis. *Am Rev Respir Dis* 1985;132:400–404.

39. Paradis IL, Dauber JH, Rabin BS. Lymphocyte phenotypes in bronchoalveolar lavage and lung tissue in sarcoidosis and idiopathic pulmonary fibrosis. *Am Rev Respir Dis* 1986;133:855–860.

40. Hance AJ, Douches S, Winchester RJ, Ferrans VJ, Crystal RG. Characterization of mononuclear phagocyte subpopulations in the human lung by using monoclonal antibodies: changes in alveolar macrophage phenotype associated with pulmonary sarcoidosis. *J Immunol* 1985;134:284–292.

41. Bitterman PB, Saltzman LE, Adelberg J, Ferrans VJ, Crystal RG. Alveolar macrophage replication. One mechanism for the expansion of the mononuclear phagocyte population in the chronically inflamed lung. *J Clin Invest* 1984;72:460–469.

42. Turner-Warwick M. *Immunology of the lung.* London: Edward Arnold, 1978;165–190.

43. Dannenberg AM Jr. Macrophages in inflammation and infection. *N Engl J Med* 1975;293:489–493.

44. Mackaness GB. The mechanisms of macrophage activation. In: Mudd S, ed. *Infectious agents and host reactions.* Philadelphia: WB Saunders, 1970;61–75.

45. Unanue ER. Antigen-presenting function of the macrophage. *Annu Rev Immunol* 1984;2:395–428.

46. Braciale TJ, Morrison LA, Sweetser MT, Sambrook J, Gething M-J, Braciale VL. Antigen presentation pathways to class I and class II MHC-restricted T lymphocytes. *Immunol Rev* 1987;98:95–114.

47. Buus S, Sette A, Grey HM. The interaction between protein-derived immunogenic peptides and Ia. *Immunol Rev* 1987; 98:115–141.

48. Harding CV, Unanue ER. Antigen processing and intracellular Ia. Possible roles of endocytosis and protein synthesis in Ia function. *J Immunol* 1989;142:12–19.

49. Paul WE. The immune system: an introduction. In: Paul WE, ed. *Fundamental immunology,* 2nd ed. New York: Raven Press, 1989;3–19.

50. Berzofsky JA. Structural basis of antigen recognition by T-lymphocytes. Implications for vaccines. *J Clin Invest* 1988;82:1811–1817.

51. Cheever AW, Byram JE, von Lichtenberg F. Immunopathology of *Schistosoma japonicum* infection in athymic mice. *Parasite Immunol* 1985;7:387–398.

52. Wahl SM, Allen JB. T lymphocytes and granuloma formation. In: Yoshida T, Torisu M, eds. *Basic mechanisms of granulomatous inflammation.* New York: Elsevier, 1989;41–59.

53. Cheever AW, Deb S, Duvall RH. Granuloma formation in *Schistosoma japonicum* infected nude mice: the effects of reconstitution with L3T4⁺ or LYT2⁺ splenic cells. *Am J Trop Med Hyg* 1989;40:66–71.

54. Kasahara K, Kobayashi K, Shikama Y, Yoneya I, Soezima K, Ide H, Takahashi T. Direct evidence for granuloma-inducing activity of interleukin-1. *Am J Pathol* 1988;130:629–638.

55. Kasahara K, Kobayashi K, Shikama Y. The role of monokines

in granuloma formation in mice: the ability of interleukin 1 and tumor necrosis factor-α to induce lung granulomas. *Clin Immunol Immunopathol* 1989;51:419–425.

56. Kobayashi K, Allred C, Cohen S, Yoshida T. Role of interleukin-1 in experimental pulmonary granuloma in mice. *J Immunol* 1985;134:358–364.

57. Kunkel SL, Chesnue SW, Plewa M, Higashi GI. Macrophage function in the *Schistosoma mansoni* egg-induced pulmonary granuloma. Role of arachidonic acid metabolites in macrophage Ia antigen expression. *Am J Pathol* 1984;114:240–249.

58. Chensue SW, Kunkel SL, Ward PA, Higashi GI. Exogenously administered prostaglandins modulate pulmonary granulomas induced by *Schistosoma mansoni* eggs. *Am J Pathol* 1983; 111:78–87.

59. Hunninghake GW, Gadek JE, Young RC, Kawanami O, Ferrans VJ, Crystal RG. Maintenance of granuloma formation in pulmonary sarcoidosis by T lymphocytes within the lung. *N Engl J Med* 1980;302:594–598.

60. Matsushima K, Larsen CG, Du Bois GC, Oppenheim JJ. Purification and characterization of a novel monocyte chemotactic and activating factor produced by a human myelomonocytic cell line. *J Exp Med* 1989;169:1485–1490.

61. Weiser WY, Temple PA, Witek-Giannotti J-AS, Remold HG, Clark SC, David JR. Molecular cloning of a cDNA encoding a human macrophage migration inhibitory factor. *Proc Natl Acad Sci USA* 1989;86:7522–7526.

62. Basham TY, Merigan TC. Recombinant interferon-γ increases HLA-DR synthesis and expression. *J Immunol* 1983;130:1492–1494.

63. Becker S. Effect of interferon-gamma on class-II antigen expression and accessory cell function. *Immunology* 1985; 4:135–145.

64. Nathan C, Yoshida R. Cytokines: interferon-γ. In: Gallin JI, Goldstein IA, Snyderman R, eds. *Inflammation.* New York: Raven Press, 1988;229–252.

65. Mahmoud AF. Schistosomiasis. In: Warren KS, Mahmoud AAF, eds. *Tropical and geographic medicine.* New York: McGraw–Hill, 1984;443–457.

66. Lammie PJ, Linette GP, Phillips SM. Characterization of *Schistosoma mansoni* antigen-reactive T cell clones that form granulomas *in vitro. J Immunol* 1985;134:4170–4175.

67. Domingo EO, Warren KS. Endogenous desensitization: changing host granulomatous response to schistosome eggs at different stages of infection with *Schistosoma mansoni. Am J Pathol* 1968;52:369–380.

68. Colley DG. Immune responses and immunoregulation in experimental and clinical schistosomiasis. In: Mansfield JM, ed. *Parasitic diseases. 1. The immunology.* New York: Marcel Dekker, 1985;1–83.

69. Ohta N, Edahiro T, Tohgi N, Ishii A, Minai M, Hosaka Y. Generation and functional characterization of T-cell lines and clones specific for *Schisotosoma japonicum* egg antigen in humans. *J Immunol* 1988;141:2445–2450.

70. Ragheb S, Boros DL. Characterization of granuloma T lymphocyte function from *Schistosoma mansoni*-infected mice. *J Immunol* 1989;142:3239–3246.

71. Warren KS. The secret of the immunopathogenesis of schistosomiasis: *in vivo* models. *Immunol Rev* 1982;61:189–213.

72. Doughty BL, Ottensen EA, Nash TE, Phillips SM. Delayed hypersensitivity granuloma formation around *Schistosoma mansoni* eggs in vitro. 3. Granuloma formation and modulation in human *Schistosoma mansoni. J Immunol* 1984;133:993–997.

73. Colley DG. Adoptive suppression of granuloma formation. *J Exp Med* 1976;143:696–700.

74. Doughty BL, Phillips SM. Delayed hypersensitivity granuloma formation and modulation around *Schistosoma mansoni* eggs *in vitro.* Regulatory T cell subsets. *J Immunol* 1982;128:37–42.

75. Chensue SW, Wellhausen SR, Boros DL. Modulation of granulomatous hypersensitivity. II. Participation of Ly 1⁺ and Ly 2⁺ T lymphocytes in the suppression of granuloma formation and lymphokine production in *Schistosoma mansoni*-infected mice. *J Immunol* 1981;127:363–367.

76. Phillips SM, Linette GP, Doughty BL, Byram JE, von Lichtenberg F. *In vivo* T cell depletion regulates resistance and

morbidity in murine schistosomiasis. *J Immunol* 1987;139:919–926.

77. Boros DL. Immunopathology of *Schisotosoma mansoni* infection. *Clin Microbiol Rev* 1989;2:250–259.

78. Phillips SM, Walker D, Abdel-Hafez SK, Linette GP, Doughty BL, Perrin PJ, el Fathelbab N. The immune response to *Schistosoma mansoni* infections in inbred rats. VI. Regulation by T cell subpopulations. *J Immunol* 1987;139:2781–2787.

79. Boros DL, Pelley RP, Warren KS. Spontaneous modulation of granulomatous hypersensitivity in *Schistosoma mansoni. J Immunol* 1975;14:1437–1441.

80. Aune TM, Freeman GL Jr, Colley DG. Production of the lymphokine soluble immune response suppressor (SIRS) during chronic experimental *Schistosomiasis mansoni. J Immunol* 1985;136:2768–2771.

81. Mathew RC, Boros DL. Regulation of granulomatous inflammation in murine schistosomiasis. III. Recruitment of antigen-specific I-J⁺ T suppressor cells of the granulomatous response by an I-J⁺ soluble suppressor factor. *J Immunol* 1986; 136:1093–1099.

82. Perrin PJ, Phillips SM. The molecular basis of granuloma formation in schistosomiasis. I. A T-cell-derived suppressor effector factor. *J Immunol* 1988;141:1714–1719.

83. Chensue SW, Boros DL, David CS. Regulation of granulomatous inflammation in murine schistosomiasis. *J Exp Med* 1983;157:219–230.

84. Olds GR, Ellner JJ. Modulation of macrophage activation and resistance by suppressor T lymphocytes in chronic murine *Schistosoma mansoni* infection. *J Immunol* 1984;133:2720–2724.

85. Chensue SW, Kunkel SL, Higashi GI, Ward PA, Borol DL. Production of superoxide anion, prostaglandins and hydroxyeicosatetraenoic acids by macrophages from hypersensitivity *Schistosoma mansoni* egg and foreign body-type granulomas. *Infect Immun* 1983;42:1116–1125.

86. Sunday ME, Stadecker MJ, Wright JA, Aoki I, Dorf ME. Induction of immune responses by schistosome granuloma macrophages. *J Immunol* 1983;130:2413–2419.

87. Denis M, Skamene E. Genetic influences on the granulomatous response with special reference to mycobacterial compounds. In: Yoshida T, Torisu M, eds. *Basic mechanisms of granulomatous inflammation.* Amsterdam: Elsevier, 1988;103–131.

88. Sternick JL, Schrier DJ, Moore VL. Genetic control of BCG-induced inflammation. *Exp Lung Res* 1983;5:217–228.

89. Modlin RL, Mehra V, Jordan R, Bloom BR, Rea TH. *In situ* and *in vitro* characterization of the cellular immune response in erythema nodosum leprosum. *J Immunol* 1986;3:883–886.

90. Modlin RL, Kato H, Mehra V, et al. Genetically restricted suppressor T-cell clones derived from lepromatous leprosy lesions. *Nature* 1986;322:459–461.

91. Kumar V, Narayanan RB, Girdhar BK. Comparison of the characteristics of infiltrates in skin and nerve of granulomas of leprosy. *Acta Leprol* 1989;7:19–24.

92. Wallach D, Flageul B, Bach MA, Cottenot F. The cellular content of dermal leprous granulomas: an immunohistological approach. *Int J Lepr* 1984;52:318–326.

93. Narayanan RB, Bhutani LK, Sharma AK, Nath I. T-cell subsets in leprosy lesions: *in situ* characterization using monoclonal antibodies. *Clin Exp Immunol* 1983;51:421–429.

94. Todd JR, West BC, McDonald JC. Human leukocyte antigen and leprosy: study in northern Louisiana and review. *Rev Infect Dis* 1990;12:63–71.

95. Kaplan G, Laal S, Sheftel G, et al. The nature and kinetics of a delayed immune response to purified protein derivative of tuberculin in the skin of lepromatous leprosy patients. *J Exp Med* 1988;168:1811–1824.

96. Nathan CF, Kaplan G, Levis WR, et al. Local and systemic effects of intradermal recombinant interferon-γ in patients with lepromatous leprosy. *N Engl J Med* 1986;315:6–15.

97. Siltzbach LE, ed. Seventh international conference on sarcoidosis and other granulomatous diseases. *Ann NY Acad Sci* 1976;278:321–333.

98. Rosen Y, Athanassiades TJ, Moon S, Lyons HA. Nongranulomatous interstitial pneumonitis in sarcoidosis: relationship to

development of epithelioid granulomas. *Chest* 1978;74:122–125.

99. Crystal RG, Roberts WC, Hunninghake GW, Gadek JE, Fulmer JD, Line BR. Pulmonary sarcoidosis: a disease characterized and perpetuated by activated lung T-lymphocytes. *Ann Intern Med* 1981;94:73–94.

100. Hunninghake GW, Crystal RG. Pulmonary sarcoidosis: a disorder mediated by excess helper T-lymphocyte activity at sites of disease activity. *N Engl J Med* 1981;305:429–434.

101. Pinkston P, Bitterman PB, Crystal RG. Spontaneous release of interleukin-2 by lung T lymphocytes in active pulmonary sarcoidosis. *N Engl J Med* 1983;308:793–800.

102. Robinson BWS, McLemore TL, Crystal RG. Gamma interferon is spontaneously released by alveolar macrophages and lung T lymphocytes in patients with pulmonary sarcoidosis. *J Clin Invest* 1985;75:1488–1495.

103. Saltini C, Crystal RG. Pulmonary sarcoidosis: pathogenesis, staging and therapy. *Internat Arch Allergy Immunol* 1985;76(suppl.):92–100.

104. Hunninghake GW, Keogh BA, Line BR, et al. Pulmonary sarcoidosis: pathogenesis and therapy. In: Boros DL, Yoshida T, eds. *Basic and clinical aspects of granulomatous diseases.* Amsterdam: Elsevier/North-Holland, 1980;275–290.

105. Semenzato G, Agostini C, Trentin L, et al. Evidence of cells bearing interleukin-2 receptor at sites of disease activity in sarcoid patients. *Clin Exp Immunol* 1984;57:331–337.

106. Costabel U, Bross KJ, Ruhle KH, Lohr GW, Matthys H. Ia-like antigens on T-cells and their subpopulations in pulmonary sarcoidosis and in hypersensitivity pneumonitis. Analysis of bronchoalveolar and blood lymphocytes. *Am Rev Respir Dis* 1985;131:337–342.

107. Saltini C, Hemler ME, Crystal RG. T-lymphocytes compartmentalized on the epithelial surface of the lower respiratory tract express the very late activation antigen complex VLA-1. *Clin Immunol Immunopathol* 1988;46:221–233.

108. Konishi K, Moller DR, Saltini C, Kirby M, Crystal RG. Spontaneous expression of the interleukin-2 receptor gene and presence of functional interleukin-2 receptors on T lymphocytes in the blood of individuals with active pulmonary sarcoidosis. *J Clin Invest* 1988;82:775–781.

109. Saltini C, Pinkston P, Lee JJ, Crystal RG. Role of T-helper cell subsets in expanding the T-cell alveolitis of active pulmonary sarcoidosis. *Clin Res* 1985;33:472A.

110. Hunninghake GW, Crystal RG. Mechanisms of hypergammaglobulinemia in pulmonary sarcoidosis: site of increased antibody production and role of T-lymphocytes. *J Clin Invest* 1981;67:86–92.

111. Saint-Remy J-MR, Mitchell DN, Cole PJ. Variation in immunoglobulin levels and circulating immune complexes in sarcoidosis. Correlation and extent of disease and duration of symptoms. *Am Rev Respir Dis* 1983;127:23–27.

112. Lawrence EC, Martin RR, Blaese RM, et al. Increased bronchoalveolar IgG secreting cells in interstitial lung diseases. *N Engl J Med* 1980;302:1186–1188.

113. Hance AJ, Saltini C, Crystal RG. Does de novo immunoglobulin synthesis occur on the epithelial surface of the human lower respiratory tract? *Am Rev Respir Dis* 1988;137:17–24.

114. Byrne EB, Evans AS, Fouts DW, Israel HL. Serological hyperactivity to Epstein–Barr virus and other viral antigens in sarcoidosis. In: Iwai K, Hosoda Y, eds. *Proceedings of the 6th international conference on sarcoidosis.* Baltimore: University Park Press, 1974;218–225.

115. Spurzem JR, Saltini C, Crystal RG. Functional significance of anti-T-lymphocyte antibodies in sarcoidosis. *Am Rev Respir Dis* 1988;137:600–605.

116. Campbell DA, du Bois RM, Butcher RG, Poulter LW. The density of HLA-DR antigen expression on alveolar macrophages is increased in pulmonary sarcoidosis. *Clin Exp Immunol* 1986;65:165–171.

117. Spurzem JR, Saltini C, Kirby M, Konishi K, Crystal RG. Expression of HLA class II genes in alveolar macrophages of patients with sarcoidosis. *Am Rev Respir Dis* 1989;140:89–94.

118. Campbell DA, Poulter LW, du Bois RM. Phenotypic analysis

of alveolar macrophages in normal subjects and in patients with interstitial lung disease. *Thorax* 1986;41:429–434.

119. Hunninghake GW. Release of interleukin-1 by alveolar macrophages of patients with active pulmonary sarcoidosis. *Am Rev Respir Dis* 1984;129:569–572.

120. Eden E, Turino GM. Interleukin-1 from human alveolar macrophages in lung disease. *J Clin Immunol* 1986;6:326–333.

121. Wewers MD, Saltini C, Sellers S, et al. Evaluation of alveolar macrophages in normals and individuals with active pulmonary sarcoidosis for the spontaneous expression of the interleukin-1 beta gene. *Cell Immunol* 1987;107:479–488.

122. Kern JA, Lamb RJ, Reed JC, Elias JA, Daniele RP. Interleukin-1-beta gene expression in human monocytes and alveolar macrophages from normal subjects and patients with sarcoidosis. *Am Rev Respir Dis* 1988;137:1180–1184.

123. Bachwich PR, Lynch JP III, Larrick J, Spengel M, Kunkel SL. Tumour necrosis factor production by human sarcoid alveolar macrophages. *Am J Pathol* 1986;125:421–425.

124. Strieter RM, Remick DG, Lynch JP III, Spengler RN, Kunkel SL. Interleukin-2-induced tumor necrosis factor-alpha (TNF-α) gene expression in human alveolar macrophages and blood monocytes. *Am Rev Respir Dis* 1989;139:335–342.

125. Saltini C, Spurzem JR, Lee JL, Pinkston P, Crystal RG. Spontaneous release of interleukin-2 by lung T-lymphocytes in active pulmonary sarcoidosis is primarily from the Leu3$^+$DR$^+$ T-cell subset. *J Clin Invest* 1986;77:1962–1970.

126. Venet A, Hance AJ, Saltini C, Robinson WS, Crystal RG. Enhanced alveolar macrophage-mediated antigen-induced T lymphocyte proliferation in sarcoidosis. *J Clin Invest* 1985;75:293–301.

127. Lem VM, Lipscomb MF, Weissler JC, Nunez G, Ball EJ, Stastny P, Toews CB. Bronchoalveolar cells from sarcoid patients demonstrate enhanced antigen presentation. *J Immunol* 1985;135:1766–1771.

128. Sanders ME, Makgoba MW, Sharrow SO, Stephany D, Springer TA, Young HA, Shaw S. Human memory T-lymphocytes express increased levels of three cell adhesion molecules (LFA-3, CD2, and LFA-1) and three other molecules (UCHL1, CDw29, and Pgp-1) and have enhanced IFN-γ production. *J Immunol* 1988;140:1401–1407.

129. Weiss A, Imboden JB. Cell surface molecules and early events involved in human T-lymphocyte activation. *Adv Immunol* 1987;41:1–38.

130. Spurzem J, Saltini C, Kirby M, Crystal RG. Compartmentalized expression of adhesion molecules on lung T-lymphocytes. *Am Rev Respir Dis* 1988;137:A46.

131. Cantrell D, Davies AA, Londei M, Feldman M, Crumpton MJ. Association of phosphorylation of the T3 antigen with immune activation of T-lymphocytes. *Nature* 1987;325:540–542.

132. Noonan DJ, Isakov N, Theofilopoulos AN, Dixon FJ, Altman A. Protein kinase C-activating phorbol esters augment expression of T-cell receptor genes. *Eur J Immunol* 1987;17:803–807.

133. du Bois RM, Balbi B, Kirby M, Crystal RG. T-lymphocyte accumulation in pulmonary sarcoidosis: evidence for persistent stimulation of sarcoid lung T-lymphocytes via the T-cell antigen receptor. *Am Rev Respir Dis* 1989;139:A61.

134. Moller DR, Konishi K, Kirby M, Balbi B, Crystal RG. Bias toward use of a specific T-cell receptor β-chain variable region in a subgroup of individuals with sarcoidosis. *J Clin Invest* 1988;82:1183–1191.

135. O'Brien RL, Happ MP, DaMas A, Palores E, Kubo R, Born WK. Stimulation of a major subset of lymphocytes expressing T-cell receptors γδ by an antigen derived from *Mycobacterium tuberculosis. Cell* 1989;57:667–672.

136. Haregewoin A, Soman G, Hom RC, Finberg RW. Human γδ$^+$ T cells respond to mycobacterial heat shock proteins. *Nature* 1989;340:309–312.

137. Balbi B, Moller DR, Kirby M, Holroyd KJ, Crystal RG. Increased numbers of T-lymphocytes with γδ$^+$ antigen receptors in a subgroup of individuals with pulmonary sarcoidosis. *J Clin Invest* 1990;85:1353–1361.

138. Tamura N, Holroyd KJ, Banks T, Kirby M, Okayama H, Crystal RG. Diversity in junctional sequences associated with the common human Vγ9 and Vδ2 gene segments in normal blood

and lung compared to the limited diversity in a granulomatous disease. *J Exp Med* 1990;172:169–181.

139. James DG, Siltzbach LE, Turiaf J. A worldwide review of sarcoidosis. *Ann NY Acad Sci* 1976;278:321–334.

140. Freiman DE, Hardy HL. Beryllium disease: the relation of pulmonary pathology to clinical course and prognosis based on a study of 130 cases from the U.S. Beryllium Case Registry. *Hum Pathol* 1970;1:25–44.

141. Jones Williams W. Beryllium disease. *Postgrad Med J* 1988; 64:511–516.

142. Williams WJ. Beryllium workers—sarcoidosis or chronic beryllium disease. *Sarcoidosis* 1989;6(suppl):34–35.

143. Jones Williams W, Wallach ER. Laser probe mass spectrometry (LAMMS) analysis of beryllium, sarcoidosis and other granulomatous diseases. *Sarcoidosis* 1989;6:111–117.

144. Williams WR, Williams WJ. Development of beryllium lymphocyte transformation tests in chronic beryllium disease. *Int Arch Allergy Appl Immunol* 1982;67:175–180.

145. Rossman MD, Kern JA, Elias JA, Cullen MR, Epstein PE, Preuss OP, Markham TN, Daniele RP. Proliferative response of bronchoalveolar lymphocytes to beryllium. *Ann Intern Med* 1988;108:687–693.

146. Maceira JM, Fukayama K, Epstein WL. Appearance of T-cell subpopulations during the time course of beryllium-induced granulomas. *J Invest Dermatol* 1984;83:314–316.

147. Saltini C, Winestock K, Kirby M, Pinkston P, Crystal RG. Maintenance of the alveolitis in patients with chronic beryllium disease by beryllium-specific helper T-cells. *N Engl J Med* 1989;320:1103–1109.

148. Pinkston P, Bitterman PB, Crystal RG. Interleukin-2 in the alveolitis of beryllium-induced lung disease. *Am Rev Respir Dis* 1984;129:A161.

149. Pepys J. Hypersensitivity disease of the lungs due to fungi and other organic dusts. *Monogr Allergy* 1969;4:1–145.

150. Stankus RP, deShazo RD. Hypersensitivity pneumonitis. In: Schwarz MI, King TE, eds. *Interstitial lung disease*. Philadelphia: BC Dekker, 1988;111–122.

151. Salvaggio J, Karr RM. Hypersensitivity pneumonitis. *Chest* 1979;75:270–276.

152. Reynolds HY. Hypersensitivity pneumonitis: correlation of cellular and immunologic changes with clinical phases of disease. *Lung* 1988;166:189–208.

153. Reyes CN, Wenzel FJ, Lawton BR, Emanuel DA. The pulmonary pathology of Farmer's lung disease. *Chest* 1982; 81:142–146.

154. Kawai T, Salvaggio J, Lake W, Harris JO. Experimental production of hypersensitivity pneumonitis with bagasse and thermophilic actinomycete antigen. *J Allergy Clin Immunol* 1972;50:276–288.

155. Hensley GT, Fink JN, Baboriak JJ. Hypersensitivity pneumonitis in the monkey. *Arch Pathol* 1974;97:33–38.

156. Bernardo F, Hunninghake GW, Gadek JE, Ferrans VJ, Crystal RG. Acute hypersensitivity pneumonitis: serial changes in lung lymphocyte subpopulations after exposure to antigen. *Am Rev Respir Dis* 1979;120:985–994.

157. Kochman S, Martin J-C, Bureau G, Dubois DE, Montreyanaud J-M. Pulmonary reactions to *Micropolyspora faeni* in sensitized rabbits. *Clin Allergy* 1972;2:307–315.

158. Schuyler MR, Kleinerman J, Pensky JR, Brandt C, Schmitt D. Pulmonary response to repeated exposure to *Micropolyspora faeni*. *Am Rev Respir Dis* 1983;128:1071–1076.

159. Schuyler M, Crocks L. Experimental hypersensitivity pneumonitis in guinea pigs. *Am Rev Respir Dis* 1989;139:996–1002.

160. Fournier E, Tonnel AB, Gosset P, Wallaert B, Amoisen JC, Voisin C. Early neutrophil alveolitis after antigen inhalation in hypersensitivity pneumonitis. *Chest* 1985;88:563–566.

161. Soler P, Nioche S, Valeyre D, et al. Role of mast cells in the pathogenesis of hypersensitivity pneumonitis. *Thorax* 1987; 42:565–572.

162. Daniele RP, Henson PM, Fantone JC III, Ward PA, Dreisin RB. Immune complex injury of the lung. *Am Rev Respir Dis* 1981;124:738–755.

163. Hunninghake GW, Gadek JE, Fales HM, Crystal RG. Human alveolar macrophage-derived chemotactic factor for neutrophils. *J Clin Invest* 1980;66:473–483.

164. Haslam PL, Dewar A, Butchers P, Primett ZS, Newman-Taylor A, Turner-Warwick M. Mast cells, atypical lymphocytes, and neutrophils in bronchoalveolar lavage in extrinsic allergic alveolitis. *Am Rev Respir Dis* 1987;135:35–47.

165. Marone G, Casolaro V, Cirillo R, Stellato C, Genovese A. Pathophysiology of human basophils and mast cells in allergic disorders. *Clin Immunol Immunopathol* 1989;50:S24–S40.

166. Bice E, Salvaggio J, Hoffman E. Passive transfer of experimental hypersensitivity pneumonitis with lymphoid cells in the rabbit. *J Allergy Clin Immunol* 1976;58:250–262.

167. Weinberger SE, Kelman JA, Elson NA, et al. Bronchoalveolar lavage in interstitial lung disease. *Ann Intern Med* 1978;89:459–466.

168. Costabel U, Bross KJ, Marxen J, Matthys H. T-lymphocytosis in bronchoalveolar lavage fluid of hypersensitivity pneumonitis. *Chest* 1984;85:514–518.

169. Semenzato G, Agostini C, Zambello R, et al. Lung T-cells in hypersensitivity pneumonitis: phenotypic and functional analyses. *J Immunol* 1986;137:1164–1172.

170. Semenzato G, Trentin L. Cellular immune responses in the lung of hypersensitivity pneumonitis. *Eur Respir J* 1990;3:357–359.

171. Costabel U. The alveolitis of hypersensitivity pneumonitis. *Eur Respir J* 1988;1:5–9.

172. Martinet Y, Pinkston P, Saltini C, Spurzem J, Muller-Querheim J, Crystal RG. Evaluation of the *in vitro* effects of cyclosporine on the lung T-lymphocyte alveolitis of active pulmonary sarcoidosis. *Am Rev Respir Dis* 1988;1242–1248.

173. Metzger J, Peterson B. Cyclosporin A enhances the pulmonary granuloma response induced by *Schistosoma mansoni* eggs. *Immunopharmacology* 1988;15:103–116.

174. Pincelli C, Fujikoa A, Suya H, Fukayama K, Epstein WL. Light and electron microscopy of experimental cutaneous granulomas in mice treated with cyclosporine. In: Grassi C, Rizzato G, Pozzi E, eds. *Sarcoidosis and other granulomatous disorders*. Amsterdam: Excerpta Medica, 1988;691–695.

THE LUNG: Scientific Foundations
edited by R.G. Crystal, J.B. West et al.
Raven Press, Ltd., New York © 1991.

CHAPTER 7.5.2

Immunoglobulin- and Complement-Mediated Immune Injury

Jeffrey S. Warren, Kent J. Johnson, and Peter A. Ward

IMMUNE-COMPLEX- AND COMPLEMENT-MEDIATED LUNG INJURY IN HUMANS

There are many inflammatory and immunologic lung diseases in which systemic complement activation and circulating immune complexes can be detected. In some cases, tissue deposits containing immune complexes and complement can be demonstrated by immunofluorescence. Despite these associations, cause-and-effect evidence linking immune-complex-mediated tissue injury [Gell and Coombs' type III hypersensitivity (1)] to human pulmonary disease remains circumstantial. Despite this caveat, these clinicopathological associations are supported by a compelling body of in vivo and in vitro experimental data suggesting that immune complexes and complement have the ability to mediate pulmonary injury.

The group of human lung diseases that have been linked to immune-complex- and complement-mediated tissue damage is extensive (2). For instance, at least some degree of parenchymal pulmonary disease can be demonstrated in the majority of patients with systemic lupus erythematosus (3). The severity of pulmonary parenchymal lupus tends to parallel that of the systemic disease and ranges from an asymptomatic and radiographically inapparent form to an acute, fulminating, hemorrhagic pneumonitis (4). Immune deposits consisting of DNA, IgG anti-DNA, and C3 have been demonstrated in the lungs of most patients with acute lupus pneumonitis (5–8). As in the case of immune-complex-mediated glomerulonephritides, electron-dense deposits have been identified subjacent to the alveolar capillary basement membrane in lung tissue from lupus pneumonitis patients (9). Conversely, immune deposits are not found within the lungs of systemic lupus patients devoid of clinically apparent pulmonary involvement (4,7).

The mechanisms by which immune complexes may mediate injury in lupus pneumonitis are not clear-cut. Traditionally, effector components of complement (e.g., C3a, C3b, C5a) have been thought to be important mediators of microvascular injury, inflammatory cell recruitment, and phagocyte activation. Inoue et al. (5) have demonstrated several of these complement-derived components in association with immunoglobulin deposits in injured lung. Eagen et al. (7) have demonstrated C1q in association with pulmonary immune deposits. Despite these observations, neither complement components nor inflammatory cells are uniformly found in lung tissue from patients with lupus pneumonitis (4,7). As will become apparent from a review of experimental studies, the pathogenesis of immune-complex-mediated pneumonitis is complicated and appears to involve a wide variety of mediators. It should be emphasized that a large number of lung diseases have been attributed to immune-complex-mediated injury (2). Among the more common or extensively characterized diseases are the idiopathic pulmonary fibrosis, rheumatoid pneumonitis, Wegener's granulomatosis, Sjogren's syndrome, hypersensitivity pneumonitis (extrinsic allergic alveolitis), and Goodpasture's syndrome.

ANIMAL MODELS OF IMMUNE-COMPLEX- AND COMPLEMENT-MEDIATED LUNG INJURY

The earliest experimental studies of immune-complex-mediated tissue injury focused on dermal blood vessels

J. S. Warren, K. J. Johnson, and P. A. Ward: Department of Pathology, University of Michigan Medical School, Ann Arbor, Michigan 48109.

and the kidneys. In the early 1960s, Kniker and Cochrane (10) described acute inflammatory changes in the walls of medium-sized pulmonary arteries in rabbits with acute serum sickness. Despite the pulmonary vascular pathology in this model, no inflammatory changes were observed in the alveoli or interstitium of the lungs. Later, Brentjens et al. (11) demonstrated irreversible damage in the alveolar interstitium and alveolar capillary basement membranes of rabbits with chronic serum sickness. Morphological and immunofluorescence studies revealed deposits of immune complexes and complement within the vascular basement membranes.

In 1974, Johnson and Ward (12) developed a model in rats, in which acute lung injury can be elicited by IgG immune complexes that form in situ at the alveolar–capillary interface. In this model, purified IgG anti-bovine serum albumin (BSA) is instilled into the alveolar air space through a tracheal cannula and antigen (BSA) is infused intravenously. Over the ensuing 4–6 hr, acute alveolitis develops. Lung injury can be quantitated by morphometric analysis, by measuring increases in lung weight or by quantitating the accumulation of iodine-125-labeled colloid in the damaged lungs. The total lung content of ^{125}I-colloid (usually nonspecific rabbit IgG) compared to the amount of ^{125}I-colloid present in 1 ml of whole blood provides a reproducible and quantitative index of lung injury, since it reflects a normalized measure of increased vascular permeability and leakage of the radioisotope-labeled colloid into the adjacent lung parenchyma. Development of lung damage in this model is largely neutrophil- and complement-dependent, thus resembling the reversed passive Arthus reaction in skin (13). Later studies also demonstrated the phlogistic potential of preformed IgG:BSA immune complexes when instilled into the lungs of rats (14). It has become clear that the physical configuration of preformed immune complexes is important in determining the intensity of subsequent lung inflammation (15). In vitro studies have suggested that this observation may be explained, at least in part, by the ability or inability of variously sized immune complexes to fix complement. Subsequent investigations have been directed towards understanding the pathogenesis of this model of acute immune-complex-mediated alveolitis. A variety of inflammatory mediator systems, including complement, appear to be necessary for the evolution of immune-complex alveolitis.

More recently, Johnson et al. (16) characterized an analogous model of immune-complex lung injury in which deposition of monoclonal murine IgA antibodies directed against dinitrophenol-substituted BSA results in acute alveolitis which develops independently of neutrophils but which is partially dependent on the presence of complement. While there is debate regarding the clinical relevance of IgA immune-complex-mediated lung injury, this model has provided insights into non-neutrophil-mediated lung injury and may have relevance to IgA immune-complex-mediated tissue injury in other organ systems such as the kidney (e.g., Berger's disease, Henoch–Schonlein purpura). The remaining portions of this chapter will outline experimental studies that have led to our current understanding of the pathogenesis of these models.

EFFECTOR CELLS AND MECHANISMS IN EXPERIMENTAL IMMUNE-COMPLEX ALVEOLITIS

Despite the fact that inflammatory cells and mononuclear inflammatory cells are often not seen in lung biopsies from patients with putative immune-complex-mediated pneumonitides, in vivo and in vitro experimental studies indicate that acute IgG immune-complex-mediated lung injury is chiefly neutrophil-dependent. Development of lung injury, quantitated by a progressive rise in microvascular permeability, is paralleled by massive neutrophil influx. In rats that have been 95% depleted of neutrophils using either rabbit anti-neutrophil serum, nitrogen mustard, or cyclophosphamide, there is a marked reduction (60–70%) in lung injury following the induction of intra-alveolar immune-complex deposition (12). Pretreatment of rats with either catalase, superoxide dismutase, hydroxyl radical scavengers, or iron chelators suppresses the development of lung injury, supporting the hypothesis that oxygen-derived metabolites play a major role in neutrophil-mediated lung injury (12). Suppression of immune-complex lung injury by superoxide dismutase (SOD) is time-dependent and, early on, is associated with reduced neutrophil influx (17). The protective effect of SOD in IgG immune-complex lung injury diminishes with delay in administration of SOD and with prolongation of the injury development period (17). This observation supports the hypothesis that oxygen-derived species play a role in neutrophil-mediated injury and that superoxide anion (O_2^-) contributes to this process not only as a precursor to other deleterious oxidant species but also as a reactant that influences neutrophil recruitment. The mechanism through which O_2^- influences neutrophil recruitment is not known with certainty but may be linked to oxidant-mediated generation of chemotactic factors. For instance, two groups of investigators have shown in vitro that exposure of plasma to xanthine/xanthine oxidase results in the generation of a chemotactic factor that amplifies the recruitment of neutrophils (18,19). Since this reaction can be blocked by SOD, O_2^- appears to be the responsible oxidant species. The biochemical identity of the resulting chemotactic factor is not known with certainty but may be an arachidonate-derived lipid. Shingu and Nobunaga (20) have observed that exposure of C5 to an oxygen-radical-generating system results in the generation of the chemotactic peptide, C5a. More recently, Vogt et al. (21) have demonstrated that exposure of purified C5 to H_2O_2 results in conformational changes leading to the formation of a C5b-9 (membrane attack complex)-like structure despite the fact that C5 cleavage does not occur. Addition of H_2O_2 to whole human plasma or serum results in complement activation with cleavage of C5 to form C5a. The importance of these *in vitro* observations to *in vivo* complement-mediated tissue injury is presently unclear, but they suggest mechanisms through which oxidants may influence neutrophil recruitment.

It has been more recent that the roles of resident alveolar macrophages as regulatory and effector cells in acute lung injury have come to be appreciated. Even in the case of nearly complete neutrophil depletion (greater than 90%), immune-complex deposition (IgG:BSA) in lung results in some degree of oxidant-dependent tissue injury (12,17). Exposure *in vitro* of isolated neutrophil or alveolar macrophages to preformed IgG-containing immune complex results in the formation of substantial quantities of oxygen-derived metabolites (O_2^- and H_2O_2) (22,23). Exposure of isolated alveolar macrophages to preformed IgA complexes causes O_2^- and H_2O_2 generation, whereas exposure of neutrophils to IgA complexes results in negligible oxidant production (23). Utilizing a cerium chloride method to ultrastructurally analyze the *in situ* elaboration of H_2O_2 in IgA immune-complex-injured rat lungs, Warren et al. (24) have recently provided direct cytochemical evidence that alveolar macrophages produce oxygen metabolites *in vivo* (Fig. 1). These observations suggest that alveolar macrophages can function as effector cells in immune-complex-mediated lung injury. The observation that IgA lung injury is partially complement-dependent yet develops fully in neutrophil-depleted rats suggests that complement components contribute to lung injury through additional mechanisms besides neutrophil recruitment and activation (16). *In vitro* studies suggest that IgA immune complexes are very inefficient activators of complement (25) but that complement components can prime alveolar macrophages, resulting in amplification of the respiratory burst (26).

There is also evidence that interactions between oxygen metabolites and lysosomal proteases may be important in the development of cell and tissue injury. Using an *ex vivo* perfused lung model, Fox and Merrigan (27) have shown that perfusion with limited concentrations of leukocytic lysosomal extracts or a cell-free oxidant-generating system (xanthine/xanthine oxidase) results in minimal lung injury, yet exposure of the lung to a combination of oxidants and proteases

results in significant lung damage. Weiss and co-workers (28,29) have shown that exposure of latent (inactive) collagenase or gelatinase (derived from secondary granules of human neutrophils) to myeloperoxidase (MPO)-H_2O_2-derived oxidant species results in activation of the enzymes. These studies illustrate several examples of oxidant–protease interaction that may have relevance to acute immune-complex-mediated lung injury. The biochemical mechanisms through which phagocyte-derived products damage biological targets have been the focus of investigation (see Chapters 7.2.1–7.2.4).

It is presently unclear what role other lung cells (besides resident alveolar macrophages and recruited neutrophils and monocytes) may play as effector cells in inflammatory lung injury in general and in immune-complex- and complement-mediated injury in particular. For instance, endothelial cells have been shown to generate low concentrations of xanthine-oxidase-derived oxidants under conditions of ischemia or exposure to activated neutrophils (30,31). In addition to their roles as effector cells, recent studies have revealed that many cells indigenous to the lungs are important in the regulation of acute inflammation through the production of cytokines, chemotactic factors, and other proinflammatory mediators.

THE ROLE OF COMPLEMENT IN EXPERIMENTAL IMMUNE-COMPLEX ALVEOLITIS

The most direct evidence implicating complement in the pathogenesis of acute immune-complex alveolitis has come from *in vivo* studies. In both the IgG and IgA immune-complex lung-injury models, C3 deposits can be demonstrated in association with alveolar septal immune-complex deposits (12,16) (Fig. 2). The requirements for an intact complement system in immune-complex alveolitis have been examined in complement-depleted rats (12,16,32). Induction of IgG immune-complex lung injury in complement-depleted rats results in markedly attenuated lung damage (approximately 80%) accompanied by diminished neutrophil influx. In the case of IgA immune-complex lung injury, complement depletion results in a 50% reduction in lung damage. In this model there is virtually no neutrophil influx regardless of the presence or absence of an intact complement system. The potency of C5a as a chemotactic factor suggests that this complement activation product is a major mediator of neutrophil influx. The lack of neutrophil recruitment in IgA immune-complex lung injury may be attributable to the relative inefficiency of IgA immune complexes in activation of the complement cascade distal to C3 (25). The capacity for IgA complexes to trigger (directly or

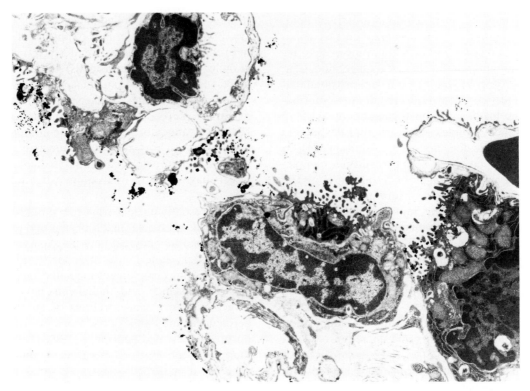

FIG. 1. Transmission electron micrograph of rat lungs instilled with CeCl$_3$ reaction buffer 3 hr after initiation of IgA immune-complex lung injury. There are numerous electron-dense cerium deposits along luminal surfaces of injured pneumocytes. Cerium-containing electron-dense deposits are also formed by alveolar macrophages and can be blocked by the intratracheal administration of catalase (24). × 8100.

indirectly) other mediators (e.g., tumor necrosis factor, interleukin-8, platelet-activating factor, leukotriene B$_4$) that appear to be involved in neutrophil recruitment is the focus of current investigation. The quantitative contributions of C3 activation products and the complement-derived membrane attack complex (C5b-9) to neutrophil recruitment are also the subject of current research. Several *in vitro* and *in vivo* studies have focused on the roles of specific complement components in inflammation. There is *in vitro* and some *in vivo* evidence which suggests that iC3b, C5a, and C5b-9 may play roles in neutrophil recruitment and phagocyte activation.

Marks et al. (33) have constructed an *in vitro* model that mimics the endothelium-associated complement deposition observed in various inflammatory states. In this model, C3 is bound to the surface of endothelial cells through a covalent linkage to the endothelium-binding lectin *Ulex europaeus*. In turn, an endothelium-associated enzyme cleaves bound C3 into iC3b, which, in turn, mediates a rapid (approximately 20 min), high-affinity neutrophil adhesion reaction. These investigators have suggested that such a mechanism could be operative very early in the acute inflammatory response. Such a mechanism would lend efficiency and directionality to complement-mediated

neutrophil recruitment. It should be emphasized that such a mechanism is not mutually exclusive of C5a-mediated neutrophil recruitment. A scenario can be envisioned in which iC3b mediates very early, high-affinity, directed neutrophil adhesion (via the neutrophil CR3 receptor), followed by a wave of C5a-depen-

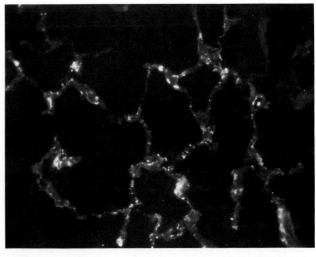

FIG. 2. Localization of C3 by immunofluorescence in acute IgG immune-complex alveolitis (12,16). × 300.

dent neutrophil chemotaxis which amplifies inflammatory cell recruitment. It will require very sensitive and precise neutrophil trafficking studies to determine the relative contributions of these mechanisms in an *in vivo* setting. It has been suggested that C3 activation products per se are insufficient to produce lung injury; moreover, small numbers of neutrophils adherent to endothelium would be very difficult to quantitate, and other mediators may be required for the cells to emigrate through capillary walls and damage target tissue.

There are relatively few data concerning the role of the membrane attack complex (C5b-9) in immune-complex-mediated lung injury. Using an antibody directed against the human membrane attack complex neoantigen, Kunkel et al. (34) have observed C5b-9 deposits in alveolar septae of rats with IgA immune-complex lung injury. *In vitro*, C5b-9 has been shown to trigger O_2^- by neutrophils, to open calcium channels in platelets, and to stimulate the release of O_2^-, prostaglandin metabolites, and interleukin-1 from peripheral blood monocytes (35). Any of these activities may play a role in immune-complex- and complement-mediated alveolitis. Presently, the relative contribution of the membrane attack complex to immune-complex-mediated alveolitis is unknown.

Many *in vitro* cell activation studies suggest that C3a, C3b, iC3b, C5a, and perhaps other complement activation products can activate neutrophils, monocytes, or macrophages (36). Most of the studies addressing complement-mediated cell activation have focused on the functional effects of these interactions or on receptor-mediated signal transduction mechanisms. The most intensively studied complement activation product in this context is C5a. Current evidence suggests that C5a engages a specific cell-membrane-associated receptor resulting in guanyl-nucleotide-binding-protein-mediated activation of phospholipase C. Activation of phospholipase C results in the generation of diacylglycerol (DAG) and inositol 1,4,5-trisphosphate (IP₃) from phosphatidylinositol 4,5-bisphosphate (PIP₂). Receptor–ligand engagement is accompanied by a rise in cytosolic calcium derived from extracellular and intracellular pools. IP₃ triggers mobilization of intracellular calcium from intracellular organelles into the cytosol, and DAG leads to the activation of protein kinase C. In concert, these metabolic activation events lead to functional responses such as directed cell movement, oxidant generation, and degranulation (37). Sophisticated biochemical analyses of cell activation have provided important information concerning effector mechanisms of phagocyte-mediated tissue injury.

Recent studies by Friedl et al. (38) have attributed a novel activity to C5a that may also have relevance to complement-mediated tissue injury. Rat pulmonary artery endothelial cells incubated with human serum that has been complement-activated by addition of cobra venom factor exhibit a pronounced conversion of xanthine dehydrogenase to xanthine oxidase. This reaction requires the presence of C5 but not C2, C6, C7, C8, or C9. The reaction can also be reproduced by the addition of recombinant human C5a to endothelial cells. Conversion of xanthine dehydrogenase to xanthine oxidase occurs rapidly (5–10 min) and can also be triggered by tumor necrosis factor and the synthetic formyl peptide, *N*-formyl-methionyl-leucyl-phenylalanine but not be interleukin-1 beta, bradykinin, or phorbol ester. This observation is somewhat analogous to that of Phan et al. (31), who have shown that activated neutrophils can also trigger conversion of xanthine dehydrogenase to xanthine oxidase in rat pulmonary artery endothelial cells. These observations have important implications in inflammatory tissue injury because of the capacity for xanthine oxidase to generate O_2^-. As alluded to previously, O_2^- may participate in the pathogenesis of inflammatory tissue injury directly, through the formation of other oxidant species, or through its effects on neutrophil recruitment.

RECENTLY RECOGNIZED MEDIATORS OF IMMUNE-COMPLEX ALVEOLITIS

Recognition that resident alveolar macrophage products and perhaps endothelial-cell-derived products may participate in the pathogenesis of alveolitis emphasizes the concept that immune-complex lung injury is not the simple result of neutrophil recruitment resulting from immunoglobulin deposition and complement activation. In the last several years it has become apparent that tumor necrosis factor (TNF), interleukin-8 (IL-8), platelet-activating factor (PAF), and perhaps interleukin-1 (IL-1) are mediators of acute immune-complex-mediated lung injury (Fig. 3).

Several investigators have observed that exposure of endothelial cell monolayers to TNF or IL-1 results in the protein-synthesis-dependent expression of various endothelial cell surface proteins (39). Among the induced endothelial molecules are endothelial–leukocyte adhesion molecule-1 (ELAM-1) and intracellular leukocyte adhesion molecule-1 (ICAM-1), which mediate endothelial-cell–neutrophil adhesive interactions, respectively (40). Warren et al. (41) have recently shown that there are markedly increased TNF levels in bronchoalveolar lavage fluid from rats with IgG immune-complex alveolitis. Neutralization of intrapulmonary TNF with a specific anti-TNF antibody greatly diminishes the lung injury. This reduction in lung injury is accompanied by a significant reduction in neutrophil influx. Recent studies have shown that the anti-TNF-mediated reduction in neutrophil influx

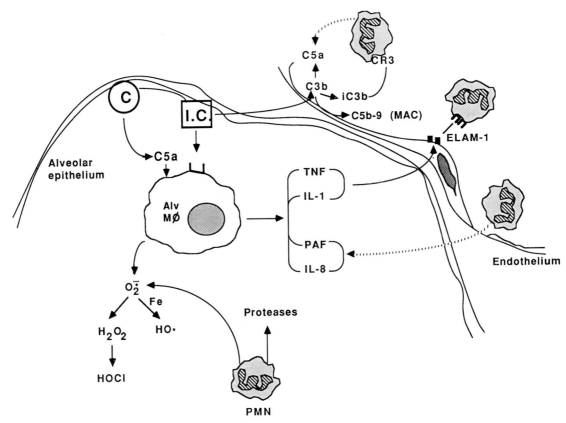

FIG. 3. Proposed pathogenesis of acute IgG immune-complex-mediated lung injury in the rat. This composite summarizes many of the putative mediators and mechanisms cogent to acute alveolitis. Alv MØ: alveolar macrophage; C: complement; C3b, C5a, iC3b, CR3: effector components of complement; C5b-9 (MAC): complement-derived membrane attack complex; ELAM-1: endothelial–leukocyte adhesion molecule-1; I.C.: immune complex; IL-1: interleukin-1; IL-8: interleukin-8; PAF: platelet-activating factor; PMN: polymorphonuclear leukocyte; TNF: tumor necrosis factor.

is time-dependent; that is, a reduction in neutrophil influx is observed 4 hr after initiation of injury but not during the early phase of alveolitis (42). While these studies clearly implicate TNF in the pathogenesis of immune-complex alveolitis, further studies will be required to dissect out the mechanisms that determine the *in vivo* relationship between intrapulmonary TNF elaboration and neutrophil influx.

Strieter et al. (43) have demonstrated that exposure of cells indigenous to the lung (endothelial cells and alveolar macrophages) to TNF results in the expression of IL-8 mRNA and secretion of biologically active IL-8. In view of the potent neutrophil chemotactic activity attributable to IL-8 (44), this may be an important neutrophil recruitment mechanism in acute alveolitis.

Intratracheal administration of the specific PAF antagonists L-652,731 and WEB-2086 also results in moderate reductions in IgG immune-complex-induced lung injury (42). This observation is analogous to studies in which PAF has been shown to play a role in dermal immune-complex vasculitis (45,46). It is presently unknown what cells are the chief sources of intrapulmonary PAF, what the triggering mechanisms are, and how PAF mediates lung damage. PAF is secreted by a wide variety of cells, is chemotactic for neutrophils, and has been shown to mediate rapid neutrophil–endothelial-cell adhesive interactions *in vitro* (47,48).

IL-1 exhibits many activities that overlap with TNF (49). Several *in vivo* studies have implicated IL-1 in neutrophil recruitment (50,51). Preliminary studies suggest that it may also play a role in IgG immune-complex alveolitis (52). It is clear that the pathogenesis of immunoglobin- and complement-mediated lung injury is complex. Unraveling the relative importance and interrelationships among various complement components, oxidants, proteases, and inflammatory mediators such as TNF, IL-8, PAF, and IL-1 should provide new insights into the pathogenesis of inflammatory tissue injury.

ACKNOWLEDGMENTS

The authors wish to thank Kimberly Drake and Jennifer Fricke for manuscript preparation, and they wish to thank Robin Kunkel for preparation of figures. This work was supported, in part, by the American Heart Association of Michigan and National Institutes of Health grants HL-45206, HL-34635, and HL-31963.

REFERENCES

1. Coombs RRA, Gell PGH. Classification of allergic reactions responsible for clinical hypersensitivity and disease. In: Gell PGH, Coombs RRA, Lachman PG, eds. *Clinical aspects of immunology*, 3rd ed. Oxford: Blackwell Scientific Publications, 1975.
2. Dreisin RB. Lung diseases associated with immune complexes. *Am Rev Respir Dis* 1981;124:748–752. In: Daniele RP, ed. *Symposium on immune complex injury of the lung. Am Rev Respir Dis* 1981;124:738–755.
3. Silberstein SL, Barland P, Grayzel A, et al. Pulmonary dysfunction in systemic lupus erythematosus. Prevalence classification and correlation with other organ involvement. *J Rheumatol* 1980;7:187–194.
4. Eagen JW, Memoli VA, Roberts JL, et al. Pulmonary hemorrhage in systemic lupus erythematosus. *J Med* 1978;57:545–560.
5. Inoue T, Kanayama Y, Ohe A, et al. Immunopathologic studies of pneumonitis in systemic lupus erythematosus. *Ann Intern Med* 1979;91:30–34.
6. Rodriquez-Iturbe B, Garcia R, Rubio L, et al. Immunohistologic findings in the lung in systemic lupus erythematosus. *Arch Pathol Lab Med* 1977;101:342–344.
7. Eagen JW, Roberts JL, Schwartz MM, et al. The composition of pulmonary immune deposits in systemic lupus erythematosus. *Clin Immunol Immunopathol* 1979;12:204–219.
8. Gamsu G, Webb WR. Pulmonary hemorrhage systemic lupus erythematosus. *J Can Assoc Radiol* 1977;29:66–68.
9. Kuhn C. Systemic lupus erythematosus in a patient with ultrastructural lesions of the pulmonary capillaries previously reported in the review as due to idiopathic pulmonary hemosiderosis. *Am Rev Respir Dis* 1972;106:931–932.
10. Kniker WT, Cochrane CG. Pathogenic factors in vascular lesions of experimental serum sickness. *J Exp Med* 1965;122:83–98.
11. Brentjens JR, O'Connell DW, Pawlowski B, Hsu KC, Andres GA. Experimental immune complex disease of the lung. The pathogenesis of a laboratory model resembling certain human interstitial diseases. *J Exp Med* 1974;140:105–125.
12. Johnson KJ, Ward PA. Acute immunologic pulmonary alveolitis. *J Clin Invest* 1974;54:49–57.
13. Cochrane CG, Janoff A. The Arthus reaction: a model of neutrophil and complement-mediated injury. In: Zweifach, Grant, McCluskey, eds. *The inflammatory process*, vol 3, 2nd ed. New York: Academic Press, 1974;59–76.
14. Scherzer H, Ward PA. Lung and dermal vascular injury produced by preformed immune complexes. *Am Rev Respir Dis* 1978;117:551–557.
15. Scherzer H, Ward PA. Lung injury produced by immune complexes of varying composition. *J Immunol* 1978;121:947–952.
16. Johnson KJ, Wilson BS, Till GO, Ward PA. Acute lung injury in rat caused by immunoglobulin A immune complexes. *J Clin Invest* 1984;74:358–366.
17. Johnson KJ, Ward PA. Role of oxygen metabolites in immune complex injury lung. *J Immunol* 1981;126:1365–1369.
18. Petrone WF, English DK, Wong K, McCord JM. Free radicals and inflammation: the superoxide dependent activation of a neutrophil chemotactic factor in plasma. *Proc Natl Acad Sci USA* 1980;77:1159–1163.
19. Perez HD, Weksler BB, Goldstein IM. Generation of a chemotactic lipid from arachidonic acid by exposure to a superoxide-generating system. *Inflammation* 1980;4:313–328.
20. Shingu M, Nobunaga M. Chemotactic activity generated in human serum from the fifth component of complement by hydrogen peroxide. *Am J Pathol* 1984;117:201–206.
21. Vogt W, Zabern I von, Hesse D, Notte R, Haller Y. Generation of an activated form of human C5 (C5b-like C5) by oxygen radicals. *Immunol Lett* 1987;14:209–215.
22. Ward PA, Duque RE, Sulavik MC, Johnson KJ. In vitro and in vivo stimulation of rat neutrophils and alveolar macrophages by immune complexes: production of O_2^- and H_2O_2. *Am J Pathol* 1983;110:297–311.
23. Warren JS, Kunkel RG, Johnson KJ, Ward PA. Comparative O_2^- responses of lung macrophages and blood phagocytic cells in the rat. Possible relevance to IgA immune complex induced lung injury. *Lab Invest* 1987;57:311–320.
24. Warren JS, Kunkel RG, Simon RH, Johnson KJ, Ward PA. Ultrastructural cytochemical analysis of oxygen radical-mediated immunoglobulin A immune complex induced lung injury in the rat. *Lab Invest* 1989;60:651–658.
25. Pffaffenback G, Lamm ME, Gigli I. Activation of the guinea pig alternative complement pathway by mouse IgA immune complexes. *J Exp Med* 1982;155:231–247.
26. Warren JS, Kunkel SL, Johnson KJ, Ward PA. In vitro activation of rat neutrophils and alveolar macrophages with IgA and IgG immune complexes. Implications for immune complex-induced lung injury. *Am J Pathol* 1987;129:578–588.
27. Fox RB, Merrigan MJ. Synergism of oxygen radicals and elastase in the pathogenesis of acute permeability pulmonary edema. *Am Rev Respir Dis* 1986;133:A153.
28. Weiss SJ, Peppin G, Ortiz H, Ragsdale C, Test SI. Oxidative autoactivation of laten collagenase by human neutrophils. *Science* 1985;227:747–749.
29. Peppin GJ, Weiss SJ. Activation of the endogenous metalloproteinase, gelatinase, by triggered human neutrophils. *Proc Natl Acad Sci USA* 1986;83:4322–4326.
30. Ratych RE, Chuknyiska RS, Bulkley GB. The primary localization of free radical generation after anoxia/reoxygenation in isolated endothelial cells. *Surgery* 1987;102:122–131.
31. Phan SH, Gannon DE, Varani J, Ryan US, Ward PA. Xanthine oxidase activity in rat pulmonary artery endothelial cells and its alteration by activated neutrophils. *Am J Pathol* 1989;134:1201–1211.
32. Tvedten HW, Till GO, Ward PA. Mediators of lung injury in mice following systemic activation of complement. *Am J Pathol* 1985;119:92–100.
33. Marks RM, Todd RJ, Ward PA. Rapid induction of neutrophil-endothelial adhesion by endothelial complement fixation. *Nature* 1989;339:314–317.
34. Kunkel RG, Warren JS, Johnson KJ, Ward PA. Demonstration of the complement membrane attack complex (MAC) in IgA-immune complex induced acute lung injury. *Fed Proc* 1988;2:A1176.
35. Muller-Eberhard HJ. The membrane attack complex. *Springer Semin Immunopathol* 1984;7:93–118.
36. Ross GD, Medof ME. Membrane complement receptors specific for bound fragments of C3. *Adv Immunol* 1985;37:217–229.
37. Shreiber RD. The chemistry and biology of complement receptors. *Springer Semin Immunopathol* 1984;7:221–234.
38. Friedl HP, Till GO, Ryan US, Ward PA. Mediator-induced activation of xanthine oxidase in endothelial cells. *FASEB J* 1989;3:2512–2518.
39. Pohlman TH, Harlan JM. Human endothelial cell response to lipopolysaccharide, interleukin-1 and tumor necrosis factor is regulated by protein synthesis. *Cell Immunol* 1989;119:41–52.
40. Luscinskas FW, Brock AF, Arnaoout MA, Gimbrone MA. Endothelial-leukocyte adhesion molecule-1-dependent and leukocyte (CD11/CD18)-dependent mechanisms contribute to polymorphonuclear leukocyte adhesion to cytokine-activated human vascular endothelium. *J Immunol* 1989;142:2257–2263.
41. Warren JS, Yabroff KR, Remick DG, Kunkel SL, Chensue SW, Kunkel RG, Johnson KJ, Ward PA. Tumor necrosis factor participates in the pathogenesis of acute immune complex alveolitis in the rat. *J Clin Invest* 1989;84:1873–1882.
42. Warren JS, Barton RA, Mandel DM, Matrasic K. Submitted for publication, 1990.
43. Strieter RM, Kunkel SL, Showell H, Remick DG, Phan SH,

Ward PA, Marks RM. Human endothelial cell gene expression of a neutrophil chemotactic factor by TNF-α, LPS, and IL-1β. *Science* 1989;243:1467–1469.

44. Walz A, Peveri P, Aschauer H, Baggiolini M. Purification and amino acid sequencing of NAF, a novel neutrophil-activating factor produced by monocytes. *Biochem Biophys Res Commun* 1987;49:755–761.

45. Hellewell PG, Williams TJ. A specific antagonist of platelet-activating factor suppresses oedema formation in an Arthus reaction but not oedema induced by leukocyte chemoattractants in rabbit skin. *J Immunol* 1986;137:302–307.

46. Warren JS, Mandel DM, Johnson KJ, Ward PA. Evidence for the role of platelet-activating factor in immune complex vasculitis in the rat. *J Clin Invest* 1989;83:669–678.

47. Benveniste J, Arnoux B. *Platelet activating factor and structurally related ether-lipids.* Amsterdam: Elsevier, 1983.

48. Zimmerman GA, McIntyre TM, Prescott SM. Thrombin stimulates the adherence of neutrophils to human endothelial cells *in vitro. J Clin Invest* 1985;76:2235–2246.

49. Le J, Vilcek J. Tumor necrosis factor and interleukin 1: cytokines with multiple overlapping biological activities. *Lab Invest* 1987;56:234–248.

50. Beck G, Habicht GS, Benach JL, Miller F. Interleukin 1: a common endogenous mediator of inflammation and the local Schwartzman reaction. *J Immunol* 1986;136:3025–3032.

51. Granstein RD, Margolis R, Mizel SB, Sauder DN. *In vivo* inflammatory activity of epidermal cell-derived thymocyte activating factor and recombinant interleukin-1 in the mouse. *J Clin Invest* 1986;77:1020–1028.

52. Warren JS, Yabroff KR, Remick DG, Kunkel SL, Kunkel RG, Johnson KJ, Ward PA. Intrapulmonary IL-1 and TNF in acute immune complex lung injury in the rat. *Fed Proc* 1989;3:A759.

THE LUNG: Scientific Foundations
edited by R.G. Crystal, J.B. West et al.
Raven Press, Ltd., New York © 1991.

CHAPTER 7.6.1

General Environment

Joe L. Mauderly and Jonathan M. Samet

Breathing exposes the lung to a complex and dynamic mixture of gaseous and particulate pollutants. The potential mechanisms of injury are diverse, as are the resulting diseases, and the adverse effects on health may be immediate or delayed. Exposures to hazardous air pollutants occur in the workplace, outdoors, indoors, and in special environments, such as vehicles. Exposures may take place voluntarily through personal activities, such as cigarette smoking or hobbies, or involuntarily through breathing contaminated air in the workplace or outdoors.

The adverse effects of inhaled pollutants have been of substantial public health and regulatory concern; consequently, investigative effort has been directed not only at understanding mechanisms of disease pathogenesis but at providing the type of data needed for regulatory purposes. For many pollutants, describing exposure–response relationships as a basis for judging acceptability of risk has been a primary focus of research. The investigative approaches for inhaled pollutants typically span from laboratory investigations of mechanisms to population studies of disease risks, and they draw on the scientific disciplines of toxicology and epidemiology. This chapter considers the methods used to investigate the health effects of inhaled pollutants. We begin by covering the concepts of exposure, dose, and susceptibility and then review the research approaches generally applied to inhaled pollutants.

Exposure to air pollutants takes place in many microenvironments, locations with relatively homogeneous air-quality characteristics (Fig. 1) (1). Total personal exposure to an air pollutant, which determines the likelihood of lung injury and the development of disease, represents the summation, across all microenvironments, of the product of the time spent in the microenvironment and the concentration of the pollutant (2). Thus, total personal exposure is determined by indoor and outdoor sources and time–activity patterns, which determine the time spent in each microenvironment. For most inhaled pollutants, the relationship between exposure and dose to target tissues is complex and is affected by physical characteristics of the inhaled agent and by biological characteristics of the exposed individual.

Throughout the world, the relative contributions of various microenvironments to total personal exposure have changed during the twentieth century. In the United States and many other developed countries, regulations have controlled pollutant concentrations in outdoor air and in workplaces. The indoor environment, where about 90% of time is spent in developed countries (3,4), has assumed increasing importance. However, outdoor air continues to make the predominant contribution for some pollutants, such as ozone. In some less developed countries, ambient pollution has increased while at the same time indoor pollution from combustion of biomass fuels remains unabated (5).

Moreover, new and unanticipated pollution problems continue to prompt research (6,7). Toxic air pollutants, many of which are carcinogens, are released into ambient air from industrial processes, both continuously and episodically. New building materials, furnishings, and household and office products have been linked to potentially hazardous indoor air pollution. Clinical clusters of nonspecific symptoms in occupants of modern office buildings, often referred to as ''sick-building'' or ''tight-building'' syndrome, have been widely reported but cannot be clearly linked to any specific air contaminant. The problem of indoor radon, evidently long-standing, was only recently rec-

J. L. Mauderly: Inhalation Toxicology Research Institute, Albuquerque, New Mexico 87185.
J. M. Samet: Pulmonary Division, Department of Medicine, University of New Mexico School of Medicine, Albuquerque, New Mexico 87131.

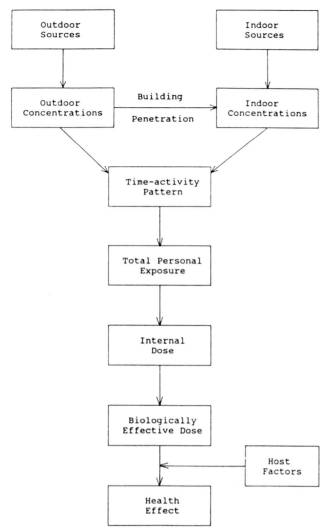

FIG. 1. Framework for considering exposure, dose, and the development of environmental respiratory disease. (From ref. 2.)

ognized. Each of these air-pollution problems has prompted research using the methods described in this chapter.

CONCEPTS OF EXPOSURE, DOSE, AND SUSCEPTIBILITY

The Respiratory Tract as a Route of Exposure

There are several excellent reviews on the role of the respiratory tract as a route of exposure to environmental agents, as well as on the field of inhalation toxicology in general (8–11). The reader is referred to these sources for detailed information; only a brief overview will be presented here.

Of all the organs, the respiratory tract presents the largest and most delicate exposure surface for contact with potentially toxic airborne materials. The surface area of the approximately 300 million alveoli in the adult human lung ranges from approximately 35 m^2 at end expiration to approximately 100 m^2 at maximum inspiration. During a lifetime, breathing brings approximately 300 million liters of air and airborne toxic agents into contact with this surface. Over most of the alveolar surface, only two cell layers, approximately 0.4–2.5 μm thick, separate the inspired air and its contaminants from the blood. Because blood leaving the lung is distributed rapidly to all parts of the body, the lung not only serves as a target organ for toxicants but also provides a route of exposure of the entire body to environmental agents.

Respiratory morbidity is common; in the United States, respiratory illness caused an estimated 657 million person-days of restricted activity and 324 million person-days of lost work during 1985 (12). Although the exact magnitude of the contribution of environmental airborne materials to this morbidity is unknown, several qualitative relationships between episodic and chronic exposures to environmental pollutants and respiratory disorders are clear. The fact that diseases of the respiratory tract account for only approximately 10% of all deaths (12) attests to the efficiency of the respiratory defenses, the repair capacity of lung tissue, and the redundancy (reserve functional capacity) inherent in the lung.

The Concept of Dose

The concept of dose is key to understanding relationships between exposures to environmental agents and adverse health effects. There are recent reviews of the dosimetry of inhaled particles (13), gases, and vapors (14,15). "Dose" might be correctly defined as the amount of the effector agent reaching the critical target site; however, the most appropriate dose term differs for different agents, different effects, and different types of studies. For some dose–effect interactions, the concentration of agent might be the controlling factor; for others, the cumulative delivery of agent (concentration × time, or C × T) might be most important. As an example of the broadest characterization of dose, epidemiological studies often employ estimates of population exposure developed from air-quality monitors located outdoors. More accurate estimates of exposure have been obtained in epidemiological studies by measurement of concentrations in the exposure environment, such as by home, workplace, or personal samplers. In most clinical and animal studies, the inhaled concentration is measured throughout defined exposure periods. Although the inhaled concentration, or C × T, is directly related to response, there is not necessarily a close mathematical relationship because of the many dosimetric variables affecting the relationship between the inhaled concentration and the amount of the effector molecules impacting on the target receptor site.

There is current effort to refine dose–response relationships by using dose terms at levels closer to the effector–receptor site and to develop dosimetric models based on physiological, morphological, pharmacological, biochemical, and molecular data. For example, modeling has been used to estimate the concentration of ozone reaching the centriacinar region (15). A further example of measurement of inhaled material at the site of response is the analysis of diesel soot in lungs of rats in order to develop lung burden–tumor incidence models for inhaled diesel exhaust (16). As the mechanisms by which an agent causes an effect are understood, the concept of dose can be carried to progressively finer (and presumably more relevant) detail. The quantification of DNA adducts from metabolites of organic compounds borne on inhaled diesel exhaust soot is an example of molecular dosimetry of an environmental pollutant (17). Clearly, the concept of dose is evolving, and the most relevant dose term must be considered to be that quantity of pollutant which can be measured and which has the greatest specificity for (most direct relationship to) the response of concern.

Respiratory Tract Defenses

Respiratory tract defenses are important determinants of the relationship between exposure and dose for many inhaled pollutants. The nasal and upper conducting airways serve to limit the dose of particles, vapors, and gases and their metabolites to the more extensive and delicate tissue of the lung. Recent findings have indicated a more important role for the defensive function of the nose than was suggested by earlier data. During nasal breathing, only approximately 20% of inhaled particles reach the deep lung, regardless of size (13). The larger particles are removed in the turbulent flow in the conducting airways by impaction and interception; however, the portion of larger particles reaching the lung increases markedly during oral breathing. It has recently been demonstrated that a much larger portion of fine particles are removed in the nose by turbulent diffusion than previously thought. In contrast to previous models in which the nasal uptake of particles below 0.5 μm in aerodynamic diameter was considered negligible (18), it is now known that the nasal uptake of particles increases with decreasing diameter below 0.1 μm (19). The importance of this finding is its implication for the deposition of radon progeny, which are preferentially attached to ultrafine particles. Similarly, it is now appreciated that most gas and vapor molecules contact the airway surface before reaching the intrathoracic airways (14). Attachment of these molecules to the surface depends upon the gas–liquid partition coefficient for each chemical species, which varies with the solubility and reactivity of each species in the airway lining fluid. Although the dynamic equilibrium between attachment and detachment of these molecules results in a portion passing deeper into the respiratory tract, the concentration of most agents reaching the lung is much lower than the concentration inhaled.

Insoluble particles deposited on the conducting airways are largely cleared (upward or downward) toward the mouth by mucociliary action and swallowed. Deposited soluble particles and gas and vapor molecules are absorbed into the airway surface liquid layer, and their fate is determined by their solubility and reactivity. Some are transformed by chemical reactions in the surface liquid or epithelial cells, whereas others are absorbed into the bloodstream. Particles reaching the alveolar region are largely cleared via phagocytosis by alveolar macrophages that transport the material to the ciliated airways. The continuous production and removal of alveolar lining and interstitial fluids also serves as a pathway for "flushing" fine particles and absorbed gas and vapor molecules from the lung. The phagocytic neutrophils also provide defense against particles deposited in the alveoli, particularly during the early phases of exposure, and immune mechanisms provide additional defenses against microorganisms and other antigenic materials.

The lung contains, as do other organs, numerous biochemical defenses against foreign materials. Antioxidant pathways, such as the glutathione system, defend against oxidants such as ozone and nitrogen dioxide. The lung is an active metabolic organ, and numerous compounds are metabolized by epithelial and endothelial cells to metabolites, some less toxic and some more toxic than the parent compound.

The respiratory tract is lined by a continuous layer of epithelium that has the defensive capacity for repair by proliferation and differentiation of cells and by scar formation in lieu of normal repopulation. Successful proliferative repair is thought to occur when the exposure to cytotoxins is not sufficient to break the epithelial basement membrane or to prevent division and differentiation of progenitor cells. An example of this reparative defense is the rapid proliferation of type II cells and subsequent differentiation into type I cells following exposure to oxidant gases (20). In addition to restoring the normal epithelium, this process acts to temporarily reduce responses to further exposure by thickening the cell layer and presenting a lower cell surface/cell mass ratio. Although the proliferation of fibroblasts and subsequent formation of fibrous scars offers a reconstructive defense if normal repair fails, this process results in a loss of normal tissue function.

The Concept of Susceptibility

The concept of susceptibility is of substantial interest from both the biological and regulatory perspectives (21,22). The Clean Air Act, which regulates concentrations of pollutants in ambient air, affords protection to all persons regardless of susceptibility. Thus, to fulfill the mandate of this far-reaching act, the effects of inhaled pollutants on the most and the least susceptible individuals must be described (23).

The term "susceptible" has most often been applied to groups who share one or more characteristics that place the group members at increased risk compared to persons lacking those characteristics. Susceptibility can be defined in biological and statistical frameworks. In a biological schema of disease pathogenesis, factors determining susceptibility modify the effects of the environmental agent of concern. In a statistical conceptualization, susceptibility might be based on the distribution of responses to exposure, with the most and least susceptible falling at the extremes of the distribution (24). Alternatively, the classification of susceptibility might hinge on the level of some characteristic for which the distributions for susceptible and non-susceptible persons are nonoverlapping.

The concept of susceptibility is readily illustrated by asthma. Asthmatics have increased airway reactivity in response to histamine, methacholine, or cold-air challenge; the distributions of airway reactivity in asthmatics and nonasthmatics are distinct and only slightly overlapping (25,26). Thus, as a group, asthmatics are widely considered as potentially susceptible to inhaled pollutants. Within asthmatics, a broad distribution of airway hyperresponsiveness can be demonstrated (25), showing that some asthmatics may be more sensitive than others.

INVESTIGATIVE TOOLS

Introduction

To characterize the health effects of inhaled pollutants, complementary lines of investigation are employed: laboratory studies, studies involving short-term exposures of human volunteers in the laboratory (generally referred to as "clinical studies"), and epidemiological studies (2). Laboratory studies are often directed at understanding mechanisms of injury; laboratory exposures may also be used to replicate biologically important patterns of human exposure while providing the capability of examining endpoints that are not accessible in human populations (e.g., bronchoalveolar lavage or lung histopathology). In clinical studies, exposure and the circumstances of exposure can be carefully controlled, and sophisticated mea-

TABLE 1. *Epidemiological study designs used to investigate the effects of inhaled pollutants*

Case–control study: An analytical design involving selection of diseased cases and nondiseased controls followed by assessment of past exposures.

Cohort study: An analytical design involving selection of exposed and nonexposed subjects with subsequent observation for disease occurrence. Short-term cohort studies of the health status of susceptible groups are often called "panel studies."

Cross-sectional study: Subjects are identified and exposure and disease status determined at one point in time.

sures of outcome can be made. However, exposures are generally brief and ethically limited to levels considered safe, and the laboratory exposures cannot fully replicate the complex mixtures inhaled in the community. Epidemiological studies address the effects of inhaled pollutants as exposure occurs in the community. The findings of epidemiological studies are often limited by errors in estimating pollutant exposure and by the difficulties of measuring and controlling for the effects of other potentially important exposures (e.g., cigarette smoking).

Research on oxidant pollution exemplifies the complementary roles of these research methods (27). Laboratory studies using *in vitro* and *in vivo* exposures have demonstrated effects of ozone on cellular structure and function, and they indicated that peroxidation of cell membranes is a key mechanism of injury (28). Long-term animal exposures have identified small airway changes at concentrations often encountered in the United States (27). Volunteers exercised at concentrations around the present National Primary Ambient Air Quality Standard experience reversible losses of ventilatory function, and the response attenuates with repeated exposure (27). Potentially susceptible populations, persons with asthma and with chronic obstructive pulmonary disease (COPD), have been included in clinical study protocols. Epidemiological studies suggest adverse effects of oxidant pollution on ventilatory function and the clinical status of asthmatics, but the findings have not been considered definitive because of the difficulty of estimating exposure.

Epidemiological Approaches

Epidemiology comprises the scientific methods used to study disease occurrence in human populations (29). Conventional epidemiological methods used to study the adverse effects of inhaled pollutants on the lung are the cross-sectional study, the cohort study, and the case–control study (Table 1). Each type of study has

TABLE 2. Data in a hypothetical cohort study or clinical trial with two exposure categories

	Exposed	Nonexposed
Involving population–time[a]		
New cases during follow-up	a	b
Population–time (person-years)	PY_1	PY_0
Involving cumulative risk[b]		
Disease during follow-up	a	b
No disease during follow-up	c	d

[a] Measure of association: ratio of incidence rates in exposed and nonexposed = $(a/PY_1)/(b/PY_0)$.

[b] Measure of association: risk ratio comparing exposed to nonexposed = $(a/a + c)/(b/b + d)$.

advantages and disadvantages for examining the effects of inhaled pollutants. The cross-sectional study is a generally economical and feasible approach, often used to investigate ambient pollution and workplace exposures. However, estimates of the effects of exposure may be biased by the tendency of more susceptible or more affected persons to reduce their level of exposure, for example, by leaving an industry or polluted area. The temporal relationship between exposure and disease may be obscured or misrepresented in cross-sectional data. For example, early cross-sectional studies of chronic airflow obstruction showed that persons with disease generally had chronic cough and sputum production, along with recurrent chest illnesses. It was hypothesized that chronic sputum production led to recurrent respiratory infections with lung injury. Subsequent cohort studies showed that this model was incorrect and that the temporal relations among chronic sputum, recurrent chest illnesses, and chronic airflow obstruction were distorted in the cross-sectional data (30,31).

Cohort and case–control studies establish the proper sequence between exposure and disease. Cohort studies represent the optimal approach for assessing the effects of rare and special exposures, such as inhalation of toxic gases or exposure to radon in underground mines. Cohort studies are prospective if the disease events will occur in the future, and retrospective if they have already taken place. The cohort design has the advantage of permitting direct estimation of disease rates for exposed and nonexposed persons and also has the capability of prospectively accumulating comprehensive exposure information (Table 2). The retrospective cohort design, often used for studying occupational exposure, can be used to rapidly evaluate the effects of a pollutant, since exposure and disease have already taken place when the investigation is initiated. Disadvantages of the cohort design include potentially high costs and losses to follow-up.

The case–control study, like the cohort study, provides a measure of association between exposure and disease (Table 3). This design has been widely used for studying lung cancer, but it has been infrequently used for nonmalignant respiratory disease. In comparison with the cohort study, the case–control study has the advantages of generally lower cost, greater feasibility, and usually shorter time frame. It is the optimum approach for studying uncommon diseases. Bias from exposure assessment and, in some circumstances, from the selection of cases and controls may limit this design.

The results of each type of epidemiological study may be affected by biases, which can alter the relationship between exposure to a pollutant and the health outcome of concern. "Selection bias" refers to distortion of the exposure–outcome relationship by differential patterns of subject participation depending on exposure and disease status. For example, subjects with airway hyperresponsiveness might be more likely to withdraw from occupational cohorts exposed to respiratory irritants.

Error in assessing either pollutant exposure or the health outcome is referred to as a "misclassification." If the error equally affects cases and controls in a case–control study or exposed and nonexposed subjects in a cohort study, the bias reduces associations towards the null value. Such nondifferential or random misclassification is of concern in most studies of inhaled pollutants and the lung; pollutant exposures are generally estimated using limited measurements or surrogates, such as propinquity to sources. Statistical power, the capability of a study to detect exposure–disease associations, declines sharply as the degree of random misclassification increases (32,33). Strategies have been proposed for assessing random misclassification in studies of inhaled pollutants and adjusting for its effects (34).

If misclassification is differential, then the bias may increase or decrease associations. Differential misclassification is of particular concern in case–control studies that assess exposures with interviews. Diseased and nondiseased subjects may not provide responses of comparable validity. For example, lung cancer cases might tend to minimize the extent of prior smoking at interview.

Confounding bias occurs when the effect of the exposure of interest is altered by another risk factor. In

TABLE 3. Data in a hypothetical case–control study[a]

	Exposed	Nonexposed
Case	a	b
Control	c	d

[a] Measure of association: relative risk of disease in exposed compared to nonexposed = $(a/b)/(c/d) = ad/bc$.

studies of inhaled pollutants, particularly for those with weak effects, confounding by cigarette smoking and occupational exposures is always of concern. The effects of confounding can be controlled through matching exposed and nonexposed subjects on potential confounding factors, or through collection of data on potential confounding factors, and use of proper analytical methods in data analysis.

The approach to studying effects of inhaled pollutants has varied with the health outcome of concern. The case–control and cohort designs have been used for respiratory and other cancers, whereas the cross-sectional and cohort designs have been used for effects other than malignancy in both the occupational and general environmental settings. For nonmalignant outcome measures, both short-term and long-term cohort approaches may be appropriate. In "panel studies," a type of short-term cohort study, subjects are enrolled and outcomes are monitored intensively. Often, daily symptom diaries are recorded, with peak flow measurements being made at least daily. Long-term cohort studies have been conducted to assess factors influencing the growth and decline of lung function across the lifespan.

For studying nonmalignant respiratory effects of inhaled pollutants, standardized methods for collecting data on symptoms and lung function should be utilized (35). The American Thoracic Society (36) and other organizations have developed and tested standardized symptom questionnaires and proposed methods for testing lung function. Use of these methods reduces bias and improves data quality.

In planning an epidemiological investigation of an inhaled pollutant, a series of complex issues must be addressed. The distribution of exposure must be described, and methods must be developed for assigning exposure to individuals as a basis for assessing exposure–disease associations and exposure–response relations, as well as for evaluating misclassification and its potential consequences. The potential health outcomes associated with exposure must be evaluated, and sensitivity and specificity of approaches for assessing the outcomes must be considered. The choice of study design is based on the temporal relationship between exposure and disease, the study populations available, and considerations of cost and feasibility.

Experimental Approaches

Clinical Studies

Clinical studies entail the short-term exposure of volunteer subjects to inhaled pollutants in the laboratory setting (37). Typically, exposure is provided through controlled contamination of the air in a chamber or through inhalation of contaminated air through a mouthpiece or mask. Thus, the duration and concentration of exposure can be controlled, serving as a basis for assessing exposure–response relationships. This method has been used most extensively for gaseous pollutants (NO_2, SO_2, and CO), but it has also been applied to particulate pollutants, such as acid aerosols. Some protocols have included multiple pollutants.

The subject groups selected for most protocols have been homogeneous, comprising either normal persons or persons with cardiac or pulmonary disease. The most widely investigated groups considered susceptible to inhaled pollutants on the basis of underlying disease have been persons with ischemic heart disease, asthma, or chronic obstructive pulmonary disease. Most often, subjects have been recruited as volunteers without reference to a defined sampling frame (38). Selection protocols have often tended to bias towards less severe disease (38).

A variety of endpoints can be monitored in a clinical study of respiratory effects: spirometric parameters, airways resistance, airways responsiveness, symptoms, and mucociliary clearance rates (39–42). Bronchoalveolar lavage may be performed following exposure, and the lavage fluid may be analyzed for markers of injury and inflammation. The development of immune responses following exposure to pollutants (e.g., NO_2) has also been evaluated (43). Clinical studies have been directed at the effects of CO on persons with ischemic heart disease; these studies have evaluated time to onset of angina during exercise as the principal outcome measure (44).

The specific exposure protocols vary with the hypothesis to be tested. Varying concentrations may be used to establish exposure–response relationships; duration and concentration may be varied to assess the comparative importance of peak exposure and total dose; and exposure may take place on multiple days to evaluate adaptation. Many protocols have included periods of exercise, which increase pollutant dose. Ethically, exposures cannot exceed levels known to be unsafe. However, protocols used for both SO_2 and ozone often produce substantial decrements in lung function in both normal persons and asthmatics (45,46).

Studies of Laboratory Animals

The most relevant information on the health effects of materials inhaled in the general environment is that obtained from humans. In the absence of such information, studies of laboratory animals can provide estimates of effects likely to occur in humans. Most of the assessments of exposure to inhaled toxicants, or the adverse effects of those exposures, can be applied to animals as well as to humans (47). Animals, on the other hand, are not humans, and the accuracy of extrapolating results from animals to humans is often difficult to assess (48). To date, although data from studies of animals have been included in criteria documents supporting standards for environmental pollutant levels, standards have been based more on data from humans than on data from animals.

The greatest advantage of animal studies is the ability to optimize experimental designs to answer specific questions and to test specific hypotheses. There are few limitations on the types or combinations of exposure materials or the range of doses in studies of animals. The experiment can be scheduled to occur at the time of the investigator's choosing. The investigator using animals can choose exposure parameters and evaluation regimens in nearly limitless combinations with a high degree of assurance that the experiment will occur according to the protocol. With few exceptions, exposures of animals can simulate any exposure pattern encountered by humans. Inhalation exposures of animals can be done once, simulating accidental or episodic exposures of humans, or can be done in a continuous or intermittent fashion, simulating chronic exposures of humans. Data can be collected from observations or measurements at any time during the study. The experiment can be designed to control for many, if not all, variables thought likely to affect the results.

One difficulty in studies of animals is the inability to expose animals for times similar to the lifespan of humans. The lifespans of commonly used animals range from 2 years for mice to 15 years for dogs, and longer for some nonhuman primates. Animals go through age-related senescent changes in all organ systems studied to date, and effects, such as cancer, which occur late in the lifespan of humans also occur late in the lifespans of animals. The question remains unanswered, however, as to whether all adverse effects that might occur late in the human lifespan can be expressed within the lifespans of laboratory animals.

The range of laboratory animal species makes it possible to address nearly all issues of human concern. No species mimics man in all characteristics. Each species has characteristics useful for addressing particular issues, and the species for each study must be chosen carefully. Summaries of the similarities and differences among animals and between animals and humans are available (49–52). A few examples of interspecies differences particularly important in studies of inhaled materials follow.

Although the lungs of all species undergo similar stages of development and senescence, the timing of these events and their relationship to birth, sexual maturation, and lifespan vary markedly among species. In

general, with regard to these processes, dogs and nonhuman primates are more similar to humans than are rodents (53,54). The lungs of rats, for example, are still growing rapidly at sexual maturation, and they continue to grow past mid-lifespan. The anatomy of the airways and intrapulmonary vessels varies among species (55). Dogs and nonhuman primates have multiple generations of respiratory bronchioles, as do humans, but respiratory bronchioles are absent or rare in rats and mice. The regional concentration gradients of inhaled gases along the respiratory tract vary among species (15). The regional deposition of inhaled particles varies among species (13), as do the time course of particle clearance from the lung and translocation to pulmonary lymph nodes (56). The behavior of alveolar macrophages toward inhaled particles varies among species (49). In general, with regard to deposition–retention characteristics, dogs and nonhuman primates are more similar to humans than are rodents. The airway responses of guinea pigs to irritants and bronchoactive drugs appear similar to those of humans; however, the airways of dogs are somewhat less reactive, and those of rats are much less reactive than those of humans. There are many differences in metabolic processes among species, both in the pathways available for metabolizing inhaled materials and in the rates of metabolism. Clearly, in designing studies using animals, the species and age of the subjects must be carefully chosen.

With few exceptions, studies of animals can be designed to accommodate the experimental designs and statistical approaches of clinical and epidemiological studies of humans. Studies of laboratory animals frequently assume designs similar to those of clinical studies of humans, in which reversible physiological changes resulting from acute (minutes to hours) inhalation exposures are measured. A common example is the use of guinea pigs to study airway responses to acute exposures to a broad range of toxicants (57). Guinea pigs have airway responses to irritants and pharmacological airway-constricting agents of the same order of magnitude as those of humans, and they also demonstrate similar degrees of intersubject variability (58). In another example, the airway responsiveness of guinea pigs, dogs, and sheep to pharmacologic bronchoconstrictors has been shown to increase after 1- to 2-hr exposures to ozone, to a degree and with a time course of recovery similar to those of humans (58). Yet another common example is the use of changes in the respiratory frequency of mice to rank the irritant potentials of chemicals during acute exposures (59). A useful correspondence has been established between the dose–response relationships for irritant effects in mice and in humans.

Nearly all types of assays of adverse effects of inhaled materials performed in humans can also be performed in animals. Clinical procedures, such as radiography, electrocardiograms, serum chemistry, and hematology, are routinely performed on dogs and nonhuman primates but are also readily applied to the smaller species. Segmental lavage by fiberoptic bronchoscopy is done in the larger species as it is in humans. Although bronchoalveolar lavage can be performed in rodents with recovery (60), it is most often performed on excised lungs (61). All respiratory function measurements used for humans have been adapted for animals, although the tests employing voluntary respiratory movements of humans (e.g., maximal forced exhalation) require anesthesia of animals (62). Challenges with bronchoactive drugs to assess airway reactivity have been done using several species (58). Skin testing and inhalation challenges with allergens are applied to animals to assess immune-mediated responses (63).

Exercise tolerance and athletic performance are more difficult to assess in animals than in humans. The willingness of animals to exercise by running (64) or swimming (65), the willingness to breathe maximally (66), and respiration and gas exchange during exercise (66) have all been evaluated. Symptomatology is difficult to assess in animals. Animals seldom express subjective symptoms that are readily classified; moreover, the investigator must rely on behavioral or functional signs, such as the respiratory pattern (59). Behavioral endpoints can be evaluated in animals, but the extrapolation to equivalent parameters in humans is often difficult (64).

Many animal studies, particularly carcinogenicity studies, take the form of prospective "epidemiological" studies of the cohort design. A population of animals is divided (usually randomly) into control and treated cohorts, health effect parameters are evaluated, and the results from the treated groups are compared statistically to those of the control group. Case–control methodology is seldom applied to studies of laboratory animals, because the exposure "history" of the animals is known from the beginning of the study and is identical for all exposed animals whether or not they express the effect of interest.

With the notable exception of a series of studies of the carcinogenicity of radioactive materials in dogs (67), most carcinogenicity studies are conducted using rats, mice, and hamsters (in order of frequency of use). The cost and length of lifespan studies using larger species, as well as the social pressures against the use of dogs and nonhuman primates, dictate the use of rodents. There are differences among species in the types and locations of lung tumors resulting from inhaled carcinogens (68). Bronchogenic carcinomas as found in humans, for example, do not occur in rodents. Despite differences in tumor type and location between rodents and humans, the benign and malignant lung tumors of rodents are thought to be useful indicators of potential pulmonary carcinogenicity in humans.

Present evidence suggests that long-term bioassays in rodents of the carcinogenicity of inhaled materials are useful for predicting the potential for pulmonary carcinogenicity in humans. Carcinogenicity assays are typically conducted using rats and/or mice exposed for a minimum of 2 years, a major portion of the lifespan. It has been shown that shorter studies may not be adequate for detecting the carcinogenic potential of inhaled agents (69). These bioassays typically use strains of rats and mice having a low spontaneous incidence of lung cancer (68). The International Agency for Research on Cancer (IARC) recently summarized current knowledge of human and animal carcinogens (70). Of the 50 agents determined to be pulmonary carcinogens in humans, there was information from studies of rats and mice on 29 agents. Of these 29 agents, 22 (76%) were conclusively shown to be pulmonary carcinogens in animals, and the limited evidence available suggested that the other seven (24%) were also carcinogens in animals. There was no known human pulmonary carcinogen for which there was conclusive evidence of a lack of carcinogenicity in animals.

Although carcinogenicity bioassays in rodents are useful for evaluating the potential for pulmonary carcinogenicity in humans, the accuracy of extrapolating results from animals to humans is limited. The limitations arise from uncertainties about the comparability of responses in animals and humans, as well as from statistical limitations due to group size. Bioassays typically employ exposures ranging from the upper limit of expected human exposures to several orders of magnitude higher, and treatment groups rarely contain more than 250 animals. Multiple exposure concentrations yield an indication of the shape of the dose–response curve at levels higher than human exposures, but the shape of the curve at levels in the range of human exposures is difficult to predict from these data (68). The sizes of populations of animals required to define exposure–response relationships at environmental levels are usually prohibitive. In lieu of this information, a linear relationship between exposure and response is typically assumed, and exposure limits for humans are set 10- to 1000-fold lower than those levels yielding no statistically significant carcinogenicity in animals (a level termed "margin of safety"). The approaches used for integrating data from bioassays and human epidemiology to estimate risks for human lung cancer from environmental exposures, and the difficulties involved, have recently been reviewed (71).

The relevance of effects at extremely high exposure levels in carcinogenicity bioassays is an important current issue. There is concern that some adverse effects which occur in animals at extremely high exposure levels may be caused by mechanisms not operative at levels to which humans are exposed. For example, statistically significant increases in lung tumor incidences in diesel-exhaust-exposed rats occur only at exposure levels causing an impairment of particle clearance from the lung, a progressive accumulation of soot, and an accompanying progressive pneumoconiosis (69). This phenomenon has been termed "lung overload," and it is not expected to occur at levels to which humans are exposed (72). Although this issue is primarily related to the carcinogenicity of inhaled particles, the principle applies to other adverse effects and to nonparticulate materials as well. The ability to design and interpret inhalation studies of animals and to extrapolate their results to humans is still evolving.

Strains of mice having particular genetic susceptibility to lung cancer are sometimes used in inhalation carcinogenesis studies, but the usefulness of this approach is questionable. These strains, such as the SENCAR (acronym for *sen*sitive to *car*cinogens) and Strain A mice, have high spontaneous rates of lung cancer, and responses to exposures are often measured by the numbers of tumors per animal rather than by the portion of animals with tumors. The ability to extrapolate these findings to predictions of carcinogenicity in humans is uncertain; the model is probably more useful for studies of the mechanisms of tumor formation. The correspondence between tumor formation in these strains and carcinogenicity in 2-year bioassays is not good (73).

Animals are used to study the influence of various host factors on susceptibility to inhaled materials. Advantage can be taken of interspecies differences (described above) to examine the influence of individual differences in the uptake, metabolism, and elimination of inhaled toxicants. Numerous differences have been shown to exist between responses of male and female animals to toxic agents. Animals have been used to study age at exposure as a susceptibility factor (54), although uncertain relationships between equivalent animal and human ages complicate the comparison.

Animal models of human lung diseases have been used to study the influence of concurrent lung disease on susceptibility to environmental exposures. There are few spontaneous animal models of human lung disease; most are induced experimentally and model only certain facets of the "equivalent" human condition (74). Animal models of asthma typically involve sensitization to antigen challenge (75,76), but it is difficult to model the range of functional and morphological changes occurring in human asthma. Animal models of emphysema are most commonly induced by instillation of proteolytic enzymes (77), and they most closely model the uncomplicated, panlobular emphysema occurring in humans with α_1-antitrypsin deficiency. Instillation of bleomycin is a common model

of pulmonary fibrosis (78); however, it is analogous only to human fibrosis, having a patchy distribution. The hyperplastic and hypersecretory characteristics of human chronic bronchitis have been difficult to model in animals. A condition resembling human chronic bronchitis has been induced in dogs by repeated, high-level exposures to sulfur dioxide (79), as well as in sensitized guinea pigs by repeated instillation of antigen (M. Schuyler, *personal communication*), but these conditions resolve upon cessation of treatment. Some models of lung disease are provided by strains of mice with genetic disorders, such as the blotchy and tight-skinned mouse models of emphysema (77) and the moth-eaten mouse model of interstitial disease (80).

Studies at the Tissue, Cellular, and Molecular Levels

Experimental studies at sub-animal levels continue to play an important role in understanding the mechanisms of the adverse health effects of inhaled airborne agents and the factors influencing individual susceptibility. These studies are generally highly focused on specific hypotheses, are often more rapid and less costly than studies of intact animals, and are currently providing a large share of the advances in our basic understanding of respiratory tract disease. Although these studies are useful for discovering and understanding fundamental phenomena, they seldom provide estimates of exposure–response relationships because of the narrowly defined and often artificial experimental conditions. Tissue, cellular, and molecular studies circumvent many host factors, defense mechanisms, and time factors operative in the intact subject. A meaningful understanding of the effects of environmental agents, therefore, requires that findings at the cellular and molecular levels be convincingly linked to findings in intact animals or in humans. A recent publication (81) gives a useful overview of current research in the cellular and molecular biology of the respiratory tract.

One current approach is the study of respiratory tract tissue transplanted into an animal host. Heterotropic tracheal grafts are used to study the effects of toxicants on tissue representative of all airways lined with respiratory epithelium. The transplanted tracheas are accessible for treatment, observation, and sampling without requiring destruction of the host. Subcutaneous rat tracheal grafts have been instilled with chemicals to test carcinogenicity in airway epithelium and to study the progression of airway cancer (82). Pollutant gases have been passed through open-ended tracheal grafts to mimic inhalation exposures (83). Denuded tracheal grafts also serve as an *in vivo* culture system for studies of the progenitorial (repopulation) capacities of different airway epithelial cells (84,85).

Normal, preneoplastic, or neoplastic rat and human airway epithelial cells have been cultured in rat tracheal grafts to study neoplastic progression (82,86,87). A similar approach is the subcutaneous injection of tumor cells into immune-deficient nude mice to allow continued tumor growth after removal from the original host (87).

Studies at the tissue level are also conducted *in vitro*. Isolated, perfused lung preparations are used for studies of pulmonary metabolism of chemicals that might be inhaled in the environment (88). Metabolic studies are also conducted using tissue homogenates (89) or cultured cells (90) incubated with chemicals, and even with microsomes isolated from lung tissue (91). Tracheal explants, sections of airway, and slices of lung parenchyma can be studied for short times in *in vitro* culture (92), but the lack of a useful transplanted or *in vitro* model for prolonged study of organized alveolar parenchyma is a current experimental limitation.

Research at the cellular level on respiratory tract responses to environmental agents is conducted using mixed primary cultures of cells isolated by enzymatic and mechanical tissue disruption, using purified populations of cells isolated by density-gradient or flow-cytometric techniques, or using cell lines derived from the respiratory tract. Cultures of normal rodent (93) or human (94) cells have been used to study the toxic and carcinogenic effects of airborne toxicants. The extrapolation of effects observed in cell cultures to those occurring *in vivo* remains a challenge. An example of a current approach to extrapolation is the estimation of *in vivo* doses by comparing cellular effects of *in vivo* exposures to those observed *in vitro*, where the dose is known (95).

Because the respiratory tract consists of many cell types, always occurring in mixed populations (96), advances in understanding phenomena at the cellular level have paralleled the ability to obtain pure populations of individual cell types. Recent developments in flow cytometry have not only provided an improved means of separating cells into relatively pure populations but have also provided measurements of normal and abnormal cell characteristics (97). An example of the usefulness of this approach is the recent separation of basal and secretory airway cells and their subsequent culture to examine their proliferative and progenitorial capacities (98). This research should help resolve current controversy about the key cell type for which radiation or chemical doses should be calculated in relation to carcinogenesis. The utility of primary cell cultures is generally limited by the loss of differentiation with succeeding cell divisions, which result in a population progressively unlike the differentiated cell of interest. An exception is the experimental system provided by the progressive differentiation of hamster tracheal epithelial cells in culture toward a mucociliary epithelium (99).

There are established lines of respiratory epithelial cells which are used in studies of the effects of environmental agents, but few have characteristics that are stable from generation to generation over a prolonged time. Preneoplastic and neoplastic epithelial cell lines allow study of the mechanisms of cancer induction (81), but these cells lose some of the characteristics of their normal counterparts *in vivo*. The lung epithelial cells (LEC) line derived from rat lung (100) has relatively stable structural and metabolic characteristics, similar to those of type II pneumocytes. These cells have been studied after exposure in culture to gas- and vapor-phase pollutants. The current use of oncogenes to immortalize epithelial cells might prove successful in providing stable cell lines (101).

Rapid advances made recently in the molecular biology of disease have included progress in understanding the genetic basis for diseases of the respiratory tract. Alterations of genes, with subsequent changes in the expression of protein gene products, have been linked to several diseases, but the greatest attention has been directed toward lung cancer. Of particular note is the study of oncogenes. Expressed in normal cells during development, these growth regulatory genes are thought to be activated by injury to DNA from physical and chemical carcinogens, and they are also thought to play a significant role in the abnormally regulated growth leading to tumor formation. The reader is referred to reviews of the molecular basis for lung cancer and the role of oncogenes (102,103).

Immunohistochemistry and *in situ* hybridization are examples of current linkages between molecular and histopathological changes. These techniques offer the identification of cells having alterations in specific genes or in gene product expression. Immunohistochemistry employs antibodies against protein products of genes to detect altered levels of protein expression. This approach has been applied to respiratory tract tissue to identify specific cell types and to determine the expression of inflammatory mediators, growth factors, and oncogene products (104). *In situ* hybridization permits the identification of RNA or DNA sequences in individual cells using specific nucleic acid probes (105). The recent development of the polymerase chain reaction technique has revolutionized the ability to detect alterations in DNA isolated from small populations of cells (106). Used together, immunohistochemistry, *in situ* hybridization, and polymerase chain reaction provide a link between molecular biology and histopathology by revealing the specific locations and natures of gene alterations in tissue. The application of these techniques is currently only limited by the availability of specific antibodies and molecular probes.

Risk Assessment

Risk assessment is increasingly utilized, particularly by governmental agencies, as a method for summarizing the extent of knowledge on inhaled pollutants. The concepts and terminology of health risk assessment were defined and described in a 1983 report by a committee of the National Research Council (107). The concept of health risk assessment is uncomplicated. The first step is hazard identification; that is, agents that pose a risk to human health are identified through epidemiological observations, animal bioassay, short-term *in vitro* tests, or other toxicological evidence. Second, the dose–response relationships, which quantify the risk per unit exposure to the agent, are established. Third, the distribution of human exposure to the agent is determined. Fourth, by combining the dose–response relationship with the information on exposure, the magnitude of the human health problem is estimated.

Health risk assessment provides a useful approach for estimating the hazard posed by pollutants to the population, as well as for identifying uncertainties in the scientific evidence which may require resolution. It may also be used to compare the hazards posed by different pollutants as a basis for establishing priorities, as well as to estimate the potential reduction in health risk that would follow intervention.

CONCLUSIONS

This chapter has reviewed complementary lines of investigation that have been used for studying the effects of inhaled pollutants on the lung. How do we employ these methods in practice? How are effects of inhaled pollutants identified and further characterized?

Some diseases associated with inhaled pollutants have been recognized as changes in occurrence were noted, and case–control and cohort studies provided subsequent evidence of an exposure–disease association. For example, during the 1940s, the increasing incidence of lung cancer prompted the performance of several case–control studies, all showing cigarette smoking to be a strong cause of lung cancer. For other pollutants, toxicological evaluation has indicated areas of concern. In the 1970s, as the numbers of diesel vehicles increased, diesel exhaust was shown to be mutagenic in short-term tests; both animal inhalation studies and epidemiological studies of diesel-exposed workers were then undertaken. Risk assessment approaches have been used to further characterize the hazard posed by diesel vehicles. Laboratory investigations of mechanisms of injury may indicate areas needing evaluation by means of animal inhalation studies or epidemiological studies.

New pollutants are regularly introduced into indoor and outdoor air. We lack effective strategies for systematically identifying these pollutants and characterizing the associated health risks. We cannot afford to evaluate each potential hazard with the full array of laboratory, animal, and human studies. Future strategies probably will involve toxicological screening with various short-term tests followed by animal inhalation studies if indicated. We also need surveillance methods for human populations.

ACKNOWLEDGMENT

Preparation of this chapter was sponsored by the U.S. Department of Energy's Office of Health and Environmental Research under Contract No. DE-AC04-76EV01013.

REFERENCES

1. Sexton K, Ryan PB. Assessment of human exposure to air pollution: methods, measurements, and models. In: Watson AY, Bates RR, Kennedy D, eds. *Air pollution, the automobile, and public health.* Washington, DC: National Academy Press, 1988;207–238.
2. National Research Council, Committee on the Epidemiology of Air Pollutants. *Epidemiology and air pollution.* Washington, DC: National Academy Press, 1985.
3. Szalai A. *The use of time: daily activities of urban and suburban populations in twelve countries.* The Hague: Moutin, 1972.
4. Chapin FS Jr. *Human activity patterns in the city.* New York: Wiley–Interscience, 1974.
5. Smith KR. *Biofuels, air pollution, and health. A global review.* New York: Plenum Press, 1987.
6. Samet JM, Marbury MC, Spengler JD. Health effects and sources of indoor air pollution. Part I. *Am Rev Respir Dis* 1987;136:1486–1508.
7. Samet JM, Marbury MC, Spengler JD. Health effects and sources of indoor air pollution. Part II. *Am Rev Respir Dis* 1988;137:221–242.
8. Kennedy GL, Trochimowicz HJ. Inhalation toxicology. In: Hayes AW, ed. *Principles and methods of toxicology.* New York: Raven Press, 1982;185–207.
9. McClellan RO, Henderson RF, eds. *Concepts in inhalation toxicology.* New York: Hemisphere Publishing, 1989.
10. Menzel DB, Amdur MO. Toxic responses of the respiratory system. In: Klaassen CD, Amdur MO, Doull J, eds. *Toxicology—the basic science of poisons,* 3rd ed. New York: Macmillan, 1986;330–359.
11. Phalen RF. *Inhalation studies: foundations and techniques.* Boca Raton, FL: CRC Press, 1984.
12. Vital and Health Statistics. *Current estimates from the National Health Interview Survey, United States, 1985.* HS (PHS) publication 86-1588, 1986.
13. Schlesinger RB. Deposition and clearance of inhaled particles. In: McClellan RO, Henderson RF, eds. *Concepts in inhalation toxicology.* New York: Hemisphere Publishing, 1989;163–192.
14. Dahl AR. Dose concepts for inhaled vapors and gases. *Toxicol Appl Pharmacol* 1990;in press.
15. Miller FJ, Overton JH, Graham RC. Regional deposition of inhaled reactive gases. In: McClellan RO, Henderson RF, eds. *Concepts in inhalation toxicology.* New York: Hemisphere Publishing, 1989;229–247.
16. Mauderly JL, Jones RK, Griffith WC, et al. Diesel exhaust is a pulmonary carcinogen in rats exposed chronically. *Fundam Appl Toxicol* 1987;9:208–221.

17. Wong D, Mitchell CE, Wolff RK, Mauderly JL, Jeffrey AM. Identification of DNA damage as a result of exposure of rats to diesel engine exhaust. *Carcinogenesis* 1986;7:1595–1597.

18. Task Group on Lung Dynamics. Deposition and retention models for internal dosimetry of the human respiratory tract. *Health Phys* 1966;12:173.

19. Yamada Y, Cheng YS, Yeh HC, Swift DL. Inspiratory and expiratory deposition of ultrafine particles in a human nasal cast. *Inhal Toxicol* 1988;1:1–11.

20. Evans MJ. Oxidant gases. *Environ Health Perspect* 1984;55:85–95.

21. Brain JD, Beck BD, Warren AJ, Shaikh RA. *Variations in susceptibility to inhaled pollutants. Identification, mechanisms, and policy implications.* Baltimore: The Johns Hopkins University Press, 1988.

22. Utell MJ, Frank R, eds. *Susceptibility to inhaled pollutants.* Philadelphia: American Society for Testing and Materials, 1989.

23. Brain JD. Introduction. In: Brain JD, Beck BD, Warren AJ, Shaikh RA, eds. *Variations in susceptibility to inhaled pollutants. Identification, mechanisms, and policy implications.* Baltimore: The Johns Hopkins University Press, 1988;1–5.

24. Bailar JC III, Louis TA. Statistical concepts and issues. In: Brain JD, Beck BD, Warren AJ, Shaikh RA, eds. *Variations in susceptibility to inhaled pollutants. Identification, mechanisms, and policy implications.* Baltimore: The Johns Hopkins University Press, 1988;30–55.

25. Cockcroft DW, Killian DN, Mellan JJA, Hargreave FE. Bronchial reactivity to inhaled histamine: a method and clinical survey. *Clin Allergy* 1977;7:235–243.

26. Hopp RJ, Bewtra AK, Nair NM, Townley RG. Specificity and sensitivity of methacholine inhalation challenge in normal and asthmatic children. *J Allergy Clin Immunol* 1984;74:154–158.

27. Lippmann M. Health effects of ozone. A critical review. *J Air Pollut Control Assoc* 1989;39:672–695.

28. Last JA. Biochemical and cellular interrelationships in the development of ozone-induced pulmonary fibrosis. In: Watson AY, Bates RR, Kennedy D, eds. *Air pollution, the automobile, and public health.* Washington, DC: National Academy Press, 1988;415–440.

29. Lilienfeld AM, Lilienfeld DE. *Foundations of epidemiology,* 2nd ed. New York: Oxford University Press, 1980.

30. Fletcher C, Peto R, Tinker C, Speizer FE. *The natural history of chronic bronchitis and emphysema.* New York: Oxford University Press, 1976.

31. U.S. Department of Health and Human Services. *The health consequences of smoking: chronic obstructive lung disease.* A report of the Surgeon General. DHHS (PHS) publication 84-50205. Washington, DC: U.S. Government Printing Office, 1984.

32. Gladen B, Rogan WJ. Misclassification and the design of environmental studies. *Am J Epidemiol* 1979;109:607–616.

33. Shy CM, Kleinbaum DG, Morgenstern H. The effect of misclassification of exposure status in epidemiological studies of air pollution health effects. *Bull NY Acad Med* 1978;54:1155–1165.

34. Armstrong BG, Oakes D. Effects of approximation in exposure assessments on estimates of exposure–response relationships. *Scand J Work Environ Health* 1982;8(suppl 1):20–23.

35. Samet JM. Definitions and methodology in COPD research. In: Hensley MJ, Saunders NA, eds. *Clinical epidemiology of chronic obstructive lung disease.* New York: Marcel Dekker, 1989;1–22.

36. Ferris BG. Epidemiology standardization project. *Am Rev Respir Dis* 1978;118(6, part 2):1–120.

37. Frank R, O'Neil JJ, Utell MJ, Hackney JD, Van Ryzin J, Brubaker PE. *Inhalation toxicology of air pollution: clinical research considerations.* Philadelphia: American Society for Testing and Materials, 1989.

38. Samet JM. Issues in the selection of subjects for clinical and epidemiological studies of asthma. In: Utell MJ, Frank R, eds. *Susceptibility to inhaled pollutants.* Philadelphia: American Society for Testing and Materials, 1989;57–67.

39. Sheppard D. Measurement of airway responsiveness in studies of health effects of air pollution. In: Frank R, O'Neil JJ, Utell MJ, Hackney JD, Van Ryzin J, Brubaker PE, eds. *Inhalation toxicology of air pollution: clinical research considerations.* Philadelphia: American Society for Testing and Materials, 1989;53–59.

40. Lippmann M. Use of aerosols for measuring airway and air space sizes and tracheobronchial mucociliary clearance rates. In: Frank R, O'Neill JJ, Utell MJ, Hackney JD, Van Ryzin J, Brubaker PE, eds. *Inhalation toxicology of air pollution: clinical research considerations.* Philadelphia: American Society for Testing and Materials, 1989;60–72.

41. Hackney JD, Linn WS. Collection and analysis of symptom data in clinical air pollution studies. In: Frank R, O'Neil JJ, Utell MJ, Hackney JD, Van Ryzin J, Brubaker PE, eds. *Inhalation toxicology of air pollutions: clinical research considerations.* Philadelphia: American Society for Testing and Materials, 1989;73–84.

42. Utell MJ. Measurements of central and peripheral pulmonary function to assess responses to air pollutants: an overview. In: Frank R, O'Neil JJ, Utell MJ, Hackney JD, Van Ryzin J, Brubaker PE, eds. *Inhalation toxicology of air pollution: clinical research considerations.* Philadelphia: American Society for Testing and Materials, 1989;43–52.

43. Goings SAJ, Kulle TJ, Bascom R, et al. Effect of nitrogen dioxide exposure on susceptibility to influenza A virus infection in healthy adults. *Am Rev Respir Dis* 1989;139:1075–1081.

44. Allred EN, Bleecker ER, Chaitman BR, et al. Short-term effects of carbon monoxide exposure on the exercise performance of subjects with coronary artery disease. *N Engl J Med* 1989;321:1426–1431.

45. Horstman DH, Folinsbee LJ. Sulfur dioxide-induced bronchoconstriction in asthmatics exposed for short durations under controlled conditions: a selected review. In: Utell MJ, Frank R, eds. *Susceptibility to inhaled pollutants.* Philadelphia: American Society for Testing and Materials, 1989;195–206.

46. McDonnell WF. Individual variability in the magnitude of acute respiratory responses to ozone exposure. In: Utell MJ, Frank R, eds. *Susceptibility to inhaled pollutants.* Philadelphia: American Society for Testing and Materials, 1989;75–89.

47. National Research Council. *Biologic markers in pulmonary toxicology.* Washington, DC: National Academy Press, 1989.

48. Calabrese EJ. *Principles of animal extrapolation.* New York: Wiley, 1983.

49. Brain JD. Species differences in inhalation toxicology: variations in exposure–dose relationships and macrophage function. In: Mohr U, Dungworth DL, Kimmele G, Lewkowski J, McClellan RO, Stober W, eds. *Inhalation toxicology: the design and interpretation of inhalation studies and their use in risk assessment.* Berlin: Springer-Verlag, 1988;11–23.

50. Hakkinen PJ, Witschi HP. Animal models. In: Witschi HP, Brain JD, eds. *Toxicology of inhaled materials.* New York: Springer, 1985;96–114.

51. Tyler WS, Coalson JJ, Stripp B. *Comparative biology of the lung.* Supplement of *Am Rev Respir Dis* 1983;128(2).

52. Warheit DB. Interspecies comparisons of lung responses to inhaled particles and gases. *Crit Rev Toxicol* 1989;20(1):1–27.

53. Mauderly JL, Hahn FF. The effect of age on lung function and structure of adult animals. In: Dungworth DL, ed. *Advances in veterinary science and comparative medicine, vol 26: Respiratory system.* New York: Academic Press, 1982;35–77.

54. Mauderly JL. Susceptibility of young and aging lungs to inhaled pollutants. In: Utell MJ, Frank R, eds. *Susceptibility to inhaled pollutants.* Philadelphia: American Society for Testing and Materials, 1989;148–161.

55. McLaughlin RF, Tyler WS, Canada RO. A study of the subgross pulmonary anatomy in various mammals. *Am J Anat* 1961;149–165.

56. Snipes MB. Species comparisons of pulmonary retention of inhaled particles. In: McClellan RO, Henderson RF, eds. *Concepts in inhalation toxicology.* New York: Hemisphere Publishing, 1989;195–221.

57. Amdur MO, Mead J. Mechanics of respiration in unanesthetized guinea pigs. *Am J Physiol* 1958;192:364–368.

58. Mauderly JL. Comparisons of respiratory function responses

of laboratory animals and man. In: Mohr U, Dungworth DL, Kimmerle G, Lewkowski J, McClellan RO, Stober, eds. *Inhalation toxicology: the design and interpretation of inhalation studies and their use in risk assessment.* Berlin: Springer-Verlag, 1988;243–261.

59. Alarie Y. Toxicological evaluation of airborne chemical irritants and allergens using respiratory reflex mechanisms. In: Leong B, ed. *Proceedings of the inhalation toxicology and technology symposium.* Ann Arbor: Ann Arbor Science Publishers, 1981;207–231.

60. Mauderly JL. Bronchopulmonary lavage of small laboratory animals. *Lab Anim Sci* 1977;27:255–261.

61. Henderson RF. Use of bronchoalveolar lavage to detect lung damage. In: Gardner DE, Crapo JD, Massaro EJ, eds. *Toxicology of the lung.* New York: Raven Press, 1988;239–268.

62. Mauderly JL. Effect of inhaled toxicants on pulmonary function. In: McClellan RO, Henderson RF, eds. *Concepts in inhalation toxicology.* New York: Hemisphere Publishing, 1989;349–404.

63. Karol MH, Hauth BA, Riley EJ, Manreni CM. Dermal contact with toluene diisocyanate (TDI) produces respiratory tract hypersensitivity in guinea pigs. *Toxicol Appl Pharmacol* 1981;58:221–230.

64. Weiss B. Behavior as an endpoint for inhaled toxicants. In: McClellan RO, Henderson RF, eds. *Concepts in inhalation toxicology.* New York: Hemisphere Publishing, 1989;475–493.

65. Dawson CA, Horvath SM. Swimming in small laboratory animals. *Med Sci Sports* 1970;2:51–78.

66. Mauderly JL, Pickrell JA, Hobbs CH, et al. The effect of inhaled 90Y fused clay aerosol on pulmonary function and related parameters of the beagle dog. *Radiat Res* 1973;56:83–96.

67. Thompson RC. *Life-span effects of ionizing radiation in the beagle dog.* Publication PNL-6822. Richland, WA: Pacific Northwest Laboratory, 1989.

68. Hahn FF. Carcinogenic responses of the lung to inhaled materials. In: McClellan RO, Henderson RF, eds. *Concepts in inhalation toxicology.* New York: Hemisphere Publishing, 1989;313–346.

69. Mauderly JL, Griffith WC, Henderson RF, et al. Evidence from animal studies for the carcinogenicity of inhaled diesel exhaust. In: *Proceedings of the Fourth International Conference on N-Substituted Aryl Compounds: Occurrence, metabolism and biological impact of nitroarenes held in Cleveland, OH, July 15–19, 1989.* New York: Plenum Press, 1990; in press.

70. IARC. *IARC monographs on the evaluation of carcinogenic risks to humans,* vols. 1–42. Overall evaluations of carcinogenicity: an updating of IARC monographs, supplement 7, 1987.

71. McClellan RO, Cuddihy RG, Griffith WC, Mauderly JL. Integrating diverse data sets to assess the risks of airborne pollutants. In: Mohr U, ed. *Assessment of inhalation hazards: integration and extrapolation using diverse data.* Berlin: Springer-Verlag, 1989;3–22.

72. Morrow PE. Possible mechanisms to explain dust overloading of the lungs. *Fundam Appl Toxicol* 1988;10:369–384.

73. Maronpot RR, Shimkin MB, Witschi HP, Smith LH, Cline JM. Strain A mouse pulmonary tumor test results for chemicals previously tested in the National Cancer Institute carcinogenicity tests. *J Natl Cancer Inst* 1986;76:1101–1112.

74. Nemery B, Dinsdale D, Verschoyle RD. Detecting and evaluating chemical-induced lung damage in experimental animals. *Bull Eur Physiopathol Respir* 1987;23:501–528.

75. Drazen JM. Pulmonary physiologic abnormalities in animal models of acute asthma. In: Lichtenstein LM, Austen KF, eds. *Asthma: physiology, immunopharmacology and treatment.* New York: Academic Press, 1977;249–264.

76. Hirshman CA. Bronchial inhalation challenge testing in dog models of asthma. In: Spector SL, ed. *Provocative challenge procedures: bronchial, oral, nasal, and exercise,* vol I. Boca Raton, FL: CRC Press, 1983;13–32.

77. Snider GL, Lucey EC, Stone PJ. Animal models of emphysema. *Am Rev Respir Dis* 1986;133:149–169.

78. Thrall RS, Swendsen CL, Shannon TH, et al. Correlation of changes in pulmonary surfactant phospholipids with compli-

ance in bleomycin-induced pulmonary fibrosis in the rat. *Am Rev Respir Dis* 1987;136:113–118.

79. Greene SA, Wolff RK, Hahn FF, Henderson RF, Mauderly JL, Lundgren DL. Sulfur dioxide-induced chronic bronchitis in beagle dogs. *J Toxicol Environ Health* 1984;13:945–958.

80. Rossi GA, Hunninghake GW, Kawanami O, et al. Motheaten mice—an animal model with an inherited form of interstitial lung disease. *Am Rev Respir Dis* 1985;131:150–158.

81. Thomassen DG, Nettesheim P, eds. *Biology, toxicology and carcinogenesis of respiratory epithelium.* New York: Hemisphere Publishing, 1990.

82. Klein-Szanto AJP, Pal BC, Terzaghi M, et al. Heterotopic tracheal transplants: techniques and applications. *Environ Health Perspect* 1984;56:75–86.

83. Klein-Szanto AJP, Marchok AC, Terzaghi M. *In vivo* studies on enhancement and promotion of respiratory tract carcinogenesis: studies with heterotopic tracheal transplants. In: Mass MJ, et al. eds. *Carcinogenesis.* New York: Raven Press, 1985;119–130.

84. Johnson NF, Hubbs AF, Thomassen DG. Epithelial progenitor cells in the rat respiratory tract. In: Thomassen DG, Nettesheim, eds. *Biology, toxicology and carcinogenesis of respiratory epithelium.* New York: Hemisphere Publishing, 1990;88–98.

85. Nettesheim P, Jetten AM, Inayama Y, et al. The role of clara cells and basal cells as epithelial stem cells of the conducting airways. In: Thomassen DG, Nettesheim P, eds. *Biology, toxicology and carcinogenesis of respiratory epithelium.* New York: Hemisphere Publishing, 1990;99–111.

86. Terzaghi M, Nettesheim P, Wiliams ML. Repopulation of denuded tracheal grafts with normal, preneoplastic, and neoplastic epithelial cell populations. *Cancer Res* 1978;38:4546–4553.

87. Baba M, Klein-Szanto AJP, Trono D, et al. Preneoplastic and neoplastic growth of xenotransplanted lung-derived human cell lines using deepithelialized rat tracheas. *Cancer Res* 1987;47:573–578.

88. Bond JA, Mauderly JL. Metabolism and micromolecular covalent binding of ^{14}C-1-nitropyrene in isolated perfused/ventilated rat lungs. *Cancer Res* 1984;44:3924–3929.

89. Bond JA, Mauderly JL, Henderson RF, et al. Metabolism of ^{14}C-1-nitropyrene in respiratory tract tissue of rats exposed to diesel exhaust. *Toxicol Appl Pharmacol* 1985;79:461–470.

90. Siegfried JM, Rudo K, Bryant BJ, et al. Metabolism of benzo(a)pyrene in monolayer cultures of human bronchial epithelial cells from a series of donors. *Cancer Res* 1986;46:4368–4371.

91. Leung HW, Henderson RF, Bond JA, et al. Studies on the ability of rat lung and liver microsomes to facilitate transfer and metabolism of benzo(a)pyrene from diesel particles. *Toxicology* 1988;51:1–9.

92. Mossman BT, Marsh JP, Dantona R, et al. Involvement of active oxygen species (AOS) in injury, repair and proliferation of tracheobronchial epithelial cells after exposure to asbestos fibers. In: Thomassen DG, Nettesheim P, eds. *Biology, toxicology and carcinogenesis of respiratory epithelium.* New York: Hemisphere Publishing, 1990;145–154.

93. Nettesheim P, Barrett JC. Tracheal epithelial cell transformation: a model system for studies on neoplastic progression. *CRC Crit Rev Toxicol* 1984;12:215–239.

94. Masui T, Lechner JF, Yoakum GH, et al. Growth and differentiation of normal and transformed human bronchial epithelial cells. *J Cell Physiol [Suppl]* 1986;4:73–81.

95. Thomassen DG. Preneoplastic transformation of rat tracheal epithelial cells in culture by alpha particles and x-rays: understanding the role of radiation in respiratory carcinogenesis and estimation of radiation dose *in vivo.* In: Chadwick KH, Seymour C, Barnhart B, eds. *Cell transformation and radiation-induced cancer.* Bristol, England: Adam Hilger, 1989;325–332.

96. Breeze RG, Wheeldon EB. The cells of the pulmonary airways. *Am Rev Respir Dis* 1977;116:705–777.

97. Shapiro HM. *Practical flow cytometry,* 7th ed. New York: Alan R. Liss, 1988.

98. Johnson NF, Wilson JS, Habbersett R, et al. Separation and

characterization of basal and secretory cells from the rat trachea by flow cytometry. *Cytometry* 1990; in press.

99. Wu R, Nolan E, Turner C. Expression of tracheal differentiated functions in serum-free hormone-supplemented medium. *J Cellular Physiol* 1985;125:167–181.

100. Li AP, Hahn FF, Zamora PO, et al. Characterization of a lung epithelial cell strain with potential applications in toxicological studies. *Toxicology* 1983;27:257–272.

101. Ke Y, Reddel RR, Gerwin BI, et al. Human bronchial epithelial cells with integrated SV40 virus T antigen genes retain the ability to undergo squamous differentiation. *Differentiation* 1988; 38:60–66.

102. Birrer MJ, Minna JD. Molecular genetics of lung cancer. *Semin Oncol* 1988;15:226–235.

103. Burck KB, Liu ET, Larrick JW. *Oncogenes: an introduction to the concept of cancer genes*. New York: Springer-Verlag, 1988.

104. Linnoila I, Petrusz P. Immunohistochemical techniques and their applications in the histopathology of the respiratory system. *Environ Health Perspect* 1984;56:131–148.

105. Pardue ML. *In situ* hybridization. In: Hames BD, Higgins SJ, eds. *Nucleic acid hybridization: a practical approach*. Oxford: IRL Press, 1985;179–202.

106. Scharf SJ, Horn GT, Erlich HA. Direct cloning and sequence analysis of enzymatically amplified genomic sequences. *Science* 1986;233:1076–1078.

107. National Research Council, Committee on the Institutional Means for Assessment of Risks to Public Health. *Risk assessment in the federal government: managing the process*. Washington, DC: National Academy Press, 1983.

THE LUNG: Scientific Foundations
edited by R.G. Crystal, J.B. West et al.
Raven Press, Ltd., New York © 1991.

CHAPTER 7.6.2

Biological Consequences of General Environmental Contaminants

Carroll E. Cross and Barry Halliwell

Much research has been directed toward elucidating the relationships between exposure to inhaled toxicants and associated lung-related health risks. Some factors which must be considered in assessing this relationship are shown in Fig. 1. Once assessments of exposure have been performed (levels 1–3 in Fig. 1), the effects of inhaled toxins on specific lung cells, as well as the consequences of these effects, must be addressed. The effects depend on (a) the amount of toxin deposited at various anatomic sites along the respiratory tract, (b) the effectiveness of the local defense mechanisms, (c) the sensitivity and intensity of neurohumoral responses, (d) the relative sensitivity to damage of the cells at risk in each location, and (e) the magnitude and nature of the resulting inflammatory and repair processes.

The airway and lung parenchyma contain numerous metabolically active and interacting individual cell types. The cells are present in varying populations in different topographic regions and are innervated in different ways (1). Considering such complexity of lung morphology and function, it is not surprising that a very wide spectrum of biological assays has been applied to describe the effects of inhaled toxins on the lung (2–6). Measured toxin-induced effects on the lung may represent pathophysiological lung defense responses (e.g., increased mucus secretion by tracheobronchial cells) or reflect indices of toxic lung cell damage (e.g., epithelial cell desquamation). Indeed, the boundary area between exposure-activated "defense"

and exposure-induced "injury" mechanisms is often indistinct, as might be exemplified by toxins eliciting (a) neuronal-mediated alterations in breathing patterns or (b) transient increases in airway reactivity. As simplistically depicted in Fig. 2, this situation becomes even more complex when one considers the inherent difficulties in distinguishing between (a) toxin-induced lung cell injury leading to secondary activation of neurohumoral–inflammatory processes and (b) primary activation of neurohumoral–inflammatory processes that leads to secondary lung cell injury. In many types of airway responses, and probably in parenchymal responses, both processes contribute to the toxin-induced biological response.

This chapter will present an overview of the interaction between inhaled environmental contaminants and the lung. No mention is made of inhaled microorganisms, allergens, or immunological responses, and only limited mention is given to the role of inhaled toxins in lung carcinogenesis. More detailed reviews of the specific effects of individual inhaled toxins and their unique reactions with the lung are enumerated elsewhere (2,3,7–9).

CLASSES OF BIOLOGICAL CONTAMINANTS

Airborne contaminants include a wide spectrum of environmental and occupational substances that can be toxic to the lung. As shown in Table 1, they can be grouped into physicochemical categories. The list of agents in each category is extensive and will not be detailed. However, some generalizations are warranted.

The physicochemical character—and, to a lesser extent, quantity—of the inhaled toxin can be expected to determine the toxin's topographic distribution,

C. E. Cross: Departments of Internal Medicine and Human Physiology, School of Medicine, University of California—Davis, Davis, California 95616.
B. Halliwell: Department of Biochemistry, King's College, University of London, London WC2R 2LS, England.

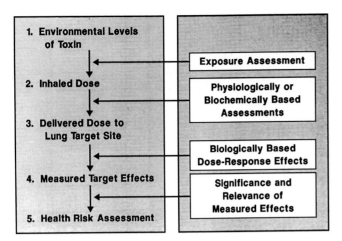

FIG. 1. Assessments of biological consequences of exposure to general environmental contaminants.

TABLE 1. *Types of inhalant toxins*

Gases (e.g., ozone, nitrogen dioxide, sulfur dioxide)
Vapors, fumes, and aerosols (e.g., chlorine gas, cadmium oxide, acid aerosol)
Inorganic particulates (e.g., nickel compounds, asbestos fibers, silica)
Organic particulates (e.g., grains, wood cedar bark, benzopyrene)
Radioactive gases (e.g., radon) and particulates (e.g., alpha- and beta-emitting radionucleotide particles)
Mixtures (e.g., cigarette smoke, diesel engine exhaust, coal tar aerosols)

thereby revealing its major site of biological effect within the respiratory tract. Large particles (over 5–10 μm in aerodynamic diameter) or highly reactive or water-soluble gases have a predilection to affect nasopharyngeal regions, whereas smaller particles (less than 3–5 μm in aerodynamic diameter) or less reactive or less soluble gases have a predilection to affect more distal lung units (10). High concentrations of inhaled toxins or the inhalation of mixtures of toxins (Table 1) can be expected to obscure these potential gradients of cell injury. Other factors to be considered include (a) toxins which are either activated or detoxified to unequal extents by cells containing uptake and metabolizing systems for the toxin in question (e.g., cytochrome P-450) (11) and (b) toxins such as particulates which could deposit selectively at airway branch points where more turbulent flow occurs (10).

Of particular interest are respirable particulates which penetrate deep into the respiratory tract and which may contain a variety of toxic elements and compounds on their surface. These would include particulates from cigarette smoke, electric utility coal combustion (fly ash), smelters and foundries, oil refineries and chemical production plants, and car exhaust, especially diesel engines. It can be expected that these particulates, deposited on airways or alveoli, would have a multitude of diverse biological effects on the lung. For example, metal dusts (such as cadmium, manganese, vanadium, and beryllium) and crystalline silica are known to interact with alveolar macrophages (AMs), although the secondary consequences are incompletely understood (12). For other toxic inhalants such as fibrous dusts, we can expect fiber type, dimensions, surface properties, including spacial configuration of surface change, and chemical composition to affect the biological consequences upon the lung.

Recent studies have suggested that normally innocuous particles of low solubility and low acute toxicity (e.g., titanium dioxide), administered at levels which overload normal lung particle clearance, can result in activation of pulmonary inflammatory and fibrogenic processes (dust overload effect) (13). Attention has also recently focused on ultrafine particles (10–40 nm) which may cross the alveolar epithelial barrier more readily than larger particles, therefore having the potential to cause a more direct interstitial lung injury. This same concept has been applied to considerations of the increased toxicity of long asbestos fiber administration observed in experimental animals, where fiber penetration to the interstitium can occur.

When considering inhalation of toxic organic materials such as bacterial cell walls and other organic products, it may be difficult to separate direct toxic mechanisms of injury (e.g., bacterial endotoxin) from immunologic responses that can occur if there has been prior sensitization to one or more antigens present.

DELIVERY TO TARGET SITES

As shown in Fig. 1, the actual dose of toxin delivered to target tissue sites depends on many factors other

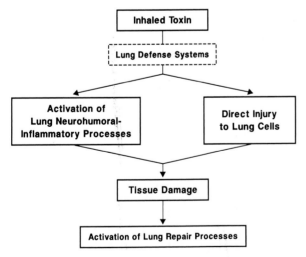

FIG. 2. Schematic diagram of toxicant-induced effects on lung cells.

than environmental concentrations. Localized respiratory tract deposition, retention, and metabolism of inhaled toxin are obvious important factors in determining the resultant biological effects on lung cells and tissue. In many instances, especially for soluble and reactive gases and for large respirable particulates and aerosols, the inhaled toxin is continuously being removed from the inhaled airstream, with the toxin concentration declining distally from the upper airway and trachea. The following factors help to determine toxicant deliveries to lung target sites: inhaled dose, solubility, and reactivity of toxin; humidity; temperature; respiratory breath profiles; total ventilation; airway mechanics; anatomic variations between species and individuals of a species; absorptive and reactive kinetics with mucus and epithelial lining fluid; and the presence or absence of disease.

The biological responses of the lung to inhaled toxins will thus depend on the pattern of deposition, dose, and time frame over which this amount persists. The regional deposition of patterns of gases, aerosols, and particulates on respiratory tract surfaces is the result of specific physical and chemical mechanisms mentioned above and detailed elsewhere (10,14,15). The accurate interpretation of lung biological effects resulting from inhaled toxins necessitates an appreciation of the factors that control and affect quantitative patterns of toxin deposition at the specific site relevant to the biological effect being measured.

MECHANISTIC CONSIDERATIONS

Many different cell-surface receptors and post-receptor transducing systems are affected by inhaled environmental toxins. The cell injury produced can be primary (i.e., a direct effect of the toxin or its metabolites). Alternatively or additionally, it can be secondary to activation of generalized inflammatory processes. In recent years, much progress has been made in developing mechanistic models as a means of investigating and improving assessment of the potential injurious effects of toxin exposures.

The identification of the mechanisms regulating pulmonary pathophysiological responses is important to understanding how biological processes are influenced by toxicological exposures. An understanding of the precise events taking place in the microenvironment at the polarized epithelial cell surface of the respiratory tract is essential. Equally important is an understanding of how host defenses and/or compensating systems intervene to prevent and/or repair toxin-induced damage if it is not too severe.

Defense Systems

The respiratory system has a number of important mechanisms to minimize the delivery and impact of inhaled toxins. These defense mechanisms include abundant reflexes, mucus production and mucociliary clearance, and cellular events involving phagocytic and immunocompetent cells (16; see also Chapters 3.1.2, 3.1.3, 3.4.1–3.4.6, 7.3.5, 7.4.1, 7.4.2, and 7.5.1). Epithelia that are frequently exposed to hostile environments often protect themselves by the secretion of mucus, and the respiratory tract exemplifies this. It is the respiratory tract mucus that represents the first lung system to encounter toxic inhalants; it thus constitutes an important lung defense system. Somewhat surprisingly, other than for the effects on the rate of mucus synthesis and secretion and mucociliary clearance (10), relatively little is known about the precise chemical interactions between toxins and mucus.

It is paradoxical that many pulmonary defensive and protective mechanisms, such as cough, mucus production, bronchoconstriction, and even phagocytic cell activation, are often measured as endpoints of lung injury by noxious substances. The use of defense system markers of endpoint effects can be considered an indicator of ongoing respiratory tract physiological processes, but it may not in and of itself constitute a toxic effect.

Particularly important for the detection of biological effects on the lung is the extensive afferent and efferent nervous system innervation of the airways (17); symptoms such as rawness, irritation, tightness, and breathlessness allow potential harm to the lung to be sensed (18). Although activation of neurohumoral responses in airways is generally recognized as being potentially injurious (to airway function), especially in asthma (17), it can be speculated that the absence of this protective network could result in more direct lung cell injury secondary to inhalation of a toxic substance, whether it be O_3 or a complex toxicant such as cigarette smoke.

The lungs also possess a sophisticated network of extracellular antiprotease (19) and antioxidant (20,21) defense mechanisms important in providing protection from both exogenous and endogenous proteolytic and oxidant stresses resulting from both primary and secondary toxic actions.

AMs play a key role in lung host defenses. They coordinate the alveolar–interstitial inflammatory and fibrotic responses to inhaled environmental toxins via their productions of various modulators of cell activity, such as chemotaxins, cytokines, and growth factors. Because they are easily obtainable in large numbers by lavage (22,23), their interactions with inhaled toxins have been extensively studied (12,23).

In the final analysis, the pathogenesis of damage caused by an inhaled toxic agent can be regarded as the result of an imbalance between (a) injurious mechanisms initiated by the toxin and (b) defensive "cytoprotective'' factors at the site where the toxicant is acting.

Epithelial Lining Fluid

The epithelial lining fluid (ELF) of the respiratory tract is the first major component of the lungs to be exposed to inhaled toxins. In proximal airways, ELF consists of a mixture of secreted mucus and the airway surface (periciliary) fluid, whereas in distal bronchiolar and alveolar regions, secretions of Clara cells and type 2 cells, including surfactant, take the place of mucus. The thickness and character of these protective fluid layers can be critical to the determination of epithelial cell ''dose'' of an inhaled toxin. These fluids contain considerable amounts of physiologically important substances capable of reacting with inhaled toxins. For example, mucus can directly scavenge certain reactive free radicals (24) and may combine directly with oxidizing agents such as NO_2 (25). It also has a substantial buffer capacity (26). Oxidation of lipid components of surfactant may damage its function and could generate cytotoxic end-products such as hydroperoxides and unsaturated aldehydes (27,28).

ELF contains low concentrations (relative to that in plasma) of plasma proteins such as ceruloplasmin and albumin (22). Albumin is a major antioxidant in plasma, because it can scavenge oxidants such as hypochlorous acid released by activated neutrophils. Both albumin and ceruloplasmin bind copper ions in ways that prevent these ions from accelerating oxidative damage to lipid and to protein (29). Hence, like other extracellular fluids (30), ELF would be expected to be more susceptible to inhaled oxidants than would plasma. This vulnerability is somewhat offset by the presence of higher concentrations (relative to that in plasma) of certain low-molecular-weight antioxidants [i.e., glutathione (31) and ascorbate (32)]. Alpha-tocopherol is also present in ELF (33). It is probable that these antioxidants represent a significant first line of defense in the lung against inhaled oxidants such as ozone, chlorine, and cigarette smoke, operating in concert with cell antioxidants and antioxidant enzymes (21). Ascorbic acid may be particularly important in this regard (34,35).

Although the antioxidant ability of plasma is fairly well characterized (34–36), the extent by which ELF protects the underlying delicate respiratory epithelium from oxidant injury is presently unclear. In fact, little is known about the specific role these fluids play in interacting with inhaled toxicants. More work is needed in this area.

Direct Effects

Few, if any, inhaled pneumotoxins directly affect receptors ''specific'' for a particular toxin; instead, they initiate biological responses by effects on numerous interacting mediator systems including nonspecific effects on cell membranes, with secondary effects on the multitude of membrane receptor and transducing cascades. The increasing development of cell culture systems that mimic *in vivo* exposure conditions will be most helpful in distinguishing between various direct and indirect toxin-induced lung cell effects, but it will require integration of information such as the role of neurohumoral and inflammatory mediator activations. The possible important role of perturbations in cell–cell and cell–matrix signaling systems must also be taken into account.

Airway Sensory Innervations and Axon Reflexes

The respiratory tract mucosa is richly innervated with sensory nerves. These well-developed sensory innervations and related reflex pathways can be considered to be a defensive mechanism designed to minimize the impact and spread of noxious inhalants (17,18). However, the end results of activation of these reflexogenic pathways are often used as ''markers'' of inhaled toxin interactions with the lung. For example, even such a frequently used index of toxin-induced epithelial damage as increase in lavage albumin concentration could be partly attributed to a neural-mediated mechanism which transiently increases epithelial and/or microvascular permeability, rather than being considered a result of a direct action of the inhaled toxin on the respiratory tract epithelial cells. Activations of these neural pathways undoubtedly represent important effector systems for many respiratory toxins, including air pollutants and cigarette smoke. Determining the extent to which activations of these normal defense pathways reflect direct nondamaging ''irritant'' activity, as opposed to activations via cell injury/damage pathways, comprises a challenge to the health scientist.

In the airways, an extensive vagal sensory nervous system has been found to be widely distributed in and beneath the airway epithelium, around blood vessels, and in the smooth muscle (17). Irritant stimuli, such as many inhaled toxins, trigger these type C, capsaicin-sensitive sensory nerves to release neuropeptides which may then initiate the process of neurogenic inflammation. These acute inflammatory responses can be produced by tachykinins, a group of neuropeptides including substance P and neurokinins A and B, which are released from unmyelinated sensory nerves. These neuropeptides stimulate mucus secretion, cause vasodilation, increase vascular permeability, cause neutrophils to adhere to vascular endothelium, may play a role in mast cell and monocyte/macrophage activa-

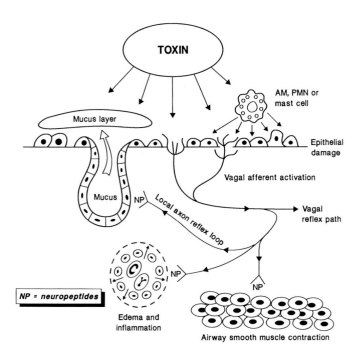

FIG. 3. Interactions of inhaled toxicants with airway neurosensory pathways.

tion, induce cough, and cause bronchoconstriction (Fig. 3) (18,37). They are capable of causing considerable epithelial cell injury and may contribute to the epithelial shedding which is characteristic of severe asthmatic reactions (17).

Stimulation of airway receptors/nerve endings may also lead to an involuntary inhibition of full inspiration, leading to reductions in total lung capacity and vital capacity and possibly leading to increased respiratory frequencies (38). Interactions between irritant toxins, inflammatory mediators, and the afferent nerve endings with their neurotransmitter release systems almost certainly play an important role in the airway inflammation seen after exposures to lung toxins such as ozone and toluene diisocyanate. Release of neurokinins by sensory nerve fibers is known to play an important role in the airway mucosal edema and inflammation caused by histamine. The precise molecular mechanisms by which neurogenic inflammatory pathways are triggered have not been fully elucidated, but it seems likely that more than one mediator–receptor system may be involved and that transient increases in intracellular free Ca^{2+} represent important events.

Inflammation-Related Effects

Inflammation is a frequent pulmonary response to inhaled toxins. The fact that the lung contains so many cell types complicates studies directed at understanding the precise cellular processes involved. The cells involved in lung inflammatory processes presumably include lung epithelial, interstitial, and endothelial cells as well as a wide spectrum of inflammatory/immune effector cells such as neutrophils (PMNs), AMs, eosinophils, basophils, lymphocytes, mast cells, platelets, and, to an extent, lung nervous system components (see Chapters 3.4.1, 3.4.5, 3.4.7, 3.4.9–3.4.11, and 7.7.1).

Lung inflammatory/immune processes initiated by inhaled toxins are capable of generating a host of mediator substances such as proteases, oxidants, eicosanoids, cytokines, and neuropeptides. Complex interactions occur between the endogenous lung cells, the inflammatory/immune effector cells, the elements of the nervous system, and the various mediators. The mediators themselves are capable of interacting synergistically or sometimes antagonistically to modulate the intensity of overall inflammatory responses. It is unlikely that any single cell type or mediator pathway is essential. There is considerable knowledge of the actions produced by individual mediators, but our understanding of their interactions is still at a rudimentary level.

The activation of lung inflammatory processes such as axon reflexes, perhaps best exemplified in asthma (17), results in a number of characteristic injurious features. These include edema, increased influxes of inflammatory cells, increased airway mucus secretion, and hyperreactivity to physical, chemical, and pharmacological stimuli. Injury to, and exfoliation of, epithelial lining cells can also occur, caused directly by inflammatory mediators and/or by cytotoxic proteins or other species (e.g., oxygen radicals) derived from inflammatory cells. Since many of these same responses are seen following direct toxin-induced cytotoxic lung cell injury, it is difficult to differentiate between (a) lung inflammatory reactions subsequent to intense activations of lung neurohumoral–mediator processes and (b) lung reactions occurring as a result of direct toxin-induced cell injury.

PMN activation and recruitment to the lung represent one important inhalant-induced toxic effect on the respiratory tract. Because this process can be assessed by bronchoalveolar lavage (22,23), attention has focused on PMNs as both markers and effectors of toxin-induced lung injury (39–41). Their precise effector role in many forms of toxin-induced lung injury remains controversial, since depletion of PMNs often does not protect fully (if at all) against lung injury in experimental animals. Of particular interest has been the hypothesis that PMNs play an important role in the airway hyperresponsiveness that occurs after exposure to some inhaled toxins, such as ozone (42,43) and isocyanates (44). It should be remembered that, to some degree, PMNs present at sites of inflammation may represent a mechanism important in the normal resolution process to a toxin-induced injury.

AMs constitute more than 95% of the cells present in the normal bronchoalveolar spaces and are known to have a variety of functions during inflammatory responses (41,45). It is almost certain that AMs play a central role in lung biological responses to inhaled toxins (41,45–47). AMs are the first lung cells to encounter inhaled particulates, and they may respond by ingesting and destroying these toxins and/or by recruiting other inflammatory cells (such as PMNs) into the lung. The rise in AM numbers appears to be a fundamental element of the lung's response to toxins. The central role of AMs is particularly clear in the case of mineral dusts, many of which activate AMs (47–49).

Activation of AMs results not only in release of several proteolytic enzymes and reactive O_2 species, but also in production of many secretory substances (e.g., macrophage elastase, which is not inhibited by α_1-antitrypsin; ref. 19). The AM secretory profile is markedly sensitive to changes in cell environment and, in particular, to injury and inflammation. Their secretory products include chemotactic factors, eicosanoids, cytokines, fibronectin, and growth-promoting and -inhibiting factors. These products are known to be capable of influencing many different cells in the alveolar compartment and to be important in influencing such processes as cell and matrix injury and repair, including fibrogenesis (41,45). AM local alveolar releases of chemotactic factors for PMNs may be of particular importance in acute injury, whereas AM-derived chemotaxins, "competence" factors, and growth factors for fibroblasts appear to play an important role in lung fibrogenic responses to toxins such as asbestosis.

It is likely that AMs demonstrate a different secretory profile for different toxins. Illustrative of the complexity of the analysis of toxin-related effects on AMs is the fact that AMs are not a homogeneous population (41,45) and that they produce over 100 secretory products (41) and at least 900 proteins, of which 45 are synthesized at a significantly increased rate and 78 at a significantly decreased rate in humans exposed to 0.4 ppm ozone for 2 hr with intermittent exercise (50).

AM responses to environmental toxins are increasingly being studied with sophisticated techniques, such as flow cytometric and molecular biology methods, to further define their toxin-induced functional changes. AMs can also down-regulate lung inflammatory reactions by the release of various inhibitor mediators (41). The balance between release of activators and inhibitors and the mechanisms regulating this release is probably often critical in determining the outcome of toxin-induced injurious processes in the lung.

Phagocytes represent only one component of a very complex network of cellular and humoral factors interacting in defense, injury, and repair of the lung (51). Lymphocytes, platelets, eosinophils, fibroblasts, mast cells, and lung epithelial and endothelial cells are all also implicated in lung injury and repair processes, often synergistically with PMNs and AMs.

Arachidonic acid metabolites may sometimes be important physiological mediators within the lung. It is probable that locally released prostaglandins are important in the control of airway secretion in a variety of disease states; as such, these eicosanoids have been implicated in the pathogenesis of a variety of lung disorders, including those secondary to inhaled toxins (51,52). It is well known that lung tissues, including epithelial cells, can release substantial amounts of eicosanoids when appropriately stimulated (52). Thus eicosanoids, along with another phospholipid-derived mediator, platelet-activating factor, are increasingly being recognized as markers of cellular responses to inhaled pollutants.

The role of cytokine and related growth-factor-mediated cascades in the control of lung inflammatory, immune, and fibrogenic reactions is now well recognized (41,45,47,53,54). For example, release of tumor necrosis factor from AMs may represent a risk factor for the development of lung fibrosis after exposure to coal dust (49). Many cytokines are being used as "state-of-the-art" markers of lung effects of inhaled toxins. A major current challenge in inhalation toxicology is to ascertain the true importance of these mediators of inflammatory processes in pulmonary responses to various environmental toxins.

Oxidant-Mediated Effects

O_2-derived species such as H_2O_2 and O_2-centered free radicals, including superoxide anion ($O_2^{\cdot-}$) and hydroxyl radical ($\cdot OH^{\cdot}$), are increasingly being implicated as an important mechanism of injury in a variety of pathologic states (55–57). These species can be produced as a direct effect of oxidizing environmental toxins, as a secondary effect of cell injury (58), or as a result of inflammation with activation and recruitment of phagocytes (59).

Examples of direct oxidant injury are provided by photochemical air pollutants (O_3 and NO_2) and cigarette smoke (56). Their toxic effects are probably mediated, in part, by reactions that involve the formation of activated O_2 species (60–62). Potentially pneumotoxic and fibrogenic mineral and metallic dusts, including crystalline silica and asbestos fibers, not only produce oxidants by activation of AMs, but many of them also contain free radical or surface iron ions that can catalyze formation of $\cdot OH$ and other reactive species (48,63–65). Many pathways for producing O_2 radicals are dependent on O_2 concentration, and it may be relevant that the lung has the highest P_{O_2} of any tissue in the human body.

The targets of oxidative damage include both cells

and extracellular components of the lung, such as constituents of ELF and lung matrix. Oxidant injury to cells is a complex event; as is the case for most toxin-related cell damage processes, the critical molecular targets for oxidant-induced cell damage are only beginning to be understood.

Several groups of investigators have reported that oxidants cause depletion of ATP in target cells, although this does not seem to explain oxidant-induced increases in epithelial cell permeability (66). DNA damage is a frequent observation (57,67,68). Cell membrane function represents an obvious potential site of peroxidative injury, thereby affecting a host of cell functions that could include membrane receptors and signal transducing systems. Cytoskeletal damage can occur by calcium ion translocation subsequent to activation of inositol lipid signaling pathways, as might alterations of intercellular tight junction activities and changes in secretory activity (48,65,67,69). Oxygen metabolites are also known to trigger arachidonic acid-dependent pathways, which may represent one basic cellular response to an oxidizing toxin (70). Oxidants might also stimulate fibrosis (71).

The harmful consequences of the generation of activated O_2 species are counterbalanced by a complex array of extracellular and intracellular antioxidant defense systems (21,55–57). Interpretation of the precise role of oxygen-derived species in toxicity is complicated by the fact that oxidant production can result from all forms of cell injury, whatever the primary inciting factor (58), and that it has been relatively difficult to demonstrate prima facie evidence of oxidant injury processes in intact biological systems, in part because of the efficiency of antioxidant defense and because of the lack of unequivocal markers of oxidant-mediated damage (72). Often a role for oxidant effects is suggested because mitigation of an effect is noted when a radical scavenger is administered to a cell culture, an animal, or a patient. Interpretation of such observations is fraught with difficulties, however (35).

Induction of membrane lipid peroxidation frequently accompanies (but is not an invariable characteristic of) oxidative stress. Many techniques have been used to measure end-products of lipid peroxidation. These have included measurements of thiobarbituric acid-reactive materials, diene conjugates, and, more recently, lipid hydroperoxides, utilizing such specialized techniques as gas liquid chromatography/mass spectrometry and high-performance liquid chromatography (HPLC) with chemiluminescence detection (73) as well as antibody methods (reviewed in ref. 74). The first two techniques have been most extensively utilized, but there are serious problems with them (72). HPLC separation of lipid hydroperoxides (identity being confirmed by sodium borohydride reduction) has proven useful in demonstrating the presence of lipid hydroperoxides in bronchoalveolar fluids (75).

The general message is that oxidant toxins (and nonoxidant toxins that create oxidative stress by cell injury or by inciting inflammatory reactions in the lung) are capable of producing many biological effects. Evaluation of these effects is still in its infancy, however (35,57).

BIOLOGICAL EFFECT MARKERS

Assessment of the pathophysiological consequences of environmental contaminants is critical to a wide variety of persons working in the fields of occupational and environmental health, including clinicians, inhalation toxicologists, and environmental health policy makers. Traditionally, the focus of the scientist has been to measure the endpoints that are reached. Nowadays, there is increasing emphasis on exploration of complex and detailed cellular and molecular mechanisms that accomplish the measured effects. The policy maker tries to relate the measured effects to the probability of significant health impairments.

An effect can be defined as a measurable marker of the interaction between a toxin and the lung (4,6). Measured endpoints can be relatively *trivial* in biological terms, such as recording subtle transient decreases in cough threshold or mild increases in airway susceptibility to nonspecific constrictor stimuli. They can also be very *serious,* such as the induction of somatic cell variants with altered phenotypes (mutagenesis). Table 2 summarizes some of the various endpoints that have been utilized to assess lung target effects elicited by inhaled toxicants.

Relationships between exposure level (applied dose), internal dose delivered to the target tissue (delivered dose), and measured biological effect are important considerations in inhalation toxicology. Major problems in this regard are: (i) the substantial uncertainties involved in distinguishing between measurement of an exposure–effect relationship where the effect measured is the transient activation of a defense system (e.g., transient bronchospasm, mucus oversecretion) and measurement of an exposure–effect relationship where the endpoint measured is physiologically significant or pathologically significant damage; (ii) the uncertainty that the most important target being damaged by the toxin is what is being measured; (iii) the fact that once an exposure has occurred, a series of events occurs at different times, some of which are detected by methodologies that have different sensitivities; and (iv) the fundamental lack of understanding of the precise physical, chemical, and biological mechanisms underlying the measured effect.

It should be noted that for the lungs, measurements

TABLE 2. *Selected evaluation techniques*

Physiological responses
Breathing profile
Routine pulmonary function tests
Lung mechanics
Nonspecific bronchial responsiveness
Mucociliary clearance rates
Airway and/or bronchiolar–alveolar permeability assessments
Respiratory tract epithelia potential difference
Airway blood flow measurements
Bronchoalveolar lavage

Pathological assessments
Quantitative histology
Bronchoalveolar lavage
Stereological (morphometric) techniques
Histochemical techniques
Radioisotopic techniques (e.g., DNA incorporation for cell turnover assessments)
In situ hybridization techniques
Measurement of DNA damage (strand breakage, chromosome aberrations or measurement of oxidative damage to DNA bases)

Biochemical systems
Organ biochemistry
Isolated perfused lung systems
Explant biochemistry (e.g., airway and parenchymal explants)
Cell culture systems
Subcellular systems

of ambient exposure concentration are frequently used in place of delivered dose to the target tissue. Because of the various processes by which the respiratory tract reacts with, filters, attenuates, degrades, and modifies inhaled toxins, it is usually difficult to know the delivered dose of a toxin.

The uncertainty of dose delivered to the target tissue leads to difficulties in comparing low-dose and high-dose exposures, resting and exercise exposures, effects of a toxin in different species, and chronic and acute exposures. In addition, pharmacokinetic considerations such as effects of duration, magnitude, and frequency of the toxin exposure must be considered (4,6). The validity of such extrapolations is critical in using response data from species other than man to predict health effect risks in humans. There must be increased emphasis on biological measurements which reflect both (a) the precise concentrations of toxins (or their metabolites) at the target site and (b) relevant mechanisms of cell damage.

After exposure to a toxin has taken place, a multiplicity of lung responses occurs. The responses depend on the delivered dose, local susceptibilities, defense systems, and the effect on the biological target being measured. Because the amount of toxin delivered will vary in different areas of the respiratory tract, the tim-

ing of measurements of effect can be of critical importance. Conventionally, the responses are classified as acute, subacute, or chronic. However, in reality a continuum exists. The fact that different responses may occur in different topographic areas of the lungs and that integrated processes of injury, inflammation, and repair occur simultaneously further confounds the precise measurement of effects and oftentimes invalidates attempts to use any simplistic index "concentration × time" to calculate equivalence of dose–response effects.

Finally, problems in extrapolating experimentally determined effects to assess risks to humans and determine health policy are many. In addition to the problems discussed above, humans are far more heterogeneous than most laboratory animals; furthermore, there are many factors that can affect individual susceptibility, such as preexisting disease, nutritional status, age, and genetic predisposition to disease. There are obvious difficulties in demonstrating low-dose health effects in humans, given the limits and expense of well-executed large-scale epidemiological studies and the conspicuous lack of truly sensitive and specific markers of lung injury.

Physiological Approaches

Pulmonary function tests have been extensively used to characterize lung responses to inhaled agents (38,76), particularly the ambient pollutants regulated by the Environmental Protection Agency (EPA). They provide a nondestructive means for evaluating the functional impact of transient or permanent alterations in respiratory control and/or structure and lend themselves to epidemiological field studies and to studies of amelioration of the pollutant effects by therapeutic agents. They are widely applicable in both humans and animals, but they have been less useful in detecting information about interactions of specific toxins with key sites and their relationships to biologic responses in the lung.

The various physiologic parameters that have been utilized to assess toxin effects on the lung are listed in Table 2. The general message of the physiological studies is that it is reasonably easy to establish time–dose physiological responses for acute exposures to single and simple combination air pollutant exposures, as has been most thoroughly done for O_3 (38). However, it is relatively difficult to delineate exposure–effect relationships (such as the acute decreased FEV_1 caused by appropriate exposurers to O_3) from chronic exposure and its potential adverse effects (exposure–disease considerations). Likewise, it has been difficult to unravel the contributions of individual toxins to overall effects ascribed to such complex toxin mixtures as cigarette smoke and "real-life" air pollutants. This is especially true with regard to assessments of synergistic interactions among the various toxin mixtures.

Pathological Assessments

The general pathological response to an inhaled toxin is epithelial cell injury and the triggering of a large variety of acute inflammatory processes. This includes an influx of inflammatory cells in concert with activation of numerous neuromediator pathways and chemotaxic, cytokine, and growth-factor release processes. The hierarchy of intraluminal, epithelial, and interstitial events has been descriptively characterized by different sets of morphologic parameters (77).

The general pattern that emerges is one of initial epithelial denudation by loss of sensitive cells (e.g., ciliary epithelium in nasal, tracheal, bronchial, and bronchiolar regions, and type I cells in alveolar regions). This is followed by variable degrees of proliferation by secretory cells and type II cells in proximal and distal regions, varying degrees of fibroblast migration, and, in some cases, sustained fibroblast proliferation and increased deposition of interstitial matrix. Temporal development and extent of toxin-induced epithelial injury and repair processes vary considerably at various sites along the respiratory tract. The intensities of the intraluminal and interstitial events are related to, but do not necessarily parallel, the degree of epithelial and underlying basement membrane injury.

Cellular and biochemical analysis of bronchoalveolar lavage fluid (BALF) is being increasingly used as an index of toxin-induced lung injury (22,23). Total lavage cell counts, differential cell counts, morphology of cells present, protein content, enzymes such as lactate dehydrogenase, and appearance of substances injected into plasma (such as radioactive albumin) have been used. Techniques such as sequential lavage sampling and the double-balloon catheter are useful for differentiating toxin-induced effects on airways from effects on more distal bronchiolar–alveolar regions.

It is generally recognized that BALF cell analysis provides useful information concerning inflammatory and fibrogenic processes and acute lung injury. For example, numerous studies have revealed that BALF cell populations from toxin-exposed lungs are physiologically different from control cells. It is also known that most forms of acute lung injury and related fibrogenic responses have a substantial component arising from inflammatory responses in air spaces (78). This has led to increasing use of lavage fluids to evaluate substances present on the respiratory epithelial surface in small concentrations, using techniques such as sensitive enzyme-linked immunoassay (ELISA) systems.

It must be noted, however, that lavage fluid and cell analysis may not accurately indicate all of the toxin-induced inflammatory events occurring in airway mucosa and lung interstitium.

BALF analysis is rapidly joining pulmonary function testing as an important diagnostic tool in quantitative investigations of toxin-related lung injury and repair processes. Assessments of toxin-induced lung fibrogenesis can be made by measuring the amounts of factors chemotactic and stimulatory for fibroblasts, and of substances such as fibronectin, vitronectin, hyaluronic acid, and procollagen and elastin-derived peptides, all of which are related to metabolism of the connective tissue matrix. Further characterization of such "markers" in BALF appears promising in trying to predict initiation, intensity, and duration of toxin-induced lung fibrogenic responses and, in some cases, these markers have already been shown to relate to the severity of fibrosis as assessed by quantitative histomorphometric analysis. As techniques become more refined, the further development of plasma markers for lung fibrosing potency can be expected.

The advent of novel pathological assessment tools over the last few years can be expected to have continuing impacts in the field of inhaled environmental pathobiology. New generations of simplified and more efficient techniques of stereological methodology, *in situ* hybridization using RNA probes for specific gene expression, and immunocytochemistry for corresponding protein distributions are being increasingly applied to the lung. Monitoring the molecular transcriptional phenotype of a cell, utilizing sensitive assays of both RNA and protein content, can now be done using a small number of cells (79), such as those obtained from lavage or punch biopsy. These and other cell and molecular biology techniques should be most useful in the further understanding of general and specific lung cell responses to inhaled toxins.

Lung cancer, widely recognized as being largely due to inhalation of toxic material (e.g., cigarette smoke), is currently the major cause of cancer deaths in the United States. A substantial body of evidence is now available to document the manifold effects of inhaled environmental contaminants in triggering hyperplastic, metaplastic, mutagenic, and carcinogenic processes in the lung (80). A toxin-induced injury/death of cells produces a cellular environment of new synthesis with constant generation of inflammatory and growth signals, including oxidants. This milieu has the potential for making the cells particularly susceptible to mutagenic and carcinogenic transformation. Endpoints being studied *in vivo* and *in vitro* include use of "markers" to reflect (a) alterations in cell proliferation pathways, (b) chromosomal damage, (c) DNA adduct formation, and (d) activation of oncogenes such as c-fos and c-myc expression (57,69).

Biochemical and Molecular Responses

In the past 50 years, much has been learned about lung response to inhaled toxins (2–9). In the main, research has focused on biochemical markers of dose–response effects, with particular attention to biochemical measurements in whole lung tissue and in respiratory tract fluids obtained by lavage. These techniques have been successful in identifying nonspecific neurogenic, inflammatory, and cellular responses to toxins and in providing some useful background information for theoretical extrapolations allowing statutory regulation of exposures. However, attempts to determine the biological effects of environmental toxins upon respiratory tract epithelium at the cellular, membrane, and molecular level are only just beginning. Although toxin-induced alterations in specific cell systems can sometimes be shown *in vivo* (e.g., Clara cell injury by substances that can be converted by cytochrome P-450 into toxic metabolites), attempts to separate the indirect effects of activation of the various neurohumoral–inflammatory mediator networks from the specific toxin-induced cell effects have not yet been successful for most toxins.

Because of the ease of access to AMs through the technique of lavage, the responses of these cells to environmental agents have been extensively studied (45,46). The respiratory tract mucosa is another potentially useful system to evaluate specific toxin effects on the lung. Several approaches are becoming available, varying from explant (81,82) and implant (83) systems to the newer techniques for harvesting epithelial mucosa cells for biochemical and morphological analysis and culture (84). It is now possible to obtain confluent primary cultures of surface epithelial cells highly enriched with mucin-secreting cells and/or ciliary cells from airways of both animals (84) and humans (85). Such systems are increasingly being used to assess toxic effects on lung cells and to define biochemical and molecular mechanisms of cell injury. Endoscopic scraping, brush, imprint, and needle biopsy techniques, which allow for repeated quantitative samplings of airway epithelium and mucosa, should increasingly provide more precise evaluations of toxic effects, although some caution must be exercised in interpreting toxin-induced effects on individual lung cells. This is because overall respiratory tract response to a given toxin usually depends on the integrated action of several types of responding and effector cells.

Combining analysis of BALF with cell culture technology represents one effective approach to further define the consequences of inhaled toxicants. More use of coculture techniques, including coculture of lung cells or tissue with inflammatory cells (86), should provide useful models to begin to understand complex cell–cell interactions associated with toxin-induced processes.

Studies using AMs, tracheal epithelial, and fibroblast cultures to evaluate cytotoxic and proinflammatory activities of a battery of mineral dusts with known *in vivo* toxicity are being increasingly utilized. Endpoints being evaluated (including oxidant generation, cytotoxicity, and collagen production) seem to differentiate particulates on the basis of their known potential to elicit adverse responses *in vivo* (87), but they have only started to define the precise cell and molecular mechanisms responsible for overall dust-induced damage processes in the lung. For example, in many bioassays, mineral dusts known to cause inflammation and pulmonary interstitial fibrosis in the lung elicit greater cytotoxic and metabolic changes in isolated lung cells than do nonfibrous, chemically similar particulates at identical concentrations.

Specific areas in which new techniques of cell and molecular biology should be exploited will need to include further definitions of toxicant interactions with (i) mediator/neuropeptide-generating pathways, (ii) cell membrane injury in relation to receptor transmodulation and signaling cascade pathways, and (iii) critical cytoplasmic and nuclear responding targets such as calcium translocations, energy generation, oxidant stress, and mechanisms of DNA damage. Methodologies such as the use of gas chromatography/mass spectrometry for fingerprinting site-specific oxidant-induced DNA damage (68) can be expected to be useful in this regard.

**PROBLEMS OF INTRASPECIES/
INTERSPECIES EXTRAPOLATIONS**

Considerable differences exist in lung structure and function between different vertebrates. Anatomical differences such as (a) degree of convolution of the nasal turbinates, (b) lengths, diameters, and branching angles of conducting airways, and (c) terminal airway–alveolar region geometry can all be expected to influence (to varying degrees) deposition, retention, and clearance patterns for inhaled toxins, particularly aerosols and particulates (88–90). In addition, the differences in cell populations in similar topographical regions of the respiratory epithelium in different species are considerable (91,92). Thus, depending on the inhaled toxin and the biological endpoint being measured, it should not be surprising to find that considerable differences in susceptibilities to toxins exist between species.

In addition to anatomical factors, differences in response to inhaled toxins can be based on mechanism (nasal, oronasal), rate, depth, and magnitude of ventilation (which together help to determine regional target site dosimetry), on the susceptibilities of the various target cell populations, and (to an unknown extent) on differences in the intensity of neurohumoral and inflammatory responses. Given these complexities, it is easy to understand the problems in performing experiments designed to administer equitoxic doses of injurious agents to the respiratory tract.

The route and speed of toxin metabolism and the extent of antioxidant defense also differ between species (21). Although comparative studies have demonstrated a shared basic repertoire of activities in PMNs and AMs from different mammalian species, they have also shown substantial variation in activation requirements and in responses (88,93), important because these cells play such a central role in responses to toxins. In addition, age, breed, strain, and sex differences in toxin susceptibility may exist. Increases in the susceptibility of the mucosa to damaging agents with age have been noted for many toxins, and diminished mucosal regenerative capacities may play a significant role. For some toxins, there is a wide spectrum of responses among healthy subjects (38). The basis for these differences is often not clear.

ADAPTATION AND TOLERANCE

"Adaptation" refers to the response of cells or cell populations to a stressful environment such that toxic effects are lessened. "Tolerance" can be broadly defined as a lessening of an observed effect with continued exposure to the toxin (e.g., a successful adaptation) (77). Interest in lung adaptation to toxins has focused on its role in causing diminished responsiveness to continued exposure to oxidant gases. The net effect is usually thought to result in a lessening of the rate at which cumulative, irreversible pulmonary damage occurs. However, care must be used in applying this generalization, because it need not apply to carcinogenesis. For example, a highly toxic agent that kills cells could potentially do less harm than a weakly cytotoxic DNA damaging agent that allows DNA damage to propagate, eventually resulting in an increased risk of carcinogenesis.

The mechanism and duration of tolerance to inhaled toxicants almost certainly relate, in part, to the dose and type of injurant and the effect being measured. Prior limited toxic insults may induce increases in antitoxic substances which confer tolerance to subsequent toxic insults, as has perhaps been best illustrated for the case of lung exposure to toxic concentrations of oxidants (21). In most instances, the precise critical cellular changes that contribute to tolerance of a toxin are not fully understood.

Many mechanisms may hypothetically give rise to adaptive processes. These include: (a) depletion or modulation of responding neurohumoral and inflammatory/immune mediator systems; (b) the replacement of sensitive epithelial cells with a more resistant, younger population of cells (e.g., during the relatively short time following proliferative repair of a toxin-damaged epithelium); (c) shift to cell types inherently more resistant to damage (e.g., type I to type II cells); and (d) induction of specific (e.g., antioxidant) or nonspecific (e.g., heat shock protein) metabolic changes conferring a degree of cellular protection against a toxin. The shift toward cells with a lower surface area/cell volume ratio (e.g., from type I cells to type II cells), caused by decreasing the membrane exposure (per cell) to a given toxin, has also been suggested as being involved (77). The importance of stress or heat shock proteins (94,95) and various cytokines (53,96–98) in inducing and maintaining lung cellular adaptations to environmental toxins remains to be more fully clarified.

CONCLUSIONS

The inhalation toxicology studies performed in the past 50 years on intact animals and humans and performed by classical anatomical, physiological, and biochemical techniques have been most helpful in drawing up an inventory of the different types of airway and parenchymal lung responses to environmental toxins. These dose–response indices have been useful in categorizing overall responses of lung to injury, in characterizing inflammatory and reparative processes in the lung, and in setting occupational and environmental health standards.

In recent years the basic understanding of lung cell biology has increased tremendously, and considerable progress has been made in applying this knowledge to the field of inhalation lung toxicology. Increasingly more emphasis is being given to the mechanisms that accomplish the previously identified endpoints. Further studies of the interactions between environmental contaminants and their impact on such basic lung tissue activities as cell membrane activation, receptor transmodulation, cell–cell signaling systems, and mediator–neuropeptide–cytokine network processes will undoubtedly soon be forthcoming. The analyses of these studies will necessarily be complex. They will involve integration of studies of intact lungs with studies of isolated tissue, cell, and molecular systems. This field represents one of the most challenging, exciting, and productive areas of modern lung biology.

ACKNOWLEDGMENTS

We are grateful to Drs. Donald L. Dungworth and Hanspeter Witschi for helpful discussions.

REFERENCES

1. Weibel ER. Lung cell biology. In: Fishman AP, Fisher AB, eds. *Handbook of physiology, Section 3: The respiratory system, vol 1.* Bethesda, MD: American Physiological Society, 1985;47–92.
2. Witschi HP, Brain JD, eds. *Toxicology of inhaled materials.* New York: Springer-Verlag, 1985.
3. Salem H, ed. *Inhalation toxicology: Research methods, applications and evaluations.* New York: Marcel Dekker, 1987.
4. *Biologic markers in pulmonary toxicology.* Washington, DC: National Academy Press, 1989.
5. McClellan RO, Henderson RF. *Concepts in inhalation toxicology.* New York: Hemisphere Publishing Corp, 1989.
6. Environmental Protection Agency. *Research to improve health risk assessments program.* Washington, DC: Publication no. EPA/600/8-88/089, September 1988.
7. Lewis LL, Nemery B. The lung as a target organ for toxicity. In: Cohen GM, ed. *Target organ toxicity,* vol II. Boca Raton, FL: CRC Press, 1986;45–80.
8. Kennedy GL. Inhalation toxicology. In: Hayers AW, ed. *Principles and methods of toxicology.* New York: Raven Press, 1989.
9. Witschi H. Responses of the lung to toxic injury. *Environ Health Perspect* 1990;85:5–13.
10. Lippman M, Yeates DB, Albert RE. Deposition, retention and clearance of inhaled particles. *Br J Ind Med* 1980;37:337–362.
11. Gram TE. The pulmonary mixed-function oxidase system. In: Witschi HP, Brain JD, eds. *Toxicology of inhaled materials.* New York: Springer-Verlag, 1985;421–470.
12. Brain JD. Toxicological aspects of alterations of pulmonary macrophage function. *Annu Rev Pharmacol Toxicol* 1986; 26:547–565.
13. Lindenschmidt RC, Driscoll KE, Perkins MA, et al. The comparison of a fibrogenic and two nonfibrogenic dusts by bronchoalveolar lavage. *Toxicol Appl Pharmacol* 1990;102:268–281.
14. Schlesinger RB. Deposition and clearance of inhaled particles. In: McClellan RO, Henderson RF, eds. *Concepts in inhalation toxicology.* New York: Hemisphere Publishing Corp, 1989;163–192.
15. Miller FJ, Overton JH, Graham RC. Regional deposition of inhaled reactive gases. In: McClellan RO, Henderson RF, eds. *Concepts in inhalation toxicology.* New York: Hemisphere Publishing Corp, 1989;229–247.
16. Brain JD. Nonimmunologic defense mechanisms. In: Fishman AP, ed. *Pulmonary diseases and disorders.* New York: McGraw-Hill, 1988;701–710.
17. Barnes PJ, Chung KF, Page CF. Inflammatory mediators and asthma. *Pharmacol Rev* 1988;40:49–84.
18. Karlsson JA, Sant' Ambrogio G, Widdicombe J. Afferent neural pathways in cough and reflex bronchoconstriction. *J Appl Physiol* 1988;65:1007–1023.
19. Janoff A. Elastases and emphysema. *Am Rev Respir Dis* 1985;132:417–433.
20. Cantin A, Crystal RG. Oxidants, antioxidants and the pathogenesis of emphysema. *Eur J Respir Dis* 1985;66(Suppl 139):7–17.
21. Heffner JE, Repine JE. Pulmonary strategies of antioxidant defense. *Am Rev Respir Dis* 1989;140:531–554.
22. Reynolds HY. Bronchoalveolar lavage. *Am Rev Respir Dis* 1987;135:250–263.
23. Henderson RF. Bronchoalveolar lavage: a tool for assessing the health status of the lung. In: *Concepts in inhalation toxicology.* New York: Hemisphere Publishing Corp, 1989;415–444.
24. Cross CE, Halliwell B, Allan A. Anti-oxidant protection: a function of tracheobronchial and gastrointestinal mucus. *Lancet* 1984;i:1328–1330.
25. Postlethwait EM, Langford SD, Bidani A. Reactive absorption kinetics of nitrogen dioxide. *FASEB J* 1990;4:A318.
26. Holma B. Effects of inhaled acids on airway mucus and its consequences for health. *Environ Health Perspect* 1989;79:109–113.
27. Akino T, Ohno K. Phospholipids of the lung in normal, toxic and diseased states. *CRC Crit Rev Toxicol* 1981;9:201–272.
28. Esterbauer H, Jurgens G, Quenhenberger O, et al. Autoxidation of human low density lipoprotein: loss of polyunsaturated fatty acids and vitamin E and generation of aldehydes. *J Lipid Res* 1987;28:495–509.
29. Halliwell B. Albumin—an important extracellular antioxidant? *Biochem Pharmacol* 1988;37:569–571.
30. Wasil M, Halliwell B, Hutchison DCS, et al. The antioxidant action of human extracellular fluids. *Biochem J* 1987;243:219–223.
31. Cantin AM, North SL, Hubbard RC, et al. Normal alveolar epithelial lining contains high levels of glutathione. *J Appl Physiol* 1987;63:152–157.
32. Suzuki Y. Reduction of hexavalent chromium by ascorbic acid in rat lung lavage fluid. *Arch Toxicol* 1988;62:116–122.
33. Pacht E, Kaseki H, Mohammed JR, et al. Deficiency of vitamin E in the alveolar fluid of cigarette smokers. *J Clin Invest* 1986;77:789–796.
34. Frei B, England L, Armes BN. Ascorbate is an outstanding antioxidant in human blood plasma. *Proc Natl Acad Sci USA* 1989;86:6377–6381.
35. Halliwell B. How to characterize a biological antioxidant. *Free Rad Res Commun* 1990;9:1–32.
36. Wayner DDM, Burton GW, Ingold KU, et al. The relative contributions of vitamin E, urate, ascorbate and proteins to the total peroxyl radical-trapping antioxidant activity of human blood plasma. *Biochim Biophys Acta* 1987;914:408–419.
37. Lotz M, Vaughan JH, Carlson DA. Effect of neuropeptides on production of inflammatory cytokines by human monocytes. *Science* 1988;241:1218–1221.
38. Hazucha MJ, Bates DV, Bromberg PA. Mechanism of action of ozone on the human lung. *J Appl Physiol* 1989;67:1535–1541.
39. Hogg JC. Neutrophil kinetics and lung injury. *Physiol Rev* 1987;67:1249–1295.
40. Okrent DG, Lichtenstein AK, Ganz T. Direct cytotoxicity of polymorphonuclear leukocyte granule proteins to human lung-derived cells and endothelial cells. *Am Rev Respir Dis* 1990; 141:179–185.
41. Sibille Y, Reynolds HY. Macrophages and polymorphonuclear neutrophils in lung defense and injury. *Am Rev Respir Dis* 1990;141:471–501.
42. O'Byrne PM, Walters EH, Gold BD, et al. Neutrophil depletion inhibits airway hyperresponsiveness induced by ozone exposure. *Am Rev Respir Dis* 1984;130:214–218.
43. Evans TW, Brokaw J, Chung KF, et al. Ozone-induced bronchial hyperreactivity in the rat. *Am Rev Respir Dis* 1988; 138:140–144.
44. Fabbri LM, Boschetto P, Zocca E, et al. Bronchoalveolar neutrophilia during late asthmatic reactions induced by toluene diisocyanate. *Am Rev Respir Dis* 1987;136:36–42.
45. Fels AOS, Cohn ZA. The alveolar macrophage. *J Appl Physiol* 1986;60:353–369.
46. Fuchs HJ, Snizek M, Shellito JE. Cellular influx and activation increase macrophage cytotoxicity and interleukin 1 elaboration during pulmonary inflammation in rats. *Am Rev Respir Dis* 1988;138:572–577.
47. Driscoll KE, Lidenschmidt RC, Mauer JK, et al. Pulmonary response to silica or titanium dioxide: inflammatory cells, alveolar-macrophage-derived cytokines, and histopathology. *Am J Respir Cell Mol Biol* 1990;2:381–390.
48. Doelman CJA, Leurs R, Oosterom WC, et al. Mineral dust exposure and free radical-mediated lung damage. *Exp Lung Res* 1990;16:41–55.
49. Born PJA, Meijers JMM, Gwaen GMH. Molecular epidemiology of coal worker's pneumoconiosis: application to risk assessment of oxidant and monokine generation by mineral dusts. *Exp Lung Res* 1990;16:57–71.
50. Devlin RB, Koren HS. The use of quantitative two-dimensional gel electrophoresis to analyze changes in alveolar macrophage proteins in humans exposed to ozone. *Am J Respir Cell Mol Biol* 1990;2:281–188.
51. Hanley SP. Prostaglandins and the lung. *Lung* 1986;164:65–77.
52. Henderson WR. Eicosanoids and lung inflammation. *Am Rev Respir Dis* 1987;135:1176–1185.
53. Kelley J. Cytokines and the lung. *Am Rev Respir Dis* 1990; 141:765–788.
54. Libby P, Freidman GB, Saloman RN. Cytokines as modulators

of cell proliferation in fibrotic diseases. *Am Rev Respir Dis* 1989;140:1114–1117.

55. Cross CE, Halliwell B, Borish ET, et al. UC Davis Conference: Oxygen radicals and human disease. *Ann Intern Med* 1987; 107:526–545.

56. Halliwell B, Gutteridge JMC. *Free radicals in biology and medicine*, 2nd ed. Oxford: Clarendon, 1989.

57. Cerutti PA, Fridovich L, McCord JM, eds. *Oxy-radicals in molecular biology and pathology*. UCLA Symposia on Molecular and Cellular Biology, vol 82, 1988.

58. Halliwell B, Gutteridge JMC. Lipid peroxidation, oxygen radicals, cell damage, and anti-oxidant therapy. *Lancet* 1984;i:1396–1398.

59. Weiss SJ. Tissue destruction by neutrophils. *N Engl J Med* 1989;320:365–376.

60. Pryor WA, Prier DG, Church, DF. Electron-spin reasonance study of mainstream and sidestream smoke: nature of the free radicals in gas-phase smoke and in cigarette tar. *Environ Health Perspect* 1983;47:345–355.

61. Menzel DB. Ozone: an overview of its toxicity in man and animals. *J Toxicol Environ Health* 1984;13:183–204.

62. Lipman M. Health effects of ozone: a critical review. *JAPCA* 1989;39:672–695.

63. Nemery B. Metal toxicity and the respiratory tract. *Eur Respir J* 1990;33:202–219.

64. Barrett C, Lamb PW, Wiseman RW. Multiple mechanisms for the carcinogenic effects of asbestos and other mineral fibers. *Environ Health Perspect* 1989;81:81–89.

65. Mossman BT, Marsh JA. Evidence supporting a role for active oxygen species in asbestosis-induced toxicity and lung disease. *Environ Health Perspect* 1989;81:91–94.

66. Winter M, Wilson JS, Bedell K, et al. The conductance of cultured epithelial cell monolayers: oxidants, adenosine triphosphate, and phorbol dibutyrate. *Am J Respir Cell Biol* 1990;2:355–363.

67. Cerutti P, Larsson R, Krupitza G, et al. Pathophysiological mechanisms of active oxygen. *Mutat Res* 1989;214:81–88.

68. Aruoma OI, Halliwell B, Dizdaroglu M. Iron ion-dependent modification of bases in DNA by the superoxide radical-generating system hypoxanthine–xanthine oxidase. *J Biol Chem* 1989;264:13024–13028.

69. Cerutti PA. Response modification in carcinogenesis. *Environ Health Perspect* 1989;81:39–43.

70. Adler KA, Holden-Stauffer WJ, Repine JE. Oxygen metabolites stimulate release of high-molecular-weight glycoconjugates by cell and organ cultures of rodent respiratory epithelium via an archidonic acid-dependent mechanism. *J Clin Invest* 1990;85:75–85.

71. Murrell GAC, Francis MJO, Bromley L. Modulation of fibroblast proliferation by oxygen free radicals. *Biochem J* 1990;265:659–665.

72. Halliwell B, Gutteridge JM. Oxygen free radicals and iron in relation to biology and medicine: some problems and concepts. *Arch Biochem Biophys* 1986;246:501–514.

73. Frei B, Yamamoto Y, Niclas D, et al. Evaluation of an isoluminol chemiluminescence assay for the detection of hydroperoxides in human blood plasma. *Anal Biochem* 1988;175:120–130.

74. Gutteridge JMC, Halliwell B. The measurement and mechanism of lipid peroxidation in biological systems. *TIBS* 1990;15:129–135.

75. Cross CE, Forte T, Stocker R, et al. Oxidative stress and abnormal cholesterol metabolism in patients with adult respiratory distress syndrome. *J Lab Clin Med* 1990;115:396–404.

76. Koenig JQ. Pulmonary reaction to environmental pollutants. *J Allergy Clin Immun* 1987;79:833–843.

77. Dungworth DL. Non-carcinogenic responses of the respiratory tract to inhaled toxicants. In: McClellan RO, Henderson RF, eds. *Concepts in inhalation toxicology*. New York: Hemisphere Publishing Corp, 1988;173–278.

78. Kuhn C, Boldt J, King TE, et al. An immunohistochemical study of architectural remodeling and connective tissue synthesis in pulmonary fibrosis. *Am Rev Respir Dis* 1989;140:1693–1703.

79. Rappolee DA, Werb Z. mRNA phenotyping for studying gene expression in small numbers of cells: platelet-derived growth factor and other growth factors in wound-derived macrophages. *Am J Respir Cell Mol Biol* 1990;2:3–10.

80. Hahn FF. Carcinogenic responses to inhaled materials. In: McClellan RO, Henderson RF, eds. *Concepts in inhalation toxicology*. New York: Hemisphere Publishing Corp, 1989;313–346.

81. Last JA, Cross CE. A new model for health effects of air pollutants: evidence for synergistic effects of mixtures of ozone and sulfuric acid aerosols on rat lungs. *J Lab Clin Med* 1978; 91:328–339.

82. Renard SI, Daughton DM, Robbins RA, et al. *In vivo* and *in vitro* methods for evaluating airway inflammation: implications for respiratory toxicology. *Toxicology* 1990;60:5–14.

83. Everitt JI, Hersterberg TW, Boreiko CJ. The use of tracheal implants in toxicology and carcinogenesis research. *Toxicology* 1990;60:27–40.

84. Wu R, Nolan E, Turner C. Expression of tracheal differentiated function in serum-free hormone-supplemented medium. *J Cell Physiol* 1985;125:167–181.

85. Wu R, Wu MMJ. Effects of retinoids on human bronchial epithelial cells: differential regulation of hyaluronate synthesis and keratin protein synthesis. *J Cell Physiol* 1986;127:73–82.

86. Yukawa T, Read RC, Kroegel C, et al. The effects of activated eosinophils and neutrophils on guinea pig airway epithelium *in vitro*. *Am J Respir Cell Mol Biol* 1990;2:341–353.

87. Mossman BT, Sesko AM. *In vitro* assays to predict the pathogenicity of mineral fibers. *Toxicology* 1990;60:53–61.

88. Brain JD, Mensah GA. Comparative toxicology of the respiratory tract. *Am Rev Respir Dis* 1983;128:S87–S90.

89. Snipes MB. Species comparisons for pulmonary retention of inhaled particles. In: McClellan RO, Henderson RF, eds. *Concepts in inhalation toxicology*. New York: Hemisphere Publishing Corp, 1989;193–227.

90. Warheit DB, Hartsky MA. Species comparisons of proximal alveolar deposition patterns of inhaled particulates. *Exp Lung Res* 1989;16:83–99.

91. Plopper CG, Dungworth DL. Structure, function, cell injury and cell renewal of bronchiolar–alveolar epithelium. In: McDowell EM, ed. *Current problems in tumour pathology, vol 3: Lung carcinomas*. Edinburgh: Churchill Livingstone, 1987;94–128.

92. Tryka AF, Witschi H, Gosslee DG, et al. Patterns of cell proliferation during recovery from oxygen injury: species differences. *Am Rev Respir Dis* 1986;133:1055–1059.

93. Styrt B. Species variation in neutrophil biochemistry and function. *J Leukocyte Biol* 1989;46:63–74.

94. Stress-induced proteins. In: Pardue ML, Feramisco R, Lindquist S, eds. *UCLA symposia on molecular and cellular biology*, vol 96. New York: Alan R Liss, 1989;1–124.

95. Storz G, Tartaglia LA, Ames BN. Transcriptional regulator of oxidative stress-inducible genes: direct activation by oxidation. *Science* 1990;248:189–194.

96. Gordon T, Sheppard D. Tumor necrosis factor inhibits a polymorphonuclear leukocyte-dependent airway edema in guinea pigs. *J Appl Physiol* 1988;64:1688–1692.

97. Tsan MF, White JE, Santana TA, et al. Tracheal insufflation of tumor necrosis factor protects rats against oxygen toxicity. *J Appl Physiol* 1990;68:1211–1219.

98. Mathison JC, Virca GD, Wolfson E, et al. Adaptation to bacterial lipopolysaccharide controls lipopolysaccharide-induced tumor necrosis factor production in rabbit macrophages. *J Clin Invest* 1990;85:1108–1118.

THE LUNG: Scientific Foundations
edited by R.G. Crystal, J.B. West et al.
Raven Press, Ltd., New York © 1991.

CHAPTER 7.6.3

The Oxidative Stress Placed on the Lung by Cigarette Smoke

Daniel F. Church and William A. Pryor

There is a large body of evidence suggesting that the major pulmonary diseases associated with cigarette smoking, including emphysema (1,2) and cancer (3,4) are (at least in part) mediated by free radicals. Cigarette smoke itself contains (a) high concentrations of free radicals (5,6) and (b) chemicals that readily react to form free radicals (6,7). It is reasonable, therefore, that the radicals present in or produced by cigarette smoke might be involved in smoking-induced pathology (8). In this chapter, we will explore the fundamental chemical and biochemical evidence supporting such a relationship. We will first briefly review the free radical chemistry associated with cigarette smoke itself; there is compelling evidence that cigarette smoke can deliver damaging radicals to the lungs of smokers. We will then present the oftentimes contradictory evidence that radical-mediated damage occurs in lungs exposed to cigarette smoke.

AN OVERVIEW OF THE FREE RADICAL CHEMISTRY OF CIGARETTE SMOKE

Cigarette smoke can be separated into two phases by the use of a glass-fiber Cambridge filter that retains 99.9% of the particulate matter in smoke with a size greater than 0.1 μm (9). The retained particulate matter is referred to as the "tar phase," whereas the material that passes through the filter is defined as the "gas phase." As we shall discuss below, each phase has its own distinctive radical chemistry.

Free radicals are formed by the high temperatures at the tip of a cigarette as the tobacco is burned; however, these radicals have lifetimes much less than a second, too short for these radicals to be inhaled by the smoker. Confirming this, we have used the electron spin resonance (ESR) spin trapping technique to detect free radicals in the gas phase of cigarette smoke and have shown that the radical concentration in fresh smoke is very low (5,8,10,11). Surprisingly, however, the concentration of highly reactive free radicals increases as cigarette smoke ages, reaching a maximum in smoke after 1–2 min (5,8). These radicals also are very short-lived, implying that they must be formed continuously by ongoing chemical processes in the smoke. That is, the radicals in smoke must exist in a steady state, being continually formed and destroyed (5,8).

The steady-state concentration of reactive organic radicals in smoke arises from reactions of the nitrogen oxides in smoke (11). Fresh cigarette smoke contains very high concentrations (~400 ppm) of nitric oxide (NO) (9). NO is a free radical, but it is relatively unreactive towards most molecules; it is slowly oxidized by dioxygen, however, to the much more reactive nitrogen dioxide (NO_2) free radical. We have shown that NO_2 can react with isoprene, a simple conjugated diene that occurs at high concentrations in smoke, to form the same types of reactive radicals (again measured using the spin trapping method) that we observe in cigarette smoke (11).

In contrast to the reactive radicals in the gas phase, the tar phase of cigarette smoke contains a much more stable radical population that is associated with a mixture of quinone (Q), semiquinone radical (QH·), and hydroquinone (QH_2) moieties held together in a polymeric matrix (6,8). These $Q/QH·/QH_2$ radicals in tar are essentially unreactive. However, we have shown that the $Q/QH·/QH_2$ radical does associate strongly with DNA in vitro (12). In addition, aqueous extracts

D. F. Church and W. A. Pryor: Biodynamics Institute, Louisiana State University, Baton Rouge, Louisiana 70803.

of tar convert dioxygen to superoxide, hydrogen peroxide (13), and the highly reactive hydroxyl radical (7); we have proposed that this reduction of dioxygen is mediated by the redox-active $Q/QH\cdot/QH_2$ tar radical system (7,13). The ability of tar components to associate with DNA and to produce the highly damaging hydroxyl radical has been shown to lead to single-strand breaks in supercoiled DNA (14) and to block DNA synthesis (15) *in vitro*. We have proposed that the tar radical can mediate the formation of highly oxidizing species (hydrogen peroxide and the hydroxyl radical) in a relatively site-specific manner.

EVIDENCE THAT CIGARETTE SMOKE PLACES AN OXIDATIVE STRESS ON THE LUNG

Lipid Peroxidation

The most widely used evidence for radical-mediated damage by an oxidative stress is an increase in the peroxidation of membrane lipids (16,17). The oxidation of membrane lipids can be monitored using a sensitive colorimetric test based on the reaction of thiobarbituric acid (TBA) with malondialdehyde (MDA), one of the minor products of lipid peroxidation (17). This methodology has been used to detect lipid peroxidation in the lung lipids of animals exposed to cigarette smoke.

Chow et al. (18) found that tar can inhibit lipid peroxidation. They exposed rats that were either vitamin E-deficient or E-supplemented to cigarette smoke daily (10 puffs/day from a standard 2R1 research cigarette). After 4 days, the levels of MDA (as measured by the TBA test) in the lung homogenates from the vitamin E-deficient group were significantly lower in the smoke-exposed animals than in the controls; in contrast, the MDA levels in the lungs from the vitamin E-supplemented group were not different in smoke-exposed and control animals (18). Furthermore, much of this inhibitory effect by cigarette smoke appeared to be associated with the tar fraction of smoke (18). Since this fraction is rich in reducing compounds such as phenols and polyphenols, it was proposed that these compounds are responsible for this apparent "protection" against lipid peroxidation by cigarette smoke (18).

Contradictory results have been reported by Gupta et al. (19), who measured the levels of TBA-reactive materials in the lungs of rats exposed to the smoke from commercial filter cigarettes having tar and nicotine values very similar to those of the 2R1 cigarettes used in the work cited above. Gupta et al. (19) found that exposure to cigarette smoke results in significant increases in the levels of MDA compared to those in sham-smoked control animals.

The initiation of lipid peroxidation by cigarette smoke has also been demonstrated by Lentz and Di Luzio (20). These investigators prepared aqueous extracts of cigarette smoke by bubbling smoke through a buffer, followed by filtration of any suspended particulate. When the membrane lipids from alveolar macrophages were then treated with this aqueous extract, a significant increase in MDA was observed.

Although these various results are somewhat contradictory, several conclusions can be reached relative to cigarette smoking and lipid peroxidation. Firstly, the results of Chow et al. (18) clearly demonstrate that the tar phase of cigarette smoke has reducing properties—in spite of the fact that aqueous solutions of tar form potent oxidants, including hydrogen peroxide and hydroxyl radicals (7,13). Secondly, the gas phase of cigarette smoke, on balance, is probably capable of initiating lipid peroxidation, consistent with the NO/NO_2-driven chemistry discussed above. Finally, the apparently inconsistent results, particularly in the animal models, presumably arise out of the differences in the smoking protocols that, in turn, alter the balance in the effects of the gas and tar phases.

Vitamin E

Antioxidants are compounds that protect against lipid peroxidation by sacrificially reacting with free radicals and thereby shortening the chain (16); vitamin E is the principal lipid-soluble antioxidant found in nature (21). Because of its critical role, the effect of manipulating vitamin E levels or the effects of a stimulus on the vitamin E pool can provide important information about the nature of an oxidative stress.

We have already described (see above) a study by Chow et al. (18) in which they found that vitamin E-supplemented rats showed less of an effect due to cigarette exposure than did vitamin E-deficient animals. In addition, this same study showed that there was a significant mortality resulting from the cigarette smoke exposure in the vitamin E-deficient group that was not observed in the vitamin E-supplemented one (18). Finally, in this same study Chow et al. (18) showed that plasma levels of vitamin E were unchanged in both vitamin E-deficient and E-supplemented animals.

The levels of vitamin E and its quinone oxidation product have been measured in bronchoalveolar lavage (BAL) fluid from human smokers and nonsmokers by Pacht et al. (22). They found that the levels of vitamin E in BAL fluid from smokers were nearly seven times lower than for nonsmokers (22). They also found that the level of vitamin E quinone was relatively larger in the BAL fluid of smokers than in that of nonsmokers. Finally, Pacht et al. (22) showed that dietary supplementation of vitamin E (2400 IU/day) significantly reduced the effects of cigarette smoking on the vitamin E levels. These results provide powerful evidence that cigarette smoke places an oxidative burden on the lungs of smokers; the much lower levels of vitamin E, and especially the relative increase in the quinone oxidation product of vitamin E, in smokers' BAL are consistent with cigarette smoke initiating lipid peroxidation and leading to the observed changes in vitamin E.

Vitamin C

Although vitamin C has not been shown to be involved in protecting the lung against cigarette smoke, it is reasonable to expect that vitamin C would be involved. For example, it is suspected that the water-soluble vitamin C interacts with the phenoxyl radical formed when vitamin E reacts with a lipid peroxyl radical, thereby regenerating the vitamin E (23). It has been reported that levels of vitamin C in the serum from cigarette smokers are lower, consistent with the involvement of vitamin C in protecting against the effects of smoking (24).

Glutathione Levels

Glutathione (GSH) is another major component of the lung's antioxidant defenses that has been shown to be dramatically affected by exposure to cigarette smoke. Once again the results are somewhat inconsistent and are difficult to interpret. Several groups have reported that the *in vivo* response to cigarette exposure is a significant increase in pulmonary GSH levels (18,20). These results suggest that there is an adaptive response to the increased oxidative load presented by smoking that is related to the detoxification of hydroperoxides and hydrogen peroxide by the GSH peroxidase enzyme system.

There is also evidence that GSH and other sulfhydryl-containing moieties may act as antioxidants by direct, sacrificial reaction with cigarette smoke constituents. Joshi et al. (25) studied the effects of acute cigarette exposure on GSH and protein sulfhydryl levels in isolated, perfused lungs from rats and rabbits. These workers found that GSH levels were significantly reduced by smoking but that there was no corresponding increase in GSH disulfide concentrations. Interestingly, however, while protein sulfhydryls in rabbit lungs were significantly reduced, protein sulfhydryls in rat lungs were unaffected, possibly reflecting species dependence of the effects of cigarette smoke (25).

There are also conflicting reports on the ability of sulfhydryl compounds to protect macrophages against the oxidative effects of cigarette smoke. Green (26) has reported that GSH, as well as other sulfhydryl species such as cysteine, protects phagocytic activity of alveolar macrophages against the effects of cigarette smoke. In contrast to these results, Lentz and Di Luzio (20) have shown that cysteine does not protect either the nuclear or supernatant fractions from alveolar macrophages against the increased lipid peroxidation initiated by cigarette smoke.

We have shown, using a simple chemical model system, that both NO and NO_2 react readily with GSH and cysteine, oxidizing them to the corresponding disulfides (27). In view of the high concentrations of these nitrogen oxides in gas-phase cigarette smoke, it is not surprising that smoke exposures would deplete the levels of lung sulfhydryl species.

Effect on Antioxidant Enzymes

In spite of the evidence cited above that cigarette smoke causes changes in lung antioxidants such as vitamin E or GSH, there is little evidence to suggest that smoke exposure causes significant changes in the activities of antioxidant enzymes. Gupta et al. (19) have reported that exposure to cigarette smoke results in no changes in the activities of any of the antioxidant enzymes, including GSH peroxidase, GSH reductase, catalase, or superoxide dismutase. This lack of effect on antioxidant enzyme activities is surprising in view of published reports of the induction of these activities as an adaptive response to oxidative stress by oxygen, ozone, and NO_2 (28,29). The activities of GSH peroxidase, GSH reductase, and glucose-6-phosphate dehydrogenase increased in the lungs of vitamin E-deficient rats exposed to cigarette smoke (18); all of these activities except for the GSH reductase were also increased by cigarette exposure of vitamin E-supplemented animals (18). These effects were generally associated with the tar phase (18). There is also a report by Joshi et al. (25) that cigarette smoke exposure reduces the activity of GSH peroxidase in the lungs from rabbits but not from rats. By contrast, York et al. (30) have reported that cigarette smoke exposure of rats results in *increased* lung GSH peroxidase activities. It has been suggested that such contradictory reports may reflect subtle differences in exposure protocols or even in animal strains (19).

Gupta et al. (31) also have demonstrated that cigarette smoke inhalation caused a marked reduction in glutathione S-transferase (GST) activity. If this is correct, then it is possible that the increased lipid peroxidation brought about by cigarette smoke inhalation results from this effect on GST (19).

Iron Deposits in Smokers' Lungs

When the lungs of long-time cigarette smokers are examined at autopsy, the tissue is typically much darker than that from a nonsmoker. It is reasonable to assume that this dark pigmentation might be partly due to the accumulation of cigarette tar in the lung tissue. However, we have recently shown that the dark pigmentation in smokers' lung tissue is associated with deposits of iron whose form is similar (based on ESR properties) to that of iron in the storage proteins ferritin and hemosiderin (32). We speculate that these iron deposits may develop as the result of the long-term oxidative insult on the lung by cigarette smoke, possibly resulting in microhemorrhaging that releases iron into the lung tissue (32). If this iron has properties similar to those of the iron in ferritin, it might be released by reducing agents such as the $Q/QH\cdot/QH_2$ tar radical or the superoxide radical (33,34). Once released, this iron would contribute to the oxidative load on the lung; for instance, reduced iron catalyzes the reduction of hydrogen peroxide to the hydroxyl radical. The consequences of the increased oxidative damage by the high levels of iron are very likely to include additional tissue damage that might well result in even more iron accumulation. Thus, these iron deposits in the smokers' lung may reflect an iron-driven "oxidative cascade" resulting from smoking (32).

ACKNOWLEDGMENTS

This was was supported by grants from the National Institutes of Health and by a contract from the National Foundation for Cancer Research.

REFERENCES

1. Janoff A. Elastases and emphysema: current assessment of the protease-antiprotease hypothesis. *Am Rev Respir Dis* 1985; 132:417–433.
2. Pryor WA. The free radical chemistry of cigarette smoke and the inactivation of alpha-1-proteinase inhibitor. In: Taylor JC, Mittman C, eds. *Pulmonary emphysema and proteolysis.* New York: Academic Press, 1987;369–392.
3. Pryor WA. Cigarette smoke and the involvement of free radical reactions in chemical carcinogenesis. *Br J Cancer* 1987;55(Suppl VIII):19–23.
4. VanDuuren BL. Carcinogens, co-carcinogens, and tumor inhibitors in cigarette smoke condensate. In: Gori GB, Bock FG, eds. *Banbury report: a safe cigarette?* New York: Cold Spring Harbor Laboratory, 1980;105–112.
5. Pryor WA, Prier DG, Church DF. An electron spin resonance study of mainstream and sidestream cigarette smoke: the nature of the free radicals in gas-phase smoke and cigarette tar. *Environ Health Perspect* 1983;47:345–355.
6. Pryor WA, Hales BJ, Premovic PI, Church DF. The nature of the free radicals in cigarette tar and suggested physiological implications. *Science* 1983;220:425–427.
7. Cosgrove JP, Borish ET, Church DF, Pryor WA. The metal-mediated formation of hydroxyl radical by aqueous extracts of cigarette tar. *Biochem Biophys Res Commun* 1985;132:390–396.
8. Church DF, Pryor WA. Free-radical chemistry of cigarette smoke and its toxicological implications. *Environ Health Perspect* 1985;64:111–126.
9. Guerin MR. Chemical composition of cigarette smoke. In: Gori GB, Bock FG, eds. *Banbury report: a safe cigarette?* New York: Cold Spring Harbor Laboratory, 1980;191–204.
10. Pryor WA, Terauchi K, Davis WH. An electron spin resonance study of cigarette smoke using spin trapping techniques. *Environ Health Perspect* 1976;16:161–175.
11. Pryor WA, Tamura M, Church DF. An ESR spin trapping study of the radicals produced in NO_x/olefin reactions: a mechanism for the production of the apparently long-lived radicals in gas-phase cigarette smoke. *J Am Chem Soc* 1984;106:5073–5079.
12. Pryor WA, Uehara K, Church DF. The chemistry and biochemistry of the radicals in cigarette smoke: ESR evidence for the binding of the tar radical to DNA and polynucleotides. In: Bors W, Saran M, Tait D, eds. *Oxygen radicals in chemistry and biology.* Berlin: Walter de Gruyter, 1984;193–201.
13. Nakayama T, Church DF, Pryor WA. Quantitative analysis of the hydrogen peroxide formed in aqueous cigarette tar extracts. *Free Rad Biol Med* 1989;7:9–15.
14. Borish ET, Cosgrove JP, Church DF, Deutsch WA, Pryor WA. Cigarette tar causes single-strand breaks in DNA. *Biochem Biophys Res Commun* 1985;133:780–786.
15. Borish ET, Pryor WA, Venugopal S, Deutsch WA. DNA synthesis is blocked by cigarette tar-induced DNA single-strand breaks in single-stranded DNA. *Carcinogenesis* 1987;8:1517–1520.
16. Pryor WA. Free radicals in autoxidation and aging. Part I. Kinetics of the autoxidation of linoleic acid in SDS micelles: calculations of radical concentrations, kinetic chain lengths and the effects of vitamin E. Part II. The role of free radicals in chronic human diseases and in aging. In: Armstrong D, Sohal RS, Cutler RG, Slater TF, eds. *Free radicals in molecular biology, aging and disease.* New York: Raven Press, 1984;13–41.
17. Chatterjee SN, Agarwal S. Liposomes as membrane models for study of lipid peroxidation. *Free Rad Biol Med* 1988;4:51–72.
18. Chow CK, Chen LH, Thacker RR, Griffith RB. Dietary vitamin E and pulmonary biochemical responses of rats to cigarette smoking. *Environ Res* 1984;34:8–17.
19. Gupta MP, Khanduja KL, Sharma RR. Effect of cigarette smoke inhalation on antioxidant enzymes and lipid peroxidation in the rat. *Toxicol Lett* 1988;41:107–114.
20. Lentz PE, Di Luzio NR. Peroxidation of lipids in alveolar macrophages: production by aqueous extracts of cigarette smoke. *Arch Environ Health* 1974;28:279–282.
21. Burton GW, Joyce A, Ingold KU. Is vitamin E the only lipid-soluble, chain-breaking antioxidant in human blood plasma and erythrocyte membranes? *Arch Biochem Biophys* 1983;221:281–290.
22. Pacht ER, Kaseki H, Mohammed JR, Cornwell DG, Davis WB. Deficiency of vitamin E in the alveolar fluid of cigarette smokers: influence on alveolar cytotoxicity. *J Clin Invest* 1986;77:789–796.
23. Niki E. Antioxidants in relation to lipid peroxidation. *Chem Phys Lipids* 1987;44:227–253.
24. Schorah CJ. Vitamin C status in population groups. In: Counsell JN, Hornig DH, eds. *Vitamin C (ascorbic acid).* Englewood, NJ: Applied Science Publishers, 1981;23–47.
25. Joshi UM, Kodavanti PRS, Mehendale HM. Glutathione metabolism and utilization of external thiols by cigarette smoke-challenged, isolated rat and rabbit lungs. *Toxicol Appl Pharmacol* 1988;96:324–335.
26. Green GM. Cigarette smoke: protection of alveolar macrophages by glutathione and cysteine. *Science* 1968;162:810–811.
27. Pryor WA, Church DF, Govindan CK, Crank G. Oxidation of thiols by nitric oxide and nitrogen dioxide: synthetic utility and toxicological implications. *J Org Chem* 1982;47:156–159.
28. Mustafa MG, Tiernay DF. Biochemical and metabolic changes in the lung with oxygen, ozone and nitrogen dioxide toxicity. *Am Rev Respir Dis* 1978;118:1061–1090.
29. Hoffman M, Stevens JB, Autor AP. Adaptation to hyperoxia in neonatal rat: kinetic parameters of the oxygen mediated induction of lung superoxide dismutase, catalase, and glutathione peroxidase. *Toxicology* 1980;16:215–226.
30. York GK, Pierce TH, Schwartz LW, Cross CE. Stimulation by

cigarette smoke of glutathione peroxidase system enzyme activities in rat lung. *Arch Environ Health* 1976;31:286–290.

31. Gupta MP, Khanduja KL, Sharma RR. Effect of cigarette smoke inhalation on certain pulmonary and hepatic drug metabolizing enzymes in vitamin A deficient rats. *Indian J Med Res* 1986; 84:301–309.

32. Church DF, Burkey TJ, Pryor WA. Preparation of human lung tissue from cigarette smokers for analysis by electron spin resonance spectroscopy. In: Packer L, Glazer AN, eds. *Oxygen Radicals in Biological Systems, Part B: Oxygen Radicals and Antioxidants. Methods Enzymol* 1990;186:665–669.

33. Aust SD. Sources of iron for lipid peroxidation in biological systems. In: Halliwell B, ed. *Oxygen radicals and tissue injury. Proceedings of the Brook Lodge Symposium.* Bethesda, MD: Federation of the American Society of Experimental Biologists, 1988;27–33.

34. Thomas CE, Morehouse LA, Aust SD. Ferritin and superoxide-dependent lipid peroxidation. *J Biol Chem* 1985;260:3275–3280.

THE LUNG: Scientific Foundations
edited by R.G. Crystal, J.B. West et al.
Raven Press, Ltd., New York © 1991.

CHAPTER 7.7.1

Injury from Inflammatory Cells

Polly E. Parsons, G. Scott Worthen, and Peter M. Henson

The widely recognized role of inflammatory cells in the injury suffered by the lungs in a wide variety of diseases has often overshadowed the role that these same cells play in protection of the lung against infection and in repair after injury. This apparent duality of function makes delineation of the specific roles of inflammatory cells in lung injury difficult. In an attempt to facilitate an understanding of the potential role of inflammatory cells in the spectrum of pulmonary diseases covered under the broad description of lung injury, we have elected to focus on a single cell type, the neutrophil—a well-studied inflammatory cell which is of critical importance in host defense and which is a prime suspect in lung injury states. While we believe that mechanisms of injury can be generalized to inflammation in many different organs and to differing types of inflammation, the unique low-pressure characteristics of the pulmonary blood supply inevitably contribute some special features to inflammatory injury in the lung, particularly with regard to capillary localization of inflammatory cells.

Before discussing lung injury, the term must be defined; this is surprisingly difficult. The definition of lung injury incorporates a range of phenomena characterized by widely differing manifestations, including, among others, functional alterations in gas exchange, excess lung water, alterations of pulmonary hemodynamics, increased vascular permeability, and lavage or histologic evidence of structural damage. To further complicate matters, inflammation and injury are often seen as synonymous. However, the fact that granulocyte emigration into the air spaces may occur without significant alteration of permeability or evi-

dence of other injury suggests that inflammation should be seen primarily as an essential protective response of tissues to insult. The injurious potential of inflammatory cells, then, is secondary, and while it may represent an alteration from the norm—and hence by some definitions, an "injury"—we would argue that in any discussion or description of lung alterations the term "injury" should be used sparingly and be accompanied by a clear description of the measurable changes that are to be used so that the reader can make up his/her own mind as to whether the effect is physiological or pathological. Indeed, for the purpose of the ensuing discussion, we will consider injury to be tissue/cell death. Although this emphasizes the process that can lead to such extreme effects, we suspect that the milder alterations are produced by mechanisms that are only different in degree and not in kind.

In an inflammatory response in the lung, circulating neutrophils accumulate in the local vasculature and migrate through the vessel wall, interstitium, and the epithelial barriers to gain access to the alveolar lumen (see Chapters 3.4.7 and 3.4.8). Each point in this sequence represents a potential site at which tissue injury may occur, but injury is not an inevitable consequence of any of these processes. During accumulation and emigration, inflammatory cells could release a variety of injurious materials, including oxygen metabolites and proteases which may also cause and potentiate injury (see Chapters 7.7.1, 7.2.1, 7.2.4, and 7.9.1). Accordingly, this chapter will focus on two specific areas of the inflammatory process: (i) the regulation of inflammatory cell accumulation in the lung and (ii) the regulation of the injurious potential of inflammatory cells.

REGULATION OF INFLAMMATORY CELL ACCUMULATION IN THE LUNG

In order for neutrophils to initiate lung injury, they must be retained within the lung. Neutrophil accu-

P. E. Parsons and G. S. Worthen: Department of Medicine, National Jewish Center for Immunology and Respiratory Disease, Denver, Colorado 80206.

P. M. Henson: Department of Pediatrcs, National Jewish Center for Immunology and Respiratory Disease, Denver, Colorado 80206.

mulation can be regulated by processes acting to alter (a) the delivery of neutrophils, (b) their retention within the microcirculation, and (c) their migration into lung parenchyma.

Regulation of Neutrophil Delivery to the Lung

It is assumed that when the inflammatory cells leave the bone marrow and enter the circulation under normal circumstances they are in a quiescent nonactivated state. This means that they can pass through the microvasculature of the lung and other organs many times without any significant effect on those vessels or the underlying tissue. Signals to induce neutrophil sequestration may occur in response to both systemic stimuli (such as mediators released into the blood) and intrapulmonary stimuli (such as the alteration of a vascular wall that passing cells can recognize). The available pools from which neutrophils are drawn include both the general circulation and a pool of neutrophils sequestered within the pulmonary vasculature. It is likely that neutrophils can be initially stimulated within the circulation. The evidence that this occurs, however, is limited because of (a) the difficulty in accessing the marginal pool for study and (b) the apparent rapidity with which neutrophils are retained within the lung following stimulation. This was demonstrated by Lien et al. (1), who found that neutrophil retention in the pulmonary capillary bed occurred within seconds of the intravascular administration of complement fragments in a canine model. Similar results have been obtained in rabbits in response to the combination of complement fragments and endotoxin (2,3).

The process of neutrophil retention in the lung involves a complex interaction between the neutrophil and vascular endothelium which is not yet clearly defined but which can be regulated at a number of levels. One regulatory level involves the control of delivery of neutrophils and other inflammatory cells to the site. Delivery may be controlled by the concentration of inflammatory cells in the circulating blood (itself under control of a variety of factors) and by the local blood flow to the inflammatory site. Because the lung receives the entire cardiac output, the latter mechanism is most efficient when the inflammatory response is localized to a small region or has a patchy distribution (4), although regional inhomogeneity has been demonstrated even in a disorder with a diffuse pattern of injury, the adult respiratory distress syndrome (ARDS) (5).

The lung appears to regulate delivery of blood to an inflammatory site through some of its own mechanisms for determining local vasoreactivity. At least two mechanisms have been suggested, perhaps the most important of which is hypoxic vasocontriction (6); see also Chapter 7.2.1.3. At an inflamed (and hence hypoxic) site, hypoxic vasoconstriction results in diversion of flow away from the involved region, thus diminishing delivery of circulating neutrophils (7) as it improves systemic oxygenation. Whether this mechanism actually limits neutrophil accumulation at the inflammatory site is unknown. A second mechanism of regulation of blood flow is through the generation of local prostanoid derivatives within the lung, and this has been demonstrated in rabbits (8) and guinea pigs (9). Under these circumstances, inflammation within a local site results in diversion of flow away from the site by a mechanism which appears to be different from that of hypoxic vasoconstriction and which rquires cyclo-oxygenase. If this cyclo-oxygenase-dependent diversion of flow is counteracted by the use of a vasodilator, the decrease in neutrophil delivery to the site is prevented and neutrophil accumulation within the lung is enhanced (8). This suggests that the diversion of blood flow limits the intensity of the inflammatory response.

Regulation of Neutrophil Retention in the Lung

Normal unstimulated neutrophils entering the lung microvascular bed to form the marginating pool are retained almost exclusively within the lung capillaries (10). Furthermore, the cells sequestered in such fashion do not pass slowly through the capillary but rather are retained at discrete sites within the lung vasculature (11), suggesting that there may be preferred sites within the lung for leukocyte sequestration. Even under normal circumstances, neutrophils which eventually transit the lung capillary may remain stationary for short periods of time, ranging from a second to as much as a few minutes. The distribution of transit times for these normal neutrophils can be affected in a number of different fashions by both (a) the hemodynamics of lung circulation (11), where increases in pulmonary artery pressure or local flow rates diminish the transit time, and (b) inflammatory stimuli (12), which dramatically increase the mean transit time. Even when stimulated, however, the cells are retained at the same site (capillary) and in the same manner (stuttering or hopping) as the normal cells, although the magnitude of the effects is much greater in an inflammatory circumstance (12). Furthermore, the cells are retained singly (12), indicating that the original suggestion that aggregation was the explanation for neutrophil accumulation in complement-induced lung injury (13) does not seem to account for sequestration in capillaries. It may, however, represent a mechanism for sequestration in arterioles.

Even though neutrophils can be shown to travel more slowly than erythrocytes in both pulmonary and systemic beds, the above data highlight an important difference between the pulmonary circulation and other circulatory beds. In the former, neutrophils may spend considerable periods of time in stationary contact with the local capillary endothelium, a condition which may greatly predispose to adhesive and other interactions (and perhaps, eventually, injury) between the neutrophil and the subjacent endothelium. In systemic vascular beds, the transit of neutrophils is prolonged, not by retention in the capillaries but by the rolling of the neutrophils along the walls of postcapillary venules (14); thus the duration of contact between the neutrophil and the vessel wall is limited.

As a function of these differences in neutrophil behavior in pulmonary and systemic microcirculations, the factors that induce initial retention of neutrophils are also under somewhat different control. The neutrophil has an average diameter of 8 μm, whereas capillaries, whether of pulmonary or systemic origin, have mean diameters of 5.5 μm (15). Thus, the neutrophil must deform in order to transit any capillary. The driving pressure for neutrophil deformation, however, must be the local capillary pressure, which is much lower in the pulmonary circuit (see Chapters 5.2.1.1, 5.2.1.3, and 5.2.2). Accordingly, the ease of neutrophil deformation may be more critical to ensure transit through the lung. Whereas neutrophils are fairly deformable at rest, they respond to chemoattractants so as to become considerably more stiff (16). In addition, the size and stiffness properties of the other circulating leukocytes, monocytes, and lymphocytes may also regulate the circulatory behavior of unstimulated cells (17). The increase in stiffness consequent to chemoattractant stimulation of neutrophils is accounted for largely by induction of cytoskeletal assembly (16) and suggests that regulation of mechanical properties of the neutrophil (and by implication, the capillary as well) may contribute to retention. It is important to restate at this point that even enhanced neutrophil retention within the pulmonary capillary bed is not necessarily associated with lung injury. For example, in a rabbit model of complement-fragment-induced neutrophil retention there were neither demonstrable changes in pulmonary permeability nor apparent histologic tissue evidence for tissue injury associated with neutrophil sequestration alone (18).

At the same time that neutrophils are apparently retained within the capillaries due to alterations in mechanical properties, however, both stimulated inflammatory and endothelial cells also express increased numbers of adhesion-related glycoproteins which may further contribute to the retention of inflammatory cells within the pulmonary microvasculature. Increased neutrophil adhesivity has been demonstrated

in response to C5a (19), tumor necrosis factor (TNF) (20), interleukin-1 (IL-1) (21), and bacterial lipopolysaccharides (LPS) (21); also, endothelial adhesivity increases in response to TNF (20,21), LPS (21), and IL-1 (22) (see Chapter 2.8 for details concerning IL-1 and TNF). Several different adherence glycoproteins have been identified on both the neutrophil and endothelial cell. The major neutrophil complexes include MAC-1, LFA-1, P150,95, and CD11/18, all of which share a common beta chain (23) against which antibodies are available. The families of adhesion molecules on the endothelial cell which have been identified include the CAM members of the immunoglobulin superfamily [ICAM-1 (24) and PECAM-1 (25)] and the members of the ELAM-related family [ELAM (26) and PADGEM (27)], and it is likely that more will be forthcoming. As yet, the corresponding molecules on the neutrophil identified by these molecules are unclear except for ICAM-1, which appears to interact with LFA-1 on the surface of the neutrophil (28). The relative importance of increased neutrophil adherence versus endothelial adherence is not yet clear. It is known that the adherence of neutrophils to the endothelium occurs quickly (29) and that the neutrophil response is rapid (19,30), whereas the maximal endothelial response can take as long as 4–6 hr (22); this suggests that the neutrophil adherence complexes may be important in the initial inflammatory response but that the endothelial response may be more important in sustaining the inflammatory response.

Whether or not neutrophil adherence is a prerequisite to lung injury is not yet clear. In patients with leukocyte glycoprotein deficiency whose neutrophils neither adhere nor migrate, localized inflammation/injury is not seen (31), suggesting that adherence is necessary. However, only a few studies have directly assessed the role of adhesion molecules in neutrophil sequestration *in vivo*. These studies suggest that antibodies directed against the common beta chain of the neutrophil adherence glycoproteins can significantly decrease neutrophil retention in the gut in an ischemia–reperfusion model (32), with minimal effect on neutrophil retention within the pulmonary microvasculature. Furthermore, in this model the antibodies decreased morbidity but did not prevent the associated pulmonary injury. It remains unclear as to whether these data reflect (as we interpret) an important role for the mechanical properties of the leukocyte, a different set of adhesion-related molecules, or a fundamentally different endothelial surface in the lung than in systemic vascular beds.

The endothelial cell may affect neutrophil adherence by producing substances that inhibit neutrophil responses. Prostacyclin (PGI2) is an important endothelial-derived arachidonic acid metabolite that has been shown to inhibit neutrophil adherence (33). The endothelial cell also contains ectoenzymes capable of converting ATP and ADP to adenosine (34), which inhibits a variety of neutrophil functions (35). Furthermore, neutrophils can cause endothelial damage (even in the absence of adherence) through the release of toxic mediators such as oxidants and elastase (36,37), although recent data indicate that endothelial cells may be able to partially protect themselves by inhibiting the production of oxidants by neutrophils (38). These new data further heighten the potential complexity of the neutrophil–endothelial interaction.

Regulation of Neutrophil Migration

To reach the alveolus from the vascular space, cells must migrate through the vascular endothelium, the basement membrane, and the alveolar epithelium. The route across the capillary endothelium appears almost exclusively along the thick segment of the alveolar capillary membrane rather than along the thin one (39), but the mechanisms responsible remain unclear. *In vitro*, it has been shown that neutrophils will migrate through endothelial monolayers without the addition of exogenous stimuli (40). The phenomenon is not seen with fibroblast, smooth muscle, or epithelial monolayers (41) and suggests that the endothelium may actually facilitate neutrophil migration, which is believed, based on ultrastructural examination, to occur between the endothelial cells (39,42–44). Recent evidence supports the early notion that the endothelium participates in the migratory process. It has been demonstrated that the up-regulation of the ICAM-1 molecule on the endothelial cell actively facilitates neutrophil migration across the endothelial cell and into the subendothelial spaces (28), and this could regulate migration *in vivo*.

Regulation of neutrophil migration appears to be exerted at a number of other levels. Chief among these appears to be the intensity of the gradient established by those chemoattractants that are present. This, however, has proved to be an extraordinarily difficult issue to settle, since the existence of a clear-cut chemoattractant gradient inferred from *in vitro* studies has not yet been unequivocally determined *in vivo*. This situation is further complicated by chemoattractants which are bound to surfaces, such as C5a (45). The magnitude of the increase in vascular permeability induced during inflammation may also effect the intensity of migratory response, perhaps by modulating the strength of the chemoattractant gradient sensed by the neutrophil (46). Finally, the chemoattractant gradient itself may wash out as a function of time unless its production is continued. This has been demonstrated

in the rabbit knee joint (47), and a variety of chemoattractant inhibitors have also been proposed which might enhance such an effect (48). However, at present the roles of these different factors in the magnitude of the migratory response to a given inflammatory signal have not been established. The effect of neutrophil migration on the integrity of the endothelium is somewhat difficult to assess because the normal permeability of an *in vivo* endothelial monolayer is not known. Work by Meyrick and co-workers (49,50) using arterial explants suggests that neutrophil migration is not associated with endothelial injury.

After migrating through the endothelium, the neutrophil must traverse the basement membrane and extravascular tissue. The mechanisms by which this occurs have been only partially elucidated. Morphologic studies suggest that the basement membrane poses a significant barrier and that the neutrophil may actually have to destroy it to traverse it (51,52). Neutrophils do produce elastase and other proteolytic enzymes which have activity against many of the constituents of the basement membrane, and thus they are capable of direct injury (53; see also Chapter 7.1.1). Furthermore, *in vitro* studies suggest that this proteolysis can occur despite the presence of antiproteases (54,55) which are known to be present in the extracellular space. Studies by Campbell and Campbell (56) have offered an explanation for this apparent dichotomy. They have shown that in the presence of protease inhibitors, neutrophil-dependent proteolysis is confined to small, sharply demarcated pericellular zones which are apparently able to restrict the access of α_1-antitrypsin inhibitor (56), thus allowing for localized proteolysis in the presence of protease inhibitors.

The last barrier to the migration into the alveolus is the alveolar epithelium. The neutrophils migrate via intercellular junctions (57), and this process can apparently occur without any associated epithelial injury. This has been demonstrated *in vitro* by many investigators (46,58) who have evaluated neutrophil migration in response to chemotactic stimuli. *In vivo*, this can be inferred from the studies of Staub et al. (59) which showed that in anesthetized sheep, neutrophil influx into the lung in response to LTB$_4$ was not associated with any persistent change in epithelial permeability. It should be noted, however, that there are circumstances in which neutrophil migration is associated with increases in epithelial permeability. For example, Sugahara et al. (60) showed that when neutrophils were stimulated with a phagocytic stimulus to migrate through type II alveolar cell monolayers, the permeability was increased (60). The explanation for these results may be that the neutrophil–epithelial interaction was prolonged in that system. Neutrophils are more adherent to alveolar type II cells than to many other cell types (including the canine kidney cell line used for most of the previously mentioned studies of epithelial permeability) (M. G. Tonnesen, *personal communication*), and prolonged contact of the neutrophil and epithelium has been associated with increased epithelial permeability (58). Whether or not this increased permeability is the result of the focal pericellular proteolysis described above is not known.

Intra-Alveolar Mediator Release

The last potential site of inflammatory cell-induced injury in the cascade is the alveolus. As described in other chapters (3.4.7, 7.1.1, 7.2.1, and 7.2.4), neutrophils produce a variety of substances (such as oxidants and proteases) which can directly cause lung injury. Although attention in acute lung injury has focused on endothelial injury, morphologic evidence to support a greater effect on the vasculature is lacking. Indeed, evidence of epithelial injury is frequently more prominent. Perhaps this is due to difficulties in recognizing injury to thin type I cells. In this regard, the use of immunocytochemical techniques to identify those cells that serve as the major target(s) may prove useful. One example of the almost total loss of alveolar epithelial cells associated with acute lung injury can be seen in a histologic section from a patient with ARDS evaluated with immunocytochemistry (Fig. 1).

The mechanisms by which neutrophils could be further activated upon arrival within the alveolus are speculative. The macrophage may play a preeminent role. In response to the neutrophil influx, macrophages may be stimulated to produce neutrophil chemoattractants causing further neutrophil recruitment and enhancing the lung injury. The macrophages can also produce cytokines such as TNF and IL-1, which are able to prime intra-alveolar neutrophils to cause lung injury (see below). The macrophage could also be responsible for the production of fibroblast growth factors which could dramatically effect the final outcome of lung injury (see Chapters 2.9, 3.4.5, and 7.8.1). This may be part of the process which differentiates the chronic fibrosis associated with some interstitial lung diseases from the more acute (and apparently transient) fibrosis seen in some patients with ARDS.

REGULATION OF THE INJURIOUS POTENTIAL OF INFLAMMATORY CELLS

We will make the simplifying assumption that the common circulating inflammatory cells exhibit more similarities than differences with regard to the mechanisms by which they can damage cells and connective tissue elements. Three major classes of injurious molecules are produced by inflammatory cells—oxygen metabolites, proteases, and cationic proteins (36)—but other toxic materials may eventually be identified. Amphipathic lipids may well be injurious, but they have not received major emphasis, perhaps because they would also be toxic to the cell that produced them. This latter feature is of interest in that the inflammatory cell itself seems relatively resistant (61) to its own toxic products—presumably an important feature in its primary role of host defense. Cytotoxic cytokines such as TNF are clearly injurious; however, their toxicity is not generalized but, rather, specific for certain cells (e.g., neoplastic cells) (62). In addition, the variety of lysosomal enzymes capable of hydrolyzing proteoglycans may contribute to alterations in connective tissue structures, including perhaps the cartilage of the airways (possibly in a manner analogous to digestive effects on cartilage in the joints).

Toxic materials are secreted/released from inflammatory cells in a regulated fashion. Prior to the 1970s, it was generally thought that inflammatory cells such as neutrophils released their contents during the process of lysis and destruction at the inflammatory site. Although this certainly happens, particularly at points of infection with strains of bacteria that produce cytocidal toxins, it is now recognized that inflammatory cells actively secrete their contents; like many other secretory processes, this is inducible and under cellular control (61,63). Neutrophil secretory products fall into three major categories: the contents of granules, lipid "mediators," and oxygen metabolites. The azurophil granules contain acid hydrolases, elastase, and many of the potentially toxic cations, and they function in many regards like classical lysosomes. The neutrophil-specific granules, on the other hand, contain materials that tend to act at neutral pH and have been considered to serve as typical secretory granules (64). Thus, discharge of the contents of these two organelles is under different control and probably occurs by different mechanisms (65,66). Specific granules (and related storage structures) appear to discharge directly at the cell surface (exocytosis) and are released either to the outside or to the phagosome earlier than are the azurophil granules (67,68). The mechanism by which the lipid mediators are released is largely unknown, and oxygen metabolites are thought either to be produced at the cell surface itself or to pass through anion channels in the membrane to gain access to the outside of the cell (69). This distinction between active secretion and passive lysis as a source of injurious materials is additionally important from a potentially therapeutic perspective. Understanding the mechanisms involved in the secretory process could allow for the design of appropriate modulating agents. It may also be sup-

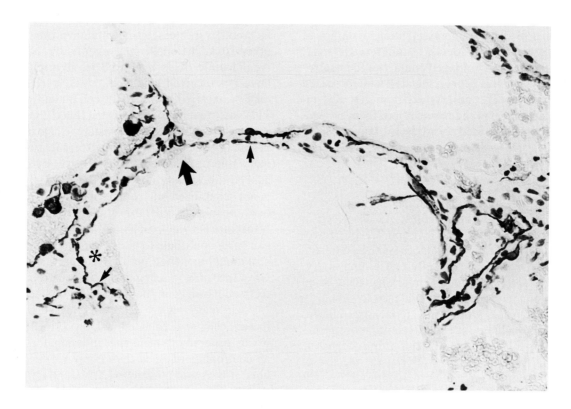

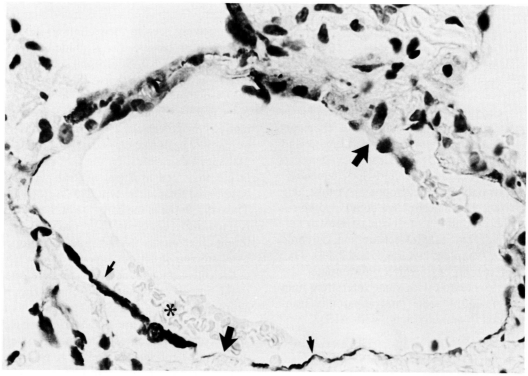

FIG. 1. Histologic sections from the lung of a patient with ARDS, stained for alveolar epithelial cells from CAM 5.2, a mouse monoclonal antibody against cytokeratins #8, 18, and 19. **A:** Areas of both intact (small arrows) and absent (large arrows) epithelial layer. In addition, areas of alveolar exudate and hemorrhage are shown (*) (×344). **B:** Higher power view of another area. Areas of dense staining for epithelial cells are shown by the black reaction product (small arrows) while absent epithelial cells are shown by large arrows. Hemorrhage and exudate are indicated by * (×688). (Courtesy of Robert J. Mason, M.D.)

posed that the secretion is significantly modulated *in vivo* in pathophysiologic events.

Priming

As discussed previously, neutrophils can migrate into the lung without producing significant damage under some circumstances whereas at other times great structural alteration ensues. Perhaps in like manner, neutrophil accumulation is sometimes considered to be the cause of severe injury and disease (e.g., ARDS) and other times thought to be associated only with protection and to be followed by normal recovery of structure and function (e.g., pneumonia). A potential explanation for these anomalies lies in the phenomenon of priming. Neutrophils (and most other inflammatory cells) can be raised to a heightened state of responsiveness by prior exposure to a priming stimulus which does not itself initiate the function in question. First shown for superoxide anion production (70), the prototypic priming agent was bacterial LPS. It is now appreciated that a wide variety of molecules [including platelet-activating factor (71; see also Chapter 2.5), TNF (72), GM-CSF (73), and IL-1 (74)] can induce this altered responsivity and that cellular responses that are enhanced include secretion, adhesiveness, and a number of synthetic functions (75). The nature of the secondary stimulus that actually induces the cell response (formyl-methionyl-leucyl-phenyalanine, C5a or immune complexes are often used experimentally) seems unimportant, suggesting the generality of the phenomenon. The mechanism is unknown but does not seem to involve alterations in number or affinity of receptors or protein synthetic mechanisms. It may reflect alterations in free cytoplasmic calcium concentrations (76). It has been further suggested in fact that complete neutrophil activation requires these two steps (priming and stimulation) even if they both occur simultaneously and thus cannot be independently detected (77).

In the context of a "normal" inflammatory response, it is likely that neutrophils can emigrate into the lung under the influence of chemotactic factors alone but, because they are not previously primed, secrete but little of their contents, perhaps just enough to accomplish the emigration itself. Encountering bacteria and/or cytokines in the inflamed alveolus, the cells would undergo priming and then the appropriate heightened responses required for removal of the infectious agents. If, on the other hand, the neutrophils are primed before or during the emigration phase, injury to the tissues through which they are migrating would be likely to ensue. Certainly, concurrent intravascular injections of LPS and chemoattractants were able to induce neutrophil-dependent increases in pulmonary vascular leakage of albumin that were not evident with either stimulus alone (2). To support the implication that this type of synergism is due to a direct priming effect on the LPS, neutrophils pretreated with LPS and washed prior to reinfusion were retained in the lung to a greater degree and for a longer time (3). In addition, generation of TNF and other cytokines would only serve to enhance the process.

Surface Effects

Although localization of inflammatory cells in the pulmonary microvasculature by itself does not produce injury, induction of the secretory events outlined above would. Another modulating factor in these circumstances is the interaction of the inflammatory cell with a surface (e.g., that of the epithelium). It has long been appreciated that neutrophils secrete more constituents when adherent (78), a phenomenon usually thought to relate to surface stimulation and to be related perhaps to the normal phagolysosome fusion in a circumstance where the "particle" to be phagocytosed is in fact the whole surface—a process called "frustrated phagocytosis." The enhanced stimulation under these circumstances is important for neutrophils (79), and in macrophages it has been shown to result not only in increased responses but also in the induction of new proteins for secretion (80,81).

A completely different effect of the surface is to provide a localized site for cell secretion that may be immune from the protective actions of plasma or tissue inhibitors. For example, the injury of endothelial cells by primed and stimulated neutrophils was unaffected by the presence of either plasma or α_1-antitrypsin, even though it was shown to be dependent on the expression of neutrophil elastase; the direct effect of purified elastase on the endothelial cells was clearly blocked by both (54). Three phenomena may explain this apparent discrepancy. First, neutrophils apparently retain some of the elastase they "secrete" on the plasma membrane (C. Fittschen and P. M. Henson, *unpublished observation*), in a manner analogous to their expression of granule membrane enzymes (such as alkaline phosphatase) as ectoenzymes after exocytosis of the granule (82). This would result in application of the toxic enzyme at the point of surface stimulation of the cell and would concentrate it at that site. Second, local concentrations of injurious materials may be very high between the inflammatory cell and its target. Levels of H_2O_2, for example, have been suggested to reach 10^{-2} M between inflammatory cells and targets (83). Third, as mentioned earlier, the interaction between a stimulated inflammatory cell and its surface target seems to be tight enough to exclude protein molecules such as α_1-antitrypsin (56). Similar effects might be expected for neutrophils encountering connective tissue surfaces during migration across the interstitium. It should also be reemphasized that if the inflammatory cell interacts with the surface for only a short time in its migratory path, it is far less likely to induce detectable alterations in this surface.

A RELEVANT MODEL: NEUTROPHILS IN ARDS

The previous sections have presented a conceptual framework of the regulation of the inflammatory process bolstered by experimental data from *in vitro* and animal systems. That animal systems are relevant to the study of the inflammatory process in humans is demonstrated by the comparison of histologic sections of a lung from a patient with ARDS and a canine lung in which inflammation was induced by the intrapulmonary administration of complement fragments (Fig.

2). As can be seen in these micrographs, the pathologic features in these two forms of injury are virtually identical: the intra-alveolar septae are edematous, the epithelial basement membrane is partially denuded, and the endothelium is essentially intact. To help put the presented data in perspective, however, it may be helpful to consider a form of lung injury, ARDS, for which there are significant data from humans on the possible role of one inflammatory cell type, the neutrophil.

There is some evidence that activation of circulating neutrophils can be detected *in vivo* in ARDS despite the apparent rapidity with which neutrophils are retained within the lung following stimulation. Zimmerman et al. (84) found that neutrophils isolated from the arterial blood of patients with ARDS were both functionally and metabolically activated as assessed by (a) an increase in the neutrophil chemotactic index, (b) stimulated chemiluminescence, (c) superoxide release,

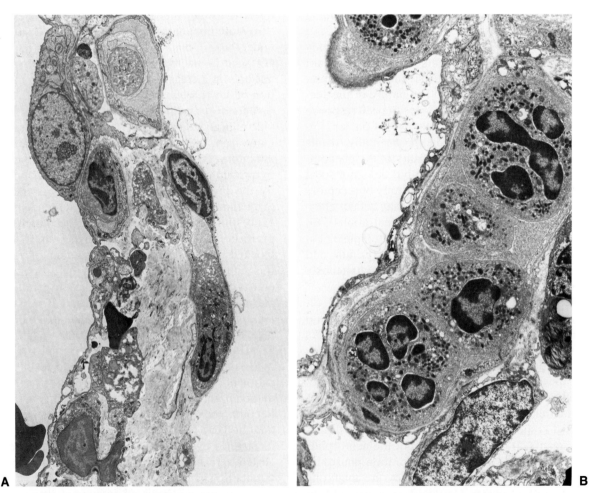

FIG. 2. Acute lung injury. **A:** Histologic section from the lung of a patient with ARDS (×1800). (From ref. 93.) **B:** Histologic section from a canine lung following the intrapulmonary administration of C5 fragments (×5400). In both micrographs there is evidence of interstitial edema and partial denudation of the alveolar epithelium with relative sparing of the endothelium.

and (d) an increase in the ratio of cyclic GMP to cyclic AMP. In a study of patients with sepsis, stimulated H_2O_2 release was significantly greater in the neutrophils isolated from the venous circulation than in those from the arterial circulation, suggesting that neutrophils could be activated in the circulation and then sequestered within the lung (85). In our laboratory we have found that circulating neutrophils from patients with ARDS (as well as in those at risk for ARDS) have changes in shape, although there is no increase in unstimulated superoxide release when compared to that in normal controls (*unpublished observations*).

There is now an increasing body of evidence that neutrophil stimuli are present in the peripheral circulation of patients who develop acute lung injury, further suggesting that neutrophils could be activated within the systemic circulation. Numerous investigators have demonstrated that the complement cascade is activated in critically ill patients with ARDS, as well as in those at risk for the development of ARDS (86–88). TNF has also been demonstrated in the plasma from patients with sepsis, and there appears to be some association with the subsequent development of ARDS (89,90). Similarly, circulating endotoxin has been shown to be associated with development of ARDS (91). The presence of these factors (both priming stimuli and chemoattractants) within the circulation may help to explain the development of lung injury in patients with an apparently distal illness (i.e., pancreatitis, abdominal trauma, nonpulmonary sepsis).

Both lung biopsy material (92,93) and bronchial lavage fluid from most patients with ARDS (94) clearly demonstrate that neutrophils are retained within the lung parenchyma and alveoli. In patients it is difficult to discern the regulatory mechanisms for the accumulation of neutrophils within the lung. There is evidence that the hypoxic vasoconstriction response is significantly dampened (5), which could allow for an enhanced neutrophil accumulation. Although there are no direct data from humans to document that the neutrophils migrate from the vasculature to the alveoli as opposed to flooding through damaged endothelium and epithelium, a study of patients at risk for developing ARDS by Fowler et al. (95) is suggestive of the former. In that study, patients who were at risk for but who did not develop ARDS were lavaged early in their disease course and found to have significant neutrophil accumulation within the alveoli despite no clinically apparent pulmonary dysfunction (95). Other supporting evidence for neutrophil migration is the presence of neutrophil chemotatic factors in bronchoalveolar lavage fluid from patients with ARDS. The source of these chemotactic factors is not definitively known, but there are multiple possibilities. One potential source of neutrophil stimuli is the lung itself, either in response to direct injury (i.e., aspiration, chest trauma,

toxic inhalation) or from the activation of resident cells (i.e., macrophages) to release chemoattractants. In support of the former possibility, Anderson and co-workers (96,97) have suggested that chemotactic factors can diffuse from sites of injury and cause the regulation of neutrophil surface glycoproteins. This could be important in the inflammatory augmentation of the lung injury which occurs following a direct pulmonary insult. There is evidence that chemoattractants are produced within the alveoli, and alveolar macrophages isolated form patients with a variety of forms of lung injury are known to produce neutrophil chemoattractants. These macrophage products include not fully characterized neutrophil chemoattractants in asthma (98), idiopathic fibrosis (99), and ARDS (94) and IL-1 patients with idiopathic interstitial fibrosis and sacoidosis (100,101). That chemoattractants generated in the alveolar space are of potential importance is suggested by the observations that the instillation of chemoattractants into the alveolus causes neutrophil sequestration within the lung. This has been demonstrated in many animal models (1,9,102) and in humans with asthma (103).

The function of intra-alveolar neutrophils in patients with ARDS has not been assessed, so it is not clear if the cells are primed and/or activated. However, toxic products of neutrophils, including oxidants, proteases, and leukotrienes, have all been demonstrated to be present in the bronchoalveolar lavage fluid of patients with ARDS, strongly suggesting that the neutrophils have been stimulated at some point in time (see Chapters 2.8, 2.10, 3.4.4, 3.4.7, 3.4.8, 7.1.1, 7.2.1, 7.2.4, 7.7.3.1, and 7.8.1).

Although each step of the inflammatory process cannot be easily demonstrated in patients with ARDS, it is clear that the *in vitro* and animal models of the role of inflammatory cells in lung injury are relevant to the events which cause human disease.

SUMMARY

In this discussion it has been suggested that inflammatory cell interaction with the lung does not inevitably result in injury. In contrast, injury results from a concatenation of events that appear to be closely regulated and that include the nature of the substrate that the cells interact with, the combination and temporal sequence of stimuli that are present, and the rates of accumulation and removal of the cells themselves. When the circumstances are ripe for injury, the cells apparently mediate the damage largely by liberation of oxygen metabolites, cations, and proteases. Potent inhibitors and inactivators are present in tissues and plasma for all of these, and thus the net result represents a balance between these factions. Injury in this scenario would be exacerbated by adhesion of the inflammatory cells to other cells or to connective tissue elements in the lung (by enhancing stimulation and by excluding access of the inhibitors) and/or by reduced vessel permeability (which would reduce the total concentration of the plasma-derived inhibitors). Although this discussion has focused on the neutrophil, it is not meant to imply that other inflammatory cells such as monocytes, eosinophils, mast cells, lymphocytes, and macrophages are not important in the inflammatory process. They not only participate independently, but they may also have important interactions with each other and with neutrophils which can both promote and regulate inflammation.

REFERENCES

1. Lien DC, Worthen GS, Capen RL, Henson JE, Wagner WW, Henson PM. The acute inflammatory process in the canine lung: direct observation of neutrophil behavior in response to C5 fragments; in preparation.
2. Worthen GS, Haslett C, Rees AJ, Gumbay RS, Henson JE, Henson PM. Neutrophil mediated pulmonary vascular injury: synergistic effect of trace amounts of lipopolysaccharide and neutrophil stimuli on vascular permeability and neutrophil sequestration in the lung. Am Rev Respir Dis 1987;136:19–28.
3. Haslett C, Worthen GS, Giclas PC, Morrison DC, Henson JE, Henson PM. The pulmonary vascular sequestration of neutrophils in endotoxemia is initated by an effect of endotoxin on the neutrophil in the rabbit. Am Rev Respir Dis 1987;136:9–18.
4. Marshall BE, Marshall C, Benumof J, Saidman LJ. Hypoxic pulmonary vasoconstriction in dogs: effects of lung segment size and oxygen tension. J Appl Physiol 1981;51:1543–1551.
5. Harris TR, Bernard GR, Brigham KL, Higgins SB, Rinaldo JE, Borovetz HS, Sibbald WJ, Kariman K, Sprung CL. Lung microvascular transport properties increased by multiple indicator dilution methods in patients with adult respiratory distress syndrome. Am Rev Respir Dis 1990;141:272–280.
6. Dawson CA. Role of pulmonary vasomotion in physiology of the lung. Physiol Rev 1984;64:544–616.
7. Fisher CJ, Wood LDH. Effect of lobar acid injury on pulmonary perfusion and gas exchange in dogs. J Appl Physiol 1980;49:150–156.
8. Downey GP, Gumbay RS, Doherty DE, Henson JE, Henson PM, Worthen GS. Enhancement of pulmonary inflammation by prostaglandin E. Evidence for a vasodilator effect. J Appl Physiol 1988;54:728–741.
9. Lien DC, Worthen GS, Capen RL, Hanson WL, Checkley LL, Henson PM, Wagner WW. Neutrophil kinetics in the pulmonary microcirculation: effects of pressure and flow in the dependent lung. Am Rev Respir Dis 1990;141:953–959.
10. Lien DC, Wagner WW, Capen RL, Haslett C, Hanson WL, Hofmeister SE, Henson PM, Worthen GS. Physiologic neutrophil sequestration in the lung: visual evidence for localization in capillaries. J Appl Physiol 1987;62:1236–1243.
11. Lien DC, Capen RL, Hanson WL, Henson JE, Wagner WW, Henson PM, Worthen GS. The acute inflammatory response in the canine lung: direct observation of neutrophil behavior in response to C5 fragments. Submitted.
12. Lien DC, Henson PM, Capen RL, Henson JE, Wagner WW Jr, Worthen GS. Neutrophil kinetics in the pulmonary microcirculation during acute inflammation. Manuscript submitted for publication.
13. Craddock PR, Hammerschmidt DE, White JG, et al. Complement (C5a)-induced granulocyte aggregation in vitro—a possible mechanism of complement-mediated leukostasis and leukopenia. J Clin Invest 1977;60:261–264.
14. Atherton A, Born GVR. Relationship between velocity of rolling granulocytes and that of blood flow in venules. J Physiol 1973;233:157–165.
15. Guntheroth WG, Luchtel DL, Kawabori I. Pulmonary microcirculation: tubules rather than sheet and post. J Appl Physiol 1982;53:510–515.
16. Worthen GS, Schwab B, Elson EL, Downey GP. Mechanics of stimulated neutrophils: cell stiffening induces retention in capillaries. Science 1989;245:183–185.
17. Downey G, Doherty DE, Schwab B, Elson EL, Henson PM, Worthen GS. Retention of leukocytes in capillaries: role of cell size and deformability. Manuscript submitted for publication.
18. Webster RO, Larsen GL, Mitchell BC, Gains AJ, Henson PM. Absence of inflammatory injury in rabbits challenged intravascularly with complement-derived chemotactic factors. Am Rev Respir Dis 1982;125:335–340.
19. Tonneson MG, Smedley LA, Henson PM. Neutrophil-endothelial cell interactions: modulation of neutrophil adhesiveness induced by complement fragments C5a and C5a des arg and formyl-methionyl-leucyl-phenylalanine in vitro. J Clin Invest 1984;74:1581–1592.
20. Gamble JR, Harlan JM, Klebonoff SJ, Vados MA. Stimulation of the adherence of neutrophils to umbilical vein endothelium by human recombinant tumor necrosis factor. Proc Natl Acad Sci USA 1985;82:8667–8671.
21. Pohlman TH, Stanness KA, Beatty PG, Ochs HD, Harlan JM. An endothelial cell surface factor(s) induced in vitro by lipopolysaccharide, interleukin 1, and tumor necrosis factor increases neutrophil adherence by a CDw18-dependent mechanism. J Immunol 1986;136(12):4548–4553.
22. Bevilacqua MP, Pher JS, Wheeler ME, Cotran RS, Gimbrone MA. Interleukin 1 acts on cultured human vascular endothelium to increase the adhesion of polymorphonuclear leukocytes, monocytes and related leukocyte cell lines. J Clin Invest 1985;76:2003–2011.
23. Hynes RO. Integrins: a family of cell surface receptors. Cell 1987;48:549–554.
24. Staunton DE, Marlin SD, Stratowa C, Duston ML, Springer TA. Primary structure of ICAM-1 demonstrates interaction between members of the immunoglobin and integrin supergene families. Cell 1988;52:925–933.
25. Neuman PJ, Berndt MC, Gorski J, et al. Cloning and relation to adhesion molecules of the immunoglobulin gene superfamily. Science 1990;247:1219–1222.
26. Bevilacqua MP, Stengelin S, Gimbrone MA Jr, Seed B. Endothelial leukocyte adhesion molecule 1: an inducible receptor for neutrophils related to complement regulatory proteins and lectins. Science 1989;243(4895):1160–1165.
27. Larsen E, Celi A, Gilbert GE, Furie BC, Erban JK, Bonfanti R, Wagner DD, Furie B. PADGEM protein: a receptor that mediates the interaction of activated platelets with neutrophils and monocytes. Cell 1989;59(2):305–312.
28. Smith CW, Macklin SD, Rothlein R, Teway C, Anderson DC. Cooperative interaction of LFA-1 and Mac-1 with intercellular adhesion molecule-1 in facilitating adherence and transepithelial migration of human neutrophils in vitro. J Clin Invest 1989;85:2008–2017.
29. Hoover RL, Briggs RT, Karnovsky MJ. The adhesive interaction between polymorphonuclear leukocytes and endothelial cells in vitro. Cell 1978;14:423.
30. Harlan JM, Killen PD, Senecal FM, et al. The role of neutrophil membrane glycoprotein GP-150 in neutrophil adherence to endothelium in vitro. Blood 1985;66(1):167–178.
31. Anderson DC, Schmalsteig FC, Arnaout MA, et al. Abnormalities of polymorphonuclear leukocyte function associated with a heritable deficiency of high molecular weight surface glycoproteins (GP-138): common relationships to diminished cell adherence. J Clin Invest 1984;74:536–551.
32. Vedder NB, Winn RK, Rice CL, Chi EY, Arfors KE, Harlan JM. A monoclonal antibody to the adherence-promoting leukocyte glycoprotein, CD18, reduces organ injury and improves survival from hemorrhagic shock and resuscitation in rabbits. J Clin Invest 1988;81:939–944.
33. Zimmerman GA, Wiseman GA, Hill HR. Human endothelial

cells modulate granulocyte adherence and chemotaxis. *J Immunol* 1985;134(3):1866–1874.

34. Chesterman CN, Ager A, Gordon J. Regulation of prostaglandin production and ectoenzyme activities in cultured aortic endothelial cells. *J Cell Physiol* 1983;116(1):45–50.
35. Grunstein BN, Rosenstein SD, Cramer S, Weissmann G, Hirshhorn R. Adenosine: a physiologic modulator of superoxide anion generation by human neutrophils. Adenosine acts via an A-2 receptor or human neutrophils. *J Immunol* 1985;135:1366–1371.
36. Henson PM, Johnston RB. Tissue injury in inflammation: oxidants, proteinases, and cationic proteins. *J Clin Invest* 1987;79:669–674.
37. Weiss SJ. Tissue destruction by neutrophils. *N Engl J Med* 1989;320(6):365–376.
38. Basford RE, Clark RL, Stiller RA, Kaplan SS, Kuhns DB, Rinaldo JE. Endothelial cells inhibit receptor-mediated superoxide production by human polymorphonuclear leukocytes via a soluble inhibitor. *Am J Respir Cell Mol Biol* 1990;2:235–243.
39. Shaw JO. Leukocytes in chemotactic fragment-induced lung inflammation: vascular emigration and alveolar surface emigration. *Am J Pathol* 1980;101:283–291.
40. Beesley JE, Pearson JD, Hutchings A, Carleton JS, Gordon JL. Granulocyte migration through endothelium in culture. *J Cell Sci* 1979;38:237–248.
41. Smedley LA, Tonneson MG, Worthen GS, Mason RJ, Henson PM. Neutrophil recognition of endothelial cells: preferential adherence and transmigration [Abstract]. *Fed Proc* 1983; 42:386.
42. Marchesi VT. The site of leukocyte emigration during inflammation. *Q J Exp Physiol* 1961;46:115–118.
43. Marchesi VT, Florey HW. Electron microscopic observations on the emigration of leukocytes. *Q J Exp Physiol* 1960;45:343–348.
44. Lipscomb MF, Onofrio JM, Nash J, Pierce AK, Towes GB. A morphologic study of the role of phagocytes in the clearance of *Staphylococcus aureus* from the lung. *J Reticuloedothel Soc* 1983;33:429–442.
45. Webster RO, Zanolari B, Henson PM. Neutrophil chemotaxis in response to surface bound C5a. *Exp Cell Res* 1980;129:55–62.
46. Milks LC, Conyers GP, Cramer EB. The effect of neutrophil migration on epithelial permeability. *J Cell Biol* 1986;103 (6):2729–2738.
47. Haslett C, Jose P, Giclas PC, Williams TJ, Henson PM. Cessation of neutrophil influx in C5a-induced acute experimental arthritis is associated with loss of chemoattractant activity from the joint space. *J Immunol* 1989;142:3510–3517.
48. Berenberg JL, Ward PA. Chemotactic factor inactivator in normal human serum. *J Clin Invest* 1973;52:1200.
49. Meyrick B, Hoffman LH, Brigham KL. Chemotaxis of granulocytes across bovine pulmonary artery intimal explants without endothelial cell injury. *Tissue Cell* 1984;16:1–16.
50. Neidermeyer ME, Meyrick B, Parl FF, Brigham KL. Facilitation of granulocyte migration into bovine pulmonary artery intimal explants by intact viable endothelium. *Am J Pathol* 1984;117:252–261.
51. Sandhaus RA, Henson PM. Elastin degradation is required for directed migration of human neutrophils through an elastin-rich barrier *in vitro. Am Rev Respir Dis* 1986.
52. Russo RG, Liotta LA, Thorgeirsson U, Brundage R, Schittman E. Polymorphonuclear leukocyte migration through human amnion membrane. *J Cell Biol* 1981;91:459–467.
53. Janoff A, Zelig JC. Vascular injury and lysis of basement membrane *in vitro* by neutral protease of human leukocytes. *Science* 1968;161:702–706.
54. Smedley LA, Tonneson MG, Sandhaus RA, et al. Neutrophil-mediated injury to endothelial cells: enhancement by LPS and essential role of neutrophil elastase. *J Clin Invest* 1986; 17:1233–1243.
55. Harlan JM, Killen PD, Harker LA, et al. Neutrophil-mediated endothelial injury *in vitro*. Mechanisms of cell detachment. *J Clin Invest* 1981;68:1394–1403.
56. Campbell EJ, Campbell MA. Pericellular proteolysis by neu-

trophils in the presence of proteinase inhibitors: effects of substrate opsonization. *J Cell Biol* 1988;106:667–676.
57. Milks LC, Brontoli MJ, Cramer EB. Epithelial permeability and the transepithelial migration of human neutrophils. *J Cell Biol* 1983;96:1241–1247.
58. Parsons PE, Sugahara K, Cott GK, Mason RJ, Henson PM. The effect of neutrophil migration and prolonged neutrophil contact on epithelial permeability. *Am J Pathol* 1987; 129(2):302–312.
59. Staub NC, Schultz EL, Koike K, Albertine KH. Effect of neutrophil migration induced by leukotriene B4 on protein permeability in sheep lung. *Fed Proc* 1985;44:30–35.
60. Sugahara K, Cott GR, Parsons PE, Mason RJ, Sandhaus RA, Henson PM. Epithelial permeability produced by phagocytosing neutrophils *in vitro. Am Rev Respir Dis* 1986;133:875–881.
61. Henson PM, Henson JE, Fittschen C, Kimani G, Bratton DL, Riches DWH. Phagocytic cells: degranulation and secretion. In: Gallin JI, Goldstein IM, Snyderman R, eds. *Inflammation: basic principles and clinical correlates.* New York: Raven Press, 1989;363–390.
62. Beutler B, Cerami A. Cachectin: more than a tumor necrosis factor. *N Engl J Med* 1987;316:379–385.
63. Henson PM. Mechanisms of exocytosis in phagocytic inflammatory cells. *Am J Pathol* 1980;101:494–511.
64. Gallin JI. Neutrophil specific granules: a fuse that ignites the inflammatory response. *Clin Res* 1984;32:320–328.
65. Lew PD, Monod A, Waldvogel FA, Dewald B, Baggiolini M. Quantitative analysis of the cytosolic free calcium dependency of exocytosis from three subcellular compartments in intact human neutrophils. *J Cell Biol* 1986;102:2197–2204.
66. Wright DG, Gallin JI. Secretory responses of human neutrophils: exocytosis of specific (secretory) granules by human neutrophils during adherence *in vitro* and during exudation *in vivo. J Immunol* 1979;123:284–294.
67. Bainton DF. Sequential degranulation of the two types of polymorphonuclear leukocyte granules during phagocytosis of microorganisms. *J Cell Biol* 1973;58:249–264.
68. Henson PM. The immunologic release of constituents from neutrophil leukocytes. II. Mechanisms of release during phagocytosis and adherence to nonphagocytosable surfaces. *J Immunol* 1971;107:1547–1557.
69. Lynch RE, Fridovich I. Permeation of the erythrocyte stroma by superoxide radical. *J Biol Chem* 1978;253:4697–4699.
70. Gunthrie LA, McPhail LC, Henson PM, Johnston RB Jr. The priming of neutrophils for enhanced release of superoxide anion and hydrogen peroxide by bacterial lipopolysaccharide: evidence for increased activity of the superoxide-producing enzyme. *J Exp Med* 1984;160:1656–1671.
71. Shalit M, Dabiri GA, Southwick FS. Platelet activating factor both stimulates and "primes" human polymorphonuclear leukocyte actin filament assembly. *Blood* 1987;70:1921–1927.
72. Berkow RL, Wang D, Larrick JW, Dodson RW, Howard TH. Enhancement of neutrophil superoxide production by pre-incubation with recombinant human tumor necrosis factor. *J Immunol* 1987;139:3783–3791.
73. DiPersio JF, Billing P, Williams R, Gasson JC. Human granulocyte–macrophage colony stimulating factor and other cytokines prime human neutrophils for enhanced arachidonic acid release and leukotriene B4 synthesis. *J Immunol* 1988;140: 4315–4322.
74. Kharazmi A, Nielsen H, Bendtzen K. Recombinant interleukin-1 alpha and beta prime human monocyte superoxide production but have no effect on chemotaxis and oxidative burst response of neutrophils. *Immunobiology* 1988;177:32–39.
75. Haslett C, Gunthrie LA, Kopaniak MM, Johnston RB, Henson PM. Modulation of multiple neutrophil functions by preparative methods and trace amounts of bacterial lipopolysaccharide. *Am J Pathol* 1985;119:101–110.
76. Forehand JR, Pabst MJ, Phillips WA, Johnston RB. Lipopolysaccharide priming of human neutrophils for an enhanced respiratory burst. Role of intracellular free calcium. *J Clin Invest* 1989;83:74–83.
77. Dewald B, Thelen M, Baggiolini M. Two transduction se-

quences are necessary for neutrophil activation receptor agonists. *J Biol Chem* 1988;263:16179–16184.

78. Henson PM, Webster RO, Henson JE. Neutrophil and monocyte activation and secretion: role of surfaces in inflammatory reactions and *in vitro*. In: Dingle JC, Gordon JL, eds. *Cellular interactions*. Elsevier/North-Holland Biomedical Press, 1981;43–56.

79. Nathan CF. Neutrophil activation on biologic surfaces. Massive secretion of hydrogen peroxide in response to products of machrophages and lymphocytes. *J Clin Invest* 1987;80:1550–1560.

80. Strunk RC, Kunke KS, Musson RA. Lack of requirement for spreading for macrophages to synthesize complement. *J Reticuloendothel Soc* 1980;28:483–493.

81. Haskill S, Johnson C, Eierman D, Becker S, Warren K. Adherence induces selective in RNA expression of monocyte mediators and proto-oncogenes. *J Immunol* 1988;140:1690–1694.

82. Henson PM. The immunologic release of constituents from neutrophil leukocytes: II. Mechanisms of release during phagocytosis and adherence to non-phagocytosable surfaces. *J Immunol* 1971;107:1547–1557.

83. Nathan CF. Secretory products of macrophages. *J Clin Invest* 1987;79:319–326.

84. Zimmerman GA, Renzetti AD, Hill HR. Functional and metabolic activity of granulocytes from patients with adult respiratory distress syndrome. *Am Rev Respir Dis* 1983;127:290–300.

85. Nahum A, Hegarty M, Wood CDH, Chamberlain WJ, Sznaider JI. Activated neutrophils are sequestered in the lungs of patients with sepsis [Abstract]. *Am Rev Respir Dis* 1989;139(4):299.

86. Weinberg PF, Matthay MA, Webster RO, Roskos KV, Goldstein IM, Murray IF. Biologically active products of complement and acute lung injury in patients with the sepsis syndrome. *Am Rev Respir Dis* 1984;130:791–796.

87. Duchateau J, Haas M, Schreyen HS, Radoux L, Sprongers I, Noel FY, Braun M, Lamy M. Complement activation in patients at risk of developing the adult respiratory distress syndrome. *Am Rev Respir Dis* 1984;130:1058–1064.

88. Parsons PE, Giclas PC. The terminal complement complex (S C5b-9) is not specifically associated with the development of the adult respiratory distress syndrome (ARDS). *Am Respir Dis* 1990;141:98–103.

89. deGroote MA, Martin MA, Densen P, Pfaller MA, Wenzel RP. Plasma tumor necrosis factor levels on patients with presumed sepsis. *JAMA* 1989;262(2):249–251.

90. Marks JD, Marks CB, Montgomery AB, Turner J, Metz CA, Murray JF. Presence of tumor necrosis factor in patients with septic shock who develop the adult respiratory distress syndrome (abstract). *Am Rev Respir Dis* 1990;141:94–97.

91. Parsons PE, Worthen GS, Moore EE, Tate RM, Henson PM. The association of circulating endotoxin with the development of the adult respiratory distress syndrome. *Am Rev Respir Dis* 1989;140:294–301.

92. Bachoten M, Weibel ER. Structural alterations of lung parenchyma in the adult respiratory distress syndrome. *Clin Chest Med* 1982;3:35–56.

93. Bachofen M, Weibel ER. Alterations of the gas exchange apparatus in adult respiratory insufficiency associated with septicemia. *Am Rev Respir Dis* 1977;116:589–615.

94. Parsons PE, Fowler AA, Hyers TM, Henson PM. Chemotactic activity in bronchoalveolar lavage fluid from patients with ARDS. *Am Rev Respir Dis* 1985;132:490–494.

95. Fowler AA, Hyerts TM, Fisher BJ, Bechard DE, Centor RM, Webster RO. The adult respiratory distress syndrome: cell populations and soluble mediators in the airspaces of patients at high risk. *Am Rev Respir Dis* 1987;136:1225–1231.

96. Anderson DC, Schmalsteig FC, Finegold MJ, Hughes BJ, Rothlein R, Miller LJ, Kohl S, Tosi MF, Jacobs RL, Waldrop TC, Goldman AS, Shearer WT, Springer TA. The severe and moderate phenotypes of heritable Mac-1, LFA-1 deficiency, their quantitative definition and relation to leukocyte dysfunction and clinical features. *J Infect Dis* 1985;152(4):668–689.

97. Anderson DC, Springer TA. Leukocyte adhesion deficiency: an inherited defect in the Mac-1, LFA-1, and p150,95 glycoproteins. *Annu Rev Med* 1987;38:175–194.

98. Gosset P, Tonnel AB, Joseph M, Prin L, Mallart A, Cheron T, Capran A. Secretion of a chemotactic factor for neutrophils and eosinophils by alveolar macrophages from asthmatic patients. *J Allergy Clin Immunol* 1984;74:827–834.

99. Hunninghake GW, Gadek JD, Lawley TJ, Crystal RG. The mechanisms of neutrophil accumulation in the lungs of patients with idiopathic pulmonary fibrosis. *J Clin Invest* 1981;68:259–269.

100. Hunninghake GW. Release of interleukin-1 by alveolar macrophages of patients with active pulmonary sarcoidosis. *Am Rev Respir Dis* 1984;129:569–572.

101. Kleinhenz ME, Fujiworn H, Rich EA. Interleukin-1 production by blood monocytes and bronchoalveolar cells in sarcoidosis. *Ann NY Acad Sci* 1986;465:91–97.

102. Shaw JD, Henson PM, Henson J, Webster RO. Lung inflammation induced by complement-derived chemotactic factors in the alveolus. *Lab Invest* 1980;42:547–558.

103. Wenzel SE, Westcott JW, Smith HR, Larsen GL. Spectrum of prostanoid release after bronchoalveolar allergen challenge in atopic asthmatics and in control groups. *Am Rev Respir Dis* 1989;139:450–457.

THE LUNG: Scientific Foundations
edited by R.G. Crystal, J.B. West et al.
Raven Press, Ltd., New York © 1991.

CHAPTER 7.7.2

Injury from Drugs

W. J. Martin II

Drug-induced lung disease is an increasingly frequent problem in clinical pulmonary medicine as more and newer therapies are being used in the treatment of human disease (1–3). The lung appears to be uniquely susceptible to injury by various drugs or toxins, and some of these adverse reactions are predictable side effects of these agents. However, in most cases, adverse drug reactions to the lung are relatively rare and often occur as a surprise to the clinician. Hence, many drug-induced lung disorders are frequently documented in the literature as isolated case reports. The relatively low incidence of lung toxicity (i.e., virtually always less than 5% for a given drug) makes modeling of drug-induced lung disease in the laboratory a difficult challenge for the investigator. Efforts to determine the mechanisms of drug toxicity using *in vitro* cellular systems or *in vivo* animal models are often frustrated by the inability to accurately model the disease as it likely occurs in human subjects. Nonetheless, our understanding of the mechanism of certain types of drug-induced lung disease has greatly improved over the past decade and will likely permit improved diagnostic and therapeutic approaches to be developed for patients who develop this iatrogenic lung disorder.

Approximately 80–100 different drugs have been associated with significant pulmonary toxicity (1–3). These drugs are frequently from pharmacologic groups such as cancer therapeutic agents, antibiotics, anti-inflammatory agents, narcotics, and cardiac medications (Table 1). Certainly, the most frequent and serious pulmonary toxicities result from the use of cancer chemotherapy and radiation therapy. These toxicities are often related to the direct cytotoxic effect of the drug

on certain cell populations in the lung. In contrast, many drugs are thought to cause lung toxicity by indirect effects often mediated by an immune response of the individual to the drug or its metabolite. Thus, drugs may injure the lung either by their direct cytotoxic effects or by eliciting an immune or inflammatory response to the lung, or possibly by both mechanisms (Table 2).

Certain populations of lung cells appear to be uniquely susceptible to injury by specific drugs or toxins. For example, the pulmonary capillary endothelium may be preferentially injured (compared to other lung cell types) by agents such as oxygen, radiation, or bleomycin (4–8); in contrast, alveolar lining epithelial cells such as type I and type II cells may be selectively injured by toxic agents such as the herbicide paraquat (9,10). Understanding the unique susceptibility of these lung cell types to drug-mediated injury may improve our insight into the specific mechanisms of toxicity. Obviously, critical injury to either side of the alveolar–capillary barrier may impair gas exchange, induce alveolar flooding, and cause alveolar collapse. If widespread injury ensues, the initial site of toxicity becomes obscured as diffuse alveolar damage develops and reparative processes are activated. The degree of initial lung injury is likely the predominant factor in predicting whether the toxic lung damage is reversible or fixed.

Repair mechanisms often can restore the normal architecture of the alveolar–capillary unit if the alveolus has an intact basement membrane. For example, if the alveolar basement membrane is destroyed during the initial phase of a drug-induced toxic reaction, it is impossible for viable lung cells to migrate to the site of injury and repopulate the damaged area (11). Fibroblasts and other mesenchymal cells recognize such extensive damage to the alveolus and initiate the process of wound repair, which unfortunately further deranges the alveolar–capillary unit and prevents any chance for restoration of normal gas-exchange function.

W. J. Martin II: Division of Pulmonary and Critical Care Medicine, Indiana University School of Medicine, Indianapolis, Indiana 46202.

TABLE 1. *Classification of drugs associated with lung toxicity*

Drug classification	Examples
Cancer therapy	Bleomycin, mitomycin C, radiation
Antibiotics	Nitrofurantoin, sulfa drugs
Anti-inflammatory agents	Aspirin, NSAIs[a]
Cardiac medications	Amiodarone, procaineamide, tocainide
Narcotics	Heroin, morphine, propoxyphene
Miscellaneous	Oxygen, tocolytics

[a] Non-steroidal anti-inflammatory agents

Similarly, widespread damage to the cellular constituents of the alveolar–capillary unit may preclude effective recovery, even with intact basement membranes. Paraquat is an example of this mechanism, since it is selectively concentrated by both type I and type II alveolar epithelial cells and induces injury of both cell types (9). Because the type I cell occupies approximately 90% of the alveolar surface and cannot replicate, paraquat-mediated damage to the type I cell is associated with significant alveolar injury. Additionally, since the type I cell is derived from the type II cell, injury of the type II cell by paraquat effectively prevents repopulation of the injured alveolar epithelial surface. Furthermore, injury to the type II cell induces a loss of surfactant production and, together with the loss of the alveolar lining cell population, causes alveolar collapse to develop. In most every case, significant paraquat toxicity results in respiratory failure and death of the patient. Thus, irreversible alveolar damage may occur if either important cell populations are irreversibly damaged or the underlying matrix of the alveolar unit is destroyed.

The timing of lung injury from toxic drugs or agents may be immediate or delayed. Radiation injury to the lung may occur within days or weeks if the dose is very high; however, radiation pneumonitis more typically occurs several months after the exposure (12). This delay in the clinical onset of lung injury suggests that radiation induces a loss of a critical cell function which only becomes apparent during cell replication several months later. The subcellular site of injury most frequently implicated in this delayed appearance of pneumonitis is nuclear DNA (12). It is presumed that the normal function of DNA in nonproliferating cells is maintained following exposure to injurious doses of radiation or cytotoxic drugs. With onset of mitosis, however, injury to the cell machinery becomes apparent and the cellular constituents of the alveolar–capillary unit can no longer maintain their normal barrier function necessary for effective gas exchange. It is likely (although not proven) that this scenario of drug injury is common to many different toxic lung reactions. The delay in appearance of injury not only results in mistaken diagnoses by clinicians, but also complicates the investigative approach to determining the mechanisms of early injury for many of these drugs.

The key to an improved understanding of drug-induced lung disease is to focus on the initial phase of injury to the alveolar capillary unit. In concept, detection and treatment of lung cell toxicity at the earliest phase of injury will result in the best opportunity to reverse the insult before widespread injury occurs and repair processes have been activated. Rather than simply listing the many drugs associated with lung injury, the remaining portion of this chapter will focus on what is known regarding the mechanism of certain types of drug-induced lung disease as examples of specific patterns of injury.

EXAMPLES OF DIRECT TOXIC INJURY

As noted, drugs may injure the lung parenchyma by either (a) direct toxic effects, (b) indirect effects mediated by inflammatory or immune-effector cells, or (c) both mechanisms. The best-studied drugs that cause lung injury by direct toxic effects are nitrofurantoin and bleomycin. Both drugs are thought to mediate toxicity by generating toxic O_2-derived species within lung cells, thereby overwhelming antioxidant defense mechanisms and eventually causing cell death (Table 3).

Nitrofurantoin

Nitrofurantoin, a urinary antiseptic, is associated with serious and sometimes fatal lung reactions (13–17). Of all the drugs that can adversely affect the lung, nitrofurantoin continues to be one of the drugs most commonly reported to induce serious lung damage (16,17). Although hypersensitivity reactions can occur, nitrofurantoin lung toxicity more typically presents as an insidious, progressive pulmonary fibrosis. Until re-

TABLE 2. *Examples of drugs that injure the lung by direct or indirect mechanisms*

Direct toxic effect	Indirect toxic effect
Bleomycin	Methotrexate
Mitomycin C	Gold
Radiation	Nitrofurantoin
Nitrofurantoin	Amiodarone
Aspirin	
Oxygen	
Amiodarone	

TABLE 3. *Balance of oxidant production and antioxidant defenses in lung cells*

Examples of oxidants generated	Method of removal by endogenous antioxidants
Single electron (e^-) transfers:	

^{a} Symbols: $O_2^{-\cdot}$, superoxide; H_2O_2, hydrogen peroxide; $\cdot OH$, hydroxyl radical; Fe^{2+}, iron.

cently, the mechanism of injury by nitrofurantoin was poorly understood.

Recent studies indicate that nitrofurantoin can undergo cyclic reduction–oxidation in a fashion similar to that of the herbicide paraquat (18–21). Under anaerobic conditions, nitrofurantoin forms an anion-free radical as detected by electron spin resonance (19); under aerobic conditions, however, it becomes reoxidized, liberating a free electron and generating toxic O_2-derived species such as superoxide, hydrogen peroxide, and hydroxyl radical (20,21). The cell employs several types of defense mechanisms to scavenge such radicals; but under conditions of oxidant stress, these mechanisms become overwhelmed, leading to a cascade of oxidant generation which eventuates in the production of the hydroxyl radical, a toxic species for which there is no adequate antioxidant protection for the cell (Table 3).

Nitrofurantoin directly injures lung tissue, specifically pulmonary endothelial cells, by generating toxic O_2 radicals within the cells (22,23). Furthermore, addition of high concentrations of O_2 accelerates nitrofurantoin toxicity in both *in vitro* and *in vivo* experiments (22–24). It has been demonstrated that cells which are genetically deficient in certain antioxidant defenses such as catalase or glutathione are unusually susceptible to injury by nitrofurantoin (25,26). Furthermore, animals depleted of selenium or α-tocopherol are also at greatly increased risk for nitrofurantoin toxicity (24,27). The ability of lung cells to withstand this injury is largely related to both the ambient O_2 concentration of the cell and the adequacy of the cell's antioxidant defenses.

Bleomycin

Bleomycin, a cancer chemotherapeutic agent derived from *Streptomyces verticillus*, represents a mixture of glycopeptides and is associated with significant pulmonary toxicity (1–3,28,29). Bleomycin is known to kill neoplastic cells by inducing DNA strand scission and interfering with DNA synthesis (30,31). Furthermore, data suggest that these effects are mediated by O_2 radicals (30–35). These O_2-derived species may result from bleomycin's property of chelating multivalent metals such as iron (30–35). Iron easily facilitates single-electron transfers to other molecules, donating and accepting electrons as it undergoes cyclic oxidation and reduction (36). The metal–drug complex likely initiates single-electron transfers within the cell and, as described for nitrofurantoin, transfers these electrons to electrophilic molecules such as O_2.

Both *in vivo* and *in vitro* studies support the hypothesis that bleomycin pulmonary toxicity is mediated, at least in part, by a bleomycin–iron complex generating toxic O_2-derived species within the lung. First, high O_2 concentrations increase the risk of bleomycin pulmonary toxicity (37–39), whereas low O_2 concentrations significantly reduce the risk of toxicity (40). Second, depletion of iron by either dietary means or use of deferoxamine, an iron chelator, has decreased the risk of bleomycin pulmonary toxicity in animals (41,42). Third, pulmonary endothelial cells, which demonstrate the earliest pathologic evidence for pulmonary toxicity by bleomycin *in vivo* (7,8), are injured *in vitro* by bleomycin by an iron-dependent process which is exacerbated by supplemental hyperoxia and which is prevented by removal of iron by deferoxamine (43). Thus, it is likely that both the therapeutic cytotoxic effect of bleomycin against cancer cells and the adverse reaction to normal lung cells are mediated, in part, by toxic O_2-derived species generated by the metal–drug complex.

Lung as a Site of Injury for Direct Drug Toxicity

Both nitrofurantoin and bleomycin share the ability to generate O_2 radicals (albeit by different mechanisms) and to cause lung damage in human subjects. Reasons for the lung being the predominant site of toxicity for these two drugs remain speculative, but one possibility relates to the role of the lung as a site of gas exchange. Lung parenchymal cells are exposed to higher concentrations of O_2 than are any other cell population in the body. It is hypothesized that the high ambient concentration of O_2 in the lung is the primary determinant in the site of injury. In support of this hypothesis is the observation that O_2 therapy in either drug-treated animals or human subjects greatly increases the risk of lung toxicity by either nitrofurantoin or bleomycin (21,24,37–39).

Additionally, oxidant-generating drugs or toxins may cause lung damage because they are preferentially concentrated within lung tissue. For example, there is evidence to indicate that the concentrations of both paraquat and bleomycin are higher in the lung than in other organ systems (9,44). Furthermore, the activity of bleomycin hydrolase, an enzyme responsible for inactivating bleomycin, is apparently deficient in certain types of lung cells and may account for the unique susceptibility of the lung to damage by this drug (45).

DRUGS ASSOCIATED WITH INDIRECT (INFLAMMATORY- OR IMMUNE-MEDIATED) TOXICITY

Many drugs that cause lung toxicity are often associated with an ''allergic'' reaction manifest as fever, chills, dyspnea, and pulmonary infiltrates with a marked peripheral eosinophilia. Oftentimes these reactions are acute, occurring within 1 or 2 days of receiving the drug and quickly dissipate with drug withdrawal. The mechanisms underlying these apparent ''allergic'' reactions are poorly understood and yet represent a sizable fraction of adverse pulmonary reactions associated with drug use.

More recently, certain drugs have also been associated with ''hypersensitivity'' reactions in the lung (1–3,46–50), similar to findings reported with hypersensitivity pneumonitis to organic antigens (51–53). Drugs such as amiodarone, nitrofurantoin, and gold have each been reported to be associated with increased numbers of inflammatory cells (neutrophils or eosinophils) and immune effector cells (typically CD8+ suppressor/cytotoxic T-lymphocytes) in the lung (46–50). Similar cell profiles have been described in the bronchoalveolar lavage (BAL) fluid from patients with farmer's lung disease and pigeon breeder's disease, which are two classic examples of hypersensitivity pneumonitis (51–53). The similarity of the cellular and pathologic profiles suggests that common mechanisms may exist to account for the clinical findings in hypersensitivity pneumonitis.

Amiodarone

Of the drugs reported to cause this abnormal immune response in the lung, the adverse pulmonary reaction associated with amiodarone therapy is the best studied. Amiodarone is a potent antidysrhythmic agent that is associated with a high incidence of serious and potentially fatal toxic lung reactions (50,54–57). Amiodarone is an example of a drug associated with both direct and indirect mechanisms of lung toxicity. The

direct mechanism of toxicity by amiodarone is beyond the scope of this chapter, but it is reviewed extensively elsewhere (57,58).

The first study which indicated that amiodarone may be associated with an abnormal inflammatory or immune response in the lung was provided by Venet et al. (48). These investigators reported that five patients with amiodarone pulmonary toxicity had a marked increase in both polymorphonuclear leukocytes (PMNs) and lymphocytes in BAL fluid (48). Of interest, the increase in BAL lymphocytes in amiodarone pulmonary toxicity represented predominantly an increase in CD8+ suppressor/cytotoxic T-lymphocytes. Similar findings in human subjects with amiodarone pulmonary toxicity have been reported by others (49,50, 57,59). The precise role of these lymphocytes in the pathogenesis of amiodarone pulmonary toxicity is unknown, but preliminary data exist which suggest that the lymphocytes are sensitized to the drug and are actively involved in an immune response (49).

Mechanism of Inflammatory Cell Recruitment

How drugs induce an increase in neutrophils or lymphocytes in the lungs is less clear; however, several mechanisms are possible. Many inflammatory disorders of the lung are thought to occur as a result of an initial deposition of immune complexes or complement within the alveolar–capillary unit. Consistent with this concept, C3 deposition has been identified in lung tissue from patients with amiodarone pulmonary toxicity (60,61). However, other investigators have failed to find evidence of complement deposition in amiodarone toxicity (54,62,63); thus, this mechanism remains poorly supported by current evidence. Furthermore, immunoglobulin deposition in the lungs of these individuals has not been clearly demonstrated to be present by immunofluorescence. However, immunoglobulin levels, specifically IgM, are markedly increased in BAL fluids from patients with amiodarone pulmonary toxicity when compared to those from normal control subjects (64). Patients receiving amiodarone, but without evidence of toxicity, also have elevated immunoglobulin levels, but they are well below those reported for patients with amiodarone pulmonary toxicity (64). The relevance of this possible marker of B-cell activation to amiodarone pulmonary toxicity remains unclear.

The most likely mechanism to account for the increase in PMNs or lymphocytes in drug-induced lung disease is the release of specific chemotactic factors from cells such as alveolar macrophages. The presence of chemotactic factors in lung tissue establishes a chemical gradient to the blood along which inflammatory cells will migrate to the source of the chemotaxins. For example, the inflammatory cell response in bleomycin pulmonary toxicity (65–67) is associated with release of chemotactic factors from alveolar macrophages for both neutrophils and lymphocytes (68). More recently, alveolar macrophages in bleomycin toxicity have been demonstrated to release interleukin 1, a well-characterized activator and chemoattractant for lymphocytes (69). Similarly, the inflammatory response in oxygen toxicity and paraquat toxicity is associated with the activation of alveolar macrophages and the release of chemotactic factors for inflammatory cells (70,71). It is probable that the alveolar macrophage is central to the control of any inflammatory or immune reaction in the lung, and significant drug-induced inflammatory responses must certainly be mediated, at least in part, by this powerful inflammatory cell.

Role of Inflammatory Cells in Disease Process

Unfortunately, there is no obvious reason or mechanism to explain how drugs such as amiodarone cause lung damage by an inflammatory or immune response in the lung. Neutrophils are often suspected as mediators of lung tissue damage in both acute and chronic inflammatory lung disorders (70–72). Activated neutrophils release toxic O_2 radicals (in response to proinflammatory signals) that may injure normal lung parenchymal cells ("innocent bystanders") in the inflammatory reaction (73,74). The role of neutrophils in drug-induced lung disease is less well established; in fact, recent studies suggest that neutrophil depletion may exacerbate bleomycin pulmonary toxicity (75,76). The influx of neutrophils into the lung is characteristically the first population of cells recruited in a hypersensitivity response to an antigenic stimulus. Thus, although their exact role remains unclear, neutrophils may serve as an early marker of an adverse drug reaction.

As previously noted, similar cell profiles of a CD8+ T-cell lymphocytosis in BAL fluid have been described in other classic hypersensitivity reactions such as farmer's lung or pigeon breeder's disease (51–53). Semenzato et al. (53) have reported that in patients with organic antigen-mediated hypersensitivity pneumonitis, the lung CD8+ lymphocyte displays significant cytotoxic and suppressor function in vitro; in contrast, CD8+ lymphocytes from asymptomatic control subjects with similar organic antigen exposure had markedly less cytotoxic and suppressor function. It is possible that CD8+ T-lymphocytes in hypersensitivity reactions have the potential to suppress the initial inflammatory response in the disorder. In possible support of this hypothesis, pulmonary fibrosis is relatively rare in hypersensitivity pneumonitis, unlike many other chronic inflammatory disorders where fibrosis is common and CD8+ lymphocytes are not present (72).

Clearly, drugs such as amiodarone, gold, or nitrofurantoin can be associated with hypersensitivity "reactions" in the lung of some patients who develop pulmonary toxicity (46–50,57–59). The pathogenesis of this reaction remains obscure for drugs, and it is equally obscure for the reaction associated with the inhalation of organic antigens. It is likely that common features exist in the pathogenic scheme for both types of reactions, and it is probable that insight into one condition will shed light on events in the other.

Lung as a Site of Injury in Indirect Toxicity

A major distinction between classic hypersensitivity pneumonitis and drug-induced hypersensitivity pneumonitis is that the former is associated with inhalation of organic antigens, whereas drugs arrive at the lung by a blood-borne pathway. It is reasonable to assume that inhaled organic antigens might elicit an immune response in the lower respiratory tract, but it is not clear as to why the lungs are targeted by drugs that are either absorbed from the gastrointestinal tract or ingested parenterally.

In part, the site of injury from drug-induced hypersensitivity reaction may relate to the concentration of the drug in the specific organ system. For example, amiodarone and its primary derivative, desethylamiodarone, are both concentrated in lung tissue and lung cells severalfold (possibly a hundredfold) above serum levels (77–79). In fact, the concentrations of amiodarone and desethylamiodarone in the lung are second only to fat tissue as a site of highest deposition of the drug. Thus, one explanation for the higher incidence of hypersensitivity reaction due to a drug may relate to its relatively high concentration in lung tissue. Unfortunately, such simple reasoning does not likely account for many of the reported drug reactions associated with inflammatory or immune-mediated responses.

INDIVIDUAL SUSCEPTIBILITY TO DRUG-INDUCED LUNG REACTION

A major area of interest for current investigation is to determine why some individuals develop pulmonary toxicity from drugs and others do not. Such differences in susceptibility to drug toxicity likely relate to (a) the diverse genetic background of individuals receiving the drug, (b) large numbers of unknown risk factors that modulate clinical expression of the drug toxicity (and, hence, modulate its diagnosis), (c) interaction of other clinical disorders such as infection or heart failure in the development of the toxicity, and (d) the probability that some drugs cause lung disease by a true hypersensitivity reaction to the drug or metabolites and thus relate to the unique immunologic response of that individual.

There are some factors that are known to affect the risk of drug-induced pulmonary disease for an individual. For example, both age and total dose of a drug often correlate with higher risks of toxicity for most drugs (1–3). Similarly, if an individual already has significant underlying lung disease, the risk of toxicity is increased (1–3). It is also known that if more than one drug or agent is used and the mechanisms of action are similar, individuals may be at significantly higher risk for a toxic reaction. This is commonly observed clinically with concomitant use of bleomycin, radiation, or O_2 therapy, all of which will increase the total oxidant stress and potentially induce a synergistic insult to the lung. *In vitro* studies support this hypothesis, indicating that higher ambient O_2 concentrations increase the risk of both bleomycin and radiation injury to lung cells (43,80).

There are many factors that may differ between individuals; this accounts for altered risk of drug toxicity. For example, Rossi and co-workers (81) suggested that mouse strain variability to bleomycin toxicity was genetically determined. However, it is not clear as to what genetically determined factors are associated with drug susceptibility or resistance. Levels of antioxidants within lung tissues or lung cells may be an important determinant for resistance to drug-induced oxidant damage. The risk of nitrofurantoin toxicity is increased markedly if endogenous cellular levels of antioxidants such as glutathione or catalase are low as a result of genetic deficiency (25,26). Our ability to screen individuals for various genetic antioxidant deficiencies within the lung is limited; however, such an approach in concept would permit determination of which individuals may be at higher risk for certain proposed therapies.

The mechanism of bleomycin-induced pulmonary fibrosis has been well studied, and the biologic effect of bleomycin appears to be related, in part, to the cellular levels of bleomycin hydrolase, an enzyme that inactivates the drug (45,82–88). Tumor sensitivity to bleomycin appears to be markedly increased if endogenous levels of the enzyme are low, whereas tumor resistance occurs when bleomycin hydrolase levels are high (85,86). The precise role of bleomycin hydrolase in the protection of lung cells from bleomycin toxicity is not known; however, it is of interest that lung cells have low levels of bleomycin hydrolase (45) and that lung injury by bleomycin is associated with the loss of bleomycin hydrolase activity (84).

Unfortunately, for the vast majority of drugs associated with pulmonary toxicity, the normal metabolism of the drug within the lung is unknown. The pathways that enhance or diminish the toxic effects of the drug within the lung are poorly understood; thus, we have little available information to suggest why some individuals exhibit severe toxicity whereas others are apparently unaffected by the drug. An improved understanding of certain common pathways such as the oxidant–antioxidant scheme may provide some insight into drug susceptibility and may suggest practical methods to screen individuals at high risk for certain therapies.

FUTURE THERAPIES

Currently, the best therapeutic approach to drug-induced lung disease is prompt recognition of the entity and withdrawal of the offending drug. The use of corticosteroids by clinicians for severe cases of toxicity remains the norm, although there are no studies that indicate the value of this regimen in reducing the toxicity of the drug.

It is likely that as our understanding of specific types of drug-induced lung disease improves, newer forms of therapy will be proposed to reduce the initial insult to the lung. Of course, the difficulty with this approach is that widespread lung injury may have occurred weeks or months prior to the clinical recognition of the adverse reaction, thus precluding an effective therapeutic intervention.

Augmentation of Endogenous Antioxidants

Drugs or agents that mediate lung injury by generating oxidants (such as O_2, nitrofurantoin, bleomycin, paraquat, and radiation) share common molecular mechanisms of tissue injury. The ability to abrogate this injury is often dependent on the successful restoration of the oxidant–antioxidant balance in the lung. Although this has not yet been accomplished in human subjects, a number of novel approaches in animal models suggest the future feasibility of such studies.

It was recognized by Frank et al. (89,90) that a small dose of endotoxin provided significant protection from oxidant injury. Similarly, sublethal exposure to hyperoxia prior to exposure to 100% O_2 also protects animals from injury (91,92). The common mechanism thought to account for this protection is that both sublethal hyperoxia and endotoxin stimulate an induction of antioxidant enzymes (such as superoxide dismutase and catalase) within the lung to levels much higher than pretreatment levels (89,90,92). Pretreatment of animals with sublethal hyperoxia or endotoxin significantly augments antioxidant defenses and potentially offers protection from damage by oxidant-generating drugs.

However, the mechanism of protection by these pretreatment regimens is not entirely clear. Endotoxin is also known to stimulate the release of two important cytokines, tumor necrosis factor (TNF) and interleukin 1 (IL-1). To test the hypothesis that these cytokines mediate the protection from oxidant injury, White et al. (93) used parenterally administered recombinant TNF and IL-1 in rats and demonstrated that these cytokines reproduced the protection afforded by endotoxin pretreatment. However, TNF and IL-1 in this study did not alter the antioxidant enzyme levels, suggesting that these cytokines mediate protection by some other yet unknown mechanism (93). Whatever the mechanism, it is clear that a variety of novel approaches may be available in future years which can be tested in human subjects to "boost" endogenous antioxidant defense mechanisms prior to initiation of therapy that has a high risk of oxidant-mediated lung damage.

Use of Exogenous Antioxidants

Typically, administration of exogenous antioxidants by conventional means will not reduce oxidant-mediated injury (21,24). This may occur because of several reasons: (a) A threshold may exist for certain antioxidants (e.g., α-tocopherol, ascorbic acid) beyond which the body decreases absorption or increases clearance of the antioxidants; (b) a short half-life exists for the antioxidants (e.g., as short as 4 min for superoxide dismutase); and (c) the antioxidants may not have adequate access to the site of tissue injury (alveolar–capillary unit) or to the site of subcellular injury (plasma or organelle membranes, nuclear DNA, or cytoplasmic sulfhydryl proteins). The pharmacologic challenge is to administer very high concentrations of antioxidants to the site of injury in the lung, with the hope that local deposition of high concentrations of antioxidants will permit diffusion to the site of oxidant injury.

Several groups of investigators have addressed this challenge in a remarkably similar fashion using liposome-encapsulated antioxidants administered either by aerosolization (94) or intravenously (95,96). These studies indicate that lung toxicity from either hyperoxia (94,95) or oxidant-generating neutrophils (96) can be significantly reduced by liposome-encapsulated antioxidants. The future potential for such a therapy in human subjects with drug-induced oxidant injury is highly intriguing and may represent a novel approach to the treatment of these disorders.

Genetic Manipulation of Drug-Induced Adverse Reactions

As our understanding of specific pathways for drug metabolism improves, the potential for genetic manipulation of this process within target organs such as the lung is greatly enhanced. For example, bleomycin toxicity occurs preferentially in the lung because of low endogenous levels of bleomycin hydrolase, the enzyme responsible for detoxifying the drug (45,84). Lazo and co-workers (88) have successfully completed molecular cloning and sequencing of rabbit lung bleomycin hydrolase. The 832-bp bleomycin hydrolase cDNA fragment encodes for a protein that contains a 15-amino-acid sequence homologous to the active site of a cysteine proteinase. The ability to clone bleomycin hydrolase may permit future therapies to be directed toward specifically augmenting lung levels of this important enzyme and potentially increasing protection to the lung prior to initiation of therapy with the drug.

The future development of novel therapeutic approaches to drug-induced lung disease will be dependent on our improved understanding of the basic mechanisms underlying pulmonary toxicity of these drugs. The potential clearly exists for future studies to utilize more specific therapies to prevent or treat adverse drug reactions in the lung. As insight is gained into the pathogenesis of these disorders, it is likely that our therapeutic approach will improve and that our understanding of individual susceptibility to drug reactions will be enhanced.

ACKNOWLEDGMENT

This work was supported, in part, by NIH grants HL-36124 and HL-36778.

REFERENCES

1. Gillett DG, Ford GT. Drug-induced lung disease. In: Thurlbeck WM, Abell MR, eds. *The lung*. Baltimore: Williams & Wilkins, 1978;21–42.
2. Rosenow EC III, Martin WJ II. Drug-induced interstitial lung disease. In: Schwarz MA, King TE, eds. *Interstitial lung disease*. Philadelphia: BC Decker, 1986;123–137.
3. Cooper JAD, White DA, Matthey RA. Drug-induced pulmonary disease. *Am Rev Respir Dis* 1986;133:321–340 (Part 1); 488–505 (Part 2).
4. Kistler GS, Caldwell PRB, Weibel ER. Development of fine structural damage to alveolar and capillary lining cells in oxygen-poisoned rat lungs. *J Cell Biol* 1967;32:605–628.
5. Bowden DH, Adamson IYR. Endothelial regeneration as a marker of the different vascular responses in oxygen-induced pulmonary edema. *Lab Invest* 1974;30:350–357.
6. Moosavi H, McDonald S, Rubin P, Cooper R, Stuard ID, Penney D. Early radiation dose–response in lung: an ultrastructural study. *Int J Radiat Oncol Biol Phys* 1977;2:921–931.
7. Adamson IYR, Drummond HB. The pathogenesis of bleomycin-induced pulmonary fibrosis in mice. *Am J Pathol* 1974;77:185–198.
8. Aso Y, Yoneda K, Kikkawa Y. Morphologic and biochemical study of pulmonary changes induced by bleomycin in mice. *Lab Invest* 1976;35:558–568.
9. Horton JK, Brigelius R, Mason RP, Bend JR. Paraquat uptake into freshly isolated rabbit lung epithelial cells and its reduction

to the paraquat radical under anaerobic conditions. *Mol Pharmacol* 1986;29:484–489.

10. Sykes BI, Purchase IFH, Smith LL. Pulmonary ultrastructure after oral and intravenous dosage of paraquat to rats. *J Pathol* 1977;121:233–241.

11. Vracko R. Significance of basal lamina for regeneration of injured lung. *Virchows Arch [A]* 1972;355:264–274.

12. Gross NJ. The pathogenesis of radiation-induced lung damage. *Lung* 1981;159:115–125.

13. Rosenow EC III, DeRemee RA, Dines DE. Chronic nitrofurantoin pulmonary reaction. *N Engl J Med* 1968;279:1258–1262.

14. Hailey FJ, Glascock HW, Hewitt WF. Pleuropneumonic reactions to nitrofurantoin. *N Engl J Med* 1969;281:1087–1090.

15. Israel KS, Brashear RE, Sharma HM, Yum MN, Glover JL. Pulmonary fibrosis and nitrofurantoin. *Am Rev Respir Dis* 1973;108:353–356.

16. Sovijarvi ARA, Lemola M, Stenius B, Idanpaan-Heikkila J. Nitrofurantoin-induced acute, subacute, and chronic pulmonary reactions: a report of 66 cases. *Scand J Respir Dis* 1977;58:41–50.

17. Holmberg L, Boman G, Bottiger LE, Eriksson B, Spross R, Wessling A. Adverse reactions to nitrofurantoin: analysis of 921 reports. *Am J Med* 1980;69:733–738.

18. Mason RP, Holtzman JL. The role of catalytic superoxide formation in the O₂ inhibition of nitroreductase. *Biochem Biophys Res Commun* 1975;67:1267–1274.

19. Mason RP, Holtzman JL. The mechanism of microsomal and mitochondrial nitroreductase. Electron spin resonance evidence for nitroaromatic free radical intermediates. *Biochemistry* 1975;14:1626–1632.

20. Sasame HA, Boyd MR. Superoxide and hydrogen peroxide production and NADPH oxidation stimulated by nitrofurantoin in lung microsomes: possible implications for toxicity. *Life Sci* 1979;24:1091–1096.

21. Boyd MR. Biochemical mechanisms in chemical-induced lung injury: role of metabolic activation. *CRC Crit Rev Toxicol* 1980;7:103–176.

22. Martin WJ II. Nitrofurantoin: evidence of the oxidant injury of lung parenchymal cells. *Am Rev Respir Dis* 1983;127:482–486.

23. Martin WJ II, Powis GW, Kachel DL. Nitrofurantoin stimulates oxidant production in pulmonary endothelial cells. *J Lab Clin Med* 1985;105:23–29.

24. Boyd MR, Catignani GL, Sasame HA, Mitchell JR, Stiko AW. Acute pulmonary injury in rats by nitrofurantoin and modification by vitamin E dietary fat and oxygen. *Am Rev Respir Dis* 1979;120:93–99.

25. Spielberg SP, Gordon GB. Nitrofurantoin cytotoxicity: *in vitro* assessment of risk based on glutathione metabolism. *J Clin Invest* 1981;67:37–41.

26. Lyng PJ, Kachel DL, Martin WJ II. Importance of hydrogen peroxide in nitrofurantoin induced cytotoxicity: experimental evidence from a genetically-defined catalase-deficient strain of mice. *J Lab Clin Med* 1988;112:301–306.

27. Peterson FJ, Mason RP, Holtzman JL. The effect of selenium and vitamin E deficiency in the toxicity of nitrofurantoin in the chick. In: Coon MJ, Cooney AH, Estabrook RW, et al., eds. *Microsomes.* New York: Academic Press, 1980;873–876.

28. Van Barneveld PWC, Van der Mark TW, Sleijfer DT, et al. Predictive factors for bleomycin-induced pneumonitis. *Am Rev Respir Dis* 1984;130:1078–1081.

29. Van Barneveld PWC, Sleijfer DT, Van der Mark TW, et al. Natural course of bleomycin-induced pneumonitis. A follow-up study. *Am Rev Respir Dis* 1987;135:48–51.

30. Lown JW, Sim SK. The mechanism of the bleomycin-induced cleavage of DNA. *Biochem Biophys Res Commun* 1977;77:1150–1157.

31. Sausville EA, Reisach J, Horwitz SB. Effect of chelating agents and metal ions on the degradation of DNA by bleomycin. *Biochemistry* 1978;17:2740–2746.

32. Oberly LW, Buettner GR. The production of hydroxyl radical by bleomycin and iron(II). *FEBS Lett* 1979;97:47–49.

33. Cunningham ML, Ringrose PS, Lokesh BR. Bleomycin cytotoxicity is prevented by superoxide dismutase *in vitro. Cancer Lett* 1983;21:149–153.

34. Solaiman D, Rao EA, Petering DH, Sealy RC, Antholine WE. Chemical, biochemical and cellular properties of copper and iron bleomycins. *Int J Radiat Oncol Biol Phys* 1979;5:1519–1521.

35. Burger RM, Kent TA, Howitz SB, Munck E, Peisach J. Mossbauer study of iron bleomycin and its activation intermediates. *J Biol Chem* 1983;258:1559–1564.

36. McCord JM, Day ED. Superoxide-dependent production of hydroxyl radical catalyzed by iron–EDTA complex. *FEBS Lett* 1978;86:139–142.

37. Goldiner PL, Carlon GC, Cvitkovic E, et al. Factors influencing postoperative morbidity and mortality in patients treated with bleomycin. *Br Med J* 1978;1:1664–1667.

38. Hakkinen PJ, Whiteley JW, Witschi HR. Hyperoxia, but not thoracic X-irradiation, potentiates bleomycin- and cyclophosphamide-induced lung damage in mice. *Am Rev Respir Dis* 1982;126:281–285.

39. Tryka AF, Skornik WA, Godleski JJ, Brain JD. Potentiation of bleomycin-induced lung injury by exposure to 70% oxygen. *Am Rev Respir Dis* 1982;126:1074–1079.

40. Berend N. Protective effects of hypoxia on bleomycin lung toxicity in the rat. *Am Rev Respir Dis* 1984;130:307–308.

41. Chandler DB, Barton JC, Briggs DD III, et al. Effect of iron deficiency on bleomycin-induced lung fibrosis in the hamster. *Am Rev Respir Dis* 1988;137:85–89.

42. Chandler DB, Fulmer JD. The effect of deferoxamine on bleomycin-induced lung fibrosis in the hamster. *Am Rev Respir Dis* 1985;131:596–598.

43. Martin WJ II, Kachel DL. Bleomycin-mediated pulmonary endothelial cell injury: protection by the iron chelator deferoxamine, but not EDTA. *J Lab Clin Med* 1987;110:153–158.

44. Ohnuma T, Holland JF, Masuda H, Waligunda JA, Goldberg GA. Microbiological assay of bleomycin: inactivation, tissue distribution, and clearance. *Cancer* 1974;33:1230–1234.

45. Lazo JS, Merrill WW, Pham ET, Lynch TJ, McCallister JD, Ingbar DH. Bleomycin hydrolase activity in pulmonary cells. *J Pharmacol Exp Ther* 1984;231:583–588.

46. Akoun GM, Mayaud CM, Milleron BJ, Perrot JY. Drug-related pneumonitis and drug-induced hypersensitivity pneumonitis [Letter]. *Lancet* 1984;1:1362–1363.

47. Ettensohn DB, Roberts NJ, Condemi JJ. Bronchoalveolar lavage in gold lung. *Chest* 1984;85:569–570.

48. Venet A, Caubarrere I, Bonan G. Five cases of immune-mediated amiodarone pneumonitis. *Lancet* 1984;1:962–963.

49. Israel-Biet D, Venet A, Caubarrere I, et al. Bronchoalveolar lavage in amiodarone pneumonitis: cellular abnormalities and their relevance to pathogenesis. *Chest* 1987;91:214–221.

50. Martin WJ II, Rosenow EC III. Amiodarone pulmonary toxicity: recognition and pathogenesis, Part I. *Chest* 1988;93:1067–1075.

51. Costabel U, Bross JK, Marxen J, Matthys H. T-lymphocytosis in bronchoalveolar lavage fluid of hypersensitivity pneumonitis: changes in profile of T-cell subsets during the course of disease. *Chest* 1984;85:514–518.

52. Leatherman JW, Michael AF, Schwartz BA, Hoidal JR. Lung T-cells in hypersensitivity pneumonitis. *Ann Intern Med* 1984;100:390–392.

53. Semenzato G, Agostini C, Zambello R, et al. Lung T-cells in hypersensitivity pneumonitis: phenotypic and functional analyses. *J Immunol* 1986;137:1164–1172.

54. Marchlinski FE, Gansler TS, Waxman HL, Josephson ME. Amiodarone pulmonary toxicity. *Ann Intern Med* 1982;97:839–845.

55. Rotmensch HH, Belhassen B, Swanson BN, et al. Steady-state serum amiodarone concentrations: relationships with antiarrhythmic efficacy and toxicity. *Ann Intern Med* 1984;101:462–469.

56. Kennedy JI, Myers JL, Plumb VJ, Fulmer JD. Amiodarone pulmonary toxicity: clinical, radiologic, and pathologic correlations. *Arch Intern Med* 1987;147:50–55.

57. Martin WJ II. Adverse pulmonary reactions induced by antiarrhythmic agents. In: Akoun GM, White JP, eds. *Treatment-induced respiratory disorders.* Amsterdam: Elsevier, 1989;88–115.

58. Martin WJ II, Rosenow EC III. Amiodarone pulmonary toxicity: recognition and pathogenesis, Part II. *Chest* 1988;93:1242–1248.

59. Akoun GM, Gautheri-Rahman S, Milleron BJ, Perrot JY, Mayaud CM. Amiodarone-induced hypersensitivity pneumonitis: evidence of an immunological cell-mediated mechanism. *Chest* 1984;85:133–135.

60. Suarez LD, Poderoso JJ, Elsner B, Bunster AM, Esteva H, Bellotti M. Subacute pneumopathy during amiodarone therapy. *Chest* 1983;83:566–568.

61. Joelson J, Kluger J, Cole S, Conway M. Possible recurrence of amiodarone pulmonary toxicity following corticosteroid therapy. *Chest* 1984;85:284–286.

62. Adams PC, Gibson GJ, Morley AR, et al. Amiodarone pulmonary toxicity: clinical and subclinical features. *Q J Med* 1986; 59:449–471.

63. Gefter WB, Epstein DM, Pietra GG, Miller WT. Lung disease caused by amiodarone, a new antiarrhythmic agent. *Radiology* 1983;147:339–344.

64. Sandron D, Israel-Biet D, Venet A, Chetien J. Immunoglobulin abnormalities in bronchoalveolar lavage specimens from amiodarone-treated subjects. *Chest* 1986;89:617–618.

65. Fahey PJ, Utell MJ, Mayewski RJ, Wandtke JD, Hyde RW. Early diagnosis of bleomycin pulmonary toxicity using bronchoalveolar lavage in dogs. *Am Rev Respir Dis* 1982;126:126–130.

66. Thrall RS, Barton RW, D'Amato DA, Sulavik SB. Differential cellular analysis of bronchoalveolar lavage fluid at various stages during the development of bleomycin-induced pulmonary fibrosis in the rat. *Am Rev Respir Dis* 1982;126:488–492.

67. White DA, Kris MG, Stover DE. Bronchoalveolar lavage cell populations in bleomycin-induced pulmonary toxicity. *Thorax* 1987;42:551–552.

68. Kaelin RM, Center DM, Bernardo J, Grant M, Snider G. The role of macrophage-derived chemoattractant activities in the early inflammatory events of bleomycin-induced pulmonary injury. *Am Rev Respir Dis* 1983;128:132–137.

69. Jordana M, Richards C, Irving LB, Glaudie J. Spontaneous *in vitro* release of alveolar macrophage cytokines after the intratracheal instillation of bleomycin in rats. *Am Rev Respir Dis* 1988;137:1135–1140.

70. Fox RB, Hoidal JR, Brown DM, Repine JE. Pulmonary inflammation due to oxygen toxicity: involvement of chemotactic factors and polymorphonuclear leukocytes. *Am Rev Respir Dis* 1981;123:521–523.

71. Schoenberger CI, Rennard SI, Bitterman PB, Fukuda Y, Ferrans VJ, Crystal RG. Paraquat-induced pulmonary fibrosis. Role of the alveolitis in modulating the development of fibrosis. *Am Rev Respir Dis* 1984;129:168–173.

72. Crystal RG, Bitterman PB, Rennard SI, Hance AJ, Keogh BA. Interstitial lung disease of unknown cause: disorders characterized by chronic inflammation of the lower respiratory tract. *N Engl J Med* 1984;310:154–166.

73. Suttorp N, Simon LM. Lung cell oxidant injury. Enhancement of polymorphonuclear leukocyte-mediated cytotoxicity in lung cells exposed to sustained *in vitro* hyperoxia. *J Clin Invest* 1982; 70:342–350.

74. Martin WJ II. Neutrophils kill pulmonary endothelial cells by a hydrogen peroxide dependent pathway: an *in vitro* model of the adult respiratory distress syndrome. *Am Rev Respir Dis* 1984; 130:209–213.

75. Thrall RS, Pham SH, McCormick JR, Ward PA. The development of bleomycin-induced pulmonary fibrosis in neutrophil-depleted and complement-depleted rats. *Am J Pathol* 1981;105:76–81.

76. Clark JG, Kuhn C III. Bleomycin-induced pulmonary fibrosis in hamsters: effect of neutrophil depletion on lung collagen synthesis. *Am Rev Respir Dis* 1982;126:737–739.

77. Canada AI, Lesko LJ, Haffajee CI, Johnson B, Asdourian GK.

78. Amiodarone for tachyarrhythmias: pharmacology, kinetics, and efficacy. *Drug Intell Clin Pharm* 1983;17:100–104.

78. Darmanata JI, van Zandwijk N, Duren DR, et al. Amiodarone pneumonitis: three further cases with review of published reports. *Thorax* 1984;39:56–64.

79. Camus P, Mehendale HM. Pulmonary sequestration of amiodarone and desethylamiodarone. *J Pharmacol Exp Ther* 1986; 237:867–873.

80. Martin WJ II, Gadek JE, Hunninghake GW, Crystal RG. Radiation pneumonitis: an *in vitro* model of lung injury. *Am Rev Respir Dis* 1981;123:140.

81. Rossi GA, Szapiel S, Ferrans VJ, Crystal RG. Susceptibility to experimental interstitial lung disease is modified by immune- and non-immune-related genes. *Am Rev Respir Dis* 1987;135:448–455.

82. Sebti SM, DeLeon JC, Lazo JS. Purification, characterization, and amino acid composition of rabbit pulmonary bleomycin hydrolase. *Biochemistry* 1987;26:4213–4219.

83. Nishimura C, Tanaka N, Suzuki H. Purification of bleomycin hydrolase with a monoclonal antibody and its characterization. *Biochemistry* 1987;26:1574–1578.

84. Filderman AE, Genovese LA, Lazo JS. Alterations in pulmonary protective enzymes following systemic bleomycin treatment in mice. *Biochem Pharmacol* 1988;37:1111–1116.

85. Sebti SM, Lazo JS. Metabolic inactivation of bleomycin analogs by bleomycin hydrolase. *Pharmacol Ther* 1988;38:321–329.

86. Lazo JS, Braun ID, Labaree DC, et al. Characteristics of bleomycin-resistant phenotypes of human cell sublines and circumvention of bleomycin resistance by liblomycin. *Cancer Res* 1989;49:185–190.

87. Sebti SM, DeLeon JC, Ma LT, Hecht SM, Lazo JS. Substrate specificity of bleomycin hydrolase. *Biochem Pharmacol* 1989; 38:141–147.

88. Sebti SM, Mignano JE, Jani JP, Srimatkandada S, Lazo JS. Bleomycin hydrolase: molecular cloning, sequencing and biochemical studies reveal membership in the cysteine proteinase family. *Biochemistry* 1989;28:6544–6548.

89. Frank L, Summerville J, Massaro D. Protection from oxygen toxicity with endotoxin. Role of the endogenous antioxidant enzymes of the lung. *J Clin Invest* 1980;65:1104–1110.

90. Frank L. Prolonged survival after paraquat. Role of the lung antioxidant enzyme systems. *Biochem Pharmacol* 1981; 30:2319–2324.

91. Massaro GD, Massaro D. Adaptation to hyperoxia. Influence on protein synthesis by lung on a granular pneumocyte ultrastructure. *J Clin Invest* 1974;53:705–709.

92. Crapo JD, Barry BE, Foscue HA, Shelburne J. Structural and biochemical changes in rat lungs occurring during exposure to lethal and adaptive doses of oxygen. *Am Rev Respir Dis* 1980; 122:123–143.

93. White CW, Ghezzi P, Dinarello CA, Caldwell SA, McMurty IF, Repine JE. Recombinant tumor necrosis factor/cachectin and interleukin 1 pretreatment decreases lung oxidized glutathione accumulation, lung injury, and mortality in rats exposed to hyperoxia. *J Clin Invest* 1987;79:1868–1873.

94. Padmanabhan R, Gudapaty R, Liemer IE, Schwartz BA, Hoidal JR. Protection against pulmonary oxygen toxicity in rats by the intratracheal administration of liposome-encapsulated superoxide dismutase or catalase. *Am Rev Respir Dis* 1985;132:164–167.

95. Turrens JF, Crapo JD, Freeman BA. Protection against oxygen toxicity by intravenous injection of liposome-entrapped catalase and superoxide dismutase. *J Clin Invest* 1984;73:87–95.

96. McDonald RJ, Berger EM, White CM, White JG, Freeman BA, Repine JE. Effect of superoxide dismutase encapsulated in liposomes or conjugated with polyethylene glycol on neutrophil bactericidal activity *in vitro* and bacterial clearance *in vivo*. *Am Rev Respir Dis* 1985;131:633–637.

THE LUNG: Scientific Foundations
edited by R.G. Crystal, J.B. West et al.
Raven Press, Ltd., New York © 1991.

CHAPTER 7.7.3.1

Biology of Acute Lung Injury

Roger G. Spragg and Robert M. Smith

Acute lung injury has been known by a variety of names, including the adult respiratory distress syndrome (ARDS), wet lung, shock lung, capillary leak syndrome, Da Nang lung, postperfusion lung, and congestive atelectasis. Many of these names recall the association between acute pulmonary disease and traumatic battlefield injuries. Thus, as noted by Major L. A. Brewer et al. (1) in 1946, "Experience gained in treating a large number of casualties . . . has shown the importance of the 'wet lung' in reference to the morbidity and mortality of patients with wounds of the chest, brain, and abdomen." These authors noted that "in the late stages of shock the capillary permeability is increased in nontraumatic regions of the body so that blood plasma escapes into the tissue spaces. That which escapes into the pulmonary alveoli results in the clinical findings of pulmonary edema." Almost a half century later, interest continues to focus on the processes by which plasma components gain access to the interstitium and alveoli of the lung through an abnormally permeable alveolar–capillary membrane. Ashbaugh et al. (2) provided definition of the syndrome in the medical setting. Catheterization of the pulmonary artery has helped to distinguish between pulmonary edema associated with elevated pulmonary vascular pressures and that associated with inflammation of the lung. The central focus of current investigation is to understand the various biologically active factors that affect permeability of the alveolar–capillary membrane, the control of expression of those factors, and their interactions.

Operational definitions of acute lung injury vary slightly. Many investigators define that injury to be lung edema that (a) occurs over a period of less than

7 days, (b) is present in the absence of pulmonary vascular pressures sufficient to be the primary cause of pulmonary edema, and (c) is diffuse in nature as reflected by panlobar infiltrates on the chest radiograph. In the presence of such edema, shunting of pulmonary blood flow and diminished lung compliance are common.

PATHOBIOLOGY AND PATHOPHYSIOLOGY OF ACUTE LUNG INJURY

Examination of pulmonary tissue and bronchoalveolar lavage (BAL) fluid from patients with ARDS suggests that a variety of inflammatory mediators may contribute to the lung injury (see Chapters 2.8, 7.1.1, 7.2.1, 7.2.4, 7.5.2, 7.7.1, 7.8.1, and 8.2.2). BAL fluid contains 1–10 mg protein/ml, and these proteins represent all classes of serum proteins (3). Polymorphonuclear leukocytes (PMNs), normally less than 2% of cells in BAL fluid, may comprise over 90% of BAL fluid cells; in addition, total cell yield is increased. Analysis of BAL fluid also reveals the presence of a variety of soluble mediators of inflammation.

Histologic examination of pulmonary tissue obtained at autopsy from patients who died after developing ARDS suggests the presence of acute and chronic stages (4). In the first few days of acute lung injury, alveoli are filled with proteinaceous fluid containing red blood cells, neutrophils, macrophages, and cell fragments. The type I epithelial cells are focally destroyed, and endothelial cells may appear swollen. Interstitial edema occurs, and cuffs of edema are seen around bronchioles and vessels. Hyaline membranes composed of fibrin strands and plasma proteins are seen predominately in alveolar ducts. The number of PMNs seen in capillaries is markedly increased; extravasated PMNs are seen in the interstitium and alveoli (5). A more chronic stage of acute lung injury is apparent after 1–2 weeks. Cuboidal epithelial cells

R. G. Spragg and R. M. Smith: Department of Medicine, Division of Pulmonary and Critical Care Medicine, University of California Medical Center, San Diego, California 92103.

TABLE 1. *Clinical conditions associated with acute lung injury*

Direct effects	Systemic effects
Aspiration	Trauma
Gastric contents	Sepsis
Hydrocarbons	Pancreatitis
Salt or fresh water	Multiple transfusions
Pneumonia	Burns
Bacterial (gram positive	Cardiopulmonary bypass
and gram negative)	Reperfusion
Fungal	Granulocytic leukemia
Mycobacterial	Drug exposure
Viral	Heroin
Mycoplasmal	Methadone
Pneumocystic	Acetylsalicylic acid
Inhalation	Placidyl
NO_2, Cl_2, SO_2, NH_3, O_2	Paraquat
Smoke	Disseminated
Embolism	intravascular
Air	coagulation
Fat	
Pulmonary contusion	
Ionizing radiation	

closely resembling type II cells cover the surfaces of alveoli and alveolar ducts. Proliferation of pericytes and fibroblasts occurs, and plasma cells, histiocytes, and lymphocytes are seen in the interstitium. Intravascular microthrombi are common (6). The acinar architecture of the lung is replaced by thick layers of fibrotic tissue. This fibrosis occurs in a pattern centered on alveolar ducts (7). Total lung collagen is increased two- to threefold after 10 or more days of illness (8). Katzenstein et al. (9) have stressed that the histopathology associated with acute lung injury is nonspecific and that it is likely to represent the effects of numerous dissimilar agents.

The physiologic changes associated with acute lung injury might be predicted from histologic examination. Compliance of the lung is low. Gas exchange is markedly impaired and is predominately due to shunt. The resistance of the pulmonary vasculature to blood flow is often increased, and airway resistance is also significantly increased (10).

CAUSES OF ACUTE LUNG INJURY

An impressive variety of insults may result in acute lung injury. These may be separated into those insults that are understood to affect directly the lung parenchyma and those insults that are distant and are hypothesized to affect the lung via systemic mechanisms (Table 1). Investigations employing animal models of acute lung injury have furthered the understanding of the pathophysiology and possible mechanisms of the

human disease. Unfortunately, none of these models is a perfect replica of that condition, as evidenced by the diversity of models that have been developed (Tables 2 and 3).

OBSERVATIONS FROM HUMAN ACUTE LUNG INJURY, WITH SELECTED REFERENCE TO ANIMAL AND *IN VITRO* EXPERIMENTS

Cell Migration

Examination of lung biopsies obtained from patients at risk for ARDS (5), of lung tissue from patients who have died with ARDS (4), and of BAL fluid from patients with ARDS (11–13) confirms a marked influx of PMNs into the lung. These observations support the hypothesis that products of PMNs may participate in the initiation and/or propagation of the lung pathology. However, examples of ARDS in profoundly neutropenic patients are described (14), suggesting that products of PMNs may not be necessary for the syndrome to develop.

Why do circulating blood PMNs enter the lung parenchyma (see Chapters 2.10, 3.4.7 and 3.4.8)? One mechanism of inflammatory cell recruitment mav be directed chemotaxis. In the initial stage of acute lung injury, cells of the lung may produce substances chemotactic for PMNs. Products of alveolar macrophages with such chemotactic activity include interleukin 1 (IL-1), interleukin 8 (IL-8), tumor necrosis factor alpha (TNF-α), platelet-derived growth factor (PDGF), and platelet-activating factor (PAF). Epithelial cells may also have the potential to produce PDGF (15), IL-8 (16), and lipoxygenase products (17). Endothelial cells synthesize IL-8 and IL-1 (18,19). Thus, a variety of chemotactic substances produced by cells of the lung may contribute to the recruitment of PMNs from the systemic circulation.

In the presence of established ARDS, a broad spectrum of substances that are known to attract PMNs is present in the inflamed lung. Studies of BAL fluid have revealed the presence of leukotriene B_4 (LTB$_4$) (20), and active components of the complement system chemotactic for neutrophils are likely to be generated (21). Monokines are certainly produced, along with fragments of proteins that participate in the coagulation cascade. One of these, fibrinopeptide B, is markedly chemotactic for PMNs (22). Phagocyte proteases may attack other lung matrix proteins, specifically elastin and collagen, and produce fragments that have chemotactic activity (23,24). Oxidized α_1-antitrypsin (α_1-AT) is present in the acutely injured lung (25) and is chemotactic for PMNs (26). Finally, chemotactic bacterial products such as the formylated peptide f-Met-

TABLE 2. *Selected animal models of acute lung injury*

Initiating stimulus	Species examined	Neutrophil-dependent?
Agents administered via the circulation		
Bacterial products		
Gram-negative endotoxin	Mouse, rabbit, sheep	Yes
Gram-negative endotoxin	Goat	No
Gram-positive bacteria	Sheep	Yes
Oleic acid	Dog, rabbit, sheep	No
Phorbol ester, f-Met-Leu-Phe	Dog, rabbit, sheep	Yes
Oxidant-generating systems	Rabbit, rat, dog	No
Eicosanoids	Rabbit, rat, sheep	Mixed
Cytokines	Rabbit, rat, sheep, others	Mixed
Fibrinopeptides	Rabbit	Unknown
Ethchlorvinyl	Dog	No
Cobra venom factor	Rat	Yes
Microembolism		
Gas bubble	Dog, sheep	Yes
Glass bead	Dog	Yes
Agents administered into the airway		
Hyperoxia	Dog, rabbit, sheep	Yes
Phorbol ester, f-Met-Leu-Phe	Rabbit	No
Immune complexes	Rat	Yes
Oxidant-generating systems	Rat	No
C5, C5a$_{Des Arg}$	Rabbit, guinea pig	Yes

Leu-Phe may be present in the lung and may participate in attracting neutrophils.

Events in the lung microvasculature may provide a second mechanism of inflammatory cell recruitment. In the face of a systemic insult, complement activation has been invoked as a specific precursor to acute lung injury (27; see also Chapter 3.4.4). Initial observations suggested that systemic complement activation results in release of C5a, or its active metabolite, C5a$_{Des Arg}$, causes intravascular aggregation of leukocytes with sequestration in the pulmonary vasculature and resultant pulmonary injury. More recently, multiple reports have documented that systemic complement activation is common in acute systemic illness and does not specifically predispose to acute lung injury (28,29).

An additional vascular event that may promote adherence of PMNs to lung endothelial cells is expression by those cells of adhesion molecules, including intercellular adhesion molecule 1 (ICAM-1) and endothelial–leukocyte adhesion molecule 1 (ELAM-1). The former is constitutively expressed, but levels increase following stimulation with IL-1, TNF, or interferon gamma (IFN-γ) (30); the latter appears following exposure of endothelial cells to TNF, lipopolysaccharides (LPS), or IL-1β (31). The CD11/CD18 complex on PMNs has increased expression after exposure of cells to IL-1 or TNF, and it may be the recognition site for ICAM-1. Finally, while endothelial cell IL-8 released in response to inflammatory mediators is chemotactic for PMNs, it may cause inhibition of PMN–endothelial-cell adhesion (32). Thus, multiple mechanisms are available to modulate PMN–endothelial-cell adherence in the acutely inflamed lung.

TABLE 3. *Organ or cell models useful for study of lung injury*

Model	Parameters examined
Hamster cheek pouch	^{125}I-albumin permeability
Isolated perfused lung	Weight gain; ^{125}I-albumin permeability; vascular resistance; organ metabolism and products
Lung explant	Cytotoxicity; cell metabolism and products
Endothelial monolayer	Cytotoxicity; phagocyte adherence; permeability; cell metabolism and products
Epithelial monolayer	Cytotoxicity; phagocyte adherence; cell metabolism and products

Therapeutic Considerations

As events that govern the multiple steps of PMN attraction, adherence to the endothelium, and migration into the interstitium of the lung become defined, it may be possible to target specific interventions to interrupt the sequence. For example, use of monoclonal antibodies directed against CD11b/CD18 prevents injury of rat lungs caused by *in vivo* activation of PMNs (33), and similar antibodies attenuate PMN-mediated injury to endothelial cell monolayers (34,35). Pentoxifylline, a methylxanthine derivative, appears to interfere with adherence of PMNs to endothelial cells mediated by cytokines (36,37). The mechanism of this effect is not know, but it may relate to pentoxifylline-induced increases in intracellular $3',5'$-cyclic adenosine monophosphate levels with subsequent effect on membrane fluidity, cell deformability, and phagocytosis (38,39). In guinea pigs, pretreatment with pentoxifylline attenuates lung injury induced by TNF or IL-2; in dogs, it attenuates lung injury induced by sepsis (36,40).

Toxic Oxygen Products

Neutrophils are known to release highly reactive reduced oxygen species such as superoxide (O_2^-) or hydrogen peroxide (H_2O_2) as one of the primary mechanisms used to kill ingested bacteria and to accomplish cytotoxic functions. Therefore it is not surprising that investigators have examined BAL fluid and tissue samples from patients with ARDS for evidence of oxidant-induced injury or effect. In human acute lung injury, evidence for the participation of oxidative processes has been found in two distinct ways. Baldwin et al. (41) documented the presence of oxidants in the lungs of patients with ARDS. They showed that breath condensate gathered from intubated patients with newly developed ARDS contained fivefold more H_2O_2 than did condensate obtained from critically ill patients without ARDS. Whether H_2O_2 contributes to the lung injury or is only a marker for the presence of metabolically active PMNs or mononuclear phagocytes is unknown. More convincing evidence for direct participation of oxidants in acute lung injury comes from examination of α_1-AT function in BAL fluid from patients with ARDS. The increased alveolar–capillary permeability—the hallmark of acute lung injury—allows the passage of increased amounts of plasma proteins into the lungs of patients with ARDS. As expected, increased amounts of α_1-AT are identified. A portion of this inhibitor is inactive, and treatment with methionine sulfoxide peptide reductase restores inhibitory activity, suggesting that the loss of activity is due to oxidation of a critical methionine residue known to exist at the substrate-binding site of α_1-AT (25,42; see also Chapter 7.1.2). Although inactive α_1-AT has not been found universally in lavage fluid from patients with ARDS (43), its presence in some studies provides evidence for oxidative processes occurring in the lungs of patients with ARDS.

That oxidants have the capacity to induce lung injury has been well documented in many different models. Using an isolated perfused blood-free rabbit lung, Tate et al. (44) showed that the enzymatic generation of O_2^- or H_2O_2 in the perfusate caused lung edema, increased alveolar–capillary membrane permeability, and pulmonary artery vasoconstriction. Similar effects on vascular permeability have been found in a hamster cheek pouch model injured by the addition of xanthine/xanthine oxidase (45), as well as in rats injured by the intratracheal instillation of oxidant-generating systems (46). In each of these studies, the manifestations of tissue injury could be prevented by the addition of oxidant scavengers. At the cellular level, reduced oxygen intermediates may incapacitate intracellular metabolism and cause direct DNA injury as well as cell death (47–50).

Despite the evidence of oxidant involvement in ARDS, the source and nature of the oxidants are not completely understood, nor are the mechanisms by which oxidants can initiate or intensify human acute lung injury. One source may be phagocytic cells (including PMNs, monocytes, macrophages, and eosinophils), which produce reactive oxygen products following stimulation. The key element in the generation of these oxidants is a single enzyme system, the respiratory-burst NADPH oxidase (NADPH is the reduced form of nicotinamide-adenine dinucleotide phosphate). This oxidase catalyzes the one-electron reduction of molecular oxygen to O_2^-, using NADPH as an intracellular substrate. Once formed, the O_2^- undergoes spontaneous dismutation to H_2O_2 in an acid environment, a reaction that is markedly accelerated in the presence of superoxide dismutase. Subsequently, these two immediate products of the respiratory burst are utilized to form more reactive oxidant species, including hydroxyl radical (OH^-), hypohalous acids (mediated by myeloperoxidase), singlet oxygen, lipid peroxides, and mono- and dichloroamines (51). Stimulation of this enzyme system in intact neutrophils results in high-permeability lung injury when PMNs are added to the perfusate of isolated lungs (52). This PMN-mediated injury does not occur when cells from subjects with chronic granulomatous disease are used. Those cells do not contain critical components of the NADPH oxidase and are incapable of generating O_2^-, but they have a normal complement of lysosomal enzymes and are otherwise functionally normal. The inability of these cells to participate in these models of acute lung injury strongly supports a pivotal role for oxygen-derived radicals. Similarly, a wide variety of animal models of acute lung injury have been shown to depend on the presence of PMNs (see Table 2) and to be attenuated by the addition of oxygen radical scavengers.

The existence of additional lung injury models that are independent of neutrophils (Table 2), coupled with the occurrence of ARDS in profoundly neutropenic patients (14), raises the possibility that non-PMN sources of oxidants may also be important in the pathogenesis of acute lung injury. Mononuclear phagocytes also contain the NADPH oxidase, but their capacity to generate oxidants varies depending on the extent of cell activation and can be augmented greatly by exposure to cytokines, including INF-γ and TNF (53,54).

Evidence that macrophages may participate in acute lung injury comes from a variety of animal models. In canine acute lung injury, Jacobs et al. (55) showed that infusion of endotoxin resulted in increased H_2O_2 production by PMA-stimulated alveolar macrophages. Similar findings were reported by Brieland et al. (56) using an antigen-antibody mediated rat lung injury model. Macrophages recovered in BAL fluid may differ substantially from the nonrecoverable macrophages, and therefore cells obtained by bronchoscopic lavage may not be representative of the entire lung macrophage population (57).

A complete understanding of the role played by PMNs or macrophage NADPH oxidase in acute lung injury is made more difficult by the complexity of the enzyme activation system. Exposure of phagocytes to subthreshold levels of one stimulating agent results in greatly augmented oxidant release in response to an alternate stimulus (58–61). This phenomenon, often referred to as "priming" (see Chapter 7.7.1), complicates the interpretation of measurements of cell oxidant production.

The endothelial cell also has oxidant-generating capacity that may contribute to tissue injury. Incubation of cultured endothelial cells with phorbol myristate acetate or calcium ionophore, ingestion by cells of polystyrene microspheres, or exposure of cells to anoxia/reoxygenation stimulates endothelial cell release of O_2^- (62–64). The formation of O_2^- by endothelial cells may result from the conversion of xanthine dehydrogenase to xanthine oxidase and the subsequent activity of that enzyme. While the maximal rates of O_2^- formation by endothelial cells are only 1–2% those of PMNs, the impact of endothelial cell O_2^- production in the microenvironment of the alveolar–capillary membrane may be of biologic significance.

O_2^--generating activity may be found in BAL fluid from experimental animals. During lung injury from influenza virus in mice, Akaike et al. (65) found a 400-fold increase in xanthine oxidase activity in alveolar lavage fluid, activity that could be abolished by treatment of the lavage fluid with allopurinol, an inhibitor of xanthine oxidase. These studies have not yet been extended to other models of lung injury, but they do illustrate the possibility that xanthine oxidase may be a significant source of superoxide radical.

Oxygen-derived radicals are an attractive target for therapeutic intervention in ARDS. Infusion of radical scavengers such as superoxide dismutase, catalase, dimethylthiourea, and mannitol has been shown to attenuate lung injury in animal models (66). Studies to evaluate these agents in human acute lung injury are in progress but may be hampered, in part, by the difficulty in delivering scavengers to the site of oxidant injury. Also, many of the reactive oxygen products that are targets of the scavengers are rapidly converted to other injurious oxidants, suggesting the need for multiple scavengers. At the present time, knowledge of the NADPH oxidase is still imperfect and it is not yet possible to target this enzyme selectively. Pentoxifylline, addressed earlier because of its effects on cell adhesion, may also inhibit receptor-mediated stimulation of the NADPH oxidase (38); it is not known whether the inhibition of lung injury seen with pentoxifylline pretreatment of animals is due to inhibition of oxidant release by PMNs, to diminished PMN adherence, or to both.

Proteases and Inhibitors

Recognizing the influx of PMNs into the lungs of patients with ARDS, investigators have sought evidence of release of proteolytic enzymes from both these phagocytes and from the alveolar macrophage. In addition, the antiprotease defenses of the acutely injured lung have been evaluated.

Activated neutrophils release a variety of neutral proteases, including collagenase, neutrophil elastase (NE), and cathepsin G (see Chapter 7.1.1). Cohen et al. (67) have shown that the concentration of enzyme-releasing peptide (ERP), a macrophage product that causes release of neutrophil proteases, is significantly greater in BAL fluid from patients with ARDS than in that from controls. ERP is the major enzyme-releasing agent in BAL fluid from patients with ARDS (67).

Collagenase released by PMNs may attack matrix proteins of the lung, including proteoglycans and collagen. The native inhibitors of this protease include α_1-AT and α_2-macroglobulin. NE, a serine protease, has the capacity to degrade a wide variety of proteins. These include elastin, proteoglycans, types III and IV collagen, and fibronectin—important structural proteins of the lung (68–70). In the distal airway of the normal lung, the major inhibitor of NE is α_1-AT, a 52-kDa protein (71). Because reactive oxygen products may oxidize α_1-AT and render it inactive, the NE–anti-NE balance in the inflamed lungs of patients with ARDS may be tipped in the direction of unchecked proteolysis.

Alveolar macrophages secrete an elastase that, as a metalloproteinase, is distinct from NE. This enzyme, capable of cleaving elastin, is inhibited in the lung parenchyma by α_2-macroglobulin and not by α_1-AT (72).

Analysis of BAL fluid from patients with established ARDS demonstrates the presence of NE. Lee et al. (11) analyzed BAL fluid samples from patients within

24 hr of clinical recognition of ARDS, and McGuire et al. (12) analyzed samples from patients with established disease. In the majority of patients, these investigators found activity in BAL fluid that was capable both of lysing low-molecular-weight synthetic substrate specific for NE and of cleaving bovine elastin; the BAL fluid also contained NE antigen. In contrast, no normals and only occasional smokers or patients with bronchitis or pneumonia had active NE in BAL fluid. Activity was inhibited by serine protease inhibitors, including α_1-AT, and was maintained in the presence of cation chelators. In all patients with significant NE activity in BAL fluid, α_1-AT function in that fluid was markedly diminished.

Loss of α_1-AT activity in BAL fluid of ARDS patients is due not only to oxidation of methionine residues critical to function of the inhibitor, but also to loss of functional activity as the inhibitor is bound to and cleaved by NE (25). In addition, metalloproteinases from PMNs may cleave and inactivate α_1-AT (73); lipid peroxidation products may also contribute to inactivation of α_1-AT.

Other investigators have also found evidence of NE antigen in BAL fluid from ARDS patients, but they have failed to find evidence of NE activity (13,43,74). In these patients, NE was predominately complexed to α_1-AT, and excess active α_1-AT was present. A small fraction of NE (<0.4%) was complexed to the 725-kDa inhibitor, α_2-macroglobulin. Whether active NE is found in BAL fluid from ARDS patients may depend on the clinical status of the patient and on sampling technique. Results of all studies indicate that NE is secreted from PMNs in the lung and that it may be available for proteolysis in the absence of inhibition by α_1-AT. Consistent with this view, elastin degradation products have been detected in serum and BAL fluid of patients with ARDS (75).

That NE may contribute to the pathology of ARDS is suggested by its ability to damage capillary endothelial cells *in vitro* and to degrade fibrinogen, coagulation factors, and components of the complement system. Intratracheal instillation of NE causes acute hemorrhagic lung injury (76).

Collagenase activity in BAL fluid from patients with ARDS is detectable by analysis of cleavage of types I and III collagen in the majority of patients with ARDS sampled within 48 hr of diagnosis (77). Activity against type I collagen is inhibited by cation chelation but not by serine protease inhibitors, consistent with a neutrophil origin for a part of the collagenase activity.

Therapeutic Considerations

For individuals with no evidence of BAL-fluid α_1-AT activity, it is rational to consider both augmentation of the antielastase defenses of the lower airway and use of antioxidant therapy to prevent further inactivation of α_1-AT. Limited experience with native or recombinant α_1-AT suggests that, either by infusion or aerosol, the protein may be delivered effectively to the noninflamed lung (78,79). Studies evaluating the potential of such treatment in patients with ARDS are in progress. As low-molecular-weight protease inhibitors that penetrate the pulmonary parenchyma become available, they may provide an attractive therapeutic potential.

Eicosanoids and Platelet-Activating Factor

As reviewed in Chapters 2.5, 3.4.5, 5.1.2.1.3, and 5.1.2.1.5, cells of the lung have the capacity to produce a variety of cyclo-oxygenase and lipoxygenase metabolites of arachidonic acid. Because several of these products have biologic activity that might reasonably contribute to the development or propagation of acute inflammatory lung injury, attention has focused on identifying the role of arachidonate metabolites in that injury.

Stephenson et al. (20) examined the levels of LTB_4, LTC_4, and LTD_4 in BAL fluid from patients with ARDS, from patients at risk for ARDS, and from controls. Levels of all three leukotrienes were greater in patients with or at risk for ARDS than in controls. LTC_4 and LTD_4 levels were greater in patients with ARDS than in patients at risk. These results are consistent with a prior observation that LTD_4 levels are increased in edema fluid from patients with ARDS compared to levels in fluid from patients with cardiogenic pulmonary edema (80). Levels of thromboxane B_2 (TxB_2) and 6-keto $PGF_{1\alpha}$ (the stable metabolite of PGI_2; PG stands for prostaglandin) in blood of patients at risk for or with ARDS are frequently, but not invariably, elevated in both groups (81).

Unfortunately, the variable uptake and metabolism of eicosanoids in the lung calls into question the usefulness of BAL fluid in evaluating the role of these mediators in acute lung injury. For example, analysis of lung tissue of rats receiving intraperitoneal endotoxin reveals levels of 6-keto $PGF_{1\alpha}$ that are approximately eight times normal. However, no elevation of BAL fluid concentration of the stable metabolite was seen (82). When known concentrations of eicosanoids are delivered to the bronchoalveolar space, removal occurs at vastly different rates; PGD_2 is rapidly removed from the alveolar space, relative to 6-keto PGF_1 (83). Analysis of BAL fluid is therefore likely to underestimate the contribution of the biologically active PGD_2 to pulmonary injury.

A variety of agents that induce acute lung injury appear to cause production of arachidonic acid metabolites during the course of that injury (reviewed in refs.

TABLE 4. *Models of acute lung injury in which eicosanoid participation is suggested*

Stimulus	Eicosanoid detected[a]	Species
Endotoxin	PGI_2, PGE_2, LTC_4, LTD_4, 5-HETE	Rat
	LTD_4, 5-HETE	Mouse
	PGI_2, TxB_2, LTD_4, 5-HETE	Sheep
Exotoxin	PGI_2, TxB_2, LTC_4	Rat
Oxidant exposure	TxB_2	Rabbit
	PGI_2, $PGF_{2\alpha}$, TxB_2, 5-HETE	Rat
Hyperoxia	LTD_4, LTE_4, PGI_2	Mouse
Phorbol ester	LTB_4, LTC_4, LTD_4	Dog
Thrombin	TxB_2, PGI_2	Sheep
Microembolism	PGI_2, TxB_2	Sheep
Ethchlorvinyl	LTC_4	Dog

[a] PGE_2, prostaglandin E_2; $PGF_{2\alpha}$, prostaglandin $F_{2\alpha}$; PGI_2, prostaglandin I_2; LTB_4; leukotriene B_4; LTC_4, leukotriene C_4; LTD_4, leukotriene D_4; TxB_2, thromboxane B_2; 5-HETE, 5-hydroxy-6,8,11,14-eicosatetraenoic acid.

20 and 82) (Table 4). Whether this response contributes to the lung injury or is merely a marker of inflammation remains unclear. Ideally, specific inhibition of eicosanoid production should modulate the pulmonary injury. Exemplifying this approach, Chang et al. (84) employed both cyclo-oxygenase and lipoxygenase inhibitors in an attempt to alter pulmonary vascular leak of protein in a rat endotoxin lung injury model. Although eicosanoid synthesis was clearly inhibited, lung vascular leak was unmodified. Such results suggest that eicosanoid production in this setting may be more a marker of cell membrane damage than an event of pathogenetic significance.

In contrast, studies of the isolated rat lung suggest a more central role for arachidonate metabolites. Oxidant or alpha-staphylotoxin exposure causes a neutrophil-independent injury of this model, and the injury is partially inhibited by inhibitors of leukotriene synthesis (82). Inhibition of thromboxane synthetase or blockade of thromboxane receptors suggests a primary role for TxA_2 in the acute bronchoconstrictor and vasoconstrictor response of the cat to endotoxin infusion (85). The effect of these interventions on the development of edema awaits investigation. Clarification of the contribution of eicosanoids to clinical acute lung injury may come with application of specific inhibitors and the ability to identify quantitatively the degree of eicosanoid production in the lung.

Several histologic and physiologic alterations seen during lung injury may reasonably follow from release of eicosanoids. LTB_4 may contribute to recruitment and degranulation of neutrophils, and a direct contribution to edema formation has been suggested. TxA_2 may contribute to the aggregation of platelets and neutrophils in the microvasculature; it may also contribute

to vasoconstriction, which accentuates edema formation. Release of PGI_2 may cause vasodilatation in the setting of hypoxic vasoconstriction and thereby contribute to mismatch of ventilation and perfusion.

While little is known of the contribution of these factors to acute lung injury, even less is known of events that stimulate and modulate their production in the setting of acute lung injury. Endotoxin, exotoxin, and oxidants, as well as physical stretching of the lung (perhaps as occurs in areas of normal lung during high-pressure mechanical ventilation), may stimulate production (86).

Oxidative inactivation of the sulfidopeptide leukotrienes (LTC_4, LTD_1, LTE_4) and of PGE_2 has been demonstrated. As reviewed by Henderson (87), such inactivation occurs in the presence of H_2O_2 (at concentrations greater than 50 mM) or at lower concentrations in the presence of H_2O_2, myeloperoxidase, and halide. Because the constituents necessary for the formation of hypohalous acids are present in the lungs of patients with ARDS (13), it is possible that oxidative inactivation of certain eicosanoids serves as an important means of limiting their biologic effects at sites of inflammation.

Therapeutic Considerations

Both inhibition of eicosanoid production and administration of vasodilatory prostaglandins have been investigated. Inhibition may occur indirectly when glucocorticoids are administered. They may modulate leukotriene synthesis by alveolar macrophages (88), and they have been shown to induce expression of lipocortin, an inhibitor of phospholipase A_2, thereby providing a mechanism by which eicosanoid production may be altered (89). Current evidence suggests that glucocorticoid treatment does not benefit patients at risk for or with ARDS (90–92). More specific inhibition with the cyclo-oxygenase inhibitor ibuprofen may provide physiologic benefit and is the subject of current clinical trials.

PGE_1 administration has been reported to improve survival of patients with ARDS. However, subsequent studies have found PGE_1 to cause pulmonary vasodilatation, with increase in shunt and decrease in arterial oxygen content (93), and have failed to confirm enhanced survival (94).

A variety of observations suggest a role for PAF in the pathogenesis of ARDS. This mediator (see Chapter 2.5) is produced by many cells of the lung, including alveolar macrophages, endothelial cells, PMNs, platelets, and mast cells. Pulmonary effects of PAF include bronchoconstriction, vasoconstriction, and edema formation. These effects may be mediated directly and by stimulating release of eicosanoids. For example,

PAF releases LTC_4 and LTD_4 from rat lungs (95) and releases LTB_4 from neutrophils (96).

PAF infusion into a variety of animals induces shock, platelet and neutrophil aggregation with thrombocytopenia and neutropenia, microvascular injury, and edema. PAF is detected in shock states induced in animals by endotoxin, and benefit accompanies administration of PAF antagonists (97). The ability of PAF to cause lung edema appears to be species-specific, and in some cases it is secondary to leukotriene generation (reviewed in ref. 98).

While PAF infusion is associated with events seen during ARDS, and PAF is detected in animals during endotoxic shock, evidence directly implicating PAF in the pathogenesis of acute lung injury in humans is not yet available.

Interleukins and TNF

An appreciation of the potent effects of peptide mediators produced by or acting upon cells of the lung has focused attention on the contribution these factors may make to acute lung injury. TNF and IL-1, -2, and -8 have been of particular interest to investigators concerned with acute lung injury.

IL-1 refers to either of two polypeptides (IL-1α and IL-1β) that, despite being distinct gene products, share the same receptor and same biologic activities (see also Chapter 2.8). IL-1 is produced by monocytes, PMNs, and alveolar macrophages. Endothelial cells also produce IL-1 when stimulated by bacterial endotoxins, thrombin, or TNF, suggesting the possibility of local amplification of inflammatory response. As summarized by Dinarello (99), IL-1 stimulates the following: hepatic synthesis of acute-phase proteins; endothelial cell production of PGI_2, PGE_2, and PAF and expression of ICAM-1 and cell-surface procoagulant activity; and fibroblast proliferation and collagen synthesis. IL-1 primes neutrophils for enhanced superoxide production in response to f-Met-Leu-Phe (100), is chemotactic for neutrophils, and stimulates degranulation of eosinophils and basophils. In addition, IL-1 promotes the expression of IL-2 receptors, the production of IL-2, and the mitogenic response of T cells.

TNF, produced principally by monocytes and macrophages, has amino acid sequence and cell receptors distinct from those of IL-1 (Chapter 2.8). Nevertheless, the biologic actions are remarkably similar. In contrast to IL-1, TNF actively stimulates the respiratory burst of PMNs. In some instances, the effects of TNF and IL-1 may be synergistic as a result of augmented second messenger signal rather than alteration of receptors. Consequently, subthreshold doses of IL-1 and TNF produce hemodynamic shock and pulmonary hemorrhage when coadministered; also, IL-1 and

TNF act synergistically in stimulating the aggregation of neutrophils and synthesis of thromboxanes (99). Thus, the many actions of IL-1 and TNF suggest that these cytokines may be involved in the neutrophil recruitment and stimulation and microvascular thrombi formation seen in acute lung injury and that they may also be involved in the fibrotic response seen in the chronic phase of that injury.

To investigate whether IL-1 activity is increased in BAL from patients with acute lung injury, Siler et al. (101) measured immunoreactive IL-1β in BAL fluids from normal individuals, from patients at risk for ARDS, and from patients with ARDS. BAL IL-1 levels were significantly and equally elevated in both patient groups compared to normal values. In addition, resting or stimulated alveolar macrophages from patients with ARDS released greater amounts of immunoreactive IL-1β than did either (a) alveolar macrophages from patients with severe pneumonia or (b) those from normal individuals (102).

A variety of experimental approaches implicate TNF in the pathogenesis of acute lung injury. First, injection of TNF into guinea pigs (103) or mice (104) results in increased pulmonary permeability and edema accompanied by neutropenia and hypotension, hallmarks of the response to endotoxin. Second, inhibition of TNF is protective in the face of an endotoxin challenge. Passive immunization of mice against TNF protects against lethal effects of subsequent injection of endotoxin (105), and administration of anti-TNF antibodies protects rabbits (106) or baboons (107) from endotoxin-induced pulmonary edema. IFN-γ and PGE_2 modulate TNF and IL-1 production (108), and antibody to IFN-γ protects mice against lethal effects of LPS injection (109).

Finally, elevated levels of TNF are seen in the blood of septic patients. Marks et al. (110) reported that 35–38% of patients with septic shock (bacteremic or not, gram-negative or gram-positive), as opposed to 8% of patients with nonseptic shock, had measurable plasma TNF levels. Patients with shock were twice as likely to develop ARDS if TNF was measurable in plasma than if it was not detected. Also worth noting is the detection of TNF in respiratory secretions (111) or BAL fluid (112) from patients with acute lung injury.

Therapeutic Considerations

The suppression of LPS-stimulated transcription and translation of TNF message by dexamethasone (113) provides rationale for the treatment of acute lung injury with corticosteroids. However, at the cellular level, dexamethasone administered 2 hr after an endotoxin stimulus fails to interrupt the post-transcriptional phase of TNF synthesis. At the clinical level, methyl prednisolone administration does not appear to affect TNF levels in plasma of septic patients (110), nor does it appear to prevent or effectively treat acute lung injury (90–92).

The protection by anti-TNF antibodies of baboons receiving an endotoxin challenge requires pretreatment (107). This finding is consistent with the observation that TNF release appears to precede, or to occur very early in the development of, septic shock and acute lung injury. Thus, anti-TNF therapies may only have a preventive role in the therapy of acute lung injury.

IL-2, a product of helper T cells (see Chapter 3.4.1), has been investigated as a cancer chemotherapeutic agent. However, side effects include pulmonary microvascular injury and edema formation. That this injury may be mediated by inflammatory cells is suggested by in vitro studies in which IL-2 stimulates the respiratory burst and degranulation of PMNs and induces alveolar macrophage and blood monocyte synthesis of TNF (reviewed in ref. 114). Pentoxifylline prevents IL-2-induced acute lung injury in guinea pigs; however, the mechanism of protection is unclear (114).

IL-8 is a peptide derived from a variety of cells, including mononuclear phagocytes, endothelial cells, epithelial cells, and fibroblasts. Expression is stimulated by exposure of cells to IL-1 and TNF-α; alveolar macrophages and endothelial cells also express IL-8 in response to LPS. IL-8 is chemotactic for PMNs, causes expression of PMN surface adhesion molecules, and stimulates release of proteases and reactive oxygen products from those cells. Baggiolini et al. (115) note the potential for IL-8 to participate in the neutrophil recruitment and activation associated with ARDS, and they suggest that the ERP recovered in BAL fluid from patients with ARDS may be IL-8 (32,67).

Growth Factors

Patients who develop acute lung injury that persists for more than several days evolve from an acute edematous inflammatory response to a chronic fibrotic state. Examination of lung obtained after 7–10 days of ARDS demonstrates massive parenchymal fibrosis with loss of normal architecture, collagen deposition, and fibroblast proliferation accompanied by an apparent marked proliferation of alveolar type II epithelial cells (4,7). Quantitative studies demonstrate a marked increase in total lung hydroxyproline content, indicative of profound collagen deposition (8). The fibrotic response accompanying acute lung injury may be the most rapid and intense reponse seen in clinical medicine. Survivors of acute lung injury frequently have complete physiologic recovery over the succeeding

12–24 months, consistent with remodeling and/or breakdown of excess collagen (116). Thus, patients with acute lung injury provide an excellent clinical example of pulmonary fibrosis and repair.

While it is rational to postulate that factors stimulating fibroblast proliferation and collagen synthesis, as well as type II cell proliferation, are produced in the acutely injured lung, few direct observations have been made. Nevertheless, a wealth of information on soluble growth factors has recently become available, and it is apparent that many of these factors may be produced and/or released in the inflamed lung (reviewed in ref. 117 and in Chapters 2.9, 3.4.5, and 7.8.1). Attention currently focuses on the participation of PDGF because of the demonstrated increased expression of that factor in lungs of hyperoxic rats prior to the onset of tissue response (118) and the enhanced expression of PDGF by macrophages of patients with more chronic pulmonary fibrosis (119). However, a multiplicity of competence and progression factors produced by macrophages, fibroblasts, and endothelial cells are likely to participate in the fibrotic response to acute lung injury.

Coagulation System

Many of the conditions that predispose to the development of ARDS (Table 1) are also associated with derangements of hemostasis and particularly with disseminated intravascular coagulation (DIC) and altered fibrinolysis (see also Chapter 3.2.3). Carvalho (120), studying serum from patients with ARDS not associated with trauma, found that virtually all had increased levels of serum fibrin(ogen) degradation products. She and others have also found reduced fibrinogen levels and shortened fibrinogen survival in patients with ARDS. Active DIC has been found in 20–60% of ARDS patients (120,121). Plasminogen activator inhibitor and Factor VIII-antigen levels are increased (122–124). Although measurement of these derangements of coagulation is proposed as predictive of the course of ARDS (120), similar abnormalities are found in critically ill patients without ARDS (124,125). Examination of lung tissue from patients with ARDS has shown the presence of (a) microvascular and large vessel thrombi, (b) platelet microemboli, and (c) diffuse endothelial injury (126,127). Platelet survival is reduced in ARDS (128), and it appears to be due to pulmonary sequestration. The potential pathways leading to the observed abnormalities in the coagulation system in ARDS are multiple and include (a) endothelial injury causing platelet adhesion and secondary activation of the coagulation cascade, (b) direct stimulation of the coagulation cascade by tissue factor released from injured lung, (c) stimulation of platelets by infectious agents, immune complexes, products of the coagulation cascade (e.g., thrombin), or products released from neutrophils (e.g., PAF), (d) impaired clearance of activated coagulation factors, and (e) abnormal activation of the coagulation cascade by proteases derived from phagocytes (120).

Fragments of coagulation factors released during the coagulation cascade or by the action of other proteases may play a role in acute lung injury. Infusion into rabbits of fibrinopeptide A, a degradation product formed by the action of plasmin on fibrinogen, results in impaired gas exchange and pulmonary hypertension (129). Infusion of fibrinopeptide D into dogs or rabbits causes acute lung injury (130,131). Elevated levels of both fibrinopeptide A and D have been found in the blood of patients with ARDS (132). Fibrinopeptides may also inhibit bacterial cell killing, oxidant production, and chemotaxis (133). Thrombin, a protease activated during coagulation, appears to elaborate chemotactic and neutrophil-aggregating factors when it is allowed to act on blood or plasma (134).

Unfortunately, as with other potential mechanisms leading to ARDS, cause and effect are difficult to distinguish. The observed alterations of the coagulation system may be secondary to other aspects of acute lung injury rather than being a cause of it. In particular, primary vascular injury may lead to *in situ* platelet deposition and thrombus formation, and it may secondarily lead to the abnormalities in circulating clotting factors (see Chapter 3.4.12). Perhaps the best evidence that the products of the disordered coagulation cascade do not participate in ARDS is the observation that heparin administration, fibrinogen depletion, or platelet depletion does not attenuate lung injury in at least one animal model (135,136).

Abnormalities of fibrinolysis appear to be present in the lungs of patients with acute lung injury. Idell et al. (137), examining lavage fluid from patients with ARDS, found that fibrinolytic activity was absent or greatly reduced in contrast to the levels measured in normal individuals or in those with interstitial fibrosis. This deficiency of fibrinolysis may be due, in part, to elevated levels of α_2-antiplasmin. Procoagulant activity was also observed in the lavage fluid from ARDS patients but not in that from control patients, and the authors suggest that these dual abnormalities may predispose to abnormal fibrin deposition in alveoli of patients with ARDS.

Surfactant System of the Lung

The surfactant system of the lung functions to maintain stability of alveolar volume during ventilation. Additional functions may include retardation of fluid flux into alveoli and modulation of alveolar macrophage

function (see Chapters 2.3, 3.1.9, and 3.1.10). Analyses of lung surfactant recovered in BAL fluid from patients with ARDS or from animal models of acute lung injury demonstrate disturbances of the lung surfactant system. The relevance of these disturbances to the pathophysiology of acute lung injury is suggested by the results of animal experiments in which treatment with exogenous lung surfactant had therapeutic effects.

Analyses of lung surfactant recovered from patients with acute lung injury indicate abnormal composition of the phospholipid fraction. Observations of Ashbaugh et al. (2) on fluid recovered from minced lung tissue obtained post-mortem from two patients with ARDS suggested surfactant dysfunction. Hallman et al. (138) demonstrated a decreased fractional composition of phosphatidylcholine (PC) and phosphatidylglycerol, a depression of the saturated PC/sphingomyelin ratio, and a profound loss of surface activity. Disaturated PC (DSPC) as a fraction of total PC was also reduced. The biochemical abnormalities were present early in the course of acute lung injury and tended to normalize during recovery. Consistent observations come from studies of polytrauma patients (139). Lung surfactant biochemical composition and function in patients with severe respiratory failure were significantly different from those in polytrauma patients with mild respiratory failure or in normal subjects. A low saturated PC/sphingomyelin ratio and undetectable phosphatidylglycerol were also found by Hallman et al. (140) in BAL fluid from two patients with lysinuric protein intolerance (LPI) who developed ARDS. LPI is an inherited disease associated with a defect in epithelial transport of the diamino acids argenine, ornithine, and lysine. Three of 41 Finnish patients with LPI have developed ARDS, strongly suggesting the possibility of a genetic predisposition for acute lung injury.

A deficiency of lung surfactant function is found in a variety of animal models of acute lung injury. Many of these have been developed for evaluation of efficacy of exogenous surfactant replacement. As described by Lachmann (141), these models include injuries secondary to (a) surfactant depletion by lavage, (b) viral and bacterial pneumonia, (c) xanthine oxidase instillation, or (d) mechanical ventilation. Anti-surfactant apoprotein antibodies and *N*-nitroso-*N*-methylurethane have been used to induce acute lung injury (142,143), and hyperoxia is accompanied by acute lung injury that exogenous lung surfactant partially prevents or treats (144). King et al. (145) have reviewed data on surfactant composition and function that come from a variety of animal models of acute lung injury. They note that in all studies using small animals, DSPC, as a fraction of total PC, is unchanged, whereas baboons with acute lung injury secondary to hyperoxia or humans with ARDS have a marked decrease in DSPC as a fraction of total PC. Such differences underscore the difficulties of interpretation of data from animal models.

There are multiple ways in which events associated with acute lung injury may affect the lung surfactant system: Quantitative and qualitative abnormalities of surfactant synthesis by injured or hyperplastic epithelial type II cells may exist; biochemical changes of lung surfactant in the alveolar space may result from lipid peroxidation or apoprotein cleavage; inhibitors of surfactant function may be present; and lung surfactant clearance mechanisms may be perturbed.

Hyperoxia is both a cause of diffuse alveolar damage and a frequent necessity in the clinical care of patients with acute lung injury (see Chapter 8.2.2). Studies of type II cells isolated from rabbits exposed to 100% O_2 demonstrate depressed phospholipid biosynthesis (146). The effect may be indirect, however, because exposure of type II cells to hyperoxia *in vitro* has only minor effects on lipid metabolism (147).

During acute lung injury, toxic oxygen products and macrophage proteases are present in the distal lung. Preliminary data suggest that oxidation of lung surfactant phospholipids may result in loss of surface activity as determined both *in vitro* and *in vivo* (148). In addition, both collagenase and human neutrophil elastase have been shown to cleave surfactant apoprotein A with *in vitro* loss of surface activity after exposure of surfactant to elastase. Neutrophil elastase may also attack hydrophobic apoproteins with associated loss of function (149,150). Given the potential for PMNs to alter lung surfactant function in the inflamed lung, it is not surprising that a preliminary report documents a decrement of surfactant surface activity induced *in vitro* by exposure to activated PMNs (151).

Although functional parameters of surface activity are abnormal in surfactant purified from lavage fluid of patients with ARDS, those parameters are markedly more abnormal when equimolar amounts of phospholipid are examined in the original lavage fluid. Multiple species that may be present in lung epithelial lining fluid have been shown to inhibit surfactant function. These include: glycolipid, albumin, hemoglobin, fibrin monomer, and bilirubin (reviewed in ref. 152).

Therapeutic Considerations

Given the many reasons to suspect surfactant dysfunction in the lungs of patients with ARDS, it is reasonable to postulate that this dysfunction may contribute to the pathophysiology of the syndrome. To overcome lack of surfactant function, both stimulation of surfactant secretion and addition of exogenous surfactant to the lung have been proposed as rational interventions. Animal experiments have not supported the former approach, and the latter efforts are currently under clinical investigation (141,152).

CONCLUSION

The study of acute lung injury has provided a fertile field for investigators from a variety of disciplines. The association between certain clinical exposures and the development of ARDS has stimulated research at many levels. For example, because exposure of animals to agents such as LPS or oxygen results in reproducible acute lung injury, it is productive to study the consequences of hyperoxia or LPS to the patient, the experimental animal, the perfused lung, the cultured cell, or the molecule in solution. Integrating the results of these studies to enhance understanding of acute lung injury is an ongoing task. The problem is complicated by the likelihood that "acute lung injury" is almost certainly not a single event, but rather a common outcome of many different biochemical events. Conversely, an apparently common stimulus may result in diverse effects. This diversity is exemplified by septic patients, who may develop diffuse pulmonary and systemic edema and multiorgan system failure, or may only experience failure of only a single organ—the lung.

Study of the products of cells present in the inflamed lung has opened a virtual Pandora's box of mediators. A central challenge to the understanding of acute lung injury is to make sense not only of the vast number of cell products that may participate in acute lung injury, but also of their potential interactions. It is likely that the profound synergistic effects of agents that prime PMNs, for example, are of true clinical importance. Thus, study of acute lung injury must heed observations from cell biology. Sensitive endpoints to evaluate the effect of complex and multiple interventions are required. Past experience has demonstrated that application of a single powerful anti-inflammatory agent is unlikely to produce a significant difference in clinical mortality. Rather, successful intervention is likely to require multiple agents to interrupt the variety of interconnected self-amplifying systems that appear to participate in acute lung injury.

REFERENCES

1. Brewer LA, Burbank B, Samson PC, Schiff CA. The "wet lung" in war casualties. *Ann Surg* 1946;123:343–362.
2. Ashbaugh DG, Bigelow DB, Petty TL, Levine BE. Acute respiratory distress in adults. *Lancet* 1967;2:319–323.
3. Holter JF, Weiland JE, Pacht ER, Gadek JE, Davis WB. Protein permeability in the adult respiratory distress syndrome: loss of size selectivity of the alveolar epithelium. *J Clin Invest* 1986;78:1513–1522.
4. Bachofen M, Weibel ER. Structural alterations of lung paren-

chyma in the adult respiratory distress syndrome. *Clin Chest Med* 1982;3:35–56.

5. Schlag G, Voigt W-H, Schnells G, Glatzl A. Vergleichende Untersuchungen der Ultrastrucktur von menschlicher Lunge und Skeletmuskulatur im Schock. II. *Anaesthesist* 1977;26:612–622.

6. Zapol WM, Jones R. Vascular components of ARDS. Clinical pulmonary hemodynamics and morphology. *Am Rev Respir Dis* 1987;136:471–474.

7. Pratt PC, Vollmer RT, Shelburne JD, Crapo JD. Pulmonary morphology in a multihospital collaborative extracorporeal membrane oxygenation project. *Am J Pathol* 1979;95:191–214.

8. Zapol WM, Trelstad RL, Coffey JW, Tsai I, Salvador RA. Pulmonary fibrosis in severe acute respiratory failure. *Am Rev Respir Dis* 1979;119:547–554.

9. Katzenstein A-L, Bloor CM, Leibow AA. Diffuse alveolar damage—the role of oxygen, shock, and related factors. *Am J Pathol* 1976;85:210–228.

10. Wright PE, Bernard GR. The role of airflow resistance in patients with the adult respiratory distress syndrome. *Am Rev Respir Dis* 1989;139:1169–1174.

11. Lee CT, Fein AM, Lippman M, Holtzmann H, Kimbel P, Wienbaum G. Elastolytic activity in pulmonary lavage fluid from patients with adult respiratory distress syndrome. *N Engl J Med* 1981;304:192–196.

12. McGuire WW, Spragg RG, Cohen AB, Cochrane CG. Studies on the pathogenesis of the adult respiratory distress syndrome. *J Clin Invest* 1982;69:543–553.

13. Weiland JE, Davis WB, Holter JF, Mohammed JR, Dorinsky PM, Gadek JE. Lung neutrophils in the adult respiratory distress syndrome: clinical and pathophysiologic significance. *Am Rev Respir Dis* 1986;133:218–225.

14. Ognibene FP, Martin SE, Parker MM, et al. Adult respiratory distress syndrome in patients with severe neutropenia. *N Engl J Med* 1986;315:547–551.

15. Sariban E, Sitaras NM, Antoniades HN, Kufe DW, Pantazis P. Expression of platelet-derived growth factor (PDGF)-related transcripts and synthesis of biologically active PDGF-like proteins by human malignant epithelial cell lines. *J Clin Invest* 1988;82:1157–1164.

16. Standiford TJ, Kunkel SL, Basha MA, Lynch JP III, Toews GB, Strieter RM. Human alveolar macrophage induced gene expression of neutrophil chemotactic factor/interleukin-8 from pulmonary epithelial cells. *Clin Res* 1990;38:139A.

17. Butler GB, Adler KB, Evans JN, Morgan DW, Szarek JL. Modulation of rabbit airway smooth muscle responsiveness by respiratory epithelium. *Am Rev Respir Dis* 1987;135:1099–1104.

18. Strieter RM, Kunkel SL, Showell HJ, et al. Endothelial cell gene expression of a neutrophil chemotactic factor by TNF-alpha, LPS, and IL-1 beta. *Science* 1989;243:1467–1469.

19. Libby P, Ordovas JM, Auger KR, Robbins AH, Birinyi LK, Dinarello CA. Endotoxin and tumor necrosis factor induce interleukin-1 gene expression in adult human vascular endothelial cells. *Am J Pathol* 1986;124:179–185.

20. Stephenson AH, Lonigro AJ, Hyers TM, Webster RO, Fowler AA. Increased concentrations of leukotrienes in bronchoalveolar lavage fluid of patients with ARDS or at risk for ARDS. *Am Rev Respir Dis* 1988;138:714–719.

21. Hetland G, Johnson E, Aasebo U. Human alveolar macrophages synthesize the functional alternative pathway of complement and active C5 and C9 *in vitro*. *Scand J Immunol* 1986;24:603–608.

22. Senior RM, Skogen WF, Griffin GL, Wilner GD. Effects of fibrinogen derivatives upon the inflammatory response. Studies with human fibrinopeptide B. *J Clin Invest* 1986;77:1014–1019.

23. Senior RM, Griffin GL, Mecham RP. Chemotactic activity of elastin-derived peptides. *J Clin Invest* 1980;66:859–862.

24. Riley DJ, Berg RA, Soltys RA, et al. Neutrophil response following intratracheal instillation of collagen peptides into rat lungs. *Exp Lung Res* 1988;14:549–563.

25. Cochrane CG, Spragg R, Revak SD. Pathogenesis of the adult respiratory distress syndrome. Evidence of oxidant activity in bronchoalveolar lavage fluid. *J Clin Invest* 1983;71:754–761.

26. Stockley RA, Shaw J, Afford SC, Morrison HM, Burnett D. Effect of alpha-1-proteinase inhibitor on neutrophil chemotaxis. *Am J Respir Cell Mol Biol* 1990;2:163–170.

27. Hammerschmidt DE, Weaver LJ, Hudson LD, Craddock PR, Jacob HS. Association of complement activation and elevated plasma-C5a with adult respiratory distress syndrome. Pathophysiological relevance and possible prognostic value. *Lancet* 1980;1:947–949.

28. Duchateau J, Haas M, Schreyen H, et al. Complement activation in patients at risk of developing the adult respiratory distress syndrome. *Am Rev Respir Dis* 1984;130:1058–1064.

29. Weinberg PF, Matthay MA, Webster RO, Roskos KV, Goldstein IM, Murray JF. Biologically active products of complement and acute lung injury in patients with the sepsis syndrome. *Am Rev Respir Dis* 1984;130:791–796.

30. Pober JS, Gimbrone MA Jr, Lapierre LA, et al. Overlapping patterns of activation of human endothelial cells by interleukin 1, tumor necrosis factor, and immune interferon. *J Immunol* 1986;137:1893–1896.

31. Bevilacqua MP, Pober JS, Mendrick DL, Cotran RS, Gimbrone MA Jr. Identification of an inducible endothelial–leukocyte adhesion molecule. *Proc Natl Acad Sci USA* 1987;84:9238–9242.

32. Gimbrone MA Jr, Obin MS, Brock AF, et al. Endothelial interleukin-8: a novel inhibitor of leukocyte–endothelial interactions. *Science* 1989;246:1601–1603.

33. Ismail G, Morganroth ML, Todd RF 3d, Boxer LA. Prevention of pulmonary injury in isolated perfused rat lungs by activated human neutrophils preincubated with anti-Mo1 monoclonal antibody. *Blood* 1987;69:1167–1174.

34. Arfors K-E, Lundberg C, Lindbom L, Lundberg K, Beatty PG, Harlan JM. A monoclonal antibody to the membrane glycoprotein complex CD18 inhibits polymorphonuclear leukocyte accumulation and plasma leakage *in vivo*. *Blood* 1987;69:338–340.

35. Diener AM, Beatty PG, Ochs HD, Harlan JM. The role of neutrophil membrane glycoprotein 150 (GP 150) in neutrophil-mediated endothelial cell injury *in vitro*. *J Immunol* 1985;135:537–543.

36. Ishizaka A, Hatherill JR, Harada H, et al. Prevention of interleukin 2-induced acute lung injury in guinea pigs by pentoxifylline. *J Appl Physiol* 1989;67:2432–2437.

37. Lilly CM, Sandhu JS, Ishizaka A, et al. Pentoxifylline prevents tumor necrosis factor-induced lung injury. *Am Rev Respir Dis* 1989;139:1361–1368.

38. Hand WL, Butera ML, King-Thompson NL, Hand DL. Pentoxifylline modulation of plasma membrane functions in human polymorphonuclear leukocytes. *Infect Immun* 1989;57:3520–3526.

39. Bessler H, Gilgal R, Djaldetti M, Zahavi I. Effect of pentoxifylline on the phagocytic activity, cAMP levels, and superoxide anion production by monocytes and polymorphonuclear cells. *J Leukocyte Biol* 1986;40:747–754.

40. Harada H, Ishizaka A, Yonemaru M, et al. The effects of aminophylline and pentoxifylline on multiple organ damage after *Escherichia coli* sepsis. *Am Rev Respir Dis* 1989;140:974–980.

41. Baldwin SR, Simon RH, Grum CM, Ketai LH, Boxer LA, Devall LJ. Oxidant activity in expired breath of patients with adult respiratory distress syndrome. *Lancet* 1986;1:11–14.

42. Johnson D, Travis J. The oxidative inactivation of human alpha 1-proteinase inhibitor: further evidence for methionine at the reactive center. *J Biol Chem* 1979;254:4022–4026.

43. Wewers MD, Herzyk DJ, Gadek JE. Alveolar fluid neutrophil elastase activity in the adult respiratory distress syndrome is complexed to alpha-2-macroglobulin. *J Clin Invest* 1988;82:1260–1267.

44. Tate RM, Vanbenthuysen KM, Shasby DM, McMurtry IF, Repine JE. Oxygen-radical-mediated permeability edema and vasoconstriction in isolated perfused rabbit lungs. *Am Rev Respir Dis* 1982;126:802–806.

45. del Maestro RF, Bjork J, Arfors KE. Increase in microvascular permeability induced by enzymatically generated free radicals. II. Role of superoxide anion radical, hydrogen peroxide, and hydroxyl radical. *Microvasc Res* 1981;22:255–270.

46. Johnson KJ, Fantone JC 3d, Kaplan J, Ward PA. *In vivo* damage of rat lungs by oxygen metabolites. *J Clin Invest* 1981;67:983–993.

47. Hyslop PA, Hinshaw DB, Halsey WA Jr, et al. Mechanisms of oxidant-mediated cell injury. The glycolytic and mitochondrial pathways of ADP phosphorylation are major intracellular targets inactivated by hydrogen peroxide. *J Biol Chem* 1988;263:1665–1675.

48. Schraufstatter IU, Hyslop PA, Hinshaw DB, Spragg RG, Sklar LA, Cochrane CG. Hydrogen peroxide-induced injury of cells and its prevention by inhibitors of poly(ADP-ribose) polymerase. *Proc Natl Acad Sci USA* 1986;83:4908–4912.

49. Spragg RG, Hinshaw DB, Hyslop PA, Schraufstatter IU, Cochrane CG. Alterations in adenosine triphosphate and energy charge in cultured endothelial and P388D1 cells after oxidant injury. *J Clin Invest* 1985;76:1471–1476.

50. Andreoli SP. Mechanisms of endothelial cell ATP depletion after oxidant injury. *Pediatr Res* 1989;25:97–101.

51. Weiss SJ. Tissue destruction by neutrophils. *N Engl J Med* 1989;320:365–376.

52. Shasby DM, Vanbenthuysen KM, Tate RM, Shasby SS, McMurtry I, Repine JE. Granulocytes mediate acute edematous lung injury in rabbits and in isolated rabbit lungs perfused with phorbol myristate acetate: role of oxygen radicals. *Am Rev Respir Dis* 1982;125:443–447.

53. Nathan CF, Murray HW, Wiebe ME, Rubin BY. Identification of interferon-gamma as the lymphokine that activates human macrophage oxidative metabolism and antimicrobial activity. *J Exp Med* 1983;158:670–689.

54. Carlsen E, Prydz H. Activation of monocytes—more than one process. Differential effect of cytokines on monocytes. *Scand J Immunol* 1988;27:401–444.

55. Jacobs RF, Kiel DP, Balk RA. Alveolar macrophage function in a canine model of endotoxin-induced lung injury. *Am Rev Respir Dis* 1986;134:745–751.

56. Brieland JK, Kunkel RG, Fantone JC. Pulmonary alveolar macrophage function during acute inflammatory lung injury. *Am Rev Respir Dis* 1987;135:1300–1306.

57. Drath DB. Enhanced superoxide release and tumoricidal activity by a postlavage, *in situ* pulmonary macrophage population in response to activation by *Mycobacterium bovis* BCG exposure. *Infect Immun* 1985;49:72–75.

58. McPhail LC, Snyderman R. Activation of the respiratory burst oxidase in human polymorphonuclear leukocytes by chemoattractants and other soluble stimuli. Evidence that the same oxidase is activated by different transductional mechanisms. *J Clin Invest* 1983;72:192–200.

59. McPhail LC, Clayton CC, Snyderman R. The NADPH oxidase of human polymorphonuclear leukocytes. Evidence for regulation by multiple signals. *J Biol Chem* 1984;259:5768–5775.

60. Vercellotti GM, Yin HQ, Gustafson KS, Nelson RD, Jacob HS. Platelet-activating factor primes neutrophil responses to agonists: role in promoting neutrophil-mediated endothelial damage. *Blood* 1988;71:1100–1107.

61. She ZW, Wewers MD, Herzyk DJ, Sagone AL, Davis WB. Tumor necrosis factor primes neutrophils for hypochlorous acid production. *Am J Physiol* 1989;257:L338–L345.

62. Matsubara T, Ziff M. Superoxide anion release by human endothelial cells: synergism between a phorbol ester and a calcium ionophore. *J Cell Physiol* 1986;127:207–210.

63. Zweier JL, Flaherty JT, Weisfeldt ML. Direct measurement of free radical generation following reperfusion of ischemic myocardium. *Proc Natl Acad Sci USA* 1987;84:1404–1407.

64. Gorog P, Pearson JD, Kakkar VV. Generation of reactive oxygen metabolites by phagocytosing endothelial cells. *Atherosclerosis* 1988;72:19–27.

65. Akaike T, Ando M, Oda T, et al. Dependence on O_2^- generation by xanthine oxidase of pathogenesis of influenza virus infection in mice. *J Clin Invest* 1990;85:739–745.

66. Heffner JE, Repine JE. Pulmonary strategies of antioxidant defense. *Am Rev Respir Dis* 1989;140:531–554.

67. Cohen AB, MacArthur C, Idell S, et al. A peptide from alveolar macrophages that releases neutrophil enzymes into the lungs

68. McDonald JA, Kelley DG. Degradation of fibronectin by human leukocyte elastase. Release of biologically active fragments. *J Biol Chem* 1980;255:8848–8858.

69. Gadek JE, Fells GA, Wright DG, Crystal RG. Human neutrophil elastase functions as a type III collagen collagenase. *Biochem Biophys Res Commun* 1980;95:1815–1822.

70. Mainardi CL, Dixit SN, Kang AH. Degradation of type IV (basement membrane) collagen by a proteinase isolated from human polymorphonuclear leukocyte granules. *J Biol Chem* 1980;255:5435–5441.

71. Gadek JE, Klein HG, Holland PV, Crystal RG. Replacement therapy of alpha 1-antitrypsin deficiency. Reversal of protease-antiprotease imbalance within the alveolar structures of PiZ subjects. *J Clin Invest* 1981;68:1158–1165.

72. Werb Z, Gordon S. Secretion of a specific collagenase by stimulated macrophages. *J Exp Med* 1975;142:346–360.

73. Vissers MC, George PM, Bathurst IC, Brennan SO, Winterbourn CC. Cleavage and inactivation of alpha-1-antitrypsin by metalloproteinases released from neutrophils. *J Clin Invest* 1988;82:706–711.

74. Idell S, Kucich U, Fein A, et al. Neutrophil elastase-releasing factors in bronchoalveolar lavage from patients with adult respiratory distress syndrome. *Am Rev Respir Dis* 1985;132:1098–1105.

75. Morgan L, Kucich U, Dershaw B, et al. Elastin degradation in the adult respiratory distress syndrome. *Am Rev Respir Dis* 1983;127:A93.

76. Senior RM, Tegner J, Kuhn C, Ohlsson K, Starcher BC, Pierce JA. The induction of pulmonary emphysema with human leukocyte elastase. *Am Rev Respir Dis* 1977;116:469–475.

77. Christner P, Fein A, Goldberg S, Lippmann M, Abrams W, Weinbaum G. Collagenase in the lower respiratory tract of patients with adult respiratory distress syndrome. *Am Rev Respir Dis* 1985;131:690–695.

78. Smith RM, Traber LD, Traber DL, Spragg RG. Pulmonary deposition and clearance of aerosolized alpha-1-proteinase inhibitor administered to dogs and to sheep. *J Clin Invest* 1989;84:1145–1154.

79. Hubbard RC, Casolaro MA, Mitchell M, et al. Fate of aerosolized recombinant DNA-produced alpha$_1$-antitrypsin: use of the epithelial surface of the lower respiratory tract to administer proteins of therapeutic importance. *Proc Natl Acad Sci USA* 1989;86:680–684.

80. Matthay MA, Eschenbacher WL, Goetzl EJ. Elevated concentrations of leukotriene D$_4$ in pulmonary edema fluid of patients with the adult respiratory distress syndrome. *J Clin Immunol* 1984;4:479–483.

81. Deby-Dupont G, Braun M, Lamy M, et al. Thromboxane and prostacyclin release in adult respiratory distress syndrome. *Intensive Care Med* 1987;13:167–174.

82. Voelkel NF, Stenmark KR, Westcott JY, Chang S. Lung eicosanoid metabolism. *Clin Chest Med* 1990;10:95–105.

83. Westcott JY, McDonnell TJ, Voelkel NF. Alveolar transfer and metabolism of eicosanoids in the rat. *Am Rev Respir Dis* 1989;139:80–87.

84. Chang SW, Westcott JY, Pickett WC, Murphy RC, Voelkel NF. Endotoxin-induced lung injury in rats: role of eicosanoids. *J Appl Physiol* 1989;66:2407–2418.

85. Parratt JR, Pacitti N, Rodger IW. Mediators of acute lung injury in endotoxaemia. *Prog Clin Biol Res* 1989;308:357–369.

86. Berry EM, Edmonds JF, Wyllie H. Release of prostaglandin E2 and unidentified factors from ventilated lungs. *Br J Surg* 1971;58:189–192.

87. Henderson WR Jr. Lipid-derived and other chemical mediators of inflammation in the lung. *J Allergy Clin Immunol* 1987;79:543–553.

88. Peters-Golden M, Thebert P. Inhibition by methylprednisolone of zymosan-induced leukotriene synthesis in alveolar macrophages. *Am Rev Respir Dis* 1987;135:1020–1026.

89. Wallner BP, Mattaliano RJ, Hession C, et al. Cloning and expression of human lipocortin: a phospholipase A$_2$ inhibitor

in patients with the adult respiratory distress syndrome. *Am Rev Respir Dis* 1988;137:1151–1158.

with potential anti-inflammatory activity. *Nature* 1986;320:77–81.

90. Bernard GR, Luce JM, Sprung CL, et al. High-dose corticosteroids in patients with the adult respiratory distress syndrome. *N Engl J Med* 1987;317:1565–1570.

91. Bone RC, Fisher CJ Jr, Clemmer TP, Slotman GJ, Metz CA, Balk RA. A controlled clinical trial of high-dose methylprednisolone in the treatment of severe sepsis and septic shock. *N Engl J Med* 1987;317:653–658.

92. Luce JM, Montgomery AB, Marks JD, Turner J, Metz CA, Murray JF. Ineffectiveness of high-dose methylprednisolone in preventing parenchymal lung injury and improving mortality in patients with septic shock. *Am Rev Respir Dis* 1988;138:62–68.

93. Mélot C, Lejeune P, Leeman M, Moraine JJ, Naeije R. Prostaglandin E1 in the adult respiratory distress syndrome benefit for pulmonary hypertension and cost for pulmonary gas exchange. *Am Rev Respir Dis* 1989;139:106–110.

94. Bone RC, Slotman G, Maunder R, et al. Randomized double-blind, multicenter study of prostaglandin E1 in patients with the adult respiratory distress syndrome Prostaglandin E1 Study Group. *Chest* 1989;96:114–119.

95. Voelkel NF, Worthen S, Reeves JT, Henson PM, Murphy RC. Nonimmunological production of leukotrienes induced by platelet-activating factor. *Science* 1982;218:286–289.

96. Lin AH, Morton DR, Gorman RR. Acetyl glyceryl ether phosphorylcholine stimulates leukotriene B4 synthesis in human polymorphonuclear leukocytes. *J Clin Invest* 1982;70:1058–1065.

97. Braquet P, Hosford D. The potential role of platelet activating factor (PAF) in shock, sepsis and adult respiratory distress syndrome (ARDS). *Prog Clin Biol Res* 1989;308:425–439.

98. McManus LM, Deavers SI. Platelet activating actor in pulmonary pathobiology. *Clin Chest Med* 1989;10:107–118.

99. Dinarello CA. Interleukin-1 and its biologically related cytokines. *Adv Immunol* 1989;44:153–205.

100. Sullivan GW, Carper HT, Sullivan JA, Murata T, Mandell GL. Both recombinant interleukin-1 (beta) and purified human monocyte interleukin-1 prime human neutrophils for increased oxidative activity and promote neutrophil spreading. *J Leukoc Biol* 1989;45:389–395.

101. Siler TM, Swierkosz JE, Hyers TM, Fowler AA, Webster RO. Immunoreactive interleukin-1 in bronchoalveolar lavage fluid of high-risk patients and patients with the adult respiratory distress syndrome. *Exp Lung Res* 1989;15:881–894.

102. Jacobs RF, Tabor DR, Burks AW, Campbell GD. Elevated interleukin-1 release by human alveolar macrophages during the adult respiratory distress syndrome. *Am Rev Respir Dis* 1989;140:1686–1692.

103. Stephens KE, Ishizaka A, Larrick JW, Raffin TA. Tumor necrosis factor causes increased pulmonary permeability and edema. *Am Rev Respir Dis* 1988;137:1364–1370.

104. Tracey KJ, Beutler B, Lowry SF, et al. Shock and tissue injury induced by recombinant human cachectin. *Science* 1986;234:470–474.

105. Beutler B, Milsark IW, Cerami A. Passive immunization against cachectin/tumor necrosis factor protects mice from the lethal effect of endotoxin. *Science* 1985;229:869–871.

106. Mathison JC, Wolfson E, Ulevitch RJ. Participation of tumor necrosis factor in the mediation of gram negative bacterial lipopolysaccharide induced injury in rabbits. *J Clin Invest* 1988;81:1925–1937.

107. Tracey KJ, Fong Y, Hesse DG. Anti-cachectin/TNF monoclonal antibodies prevent septic shock during lethal bacteremia. *Nature* 1987;330:662–664.

108. Hart PH, Whitty GA, Piccoli DS, Hamilton JA. Control by IFN- and PGE2 of TNF and IL-1 production by human monocytes. *Immunology* 1989;66:376–383.

109. Billiau A. Not just cachectin is involved in toxic shock. *Nature* 1988;331:665–668.

110. Marks JD, Berman C, Luce JM, et al. Plasma tumor necrosis factor in patients with septic shock. *Am Rev Respir Dis* 1990;141:94–97.

111. Millar AB, Singer M, Meager A, Foley NM, Johnson NM, Rook GAW. Tumour necrosis factor in bronchopulmonary secretions of patients with adult respiratory distress syndrome. *Lancet* 1989;2:712–714.

112. Roberts DJ, Davies JM, Evans CC, Bell M, Mostafa SM. Tumour necrosis factor and adult respiratory distress syndrome. *Lancet* 1989;2:1043–1044.

113. Beutler B, Krochin N, Milsark IW, Luedke C, Cerami A. Control of cachectin (tumor necrosis factor) synthesis: mechanisms of endotoxin resistance. *Science* 1986;232:977–980.

114. Ishizaka A, Hatherill JR, Harada H, et al. Prevention of interleukin 2-induced acute lung injury in guinea pigs by pentoxifylline. *J Appl Physiol* 1989;67:2432–2437.

115. Baggiolini M, Walz A, Kunkel SL. Neutrophil-activating peptide-1/interleukin-8, a novel cytokine that activates neutrophils. *J Clin Invest* 1989;84:1045–1049.

116. Pontoppidan J, Huttemeier PC, Quinn DA. Etiology, demography, and outcome. In: Zapol WM, Falke KJ, eds. *Acute respiratory failure.* New York: Marcel Dekker, 1985;1–22.

117. King RJ, Jones MB, Minoo P. Regulation of lung cell proliferation by polypeptide growth factors. *Am J Physiol* 1989;257:L23–L38.

118. Fabisiak JP, Evans JN, Kelley J. Increased expression of PDGF-B (c-sis) mRNA in rat lung precedes DNA synthesis and tissue repair during chronic hyperoxia. *Am J Respir Cell Mol Biol* 1989;1:181–189.

119. Martinet Y, Rom WN, Grotendorst GR, Martin GR, Crystal RG. Exaggerated spontaneous release of platelet-derived growth factor by alveolar macrophages from patients with idiopathic pulmonary fibrosis. *N Engl J Med* 1987;317:202–209.

120. Carvalho AC. Blood alterations during ARDS. In: Zapol WM, Falke KJ, eds. *Acute respiratory failure.* New York: Marcel Dekker, 1985;303–346.

121. Bone RC, Francis PB, Pierce AK. Intravascular coagulation associated with the adult respiratory distress syndrome. *Am J Med* 1976;61:585–589.

122. Bagge L, Haglund O, Wallin R, Borg T, Modig J. Differences in coagulation and fibrinolysis after traumatic and septic shock in man. *Scand J Clin Lab Invest* 1989;49:63–72.

123. Carvalho AC, DeMarinis S, Scott CF, Silver LD, Schmaier AH, Colman RW. Activation of the contact system of plasma proteolysis in the adult respiratory distress syndrome. *J Lab Clin Med* 1988;112:270–277.

124. Moalli R, Doyle JM, Tahhan HR, Hasan FM, Braman SS, Saldeen T. Fibrinolysis in critically ill patients. *Am Rev Respir Dis* 1989;140:287–293.

125. Garcia Frade LJ, Landin L, Avello AG, et al. Changes in fibrinolysis in the intensive care patient. *Thromb Res* 1987;47:593–599.

126. Hill JD, Ratliff JL, Parrott JCW, et al. Pulmonary pathology in acute respiratory insufficiency: lung biopsy as a diagnostic tool. *J Thorac Cardiovasc Surg* 1976;71:64–72.

127. Tomashefski JF Jr, Davies P, Boggis C, Greene R, Zapol WM, Reid LM. The pulmonary vascular lesions of the adult respiratory distress syndrome. *Am J Pathol* 1983;112:112–126.

128. Schneider RC, Zapol WM, Carvalho AC. Platelet consumption and sequestration in severe acute respiratory failure. *Am Rev Respir Dis* 1980;122:445–451.

129. Bayley T, Clements JA, Osbahr AJ. Pulmonary and circulatory effects of fibrinopeptides. *Circ Res* 1967;21:469–485.

130. Manwaring D, Curreri PW. Platelet and neutrophil sequestration after fragment D-induced respiratory distress. *Circ Shock* 1982;9:75–80.

131. Manwaring D, Thorning D, Curreri PW. Mechanisms of acute pulmonary dysfunction induced by fibrinogen degradation product D. *Surgery* 1978;84:45–54.

132. Haynes JB, Hyers TM, Giclas PC, Franks JJ, Petty TL. Elevated fibrin(ogen) degradation products in the adult respiratory distress syndrome. *Am Rev Respir Dis* 1980;122:841–847.

133. Kazura JW, Wenger JD, Salata RA, Budzynski AZ, Goldsmith GH. Modulation of polymorphonuclear leukocyte microbicidal activity and oxidative metabolism by fibrinogen degradation products D and E. *J Clin Invest* 1989;83:1916–1924.

134. Lo SK, Lai L, Cooper JA, Malik AB. Thrombin-induced gen-

eration of neutrophil activating factors in blood. *Am J Pathol* 1988;130:22–32.

135. Binder AS, Kageler W, Perel A, Flick MR, Staub NC. Effect of platelet depletion on lung vascular permeability after microemboli in sheep. *J Appl Physiol* 1980;48:414–420.

136. Binder AS, Nakahara K, Ohkuda K, Kageler W, Staub NC. Effect of heparin or fibrinogen depletion on lung fluid balance in sheep after emboli. *J Appl Physiol* 1979;47:213–219.

137. Idell S, James KK, Levin EG, et al. Local abnormalities in coagulation and fibrinolytic pathways predispose to alveolar fibrin deposition in the adult respiratory distress syndrome. *J Clin Invest* 1989;84:695–705.

138. Hallman M, Spragg RG, Harrell JH, Moser KM, Gluck L. Evidence of lung surfactant abnormality in respiratory failure: study of bronchoalveolar lavage phospholipids, surface activity, phospholipase activity, and plasma myoinositol. *J Clin Invest* 1982;70:673–683.

139. Pison U, Seeger W, Buchhorn R, et al. Surfactant abnormalities in patients with respiratory failure after multiple trauma. *Am Rev Respir Dis* 1989;140:1033–1039.

140. Hallman M, Maasilta P, Sipila I, Tahvanainen J. Composition and function of pulmonary surfactant in adult respiratory distress syndrome. *Eur Respir J [Suppl]* 1989;3:104s–108s.

141. Lachmann B. Surfactant replacement in acute respiratory failure: Animal studies and first clinical trials. In: Lachmann B, ed. *Surfactant replacement therapy.* New York: Springer-Verlag, 1987;212–223.

142. Suzuki Y, Robertson B, Fujita Y, Grossmann G. Respiratory failure in mice caused by a hybridoma making antibodies to the 15 kDa surfactant apoprotein. *Acta Anaesthesiol Scand* 1988;32:283–289.

143. Liau DF, Barrett CR, Bell AL, Ryan SF. Normal surface prop-erties of phosphatidylglycerol-deficient surfactant from dog after acute lung injury. *J Lipid Res* 1985;26:1338–1344.

144. Holm BA, Matalon S. Role of pulmonary surfactant in the development and treatment of adult respiratory distress syndrome. *Anesth Analg* 1989;69:805–818.

145. King RJ, Coalson JJ, Seidenfeld JJ, Anzueto AR, Smith DB, Peters JI. O_2- and pneumonia-induced lung injury. II. Properties of pulmonary surfactant. *J Appl Physiol* 1989;67:357–365.

146. Holm BA, Matalon S, Finkelstein JN, Notter RH. Type II pneumocyte changes during hyperoxic lung injury and recovery. *J Appl Physiol* 1988;65:2672–2678.

147. Haagsman HP, Schuurmans EA, Batenburg JJ, van Golde LM. Phospholipid synthesis in isolated alveolar type II cells exposed *in vitro* to paraquat and hyperoxia. *Biochem J* 1987;245:119–126.

148. Gilliard N, Heldt G, Merritt TA, Pappert D, Spragg RG. Functional consequences of porcine lung surfactant oxidation. *Am Rev Respir Dis* 1990;141:A365.

149. Pison U, Tam EK, Caughey GH, Hawgood S. Proteolytic inactivation of dog lung surfactant-associated proteins by neutrophil elastase. *Biochim Biophys Acta* 1989;992:251–257.

150. Haagsman HP, Hawgood S, Sargeant T, et al. The major lung surfactant protein, SP 28–36, is a calcium-dependent, carbohydrate-binding protein. *J Biol Chem* 1987;262:13877–13880.

151. Ryan S, Ghassibi Y, Liau D. Effects of neutrophils on surfactant. *Chest* 1989;95(Suppl):30A.

152. Spragg RG, Richman P, Gilliard N, Merritt TA. The future for surfactant therapy of the adult respiratory distress syndrome. In: Lachmann B, ed. *Surfactant replacement therapy.* New York: Springer-Verlag, 1987;203–211.

THE LUNG: Scientific Foundations
edited by R.G. Crystal, J.B. West et al.
Raven Press, Ltd., New York © 1991.

CHAPTER 7.7.3.2

Parenchymal Changes

Marianne Bachofen and Hans Bachofen

The deliberately chosen nonspecific term "acute lung injury" denotes diffuse alterations of lung parenchyma showing rather uniform clinical and morphologic features regardless of a large variety of different etiologies (1–5). In the early state, the hallmark is an interstitial and alveolar edema owing to damage of the delicate endothelial and epithelial cell layers of the gas-exchange apparatus (i.e., a leaky air–blood barrier) (3,6). This high-permeability edema is associated with signs (in particular, a conspicuous accumulation and sequestration of leukocytes) of an inflammatory process of variable intensity (2,7–9). The analysis of lung pathomorphology does not reveal whether the overt damage of the air–blood barrier is caused or followed by an inflammatory process involving leukocytes, platelets, complement, proteolytic enzymes, oxygen free radicals, products of arachidonic acid, and probably many other mechanisms. Both tissue injury and inflammation impair lung function: If eventually the functional derangements meet the so far stringent clinical criteria, and congestive heart failure can be excluded, the term "adult respiratory distress syndrome" (ARDS) will be used (10,11).

The acute lung injury may subside by swift repair of the damage, especially in patients without multiple organ failure. Often, however, it is followed by subacute or chronic stages that mirror the ongoing inflammatory process and tissue reaction to injury. Epithelial transformation, distinct alveolar septal thickening by cell proliferation, and infiltration with a variety of in-

terstitial cells are characteristic, finally ending up in a progressive interstitial and intra-alveolar fibrosis.

Yet the transition from the acute to the subacute pattern of changes is gradual and sometimes delayed: Cell proliferation starts while signs of a leaky barrier still prevail; even in far advanced stages, edematous areas may be observed side by side with fibrotic regions. The reasons for the differences in the course and evolution of the pathologic process are as yet enigmatic. Possibly, the extent of the initial damage plays a role (12); in human disease, more likely the perpetuation of a vicious circle between inflammation and tissue injury is the predominant mechanism responsible for a delayed and often fatal outcome.

The observations reported on are mainly based on human lung tissue samples (1–3,5,6). This partiality is not to underrate the wealth of information obtained from animal experiments (3,8,13), including possible species differences in the reaction to injurious agents (3,8,14,15), but, instead, to comprehensively illustrate the spectrum of tissue damage underlying human disease.

EARLY PARENCHYMAL CHANGES

The Leaky Air–Blood Barrier

Basic Morphologic Pattern

In tissue samples obtained within 1 or 2 days after manifestation of respiratory failure, the gross architecture of fine lung parenchyma is not seriously deranged. Focal alveolar collapses may occur; predominant, however, are the signs of pulmonary edema and, in many cases, a conspicuous accumulation of inflam-

M. Bachofen: Department of Anesthesiology and Intensive Care, Inselspital, CH-3010 Berne, Switzerland.

H. Bachofen: Department of Medicine, Inselspital, CH-3010 Berne, Switzerland.

matory cells in the intravascular, interstitial, and intra-alveolar spaces.

Alveolar Spaces

The alveoli are inhomogeneously filled with protein-aceous fluid, blood cells, macrophages, cell debris, and remnants of surfactant. In order to appreciate the uneven distribution of edema and the changes in alveolar architecture, the lung tissue must be fixed by vascular perfusion—for example, by introducing the fixative via a Swan–Ganz catheter into the lung (16). At sites with slight or moderate edema, the alveolar exudate accumulates in alveolar corners and in pools between capillaries and folded-up septa (Fig. 1). With increasing edema, alveolar fluid menisci are found which expand between alveolar entrance rings (17). Notably, the free surface is covered by an osmiophilic layer (surfactant)

(Fig. 1), and dense spots of tubular myelin can be observed. Eventually, there are patchy areas of completely filled alveoli, suggesting spatial differences in barrier permeability in spite of diffuse distribution of air- or blood-borne noxious agents. Occasionally, condensed strands of amorphous, fibrin-containing material cover alveolar surfaces, with a predilection for alveolar entrance rings. These so-called hyaline membranes firmly stick to the septum wherever the epithelial lining is destroyed.

Interstitial Spaces

In the acute stage, most interstitial spaces are enlarged by accumulation of a cell-rich fluid, though a difference becomes apparent between the interstitial spaces of the peripheral and the axial connective tissue systems on the one hand and those of the alveolar septa on the

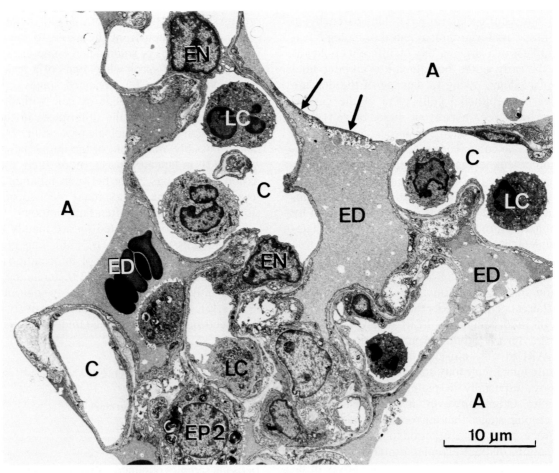

FIG. 1. Electron-microscopic view of perfusion fixed lung parenchyma in a young boy dying with signs of acute ARDS. Alveolar edema (ED) is collected in septal corners and between folded-up septa. Capillaries (C) are devoid of blood, with the exception of sticking leukocytes (LC). Note remnants of surfactant forming a fine osmiophilic layer on the free fluid surface (*arrows*). A, alveolus; EN, endothelial cell; EP2, epithelial type II cell with lamillated bodies. (We are indebted to Dr. G. Wolff for the tissue sample.)

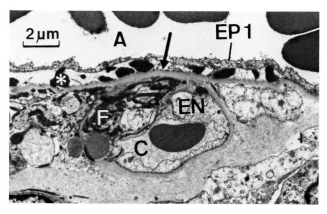

FIG. 2. Section of alveolar septum in the acute stage of ARDS. Fibrin depositions (*asterisk*) remove a squamous epithelial cell extension (EP1) from its fused epithelial and endothelial basement membrane (*arrow*) overlying a capillary (C) with swollen endothelial cells (EN) and sub-endothelial fibrin strands (F).

other hand. In the former, particularly in the connective tissue cuffs around larger vessels and bronchioles, the abundant edema fluid rarely includes migrated blood cells or scraps of fibrin; the parenchymatous connective tissue of the alveolar septum, on the other hand, is engorged predominantly by the extravasation of cellular components. Local fibrin depositions give evidence of an activated coagulation process. Characteristically, the exudate is confined to the thicker part of the septal interstitium, where the endothelial and epithelial basement membranes are separated. In severely damaged lungs, fibrin strands may also be interposed between capillary endothelium or alveolar epithelium and fused basement membrane (Fig. 2); this observation is discussed in more detail below.

Epithelial and Endothelial Cell Layers

Both capillary endothelial and alveolar epithelial cell layers constitute the barrier which, under normal conditions, keeps the lung "dry," whereas the basement membrane is very permeable to liquids, macromolecules, and even cells (18,19). Abundant exudate in the interstitial space suggests an increased endothelial permeability, alveolar edema an additional epithelial leakage. The direct morphologic evidence turns out to be easily obtained for the alveolar lining (Fig. 3). Usually all stages of epithelial damage are visible, ranging from mere cytoplasmic swelling to total cellular destruction, leaving a bare or hyaline-membrane-covered basement membrane. Overt endothelial defects, on the other hand, are much less evident. Even in the immediate vicinity of completely destroyed epithelial cell extensions, separated by the basement membrane only, endothelial linings are usually continuous with

morphologically intact cell junctions (Fig. 3). Focal irregularities of the luminal surface due to cytoplasmic swelling and large vacuoles can be observed. Occasional endothelial defects are usually covered with fibrin depositions alongside complete capillary destructions caused by occluding microthrombi (Fig. 4a). Rarely, endothelial gaps can be observed at sites where blood cells—in particular, leukocytes—are about to escape into the extravascular space (1). The conspicuous discrepancy between the extent of epithelial and endothelial damage is explained by different repair potentials of the two lining layers rather than by a dissimilar reaction to injury. This hypothesis is supported by findings in lung biopsies of patients after severe hypovolemic–traumatic shock, but prior to the development of respiratory distress (20): In these biopsy specimens obtained very shortly after injury, widespread lesions of endothelial cells have been observed, including cytoplasmic swelling, loss of cell organelles, and focal necrosis. The enormous plasticity and high repair capacity of endothelial cells have been demonstrated in numerous animal experiments (21–23); these characteristics are likewise supported by observations in human tissue samples. Focal fibrin deposits and small microthrombi are generally covered by tentacular endothelial cell extensions, and conspicuous fragmentations of endothelial cell layers into multiple, tightly joined segments may be suggestive of a prompt repair of endothelial gaps. In view of the swift endothelial repair documented in animal experiments, it is likely that in our human tissue samples the stage of early lesions and capillary leakage had passed long before the patient died. Nevertheless, the disparity between endothelial and epithelial lesions in human lungs is remarkable, and one might ask whether type I cells of humans are more sensitive than those of sheep and rodents, or whether particular pathways of inflammation or metabolism play a role in humans (24–26).

Alterations Within the Vascular Bed

Small Arteries

Detailed examination of the vascular bed of lungs of patients with acute respiratory failure has shown that the vascular lesions are not restricted to the microvasculature, but that extensive alterations also occur in small extra-alveolar vessels (both arteries and veins) (27–29). Vascular casts revealed widespread stenosis and occlusion of small arteries, resulting in uneven perfusion of lung parenchyma. Interestingly, within the patchy regions with sparse perfusion the peripheral airways and air spaces were patent, suggesting that the obliteration of small vessels might have occurred very early in the disease (i.e., before the development of

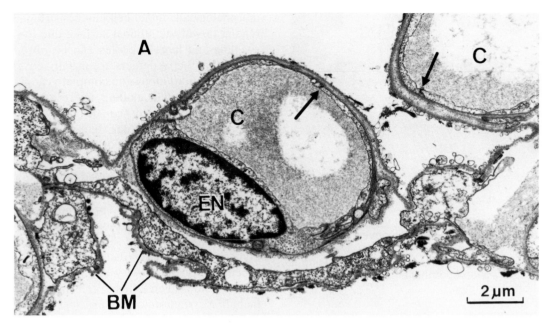

FIG. 3. Alveolar septum of acute ARDS, showing a totally denuded basement membrane (BM) opposite to a well-preserved capillary (C) with morphologically intact endothelial cell junctions (*arrows*). A, alveolar space; EN, endothelial cell.

diffuse damage to the microvasculature which inevitably results in alveolar flooding). In addition to thromboembolic alterations, other factors may cause narrowing and obstruction of small arteries, such as (a) endothelial swelling, (b) compression by perivascular hemorrhage and edema in the early stage (27), and (c) compression by diffuse necrotizing vasculitis and sclerosis of the vessel wall in the subacute stage. Finally, in the chronic stage an extensive vascular remodeling and destruction can be observed in association with fibrotic tissue alterations (2,27).

Not yet clarified is the origin of the thromboembolic lesions of small arteries in the acute stage. A possible mechanism is an endothelial cell injury inducing *in situ* thrombosis (27,29). On the other hand, since the organizing microthrombi in the preacinar arteries are predominantly composed of red and white cells and layered with fibrin, they may as well originate from systemic microemboli. Especially in the course of major surgery, intravascular microaggregates are formed (30), and exogenous microembolic material may be derived from mass transfusion of stored blood (31,32).

Microvasculature

At the early stage of the disease, the tissue compartment with the least spectacular structural alterations often is the capillary network. Occasional obliterations due to microthrombi or capillary narrowing by voluminous interstitial edema result, at best, in a moderate capillary volume reduction. The entire septum volume and its components are not substantially different from normal as confirmed by morphometry (1,2) (Fig. 5). Noteworthy, though, are increased numbers of intravascular granulocytes, which sometimes may even exceed the amount of red blood cells, especially in cases of septicemia (Fig. 4b). At the worst, numerous capillaries are completely plugged by thrombi of sequestered leukocytes, seriously impairing capillary perfusion. Another, more indirect sign of a disturbed microcirculation is conspicuous differences in capillary hematocrit, possibly as a consequence of capillary and precapillary microthrombi (Fig. 5).

Differences in Morphology: Clue to Damaging Mechanisms?

As mentioned above, the basic pattern of tissue injury accounting for the abundant extravasation of plasma and blood cells is rather uniform. Yet, some differences do exist in different lungs with regard to number and types of intra- and extravascular cells or with regard to the amount of fibrin deposition and microthrombi. The question is whether these particular alterations within and around the microvascular bed reflect different pathogenetic pathways of tissue injury. On careful consideration of all the evidence obtained by animal and *in vitro* experiments, three initiating mechanisms still appear attractive: (i) primary and direct damage to the cell barriers by humoral factors and toxic agents (33–35); (ii) injury mediated by

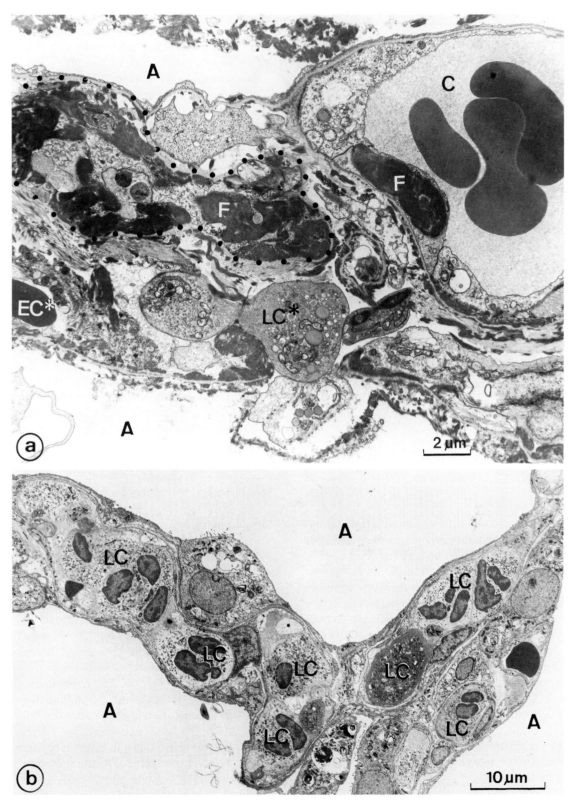

FIG. 4. (**a**) Section of alveolar septum with vast capillary destruction in acute ARDS. Note preserved capillary cross-section (C) with intra- and subendothelial fibrin depositions (F); note also the completely obliterated capillary, the contour of which is indicated by its basement membrane only (*dotted outline*). LC*, extravascular leukocyte; EC*, extravascular erythrocyte; A, alveolar space. (**b**) Alveolar septum of patient with acute septicemia. Capillaries are plugged with leukocytes (LC). A, alveolar space.

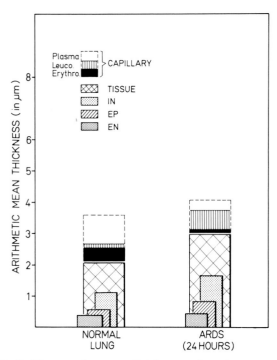

FIG. 5. Changes in mean thickness of septum components (volume per unit area of epithelial basement membrane), relative tissue and capillary volumes, and intravascular constituents in acute ARDS compared to normal lung.

products of intra- and extravascular coagulation (13,36–42); and (iii) sequestration and activation of neutrophils in the pulmonary microvasculature (8,9,21,43–49).

We found derangements consistent with the first hypothetical mechanism in the early stages of ARDS after traumatic injuries (Fig. 3), in neurogenic lung edema, and after inhalation of toxic gases (H₂S). In these conditions, signs of widespread barrier damages were not accompanied by a significant inflammatory reaction (i.e., by a striking accumulation of leukocytes). In both compartments (namely, the interstitial and alveolar spaces), erythrocytes prevailed. However, with numerous fibrin depositions and occasional microthrombi present, an interaction of several factors cannot be excluded.

In fact, signs of activation of coagulation are a common finding in the early stage of acute lung injury regardless of the precipitating injury. Fibrin depositions may be found everywhere on the path from the capillary lumen to the alveolar space (Figs. 2 and 4a). Large fibrin clots and microthrombi completely obliterating the capillary lumen at sites of destroyed endothelial cells are found less frequently. However, the micrographs are inconclusive of whether microthrombi and fibrin clots are pathogenetic agents or mere markers of capillary injury, and also the results of ex-

perimental studies are equivocal (38,50,51). There is increasing evidence that, in particular, extravascular fibrin depositions may potentiate and perpetuate the inflammatory process (40–42,52,53).

The conspicuous accumulation of polymorphonuclear leukocytes in the intra- and extravascular spaces of lung parenchyma is almost invariably present in acute lung injury associated with septicemia or with localized suppurative processes such as intra- and retroperitoneal abscesses, which often require repeated surgical interventions. There is overwhelming evidence that implicates activated neutrophils as mediators of acute lung injury by the release of free oxygen radicals, proteolytic enzymes, and other agents (43–49). Two observations are interesting, however: (i) The extent of damage to the sensitive endothelial and epithelial cell layers does not necessarily correlate with the local amount of leukocytes, and (ii) acute lung injury does occur in neutropenic patients (54,55).

In conclusion, morphologic variations do exist in the acute stage of the disease, but their significance with regard to the etiology and the further course of the disease is difficult to assess, and the risk of overinterpretation is real. Subsequently, these differences soon disappear, and ubiquitous infiltrations with leukocytes and other inflammatory cells are the invariable finding, presumably reflecting the ensuing vicious circle of tissue injury and inflammation.

Morphometry: Structure–Function Relationship

Morphometric analyses support the qualitative impression that in the early stage of acute lung injury (i.e., within about 24 hr), the changes in septal architecture and capillary volume are not substantial. In most cases there is a small increase in tissue volume predominantly due to interstitial exudate, and about an equivalent decrease in capillary volume (Fig. 5). However, these alterations in no way explain the functional disturbances, and even the amount of alveolar edema does not closely correlate with the impairment of pulmonary gas exchange (33). The reasons for the apparent mismatch between structure and function are manifold. First, as mentioned above, not only the fine lung parenchyma, but also extra-alveolar vessels, may be affected. Second, changes in lung mechanics may further impair the matching of ventilation and perfusion in different lung regions. And third, vasoactive metabolites of inflammation (33)—in particular, microthrombi and leukocyte plugs—may seriously disturb the microcirculation, which is a determinant of pulmonary gas exchange. There is even some morphometric evidence of microcirculatory dysfunction, because the capillary hematocrit is found to be considerably lower than the large vessel hematocrit (1). However, since many factors evade a morphologic analysis, attempts to correlate structural with functional impairments are futile at this stage of the disease.

REACTIONS TO TISSUE INJURY

Resorption of Exudate

Clinical experience shows that the course of life-threatening acute lung injury, as judged by clinical and pathophysiological criteria, is highly variable. At best, resorption of protein-rich alveolar edema takes place within a few days, and further signs of tissue damage rapidly subside without sequelae. Arbitrary definitions of ARDS are often responsible for disregarding these benign courses of the disease. As a rule, the resorption of permeability edema fluid takes considerably longer than that of hemodynamic edema fluid: The delay can be explained by the high osmotic pressure of the exudate (6,56), by the abundant amount of protein and particulate matter to be cleared by macrophages, and probably by the persistence of barrier leaks as demonstrated by radiological examinations (57). Evidently, in these cases the tissue reaction is restricted to a swift repair of the leaky barrier without excessive cellular proliferation and generalized inflammation. As a supportive factor, the rapid replenishment with normally functioning surfactant might play an important role (58). At worst, edema persists or recurs several times, and a gradual transition of the edematous phase into a subacute injury phase promoted by ongoing inflammation and tissue reaction can be observed.

Subsequent Tissue Alterations

As a rule, severe acute lung injury is followed by subacute tissue alterations that can be categorized into three different patterns of injury, namely, a *distortion-type injury*, a *fibrosis-type injury*, and a *destruction-type injury* (59,60), all of which may concur in the same lung weeks after the initial damage. The causes for the differences in type and course of injuries are not clear. Probably they are related to the intensity and duration of the initial noxious agent (12), to the intensity and the extent of inflammation, and to damaging influences and complications associated with treatment (ventilation with high oxygen concentrations and excessive pressures, drug therapy, secondary infections, etc.). The distinction seems reasonable, since the type of injury may be crucial to the outcome and, in particular, to the degree of reversibility and repair of the damage.

Distortion-type injury is characterized by the further accumulation of inflammatory cells in the extravascular space, by the proliferation of lung cells (in particular, the type II pneumocytes), and probably, in part, by the deficiency of surfactant. Epithelial defects with segments of denuded basement membrane become covered by proliferating type II cells: There is firm evidence that type II cell growth and division are essential for the renewal of type I epithelium (61–63). However, the augmentation of cuboidal alveolar epithelial cells varies considerably among patients. As fast as within 2 weeks, a generalized transformation of these bulky cuboidal cells, characterized by poorly developed lamellated bodies, can be observed (Fig. 6). Occasionally, the newly formed cell layers not only

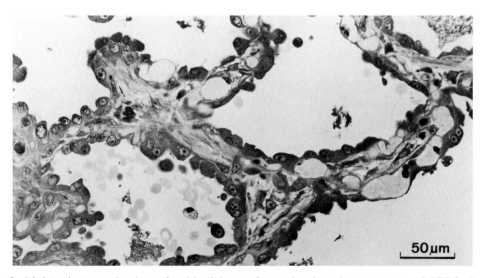

FIG. 6. Light-microscopic view of epithelial transformation in subacute stage of ARDS. A continuous layer of type II cuboidal epithelial cells replaces most of the destroyed squamous type I epithelial cells.

cover the epithelial basement membranes that serve as a scaffold for organized repair (64), but also cover strands of coagulated exudate (hyaline membranes), reflecting the complex cell–cell and cell–matrix interactions (4,63,65). In parallel with the proliferation of type II cells, the volume of the interstitial space increases to a variable but often very large extent by interstitial edema, further infiltration of blood-borne inflammatory cells (in particular, macrophages, lymphocytes, and plasma cells), and proliferation of local interstitial cells, including typical fibroblasts, myofibroblasts, and pericytes (66). In contrast to fibrotic and destructive lesions, these alterations are probably reversible and hence do not preclude a favorable outcome.

Fibrosis-type injury results in a profound rearrangement and disorganization of the acinar architecture which can be recognized best on light micrographs. The volume of the interstitial spaces increases to a variable but often very large extent by immigrated in-

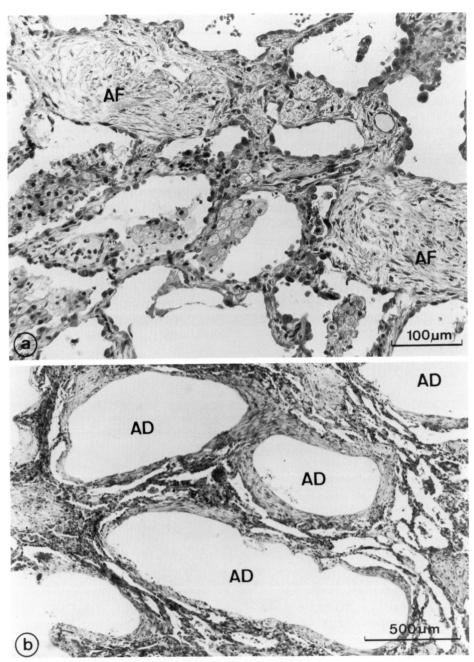

FIG. 7. (**a**) Intra-alveolar fibrosis (AF) and (**b**) alveolar duct (AD) fibrosis in a patient who died 2 weeks after the onset of ARDS due to septicemia.

flammatory cells as well as by rapidly proliferating mesenchymal cells and their connective tissue products. Bulky masses consisting of fibrotic tissue plates and folded-up septa of collapsed alveoli surround unusually wide air spaces, mostly widened alveolar ducts or even respiratory bronchioles. At some sites, the protein and cell-rich alveolar edema becomes organized by loose fibrous connective tissue, resulting in intra-alveolar fibrosis (Fig. 7a) (2,4,67,68). Frequently, entire alveolar ducts are ensheathed by a thick layer of fibrotic tissue, appropriately termed "alveolar duct fibrosis" (Fig. 7b) (68).

A most impressive alteration with regard to pulmonary gas exchange in this fibrosis-type injury is the drastic rarefaction of the microvasculature. The capillaries are found to be reduced in number and volume: Sometimes they are collapsed or seem compressed by surrounding edema, accumulations of cells, and broad fiber bundles. The irreversible damage to the microvasculature is accompanied by a profound vascular remodeling of extra-alveolar vessels (27–29).

Destruction-type injury is seen in the later stage of the disease, resembling the bronchopulmonary dysplasia in the neonate (69). There are obliterations or marked epithelial dysplasia of bronchioles, and large cystic air spaces with thick fibrotic walls are formed. On chest x-rays and lung slices, a conspicuous "honeycombing pattern" becomes predominant, reflecting extensive and irreversible damage of lung parenchyma.

Structure–Function Relationship

The quantitative importance of the morphologic appearance is best illustrated by morphometric data. Figure 8 shows the average results obtained in lungs from two patients who succumbed to the disease several weeks after its onset. The left-hand histogram demonstrates (a) the reduced surfaces and the increased thickness of the blood–gas barrier and (b) the profound effect of the disease on the microcirculation. Not only is there a substantial reduction in capillary volume, but the extremely low capillary hematocrit indicates that the remaining capillaries are no longer adequately perfused. The histogram in the middle of the figure illustrates (a) the considerably increased tissue components of alveolar septa and (b) the reduced capillary bed. The right-hand histogram depicts one functional consequence of the structural alterations: The morphometrically estimated diffusing capacity (D_L: right-hand column), an index of the gas-exchanging capacity of the lung (70), is critically reduced. For the calculation of this value, all measurement data of the entire alveolar surface have been considered. If only those parts of the parenchyma are included with free alveolar surfaces that have been cleared from edema fluid, the

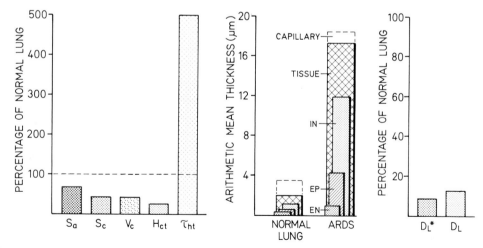

FIG. 8. Morphometric data obtained from lungs of two patients who died in respiratory failure several weeks after acute lung injury due to septicemia. The left-hand histogram depicts the alveolar surface area (S_a), the capillary surface area (S_c), the capillary volume (V_c), the intra-capillary hematocrit (H_{ct}), and the harmonic mean thickness of the blood–gas barrier (τ_{ht}), expressed as a percentage of the normal lung. The middle histogram depicts the changes in the mean thickness of the individual septum components (volume per unit area of epithelial basement membrane) and relative capillary and tissue volume. EN, endothelium; EP, epithelium; IN, interstitium. The right-hand histogram depicts the morphometrically estimated diffusing capacity for the total alveolar surface D_L and for the free alveolar surface D_L·, expressed as a percentage of the normal lung.

estimated diffusing capacity (D_L^*: left-hand column) is even more reduced, to less than 10% of the value measured in normal human lungs. Since D_L estimated by morphometry reflects the maximum gas-transfer capacity of the lung, the observed reduction reaches a dangerous limit, where an additional impairment of gas exchange by diffusion–perfusion or ventilation–perfusion inequalities and right-to-left shunts is likely to result in an arterial O_2 deficit incompatible with life. It has to be emphasized that the increase in tissue volume, the progression of fibrosis, and the degree of tissue derangement do not correlate with the duration of the disorder. In addition, the total tissue increase appears to be a less reliable index of functional impairment than the capillary volume/tissue volume ratio, which, in the normal lung, is close to 1. In patients with severe loss of gas-exchanging function, this ratio was decreased to approximately 10% of the normal value.

REPAIR AND PERSISTENT DAMAGES

The material presented illustrates the pattern of tissue injury, consequences of the ensuing inflammatory process, and some aspects of tissue reaction that might be considered the first step of repair. These include (a) the swift closure of endothelial leaks and (b) the substitution of destroyed squamous alveolar epithelial cells by proliferated type II pneumocytes, which, in turn, are able to transform into squamous type I cells (5,61–63). In patients, the further process of repair, resolution of pulmonary inflammation, and restoration of functional structures remains hypothetical (71). Obviously, analyses of lung tissue from patients who succumbed to the disease are biased, and randomized tissue sampling from recovering patients is precluded for obvious ethical reasons. Some indirect evidence can be obtained by a close follow-up of clinical, radiological, and pathophysiological signs. Accordingly, many survivors show a slow evolution back to normal or near-normal conditions. In others, tissue repair appears to be far from complete (72,73): Persisting pulmonary hypertension points to an irreversibility of the vascular remodeling (27), or to a definitive and substantial destruction of the microvasculature; a restrictive ventilatory defect associated with radiological evidence of multiple scars suggests end-stage fibrosis, whereas bullous emphysema mirrors local destruction of lung tissue probably caused by proteolytic enzymes (69,74).

REFERENCES

1. Bachofen M, Weibel ER. Alterations of the gas exchange apparatus in adult respiratory insufficiency associated with septicemia. *Am Rev Respir Dis* 1977;116:589–615.
2. Bachofen M, Weibel ER. Structural alterations of lung parenchyma in the adult respiratory distress syndrome. *Clin Chest Med* 1982;3:35–56.
3. Albertine KH. Ultrastructural abnormalities in increased-permeability pulmonary edema. *Clin Chest Med* 1985;6:345–369.
4. Trelstad RL, Martin EG, Zapol WM. Interstitial alterations following acute lung injury. In: Zapol WM, Falke KJ, eds. *Acute respiratory failure*. New York: Marcel Dekker, 1985;185–207.
5. Bachofen M, Weibel ER. Basic pattern of tissue repair in human lungs following unspecific injury. *Chest* 1974;65(Suppl):14–19.
6. Bachofen M, Bachofen H, Weibel ER. Lung edema in the adult respiratory distress syndrome. In: Fishman AP, Renkin EM, eds. *Pulmonary edema*. Bethesda, MD: American Physiological Society, 1979;241–252.
7. Hogg JC. Neutrophil kinetics and lung injury. *Physiol Rev* 1987;67:1249–1295.
8. Brigham KL, Meyrick B. Endotoxin and lung injury. *Am Rev Respir Dis* 1986;133:913–927.
9. Worthen GS, Haslett C, Rees AJ, et al. Neutrophil-mediated pulmonary vascular injury. *Am Rev Respir Dis* 1987;136:19–28.
10. Petty TL. Adult respiratory distress syndrome: definition and historical perspective. *Clin Chest Med* 1982;3:3–7.
11. Hudson LD. Causes of the adult respiratory distress syndrome—clinical recognition. *Clin Chest Med* 1982;3:195–212.
12. Shen AS, Haslett C, Feldsien DC, Henson PM, Cherniack RM. The intensity of chronic lung inflammation and fibrosis after bleomycin is directly related to the severity of acute injury. *Am Rev Respir Dis* 1988;137:564–571.
13. Malik AB, Staub NC. Mechanisms of lung microvascular injury. *Ann NY Acad Sci* 1982;384:1–562.
14. Warner AE, DeCamp MM Jr, Molina RM, Brain JD. Pulmonary removal of circulating endotoxin. Results in acute lung injury in sheep. *Lab Invest* 1988;59:219–230.
15. Winn R, Manuder R, Chi E, Harlan J. Neutrophil depletion does not prevent lung edema after endotoxin infusion in goat. *J Appl Physiol* 1987;62:116–121.
16. Bachofen M, Bachofen H. Fixation of human lungs. In: Gil J, Kleinermann J, eds. *Structural methods in experimental lung research*. New York: Marcell Dekker, 1990; in press.
17. Bachofen H, Bachofen M, Weibel ER. Ultrastructural aspects of pulmonary edema. *J Thorac Imag* 1988;3:1–7.
18. Gonzales-Crussi F, Boston RW. The absorption function of the neonatal lung. Ultrastructural study of horseradish peroxidase uptake at the onset of ventilation. *Lab Invest* 1972;26:114–121.
19. Lauweryns JM, Baert JH. The role of pulmonary lymphatics in the defenses of the distal lung: morphological and experimental studies of the transport mechanisms of intratracheally instilled particles. *Ann NY Acad Sci* 1974;221:244–275.
20. Schlag G, Redl HR. Morphology of the human lung after traumatic injury. In: Zapol WM, Falke KJ, eds. *Acute respiratory failure*. New York: Marcel Dekker, 1985.
21. Till GO, Johnson KJ, Kinkel R, Ward PA. Intravascular activation of complement and acute lung injury—dependency on neutrophils and toxic oxygen metabolites. *J Clin Invest* 1982;69:1126–1135.
22. Reidy MA, Schwartz SM. Endothelial regeneration. III. Time course of intimal changes after small defined injury to rat aortic endothelium. *Lab Invest* 1981;44:301–308.
23. Cunningham AL, Hurley JV. Alpha-naphthyl-thiourea-induced pulmonary edema in the rat: a topographical and electron-microscope study. *J Pathol* 1972;106:25–35.
24. Cohen AB, MacArthur C, Idell S, et al. A peptide from alveolar macrophages that releases neutrophil enzymes into the lungs in patients with the adult respiratory distress syndrome. *Am Rev Respir Dis* 1988;137:1151–1158.
25. Niewoehner JE, Rice K, Duane P, et al. Induction of alveolar epithelial injury by phospholipase A2. *J Appl Physiol* 1989;66:261–267.
26. Millar AB, Singer M, Meager A. Tumor necrosis factor in bronchopulmonary secretions of patients with adult respiratory distress syndrome. *Lancet* 1989;II:712–713.
27. Jones R, Zapol WM, Tomashefsky JF Jr, Kirton OC, Kobayashi K, Reid LM. Pulmonary vascular pathology: human and ex-

perimental study. In: Zapol WM, Falke KJ, eds. *Acute respiratory failure.* New York: Marcel Dekker, 1985;23–160.

28. Snow RL, Davies P, Pontoppidan H, Zapol WM, Reid L. Pulmonary vascular remodelling in adult respiratory distress syndrome. *Am Rev Respir Dis* 1982;126:887–892.
29. Tomashefski JF Jr, Davies P, Boggis C, Greene R, Zapol WM, Reid L. The pulmonary vascular lesion of the adult respiratory distress syndrome. *Am J Pathol* 1983;112:112–126.
30. McCollum CN, Poskitt KR. Intravascular microaggregates and pulmonary embolization in shock and surgery. In: Kox W, Bihari D, eds. *Shock and the adult respiratory distress syndrome.* Berlin: Springer, 1988;43–64.
31. Brown C, Dhurandhar HN, Barrett J, Litwin MS. Progression and resolution of changes in pulmonary function and structure due to pulmonary microembolism and blood transfusion. *Ann Surg* 1977;185:92–99.
32. Geelhoed GW, Bennett SH. "Shock lung" resulting from perfusion of canine lungs with stored bank blood. *Am Surg* 1975;41:661–682.
33. Brigham KL. Mechanisms of lung injury. *Clin Chest Med* 1982;3:9–24.
34. Jenkinson SG. Free radical effects on lung metabolism. *Clin Chest Med* 1989;10:37–47.
35. Chang S, Feddersen CO, Henson PM, Voelkel NF. Platelet-activating factors mediate hemodynamic changes and lung injury in endotoxin-treated rats. *J Clin Invest* 1987;79:1498–1509.
36. Rowland FN, Donovan MD, Picciano PT, Wilner DG, Kreutzer DL. Fibrin-mediated vascular injury. *Am J Pathol* 1984;117:418–428.
37. Malik AB. Pulmonary microembolism. *Physiol Rev* 1983;63:1114–1207.
38. Heffner JE, Steven A, Repine JE. The role of platelets in the adult respiratory distress syndrome: culprits or bystanders? *Am Rev Respir Dis* 1987;135:482–492.
39. Idell S, Peterson BT, Gonzales KK, et al. Local abnormalities of coagulation and fibrinolysis and alveolar fibrin deposition in sheep with oleic acid-induced lung injury. *Am Rev Respir Dis* 1988;138:1282–1294.
40. Cooper JA, Lo SK, Malik AB. Fibrin is a determinant of neutrophil sequestration in the lung. *Circ Res* 1988;63:735–741.
41. Ferro TJ, Lynch JJ, Malik AB. Macrophages activated by fibrin increase albumin permeability across pulmonary artery endothelial monolayers. *Am Rev Respir Dis* 1989;139:940–945.
42. Idell S, James KK, Levine EG, et al. Local abnormalities in coagulation and fibrinolytic pathways predispose to alveolar fibrin deposition in the adult respiratory distress syndrome. *J Clin Invest* 1989;84:695–705.
43. Craddock PR, Fehr J, Brigham KL, et al. Complement and leukocyte-mediated pulmonary dysfunction in hemodialysis. *N Engl J Med* 1977;296:769–774.
44. Hosea S, Brown E, Hammer C, et al. Role of complement activation in a model of adult respiratory distress syndrome. *J Clin Invest* 1980;66:375–382.
45. Martin WJ II. Neutrophils kill pulmonary endothelial cells by a hydrogen-peroxide-dependent pathway. *Am Rev Respir Dis* 1984;130:209–213.
46. Haslett C, Worthen GS, Giclas PC, et al. The pulmonary vascular sequestration of neutrophils in endotoxemia is initiated by an effect of endotoxin on the neutrophil in the rabbit. *Am Rev Respir Dis* 1987;136:9–18.
47. Stephens KE, Ishizaka A, Wu Z, et al. Granulocyte depletion prevents tumor necrosis factor-mediated acute lung injury in guinea pigs. *Am Rev Respir Dis* 1988;138:1300–1307.
48. Antony VB, Owen CL, English D. Polymorphonuclear leucocyte cytoplasts mediate acute lung injury. *J Appl Physiol* 1988;65:706–713.
49. Worthen GS, Schwab B, Elson EL, Downey GP. Mechanics of stimulated neutrophils: cell stiffening induces retention in capillaries. *Science* 1989;245:183–186.
50. Snapper JR, Hinson JM Jr, Hutchison AA, Lefferts PL, Ogletree ML, Brigham KL. Effects of platelet depletion on the unanesthetized sheep's pulmonary response to endotoxemia. *J Clin Invest* 1984;74:1782–1791.
51. Fantone JC, Kunkel RG, Kinnes DA. Potentiation of alpha-naphthyl-thiourea-induced lung injury by prostaglandin E$_1$ and platelet depletion. *Lab Invest* 1984;50:703–710.
52. Dang CV, Bell WR, Kaiser D, Wong A. Disorganisation of cultured vascular endothelial cell monolayers by fibrinogen fragments. *Science* 1985;227:1487–1490.
53. Senior RM, Skodgen WF, Griffen GL, Wilner GD. Effects of fibrinogen derivatives upon the inflammatory response. *J Clin Invest* 1986;77:1014–1019.
54. Maunder RJ, Hackman RC, Ritt E, et al. Occurrence of the adult respiratory distress syndrome in neutropenic patients. *Am Rev Respir Dis* 1986;133:313–317.
55. Ognibene FP, Martin SE, Parker MM, et al. Adult respiratory distress syndrome in patients with severe neutropenia. *N Engl J Med* 1986;315:547–551.
56. Vreim CE, Staub NC. Protein composition of lung fluids in acute alloxan edema in dogs. *Am J Physiol* 1976;230:376–379.
57. Pinet F, Tabib A, Clermont A, et al. Post-traumatic shock lung: postmortem microangiographic and pathologic correlation. *AJR* 1982;139:449–454.
58. Harris JB, Jackson F Jr, Moxley MA, Longmore WJ. Effect of exogenous surfactant instillation on experimental acute lung injury. *J Appl Physiol* 1989;66:1846–1851.
59. Crystal RG, Ferrans VJ. Reactions of the interstitial space to injury. In: Fishman AP, ed. *Pulmonary diseases and disorders.* New York: McGraw-Hill, 1988;711–738.
60. Basset F, Ferrans JV, Soler P, et al. Intraluminal fibrosis in interstitial lung disorders. *Am J Pathol* 1986;122:443–461.
61. Adamson IYR, Bowden DA. The type 2 cell as progenitor of alveolar epithelial regeneration: a cytodynamic study in mice after exposure to oxygen. *Lab Invest* 1974;30:35–42.
62. Evans MJ, Cabral LJ, Stephens RJ, Freeman G. Transformation of alveolar type 2 cells to type 1 cells following exposure to NO$_2$. *Exp Mol Pathol* 1975;22:142–150.
63. Rannels DE, Rannels SR. Influence of the extracellular matrix on type 2 cell differentiation. *Chest* 1989;96:165–173.
64. Vracko R. Significance of the basal lamina for regeneration of injured lung. *Virchows Arch* 1972;355:264–274.
65. Crouch EC, Moxley MA, Longmore W. Synthesis of collagenous proteins by pulmonary type II epithelial cells. *Am Rev Respir Dis* 1987;135:1118–1123.
66. Adler KB, Low RB, Leslie KO, et al. Biology of disease. Contractile cells in normal and fibrotic lung. *Lab Invest* 1989;60:473–485.
67. Thurlbeck W, Thurlbeck SM. Pulmonary effects of paraquat poisoning. *Chest* 1976;69(Suppl):276–280.
68. Pratt PC, Vollmer RT, Shelburne JD, et al. Pulmonary morphology in a multihospital collaborative extracorporal membrane oxygenation project. *Am J Pathol* 1979;95:191–214.
69. Churg A, Golden J, Fligiel S, Hogg JC. Bronchopulmonary dysplasia in the adult. *Am Rev Respir Dis* 1983;127:117–120.
70. Weibel ER. *Stereological methods: practical methods for biological morphometry,* vol 1. London: Academic Press, 1979.
71. Henson PM, Larsen GL, Henson JE, Newman SL, Musson RA, Leslie CC. Resolution of pulmonary inflammation. *Fed Proc* 1984;43:2799–2806.
72. Bachofen M, Bachofen H. Der Heilungsverlauf des schweren "adult respiratory distress syndrome". *Schewiz Med Wochenschr* 1979;109:1982–1989.
73. Peters JI, Bell RC, Rrikoda TJ, et al. Clinical determinants of abnormalities in pulmonary functions in survivors of the adult respiratory distress syndrome. *Am Rev Respir Dis* 1989;129:1163–1168.
74. Cochrane C, Spragg RG, Revak SD. Oxidative inactivation of alpha-1-proteinase inhibitor in broncho-alveolar lavage fluid of patients with the adult respiratory distress syndrome. *J Clin Invest* 1982;71:754–761.

THE LUNG: Scientific Foundations
edited by R.G. Crystal, J.B. West et al.
Raven Press, Ltd., New York © 1991.

CHAPTER 7.8.1

Biologic Basis of Pulmonary Fibrosis

Ronald G. Crystal, Victor J. Ferrans, and Francoise Basset

The fibrotic lung disorders include a diverse group of disorders of the lower respiratory tract characterized by injury to the lung parenchyma and by replacement of the normal architecture by mesenchymal cells and the connective tissue matrix secreted by these cells (1–5). Until recently, these disorders were conceptualized as the "interstitial" lung disorders, reflecting the concept that the fibrosis appeared to be confined to the interstitium of the alveolar walls (see Chapter 3.3.1) (3,5). It is now recognized, however, that most fibrotic lung disorders are "intra-alveolar" as well as "interstitial," with injury to the epithelial surface often associated with (a) the interstitial contents moving through rents in the epithelial basement membrane and (b) mesenchymal cells and their products accumulating in spaces normally occupied by air (6).

The purpose of this chapter is to provide an overview of the biologic processes underlying the development of pulmonary fibrosis. The fundamental concept underlying these processes is relatively simple: The fibrotic lung disorders are chronic inflammatory disorders in which inflammatory processes in the lower respiratory tract injure the lung and modulate the proliferation of mesenchymal cells that form the basis of the fibrotic scar (Figs. 1 and 2) (1,2,7). In this regard, the biologic basis of pulmonary fibrosis is akin to the process of normal wound-healing, in which injury to normal tissues is followed by inflammation and then repair by the mechanism of scar formation (4). However, whereas wound-healing is normally localized in space and confined in time, the fibrotic lung diseases generally involve the entire organ and are chronic, on-going processes. Furthermore, whereas wound-healing typically follows the same pattern and results in the same consequences, there is a broad diversity among the various types of fibrotic lung disease (1–5). Consistent with the concept that it is the inflammation that drives the process of fibrosis, the basis for the differences among the fibrotic lung disorders is centered in the differences in the types of inflammation that characterize each disorder (1,2,5). In this regard, the inflammation of some interstitial lung disorders is dominated by alveolar macrophages, whereas in others the inflammation has major components of neutrophils, lymphocytes, and/or eosinophils (2,8,9). Since each of the different inflammatory cells has a different armamentarium of available mediators, the effect of each cell type is quite different.

THE "ALVEOLITIS" OF FIBROTIC LUNG DISEASE

In the context that the inflammation associated with fibrotic lung disease is confined to the alveolar structures, the inflammation is referred to as an "alveolitis" (9). Several lines of evidence support the concept that the alveolitis precedes the injury and fibrosis of fibrotic lung disease. First, in early disease, areas of alveolitis are found without evidence of derangements of the alveolar architecture (1,2,7) (Fig. 3). Second, in familial cases of idiopathic pulmonary fibrosis, the children of individuals with fibrotic lung disease have alveolitis without clinical evidence of disease, suggesting that the alveolitis comes first (10). Third, in animal models of pulmonary fibrosis, induction of the alveolitis is followed by fibrotic lung disease (see Chapter 7.8.2). Finally, in both experimental animal models and human disease, suppression of the alveolitis is associated with a stabilization of the disease (11,12).

Evaluation of the character of the alveolitis of the

R. G. Crystal: Pulmonary Branch, National Heart, Lung and Blood Institute, National Institutes of Health, Bethesda, Maryland 20892.

V. J. Ferrans: Pathology Branch, National Heart, Lung and Blood Institute, National Institutes of Health, Bethesda, Maryland 20892.

F. Basset: INSERM U82, Faculté Xavier Bichart, Paris, France 75017.

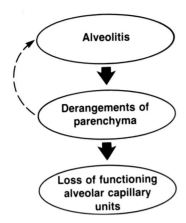

FIG. 1. General concepts of the pathogenesis of fibrotic lung disease. Independent of the cause, the fibrotic lung diseases are inflammatory disorders in which inflammation in the lower respiratory tract (the "alveolitis") causes the derangements of the lung parenchyma, eventually leading to loss of functioning alveolar capillary units. In some cases, the derangements to the parenchyma amplify the inflammation. The alveolitis is responsible for the injury to the lung parenchyma as well as for the replacement of the normal architecture with mesenchymal cells and their connective tissue products.

different fibrotic lung diseases has led to general concepts of the relative "danger" of different types of inflammation to the alveolar structures. The danger relates to the potential of the inflammatory cells to derange the alveolar architecture. In this regard, neutrophils can cause the most damage, with alveolar macrophages and eosinophils next; lymphocytes have the least potential to cause damage. For a discussion of this general concept see refs. 1–3, 5, 8, and 9; for de-

tails concerning the potential of inflammatory cells to injure the alveolar walls, see Chapters 3.4.7 (neutrophils), 3.4.9 (eosinophils), 3.4.5 (alveolar macrophages), 3.4.1 (lymphocytes), 3.4.10 (basophils), and 3.4.11 (mast cells). Many of the differences among these cells relates to the specific mediators they are capable of releasing. In this regard, all available evidence suggests that most damage in the fibrotic lung disease comes from oxidants—hence the danger of

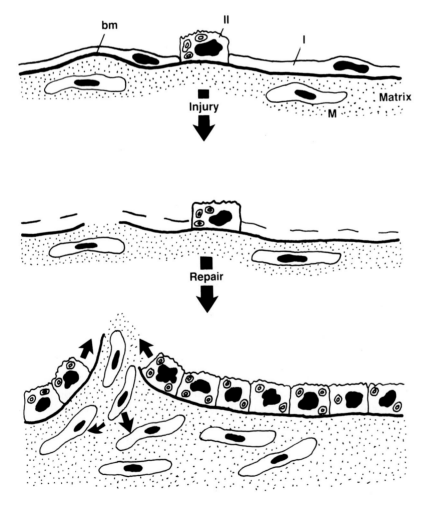

FIG. 2. Sequential processes of injury and repair of the alveolar wall in fibrotic lung disease. **Top:** The normal alveolar wall, with type I epithelial cells (I), type II epithelial cells (II), the epithelial basement membrane (bm), mesenchymal cells (M), and connective tissue matrix. For simplicity, the alveolar capillaries are omitted. **Middle:** Injury causes the loss of type I cells and also causes breaks in the basement membrane. **Bottom:** The repair process includes proliferation of mesenchymal cells along with the deposition of connective tissue. Some interstitial contents move into the alveolar airspaces through rents in the basement membrane, causing intra-alveolar fibrosis. The damaged type I cells are replaced by proliferating type II cells (and sometimes by bronchiolar epithelial cells migrating down from small airways). The intra-alveolar fibrosis is re-epithelialized, and the fibrotic mass is incorporated into the alveolar wall (see refs. 6 and 30 for details).

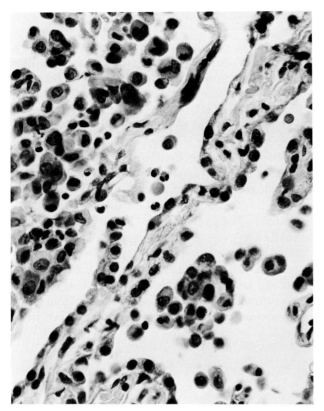

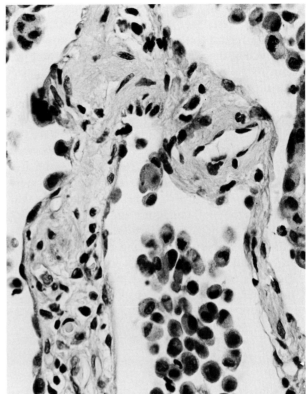

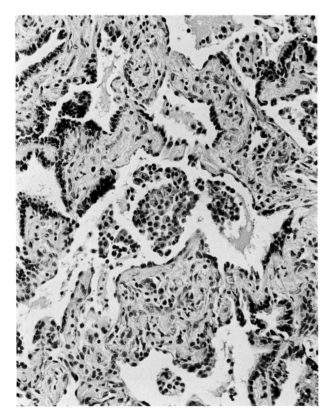

FIG. 3. Sequential biologic processes in the development of pulmonary fibrosis. Shown are three micrographs from the lung of an IPF patient. **A:** Early IPF. There is an alveolitis dominated by alveolar macrophages, with fewer numbers of neutrophils, lymphocytes, and eosinophils. The alveolar walls are close to normal, although there are changes in the epithelium with relatively more type II cells than normal. Hematoxylin and eosin, ×400. **B:** Mid-course IPF. The alveolitis persists, but there are now changes in the epithelium and thickening of the alveolar walls with fibrosis. Hematoxylin and eosin, ×400. **C:** Late IPF. There is marked derangement of the architecture, with inflammation, changes in the epithelial cells, and marked widening of the alveolar walls with fibrosis. Hematoxylin and eosin, ×180. (All micrographs are from ref. 7.)

neutrophils, the most potent oxidant producer of all inflammatory cells (see Chapters 3.4.7, 7.2.1, and 7.4.2). With regard to the development of fibrosis per se, the alveolar macrophage is the most important because of its ability to release growth signals for mesenchymal cells (see Chapters 2.9 and 3.4.5).

The acceptance of the alveolitis concept as the central mechanism in the pathogenesis of the fibrotic lung disease does not mean that inflammatory cells are the only biologic players in the development of pulmonary fibrosis. There is increasing evidence that parenchymal cells, including epithelial, endothelial, and mesenchymal cells, are capable of releasing cytokines that contribute to the "inflammatory" milieu (see Chapters 2.8, 2.10, 3.1.1, and 3.2.2). Furthermore, matrix components are capable of enhancing inflammatory processes by virtue of their ability (as intact molecules or as fragments, or combined with other molecules) to act as chemoattractants to expand the inflammation (see Chapters 3.3.2–3.3.4, and 3.3.6)

IDIOPATHIC PULMONARY FIBROSIS

As a clinical paradigm of the processes responsible for the changes to the alveolar architecture that characterizes the fibrotic lung disorders, we will focus on the "classic" fibrotic lung disease, idiopathic pulmonary fibrosis (IPF) (1,2,14,15). Although the term "idiopathic" suggests that IPF may be a collection of fibrotic lung disorders of unknown etiology, IPF is believed to be a specific disorder with characteristic features (1–3). In Great Britain, IPF is referred to as "cryptogenic fibrosing alveolitis" (13).

IPF is a chronic, usually fatal disorder affecting only the lower respiratory tract (14). It usually begins in middle age, presenting with dyspnea with exercise, and has a 4- to 5-year course from the onset of symptoms to death. As the disease progresses, the lung becomes less and less able to transfer oxygen from air to blood in a normal fashion. Typically, an individual with IPF in mid-course has mild hypoxemia at rest which wors-

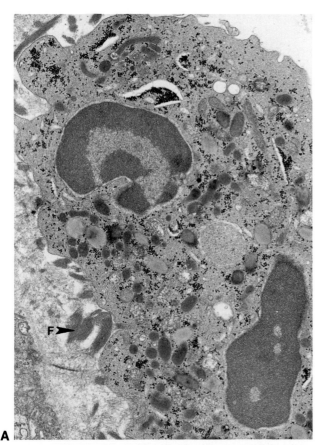
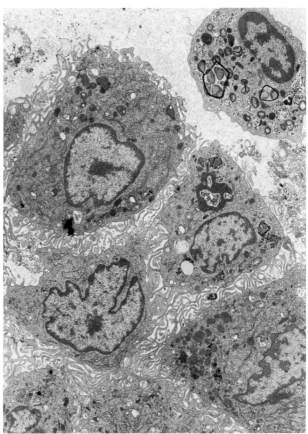

FIG. 4. Alveolitis of IPF. **A:** Neutrophil in the alveolar wall adjacent to strands of fibrin (F) and collagen fibrils (*upper right*). At the far left is the basal portion of an epithelial cell with its basement membrane. Transmission electron micrograph, ×17,600. **B:** Intra-alveolar inflammation. Alveolar macrophages dominate this view, with one eosinophil at the top right. The alveolar macrophages appear activated with marked filopodia and abundant cytoplasmic organelles. Transmission electron micrograph, ×5950. (Both micrographs are from ref. 7.)

ens markedly with exercise (16). Late in the disease, there is a progressive limitation in physical activity, because vital organs are relatively "starved" of O_2 (1,2). The dyspnea and problems with oxygen transfer result from derangements to the lung parenchyma that include injury to all of the cellular components of the alveolar wall and the accumulation of mesenchymal cells and their connective tissue products within the alveolar walls and the alveolar air-spaces (see below and refs. 1 and 2).

The derangements to the lung parenchyma in IPF are caused by a chronic alveolitis which is dominated by alveolar macrophages and neutrophils but which also includes lymphocytes and eosinophils and, to a much lesser extent, basophils and mast cells (Fig. 4) (2,8,9,14,15,17–25). As the name suggests, the etiology of IPF is unknown. It is likely, however, that the inflammatory process is driven, at least in part, by immune complexes produced within the lower respiratory tract (17,26,27). These immune complexes interact with alveolar macrophages and help to maintain these cells in a chronic state of activation. As such, the alveolar macrophages are releasing mediators that amplify the inflammation by recruiting other inflammatory cells (particularly neutrophils). Together, the mass of activated inflammatory cells in the lower respiratory tract causes progressive injury to the lung parenchyma and stimulates mesenchymal cells to accumulate.

CHANGES IN THE LUNG PARENCHYMA IN IDIOPATHIC PULMONARY FIBROSIS

In the context that the alveolitis mediates the derangements to the lung parenchyma that characterize IPF and results in the progressive loss of functioning alveolar–capillary units, it is helpful to define the actual changes in the lung architecture that typify this disease. These changes are localized primarily in the alveoli. Although small airways are also involved in the disease process (28), the dominant abnormalities in lung function result from processes based in the alveoli (2,16).

Epithelial Cells

In the normal lung the alveolar epithelium consists of type I and type II epithelial cells (Fig. 2). Although type I cells cover more than 90% of the epithelial surface, there are actually 1.9-fold more type II cells than type I cells (29). Type II cells can proliferate and differentiate into type I cells, whereas type I cells are terminally differentiated cells that cannot replicate (see Chapter 3.1.1).

IPF is characterized by damage to the normal alveolar epithelium, including cytoplasmic swelling, degeneration, and necrosis (30). There is a marked loss of type I cells (Fig. 2). If the epithelial basement membrane is intact, the epithelial surface is re-epithelialized by the remaining type II cells (Figs. 5–7). If the damage includes the proximal portion of the acini and the terminal bronchioles, epithelial renewal also includes bronchial epithelial cells with cuboidal cells, Clara cells, and occasional ciliated cells. In some areas, the regenerating epithelial cells stack upon one another and show evidence of squamous metaplasia (Figs. 3 and 5–7). Consistent with these marked epithelial changes, IPF is associated with an increased risk for bronchogenic carcinoma, particularly in IPF patients who also smoke cigarettes (31,32).

Endothelial Cells

The endothelium of the alveolar capillaries of the normal lung forms a continuous surface lining the endothelial basement membrane (33). In the regions away from the cell nucleus, the cytoplasm is very attenuated, such that the plasma membranes of the luminal and basal surfaces almost abut each other. In contrast to the tight junctions between the epithelial cells, the normal junctions between the endothelial cells are relatively loose. Despite this, the surface is continuous, with no evidence of fenestra as observed normally in capillaries of the nose and bronchial walls (35).

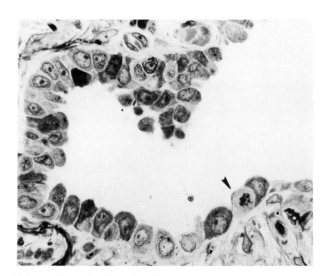

FIG. 5. "Repaired" epithelium in IPF. The normal alveolar epithelium is replaced by cuboidal cells, one of which is undergoing mitosis (*arrow*). Some of the cuboidal cells are type II cells, whereas others are bronchiolar epithelial cells. Note the multiple layers of the epithelial cells on the left, marked departure from the normal epithelium. Plastic-embedded (0.5 μm) tissue, alkaline toluidine blue, ×480. (From ref. 30.)

In IPF there is evidence of capillary endothelial cell injury, with cytoplasmic changes, degeneration, and, in some cases, necrosis. It is not known to what extent the endothelium is actually capable of regenerating in this disease; unlike the exaggerated proliferation of epithelial cells (see above) and mesenchymal cells (see below) observed in the IPF lung, ultrastructural evaluation of the endothelium does not show evidence of mitoses. The alveolar capillary endothelium in IPF takes on the appearance of bronchiolar endothelium with regions of fenestrations, a marked morphologic change from the normal continuous layer of endothelium observed in the normal lung; this is compatible with the concept that the IPF lung is relatively "leaky" compared to normal (O. Kawanami, Nippon Medical School, Kawasaki, Japan, *personal communication*).

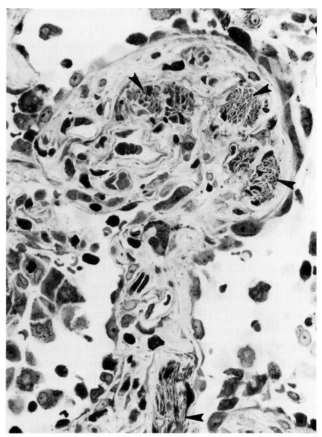

FIG. 7. Fibrosis in IPF. The epithelium has been "repaired" with mostly cuboidal cells; in addition, the alveolar wall is thickened with masses of smooth muscle cells (*arrows*), other mesenchymal cells, and masses of connective tissue. There is a macrophage-dominated alveolitis in the air-spaces and interstitium. Plastic-embedded tissue (0.5 μm), alkaline toluidine blue, ×1000. (From ref. 7.)

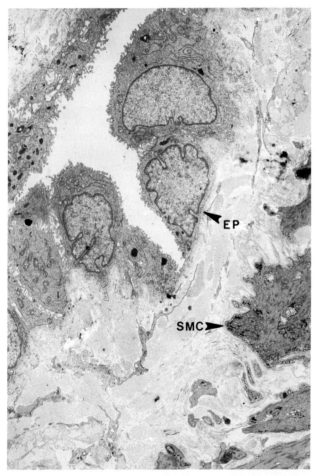

FIG. 6. Alveolar wall in IPF in mid-course showing changes in the epithelium and also showing fibrosis of the alveolar wall. The view is similar to that in Fig. 5, except that Fig. 6 is a transmission electron micrograph with higher magnification (×5480) showing more detail. The epithelium is repopulated mostly by cuboidal cells (EP), and smooth muscle cells (SMC) are observed in the interstitium. Below the epithelium is a region of thickened, disordered fibrous connective tissue, typical of this disorder. (From ref. 7.)

Basement Membranes

The normal alveolar epithelial and endothelial basement membranes are thin and continuous (see Chapter 3.3.6). In IPF the epithelial basement membranes are thickened and often duplicated, and in many places are fragmented or lost entirely (6,30). In some areas the basement membrane is intact, but it is denuded of all epithelium. Like the epithelial basement membrane, the endothelial basement membrane in the IPF lung has areas of disruptions, but duplications are infrequent (O. Kawanami, *personal communication*).

"Interstitial" Versus "Intraluminal" Fibrosis

As discussed above, the classic concepts of the fibrotic lung disorders held that the fibrotic process was contained within the alveolar interstitium. It is now recognized that intraluminal fibrosis is an important component in the pattern of injury and repair in a disorder such as IPF (6). The intraluminal fibrosis appears in several forms, including: (a) intraluminal buds, which partially fill the alveoli, alveolar ducts, and/or distal bronchioles; (b) obliterative changes, in which loose connective tissue masses obliterate the distal airspaces; and (c) mural incorporation of previously intraluminal connective tissue masses, which fuse with the alveolar, alveolar ductal, or bronchiolar structures and frequently become reepithelialized.

The relevance of intraluminal fibrosis to the pathogenesis of IPF relates to two important concepts. First, to develop within the air-spaces, intraluminal fibrosis of any kind must involve processes causing defects in the epithelium and epithelial basement membranes through which mesenchymal cells can migrate from the interstitium into the intraluminal compartment (Fig. 2). Second, intraluminal fibrosis, particularly the obliterative changes and mural incorporation, play an important role in pulmonary remodeling. This is particularly true when adjacent alveoli become fused, forming the masses of connective tissue that characterize the late stages of IPF (Fig. 3).

Mesenchymal Cells

The mesenchymal cell population in the normal alveolar interstitium is heterogeneous and includes fibroblasts, myofibroblasts, pericytes, smooth muscle cells, and undifferentiated cells (see Chapter 3.3.1). In the

IPF lung there are more mesenchymal cells, and although the same subpopulations are present, they are in different relative proportions to one another as compared to those in the normal lung.

In the normal alveolar walls, mesenchymal cells represent approximately 29% of all parenchymal cells (F. Basset, V. Ferrans, P. Fouret, P. Soler, R. G. Crystal, *unpublished observations*). Among the mesenchymal cells, myofibroblasts, fibroblasts, and pericytes dominate, with few smooth muscle cells or undifferentiated cells. In contrast, in the IPF lung there is a 1.8-fold increase in the proportion of parenchymal cells that are mesenchymal cells. Furthermore, whereas mesenchymal cells in the normal lung proliferate at a slow rate, in the IPF lung the rate of mesenchymal cell proliferation is increased, particularly among the fibroblast subpopulation (Fig. 8). Not only are there increases in the numbers of mesenchymal cells in the IPF lung, but the relative proportions of the various subtypes are different than in the normal lung. Most strikingly, there is a 10-fold increase in the relative proportion of smooth muscle cells in the IPF lung (Figs. 6 and 7).

Interstitial Connective Tissue Matrix

The classification of IPF as a "fibrotic lung disease" was originally based on the light-microscopic observation of thick bundles of collagen within the alveolar walls. Ultrastructural evaluation shows that the collagen bundles not only are increased in number, but

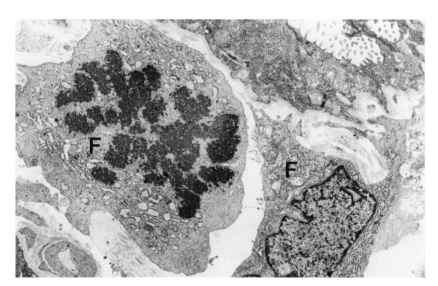

FIG. 8. Mitosis of mesenchymal cells in IPF. Shown is an alveolar wall lined by cuboidal epithelial cells. Two fibroblasts (F) are seen; the fibroblast on the left is undergoing mitosis. Transmission electron micrograph, ×5200.

are oftentimes twisted and frayed as well (7). Biochemical evidence supports the concept that there is more collagen in the IPF lung than in the normal lung (36–41). Early in the disease there may be more type III collagen deposited; later on, however, type I dominates, resulting in an increased ratio of type I to type III collagen (42). Initially, the intra-alveolar fibrosis of IPF is characterized by a loosely formed matrix (6). The collagen bundles are poorly formed or are composed of thin, separate collagen fibrils, mostly comprised of type III collagen (42).

Very little attention has been focused on matrix components other than collagen in the IPF lung, although it is likely that there are changes in the form, quantity, and types of each component. Foci of fibronectin deposits are observed within the interstitium and the air-spaces (42). The intra-alveolar connective tissue appears to be superimposed on a base of fine, fibrillar material in a network of small stellate electron-dense spicules; it is likely that these components are fibrin and proteoglycans, respectively (6).

PATHOGENESIS OF IDIOPATHIC PULMONARY FIBROSIS

As the name of the disease suggests, the etiology of IPF is unknown. Although all available evidence is consistent with the concept that the disease results from an uncontrolled, chronic inflammatory process in the lower respiratory tract, it is not clear what initiates and maintains the alveolitis. The most plausible hypothesis suggests that the inflammation follows a variety of insults to the alveoli, but only in susceptible individuals (15). For example, a viral pneumonitis that is self-limiting for most individuals may trigger anti-self immune processes in a subgroup of individuals with the appropriate (as yet unidentified) hereditary background (10).

Consistent with the concept that immune processes initiate the inflammation, immune complexes are found in the epithelial lining fluid of individuals with IPF (17,43). Most of these immune complexes utilize IgG (43). The antigens for the immune complexes are unknown, but they may well be "self" antigens, where the immune system inappropriately recognizes normal (or deranged) lung tissue as being "foreign." Support for such a scenario includes the observations that IPF patients have T-cells that are activated by connective tissue matrix components (44) and have circulating antibodies directed toward type II alveolar epithelial cells (45). Although the ratio of CD4$^+$ (helper/inducer) T-cells to CD8$^+$ (suppressor/inducer) T-cells in the IPF lung is normal, there may be compartments of lymphocyte subtypes with nodular collection of CD4$^+$ T-cells within the alveolar walls (46). Furthermore, enhanced helper T-cell function has been observed among blood T-cells in these individuals (47).

Alveolitis of IPF

Independent of the etiology of IPF, there is no question that it is a chronic inflammatory disease (see ref. 2 for review). The alveolitis is found throughout the lung parenchyma, but the intensity is patchy. The inflammatory cells are present in the alveolar walls and on the alveolar epithelial surface; on the average, the composition of the alveolitis in these locations is similar (1–3,15–25).

The alveolitis of IPF is dominated by alveolar macrophages, but the most striking component is the increased numbers of neutrophils (Fig. 4) (17,18). In the normal lung, neutrophils are present but are in low numbers, representing at most 1–2% of the inflammatory cells on the epithelial surface (8). In contrast, in IPF, neutrophils represent 5–20% of the inflammatory cells present on this surface (14,17,18,22,24, 25,48). Put in the context that neutrophils have a lifespan of only 1–2 days after leaving the circulation (see Chapter 3.4.8), the lung in IPF must contend with a chronic burden of neutrophils and a powerful array of mediators. In addition to alveolar macrophages and neutrophils, the inflammation includes increases in the total numbers of lymphocytes (see above), eosinophils, basophils, and mast cells (19–21,23).

The major components of the alveolitis of IPF accumulate by a combination of (a) recruitment of inflammatory cells from blood and (b) the increased proliferation of inflammatory cells in the lung parenchyma. The alveolar macrophage plays a central role in this process by releasing chemotactic factors for neutrophils (17,49–55) (Fig. 9). It is likely that leukotriene B$_4$ is the dominant neutrophil chemotactic factor, although alveolar macrophages can also release interleukin 8, an 8-kDa cytokine with neutrophil chemotactic activity (49–56). Immune complexes in the lower respiratory tract in IPF are believed to be the major stimuli that are chronically activating the alveolar macrophages to release these neutrophil chemotactic factors (2,17,49,50,57,58).

The alveolar macrophages accumulate in the IPF lung as a result of two mechanisms: enhanced recruitment and local proliferation. The specific chemotactic factor for recruiting monocytes to the IPF lung is not known, but evaluation of the alveolar macrophage population with specific monoclonal antibodies suggests increased numbers of young, newly recruited alveolar macrophages (59). Exaggerated local proliferation of alveolar macrophages is also ongoing in IPF, with these cells replicating at a three- to fourfold greater

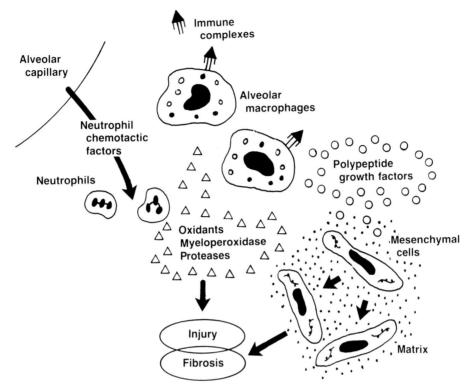

FIG. 9. Major biologic processes associated with injury and fibrosis of the lower respiratory tract in IPF. Immune complexes stimulate alveolar macrophages to release neutrophil chemotactic factors that attract neutrophils in alveolar capillaries. Together, the activated alveolar macrophages and neutrophils produce a burden of oxidants, myeloperoxidase, and proteases that injure the alveolar wall. The activated alveolar macrophages also release polypeptide growth factors that stimulate mesenchymal cells to proliferate. The result is more mesenchymal cells, and hence a larger mass of connective tissue matrix.

rate than normal (60). The mechanisms of accumulation of eosinophils, lymphocytes, basophils, and mast cells are unknown.

Mechanisms of Injury

IPF is an excellent example of the two-edged sword of the inflammatory/immune cells in the lung. Whereas the inflammatory cells play a central role in pulmonary host defense, these same populations of inflammatory cells, if present in sufficient numbers and if activated, can markedly derange the fragile alveolar walls (Fig. 9) (see Chapters 3.4.5, 3.4.7, 7.3.5, 7.7.1, and 7.7.3.1 and refs. 61–63). Although the inflammatory cells that comprise the alveolitis of IPF have the potential to release a broad array of mediators capable of injuring the lung parenchyma, analysis of the types of derangements observed in the parenchyma helps to sort out which classes of mediators may play a dominant role. Since the dominant morphologic evidence of injury in IPF is damage to the epithelium and endothelium,

breaks in basement membranes, and fraying of interstitial collagen (see above and Figs. 3 and 5–7), it is rational to hypothesize that mediators capable of causing this kind of damage likely play a major role in the pathogenesis of IPF.

Oxidants

Several lines of evidence strongly suggest that the exaggerated release of oxidants by alveolar macrophages, neutrophils, and possibly eosinophils plays a major role in the injury to the epithelium and endothelium. First, all of these cells are capable of releasing oxidants, including superoxide anion, hydrogen peroxide, and the hydroxyl radical (see Chapters 3.4.5, 3.4.7, and 3.4.9). Second, inflammatory cells recovered from the lung of individuals with IPF are releasing exaggerated amounts of superoxide anion and hydrogen peroxide (62,64). Third, neutrophils contain myeloperoxidase, an enzyme capable of converting hydrogen peroxide to the very toxic hypohalide radical (see Chapter 3.4.7). Consistent with this knowledge, and with the knowledge that neutrophils participate in the alveolitis of IPF, there is a high concentration of myeloperoxidase in epithelial lining fluid of individuals with IPF (62). Fourth, when lung epithelial cells are exposed to inflammatory cells and to epithelial lining fluid recovered from the lung of individuals with IPF, there is a synergistic cytotoxic effect (62). Finally, the antioxidant glutathione (GSH) is normally present in high concentrations in epithelial lining fluid and thus helps to protect the epithelium of the lower respiratory tract from oxidants (65). In IPF, for reasons that are not understood, the levels of GSH are decreased four-fold, further placing the epithelium at marked risk for oxidant injury (66).

Proteases

The fragmentation of interstitial collagen fibers and basement membrane components observed in IPF strongly suggests that proteases play a role in the injury process. The most direct evidence for this is the finding of large concentrations of collagenase, likely neutrophil-derived, in epithelial lining fluid of individuals with IPF (67). Importantly, no active neutrophil elastase is detected in the IPF lung, despite the fact that neutrophils are present and are likely releasing this potent protease. Consistent with this concept, elastic fibers in the alveolar interstitium do not appear deranged in IPF. The most likely explanation for these observations is that the neutrophil elastase is released but is subsequently inhibited by α_1-antitrypsin, the natural inhibitor of this enzyme (see Chapters 7.1.1 and 7.1.2). In contrast, the lung has very little defense against collagenase (at least on the epithelial surface; see Chapter 7.1.2) and is thus susceptible to collagenolytic enzymes, even though they are generally less potent than proteolytic enzymes such as neutrophil elastase.

Interestingly, *in vitro* evaluation of fragments of lung parenchyma from IPF patients has demonstrated a relative decrease in collagenolytic activity compared to that in the normal lung (41,68). While this observation appears to contradict the observation of increased levels of a neutrophil-derived collagenase on the epithelial surface in IPF, the decreased collagenolytic activity observed in the lung fragments likely represents a different class of collagenase. In this regard, fibroblasts produce a collagenase that likely plays an important role in the normal turnover of interstitial collagen (see Chapter 7.1.1). It may be this class of collagenase that is reduced in the IPF lung (thus permitting newly synthesized collagen to accumulate at a rate faster than normal, thereby contributing to the fibrotic process), whereas the neutrophil-

derived collagenase may cause fragmentation of the collagen once it is deposited.

Other Mediators

It is possible to hypothesize a potential role for many inflammatory mediators as participants in the process of lung injury in IPF, but other than the oxidants myeloperoxidase and collagenase, the role of other mediators is unclear. For example, eosinophil cationic protein (ECP) has been observed in IPF epithelial lining fluid (21). ECP is toxic to parasites, it is neurotoxic, and it can damage cell membranes (see Chapter 3.4.9), but it is not known whether ECP will damage the lung parenchyma. Histamine levels are also increased (69,70), likely reflecting the increase in mast cells in the alveolar walls (20). This might be the mechanism of the mild increased permeability observed in the lung parenchyma in IPF.

Mechanisms of Fibrosis

The classic concept of the "fibrosis" of pulmonary fibrosis, evolving from light-microscopic evaluation of lung biopsy and autopsy specimens, focused on the apparent increased numbers of collagen fibers in the thickened alveolar walls. From this, it was assumed that the collagen accumulated because the mesenchymal cells were producing more collagen; that is, the central "repair" process following injury was conceptualized as the up-regulation of synthesis and secretion of connective tissue matrix components, particularly collagen.

Although the up-regulation of collagen production by mesenchymal cells can be demonstrated *in vitro* (71), and such a process may be ongoing in the lung in IPF, it is now recognized that the dominant "repair" mechanism following alveolar injury is mesenchymal cell proliferation (2,72–85). This concept has developed from several lines of evidence. First, the parenchyma of the lung in IPF contains a relatively greater number of mesenchymal cells than of other parenchymal cells (see discussion of the morphologic changes in IPF, above). This observation is even more striking in the context that other cells, such as epithelial cells, are also increased in number (Figs. 5–7) (30). Second, whereas mitoses of mesenchymal cells within the alveolar wall are rarely observed, such events can be found in the IPF lung (Fig. 8), suggesting that mesenchymal cells in the IPF lung are proliferating at a rate higher than normal. Finally, alveolar macrophages removed from the lung of individuals with IPF are releasing potent polypeptide growth factors for mesenchymal cells, the same growth factors that will stimulate mesenchymal cells to proliferate *in vitro* (72,73,76,78–85).

From these considerations, an overall understanding of the fibrotic process has emerged: In the milieu of injury of the normal alveolar architecture, activated alveolar macrophages release potent growth factors that instruct mesenchymal cells to proliferate (Fig. 9). Since mesenchymal cells usually produce large amounts of collagen [approximately 6×10^5 collagen chains/cell-hr is typical for a human lung fibroblast population in culture (86)], the consequences of having an increased number of mesenchymal cells in the alveolar walls and alveolar air spaces is the deposition of a larger mass of collagen in the lung parenchyma than occurs in the normal lung in the same time period. Superimposed on this concept is the understanding of the importance of intra-alveolar fibrosis in the overall process (6). Through breaks in the basement membrane, mesenchymal cells and their connective tissue products accumulate in the air spaces, and there is subsequent re-epithelialization to incorporate these intra-alveolar masses into the alveolar wall. The overall result of these biologic processes is what is observed by histology: Alveolar walls are thickened with collagen fibers. Furthermore, it is important to recognize that each of the individual processes involved in the development of fibrosis is a normal biologic process, and it is the combination of these many normal processes that leads to the overall "abnormal" process of fibrosis.

Polypeptide Growth Factors

The alveolar macrophage is capable, when appropriately activated, of releasing a number of potent polypeptide growth factors (see Chapters 2.9 and 3.4.5). Evaluation of alveolar macrophages recovered from the epithelial surface of the lung of individuals with IPF has demonstrated they are spontaneously releasing three of these growth factors: platelet-derived growth factor (PDGF), fibronectin, and alveolar macrophage insulin-like growth factor 1 (IGF-1, formally called "alveolar macrophage-derived growth factor") (72,73,76,78–85). It is possible that cells other than alveolar macrophages are releasing such growth factors in the IPF lung and/or that other polypeptide growth factors play a role in IPF, but no other sources or molecules have been clearly identified.

PDGF, a 30-kDa dimer, is the most potent of the growth factors, with the ability to attract mesenchymal cells and stimulate them to enter the growth cycle (i.e., act as a stimulus to enter the G1 phase of the cell cycle; see Chapter 2.9). In IPF, the alveolar macrophages are releasing fourfold more PDGF than normal (81). Immune complexes (the putative alveolar macrophage ac-

tivating signals in IPF) are capable of activating normal alveolar macrophages *in vitro* to release PDGF (81). Evaluation of IPF alveolar macrophages has demonstrated an increased rate of transcription of the genes for the PDGF A and B chains (85). However, quantitation of mRNA levels shows that the B-chain transcripts dominate, suggesting that the PDGF molecules being synthesized and released by IPF alveolar macrophages are B–B homodimers, the most potent form of PDGF (85). This observation is also important conceptually because the PDGF B-chain gene is the *c-sis* proto-oncogene, the human equivalent of the *s-cis* viral gene of the simian sarcoma virus (87,88). Thus, IPF is one of the few examples in which there has been clear demonstration of the exaggerated local expression of an oncogene in a non-neoplastic disease state; that is, the biologic processes involved in the development of pulmonary fibrosis include a process central to the development of some neoplasms.

Fibronectin, a 440-kDa dimer, is generally considered to be a matrix component, with a variety of functions relevant to cell–cell and cell–matrix interactions (see Chapter 3.3.4). However, fibronectin can also act as a growth factor, initiating mesenchymal cells to enter G1 (75). In IPF, alveolar macrophages express increased amounts of fibronectin mRNA transcripts and release increased amounts of fibronectin, and there are increased levels of fibronectin in the epithelial lining fluid of these individuals (72,74,80,82). It is not clear what stimulates the alveolar macrophages to up-regulate the fibronectin gene in IPF, since attempts to modulate the fibronectin gene in normal alveolar macrophages *in vitro* have been unsuccessful.

The alveolar macrophage form of IGF-1 is 20–25 kDa, much larger than the serum form of IGF-1 (7–6 kDa, referred to as "somatomedin C") (83,89). IGF-1 acts late in G1 to take PDGF- or fibronectin-stimulated mesenchymal cells through to the S phase and subsequent proliferation (79,83,89). Early studies with IPF alveolar macrophages showed the spontaneous release of "alveolar macrophage-derived growth factor," a molecule now recognized to be IGF-1 (73,76,79,83,89). It is not known if IGF-1 or equivalent late-G1-acting growth signal is mandatory to drive mesenchymal cells to proliferate in the lung in IPF, since PDGF is capable of stimulating mesenchymal cells to proliferate in the absence of such signals. However, the fact that IGF-1 is likely present in excess in the IPF lung is consistent with the overall concept of the central role of exaggerated mesenchymal cell proliferation in the pathogenesis of pulmonary fibrosis.

Although the release of these polypeptide growth factors explains the exaggerated mesenchymal cell proliferation in the IPF lung, it does not explain the alterations in the relative proportions of the subpopulations of mesenchymal cells observed in IPF (see discussion of the morphology of IPF, above; for example, note the islands of accumulated smooth muscle cells in the IPF lung in the context of the rarity of smooth muscle cells in the normal alveolar walls (Figs. 6 and 7). It is not clear why there are changes in the proportions of mesenchymal cell subpopulations in IPF, but possible mechanisms include the following: (a) Different subtypes of mesenchymal cells have different relative densities of receptors for the polypeptide growth factors released by alveolar macrophages, resulting in a differential rate of subpopulation proliferation; (b) different subtypes have different inherent relative growth rates; (c) the subtypes differentiate into smooth muscle cells at an increased rate; and (d) some subtypes are attracted from the terminal bronchioles by chemotactic factors released in the alveolar walls (81).

Modulation of Connective Tissue Production and Degradation

There is no clear evidence that changes in connective tissue synthesis of degradation are important biological processes in the pathogenesis of pulmonary fibrosis in IPF, but there are observations consistent with the concept that such processes may be ongoing. Three classes of molecules—transforming growth factor β (TGF-β), prostaglandin E (PGE), and collagenases—have been implicated.

TGF-β, a 25-kDa molecule now recognized to be a family of several similar molecules, has dual effects in relation to fibrosis (90–92). In some *in vitro* systems TGF-β decreases the rate of proliferation of mesenchymal cells, whereas in others it has the opposite effect. There is no question, however, that TGF-β is capable of up-regulating genes for type I collagen and fibronectin, suggesting that it may play a role in stimulating mesenchymal cells in the lung parenchyma to produce more connective tissue (71,93). Whereas a role for TGF-β in IPF (or any human fibrotic lung disorder) has not been shown, it is known that respiratory epithelial lining fluid of the normal human lung contains large amounts of TGF-β and that alveolar macrophages are capable of expressing the TGF-β gene and releasing TGF-β (90,94). Thus, a scenario can be hypothesized whereby TGF-β in epithelial lining fluid gains access to mesenchymal cells following lung injury and breaks in the alveolar basement membrane, causing increased connective tissue deposition in the lung parenchyma.

PGE, a metabolite of arachidonic acid, has dual effects relevant to pulmonary fibrosis, including the following: (a) PGE causes increased intracellular degradation of collagen as it is being synthesized by mesenchymal cells, and (b) PGE suppresses the rate of mesenchymal cell proliferation in response to polypeptide growth factors (95). In the normal lung, there are large amounts of PGE in respiratory epithelial lining fluid; that is, PGE may normally serve as a counterbalance to signals for mesenchymal cell production of collagen and/or proliferation. However, in IPF, the levels of PGE in respiratory epithelial lining fluid are decreased significantly (T. Ozaki, S. Rennard, and R. Crystal, *unpublished observation*). Although mechanisms causing this are unknown, the consequences may be to release mesenchymal cells to respond to exogenous signals that ultimately result in the accumulation of mesenchymal cells and their connective tissue products.

Not much is known about the normal turnover of collagen in the human lung, although the fact that the normal human lung parenchyma continually synthesizes and secretes collagen but does not accumulate collagen implies that there must be ongoing mechanisms to balance synthesis with degradation of extracellular collagen (37). Collagenase has been observed in the normal human lung, and it is produced by cells such as mesenchymal cells and inflammatory cells (see Chapter 7.1.1). Studies with fragments of lung from IPF imply a decrease in collagenase activity, but it is not clear what role this may have in the enhanced collagen accumulation observed as part of the fibrotic process (see above for a discussion of this in relation to the increased amounts of collagenase activity also observed in IPF) (41,67).

APPROACHES TO THERAPY

With the understanding that the pathogenesis of fibrosis in IPF involves a variety of normal but exaggerated biologic processes, it follows that rational therapy for IPF should be directed toward suppressing these processes. Current strategies are directed toward nonspecific suppression of the inflammation, defending the parenchyma against injury, and suppressing the response of mesenchymal cells to exogenous growth signals.

Nonspecific Suppression of Inflammation

The classic therapy for IPF is the chronic administration of glucocorticoids (2,96,97). Although there is anecdotal evidence of responses to these agents, there have been no controlled trials to demonstrate their effectiveness; in addition, IPF patients treated with glucocorticoids often develop a range of adverse effects typical of these agents. Furthermore, although human alveolar macrophages have receptors for glucocorticoids, IPF patients treated with glucocorticoids generally release the same exaggerated amounts of polypeptide growth factors as do untreated IPF patients (98).

Cyclophosphamide is capable of reducing the burden of neutrophils in the IPF lung (99). There is some evidence that cyclophosphamide alone or in combination with glucocorticoids is more effective than glucocorticoids alone in the treatment if IPF, but the evidence is not definitive (100).

Defense of the Parenchyma Against Injury

In the context that oxidants and proteases play a role in the injury to the lung in IPF, enhancing antioxidant and antiprotease defense against this onslaught is a rational approach to this disease. As a first approach to this concept, reduced GSH has been delivered by aerosol to individuals with IPF, demonstrating (a) a subsequent increase in oxidized GSH in respiratory epithelial lining fluid and (b) a decrease in superoxide anion release by inflammatory cells recovered from the epithelial surface (101,102). With regard to proteases, the most rational approach would be to augment anticollagenase levels to protect against the fragmentation of collagen by neutrophil collagenase. One such approach would be administration of the tissue inhibitor of metalloproteinases, a known collagenase inhibitor (see Chapter 7.1.2). Such studies have not been attempted, and there is the possible risk that enhancing anticollagenase activity may permit collagen to accumulate at a more rapid rate.

Suppression of the Response of Mesenchymal Cells to Exogenous Signals

The first approach to this strategy was to use colchicine, an inhibitor of protein secretion, in an attempt to suppress the release of growth factors by alveolar macrophages (103). However, while possible *in vitro*, the levels required for *in vivo* suppression would not be tolerated without adverse effects. Presently, efforts are being focused on ways to augment PGE levels in the lung. Since PGE both suppresses collagen production by mesenchymal cells and decreases the ability of mesenchymal cells to respond to exogenous growth signals, it may be a useful agent in preventing the fibrotic process in IPF. Strategies have been developed to deliver PGE directly to the epithelal surface of the lower respiratory tract by aerosol. Studies in sheep have shown that the respiratory epithelial lining fluid PGE levels can be enhanced by this approach, although interstitial levels (as reflected by measurements in lung lymph) are not significantly increased (104). Thus, this approach may be useful for suppressing the

intra-alveolar component of the fibrosis of IPF but not for suppressing the interstitial component.

REFERENCES

1. Crystal RG, Gadek JE, Ferrans VJ, Fulmer JD, Line BR, Hunninghake GW. Interstitial lung disease: current concepts of pathogenesis, staging, and therapy. *Am J Med* 1981;70:542–568.
2. Crystal RG, Bitterman PB, Rennard SI, Hance A, Keogh BA. Interstitial lung disease of unknown cause: disorders characterized by chronic inflammation of the lower respiratory tract. *N Engl J Med* 1984;310:154–166, 235–244.
3. Davis WB, Crystal RG. Chronic interstitial lung disease. In: Simmons D, ed. *Current pulmonology*, vol V. New York: Wiley, 1984;347–473.
4. Rennard SI, Bitterman PB, Crystal RG. Current concepts of the pathogenesis of fibrosis: lessons from pulmonary fibrosis. In: Berk P, ed. *Myelofibrosis and the biology of connective tissue*. New York: Alan R. Liss, 1984;359–377.
5. Crystal RG, Ferrans VJ. Reactions of the interstitial space to injury. In: Fishman AP, ed. *Pulmonary diseases and disorders*. New York: McGraw–Hill, 1988;711–738.
6. Basset F, Ferrans VJ, Soler P, Takemura T, Fuduka Y, Crystal RG. Intraluminal fibrosis in interstitial lung disorders. *Am J Pathol* 1986;122:443–461.
7. Crystal RG, Fulmer JD, Baum BJ, Bernardo J, Bradley KH, Breul SD, Elson NA, Fells GA, Ferrans VJ, Gadek JE, Hunninghake GW, Kawanami O, Kelman JA, Line BR, McDonald JA, McLees BD, Roberts WC, Rosenberg DM, Tolstoshev P, Von Gal E, Weinberger SE. Cells, collagen and idiopathic pulmonary fibrosis. *Lung* 1978;155:199–224.
8. Hunninghake GW, Gadek JE, Kawanami O, Ferrans VJ, Crystal RG. Inflammatory and immune processes in the human lung in health and disease: evaluation by bronchoalveolar lavage. *Am J Pathol* 1979;97:149–206.
9. Koegh BA, Crystal RG. Alveolitis: the key to the interstitial lung disorders. *Thorax* 1982;37:1–10.
10. Bitterman PB, Rennard SI, Keogh BA, Wewers MD, Adelberg S, Crystal RG. Familial idiopathic pulmonary fibrosis: evidence of lung inflammation in unaffected family members. *N Engl J Med* 1986;314(21):1343–1347.
11. Snider GL. Interstitial pulmonary fibrosis. *Chest* 1986;89(Suppl 3):115S–121S.
12. Reiser KM, Last JA. Early cellular events in pulmonary fibrosis. *Exp Lung Res* 1986;10(4):331–355.
13. Scadding JG, Hinson KFW. Diffuse fibrosing alveolitis (diffuse interstitial fibrosis of the lungs): correlation of histology at biopsy with prognosis. *Thorax* 1967;22:291–304.
14. Crystal RG, Fulmer JD, Roberts WC, Moss ML, Line BR, Reynolds HY. Idiopathic pulmonary fibrosis: clinical, histologic, radiographic, physiologic, scintigraphic, cytologic, and biochemical aspects. *Ann Intern Med* 1976;85:769–788.
15. Hance A, Crystal RG. Idiopathic pulmonary fibrosis. In: Flenley DC, Petty TL, eds. *Recent advances in respiratory medicine*, vol 3. Edinburgh: Churchill Livingstone, 1983;249–287.
16. Fulmer JD, Roberts WC, Von Gal ER, Crystal RG. Morphologic–physiologic correlates of the severity of fibrosis and degree of cellularity in idiopathic pulmonary fibrosis. *J Clin Invest* 1979;63:665–676.
17. Borok Z, Trapnell BC, Crystal RG. Neutrophils and the pathogenesis of idiopathic pulmonary fibrosis. In: Baggiolini M, Pozzi E, Semenzato G, eds. *Pathophysiology of pulmonary cells: neutrophils and lymphocytes*. Milan: Masson Italia, 1990; in press.
18. Reynolds HY, Fulmer JD, Kazmierowski JA, Roberts WC, Frank MM, Crystal RG. Analysis of bronchoalveolar lavage fluid from patients with idiopathic pulmonary fibrosis and chronic hypersensitivity pneumonitis. *J Clin Invest* 1977; 59:165–175.
19. Davis WB, Fells GA, Sun X, Gadek JE, Venet A, Crystal RG. Eosinophil-mediated injury to lung parenchymal cells and in-

terstitial matrix: a possible role for eosinophils in chronic inflammatory disorders of the lower respiratory tract. *J Clin Invest* 1984;74:269–278.

20. Kawanami O, Ferrans VJ, Fulmer JD, Crystal RG. Ultrastructure of pulmonary mast cells in patients with fibrotic lung disorders. *Lab Invest* 1979;40:717–734.

21. Hällgren R, Bjermer L, Lundgren R, Venge P. The eosinophil component of the alveolitis in idiopathic pulmonary fibrosis. Signs of eosinophil activation in the lung are related to impaired lung function. *Am Rev Respir Dis* 1989;139(2):373–377.

22. Shindoh Y, Shimura S, Tomioka M, Aikawa T, Sasaki H, Takishima T. Cellular analysis in bronchoalveolar lavage fluids in infiltrative and fibrotic stages of idiopathic pulmonary fibrosis. *Tohoku J Exp Med* 1986;149(1):47–60.

23. Shindoh Y, Tanno Y, Ida S, Takishima T. Morphological characterization off basophilic cells in bronchoalveolar lavage fluids from patients with bronchial asthma and idiopathic pulmonary fibrosis. *Tohoku J Exp Med* 1987;152(1):101–102.

24. Haslam PL, Turton CWG, Lukoszek A, Salsbury AJ, Dawar A. Bronchoalveolar lavage fluid cell counts in cryptogenic fibrosing alveolitis and their relation to therapy. *Thorax* 1980;35:328–339.

25. Turner-Warwick M, Burrows B, Johnson A. Cryptogenic fibrosing alveolitis: clinical features and their influence on survival. *Thorax* 1980;35:171–180.

26. Dreisin RB, Schwarz MI, Theofilopoulos AN, Stanford RE. Circulating immune complexes in the idiopathic interstitial pneumonias. *N Engl J Med* 1978;298:353–357.

27. Martinet Y, Haslam PL, Turner-Warwick M. Clinical significance of circulating immune complexes in 'lone' cryptogenic fibrosing alveolitis and those with associated connective tissue disorders. *Clin Allergy* 1984;14:491–497.

28. Fulmer JD, Roberts WC, Von Gal ER, Crystal RG. Small airways in idiopathic pulmonary fibrosis: comparison of morphologic and physiologic observations. *J Clin Invest* 1977;60:595–610.

29. Crapo JD, Barry BE, Gehr P, Bachofen M, Weibel ER. Cell number and cell characteristics of the normal human lung. *Am Rev Respir Dis* 1982;125:332–337.

30. Kawanami O, Ferrans VJ, Crystal RG. Structure of alveolar epithelial cells in patients with fibrotic lung disorders. *Lab Invest* 1982;46:39–53.

31. Ohtsuka Y, Tanimura K, Munakata M, Ukita H, Homma H, Kawakami Y. Idiopathic interstitial pneumonia (IIP) as a risk factor for a lung cancer—a prospective study. *Am Rev Respir Dis* 1990;141(Suppl):A61.

32. Nukiwa T, Sakuraba S, Aiba M, Dambara T, Kira S. Does the chronic inflammatory milieu in the peripheral airspace act as a promoter for the high incidence carcinogenesis in patients with idiopathic interstitial pneumonia (IIP)? *Am Rev Respir Dis* 1990;141(Suppl):A61.

33. Weibel ER. Morphologic basis of alveolar–capillary gas exchange. *Physiol Rev* 1973;53:419–495.

34. Grevers G, Herrmann U. Fenestrated endothelia in vessels of the nasal mucosa: an electron-microscopic study in the rabbit. *Arch Otorhinolaryngol* 1987;244:55–60.

35. Hirabayashi M, Yamamoto T. An electron-microscopic study of the endothelium in mammalian bronchial microvasculature. *Cell Tissue Res* 1984;236:19–25.

36. Bradley K, McConnell-Breul S, Crystal RG. Lung collagen heterogeneity. *Proc Natl Acad Sci USA* 1974;71:2828–2832.

37. Bradley K, McConnell-Breul S, Crystal RG. Collagen in the human lung: quantitation of rates of synthesis and partial characterization of composition. *J Clin Invest* 1975;55:543–550.

38. Fulmer JD, Bienkowski RS, Cowan MJ, Breul SD, Bradley KM, Ferrans VJ, Roberts WC, Crystal RG. Collagen concentration and rates of synthesis in idiopathic pulmonary fibrosis. *Am Rev Respir Dis* 1980;122:289–301.

39. Kirk JM, Da Costa PE, Turner-Warwick M, Littleton RJ, Laurent GJ. Biochemical evidence for an increased and progressive deposition of collagen in lungs of patients with pulmonary fibrosis. *Clin Sci* 1986;70(1):39–45.

40. Saldiva PH, Delmonte VC, de Carvalho CR, Kairalla RA, Auler JO Jr. Histochemical evaluation of lung collagen content in acute and chronic interstitial diseases. *Chest* 1989;95(5):953–957.

41. Selman M, Montano M, Ramos C, Chapela R. Concentration, biosynthesis and degradation of collagen in idiopathic pulmonary fibrosis. *Thorax* 1986;41(5):355–359.

42. Kuhn C 3d, Boldt J, King TE Jr, Crouch E, Vartio T, McDonald JA. An immunohistochemical study of architectural remodeling and connective tissue synthesis in pulmonary fibrosis. *Am Rev Respir Dis* 1989;140(6):1693–1703.

43. Dall'Aglio PP, Pesci A, Bertorelli G, Brianti E, Scarpa S. Study of immune complexes in bronchoalveolar lavage fluids. *Respiration* 1988;54(Suppl 1):36–41.

44. Kravis TC, Ahmed A, Brown TE, Fulmer JD, Crystal RG. Pathogenic mechanisms in pulmonary fibrosis: collagen-induced migration inhibition factor production and cytotoxicity mediated by lymphocytes. *J Clin Invest* 1976;58:1223–1232.

45. Baumgartner U, Scholmerich J, Becher S, Costabel U. Detection of antibodies in serum of patients with idiopathic pulmonary fibrosis against isolated rat alveolar type II cells. *Respiration* 1987;52(2):122–128.

46. Paradis IL, Dauber JH, Rabin BS. Lymphocyte phenotypes in bronchoalveolar lavage and lung tissue in sarcoidosis and idiopathic pulmonary fibrosis. *Am Rev Respir Dis* 1986;133(5):855–860.

47. Cathcart MK, Emdur LI, Ahtiala-Stewart K, Ahmad M. Excessive helper T-cell function in patients with idiopathic pulmonary fibrosis: correlation with disease activity. *Clin Immunol Immunopathol* 1987;43(3):382–394.

48. Weinberger SE, Kelman JA, Elson NA, Young RC Jr, Reynolds HY, Fulmer JD, Crystal RG. Bronchoalveolar lavage in intersitital lung disease. *Ann Intern Med* 1978;89:459–466.

49. Hunninghake GW, Gadek JE, Fales HM, Crystal RG. Human alveolar macrophage-derived chemotactic factor for neutrophils: stimuli and partial characterization. *J Clin Invest* 1980;66:473–483.

50. Hunninghake GW, Gadek JE, Lawley TJ, Crystal RG. Mechanisms of neutrophil accumulation in the lungs of patients with idiopathic pulmonary fibrosis. *J Clin Invest* 1981;68:259–269.

51. Merrill WW, Naegel GP, Matthay RA, Reynolds HY. Alveolar macrophage-derived chemotactic factor: kinetics of *in vitro* production and partial characterization. *J Clin Invest* 1980;65:268–276.

52. Fels AOS, Pawlowski NA, Cramer EB, King TKC, Cohn ZA, Scott WA. Human alveolar macrophages produce leukotriene B$_4$. *Proc Natl Acad Sci USA* 1982;79:7866–7870.

53. Martin TR, Raugi G, Merritt TL, Henderson WR Jr. Relative contribution of leukotriene B$_4$ to the neutrophil chemotactic activity produced by the resident human alveolar macrophage. *J Clin Invest* 1987;80:1114–1124.

54. Strieter RM, Kunkel SL, Showell HJ, Remick DG, Phan SH. Endothelial cell gene expression of a neutrophil chemotactic factor by TNF-α, LPS, and IL-1β. *Science* 243:1467–1469.

55. Baggiolini M, Walz A, Kunkel SL. Neutrophil-activating peptide-1/interleukin 8, a novel cytokine that activates neutrophils. *J Clin Invest* 1989;84:1045–1049.

56. Wardlaw AJ, Hay H, Cromwell O, Collins JV, Kay AB. Leukotrienes, LTC$_4$ and LTB$_4$, in bronchoalveolar lavage in bronchial asthma and other respiratory diseases. *J Allergy Clin Immunol* 1989;84:19–26.

57. Gadek JE, Hunninghake GW, Zimmerman RL, Crystal RG. Regulation of the release of alveolar macrophage-derived neutrophil chemotactic factor. *Am Rev Respir Dis* 1980;121:723–733.

58. Du Bois RM, Townsend PJ, Cole PJ. Alveolar macrophage lysosomal enzyme and C3b receptors in cryptogenic fibrosing alveolitis. *Clin Exp Immunol* 1980;40:60–65.

59. Hoogsteden HC, van Dongen JJ, van Hal PT, Delahaye M, Hop W, Hilvering C. Phenotype of blood monocytes and alveolar macrophages in interstitial lung disease. *Chest* 1989;95(3):574–577.

60. Bitterman PB, Saltzman LE, Adelberg S, Ferrans VJ, Crystal RG. Alveolar macrophage replication: one mechanism for the expansion of the mononuclear phagocyte population in the chronically inflamed lung. *J Clin Invest* 1984;74:460–469.

61. Martin WJ II, Gadek JE, Hunninghake GW, Crystal RG. Oxidant injury of lung parenchymal cells. *J Clin Invest* 1981;68:1277–1288.

62. Cantin AM, North SL, Fells GA, Hubbard RC, Crystal RG. Oxidant mediated epithelial cell injury in idiopathic pulmonary fibrosis. *J Clin Invest* 1987;79:1665–1675.

63. Reynolds HY. Lung inflammation: normal host defense or a complication of some diseases? *Annu Rev Med* 1987;38:295–323.

64. Strausz J, Muller-Quernheim J, Steppling H, Ferlinz R. Oxygen radical production by alveolar inflammatory cells in idiopathic pulmonary fibrosis. *Am Rev Respir Dis* 1990;141(1):124–128.

65. Cantin A, North SL, Hubbard RC, Crystal RG. Normal alveolar epithelial lining fluid contains high levels of glutathione. *J Appl Physiol* 1987;63:152–157.

66. Cantin AM, Hubbard RC, Crystal RG. Glutathione deficiency in the epithelial lining fluid of the lower respiratory tract of patients with idiopathic pulmonary fibrosis. *Am Rev Respir Dis* 1989;139:370–372.

67. Gadek JE, Kelman JA, Fells GA, Weinberger SE, Horwitz AL, Reynolds HY, Fulmer JD, Crystal RG. Collagenase in the lower respiratory tract of patients with idiopathic pulmonary fibrosis. *N Engl J Med* 1979;301:737–742.

68. Montano M, Ramos C, Gonzalez G, Vadillo F, Pardo A, Selman M. Lung collagenase inhibitors and spontaneous and latent collagenase activity in idiopathic pulmonary fibrosis and hypersensitivity pneumonitis. *Chest* 1989;96(5):1115–1119.

69. Rankin JA, Kaliner M, Reynolds HY. Histamine levels in bronchoalveolar lavage from patients with asthma, sarcoidosis, and idiopathic pulmonary fibrosis. *J Allergy Clin Immunol* 1987;79(2):371–377.

70. Casale TB, Trapp S, Zehr B, Hunninghake GW. Bronchoalveolar lavage fluid histamine levels in interstitial lung diseases. *Am Rev Respir Dis* 1988;138(6):1604–1608.

71. Fine A, Goldstein RH. The effect of transforming growth factor-beta on cell proliferation and collagen formation by lung fibroblasts. *J Biol Chem* 1987;262(8):3897–3902.

72. Rennard SI, Hunninghake GW, Bitterman PB, Crystal RG. Production of fibronectin by the human alveolar macrophage: mechanism for the recruitment of fibroblasts to sites of tissue injury in interstitial lung diseases. *Proc Natl Acad Sci USA* 1981;78:7147–7151.

73. Bitterman PB, Rennard SI, Hunninghake GW, Crystal RG. Human alveolar macrophage growth factor for fibroblasts: regulation and partial characterization. *J Clin Invest* 1982;70:806–822.

74. Rennard SI, Crystal RG. Fibronectin in human bronchopulmonary lavage fluid: elevation of patients with interstitial lung disease. *J Clin Invest* 1982;69:113–122.

75. Bitterman PB, Rennard SI, Adelberg S, Crystal RG. Role of fibronectin as a growth factor for fibroblasts. *J Cell Biol* 1983;97:1925–1932.

76. Bitterman PB, Adelberg S, Crystal RG. Mechanisms of pulmonary fibrosis: spontaneous release of the alveolar macrophage derived growth factor in the interstitial lung disorders. *J Clin Invest* 1983;72:1801–1813.

77. Martinet Y, Bitterman PB, Mornex J-F, Grotendorst GR, Martin GR, Crystal RG. Activated human monocytes express the c-sis proto-oncogene and release a mediator showing PDGF-like activity. *Nature* 1986;319(9):158–160.

78. Mornex J-F, Martinet Y, Yamauchi K, Bitterman P, Grotendorst GR, Chytil-Weir A, Martin GR, Crystal RG. Spontaneous expression of the c-sis gene and release of a platelet-derived growth factor-like molecule by human alveolar macrophages. *J Clin Invest* 1986;78:61–66.

79. Bitterman PB, Wewers MD, Rennard SI, Adelberg S, Crystal RG. Modulation of alveolar macrophage-driven fibroblast proliferation by alternative macrophage mediators. *J Clin Invest* 1986;77(3):700–708.

80. Yamauchi K, Martinet Y, Crystal RG. Modulation of fibronectin gene expression in human mononuclear phagocytes. *J Clin Invest* 1987;80(6):1720–1727.

81. Martinet Y, Rom WN, Grotendorst GR, Martin GR, Crystal RG. Exaggerated spontaneous release of a platelet-derived

growth factor by alveolar macrophages from patients with idiopathic pulmonary fibrosis. *N Engl J Med* 1987;317(4):202–209.

82. Adachi K, Yamauchi K, Bernaudin J-F, Ferrans VJ, Crystal RG. Evaluation of fibronectin gene expression by *in situ* hybridization: differential expression of the fibronectin gene among populations of human alveolar macrophages. *Am J Pathol* 1988;138:193–203.

83. Rom WN, Basset P, Fells GA, Nukiwa T, Crystal RG. Alveolar macrophages release an insulin-like growth factor I-type molecule. *J Clin Invest* 1988;82:1685–1693.

84. Trapnell BC, Crystal RG. Pathogenesis of tissue fibrosis: growth factor gene expression in mononuclear phagocytes. In: Melchers F, ed. *Progress of immunology*. Berlin: Springer-Verlag, 1989;754–764.

85. Nagaoka I, Trapnell BC, Crystal RG. Up-regulation of platelet-derived growth factor-A and -B gene expression in alveolar macrophages of individuals with idiopathic pulmonary fibrosis. *J Clin Invest* 1990;85:2023–2027.

86. Breul SK, Bradley KH, Hance AJ, Schafer MP, Berg RA, Crystal RG. Control of collagen production by human diploid lung fibroblasts. *J Biol Chem* 1980;255:5250–5260.

87. Waterfield MD, Scarce GT, Whittle N, Stroobant P, Johnsson A, Wasteson A, Westermak B, Heldin CH, Huang JS, Deuel TF. Platelet-derived growth factor is structurally related to the putative transforming protein p28^sis of simian sarcoma virus. *Nature* 1983;304:35–39.

88. Doolittle RF, Hunkapiller MW, Hood LE, Devare SG, Robbins KC, Aaronson SA, Antoniades HN. Simian sarcoma virus onc gene, v-sis, is derived from the gene (or genes) encoding a platelet-derived growth factor. *Science* 1983;21:275–277.

89. Nagoka I, Trapnell BC, Crystal RG. Regulation of insulin-like growth factor-I expression in mononuclear phagocytes. *J Clin Invest* 1990;85:445–448.

90. Yamauchi K, Martinet Y, Basset P, Fells GA, Crystal RG. High levels of transforming growth factor-β are present in the epithelial lining fluid of the normal human lower respiratory tract. *Am Rev Respir Dis* 1988;137:1360–1363.

91. Roberts AB, Anzano MA, Wakefield LM, Roche NS, Stern DF, Sporn MB. Type β transforming growth factor: a bifunctional regulator of cellular growth. *Proc Natl Acad Sci USA* 1985;82:119–123.

92. Hill DJ, Strain AJ, Elstow SF, Swenne I, Milner RD. Bi-functional action of transforming growth factor-β on DNA synthesis in early passage human fetal fibroblasts. *J Cell Physiol* 1986;128:322–328.

93. Roberts CJ, Birkenmeier TM, McQuillan JJ, Akiyama SK, Yamada SS, Chen WT, Yamada KM, McDonald JA. Transforming growth factor beta stimulates the expression of fibronectin and of both subunits of the human fibronectin receptor by cultured human lung fibroblasts. *J Biol Chem* 1988;263(10):4586–4592.

94. Yamauchi K, Basset P, Martinet Y, Crystal R. Normal human alveolar macrophages express the gene coding for transforming growth factor-β, a protein with a capacity to suppress fibroblast growth. *Am Rev Respir Dis* 1987;135(4):A66.

95. Ozaki T, Rennard SI, Crystal RG. Cyclooxygenase metabolites are compartmentalized in the human lower respiratory tract. *J Appl Physiol* 1987;62(1):219–222.

96. Crystal RG. Therapy of idiopathic pulmonary fibrosis. In: Fauci A, Lichtenstein L, eds. *Current therapy in allergy and immunology*. Philadelphia: BC Decker, 1983;197–203.

97. Keogh BA, Bernardo J, Hunninghake GW, Line BR, Price D, Crystal RG. Effect of intermittent high dose parenteral corticosteroids on the alveolitis of idiopathic pulmonary fibrosis. *Am Rev Respir Dis* 1983;127:18–27.

98. Lacronique JG, Rennard SI, Bitterman PB, Ozaki T, Crystal RG. Alveolar macrophages in idiopathic pulmonary fibrosis have glucocorticoid receptors, but glucocorticoid therapy does not suppress alveolar macrophage release of fibronectin and alveolar macrophage derived growth factor. *Am Rev Respir Dis* 1984;130:450–456.

99. O'Donnell K, Keogh B, Cantin A, Crystal RG. Pharmacologic suppression of the neutrophil component of the alveolitis in

idiopathic pulmonary fibrosis. *Am Rev Respir Dis* 1987; 136(2):288–292.

100. Johnson MA, Kwan S, Snell NJC, Nunn AJ, Darbyshire JH, Turner-Warwick M. Randomised controlled trial comparing prednisolone alone with cyclophosphamide and low dose prednisolone in combination in cryptogenic fibrosing alveolitis. *Thorax* 1989;44:280–288.

101. Buhl R, Vogelmeier C, Crittenden M, Hubbard RC, Hoyt RF, Wilson EM, Cantin AM, Crystal RG. Augmentation of reduced glutathione levels in the epithelial lining fluid of the lower respiratory tract by direct aerosol administration of glutathione. *Proc Natl Acad Sci USA* 1990; in press.

102. Borok Z, Buhl R, Grimes G, Bokser A, Hubbard R. Glutathione aerosol therapy to augment the alveolar epithelial antioxidant screen in idiopathic pulmonary fibrosis. *Am Rev Respir Dis* 1990;141(4):A320.

103. Rennard SI, Bitterman PB, Ozaki T, Crystal RG. Colchicine suppresses the release of fibroblast growth factors from alveolar macrophages *in vitro:* the basis of a possible therapeutic approach to the fibrotic disorders. *Am Rev Respir Dis* 1988;137:181–185.

104. Borok Z, Gillissen A, Buhl R, Hoyt RF, Hubbard RC, Crystal RG. Augmentation of functional prostaglandin E levels on the respiratory epithelial surface by aerosol administration. *Clin Res* 1990;38(2):485A.

THE LUNG: *Scientific Foundations*
edited by R.G. Crystal, J.B. West et al.
Raven Press, Ltd., New York © 1991.

CHAPTER 7.8.2

Animal Models of Pulmonary Fibrosis

Alan Fine, Ronald H. Goldstein, and Gordon L. Snider

Pulmonary fibrosis may be defined as an inflammatory process involving all components of the alveolar wall which results in the disordering of the lung architecture with deposition of excess connective tissue elements; fibrosis need not be present at all stages of the process (1–4). The initial inflammatory process may be granulomatous or nongranulomatous and may completely resolve without apparent sequelae. Pulmonary fibrosis may be considered a subset of the interstitial lung diseases.

Diverse exposures and conditions are believed to cause pulmonary fibrosis in humans. Examples are inhalation of (a) particulate agents such as silica, asbestos, or organic dusts and (b) gaseous agents such as cadmium fumes, (c) physical agents such as ionizing radiation and (d) infectious agents may also give rise to pulmonary fibrosis (1,3,4). In many cases, an etiology cannot be identified; such cases are referred to as "idiopathic." About 15% of the idiopathic cases are associated with systemic diseases such as rheumatoid arthritis (3,4). Most patients with pulmonary fibrosis develop symptoms insidiously and deteriorate progressively over several years (4,5). Pulmonary fibrosis may also result from a fulminant lung injury such as that observed in patients with the adult respiratory distress syndrome (ARDS) who have survived into the 2nd week of their disease (6). A subgroup of those patients with ARDS develop fibrosis and become symptomatic over the course of weeks to months (6). Hamman and Rich (7) described a rapidly progressive form of pulmonary fibrosis that ran its course over a period of months.

Whether the acute fulminant form or the idiopathic variety is part of the spectrum of a single disease or represents distinct disease entities is unclear. To gain insight into mechanisms which determine the outcome of lung injury, a variety of animal models of pulmonary fibrosis have been developed and studied. In these models, acute lung injury is induced through administration of a noxious agent in a single dose. A massive inflammatory reaction ensues, which may resolve in some cases or may rapidly progress to fibrosis in other cases. The outcome of the injury depends on a complex interaction of the extent of initial injury, the nature of the subsequent inflammatory reaction, and other poorly understood factors. These models seem to more closely parallel the forms of human pulmonary fibrosis which follow ARDS or typify the Hamman–Rich syndrome (6,7) rather than the insidious, chronic form of human pulmonary fibrosis. The progressive form can be simulated in animals by the repeated administration of a noxious agent (8).

Numerous distinct noxious substances produce animal pulmonary fibrosis in a variety of different species (9–22). These agents include: bleomycin (9–11), ionizing radiation (12–14), paraquat (15), toxic oxygen products (16,17), phorbol myristate acetate (18), silica (19), asbestos (20), butylated hydroxytoluene (21,22), and others. Rather than survey the literature on each of these injurious agents, our goal in this review is to summarize the factors which determine the outcome of an acute lung injury, regardless of the precipitating etiology (see also Chapters 7.2.1, 7.2.4, 7.3.5, 7.5.2, 7.7.1, 7.7.2, 7.7.3.1, and 7.8.1).

HISTOPATHOLOGICAL CHANGES IN ANIMAL PULMONARY FIBROSIS

The development of fibrosis seems to relate primarily to the events which subserve the reparative process rather than the injury per se (Table 1). Although the process is initiated by exposure to an injurious agent, additional injury appears to be associated with the in-

A. Fine, R. H. Goldstein, and G. L. Snider: Pulmonary Section, Boston D.V.A. Medical Center, Boston, Massachusetts 02130.

TABLE 1. *Characteristic features of experimental interstitial fibrosis in animals*

Initial injury
Focal distribution
Leakage of serum proteins and cells into the alveolar space
Damage to epithelial and endothelial cells
Increased procoagulant activity
Decreased fibrinolytic activity

Reparative phase
Increased fibroblast proliferation
Increased connective tissue production
Loss of alveolar units

flux of inflammatory cells. In particular, toxic oxygen derivatives and proteolytic enzymes are released by inflammatory cells, which cause further cellular damage and disruption of the associated extracellular matrix (23,24; see also Chapters 7.1.1 and 7.1.2).

Initial Injury

Various agents damage either pulmonary epithelium or capillary endothelium, and abnormalities in one or both cell types are usually the first observable change (25). The lesion is typically focal and inhomogeneous in distribution, even when the process is widespread. This may reflect distribution of the injurious agent during administration. Regardless of the initial site of injury, alterations in capillary permeability rapidly ensue (26). Leakage of serum proteins, cells, and platelets into the interstitial and alveolar space is apparent several hours after injury (10). Marked increases in total DNA content soon after injury reflect the dramatic increases in inflammatory cells that are seen in the lungs or noted by bronchoalveolar lavage (27). Dramatic increases in surfactant production have been noted in several models, particularly following instillation of silica (28–30).

The coagulation system is activated early, and fibrinogen in the intra-alveolar space is converted to fibrin (31–34). Fibroblasts contain receptors for fibrinogen–fibrin (35,36). These proteins could function as a nascent extracellular substrate for adhesion, since fibroblasts adhering to a fibrin meshwork *in vitro* synthesize collagen (35,36). Several studies have shown that lavage fluid obtained soon after acute injury contains a significant increase in procoagulant activity and a significant decrease in fibrinolytic activity (31–34). With resolution of injury, these abnormalities resolve (33). In contrast, if fibrosis ensues, a persistent predisposition to fibrin formation can be documented (33).

The exudation of inflammatory cells into the interstitium and the alveolar space continues for at least 24–48 hr (10). Similar to other acute inflammatory reactions, there is an initial predominance of neutrophils (37,38). Over the next several days, the neutrophils begin to recede, but overall increases in neutrophils may persist for several months (39). Macrophages and lymphocytes then become the predominant cell type (38). Several investigators have also shown that there is an increased number of eosinophils and mast cells in the interstitium (40–42). Eosinophils contain proteases and other substances which have been shown to degrade matrix molecules (41), indicating that these cells could function to remodel newly synthesized scar tissue.

In asbestos-induced lung injury, macrophages may first predominate because of migrations to sites of alveolar duct bifurcations, the initial site of fiber deposition (43,44). The overwhelming majority of lymphocytes which migrate into sites of lung injury are T cells (38). In contrast to circulating blood and lymph, where helper cells predominate, there is an equal proportion of helper and suppressor T-cell subsets in an injured lung (38). The role of specific cell-surface adhesion molecules mediating the migration of specific T-cell subsets into an injured lung is not certain. Overall, the fact that mononuclear cells synthesize and secrete a wide variety of effector molecules which affect the growth and remodeling of the extracellular matrix suggests a critical role for these cells in the reparative process (45–48).

Denudation of the epithelium and disruption of the epithelial basement membrane are common early features (25,37,49–51). Type I cells, forming approximately 80% of the surface area of alveoli, are more susceptible to injury than are type II cells (50,51). Within several days of injury, dedifferentiation and replication of type II cells occur as these cells spread out to replace the damaged type I cells (25,29,30,52–54). Ultrastructural studies have demonstrated marked alterations in the epithelial basement membrane (49). Disruptions in the basement membrane result in direct contact between alveolar epithelial cells and underlying mesenchymal cells (37). The function of such contacts is not clear; epithelial–mesenchymal contacts have been noted in carcinomas when there is an accompanying local fibrotic reaction (55). Progressive folding, thickening, and duplication of the epithelial basement membrane occur, most marked in regions of fibrosis (49). These most likely represent denuded basement membranes for alveoli that have collapsed.

Reparative Phase

The repair of the injury usually involves an increase in fibroblast proliferation, deposition of connective tissue, and alteration in lung architecture. A marked increase in interstitial myofibroblasts has been shown in several different models (25,56–59). These cells have characteristics of both smooth muscle cells and fibroblasts (57,58; see also Chapter 3.3.1). Myofibroblasts are found during repair of injured tissues (59), may function to synthesize type III collagen (60), and may mediate the increased contractile properties of injured lung parenchyma (57). If the inflammatory reaction does not completely resolve, histological and biochemical confirmation of fibrosis is noted several weeks after induction of injury (61–64).

Loss of alveolar units occurs with either (a) proliferation of fibroblasts within the interstitium or (b) migration and proliferation of fibroblasts within an organizing exudate in the alveolar space (65,66). This process results in increases in collagen, elastin, and glycosaminoglycans in the lung (2,67; see also Chapters 3.3.2, 3.3.3, and 3.3.5). Variations in the amount of connective tissue deposited, as well as changes in lung architecture, may relate to the site of injury or extent of cellular damage (2,67–72). Some injuries result in a mixed pattern of pulmonary fibrosis with air-space disease. Cadmium chloride will induce an acute lung injury which culminates in pulmonary fibrosis (73), although air-space enlargement also occurs. With the concomitant administration of a lathyrogen (β-aminoproprionitrile), cadmium chloride induces a lesion typical of bullous emphysema (73). Thus the reparative process following injury by different agents has some similar themes and some special features.

Recent data would suggest that multiple distinct cellular pathways can be individually activated by specific effector molecules (74). For example, the insulin-like growth factors and transforming growth factor beta (TGF-β) activate collagen formation in human lung fibroblasts through two clearly distinguishable mechanisms (74). Such results would indicate that although the morphological characteristics of lung injury may follow a defined set of events, the molecular pathways activated may differ in different types of injury.

PHYSIOLOGICAL RESPONSE OF THE LUNG TO INJURY

Animals exposed to substances which induce fibrosis display abnormalities on pulmonary function tests characteristic of human pulmonary fibrosis (11,27, 70,75). The diffusion capacity for carbon monoxide decreases as do lung volumes and compliance (11,70). Widened alveolar–arterial oxygen gradients develop after several weeks (11). Importantly, no clear relationship between physiological abnormalities and changes in the cellular and connective tissue elements in animal pulmonary fibrosis has been elucidated (70). These studies suggest a complex, multifactorial rela-

tionship between alterations in lung structure, the biochemical composition of the injured lung, and lung function abnormalities.

ROLE OF INDIVIDUAL CELLS IN ANIMAL PULMONARY FIBROSIS

There has been considerable interest in determining whether a particular cell type functions as the critical mediator of fibrosis (67,76). Investigators have focused their attention on parenchymal lung cells and on the immune and effector cells which migrate to the lung during injury and repair. Information derived from *in vitro* studies indicates that a variety of cell types have the capacity to release factors which regulate the growth and function of other cells. Such findings suggest that there is considerable overlap with regard to the roles that particular cells play in the evolution of fibrosis.

Platelets

Little information is available regarding the role of platelets in the development of fibrosis (see Chapter 3.4.12). Increased numbers of platelets in pulmonary capillaries, exudation of these cells into the interstitial and alveolar space, and clot formation accompany early stages of lung injury (31–34,77). Platelet-activating factor (1-*O*-octadecyl-2-acetyl-*sn* glycerol-3 phosphorylcholine) can cause animal pulmonary fibrosis in a dose-dependent manner (78). Whether this is due to its effects on platelets or other effector cells is not clear. Investigators have speculated that platelets release substances which regulate the subsequent migration of neutrophils (77). Platelets are known to secrete platelet-derived growth factor (PDGF), TGF-β, and other molecules which regulate mesenchymal cell growth and synthesis of matrix proteins (79,80).

Endothelial Cells

Alterations in capillary permeability with associated ultrastructural changes in endothelial cells and underlying basement membrane have been noted during early phases of a variety of lung injuries (14,81; see also Chapter 3.2.2). These alterations include cell swelling and disruptions of the basement membrane (14). The extent of these changes and their reversibility may be critical to the outcome of lung injury. Irradiation-induced pulmonary fibrosis is the lesion classically associated with early injury confined to the endothelium (14). Surface molecules (including heparan sulfate and factor VIII) and secreted products of endothelial cells affect hemostasis (82,83). Activation or disruption of these functions may contribute to the increased procoagulant activity and decreased fibrinolytic activity which accompany early phases of lung injury (33,34). Moreover, endothelial cell surface proteins mediate the migration of inflammatory cells into the walls of airways in an animal model of asthma (84). Similar to platelets, endothelial cells possess the capacity to release a host of substances which modulate mesenchymal cell growth and synthesis of matrix proteins (85,86). These include TGF-β and PDGF (85,86). Overall, the precise role of endothelial cells in mediating the outcome of lung injury has not been clearly elucidated. However, their function in limiting the exudation of serum proteins into the alveolar space, combined with their ability to synthesize important regulatory substances, suggests a critical role.

Alveolar Epithelium

Necrosis of type I cells with alterations in the underlying basement membrane is a prominent feature of lung injury (67). As the lesion progresses, type II cells dedifferentiate into type I cells and repopulate the alveolar basement membrane. The ability of this process to restore the alveolar epithelium to normal is dependent, at least in part, on the extent of the initial damage to type I epithelium (87). Investigators have speculated that these events in some manner trigger mechanisms which results in the development of pulmonary fibrosis (87).

Neutrophils

The observations that neutrophils release toxic oxygen metabolites and proteases resulted in the suggestion that these cells may initiate and amplify the early lung injury (23,24; see also Chapter 3.4.7). However, ARDS occurs in humans who are neutropenic (88). Accumulated experimental evidence has shown that depletion of neutrophils prior to induction of lung injury results in an increased collagen content and synthetic rates (89,90). Beige mice have a congenital defect in neutrophil degranulation and have an increased collagen content following lung injury (91). When rabbits are administered phorbol myristate acetate (a potent neutrophil activator), neutrophils accumulate in the alveolar space (18). This injury may heal without fibrosis. Taken together, these studies would suggest that neutrophils may participate in limiting the extent of fibrosis.

Macrophages

Similar to neutrophils, macrophages release toxic oxygen metabolites and a variety of proteases which de-

grade extracellular matrix proteins (92,93; see also Chapters 3.4.5 and 7.1.1). These findings suggest a role for macrophages in mediating the extent of tissue injury. In addition, these cells play a key role in resolution of injury. In classic studies of skin injury, Leibovich and Ross (94) found that macrophages regulate fibroblast growth. It is likely that the continuous influx of these cells into lung has a significant effect on tissue repair. Macrophages may play a special role in inorganic-dust-associated pulmonary fibrosis (43,44,95). There is an early association between dust particles and macrophages (95). Exposure of macrophages to silica causes release of lysosomal enzymes and a fibrogenic factor (95,96). Additional studies have shown that macrophages release many different types of effector molecules which stimulate or inhibit mesenchymal cell growth and production of matrix proteins (97–100). These include PDGF, TGF-β, insulin-like growth factors, and others (97–100). During the resolution of lung injury, macrophages may also secrete prostaglandins which inhibit fibroblast function, thus limiting the extent of fibrosis (101). Because macrophages are multifunctional, it is difficult to define the exact role they play in the fibrotic process.

Lymphocytes

Increased levels of lymphocytes are first noted several days after induction of lung injury (95). Evidence for a distinct role in animal pulmonary fibrosis is not entirely clear. The extent of fibrosis following bleomycin injury in athymic T-cell-deficient mice is either unchanged or slightly decreased as compared with that in normal animals (47,102). T-cell activity may be involved in the diminished fibrotic response in BALB/c mice following bleomycin treatment (46). Alterations in cellular immunity have been noted to accompany lung injury (103). The development of immune reactivity to type I collagen is mediated by altered T-cell function (103). Whether such observations are epiphenomena or contribute to the fibrotic response is uncertain. Similar to other cell types, lymphocytes release effector molecules (such as TGF-β) which affect mesenchymal function (104).

Mesenchymal Cells

The lung interstitial cells are situated in the thick portion of the alveolar wall between the epithelium and the capillary endothelium (105; see also Chapter 3.3.1). During lung injury, these cells are stimulated to proliferate and increase their production of connective tissue proteins (1,2). It appears that fibroblasts migrate through discontinuities in the epithelial basement membrane and then proliferate in the alveolar space

(25). Current information indicates that interstitial fibroblasts proliferate and synthesize matrix proteins in response to stimulation by effector molecules released during lung injury. These effector molecules activate fibroblast functions through distinct and distinguishable pathways (74). *In vitro* studies have shown that toxic agents may directly activate fibroblasts (106,107).

Fibroblasts within the pulmonary interstitium are heterogeneous with respect to morphology and function, although these differences have not been fully characterized. Heterogeneity is demonstrated by the increased numbers of myofibroblasts which are noted early after lung injury (25,57,58). Distinct subpopulations of cells may be responsible for different aspects of the fibrotic response and may differentially respond to inflammatory mediators. The growth characteristics of cultured lung fibroblasts derived from fibrotic lungs have been shown to be abnormal (108,109). Both increased and decreased rates of proliferation have been noted (108,109). Such studies are complicated by effects of cell isolation procedures, which may preferentially permit selective outgrowth of distinct subpopulations (2).

ROLE OF CYTOKINES IN LUNG INJURY

The isolation, characterization, and cloning of numerous distinct effector molecules demonstrate that a variety of cytokines may participate in the fibrotic response (110; see also Chapters 2.8, 2.9, and 7.8.1). The biological effect of individual cytokines may be modulated, and even reversed, by the presence of other cytokines (111). These observations illustrate the difficulties in ascribing a particular function to a single cytokine based on properties that have been defined *in vitro.*

Nevertheless, in several animal models of pulmonary fibrosis, critical roles for individual cytokines have been demonstrated. Several studies have shown that chemoattractants are released during the course of lung injury (112–117). Factors which activate neutrophils, lymphocytes, and macrophages are found at various times after injury. The presence of these factors over time tends to correlate with the cellular profile of the inflammatory reaction (113). These factors are derived from pulmonary macrophages and from activation of complement proteins (112–117). The serum-derived complement protein C5A is found in lavages from injured lungs and may be related to the migration of macrophages to sites of tissue damage (116,117). Interestingly, complement depletion by administration of cobra venom decreases the amount of fibrosis that follows lung injury (118; see also Chapter 7.5.2).

Recent studies suggest that TGF-β and tumor necrosis factor (TNF) are important mediators of fibrosis (119–123). Several studies have shown that TGF-β is a potent activator of matrix formation *in vitro* (119,120,123). TGF-β derived from numerous cell types increases production of collagen (119,120), fibronectin (123), and cell-surface matrix protein receptors (integrins) (124) and causes inactivation of metalloproteinases (125). TGF-β appears to activate synthesis of these molecules through complex mechanisms which involve both transcriptional and post-transcriptional processes (126,127). In addition, subcutaneous administration of TGF-β results in a localized fibrosis (120). Increases in total lung TGF-β mRNA and TGF-β protein are found early after bleomycin injury, preceding the increase in matrix gene expression (99,128). Immunohistochemical studies indicated that TGF-β was localized to sites of increased cellularity and matrix formation (99). Increases in total lung TGF-β mRNA do not occur during the course of silica-induced lung injury (122). These results suggest that the profile of effector molecules mediating the fibrotic response may be specific for each agent which induces lung injury.

An increase in the total lung TNF mRNA accompanies lung injury induced by silica and bleomycin (45,122). The source of the TNF has been reported to be T-lymphocytes in the bleomycin model and to be pulmonary macrophages in the silica model (45,122). Collagen deposition in silica-induced lung injury can be markedly decreased by administration of an anti-TNF antibody, indicating that the effects of TNF are critical to the pathogenesis of these lesions (122). The addition of TNF to fibroblast cultures inhibits collagen formation (129), suggesting that the effect of TNF on collagen formation, *in vivo,* is indirect. Perhaps, TNF increases capillary permeability or must act in concert with other effector substances to exert its effects. The dissociation between the effects of TNF *in vivo* and *in vitro* is of considerable interest. It points to the hazards involved in extending observations derived from tissue culture experiments to the complex inflammatory reaction that occurs *in vivo.*

Other well-defined inflammatory mediators may be involved in the development of animal pulmonary fibrosis. Increases in total lung platelet-derived-growth-factor B-chain mRNA levels have been noted during hyperoxic lung injury (130). Interleukin 1 is released by macrophages as a result of exposure to inorganic dusts (131). Interleukin 1 increases prostaglandin synthesis by activating cyclo-oxygenase activity in mesenchymal cells (132). Effector molecules which inhibit mesenchymal cell function may play a role in restraining the extent of the fibrotic response. Macrophages release a factor which inhibits collagen formation through a prostaglandin-E_2-dependent mechanism (133,134). In addition, interleukin 6 is produced by several cell types found in inflammatory reactions in the lung (135).

CONNECTIVE TISSUE SYNTHESIS

In vivo and organ culture studies have shown increases in total amounts of connective tissue in lungs 7–10 days after induction of injury, along with increased rates of connective tissue synthesis (19,61,62,136). Current information suggests that increased rates of matrix synthesis result from the activation of interstitial fibroblasts by effector molecules released at sites of injury (121,122), although several investigators have suggested that injurious agents may be direct activators of matrix formation (106,107). Other lung cells have the capacity to synthesize connective tissue elements; for example, type II cells synthesize type IV collagen, fibronectin, and thrombospondin (137). Synthesis of collagen types I, III, and V (63,68,109,138), elastin (71,139), fibronectin (128,140), and glycosaminoglycans (GAGs) (72,141) has all been shown to be seen following lung injury. Increases in enzymes critical to connective tissue synthesis are also seen (62,142–144). Prolyl hydroxylase and lysyl oxidase (which are involved in the post-translational modification of collagen and elastin) are increased, as is glucosamine-6-phosphate (which is involved in GAG synthesis) (62,142–144). Sustained increases in rates of connective tissue formation may occur up to several weeks after injury (145).

Increased levels of collagen mRNAs are noted 7–14 days after injury and decline to control levels by 4 weeks (128). The rate of $\alpha 1(I)$ gene transcription is elevated at this time, indicating that the increase in collagen formation in acute fibrotic reactions is due to activation of transcription (146,147). There is an increase in the ratio of type I to type III collagen (63,138), similar to that found in human pulmonary fibrosis (148,149). Investigators have reported that the physical properties of collagen synthesized during resolution of acute injury may be altered (107), and there is conflicting information regarding changes in collagenolytic activity (64,150).

Increased elastin synthesis (which appears related to activation of transcription) and increased formation of elastin cross-links are also found (71,139,147). These events seem to follow the observed increase in collagen formation (139,147). There is a relative increase in dermatan sulfate production over that of other GAGs (141). Increased fibronectin production is also related to activation of transcription (147). Numerous cell types found in the lung synthesize this molecule, and it is also found in serum (123,137,151). It has diverse biological effects, including possible roles in regulating fibroblast growth (152), forming nascent extracellular matrices (153), and functioning as a cell adhesion molecule (151).

THERAPEUTIC APPROACHES TO ANIMAL PULMONARY FIBROSIS

Various agents have been tested for efficacy in decreasing the fibrotic response which follows lung injury (142,154–158). Many of these agents show beneficial effects in terms of improving physiologic function or decreasing collagen accumulation. However, because of the complex nature of pulmonary fibrosis, it is difficult to elucidate their exact mode of action. Administration of steroids decreases the extent of collagen formation (154–157). Steroids have been shown to diminish the degree of endothelial cell and type I cell damage without affecting the extent of the subsequent inflammatory reaction (157). Agents such as *d*-penicillamine and *p*-aminobenzoic acid inhibit levels of collagen formation in insoluble fractions, indicating an effect of incorporation of newly synthesized collagen into the extracellular matrix (158). There is evidence that both cyclo-oxygenase and lipoxygenase inhibitors diminish fibrosis (159,160). Proline analogues, such as dehydroproline, inhibit collagen production in animal pulmonary fibrosis (142). Cyclosporin, an inhibitor of T-lymphocyte function, may have beneficial effects in animal pulmonary fibrosis (161).

As discussed above, cytokine-specific antibodies such as anti-TNF have had dramatic effects in several different models of animal pulmonary fibrosis (122). Such studies indicate the potential of utilizing monoclonal antibodies directed at critical molecules of the fibrotic reaction. Employing these tools to inhibit an essential early event in the pathogenesis of animal pulmonary fibrosis might be particularly efficacious. For example, antibodies directed to endothelial cell surface molecules which mediate the migration of inflammatory cells from the vascular space to the interstitium could prevent activation of interstitial fibroblasts. Similarly, intervention directed at preventing early endothelial cell or type I cell damage would likely be effective in decreasing fibrosis.

FUTURE DIRECTIONS

The application of molecular techniques to studying animal pulmonary fibrosis should permit a more detailed understanding of the pathogenesis of this disease (Table 2). *In situ* hybridization can identify distinct cell populations responsible for synthesizing specific proteins involved in mediating the resolution of lung injury. Employing this technique, the cell of origin for specific matrix proteins can be identified. In addition, this technique would permit a detailed genetic analysis

TABLE 2. *Future directions*

Application of new techniques
  In situ hybridization
  Polymerase chain reaction
  Reverse genetics
Monoclonal antibodies against specific inflammatory
  mediators
Development of transgenic animals

of inflammatory cells, identifying distinct subtypes responsible for synthesizing specific effector molecules.

The polymerase chain reaction (PCR) is a powerful technique which can be utilized to generate a profile of the genes that are activated during the course of an inflammatory reaction, as in lung injury (162,163). PCR is a method which rapidly amplifies specific regions of DNA (163). Protocols have been devised so that small amounts of mRNA may be used as starting material. Following isolation of mRNA, cDNAs are synthesized. Employing synthetic extension primers which flank a segment of the specific DNA of interest, repeated automated cycles of PCR-catalyzed synthesis generate greater than a millionfold amplification of the flanked DNA segment. This powerful tool can be used to analyze expression of genes that are expressed at low levels. Moreover, the method is automated and rapid and requires no radioactivity. This technique is best used for a qualitative analysis of gene expression.

Reverse genetics has been employed to identify the genetic abnormalities in human diseases such as cystic fibrosis and muscular dystrophy (164–167). Sophisticated genetic and chromosomal analyses permitted identification of the abnormal gene prior to identification of the abnormal protein (164–167). In terms of the genetics of pulmonary fibrosis, sporadic familial outbreaks of human pulmonary fibrosis have been documented but not well characterized (168). The motheaten mouse is a genetic disorder in mice in which homozygotes develop interstitial lung disease several weeks after birth (169). Employing reverse genetics, a detailed analysis of the genetic abnormality in this inherited form of animal pulmonary fibrosis is possible and would likely advance the understanding of the pathogenesis of this disease.

The ability to insert specific genes into the embryo— and, as a result, into the germ-line—is now feasible (170). The new gene (the transgene) can be transmitted to their offspring. This tool has been used to identify the role of specific genes in development (171), to induce malignancies through insertion of oncogenes (170), and to develop animal models of genetic diseases such as sickle cell anemia, through the insertion of an abnormal human allele (172). This technique can also be employed to analyze the function of discrete DNA elements which regulate the transcription of a specific gene *in vivo*. The promoter of a gene can be attached to an indicator gene not present in the eukaryotic genome, such as chloramphenicol acetyltransferase (CAT). This hybrid gene can be introduced into an animal, and a rapid assay for CAT activity can be employed to analyze the effects of various regions of the promoter on CAT expression *in vivo*. Induction of lung injury in transgenic animals containing regulatory DNA elements linked to CAT would permit an analysis of critical regions of a gene which affect its expression during fibrosis. Such an approach using the collagen promoter linked to CAT is under way in several laboratories.

REFERENCES

1. Crystal RG, Bitterman PB, Rennard SI, Hance AS, Keough BA. Interstitial lung diseases of unknown cause. *N Engl J Med* 1984;31:154–161 and 235–244.
2. Goldstein RH, Fine A. Fibrotic reactions in the lung: the activation of the lung fibroblast. *Exp Lung Res* 1986;11:245–261.
3. Weg JG. Chronic noninfectious parenchymal diseases. In: Guenter CA, Welch MH, eds. *Pulmonary medicine*, 2nd ed. Philadelphia: JB Lippincott, 1982;607–662.
4. Crystal RG. Interstitial lung disease. In: Wyngaarden JB, Smith LH Jr, eds. *Cecil textbook of medicine*. Philadelphia: WB Saunders, 1980;421–435.
5. Crystal RG, Fulmer JD, Roberts WC, Moss ML, Line BR, Reynolds HY. Idiopathic pulmonary fibrosis: clinical, histologic, radiographic, physiologic, scintigraphic, cytologic, and biochemical aspects. *Ann Intern Med* 1976;65:769–788.
6. Coalson JJ. The ultrastructure of human fibrosing alveolitis. *Virchows Arch [Pathol Anat]* 1982;395:181–199.
7. Hamman L, Rich AR. Fulminating diffuse interstitial fibrosis of the lungs. *Trans Am Clin Climatol Assoc* 1935;51:154–163.
8. Willoughby WF, Willoughby JB, Cantrell BB, Wheelis R. *In vivo* responses to inhaled proteins. II. Induction of interstitial pneumonitis and enhancement of immune complex-mediated alveolitis by inhaled concanavalin A. *Lab Invest* 1979;40:399–414.
9. Adamson IY, Bowden DH. The pathogenesis of bleomycin-induced pulmonary fibrosis in mice. *Am J Pathol* 1974;77:185–197.
10. Snider GL, Hayes JA, Korthy AL. Chronic interstitial pulmonary fibrosis produced in hamsters by endotracheal bleomycin: pathology and stereology. *Am Rev Respir Dis* 1978;177:1099–1108.
11. Snider GL, Celli BR, Goldstein RH, O'Brien JJ, Lucey EC. Chronic interstitial pulmonary fibrosis produced in hamsters by endotracheal bleomycin: lung volumes, volume–pressure relations, carbon monoxide uptake and arterial blood gas studies. *Am Rev Respir Dis* 1978;117:289–297.
12. Slausen DO, Hahn FF, Chiffelle TL. The pulmonary vascular pathology of experimental radiation pneumonitis. *Am J Pathol* 1977;88:635–654.
13. Collins JF, Johanson WG Jr, McCullough B, Jones MA, Waugh HJ Jr. Effects of compensatory lung growth in irradiation-induced regional pulmonary fibrosis in the baboon. *Am Rev Respir Dis* 1978;117:1079–1089.
14. Adamson IY, Bowden DH. Endothelial injury and repair in radiation-induced pulmonary fibrosis. *Am J Pathol* 1983;112:224–230.
15. Smith P, Heath D, Kay JM. The pathogenesis and structure of paraquat-induced pulmonary fibrosis in rats. *J Pathol* 1974;114:57–67.
16. Phan SH, Armstrong G, Sulavik MC, Scrier D, Johnson KJ, Ward PA. A comparative study of pulmonary fibrosis induced

by bleomycin and an O_2 metabolic-producing enzyme system. *Chest* 1983;83(Suppl):44–45.

17. Fantone JC, Johnson KJ, Till GO, Ward PA. Acute and progressive lung injury secondary to toxic oxygen products from leukocytes. *Chest* 1983;83(Suppl):46–48.

18. Taylor RG, McCall CE, Thrall RS, Woodruff RD, O'Flaherty JT. Histopathologic features of phorbol myristate acetate-induced lung injury. *Lab Invest* 1985;52:61–70.

19. Reiser KM, Hesterberg TW, Haschek WM, Last JA. Experimental silicosis. I. Acute effects of intratracheally instilled quartz on collagen metabolism and morphologic characteristics of rat lungs. *Am J Pathol* 1982;107:176–185.

20. Begin R, Masse S, Bureau MA. Morphologic features and function of the airways in early asbestosis in the sheep model. *Am Rev Respir Dis* 1982;126:870–876.

21. Haschek WM, Brody AR, Klein-Szanto AJ, Witschi H. Animal model of human disease: diffuse interstitial pulmonary fibrosis: pulmonary fibrosis in mice induced by treatment with butylated hydroxytoluene and oxygen. *Am J Pathol* 1981;105:333–335.

22. Haschek WM, Klein-Szanto AJ, Last JA, Reiser KM, Witschi H. Long-term morphological and biochemical features of experimentally induced lung fibrosis in the mouse. *Lab Invest* 1982;46:438–449.

23. Johnson KJ, Fantone JC, Kaplan J, Ward PA. In vivo damage of rat lungs by oxygen metabolites. *J Clin Invest* 1981;67:983–993.

24. Weiss SJ. Tissue destruction by neutrophils. *N Engl J Med* 1989;320:365–376.

25. Thet LA, Parra SC, Shelbourne JD. Sequential changes in lung morphology during the repair of acute oxygen-induced lung injury in adult rats. *Exp Lung Res* 1986;11:209–228.

26. Brigham KL, Meyrick B. Interactions of granulocytes with the lungs. *Circ Res* 1985;54:623–635.

27. McCullough B, Collins JF. Bleomycin-induced diffuse interstitial pulmonary fibrosis in baboons. *J Clin Invest* 1978;61:79–88.

28. Davis GS. Pathogenesis of silicosis: current concepts and hypothesis. *Lung* 1986;164:139–154.

29. Miller BE, Dethloff LA, Gladen BC, Hook GER. Progression of type II cell hypertrophy and hyperplasia during silica-induced pulmonary inflammation. *Lab Invest* 1987;57:546–554.

30. Miller BE, Dethloff LA, Hook GER. Silica-induced hypertrophy of type II cells in the lungs of rats. *Lab Invest* 1986;55:153–163.

31. Tryka AF, Godleski JJ, Brain JD. Differences in effects of immediate and delayed hyperoxia exposure on bleomycin-induced pulmonary injury. *Cancer Treat Rep* 1984;68:759–764.

32. Berend N. The effect of bleomycin and oxygen on rat lung. *Pathol* 1984;16:136–139.

33. Idell S, James KK, Giles C, Fair DS, Thrall RS. Abnormalities of pathways of fibrin turnover in lung lavage of rats with oleic acid and bleomycin-induced lung injury support alveolar fibrin deposition. *Am J Pathol* 1989;135:387–399.

34. Sitrin RG, Brubaker PG, Fantone JC. Tissue fibrin deposition during acute lung injury in rabbits and its relationship to procoagulant and fibrinolytic activities. *Am Rev Respir Dis* 1987;135:930–936.

35. Colvin RB, Gardner PI, Robbin RO, Verderber EL, Lanigan JM, Mosesson MW. Cell surface fibrinogen–fibrin receptors on cultured human fibroblasts. *Lab Invest* 1979;41:464–472.

36. Grinnel F, Feld M, Minter D. Fibroblast adhesion to fibrinogen and fibrin: requirement for cold-insoluble globulin (plasma fibronectin). *Cell* 1980;19:517–525.

37. Brody AR, Soler P, Basset F, Haschek WM, Hanspeter W. Epithelial–mesenchymal associations of cells in human pulmonary fibrosis and BHT–oxygen-induced fibrosis in mice. *Exp Lung Res* 1981;2:207–220.

38. Thrall RS, Barton RW, D'Amato DA, Sulavik SB. Differential cellular analysis of bronchoalveolar lavage fluid obtained at various stages during the development of bleomycin-induced pulmonary fibrosis in the rat. *Am Rev Respir Dis* 1982;126:488–492.

39. Glassroth JL, Bernardo J, Lucey EC, Center DM, Jung-Legg Y, Snider GL. Interstitial pulmonary fibrosis induced in ham-

sters by intratracheally administered chrysotile asbestosis. *Am Rev Respir Dis* 1984;130:242–248.

40. Chandler DB, Hyde DM, Giri SN. Morphometric estimates of infiltrative cellular changes during the development of bleomycin-induced pulmonary fibrosis in hamsters. *Am J Pathol* 1983;112:170–177.

41. Sun XH, Davis WB, Fukuda Y, Ferrans VJ, Crystal RG. Experimental Polymixin B-induced interstitial lung disease characterized by an accumulation of cytotoxic eosinophils in the alveolar structures. *Am Rev Respir Dis* 1985;131:103–108.

42. Watanabe S, Watanabe K, Ohishi T, Aiba M, Kageyama K. Mast cells in the rat alveolar septa undergoing fibrosis after ionizing irradiation. *Lab Invest* 1974;31:555–567.

43. Bozelka BE, Sestini P, Gaumer HG, Hamad Y, Heather CJ, Salvaggio JE. A murine model of asbestosis. *Am J Pathol* 1983;112:326–337.

44. Warheit DB, Chang LY, Hill LH, Hook GER, Crapo JD, Brody AR. Pulmonary macrophage accumulation and asbestos-induced lesions at sites of fiber deposition. *Am Rev Respir Dis* 1984;129:301–310.

45. Piguet PF, Collart MA, Grau GE, Kapanci Y, Vassalli P. Tumor necrosis factor/cachectin plays a key role in bleomycin-induced pneumopathy and fibrosis. *J Exp Med* 1989;170:655–663.

46. Schrier DJ, Phan SH. Modulation of bleomycin-induced pulmonary fibrosis in the BALB/c mouse by cyclophosphamide-sensitive T cells. *Am J Pathol* 1984;116:270–278.

47. Schrier DJ, Phan SH, McGarry BM. The effects of the nude (nu/nu) mutation on bleomycin-induced pulmonary fibrosis. *Am Rev Respir Dis* 1983;127:614–617.

48. Hubbard AK. Role for T lymphocytes in silica-induced pulmonary inflammation. *Lab Invest* 1989;61:46–52.

49. Vaccaro CA, Brody JS, Snider GL. Alveolar wall basement membranes in bleomycin-induced pulmonary fibrosis. *Am Rev Respir Dis* 1985;132:905–912.

50. Evans MJ, Cabral LJ, Stephens RJ, Freeman G. Renewal of alveolar epithelium in the rat following exposure to NO_2. *Am J Pathol* 1973;70:175–198.

51. Kapanci Y, Weibel ER, Kaplan HP, Robinson FR. Pathogenesis and reversibility of the pulmonary lesions of oxygen toxicity in monkeys. II. Ultrastructural and morphometric studies. *Lab Invest* 1969;20:101–118.

52. Adamson IY, Bowden DH. Bleomycin-induced injury and metaplasia of alveolar type 2 cells. *Am J Pathol* 1979;96:531–544.

53. Haschek WM, Reiser KM, Klein-Szanto AJP, Kehrer JP, Smith LH, Last JA, Witschi HP. Potentiation of butylated hydroxytoluene-induced acute lung damage by oxygen. *Am Rev Respir Dis* 1983;127:28–34.

54. Haschek WM, Klein-Szanto AJP, Last JA, Reiser KM, Witschi H. Long-term morphologic and biochemical features of experimentally induced lung fibrosis in the mouse. *Lab Invest* 1982;46:438–449.

55. Schurch W, Seemayer TA, Lagace R. Stromal myofibroblasts in primary invasive and metastatic carcinomas. *Virchows Arch [Pathol Anat]* 1981;391:125–139.

56. Callahan LM, Evans JN, Alder KB. Alterations in the cellular population of the alveolar wall in an animal model of fibrosis. *Chest* 1986;89:188S–189S.

57. Evans JN, Kelley J, Low RB, Alder KB. Increased contractility of isolated lung parenchyma in an animal model of pulmonary fibrosis induced by bleomycin. *Am Rev Respir Dis* 1982;125:89–94.

58. Low RB, Woodcock-Mitchell J, Evans JN, Adler KB. Actin content of normal and of bleomycin-fibrotic rat lung. *Am Rev Respir Dis* 1984;129:311–316.

59. Gabbiani G, Le Lous M, Bailey AJ, Bazin S, Delauney A. Collagen and myofibroblasts, a chemical, ultrastructural, and immunologic study. *Virchows Arch [Cell Pathol]* 1976;21:133–145.

60. Bateman E, Turner-Warwick M, Adelmann-Grill BC. Immunohistochemical study of collagen types in human foetal lung fibrotic lung disease. *Thorax* 1981;36:645–653.

61. Phan SH, Thrall RS, Ward PA. Bleomycin-induced pulmonary

fibrosis in rats: biochemical demonstration of increased rate of collagen synthesis. *Am Rev Respir Dis* 1980;121:501–506.

62. Clark JG, Overton JE, Marino BA, Uitto J, Starcher BC. Collagen biosynthesis in bleomycin-induced pulmonary fibrosis in hamsters. *J Lab Clin Med* 1980;96:943–953.

63. Reiser KM, Last JA. Pulmonary fibrosis in experimental acute respiratory disease. *Am Rev Respir Dis* 1981;123:58–63.

64. Laurent GJ, McAnulty RJ. Protein metabolism during bleomycin-induced pulmonary fibrosis in rabbits: *in vivo* evidence for collagen accumulation because of increased synthesis and decreased degradation of the newly synthesized collagen. *Am Rev Respir Dis* 1983;128:82–88.

65. Fukuda Y, Ishizaki M, Masuda Y, Kimura G, Kawanami O, Masugi Y. The role of intraalveolar fibrosis in the process of pulmonary structural remodeling in patients with diffuse alveolar damage. *Am J Pathol* 1987;126:171–182.

66. Fukuda Y, Ferrans VJ, Schoenberger CI, Rennard SI, Crystal RG. Patterns of pulmonary structural remodeling after experimental paraquat toxicity. *Am J Pathol* 1985;118:452–475.

67. Snider GL. Interstitial pulmonary fibrosis. *Chest [Suppl]* 1986;89:115S–121S.

68. Phan SH. Diffuse interstitial fibrosis. In: Massaro D, ed. *Lung cell biology.* New York: Marcel Dekker, 1989;907–980.

69. Laurent GJ, McNulty RJ, Corrin B, Cockerill P. Biochemical and histological changes in pulmonary fibrosis induced in rabbits with intratracheal bleomycin. *Eur J Clin Invest* 1981; 11:441–448.

70. Goldstein RH, Lucey EC, Franzblau C, Snider GL. Failure of mechanical properties to parallel changes in lung connective tissue composition in bleomycin-induced pulmonary fibrosis in hamsters. *Am Rev Respir Dis* 1979;120:67–73.

71. Starcher BC, Kuhn C, Overton JE. Increased elastin and collagen content in the lungs of hamsters receiving an intratracheal injection of bleomycin. *Am Rev Respir Dis* 1978;117:299–305.

72. Karlinsky J. Glycosaminoglycans in emphysematous and fibrotic hamster lungs. *Am Rev Respir Dis* 1982;125:85–88.

73. Niewoehner DE, Hoidal JR. Lung fibrosis and emphysema: divergent responses to a common injury. *Science* 1982;217: 359–360.

74. Fine A, Poliks CF, Donahue LP, Smith BD, Goldstein RH. The differential effect of prostaglandin E$_2$ on transforming growth factor-β and insulin-induced collagen formation in lung fibroblasts. *J Biol Chem* 1989;264:16989–16991.

75. Berend N, Feldsien D, Cederbaums D, Cherniak RM. Structure–function correlation of early stages of lung injury induced by intratracheal bleomycin in the rabbit. *Am Rev Respir Dis* 1985;132:582–589.

76. Snider GL. Interstitial pulmonary fibrosis—which cell is the culprit? [Editorial] *Am Rev Respir Dis* 1983;127:535–539.

77. Barry BE, Crapo JD. Patterns of accumulation of platelets and neutrophils in rat lungs during exposure to 100% and 85% oxygen. *Am Rev Respir Dis* 1985;132:548–555.

78. Camussi G, Pawlowski I, Tetta C, Rofinello C, Albeton M, Brentjens J, Andres G. Acute inflammation induced in the rabbit by local instillation of 1-*O*-octadecyl-2-acetyl-*sn*-glycerol-3-phosphorylcholine or of native platelet-activating factor. *Am J Pathol* 1983;112:78–88.

79. Deuel TF, Huang JS. Platelet-derived growth factor: purification, properties, and biological activities. *Prog Hematol* 1983;13:201–221.

80. Assoian RK, Komoriya A, Meyers CA, Sporn MB. Transforming growth factor-β in human platelets: identification of a major storage site, purification, and characterization. *J Biol Chem* 1983;80:7155–7160.

81. Catravas JD, Lazo JS, Dobuler KJ, Mills LR, Gillis CN. Pulmonary endothelial dysfunction in the presence or absence of interstitial injury induced by intratracheally injected bleomycin in rabbits. *Am Rev Respir Dis* 1983;128:740–746.

82. Marcum JA, Rosenberg RD. Anticoagulantly active heparan sulfate proteoglycan and the vascular endothelium. *Semin Thromb Hemost* 1987;13:464–474.

83. Farber HW, Fairman P, Milan JE, Rounds S, Glauser F. Pulmonary response to foreign body microemboli in dogs: release

of neutrophil chemoattractant activity by vascular endothelial cells. *Am J Respir Mol Biol* 1989;1:27–35.

84. Wegner CD, Gundel RH, Reilly P, Haynes N, Letts GL, Rothlein R. Intercellular adhesion molecule-1 (ICAM-1) in the pathogenesis of asthma. *Science* 1990;247:456–459.

85. Antonelli-Orlidge A, Saunders KB, Smith SR, D'Amore PA. An activated form of transforming growth factor β is produced by cocultures of endothelial cells and pericytes. *Proc Natl Acad Sci USA* 1989;86:4544–4548.

86. DiCorleto PE, Bowen-Pope DF. Cultured endothelial cells produce a platelet-derived growth factor. *Proc Natl Acad Sci USA* 1983;80:1919–1923.

87. Bowden DH. Unraveling pulmonary fibrosis: the bleomycin model [Editorial]. *Lab Invest* 1984;50:487–488.

88. Ognibene FP, Martin SE, Parker MM, Schlesinger T, Roach P, Burch C, Shelhamer JH, Parrillo JE. Adult respiratory distress syndrome in patients with severe neutropenia. *N Engl J Med* 1986;315:547–551.

89. Thrall RS, Phan SH, McCormick JR, Ward PA. The development of bleomycin-induced pulmonary fibrosis in neutrophil-depleted and complement-depleted rats. *Am J Pathol* 1981; 105:76–81.

90. Clark JG, Kuhn C III. Bleomycin-induced pulmonary fibrosis in hamsters: effect of neutrophil depletion on lung collagen synthesis. *Am Rev Respir Dis* 1982;126:737–739.

91. Phan SH, Schrier D, McGarry B, Duque RE. Effect of the beige mutation on bleomycin-induced pulmonary fibrosis in mice. *Am Rev Respir Dis* 1983;127:456–459.

92. Johnson KJ, Ward PA. Acute and progressive lung injury after contact with phorbol myristate acetate. *Am J Pathol* 1983; 107:29–35.

93. Mass B, Ikeda T, Meranze DR, Weinbaum G, Kimbel P. Induction of experimental emphysema, cellular and species specificity. *Am Rev Respir Dis* 1972;106:384–391.

94. Leibovich SJ, Ross R. A macrophage-dependent factor that stimulates the proliferation of fibroblasts *in vitro*. *Am J Pathol* 1976;84:501–514.

95. Reiser KM, Last JA. Early cellular events in pulmonary fibrosis. *Exp Lung Res* 1986;10:331–355.

96. Heppleston AG, Styles JA. Activity of a macrophage factor in collagen formation by silica. *Nature* 1967;214:521–522.

97. Martinet YP, Bitterman PB, Mornex JF, Grotendorst GR, Martin GR, Crystal RG. Activated monocytes express the c-sis proto-oncogene and release a mediator showing PDGF-like activity. *Nature* 1986;319:158–160.

98. Assoian RK, Fleurdelys BE, Stevenson HC, Miller PJ, Madtes DK, Raines EW, Ross R, Sporn MB. Expression and secretion of type β transforming growth factor by activated human macrophages. *Proc Natl Acad Sci USA* 1987;84:6020–6024.

99. Khalil N, Bereznay O, Sporn MB, Greenberg AH. Macrophage production of transforming growth factor β and fibroblast collagen synthesis in chronic pulmonary inflammation. *J Exp Med* 1989;170:727–737.

100. Nagaoka I, Trapnell BC, Crystal RG. Regulation of insulin-like growth factor gene expression in the human macrophage-like cell line U937. *J Clin Invest* 1990;85:448–455.

101. Humes JL, Bonney RJ, Pelus L, Dahlgren ME, Sadowski SJ, Kuehl FA Jr, Davies P. Macrophages synthesize and release prostaglandins in response to inflammatory stimuli. *Nature* 1977;269:149–150.

102. Szapiel SV, Elson NA, Fulmer JD, Hunninghake GW, Crystal RG. Bleomycin-induced interstitial pulmonary disease in the nude athymic mouse. *Am Rev Respir Dis* 1979;120:893–899.

103. Schrier DJ, Phan SH, Ward PA. Cellular sensitivity to collagen in bleomycin-treated rats. *J Immunol* 1982;129:2156–2159.

104. Kehrl JH, Wakefield LM, Roberts AB, et al. Production of transforming growth factor β by human T lymphocytes and its potential in the regulation of T cell growth. *J Exp Med* 1986;163:1037–1050.

105. Kapanci Y, Assimacopoulos A, Irle C, Zwahlen A, Gabbiani G. Contractile interstitial cells in pulmonary alveolar septa: a possible regulation of ventilation/perfusion ratio? *J Cell Biol* 1974;60:375–392.

106. Clark JG, Starcher BC, Uitto J. Bleomycin-induced synthesis

of type I procollagen by human lung and skin fibroblasts in culture. *Biochim Biophys Acta* 1980;631:359–370.

107. Richards RJ, Curtis CG. Biochemical and cellular mechanisms of dust-induced lung fibrosis. *Environ Health Perspect* 1984; 55:393–416.

108. Absher M, Hildebran J, Trombley L, Woodcock-Mitchell J, Marsh J. Characteristics of cultured lung fibroblasts from bleomycin-treated rats. *Am Rev Respir Dis* 1984;129:125–129.

109. Phan SH, Varani J, Smith D. Rat lung fibroblast collagen metabolism in bleomycin-induced pulmonary fibrosis. *J Clin Invest* 1985;76:241–247.

110. Kelley J. Cytokines of the lung. *Am Rev Respir Dis* 1990; 141:765–788.

111. Anzano MA, Roberts AB, Sporn MB. Anchorage-independent growth of primary rat embryo cells is induced by platelet-derived growth factor and inhibited by type-β transforming growth factor. *J Cell Physiol* 1986;126:312–318.

112. Lugano EM, Dauber JH, Daniele RP. Acute experimental silicosis. *Am J Pathol* 1982;109:27–36.

113. Kaelin RM, Center DM, Bernardo J, Grant M, Snider GL. The role of macrophage-derived chemoattractant activities in the early inflammatory events of bleomycin-induced pulmonary injury. *Am Rev Respir Dis* 1983;128:132–137.

114. Kagan E. Oghiso Y, Hartman DP. Enhanced release of a chemoattractant for alveolar macrophages after asbestos inhalation. *Am Rev Respir Dis* 1983;128:680–687.

115. Fox RB, Hoidal JR, Brown DM, Repine JE. Pulmonary inflammation due to oxygen toxicity: involvement of chemotactic factors and polymorphonuclear leukocytes. *Am Rev Respir Dis* 1981;123:521–523.

116. Warheit DB, Hill LH, George G, Brody AR. Time course of chemotactic factor generation and the corresponding macrophage response to asbestos inhalation. *Am Rev Respir Dis* 1986;134:128–133.

117. Warheit DB, George G, Hill LH, Snyderman R, Brody AR. Inhaled asbestos activates a complement-dependent chemoattractant for macrophages. *Lab Invest* 1985;52:505–514.

118. Phan SH, Thrall RS. Inhibition of bleomycin-induced pulmonary fibrosis by cobra venom factor. *Am J Pathol* 1982;107:25–28.

119. Fine A, Goldstein RH. The effect of transforming growth factor-β on cell proliferation and collagen formation by lung fibroblasts. *J Biol Chem* 1987;262:3897–3902.

120. Roberts AB, Sporn MB, Assoian RK, et al. Transforming growth factor type β: rapid induction of fibrosis and angiogenesis *in vivo* and stimulation of collagen formation *in vitro*. *Proc Natl Acad Sci USA* 1986;83:4167–4171.

121. Raghow R, Irish P, Kang AH. Coordinate regulation of transforming growth factor β gene expression and cell proliferation in hamster lungs undergoing bleomycin-induced pulmonary fibrosis. *J Clin Invest* 1989;84:1836–1842.

122. Piguet PF, Collart MA, Grau GE, Sappino AP, Vassalli P. Requirement of tumour necrosis factor for development of silica-induced pulmonary fibrosis. *Nature* 1990;344:245–247.

123. Ignotz R, Massague J. Transforming growth factor-beta stimulates the expression of fibronectin and collagen and their incorporation into the extracellular matrix. *J Biol Chem* 1986; 261:4337–4345.

124. Ignotz RA, Massague J. Cell adhesion protein receptors as targets for transforming growth factor-β action. *Cell* 1987;51:189–197.

125. Laiho, M, Saksela O, Andreasen PA, Keski-Oja J. Enhanced production and extracellular deposition of the endothelial-type plasminogen activator in cultured human lung fibroblasts by transforming growth factor-beta. *J Cell Biol* 1986;103:2403–2410.

126. Raghow R, Postlewaite AE, Keski-Oja J, Moses HL, Kang AH. Transforming growth factor-β increases steady state levels of type I procollagen and fibronectin messenger RNAs posttranscriptionally in cultured human dermal fibroblasts. *J Clin Invest* 1987;79:1285–1288.

127. Rossi P, Karsenty G, Roberts A, Roche NS, Sporn MB, de Crombrugghe B. A nuclear factor 1 binding site mediates the transcriptional activation of a type I collagen promoter by TGF-β. *Cell* 1988;52:405–414.

128. Hoyt DG, Lazo JS. Alterations in pulmonary mRNA encoding procollagens, fibronectin, and transforming growth factor-β precede bleomycin-induced pulmonary fibrosis in mice. *J Pharmacol Exp Ther* 1988;246:765–771.

129. Solis-Herruzo JA, Brenner DA, Cholkier M. Tumor necrosis factor α inhibits collagen gene transcription and collagen synthesis in cultured human fibroblasts. *J Biol Chem* 1988; 263:5841–5845.

130. Fabisiak JP, Evans JN, Kelley J. Increased expression of PDGF-B (c-sis) mRNA in rat lung precedes DNA synthesis and tissue repair during chronic hyperoxia. *Am J Respir Cell Mol Biol* 1989;1:181–189.

131. Hartman DP, Georgian MM, Oghiso Y, Kagan E. Enhanced interleukin activity following asbestos inhalation. *Clin Exp Immunol* 1984;55:643–650.

132. Dayer JM, de Rochemonteix B, Burrus B, Demcauk S, Dinarello CA. Human recombinant interleukin 1 stimulates collagenase and prostaglandin E_2 production by human synovial cells. *J Clin Invest* 1986;77:645–648.

133. Clark JG, Kostal KM, Marino BA. Modulation of collagen production following bleomycin-induced pulmonary fibrosis in hamsters. *J Biol Chem* 1982;257:8098–8105.

134. Clark JG, Kostal KM, Marino BA. Bleomycin-induced pulmonary fibrosis in hamsters. An alveolar macrophage product increases fibroblast prostaglandin E_2 and cyclic adenosine monophosphate and suppresses fibroblast proliferation and collagen production. *J Clin Invest* 1983;72:2082–2091.

135. Wong GG, Clark SC. Multiple actions of interleukin 6 within a cytokine network. *Immunol Today* 1988;5:137–139.

136. Kehrer JP, Witschi H. *In vivo* collagen accumulation in an experimental model of pulmonary fibrosis. *Exp Lung Res* 1980; 1:259–270.

137. Sage H, Farin FM, Striker GE, Fisher AB. Granular pneumocytes in primary culture secrete several major components of the extracellular matrix. *Biochemistry* 1983;22:2148–2155.

138. Raghu G, Striker LJ, Hudson LD, Striker GE. Extracellular matrix in normal and fibrotic human lungs. *Am Rev Respir Dis* 1985;131:281–289.

139. Cantor JO, Keller OS, Cerreta JM, Mandl I, Turino GM. Measurement of cross-linked elastin synthesis in bleomycin-induced pulmonary fibrosis using a highly sensitive assay for desmosine and isodesmosine. *J Lab Clin Med* 1984;103:384–392.

140. Schoenberger CI, Rennard SI, Bitterman PB, Fukuda Y, Ferrans VJ, Crystal RG. Paraquat-induced pulmonary fibrosis. Role of the alveolitis in modulating the development of fibrosis. *Am Rev Respir Dis* 1984;129:168–173.

141. Cantor JO, Osman M, Cereta JM, Mandl I, Turino GM. Glycosaminoglycan synthesis in explants derived from bleomycin-treated fibrotic hamster lungs. *Proc Soc Exp Biol Med* 1983; 173:362–366.

142. Kelley J, Newman RA, Evans JN. Bleomycin-induced pulmonary fibrosis in the rat. Prevention with an inhibitor of collagen synthesis. *J Lab Clin Med* 1980;96:954–964.

143. Counts DF, Evans JN, Dipetrillo TA, Sterling KM Jr, Kelley J. Collagen lysyl oxidase activity in the lung increases during bleomycin-induced pulmonary fibrosis in hamsters. *J Pharmacol Exp Ther* 1981;219:675–678.

144. Yoshida A, Hiramatsu M, Hatakeyama K, Minami N. Elevation of glucosamine 6-phosphate synthetase activity in bleomycin-induced pulmonary fibrosis in hamsters. *J Antibiot (Tokyo)* 1982;35:882–885.

145. Last JA, Greenberg DB, Castleman WL. Ozone-induced alterations in collagen metabolism of rat lungs. *Toxicol Appl Pharmacol* 1979;51:247–258.

146. Kelley J, Chrin L, Shull S, Rowe DW, Cutroneo KR. Bleomycin selectively elevates mRNA levels for procollagen and fibronectin following acute lung injury. *Biochem Biophys Res Commun* 1985;131:836–843.

147. Raghow R, Lurie S, Sayer JM, Kang AH. Profiles of steady state levels of messenger RNAs coding for type I procollagen, elastin, and fibronectin in hamster lungs undergoing bleomycin-

induced interstitial pulmonary fibrosis. *J Clin Invest* 1985; 76:1733–1739.

148. Madri JA, Furthmayr H. Collagen polymorphism in the lung: an immunohistochemical study of pulmonary fibrosis. *Hum Pathol* 1980;11:353–366.

149. Seyer JM, Hutcheson ET, Kang AH. Collagen polymorphism in idiopathic chronic pulmonary fibrosis. *J Clin Invest* 1976; 57:1498–1507.

150. Gadek JE, Kelman JA, Fells G, Weinberger ST, Horwitz AL, Reynolds HY, Fulmer JD, Crystal RG. Collagenase in the lower respiratory tract of patients with idiopathic pulmonary fibrosis. *N Engl J Med* 1979;301:737–742.

151. Singer II, Kawka DW, Scott S, Mumford RA, Lark MW. The fibronectin cell attachment sequence arg-gly-asp-ser promotes focal contact formation during early fibroblast attachment and spreading. *J Cell Biol* 1987;104:573–584.

152. Bitterman PB, Rennard SI, Crystal RG. Role of fibronectin as a growth factor for fibroblasts. *J Cell Biol* 1983;97:1925–1932.

153. Kurkinen M, Vaheri A, Roberts PJ, Stenman S. Sequential appearance of fibronectin and collagen in experimental granulation tissue. *Lab Invest* 1980;43:47–51.

154. Phan SH, Thrall RS, Williams C. Bleomycin-induced pulmonary fibrosis. Effects of steroid on lung collagen metabolism. *Am Rev Respir Dis* 1981;124:428–434.

155. Hesterberg TW, Last JA. Ozone-induced acute pulmonary fibrosis in rats. Prevention of increased rates of collagen synthesis by methylprednisolone. *Am Rev Respir Dis* 1981;123:47–52.

156. Cheney FW, Huang TH, Gronka R. Effects of methylprednisolone on experimental pulmonary injury. *Ann Surg* 1979; 190:236–242.

157. Smith LJ. The effect of methylprednisolone on lung injury in mice. *J Lab Clin Med* 1983;101:629–640.

158. Zuckerman JE, Mannfred AH, Giri S. Evaluation of antifibrotic drugs in bleomycin-induced pulmonary fibrosis in hamsters. *J Pharmacol Exp Ther* 1980;213:425–431.

159. Thrall RS, McCormic JR, Jack RM, McReynolds RA, Ward PA. Bleomycin-induced pulmonary fibrosis in the rat. *Am J Pathol* 1979;95:117–130.

160. Phan SH, Kunkel SL. Inhibition of bleomycin-induced pulmonary fibrosis by nordihydroguaiaretic acid. *Am J Pathol* 1986;124:343–352.

161. Sendelbach LE, Lindenschmidt RC, Witschi HP. The effect of cyclosporine A on pulmonary fibrosis induced by butylated hydroxytoluene, bleomycin and beryllium sulfate. *Toxicol Lett* 1985;26:169–173.

162. Rappolee DA, Mark D, Banda MJ, Werb Z. Wound macrophages express TGF-alpha and other growth factors in vivo: analysis of mRNA phenotyping. *Science* 1988;241:708–710.

163. Saiki RK, Gelfand DH, Stoffel S, Scharff SJ, Higuchi RG, Horn GT, Mullis KB, Ehrlich HA. Primer-directed enzymatic amplification of DNA with a thermostable DNA polymerase. *Science* 1988;239:487–491.

164. Rommens JM, Iannuzzi MC, Kerem B, et al. Identification of the cystic fibrosis gene: chromosome walking and jumping. *Science* 1989;245:1059–1065.

165. Riordan JR, Rommens JM, Kerem BS, et al. Identification of the cystic fibrosis gene: cloning and characterization of complementary DNA. *Science* 1989;245:1066–1072.

166. Kerem BS, Rommens JM, Buchanan JA, et al. Identification of the cystic fibrosis gene: genetic analysis. *Science* 1989; 245:1073–1080.

167. Koenig M, Monaco AP, Kunkel LM. The complete sequence of dystrophin predicts a rod-shaped protein. *Cell* 1988;53:219–228.

168. Sandoz E. Uber zwei falle von "fotaler bronchektasie." *Beitr Pathol Anat* 1907;41:495–516.

169. Rossi GA, Hunninghake GW, Kawanami O, Ferrans VJ, Hansen CT, Crystal RG. Motheaten mice—an animal model with an inherited form of interstitial lung disease. *Am Rev Respir Dis* 1985;131:150–158.

170. Hanahan D. Transgenic mice as probes into complex systems. *Science* 1989;246:1265–1275.

171. Braun RE, Behringer RR, Peschon JJ, Brinster RL, Palmiter RD. Genetically haploid spermatids are phenotypically diploid. *Nature* 1989;337:373–376.

172. Ryan TM, Townes TM, Reilly MP, Asakura T, Palmiter RD, Brinster RL, Behringer RR. Human sickle hemoglobin in transgenic mice. *Science* 1990;247:566–568.

THE LUNG: Scientific Foundations
edited by R.G. Crystal, J.B. West et al.
Raven Press, Ltd., New York © 1991.

CHAPTER 7.9.1

Vulnerability of the Lung to Proteolytic Injury

Richard C. Hubbard and Ronald G. Crystal

In order to function as the gas exchanger, the alveoli, by necessity, bring air and blood into as close proximity as possible. To accomplish this, the alveolar walls are relatively thin and depend on the extracellular matrix of connective tissue to define the architecture and provide mechanical support during respiration (see Chapter 3.3.1). Although this design is efficient, one consequence is the vulnerability of the lung to proteolytic attack by enzymes capable of destroying connective tissue proteins. In this regard, destruction of the interstitial matrix leads to loss of the alveolar unit; if sufficient numbers of alveoli are so affected, the result is the clinical disorder emphysema.

The current understanding of the vulnerability of the lung to proteases, and of the clinical consequences of uncontrolled proteolysis of the alveolar walls, evolved from the discovery in 1963 by Laurell and Eriksson [1] of the hereditary disorder α_1-antitrypsin (α_1AT) deficiency and its association with a high risk for emphysema. In this chapter, we will use α_1AT deficiency as a "model" to develop the concept of how the vulnerability of the lung to proteolytic damage leads to emphysema when the normal antiprotease protective screen of the alveolar structures is inadequate to deal with its burden of proteases. The central concept is simply stated: Since α_1AT normally provides the major protection of the alveolar walls against the powerful protease neutrophil elastase (NE), a deficiency of α_1AT leaves the alveolar walls unable to contend with a chronic burden of NE released by neutrophils that traffic to the lung. For details concerning various aspects of this process, see chapters on proteases (7.1.1), antiproteases (7.1.2), structure and organization of the interstitium (3.3.1), the connective tissue components

of the interstitium (3.3.1–3.3.6), neutrophils, neutrophil traffic, and chemotaxis (3.4.7, 3.4.8, and 2.10, respectively), consequences of proteolytic injury (7.1.3), and the oxidative stress placed on the lung by cigarette smoke (7.6.3). Although α_1AT deficiency can also be associated with hepatic, hematologic, and skin disease, we will focus only on those aspects of α_1AT deficiency relevant to the enhanced vulnerability of the lung to proteolytic attack; for details concerning other aspects of this disease, see refs. 2–10.

α_1-ANTITRYPSIN DEFICIENCY

The typical α_1AT-deficient individual develops symptoms referable to the lungs between ages 25 and 40 (3,8,11). The earliest symptom is usually dyspnea on exertion. Although infrequent as an initial symptom, about 50% develop a productive cough and frequent pulmonary infections. A significant proportion manifest airway reactivity with wheezing. As the disease progresses, there is progressive limitation in physical activity, due in part to the worsening dyspnea and in part to systemic oxygen deprivation.

Estimates of the allelic frequency of the α_1AT deficiency alleles suggest that there are 20,000 to 40,000 α_1AT-deficient individuals in the United States, making it the second most common lethal hereditary disorder affecting Caucasians (see below) (3,5,8). The disease is accelerated by cigarette smoking, and thus it is common for surveys to find males outnumbering females 2 to 1 due to patterns of cigarette smoking (8,11).

Longitudinal studies of adults with α_1AT deficiency suggest that their lifespan is shortened by 10–15 years compared to that of the normal population (11,12). In the United States, individuals with α_1AT deficiency who are known to have emphysema and who are at least 18 years of age have a 52% chance of being alive at age 50 (compared to 93% for the general population)

R. C. Hubbard and R. G. Crystal: Pulmonary Branch, National Heart, Lung and Blood Institute, National Institutes of Health, Bethesda, Maryland 20892.

and a 16% chance of being alive at age 60 (compared to 85%) (11).

Physical examination typically reveals evidence of emphysema with decreased breath sounds, particularly at the bases. The chest roentgenogram, computed tomography, and ventilation–perfusion scans show the lung destruction, primarily in lower lung zones and commonly associated with bullae. Lung function abnormalities are also typical of emphysema and include airflow limitation, increase in total lung capacity, and reduction in the diffusing capacity for carbon monoxide.

Relationship Between α_1AT Levels and Risk for Lung Destruction

The emphysema of α_1AT deficiency results from an inadequate anti-NE screen of the lower respiratory tract due to low levels of α_1AT. The major function of α_1AT is to inhibit NE, a powerful, destructive proteolytic enzyme produced in myelocytic bone marrow precursor cells and stored in circulating neutrophils (Fig. 1) (13–15). The liver is the major site of α_1AT gene expression, releasing approximately 2 g of α_1AT into the circulation daily (16,17). With its molecular mass of 52 kDa, α_1AT diffuses throughout the body, protecting the extracellular matrix from attack by NE released by neutrophils (18–20). The alveolar walls are particularly vulnerable to a deficiency of α_1AT for several reasons: their relatively fragile architecture (Chapter 3.3.1); the major role played by α_1AT in forming a protective anti-NE screen at this site (Chapter 7.1.2); and the chronic trafficking of neutrophils to the lung (Chapter 3.4.8).

The amount of α_1AT necessary to provide adequate protection of the lower respiratory tract can be conceptualized as the "threshold" level above which sufficient amounts of α_1AT are available to provide adequate anti-NE protection to alveolar tissues. Since levels of α_1AT in the lower respiratory tract are determined by the serum α_1AT level, epidemiologic studies of the relationships among α_1AT levels, phenotypes, and the rates of development of emphysema have led to the establishment of the "threshold" serum α_1AT level which is protective against developing emphysema (Fig. 2). In this regard, serum α_1AT levels of less than 6.9 μM (50 mg/dl based on previously used standards; see ref. 20) are associated with a high risk for developing emphysema, and levels of 6.9 to 11 μM (50–80 mg/dl) are at a mildly increased risk, whereas levels of more than 11 μM have no increased risk compared to the background risk of the general population (21). By extrapolation from the serum α_1AT threshold of 11 μM, an alveolar epithelial lining fluid (ELF) α_1AT level of 1.2 μM and interstitial fluid levels of 5–7 μM

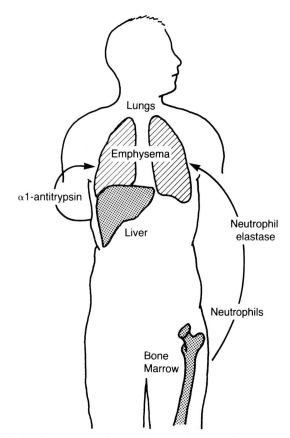

FIG. 1. Organs involved in the pathogenesis of the emphysema associated with α_1-antitrypsin (α_1AT) deficiency. The liver is the primary source of α_1AT. Neutrophils, derived from bone marrow precursor cells, carry neutrophil elastase (NE), a destructive enzyme capable of destroying the fragile walls of the pulmonary alveoli. The lung is normally protected from NE by α_1AT. If mutations of the α_1AT gene result in insufficient amounts of functional α_1AT to protect the lung from NE, the eventual result is emphysema.

constitute the threshold for adequate lower respiratory tract α_1AT anti-elastase protection (7,22).

Neutrophil Elastase–Antineutrophil Elastase Balance in the Lower Respiratory Tract

There is normally a mild, chronic burden of NE in the lower respiratory tract as a result of its release by neutrophils present in pulmonary capillaries, within the interstitium, or on the epithelial surface of the alveoli (23,24; see also Chapter 3.4.8). The number of these neutrophils may increase substantially in the presence of infection or as a result of the release of chemotactic mediators for neutrophils in lung inflammation, such as with cigarette smoking (23). The NE burden is normally balanced by an excess of antiproteases, principally α_1AT, which provides ample anti-NE protection to lung parenchyma (see Chapter 7.1.2). In the pres-

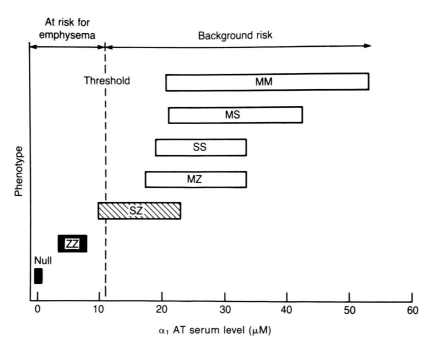

FIG. 2. Relationship between serum α_1-antitrypsin (α_1AT) levels, α_1AT phenotype, and the risk for developing emphysema. Epidemiologic studies suggest that a "threshold" serum α_1AT level of 11 μM is necessary to provide sufficient α_1AT to protect the alveolar walls from destruction by neutrophil elastase. Individuals with serum α_1AT level greater than 11 μM (phenotypes MZ, SS, MS, and MM) have the normal, low "background" risk for emphysema of the general population. Individuals with serum α_1AT levels less than 11 μM (Null, ZZ, and other rare deficiency phenotypes) are at increased risk for emphysema. Individuals with the SZ phenotype may be at slightly increased risk. See refs. 20 and 21 for details.

ence of excess active α_1AT, the NE released by neutrophils combines in a 1:1 ratio with α_1AT and is thus prevented from attacking and degrading proteins of the extracellular matrix.

Based on the concept of the protective "threshold" (see above), an ELF α_1AT level of 1.2 μM constitutes the minimal adequate antiprotease level necessary to counterbalance the normal elastase burden. Reductions in the total level of α_1AT below the threshold (as occurs with α_1AT deficiency) or in the amount of normally functional α_1AT, due to oxidative inactivation of α_1AT within the lung (e.g., as occurs in association with cigarette smoking; see below) tips the NE–anti-NE balance in favor of NE, leaving the lung vulnerable to parenchymal destruction.

Effect of Cigarette Smoking

Cigarette smoking is associated with the development of emphysema in individuals with normal serum and lung levels of α_1AT, as well as with the accelerated emphysema development in individuals who have α_1AT deficiency. α_1AT-deficient cigarette smokers develop symptoms of emphysema 10–15 years earlier than do their nonsmoking counterparts (12).

Cigarette smoking affects the NE–anti-NE balance because it is associated with markedly increased levels of oxidants within the lower respiratory tract. The oxidants present in smokers' lungs are derived from several sources. Cigarette smoke itself contains a large amount of free radicals (see Chapter 7.6.3). In addition, oxidants are chronically produced in exaggerated amounts by inflammatory cells in the lower respiratory tract of the cigarette smoker (25,26). These oxidants interact with the active-site Met^{358} residue of the α_1AT molecule, converting it from the native to the sulfoxide form, resulting in a loss of the normal inhibitory activity of the α_1AT molecule against NE (26–28). *In vitro* studies have demonstrated that oxidized α_1AT is approximately 2000-fold less active against NE than is native α_1AT (29), and *in vivo* studies have shown (a) the presence of oxidized α_1AT in smokers' lungs (27) and (b) a significant reduction of the anti-NE activity of α_1AT in the epithelial lining fluid of cigarette smokers compared to normal (30–32).

Cigarette smoking also affects the NE–anti-NE balance by increasing the number of neutrophils, and hence the level of NE, within the lower respiratory tract (23). The increased numbers of neutrophils in the lower respiratory tract of the cigarette smoker as compared to those of normal individuals is due to the attraction by chemotactic molecules for neutrophils (a) released by alveolar macrophages, (b) nicotine, (c) fragments of connective tissue, and (d) α_1AT fragments, coupled with the overall increase in circulating neutrophils in cigarette smokers (23,33–36). Thus, cigarette smoking is associated with an alteration in the normal NE–anti-NE balance as a result of both (a) reducing the function of α_1AT which is present in the lung and (b) increasing the amount of NE which must be inactivated; the net result is that smokers are at a higher risk for developing lung destruction than are nonsmokers. These observations regarding the impact of cigarette smoking on the NE–anti-NE balance help to explain the occurrence of emphysema in normal individuals who smoke, its rarity in nonsmokers, and the accelerated development of emphysema in α_1AT-deficient individuals who smoke.

α_1-ANTITRYPSIN ALLELES "AT RISK" FOR EMPHYSEMA

Categorization

The α_1AT gene locus is pleomorphic, with at least 75 alleles identified. Conceptually, the α_1AT alleles are conveniently classified as "normal" (alleles coding for α_1AT proteins present in normal amounts and with normal function; for details concerning the normal α_1AT alleles, see Chapter 7.1.2 and refs. 3,5–8) and "at risk" (alleles that cause the individual to become "at risk" for disease). Subgroups of the "at risk" class include (a) the "deficiency" alleles (coding for α_1AT molecules detectable in serum but at levels lower than

normal), (b) the "null" alleles (no α_1AT is detectable in serum), and (c) the "altered function" subgroup (coding for an α_1AT protein that functions other than as an inhibitor of NE).

Identification

Classically, identification of α_1AT phenotypes capitalizes on two facts: (i) Most α_1AT alleles code for α_1AT proteins that differ from one another by charge, and thus can be identified by isoelectric focusing (IEF) analysis of serum; and (ii) the α_1AT allele dictates the serum α_1AT level (3,8,37). Thus, the α_1AT phenotype is traditionally determined by analyzing the serum for the α_1AT IEF pattern, by measurement of serum α_1AT levels, and, if necessary, by family studies.

Except for the null alleles and a few rare alleles, the nomenclature for the α_1AT alleles is based on a letter code (A to Z) relating to the position of migration of the α_1AT protein in IEF of plasma between pH 4 and 5 (Fig. 3) (3,8,37). The common normal variants migrate in the middle and are thus referred to as the "M-family" alleles, whereas the deficiency variant originally described by Laurell and Eriksson (1) migrates toward the cathode and is referred to as "Z." When two alleles have an identical IEF pattern, and the sequence difference is known, the relevant residue is specifically indicated [e.g., M1(Ala^{213}) and M1(Val^{213}) migrate in the identical position on IEF]. Some rare alleles are labeled by a letter indicating the IEF position together with the birth site of the index case carrying the allele [e.g., M$_{procida}$]. The null alleles are labeled "Null" together with the birthplace of the index case (e.g., Null$_{bellingham}$).

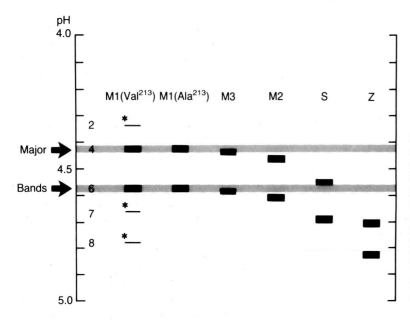

FIG. 3. Illustration of the major α_1-antitrypsin (α_1AT) bands observed by isoelectric focusing of serum at pH 4.0 (anode) to 5.0 (cathode). Shown are the patterns for each of the common alleles. For each allele there are at least five forms of α_1AT circulating in serum, including the two major bands ("4" and "6," indicated by arrows and shaded boxes) and three minor bands [indicated only for the M1(Val^{213}) allele, with "*" denoting the "2," "7," and "8" bands]. The various bands result from post-translational modification of the α_1AT protein. See refs. 3, 5, and 8 for details.

As more α_1AT genes are sequenced, it has become clear that this approach does not identify all alleles. Furthermore, when family analysis is not possible, it is difficult to identify "null" heterozygotes. The adaptation of recombinant DNA methodologies to the analysis of the α_1AT alleles has led to the development of rapid, accurate methods of genotyping. As a result, several approaches are now available to identify α_1AT alleles in genomic DNA. The most powerful of these, now widely available, is the use of the polymerase chain reaction to amplify individual segments of the α_1AT coding exons. This permits rapid evaluation using labeled oligonucleotide probes; or, using allele-specific primers combined with polymerase chain reaction, only those α_1AT alleles specific for the probe are amplified (37–40).

The "At Risk" Alleles

The "at risk" alleles occur most commonly in Caucasians of northern European descent (2,8). α_1AT deficiency is rare in Blacks or Asians. Two "at risk" alleles must be inherited to confer risk for clinically significant disease (2,8). Most "at risk" mutations are single base substitutions causing single amino acid modifications in the mature protein. Others are either (a) nonsense mutations inserting a premature stop codon into the normal coding sequence, (b) single or double base deletions or insertions causing frameshifts resulting in distal premature stop codons, (c) deletions of one codon in the coding sequence, or (d) deletion of all coding exons (Table 1 and Fig. 4).

There are five different mechanisms by which these

TABLE 1. *Mutations of the α_1-antitrypsin gene associated with an increased risk for emphysema[a]*

Relative frequency[b]	Allele	Base allele[c]	Mutation site (exon)	Sequence compared to base allele	Reference
Common	Z	M1(Ala[213])	V	Glu[342] GAG-→Lys AAG	55
	S	M1(Val[213])	III	Glu[264] GAA-→Val GTA	58
Rare	M$_{heerlen}$	M1(Ala[213])	V	Pro[369] CCC-→Leu CTC	91
	M$_{malton}$	M2	II	Phe[52] TTC-→delete TTC	49,92
	M$_{mineral\ springs}$	M1(Ala[213])	II	Gly[67] GGG-→Glu GAG	39
	M$_{procida}$	M1(Val[213])	II	Leu[41] CTG-→Pro CCG	93
	M$_{nichinan}$[d]	Unknown	II	Phe[52] TTC-→delete TTC Gly[148] GGG-→Arg AGG	94
	M$_{iiyama}$	Unknown	II	Ser[53] TCC-→Phe TTC	95
	I	M1(Val[213])	II	Arg[39] CGC-→Cys TGC	7, 92
	P$_{lowell}$	M1(Val[213])	III	Asp[256] GAT-→Val GTT	52
	W$_{bethesda}$	M1(Ala[213])	V	Ala[336] GCT-→Thr ACT	53
	Null$_{granite\ falls}$	M1(Ala[213])	II	Tyr[160] TAC-→delete C-→5′shift-→stop[160] TAG	44
	Null$_{bellingham}$	M1(Val[213])	III	Lys[217] AAG-→stop[217] TAG	43
	Null$_{mattawa}$	M1(Val[213])	V	Leu[353] TTA-→insert T→Phe[353] TTT-→3′shift-→stop[376] TAG	96
	Null$_{isola\ de\ procida}$	Unknown	II–V	Delete 10 kb, including exons II–V	41
	Null$_{hong\ kong}$	M2	IV	Leu[318] CTC-→delete TC-→5′shift-→stop[334] TAA	50
	Null$_{bolton}$	M1(Val[213])	V	Pro[362] CCC-→delete C-→5′ shift-→stop[373] TAA	97
	Null$_{devon}$	Unknown	II	Gly[115]-→Ser	98
	Null$_{ludwigshafen}$	M2	II	Ile[92] ATC-→Asn AAC	98
	Null$_{clayton}$	M1(Val[213])	V	Phe[362] CCC-→insert T-→3′shift-→stop[376] TAG	e

[a] List of α_1AT alleles associated with an increased risk for emphysema for which a partial or complete sequence is known at the gene level. Details can be found in the references listed and in reviews (3,5–8,98). There have been other "at risk" alleles identified by isoelectric focusing, but the sequence is unknown (see ref. 5). For the affected individual to be at risk, both parental alleles must be in the "at risk" category (see text).

[b] Relative frequency for that category. "Common" alleles are those with allelic frequencies greater than 1%.

[c] "Base allele" represents the common, normal allele upon which the mutation developed; M1(Ala[213]) is believed to be the oldest human α_1AT allele from which all other alleles derived (see Chapter 7.1.2 and ref. 99 for review). "Unknown" indicates that only a partial sequence is known and that the base allele therefore cannot be determined.

[d] For M$_{nichinan}$, there are two mutations distinguishing the α_1AT allele from its respective base allele, suggesting that there may be intermediate, as yet unidentified, allele.

[e] M. Brantly and R. Crystal, *unpublished observation*.

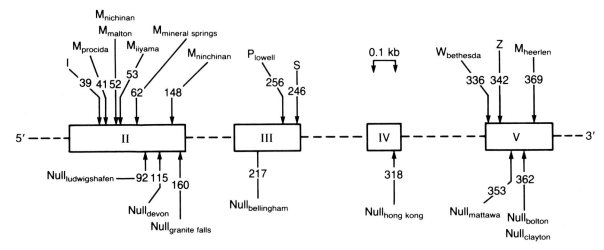

FIG. 4. Locations of the "at risk" mutations of the α_1-antitrypsin (α_1AT) gene associated with α_1AT deficiency and emphysema. Exons II, III, IV, and V are indicated by rectangles; for details concerning the entire normal gene, see Chapter 7.1.2. The location of each mutation is indicated by an arrow and also by the number of the amino acid codon where the mutation has been identified. Mutations above the gene are those in which the α_1AT protein can be detected in serum (the "deficiency" and "dysfunctional" groups of "at risk" alleles); those below are characterized by no α_1AT protein detectable in serum (the "null" group of "at risk" alleles). Note that the various mtutations are actually on different "base" normal α_1AT alleles; see Table 1 and Fig. 6 for details.

"at risk" mutations result in "α_1-antitrypsin deficiency," although there is some overlap; that is, some mutations result in more than one process contributing to the deficiency state. Since the hepatocyte is the major source of α_1AT in the body, most of these mechanisms affect the processes by which the hepatocyte synthesizes and secretes α_1AT (Fig. 5).

First, the α_1AT gene may be deleted. There is one example of this, Null$_{\text{isola de procida}}$, an allele in which the four coding exons are deleted (41).

Second, the α_1AT mRNA is degraded, as likely occurs with Null$_{\text{bellingham}}$ and Null$_{\text{granite falls}}$ (42–44). The mechanism for this is not known, but it likely relates to instability of the mRNA secondary to stop codons in coding exons.

Third, the newly synthesized α_1AT molecule accumulates within the hepatocyte. This likely results from modifications in charge and/or three-dimensional configuration of the newly synthesized molecule, and it may involve the processes of translocation of α_1AT from the rough endoplasmic reticulum to the Golgi complex. This mechanism is responsible for α_1AT deficiency associated with the Z, M$_{\text{malton}}$, and Null$_{\text{hong kong}}$ mutations (45–50).

Fourth, the newly synthesized α_1AT molecule is degraded within the synthesizing cell, probably because the molecule is unstable prior to folding into its final form. This mechanism is associated with the S, P$_{\text{lowell}}$, and W$_{\text{bethesda}}$ alleles (51–53).

Finally, the molecule is secreted, but the secreted form does not function normally as an inhibitor of NE.

There is only one example (39) where this is associated with emphysema (M$_{\text{mineral springs}}$), although the "Pittsburgh" mutation (Met^{358} --> Arg; a mutation that causes a coagulation problem because of the conversion of the molecule to a "thrombin-like molecule"; see ref. 54) would likely result in emphysema if inhibited in a homozygous form.

The most common deficiency alleles are Z and S (see below). For details concerning the rare deficiency and null alleles, see refs. 6–8 and 39–54.

The Z Mutation

The Z allele is the most common cause of the clinically recognized α_1AT deficiency, with Z homozygotes representing more than 90% of all cases (11). The allelic frequency is 1–2% in Caucasians of northern European descent, leading to the estimate of 20,000 to 40,000 Z homozygotes in the United States. The Z mutation is a single base substitution in exon V of the normal M1(Ala^{213}) allele causing a Glu^{342} --> Lys substitution in the molecule (55). Despite normal levels of α_1AT mRNA transcripts in the α_1AT-synthesizing cells of Z homozygotes, protein secretion is only 15% of that in normal individuals (17), because the newly synthesized α_1AT molecules accumulate in the rough endoplasmic reticulum.

The mechanisms responsible for the intracellular accumulation of α_1AT in association with the Z allele are unclear (45–48). The change in the amino acid se-

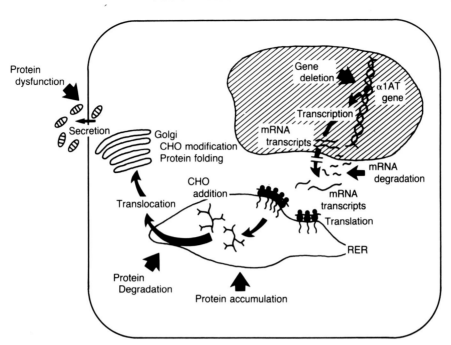

FIG. 5. Categorization of the "at-risk" mutations of the α_1-antitrypsin (α_1AT) gene based on the mechanisms by which they cause α_1AT deficiency. Shown is a hepatocyte with the normal pathway of α_1AT transcription, translation, post-translational modification with the addition of carbohydrates (CHO), protein folding and carbohydrate modification, and secretion of α_1AT. Mechanisms which result in α_1AT deficiency include gene deletion, degradation of mRNA transcripts, protein accumulation in the rough endoplasmic reticulum (RER), protein degradation prior to translocation to the Golgi complex, and release of dysfunctional α_1AT. See text and ref. 7 for details.

quence in the Z α_1AT molecule (Glu^{342} --→ Lys) results in the loss of an internal salt bridge between Glu^{342} and Lys^{290} which normally functions to stabilize the α_1AT molecule as it is synthesized (45–47). Other data suggest that the insertion of a positive charge at residue 342 causes the α_1AT to accumulate, independent of the charge of the residue at 290 (48). Alternatively, the Z mutation might cause a loss of a translocation signal recognition site within the α_1AT molecule. Whatever the mechanism, the consequences are (a) prevention of normal α_1AT translocation to the Golgi and (b) subsequent secretion.

There is also evidence that the Z molecule does not function normally as an inhibitor of NE. At the concentrations found in the lung, inhibition of NE by the Z form of α_1AT takes 12-fold longer than does normal α_1AT (56,57). Thus, the Z deficiency is a combined defect consisting of reduced amounts of a partially incompetent molecule, leaving the lung of the Z homozygote almost defenseless against NE.

S Mutation

The S allele is more common than Z, with an allelic frequency of 2–4% in Caucasians of northern Euro-

pean descent (2,3,8). Because the deficiency is relatively mild, and since the S molecule functions reasonably well as an inhibitor of NE, the S homozygote is not at increased risk (57). However, inheritance of the S allele along with an allele causing a profound deficiency of α_1AT (e.g., Z) puts the individual at mild risk.

Like the Z mutation, the S mutation (Glu^{264} --→ Val) modifies the internal architecture of α_1AT by disruption of a normal salt bridge (Glu^{264} --→ Lys^{387}) (47,58). Despite this similarity, the consequences of the S mutation are very different from those of the Z mutation. In S homozygotes, α_1AT mRNA is transcribed in normal form and amount, but some of the newly synthesized S molecules are probably shunted from the rough endoplasmic reticulum into lysosomes, where they are degraded (51).

Evolution of the "At Risk" Alleles

As discussed in Chapter 7.1.2, the α_1AT gene belongs to a group of serine antiproteases referred to as the "serpins." The oldest human α_1AT gene is M1(Ala^{213}); the other common normal α_1AT alleles (M1(Val^{213}), M3, and M2, likely evolved from the

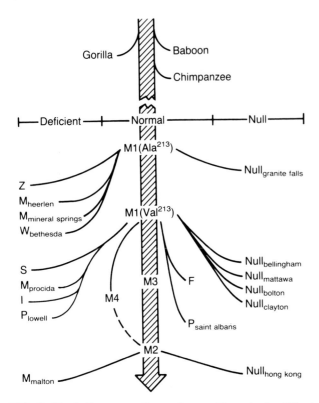

FIG. 6. Evolutionary pattern of α_1-antitrypsin (α_1AT) alleles. Shown is the likely evolutionary pattern of the normal, deficient, and null α_1AT alleles for which the gene sequence is known. *Top*: The nonhuman primate alleles (see Chapter 7.1.2 for details). *Middle* and *bottom*: The normal human alleles. *Left*: The deficiency alleles. *Right*: The null alleles. M1(Ala^{213}) is the closest allele in sequence to the chimpanzee and is thus likely the "oldest." The other common normal alleles are derived from M1(Ala^{213}) by single base substitutions and corresponding amino acids (see Chapter 7.1.2 and ref. 99). The substitution defining the uncommon normal M4 allele could have been derived from either M1(Val^{213}) or M2 (100). All of the deficiency and null alleles shown are derived from different normal alleles by base substitutions, deletions, or additions (see Table 1).

M1(Ala^{213}) gene by single base mutations (see discussion and Table 2 of Chapter 7.1.2). Evaluation of the coding sequence of all of the known "at risk" α_1AT alleles permits the construction of a putative pattern of evolution of the "at risk" alleles from the normal alleles (Fig. 6).

There are conflicting opinions as to whether there may have been selection pressures on the α_1AT gene during evolution. It is unlikely that the development of emphysema associated with the Z homozygote state of α_1AT deficiency produced any "negative" selection, since most offspring are produced before the emphysema becomes clinically manifest. Furthermore, although cigarette smoking markedly accelerates α_1AT deficiency, the gene pool of northern European Caucasions was not exposed to this "environmental"

factor until the 16th century. However: (a) α_1AT does inhibit acrosein (the protease sperm used to enter the ovum), and there is some evidence of an increased incidence of multiple births among α_1AT-deficient individuals; and (b) in the pre-antibiotic era, individuals with α_1AT deficiency might have had an advantage in dealing with infection with *Mycobacterium tuberculosis*; with less α_1AT available, neutrophils may have greater access to cavities of chronic infection (because the neutrophil elastase would not be inhibited in the local milieu), thus helping to suppress the infection.

STRATEGIES TO CORRECT THE α_1AT DEFICIENCY STATE

Strategies to prevent lung destruction in α_1AT deficiency are based upon the understanding that the NE–anti-NE imbalance in the lower respiratory tract must be corrected either by reducing the levels of NE or by increasing the level of antiproteases available to inhibit NE. At present there are no known methods of chronically safely reducing numbers of neutrophils, and hence the NE burden, in the lung. Strategies for increasing the level of antiproteases in the lower respiratory tract can be classified into six groups, including: (i) modulation of α_1AT gene expression; (ii) augmentation with purified human plasma α_1AT; (iii) use of recombinant forms of α_1AT; (iv) use of other naturally occurring proteases; (v) use of chemical antiproteases; and (vi) gene therapy.

Modulation of α_1AT Gene Expression

Strategies to modulate endogenous expression of the α_1AT gene have been directed toward the hepatocyte, the cell responsible for producing greater than 95% of serum α_1AT. It has been recognized for some time that an individual's serum α_1AT level varies to some degree; α_1AT is an acute phase reactant, and serum α_1AT levels rise with fever, trauma, shock, and pregnancy (see ref. 4 for review). Although the understanding of the genetic control mechanisms responsible for the modulation of α_1AT levels is limited (see Chapter 7.1.2), attempts have been made to modulate serum α_1AT levels *in vivo* through the use of pharmacologic agents. Success, however, has been limited. For example, typhoid vaccine administration to normal or MZ heterozygotes transiently increases α_1AT levels, but it does not increase levels in Z homozygotes. Likewise, use of estrogen–progesterone combinations to mimic the hormonal milieu of pregnancy has been equally unsuccessful. Other hormonal manipulations have been tried to increase serum α_1AT levels. Danazol, a derivative of 17α-ethinyl testosterone, is known to increase hepatic production of the antiprotease C1-

esterase in hereditary angioedema, but in α_1AT deficiency the α_1AT levels achieved are far below the protective threshold (59,60). Finally, tamoxifen, an agent which binds to estrogen receptors and which theoretically might increase serum α_1AT levels in a manner analogous to that which occurs in pregnancy, has little effect on serum α_1AT levels in ZZ individuals (61). Interestingly, tamoxifen does increase serum α_1AT levels in association with alleles such as S and P_{lowell} (52,62); that is, tamoxifen probably has an effect on α_1AT gene expression, but the post-translational abnormalities associated with the Z allele prevent tamoxifen from having a useful therapeutic effect in Z homozygotes.

Augmentation with Purified Human Plasma α_1AT

As demonstrated by Gadek et al. (19) in 1981, and in a large-scale study by Wewers et al. (20) in 1987, direct augmentation of serum and lung α_1AT levels is possible through the administration of human plasma-purified α_1AT. Plasma-purified α_1AT is now available as a commercially prepared preparation obtained from pooled human plasma, which has been heat-treated to reduce the risk of transmitting viral pathogens. When given intravenously at a dose of 60 mg/kg weekly (20) or 250 mg/kg monthly (63), human plasma-purified α_1AT is an effective means of augmenting lung α_1AT concentrations to above threshold protective levels.

Weekly infusion is accompanied by a rapid rise in the serum α_1AT level to greater than 40 μM, followed by a gradual decline consistent with the normal rate of clearance of α_1AT (4.5 days) (20). The serum α_1AT level averages approximately 22 μM during weekly therapy, a value which is five- to sevenfold higher than in untreated Z individuals and which is more than twofold greater than the estimated serum threshold level. Importantly, the infused α_1AT diffuses from plasma into the lung, where it raises the epithelial lining fluid α_1AT concentration significantly above the threshold level of 1.2 μM. In addition, the ELF anti-NE capacity, a measure of the active anti-NE protection of the lower respiratory tract, increases in a parallel manner.

Monthly infusions of α_1AT produce similar results (63). Peak serum levels approach 200 μM immediately following infusion, and they decline over time at much the same rate as in weekly therapy. Nadir serum α_1AT levels on monthly therapy are generally somewhat lower than those observed on weekly therapy, but, importantly, lung levels of α_1AT and anti-NE capacity are comparable. Thus, like weekly augmentation therapy, monthly administration results in a sustained increase in both serum and lung anti-NE protective levels to well above threshold and approaching levels of normal individuals.

While effective, intravenous augmentation therapy is inefficient. Only an estimated 2% of the total infused α_1AT eventually reaches the lung—in effect, 98% of the drug is wasted. To evaluate the feasibility of directly targeting therapy to the lower respiratory tract, where it is needed to prevent NE-mediated lung destruction, α_1AT was administered by aerosol to α_1AT-deficient individuals (64). Utilizing an aerosol generator capable of developing α_1-antitrypsin droplets sufficiently small ($\leq$3 μM mass median diameter), to reach the alveoli (see Chapter 7.3.1) when administered at a dose of 200 mg twice daily, aerosolized plasma α_1AT effectively raised ELF α_1AT levels and anti-NE capacity to the normal range. Aerosol therapy appears to be safe, with no evidence of allergic reactions or change in lung function in association with repeated aerosol administration of α_1AT. From studies in sheep, it is clear that aerosolized plasma α_1AT reaches the interstitium, and studies in humans demonstrate that it reaches the plasma (64). The major experimental hurdle to overcome with plasma α_1AT aerosol therapy is to demonstrate that it effectively raises α_1AT levels in the interstitium to 5–7 μM, the level estimated to be the interstitial protective "threshold" (7,22).

Augmentation with Recombinant Forms of α_1AT

Using recombinant DNA techniques, α_1AT has been produced in *Escherichia coli* and in the yeast *Saccharomyces cerevisiae* (65–67). These recombinant forms of α_1AT (rAAT) are similar to the naturally occurring plasma α_1AT except they lack the three carbohydrate side chains. rAAT has a molecular mass of 45-kDa and also has normal anti-NE function, with an association rate constant for NE of approximately 10^7 M^{-1} sec^{-1} (67–69). However, the lack of carbohydrate side chains has a serious consequence: When given intravenously (to primates), it is rapidly cleared from the plasma and has a half-life of approximately 90 min, with much of the infused material undergoing rapid renal excretion, thus obviating the intravenous route for human therapy (67).

To circumvent the problem of rapid clearance, rAAT has been given successfully to α_1AT-deficient individuals by the aerosol route (70). As with plasma α_1AT, *in vitro* studies have demonstrated that rAAT structure and function are not altered by the process of aerosolization. Aerosolized rAAT increased ELF levels of α_1AT and anti-elastase capacity in a dose-dependent fashion, in a manner which suggested that a dose of 200 mg daily would result in elevation of α_1AT levels to above threshold levels in the lung. Importantly, aerosolized rAAT is able to pass through alveolar epithelium to gain access to the interstitium. Like the plasma form of α_1AT, the major hurdle to overcome with aerosol therapy with rAAT is to demonstrate that it can raise interstitial levels to above the protective threshold.

Other forms of recombinant α_1AT have been synthesized, taking advantage of the knowledge that alterations in the active-site amino acid residue confer different properties to the α_1AT molecule. In the naturally occurring form of α_1AT, the Met[358] at the active inhibitory site can be easily oxidized, and thus α_1AT can be rendered impotent in the milieu of cigarette smoke and in inflammation (see above and Chapter 7.1.2). When Val, Ala, or Ile is substituted for the active-site Met[358], the recombinant α_1AT retains its ability to inhibit NE, yet it is resistant to oxidation (26,65,66,69,71). The recombinant variant Leu[358] inhibits NE, is resistant to oxidation, and also inhibits cathepsin G, another neutrophil protease which may play a role in proteolytic lung injury (see Chapter 7.1.1). The ability to withstand oxidation makes the modified forms of α_1AT attractive alternatives for potential use in conditions characterized by excessive burden of NE and oxidants.

Site-directed mutagenesis has been used to selectively remove one or more of the three Asn glycosylation sites on the α_1AT molecule to analyze the effect of carbohydrates on the rate of clearance of α_1AT from plasma (72). Fully glycosylated α_1AT molecules are cleared much less rapidly than are molecules containing deletions of single or a pair of carbohydrate side chains, whereas α_1AT molecules completely lacking carbohydrates are cleared most rapidly.

Other Naturally Occurring Antiproteases

Several other human, experimental animal, and plant antiproteases have been considered for possible augmentation therapy in α_1AT deficiency. The most important of these is secretory leukoprotease inhibitor (SLPI), a 12-kDa nonglycosylated protein synthesized and secreted by human respiratory tract mucosal cells (see Chapter 7.1.2). SLPI inhibits NE nearly as effectively as α_1AT, with an association rate constant of 10^7 M^{-1} sec^{-1}. Its concentration in ELF is highest in the airways, the site of its synthesis; overall, SLPI contributes less than 10% to the overall anti-NE protective screen of the lower respiratory tract (18,73,74). Recombinant SLPI has been produced in *E. coli* and, when introduced intratracheally, is able to prevent elastase from causing emphysema in hamsters (75; see Chapter 7.1.3). Recombinant SLPI can be aerosolized, and it effectively augments the ELF anti-NE capacity following aerosolization in sheep (76).

Eglin-c, a single-chain 8.1-kDa polypeptide originally purified from the medicinal leech *Hirudo medicinalis*, has been cloned and produced in *E. coli* (77–79). Eglin-c inhibits both NE and cathepsin G, as well as several other proteases. Like SLPI, intratracheal instillation of eglin-c reduces the severity of elastase-induced emphysema in hamsters. However, as might be expected from a protein from a nonhuman source, eglin-c is allergenic to humans and therefore cannot be used clinically in its present form.

NE is markedly inhibited by *cis*-unsaturated fatty acids, such as oleic acid (80). A family of serine protease inhibitors has been identified in the seeds of squash (*Curcurbita maxima*), several of which might be potentially useful (81). A number of NE inhibitors have been isolated from microorganisms, including elasnin, elasninal, chymostatin, leupeptin, valinal, and antipain (80). Although some of these molecules inhibit the development of emphysema in animal studies (80), it is unlikely that they will be useful for humans because of the danger of immune reactions associated with chronic administration.

Chemical Antiproteases

There are more than 40 synthetic serine protease inhibitors which have varying activities against NE (see ref. 80 for a comprehensive review of these agents). For the most part, the potential toxicity of these agents will prevent their use in humans, but they serve as useful models for the development of useful therapeutic agents. These molecules fall into several broad categories. The most widely used are the peptide aldehydes, which tend to be highly reactive and easily oxidized. Boroval [methoxy-succinyl-alanyl-alanyl-prolyl-boronyl-valyl-pinacol ester] is one such agent which reversibly inhibits NE and which has been evaluated for its ability to ameliorate elastase-induced emphysema in hamsters (82). However, contrary to expectations, boroval not only failed to reduce tissue injury, but also exacerbated the emphysema—possibly because as NE–boroval complexes gained access to the interstitium, they dissociated, thereby freeing NE to degrade extracellular proteins. This finding illustrates one potential problem of reversible synthetic inhibitors: Whereas the naturally occurring antiproteases such as α_1AT and SLPI interact with NE in an essentially irreversible fashion, reversible inhibitors can release NE, allowing it to destroy lung tissue.

Another broad group of synthetic antiproteases are the peptide chloromethyl ketones, molecules which irreversibly inhibit serine proteases (80). Chloromethyl ketones are capable of preventing many of the effects of intratracheally instilled NE (83), but the toxicity of chloromethyl ketones prevents them from being used clinically.

Beta-lactam-based compounds have recently been identified as specific potent inhibitors of NE (84).

When given intratracheally, these agents prevent hemorrhagic air-space damage in marmosets challenged with intratracheal NE. These molecules are rapidly cleared from the circulation following intravenous injection, and thus their use may be limited to aerosol therapy. Another chemical pharmaceutical agent, a reversible inhibitor, also prevents elastase-induced emphysema in animals when administered intratracheally, by aerosol, subcutaneously, or orally (85).

One theoretical advantage, and danger, of these small molecules is that they can gain access to tissue sites inaccessible to a large naturally occurring NE inhibitor such as α_1AT (86). This is an advantage because they may be able to prevent NE from attacking connective tissue in confined areas (such as beneath the surface of a neutrophil). This advantage, however, is theoretically a danger, because these molecules may inhibit NE-like proteases in sites where they are vital. The only way these theoretical questions can be answered is by long-term safety studies in humans.

GENE THERAPY

Because α_1AT functions in the extracellular milieu, gene therapy for the prevention of emphysema in α_1AT deficiency is conceptually a straightforward problem. All that is needed is to have the normal gene safely introduced into sufficient numbers of cells to produce and secrete enough α_1AT to protect the lung. Several different cell types are possible targets for gene therapy of α_1AT deficiency.

First, since alveolar macrophages normally express the α_1AT gene (17) and are derived from circulating blood monocytes, it should be possible to provide augmentation of α_1AT produced within the lung by inserting the normal α_1AT cDNA into bone marrow monocyte precursor cells, with subsequent eventual repopulation of the alveolar macrophages producing α_1AT in the lower respiratory tract.

Second, fibroblasts have been used experimentally to demonstrate the feasibility of introducing the normal α_1AT cDNA into cells not normally expressing this gene. The N2 retroviral shuttle vector has been used to integrate the normal human cDNA into murine fibroblasts, which then has produced and secreted normal, glycosylated human α_1AT (87). When these cells were transplanted into the peritoneal cavity of nude mice, human α_1AT was detectable in plasma and, importantly, in ELF; that is, in effect the mice had received the therapeutic equivalent of a human liver transplant secreting one protein—α_1AT (88).

Third, T-lymphocytes are attractive targets because of their ability to be grown rapidly with interleukin-2 and their ability to be manipulated to permit *in vivo* expansion through the T-cell antigen receptor (89).

Finally, the epithelial surface of the lower respiratory tract is an inviting target for gene therapy because of the accessibility of these cells by the air route. In this regard, a retroviral vector has been used to transfer the α_1AT gene into airway epithelial cells *in vitro* (90), and an adenoviral vector has been successfully used to transfer a functional human α_1AT cDNA to respiratory tract epithelial cells of experimental animals *in vitro* and *in vivo*.

REFERENCES

1. Laurell CB, Eriksson S. The electrophoretic α1-globulin pattern of serum in α1-antitrypsin deficiency. *Scand J Clin Lab Invest* 1963;15:132–140.
2. Gadek JE, Crystal RG. α-1 antitrypsin deficiency. In: Stanbury JB, Wyngaarden JB, Fredrickson DS, Goldstein JL, Brown MS, eds. *The metabolic basis of inherited disease.* New York: McGraw-Hill, 1982;1450–1467.
3. Brantly M, Nukiwa T, Crystal RG. Molecular basis of α1-antitrypsin deficiency. *Am J Med* 1988;84:13–31.
4. Hubbard RC, Crystal RG. Alpha 1-antitrypsin augmentation therapy for alpha 1-antitrypsin deficiency. *Am J Med* 1988; 84:52–62.
5. Crystal RG, Brantly ML, Hubbard RC, Curiel DT, States DJ, Holmes MD. The α1-antitrypsin gene and its mutations: clinical consequences and strategies for therapy. *Chest* 1989;95:196–208.
6. Crystal RG. The α1-antitrypsin gene and its deficiency states. *Trends Genet* 1989;5:411–417.
7. Crystal RG. α1-Antitrypsin deficiency, emphysema and liver disease: genetic basis and strategies for therapy. *J Clin Invest* 1990;85:1343–1352.
8. Cox DW. α1-Antitrypsin deficiency. In: Scriver CR, Beaudet AL, Sly WS, Valle D, eds. *The metabolic basis of inherited disease.* New York: McGraw–Hill, 1989;2409–2437.
9. Carrell RW. α1-Antitrypsin: molecular pathology, leukocytes, and tissue damage. *J Clin Invest* 1986;78:1427–1431.
10. Carrell RW, Owen MC. α1-Antitrypsin: structure, variation and disease. *Essays Med Biochem* 1979;4:83–119.
11. Brantly ML, Paul LD, Miller BH, Falk RT, Wu M, Crystal RG. Clinical features and natural history of the destructive lung disease associated with alpha 1-antitrypsin deficiency of adults with pulmonary symptoms. *Am Rev Respir Dis* 1988;138:327–336.
12. Larsson C. Natural history and life expectancy in severe alpha$_1$-antitrypsin deficiency, PiZ. *Acta Med Scand* 1978; 204:345–351.
13. Barrett AJ. An introduction to proteases. In: Barrett AJ, Salvesen G, eds. *Protease inhibitors.* New York: Elsevier, 1986; 1–22.
14. Travis J, Salvesen GS. Human plasma proteinase inhibitors. *Annu Rev Biochem* 1983;52:655–709.
15. Fouret P, du Bois RM, Bernaudin J-F, Takahashi H, Ferrans VJ, Crystal RG. Expression of the neutrophil elastase gene during human bone marrow cell differentiation. *J Exp Med* 1989;169:833–845.
16. Jones EA, Vergalla J, Steer CJ, Bradley-Moore PR, Vierling JM. Metabolism of intact and desialylated α1-antitrypsin. *Clin Sci Mol Med* 1978;55:139–148.
17. Mornex JF, Chytil-Weir A, Martinet Y, Courtney M, LeCocq JP, Crystal RG. Expression of the alpha 1-antitrypsin gene in mononuclear phagocytes of normal and alpha 1-antitrypsin deficient individuals. *J Clin Invest* 1986;77:1952–1961.
18. Gadek JE, Zimmerman RL, Fells GA, Rennard SI, Crystal RG. Antielastases of the human alveolar structures: implications for the protease–antiprotease theory of emphysema. *J Clin Invest* 1981;68:889–898.
19. Gadek JE, Klein H, Holland PV, Crystal RG. Replacement

therapy of alpha 1-antitrypsin deficiency: reversal of protease–antiprotease imbalance within the alveolar structures of PiZZ subjects. *J Clin Invest* 1981;68:1158–1165.

20. Wewers MD, Casolaro MA, Sellers SE, Swayze SC, McPhaul KM, Crystal RG. Replacement therapy for alpha 1-antitrypsin deficiency associated with emphysema. *N Engl J Med* 1987;316:1055–1062.

21. Buist AS, Burrows B, Cohen A, Crystal RG, Fallat R, Gadek J, Turino G. Guidelines for the approach to the individual with severe hereditary alpha 1-antitrypsin deficiency. *Am Rev Respir Dis* 1989;140:1494–1498.

22. Hubbard RC, Crystal RG. Strategies for aerosol therapy of α1-antitrypsin deficiency by the aerosol route. *Eur J Respir Dis* (Suppl)1990;9:445–525.

23. Hunninghake GW, Crystal RG. Cigarette smoking and lung destruction: accumulation of neutrophils in the lungs of cigarette smokers. *Am Rev Respir Dis* 1983;128:833–838.

24. Rennard SI, Basset G, Lecossier D, O'Donnell KM, Martin PG, Crystal RG. Estimation of the apparent volume of epithelial lining fluid recovered by bronchoalveolar lavage using urea as an endogenous marker of dilution. *J Appl Physiol* 1986;60(2):532–538.

25. Hoidal JR, Fox RB, LeMarbe PA, Perri R, Repine JE. Altered oxidative metabolic responses *in vitro* of alveolar macrophages from asymptomatic cigarette smokers. *Am Rev Respir Dis* 1981;123:85–89.

26. Hubbard RC, Ogushi F, Fells GA, Cantin AM, Courtney M, Crystal RG. Oxidants spontaneously released by alveolar macrophages of cigarette smokers can inactivate the active site of α1-antitrypsin, rendering it ineffective as an inhibitor of neutrophil elastase. *J Clin Invest* 1987;80(5):1289–1295.

27. Carp H, Miller F, Hoidal JR, Janoff A. Potential mechanism of emphysema: α1-proteinase inhibitor recovered from lungs of cigarette smokers contains oxidized methionine and has a decreased elastase inhibitory capacity. *Proc Natl Acad Sci USA* 1982;79:2041–2045.

28. Johnson D, Travis J. The oxidative inactivation of human α-1-proteinase inhibitor—further evidence for methionine at the reactive center. *J Biol Chem* 1979;254:4022–4026.

29. Beatty K, Bieth J, Travis J. Kinetics of association of serine proteinases with native and oxidized α-1-proteinase inhibitor and α-1-antichymotrypsin. *J Biol Chem* 1980;255:3931–3934.

30. Gadek JE, Fells GA, Crystal RG. Cigarette smoking induces functional antiprotease deficiency in the lower respiratory tract of humans. *Science* 1979;206:1315–1316.

31. Fells G, Ogushi F, Hubbard R, Crystal R. α1-Antitrypsin in the lower respiratory tract of cigarette smokers has a decreased association rate constant for neutrophil elastase. *Am Rev Respir Dis* 1987;135(4):A291.

32. Wewers MD, Herzyk DJ, Gadek JE. Comparison of smoker and nonsmoker lavage fluid for the rate of association with neutrophil elastase. *Am J Respir Cell Mol Biol* 1989;1:423–429.

33. Totti N, McCusker RT, Campbell EJ, Griffin GL, Senior RM. Nicotine is chemotactic for neutrophils and enhances neutrophil responsiveness to chemotactic peptides. *Science* 1984;223:169–171.

34. Senior RM, Griffin GL, Mecham RP. Chemotactic activity of elastin derived peptides. *J Clin Invest* 1980;66:859–862.

35. Banda MJ, Rice AG, Griffin GL, Senior RM. The inhibitory complex of human α1-proteinase inhibitor and human leukocyte elastase is a neutrophil chemoattractant. *J Exp Med* 1988;167:1608–1615.

36. Janoff A. Elastases and emphysema. *Am Rev Respir Dis* 1985;132:417–433.

37. Cox DW, Johnson AM, Fagerhol MK. Report of nomenclature meeting for α1-antitrypsin: INSERM, Rouen Bois-Guillaume. *Hum Genet* 1980;53:429–433.

38. Okayama H, Curiel DT, Brantly ML, Holmes MD, Crystal RG. Rapid, nonradioactive detection of mutations in the human genome by allele specific amplification. *J Lab Clin Med* 1989;114:105–113.

39. Curiel DT, Stier LE, Crystal RG. Molecular basis of α1-antitrypsin deficiency and emphysema associated with the α1-antitrypsin M$_{mineral\ springs}$ allele. *Mol Cell Biol* 1990;10:47–56.

40. Holmes MD, Brantly ML, Curiel DT, Weidinger S, Crystal RG. Characterization of the normal α1-antitrypsin allele V$_{munich}$: a variant associated with a unique protein isoelectric focusing pattern. *Am J Hum Genet* 1990;46:810–816.

41. Takahashi H, Crystal RG. α1-Antitrypsin Null$_{isola\ de\ procida}$: a novel sub-class of α1-antitrypsin deficiency alleles caused by deletion of all α1-antitrypsin coding of exons. *Am J Hum Genet* 1990;47:403–413.

42. Garver RI Jr, Mornex J-F, Nukiwa T, Brantly M, Courtney M, LeCocq J-P, Crystal RG. Alpha 1-antitrypsin deficiency and emphysema caused by homozygous inheritance of non-expressing alpha 1-antitrypsin genes. *N Engl J Med* 1986;314(12):762–766.

43. Satoh K, Nukiwa T, Brantly M, Garver RI, Courtney M, Crystal RG. Emphysema associated with complete absence of α1-antitrypsin in serum and the homozygous inheritance of a stop codon in an α1-antitrypsin-coding exon. *Am J Hum Genet* 1988;42:77–83.

44. Holmes M, Curiel D, Brantly M, Crystal RG. Characterization of the intracellular mechanism causing the alpha 1-antitrypsin Null$_{granite\ falls}$ deficiency state. *Am Rev Respir Dis* 1989;140:1662–1667.

45. Brantly ML, Courtney M, Crystal RG. Repair of the secretion defect in the Z form of α1-antitrypsin by addition of a second mutation. *Science* 1988;242:1700–1702.

46. McCraken AA, Kruse KB, Brown JL. Secretion of mutant alpha-1-proteinase inhibitors. *J Cell Biochem* 1988;Suppl 12B:286.

47. Loebermann H, Tokuoka R, Deisenhofer J, Huber R. Human α1-proteinase inhibitor. *J Mol Biol* 1984;177:531–556.

48. Sifers RN, Hardick CP, Woo SLC. Disruption of the 290–342 salt bridge is not responsible for the secretory defect of the PiZ α1-antitrypsin variant. *J Biol Chem* 1989;264:2997–3001.

49. Curiel DT, Holmes MD, Okayama H, Brantly ML, Vogelmeier C, Travis WD, Stier L, Perks WH, Crystal RG. Molecular basis of the lung and liver disease associated with the α1-antitrypsin deficiency allele M$_{malton}$. *J Biol Chem* 1989;264:13938–13945.

50. Sifers RN, Brashears-Macatee S, Kidd VJ, Muensch H, Woo SLC. A frameshift mutation results in a truncated α1-antitrypsin that is retained within the rough endoplasmic reticulum. *J Biol Chem* 1988;263:7330–7335.

51. Curiel DT, Chytil A, Courtney M, Crystal RG. Serum α1-antitrypsin deficiency associated with the common S-type (Glu^{264} → Val) mutation results from exaggerated preglycosylation intracellular degradation of α1-antitrypsin prior to secretion. *J Biol Chem* 1989;264:10477–10485.

52. Holmes M, Brantly M, Wurts L, Crystal RG. Characterization of the sequence differences among the P-family of α1-antitrypsin alleles. *Am Rev Respir Dis* 1989;139:A369.

53. Holmes M, Brantly M, Fells G, Crystal RG. Molecular basis of the W$_{bethesda}$ α1-antitrypsin deficiency variant. *Aust NZ J Med* 1990;170:1013–1020.

54. Owen MC, Brennan SO, Lewis JH, Carrell RW. Mutation of antitrypsin to antithrombin: α1-antitrypsin Pittsburgh (358 Met → Arg), a fatal bleeding disorder. *N Engl J Med* 1983;309:694–698.

55. Nukiwa T, Satoh K, Brantly ML, Ogushi F, Fells GA, Courtney M, Crystal RG. Identification of a second mutation in the protein coding sequence of the Z-type alpha 1-antitrypsin gene. *J Biol Chem* 1986;261:15989–15994.

56. Ogushi F, Fells GA, Hubbard RC, Straus SD, Crystal RG. Z-type α1-antitrypsin is less competent than M1-type α1-antitrypsin as an inhibitor of neutrophil elastase. *J Clin Invest* 1987;80(5):1366–1374.

57. Ogushi F, Hubbard RC, Fells GA, Casolaro MA, Curiel DT, Brantly ML, Crystal RG. Evaluation of the S-type of alpha-1-antitrypsin as an *in vivo* and *in vitro* inhibitor of neutrophil elastase. *Am Rev Respir Dis* 1987;137:364–370.

58. Long GL, Chandra T, Woo SLC, Davie EW, Kurachi K. Complete sequence of the cDNA for human α1-antitrypsin and the gene for the S variant. *Biochemistry* 1984;23:4828–4837.

59. Gadek JE, Fulmer JD, Gelfand JA, Frank MM, Petty TL, Crystal RG. Danazol-induced augmentation of serum α1-antitrypsin

levels in individuals with marked deficiency of this antiprotease. *J Clin Invest* 1980;66:82–87.

60. Wewers M, Gadek JE, Keogh BA, Fells GA, Crystal RG. Evaluation of danazol therapy for patients with PiZZ alpha 1-antitrypsin deficiency. *Am Rev Respir Dis* 1986;134:476–480.

61. Wewers MD, Brantly ML, Casolaro MA, Crystal RG. Evaluation of tamoxifen as a therapy to augment alpha 1-antitrypsin concentrations in Z homozygous alpha 1-antitrypsin deficient subjects. *Am Rev Respir Dis* 1987;135:401–402.

62. Eriksson S. The effect of tamoxifen in intermediate alpha$_1$-antitrypsin deficiency associated with the phenotype P$_i$SZ. *Ann Clin Res* 1983;15:95–98.

63. Hubbard R, Sellers S, Czerski D, Stephens L, Crystal RG. Biochemical efficacy and safety of monthly augmentation therapy for α1-antitrypsin deficiency. *JAMA* 1988;260:1259–1264.

64. Hubbard RC, Brantly ML, Sellers SE, Mitchell ME, Crystal RG. Delivery of proteins for therapeutic purposes by aerosolization: direct augmentation of anti-neutrophil elastase defenses of the lower respiratory tract in α1-antitrypsin deficiency with an aerosol of α1-antitrypsin. *Ann Intern Med* 1989; 111:206–212.

65. Courtney M, Jallat S, Tessier LH, Benavente A, Crystal RG, LeCocq JP. Synthesis in *E. coli* of alpha 1-antitrypsin variants with potential in the therapy of emphysema and thrombosis. *Nature* 1985;313:149–151.

66. Rosenberg S, Barr PJ, Najarian RC, Hallewell RA. Synthesis in yeast of a functional oxidation-resistant mutant of human α$_1$-antitrypsin. *Nature* 1984;312:77–80.

67. Casolaro MA, Fells G, Wewers M, Pierce JE, Ogushi F, Hubbard R, Sellers S, Forstrom J, Lyons D, Kawasaki G, Crystal RG. Augmentation of lung antineutrophil elastase capacity with recombinant human α1-antitrypsin. *J Appl Physiol* 1987; 63(5):2015–2023.

68. Straus SD, Fells GA, Wewers MD, Courtney M, Tessier L-H, Tolstoshev P, LeCocq J-P, Crystal RG. Evaluation of recombinant DNA-directed *E. coli* produced α1-antitrypsin as an anti-neutrophil elastase for potential use as replacement therapy of α1-antitrypsin deficiency. *Biochem Biophys Res Commun* 1985;130:1177–1185.

69. Travis J, Owen M, George P, Carrell R, Rosenberg S, Hallewell RA, Barr PJ. Isolation and properties of recombinant DNA produced variants of human α$_1$-proteinase inhibitor. *J Biol Chem* 1985;260:4384–4389.

70. Janoff A, George-Nasciemento C, Rosenberg S. A genetically engineered, mutant human α1-proteinase inhibitor is more resistant than the normal inhibitor to oxidative inactivation by chemicals, enzymes, cells, and cigarette smoke. *Am Rev Respir Dis* 1986;133:353–356.

71. Jallat S, Carvallo D, Tessier LH, Roecklin D, Roitsch C, Ogushi F, Crystal RG, Courtney M. Altered specificities of genetically engineered α$_1$ antitrypsin variants. *Protein Eng* 1986;1:29–35.

72. Satoh K, Takahashi H, Crystal RG. Influence of the number of carbohydrate side chains on the *in vivo* behavior of α1-antitrypsin. *Am Rev Respir Dis* 1989;139:A202.

73. Wewers MD, Casolaro MA, Crystal RG. Comparison of alpha 1-antitrypsin levels and anti-neutrophil elastase capacity of blood and lung in an individual with the alpha 1-antitrypsin phenotype null–null before and during alpha 1-antitripsin augmentation therapy. *Am Rev Respir Dis* 1987;135:539–543.

74. Vogelmeier C, Hubbard R, Geiger R, Fritz H, Crystal RG. Secretory leukoprotease inhibitor levels in normal upper and lower respiratory tract epithelial lining fluid of normals. *Am Rev Respir Dis* 1989;139:A200.

75. Lucey EC, Stone PJ, Ciccolella DE, Breuer R, Christenson TG, Thompson RC, Snider GL. Recombinant human secretory leukoprotease inhibitor: In vitro properties, and amelioration of human neutrophil elastase-induced emphysema and secretory cell metaplasia in the hamster. *J Lab Clin Med* 1990; 115:224–232.

76. Vogelmeier C, Buhl R, Hoyt RF, Wilson E, Fells GA, Hubbard RC, Schnebli HP, Thompson RC, Crystal RG. Aerosolization of recombinant secretory leukoprotease inhibitor as a strategy to augment the anti-neutrophil elastase protective screen of the

77. Snider GL, Stone SJ, Lucey EC, Breuer RA, Calove JD, Seshadri T, Catanese A, Maschler R, Schnebli HP. Eglin-c, a polypeptide derived from the medicinal leech, prevents human neutrophil elastase-induced emphysema and bronchial cell secretory cell metaplasia in the hamster. *Am Rev Respir Dis* 1985;132:1155–1161.

78. Lucey EC, Store DJ, Christensen TG, Breuer R, Calore JD, Snider GL. Effect of varying the time interval between intratracheal administration of eglin-c and human neutrophil elastase on prevention of emphysema and secretory cell metaplasia in hamsters. *Am Rev Respir Dis* 1986;134:471–475.

79. Nick HP, Probst A, Schnebli HP. Development of eglin-c as a drug: pharmacokinetics. In: Horl H, Heidland A, eds. *Proteases II*. New York: Plenum Press, 1988;83–88.

80. Powers JC, Harper JW. Inhibitors of serine proteinases. In: Barrett AJ, Salvesen G, eds. *Proteinase inhibitors*. New York: Elsevier, 1986;55–152.

81. McWherter CA, Walkenhorst WA, Campbell EJ, Glover GI. Novel inhibitors of human leukocyte elastase and cathepsin G. Sequence variants of squash seed protease inhibitors with altered protease specificity. *Biochemistry* 1989;28:5708–5714.

82. Stone PJ, Lucey EC, Snider GL. Induction and exacerbation of emphysema in hamsters with human neutrophil elastase reversibly inhibited by a peptide boronic acid. *Am Rev Respir Dis* 1990;141:47–52.

83. Lucey EC, Stone PJ, Powers JC, Snider GL. Amelioration of human neutrophil elastase-induced emphysema in hamsters by pretreatment with an oligopeptide chloromethyl ketone. *Eur Respir J* 1989;2:421–427.

84. Bonney RJ, Ashe B, Mayock A, Dellea P, Hand K, Osinga D, Fletcher D, et al. Pharmacologic profile of the substituted beta-lactam L659,286: a member of a new class of human PMN elastase inhibitors. *J Cell Biochem* 1989;39:47–53.

85. Williams JC, Stein RL, Knee C, Egan J. Pharmacologic characterization of ICI 200,880: a novel potent and selective inhibitor of human neutrophil elastase. *Am Rev Respir Dis* 1990; 141(4):A206.

86. Campbell EJ, Senior RM, McDonald JA, Cox DL. Proteolysis by neutrophils: relative importance of cell–substrate contact and oxidative inactivation of protease inhibitors *in vitro*. *J Clin Invest* 1982;70:845–852.

87. Garver RI, Chytil A, Karlsson S, Fells GA, Brantly ML, Courtney M, Kantoff PW, Nienhuis AW, Anderson WF, Crystal RG. Production of glycosylated, physiologically "normal" human α1-antitrypsin by mouse fibroblasts modified by insertion of a human α1-antitrypsin cDNA using a retroviral vector. *Proc Natl Acad Sci USA* 1987;84(4):1050–1054.

88. Garver RI, Chytil A, Courtney M, Crystal RG. Clonal gene therapy: transplanted mouse fibroblast clones express human α1-antitrypsin gene *in vivo*. *Science* 1987;237:762–764.

89. Curiel D, Stier L, Crystal RG. Gene therapy for α1-antitrypsin deficiency using lymphocytes as vehicles for α1-antitrypsin delivery. *Clin Res* 1989;37(2):578A.

90. Chytil A, Garver R, Crystal R. Human α1-antitrypsin production by human epithelial cells infected with a retroviral vector containing the human α1-antitrypsin gene. *Am Rev Respir Dis* 1988;137(4):371.

91. Hofker MH, Nukiwa T, van Paassen HMB, Nelen M, Frants RR, Kramps JA, Klasen EC, Crystal RG, A pro --→ leu substitution in codon 369 in the α1-antitrypsin deficiency variant PI MHeerlen. *Hum Genet* 1989;81:264–268.

92. Graham A, Kalsheker NA, Newton CR, Bauforth FJ, Powell SJ, Markham AF. Molecular characterization of three alpha 1-antitrypsin deficiency variants: proteinase inhibitor (Pi), Null$_{cardiff}$(Asp^{256} → Val), PiM$_{malton}$(Phe^{51} → deletion) and PiI(Arg^{39} → Cys). *Hum Genet* 1989;84:55–58.

93. Takahashi H, Nukiwa T, Satoh K, Ogushi F, Brantly M, Fells G, Stier L, Courtney M, Crystal RG. Characterization of the gene and protein of the α1-antitrypsin "deficiency" allele M$_{procida}$. *J Biol Chem* 1988;263:15528–15534.

94. Matsunaga E, Shiokawa S, Nakamura H, Maruyama T, Tsuda K, Fukumaki Y. Molecular analysis of the gene of the alpha

1-antitrypsin deficiency variant M$_{nichinan}$. *Am J Hum Genet* 1990;46:602–612.

95. Seyama K, Takabe K, Miyake K, Miyahara Y, Takahashi H, Nukiwa T, Kira S. $_{miiyama}$ (Ser^{53}(TCC) to Phe^{53}(TTC)), a new α1-antitrypsin deficient variant in Japan. *Am Rev Respir Dis* 1990;141(4, part 2 of 2):A355.

96. Curiel D, Brantly M, Curiel E, Hubbard R, Stier L, Sellers S, Crystal RG. α1-Antitrypsin deficiency caused by the α1-antitrypsin Null$_{mattawa}$ gene: an insertion mutation rendering the α1-antitrypsin gene incapable of producing α1-antitrypsin. *J Clin Invest* 1989;83:1144–1152.

97. Frazier GC, Siewertsen M, Harrold TR, Cox DW. Deletion/ frameshift mutation in the α1-antitrypsin null allele, PI*QO$_{bolton}$. *Hum Genet* 1989;83:377–382.

98. Carrell RW, Aulak KS, Owen MC. Molecular pathology of the serpins. *Mol Biol Med* 1989;6:35–42.

99. Nukiwa T, Brantly M, Ogushi F, Fells G, Satoh K, Stier L, Courtney M, Crystal RG. Characterization of the M1(Ala^{213}) type of α1-antitrypsin, a newly recognized, common "normal" α1-antitrypsin haplotype. *Biochemistry* 1987;26:5259–5267.

100. Okayama H, Holmes MD, Brantly ML, Crystal RG. Characterization of the coding sequence of the normal M4 α1-antitrypsin gene. *Biochem Biophys Res Commun* 1989;162:1560–1570.

THE LUNG: Scientific Foundations
edited by R.G. Crystal, J.B. West et al.
Raven Press, Ltd., New York © 1991.

CHAPTER 7.9.2

Abnormal Chloride and Sodium Channel Function in Cystic Fibrosis Airway Epithelia

Michael J. Welsh

Cystic fibrosis (CF), an autosomal recessive disorder, is the most common lethal genetic disease in Caucasians (1). In the last few years we have seen considerable progress toward an understanding of the metabolic abnormalities in CF, primarily because of advances in two areas: Studies of several epithelia involved in CF have demonstrated defective electrolyte transport, and the CF gene has been discovered.

Although CF is a disease that affects multiple organ systems, respiratory disease is the major cause of morbidity and mortality: 95% of CF patients die of respiratory failure. The clinical manifestations of CF lung disease were important in leading investigators to study electrolyte transport by CF airway epithelia. The basic research observations on epithelial function have, in turn, provided a plausible explanation for the pathogenesis and pathophysiology of the disease. This chapter will focus on electrolyte transport by the airway epithelium and on its defective regulation in CF. The major focus will be on recent studies of Cl^- and Na^+ channels. The reader may turn to other sources for an in-depth discussion of the clinical manifestations of CF (1) and for a general discussion of electrolyte transport by airway epithelia (2).

TRANSEPITHELIAL ELECTROLYTE TRANSPORT

Transport by Normal Airway Epithelia

Electrolyte transport by the airway epithelium controls, in part, the quantity and composition of respiratory tract fluid. Thus, it helps to effect normal mucociliary clearance, the normal pulmonary defense mechanism that removes inhaled particulate material from the airways. In CF, the mucociliary clearance process is defective, most likely as a result of the abnormal electrolyte transport.

The airway epithelium can either actively transport Cl^- from the submucosal to the mucosal surface, thereby driving fluid secretion, or it can absorb Na^+, driving fluid in the opposite direction. In both cases, the counterion is thought to move passively through the paracellular pathway. The relative magnitude of the two active transport processes is determined by the species, the airway region, and the neurohumoral environment.

Figure 1 shows a cellular model that describes our current understanding of how airway epithelial cells secrete Cl^- and absorb Na^+ (2). The main features of the model are as follows: (a) Cl^- ions enter the cell across the basolateral membrane via an electrically neutral cotransport process, coupled to Na^+ and possibly to K^+. The entry of Na^+ ions provides the driving force for accumulation of Cl^- against its electrochemical gradient. (b) Cl^- ions exit passively through an apical membrane Cl^- conductance, moving down a favorable electrochemical gradient. The regulation of the apical membrane Cl^- permeability controls, in part, the rate of transepithelial secretion. (c) Na^+, which enters the cell at the basolateral membrane coupled to Cl^-, exits across the basolateral membrane via the Na^+,K^+-adenosine-triphosphatase (ATPase). This enzyme provides the energy for transepithelial Cl^- secretion by maintaining a low intracellular Na^+ concentration. The Na^+,K^+-ATPase also accumulates K^+ inside the cell. (d) K^+ exits passively through a basolateral membrane K^+ channel. The basolateral K^+ conductance and the K^+ gradient hyperpolarize

M. J. Welsh: Howard Hughes Medical Institute and Departments of Internal Medicine and of Physiology and Biophysics, University of Iowa College of Medicine, Iowa City, Iowa 52242.

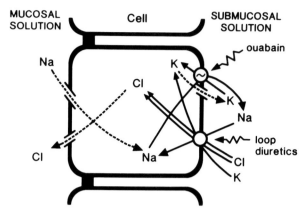

FIG. 1. Cellular model of the mechanism of transepithelial Cl⁻ and Na⁺ transport by the airway epithelium. See text for details.

the cell, providing the electrical driving force for Cl⁻ exit and also providing part of the driving force for Na⁺ entry at the apical membrane. (e) Na⁺ enters the cell passively through an apical membrane Na⁺ channel, moving down a favorable electrochemical gradient.

The rate of transepithelial Cl⁻ secretion is regulated by several neurotransmitters, autacoids, and hormones (2). Many of the agents appear to stimulate Cl⁻ secretion by increasing cellular levels of cAMP, although an increase in the cellular concentration of Ca^{2+} ($[Ca^{2+}]_c$) also stimulates secretion. Prostaglandins may be particularly important in regulating secretion, because they are produced by the epithelial cells and secreted into the submucosal space where they interact with basolateral prostaglandin receptors to stimulate an accumulation of intracellular cAMP. Several agents that stimulate secretion, particularly inflammatory neuropeptides such as bradykinin, appear to stimulate secretion via a stimulation of prostaglandin synthesis.

Less is known about how the rate of Na⁺ absorption is controlled. Many agents that stimulate Cl⁻ secretion decrease Na⁺ absorption. As in a variety of other Na⁺-absorbing epithelia, aldostrone may also regulate Na⁺ absorption, although the effects appear to be variable.

Transport by CF Airway Epithelia

The clinical observation that CF airway secretions appear thick and dehydrated led Knowles et al. (3) to study electrolyte transport by CF respiratory epithelia. They found that *in vivo* the voltage across upper and lower airway epithelia was higher in CF patients than in normal subjects or in disease controls. This observation suggested a defect in electrolyte transport. The results of subsequent *in vivo* Cl⁻ substitution studies,

along with the observation that transepithelial Cl⁻ fluxes are decreased in excised airway epithelia as well as in CF airway epithelia cultured on permeable supports, indicated that CF airway epithelium is relatively impermeable to Cl⁻ (4–8). Intracellular microelectrode measurements, combined with ion substitution studies, localized the CF Cl⁻ impermeability to the cellular pathway—specifically, to the apical membrane (7,9).

CF airway epithelia also showed an abnormality in Na⁺ absorption. In excised nasal epithelia and airway epithelial cells grown on permeable supports, the rate of transepithelial Na⁺ absorption was two- to threefold greater than in non-CF epithelia (10). In addition, β-adrenergic agonists and forskolin, both of which increase cellular concentrations of cAMP, stimulated Na⁺ absorption in CF epithelia. As indicated above, the opposite was found in normal epithelia: cAMP either decreased the rate of Na⁺ absorption or did not change it.

APICAL MEMBRANE CHLORIDE CHANNELS IN AIRWAY EPITHELIA

Types of Chloride Channels

To understand the reason for the decreased apical membrane Cl⁻ permeability in CF, several investigators applied the patch-clamp technique to primary cultures of airway epithelial cells. The patch-clamp technique employs a glass microelectrode to form a high-resistance seal between the glass pipette and the cell membrane (11). It thereby allows one to record the opening and closing of single ion channels and measure the current flowing through them.

Airway epithelia contain several Cl⁻ channels; however, the most extensively studied Cl⁻ channel shows a characteristic outwardly-rectifying current–voltage relationship (12–17). The current–voltage relationship rectifies in excised, inside-out patches even in the presence of symmetrical Cl⁻ concentrations (Fig. 2). Because of the outward rectification, there is no unique value of single-channel conductance; however, most reports suggest a slope conductance of 25–40 pS (estimated at 0 mV in symmetrical Cl⁻ solutions). The channel is 7–12 times more selective for Cl⁻ than for Na⁺.

The outwardly-rectifying Cl⁻ channel has several properties which suggest that it is responsible, at least in part, for the apical membrane Cl⁻ permeability:

1. *Location.* The channel was found in patches of membrane obtained from confluent sheets of cells where only the apical membrane was accessible to the recording pipette (12–14). In contrast, basolateral K⁺

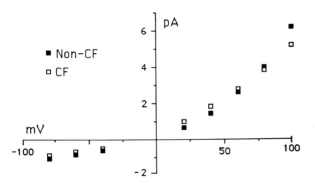

FIG. 2. Single-channel current–voltage relationship of outwardly-rectifying Cl⁻ channels from a normal cell (■) and a CF cell (□). (From ref. 13.)

channels were not observed in the apical membrane of confluent sheets of cells (18).

2. *Anion selectivity.* The anion selectivity sequence of the channel (SCN⁻ > I⁻ > Br⁻ = Cl⁻ > SO₄²⁻ = gluconate) (19,20) is the same as the anion permeability sequence of the apical membrane.

3. *Effect of blockers.* Several agents block both the apical Cl⁻ conductance and the outwardly rectifying Cl⁻ channel, including: anthracene-9-carboxylic acid, diphenalamine-2-carboxylate, and NPPB (12,15, 20,21).

4. *Regulation.* Several hormones and neurotransmitters (2) increase the apical Cl⁻ conductance and activate outwardly-rectifying Cl⁻ channels (discussion below).

5. *Defective regulation in CF.* As discussed below, the outwardly-rectifying Cl⁻ channel is defectively regulated in CF airway epithelia, in which the apical membrane is Cl⁻-impermeable.

Lower-conductance Cl⁻ channels (approximately 10 pS and 20 pS with linear current–voltage relationships) have also been observed in normal and CF airway epithelial cells (14,22); however, less is known about their properties and regulation. Outwardly-rectifying Cl⁻ channels, as well as smaller Cl⁻ channels with linear current–voltage relationships, have also been observed in other epithelial cells involved in CF.

Chloride Channel Activation by Depolarization

Early studies of the outwardly-rectifying Cl⁻ channel showed that when quiescent patches of membrane were excised from normal and CF cells, the channels became activated[1] (12–14). Subsequent studies

showed that activation was, at least in part, due to membrane depolarization (23,24): Large, sustained depolarizing voltages (+80 to +140 mV) activated Cl⁻ channels in excised inside-out patches (23,24). Activation depended upon both the absolute membrane voltage and the duration of depolarization: As both increased, the chance of activation increased (25). Activation by depolarization was a relatively slow process, requiring seconds or minutes; thus, it is different from the effects of voltage observed in other "voltage-dependent" ion channels. Depolarization-dependent activation was also different from the effect of voltage on other channels, because the channel remained in the activated state even when the membrane voltage was reduced to less depolarizing values. However, activation by depolarization proved to be reversible by membrane hyperpolarization (25).

Voltage-induced changes in activation state do not represent physiologic processes, because depolarization does not activate outwardly-rectifying Cl⁻ channels in cell-attached patches. Measurements of apical membrane voltage also suggest that depolarization is unlikely to activate apical membrane Cl⁻ channels (2). Secretagogues such as β-adrenergic agonists produce only relatively small changes in apical membrane voltage. More importantly, the change in voltage is caused by the activation of Cl⁻ channels, not the converse. Alteration of apical voltage by the passage of transepithelial currents also failed to affect apical conductance in native airway epithelia.[2] Although depolarization-dependent activation of Cl⁻ channels in excised patches was unexpected, and the mechanisms involved are unknown, the phenomenon has proven to be of value in studies designed to study channel regulation: Membrane depolarization provides an independent way of activating outwardly-rectifying Cl⁻ channels following other experimental maneuvers.

PHOSPHORYLATION-DEPENDENT REGULATION OF CHLORIDE CHANNELS

Activation of Chloride Channels by cAMP-Dependent Protein Kinase

The conductive properties of outwardly-rectifying Cl⁻ channels in excised cell-free patches of membrane from normal and CF airway epithelial cells were identical (Fig. 2) (13–16). However, the regulation of Cl⁻ channels in normal and CF cells was different. Iso-

---

[1] The outwardly-rectifying Cl⁻ channel functions in at least two modes. I refer to an "inactivated" channel as one that is unstimulated or quescient and always in the closed state; that is, the probability of being in the open state, P_o, is 0. An "activated" channel is one that has been stimulated and that spontaneously flickers back and forth between the open and closed states ($P_o > 0$).

[2] Although there have been varying reports about the influence of voltage on open-state probability (P_o) of the channel studied in excised patches, voltage probably plays little role in physiologic regulation.

A. Control

B. PKA and ATP

C. PKA, ATP, PKC, and DiC8

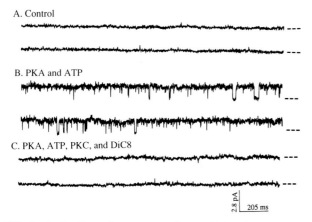

2.8 pA | 205 ms

FIG. 3. Activation of an outwardly-rectifying Cl⁻ channel by cAMP-dependent protein kinase A (PKA) followed by inactivation with protein kinase C (PKC). Dashed line indicates zero current level. **A:** Baseline conditions. **B:** PKA plus ATP (1 mM). **C:** Addition of PKC plus dioctanoylglycerol (DiC8, 1 µg/M). Bath $[Ca^{2+}]_c$ was 1 µM. (From ref. 29.)

proterenol and other agents that increase intracellular levels of cAMP activated Cl⁻ channels in cell-attached patches of membrane from normal cells (12–14). In contrast, such secretagogues failed to activate Cl⁻ channels in CF cells. Failure to activate Cl⁻ channels was not due to the absence of outwardly-rectifying Cl⁻ channels: They were present in the membrane, as demonstrated by depolarization-dependent activation once the patches of membrane were excised. Such studies indicated that outwardly-rectifying Cl⁻ channels were activated by an intracellular second messenger, most likely cAMP. Other studies showed that intracellular levels of cAMP are regulated in a similar manner in normal and CF cells (13,22,26) and that cAMP-dependent protein kinase A (PKA) was normal in CF cells (27,28). These observations indicated that the defect in CF Cl⁻ channel regulation lay at a site distal to cAMP accumulation.

As a result of those studies, attention turned to an examination of the effect of PKA on outwardly-rectifying Cl⁻ channels studied in cell-free membrane patches. In many cells, cAMP exerts its effect by activating PKA, which then produces the biologic effect by protein phosphorylation. Direct evidence that cAMP regulates the Cl⁻ channel came from studies in which the purified catalytic subunit of PKA plus ATP was applied to the internal (cytosolic) surface of excised patches (16,23,24,29) (see Fig. 3 for an example). Figure 3A shows the channel in an inactivated state (no openings were observed). When PKA and ATP were added, the channel became activated (Fig. 3B and 3C). Activation required both ATP and PKA; neither alone was sufficient. Moreover, neither heat-inactivated catalytic subunit nor PKA added in the presence

of the peptide protein kinase inhibitor of PKA caused activation. Thus, the addition of PKA under phosphorylating conditions to excised Cl⁻ channels mimicked the effect of secretagogues added to cell-attached Cl⁻ channels. These results indicate that phosphorylation of the channel itself or of an associated regulatory protein activates the channel.³

When similar studies were performed in CF cells, the catalytic subunit of PKA failed to activate Cl⁻ channels, even though channels were present, as demonstrated by subsequent activation with strong membrane depolarization (16,23,24). The failure of PKA to activate CF Cl⁻ channels in excised, cell-free patches indicated that the CF defect lay distal to PKA, either in the channel itself or in an associated regulatory protein. These results suggest a model for Cl⁻-channel regulation by phosphorylation (Fig. 4).

Activation of Chloride Channels by Protein Kinase C

Protein kinase C (PKC) plays an important role in regulating secretion and ion channels in several cell types. Evidence suggesting that PKC might also be important in regulating Cl⁻ channels in airway epithelial cells came from two types of study: (i) Several Cl⁻ secretagogues, including bradykinin and isoproterenol, increased the cellular mass of diacylglycerol in airway epithelial cells (30). Diacylglycerol is a physiologic activator of PKC. (ii) Tumor-promoting phorbol esters, [such as phorbol 12-myristate 13-acetate (PMA)], which are membrane-permeant activators of PKC, altered Cl⁻ secretion (27,31,32). However, the response to phorbol esters was complex. On the one hand, phorbol esters caused a transient stimulation of Cl⁻ secretion. On the other hand, phorbol esters inhibited cAMP-induced Cl⁻ secretion. This dual effect resulted (at least in part) from an effect on the Cl⁻ channel, because ¹²⁵I⁻ efflux (an assay of Cl⁻ channel function in intact cells which is not dependent on the activity of other transport processes) showed a similar response to PMA (29).

Studies using purified PKC in excised cell-free patches of membrane provided more direct evidence that the Cl⁻ channel can be regulated by PKC (16,29). Addition of PKC to the cytosolic (internal) surface activated Cl⁻ channels. Activation required PKC, a diacylglycerol, and ATP; addition of only two of the three was insufficient. Activation was usually seen at

---

³ In discussing regulation of the Cl⁻ channel, I often refer to the channel as a single entity, but based on observations of other channels, it may consist of a channel complex with multiple subunits and associated proteins.

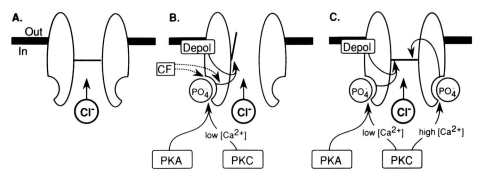

FIG. 4. Model of Cl⁻-channel regulation by phosphorylation. Inner and outer surface of the membrane are indicated in **A**. Channel is defined as "inactivated" when the "gate" is closed (**A** and **C**) and "activated" when it is opened (**B**) (see footnotes 1 and 3 in the text). The gate may involve different molecular steps. "Depol" refers to strong, sustained membrane depolarization. At high [Ca²⁺], PKC may also phosphorylate the low Ca²⁺ site. (Adapted from ref. 29.)

a low internal (bath) [Ca²⁺] (< 10 nM), although activation could sometimes be seen at approximately 100–150 nM. These observations indicate that PKC phosphorylates and activates the channel (or an associated protein) at a low internal [Ca²⁺] (Fig. 4).

In contrast to the results obtained in normal cells, Cl⁻ channels in excised patches of membrane from CF cells were not activated by PKC at a low internal [Ca²⁺]. The failure of both PKA and PKC to activate CF Cl⁻ channels suggests that both enzymes might phosphorylate in a similar region or domain of the channel or in an associated membrane protein. The data also suggested that the CF defect might lie either in defective phosphorylation or in the mechanism that links phosphorylation to the change in channel conformation that causes activation.

Inactivation of Chloride Channels by Protein Kinase C

When PKC was added to excised patches in the presence of a high internal [Ca²⁺], different results were obtained: No channels were activated, and subsequent depolarization failed to activate Cl⁻ channels (29). Addition of PKC, a diacylglycerol or phorbol ester, and ATP at a high [Ca²⁺] (≥ 1 μM) inactivated Cl⁻ channels that had first been activated by PKA (see Fig. 3), by PKC at a low internal [Ca²⁺], or by depolarization (Fig. 5).

Protein phosphorylation is controlled by both kinases and phosphatases. The observation that inactivation was reversible in most cases (Fig. 5) suggested that a membrane-associated phosphatase was present

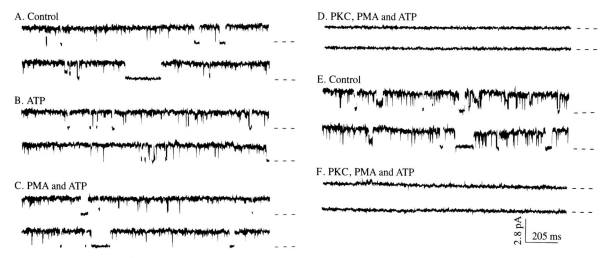

FIG. 5. PKC-dependent inactivation of a depolarization-activated Cl⁻ channel at 1 μM Ca²⁺. Holding voltage was −40 mV, and tracings were obtained at +40 mV. Recordings were made under the following conditions: (**A**) control, no additions; (**B**) ATP 1 mM; (**C**) PMA (100 nM) and ATP; (**D**) PKC, PMA, and ATP; (**E**) control conditions after removal of PKC, PMA, and ATP from the internal solution; (**F**) readdition of PKC, PMA, and ATP. (From ref. 29 with permission.)

in the cell-free membrane patch (29). At least one of the phosphatases involved is likely to be calcineurin, because Ca^{2+} was usually required to reverse the effects of PKC; in addition, the calmodulin antagonist, W7, prevented reactivation (33).

At a high internal $[Ca^{2+}]$, PKC inactivated both normal and CF Cl^- channels. These observations suggest that the channel has two different phosphorylation sites: one activating and one inactivating, one with defective function in CF and one with normal function in CF (Fig. 4).

There are several possible ways to explain the two opposite effects of PKC on the Cl^- channel (29): Different responses may be due to an effect of Ca^{2+} on the channel, on PKC, or on the interaction between the two. First, Ca^{2+} might change channel conformation, making different sites accessible for PKC-dependent phosphorylation. Second, the Ca^{2+} dependence of PKC might be influenced by the nature of the substrate, so that one phosphorylation site might not require Ca^{2+} for an effect, whereas the other would. Third, the interaction of PKC with the membrane might be Ca^{2+}-dependent; for example, in the absence of Ca^{2+}, PKC might phosphorylate an extrinsic site on the channel, and in the presence of Ca^{2+}, PKC might phosphorylate a site on the channel associated with the membrane. Alternatively, different effects of PKC could be caused by isozymes that phosphorylate different sites: (a) a Ca^{2+}-independent form that activates the channel and (b) a Ca^{2+}-dependent form that inactivates the channel. This hypothesis is possible because the PKC preparations that were used probably contain more than one isozyme (16,29). In any case, each of these alternatives requires that PKC show substrate specificity for two different phosphorylation sites on the channel or associated protein.

ACTIVATION OF CHLORIDE CHANNELS BY AN INCREASE IN CELL CALCIUM

In many cells, including epithelial cells, an increase in the cytosolic free Ca^{2+} concentration ($[Ca^{2+}]_c$) stimulates secretion. A suggestion that an increase in $[Ca^{2+}]_c$ might be involved in activation of Cl^- channels and stimulation of Cl^- secretion in airway epithelia was supported by the observation that secretagogues such as bradykinin and isoproterenol increase $[Ca^{2+}]_c$ in airway epithelia (27,36). Such agonist-induced changes in $[Ca^{2+}]_c$ appear to be normal in CF epithelial cells (27).

There is less information about how an increase in $[Ca^{2+}]_c$ regulates Cl^- channels. Evidence that $[Ca^{2+}]_c$ regulates apical Cl^- channels comes from the observation that Ca^{2+} ionophores, A23187 and ionomycin, activate apical membrane Cl^- channels in intact cells

as measured in several assay systems: They stimulate transepithelial Cl^- secretion and increase apical Cl^- conductance (26,35), they activate Cl^- channels studied with the cell-attached patch-clamp technique (14), and they stimulate $^{125}I^-$ efflux (34). However, changes in $[Ca^{2+}]_c$ were temporally dissociated from changes in channel activation: A transient increase in $[Ca^{2+}]_c$ produced a prolonged activation of Cl^- channels, as assayed with $^{125}I^-$ efflux (34,36). This observation suggested that Ca^{2+}-dependent activation might be indirect. This suggestion was supported by the observation that in excised, cell-free patches, changes in the $[Ca^{2+}]$ bathing the cytosolic surface of the patch did not change open-state probability nor did they influence activation of outwardly-rectifying Cl^- channels immediately following excision (12,15, 17,34). At present the mechanism of activation is unknown, but activation by an increase in $[Ca^{2+}]_c$ does not appear to involve a kinase-dependent phosphorylation: Ca^{2+} ionophores activated Cl^- channels even in cells in which ATP levels had been depleted and in the presence of nonspecific kinase inhibitors (37).

Many questions remain about how $[Ca^{2+}]_c$ controls Cl^- channels in airway epithelia. For example, are Cl^- channels regulated by $[Ca^{2+}]_c$ the same as those regulated by phosphorylation? What are the intermediates between an increase in $[Ca^{2+}]_c$ and activation of Cl^- channels? Such questions are important because Ca^{2+}-dependent regulation of Cl^- channels and secretion remains intact in CF (26,35). The fact that Ca^{2+}-dependent Cl^- channel activation is normal in CF suggests a strategy for bypassing the cAMP-dependent defects in CF.

REGULATION OF CHLORIDE CHANNELS BY OTHER FACTORS

Several other factors have been observed to regulate outwardly-rectifying Cl^- channels; they include the following.

Changes in Osmolarity

Changes in cell volume may also regulate the outwardly-rectifying Cl^- channel. When extracellular osmolarity was decreased, outwardly-rectifying Cl^- channel current increased in whole-cell patch-clamp studies (21). The current appeared to flow through apical Cl^- channels, because a reduction of bath osmolarity also stimulated transepithelial Cl^- secretion (activation of basolateral Cl^- channels would not cause secretion). Although a reduction in bath osmolarity probably causes cell swelling, the mechanism of signal transduction and the second messengers involved are presently unknown. It would be interesting to know whether osmotic changes play a physiologic role in controlling Cl$^-$ secretion and Cl$^-$ channels.

Temperature

When patches of membrane are excised from the cell, Cl$^-$ channels sometimes activate spontaneously; but in most cases, depolarization is required for activation. However, when studies were done at 37°C, Cl$^-$ channels activated on excision much more frequently, without requiring depolarization (15). Evidence that bath temperature had an effect came in studies of excised cell-free patches; an increase in the temperature of the bath solution from 23°C to 37°C activated outwardly-rectifying Cl$^-$ channels (25). When the bath temperature was reduced to 23°C the channel remained in the activated state, but it could then be inactivated by membrane hyperpolarization. A subsequent increase in bath temperature to 37°C would then once again activate channels. Activation by temperature is not a physiologic process, because it only occurs in excised patches. The ability of an increased temperature to activate Cl$^-$ channels multiple times in some patches, combined with the interaction between temperature and voltage, suggests that the effect of temperature is not mediated by an enzymatic reaction.

Proteolysis

In excised, inside-out patches, addition of trypsin (0.05%) to the internal surface activated outwardly-rectifying Cl$^-$ channels (25). Once activated, the Cl$^-$ channels had the same conductive and ion selectivity properties as did channels activated by other methods. This result suggests that proteolysis in a regulatory domain of the channel, or in an associated protein, relieves inhibition. Channels activated by trypsin could not be inactivated by phosphorylation with PKC at a high internal [Ca^{2+}] or by hyperpolarization, suggesting that trypsin produced an irreversible change in the channel.

Arachidonic Acid

Several inflammatory peptides and neurotransmitters release arachidonic acid, which increases the production of prostaglandins. Several prostaglandins, in turn, increase cellular levels of cAMP (2), thereby stimulating Cl$^-$ secretion. However, studies using cell-free membrane patches suggest that arachidonic acid itself may also regulate Cl$^-$ channels (38,39). Arachidonic acid inactivated Cl$^-$ channels at a free concentration of 5 μM. Inhibition only occurred when arachidonic

acid was added to the internal (cytosolic) side of the membrane. Inhibition was reversed when arachidonic acid was washed away. The data suggest that arachidonic acid, rather than a cyclo-oxygenase or lipoxygenase metabolite, inhibited the channel: (a) Inhibitors of these enzymes, indomethacin and nordihydroguarietic acid, did not prevent the response; (b) fatty acids, which are not substrates, also inhibited the channel; and (c) metabolites of arachidonic acid were not as effective as arachidonic acid. Arachidonic acid also inhibited CF Cl$^-$ channels. These results suggest that fatty acids directly inhibit outwardly-rectifying Cl$^-$ channels in excised patches and that arachidonic acid might be a negative modulator of Cl$^-$ channels during some receptor-mediated stimulation of Cl$^-$ secretion. However, this hypothesis is difficult to prove because arachidonic acid metabolites also regulate the Cl$^-$ channel in the intact cell.

Mechanisms of Chloride Channel Activation and Inactivation

Large membrane depolarization, an increase in bath temperature, an increase in [Ca^{2+}]$_c$, a reduction in bath osmolarity, and internal trypsin all activate Cl$^-$ channels in both normal and CF cells (Fig. 6). Likewise, phosphorylation by PKC at a high internal [Ca^{2+}] and internal arachidonic acid inactivate Cl$^-$ channels in both normal and CF cells. The only difference between Cl$^-$ channels from normal and CF cells is in activation by phosphorylation: Phosphorylation by PKA or by PKC at a low internal [Ca^{2+}] fails to activate CF channels.

The multiple modes of regulation raise several questions. Are different types of Cl$^-$ channels activated by the various maneuvers shown in Fig. 6? Do several regulatory mechanisms activate a single type of channel? Is only a single type of Cl$^-$ channel defectively regulated in CF? These questions are important but

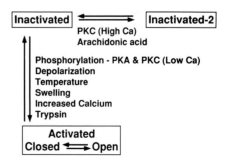

FIG. 6. Mechanisms of channel activation and inactivation. The channel can be activated by the indicated maneuvers, or it can be taken to a second inactivated state by PKC at a high internal [Ca^{2+}] or arachidonic acid. See text for details.

are not completely answered. As discussed above, there is evidence for more than one type of Cl⁻ channel in airway epithelia. However, most studies of regulation have focused on outwardly-rectifying Cl⁻ channels. Even in that case, it is not yet certain whether all outwardly-rectifying Cl⁻ channels are the same in terms of regulation. Another related question concerns the presence, regulation, and types of Cl⁻ channels that exist on intracellular organelles. Unfortunately, to date, we have no sequence information on the Cl⁻ channels involved in epithelial transport. Such information, combined with an understanding of Cl⁻ channel function, may give us further insights into normal and defective Cl⁻ transport.

EPITHELIAL SODIUM CHANNELS

As discussed above, CF airway epithelia also have an increased rate of transepithelial Na⁺ absorption (10). The increased Na⁺ absorption contributes to the increased transepithelial voltage and may have an important effect on the quantity and composition of the respiratory tract fluid (3,6,10). In most Na⁺-absorbing epithelia, Na⁺ entry into the cell occurs through an amiloride-inhibitable apical membrane Na⁺ channel. The Na⁺ channel controls, in part, the rate of transepithelial Na⁺ absorption. Thus, in CF airway epithelia, defective regulation of apical membrane Na⁺ channels is likely to be responsible for the increased rate of Na⁺ absorption. This suggestion is supported by the observation that amiloride inhibits Na⁺ absorption in both normal and CF airway epithelia (4,6,10).

There are at least three possible alterations in Na⁺-channel function that could explain an increased rate of absorption: The number of functional Na⁺ channels could be increased, open-state probability in individual Na⁺ channels could be increased, or there could be some combination of the above. At present it is difficult to choose between these possibilities. One preliminary study suggested that the number of cation channels found in CF airway epithelial cells was increased (22). Another study suggested that the number of Na⁺ channels was the same in CF epithelia, but the open-state probability was increased (40). It is apparent that we have much to learn about the regulation of Na⁺ channels and the relationship between the rate of Na⁺ absorption and the rate of Cl⁻ secretion in airway epithelia. Insight into these problems will be important in understanding the pathogenesis and pathophysiology of CF airway disease.

RELATION OF THE CF GENE PRODUCT TO THE ION CHANNEL ABNORMALITIES

Although the CF gene has recently been identified (41–43), the relationship between the CF gene product [named the "cystic fibrosis transmembrane conductance regulator" (CFTR)] and the abnormal electrolyte transport is unknown. At least three areas of questions about the relationship need to be addressed.

The first area relates to the function and location of the normal CFTR protein. The predicted amino acid sequence of CFTR suggests a protein structure which contains a membrane-spanning domain (containing six membrane-spanning sequences), followed by a possible nucleotide-binding domain (which resembles nucleotide-binding regions in several other prokaryotic and eukaryotic proteins), a "regulatory domain" (which contains multiple putative phosphorylation sites for both PKA and PKC), a second membrane-spanning domain, and then a second nucleotide-binding domain (42). At a superficial level, two structural predictions are consistent with what we know about abnormal electrolyte transport in CF. First, CFTR is likely to be a membrane protein, and the CF biologic defect is observed in isolated, cell-free membrane preparations. Second, the CFTR contains multiple consensus phosphorylation sequences for PKA and PKC, and the Cl⁻ channel involved by CF is regulated by phosphorylation with these two enzymes. There has been substantial speculation about whether the gene product is an ion channel or a protein that might regulate ion channels. In either case, it is not clear why this protein would have domains that resemble nucleotide-binding domains. Much work will be required to understand the function of CFTR.

The second area relates to the abnormal function of the mutant form of CFTR. The most common mutation in CFTR is a deletion of phenylalanine in position 508 (44). Given our current lack of knowledge about the function of this protein, it is impossible to understand how such a defect in a putative nucleotide-binding domain might cause abnormal Na⁺ absorption and defective phosphorylation-dependent regulation of Cl⁻ channels. Perhaps this suggests that phosphorylation is intact in CF cells but that some conformational change secondary to phosphorylation is defective.

The third area relates to the issue of how a defect in CFTR, and the resulting electrolyte transport abnormalities cause the phenotypic characteristics so commonly observed in CF. At present, the pathophysiologic manifestations of CF are only observed at the tissue or organ level; no adverse effects of the CF gene have been described at the cellular level. Insight into these problems is required if we are to understand the cause of the morbidity and mortality and if we are to alter the prognosis of this fatal disease.

ACKNOWLEDGMENTS

Work from the author's lab was supported, in part, by grants from the National Heart, Lung and Blood Institute (HL-42385 and HL-29851) and the National Cystic Fibrosis Foundation. I thank Theresa Mayhew for excellent assistance.

REFERENCES

1. Boat TF, Welsh M, Beaudet AL. Cystic fibrosis. In: Scriver CR, Beaudet AL, Sly WS, Valle D, eds. *The metabolic basis of inherited disease*, 6th ed. New York: McGraw–Hill, 1989;2649–2680.
2. Welsh MJ. Electrolyte transport by airway epithelia. *Physiol Rev* 1987;67:1143–1184.
3. Knowles M, Gatzy J, Boucher R. Increased bioelectric potential difference across respiratory epithelia in cystic fibrosis. *N Engl J Med* 1981;305:1489–1495.
4. Knowles M, Gatzy J, Boucher R. Relative ion permeability of normal and cystic fibrosis nasal epithelium. *J Clin Invest* 1983;71:1410–1417.
5. Knowles MR, Stutts MJ, Spock A. Abnormal ion permeation through cystic fibrosis respiratory epithelium. *Science* 1983; 221:1067–1070.
6. Yankaskas JR, Cotton C, Knowles M, Gatzy JT, Boucher RC. Culture of human nasal epithelia cells on collagen matrix supports: a comparison of bioelectric properties of normal and cystic fibrosis epithelia. *Am Rev Respir Dis* 1985;132:1281–1287.
7. Widdicombe JH, Welsh MJ, Finkbeiner WE. Cystic fibrosis decreases the apical membrane chloride permeability of monolayers cultured from cells of tracheal epithelium. *Proc Natl Acad Sci USA* 1985;82:6167–6171.
8. Yankaskas JR, Gatzy J, Knowles MR, Boucher RC. Persistence of abnormal chloride ion permeability in cystic fibrosis nasal epithelial cells in heterologous culture. *Lancet* 1985;8435:954–956.
9. Cotton CU, Stutts MJ, Knowles MR, Gatzy J, Boucher RC. Abnormal apical cell membrane in cystic fibrosis respiratory epithelium. An *in vitro* electrophysiologic analysis. *J Clin Invest* 1987;79:30–85.
10. Boucher RC, Stutts MJ, Knowles MR, Cantley L, Gatzy JT. Na⁺ transport in cystic fibrosis respiratory epithelia. Abnormal basal rate and response to adenylate cyclase activation. *J Clin Invest* 1986;78:1245–1252.
11. Hamill OP, Marty A, Neher E, Sakmann B, Sigworth FJ. Improved patch-clamp techniques for high-resolution current recording from cells and cell-free membrane patches. *Pflügers Arch* 1981;391:85–100.
12. Welsh MJ. An apical membrane chloride channel in human tracheal epithelium. *Science* 1986;232:1648–1650.
13. Welsh MJ, Liedtke CM. Chloride and potassium channels in cystic fibrosis airway epithelium. *Nature* 1986;322:467–470.
14. Frizzell RA, Rechkemmer G, Shoemaker RL. Altered regulation of airway epithelial cell chloride channels in cystic fibrosis. *Science* 1986;233:558–560.
15. Kunzelmann K, Pavenstadt H, Greger R. Properties and regulation of chloride channels in cystic fibrosis and normal airway cells. *Pflügers Arch* 1989;415:172–182.
16. Hwang, T-C, Lu L, Zeitlin PL, et al. Cl⁻ channels in CF: lack of activation by protein kinase C and cAMP-dependent protein kinase. *Science* 1989;244:1351–1353.
17. Hanrahan JW, Tabcharani JA. Possible role of outwardly rectifying anion channels in epithelial transport. In: Durham JH, Hardy MA, eds. *Bicarbonate, chloride, and proton transport systems*, vol 574. New York: New York Academy of Sciences, 1989;30:30–43.
18. Welsh MJ, McCann JD. Intracellular calcium regulates basolateral potassium channels in a chloride-secreting epithelium. *Proc Natl Acad Sci USA* 1985;82:8823–8826.
19. Frizzell RA. Cystic fibrosis: a disease of ion channels? *Trends Neurosci* 1987;10(5):190–193.
20. Li M, McCann JD, Welsh MJ. Apical membrane Cl⁻ channels in airway epithelia: anion selectivity and effect of an inhibitor. *Am J Physiol (Cell Physiol)* 1989;259(28):C295–C301.

21. McCann JD, Li M, Welsh MJ. Identification and regulation of whole-cell chloride currents in airway epithelium. *J Gen Physiol* 1989;94(6):1015–1036.
22. Duszyk M, French AS, Man SFP. Cystic fibrosis affects chloride and sodium channels in human airway epithelia. *Can J Physiol Pharmacol* 1989;67:1362–1365.
23. Li M, McCann JD, Liedtke CM, et al. cAMP-dependent protein kinase opens chloride channels in normal but not cystic fibrosis airway epithelium. *Nature* 1988;331:358–360.
24. Schoumacher RA, Shoemaker RL, Halm DR, et al. Phosphorylation fails to activate chloride channels from cystic fibrosis airway cells. *Nature* 1987;330:752–754.
25. Welsh MJ, Li M, McCann JD. Activation of normal and cystic fibrosis Cl⁻ channels by voltage, temperature, and trypsin. *J Clin Invest* 1989;84:2002–2007.
26. Widdicombe JH. Cystic fibrosis and β-adrenergic response of airway epithelial cell cultures. *Am J Physiol (Regul Integrative Comp Physiol)* 1986;251:R818–R822.
27. Boucher RC, Cheng EHC, Paradiso AM, et al. Chloride secretory response of cystic fibrosis human airway epithelia. *J Clin Invest* 1989;84:1424–1431.
28. Barthelson R, Widdicombe J. Cyclic adenosine monophosphate-dependent kinase in cystic fibrosis tracheal epithelium. *J Clin Invest* 1987;80:1799–1802.
29. Li M, McCann JD, Anderson MP, Clancy JP, et al. Regulation of chloride channels by protein kinase C in normal and cystic fibrosis airway epithelia. *Science* 1989;244:1353–1356.
30. Anderson MP, Welsh MJ. Isoproterenol, cyclic AMP and bradykinin stimulate diacylglycerol production in airway epithelium. *Am J Physiol (Lung Cell Mol Physiol)* 1990;258:L294–L300.
31. Welsh MJ. Effect of phorbol ester and calcium ionophore on chloride secretion in cultured canine tracheal epithelium. *Am J Physiol (Cell Physiol)* 1987;253:C828–C834.
32. Barthelson RA, Jacoby DB, Widdicombe JH. Regulation of chloride secretion in dog tracheal epithelium by protein kinase C. *Am J Physiol (Cell Physiol)* 1987;253:C802–C808.
33. Anderson MP, Welsh MJ. An endogenous calcium-dependent phosphatase regulates airway epithelial chloride channels. *Clin Res* 1989;37(4):917A.
34. Clancy JP, McCann JD, Li M, Welsh MJ. Calcium-dependent regulation of airway epithelial chloride channels. *Am J Physiol (Lung Cell Mol Physiol)* 1990;258:L25–L32.
35. Willumsen NJ, Boucher RC. Activation of an apical Cl⁻ conductance by Ca²⁺ ionophores in cystic fibrosis airway epithelia. *Am J Physiol (Cell Physiol)* 1989;256:C226–C233.
36. McCann JD, Bhalla RC, Welsh MJ. Release of intracellular calcium by two different second messengers in airway epithelium. *Am J Physiol (Lung Cell Mol Physiol)* 1989;257:L116–L124.
37. Clancy JP, McCann JD, Welsh MJ. Evidence that calcium-dependent activation of airway epithelia chloride channels is not dependent on phosphorylation. *Am J Physiol (Lung Cell Mol Physiol)* 1990;in press.
38. Anderson MP, Welsh MJ. Fatty acids inhibit apical membrane chloride channels in airway epithelia. *Proc Natl Acad Sci USA* 1990;in press.
39. Hwang TC, Guggino SE, Guggino WB. Arachidonic acid block of epithelial Cl⁻ channels in tracheal airway cells. *Biophys J* 1990;57:88a.
40. Disser J, Fromter E. Properties of Na⁺ channels of respiratory epithelium from CF and non CF patients. *Pediatr Pulmonol Suppl* 1989;4:115.
41. Rommens JM, Iannuzzi MC, Kerem B-S, et al. Identification of the cystic fibrosis gene: chromosome walking and jumping. *Science* 1989;245:1059–1065.
42. Riordan JR, Rommens JM, Kerem B-S, et al. Identification of the cystic fibrosis gene: cloning and characterization of complementary DNA. *Science* 1989;245:1066–1073.
43. Kerem B-S, Rommens JM, Buchanan JA, et al. Identification of the cystic fibrosis gene: genetic analysis. *Science* 1989;245:1073–1080.
44. Lemna WK, Feldman GL, Kerem B-S, et al. Mutation analysis for heterozygote detection and the prenatal diagnosis of cystic fibrosis. *N Engl J Med* 1990;322:291–296.

THE LUNG: Scientific Foundations
edited by R.G. Crystal, J.B. West et al.
Raven Press, Ltd., New York © 1991.

CHAPTER 7.9.3

Ciliary Dysfunction

Björn A. Afzelius

The mucociliary clearance mechanism is described in Chapter 7.3.2, and it suffices to mention here that its two main components are the mucous blanket, which traps inhaled bacteria and dust, and the ciliated epithelium, which propels the mucous blanket toward the pharynx. The mucus is then unconsciously swallowed. Undoubtedly, it is an important first barrier against infection, although the degree to which it is essential has been debated. The following quotation from Hilding (1) probably is representative of the older investigators: "Death may occur from failure of the ciliary system within the respiratory tract, the cilia become destroyed and the ciliary function lost. Secretions collect, as a result, in such large quantities that the patients die of asphyxia."

It has hence come as a surprise that a disease exists in which the cilia are immotile, dysmotile, or even missing altogether, and that the patients suffering from it can live a fairly normal life, can work in physically and mentally demanding occupations, and seem to have a normal life span (2). The disease has been termed "immotile-cilia syndrome," but several other terms have also been proposed for it or for some subgroup of it—for instance, "primary ciliary dyskinesia" or "acilia syndrome." The syndrome will be presented here in some detail in the first five sections of this chapter. The sixth section contains a description of a few related diseases, and the seventh section deals with some acquired ciliary dysfunctions.

CLINICAL CHARACTERISTICS
OF THE IMMOTILE-CILIA SYNDROME

The clinical symptoms differ in severity at different stages of life. In the neonatal stage, respiratory distress is common and some newborns have to be kept in an incubator. The baby is born with a running nose. In childhood, frequent ear infections are problematic as well as polyposis and infections in the respiratory tract. Bronchiectases probably are not present at birth but may develop early, sometimes even in childhood. After puberty it is usually the infertility problem which brings the patients to the clinic; most men are sterile, and many women have a lowered fertility. Another common complaint is headache, which might be secondary to chronic sinusitis. Bronchitis and rhinitis are constant findings. Lung function may be normal but more often shows by the third decade an impaired ventilation, which at times may be severe. Radiologically, the disease progresses from bronchial wall thickening, with or without hyperinflation, to increasing hyperinflation plus parenchymal changes such as segmental atelectasis, consolidation, and bronchiectasis (3).

Nearly all the clinical symptoms listed above can be explained by the fact that the mucociliary clearance in nose, sinuses, middle ear, and oviducts is absent or insufficient. Male sterility is due to the sperm tail being immotile or poorly motile; the sperm tail can be said to be an elongated, somewhat modified cilium. A further characteristic of the immotile-cilia syndrome is more enigmatic: A high percentage of the cases—perhaps 50%—have situs inversus viscerum. This subgroup of the immotile-cilia syndrome usually conforms to a disease that has been known for over 50 years, namely, Kartagener syndrome or Kartagener's triad (i.e., situs inversus, bronchiectasis, and chronic sinusitis) (4). It has been speculated that cilia of some epithelia in normal embryos push the heart to the left side, whereupon the liver will shift to the right, whereas with immotile cilia, situs determination is random (2). For a more detailed description of the immotile-cilia syndrome, see reviews in refs. 5 and 6.

B. Afzelius: Department of Ultrastructure Research, The Wenner–Gren Institute, University of Stockholm, S-106 91 Stockholm, Sweden.

DIAGNOSIS OF THE IMMOTILE-CILIA SYNDROME

Vital Microscopy

The cardinal criterion of the immotile-cilia syndrome is inborn immotility, dysmotility, or absence of cilia. In most (but not all) cases, the defect is generalized. The exceptional cases might be those where the upper and lower respiratory tract have defective cilia, whereas the sperm tail has a normal motility (7). Sperm tails and respiratory cilia have protein compositions that differ to some degree (8). There are also cases where only some of the ciliated epithelia are affected but not others, and the explanation could then either be that cilia from different epithelia differ somewhat in their composition or that there are cases of mosaicism.

The logical way to diagnose the immotile-cilia syndrome would seem to be to examine the motility or immotility of the cilia. For various reasons, this is not easy, except in certain cases. Examination of the motility or immotility of ejaculated spermatozoa, on the other hand, is a standard procedure to be recommended whenever immotile-cilia syndrome is suspected in an adult man. Immotile spermatozoa would indicate that the patient suffers from immotile-cilia syndrome, whereas a lack of spermatozoa in the ejaculate would indicate that he has Young's syndrome (see the section on related genetic diseases, and see also refs. 9 and 10).

Respiratory tract cilia normally are covered by a mucous blanket, and their movements are thus hidden to the investigator, unless the mucus can be washed off. The frequency of the ciliary beatings can be studied in epithelia *in situ* by the reflections from the mucous layer of a projected light beam. However, frequency is of much less importance than geometry of effective stroke and recovery stroke of the cilia (see below and Chapter 3.1.2).

Ciliated epithelia from the respiratory tract can be excised from their normal sites and examined in the light microscope (11). It is not known to what degree the ciliary beat pattern changes when the mucous layer is washed off. Ciliary beat frequency at body temperature is 10–15 Hz in a healthy person, which is too high to be determined by the unaided eye. The shape of the ciliary strokes can be evaluated to even a lesser degree. In order to detect whether the ciliary strokes have a normal or an abnormal configuration, it is necessary to study them aided by oscillography or video recording (12,13). Many patients with clinical symptoms of the immotile-cilia syndrome have some kind of ciliary motility, albeit an erratic one; these have been described as resembling symmetric metronome-like to-and-fro movements, multiplanar eggbeater-like rotations of the midsection of the cilium, displays of slow grabbing movements, rapid low-amplitude vibrations, or rotational waves in a corkscrew-like motion (12,13).

An examination of biopsies by phase contrast microscopy or interference contrast microscopy can give rise to some false-positive results, unless the observer is trained in analyzing the ciliary waveforms. There may also be incidents of a false-negative diagnosis in cases where the ciliated epithelium either has been exposed to cold temperature or has been damaged during handling. Yet examination of ciliary beatings is so quick and simple that it is recommended as a first screening method. For a more complete examination of the living epithelium, the test battery by Van der Baan et al. (14) can be employed; these authors base their diagnosis on a combination of data from ciliary beat frequency, ciliary beat coordination, and ciliary beat amplitude.

Electron-Microscopic Investigations of Cilia

The first cases of immotile-cilia syndrome were diagnosed by electron microscopy of ultrathin sections through bronchial or nasal mucosa and showed the cilia to lack dynein arms (Fig. 1) (2,15). Because the dynein arms provide the motor force during ciliary beatings, the data were interpreted as indicating ciliary immotility. Spermatozoa lacking dynein arms had also been observed at that time and were found to be completely immotile (16,17). Several investigators have later confirmed that cilia from persons with Kartagener syndrome and related diseases may lack dynein arms and may be motionless (18–20).

Whereas a partial or total lack of dynein arms seems to be the most common finding when examining cilia from persons with symptoms of the immotile-cilia syndrome, this ciliary defect is far from the only one. Other subgroups include disorganized axoneme, defective spokes, transposed microtubules, and other forms (5,18–21). Cilia in these latter groups usually are motile, although the motility pattern is erroneous and the cilia is evidently unable to perform effective mucociliary clearance. There is even a group with total lack of cilia on those cells in the respiratory tract and middle ear that normally would carry cilia (22–24). In this latter subgroup the cells are provided with long microvilli (or cytofila) and sometimes have numerous fibrogranular complexes (i.e., basal body precursors). Evidently the immotile-cilia syndrome (including the dyskinetic varieties as well as the varieties without cilia) is a heterogeneous disease. In spite of this, the clinical picture is uniform and it appears impractical

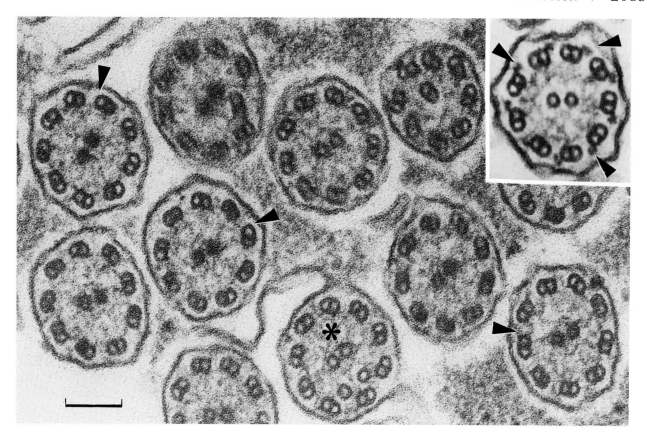

FIG. 1. Cross-sectioned cilia from a person suffering from the immotile-cilia syndrome. The dynein arms are missing (*arrowheads*), the orientation of the cilia is poor, and there is an increased percentage of cilia that have supernumerary microtubulues (*asterisk*). The inset shows a normal cilium with dynein arms (*arrowhead*). Scale marker: 0.1 μm.

to have different names for the different subgroups. The term "immotile-cilia syndrome" is descriptive and has priority. Situs inversus may be present only in those subgroups of the syndrome that have a deficiency of dynein arms (20).

One subgroup of the disease is of particular interest in this connection. Its epithelial cells carry cilia with a normal ultrastructure, yet the cilia seem to be nonfunctioning (25). An ultrastructural examination will give a false-negative diagnosis in these few and exceptional cases. Whether there also are cases of false-positive diagnosis is not settled. Corbeel et al. (26) have reported on a patient who, in an acute phase of bronchiectasis, had cilia with a decreased number of dynein arms but who, after antibiotic treatment and recovery, had a normal number of dynein arms. It would thus seem that the dynein arm deficiency is not necessarily an unfailing criterion of the immotile-cilia syndrome, although in most cases it certainly is diagnostic.

The subgroup of dynein arm-deficient cilia is usually combined with two further characteristics: (a) An increased percentage of cilia (over 5%) have either supernumerary microtubules or missing ones, and (b) the alignment of the cilia is not as good as it is in healthy epithelia (27,28). Cilia with a very poor alignment cannot be expected to act as a good mucociliary escalator.

The scanning electron microscope, which is capable of imaging the surface topography, may also be used for diagnostic work of the immotile-cilia syndrome. The main problem is the difficulty of ridding the epithelium of mucus. In suitable preparations the degree of ciliary alignment can be evaluated, since the tips of the respiratory tract cilia have been found to be somewhat bent in the direction of the effective stroke. Thus it is, at least in principle, possible to determine the direction of the effective stroke and to judge whether a certain field of cilia consists of well-aligned members or poorly aligned ones (29).

Mucociliary Clearance

Ciliary motility as such is of limited interest when studying the functions of the lung. It is the work performed by the cilia that is important. The collective work by the cilia in a portion of the respiratory tract can be estimated by measuring the mucociliary clearance (see also Chapter 7.3.2). Different methods to measure this parameter are known, and many of them have been employed in diagnostics.

The simplest method is the saccharine test, in which small saccharine particles are placed on the nasal mucosa and the subject is asked to inform the investigator when a bitter taste is noticed near the pharynx. Under standardized conditions (avoidance of sneezing, sniffing, coughing, etc.) and with adult test subjects, this method will give a figure for the transport rate of the mucous layer in the nasal cavity. This transport rate may not necessarily be identical to that in the trachea, bronchi, or bronchioles; in fact, there is only a weak correlation between clearance rate in nasal and trach-eobronchial mucosa (30,31). Although the saccharine test alone cannot solve the diagnostic problems of the immotile-cilia syndrome, it is so simple that it can be recommended as a first screening method. A greatly prolonged transport time, together with typical clinical data, often will suffice. The saccharine test is, however, difficult to perform, and it is unreliable for patients under 10 years of age.

Other methods require the use of either radioactive markers (usually ^{99}Tc-tagged Teflon spheres) or radio-opaque deposits studied radiologically. The former method is preferable. The test is to be used on adult patients only. The techniques to measure the trach-eobronchial or nasal clearance differ in different laboratories (31–34), but they seem to give a good and reliable value of the efficacy of the mucociliary apparatus. It should be noted, however, that coughing during the measuring period will result in a clearance that can be termed "coughing clearance" rather than "mucociliary transport" (35).

Mucociliary clearance is also slow or absent in a number of conditions other than the immotile-cilia syndrome (e.g., in asthma and other forms of obstructive lung disease or infections by mycoplasma or *Bordetella*) (36,37).

Biochemical and Histochemical Investigations of Ciliary Proteins

If it is suspected or documented that dynein arms are lacking in a certain sample of cilia or sperm tails, a logical (next) step would be to determine whether these organelles contain dyneins. The dynein molecules are located in the dynein arms, but some dynein species might theoretically be found elsewhere in the axoneme (Chapter 3.1.2). The amount of proteins (in general) and dyneins (in particular) within an ejaculate is sufficient for such an electrophoretic investigation, whereas a curette biopsy or brushing from the nasal

mucosa probably would be insufficient with present-day techniques. It has been noted that most dynein species are absent in the ejaculates from men with the immotile-cilia syndrome and lacking dynein arms (38; and Pallini, *unpublished data*). This finding would rule out the possibility that the dyneins are present in the axoneme at a wrong location or that the dyneins are present in an inactive form.

Localization of the Dynein Gene

Garber et al. (39) have isolated the cDNA of the gene to the heavy chain of dynein. They have also demonstrated that there is a low, if not single, copy number of this gene and that there is a considerable conservation of this domain in other vertebrates. With this cDNA as a probe, it should be possible to find out where the dynein gene is located in the genome of a healthy person and whether the gene is lost in a person who has no dynein arms in the cilia.

GENETIC ASPECTS

A striking feature of the immotile-cilia syndrome is its heterogeneity. There are evidently a large number of genes which, when mutated, can be responsible for the manifestations of the disease. Published pedigrees indicate that the disease in all (or nearly all) its forms has a recessive mode of inheritance. Because persons suffering from the syndrome usually are infertile, nearly all the affected children are born to parents who are healthy but who evidently are carriers. The ratio between affected and healthy siblings to persons with the immotile-cilia syndrome is close to 1:3, which is to be expected with recessive traits (40,41).

PREVALENCE

The prevalence of the immotile-cilia syndrome can be estimated from these figures: Situs inversus has a prevalence of about 1:10,000 in many countries; a little over 20% of these also have bronchiectasis (42). If it is correct that equally many cases with immotile-cilia syndrome have situs inversus as have (the normal) situs solitus, then its prevalence would be twice that of Kartagener syndrome or around 1:25,000. If other categories with a much lower incidence of situs inversus are included (ciliary dyskinesia and lack of cilia), then the prevalence of the syndrome will be greater.

These considerations lead to the question of whether there might be a whole spectrum ranging from completely immotile (and totally useless) cilia to those that are partly functioning and, ultimately, to the fully active and useful ones. This appears probable *a priori,* and some support hereof can be found in studies on mucociliary clearance rates in monozygotic twins and in various inbred mouse strains (43,44). Such studies have shown that the tracheobronchial clearance rate is, to a great extent, constitutionally determined.

TREATMENT AND PROGNOSIS

Treatment is symptomatic and is directed against complications in the respiratory tract: antibiotics during infections, bronchodilators when there is airway obstruction, and physiotherapy with postural drainage and abandonment of smoking (5,6). Coughing should not be suppressed, since it acts as a substitute for mucociliary clearance. Thoracic surgical intervention against bronchiectasis is sometimes indicated. Situs inversus, when present, is usually total and is not combined with any congenital malformations.

RELATED GENETIC DISEASES

A number of other diseases have characteristics that, in some respects, resemble those of the immotile-cilia syndrome. Young's syndrome, which has been mentioned above (see subsection on vital microscopy), is characterized by chronic sinusitis and bronchitis and often by bronchiectasis and azoospermia. The cilia and the (testicular) spermatozoa have normal ultrastructure and motility (9,10). The site of the primary defect is unknown.

In cystic fibrosis there is chronic bronchitis, male infertility, and an ion composition of secretions that is abnormal and that causes the mucus to become unduly viscous. In fact, neither the ciliary activity nor coughing is effective in clearing the mucus, and cystic fibrosis is a much more severe disease than is immotile-cilia syndrome. Cilia have a normal ultrastructure (45). The gene of the disease has been isolated by F. Collins and L. C. Tsui (*unpublished data,* August 1989), and corresponding protein probably acts in ion channelling over the cell membrane.

Immunoglobulin deficiency (Chapter 7.4.2) is characterized by frequent bacterial infections in the airways and is usually also characterized by a defective mucociliary clearance. Cilia have a normal ultrastructure, and after a prolonged treatment with antibiotics and gamma globulins, the mucociliary clearance rate may return to normal values (46).

Retinitis pigmentosa is a progressive retinal degeneration that eventually leads to blindness. It is genetically heterogeneous. The fertility is lowered, but the functions of the respiratory tracts are normal. It has been found by Fox et al. (47) and confirmed by others (48,49) that nasal cilia and sperm tails show a somewhat increased incidence of axonemal abnormalities. This is the only genetic disease, apart from the immotile-cilia syndrome, in which defective ciliary ultrastructure has been described.

ACQUIRED CILIARY DYSFUNCTIONS

Most of this chapter has dealt with a primary ciliary error, the immotile-cilia syndrome. It is important, however, to realize that changes in the ciliary structure and function may develop also as a consequence of infection or injury. In such cases of secondary ciliary lesions, the structural changes have turned out to be manifold but of kinds that can be regarded as unspecific. Fusion of several cilia into so-called compound cilia, disorganization of the axoneme, swollen cilia, and increased numbers of cilia with extra or missing microtubules (over 5% of the ciliary population) are often seen after infection with viruses, bacteria, and mycoplasma, in asthma, or in smokers (50,51). Similarly, both virus infection and benzo[*a*]pyrene exposure may affect the epithelia so that some cilia are internalized (i.e., projecting into the cytoplasm rather than into the lumen). A release of elastase or protease may cause the ciliary membrane and the central microtubules of the axoneme to degenerate. Because these various acquired ciliary defects are so commonly seen (sometimes also seen in normal subjects), they have little or no diagnostic value. Substances such as lipophilic or mercuric preservatives, local anesthetics and antihistamines, adsorption enhancers (such as bile salts), and many bacterial substances are ciliotoxic, although they do not necessarily influence ciliary ultrastructure (52,53). A diet deficient in vitamin A will give rise to metaplastic changes in the respiratory tract in that the ciliated epithelium is replaced by a squamous epithelium (54).

CONCLUSIONS

The immotile-cilia syndrome provides a unique insight into the role of cilia (as opposed to the role of mucus-plus-cilia) in the human body. It has been established that the existence of functioning cilia is an important factor, although it is not of vital importance. It is evident that various other defense mechanisms can act as substitutes for a faulty mucociliary escalator. Coughing seems to be foremost among these substitute mechanisms (55). The immotile-cilia syndrome has turned out to be a heterogeneous disease. Diagnosis can be a problem. One of the difficulties is to differentiate between (a) the inherited diseases of immotile, dysmotile, or missing cilia and (b) acquired ciliary diseases. The most reliable criteria of the immotile-cilia syndrome seem to be the clinical picture and the early onset of the symptoms.

REFERENCES

1. Hilding AC. The relation of ciliary insufficiency to death from asthma and other respiratory diseases. *Ann Otol Rhinol Laryngol* 1943;52:5–19.
2. Afzelius BA. A human syndrome caused by immotile cilia. *Science* 1976;193:317–319.
3. Nadel HR, Stringer DA, Levison H, Turner JAP, Sturgess JM. The immotile cilia syndrome: radiological manifestations. *Radiology* 1985;154:651–655.
4. Kartagener M. Zur Pathologie der Bronchiektasien: Bronchiektasien bei Situs viscerum inversus. *Beitr Klin Tuberk* 1933; 83:489–501.
5. Afzelius BA, Mossberg B. Immotile-cilia syndrome (primary ciliary dyskinesia) including Kartagener syndrome. In: Scriver CR, Beaudet AL, Sly WS, Valle D, eds. *The metabolic basis of inherited disease*, 6th ed. New York: McGraw-Hill, 1989;2739–2750.
6. Sturgess J, Turner JAP. Ultrastructural pathology of cilia in the immotile cilia syndrome. *Perspect Pediatr Pathol* 1984;8:133–161.
7. Jonsson MS, McCormick JR, Gillies CG, Gondos B. Kartagener's syndrome with motile spermatozoa. *N Engl J Med* 1982; 307:1131–1133.
8. Pallini V, Bugnoli M, Mencarelli C, Scapigliati G. Biochemical properties of ciliary, flagellar and cytoplasmic dyneins. *Symp Soc Exp Biol* 1982;35:399–419.
9. Handelsman DJ, Conway AJ, Boyland LM, Turtle JR. Young's syndrome. Obstructive azoospermia and chronic sinopulmonary infections. *N Engl J Med* 1984;310:3–9.
10. Greenstone MA, Rutman A, Hendry WF, Cole PJ. Ciliary function in Young's syndrome. *Thorax* 1988;43:153–154.
11. Rutland J, Cole PJ. Non-invasive sampling of nasal cilia for measurement of beat frequency and study of ultrastructure. *Lancet* 1980;2:564–565.
12. Pedersen M, Nielsen MH. Abnormal ciliary motility as a cause of chronic airway disease. *Prog Respir Dis* 1981;17:190–196.
13. Rossman CM, Forrest JB, Lee RMKW, Newhouse AF, Newhouse MT. The dyskinetic cilia syndrome. *Chest* 1981;80:860–864.
14. Van der Baan S, Veerman AJP, Wulffraat N, Bezemer PD, Feenstra L. Primary ciliary dyskinesia. *Acta Otolaryngol (Stockh)* 1986;102:274–281.
15. Pedersen H, Mygind N. Absence of axonemal arms in nasal mucosa cilia in Kartagener's syndrome. *Nature* 1976;262:494–495.
16. Afzelius BA, Eliasson R, Johnsen O, Lindholmer C. Lack of dynein arms in immotile human spermatozoa. *J Cell Biol* 1975;66:225–232.
17. Pedersen H, Rebbe H. Absence of arms in the axoneme of immobile human spermatozoa. *Biol Reprod* 1975;12:541–544.
18. Turner JAP, Corkey CWB, Lee JYC, Levison H, Sturgess J. Clinical expression of immotile cilia syndrome. *Pediatrics* 1981;67:805–810.
19. Salomon JL, Grimfeld A, Tournier G, Baculard A, Escalier D, Jouannet P, David G. Ciliary disorders of the bronchi in children. *Rev Fr Mal Respir* 1983;11:645–656.
20. Escalier D, Jouannet P, David G. Abnormalities of the ciliary axonemal complex in children. *Biol Cell* 1982;44:271–282.
21. Afzelius BA. The immotile cilia syndrome—a microtubule-associated defect. *Crit Rev Biochem* 1985;19:63–87.
22. Gordon RE, Kattan M. Absence of cilia and basal bodies with predominance of brush cells in the respiratory mucosa from a patient with immotile cilia syndrome. *Ultrastruct Pathol* 1984; 6:45–49.
23. Welch MJ, Stiehm ER, Dudley JP. Isolated absence of nasal cilia. *Ann Allergy* 1984;52:32–34.
24. De Santi MM, Gardi C, Barlocco G, Canciani M, Mastella G,

25. Lungarella G. Cilia-lacking respiratory cells in ciliary aplasia. *Biol Cell* 1988;64:67–70.
25. Herzon FS, Murphy S. Normal ciliary ultrastructure in children with Kartagener's syndrome. *Ann Otol Rhinol Laryngol* 1980;89:81–83.
26. Corbeel L, Cornille F, Lauweryns J, Boel M, Van der Berghe G. Ultrastructural abnormalities of bronchial cilia in children with recurrent airway infections and bronchiectasis. *Arch Dis Child* 1981;56:929–933.
27. Holley MC, Afzelius BA. Alignment of cilia in immotile-cilia syndrome. *Tissue Cell* 1986;18:521–529.
28. Rautiainen M, Collan J, Nuutinen J, Afzelius BA. The variation of beat direction in immotile-cilia syndrome. *Arch Otolaryngol* 1989;247: in press.
29. Veerman AJP, Van Delden L, Feenstra L, Leene W. Scanning and transmission electron microscopy in the immotile cilia syndrome. *Ultramicroscopy* 1979;4:133–134.
30. Andersen I, Camner P, Jensen PL, Philipson K, Proctor DF. A comparison of nasal and tracheobronchial clearance. *Arch Environ Health* 1974;29:290–293.
31. Andersen I, Proctor DF. Measurement of nasal mucociliary clearance. *Eur J Respir Dis* 1983;64(Suppl 127):37–40.
32. Camner P. The production and use of test aerosols for studies of human tracheobronchial clearance. *Environ Physiol* 1971; 1:137–154.
33. Pavia D, Sutton PP, Agnew JE, Lopez-Vidriero MT, Newman SP, Clarke SW. Measurements of bronchial mucociliary clearance. *Eur J Respir Dis* 1983;64(Suppl 127):41–56.
34. Puchelle E, Aug F, Pham QT, Bertrand A. Comparison of three methods for measuring nasal mucociliary clerance in man. *Acta Otolaryngol (Stockh)* 1981;91:297–303.
35. Camner P, Mossberg B, Philipson K. Tracheobronchial clearance and chronic obstructive lung disease. *Scand J Respir Dis* 1973;54:272–281.
36. Jarstrand C, Camner P, Philipson K. *Mycoplasma pneumoniae* and tracheobronchial clearance. *Am Rev Respir Dis* 1974; 110:415–419.
37. Bemis DA, Kennedy JR. An improved system for studying the effect of *Bordetella bronchiseptica* of the ciliary activity of canine tracheal epithelial cells. *J Infect Dis* 1981;144:349–357.
38. Baccetti B, Burrini AG, Pallini V. Spermatozoa and cilia lacking axoneme in an infertile man. *Andrologia* 1980;12:525–532.
39. Garber AT, Retief JT, Dixon GH. Isolation of dynein heavy chain cDNAs from trout testis which predict an extensive carboxyl-terminal α-helical coiled-coil domain. *EMBO J* 1989; 8:1727–1734.
40. Afzelius BA. Genetical and ultrastructural aspects of the immotile-cilia syndrome. *Am J Hum Gen* 1981;33:852–864.
41. Sturgess JM, Thompson MW, Czegledy-Nagy E, Turner JAP. Genetic aspects of immotile cilia syndrome. *Am J Med Genet* 1986;25:149–160.
42. Adams R, Churchill ED. Situs inversus, sinusitis and bronchiectasis. *J Thorac Surg* 1937;7:206–217.
43. Camner P, Philipson K, Friberg L. Tracheobronchial clearance in twins. *Arch Environ Health* 1972;24:82–87.
44. Brownstein DG. Tracheal mucociliary transport in laboratory mice. Evidence for genetic polymorphism. *Exp Lung Res* 1987;13:185–191.
45. Kollberg H, Mossberg B, Afzelius BA, Philipson K, Camner P. Cystic fibrosis compared with the immotile-cilia syndrome. *Scand J Respir Dis* 1978;59:297–306.
46. Mossberg B, Björkander J, Afzelius BA, Camner P. Mucociliary clearance in patients with immunoglobulin deficiency. *Eur J Respir Dis* 1982;63:570–578.
47. Fox B, Bull TB, Arden GB. Variations in the ultrastructure of human nasal cilia including abnormalities found in retinitis pigmentosa. *J Clin Pathol* 1980;33:327–335.
48. Finkelstein D, Reissig M, Kashima H, Massof R, Hillis A, Proctor D. Nasal cilia in retinitis pigmentosa. *Birth Defects* 1982;18:197–208.
49. Hunter DG, Fishman GA, Kretzer FL. Abnormal exonemes in X-linked retinitis pigmentosa. *Arch Ophthalmol* 1988;106:362–368.
50. Afzelius BA. "Immotile-cilia syndrome" and ciliary abnormal-

ities induced by infection and injury. *Am Rev Respir Dis* 1981;124:107–109.

51. Wilson R. Secondary ciliary dysfunction. *Clin Sci* 1988;75:113–120.

52. Hermens WAJJ, Merkus FWHM. The influence of drugs on nasal ciliary movement. *Pharmacol Res* 1987;4:445–449.

53. Wilson R, Cole P. The effect of bacterial products on ciliary function. *Am Rev Respir Dis* 1988;138(Suppl):49–53.

54. McDowell EM, Keenan KP, Huang M. Effects of vitamin A-deprivation on hamster tracheal epithelium. *Virchows Arch [Cell Pathol]* 1984;45:197–219.

55. Mossberg B, Afzelius BA, Eliasson R, Camner P. On the pathogenesis of obstructive lung disease. *Scand J Respir Dis* 1978;59:55–65.

SECTION 8

Special Environments and Interventions

The final section of this book deals with special situations of importance in pulmonary science. There are several environments in which the lung and the process of respiration in general play a dominant role. The first of these is high altitude, which has historically been regarded as one of the best models for demonstrating the adaptability of human beings to a potentially hostile environment. It is a remarkable fact that after a suitable period of acclimatization, human beings can reach the summit of Mount Everest without supplementary oxygen, whereas someone acutely exposed to the oxygen deprivation of that altitude loses consciousness in a minute or two. In spite of the long history of advances in high-altitude medicine, some of the most important observations have been made in the past 10 years, and indeed many unanswered questions still remain. The topic is not only of interest to lowlanders who go to high altitude for recreational purposes and the very large number of people who live at high altitude in the Andes and the Tibetan plateau. A better understanding of the effects of chronic oxygen deprivation is clearly important for the management of many patients with lung disease.

The next two chapters, on diving and hyperbaric environments, have both important economic and therapeutic overtones. Extensive deep sea diving occurs in connection with oil exploration on the Continental Shelf, and recreational scuba diving is as popular as ever. Both environments are associated with substantial hazards, and accidents are distressingly common. Hyperbaric medicine has a long history but only recently has attained respectability. Even now the topic generates controversy in some quarters, but it is clear that the ability to raise a partial pressure of oxygen in the blood to very high levels definitely has its uses.

Space medicine is one of the more colorful topics in environmental medicine, and it will become increasingly important as astronauts and cosmonauts spend longer periods in space. Scientists not familiar with this field are often surprised to learn that the amount of medical research that has been carried out in space is very small in spite of man's 30-year history in the environment. The fact is that most of the time that astronauts have spent in space has been devoted to operational needs, and the general attitude has been that if the astronauts return safely, the work should continue. However, weightlessness causes a host of physiological changes in the body (particularly in the lungs), and several important experiments will shortly be performed on astronauts while in orbit.

In the second part of this section, a number of interventions of importance in pulmonary science are considered, including (a) oxygen therapy with its potential hazard of oxygen toxicity, (b) mechanical ventilation, (c) anesthesia, (d) extracorporeal oxygenation, and (e) lung transplantation. Some of these topics—for example, oxygen therapy and anesthesia—are day-by-day procedures, but important advances are continually being made. For example, while the arterial hypoxemia that accompanies anesthesia has been recognized for some 30 years, only in the past two or three have the mechanisms been clearly elucidated. Other interventions such as mechanical ventilation have been extensively used since the poliomyelitis epidemics of the 1940s, but again novel methods of ventilation with intriguing physiological aspects have recently been introduced. Both oxygen therapy and mechanical ventilation are frequently used in the intensive care environment, but our knowledge of how these critically important procedures affect very sick lungs is often rudimentary. This is an area where the physician often operates intuitively because the physiological mechanisms are so obscure.

While interventions such as oxygen therapy, mechanical ventilation, and anesthesia are everyday events, extracorporeal oxygenation and transplantation are still rather exotic. However, there is little doubt that with improvements in knowledge, both of these interventions will become important in pulmonary medicine. Lung transplantation in particular is at a very exciting point in time, partly because of great improvements in immunosuppressive drugs. This is an area where the future is bound to bring dramatic advances.

The Editors

THE LUNG: Scientific Foundations
edited by R.G. Crystal, J.B. West et al.
Raven Press, Ltd., New York © 1991.

CHAPTER 8.1.1

High Altitude

John B. West

There have been considerable advances in high-altitude medicine and physiology over the last few years, and many aspects fall within the province of pulmonary science. One of the reasons for the growing interest is the large number of people who now live at high altitude, and another reason is the increasing economic importance of these regions. As an example, some 2.5 to 3 million people live at altitudes over 3000 m (approximately 10,000 ft) on the Tibetan Plateau; many mines are situated above this altitude in the South American Andes, which extend from Colombia (to the north) to central Chile (to the south).

Another reason for the burgeoning interest in high altitude is the large number of people who ski, trek, or climb in high places. The cable cars at some modern skiing resorts go up to over 3300 m (11,000 ft), and large numbers of visitors develop some degree of acute mountain sickness; occasionally, high-altitude pulmonary edema and high-altitude cerebral edema are seen. Mountaineers reach much higher altitudes. For example, 30 climbed to the summit of Mt. Everest in the post-monsoon season of 1988, and there were no less than nine deaths on the mountain.

Finally, there are important lessons from high altitude in improving our understanding of the severe hypoxia of lung disease. A climber near the summit of Mt. Everest who is breathing air is exposed to extremes of hypoxic stress that normal subjects never encounter in other circumstances. In fact, humans appear to be right at the limit of tolerance to hypoxia under these conditions. There is no better way of studying human responses to prolonged extreme hypoxia than making observations at very high altitude (1).

J. B. West: Department of Medicine, University of California—San Diego, La Jolla, California 92093.

ATMOSPHERE

The barometric pressure decreases with distance above the earth's surface in an approximately exponential manner (Fig. 1). Indeed, if air temperature did not decline with altitude, the relationship would be strictly exponential. At an altitude of 5500–5800 m (18,000–19,000 ft), barometric pressure is half the sea level value of 760 torr. On the summit of Mt. Everest at an altitude of 8848 m (29,028 ft), the barometric pressure is about 250 torr. At altitudes approaching 20,000 m (about 65,000 ft), the barometric pressure falls below the water vapor pressure at 37°C and tissues vaporize or "boil."

The relationship between barometric pressure and altitude causes frequent confusion. As long ago as 1878, Paul Bert, in his monumental *La Pression Barométrique*, predicted a barometric pressure of 248 torr on the summit of Mt. Everest, based on a number of measurements reported at lower altitudes, mainly in the Andes. Additional measurements were made by other travelers to high mountains (2,3), and these were all consistent. However, confusion arose in the 1920s and 1930s when the Standard Atmosphere was introduced by the aviation industry for calibrating altimeters and low-pressure chambers. The Standard Atmosphere model was never meant to be used to predict the actual barometric pressure at a particular location. Rather, it was developed as a model of more or less average conditions over the surface of the world (4).

In fact, barometric pressure at high altitude depends on latitude, and it turns out that most high mountains—for example, in the Himalayas, South American Andes, and European Alps—are at latitudes relatively near the equator. The result is that the barometric pressures predicted from the Standard Atmosphere are too low for these regions (5,6). The point is emphasized here because whenever physiologists have used the Standard Atmosphere to predict barometric pressures

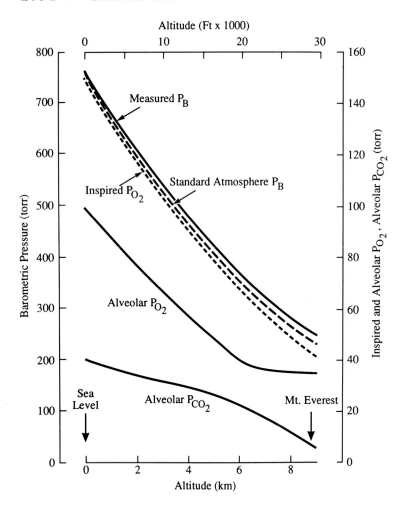

FIG. 1. Barometric pressure, P_{O_2} of moist inspired gas, alveolar P_{O_2}, and alveolar P_{CO_2} versus altitude. The barometric pressures for the Standard Atmosphere are shown, along with typical values measured on high mountains in the Himalayas and Andes. The alveolar gas values are for acclimatized subjects and are only approximate. At moderate altitudes (3000–4500 m), permanent residents have lower values of alveolar P_{O_2} and higher P_{CO_2} values than do acclimatized lowlanders.

at extreme altitudes, the results were seriously in error. For example, the Standard Atmosphere predicts a pressure of 236 torr on the summit of Mt. Everest, whereas the pressure is close to 250 torr (6). This increase of 14 torr makes all the difference between whether a climber breathing air can reach the summit or not (7).

VENTILATION

When a person who normally lives near sea level (lowlander) spends a period of time at high altitude, a whole series of compensatory responses takes place, a process known as *acclimatization*. The effectiveness of these responses is remarkable. For example, acclimatized individuals can do small amounts of work at altitudes where the barometric pressure is so low that an unacclimatized person, acutely exposed, would lose consciousness within a minute or so.

One of the most important features of acclimatization is hyperventilation. Its physiological value can be seen by considering the effects of very high altitude. For example, the P_{O_2} of moist inspired gas on the sum-

mit of Mt. Everest is about 43 torr (Fig. 1). If the climber maintained his sea level ventilation unchanged, the alveolar P_{CO_2} would be 40, and therefore the alveolar (and arterial) P_{O_2} would be close to zero. However, by increasing his ventilation some fivefold, he reduces his arterial P_{CO_2} to about 7.5 torr and thus maintains an arterial P_{O_2} of about 35 torr (Fig. 1). A more modest degree of hyperventilation is seen at less extreme altitudes. For example, the arterial P_{CO_2} in permanent residents at 4600 m (15,000 ft) in the South American Andes is about 33 torr (8).

The cause of the hyperventilation is hypoxic stimulation of the peripheral chemoreceptors, including the carotid and aortic bodies but chiefly the former (see Chapters 5.4.2 and 5.4.3). The ventilation increases abruptly during the first 2 hr following ascent, and then more slowly over several days (9). The slow secondary rise in ventilation can be partly explained by increased renal elimination of bicarbonate. This reduces the initial respiratory alkalosis, which tends to inhibit ventilation. However, other factors may be (a) a loss of bicarbonate from the cerebrospinal fluid and (b) an increased sensitivity of the carotid body as a result of the chronic hypoxia (10).

There is some evidence that the greater the hypoxic ventilatory response (HVR), the better the performance of climbers at extreme altitude (11,12). This is not surprising because the climbers with the highest HVR will maintain a better alveolar and therefore arterial Po_2, other things being equal. However, there are certainly exceptions, and a number of elite mountain climbers have been shown to have only moderate values of HVR (13). The inverse is probably true; that is, a lowlander with a very low HVR will have a poor tolerance for extreme altitude.

Paradoxically, permanent residents of high altitude (highlanders) have been shown to have a low (blunted) HVR (14–16). Perhaps this reflects a difference between *acclimatization* (which is the process that occurs in lowlanders who ascend to high altitude) and true genetic *adaptation* (which occurs over many generations at high altitude). Presumably the native highlanders have other cellular responses that allow them to tolerate the high altitude well in spite of a lower arterial Po_2.

However, there is some evidence that the blunted hypoxic ventilatory response is not due to natural selection. For example, children born at sea level with severe hypoxemia caused by cyanotic congenital heart disease have been shown to have a low hypoxic ventilatory response (17), and lowlanders living for up to 39 years at an altitude of 3100 m have been shown to develop gradual blunting of their HVR (18). Furthermore, Lahiri et al. (19) reported that the children of Andean Indians had a normal HVR which only became blunted as they grew into adulthood at high altitude.

BLOOD CHANGES

Polycythemia

One of the best known physiological responses to high altitude is the increase in red blood cell concentration of the blood. The resulting rise in hemoglobin concentration, and therefore oxygen-carrying capacity, means that although the arterial Po_2 and oxygen saturation are diminished, the oxygen concentration of the arterial blood may be normal or even above normal.

The value of polycythemia in maintaining the arterial oxygen concentration can be seen by looking at permanent residents of Morococha in the Peruvian Andes [altitude 4540 m (14,900 ft), barometric pressure 446 torr]. The arterial Po_2 is only 45 torr, and the corresponding arterial oxygen saturation is 81%. Ordinarily, this would considerably decrease the arterial oxygen concentration; however, because of the polycythemia, the hemoglobin concentration is increased to 19.8 g/dl, giving an arterial oxygen concentration of 22.4 ml/

dl, which is above the normal sea level value (8). The polycythemia also tends to maintain the Po_2 of mixed venous blood because the normal extraction of oxygen by the tissues is accomplished for a smaller fall in peripheral capillary Po_2, and typically at this altitude the Po_2 of mixed venous blood is only 7 torr below normal.

Even higher levels of hemoglobin concentration are seen in climbers at very high altitudes. For example, Pugh (20) reviewed results from five expeditions (51 observations in 40 subjects) and concluded that the hemoglobin concentration after about 6 weeks at high altitude averaged 20.5 g/dl and was independent of altitude above 5500 m. This corresponds to a mean hematocrit of about 60–62%.

The polycythemia occurs in response to an increased production of erythropoietin from the kidney as a consequence of the tissue hypoxia (Fig. 2). Increased levels of blood erythropoietin have been demonstrated in lowlanders after rapid ascent to high altitude (21,22). However, in one study of lowlanders who ascended to

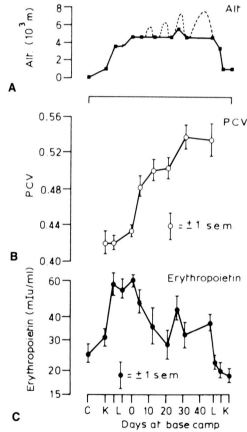

FIG. 2. Effect of ascent to high altitude on packed cell volume and serum erythropoietin. (**A**) Altitude–time profile for the eight subjects. The dashed line indicates ascent above base camp between blood samples. (**B**) Graph showing mean packed cell volume (PCV). (**C**) Graph showing mean erythropoietin concentration. C, control at sea level; K, Kashgar (1200 m); L, Karakol Lakes (3500 m). (From ref. 21.)

4360 m (14,300 ft) in 2 hr, the serum erythropoietin level remained significantly elevated for 9 days but then returned to the normal level before any significant change in hemoglobin concentration was seen (22). This observation is difficult to explain. By contrast, native highlanders of Peru have an elevated steady-state erythropoietin concentration. In one remarkable experiment, pooled plasma from natives of Morococha (4540 m) was injected into volunteers in Lima at sea level who then developed a pronounced reticulocytosis compared with control recipients of normal plasma (23).

In lowlanders who ascend to high altitude, the increase in red blood cell concentration continues for some 6 weeks before it levels out. The resulting increase in red blood cell mass is accompanied by a fall in plasma volume with the result that total circulating blood volume is little changed (24). Sometimes an increase in hematocrit is seen within a day or two of ascent, but this is caused by dehydration.

An interesting question is whether the marked polycythemia of very high altitude is really a useful physiological response, in spite of the increased oxygen-carrying capacity of the blood. It is known that high hematocrits are associated with uneven blood flow in peripheral capillaries as a result of rouleaux formation and sludging, and that these flow phenomena may interfere with efficient oxygen unloading. As a result, some physicians, especially in Europe, have advocated hemodilution of climbers at extreme altitude, claiming that this reduces the incidence of illnesses such as frostbite, which is believed to be caused by a combination of cold and tissue hypoxia.

To obtain data on this issue, a pilot study of hemodilution was carried out on four climbers who were well acclimatized to an altitude of 5400 m (17,700 ft). Approximately 15% of the blood volume was removed and replaced with human serum albumin, thus reducing the hematocrit from about 58% to 50%. It was found that exercise tolerance did not change, suggesting that the polycythemia conferred little advantage (25). Along similar lines, Winslow and Monge (26) actually showed improvement of exercise tolerance in high-altitude Andean natives whose very high hematocrits were reduced by the removal of blood over several weeks.

It should be pointed out that the evolutionary pressure for the increase in red cell production in response to tissue hypoxia was developed over thousands of years at sea level, where it performs an important role in replacing cells if these are lost as a result of trauma, malnutrition, or parasite infection. However the tissue hypoxia of extreme altitude is caused by an entirely different mechanism, and it may well be that the severe polycythemia of very high altitude actually confers no advantage.

Acid–Base Status

We have seen that marked hyperventilation occurs during high-altitude acclimatization, and it is not surprising that this results in a respiratory alkalosis. However, the extent of the alkalosis at extreme altitude is remarkable. For example, based on measurements of the alveolar P_{CO_2} on the summit of Mt. Everest, and values of base excess measured slightly below this, the arterial pH on the summit apparently exceeded 7.7 (27). In climbers living at an altitude of 6300 m (20,700 ft), the mean arterial pH was 7.47. There is even some evidence that high-altitude natives who have been at the same altitude for generations have a mild respiratory alkalosis. For example, Winslow et al. (28) reported a mean plasma pH of 7.439 ± 0.065 in 46 high-altitude natives of Morococha (4540 m).

The respiratory alkalosis of high altitude is apparently advantageous for oxygen transfer from the air to the mitochondria because it increases the oxygen affinity of hemoglobin and thus enhances the loading of oxygen by the pulmonary capillary (see next section). It can be argued that the increased affinity also interferes with the unloading of oxygen from peripheral capillaries. However, there is both experimental (29–31) and theoretical (32,33) evidence that the increased oxygen affinity is beneficial at high altitude. Indeed it is of interest that an increased oxygen affinity is frequently seen in animals who live in low-oxygen environments (34).

An intriguing question is why climbers at extreme altitude do not increase the elimination of bicarbonate by the kidney to return the arterial pH near to the normal value. The fact is that metabolic compensation appears to be extremely slow at very high altitudes. This is possibly because of chronic volume depletion, which has been demonstrated in climbers living at 6300 m (35). It is known that the kidney is slow to correct a respiratory alkalosis in the presence of chronic volume depletion because further elimination of bicarbonate exaggerates the dehydration through the loss of a corresponding cation. On the other hand, renal function was apparently well maintained in a group of normal subjects living at 5800 m because they were able to concentrate and dilute urine normally and respond normally to an induced metabolic acidosis and alkalosis (36).

PULMONARY GAS EXCHANGE

As indicated earlier, hyperventilation helps to maintain the alveolar P_{O_2} in the face of the falling inspired value. For example, at the extreme on the summit of Mt. Everest, the alveolar P_{O_2} is about 35 torr, only 7 or 8 torr lower than the P_{O_2} of moist inspired gas (Fig. 1).

However, the arterial P_{O_2} can be lower than the alveolar value because of either (a) diffusion-limitation across the blood–gas barrier or (b) the presence of ventilation–perfusion inequality.

Diffusion

Acclimatized lowlanders have little, if any, increase in pulmonary diffusing capacity for carbon monoxide at high altitude (37–40). In one study on exercising subjects at altitudes up to 5800 m after 7–10 weeks of acclimatization, there was a small increase (15–20%) in pulmonary diffusing capacity. However, this small change could be wholly accounted for by the increased rate of reaction of carbon monoxide with hemoglobin due to hypoxia, as well as by the increased blood hemoglobin concentration (41).

On the other hand, high-altitude natives have been shown to have pulmonary diffusing capacities that are about 20–25% higher than predicted, or higher than in normal lowlander controls (38,39,42). The increased diffusing capacities were demonstrated during both rest and exercise. Although there is a potential problem in such studies with the appropriateness of the predicted values for diffusing capacity, it is likely that the higher values can be explained by the development of larger lungs therefore causing an increased alveolar surface area and capillary blood volume. Early visitors to high altitude, such as Barcroft et al. (43), commented on the remarkable chest development of the Peruvian high-altitude natives.

Subsequently it has been shown that animals exposed to low-oxygen partial pressures during their active growth phase develop larger lungs and greater diffusing capacities than do animals reared in a normoxic environment (44,45). The opposite is also true; animals reared in a hyperoxic environment develop small lungs (44).

At high altitude, there is good evidence that diffusion-limitation of oxygen transfer across the blood–gas barrier in the lung results in an alveolar–arterial P_{O_2} difference at rest, and that this is exaggerated on exercise. Diffusion-limitation is probably only seen at rest at extreme altitudes, but it occurs during exercise at even moderate altitudes. Barcroft et al. (43) showed that the arterial oxygen saturation fell as a result of exercise in Cerro de Pasco [altitude 4330 m (14,200 ft)], and they correctly attributed the desaturation to failure of the P_{O_2} to equilibrate between alveolar gas and pulmonary capillary blood. These observations were confirmed during the 1960–1961 Himalayan Scientific and Mountaineering Expedition when a striking fall in arterial oxygen saturation was seen during severe exercise at an altitude of 5800 m (19,000 ft) (46). Similar observations were made during the 1981 Amer-

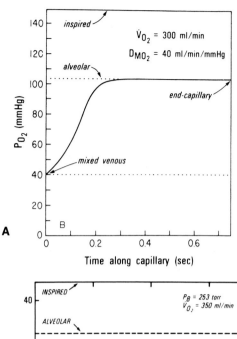

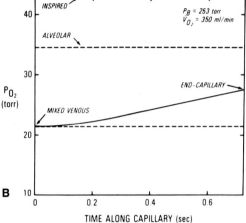

FIG. 3. (A) Calculated time course for P_{O_2} in the pulmonary capillary at sea level in the resting human. Note that there is ample time for equilibration of the P_{O_2} between alveolar gas and end-capillary blood. (From ref. 49.) (B) Similar calculations for a climber at rest on the summit of Mt. Everest. Note that there is considerable diffusion-limitation of oxygen uptake with a large alveolar end-capillary P_{O_2} difference. (From ref. 50.)

ican Medical Research Expedition to Everest (47) and the low-pressure-chamber simulation, Operation Everest II (48).

Figure 3a shows the calculated time course for P_{O_2} in the pulmonary capillary at sea level in the resting human. Note that there is ample time for equilibration of P_{O_2} between alveolar gas and end-capillary blood (49). In contrast, Fig. 3b shows the calculated time course for a climber at rest on the summit of Mt. Everest. Note that the blood comes into the lung with a P_{O_2} of only about 21 torr and that the P_{O_2} rises very slowly along the pulmonary capillary, reaching a value of only about 28 torr at the end (50). There is a large P_{O_2} difference between alveolar gas and end-capillary blood. This is the hallmark of diffusion-limitation of oxygen transfer.

The reason for the slow rate of rise of Po_2 along the pulmonary capillary is the large change in arterial oxygen concentration per unit change of Po_2 of the blood. This, in turn, results from two factors. First, oxygen loading is taking place very low on the oxygen dissociation curve, where it is very steep; and second, there is substantial polycythemia. Piiper and Scheid (51) have clarified the factors responsible for diffusion-limitation of gas transfer across the blood–gas barrier. This depends on the factor $D/Q\beta$, where D is the diffusing capacity, Q is the blood flow, and β is the effective "solubility" of the gas in blood. For oxygen, this is the slope of the dissociation curve. Diffusion-limitation becomes likely when this factor becomes small, and this occurs for oxygen at high altitude because of the large increase in β. Indeed, oxygen is beginning to take on some of the characteristics of carbon monoxide, which is the diffusion-limited gas par excellence. During exercise, the time available for oxygen loading is decreased because of the increased cardiac output, and the situation shown in Fig. 3b is even further exaggerated. Naturally, if a patient with thickening of the blood–gas barrier caused by interstitial lung disease (for example) goes to high altitude, the diffusion-limitation of oxygen will be even more severe.

Ventilation–Perfusion Relationships

There is evidence that the topographical distribution of ventilation–perfusion ratios in the normal lung improves at high altitude as a result of the more uniform distribution of blood flow resulting from the increased pulmonary arterial pressure (52). However, the topographical inequality of ventilation–perfusion ratios is such a minor factor in overall gas exchange that the effect of this change is relatively trivial.

Recent measurements by Wagner et al. (48) during Operation Everest II indicate that ventilation–perfusion inequality may be worsened at rest as altitude increases and that it may deteriorate further during exercise. These measurements were made using the multiple inert-gas elimination technique (53) and exploiting the fact that inert-gas exchange is not diffusion-limited, even during maximal exercise. These investigators reported that the log standard deviation of blood flow (a measure of ventilation–perfusion inequality) tended to increase at rest as the simulated altitude increased from sea level to the summit of Mt. Everest. During exercise at any barometric pressure, ventilation–perfusion inequality worsened, with the most severe impairment being seen during a maximal oxygen uptake of 1.75 liters/min at a barometric pressure of 347 torr, equivalent to an altitude of about 6300 m (20,800 ft).

In this study, it was also possible to partition the observed alveolar–arterial Po_2 difference caused by diffusion-limitation on the one hand and by ventilation–perfusion inequality on the other. The results showed that at sea level, essentially all the alveolar–arterial Po_2 difference was attributable to ventilation–perfusion inequality up to an oxygen consumption of nearly 3 liters/min; but above sea level, some diffusion-limitation apparently occurred. At a barometric pressure of 429 torr (altitude approximately 5200 m), diffusion-limitation apparently occurred when the oxygen uptake exceeded 1 liter/min. At the highest simulated altitudes (i.e., above 8000 m), almost all the observed alveolar–arterial Po_2 difference during exercise could be ascribed to diffusion-limitation.

CARDIOVASCULAR SYSTEM

Cardiac Output and Function

Compared with normoxia, acute exposure to hypoxia causes an increase in cardiac output both at rest and for a given level of exercise (54–56). The physiological value of this response is that it increases the oxygen delivery to the periphery.

In acclimatized lowlanders at high altitude, as well as in high-altitude natives, this increase in cardiac output is not seen. Instead, the relationship between cardiac output and oxygen uptake (or work rate) returns to the sea level value. This was shown by Pugh (57) and confirmed by more recent studies (58–60). The reason for the return of the cardiac output/work rate relationship to the sea level value is obscure. It should be pointed out that because of the polycythemia in well-acclimatized subjects, hemoglobin flow is increased. Nevertheless, it seems paradoxical that the body does not make use of the increase in oxygen delivery to the peripheral tissues that could be accomplished by a raised cardiac output. After all, the other great oxygen convective system, ventilation, shows an enormous increase at high altitude, as we have seen.

Although the cardiac output/work rate relationship is unchanged in acclimatized subjects at high altitude, heart rate is increased and stroke volume is correspondingly reduced. The reasons for this are unclear, although reflex activity from the carotid body and an increase in circulating catecholamines may be factors. It has been suggested that the reduced stroke volume might be related to impaired myocardial contractility. However, measurements made during Operation Everest II showed that myocardial contractility was maintained up to extremely high altitudes; indeed there was even a suggestion that it was actually improved

(60,61). The measurements were made by cardiac catheterization and two-dimensional echocardiography and showed that ventricular ejection fraction, the ratio of peak systolic pressure to end-systolic volume, and mean normalized systolic volume at rest were all sustained at a barometric pressure of 282 torr, corresponding to an altitude of about 8000 m.

These remarkable results emphasize the difference between myocardial hypoxemia and ischemia. Of course, they should not be taken to imply that a patient with coronary artery disease is not at increased risk at high altitude, although this has been suggested (62). It is difficult to think of an organ system whose function is not impaired at these extreme altitudes, and this makes it all the more remarkable that the myocardium is so tolerant to severe hypoxia.

Pulmonary Circulation

Pulmonary hypertension occurs at high altitude as a result of hypoxic pulmonary vasoconstriction (see Chapter 5.2.1.3). For example, acclimatized lowlanders increase their mean pulmonary artery pressure from about 12 to 18 torr at an altitude of 4540 m (63,64). The pressure increases considerably during exercise. In Operation Everest II, the mean pulmonary artery pressure was about 34 torr at rest at a barometric pressure of 282 torr (altitude about 8000 m), and it rose to a mean of 54 torr on exercise (65). Additional measurements of pulmonary wedge pressure and cardiac output confirmed that the pulmonary hypertension was caused by an increased pulmonary vascular resistance (Fig. 4).

An interesting feature of the Operation Everest II results was that the pulmonary vascular resistance did not return to normal when 100% oxygen was breathed.

This indicates that after only 2 or 3 weeks of hypoxia, there was a substantial degree of irreversibility of the increased pulmonary vascular resistance. Presumably, there were structural changes in the pulmonary blood vessels in addition to simple contraction of vascular smooth muscle (see Chapter 4.2.5).

PERIPHERAL TISSUES

Traditionally, the features of high-altitude acclimatization that have attracted most study have been the increase in ventilation and the development of polycythemia. However, there is increasing evidence that important changes take place at the tissue level, although naturally these are more difficult to measure. One of the first studies showing intracellular changes was that by Hurtado et al. (66); they showed that dogs born and raised in Morococha (4540 m) had increased concentrations of myoglobin in diaphragm, adductor muscles of the leg, pectoral muscles of the chest, and myocardium when compared with control dogs in Lima at sea level. More recently, it has been shown that the myoglobin concentrations in the sartorius muscle of high-altitude natives of Cerro de Pasco (4400 m) were higher than in sea level controls (67). Other studies have also shown increases in myoglobin in skeletal muscle, myocardium, and diaphragm (68–70). Thus, just as the concentration of hemoglobin in the blood increases at high altitude, so does the concentration of myoglobin in skeletal muscle. The physiological advantages of myoglobin include facilitating oxygen diffusion, buffering regional differences of P_{O_2}, and providing an oxygen store for short periods of very severe oxygen deprivation.

Another change in peripheral tissues is an increase in density of capillaries which, other things being

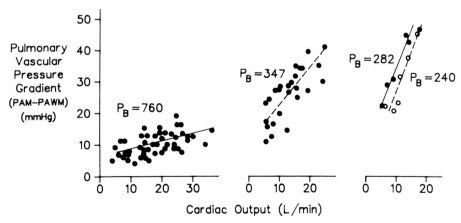

FIG. 4. Mean pulmonary artery pressure minus mean pulmonary wedge pressure plotted against cardiac output (by thermodilution) at various barometric pressures (P_B) during Operation Everest II. For the measurements at 240 torr, the subjects breathed an oxygen mixture to give an inspired P_{O_2} of 43 torr. (Modified from ref. 65.)

equal, would enhance oxygenation by reducing the diffusion pathway for oxygen. A number of early studies reported increased vascularization of the brain, retina, skeletal muscle, and liver of experimental animals exposed to low barometric pressures over several weeks (71–74). In addition, it was shown that the rate of absorption of gas from subcutaneous gas pockets in rats was increased, implying an increase in capillary number (75).

However, in skeletal muscle the consensus now seems to be that although capillary density (number of capillaries per unit volume of tissue) is increased at high altitude, this is not caused by the formation of new capillaries but by a reduction in size of the muscle fibers. For example, Banchero (76) studied four groups of guinea pigs; these included animals at sea level, animals in Denver (1610 m), animals native to the Andes (3900 m), and animals exposed to a simulated altitude of 5100 m. All the results were consistent with the increase in capillary density being caused by decrease in cross-sectional area of the fibers.

Recent results obtained from muscle biopsies in humans are in accordance with these findings in experimental animals. For example, Cerretelli obtained muscle biopsies on climbers after they had returned from an attempt to climb Lhotse Shar (8398 m) and found that although capillary density was somewhat raised, the increase could be wholly accounted by a reduction of muscle fiber size. Similar results were found in Operation Everest II. Parenthetically, the loss of muscle fiber mass at these extreme altitudes might better be regarded as an example of high-altitude deterioration rather than acclimatization.

The number of mitochondria in myocardium was reported to be higher in cattle born and raised at 4250 m than in those born and raised at sea level (77). The investigators argued that the increase in mitochondrial number was advantageous because it reduced the dif-

fusion distance of intracellular oxygen. However, in another study of mitochondrial density of myocardium of rabbits and guinea pigs, the values reported at 4330 m were similar to those reported at sea level (78). At extreme altitude the mitochondrial volume of human skeletal muscle apparently decreases, and again this can probably be explained by the muscle atrophy.

There is also evidence of changes in intracellular oxidative enzymes at high altitude. In an early study, Reynafarje (67) reported that the concentrations of three of the enzymes in the electron transport chain (NADH-oxidase, cytochrome C reductase, and NAD[P]$^+$ transhydrogenase) were higher in the biopsies of sartorius muscle of high-altitude natives from Cerro de Pasco (4400 m) than in the biopsies from residents of Lima at sea level. Since then, other investigators have confirmed increases in enzymes of the electron transport chain (and also in those of the Krebs cycle) in myocardium of various animals (77,79). However, in contrast to these findings at moderately high altitudes (3500–5000 m), measurements made on muscle biopsies taken from subjects exposed to extreme altitudes apparently showed a reduction of enzymes of both the Krebs cycle and the electron transport chain (80). Again these results may reflect the muscle atrophy which is a feature of exposure to extreme altitude.

SLEEP

Sleep is typically impaired at high altitude. Climbers frequently complain that they do not feel refreshed when they awake in the morning after a night at high altitude, and an increase in the frequency of arousals from sleep has been documented (81,82). A striking feature of sleep at high altitude is the great incidence of periodic breathing. Figure 5 shows an example obtained during the 1981 American Medical Research Ex-

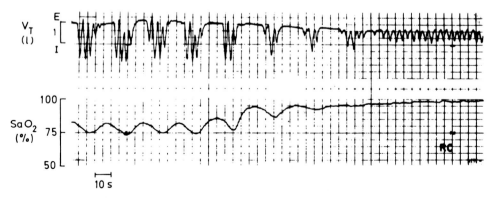

FIG. 5. Periodic breathing in a lowlander during sleep at 5400 m. Halfway through the tracing, oxygen was added to the inspired gas. This raised the arterial oxygen saturation, eliminated the apneic periods, and reduced the strength of period breathing. V_T, tidal volume; S_aO_2 arterial oxygen saturation by ear oximeter. (From ref. 83.)

pedition to Everest (83). The waxing and waning of breathing is clearly seen with apneic periods of 10–15 sec in duration. The arterial oxygen saturation (as measured by ear oximetry) fluctuated with the same frequency. Halfway through the record the subject was given 100% oxygen to breathe; this caused a rise in arterial oxygen saturation and a striking decrease in the strength of the periodic breathing.

Virtually all lowlanders develop periodic breathing at an altitude of 5400 m, but the phenomenon is seen at much lower altitudes and indeed occasionally occurs to a minor degree at sea level (84,85). Interestingly, Sherpas do not generally show periodic breathing at altitudes such as 5400 m (83), and it has been suggested that the difference in behavior is related to the Sherpas' blunted hypoxic ventilatory response. The hypothesis is that the periodic breathing in the lowlanders is related to the very high gain of the feedback system controlling ventilation as a result of the severe hypoxia. Control systems with very high gains frequently show instability. However, because Sherpas have a reduced hypoxic ventilatory response, the gain of the system is less, and as a result the instability is avoided. This may have a selective advantage because the very low values of arterial oxygen saturation which follow the apneic periods probably represent the most severe hypoxic stress of the 24-hr period (86). Administration of the carbonic anhydrase inhibitor, acetazolamide, reduces periodic breathing at high altitude (87,88).

OTHER PHYSIOLOGICAL CHANGES

Reference has already been made to the muscle atrophy which is a striking feature of residence at extreme altitude (5800 m and above). For example, during the 1960–1961 Himalayan Scientific and Mountaineering Expedition, the wintering party had ample food and a relatively normal lifestyle but suffered a relentless loss of weight, which averaged 0.5 to 1.5 kg/week (20). Reduction of appetite may play a role in the weight loss, but during that study, measurements of calorie intake showed that these were adequate for the degree of physical activity. There is evidence of impaired gastrointestinal absorption at high altitude, including reduced xylose and fat absorption (89). However, it is likely that there is some fundamental change in muscle protein metabolism at high altitude. Acute hypoxia, which occurs at an altitude of 4550 m, has been shown to result in a net loss of amino acids from human muscles, probably due to fall in muscle protein synthesis (90).

There is good evidence of impaired fluid balance at high altitude. Trekkers sometimes develop marked peripheral edema including swelling of the periorbital tissues, hands, and feet, and the diseases of high altitude

include pulmonary edema and cerebral edema (see below). There are several reports of suppression of aldosterone at high altitude (91–94). However, studies of the effects of altitude on plasma renin activity have given conflicting results. Preliminary results from a study of atrial natriuretic peptide in humans have shown a rise on ascent to high altitude (95). There is also evidence of (a) stimulation of the adrenal cortex by adrenocorticotropic hormone (ACTH) and (b) increased cortisol excretion. Increased catecholamines have been reported (96–98), and exercise exaggerates this rise. The increase is chiefly due to noradrenaline.

Thyroid activity is increased in humans at high altitude. Elevated levels of thyroxine-binding globulin and free T4 (thyroxine) have been reported (99). Exercise at high altitude increases both T3 (triiodothyronine) and T4 to a greater extent than does exercise at sea level. The basal metabolic rate (BMR) is elevated during the first 2 weeks at moderate altitude, and this correlates with the free T4 level (100). At higher altitudes (above 5500 m), BMR remains elevated for months (101) as does T4 (102). Goiter is common in mountainous regions primarily because of iodine deficiency, although, as indicated above, altitude hypoxia stimulates thyroid function.

Fasting blood glucose is lower in subjects acclimatized to high altitude than in those acclimatized to sea level (103–105), and the rise in both blood glucose and insulin levels following glucose loading is less at high altitude (103,105). The reasons are not clear; however, glucose may be absorbed less rapidly above 5500 m, and liver glycogen synthesis may be enhanced at high altitude (106). There are reports of reductions in testosterone and luteinizing hormone at 3500 m (107). Renal function appears to be maintained up to altitudes of 5800 m as measured by the ability to concentrate urine, eliminate a water load, and respond appropriately to ingestion of bicarbonate or ammonium chloride (36). However, as indicated above, it appears that metabolic compensation for respiratory alkalosis is very slow at extreme altitude.

There is evidence of impairment of central nervous system (CNS) function at very high altitude; more remarkably, there is residual impairment when climbers return to sea level. For example, following the 1981 American Research Expedition to Everest, both short-term memory and a test of manipulative skill (finger tapping) showed changes after the expedition as compared with before. Short-term memory returned over the next 12 months, but the finger-tapping test remained abnormal in most members of the expedition for at least a year (108). Interestingly, the climbers with the highest hypoxic ventilatory response developed the most severe CNS changes, possibly because the greater decrease in arterial P_{CO_2} caused more severe cerebral vasoconstriction and therefore greater cerebral hypoxia.

ACUTE MOUNTAIN SICKNESS

Newcomers to high altitude frequently develop a syndrome characterized by headache, fatigue, dizziness, palpitations, nausea, loss of appetite, and insomnia. A very early description was given by Acosta in 1590 (109), and a particularly detailed account was given by Ravenhill in 1913 (110). The lowest altitude at which some individuals are affected is about 2500 m (8200 ft), and an incidence of 43% in trekkers at an altitude of 4343 (14,300 ft) was reported (111). Frequently, there is a period of some 6–12 hr before symptoms occur, though this may be longer. The condition is most severe on the second or third day after ascent, and by the fourth or fifth day, recovery is usually complete. Physical examination often reveals crackles in the chest, some peripheral edema, and, occasionally, retinal hemorrhages (111).

The etiology of acute mountain sickness is poorly understood. Presumably, the underlying cause is hypoxia, possibly complicated by the hypocapnia and respiratory alkalosis. People whose ventilation increases most at high altitude seem to be less at risk (112,113). The role of hypocapnia is uncertain, but in a hypobaric chamber study, adding carbon dioxide to the inspired gas exaggerated the symptoms, possibly because of the increased cerebral blood flow (114).

It is tempting to link acute mountain sickness with some abnormality of fluid balance. The signs of crackles in the chest and peripheral edema suggest this, and the headache (which is often the most prominent symptom) may be due to mild cerebral edema. The two major complications of acute mountain sickness—high-altitude pulmonary edema and high-altitude cerebral edema—are presumably related to abnormal fluid control. Trekkers and soldiers who gain weight at high altitude because of an antidiuresis are more prone to develop acute mountain sickness (112,115). However, there is apparently no increase in antidiuretic hormone (ADH) in patients with acute mountain sickness (116,117).

The renin–aldosterone system may play a role. As indicated earlier, ascent to high altitude usually reduces aldosterone levels (91–94). However, exercise stimulates the release of renin, which, in turn, via angiotensin, stimulates aldosterone release, and this may cause salt and water retention. A correlation among acute mountain sickness symptoms scores, aldosterone levels, and reduced 24-hr urine sodium output has been reported (118). However, other investigators have found lower aldosterone concentrations in subjects with acute mountain sickness (119).

There is a tremendous variation in individual vulnerability to acute mountain sickness. Physical fitness at sea level is no guarantee of immunity. There is some evidence that young people are more at risk than are the elderly (120). It is clear that rate of ascent is an important factor. A suggested rule of thumb is that above 3000 m (about 10,000 ft), each night should be spent not more than 300 m (about 1,000 ft) above the last, with a rest day (two nights at the same altitude) every 2 or 3 days. In addition, anyone who experiences symptoms of acute mountain sickness should go no higher until he or she improves. Sometimes descent is the only sensible option.

The carbonic anhydrase inhibitor, acetazolamide (Diamox), has been shown to reduce the incidence of acute mountain sickness in double-blind trials in the field (121–123). In addition, this drug improves sleep and helps to prevent the severe oxygen desaturation associated with periodic breathing (87). One or two 250-mg tablets per day are sufficient; a slow-release form of the drug is available. Side effects include paresthesia of the fingers and toes, and some people have gastric upsets. Carbonated drinks such as beer taste flat. In most studies the drug has been taken for a day prior to ascent, but recent reports suggest that it is valuable if taken when the symptoms develop. Dexamethasone (124) and spironolactone (125) have also been reported to reduce the incidence of acute mountain sickness.

As indicated above, the condition is usually self-limiting. If symptoms persist, the best treatment is descent. Dexamethasone is useful for the emergency treatment of the condition (126), and aspirin may relieve the headache. Inhalation of 3% carbon dioxide in air has been shown to reduce symptoms (127), presumably through the increase in arterial P_{O_2} caused by the hyperventilation.

HIGH-ALTITUDE PULMONARY EDEMA

This potentially fatal condition is often regarded as a complication of acute mountain sickness, but it may develop with few, if any, of the symptoms described above. A typical history is as follows. The subject ascends rapidly to high altitude and is very active in getting there (or very active on arrival). He or she becomes increasingly short of breath and fatigued and may develop a dry cough. Orthopnea is common. The physical signs include tachypnea, tachycardia, and crackles at the lung bases. The condition may progress until he or she coughs up copious pink frothy sputum and dies.

The incidence of high-altitude pulmonary edema is difficult to determine because it depends on rate of ascent and altitude. Hackett and Rennie (120) found seven cases in 278 trekkers to Pheriche (4234 m, or 13,900 ft) on their way to the Everest Base Camp. This is an incidence of 2.5%. However, lower incidences have been reported in other studies.

The etiology of high-altitude pulmonary edema is not fully understood and is presently an area of active investigation. Several studies by cardiac catheterization have shown high pulmonary artery pressures, up to 144 torr systolic (128). This indicates that the patients have severe hypoxic pulmonary vasoconstriction. However, the pulmonary artery wedge pressure is normal (128–131). This implies that pulmonary capillary pressure is not raised as a result of an increase in pulmonary venous pressure, contrary to what occurs in left ventricular failure.

An interesting hypothesis was put forward by Hultgren (132), who suggested that the pulmonary vasoconstriction that occurs in response to the alveolar hypoxia is uneven. As a result, those capillaries that are not protected from the high pulmonary artery pressure by arteriolar constriction are exposed to very high pressures and leak fluid. The fact that the radiographic appearance of the edema is often patchy is consistent with this hypothesis. In addition, Hackett et al. (133) reported four cases of high-altitude pulmonary edema at modest altitudes (2000–3000 m) where there was a congenital absence of the right pulmonary artery. This diversion of all the blood flow through one lung would exaggerate the effect of any hypoxic pulmonary vasoconstriction.

However, Hackett et al. (134) and Schoene et al. (135) have made the surprising observation that the alveolar fluid has a very high protein content. The fluid was obtained by enterprisingly bronchoscoping climbers with high-altitude pulmonary edema on Mt. McKinley. At first sight, it is difficult to reconcile this high permeability type of edema with an increased pulmonary capillary pressure. However, recent work in our laboratory has shown that when the pulmonary capillary pressure is raised to 40 torr in anesthetized rabbits, disruption of capillary endothelial and alveolar epithelial cells occurs (136). This observation prompted an analysis of the mechanical stresses to which the capillaries are subjected, and these were shown to be extremely high, indeed as high as in the normal human aorta wall (137). The cellular disruption would explain the high-protein pulmonary edema. Thus, our conclusion is that the mechanism of high-altitude pulmonary edema is stress failure of pulmonary capillaries when their pressure rises to high values.

Rapid ascent and heavy exercise appear to be risk factors, although the condition can certainly occur in the absence of hard physical exertion. The best treatment by far is rapid descent, and often a reduction of altitude of as little as 300 m (about 1000 ft) may result

in a dramatic improvement. Oxygen should be given if it is available, but often the relief is only partial and the patient may continue to deteriorate. Diuretics such as furosemide should be used with caution because these patients are often dehydrated. Positive airway pressure may give temporary respite. An interesting recent development is the Gamow bag, in which the patient is placed and exposed to increased pressure by means of a foot pump. This is equivalent to a rapid descent of altitude.

HIGH-ALTITUDE CEREBRAL EDEMA

Some patients with acute mountain sickness progress to this much more serious condition characterized by photophobia, ataxia, hallucinations, clouding of consciousness, coma, and eventually death. Examination of the retina usually shows papilledema; also, there may be concurrent evidence of high-altitude pulmonary edema, though not always. It is often difficult to identify the point at which severe acute mountain sickness progresses to high-altitude cerebral edema.

Lumbar puncture usually shows an increased pressure (138), and computerized tomography reveals evidence of cerebral edema (139). Autopsy findings confirm the presence of cerebral edema with swollen, flattened gyri, compression of the sulci, and, frequently, widespread petechial hemorrhages (138,140, 141).

The incidence of the condition is less than that of high-altitude pulmonary edema but is difficult to determine accurately. The precise etiology is unclear but may be related to the increased cerebral blood flow caused by the hypoxia, resulting in cerebral vasodilatation (see Chapter 5.5.3.2). The most important aspect of treatment is rapid descent; oxygen should be given if this is available.

High-altitude retinal hemorrhage is a related condition. Frayser et al. (142) found retinal hemorrhages in 35% of subjects flown to 5330 m (17,500 ft). Usually, the hemorrhages are multiple and are near vessels; often they are flame-shaped. There is generally no interference with vision unless the hemorrhage is near the optic disk. Recovery occurs on descent. The condition is presumably caused by the greatly increased retinal blood flow; measurements have shown this to be increased by 105% (142).

CHRONIC MOUNTAIN SICKNESS

This is sometimes known as Monge's disease; it was named after Carlos Monge, who described the condition in Peru. Long-term residents of high altitude sometimes develop an ill-defined syndrome characterized by fatigue, reduced exercise tolerance, headache, dizziness, somnolence, loss of mental acuity, marked polycythemia, and severe hypoxemia. The combination of severe oxygen desaturation and polycythemia results in a dramatic cyanotic appearance. The most striking findings are an increased red blood cell count, hemoglobin saturation, hematocrit with hemoglobin concentrations as high as 28 g/dl, and hematocrits of up to 83% (143). There is no increase in white blood cells. Blood gases show a lower arterial P_{O_2} and higher arterial P_{CO_2} than the rest of the population at the same altitude. The reduced arterial P_{O_2} is caused by a relative hypoventilation, and the resulting tissue hypoxia is presumably responsible for increased red blood cell production. Because of the very high hematocrit, the viscosity of the blood is greatly increased and this is presumably a factor in the high pulmonary artery pressures that are found. Right ventricular hypertrophy occurs, along with appropriate electrocardiographic changes.

A feature of the condition is that the symptoms and signs regress when the patient goes to a lower altitude. However, often this is not possible for economic reasons, and venesection has been shown to be beneficial. This improves exercise performance (in some patients) (26), pulmonary gas exchange (144), and many of the neuropsychological symptoms.

Patients with chronic mountain sickness have been shown to have a low hypoxic ventilatory response when compared with healthy controls at the same altitude (14). However, it is not clear whether these patients represent a clearly defined subset of highlanders or whether they are simply at the bottom of the normal distribution. In early studies of chronic mountain sickness, many of the patients were miners and there was controversy about whether the hypoxemia and polycythemia were secondary to lung disease. However, it is now established that the condition can exist in patients with essentially normal lungs.

REFERENCES

1. Ward MP, Milledge JS, West JB. *High altitude medicine and physiology.* London: Chapman & Hall Medical, 1989.
2. Zuntz N, Loewy A, Muller F, Caspari W. Atmospheric pressure at high altitudes. In: *Hohenklima und Bergwanderungen in ihrer Wirkung auf den Menschen.* Berlin: Bong, 1906;37–39. Translation of relevant pages. In: West JB, ed. *High altitude physiology* Stroudsburg, PA: Hutchinson Ross, 1981.
3. FitzGerald MP. The changes in the breathing and the blood of various altitudes. *Philos Trans R Soc Lond Ser B* 1913;203:351–371.
4. International Civil Aviation Organization. *Manual of the ICAO standard atmosphere,* 2nd ed. Montreal, Quebec: International Civil Aviation Organization, 1964.
5. Pugh LGCE. Resting ventilation and alveolar air on Mt. Everest: with remarks on the relation of barometric pressure to altitude in mountains. *J Physiol (Lond)* 1957;135:590–610.
6. West JB, Lahiri S, Maret KH, Peters RM Jr, Pizzo CJ. Barometric pressures at extreme altitudes on Mt. Everest: phys-

iological significance. *J Appl Physiol: Respir Environ Exercise Physiol* 1983;54:1188–1194.
7. West JB. Climbing Mt. Everest without supplementary oxygen: an analysis of maximal exercise during extreme hypoxia. *Respir Physiol* 1983;52:265–279.
8. Hurtado A. Animals in high altitudes: resident man. In: Dill DB, ed. *Handbook of physiology, Section 4: Adaptation to the environment.* Washington, DC: American Physiological Society, 1964, 843–860.
9. Rahn H, Otis AB. Man's respiratory response during and after acclimatization to high altitude. *Am J Physiol* 1949;157:445–449.
10. Barnard P, Andronikou S, Pokorski M, Smatresk N, Mokashi A, Lahiri S. Time-dependent effect of hypoxia on carotid body chemosensory function. *J Appl Physiol* 1987;63:685–691.
11. Schoene RB, Lahiri S, Hackett PH, Peters RM Jr, Milledge JS, Pizzo CJ, Sarnquist FH, Boyer SJ, Graber DJ, Maret KH, West JB. Relationship of hypoxic ventilatory response to exercise performance on Mount Everest. *J Appl Physiol: Respir Environ Exercise Physiol* 1984;56:1478–1483.
12. Musuyama S, Kimura H, Sugita T, Kuriyama T, Tatsumi K, Kunitomo F, Okita S, Tojima H, Yuguchi Y, Watanabe S, Honda Y. Control of ventilation in extreme-altitude climbers. *J Appl Physiol* 1986;61:500–506.
13. Oelz O, Howald H, diPrampero PE, Hoppeler H, Claassen H, Jenni R, Bühlmann A, Ferretti G, Bruckner JC, Veicsteinas A, Gussoni M, Certetelli P. Physiological profile of world-class high-altitude climbers. *J Appl Physiol* 1986;60:1734–1742.
14. Severinghaus JW, Bainton CR, Carcelen A. Respiratory insensitivity to hypoxia in chronically hypoxic man. *Respir Physiol* 1966;1:308–334.
15. Lahiri S, Milledge JS. Sherpa physiology. *Nature* 1965;207:10–12.
16. Milledge JS, Lahiri S. Respiratory control in lowlanders and Sherpa highlanders at altitude. *Respir Physiol* 1967;2:310–322.
17. Edelman NH, Lahiri S, Bruado L, Cherniack NS, Fishman AP. The blunted ventilatory response to hypoxia in cyanotic congenital heart disease. *N Engl J Med* 1970;282:405–411.
18. Weil JV, Byrne-Quinn E, Sodal IE, Filley GF, Grover RF. Acquired attenuation of chemoreceptor function in chronically hypoxic man at high altitude. *J Clin Invest* 1971;50:186–195.
19. Lahiri S, Delaney RG, Brody JS, Simpser M, Velasquez T, Motoyama EK, Polgar C. Relative role of environmental and genetic factors in respiratory adaptation to high altitude. *Nature* 1976;261:133–135.
20. Pugh LGCE. Animals in high altitudes: man above 5000 m—mountain exploration. In: Dill DB, Adolph EF, Wilber CG, eds. *Handbook of physiology, Section 4.* Washington, DC: American Physiological Society, 1964, 861–868.
21. Milledge JS, Cotes PM. Serum erythropoietin in humans at high altitude and its relation to plasma renin. *J Appl Physiol* 1985;59:360–364.
22. Abbrecht PH, Littell JK. Plasma erythropoietin in men and mice during acclimatization to different altitudes. *J Appl Physiol* 1964;32:54–58.
23. Merino CF. The plasma erythropoietic factor in the polycythemia of high altitude. In: Report 56-103 to Air Force University School of Aviation Medicine, USAF, Randolph AFB, Texas, 1956;103.
24. Pugh LGCE. Blood volume and haemoglobin concentration at altitudes above 18000 ft (5500 m). *J Appl Physiol* 1964;170:344–354.
25. Sarnquist FH, Schoene RB, Hackett PH, Townes BD. Hemodilution of polycythemic mountaineers: effects on exercise and mental function. *Aviat Space Environ Med* 1986;57:313–317.
26. Winslow RM, Monge CC. *Hypoxia, polycythemia, and chronic mountain sickness.* Washington, DC: Johns Hopkins University Press, 1987;184–196.
27. Winslow RM, Samaja M, West JB. Red cell function at extreme altitude on Mount Everest. *J Appl Physiol: Respir Environ Exercise Physiol* 1984;56:109–116.
28. Winslow RM, Monge CC, Statham JJ, Gibson CG, Charache S, Whittembury J, Moran O, Berger RL. Variability of oxygen

affinity of blood: human subjects native to high altitude. *J Appl Physiol* 1981;51:1411–1416.

29. Eaton JW, Skeleton TD, Berger E. Survival at extreme altitude: protective effect of increased hemoglobin–oxygen affinity. *Science* 1974;183:743–744.

30. Turek Z, Kruezer F, Ringnalda BEM. Blood gases at several levels of oxygenation in rats with a left shifted blood oxygen dissociation curve. *Pflügers Arch* 1978;376:7–13.

31. Hebbel RP, Eaton JW, Kronenberg RS, Zanjani ED, Moore LG, Berger EM. Human llamas: adaptation to altitude in subjects with high hemoglobin oxygen affinity. *J Clin Invest* 1978;62:593–600.

32. Bencowitz HZ, Wagner PD, West JB. Effect of change in P50 on exercise tolerance at high altitude: a theoretical study. *J Appl Physiol: Respir Environ Exercise Physiol* 1982;53:1487–1495.

33. Turek Z, Kreuzer F, Hoofd LJC. Advantage or disadvantage of a decrease of blood oxygen affinity for tissue oxygen supply at hypoxia: a theoretical study comparing man and rat. *Pflügers Arch* 1973;342:185–197.

34. Hall FG, Dill DB, Guzman-Barron ES. Comparative physiology at high altitudes. *J Cell Comp Physiol* 1936;8:301–313.

35. Blume FD, Boyer SJ, Braverman E, Cohen A, Dirkse J, Mordes JP. Impaired osmoregulation at high altitude. *JAMA* 1984;252:524–526.

36. Pugh LGCE. Physiological and medical aspects of the Himalayan scientific and mountaineering expedition 1960–61. *Br Med J* 1962;2:621–633.

37. Kreuzer F, Van Lookeren, Campagne P. Resting pulmonary diffusing capacity for CO and O_2 at high altitude. *J Appl Physiol* 1965;20:519–524.

38. DeGraff AC, Grover RF, Johnson RL, Hammond JW, Miller JM. Diffusing capacity of the lung in Caucasians native to 3100 m. *J Appl Physiol* 1970;29:71–76.

39. Dempsey JA, Reddan WG, Birnbaum ML, Forster HV, Thoden JS, Grover RF, Rankin J. Effects of acute through lifelong hypoxic exposure on exercise pulmonary gas exchange. *Respir Physiol* 1971;13:62–89.

40. Guleria JS, Pande JN, Sethi PK, Roy SB. Pulmonary diffusing capacity at high altitude. *J Appl Physiol* 1971;31:536–543.

41. West JB. Diffusing capacity of the lung for carbon monoxide at high altitude. *J Appl Physiol* 1962;17:421–426.

42. Remmers JE, Mithoefer JC. The carbon monoxide diffusing capacity in permanent residents at high altitudes. *Respir Physiol* 1962;43:357–364.

43. Barcroft J, Binger CA, Bock AV, Doggart JH, Forbes HS, Harrop G, Meakins JC, Redfield AC. Observations upon the effect of high altitude on the physiological processes of the human body, carried out in the Peruvian Andes, chiefly at Cerro de Pasco. *Philos Trans R Soc Ser B* 1923;211:351–480.

44. Burri PH, Weibel ER. Morphometric estimation of pulmonary diffusion capacity. II. Effect of environmental P_{O_2} on the growing lung. *Respir Physiol* 1971;11:247–264.

45. Bartlett D Jr, Remmers JE. Effects of high altitude exposure on the lungs of young rats. *Respir Physiol* 1971;13:116–125.

46. West JB, Lahiri S, Gill MB, Milledge JS, Pugh LGCE, Ward MP. Arterial oxygen saturation during exercise at high altitude. *J Appl Physiol* 1962;17:617–621.

47. West JB, Boyer SJ, Graber DJ, Hackett PH, Maret KH, Milledge JS, Peters RM Jr, Pizzo CJ, Samaja M, Sarnquist FH, Schoene RB, Winslow RM. Maximal exercise at extreme altitudes on Mount Everest. *J Appl Physiol: Respir Environ Exercise Physiol* 1983;55:688–698.

48. Wagner PD, Sutton JR, Reeves JT, Cymerman A, Groves BM, Malconian MK. Operation Everest II. Pulmonary gas exchange throughout a simulated ascent of Mt. Everest. *J Appl Physiol* 1987;63:2348–2359.

49. West JB, Wagner PD. Predicted gas exchange on the summit of Mt. Everest. *Resp Physiol* 1980;42:1–16.

50. West JB, Hackett PH, Maret KH, Milledge JS, Peters RM Jr, Pizzo CJ, Winslow RM. Pulmonary gas exchange on the summit of Mt. Everest. *J Appl Physiol: Respir Environ Exercise Physiol* 1983;55:678–687.

51. Piiper J, Scheid P. Blood–gas equilibration in lungs. In: West JB, ed. *Pulmonary gas exchange, vol 1: Ventilation, blood flow, and diffusion.* New York: Academic Press, 1980;131–171.

52. Dawson A. Regional lung function during early acclimatization to 3100 m altitude. *J Appl Physiol* 1972;33:218–223.

53. Wagner PD, Saltzman HA, West JB. Measurement of continuous distributions of ventilation–perfusion ratios: theory. *J Appl Physiol* 1974;36:588–599.

54. Asmussen E, Consolazio FC. The circulation in rest and work on Mount Evans (4300 m). *Am J Physiol* 1941;32:555–563.

55. Kontos HA, Levasseur JE, Richardson DW, Page Mauck H Jr, Patterson JL Jr. Comparative circulatory responses to systemic hypoxia in man and in unanesthetized dog. *J Appl Physiol* 1967;23:381–386.

56. Vogel JA, Harris CW. Cardiopulmonary responses of resting man during early exposure to high altitude. *J Appl Physiol* 1967;22:1124–1128.

57. Pugh LGCE. Cardiac output in muscular exercise at 5,800 m (19,000 ft). *J Appl Physiol* 1964;19:441–447.

58. Cerretelli P. Limiting factors to oxygen transport on Mt. Everest. *J Appl Physiol* 1976;40:658–667.

59. Vogel JA, Hartley LH, Cruz JC. Cardiac output during exercise in altitude natives at sea level and high altitude. *J Appl Physiol* 1974;36:173–176.

60. Reeves JT, Groves BM, Sutton JR, Wagner PD, Cymerman A, Malconian MK, Rock PB, Young PM, Houston CS. Operation Everest II: preservation of cardiac function at extreme altitude. *J Appl Physiol* 1987;63:531–539.

61. Suarez J, Alexander JK, Houston CS. Enhanced left ventricular systolic performance at high altitude during Operation Everest II. *Am J Cardiol* 1987;60:137–142.

62. Rennie D. Will mountains trekkers have heart attacks? *JAMA* 1989;261:1045–1046.

63. Rotta A, Canepa A, Hurtado A, Velasquez T, Chavez R. Pulmonary circulation at sea level and at high altitudes. *J Appl Physiol* 1956;9:328–336.

64. Sime F, Pe aloza D, Ruiz L, Gonzales N, Covarrubias E, Postigo R. Hypoxemia, pulmonary hypertension, and low cardiac output in newcomers at low altitude. *J Appl Physiol* 1974;36:561–571.

65. Groves BM, Reeves JT, Sutton JR, Wagner PD, Cymerman A, Malconian MK, Rock PB, Young PM, Houston CS. Operation Everest II: elevated high-altitude pulmonary resistance unresponsive to oxygen. *J Appl Physiol* 1987;63:521–530.

66. Hurtado A, Rotta A, Merino C. Studies of myohemoglobin at high altitudes. *Am J Med Sci* 1937;194:708–713.

67. Reynafarje B. Myoglobin content and enzymatic activity of muscle and altitude adaptation. *J Appl Physiol* 1962;17:301–305.

68. Clark RT Jr, Criscuolo D, Coulson DK. Effects of 20,000 feet simulated altitude on myoglobin content of animals with and without exercise. *Fed Proc* 1952;11:25.

69. Vaughan BE, Pace N. Changes in myoglobin content of the high altitude acclimatized rat. *Am J Physiol* 1956;185:549–556.

70. Tappan DV, Reynafarje BD. Tissue pigment manifestation of adaptation to high altitudes. *Am J Physiol* 1957;190:99–103.

71. Mercker H, Schneider M. ber Capillarveranderungen des Gehirns bei Hohenanpassung. *Pflügers Arch* 1949;251:49–55.

72. Opitz E. Increased vascularization of the tissue due to acclimatization to high altitude and its significance for oxygen transport. *Exp Med Surg* 1951;9:389–403.

73. Valdivia E. Total capillary bed in striated muscle of guinea pigs native to the Peruvian mountains. *Am J Physiol* 1958;194:585–589.

74. Cassin SR, Gilbert D, Bunnell CF, Johnson EM. Capillary development during exposure to chronic hypoxia. *Am J Physiol* 1971;220:448–451.

75. Tenney SM, Ou LC. Physiological evidence for increased tissue capillarity in rats acclimatized to high altitude. *Respir Physiol* 1970;8:137–150.

76. Banchero N. Long-term adaptation of skeletal muscle capillarity. *Physiologist* 1982;25:385–389.

77. Ou LC, Tenney SM. Properties of mitochondria from hearts of cattle acclimatized to high altitude. *Respir Physiol* 1970;8:151–159.

78. Kearney MS. Ultrastructural changes in the heart at high altitude. *Pathol Microbiol* 1973;39:258–265.

79. Harris P, Castillo Y, Gibson K, Heath D, Arias-Stella J. Succinic and lactic dehydrogenase activity in myocardial homogenates from animals at high and low altitude. *J Mol Cell Cardiol* 1970;1:189–193.

80. Green HJ, Sutton J, Young P, Cymerman A, Houston CS. Operation Everest II: muscle energetics during maximal exhaustive exercise. *J Appl Physiol* 1989;66:142–150.

81. Reite M, Jackson D, Cahoon RL, Weil JV. Sleep physiology at high altitude. *Electroencephalogr Clin Neurophysiol* 1975;38:463–471.

82. Weil JV, Kryger MH, Scoggin CH. Sleep and breathing at high altitude. In: Guilleminault C, Dement W, eds. *Sleep apnea syndromes.* New York: Alan R Liss, 1978, 119–136.

83. Lahiri S, Barnard P. Role of arterial chemoreflexes in breathing during sleep at high altitude. In: Sutton JS, Houston CS, Jones NL, eds. *Hypoxia, exercise, and altitude.* New York: Alan R Liss, 1983, 75–85.

84. Lenfant C. Time-dependent variations of pulmonary gas exchange in normal men at rest. *J Appl Physiol* 1967;22:675–684.

85. Priban I. An analysis of some short term patterns of breathing in man at rest. *J Appl Physiol* 1963;166:425–434.

86. West JB, Peters RM Jr, Aksnes G, Maret KH, Milledge JS, Schoene RB. Nocturnal periodic breathing at altitudes of 6300 m and 8050 meters. *J Appl Physiol* 1986;61:280–287.

87. Sutton JR, Houston CS, Mansell AL, McFadden M, Hackett P, Powles CP. Effect of acetazolamide on hypoxemia during sleep at high altitude. *N Engl J Med* 1979;301:1329–1331.

88. Hackett PH, Roach RC, Harrison GL, Schoene RB, Mills WJ Jr. Respiratory stimulants and sleep periodic breathing at high altitude. *Am Rev Respir Dis* 1987;135:896–898.

89. Boyer SJ, Blume FD. Weight loss and changes in body composition at high altitude. *J Appl Physiol: Respir Environ Exercise Physiol* 1984;57:1580–1585.

90. Rennie MJ, Babij P, Sutton JR, Tonkins WJ, Read W, Ford C, Haliday D. Effects of acute hypoxia on forearm leucine metabolism. In: Sutton JR, Houston CS, Jones NL, eds. *Hypoxia, exercise and altitude.* New York: Alan R Liss, 1983.

91. Williams ES. Salivary electrolyte composition at high altitude. *Clin Sci* 1961;21:37–42.

92. Tuffley RE, Rubenstein D, Slater JDH, Williams ES. Serum renin activity during exposure to hypoxia. *J Endocrinol* 1970;48:497–510.

93. Sutton JR, Viol GW, Gray GW, McFadden M, Keane PM. Renin, aldosterone, electrolyte, and cortisol responses to hypoxic decompression. *J Appl Physiol: Respir Environ Exercise Physiol* 1977;43:421–424.

94. Milledge JS, Catley DM, Ward MP, Williams ES, Clarke CRA. Renin-aldosterone and angiotensin-converting enzyme during prolonged altitude exposure. *J Appl Physiol: Respir Environ Exercise Physiol* 1983;55:699–702.

95. Milledge JS, Beeley JM, McArthur S, Morice AH. Atrial natriuretic peptide, altitude and acute mountain sickness. *Clin Sci* 1989;77:509–514.

96. Cunningham WL, Becker EJ, Kreuzer F. Catecholamines in plasma and urine at high altitude. *J Appl Physiol* 1965;20:607–610.

97. Pace N, Griswold RL, Grunbaum BW. Increase in urinary norepinephrine excretion during 14 days sojourn at 3800 m elevation [Abstract]. *Fed Proc* 1964;23:521.

98. Maher JT, Jones LG, Hartley LH, Williams GH, Rose LI. Aldosterone dynamics during graded exercise at sea level and high altitude. *J Appl Physiol* 1975;39:18–22.

99. Surks MI. Elevated PBI, free thyroxine, and plasma protein concentration in man at high altitude. *J Appl Physiol* 1966;21:1185–1190.

100. Stock MJ, Morgan NG, Ferro-Luzzi A, Evans E. Effect of altitude on dietary-induced thermogenesis at rest and during light exercise in man. *J Appl Physiol: Respir Environ Exercise Physiol* 1978;45:345–349.

101. Gill MB, Pugh LGCE. Basal metabolism and respiration in men living at 5800 m (1900 ft). *J Appl Physiol* 1964;19:949–954.

102. Mordes JP, Blume FD, Boyer S, Zheng M, Braverman LE. High altitude pituitary–thyroid dysfunction on Mount Everest. *N Engl J Med* 1983;308:1135–1138.

103. Stock MJ, Chapman C, Stirling JL, Campbell IT. Effects of exercise, altitude, and food on blood hormone and metabolite levels. *J Appl Physiol: Respir Environ Exercise Physiol* 1987;45:350–354.

104. Blume FD, Pace N. Effect of translocation to 3800 m altitude on glycolysis in mice. *J Appl Physiol* 1967;23:75–79.

105. Blume FD. Metabolic and endocrine changes at altitude. In: West JB, Lahiri S, eds. *High altitude and man.* Bethesda, MD: American Physiological Society, 1984.

106. Blume FD, Pace N. The utilization of ^{14}C-labeled palmitic acid, alanine and aspartic acid at high altitude. *Environ Physiol* 1971;1:30–36.

107. Sawhney RC, Chabra PC, Malhotra AS, Singh T, Riar SS, Rai RM. Hormone profiles at hugh altitude in man. *Andrologia* 1985;17:178–184.

108. Townes BD, Hornbein TF, Schoene RM, Sarnquist FH, Grant I. Human cerebral function at extreme altitude. In: West JB, Lahiri S, eds. *High altitude and man.* Washington, DC: American Physiological Society, 1984, 31–36.

109. Acosta J de. *Historia Natural y Moral de las Indias.* Iuan de Leon, Seville, Lib. 3, Cap. 9, 1590.

110. Ravenhill TH. Some experiences of mountain sickness in the Andes. *J Trop Med Hyg* 1913;16:314–320.

111. Hackett PH, Rennie D. Rales, peripheral edema, retinal hemorrhage and acute mountain sickness. *Am J Med* 1979;67:214–218.

112. Hackett PH, Rennie D, Hofmeister SE, Grover RF, Grover EB, Reeves JT. Fluid retention and relative hypoventilation in acute mountain sickness. *Respiration* 1982;43:321–329.

113. Hu ST, Huang WY, Chu SC, Pa CF. Chemoreflexive ventilatory response at sea level in subjects with past history of good acclimatization and severe acute mountain sickness. In: Brendel W, Zink RA, eds. *High altitude physiology and medicine.* New York: Springer-Verlag, 1982.

114. Maher JT, Cymerman A, Reeves JA, Cruz JC, Denniston JC, Grover RF. Acute mountain sickness: increased severity in eucapnic hypoxia. *Aviat Space Environ Med* 1975;46:826–829.

115. Singh I, Khanna PK, Srivastava MC, Lal M, Roy SB, Subramanyam CSV. Acute mountain sickness. *N Engl J Med* 1969;280:175–184.

116. Hackett PH, Forsling ML, Milledge J, Rennie D. Release of vasopressin in man at altitude. *Horm Metab Res* 1978;10:571.

117. Harber MJ, Williams JD, Morton JJ. Antidiuretic hormone excretion at high altitude. *Aviat Space Environ Med* 1981;52:38–40.

118. Milledge JS, Beeley JM, McArthur S, Morice AH. Atrial natriuretic peptide and acute mountain sickness. *Clin Sci* 1988;75:26.

119. Hogan RP, Kotchen TA, Boyd AE, Hartley LH. Effect of altitude on the renin–aldosterone system and metabolism of water and electrolytes. *J Appl Physiol* 1973;35:385–390.

120. Hackett PH, Rennie D. Rales, peripheral edema, retinal hemorrhage and acute mountain sickness. *Am J Med* 1979;67:214–218.

121. Forwand SA, Landowne M, Follansbee JN, Hansen JE. Effect of acetazolamide on acute mountain sickness. *N Engl J Med* 1968;279:839–845.

122. Birmingham Medical Research Expeditionary Society Mountain Sickness Study Group. Acetazolamide in control of acute mountain sickness. *Lancet* 1981;1:180–183.

123. Larsen EB, Roach KRC, Schoene RB, Hornbein TF. Acute mountain sickness and acetazolamide. Clinical efficacy and effect on ventilation. *JAMA* 1982;248:328–332.

124. Johnson TS, Rock PB, Fulco CS, Trad LA, Spark RF, Maher JT. Prevention of acute mountain sickness by dexamethasone. *N Engl J Med* 1984;310:683–686.

125. Currie TT, Carter PH, Champion WL, Fong G, Francis JK, McDonald IH, Newing RK, Nunn IN, Sisson RN, Sussex MK, Zacharin RF. Spironolactone and acute mountain sickness. *Med J Aust* 1976;2:168–170.

126. Ferrazzini G, Maggiorini M, Kriemler S, Bartsch P, Oelz O.

Successful treatment of acute mountain sickness with dexamethasone. *Br Med J* 1987;294:1380–1382.

127. Harvey TC, Raichle ME, Winterborn MH, Jensen J, Lassen NA, Richardson NV, Bradwell AR. Effect of carbon dioxide in acute mountain sickness: a rediscovery. *Lancet* 1988;2:639–641.

128. Hultgren HN, Lopez CE, Lundberg E, Miller H. Physiologic studies of pulmonary edema at high altitude. *Circulation* 1964;29:393–408.

129. Paneloza D, Sime F. Circulatory dynamics during high altitude pulmonary edema. *Am J Cardiol* 1969;23:369–378.

130. Antezana G, Leguia G, Guzman AM, Coudert J, Spielvogel H. Hemodynamic study of high altitude pulmonary edema (12,200 ft). In: Bredel W, Zink RA, eds. *High altitude physiology and medicine*. New York: Springer-Verlag, 1982, 232–241.

131. Fred HL, Schmidt AM, Bates T, Hecht HH. Acute pulmonary edema of altitude. Clinical and physiologic observations. *Circulation* 1962;25:929–937.

132. Hultgren HN. High altitude pulmonary edema. In: Hegnauer AH, ed. *Biomedicine problems of high terrestrial altitude*. New York: Springer-Verlag, 1969.

133. Hackett PH, Crerg CE, Grover RF, Honigman KB, Houston CS, Reeves JT, Sophocles AM, Van Hardenbrock M. High altitude pulmonary edema in persons without the right pulmonary artery. *N Engl J Med* 1980;302:1070–1072.

134. Hackett PH, Bertman J, Rodriguez G. Pulmonary edema fluid protein in high-altitude pulmonary edema. *JAMA* 1986;256:36.

135. Schoene RB, Hackett PH, Henderson WR, Sage EH, Chow M, Roach RC, Mills WJ, Martin TR. High-altitude pulmonary edema. Characteristics of lung lavage fluid. *JAMA* 1986;256:63–69.

136. Tsukimoto K, Mathieu-Costello O, Prediletto R, West JB. Ultrastructural appearances of pulmonary capillaries at high distending pressures. *FASEB J* 1990;4:A969.

137. West JB, Tsukimoto K, Mathieu-Costello O, Prediletto R. Stress failure in pulmonary capillaries. *FASEB J* 1990;4:A1276.

138. Houston CS, Dickinson J. Cerebral form of high-altitude illness. *Lancet* 1975;2:758–761.

139. Koyama S, Kobayashi T, Kubo K, Fukushima M, Yoshimura K, Shibamoto T, Yagi H, Handa K, Kusama S. Catecholamine metabolism in patients with high altitude pulmonary edema (HAPE). *Jpn J Mount Med* 1984;4:119.

140. Singh I, Khanna PK, Srivastava MC, Lah M, Roy SB, Subramanyam CSV. Acute mountain sickness. *N Engl J Med* 1969;280:175–184.

141. Dickinson J, Heath D, Gosney J, Williams D. Altitude related deaths in seven trekkers in the Himalayas. *Thorax* 1983;38:646–656.

142. Frayser R, Houston CS, Bryan AC, Rennie ID, Gray G. Retinal haemorrhage at high altitude. *N Engl J Med* 1970;282:1183–1184.

143. Hurtado A. Chronic mountain sickness. *JAMA* 1942;120:1278–1282.

144. Cruz JC, Diaz C, Marticorena E, Hilario V. Phlebotomy improves pulmonary gas exchange in chronic mountain polycythemia. *Respiration* 1979;38:305–313.

THE LUNG: Scientific Foundations
edited by R.G. Crystal, J.B. West et al.
Raven Press, Ltd., New York © 1991.

CHAPTER 8.1.2

Diving

Claes Lundgren

Respiratory function is challenged in several ways in diving and in high-pressure environments. Some problems arise from the change in pressure as the depth increases or decreases, and some are caused by the absolute pressure level (depth) that is reached. Even the small pressure difference across the chest wall that is generated by head-out immersion may have profound effects on lung function. Some of the respiratory problems in diving may be due to the effects of the breathing gear; for a review of this topic, see ref. 1.

The pressure that the water exerts is caused by its density; because water is largely incompressible, the pressure increases at a constant rate as depth increases. This rate is 1.0 atmosphere, or 760 mmHg or 101.3 kilopascals, per 10 m (33 ft) of depth.[1] Consequently, the total pressure at 10 m is 2 atmospheres absolute (ATA) (i.e., 1.0 ATA due to the water column and 1.0 ATA due to the gaseous atmosphere above the water), at 20 m (66 ft) the pressure is 3.0 ATA, and so on.

Research into the respiratory physiology of diving humans is typically performed in three settings: (a) in actual dives in the sea, (b) in hyperbaric chambers where the subject is surrounded by mixtures of compressed gases of varying composition and where the total pressure is set to equal a given depth in the sea (these are known as "simulated dry dives"), and (c) in a water-filled compartment in a hyperbaric chamber where submersion effects can be studied at any simulated depth by controlling the pressure of the gas above the water interphase (these are known as "simulated wet dives").

This chapter will deal primarily with the respiratory function of the lungs in the diving environment. The lung may also play a role as a target organ for, or as an origin of, certain injury mechanisms in diving. Specifically, it may receive gas emboli giving rise to the pain and respiratory distress known as "chokes" in decompression sickness, or it may be the origin of arterial gas embolism as a result of pulmonary barotrauma during ascent. In the latter case, as ambient pressure is falling, gas that is trapped in the lung expands to the point of rupturing lung tissue and invading the pulmonary circulation. These types of dysbarism have recently been reviewed by Lundgren and Farhi (2).

BREATH-HOLD DIVING

Some of the most dramatic effects of diving on respiratory function occur in conjunction with the simplest and most primitive form of diving, namely, breath-hold diving. This activity is still being practiced as a profession by thousands of Korean and Japanese female divers collecting edibles at depths down to about 20 m (66 ft); a small group of competitive breath-hold divers have gradually brought the world depth record to 112 m (370 ft), requiring about 3 min of submersion. Given these amazing figures, the following question arises: What is the maximum depth and duration that can be achieved in breath-hold diving, and what are the limiting factors?

The Depth Limit

The depth limit is set by respiratory and circulatory mechanics as well as by the adequacy of gas exchange. It has earlier been held that the depth limit in terms of chest wall mechanics would be set by the relationship between an individual's total lung capacity (TLC) and his or her residual volume (RV). It follows that for

C. Lundgren: Center for Research in Special Environments, Department of Physiology, State University of New York—Buffalo, Buffalo, New York 14214.

[1] Disregarding small variations in the density of water, depending on salinity and temperature.

the average young adult who starts a dive after inhaling maximally, the highest tolerable pressure would, according to Boyle's law, be calculated as follows:

$$TLC \times P_1 = RV \times P_2$$

where $P_1 = 1.0$ ATA and P_2 is the pressure at maximum depth.

Disregarding, for the sake of simplicity, volume changes due to gas exchange during the descent and inserting reasonable figures:

$$P_2 = \frac{6.0 \times 1.0}{1.5} = 4 \text{ ATA}$$

That is, a pressure increase to 4 ATA which is reached at 30 m (99 ft) would reduce the TLC volume to RV.

This theoretical projection contrasts sharply with the above-mentioned record depth of about 110 m (12 ATA). Again, according to Boyle's law, at this great depth the initial TLC volume of 6 liters would be reduced to about 0.5 liter. The explanation for how this can occur without the chest being crushed was presented by Craig (3), whose study indicated that air space vacated by compression can be made up for by redistribution of blood from the periphery into the chest. In experiments performed on himself, Craig descended under water after first having expired to RV. The esophageal pressure, properly referenced, showed no drop as he proceeded down to a maximum depth of 4.5 m. This was taken to indicate that the lung air was being compressed to pressure equilibrium with the surrounding water by 600 ml of blood entering the chest. Although prone to methodological uncertainties, measurements of electrical impedance of the chest in a subject performing breath-hold dives to 90 and 130 ft have indicated blood volume increases in the chest of 1047 and 850 ml, respectively (4).

That a considerable volume of blood can indeed be translocated into the blood-containing structures of the chest has been demonstrated by other types of measurements. Mere immersion with the head above the water is sufficient to redistribute about 700 ml of blood into the chest as measured by dye-dilution technique (5). In this situation the vital capacity (VC) has been found to be reduced by about 5.5% in water of thermoneutral (35°C) temperature and by as much as 12% in water at 20°C; in warm water (40°C) it was not significantly reduced (6). This indicates that the peripheral circulatory effects of the temperature of the water are somewhat independent of its hydrostatic effects. It would appear then that, for optimal mechanical benefit from blood redistribution, a breath-hold dive should be started with a maximal inspiration before getting into the water, and the dive should be performed in cool water.

There are no reports in the literature that identify, with certainty, the failure mode that ultimately sets the depth limit for breath-hold dives. It may, in analogy with what has been suggested for deep snorkel breathing, be cardiac damage, or it could be rupture of pulmonary vessels and/or pulmonary edema. A couple of reports on fatalities in conjunction with breath-hold diving to 80 ft and 100 ft, respectively, are somewhat supportive of the so-called lung-squeeze hypothesis. Autopsy findings included intravascular congestion, interstitial edema, vascular injury, and intra-alveolar hemorrhage (7,8).

The Time Limit

The maximum duration of the dive depends on metabolic rate and on the ability of the diver to store CO_2 and O_2. Either CO_2 or O_2 handling may become the limiting function. The breath-hold diver's safety depends on a delicate balance: The arterial P_{CO_2} must not reach the breaking point, typically at about 55 mmHg, before the diver reaches the surface, yet the buildup of P_{CO_2} must proceed at a pace that is rapid enough relative to the fall in P_{O_2} so as to make the diver aware of the need to return to the surface before loss of consciousness is caused by hypoxia.

The Danger of Hyperventilation

Voluntary hyperventilation is sometimes practiced in order to prolong the duration of a breath-hold dive. The method has proven at times to be inordinately effective: The ensuing breath-hold may last forever. The pathophysiology of such a mishap, as well as its practical significance, was underscored by Craig (9), who collected information on 58 cases of loss of consciousness during underwater swimming, the majority of which could be tied to hyperventilation before the swim. Craig's interpretation of the physiological event was that hyperventilation will reduce body CO_2 stores as a function of excess alveolar ventilation and duration of the hyperventilation. It will then take a proportionately longer time before the stores are replenished with CO_2 so that the breaking point P_{CO_2} is reached. Since the oxygen stores of the body are only enhanced to a very small extent by hyperventilation, the P_{O_2} will have time to become reduced to dangerously low levels.

The CO_2–O_2 Paradox

When breath-holding is combined with dives to great depths, remarkable alterations occur in the exchange of CO_2 and O_2 between alveolar air and blood. During descent, the air in the lungs is compressed, thereby causing a rise in both CO_2 and O_2 partial pressures. A total pressure increase of merely 90 mmHg in the lung air is sufficient for the alveolar CO_2 pressure (P_{ACO_2}) (normally at 40 mmHg) to increase to the venous Pco_2 (P_{VCO_2}) level of 45 mmHg. This occurs when the depth of 1.2 m (4 ft) is reached.

As depth increases further, P_{ACO_2} will increase and tend to exceed P_{VCO_2}, even as the latter climbs as a result of recirculation. As a result, CO_2 from the alveolar gas is being reabsorbed into the blood passing the lung. This paradoxical reversal of CO_2 flow, first described by Lanphier and Rahn (10), is illustrated in Figs. 1 and 2. As the diver ascends toward the surface, the alveolar air expands, its pressure drops, and therefore the P_{ACO_2} falls, allowing CO_2 unloading to occur again from the blood into the alveolar air. This might help to relieve respiratory CO_2 drive towards the end of the ascent. The P_{AO_2}, also being influenced by changes in lung gas pressure, will increase as the depth increases, thus probably reducing the respiratory drive from CO_2 during the deep phase of the dive (Fig. 1). It will also provide a larger amount of absorbable oxygen (at physiologically acceptable P_{AO_2} levels) than would be available if the breath-hold, with the same amount of alveolar gas, were performed at 1.0 ATA (see below).

During ascent there are two remarkable aspects to O_2 exchange. The first is that, in analogy with what happens for CO_2, the P_{AO_2} will fall. This is the cause of the so-called hypoxia of ascent. The potential se-

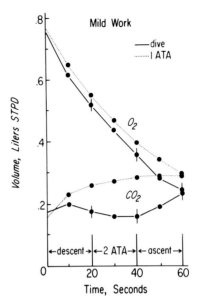

FIG. 2. Volumes of CO_2 and O_2 (corrected to standard conditions) in the lung space during the same experimental conditions as in Fig. 1. (From ref. 10.)

verity of the condition is appreciated if one assumes that a breath-hold diver were to linger at the bottom in, for instance, a 30-m (4 ATA, 99 ft) dive until his or her alveolar oxygen concentration has gone down to 3.1% as a result of metabolic oxygen uptake. This still allows for adequate oxygenation of the blood, since at 4 ATA the P_{AO_2} would be

$$P_{AO_2} = 0.03(4 \times 760 - 47) = 90 \text{ mmHg}$$

However, as pressure falls during ascent, the critical level of P_{AO_2} (and hence arterial Po_2, P_{aO_2}) of 30 mmHg, at which loss of consciousness generally occurs, will be encountered at a pressure P which may be calculated as follows:

$$(P \times 760 - 47) \times 0.03 = 30; \text{ i.e., } P = 1.32 \text{ ATA}$$

That is, a dangerously low P_{aO_2} will be reached 3.2 m (10.6 ft) below the surface or even deeper because, in addition to the effects on the lung gas pressure by the ascent, there is continued metabolic O_2 consumption. Whether or not the diver will reach the surface without losing consciousness will depend on rate of ascent, metabolism, circulation time from lungs to brain, and P_{VO_2}. The importance of the P_{VO_2} has to do with the second aspect of the O_2 exchange during ascent. In conjunction with the drop in alveolar air pressure, the P_{AO_2} may reach a level below that of the venous blood. A paradoxical flow of oxygen into the alveolar air will then result. This phenomenon, as well as its potential importance for the safety of the breath-hold diver, has been analyzed by Olszowka and Rahn (11). Employing a computer model of the gas exchange in the body, they investigated a typical 100-m dive last-

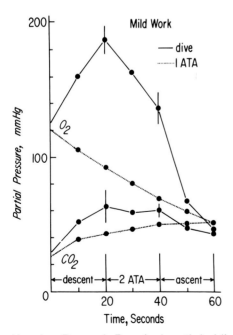

FIG. 1. Alveolar Po_2 and Pco_2 in breath-holding, preceded by air breathing, at 1 ATA and during dry dives to 2 ATA (33 ft). (From ref. 10.)

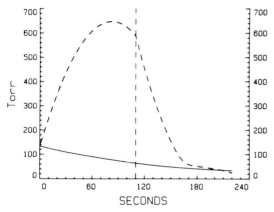

FIG. 3. Alveolar P_{O_2} versus time during computer-simulated breath-holds. The solid line represents breath-holding at 1 ATA. The dashed curve represents the same subject breath-hold diving, reaching the depth of 100 m at 110 sec (dashed line: end of descent, beginning of ascent) and returning to the surface at 220 sec. (From ref. 11.)

ing 220 sec. The $P_{A_{O_2}}$ in the dive, as well as that in a breath-hold of equal duration at the surface, is shown in Fig 3. Clearly, the gain in $P_{A_{O_2}}$ from gas compression gives the diver access to oxygen at considerably more advantageous P_{O_2} levels throughout most of the dive than is the case for the surface breath-holder. Towards the end of the ascent, this advantage is lost and the dive curve dips under the surface curve and becomes gradually lower during the last 50 sec of the breath-hold. However, as shown in Fig. 4, which illustrates events during this time period in more detail, the rapid decline of the $P_{A_{O_2}}$, which would be the result if reduction of alveolar gas pressure alone dictated its course, is mitigated by a paradoxical flow of oxygen

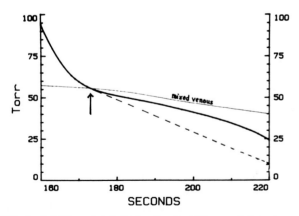

FIG. 4. Additional details for the last 60 sec of dive shown in full in Fig. 3. The heavy solid line represents $P_{A_{O_2}}$, and the light solid line represents $P_{V_{O_2}}$. The arrow at 173 sec indicates cross-over point after which $P_{V_{O_2}}$ exceeds $P_{A_{O_2}}$. The dashed line indicates change of $P_{A_{O_2}}$ because of lung expansion in the hypothetical case of no O_2 transfer after 173 sec. (From ref. 11.)

from the venous blood into the alveolar gas. This may be an important mechanism that preserves $P_{A_{O_2}}$, and hence $P_{a_{O_2}}$, at a level compatible with retained consciousness throughout the ascent (11).

The Dive Response

The dive response consists of bradycardia, reduced cardiac output, and peripheral vasoconstriction elicited by breath-holding and submersion. It has been suggested that the dive response enhances human tolerance to asphyxia, at least in near-drowning situations in cold water; this response presumably explains cases of survival after submersions lasting up to 40 min (12). The role of the dive response would be to conserve blood-borne oxygen primarily for use by the heart and central nervous system (CNS), by vasoconstriction in other tissues. However, measurements of maximal breath-hold duration have failed to demonstrate any gains when the diving response was elicited in volunteer subjects by whole-body immersion (13). In fact, whole-body immersion in cool water, which is more effective in eliciting the dive response, was associated with shorter breath-holds than was submersion in warmer water. This was attributed to a cold-induced stimulation of metabolism which speeded up the arrival at the breaking point $P_{A_{O_2}}$ and $P_{A_{CO_2}}$ levels (13). When induced by cold-water face immersion alone, the diving response has been variously described as being connected with a decrease (14), no change (15), or a modest increase in maximal breath-hold duration (16). Observations in expert divers have indicated that when they perform deep breath-hold dives, high lactic acid levels are present in the blood immediately after the dive, whereas the alveolar gas composition shows only moderately asphyxic O_2 and CO_2 concentrations (17). This was taken to indicate that, during the dives, a considerable amount of shunting of blood flow, past major peripheral vascular beds, occurred.

BREATHING UNDERWATER

Immersion/Submersion

The simplest form of breathing device for diving is the snorkel. However, this breathing tube, typically connected with a mouthpiece, is extremely limited in terms of the diving depth that can safely be attained, because a pressure imbalance is created across the chest. The mean alveolar gas pressure remains 1 ATA, mediated from the surface air via the tube, whereas the water pressure is added on the chest and abdomen. The greatest pressure a maximal inspiratory effort can generate is on the order of 100–150 cmH$_2$O; this places the theoretical depth limit at about 1 m (3 ft), and the inspiratory effort will be extremely taxing. In addition, the low pressure in the chest is, as mentioned earlier, conducive to forceful redistribution of blood from the periphery into the blood-containing structures of the chest. The early literature on "diving physiology" contains a description of a remarkable case of acute cardiac dilatation suffered by an investigator (18) when, for the purpose of measuring the force of the inspiratory muscles, he descended to a depth of 2 m (6.5 ft) while breathing through a snorkel.

A diver's breathing gear must provide breathing gas at the appropriate pressure and with a suitable composition. From what has been said earlier, it follows that the pressure should be near the average water pressure prevailing on the chest. The necessary high gas pressure is typically achieved either by pumping breathing gas down to the diver through a hose from the surface or by supplying it from the compressed gas bottles of a self-contained underwater breathing apparatus (scuba). Various valve mechanisms provide the diver with gas at the "ambient" water pressure. However, there is some debate as to what is exactly the reference pressure to which the breathing gas pressure should be balanced (1). The pressure centroid of the chest is a reference point often referred to in discussing this topic. In the upright position it is located 14 cm below the sternal notch, and in the prone posture it is about 7 cm behind the sternal angle. When the breathing gas pressure equals water pressure at the centroid, the expiratory reserve volume is the same as in the nonsubmersed condition. Deviations in breathing gas pressure, sometimes referred to as "static lung loading," frequently occur because the devices controlling breathing gas pressure according to water pressure are not always located at exactly the same depth as the chest pressure centroid (Fig. 5). Static lung loading by as little as -10 to -20 cmH$_2$O is conducive to

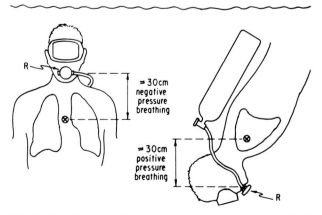

FIG. 5. Relative positions of chest pressure centroid (X) and scuba regulator (R) during head-up and head-down postures under water determine exposure to negative and positive static lung loading, respectively.

dyspnea, especially when exercise and high gas densities are factors in the dive (19,20). A positive pressure of about 10 cmH$_2$O, on the other hand, was found to be connected with the least dyspnea during air-breathing and heavy exercise at 6.76 ATA (190 ft) (19,20). This is in agreement with observations in helium–oxygen-breathing subjects at much greater depths in wet dives. Both the subjects of Dwyer et al. (21) at 43.4 ATA (1400 ft) and of Spaur et al. (22) at 49.5 ATA (1600 ft) experienced work-limiting dyspnea primarily of inspiratory nature. Positive-pressure breathing would tend to reduce the strain on inspiratory muscles and should consequently be expected to relieve such dyspnea as has also been confirmed by Thalmann and Piantadosi (23). Despite the dyspnea, no marked disturbances in overall oxygen and carbon dioxide exchange were found in the five studies just mentioned. The mechanism behind exertional dyspnea in diving is unclear.

Negative static lung loading during exercise has been shown to be less conducive to expiratory flow limitation in the prone than in the upright posture, and this was attributed to a larger end-expiratory lung volume in the former posture (24). Those experiments were performed in subjects immersed immediately beneath the surface. In contrast, at 190 ft the combination of negative static lung loading, submersion, and exercise in air-breathing subjects caused more dyspnea in the prone than in the upright posture (19,20). The possible role of extrathoracic airway compression in this context is mentioned later.

The disturbances in lung function in the diver exposed to negative static lung loads are likely to be similar to those observed in subjects undergoing head-out immersion. Changes in ventilation–perfusion distribution occur for several reasons, but to varying degrees in different individuals. The main factors involved, all mutually interacting, are (a) respiratory mechanics, (b) pulmonary circulation, and (c) breathing pattern.

The negative static lung loading reduces the functional residual capacity (FRC) by lowering the expiratory reserve volume (ERV). Reduced FRC, combined with the intrathoracic accumulation of about 700 ml of blood (5), has two notable effects: airway closure and reduced pulmonary compliance (25,26). The airway closure has been ascribed to two possible mechanisms: vascular engorgement in airway mucosa and an increased lung weight causing a preferential closing of airways in dependent regions (25). Coupled with the tendency for airway closure is that closing volume increases (25,27). When the diver uses oxygen-breathing gear, the airway closure is conducive to the formation of absorption atelectases and reductions in VC of between 24% and 42% (28,29).

The reduction in compliance may be due to an erectile effect of the lung capillaries being engorged with blood—a mechanism first demonstrated in excised animal lungs by von Basch (30) in 1887. In addition, it has been suggested that a slow component in the development of a stiffer lung during immersion may be due to an increased interstitial fluid volume (26).

The distribution of ventilation as evident from radioactive xenon spirometry is shifted towards the apical lung regions, making for a somewhat more even distribution of lung ventilation than in the nonimmersed state. At the same time, an apical shift of perfusion was also evident (31). This increase in apical perfusion would be expected from the fourfold increase in mean pulmonary arterial pressure which occurred as a result of the immersion (5). In the latter paper it was also pointed out that increased air trapping in the dependent parts of the lungs may cause local hypoxia that would tend to cause redistribution of blood flow towards apical, better-ventilated regions. A higher perfusion in apical regions than in the lung bases, due to immersion in erect standing subjects, was observed by Prefaut et al. (32) and was ascribed to a high pleural pressure at the lung bases causing vascular narrowing and higher flow resistance.

The possibility that gas exchange may be influenced by the changes in ventilation–perfusion matching that immersion causes has been considered in some studies. A drop in P_aO_2 by 10 mmHg during head-out immersion was observed by Cohen et al. (33), whereas Arborelius et al. (31) saw no P_aO_2 changes. These discrepancies may be looked upon in light of the studies of Prefaut et al. (34). They related changes in the alveolar–arterial oxygen pressure difference (P_{A-aO_2}) and diffusing capacity to the respiratory pattern of their immersed subjects. Three types of subjects were identified with regard to how large their FRC was, relative to the CV: (i) relatively young and lightly built persons who, even during immersion, breathe outside their CV, (ii) persons of intermediate age and/or body weight whose tidal volumes partly overlap with CV, and (iii) older and/or heavier persons whose tidal volumes are confined within the CV. With immersion, improvement of diffusing capacity dominated in the first type of subject and the P_{A-aO_2} became reduced. With the third type, the ventilation–perfusion mismatch dominated and the P_{A-aO_2} deteriorated by as much as 15 mmHg in some individuals (34).

Ventilatory Requirements

Because of the compression that gases undergo with increasing depth, the molar concentrations of the respective components in a breathing gas mixture increase. One aspect of the increase in oxygen partial pressure is that it introduces the risk of oxygen intoxi-

ication for which the lungs are among the primary targets. Chapter 8.1.3 addresses this topic. With regard to oxygen availability, the compression means that a larger proportion of the oxygen in the respired air can be used for metabolism at depth than at 1.0 ATA. For instance, of the 1.7 liters STPD of oxygen contained in 10 liters BTPS of air providing alveolar ventilation at the surface, typically about 0.6 liter STPD is available for metabolic use if a normal P_{AO_2} of about 100 mmHg is to be retained.[2] However, when the same air mass is inspired at 30 m (4 ATA, 99 ft), the amount of the oxygen (now compressed to 0.5 liter BTPS) that can be metabolized is about 1.5 liters STPD. Clearly, this is of little practical value in open breathing systems, since the ventilation requirements depend on the need for CO_2 elimination. Only in the case of so-called rebreathing apparatus with built-in CO_2 absorption can a larger proportion of the oxygen fraction be used for the diver's metabolism.

To keep the P_{ACO_2} at a physiologically acceptable level, the alveolar ventilation ($\dot{V}_A$) is guided by the well-known relationship

$$\dot{V}_A = \frac{863 \cdot \dot{V}_{CO_2}}{P_{ACO_2}}$$

where $\dot{V}_A$ is expressed in liters BTPS and $\dot{V}_{CO_2}$ (carbon dioxide elimination) is expressed in liters STPD; 863 is a factor correcting for the BTPS–STPD discrepancy.

In other words, the ventilation requirement depends on metabolism and P_{ACO_2}, not on absolute pressure. Since the amount of gas in a breath depends on the pressure, it follows that a given lung ventilation will drain the scuba diver's bottled air supply at a rate that is directly proportional to the depth, thereby vasting correspondingly increasing amounts of oxygen.

Inadequate CO_2 elimination is a common and potentially serious problem in diving. Cases of loss of consciousness under water, apparently due to hypoventilation and hypocapnea, have been described. Two divers who had had such experiences were shown to have unusually low responses to inspired carbon dioxide (35), a trait that apparently distinguishes divers (active divers as well as ex-divers) from non-divers in general (36).

Whether the divers' low CO_2 response is inherent or acquired is still an open question. However, it is apparently produced by several factors, including the high inspired P_{O_2}, high gas density, and exercise (for a detailed discussion, see ref. 37).

The increased gas pressure at greater depths puts a mechanical limitation to the level of ventilation that can be achieved. This limitation is linked to the increase in density of the gas inhaled; this is true whether

---

[2] STPD stands for standard temperature and pressure, dry; BTPS stands for body temperature and pressure, saturated.

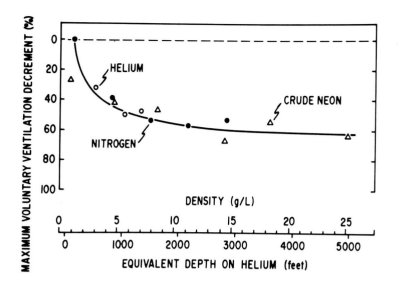

FIG. 6. Maximum voluntary ventilation as a function of breathing gas density. Results from measurements in two subjects. The respiration of crude neon at a 1200-ft depth equivalent was used to simulate density effects to be expected with helium at greater depths to 5000 ft. (From ref. 39.)

the density increase is due to high pressure or to the composition of the gas mixture (38). This is illustrated in Fig. 6, which relates maximal voluntary ventilation (MVV) to gas density. A range of gas densities was achieved by varying the composition of respired gas mixtures and environmental pressure (39). In the latter paper it is pointed out that as gas density becomes progressively higher, the additional depression of MVV becomes relatively less pronounced. The relationship between the MVVs that an individual may achieve at 1.0 ATA and at depth, respectively, is given by Lanphier and Camporesi (37):

$$MVV_{(depth)} = MVV_0 \times \rho^{-k}$$

where ρ is the gas density, k is a best-fit regression exponent (typically between 0 and 0.5), and MVV_0 is the MVV measured when $\rho = 1$. Remarkably, exercise-ventilation levels at simulated depth have in some studies been found to approach the resting 15-sec MVV measured at the same depth (39–41) or even to exceed it (19). Other reports hold, however, that exercise ventilation at depth is limited to the same level relative to MVV as at 1 ATA (21,42,43). These differences may depend on methodological factors. However, it has been shown that exercise per se tends to counteract MVV limitation at depth. Measurements of MVV during exercise at 200 W and 6.76 ATA yielded values up to 17% higher than during rest, and expiratory flow was increased up to 48% (44). This exercise effect, also present at 1 ATA, has primarily been ascribed to altered autonomic control of airway resistance (45). The usefulness of MVV, measured at depth, as a predictor for attainable exercise performance has been questioned because of considerable increase in physiological dead space observed at great depths (46).

The limitation to pulmonary gas flow at depth is mainly on expiration and has been ascribed to high gas

density causing dynamic airway collapse (41,47). Maximal expiratory flow in this condition (at lung volumes larger than 25% VC) is proportional to the gas density raised to about the −0.4 to −0.45 power (41,44,48). In view of this, it is remarkable that, as mentioned earlier, the dyspnea experienced during exertion at depth is usually linked to inspiration. It has been proposed that this might reflect inspiratory muscle fatigue (47). The notion is that, since FRC tends to become enlarged during exercise at high pressure (41,48–50), more elastic work is required during inspiration while, in addition, the inspiratory muscles are placed at a mechanical disadvantage. Thus, the inspiratory muscles may become fatigued. However, measurements directly supporting this hypothesis are still lacking.

The possibility of dynamic compression of the extrathoracic trachea during inspiration at depth has recently been brought to light (51). This would occur due to a negative transmural pressure below the vocal cords when sufficiently high flow rates and gas densities are present. During maximum inspirations at 300 m with gas at a density of 5.9 g/liter, divers showed evidence of sudden inspiratory limitation (51). In the same vein, a higher tolerance for negative static lung loading imposed by breathing gear in the upright than in the prone posture under water has been suggested to be due to the lesser water pressure on the neck in the upright posture (50).

Although the gas-density effect becomes less pronounced with increasing depth as illustrated in Fig. 6 and as formulated in the earlier-mentioned power function of gas density, the notion was long held that this effect would make exercise ventilation gradually more restricted to the point where the diver would be unable to do useful work. Based on various measures of maximal expiratory flows on subjects in dry-chamber dives, Varene et al. (52) predicted that the exercise performance in helium–oxygen atmospheres would be limited to 150–225 W at 40 ATA, 135–215 W at 50 ATA, and 125–200 W at 60 ATA. Given that mean maximal expiratory flow rates recorded by Vorosmarti et al. (53) showed very little deterioration at relative gas densities above 5 (air at 1 ATA being set at 1.0) and up to 15, they predicted that, using helium–oxygen mixtures, divers should not be unduly limited by pulmonary mechanics in doing moderate work (125 W) at pressures in the range of 100 ATA. Exercise has been performed in dry dives at an intensity of about 100 W while respiring a crude-neon–oxygen mixture at 1200-ft equivalent pressure (39). The gas density of about 25 g/liter, corresponding to helium–oxygen breathing at 5000 ft, still did not render ventilatory function symptomatically difficult and allowed alveolar (end-tidal) levels of P_{CO_2} below 50 mmHg. Attempts at performing 200 W were thwarted by inadequate ventilation.

Control of Ventilation

One element in reduced ventilation at depth is, as mentioned earlier, high oxygen pressures (37). However, the CNS-depressing effect of nitrogen at high air pressures appears not to involve central respiratory response as far as CO_2 sensitivity is concerned. Linnarsson and Hesser (54) found no change in inspiratory occlusion pressure in subjects breathing air at 6.1 bar (P_{O_2} = 1.3 bar) with increasing inhaled CO_2 concentrations. Controls were performed during O_2–CO_2 inhalation at 1.3 bar. In contrast, the ventilatory response to CO_2 was reduced by 39%. The investigators concluded that the depression in ventilation was due to increased airway resistance, caused in turn by increased gas density, and that possibly the resistance-induced stimulation of intrathoracic receptors resulted in a reflex increase in central inspiratory activity. A reduction in ventilatory response to CO_2 rebreathing with increasing gas density has also been recorded in experiments with nitrogen, helium, and crude neon up to a maximal density of about 25 g/liter (39). The conclusion from those observations, too, was that the ventilatory depression was related to increased gas density and work of breathing and not to the narcotic actions of the inhaled inert gas. The possibility that divers as a group exhibit low CO_2 sensitivity has already been mentioned.

Remarkably, resting hypoventilation and hypercapnia due to increased gas density at intermediate depths was replaced at greater depths by a higher ventilation and lower end-tidal CO_2 pressure than at the surface and was ascribed to a stimulation of respiratory control centers by hydrostatic pressure per se (55). Such an effect, akin to the so-called high-pressure nervous syndrome, may have acted in the subjects of Salzano et al. (46), who, while at simulated depths of 1509 and 2132 ft, were breathing gases at densities of between 7.9 and 17.1 g/liter and exhibited larger V_E during both rest and mild exercise than when at 1.0 ATA with a gas density of 1.1 g/liter. Another explanation favored by the latter investigators (46) was that the increased breathing at depth was in response to increased physiological dead space. The dead space may increase at high gas densities as a result of hindered intrapulmonary diffusion. For a discussion of this topic, see ref. 47. However, it is noteworthy that over the density range studied, Salzano et al. (46) saw no deterioration in P_{aO_2}.

The P_{aO_2}–Density Paradox

Early observations of signs of hypoxia in animals at helium pressures of about 100 ATA were taken to indicate impaired oxygen diffusion in the gas phase of the lungs; for a review, see ref. 56. However, several investigators have since noted a decreased P_{A-aO_2} with increasing respired gas density. This phenomenon has been attributed to a reduced variance in ventilation–perfusion ($\dot{V}_A/\dot{Q}$) ratio (57). This reduction was thought to be due to an enhanced effect of cardiogenic mixing in peripheral lung units that, in the presence of an increased gas density, exhibit parallel inhomogeneity.

Direct measurements of $\dot{V}_A/\dot{Q}$ distribution during respiration of air, as well as helium–oxygen measurements, failed to show any differences, although again the P_{A-aO_2} was lowered with helium (58). The proposed mechanism is one of changing interaction between diffusion and convection on inspiration. The implication of the latter was, furthermore, that gases eliminated from the blood could behave differently than gases absorbed. This would account for the opposite behavior of O_2 and CO_2 reported by Wood et al. (57) and Salzano et al. (46), who, among others, reported increasing physiological CO_2 dead space in the face of improved or unaltered P_{aO_2} with increasing density of the inspired gas.

INERT-GAS EXCHANGE

The processes of uptake and elimination of inert gases are intimately linked to human adaptation and maladaptation to the diving environment. The inert gases most frequently used in breathing gas mixtures for diving are nitrogen (usually in air), helium, and, less frequently, hydrogen and neon. They are important because of the roles they may play with regard to respiratory impediment, narcosis, counterdiffusion phenomena, and decompression sickness.[3] The effects of the density of the breathing medium were dealt with earlier. The other phenomena are linked to differences in diffusibility and solubility of the respective gases in blood and other tissues.

DECOMPRESSION SICKNESS

Central to the etiology of decompression sickness (DS) is that gases that are inspired will enter into physical solution in body tissues. When the hydrostatic pressure in the tissues is reduced as a reflection of lower ambient pressure, sufficient amounts of gas may, under certain circumstances, be liberated and cause DS. The amount of a gas that can be held in the tissues depends on its solubility in the tissues, its partial pressure, and the hydrostatic pressure in the tissues. The rate at which a gas will enter or leave the tissues once its partial pressure in the lungs is changed relative to tissue gas pressure depends primarily on the blood perfusion and blood solubility but also on its diffusibility. The dependence of inert-gas exchange on circulation is exemplified by the observation that whole-body nitrogen elimination during oxygen breathing was considerably faster when the subjects were immersed in water to the neck than when sitting nonimmersed (60). Elimination of a deposit of radioactive xenon in a leg muscle was similarly increased (61). These changes could be linked to a more than 30% increase in cardiac output resulting from the earlier-mentioned redistribution of blood into the chest caused by immersion (5). In the same vein, breathing oxygen at high pressures depresses the circulation and reduces the rate of nitrogen washout below the level that can be achieved inhaling normoxic (and nitrogen-free) gas mixtures (62). It is noteworthy that transport of gases that (like the ones just mentioned) are relatively poorly soluble in blood is (for all practical purposes) exclusively dependent on perfusion and independent of lung ventilation (63).

During ascent (decompression) the ambient pressure falls, and with it goes the hydrostatic pressure in the tissues. This reduces the ability of the tissues to hold inert gas in solution. If the decompression is conducted at an appropriately slow rate, the emerging overload of inert gas in the tissues will be transported (while still in solution) via the circulation to the lungs and exhaled. If, on the other hand, decompression is too rapid, the inert gas (and, secondarily, oxygen and carbon dioxide) will be released as bubbles. Depending on their size, number, and location, these bubbles can cause a

host of symptoms and malfunctions. These include, but are not limited to, joint pains (the bends), chest pain and coughing (the chokes), paresthesias and paralysis due to spinal cord involvement, catastrophic circulatory failure, and, ultimately, death. In order for a decompression to be conducted, a gradient of inert-gas pressure from the tissues to the alveoli must be established; furthermore, in order for the decompression to be carried out as rapidly as possible, this gradient should be as high as it can safely be. The concept of gas supersaturation in the tissues (i.e., a condition in which the tissue gas pressure may, without bubble formation, exceed the hydrostatic pressure by a given amount or ratio) has been central to decompression theory and practice since the days of J. S. Haldane and co-workers (64). However, since that time, the supersaturation ratios compatible with safe decompression have repeatedly undergone revision in the conservative direction. Haldane originally recommended as safe a decompression performed so as to establish a tissue-gas-pressure/ambient-pressure ratio of about 1.78:1 (64). Recent observations indicate that gas liberation occurs at nitrogen supersaturation ratios as low as 1.1:1 (65) or even 1.05:1 (R. Eckenhoff, *personal communication*, 1990).

These observations again bring into focus the old concept of inherent unsaturation in the tissues. As pointed out by Rahn (66), the sum of gas pressures in metabolizing tissues is always less than that of the atmosphere. This depends on the fact that in the tissues the drop in P_{O_2} (relative to alveolar air P_{O_2}) is always greater than the rise in P_{CO_2} (see Table 1). Note that, assuming a bubble is surrounded by soft tissues that transmit the ambient pressure, the total gas pressure in the bubble is always the same as the pressure of the environment of the body (plus tissue pressure and pressure due to surface tension).

It follows from the above that the tissue nitrogen pressure can, for the purpose of providing a gradient for nitrogen flow from tissues to alveolar air, be in-

TABLE 1. *Gas tensions (mmHg) when breathing air at 1.0 atmosphere*

	Alveolar air and arterial blood	Tissue	Bubble
H_2O	47	47	47
O_2	103	40	40
CO_2	40	45 ⎫ 655[a]	45
N_2	570	570 ⎭	628
Total	760 ⟷ 702		760[b]
	Δp = 58 mmHg		

[a] N_2–O_2–CO_2 supersaturation ratio is $\dfrac{655}{760}$ = 0.86:1.

[b] Disregarding compression effects of tissue pressure and surface tension of bubble.

---

[3] For a major, current overview of the physiology and pathophysiology of decompression sickness and related phenomena, see ref. 59.

creased by 58 mmHg without exceeding a supersaturation quotient of unity, a condition that will ensure freedom from gas liberation. Moreover, exchanging oxygen for air as breathing medium will maximize the nitrogen pressure difference between tissues and alveolar gas, thus enhancing nitrogen washout. This advantage is even further increased when, during recompression treatment of DS, the ambient pressure—and therefore the gas pressure (and nitrogen pressure) in bubbles—is raised.

The Bubble Filter

Decompression schedules that currently are widely used allow supersaturation levels well above the ones just mentioned. It is therefore not surprising that when the ultrasound Doppler technique was employed for detection of intravenous gas bubbles, it soon became clear that dives that are carried out according to widely accepted decompression standards and that are symptom-free may well result in relatively intense venous gas embolism (67). This brings attention to the role of the lungs as a bubble filter.

In experiments on dogs, the size of bubbles generated by decompression stress has been recorded as ranging from 19 to 700 μm (68). The lungs have been demonstrated to effectively filter bubbles of sizes down to the smallest just mentioned (69). Large amounts of bubbles could, however, overload the lungs' filter function, and (pharmacological) vasodilatation also made bubbles appear on the arterial side. It is noteworthy that arterial bubbles have been recorded in systemic arteries in humans undergoing symptom-free decompressions (70). An open foramen ovale as an alternative route for movement of bubbles from the venous to the arterial side has recently come into focus; this mechanism has been suggested as important in the etiology of severe (spinal cord) DS (71).

While it is evident that gas liberation in the body is essential for the development of DS, bubbles on the venous side of the circulation are, as already mentioned, not necessarily connected with overt symptoms. It has even been proposed that clinically silent venous gas emboli may serve to enhance inert-gas elimination from the tissues. Thus, nitrogen elimination by helium–oxygen breathing after dives to 100 ft was more rapid if the measurements were performed during decompression stops at 10 or 50 ft of depth than at 100 ft (72). This was taken to indicate that bubbles (containing a hundred times more nitrogen than an equivalent volume of blood) would form and that once they became lodged in the pulmonary capillaries, they would give up their nitrogen by diffusion to the alveolar space (72). However, this proposed mechanism is rendered less likely by experiments in which inert-gas em-

bolization of the lungs blocked nitrogen clearance of the blood, causing it to retain twice as much nitrogen as when it perfused lungs which were free of emboli (73). Moreover, it is possible that once bubbles lodge in systemic capillaries, they may interfere with perfusion and, thus, interfere with inert-gas washout. In addition, they will serve as a sink for further gas transfer from the tissues, thus slowing gas elimination via circulatory washout even more (cf. ref. 74).

Finally, although gas liberation is the necessary first step in decompression sickness, recent work on bubble-induced complement activation indicates that this is an important secondary factor determining the morbidity of DS (75).

COUNTERDIFFUSION

A remarkable aberration of normal gas exchange while at constant pressure may be observed during conditions of so-called counterdiffusion. Clinical manifestations of this phenomenon were first observed in experimental chamber dives in which the subjects breathed a nitrogen–oxygen or neon–oxygen mixture while surrounded by a helium–oxygen mixture. They developed itching maculopapular skin lesions and severe vestibular disturbances (76,77). Some of these phenomena have been explained as being caused by gas liberation due to diffusion of two gases (with different diffusion characteristics) in opposite direction through a lipid–aqueous bilayer (in the actual case the skin and underlying tissue) (77). Given that the diffusional resistance for each gas is less when it enters the first layer than when it enters the second layer in its diffusion path, it can be shown that the sum of the gases' partial pressures at the bilayer interphase can provide for a substantial supersaturation. Pigs, experimentally exposed to helium in the surrounding atmosphere while breathing a high concentration of nitrous oxide, developed fatal gas embolism at an ambient pressure of 1.0 ATA (78).

Another situation that may lead to remarkable changes in inert-gas tensions in the tissues at stable environmental pressure is when a sequence of two or more inert gases is inhaled. Depending on the properties of the gases, a condition of transitory sub- or supersaturation may be generated. Among the proposed mechanisms, the simplest is based on the strictly perfusion-limited Haldanian gas-exchange model; an alternative, more sophisticated one recognizes the possibility of diffusion limitation of gas transportation to the tissues (79). The Haldanian concept of inert-gas exchange of the tissues being determined by the rate of blood perfusion and the blood–tissue partition coefficient is of particular relevance to fatty tissue. An example offered by Tepper et al. (79) considers a fatty tissue that is saturated with nitrogen by inhaling air (~80% N$_2$) at a pressure of 1 atmosphere. The blood-fat solubility ratio that pertains to the lipid fraction of this tissue is 0.2. If a sudden shift is made to helium (80%)–oxygen (20%) breathing, nitrogen will be washed out and helium will at the same time enter the tissue. The nitrogen pressure in the fat will fall more slowly than the helium pressure will increase because the blood–fat partition coefficient of nitrogen at 0.214 is considerably lower than that of helium at 0.556. As a consequence, there will be a transitory increase in total inert-gas pressure (N$_2$ plus He) in the fat that will result in supersaturation.

Reversal of the sequence—that is, helium–oxygen being followed by nitrogen–oxygen breathing—may be expected to create a temporary condition of sub-saturation. Such shifts in inert-gas exposures have been employed with some apparent success to shorten the decompression time in diving (80).

PULMONARY BAROTRAUMA

When a diver ascends, the gas in his/her lungs expands according to Boyle's law. Excess gas is normally exhaled, but if the breath is inadvertently held or if, due to some localized lung pathology, the airway of a part of the lung is closed off, the expanding gas cannot escape and the lung tissue may become overexpanded to the point of rupture. Typically, the air then takes either one of two routes: It dissects into the mediastinum, it may cause a pneumopericardium, and it may show up as a pneumothorax or subcutaneous emphysema, particularly in the neck region; alternatively, it enters the circulation and causes cerebral embolism, often resulting in sudden dramatic symptoms. However, in a group of submarine escape trainees, 3.5% showed focal electroencephalographic changes suggestive of subclinical cerebral embolism (81).

Pulmonary barotrauma has not been definitely connected with any one single predisposing factor, although Colebatch et al. (82) recorded abnormally low static lung compliance in six young divers who had contracted this condition. The investigators suggested that unevenly distributed lung elastance may predispose low-elastance lung areas to overstretch and rupture.

Arterial gas embolism is primarily treated by urgent recompression in a hyperbaric chamber aimed at reducing the size of emboli and eventually bringing them into solution.

INERT-GAS NARCOSIS

The gases that are used for dilution of oxygen in breathing gas mixtures for divers are all chemically inert during physiological conditions. Nonetheless, they are, to varying degrees, capable of inducing narcosis. The narcotic action of these gases in order of declining potency is argon, nitrogen, hydrogen, neon, and helium (for helium and neon, narcotic effects are not a practical concern). This hierarchy is closely related to fat solubility of the gases as shown in Table 2.

The inert-gas narcosis involves both higher mental functions and psychomotor performance, although the latter typically is involved to a lesser degree. As an example, air breathing at 10 ATA reduced the average performance in terms of arithmetic calculations in a group of 14 subjects by about 25%, whereas their manual dexterity was reduced by about 10% (10 subjects) (84). Sensations and behavior reminiscent of drunkenness are also common.

An important practical and theoretical aspect of the narcotic action of inert gases in diving is that this action is antagonistic to some expressions of the high-pressure nervous syndrome (for an overview, see ref. 85).

TABLE 2. *Correlation of narcotic potency of the inert gases, hydrogen, oxygen, and carbon dioxide with lipid solubility and other physical characteristics[a]*

Gas	Molecular weight	Solubility in lipid	Temperature (°C)	Oil–water solubility ratio	Relative narcotic potency
					(Least narcotic)
He	4	0.015	37	1.7	4.26
Ne	20	0.109	37.6	2.07	3.58
H$_2$	2	0.036	37	2.1	1.83
N$_2$	28	0.067	37	5.2	1
A	40	0.14	37	5.3	0.43
Kr	83.7	0.43	37	9.6	0.14
Xe	131.3	1.7	37	20.0	0.039
					(Most narcotic)
O$_2$	32	0.11	40	5.0	
CO$_2$	44	1.34	40	1.6	

[a] From ref. 83.

The latter is a condition due to high hydrostatic pressure per se which first was observed in humans breathing helium–oxygen mixtures at 600 ft and deeper. The symptoms and signs consisted of reduced mental and psychomotor performance, dizziness, nausea, vomiting, tremor, and electrocardiographic changes. In animals, deeper exposures led to generalized convulsions. Remarkably, addition of small amounts of the more narcotic gases to the basic helium–oxygen breathing mixture could ameliorate some of these problems. This antagonism between pressure effects and narcosis has led to a fruitful line of ongoing studies into their fundamental mechanisms of cellular action, and it has also led to the use of three-component gas mixtures in deep diving (86,87)

ACKNOWLEDGMENT

This work was supported, in part, by U.S. Naval Medical R & D Command Contract no. N0001489J1702.

REFERENCES

1. Physiological and human engineering aspects of underwater breathing apparatus. In: Lundgren C, Warkander D, eds. *Proceedings of an Undersea and Hyperbaric Medical Society workshop*. Bethesda, MD: Undersea and Hyperbaric Medical Society, 1989;270.
2. Lundgren CEG, Farhi LE. Pulmonary circulation in diving and hyperbaric environment. In: Weir EK, Reeves JT, eds. *Pulmonary vascular physiology and pathophysiology. Lung biology in health and disease*. New York: Marcel Dekker, 1989;199–240.
3. Craig AB Jr. Depth limits of breath-hold diving (an example of Fennology). *Respir Physiol* 1968;5:14–22.
4. Schaefer KE, Allison RD, Dougherty JH Jr, Carey CR, Walker R, Yost F, Parker D. Pulmonary and circulatory adjustments determining the limits of depths in breathhold diving. *Science* 1968;162:1020–1023.
5. Arborelius M Jr, Balldin UI, Lilja B, Lundgren CEG. Hemodynamic changes in man during immersion with the head above water. *Aerosp Med* 1972;43:592–598.
6. Kurss DI, Lundgren CEG, Pasche AJ. Effect of water temperature on vital capacity in head out immersion. In: Bachrach AJ, Matzen MM, eds. *Underwater physiology VII*. Bethesda, MD: Undersea and Hyperbaric Medical Society, 1981;297–301.
7. Strauss MB, Wright PW. Thoracic squeeze diving casualty. *Aerosp Med* 1971;42:673–675.
8. Kahn M. Fatal thoracic squeeze. *J Indian Med Assoc* 1979;73:38–39.
9. Craig AB Jr. Summary of 58 cases of loss of consciousness during underwater swimming and diving. *Med Sci Sports* 1976;8:171–175.
10. Lanphier EH, Rahn H. Alveolar gas exchange during breath-hold diving. *J Appl Physiol* 1963;18:471–477.
11. Olszowka AJ, Rahn H. Breath hold diving. In: Sutton JR, Houston CS, Coates G, eds. *Hypoxia and cold*. New York: Praeger, 1987;417–428.
12. Nemiroff MJ, Saltz GR, Weg JG. Survival after cold-water near-drowning: the protective effect of the diving reflex. *Am Rev Respir Dis* 1977;115:145.
13. Sterba JA, Lundgren CEG. Diving bradycardia and breath-holding time in man. *Undersea Biomed Res* 1985;12:139–150.
14. Whayne TF, Killip T III. Simulated diving in man: comparison of facial stimuli and response in arrhythmia. *J Appl Physiol* 1967;22:800–807.
15. Sterba JA, Lundgren CEG. Breath-hold duration in man and the diving response induced by face immersion. *Undersea Biomed Res* 1988;15:361–375.
16. Mukhtar MR, Patrick JM. Ventilatory drive during face immersion in man. *J Physiol (Lond)* 1986;370:13–24.
17. Cerretelli P, Costa M, Ferretti G, Ferrigno M, Lundgren CEG, Marconi C. Gas exchange and energy metabolism during deep breath-hold diving in elite divers. Submitted for publication.
18. Stigler R. Die Kraft unserer Inspirations Muskulatur. *Pflügers Arch* 1911;139:234–254.
19. Thalmann ED, Sponholtz DK, Lundgren CEG. Effects of immersion and static lung loading on submerged exercise at depth. *Undersea Biomed Res* 1979;6:259–290.
20. Hickey DD, Norfleet WT, Pasche AJ, Lundgren CEG. Respiratory function in the upright working diver at 6.8 ATA (190 fsw). *Undersea Biomed Res* 1987;14:241–262.
21. Dwyer J, Saltzman HA, O'Bryan R. Maximal physical work capacity of man at 43.4 ATA. *Undersea Biomed Res* 1977;4:359–372.
22. Spaur WH, Rahmond LW, Knott MM, Crothers JC, Braithwaite WR, Thalmann ED, Uddin DF. Dyspnea in divers at 49.5 ATA: Mechanical, not chemical, in origin. *Undersea Biomed Res* 1977;4:183–198.
23. Thalmann ED, Piantadosi CA. Submerged exercise at pressure up to 55.55 ATA. *Undersea Biomed Res* 1981;8:25.
24. Derion T, Reddan WG, Lanphier EH. Effects of body position and static lung loading during immersion on end-expiratory lung volume and peak expiratory flow. *Undersea Biomed Res* 1988;15:Abstract 69.
25. Dahlbäck GO. Lung mechanics during immersion in water. Thesis, Laboratory of Aviation and Naval Physiology, Institute of Physiology and Biophysics. University of Lund, Lund, Sweden, 1978.
26. Baer R, Dahlbäck GO, Balldin UI. Pulmonary mechanics and atelectasis during immersion in oxygen breathing subjects. *Undersea Biomed Res* 1987;14:229–240.
27. Bondi KR, Murray Young J, Bennett RM, Bradley ME. Closing volumes in man immersed to the neck in water. *J Appl Physiol* 1976;40:736–740.
28. Balldin UI, Dahlbäck GO, Lundgren CEG. Changes in vital capacity produced by oxygen breathing during immersion with the head above water. *Aerosp Med* 1971;42:384–387.
29. Dahlbäck GO, Balldin UI. Positive-pressure oxygen breathing and pulmonary atalectasis during immersion. *Undersea Biomed Res* 1983;10:39–44.
30. von Basch S. Über eine Funktion des Capillar Druckes in den Lungenalveolen. *Wiener Med Blätter* 1887;15:465–467.
31. Arborelius M Jr, Balldin UI, Lilja B, Lundgren CEG. Regional lung function in man during immersion with the head above water. *Aerosp Med* 1972;43:701–707.
32. Prefaut C, Dubois F, Roussos C, Amaral-Marques R, Macklem PT, Ruff F. Influence of immersion to the neck in water on airway closure and distribution of perfusion in man. *Respir Physiol* 1979;37:313–323.
33. Cohen R, Bell WH, Saltzman HA, Kylstra JA. Alveolar-arterial oxygen pressure difference in man immersed up to the neck in water. *J Appl Physiol* 1971;30:720–723.
34. Prefaut C, Ramonatxo M, Boyer R, Chardon G. Human gas exchange during water immersion. *Respir Physiol* 1978;34:307–318.
35. Morrison JB, Florio JT, Butt WS. Observations after loss of consciousness under water. *Undersea Biomed Res* 1978;5:179–187.
36. Sherman D, Eilender E, Shefer A, Kerem D. Ventilatory and occlusion pressure responses to hypercapnia in divers and nondivers. *Undersea Biomed Res* 1980;7:61–74.
37. Lanphier EH, Camporesi EM. Respiration and exercise. In: Bennett PB, Elliott DH, eds. *Physiology and medicine of diving*. San Pedro, CA: Best, 1982;99–156.
38. Maio DA, Farhi LE. Effect of gas density on mechanics of breathing. *J Appl Physiol* 1967;23:687–693.

39. Lambertsen CJ, Gelfand R, Peterson R, Strauss R, Wright WB, Dickson JG Jr, Puglia C, Hamilton RW Jr. Human tolerance to He, Ne, and N_2 at respiratory gas densities equivalent to He–O_2 breathing at depths to 1200, 2000, 3000, 4000, and 5000 feet of sea water (Predictive Studies III). *Aviat Space Environ Med* 1977;48:843–855.

40. Miller JN, Wangensteen OD, Lanphier EH. Respiratory limitations to work at depth. In: Fructus X, eds. *Proceedings of the third international conference on hyperbaric and underwater physiology.* Paris: Doin, 1972;118–123.

41. Wood LDH, Bryan AC. Exercise ventilatory mechanics at increased ambient pressure. *J Appl Physiol: Respir Environ Exercise Physiol* 1978;44:231–237.

42. Fagraeus L, Linnarsson D. Maximal voluntary and exercise ventilation at high ambient air pressures. *Forsvarsmedicin* 1973;9:275–278.

43. Anthonisen NR, Utz G, Kruger MH, Urbanetti JS. Exercise tolerance at 4 and 6 ATA. *Undersea Biomed Res* 1976;3:95–102.

44. Hickey DD, Lundgren CEG, Pasche AJ. Influence of exercise on maximal voluntary ventilation and forced expiratory flow at depth. *Undersea Biomed Res* 1983;10:241–254.

45. Lewis BM, Morton JW. Effects of inhalation of CO_2, muscular exercise and epinephrine on maximal breathing capacity. *J Appl Physiol* 1954;7:309–312.

46. Salzano JV, Camporesi EM, Stolp BW, Moon RE. Physiological responses to exercise at 47 and 66 ATA. *J Appl Physiol: Respir Environ Exercise Physiol* 1984;57:1055–1068.

47. Van Liew HD. Mechanical and physical factors in lung function during work in dense environments. *Undersea Biomed Res* 1983;10:255–264.

48. Hesser CV, Lind F, Faijerson B. Effects of exercise and raised air pressures on maximal voluntary ventilation. In: Grimstad J, ed. *Proceedings of the European Underwater Biomedical Society 5th annual scientific meeting,* July 5–6, 1979. Bergen, Norway: European Undersea Biomedical Society, Bergen, 1979; pp. 203–212.

49. Van Liew HD, Sponholtz DK. Effectiveness of a breath during exercise in a hyperbaric environment. *Undersea Biomed Res* 1981;8:147–161.

50. Hickey DD, Norfleet WT, Pasche AJ, Lundgren CE. Respiratory function in the upright, working diver at 6.8 ATA (190 fsw). *Undersea Biomed Res* 1987;14:241–262.

51. Flook V, Fraser IM. Inspiratory flow limitation in divers. *Undersea Biomed Res* 1989;16:305–311.

52. Varene P, Vieillefond H, Lemaire C, Saumon G. Expiratory flow volume curves and ventilatory limitation of muscular exercise at depth. *Aerosp Med* 1974;45:161–166.

53. Vorosmarti J, Bradley ME, Anthonisen NR. The effects of increased gas density on pulmonary mechanics. *Undersea Biomed Res* 1975;2:1–10.

54. Linnarsson D, Hesser CM. Dissociated ventilatory and central respiratory responses to CO_2 and raised N_2 pressure. *J Appl Physiol: Respir Environ Exercise Physiol* 1978;45:756–761.

55. Gelfand R, Lambertsen CJ, Strauss R, Clark JM, Puglia CD. Human respiration at rest in rapid compression and at high pressures and gas densities. *J Appl Physiol: Respir Environ Exercise Physiol* 1983;54:290–303.

56. Lanphier EH. Human respiration under increased pressures. In: Sleigh M, Macdonald A, eds. *The effects of pressure on organisms (Symposia of the Society for Experimental Biology, No. XXVI).* Cambridge: Cambridge University Press, 1972;379–394.

57. Wood LDH, Bryan AC, Bau SK, Weng TR, Levison H. Effect of increased gas density on pulmonary gas exchange in man. *J Appl Physiol* 1976;41:206–210.

58. Christopherson S, Hlastala MP. Pulmonary gas exchange during altered density gas breathing. *J Appl Physiol: Respir Environ Exercise Physiol* 1982;52:221–225.

59. The physiological basis of decompression. In: Vann RD, ed. *Thirty-eighth Undersea and Hyperbaric Medical Society workshop.* Bethesda, MD: Undersea and Hyperbaric Medical Society, 1989;437 pp.

60. Balldin UI, Lundgren CEG. Effects of immersion with the head above water on tissue nitrogen elimination in man. *Aerosp Med* 1972;42:1101–1108.

61. Balldin UI, Lundgren CEG, Lundwall J, Mellander S. Changes in the elimination of ^{133}xenon from the anterior tibial muscle in man induced by immersion in water and by shifts in body position. *Aerosp Med* 1971;42:489–493.

62. Anderson D, Nagasawa GK, Norfleet WT, Olszowka A, Lundgren CEG. High partial pressures of inspired O_2 decrease tissue perfusion and N_2 elimination. *Undersea Biomed Res* 1989;16(Suppl):151.

63. Farhi LE. Elimination of inert gas by the lung. *Respir Physiol* 1967;3:1–11.

64. Boycott AE, Damant GCC, Haldane JS. The prevention of compressed-air illness. *J Hyg (Lond)* 1908;8:343–443.

65. Hills BA. Concepts of inert gas exchange in tissues during decompression. In: Lambertsen CJ, ed. *Underwater physiology; Proceedings of the fourth symposium on underwater physiology.* New York: Academic Press, 1971;115–122.

66. Rahn H. Gasometric method for measurement of tissue oxygen tension. *Fed Proc* 1957;16:685–688.

67. Spencer MP. Decompression limits for compressed air determined by ultrasonically detected blood bubbles. *J Appl Physiol* 1976;40:229–235.

68. Hills BA, Butler BD. Size distribution of intravascular air emboli produced by decompression. *Undersea Biomed Res* 1981;8:163–170.

69. Butler BD, Hills BA. The lung as a filter for microbubbles. *J Appl Physiol* 1979;47:537–543.

70. Brubakk AD, Grip A, Holland B, Onarheim J, Tønjum S. Arterial gas bubbles following ascending excursions during He–O_2 saturation diving. In: Program and Abstracts, Undersea Medical Society Annual Scientific Meeting, May 25–29, 1981. *Undersea Biomed Res* 1981:8:A6.

71. Moon RE, Camporesi EM, Kisslo JA. Patent foramen ovale and decompression sickness in divers. *Lancet* 1989;1:513–514.

72. Kindwall EP, Baz A, Lightfoot EN, Lanphier EM, Seireg A. Nitrogen elimination in man during decompression. *Undersea Biomed Res* 1975;2:285–297.

73. Hlastala MP, Robertson HT, Ross BK. Gas exchange abnormalities produced by venous gas emboli. *Respir Physiol* 1979;36:1–17.

74. D'Aoust BG, Swanson HT, White R, Dunford R, Mahoney J. Central venous bubbles and mixed venous nitrogen in goats following decompression. *J Appl Physiol: Respir Environ Exercise Physiol* 1981;51:1238–1244.

75. Ward CA, McCullough D, Yee D, Stanga D, Fraser WD. Complement activation involvement in decompression sickness of rabbits. *Undersea Biomed Res* 1990;17:51–66.

76. Blenkarn GD, Aquadro C, Hills BA, Salzman HA. Urticaria following the sequential breathing of various inert gases at a constant ambient pressure of 7 ATA: a possible manifestation of gas-induced osmosis. *Aerosp Med* 1971;42:141–146.

77. Graves DJ, Idicula J, Lambertsen CJ, Quinn JA. Bubble formation resulting from counterdiffusion supersaturation: a possible explanation for inert gas urticaria and vertigo. *Phys Med Biol* 1973;18:256–264.

78. Pisarello JM, Fried M, Fisher DG, Lambertsen CJ. Superficial isobaric counterdiffusion gas lesion disease: effects leading to mortality. In: Bachrach AJ, Matzen MM, eds. *Underwater physiology VIII.* Bethesda, MD: Undersea and Hyperbaric Medical Society, 1984;101–106.

79. Tepper RS, Lightfoot EN, Baz A, Lanphier EH. Inert gas transport in the microcirculation: risk of isobaric supersaturation. *J Appl Physiol: Respir Environ Exercise Physiol* 1979;46:1157–1163.

80. Keller H, Bühlmann A. Deep diving and short decompression by breathing mixed gases. *J Appl Physiol* 1965;20:1267–1270.

81. Ingvar DH, Adolfson J, Lindemark CO. Cerebral gas embolism during training of submarine personnel in free escape: an electroencephalographic study. *Aerosp Med* 1973;44:628–635.

82. Colebatch HJH, Smith MM, Ng CKY. Increased elastic recoil

as a determinant of pulmonary barotrauma in divers. *Respir Physiol* 1976;26:55–64.

83. Bennett PB. Inert gas narcosis. In: Bennett PB, Elliott DH, eds. *The physiology and medicine of diving,* 3rd ed. San Pedro, CA: Best, 1982;239–261.

84. Adolfson J. Human performance and behavior in hyperbaric environments. Thesis, Department of Psychology, University of Gothenburg, Gothenburg, Sweden. *Acta Psychol Gothoburgensia* 1967;1:1–74.

85. Bennett PB. The high pressure nervous syndrome in man. In: Bennett PB, Elliott DH, eds. *The physiology and medicine of diving,* 3rd ed. San Pedro, CA: Best, 1982;262–296.

86. Bennett PB, Blenkarn GD, Roby J, Youngblood D. Suppression of the high pressure nervous syndrome in human deep dives by He–N$_2$–O$_2$. *Undersea Biomed Res* 1974;1:221–237.

87. Rostain JC, Gardette-Chauffour MG, Lemaire C, Naquet R. Effects of a H$_2$–He–O$_2$ mixture on the HPNS up to 450 msw. *Undersea Biomed Res* 1988;15:257–270.

THE LUNG: Scientific Foundations
edited by R.G. Crystal, J.B. West et al.
Raven Press, Ltd., New York © 1991.

CHAPTER 8.1.3

Therapeutic and Toxic Effects of Hyperbaric Oxygenation

James M. Clark

The usefulness of breathing oxygen at increased ambient pressures has been established in medicine and diving (1–4). Therapeutic administration of oxygen in a compression chamber represents in many ways an extension of normobaric oxygen therapy as given in the normal hospital environment. The chamber is used to administer oxygen doses that cannot be achieved at 1.0 atmosphere absolute (ATA). Similarly, the diver breathing oxygen in the hyperbaric underwater environment is exposed to a range of oxygen doses that represent a continuum of the lower levels of hyperoxia encountered by the aviator or astronaut in the hypobaric aerospace environment. In both the hyperbaric chamber and undersea environment, the lung is the point of entry for delivery of increased oxygen pressures to all organs and tissues of the body.

The patient or diver who breathes oxygen at increased ambient pressure can benefit from the many desirable effects of hyperoxia concurrently with exposure to accelerated development of adverse effects on cellular metabolic processes. Both the beneficial and adverse effects of hyperoxia will be considered in this chapter, with particular emphasis on those effects that occur uniquely or that are significantly enhanced in the hyperbaric environment. Because the increased oxygen pressures that are administered via the lung are delivered in varying doses by the arterial circulation to all organs and tissues, beneficial and adverse effects of hyperoxia at extrapulmonary sites will be considered as well as those on the lung itself.

J. M. Clark: Departments of Environmental Medicine and Pharmacology, Institute for Environmental Medicine, University of Pennsylvania Medical Center, Philadelphia, Pennsylvania 19104.

PHYSIOLOGICAL BASIS OF HYPERBARIC OXYGEN THERAPY

The oxygen environment of any organ or tissue is determined by several interacting factors that influence the balance between oxygen supply and its metabolic utilization. Arterial oxygen content is influenced by oxygen partial pressure, hemoglobin concentration, and oxyhemoglobin percent saturation. In addition, organ oxygen supply is highly dependent on arterial blood flow. Capillary network density determines the diffusion distance from the nearest capillary to any individual cell. At the mitochondrial end of the oxygen pathway, tissue demands for oxygen are determined by the level of metabolic activity.

Many of the therapeutic benefits of hyperbaric oxygenation are associated with its capacity for increasing oxygen delivery to hypoxic tissues (Fig. 1). Although hemoglobin is 97–98% saturated at normal arterial P_{O_2} and therefore can hold little additional oxygen, the quantity of physically dissolved oxygen increases linearly with arterial P_{O_2} elevation by about 2.4 ml O_2 per 100 ml blood per atmosphere of inspired P_{O_2} (6). This important increment in arterial oxygen content is associated with an even larger elevation of the oxygen partial pressure gradient from capillary blood to metabolizing cell. The concurrent increments in oxygen content and diffusion gradient facilitate oxygen delivery to tissues that, from ischemia or some other cause, remain hypoxic during air breathing. Although oxygen breathing at 1.0 ATA would also be beneficial in some of these states, the associated increments in oxygen content and P_{O_2} are often insufficient to ensure restoration of normal metabolic function in ischemic tissues. In addition to enhancing oxygen delivery, hyperbaric oxygenation has other

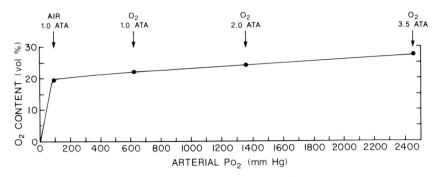

FIG. 1. Relationship of arterial oxygen content to arterial P_{O_2} in normal men. Oxygen content values represent combinations of hemoglobin-bound and physically dissolved oxygen in the arterial blood of men breathing air at 1.0 ATA and breathing oxygen at 1.0, 2.0, and 3.5 ATA. Arterial P_{O_2} values are averages for 10 men at 1.0 and 2.0 ATA and for a subgroup of 6 men at 3.5 ATA (5). Of each oxygen content value, 20 ml of O_2 per 100 ml blood (vol %) is bound to hemoglobin and the remainder is physically dissolved. A solubility factor of 0.0031 ml O_2 per mmHg P_{O_2} per 100 ml blood (6) was used to calculate volumes of physically dissolved oxygen.

therapeutic effects that will be discussed in relation to the specific disease states in which they occur.

CURRENT INDICATIONS FOR HYPERBARIC OXYGEN THERAPY

Clinical applications of hyperbaric oxygenation now extend considerably beyond its initial use in diving medicine (1–3). Several conditions in which there is a rational basis for its use and in which its clinical efficacy has been demonstrated are listed in Table 1. Experimental and clinical evidence in support of these applications has recently been summarized by the Hyperbaric Oxygen Committee of the Undersea and Hyperbaric Medical Society (2). A succinct, comprehensive review (3) that summarizes much of what is known about mechanisms for therapeutic effects of hyperoxia has also been published recently.

TABLE 1. *Current indications for hyperbaric oxygen therapy approved by the Hyperbaric Oxygen Committee of the Undersea and Hyperbaric Medical Society*

Gas lesion diseases
  Decompression sickness
  Gas embolism
Vascular insufficiency states
  Radiation necrosis of bone or soft tissue
  Healing enhancement in problem wounds
  Compromised skin grafts or flaps
  Acute traumatic ischemias
  Thermal burns
Infections
  Clostridial myonecrosis
  Necrotizing soft-tissue infections
  Chronic refractory osteomyelitis
Defects in oxygen transport
  Carbon monoxide poisoning

POSSIBLE MECHANISMS FOR BENEFITS OF HYPERBARIC OXYGENATION

Gas Lesion Diseases

Arterial gas embolism and decompression sickness have been referred to as "gas lesion diseases" to emphasize the primary role of gas bubbles in causing circulatory obstruction and/or tissue distortion (7). Arterial gas embolism is caused by intra-arterial injection of gas (usually air) from an external source such as a ruptured lung or a surgical accident, often involving a cardiovascular or neurosurgical procedure (8). Decompression sickness arises from bubbles formed in tissues or the venous circulation when ambient pressure is reduced too rapidly to permit circulatory and pulmonary elimination of excess nitrogen dissolved in tissues during a prior exposure to increased pressure. Arterial gas embolism and decompression sickness can occur together when intravenous bubbles arising from inadequate decompression traverse the pulmonary circulation via intracardiac or intrapulmonary shunts to enter the systemic arterial circulation.

Regardless of the source of bubbles, the primary aims of therapy are reduction in bubble size, acceleration of bubble resolution, and maintenance of tissue oxygenation (9). All of these aims can be achieved simultaneously by administration of 100% O_2 at an increased ambient pressure (Fig. 2). In both arterial gas embolism and decompression sickness, increased blood viscosity, hypovolemia, and other systemic effects of bubble interactions with blood components and vessels occur concurrently with the localized tissue ischemia caused by mechanical vascular obstruction. Prognosis for a full recovery is enhanced by avoiding delay between onset of symptoms and initiation of hyperbaric oxygen therapy to minimize both

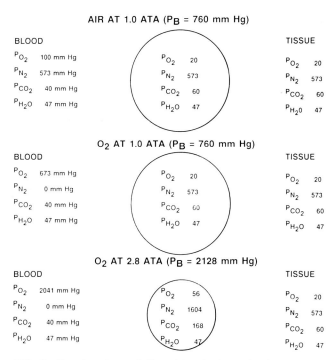

FIG. 2. Gas tension relationships in hyperbaric oxygen therapy of gas embolism and decompression sickness. Initial relationships for gas tensions in blood, tissue, and an embolic bubble are shown. Breathing O_2 at 1.0 ATA hastens bubble resolution by providing an outward diffusion gradient for N_2. Compression to 2.8 ATA decreases bubble size immediately and greatly increases the outward diffusion gradient for N_2.

the period of tissue ischemia and the activation of secondary bubble effects. Administration of 100% O_2 at 1.0 ATA will provide some benefit, especially if definitive therapy must be delayed, by hastening the elimination of inert gas.

Vascular Insufficiency States

Clinical states in which wound healing may be delayed or arrested secondary to ischemic hypoxia include radiation necrosis of bone or soft tissue, diabetic microangiopathy, compromised skin grafts or myocutaneous flaps, crush wounds or other acute traumatic ischemias, and thermal burns (Table 1). Clinical experience and, in some cases, animal models indicate that hyperbaric oxygen therapy can enhance wound healing in each of these states. Although underlying mechanisms are not defined in detail, many known effects of hyperbaric oxygenation have potential for therapeutic benefit.

Radiation Necrosis

A delayed injury response to high-dose radiation therapy is characterized by the development of tissues that

have a reduced density of capillaries, decreased numbers of fibroblasts, and delayed or arrested healing in response to accidental or surgical trauma (10,11). These vascular, cellular, and metabolic deficits appear to be caused by the progressive loss of microcirculation secondary to obliterative radiation endarteritis (3,12). As a result of the widespread and effective use of irradiation in the therapy of oral malignancies, clinical sequelae of radiation damage are relatively common in these patients. In its fully developed state, osteoradionecrosis of the jaws consists of nonhealing exposed bone in association with a variable incidence of pain, orocutaneous fistulae, and pathologic fractures (10,11,13).

Adjunctive use of hyperbaric oxygenation in the therapy of mandibular or maxillary radionecrosis has greatly reduced the incidence of postoperative complications after the surgical resection of necrotic bone to arrest the disease process (13,14). This sometimes debilitating surgery can then be followed, when necessary, by reconstructive procedures to restore jaw function and improve facial appearance. The increased capacity for healing of irradiated tissues after a series of hyperbaric oxygen therapies is associated with induction of capillary angiogenesis and increased numbers of fibroblasts (10,11). Oxygen stimulation of collagen synthesis by fibroblasts is thought to provide a matrix for ingrowth of capillaries.

In patients who have received at least 6500 rad of external radiation for oral malignancy, measurements of transcutaneous Po_2, which correlates with vascular density of the underlying tissues, show that Po_2 values in the center of the radiation field average about 30% of the values over a comparable nonirradiated reference tissue (11–13). After six to eight daily hyperbaric oxygen therapies, the Po_2 of the irradiated area rises progressively to plateau at about 80% of the reference tissue value within a total of 18–20 therapies. Transcutaneous Po_2 measurements in a few patients up to 3 years after receiving a series of hyperbaric oxygen therapies appear to indicate that the partially restored vascular density of the irradiated tissue is persistent. In a group of 74 patients who required extractions of one or more teeth from a mandibular segment that had received a radiation dose of at least 6000 rad, a prospectively randomized trial comparing adjunctive hyperbaric oxygen therapy and systemic antibiotics showed a significant reduction of postoperative osteoradionecrosis in the oxygen group (15).

Acute Traumatic Ischemias

In cases of crush injury and other acute traumatic ischemias, it is rational to use hyperbaric pressures to provide gradients that will increase oxygen diffusion into ischemic areas. However, this benefit must be provided intermittently to prevent the development of oxygen poisoning. Although appropriately controlled studies are lacking, extensive clinical experience indicates that tissue salvage is increased in areas of marginal perfusion (3,16).

Possible benefits of hyperbaric oxygenation in acute ischemia have been evaluated in two animal models. In one model, consisting of a dog hindlimb compartment syndrome, intermittent hyperbaric oxygen therapy significantly reduced muscle edema and necrosis, with a concurrent improvement in muscle viability (17). Hyperbaric oxygenation also reduced post-ischemic edema in a rat model of ischemia–reperfusion injury (18). Subsequent metabolic studies showed that a single therapy significantly increased cellular levels of adenosine triphosphate and phosphocreatine and reduced lactate concentration (19).

Animal Models of Vascular Insufficiency States

Stimulation of capillary proliferation by hyperbaric oxygenation has also been demonstrated in a rat burn model in which 20% full thickness wounds were produced by scalding a depilated area of the back for 10 sec (20). Angiographic and histologic examinations of the burned areas showed that rats that received intermittent hyperbaric oxygen therapy had much more extensive capillary proliferation than did control animals that breathed air.

In a variety of animal models of compromised grafts and flaps, responses to adjunctive hyperbaric oxygenation are characterized by improved tissue oxygenation, increased capillary density, and enhanced viability (3,21–23). Other studies using animal models show no benefit with hyperbaric oxygenation (24,25). However, procedural flaws in these studies have been noted (3). The fact that an experimental graft or flap can be compromised so severely that it does not respond favorably to hyperbaric oxygenation should not detract from the observation of improved viability with hyperbaric oxygenation while using another model in which the initial degree of tissue ischemia is less severe.

Infections

Infectious diseases in which hyperbaric oxygenation has been used adjunctively include clostridial myonecrosis (gas gangrene) (26–28), a variety of necrotizing soft tissue infections (29,30), and chronic refractory osteomyelitis (31,32). Although there are no prospective, randomized clinical trials that validate the use of hyperbaric oxygen therapy in any of these conditions, supporting evidence is provided by a combination of clinical reports, animal models, and accumulating information about potential mechanisms for therapeutic actions of hyperoxia. Addition of hyperbaric oxygenation to the standard application of surgical and antibiotic therapy in clostridial myonecrosis is reported to increase tissue salvage and decrease mortality (33,34). Using animal models of clostridial myonecrosis in dogs, rabbits, and guinea pigs, the combination of surgery, antibiotics, and hyperbaric oxygenation significantly improved survival beyond that provided by any combination of only two modalities (35,36).

Direct Effects of Hyperoxia Against Infections

In vitro studies have demonstrated that sufficiently high oxygen pressures can kill a wide variety of bacteria (37), but bactericidal doses of oxygen are not achieved in most infected tissues while using oxygen pressure–exposure duration combinations that are tolerable for the patient (38,39). It is possible that bactericidal doses for strict anaerobes and bacteriostatic doses for facultative and aerobic organisms are reached in tissues that have a relatively intact blood supply. In the special case of gas gangrene infections, oxygen doses achieved in at least the margins of advancing infection are sufficiently high to block production of the lethal alpha exotoxin produced by Clostridium species (40). This action probably represents the most significant benefit of adjunctive hyperbaric oxygenation in the therapy of clostridial myonecrosis, because toxemia (rather than septicemia) is known to be the primary cause of systemic toxicity in this disease.

Indirect Effects of Hyperoxia Against Infections

Under hypoxic conditions, the bactericidal efficiency of polymorphonuclear leucocytes is decreased (41), presumably by an impaired generation of oxygen radicals. Leucocyte function in hypoxic areas is improved when oxygen tension is elevated to normal or slightly increased levels (42,43). Improved antibiotic efficacy by restoration of normal P_{O_2} levels has also been demonstrated in a rabbit osteomyelitis model (44). In a recently reported model of polymicrobial sepsis in the rat, mortality was significantly reduced by early administration of intermittent hyperbaric oxygen therapy (45). Positive cultures of blood and peritoneal fluids from surviving animals were not consistent with a direct antibacterial action of hyperoxia, leaving enhancement of host defenses as the most likely basis for the observed reduction in mortality.

Defects in Oxygen Transport

Carbon Monoxide Poisoning

Defective indoor heaters and automobile exhaust systems combine with smoke inhalation to make carbon monoxide (CO) the leading cause of death by poisoning in the United States (3). Severity of intoxication is determined by both the level and duration of CO exposure. For a given concentration of carboxyhemoglobin, a long exposure to a relatively low CO partial pressure causes greater morbidity than does a shorter exposure to a higher CO pressure, because vital organs are hypoxic for longer periods of time. The severity of neurological intoxication is apparently exacerbated when cerebral hypoxia caused by impairment of arterial oxygen transport is combined with ischemia induced by concurrent cardiac dysfunction (46,47). Although mechanisms are not known, the occurrence of mild to severe neurological sequelae for up to 4 weeks after apparent recovery from acute intoxication is well documented (3).

Administration of oxygen reduces the half-time for carboxyhemoglobin dissociation from over 5 hr on air to 90 min on O_2 at 1.0 ATA or to 23 min on O_2 at 3.0 ATA (3). In addition, hyperbaric oxygenation provides (a) an increased arterial content of physically dissolved oxygen and (b) an increased pressure gradient for driving oxygen into ischemic tissues. Several investigators have reported that severe, CO-induced deficits in neurological and cardiovascular function can be reversed by administration of hyperbaric oxygen therapy (3,48,49). Reduction in the incidence of delayed neurological sequelae by prompt administration of hyperbaric oxygenation at the time of acute intoxication has also been reported (50,51). However, appropriately

controlled clinical trials are needed to confirm these apparent benefits beyond reasonable doubt.

A recently developed *in vivo* model, showing hyperoxic reversal of CO effects in the rat brain (52), has provided a potential mechanism for a therapeutic action of hyperbaric oxygenation that is independent of an increased rate of carboxyhemoglobin dissociation. Brain lipid peroxidation occurred in this model following a CO exposure that was sufficiently severe to cause a brief period of hypotension and syncope. The onset of lipid peroxidation following CO exposure was prevented by O_2 administration at 3.0 ATA, but not by O_2 breathing at 1.0 ATA. The observed antagonism of lipid peroxidation appeared to be mediated by an O_2-induced production of H_2O_2. Direct antagonism of lipid peroxidation by H_2O_2 has been reported previously (53,54). The related implication that at least some manifestations of CO poisoning are caused by a form of ischemia–reperfusion injury, and that hyperbaric oxygenation can ameliorate these effects, has great potential significance in the therapy of any disease state in which such an injury is involved.

LIMITATIONS IMPOSED BY OXYGEN TOXICITY

The severity of oxygen poisoning increases progressively with elevation of inspired P_{O_2} and with greater duration of exposure (55,56). At sufficient pressure and exposure duration, oxygen will cause initial functional impairment and final chemical destruction of any living cell. Many of the diverse manifestations of oxygen poisoning are summarized in Fig. 3.

There is extensive evidence that formation of active radicals is an intermediate event in the production of

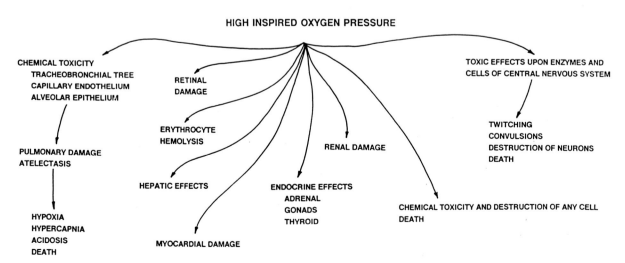

FIG. 3. Diversity and progression of toxic effects produced by exposure to increased oxygen pressures. (Modified from ref. 56.)

oxidant damage to cell membranes and constituents (57). Antioxidant defense mechanisms have also been identified (58). Although exact mechanisms are not known, the number and complexity of possible interactions between active species and antioxidant defenses provide many potential sites and pathways for influencing both the nature and the severity of toxic effects.

A remarkable capacity for reversal of toxic effects and recovery from severe oxygen poisoning has been demonstrated in animals and in humans (55,56). Complete recovery from milder degrees of oxygen poisoning occurs even more rapidly. The inherent capacity for reversal of toxic effects and recovery from clinically effective oxygen doses makes administration of hyperbaric oxygenation one of the safest therapeutic modalities in modern medicine.

Pulmonary Tolerance to Hyperbaric Oxygen Pressures

Although pulmonary effects of oxygen toxicity found during prolonged exposure at 1.0 ATA (Chapter 8.2.2) occur more rapidly at higher pressures, there is still a period of time during which no toxic effects are evident; moreover, recovery is complete between exposures that are sufficiently spaced (56,59). Accordingly, pulmonary symptoms or signs are not produced by the hyperbaric oxygen therapy protocols used for most elective conditions. However, symptoms of pulmonary oxygen poisoning [i.e., substernal discomfort, chest tightness, cough, and dyspnea (6,55,56,60)] are sometimes experienced in varying combinations by patients who undergo aggressive hyperbaric oxygen therapy for conditions such as severe decompression sickness or arterial gas embolism.

In studies designed to define limits of tolerance to continuous oxygen exposure over a range of useful pressures, normal men breathed oxygen at pressures of 3.0, 2.5, 2.0, and 1.5 ATA for average durations of 3.4, 5.7, 9.0, and 17.7 hr, respectively (60). Pulmonary mechanical function was significantly impaired by all four exposure combinations, and the single-breath CO diffusing capacity was reduced by all combinations except 3.4 hr at 3.0 ATA. Arterial oxygenation was detectably impaired only after exposure for 17.7 hr at 1.5 ATA, and then only during exercise. Overall, these results indicated that pulmonary mechanical function was impaired earlier and more prominently than gas exchange function during continuous exposures over the entire range of pressures used in hyperbaric oxygen therapy. All pulmonary function decrements were fully reversible, even after exposure durations that were much longer than current therapeutic applications (60).

TABLE 2. *Signs and symptoms of CNS oxygen poisoning in normal men[a]*

Facial pallor	Diaphragmatic spasms
Sweating	Nausea
Bradycardia	Spasmodic vomiting
Palpitations	Fibrillation of lips
Apprehension	Lip twitching
Visual field constriction	Twitching of cheek, nose,
Auditory hallucinations	eyelids
Tinnitus	Syncope
Vertigo	Convulsions
Respiratory changes	

[a] Adapted from ref. 61.

Central Nervous System Effects of Oxygen Toxicity

Overt manifestations of central nervous system (CNS) oxygen poisoning are characterized by the diverse symptoms and signs (Table 2) that were observed in divers who breathed oxygen at pressures of 3.0 ATA or higher until they experienced one or more of these effects (61). Despite extensive efforts to develop reliable methods for detecting the onset of CNS intoxication prior to the occurrence of convulsions, no consistent preconvulsive index could be identified. Minor symptoms did not always precede the onset of convulsions, and even when a preconvulsive aura did occur, it was often followed so quickly by seizures that it had little practical value. Electroencephalography also proved to be a poor index of incipient CNS intoxication, because brain electrical activity was not altered prior to seizure onset. More recent studies have confirmed that electroencephalographic changes in humans occur only upon initiation of the actual seizure (62). Mental performance is also maintained during the period immediately before seizure onset.

The onset of oxygen convulsions is hastened by the presence of acute hypercapnia, whether it be induced by elevation of inspired P_{CO_2}, increased breathing resistance, or narcotic depression of ventilation. The adverse effects of acute hypercapnia are mediated by cerebral vasodilation and delivery of a higher oxygen dose to the brain (6,56). When care is taken to avoid such factors, the incidence of oxygen convulsions during therapeutic exposures is about 1 per 10,000 patient therapies (3,59). Even when a convulsion does occur, there are no residual effects if trauma is prevented (6,56,61).

Toxic Effects on Visual Function

Ocular effects of oxygen toxicity are influenced by many variables in addition to oxygen dose (56,63). Examples of these variable influences include (a) the production of retrolental fibroplasia in a premature infant exposed to hyperoxia (6,56,63) and (b) the reversible, unilateral loss of vision during a 2.0-ATA oxygen exposure of an individual who had a past history of retrobulbar neuritis in the same eye (64). The former example involves a unique condition caused by exposure of the premature retina to any level of hyperoxia, whereas the latter involves an individual predisposition to oxygen toxicity in one eye.

When normal men breathe oxygen at 3.0 ATA, loss of peripheral vision starts at 2.5–3.0 hr of exposure and progresses to an average loss of about 50% of the visual field area at 3.5 hr, with individual losses as great as 90% (62). Central visual acuity is not significantly altered. Recovery of peripheral vision is essentially complete within 30–45 min after exposure termination. Continuous oxygen exposure for 8–10 hr at 2.0 ATA significantly reduces the electrical response of retinal glial cells to a light flash, with complete recovery post-exposure over a period of several hours (62,65). Concurrent changes in peripheral vision are smaller and less consistent. During oxygen exposure for 16–19 hr at 1.5 ATA, neither visual fields nor retinal electrical activity is altered consistently (62).

Therapy protocols used for elective conditions by most practitioners involve daily exposures of the patient for 5 or 6 days per week to oxygen pressures of 2.4 or 2.0 ATA for durations of 90 or 120 min, respectively. About one-third of these patients, with indications of a higher incidence in elderly patients, develop some degree of myopia that usually starts within 2–4 weeks of therapy, is progressive thereafter, and reverses completely within a few days to several weeks after completion of the therapy series (66,67). Although the exact mechanism is unknown, systematic elimination of other possible causes implicates a reversible change in lens shape or metabolism (68). In a group of 25 patients who received an extremely prolonged series of 150–850 daily therapies, 7 of 15 patients who had clear lens nuclei at the start of therapy developed cataracts that persisted or were only partly reversible after termination of the series (69). The myopia associated with the lens changes was also only partly reversible. Most clinical conditions that respond favorably to hyperbaric oxygenation require a cumulative series of 60 therapies or less (2,3).

EXTENSION OF OXYGEN TOLERANCE

Any agent that significantly delays the onset and progression of oxygen poisoning would be extremely useful in therapeutic and diving operational applications of hyperoxia. Such an agent would have to be distributed throughout all body tissues to counteract effectively the multiple and diverse effects of oxygen toxicity (Fig. 3). In addition to wide distribution across

cellular membrane barriers, the agent would have to oppose inhibitory actions against a variety of enzymatic targets within the same cellular location. For all of these reasons, the chemical protective agents that have been developed thus far have only limited potential for practical applications (6,70).

At the present time, the most effective and practical means for extension of oxygen tolerance in humans is the systematic alternation of oxygen exposure periods with normoxic intervals to exploit the empirical observation that rates of reversal for many effects of oxygen toxicity are more rapid during the normoxic intervals than their rates of development during the oxygen periods. The efficacy of this procedure has been demonstrated in animals and in humans (6,55,56,70,71). Intermittent oxygen exposure delays the onset of toxic effects in all organs and tissues, and it has none of the limitations associated with chemical protective agents. The basis for the inherent superiority of this procedure resides in its dependence upon the periodic, sequential elevation and reduction of oxygen tension rather than the passage of a chemical agent across cellular membrane barriers (70). The principle of intermittent oxygen exposure has been empirically incorporated into most of the oxygen therapy tables that are in current use, and studies designed to obtain information that will allow more effective exploitation of this principle are under way (72).

ACKNOWLEDGMENTS

This work was supported, in part, by Naval Medical Research and Development Command Contract N00014-88-K-0270 and National Aeronautics and Space Administration Research Contract NAG 9-342.

REFERENCES

1. Davis JC, Hunt TK, eds. *Problem wounds. The role of oxygen.* New York: Elsevier, 1988.
2. Mader JT, ed. *Hyperbaric oxygen therapy committee report.* Bethesda, MD: Undersea and Hyperbaric Medical Society, 1989.
3. Thom SR. Hyperbaric oxygen therapy. *J Intensive Care Med* 1989;4:58–74.
4. Lambertsen CJ. Basic requirements for improving diving depth and decompression tolerance. In: Lambertsen CJ, ed. *Underwater physiology.* Baltimore: Williams & Wilkins, 1967;223–240.
5. Clark JM, Lambertsen CJ. Alveolar–arterial O_2 differences in man at 0.2, 1.0, 2.0, and 3.5 Ata inspired Po_2. *J Appl Physiol* 1971;30:753–763.
6. Lambertsen CJ. Effects of hyperoxia on organs and their tissues. In: Robin ED, ed. *Extrapulmonary manifestations of respiratory disease. Lung biology in health and disease,* vol 8 (Lenfant C, series ed.). New York: Marcel Dekker, 1978;239–303.
7. Lambertsen CJ, Idicula J. A new gas lesion syndrome in man, induced by "isobaric gas counterdiffusion." *J Appl Physiol* 1975;39:434–443.
8. Peirce EC. Cerebral gas embolism (arterial) with special refer-

ence to iatrogenic accidents. *Hyperbaric Oxygen Rev* 1980; 1:161–184.

9. Davis JC, Elliott DH. Treatment of the decompression disorders. In: Bennett PB, Elliott DH, eds. *The physiology and medicine of diving*, 3rd ed. San Pedro, CA: Best, 1982;473–487.

10. Marx RE. A new concept in the treatment of osteoradionecrosis. *J Oral Maxillofac Surg* 1983;41:351–357.

11. Marx RE. Osteoradionecrosis of the jaws: review and update. *Hyperbaric Oxygen Rev* 1984;5:48–126.

12. Marx RE, Johnson RP. Studies in the radiobiology of osteoradionecrosis and their clinical significance. *Oral Surg Oral Med Oral Pathol* 1987;64:379–390.

13. Marx RE, Johnson RP. Problem wounds in oral and maxillofacial surgery: the role of hyperbaric oxygen. In: Davis JC, Hunt TK, eds. *Problem wounds. The role of oxygen*. New York: Elsevier, 1988;65–123.

14. Marx RE, Ames JR. The use of hyperbaric oxygen therapy in bony reconstruction of the irradiated and tissue-deficient patient. *J Oral Maxillofac Surg* 1982;40:412–420.

15. Marx RE, Johnson RP, Kline SN. Prevention of osteoradionecrosis: a randomized prospective clinical trial of hyperbaric oxygen versus penicillin. *J Am Dent Assoc* 1985;111:49–54.

16. Strauss MB, Hart GB. Crush injury and the role of hyperbaric oxygen. *Top Emerg Med* 1984;6:9–24.

17. Strauss MB, Hargens AR, Gershuni DH, et al. Reduction of skeletal muscle necrosis using intermittent hyperbaric oxygen in a model compartment syndrome. *J Bone Joint Surg* 1983; 65A:656–662.

18. Nylander G, Lewis D, Nordstrom H, Larsson J. Reduction of the post ischemic edema with hyperbaric oxygen. *Plast Reconstr Surg* 1985;76:596–603.

19. Nylander G, Nordstrom H, Lewis D, Larsson J. Metabolic effects of hyperbaric oxygen in post-ischemic muscle. *Plast Reconstr Surg* 1987;79:91–96.

20. Ketchum SA, Thomas AN, Steer M, Hall AD. Angiographic studies of the effects of hyperbaric oxygen on burn wound revascularization. In: Wada J, Iwa T, eds. *Proceedings of the fourth international congress on hyperbaric medicine*. Baltimore: Williams & Wilkins, 1970;383–394.

21. Shulman AG, Krohm HL. Influence of hyperbaric oxygen and multiple skin allografts on the healing of skin wounds. *Surgery* 1967;62:1051–1058.

22. Jurell G, Kaijser L. The influence of varying pressure and duration of treatment with hyperbaric oxygen on the survival of skin flaps: an experimental study. *Scand J Plast Reconstr Surg* 1973;7:25–28.

23. Nemiroff PM, Lunger AL. The influence of hyperbaric oxygen and irradiation on experimental skin flaps: a controlled study. *Surg Forum* 1987;38:565–567.

24. Kernaham DA, Zingg W, Kay CW. The effect of hyperbaric oxygen on the survival of experimental skin flaps. *Plast Reconstr Surg* 1965;36:19–25.

25. Caffee HA, Gallagher TJ. Experiments on the effect of hyperbaric oxygen on flap survival in the pig. *Plast Reconstr Surg* 1988;81:751–754.

26. Bakker DJ. Clostridial myonecrosis. In: Davis JC, Hunt TK, eds. *Problem wounds. The role of oxygen*. New York: Elsevier, 1988;153–172.

27. Hart GB, Lamb RC, Strauss MB. Gas gangrene. I. A collective review. *J Trauma* 1983;23:991–995.

28. Hart GB, Lamb RC, Strauss MB. Gas gangrene. II. A 15-year experience with hyperbaric oxygen. *J Trauma* 1983;23:995–1000.

29. Bakker DJ. Pure and mixed aerobic and anaerobic soft tissue infections. *Hyperbaric Oxygen Rev* 1985;6:65–96.

30. Zanetti CL. Necrotizing soft tissue infection and adjunctive hyperbaric oxygen. *Chest* 1988;92:670–671.

31. Davis JC, Heckman JD, DeLee JC, Buckwald FJ. Chronic nonhematogenous osteomyelitis treated with adjuvant hyperbaric oxygen. *J Bone Joint Surg* 1986;68A:1210–1217.

32. Strauss MB. Refractory osteomyelitis. *J Hyperbaric Med* 1987; 2:147–159.

33. Caplan ES, Kluge RM. Gas gangrene. *Arch Intern Med* 1976; 136:788–791.

34. Sweigal JF, Shim SS. A comparison of the treatment of gas gangrene with and without hyperbaric oxygen. *Surg Gynecol Obstet* 1973;136:969–970.

35. Demello FJ, Haglin JJ, Hitchcock CR. Comparative study of experimental *Clostridium perfringins* infection in dogs treated with antibiotics, surgery, and hyperbaric oxygen. *Surgery* 1973; 73:936–941.

36. Demello FJ, Hitchcock CR, Haglin JJ. Evaluation of hyperbaric oxygen, antibiotics and surgery in experimental gas gangrene. In: Trapp WG, Banister EW, Davison AJ, Trapp PA, eds. *Fifth international hyperbaric congress proceedings*. Vancouver: Simon Fraser University, 1974;554–561.

37. Gottlieb SF. Oxygen under pressure and microorganisms. In: Davis JC, Hunt TK, eds. *Hyperbaric oxygen therapy*. Bethesda, MD: Undersea Medical Society, 1977;79–99.

38. McAllister TA, Stark JM, Norman JN, Ross RM. Inhibitory effects of hyperbaric oxygen on bacteria and fungi. *Lancet* 1963;2:1040–1042.

39. Brown GL, Thomson PD, Mader JT, Hilton JG, Browne ME, Wells CH. Effects of hyperbaric oxygen upon *S. aureus*, *Ps. aeruginosa*, and *C. albicans*. *Aviat Space Environ Med* 1979;50:717–720.

40. Van Unnik AJM. Inhibition of toxin production in *Clostridium perfringins in vitro* by hyperbaric oxygen. *Antonie Van Leeuwenhoek* 1965;31:181–186.

41. Mandell G. Bactericidal activity of aerobic and anaerobic polymorphonuclear neutrophils. *Infect Immun* 1974;9:337–341.

42. Knighton DR, Halliday B, Hunt TK. Oxygen as an antibiotic: the effect of inspired oxygen on infection. *Arch Surg* 1984; 119:199–204.

43. Mader JT, Brown GL, Guckian JC, Wells CH, Reinarz JA. A mechanism for the amelioration by hyperbaric oxygen of experimental staphylococcal osteomyelitis in rabbits. *J Infect Dis* 1980;142:915–922.

44. Mader JT, Adams KR, Sutton TE. Infectious diseases: pathophysiology and mechanisms of hyperbaric oxygen. *J Hyperbaric Med* 1987;2:133–140.

45. Thom SR, Lauermann MW, Hart GB. Intermittent hyperbaric oxygen therapy for reduction of mortality in experimental polymicrobial sepsis. *J Infect Dis* 1986;154:504–510.

46. Ginsberg MD, Myers RE, McDonagh BF. Experimental carbon monoxide encephalopathy in the primate. *Arch Neurol* 1974; 30:209–216.

47. Okeda R, Funata N, Song J, Higashino F, Takano T, Yokoyama K. Comparative study on pathogenesis of selective cerebral lesions in carbon monoxide poisoning and nitrogen hypoxia in cats. *Acta Neuropathol* 1982;56:265–272.

48. Goulon M, Barios A, Rapin M. Intoxication oxycarbonee et anoxie aigue par inhalation de gay de charbon et d'hydrocarbures. *Ann Med Interne (Paris)* 1969;120:335–349.

49. Yee IM, Brandon GK. Successful reversal of presumed carbon monoxide induced semicoma. *Aviat Space Environ Med* 1983; 54:641–643.

50. Myers RAM, Snyder SK, Emhoff TA. Subacute sequelae of carbon monoxide poisoning. *Ann Emerg Med* 1985;14:1163–1167.

51. Mathieu D, Nolf M, Durocher A, Saulnier F. Acute carbon monoxide poisoning risk of late sequelae and treatment by hyperbaric oxygen. *Clinical Toxicology* 1985;23:315–324.

52. Thom SR. Antagonism carbon monoxide-mediated brain lipid peroxidation by hyperbaric oxygen. *Toxicol Appl Pharmacol*, in press.

53. Morehouse LA, Tien M, Bucher JR, Aust SD. Effect of hydrogen peroxide on the initiation of microsomal lipid peroxidation. *Biochem Pharmacol* 1983;32:123–127.

54. Imlay JA, Linn S. DNA damage and oxygen radical toxicity. *Science* 1988;240:1302–1309.

55. Clark JM, Lambertsen CJ. Pulmonary oxygen toxicity: a review. *Pharmacol Rev* 1971;23:37–133.

56. Clark JM. Oxygen toxicity. In: Bennett PB, Elliott DH, eds. *The physiology and medicine of diving*, 3rd ed. San Pedro, CA: Best, 1982;200–238.

57. Jamieson D. Oxygen toxicity and reactive oxygen metabolites in mammals. *Free Radical Biol Med* 1989;7:87–108.

58. Forman HJ, Fisher AB. Antioxidant defenses. In: Gilbert DL, ed. *Oxygen and living processes*. New York: Springer-Verlag, 1981;235–249.

59. Davis JC, Dunn JM, Heimbach RD. Hyperbaric medicine: patient selection, treatment procedures, and side-effects. In: Davis JC, Hunt TK, eds. *Problem wounds. The role of oxygen*. New York: Elsevier, 1988;225–235.

60. Clark JM. Pulmonary limits of oxygen tolerance in man. *Exp Lung Res* 1988;14:897–910.

61. Donald KW. Oxygen poisoning in man. I and II. *Br Med J* 1947;1:667–672, 712–717.

62. Lambertsen CJ, Clark JM, Gelfand R, et al. Definition of tolerance to continuous hyperoxia in man. An abstract report of Predictive Studies V. In: Bove AA, Bachrach AJ, Greenbaum LJ Jr, eds. *Underwater and hyperbaric physiology IX*. Bethesda, MD: Undersea and Hyperbaric Medical Society, 1987;717–735.

63. Nichols CW, Lambertsen CJ. Effects of high oxygen pressures on the eye. *N Engl J Med* 1969;281:25–30.

64. Nichols CW, Lambertsen CJ, Clark JM. Transient unilateral loss of vision associated with oxygen at high pressure. *Arch Ophthalmol* 1969;81:548–552.

65. Clark JM, Lambertsen CJ, Montabana DJ, Gelfand R, Cobbs WH. Comparison of visual function effects in man during continuous oxygen exposures at 3.0 and 2.0 ATA for 3.4 and 9.0 hours (in Predictive Studies V). *Undersea Biomed Res* 1988;15(Suppl):32.

66. Anderson B Jr, Farmer JC Jr. Hyperoxic myopia. *Trans Am Ophthalmol Soc* 1978;76:116–124.

67. Lyne AJ. Ocular effects of hyperbaric oxygen. *Trans Ophthalmol Soc UK* 1978;98:66–68.

68. Anderson B Jr, Shelton DL. Axial length in hyperoxic myopia. In: Bove AA, Bachrach AJ, Greenbaum LJ Jr, eds. *Underwater and hyperbaric physiology IX*. Bethesda, MD: Undersea and Hyperbaric Medical Society, 1987;607–611.

69. Palmquist BM, Philipson B, Barr PO. Nuclear cataract and myopia during hyperbaric oxygen therapy. *Br J Ophthalmol* 1984;68:113–117.

70. Lambertsen CJ. Extension of oxygen tolerance in man: philosophy and significance. *Exp Lung Res* 1988;14:1035–1058.

71. Hendricks PL, Hall DA, Hunter WH Jr, Haley PJ. Extension of pulmonary O_2 tolerance in man at 2 ata by intermittent O_2 exposure. *J Appl Physiol: Respir Environ Exercise Physiol* 1977;42:593–599.

72. Clark JM, Lambertsen CJ. Principles of oxygen tolerance extension defined in the rat by intermittent oxygen exposure at 2.0 and 4.0 ATA. *Undersea Biomed Res* 1989;16(Suppl):99.

THE LUNG: Scientific Foundations
edited by R.G. Crystal, J.B. West et al.
Raven Press, Ltd., New York © 1991.

CHAPTER 8.1.4

Space

John B. West

Human beings entered the space environment only 30 years ago. Nevertheless, it has become clear that this adventure has brought a whole series of new challenges to medicine and biology. The chief hazards of space include (a) the effects of microgravity (weightlessness) on the body, (b) possible exposure to high levels of ionizing radiation including exotic particles not present in the earth's environment, and (c) the consequences of living in a confined space for long periods (1). This last aspect of the space environment has spawned a whole area of research known as "closed environment life support systems" (CELSS), in which human beings and plants live symbiotically. In addition to these problems of human space biology and medicine, space life science extends to other, broader issues such as the origins and evolution of life, the detection of extant or extinct life on other planets, and the search for extraterrestrial intelligence (SETI).

Hypoxia is not a feature of the space environment, because the astronaut or cosmonaut takes his atmosphere with him. Indeed, the early U.S. manned space flights, including the Apollo flights to the moon, were characterized by hyperoxia because the astronauts were breathing 100% oxygen at a reduced barometric pressure, giving an inspired P_{O_2} of about 260 torr (normal sea level value is 149 torr). However, even when the astronauts are breathing 21% oxygen in nitrogen at 760 torr (as at sea level), there are concerns about the buildup of toxic contaminant gases in the closed spacecraft.

In the context of pulmonary science, the most important factor of the space environment is microgravity, and this affects pulmonary function in a number of ways. However, first it should be pointed out that weightlessness affects many organ systems of the body and that these disturbances of function are generally more important than in the case of the lung. The effects of weightlessness in humans include the following:

1. *Altered vestibular function leading to space sickness.* This is particularly important in the present relatively short (7–9 day) flights of the Shuttle.

2. *Bone decalcification.* This principally affects weight-bearing bones, and there is some evidence that the abnormality is not completely corrected when the astronaut or cosmonaut returns to earth. Some people believe that this problem may ultimately limit the duration of long-term space flight.

3. *Muscle atrophy.* This is presumably related to disuse and causes loss of strength. Histological changes are seen within a few days in skeletal muscles of experimental animals.

4. *Cardiovascular system.* The astronaut develops postural hypotension when he returns to the $1g$ environment, and he is unduly sensitive to lower-body negative pressure while in orbit. The mechanism of this so-called deconditioning is poorly understood.

5. *Blood.* There is a loss of both red blood cell mass and plasma volume.

6. *Renal and endocrine.* There are alterations in the amount and distribution of body fluid volume.

Several experiments designed to elucidate the mechanisms of these changes will fly on Spacelab SLS-1, scheduled for late-1990 (2).

TOPOGRAPHICAL DIFFERENCES OF PULMONARY STRUCTURE AND FUNCTION

The normal lung is exquisitely sensitive to gravity, which causes regional differences in blood flow, ventilation, gas exchange, alveolar size, intrapleural pressure, and mechanical stress (3). Presumably all of these will be greatly reduced, and even abolished, in the microgravity environment (Fig. 1).

J. B. West: Department of Medicine, University of California–San Diego, La Jolla, California 92093.

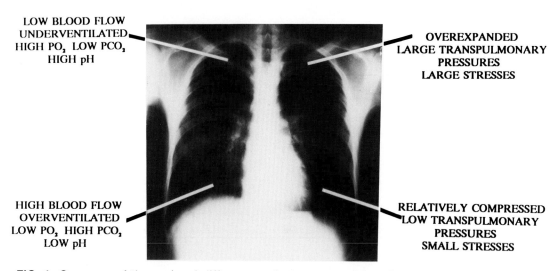

LOW BLOOD FLOW
UNDERVENTILATED
HIGH PO₂ LOW PCO₂
HIGH pH

OVEREXPANDED
LARGE TRANSPULMONARY
PRESSURES
LARGE STRESSES

HIGH BLOOD FLOW
OVERVENTILATED
LOW PO₂ HIGH PCO₂
LOW pH

RELATIVELY COMPRESSED
LOW TRANSPULMONARY
PRESSURES
SMALL STRESSES

FIG. 1. Summary of the regional differences of structure and function caused by gravity. Presumably these will be greatly reduced, or even abolished, in microgravity.

Blood Flow

The effects of gravity on the regional distribution of blood flow were discussed in Chapter 5.2.3. Blood flow decreases up the upright human lung, reaching very low values at the apex. The inequality of blood flow is altered by change of posture; thus in the supine position, apical and basal blood flow are the same, but there is an increase in blood flow from the anterior to posterior (dependent) region of the lung. During upright exercise, both apical and basal blood flows increase, and the distribution becomes more uniform (4).

The regional differences in blood flow can be explained by the effects of the pulmonary arterial, venous, and alveolar pressures on the pulmonary capillaries (5). Basically, the gradient can be attributed to the hydrostatic pressures in the column of blood in the lung which are not balanced by similar pressures in the alveoli. In addition, lung volume plays a role because when the expansion of the lung is decreased, the extra-alveolar vessels narrow, and this contributes to an increase in vascular resistance (6). The result is a region of reduced blood flow at the lung base.

It is known that increased acceleration exaggerates the normal regional inequality of blood flow. Extensive centrifuge studies of $+g_z$ acceleration (headward) and $+g_x$ (forward acceleration) have been carried out (7). Pilots are subjected to $+g_z$ accelerations during tight turns in high-performance aircraft, and astronauts lie supine in the spacecraft during lift-off ($+g_x$) because tolerance to acceleration is better in this position. The only studies of the effects of microgravity on blood-flow distribution to date are those carried out in aircraft performing Keplerian arcs (see below).

Ventilation

Gravity-induced regional inequality of ventilation was discussed in Chapter 5.1.2.6. Because the lung distorts under its own weight, the alveoli at the base of the upright lung are relatively compressed compared with the apical alveoli; and because poorly expanded lung is more compliant, ventilation increases down the upright human lung (8). Thus the changes in ventilation are in the same direction as those for blood flow, but the magnitude of the inequality of ventilation is less.

A striking change in the regional distribution of ventilation occurs at low lung volumes because the basal airways close; and for small inspirations from residual volume, no gas enters the basal regions. Therefore under these conditions, the normal pattern of ventilation is reversed, with the apex being ventilated best.

Increased acceleration has been shown to exaggerate the normal regional differences in ventilation, as for blood flow. At high $+g_z$ levels (aircraft in a tight turn) an interesting dissociation of ventilation and blood flow can occur. Blood flow is confined to the base of the lung because of hydrostatic effects, whereas ventilation is confined to the upper regions because of basal airway closure. As a result there is little meeting of the two, and gas exchange is greatly impaired (7). Studies of the effects of weightlessness on the distribution of ventilation have been confined so far to parabolic flights (see below).

Gas Exchange

Because gas exchange in any region of the lung is determined by the ventilation–perfusion ratio (see Chapter 5.3.4), the regional differences of blood flow and ventilation imply regional differences of gas exchange. For example, because the ventilation–perfusion ratio is relatively high at the apex of the lung, this region has a high P_{O_2}, low P_{CO_2}, and high pH (9). Furthermore, the uptake of oxygen and elimination of carbon dioxide by the upper regions of the lung are relatively small because of the reduced blood flow and ventilation to that region. On exercise, when the pulmonary artery pressure rises and the distribution of blood flow becomes more uniform, the upper regions of the lung take on a larger proportion of total gas exchange.

Alveolar Size

Because the lung distorts under its own weight, the basal alveoli are less well expanded than the apical alveoli (Chapter 5.1.2.6). In anesthetized dogs frozen in the head-up position, the apical alveoli are four times larger by volume than those at the base (10,11). However, when the animals were frozen in the supine position, the size of the apical and basal alveoli were the same, confirming that gravity was responsible for the differences. These differences in alveoli size are closely related to the regional differences in ventilation described above.

Intrapleural Pressures

The weight of the lung is supported, to a large extent, by the rib cage and diaphragm. As a result of the downward-acting weight force, the pressure near the bottom of the lung must be greater than the pressure near the top. This means that the intrapleural pressure is less negative at the bottom of the lung than at the top. Regional differences in intrapleural pressure were first demonstrated in head-up anesthetized dogs (12) and subsequently in many other animals (13). Early evidence in humans was obtained by measuring esophageal pressure at different levels (14).

Parenchymal Stresses

Just as the relative overexpansion of the lung at the apex is associated with very low intrapleural pressures, it also causes large mechanical parenchymal stresses. Because of technical difficulties, these have not been measured directly, but the pattern of stress distribution has been analyzed by finite element techniques (15,16). The higher stresses near the apex may explain the pattern of development of centrilobular emphysema, spontaneous pneumothorax, and other diseases (17). Figure 1 summarizes the topographical dif-

ferences of pulmonary structure and function discussed above.

Effects of Microgravity on Topographical Differences

All the regional differences of structure and function referred to above are caused by gravity. The weight of the column of blood in the lung is responsible for the regional differences of blood flow, whereas the distortion of the lung itself by its own weight causes the regional differences in ventilation, alveolar size, intrapleural pressure, and parenchymal stress. Therefore, presumably the regional differences will be greatly reduced by weightlessness, though there are reasons to think that they might not be completely abolished (see below).

To date, the only measurements of the effects of microgravity on these topographical differences are those that were carried out in 1978 on a Learjet aircraft during Keplerian arcs (18). The measurements were made with prototype equipment being developed for the upcoming experiment on Spacelab SLS-1, and data were obtained from four normal subjects during 112 weightless periods lasting up to 27 sec.

The inequality of ventilation was measured from single-breath nitrogen washouts which were performed with a test inspiration containing an initial bolus of argon at residual volume. Striking alterations in the pattern were seen during weightlessness compared with the measurements obtained at $1g$ flying straight and level (Fig. 2). Note that the cardiogenic oscillations (19) on the alveolar plateau were greatly diminished at $0g$, and that there was a striking reduction of terminal rises for both nitrogen and argon. The cardiogenic oscillations are caused by preferential emptying of the lung bases due to movement of the beating heart, whereas the terminal rises of nitrogen and argon are the result of basal airway closure. These measurements provided strong evidence that under weightless conditions, the topographical differences of lung expansion and ventilation were dramatically reduced.

An interesting feature of these studies is that the nitrogen tracings for $0g$ showed larger cardiogenic oscillations and terminal rises (though these were both small) than did the argon tracings. The probable reason for this is the compression of the base of the lung caused by a period of increased g forces prior to the weightless parabolic arc, along with the fact that the lung takes a few seconds to recover from this distortion. The point is mentioned here partly to bring out a limitation of parabolic profile maneuvers in that these are preceded and succeeded by periods of increased gravitational loading. This factor, along with the short duration of the microgravity, limits the value of this

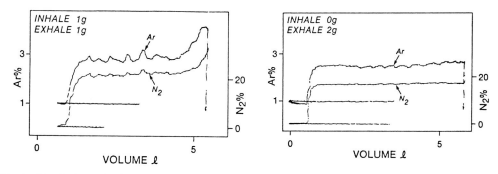

FIG. 2. Single-breath nitrogen washouts following a vital capacity inspiration of pure oxygen. An argon bolus was added at the beginning of inspiration. Note that the tracings at 1g showed prominent cardiogenic oscillations and terminal rises, indicating topographical inequality of ventilation. These were greatly reduced in the measurements at 0g. (From ref. 18.)

type of measurement. However, flying Keplerian arcs is the only way to generate the microgravity state for more than 2 or 3 sec (free fall) in the absence of orbital flight.

At the time that these measurements were made, there was disagreement on whether the topographical inequality of ventilation was caused by distortion of the lung by its own weight, or whether it was due to distortion of the chest wall by gravity. To answer this question, chest radiographs were taken in both the 1g and 0g states, and the shape of the rib cage and diaphragm was traced. The results showed that there was very little change, although during microgravity there was a tendency for the diaphragm to be higher and for the rib cage to be slightly wider (20).

Information was also obtained on the topographical distribution of pulmonary blood flow in these experiments (Fig. 3). For these measurements, the subject first hyperventilated for about 5 sec, and then he held his breath at total lung capacity for approximately 15 sec. Subsequently, expired P_{O_2} and P_{CO_2} were measured with the mass spectrometer during a steady flow

exhalation to residual volume. The size of the cardiogenic oscillations on the alveolar plateau was determined by how rapidly the P_{O_2} and P_{CO_2} had changed during the breathhold period, and this was a measure of blood flow per unit lung volume. As Fig. 3 shows, the cardiogenic oscillations were exaggerated by increased acceleration, but they were almost abolished under weightless conditions. Again, this was strong evidence that the topographical inequality of blood flow is grossly reduced in the microgravity environment.

An interesting question is whether there will be residual topographical differences in structure and function in the weightless state. There are some reasons to expect this. For example, as far as ventilation is concerned, the peculiar intrinsic shape of the lung, coupled with the way in which the chest wall expands (the diaphragm descends more than the rib cage widens), certainly suggests that the weightless lung may not be uniformly expanded during inspiration, and the resulting intrapleural pressures may not be the same everywhere. It should also be remembered that there are various mechanisms of uneven ventilation in addition to the topographical inequality caused by the weight of the lung; these are discussed in Chapter 5.1.2.5, where it was pointed out that there is some uncertainty about the relative importance of gravity-dependent and gravity-independent causes of ventilatory inequality. By making measurements of the distribution of ventilation in the absence of gravity, it should be possible to determine the importance of this factor.

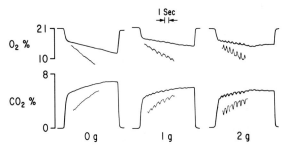

FIG. 3. Information on changes in the topographical inequality of blood flow during microgravity. This was determined from the height of the cardiogenic oscillations in the exhaled O_2 and CO_2 following a brief hyperventilation and 15-sec breath-hold at total lung capacity (see text). Note that the oscillations were almost absent at 0g, indicating a nearly uniform topographical distribution of blood flow. (From ref. 18.)

MECHANICS OF BREATHING

As indicated above, it is known that gravity affects the topographical distribution of alveolar size, intrapleural pressure, and parenchymal stress within the lung. All these topics fall within the province of lung mechanics.

In addition, it has been shown that changes of posture in the normal 1g environment alter functional residual capacity, the position of the diaphragm, and the relative displacements of the rib cage and abdominal compartments during normal tidal breathing (21). Finally, there is evidence that change of posture alters the flow–volume curves obtained during a maximal forced expiration (22). Thus although very few measurements have been made in the microgravity environment, it is likely that there will be a number of changes in the mechanics of breathing.

Lung Volume and Chest Wall Configuration

Few studies have been made on the changes of lung volume caused by microgravity. In an early analysis, Agostoni and Mead (21) predicted that the functional residual capacity in the weightless state would be about 10% less than in the upright posture at 1g. Baumgarten et al. (23) recorded the circumferences of the rib cage and abdomen during "roller coaster" flight patterns in which increased and decreased g_z levels were obtained, and they reported that there was a tendency for the mean respiratory level to move towards expiration during the low-g_z phase and towards inspiration during the high-g_z phase. However, subsequent studies by the same group (24,25) apparently did not confirm these findings.

As indicated above, Michels et al. (20) took chest radiographs at residual volume, functional residual capacity, and total lung capacity in five subjects in an aircraft flying in a Keplerian arc. There was a tendency for the diaphragm to move up and the rib cage to widen at 0g, but no direct measurements of lung volume were made.

Recently, Paiva et al. (26) studied lung volume and chest wall configuration in five seated normal subjects during Keplerian arcs performed in a NASA KC-135 aircraft during three flights on consecutive days. Flow rates at the mouth were measured with a Fleisch pneumotachograph, and these were integrated to give changes in lung volume. Rib cage and abdominal motion were obtained from an inductance plethysmograph (Respitrace) with two bands placed at the level of the nipples and umbilicus, respectively. Special attention was given to calibration, including the errors introduced by changes of pressure within the aircraft cabin. In addition to making measurements during microgravity in a Keplerian arc, further observations were made with the aircraft performing "a roller coaster" maneuver.

The major findings of this study were as follows:

1. There was a consistent relationship between the functional residual capacity measured from the flowmeter tracing, the thoraco-abdominal volume mea-

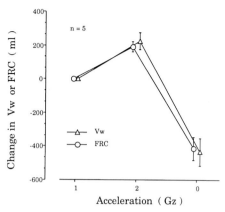

FIG. 4. Change in functional residual capacity (FRC) and end-expiratory thoraco-abdominal volume (V_w). Bars show standard errors. Note the almost equal decline of both variables at 0g. (From ref. 26.)

sured from the inductance phethysmograph, and the gravitational acceleration ($+g_z$). In other words, during microgravity, both volumes decreased, while during increased g_z the volumes increased (Fig. 4). The functional residual capacity and thoraco-abdominal volume decreased to the same extent during microgravity, suggesting that the changes were not caused by an increase in thoracic blood volume.

2. These volume changes were almost entirely due to changes in the abdominal compartment. The volume of the rib cage showed only minor and inconsistent changes (Fig. 5).

3. The abdominal contribution to tidal breathing increased substantially under conditions of microgravity. In contrast, when the gravitational acceleration was nearly doubled, the abdominal contribution to tidal breathing decreased slightly.

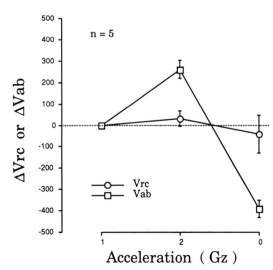

FIG. 5. Change in end-expiratory rib cage (V_{rc}) and abdominal (V_{ab}) volumes at different g levels. Note the substantial fall in abdominal volume at 0g. (From ref. 26.)

4. In spite of the changes in thoraco-abdominal volume and configuration, the temporal pattern of breathing (i.e., tidal breathing frequency) and the relative duration of inspiration and expiration were unaffected by changes in acceleration.

Vital capacity was also measured in this study, and there was a suggestion of small (approximately 8%) decrease during microgravity. A decrease had also been reported during Skylab 4 (27), but this was probably partly due to the reduced ambient pressure and the high oxygen concentration within the spacecraft, because ground-based simulations also showed a slight fall. In another study performed during Keplerian arcs, no consistent changes in vital capacity between $1g_z$ and $0g_z$ conditions were found in four seated normal subjects (18).

Flow–Volume Curves

Castile et al. (22) showed that change of posture from the upright to the supine position frequently altered the shape of the maximum expiratory flow–volume curve. A common pattern was that flow was higher at large lung volumes and lower at small lung volumes in the supine as opposed to the upright position. They attributed the changes to alterations in the distribution of parenchymal stresses which altered the location of airway choke points. These choke points are believed to determine the flow rates under conditions of dynamic compression.

Recently, Guy et al. (28) recorded maximum expiratory flow–volume curves in nine seated subjects during exposure to short periods of microgravity. These were obtained during Keplerian arcs on a NASA KC-135 aircraft and then compared with measurements made during level (1g) flight. The data were digitally filtered and then ensemble-averaged after alignment at residual volume. The results showed a tendency for expired volume (forced vital capacity, FVC) to decrease by an average of 2.4%. Peak expiratory flow rate also fell slightly (average 2.6%) at 0g compared to 1g. However, these small changes were not statistically significant.

Individual changes in the shape of the descending limb of the curves were found (Fig. 6). Four subjects had significant reductions in maximum flow at low lung volumes, a pattern similar to that found at 1g when changing from the upright to the supine position. Subjects with readily identifiable features (such as bumps) in their curves retained those features at 0g, although their position on the volume axis was altered.

The fact that the flow rates were reduced at low lung volumes, at least in a subgroup of subjects, was interesting. It indicated that the removal of the gravitational stresses, along with the resulting reduction in

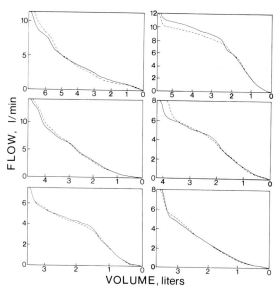

FIG. 6. Maximum expiratory flow–volume curves obtained at 1g and 0g. Note that in four subjects at 0g, there was a reduced flow rate at low lung volumes, indicating that removal of the gravitational distortion of the lung did not increase flow rates. Dashed lines, 0g; solid lines, 1g. (From ref. 28.)

gravitational inhomogeneity of lung expansion, did not result in an increased expiratory flow. Since change of posture from the upright to supine position results in reduced flow rates at low lung volumes, at least in a subset of subjects (22), we reasoned that the upright lung had a more favorable distribution of stresses, and therefore choke points, than did the supine lung. Our expectation was that we might find the highest expiratory flow rates in the gravitationally unstressed lung, but this was not the case. The results suggest that the lung has adapted to the most efficient configuration for expiratory flow in the upright position, and that although parenchymal expansion is more homogeneous in microgravity, this does not enhance expiratory flow rates.

INCREASED PULMONARY VASCULAR PRESSURES

There is evidence that when a subject enters the microgravity of orbital flight, there is a headward shift of blood and tissue fluids, vascular congestion of the head and neck, and eventually a reduction in total fluid volume. The initial fluid shift is believed to be 1.5–2 liters, the major portion of which expands the pulmonary blood vessels and heart. Astronauts have experienced a sensation of fullness in the head, stuffy noses, nasal voices, and slender legs (29,30). Photographs taken during orbital flight frequently show evidence of facial edema with periorbital swelling. Soviet studies have apparently shown a sustained increase in jugular vein pressure and a reduction in venous pressure in the legs during space flight (31).

This substantial headward shift of blood volume is believed to be caused by the lack of gravitational pooling of blood in the lower extremities. There is some evidence that the increased intrathoracic blood volume rapidly induces a diuresis as a result of the corresponding increase in right atrial pressure. This is thought to lead to a reduction in plasma volume which contributes to the postflight orthostatic intolerance and impaired exercise capacity (32). Although the fluid volume changes have not impaired crew efficiency or well-being during flight, it is possible to show abnormal responses to the reduction in blood volume using lower-body negative pressure in flight (33). It should be added that some recent measurements have failed to show the initial diuresis upon orbital insertion. However, this may be partly because the astronauts are placed in the supine position with the legs slightly raised for several hours prior to lift-off, and also because there is some fluid deprivation during this time.

To date, there have been very few measurements of the effects of these fluid shifts on pulmonary function. As indicated above, data obtained on Skylab 4 indicated a decrease in vital capacity, although whether this was due to a cephalad shift of the diaphragm during weightlessness or due to body fluid redistribution into the thoracic cavity was not determined (29). However, changes in pulmonary function would certainly be expected as a result of the engorgement of pulmonary blood vessels. These would include (a) increases in the diffusing capacity of the lung for carbon monoxide and (b) increases in pulmonary capillary blood volume. Measurements of these variables will be made during Spacelab SLS-1, scheduled for late-1990.

An intriguing possibility is that the increase in pulmonary vascular pressures may increase fluid filtration and lead to interstitial pulmonary edema. It is now known that any increase in pulmonary capillary pressure increases the rate of movement of fluid out of the capillaries into the interstitial space, accompanied by a corresponding increase in lymph flow (34). The development of radiological pulmonary edema has been described in a man who was accidentally suspended upside down for several hours following an accident in which he fell off a ladder and was held by his leg. Presumably the edema was caused by increased pressures in the pulmonary vasculature.

The development of interstitial pulmonary edema would be expected to increase pulmonary tissue volume and vascular resistance (35), cause uneven ventilation (36), and increase residual volume as a result of premature small airway closure (37). Such changes are particularly likely to occur during exercise, when pulmonary artery and pulmonary venous pressures in-crease along with the rise in pulmonary blood flow. Surprisingly, the lungs of animals which have been exposed to orbital flight have not apparently been examined histologically for evidence of interstitial pulmonary edema. This is presently being done on rats flown in the Soviet Cosmos mission of the summer of 1989.

PULMONARY RETENTION OF INHALED AEROSOL

The term "aerosol" refers to a collection of small particles which remain airborne for a substantial amount of time. Many pollutants exist in this form, and there is evidence of a substantial concentration of aerosol in the spacecraft environment. The pattern of deposition in the lung depends on particle size (38), and gravity plays an important role (see Chapter 7.3.1). The largest inhaled particles deposit by impaction which occurs when the particles fail to turn the corners of the nasal passages or upper respiratory tract and impinge on the wet mucous surfaces where they are trapped. The nose is remarkably efficient at removing the largest particles by this mechanism.

Medium-sized particles gradually settle out through the process of sedimentation, which is gravity-dependent. This is particularly important for particles of aerodynamic diameter of 1–5 μm, because the larger particles are removed by impaction and the smaller particles settle so slowly. Deposition by sedimentation occurs extensively in the small airways, including the terminal and respiratory bronchioles, because the dimensions of these airways are small and thus the particles have a shorter distance to fall. However, sedimentation also occurs in other regions of the lung.

Diffusion is the random movement of particles as a result of their continuous bombardment by gas molecules; this only occurs to a significant extent in the smallest particles, which are less than 0.1 μm in diameter. Deposition by diffusion chiefly takes place in the small airways and alveoli, where the distances to the wall are the shortest. However, some deposition by this mechanism also occurs in the larger airways.

Because sedimentation will be abolished in the microgravity environment, it is clear that the pattern of aerosol retention will be altered (39). Indeed, measurements by Hoffman and Billingham (40) have already shown reduced deposition of 2-μm inhaled particles during short periods of weightlessness obtained by flying an aircraft in a Keplerian arc. This means that these particles will penetrate further into the lung, with the increased possibility of infection.

Preliminary measurements of the Shuttle Orbiter air environment have demonstrated a substantial increase in microbial counts during flights (41). A variety of airborne particles have been found in the mid and flight decks, including synthetic fibers, hair, food, and paint chips. It is not yet known what sized particles carry bacterial, spore, and viral contaminants, but these are frequently in the range of 0.1–10 μm in diameter.

Because of the absence of normal sedimentation, it is relatively difficult to remove dust from an orbiting spacecraft. Indeed, the only effective mechanism is to pass the air through filters with direct impaction of the particles. There is anecdotal evidence that use of the waste collection system by the Shuttle Orbiter crew has resulted in an increase in aerosol concentration which presumably contains pathogenic bacteria. For example, the crew of Spacelab 1 referred to a "brown cloud" in the vicinity of the waste collection system after use. Although the operation of this will no doubt be improved, the possibility of contaminated aerosol in a spacecraft environment remains. Experiments have been proposed to measure the pattern of retention of aerosol of different sizes during an upcoming Spacelab.

NITROGEN WASHOUT FOR EXTRAVEHICULAR ACTIVITY

In order for the astronaut to work outside the spacecraft (extravehicular activity, or EVA) to repair equipment, etc., he must don a pressure suit to protect him from the hard vacuum of space. Current U.S. pressure suits contain pure oxygen at a pressure of only 4.1 psi (212 torr; sea level normal is 14.7 psi), because higher pressures cause the suit to become very stiff, thereby restricting maneuverability. Since the normal atmosphere of the shuttle is 21% oxygen and 79% nitrogen at 760 torr, an astronaut who puts on the suit and is exposed to the low pressure has a considerable risk of decompression sickness ("bends") as described in Chapter 8.1.2. The only way to prevent this is to wash out much of the nitrogen in the body tissues, and the most convenient way to do this is for the astronaut to breathe pure oxygen for a period prior to EVA.

Decompression schedules have been developed for diving, based on a combination of theoretical and empirical data (Chapter 8.1.2). However, the denitrogenation rate depends on the distribution of cardiac output to various tissues; it also depends on the nitrogen capacity of the tissues, which is partly determined by their adipose content. These factors almost certainly change during long-term space flight. For example, skeletal muscle atrophy occurs, particularly in the legs, because these muscles are rarely used in the microgravity environment. As a result, the optimal times for safe denitrogenation are uncertain.

Although at first sight this may appear to be a relatively trivial operational problem, in fact it causes great concern. First, there is good evidence that astronauts have developed bends during EVA in previous missions. Furthermore, the situation could easily become very dangerous; it is easy to imagine a scenario where an astronaut is so disabled that he is not able to reenter the spacecraft. In addition, the period required for denitrogenation (several hours) consumes much of the astronauts' working time. This is particularly important in the context of the proposed orbiting Space Station where substantial amounts of EVA time are envisaged. This problem is so important that there have been strong arguments to reduce the total pressure inside the Space Station to 630 torr (approximate barometric pressure of Denver), for example. This would substantially reduce the time required for denitrogenation. Another solution is to develop a pressure suit which has improved maneuverability at a higher pressure, but this is technically very difficult. Finally, it may be possible for the astronaut to sleep in a special low-pressure compartment of the Space Station prior to EVA and thus not waste working time.

GENERAL CONSIDERATIONS

A number of general problems arise in connection with managing pulmonary problems and monitoring lung function during long-term space flight. Because a spacecraft is a closed environment to which oxygen is added and carbon dioxide is removed, the possibility of toxic contaminants building up is real. This can occur, for example, by outgassing of materials which do not appear to provide any hazard under normal conditions. In particular, some plastic materials are hazardous for this reason.

The spacecraft atmosphere must be continually monitored for oxygen and carbon dioxide levels. There is little point in trying to reduce the carbon dioxide concentration to the levels in terrestrial air, because this requires such extensive scrubbing. Instead, the carbon dioxide concentration is allowed to rise slightly, as in a submarine, to a point where a balance is obtained between (a) the astronauts' comfort and safety and (b) the requirement for additional carbon dioxide absorbers. At least one example of contamination of the spacecraft atmosphere has occurred. This was following the Apollo–Soyuz Test Project when the U.S. crew developed acute pneumonitis following reentry as a result of inadvertent exposure to N_2O_4 from the reaction control jets; as a result, the crew required hospitalization.

It will be important to have equipment for monitoring function on a long-term space flight such as the orbiting Space Station. A packet of noninvasive single-breath tests has been developed for Spacelab SLS-1 and might form a suitable basis for a long-term facility.

REFERENCES

1. Nicogossian AE, Parker JF. *Space physiology and medicine*, 2nd ed. Washington, DC: National Aeronautics and Space Administration, 1987.
2. West JB. Spacelab—the coming of age of space physiology research. *J Appl Physiol: Respir Environ Exercise Physiol* 1984;57:1625–1631.
3. West JB, ed. *Regional differences in the lung*. New York: Academic Press, 1977.
4. West JB, Dollery CT. Distribution of blood flow and ventilation-perfusion ratio in the lung, measured with radioactive CO_2. *J Appl Physiol* 1960;15:405–410.
5. West JB, Dollery CT, Naimark A. Distribution of blood flow in isolated lung: relation to vascular alveolar pressures. *J Appl Physiol* 1964;19:713–724.
6. Hughes JMB, Glazier JB, Maloney JE, West JB. Effect of lung volume on the distribution of pulmonary blood flow in man. *Respir Physiol* 1968;4:58–72.
7. Glaister DH. Effect of acceleration. In: West JB, ed. *Regional differences in the lung*. New York: Academic Press, 1977, 323–379.
8. Milic-Emili J, Henderson AM, Dolovich MB, Trop D, Kaneko K. Regional distribution of inspired gas in the lung. *J Appl Physiol* 1966;21:749.
9. West JB. Regional differences in gas exchange in the lung of erect man. *J Appl Physiol* 1962;17:893–898.
10. Glazier JB, Hughes JMB, Maloney JE, West JB. Vertical gradient of alveolar size in lungs of dogs frozen intact. *J Appl Physiol* 1967;23:694–705.
11. Hogg JC, Nepszy S. Regional lung volume and pleural pressure gradient estimated from lung density in dogs. *J Appl Physiol* 1969;27:198–203.
12. Krueger JJ, Bain T, Patterson JL Jr. Elevation gradient of intrathoracic pressure. *J Appl Physiol* 1961;16:465–468.
13. Agostoni E. Transpulmonary pressure. In: West JB, ed. *Regional differences in the lung*. New York: Academic Press, 1977, 245–280.
14. Milic-Emili J, Mead J, Turner JM. Topography of esophageal pressure as a function of posture in man. *J Appl Physiol* 1964;19:212–216.
15. West JB, Matthews FL. Stresses, strains, surface pressures in the lung caused by its weight. *J Appl Physiol* 1972;31:332–345.
16. Vawter DL, Matthews FL, West JB. Effect of shape size of lung chest wall on stresses in the lung. *J Appl Physiol* 1975;39:9–17.
17. West JB. Distribution of mechanical stress in the lung, a possible factor in localization of pulmonary disease. *Lancet* 1971;1:839–841.
18. Michels DB, West JB. Distribution of pulmonary ventilation perfusion during short periods of weightlessness. *J Appl Physiol* 1978;45:987–998.
19. Fowler KT, Reid J. Cardiac oscillations in expired gas tensions, and regional pulmonary blood flow. *J Appl Physiol* 1961;16:863–868.
20. Michels DB, Friedman PJ, West JB. Radiographic comparison of human lung shape during normal gravity weightlessness. *J Appl Physiol* 1979;47:851–857.
21. Agostoni E, Mead J. Statics of the respiratory system. In: Fenn WO, Rahn H, eds. *Handbook of physiology, Section 3: Respiration, vol 1*. Washington, DC: American Physiological Society, 1964;387–409.
22. Castile R, Mead J, Jackson A, Wohl ME, Stokes D. Effects of posture on flow–volume curve configuration in normal humans. *J Appl Physiol* 1982;53:1175–1183.
23. Baumgarten RJ von, Baldrighi G, Vogel H, Thumler R. Physiological response to hyper- and hypogravity during rollercoaster flight. *Aviat Space Environ Med* 1980;51:145–154.
24. Wetzig J. Respiration measurements in the weightlessness of parabolic flight. In: Frimond D, Confalone A, Pletser V, eds. *ESTEC working paper 1457*. Noordwijk, 1986.
25. Wetzig J, Baumgarten R von. Respiratory parameters aboard an aircraft performing parabolic flights. *Proc Third Eur Symp Life Sci Res Space* 1987;271:47–50.
26. Paiva M, Estenne M, Engel LA. Lung volumes, chest wall configuration and pattern of breathing in microgravity. *J Appl Physiol* 1989;67:1542–1550.
27. Sawin CF, Nicogossian AE, Rummel JA, Michel EL. Pulmonary function evaluation during the Skylab and Apollo–Soyuz missions. *Aviat Space Environ Med* 1976;47:168–172.
28. Guy HJB, Prisk GK, Elliott AR, West JB. Maximum expiratory flow-volume curves during short periods of microgravity. *J Appl Physiol* 1990;in press.
29. Johnston RS, Dietlein LF, eds. *Proceedings of the Skylab life sciences symposium*. Washington, DC: National Aeronautics and Space Administration, 1977.
30. Money KE. Biological effects of space travel. *Can Aeronaut Space J* 1981;27:195–201.
31. Gazenko OG, Genin AM, Egorov AD. Major medical results of the Salyut-6–Soyuz 195-day space flight. *Congr Int Astronaut Fed. 32 Sess D-5*, vol 2. Rome, 1981.
32. Blomqvist CG, Stone HL. Cardiovascular responses to gravitational stress. In: Shepherd JT, Abbound FM, eds. *Handbook of physiology, Section 2: The cardiovascular system, vol 3*. Bethesda, MD: American Physiological Society, 1983;1025–1063.
33. Johnson RL, Hoffler GW, Nicogossian AE, Bergman SA Jr, Jackson MM. Lower body negative pressure: third manned Skylab mission. In: Johnston RS, Dietlein LR, eds. *Biomedical results from Skylab*. Washington, DC: National Aeronautics and Space Administration, 1977.
34. Staub NC. New concepts about the pathophysiology of pulmonary edema. *J Thorac Imag* 1988;3:8–14.
35. West JB, Dollery CT, Heard BE. Increased pulmonary vascular resistance in the dependent zone of the isolated dog lung caused by perivascular edema. *Circ Res* 1965;17:191–206.
36. Ruff F, Hughes JMB, Stanley N, McCarthy D, Greene R, Aronoff A, Clayton L, Milic-Emili J. Regional lung function in patients with hepatic cirrhosis. *J Clin Invest* 1971;50:2403–2413.
37. Milic-Emili J, Ruff F. Effects of pulmonary congestion and edema on small airways. *Bull Physiol Pathol* 1971;7:1181–1196.
38. Dautreband L, Beckmann H, Walkerhorst W. Lung deposition of fine dust particles. *AMA Arch Ind Health* 1957;16:179–187.
39. Muir DCF. Influence of gravitational changes on the deposition of aerosols in the lungs of man. *Aerospace Med* 1967;159–161.
40. Hoffman RA, Billingham J. Effect of altered G levels on deposition of particulates in the human respiratory tract. *J Appl Physiol* 1975;38:955–960.
41. Henney MR, Kropp KD, Pierson DL. Microbial monitoring of orbiter air. In: *Scientific program of the 55th Annual Scientific Meeting of the Aerospace Medical Association*, May 6–10, San Diego, CA, 1984.

THE LUNG: Scientific Foundations
edited by R.G. Crystal, J.B. West et al.
Raven Press, Ltd., New York © 1991.

CHAPTER 8.2.1

Oxygen Therapy

Jesse Hall and Lawrence D. H. Wood

Joseph Priestley, independent codiscoverer (with Carl Wihelm Steele) of oxygen in the latter portion of the eighteenth century, almost immediately speculated upon the medicinal applications of this substance. Yet it was almost 150 years later that Dr. Alvan Barach routinely administered oxygen to hospitalized patients with acute and chronic lung disease, observing that supplemental oxygen relieved dyspnea, improved function, and resolved peripheral edema. Since the advent of Dr. Barach's innovative therapy and empiric observations, considerable information has been generated in the investigation of the physiology of oxygen transport, the mechanisms of hypoxemia, and the effects of oxygen therapy. This chapter reviews the current scientific basis for the rationales and benefits of oxygen therapy. After brief description of the goals and techniques of oxygen therapy, we discuss clinical applications, including long-term therapy in chronic airflow obstruction, nocturnal oxygen therapy, and oxygen administration in acute hypoxemic respiratory failure. In addition, unusual but important applications such as oxygen–helium mixtures in airway obstruction, oxygen therapy during high-altitude exposure, and hyperbaric oxygen in carbon monoxide poisoning are commented upon.

GOALS OF OXYGEN THERAPY

Enrichment of the oxygen fraction in inspired air (F_IO_2) is a potential treatment for disorders induced by both alveolar and tissue hypoxia. Alveolar hypoxia (low $P_{A}O_2$) occurs most commonly in chronic lung diseases [chronic obstructive pulmonary disease (COPD), asthma, sleep-disordered breathing] in which large

numbers of air spaces are poorly ventilated in relation to their perfusion. Air inspired with a P_IO_2 of about 140 torr into alveoli with low V_A/Q has sufficient oxygen removed to approach the mixed venous P_{O_2} of 40 torr, whereas less CO_2 is added to the alveolar gas as it approaches mixed venous P_{CO_2} of 50 torr. Low $P_{A}O_2$ stimulates hypoxic pulmonary vasoconstriction (HPV), with consequent pulmonary hypertension, right heart dysfunction, and reduced cardiac output (Q_t). Alveolar hypoxia also causes incomplete saturation of arterial hemoglobin (S_aO_2), thereby reducing arterial O_2 content (C_aO_2) and oxygen delivery ($QO_2 = C_aO_2 \times Q_t$) to systemic organs which may cause tissue hypoxia. Increasing F_IO_2 from 0.2 to 0.4 raises P_IO_2 to 280 torr and virtually eliminates alveolar hypoxia and desaturation in all but the very low V_A/Q units. Accordingly, one effective, achievable goal for O_2 therapy in these chronic lung diseases provides sufficient O_2 enrichment at home or in the hospital to ensure that S_aO_2 is greater than 90%, usually at a P_aO_2 of 65–70 torr, in a cost-efficient, convenient manner (1).

Other lung diseases (pulmonary edema, pneumonia, lung hemorrhage) result from the filling of air spaces with liquid or cellular elements from the circulation. Then, even large and toxic increases in F_IO_2 are ineffective in increasing P_aO_2 and C_aO_2 because the inspired oxygen is excluded from the pulmonary blood perfusing the flooded air spaces, causing intrapulmonary shunt (Q_s/Q_t). Acute hypoxia in these shunt lung diseases seems less well tolerated than the hypoxia of chronic lung diseases (1). Furthermore, the acute lung injury which led to shunt may be more vulnerable to toxicity from the high F_IO_2, a topic discussed in detail elsewhere in this book. As a result, effective oxygen therapy requires several adjuncts which seek to minimize the toxic F_IO_2 required to maintain aerobic tissue metabolism. Positive end-expiratory pressure (PEEP) reduces Q_s/Q_t and Q_t, reduced pulmonary artery wedge pressure (P_{pw}) reduces edema and Q_t, and va-

J. Hall and L. D. H. Wood: Section of Pulmonary and Critical Care Medicine, University of Chicago, Chicago, Illinois 60637.

soactive drugs or red blood cell transfusions maintain or raise Q_{O_2} but increases Q_s/Q_t (2). Since these adjunctive therapies have the potential to relieve or aggravate tissue hypoxia, the goals of O_2 therapy in shunt lung disease are to seek (a) the lowest PEEP providing 90% saturation of an adequate circulating hemoglobin on a nontoxic F_IO_2 and (b) the lowest P_{pw} compatible with adequate Q_t and Q_{O_2} (2).

TECHNIQUES OF OXYGEN ADMINISTRATION AND MONITORING

Oxygen Delivery Systems

The ubiquitous need for oxygen in the modern acute-care hospital requires these facilities to have bulk storage with oxygen piped to all patient-care areas. Long-term oxygen therapy in the outpatient setting is achieved by the use of compressed gas, liquid oxygen, or oxygen concentrators. Tanks of compressed gas are widely used but require frequent refilling and are minimally transportable for extended periods of time. Liquid oxygen may be stored at home in insulated reservoirs at $-300°C$ for direct use by the nonambulatory patient, and transfilling of portable devices by the patient allows up to 8 hr of continuous oxygen delivery at a rate of 2 liters/min, thus facilitating out-of-home activities. Disadvantages of liquid systems include increased cost in some care settings (3); in at least one study (4) there was a high incidence of inaccurate oxygen delivery, creating a potential for inadequate treatment of hypoxemia.

Oxygen concentrators extract oxygen from atmospheric gas and employ either a molecular sieve or membrane concentration design (3). The former is capable of generating low flows at high oxygen concentration (>90%), and the latter is capable of doubling ambient oxygen concentration. Accordingly, higher flows will be required with membrane concentrators for correction of any given degree of hypoxemia; occasionally, very high flows may be necessary such that patient compliance is compromised. Concentrators are relatively cheap and eliminate the need for transport of oxygen to the patient's home, but they require a constant electric source, consume considerable power, and are not presently portable.

Oxygen Conservation Devices

The cost of home oxygen therapy is considerable, with one recent estimate based upon Congressional Budget Office data indicating that 500,000 to 800,000 individuals used home oxygen in the United States at an annual cost of two to three billion dollars, 60% of which was paid by the federal government through Medicare

reimbursement (5). Such tremendous expenditures have fueled governmental overview of indications for oxygen therapy as well as creation of guidelines to promote the use of devices to conserve oxygen and reduce cost. These devices may be classified as reservoirs, demand or pulse systems, and transtracheal catheters.

Reservoir devices provide approximately 20 ml of oxygen stored during noninspiratory portions of the respiratory cycle, thereby permitting a 40–75% reduction in flow rates (6). The reservoirs are directly attached to a nasal cannula or may be worn as a pendant around the neck. These devices may be beneficial in preventing arterial desaturation during muscular exercise in COPD (7). The magnitude of oxygen conservation is extremely variable and difficult to predict for a given patient, and patient acceptance of these devices is not high (8). Demand systems, which provide respiratory-phased oxygen delivery, are most often actuated by (a) abdominal or chest motion detected by an impedance device, (b) nasal temperature change sensed by a thermistor, or (c) valves sensitive to inspiratory or expiratory airway pressure excursions (6). Although they are theoretically appealing and have potential advantages such as modification of oxygen supply during exercise to meet increased demand, these devices have not gained wide acceptance due to considerable initial cost and maintenance difficulties.

Transtracheal Oxygen Administration

Heimlich and Carr (9) first demonstrated that continuous transtracheal delivery of oxygen at low flow rates could correct hypoxemia in patients with chronic lung disease, and this approach is now widely employed. This technology reduces oxygen requirement substantially, decreases costs, and is tolerated by most patients, with an acceptable incidence of complications (10,11). Transtracheal delivery of oxygen may be the preferred route for patients who cannot be adequately saturated with high flows via nasal cannula (10). Of interest is the marked decrease in dyspnea and increased exercise tolerance noted by several investigators (11,12). In patients with COPD and restrictive lung disease, transtracheal gas flow of 6 liters/min was associated with a decrease in inspired minute ventilation of 50% (12). This reduction in ventilation and associated improvement in dyspnea appeared to be unrelated to changes in oxygen delivery or arterial hemoglobin saturation, since transtracheal air administration resulted in similar effects. These findings were consistent with the notion that patients receiving transtracheal oxygen therapy have decreased inspiratory work as a mechanism explaining improved dyspnea and exercise capacity, and they alert clinicians to the possibility that benefits derived from oxygen therapy may in some cases be due to effects apart from correction of hypoxemia.

F_IO_2 in the Nonintubated Patient

The use of a low-flow oxygen system necessarily results in mixing of ambient air to meet inspiratory flow demand. The development of high-flow mask systems was propelled not only by a desire to achieve a high F_IO_2, but also by a need to have mixing occur in a predictable fashion such that F_IO_2 could be determined by the clinician. This would permit "controlled" oxygen therapy in patients who might have adverse consequences from even small increments in F_IO_2, a concept to be discussed at length below. Additionally, a known F_IO_2 would permit calculation of the alveolar-arterial oxygen difference and would thus facilitate the clinical assessment of lung pathology and associated gas-exchange abnormalities. Although the concentration of oxygen achieved by many of these devices can vary considerably when tested on simulators, striking deviation from predicted F_IO_2 is observed when tracheal oxygen concentrations are measured in volunteers with hyperventilatory breathing patterns (13). We find that under typical clinical conditions in nonintubated patients with respiratory distress, the following statements apply: (a) F_IO_2 cannot be accurately determined and lung gas-exchange efficiency cannot be assessed unless the patient is breathing room air; (b) it is not necessary to know F_IO_2 for prevention of depressed drive to breathe; and (c) even with high-flow systems with rebreathing reservoirs, F_IO_2 will often be considerably less than 0.5 and vary widely in different clinical settings, so monitoring S_aO_2 is important.

Monitoring Oxygen Therapy

To the extent that the endpoint of oxygen therapy is resolution of hypoxemia, direct measurement of P_O2 or hemoglobin saturation would provide the most reasonable monitors of efficacy. Arterial blood gas analysis has become routine and is useful in the setting of critical illness in view of the information regarding ventilatory and acid–base status that it additionally provides. Yet it is invasive, costly, and does not provide continuous information concerning gas exchange. This last point is important in several settings of oxygen therapy, particularly during exercise or sleep in patients with chronic lung disease.

The development of pulse oximetry in the past decade has improved the ability to assess saturation on an ongoing basis. By analyzing the pulsatile component of the absorbance of hemoglobin in red and infrared light, these devices eliminate much of the difficulty in calibration and operation of the older-generation oximeters; also, measurements compare favorably with direct arterial oximetry. Errors in measurement of saturation will occur in the presence of elevated bilirubin levels, carboxyhemoglobinemia, or methemoglobinemia; in clinical practice, however, light and motion artifact are the most commonly encountered problems (14). Because patients with chronic lung disease commonly exhibit significant fluctuations in arterial oxygen saturation (particularly during sleep), these devices are likely to find increasing clinical application, particularly prototypes which allow continuous monitoring in the ambulatory patient.

OXYGEN THERAPY IN AIRFLOW OBSTRUCTION AND SHUNT LUNG DISEASES

Long-Term Oxygen Therapy

Early uncontrolled series reported that long-term oxygen therapy (LTOT) in patients with COPD resulted in: (a) correction of erythrocytosis in most (if not all) patients, with hematocrit decreasing gradually over 4–6 weeks after institution of therapy; (b) diminished pulmonary artery pressure and resistance in many patients (this potentially beneficial hemodynamic effect could occur with as little as 12–15 hr of oxygen per day); (c) decreased admission to hospital for exacerbations characterized by cor pulmonale; and (d) improved central nervous system function. These and other clinical observations suggesting improved function and survival resulted in frequent use of LTOT, despite the expense of this therapy and the frequency of COPD. This therapeutic dilemma was addressed by the Medical Research Council of the United Kingdom and by the National Institutes of Health in the United States, with prospective randomized trials to determine long-term benefit (15,16).

The British study (15) enrolled 87 patients, randomized between no oxygen therapy and 2 liters/min for at least 15 hr/day, including the sleeping hours. Patients were followed for 5 years. The American study (16) recruited 203 patients at six centers who were randomized to receive oxygen either nightly for 12 hr or continuously for at least 19 hr/day. The dose of oxygen used was the amount necessary to raise the arterial P_O2 to 65 torr, with 1 liter/min additional oxygen flow at night. Both studies showed a clear difference in survival between the groups (Fig. 1); together, these studies strongly supported the notion that LTOT improved survival in COPD and that more continuous therapy was preferable. The American study also attempted to assess the effects of LTOT on neuropsychological, emotional, and social function. Although both patient groups showed improvement in social and emotional

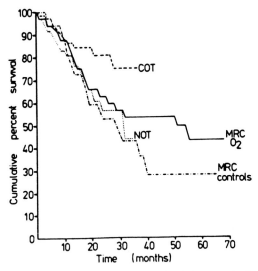

FIG. 1. Survival data for the Medical Research Council (MRC) and North American (NOT, COT) long-term oxygen therapy trials. Note that in the MRC study, patients receiving nocturnal oxygen therapy had improved survival over controls receiving none. In the North American trial, patients receiving continuous oxygen therapy (COT) had improved survival over patients receiving only nocturnal oxygen therapy (NOT). (From ref. 3.)

function after 6 months of treatment, significant differences could not be demonstrated between the two groups.

It is clear from these studies that oxygen improves survival in hypoxemic patients with COPD. Pulmonary hypertension with cor pulmonale has long been recognized as a poor prognostic sign in COPD, with a mortality in excess of 65% over 4 years (17). Conceivably, oxygen therapy relieves or prevents the progression of pulmonary hypertension with associated right heart failure. In analysis of the British trial, no difference in pulmonary artery pressure or pulmonary vascular resistance was noted between the two groups. In the North American series (18), neither group normalized baseline elevations of pulmonary artery pressure and resistance while on supplemental oxygen, but the group receiving continuous therapy did exhibit a fall in resting pulmonary artery pressure of about 3 torr with a 20% decrease in pulmonary vascular resistance associated with an increase in stroke volume index; hemodynamics were slightly more improved during exercise. For both groups, the early change in pulmonary artery pressure was associated with subsequent survival. Of note, oxygen therapy was most effective in reducing mortality in patients with an initial low pulmonary artery pressure and resistance, suggesting that early therapy to prevent more severe pulmonary vascular disease may be a desirable goal. The hemodynamic response to 24 hr of oxygen therapy might be

useful as a means for selecting patients for LTOT. In 28 patients with COPD and cor pulmonale, responders, defined as those with a greater than 5 torr drop in mean pulmonary artery pressure, had an 85% survival over 2 years, compared to only 22% in nonresponders (19). The progressive rise in pulmonary arterial pressure and resistance in these patients can be halted and partially reversed by LTOT (see Fig. 2), although normalization of these values is rarely observed (20). When oxygen was removed from patients receiving LTOT, pulmonary vascular resistance increased 31% during rest and 29% during exercise, with no change in the pulmonary capillary wedge pressure and a fall in stroke volume (21). Although these findings are consistent with a view that resolution of hypoxia-mediated pulmonary hypertension explains survival benefit in LTOT, other studies suggest that improved oxygen delivery to peripheral tissues may be an alternative and independent mechanism to explain this finding (22–24).

These studies do not clarify if, in a given patient, benefit from LTOT is conferred by prevention of progression of pulmonary vascular disease or by augmentation of oxygen delivery to key tissues, or by both. Nonetheless, it is well demonstrated that LTOT in hypoxemic patients with COPD will improve survival. Analysis of data combined from prospective studies indicates that nocturnal oxygen therapy is preferable to no therapy, and that continuous therapy (>19 hr/day) is better still for patient survival (15,16). Incremental benefit to be derived from 24-hr-a-day use of oxygen has not been determined. Current recommendations (25) are that LTOT be prescribed when $P_{O_2} <$ 55 torr at rest in a patient with COPD who is stable and receiving optimal therapy, or when $P_{O_2} = 56$–59 torr and cor pulmonale, erythrocytosis, or peripheral edema is present. Ideally, the dose of oxygen prescribed should be determined for exercise, sleep, and the awake resting state separately, as determined by some measure of continuous saturation such as pulse oximetry. The utility of beginning LTOT at an earlier point in the course of COPD, as well as the usefulness of oxygen during exercise in patients who desaturate only during activity, remains to be defined. Also, these guidelines for LTOT in COPD have generally been used for patients with chronic lung disease of all types, despite the lack of large reported series of other patient groups.

Nocturnal Oxygen Therapy

Normal sleep is characterized by depressed ventilation with an elevated P_{CO_2} and a decreased arterial P_{O_2}, but these changes are not extreme. Significant noc-

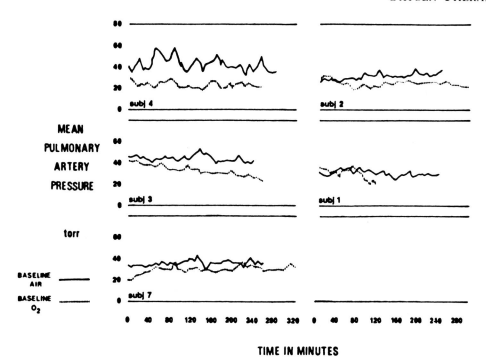

MEAN
PULMONARY
ARTERY
PRESSURE

torr

BASELINE
AIR

BASELINE
O₂

FIG. 2. Response of pulmonary artery pressure to nocturnal oxygen therapy in patients with COPD. Several representative tracings of continuously monitored pulmonary artery pressure are shown. (From ref. 34.)

turnal desaturation is a feature of individuals with sleep-disordered breathing (SDB), neuromuscular disease, and COPD. In the former instance, hypoxemia is related to episodes of either upper-airway obstruction or central apnea. Although primary therapy is directed at the obstructive or central apneic events directly or at precipitating factors such as obesity or hypothyroidism (26), a number of studies have investigated the utility of oxygen therapy in this setting. Acute and chronic hyperoxia decreased the number and total time of apneas in a group of patients with obstructive sleep apnea (OSA), although individual apneas were prolonged (27). Of clinical significance, a subset of patients improved symptomatically, whereas another subset worsened. Other investigators have reported improvement of central apneic events (28) and sleep architecture in OSA (29) with oxygen therapy. Conceivably, chronic intermittent nocturnal hypoxemia results in central nervous system dysfunction that potentiates underlying sleep apnea over time. Although oxygen may benefit some patients, there is (a) difficulty predicting who will benefit and (b) little information as to effect on the course of SDB. Accordingly, before nocturnal oxygen therapy is used in SDB, correction of untoward desaturation should be confirmed by oximetry.

Nocturnal desaturation has been described in a number of neuromuscular diseases (diaphragmatic paral-

ysis, myasthenia gravis, and muscular dystrophy), particularly when diaphragm involvement is prominent (30). Weakness of upper airway muscles may predispose these patients to OSA, whereas respiratory muscle weakness can result in worsening of nocturnal hypoventilation sufficient to produce desaturation. In view of the limited experience with such patients, attempts at correction of nocturnal desaturation with oxygen therapy should be done only with careful documentation of benefit with polysomnographic or continuous oximetric monitoring.

In COPD, nocturnal desaturation results from (a) associated SDB, (b) the usual reduction in ventilation and P_{AO_2} during non-rapid eye movement (NREM) sleep combined with hypoxemia due to COPD while awake, or (c) increases in ventilation–perfusion mismatching associated primarily with rapid eye movement (REM) sleep (31). The incidence of significant desaturation is extremely high in patients whose baseline awake P_{O_2} is <60 torr (32). The clinical relevance of periodic desaturation is not certain but has been demonstrated to be associated with worsening pulmonary hypertension and ischemic electrocardiographic changes and arrhythmias (33,34). Cor pulmonale in COPD may begin with nocturnal desaturation producing episodic pulmonary hypertension which progresses over time to become ultimately irreversible, and a fall in pulmonary artery pressures may be seen in patients with COPD treated with nocturnal oxygen (34) (see Fig. 2).

Oxygen for Acute-on-Chronic Respiratory Failure

Patients with COPD often experience acute deteriorations characterized by worsened hypoxemia and hypoventilation, a phenomenon termed "acute-on-chronic respiratory failure" (ACRF). As in chronic stable lung disease, this hypoxemia is due to mismatching of ventilation and perfusion and is corrected with modest oxygen enrichment of inspired air (35). Yet the notion became pervasive that excessive oxygen administration in ACRF could precipitate a need for mechanical ventilatory support, since patients with COPD might rely upon a hypoxic drive to breath (36). When this possibility was tested, a further increase in P_{CO_2} was almost always seen in patients with ACRF at the initiation of oxygen therapy, but this increment in hypercarbia was not explained on the basis of worsened hypoventilation (37,38). A large component of the observed elevation in P_{CO_2} was explained by an increase in dead space (37,38), a ventilation–perfusion alteration that could occur as a result of oxygen-mediated relaxation of airways (39) or alteration of blood flow (40). Of note, drive to breath measured by mouth occlusion pressure ($P = 0.1$) was three times normal despite abolition of hypoxic drive by oxygen therapy, and minute ventilation was not reduced (37).

These observations are consistent with a view that hypercarbia following oxygen therapy in ACRF does not necessarily signal worsened respiratory failure secondary to diminished drive to breathe. Indeed, attention in this disorder has increasingly turned toward respiratory muscle fatigue (resulting from the excessive mechanial load of ACRF) as an explanation for failure in these patients (41). Unwarranted reluctance to provide oxygen might actually contribute to ventilatory failure by adverse effects on muscle function (42) or through hypoxic impairment of the patient's compliance with other therapies aimed at reversible causes of ACRF (41), including the drive to breathe (43). Our own approach is to use sufficient amounts of supplemental oxygen to achieve 90% arterial saturation, titrated by applying nasal prongs and increasing flow while saturation is measured by pulse oximetry. If bedside measures of airflow obstruction and respiratory muscle function (respiratory rate, use of accessory muscles, pulsus paradoxus, chest auscultation) indicate improvement with oxygen and other therapies, we discourage the measurement of blood gases because hypercapnia is not likely to signal a deteriorating course (41). This titrated therapy should be conducted in a closely monitored setting, since progression of ventilatory failure may occur despite correction of hypoxemia (41).

Oxygen Therapy in Asthma

As discussed elsewhere in this book, asthma is a disease of episodic reversible bronchospasm, ranging in severity from a chronic asymptomatic state to episodes necessitating mechanical ventilation. Arterial hypoxemia is a feature of the whole range of severity of the asthmatic episode, and it is almost entirely attributable to a large fraction of the pulmonary blood flow going to low V_A/Q units in the absence of much true shunt. As a result, modest enrichment of the inspired air corrects the hypoxemia even in patients with status asthmaticus. In eight such patients, P_{aO_2} was 95 ± 20 torr during ventilation, with $F_{I O_2}$ ranging from 0.3 to 0.5; the large alveolar–arterial P_{O_2} difference was due to 17% venous admixture, of which only 1.5% was due to true shunt. Most of the hypoxemia could be attributed to 28% of the pulmonary blood flow perfusing units with $V_A/Q < 0.1$ (44). In asymptomatic asthmatics whose FEV_1 values were about 80% of predicted values, arterial P_{O_2} ranged from 70 to 100 torr; hypoxemia, when present, was attributable to increased perfusion to units with low V_A/Q (45). Between these extremes, blood gases of patients during acute bronchospasm showed P_{aO_2} of 70 ± 10 torr and P_{CO_2} of 34 ± 4 torr; in these 101 patients, hypoxemia correlated with the severity of airflow obstruction as measured by FEV_1, and the hypoxemia was easily corrected with oxygen therapy because all values of Q_s/Q_t were less than 10% (46). In 10 other asthmatics hospitalized for treatment of their acute severe asthma, P_{aO_2} was 51 ± 3 torr; this hypoxia was again due to perfusion of a large number of units with low V_A/Q, and it did not correlate with the degree of spirometric abnormality until quite late in the resolution of the acute asthmatic attack (47). Taken together, these results suggest that arterial hypoxemia is a marker of the severity of chronic asymptomatic asthma, but it does not warrant oxygen therapy unless associated with other abnormalities such as nocturnal desaturation as discussed above; in asthmatic patients with acute bronchospasm, arterial hypoxemia is easily corrected with enriched oxygen, but the severity of hypoxemia contributes little further to the many other symptomatic and objective evaluations of airflow obstruction contributing to the prediction of their need for hospitalization.

Oxygen Therapy in Lung Diseases Characterized by Shunt

A variety of clinical conditions are characterized by relatively acute filling of air spaces with elements of the pulmonary blood to cause arterial hypoxemia as a consequence of the intrapulmonary shunt (48). Desaturation of the circulating hemoglobin causes (a) reduced delivery of oxygen to the peripheral tissues (Q_{O_2}), (b) tissue hypoxia characterized by reduced oxygen consumption (V_{O_2}), and (c) anaerobic metabolism when the limits of oxygen extraction from desaturated blood are exceeded (49). Accordingly, arterial and tissue hypoxia are cardinal features of these shunt lung diseases, yet oxygen therapy provides only limited relief because even 100% oxygen is excluded from the pulmonary blood flow by air-space liquid, while non-flooded alveoli are perfused with blood which is nearly completely saturated even during air breathing. This is illustrated in the left panel of Fig. 3, where a small increase in $F_{I_{O_2}}$ increases $P_{a_{O_2}}$ considerably when the shunt is small, yet when Q_s/Q_t is 50%, changing the inspired gas from air to oxygen only raises the $P_{a_{O_2}}$ from 38 to 48 torr (48). The right panel of Fig. 3 illustrates an often overlooked feature of this small increase in P_{O_2}. The arterial oxygen content increases more between an $F_{I_{O_2}}$ of 0.21 and 1.0 when the shunt is 50% than when Q_s/Q_t is 10%. At the higher value of Q_s/Q_t, the largest part of the increment occurred between 20% and 50% inspired oxygen, all as a consequence of the shape of the oxyhemoglobin dissociation curve (48).

Yet, physicians prefer to keep $P_{a_{O_2}} > 50$ torr even if it requires toxic $F_{I_{O_2}}$, because the limits of acute hypoxia for vital organs are not yet well defined and the consequences of excessive hypoxia seem quick and irreversible. For example, one evaluation of canine cardiac dysfunction during progressive hypoxemia demonstrated that ventricular contractility first became significantly depressed at $P_{a_{O_2}}$ values of about 40 torr and saturation values of about 70% (50). Relatively minor further reductions in $P_{a_{O_2}}$ (36 torr) and saturation (63%) were associated with progressive anaerobic myocardial metabolism, dilated cardiomyopathy, bradycardia, shock, and death. Such data lend support to the inclination of physicians to maintain arterial saturation close to 90%. Greater than 90% saturation achieves little further $S_{a_{O_2}}$ and Q_{O_2} along the relatively flat slope of the oxyhemoglobin dissociation curve, whereas less than 90% saturation exposes the patient to larger drops in Q_{O_2} along the steep portion of the dissociation curve (2,48).

Because oxygen therapy for shunt lung diseases confers relatively small relief to tissue hypoxia, diverse interventions may be thought of as adjuncts to oxygen therapy designed to maximize beneficial effects while minimizing the toxic effects of oxygen. Of course, each of these interventions has its own adverse effects, so a recurring theme of oxygen therapy for diseases with shunt is to use the least adjunctive therapy achieving a predefined endpoint so as not to tip the therapeutic balance in the direction of complications (51). A partial list of adjunctive oxygen therapies includes: (a) PEEP; (b) increased circulating hemoglobin concentration and increased cardiac output; (c) reduced oxygen consumption and avoiding or treating defects in peripheral oxygen extraction; (d) vasoactive drugs which increase cardiac output but do not block HPV; (e) avoidance of secondary lung damage or reduced venous return using optimal ventilator settings; and (f) avoiding atelectasis, along with positioning the patient for optimal

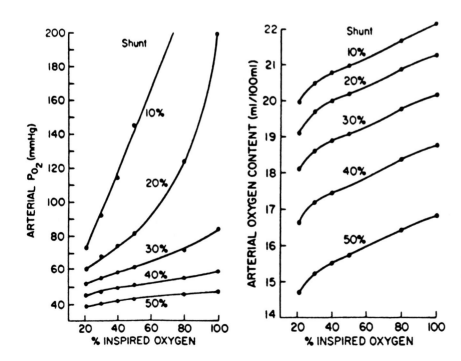

FIG. 3. Left panel: Arterial P_{O_2} as a function of inspired oxygen percentage at various degrees of shunt. **Right panel:** Increase in arterial oxygen content with increased percent of inspired oxygen at various degrees of shunt. See text for further details. (From ref. 48.)

O_2 exchange. The relative importance of each of these adjunctive measures varies with the causes of air-space filling. One common cause of shunt is the adult respiratory distress syndrome (ARDS), which may present different challenges to oxygen therapy between (a) the acute, exudative stage dominated by increased Q_s/Q_t (48) and (b) the later, proliferative phase dominated by fibrosis and a potential for large numbers of very low V_A/Q units which may themselves be more responsive to altered $F_{I}O_2$ than to large Q_s/Q_t. Other causes of diffuse air-space filling are cardiogenic pulmonary edema due to left ventricular dysfunction or fluid overload (51), whereas localized air-space filling occurs in pneumonia, in lung contusion with or without flail chest, and in atelectasis of dependent lung regions.

Each of these specific pulmonary diseases is described elsewhere in this book, so our goal here is to describe briefly the finesse of employing the adjuncts to optimize O_2 therapy for lung diseases having large Q_s/Q_t. PEEP reduces Q_s/Q_t by redistributing the alveolar edema to the peribronchovascular interstitium (52). It is not uncommon for PEEP <12 torr to reduce Q_s/Q_t from 50% to 30% in ARDS (53). As indicated by the left panel of Fig. 3, such an outcome allows the $F_{I}O_2$ to be reduced from 100% to 50% while increasing the P_aO_2 from 40 torr to 60 torr, associated with an increase in C_aO_2 from 16.8 to 19 vol % (see Fig. 3, right panel). Yet, PEEP also reduces venous return and cardiac output by raising pleural and right atrial pressures (2). Of course, this reduced blood flow and Q_{O_2} can then be treated with infusions of blood or other volume expanders, but this volume expansion can potentially increase P_{pw} and thus increase edema (2,51,54). Alternatively, vasoactive drugs can increase cardiac output at lower P_{pw} and thus reduce edema while increasing Q_{O_2} (2,54), provided that the pulmonary vasoactivity does not increase Q_s/Q_t excessively (2,51,54,55). Finding the optimal balance between the beneficial and adverse effects of these interdependent interventions is aided by keeping the goals of O_2 therapy clear: (a) Seek the lowest PEEP giving 90% saturation of an adequate circulating hemoglobin on nontoxic $F_{I}O_2$, and (b) seek the lowest P_{pw} giving adequate cardiac output and Q_{O_2} to meet peripheral O_2 demand (2).

Achieving these goals is facilitated by (a) judicious lowering of the patient's O_2 consumption, (b) elective intubation and mechanical ventilation during respiratory muscle relaxation, (c) treating sepsis and hyperthermia, and (d) avoiding excess carbohydrate intake (49,51,56). These measures reduce the Q_{O_2} and cardiac output required to maintain aerobic metabolism. In addition, cardiac output may be depressed less for a given PEEP by reducing the tidal volume and frequency to the lowest combination preventing excess CO_2 retention (56). In unilateral lung diseases with large Q_s/Q_t

such as early untreated pneumonia, ventilating the patient in the lateral decubitus position with the diseased lung uppermost uses gravity to reduce shunt (57), whereas PEEP is less effective (58). In other unilateral lung diseases such as pulmonary contusion, the severe hypoxemia during air breathing is easily correctable with lesser amounts of oxygen coupled with pain control because pulmonary blood flow to the consolidated lung regions is reduced, and shunt is small despite extensive air-space consolidation (59,60).

SPECIAL APPLICATIONS OF OXYGEN THERAPY

Oxygen Therapy During Altitude Exposure

The ascent of Mt. Everest (8848 m) without supplemental oxygen by Habeler and Messner resolved a long-standing debate concerning man's physiologic limits. This remarkable feat required ability and conditioning to permit mountaineering in an environment with a barometric pressure of 253 torr, an inspired oxygen of 43 torr, and an alveolar oxygen tension of 35 torr (61). Without acclimatization, tolerance to high-altitude exposure is poor, with an incidence of acute mountain sickness (AMS) estimated to be as high as 70% in poorly adapted trekkers in Nepal at substantially lower elevations. Oxygen therapy on ascent prevents AMS, but it is interesting that it does not completely relieve all symptoms of this syndrome when instituted after onset and, in the view of some authorities, does not cause as rapid a resolution of symptoms as descent (62).

A more common problem for most clinicians is the potential for altitude exposure during air travel for patients with chronic cardiopulmonary disease, thus risking hypoxemia. Cabin pressure on commercial aircraft ranges from 560 to 700 torr, correlating to pressures at approximately 900 to 2400 m. Schwartz et al. (63) studied 13 patients with COPD and found a mean fall in arterial P_{O_2} of 17 torr at 1650 m and of 23 torr at 2250 m. Interestingly, observed P_{O_2} could not be easily predicted by extrapolation of earlier measured sea-level arterial blood gases and A–a gradient. These investigators concluded that the best determination of patient response and oxygen requirement could be made by blood gas analysis with the patient breathing a hypoxic gas mixture to simulate his or her altitude exposure (63).

Carbon Monoxide Poisoning

Exposure to products of combustion is often associated with the inhalation and absorption of toxic amounts of carbon monoxide (CO). CO has 250 times greater affinity than O_2 for hemoglobin (64), so exposure to low levels in the atmosphere (0.4–1%) can cause levels of circulating carboxyhemoglobin (COHb) greater than 50% (65). This causes anaerobic metabolism and severe metabolic acidosis, leading to death without effective oxygen therapy and to delayed neurologic sequelae even with optimal treatment (65). The tissue hypoxia arises, in part, from the reduced oxygen flow to the tissues when COHb does not transport oxygen, but even lethal levels of 50% COHb still allow values of Q_{O_2} which are half normal and which are thus quite able to meet tissue metabolic needs if the O_2 extraction fraction were able to increase to 0.5. A second and more important mechanism is reduced P_{50} such that the release of 50% of the transported oxygen does not occur until the tissue P_{O_2} becomes closer to 10 torr than to the normal P_{50} of 27 torr (64). These two mechanisms alone may be sufficient to cause tissue hypoxia, but it seems that a poisoning of the cytochrome chain by high levels of CO adds to the anaerobic metabolism (66).

Once exposure to inhaled CO is terminated, a spontaneously breathing patient will eliminate half the CO in about 6 hr (67). Intubation and ventilation with 100% oxygen shorten the half-time to about 1.5 hr and may ameliorate some of the tissue hypoxia through delivery of increased oxygen in solution. One utilization of hyperbaric oxygenation (HBO) available is to further reduce the half-time of CO elimination to 23 min during ventilation with 100% oxygen at 3 atm absolute (67). There is some evidence that once this HBO therapy has reduced CO levels to less than 10% after a relatively brief 2-hr treatment, it is necessary to treat the patient some 8 hr later when the CO levels may have risen again as a result of the release of myoglobin-bound CO which had not been eliminated (68). A point of emphasis is that early and potentially lethal CO intoxication is associated with normal values of P_{O_2} during room air breathing, so the reason for early oxygen therapy is to enhance the elimination of the poison in order to treat the tissue hypoxia arising from inability of the tissues to extract oxygen from blood having normal $P_{a}O_2$. Other potential uses of HBO—including the treatment of deep anaerobic infections, enhanced wound and burn healing, and chronic osteomyelitis—are currently under extensive investigation to evaluate their efficacy, and thus they are outside the scope of this review of established oxygen therapy (68).

Heliox for Upper Airway Obstruction

A rare but dramatic cause of respiratory distress is associated with diverse forms of obstruction of the upper airway. These patients complain of dyspnea associated with obvious respiratory distress and use of the accessory muscles of respiration; frequently, inspiratory stridor is evident. Whenever blood gases are obtained, they confirm acute respiratory acidosis (usually without hypoxemia) in patients breathing oxygen-enriched gas (69). Several reports indicate immediate diminution of the signs and symptoms within minutes of breathing heliox, a gas consisting of 21% oxygen in helium (69).

The mechanism for this beneficial effect resides in the density dependence of the flow-related pressure drop across the upper airway. In normal airways there is a minimal cross-sectional area at the glottic aperture of about 2 cm^2, where the pressure drop is about 1 cm of H_2O and varies directly with the gas density and inversely with the square of the cross-sectional area. When tumor or other upper airway masses narrow the cross-sectional area to as small as 0.5 cm^2, the pressure drop across the orifice increases 16-fold, sufficient to cause moderate distress in the patient with normal inspiratory muscle function. Very minor further decreases in cross-sectional area to 0.4 cm^2 or less can cause hypoventilation associated with a pressure drop of 25–50 cm H_2O liter^{-1} sec^{-1} inspiratory flow. This very large pressure drop is reduced by a factor of 3 in accord with the reduced gas density when heliox is substituted, accounting for the dramatic and sustained relief in patients with upper airway obstruction (69). Note that heliox has no beneficial effect in the much more common lower airway obstruction because the resistance to airflow is much less dependent on gas density beyond the lobar bronchi where chronic airflow obstruction resides. Despite a number of anecdotal case reports and small series indicating the utility of this gas mixture, its availability to emergency rooms or inpatient services is sporadic (69). Accordingly, it is mentioned here as a variant of oxygen therapy, because the provision of emergency oxygen supplies in health institutions should include the provision of this special gas for this unique condition and therapy (70).

REFERENCES

1. Fulmer JD, Snider GL. American College of Chest Physicians (ACCP)—National Heart, Lung and Blood Institute (NHLBI) Conference on Oxygen Therapy. *Arch Int Med* 1984;144:1645–1655.
2. Wood LDH, Prewitt RM. Cardiovascular management in acute hypoxemic respiratory failure. *Am J Cardiol* 1981;47:963–972.
3. Flenley DC. Long-term home oxygen therapy. *Chest* 1985;87(1):99–103.
4. Massey LW, Hussey JD, Albert RK. Inaccurate oxygen delivery in some portable liquid oxygen devices. *Am Rev Respir Dis* 1988;137:204–205.
5. O'Donohue WJ Jr. The future of home oxygen therapy. *Respir Care* 1988;33(12):1125–1130.
6. Tiep BL, Lewis MI. Oxygen conservation and oxygen-conserving devices in chronic lung disease. *Chest* 1987;92(2):263–272.
7. Arlati S, Rolo J, Micaleff E, et al. A reservoir nasal cannula improves protection given by oxygen during muscular exercise in COPD. *Chest* 1988;93(6):1165–1169.

8. Claiborne RA, Paynter DE, Dutt AK, et al. Evaluation of the use of an oxygen conservation device in long-term oxygen therapy. *Am Rev Respir Dis* 1987;136:1095–1098.

9. Heimlich JH, Carr GC. Transtracheal catheter technique for pulmonary rehabilitation. *Ann Otol Rhinol Laryngol* 1985;94:502–504.

10. Christopher KL, Spofford BT, Brannin PK, et al. Transtracheal oxygen therapy for refractory hypoxemia. *JAMA* 1986;256:494–497.

11. McCarty DC, Goodman JR, Petty TL. A program for transtracheal oxygen delivery: assessment of safety and efficacy. *Ann Intern Med* 1987;107:802–808.

12. Couser JI Jr, Make BJ. Transtracheal oxygen decreases inspired minute ventilation. *Am Rev Respir Dis* 1989;139:627–631.

13. Gibson RL, Comer PB, Beckham RW, et al. Actual tracheal oxygen concentrations with commonly used oxygen equipment. *Anesthesiology* 1976;44(1):71–73.

14. Tremper KK. Pulse oximetry. *Chest* 1989;95(4):713–715.

15. Stuart-Harris C, Bishop JM, Clark TJH, Dornhorst AC, Cotes JE, Flenley DC, Howard P, Oldham PD. Long term domiciliary oxygen therapy in chronic hypoxic cor pulmonale complicating chronic bronchitis and emphysema. *Lancet* 1981;181–685.

16. Kvale PA, Anthonisen NR, Cugell W, Petty TL, Boylem T. Continuous or nocturnal oxygen therapy in hypoxemic chronic obstructive lung disease. *Ann Intern Med* 1980;93:391–398.

17. Renzetti AD, McClement JH, Litt BD. The Veterans Administration cooperative study of pulmonary function. III. Mortality in relation to respiratory impairment in chronic obstructive pulmonary disease. *Am J Med* 1966;41:115–129.

18. Timms RM, Khaja FU, Williams GW. The Nocturnal Oxygen Therapy Trial Group. Hemodynamic response to oxygen therapy in chronic obstructive pulmonary disease. *Ann Intern Med* 1985;102:29–36.

19. Ashutosh K, Mead G, Dunsky M. Early effects of oxygen administration and prognosis in chronic obstructive pulmonary disease and cor pulmonale. *Am Rev Respir Dis* 1983;127:399–404.

20. Weitzenblum E, Sautegeau A, Ehrhart M, Mammosser M, Pelletier A. Long-term oxygen therapy can reverse the progression of pulmonary hypertension in patients with chronic obstructive pulmonary disease. *Am Rev Respir Dis* 1985;131:493–498.

21. Selinger SR, Kennedy TP, Buescher P, Terry P, Parham W, Gofreed D, Medinger A, Spagnolo V, Michael JR. Effects of removing oxygen from patients with chronic obstructive pulmonary disease. *Am Rev Respir Dis* 1987;136:85–91.

22. Kawakami Y, Kishi F, Yamamoto H, Miyamoto K. Relation of oxygen delivery, mixed venous oxygenation, and pulmonary hemodynamics to prognosis in chronic obstructive pulmonary disease. *N Engl J Med* 1983;308(18):1046–1049.

23. Douglass A, Morrison RH, Goldman S. Preliminary study of the effects of low flow oxygen on oxygen delivery and right ventricular function in chronic lung disease. *Am Rev Respir Dis* 1986;133:390–395.

24. Macnee W, Wathen CG, Flenley DC, Muir AD. The effects of controlled oxygen therapy on ventricular function in patients with stable and decompensated cor pulmonale. *Am Rev Respir Dis* 1988;137:1289–1295.

25. Levin DC, Neff TA, O'Donohue WJ, Pierson DJ, Petty TL, Snider GL. Conference report: further recommendations for prescribing and supplying long-term oxygen therapy. *Am Rev Respir Dis* 1988;138:745–747.

26. Strohl KP, Cherniack NS, Gothe B. Physiologic basis of therapy for sleep apnea. *Am Rev Respir Dis* 1986;134:791–802.

27. Martin RJ, Sanders MH, Gray BA, et al. Acute and long-term ventilatory effects of hyperoxia in the adult sleep apnea syndrome. *Am Rev Respir Dis* 1982;125:175–180.

28. McNicholas WT, Carter JL, Rutherford R, et al. Beneficial effect of oxygen in primary alveolar hypoventilation with central sleep apnea. *Am Rev Respir Dis* 1982;125:773–775.

29. Smith PL, Haponik EF, Bleecker ER. The effects of oxygen in patients with sleep apnea. *Am Rev Respir Dis* 1984;130:958–963.

30. Skatrud J, Iber C, McHugh W, et al. Determinants of hypoventilation during wakefulness and sleep in diaphragmatic paralysis. *Am Rev Respir Dis* 1980;121:587–593.

31. Catterall JR, Douglas NJ, Calverely PMA, Shapiro CM, Brezinova V, Brash HM, Flenley DC. Transient hypoxemia during sleep in chronic obstructive pulmonary disease is not sleep apnea syndrome. *Am Rev Respir Dis* 1983;128:24–29.

32. Koo KW, Sax DS, Snider GL. Arterial blood gases and pH during sleep in chronic obstructive pulmonary disease. *Am J Med* 1975;58:663–670.

33. Tirlapur VG, Mir MA. Nocturnal hypoxemia and associated electrocardiographic changes in patients with chronic obstructive airways disease. *N Engl J Med* 1982;306:125–130.

34. Fletcher EC, Levin DC. Cardiopulmonary hemodynamics during sleep in subjects with chronic obstructive pulmonary disease: the effect of short and long term oxygen. *Chest* 1984;85:6–14.

35. Wagner P, Dantzker D, Dueck D, et al. Ventilation–perfusion inequality in chronic obstructive pulmonary disease. *J Clin Invest* 1977;59:203–216.

36. Campbell EJM. The J Burns Amberson Lecture. The management of acute respiratory failure in chronic bronchitis and emphysema. *Am Rev Respir Dis* 1967;96:626–639.

37. Aubier M, Murciano D, Fournier M, et al. Central respiratory drive in acute respiratory failure of patients with chronic obstructive pulmonary disease. *Am Rev Respir Dis* 1980;122:191–199.

38. Aubier M, Murciano D, Milic-Emili J, et al. Effects of administration of O₂ on ventilation and blood gases in patients with chronic obstructive pulmonary disease during acute respiratory failure. *Am Rev Respir Dis* 1980;122:147–154.

39. Libby DM, Briscoe WA, King TKC. Relief of hypoxia-related bronchoconstriction by breathing 30 per cent oxygen. *Am Rev Respir Dis* 1981;123:171–175.

40. Lee J, Read J. Effect of oxygen breathing on distribution of pulmonary blood flow in chronic obstructive lung disease. *Am Rev Respir Dis* 1967;96:1173–1180.

41. Schmidt GA, Hall JB. Acute or chronic respiratory failure. Assessment and management of patients with COPD in the emergent setting. *JAMA* 1989;261:3444–3453.

42. Bye PTP, Esau SA, Levy RD, Shiner RJ, Macklem PT, Martin JG, Pardy RL. Ventilatory muscle function during exercise in air and oxygen in patients with chronic air-flow limitation. *Am Rev Respir Dis* 1985;132:236–240.

43. Yanos J, Keamy MF, Leisk L, Hall JB, Walley KR, Wood LDH. The mechanism of respiratory arrest in inspiratory loading and hypoxemia. *Am Rev Respir Dis* 1990;141:933–937.

44. Rodriguez-Roisin R, Ballester E, Roca J, Torres A, Wagner PD. Mechanisms of hypoxemia in patients with status asthmaticus requiring mechanical ventilation. *Am Rev Respir Dis* 1989;139:732–739.

45. Wagner PD, Hedenstierna G, Bylin G. Ventilation perfusion inequality in chronic asthma. *Am Rev Respir Dis* 1987;1336:605–612.

46. McFadden ER, Lyons HA. Arterial blood gas tension in asthma. *N Engl J Med* 1968;278:1027–1032.

47. Roca J, Ramis L, Rodriguez-Roisin R, Ballester E, Montserrat JM, Wagner PD. Serial relationships between ventilation perfusion inequality and spirometry in acute severe asthma requiring hospitalization. *Am Rev Respir Dis* 1988;137:1055–1061.

48. Dantzker RM. Gas exchange in the adult respiratory distress syndrome. *Clin Chest Med* 1982;3:57–67.

49. Schumacker PT, Samsel RW. Oxygen delivery and uptake by peripheral tissues: physiology and pathophysiology. *Crit Care Clin* 1989;5:255–269.

50. Walley KR, Becker CJ, Hogan RA, Teplinsky K, Wood LDH. Progressive hypoxemia limits oxygen consumption and left ventricular contractility. *Circ Res* 1988;63:849–859.

51. Hall JB, Wood LDH. Pulmonary edema. In: Cherniack R, ed. *Current therapy and respiratory medicine*. Toronto: BC Becker, 1989;275–280.

52. Malo J, Ali J, Wood LDH. How does positive end expiratory pressure reduce intrapulmonary shunt in canine pulmonary edema? *J Appl Physiol* 1984;57:1002–1010.

53. Ralph DB, Robertson HT, Weaver LJ, Hlastala MP, Carrico CJ, Hudson LD. Distribution of ventilation and perfusion during positive end expiratory pressure in the adult respiratory distress syndrome. *Am Rev Respir Dis* 1985;131:54–60.

54. Long GR, Breen PH, Meyers I, Wood LDH. Treatment of ca-

nine aspiration pneumonitis: fluid volume reduction vs. fluid volume expansion. *J Appl Physiol* 1988;65:1736–1744.

55. Melot C, Lejeune P, Leeman M, Morain J, Naeije R. Prostaglandin E1 in the adult respiratory distress syndrome. *Am Rev Respir Dis* 1989;139:106–110.

56. Hall JB, Wood LDH. Liberation of the patient from mechanical ventilation. *JAMA* 1987;257:1621–1628.

57. Remolina C, Khan AU, Santiago TV, Edelman NH. Positional hypoxemia in unilateral lung disease. *N Engl J Med* 1981; 304:523–525.

58. Mink SN, Light RB, Cooligan T, Wood LDH. The effect of PEEP on gas exchange and pulmonary perfusion in canine lobar pneumonia. *J Appl Physiol* 1981;50:517–523.

59. Oppenheimer L, Craven KD, Forkert L, Wood LDH. Pathophysiology of pulmonary contusion in dogs. *J Appl Physiol* 1979;47:718–728.

60. Shorr RM, Crittenden M, Indeck M. Lung thoracic trauma: analysis of 515 patients. *Ann Surg* 1987;206:200–205.

61. West JB, Hackett PH, Maret KH, Milledge JS, Peters RM Jr, Pizzo CJ, Winslow RM. Pulmonary gas exchange on the summit of Mt. Everest. *J Appl Physiol* 1983;55:678–687.

62. Hackett PH, Rennie D. Acute mountain sickness. *Semin Respir Med* 1983;5(2):132–140.

63. Schwartz JS, Bencowitz HZ, Moser KM. Air travel hypoxemia with chronic obstructive pulmonary disease. *Ann Intern Med* 1984;100(4):473–477.

64. Roughton FJW, Darling RC. The effect of carbon monoxide on the oxyhemoglobin dissociation curve. *Am J Physiol* 1940; 141:17–31.

65. Fink PA. Exposure to carbon monoxide: review of the literature and 567 autopsies. *Milit Med* 1966;131:1513–1539.

66. King CE, Dodd SL, Cain SM. O_2 delivery to contracting muscle during hypoxic or CO hypoxia. *J Appl Physiol* 1987;63:726–732.

67. Peterson JE, Stewart RD. Absorption and elimination of carbon monoxide by inactive young men. *Arch Environ Health* 1970; 21:165–171.

68. Thom SR. Hyperbaric oxygen therapy. *J Intensive Care Med* 1989;4:58–74.

69. Curtis JL, Mahlmeister M, Fink JB, Lampe G, Matthay MA, Stulbarg MS. Helium oxygen gas therapy: use and availability for the emergency treatment of inoperable airway obstruction. *Chest* 1986;90:455–457.

70. Stillwell PC, Qick JD, Munro PR, Mallory JB. Effectiveness of open circuit and oxyhood delivery of helium oxygen. *Chest* 1989;95:1222–1224.

THE LUNG: Scientific Foundations
edited by R.G. Crystal, J.B. West et al.
Raven Press, Ltd., New York © 1991.

CHAPTER 8.2.2

Oxygen Toxicity

Philip J. Fracica, Claude A. Piantadosi, and James D. Crapo

Supplemental oxygen is perhaps the most rapid and effective therapeutic strategy to reverse arterial hypoxemia from any etiology except veno-arterial shunt. Impairment of gas exchange in almost all pulmonary disease processes is a common consequence of disordered respiratory structure and function. Thus, oxygen therapy is widely employed and usually provides the expected benefit without toxicity. Unfortunately, with progressive pulmonary dysfunction, increasing concentrations of oxygen are required, and as the oxygen concentration is increased, so is the likelihood that the oxygen itself produces additive pulmonary injury. This may lead to the establishment of a self-perpetuating cycle in which increasing injury results in greater oxygen requirements, thereby producing further damage.

Uninterrupted exposure to nearly pure oxygen environments at 1 atmosphere has been demonstrated repeatedly to cause death in many mammalian species (1–3). High inspired concentrations of oxygen have been identified as a significant contributing factor to respiratory failure in humans with severe lung injury. The overall clinical importance of oxygen toxicity in humans has been obscured by the coexistence of severe underlying pulmonary pathology in individuals receiving high concentrations of oxygen for therapeutic purposes. There are substantial gaps in our understanding of the interaction between various underlying disease processes with hyperoxia and the amount of oxygen required for development of toxic effects. It is hoped that current research on mechanisms of hyperoxic lung damage as a single injury will form the basis for understanding the impact of hyperoxia on the course of concomitant pulmonary disease.

OXYGEN RADICALS

The basic mechanism underlying oxygen toxicity appears to be the generation of highly reactive, partially reduced oxygen compounds (4–6). During normal cellular respiration, oxygen is reduced fully by the acceptance of four electrons and the production of water. When the transfer of electrons to oxygen is incomplete (e.g., one or two electrons transferred), partially reduced species of oxygen such as superoxide anion and hydrogen peroxide are formed. These partially reduced species of oxygen can further react to produce both singlet oxygen and hydroxyl radical and can lead to formation of lipid peroxides. The primary intracellular sites of oxygen radical production are not well defined; however, there is evidence that both mitochondria and microsomes play important roles in this process (7–9).

Oxygen radicals have the ability to react with and damage many important biomolecules, including enzymes, membrane lipids, and nucleic acids. It is believed that the resultant loss of cell function eventually results in lethal cytotoxicity (10). The direct toxic effects of oxygen radicals are difficult to assess *in vivo* because of the inflammatory responses that develop during the injury and produce additional damage. Not only are inflammatory responses initiated by hyperoxia, but they appear to be modified and intensified synergistically by ongoing hyperoxia. This interaction appears to involve increased activity of leukocytic proteases and inhibition of antiproteases in a hyperoxic environment. Furthermore, exposure of inflammatory cells to proteases can result in enhanced production of oxygen radicals by the inflammatory cells (11–14).

PATHOLOGIC RESPONSES TO HYPEROXIC EXPOSURE

Although the pathologic response to prolonged hyperoxic exposure produces changes throughout the respi-

P. J. Fracica, C. A. Piantadosi, and J. D. Crapo: Division of Allergy, Critical Care, and Respiratory Medicine, Duke University Medical Center, Durham, North Carolina 27710.

ratory system from the epithelium of conducting airways to the pleural space, the alveolar septum has been a primary focus of attention as a result of the extensive structural changes that occur at this site. The implications of these changes for disruption of normal gas-exchange function are obvious. The temporal sequence of progressive histologic injury has been well studied in the rat (15,16). The survival of rats during continuous 100% oxygen exposure averages 60–66 hr. At death the lungs are edematous and substantial pleural effusions are present. With severe hyperoxic injury, significant endothelial cell injury is present, characterized by diminished capillary surface area and reduced numbers of endothelial cells. Intracapillary neutrophil content is increased substantially, as are the volume and cellularity of the alveolar septal interstitium. With lethal hyperoxic exposure there are no significant quantitative changes in numbers of alveolar epithelial cells; however, ultrastructural changes such as membrane ruffling of the type I pneumocyte and blunting of microvilli on the type II cell are present. At death, oxygen-poisoned rats show prominent injury to the capillary endothelial cells, interstitial edema, and increased cellularity, with relative sparing of structural injury to the epithelial cells.

Pathologic descriptions of human oxygen toxicity have been limited by the presence of coexisting pulmonary disease as well as by variability in the concentration–time profile of oxygen exposure. Pathologic changes ascribed to oxygen toxicity in humans include abnormalities of alveolar epithelial cells, endothelial cell injury, and septal thickening. Epithelial changes have been prominent, with extensive areas of epithelial cell sloughing and denuded basement membrane covered by hyaline membranes (3). In lower pri-

mates, quantitative electron microscopy has revealed significant changes across the alveolar septum with type I epithelial cell destruction, type II cell proliferation, increased interstitial thickness, and endothelial cell injury and destruction (2). More recent structural data have been obtained on the pattern of hyperoxic injury in the baboon (17). Morphometric analysis has been applied to tissues from primates exposed to hyperoxia, and the analysis has been used for precise sequencing of the cellular injury patterns, providing a detailed, quantitative paradigm of the adverse effects of hyperoxia on the lungs. Figure 1 provides a summary of the development of morphologic changes in lungs of baboons continuously exposed to a >98% oxygen environment.

STAGES IN OXYGEN TOXICITY

Early Injury

The earliest significant histologic changes are endothelial cell swelling and neutrophil aggregation (Figs. 2 and 3). In baboons, this occurs between 40 and 66 hr of exposure to 100% O_2 at 1 atmosphere absolute (ATA). At this point a significant reduction in pulmonary endothelial cell numbers does not occur. In fact, there is a nonsignificant trend towards proliferation of endothelial cells with early injury. Endothelial cell swelling occurs early and is associated with an increased cytoplasmic vacuolation. The simultaneous findings of endothelial cell changes and increased intravascular neutrophil content raise the issue of whether the endothelial cell injury is due to neutrophil activity or whether a primary hyperoxic endothelial

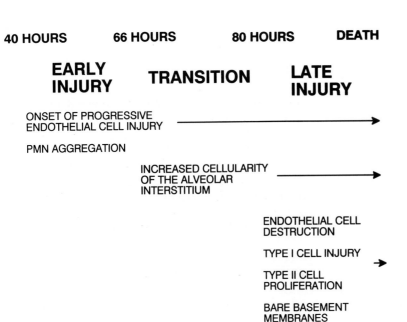

FIG. 1. Schematic presentation of the sequence of development of pulmonary morphologic changes during prolonged exposure of baboons to >98% oxygen. PMN, polymorphonuclear leukocyte.

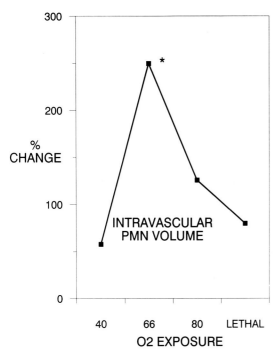

FIG. 2. Morphometrically determined changes in the volume of intravascular neutrophils (compared to matched control lung samples) in lung tissue from hyperoxic baboons after 40-, 66-, and 80-hr exposures and after lethal hyperoxic exposures. Asterisk denotes $p < 0.05$. PMN, polymorphonuclear leukocyte.

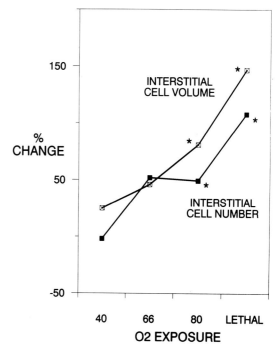

FIG. 4. Morphometrically determined changes in alveolar interstitial cell average volume and cell number during hyperoxic exposure of baboons. Asterisk denotes $p < 0.05$.

cell injury results in increased neutrophil aggregation. The observation that the endothelial cell swelling is not confined to areas with adjacent neutrophils provides some evidence of a primary endothelial cell injury as one of the early steps in hyperoxic lung injury.

Transition Phase from Early to Late Injury

As the hyperoxic injury progresses, the alveolar septal interstitium develops increased cellularity, largely due to an increase in inflammatory cell content (Figs. 4 and 5). Additional endothelial cell swelling occurs during this phase, whereas the epithelial cells remain relatively unaffected morphologically. Studies of epithelial cell function during this transitional phase suggest that there are significant changes such as enhanced permeability to solutes (18,19). The changes that occur in this period are probably an extension of the events occurring during early injury. As endothelial cell injury progresses, inflammatory cells recruited into the microvasculature can enter the interstitial space.

Late Injury

The final stages of hyperoxic injury are notable for widespread destruction among most cell populations and for the onset of overt epithelial cell structural changes. At this point, decreased numbers of endo-

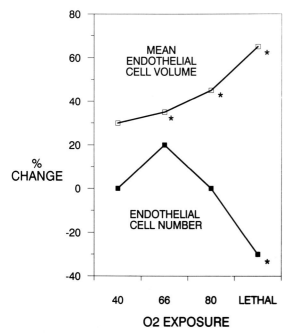

FIG. 3. Morphometrically determined changes in endothelial cell number and mean cell volume during hyperoxic exposure of baboons. Asterisk denotes $p < 0.05$.

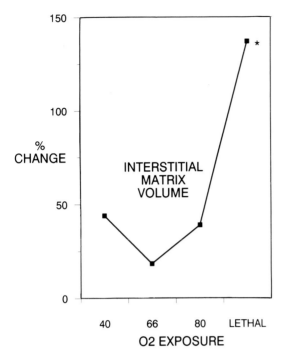

FIG. 5. Morphometrically determined changes in the alveolar septal interstitial matrix volume during baboon hyperoxic exposure. Asterisk denotes $p < 0.05$.

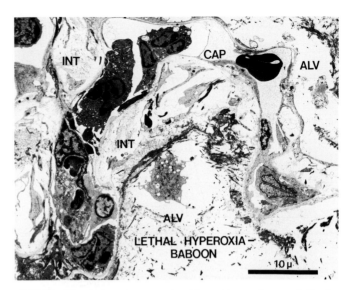

FIG. 6. Electron micrograph of lung tissue from a lethal-oxygen-exposed baboon. The alveolar spaces (ALV), septal interstitium (INT), and capillary lumen (CAP) are labeled. Extensive tissue injury is present, illustrating many of the features of the late phase of hyperoxic injury. The capillary endothelial cells are badly damaged, and in some areas they are destroyed. The type I epithelial cells are also injured, with small areas of denuded basement membrane. A widened interstitial space and neutrophils in a capillary remnant are present.

thelial cells are present, and those that remain show even further swelling (Fig. 3). Extensive capillary injury is present with areas of discontinuous endothelial cell lining. Many capillaries appear densely packed with cellular debris, neutrophils, monocytes, platelets, and erythrocytes. Little or no plasma is seen in many capillaries. It is probable that such capillaries are no longer adequately perfused. Neutrophils can be seen throughout the interstitium, and in some areas they can be found between epithelial cells and subjacent basement membranes. The interstitium is widened greatly from both cellular infiltration and a significant increase in the volume of the interstitial matrix (Figs. 4 and 5). The latter finding reflects increased water and protein content. This interstitial edema is probably due to extensive endothelial cell destruction. Figure 6 shows many of the histologic features of advanced hyperoxic injury.

It is not until the late injury stage that epithelial cell destruction is observed with areas of the alveolar surface denuded of cellular lining. In these areas, the bare basement membrane is covered only by adherent fibrinous materials and fragments of cells. There is marked injury of type I cells, with a concomitant proliferation of type II cells (Figs. 7 and 8). A major consequence of these changes is a shift in the composition of the epithelium lining the alveoli, with a substantially greater proportion of surface covered by type II cells.

The progression of the histologic pattern of injury represents an interaction between (a) oxygen re-

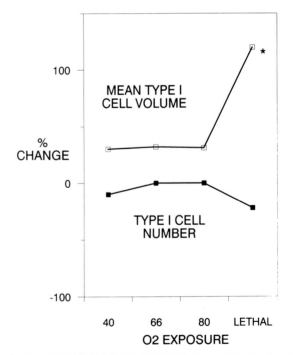

FIG. 7. Morphometrically determined changes in pulmonary type I epithelial cell mean volume and cell number during baboon hyperoxic exposure. Asterisk denotes $p < 0.05$.

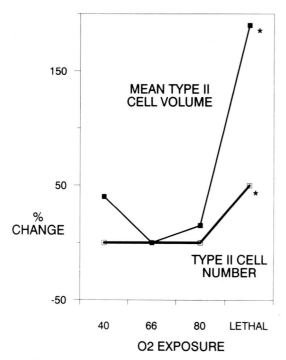

FIG. 8. Morphometrically determined changes in pulmonary type II epithelial cell mean volume and cell number during baboon hyperoxic exposure. Asterisk denotes $p < 0.05$.

sponses by individual cell types, (b) migration of inflammatory cells, and (c) fluid shifts due to disruption of normal permeability barriers. It is difficult to determine how much of the cellular injury results directly from hyperoxia and which aspects of injury are due to inflammatory cell actions. The sequence of injury and neutrophil migration commences at the vascular surface and moves outward through the interstitium to the epithelial cells. Regardless of the final mediators responsible for injury, two broad patterns of cellular response can be identified. Both the type I cell and the endothelial cell are damaged and destroyed with hyperoxia, with the endothelial cell succumbing to early injury and the type I cell showing initial resistance to structural injury followed later by destruction. The relatively normal appearance of type I epithelial cells during early hyperoxic injury illustrates a limitation of morphologic analysis in identifying some injury processes, since there is considerable evidence that the permeability of the alveolar epithelium is substantially disrupted relatively early during hyperoxic exposures in most species, including man (18,19). Type II epithelial cells are unusual in their response to hyperoxic exposure, since they proliferate while other cells are being destroyed. This late proliferation may be a response to the destruction of type I cells and the exposure of denuded basement membranes, rather than being a direct consequence of hyperoxia on type II cells.

PROTECTIVE MECHANISMS

Even at ambient oxygen concentrations, oxygen-derived free radicals are probably produced in tissue. However, oxygen radical production under normoxic conditions is sufficiently small that cellular defense mechanisms can prevent the occurrence of substantial injury (10). Cellular defense mechanisms include both enzymatic and nonenzymatic components. Superoxide dismutases (SODs) are metalloenzymes that catalyze the conversion of superoxide anions to hydrogen peroxide. Intracellular SOD occurs as an intracytoplasmic enzyme containing dimeric copper and zinc. A tetrameric manganese form of the enzyme is localized predominantly to the mitochondria (20). A third form of SOD, with a primarily extracellular localization, has been described recently in several mammalian species (21). Hydrogen peroxide produced by the action of SOD is eliminated by the action of catalase in reactions that yield water and oxygen (22). Glutathione peroxidase catalyzes the reduction of hydrogen peroxide to water by removing electrons from glutathione, thus producing glutathione disulfide (23). Nonenzymatic free-radical defenses include alpha-tocopherol, which acts as a radical scavenger and can terminate a chain of successive radical formation (24). Other well-known oxygen radical scavengers include glutathione, ascorbic acid, and beta-carotene (25,26). Cellular repair mechanisms may also be considered a form of cellular antioxidant defense, since cells with well-developed repair mechanisms may be able to tolerate more oxidant injury before dying.

OXYGEN TOLERANCE

In many species, exposure to several stimuli can cause changes that allow animals to tolerate subsequent hyperoxic exposure with reduced injury. Oxygen tolerance is usually demonstrated by increased survival time during continuous exposure to a 100% oxygen environment. Administration of endotoxin and previous exposure to sublethal hyperoxia (0.8–0.85 ATA) are two well-described means of producing oxygen tolerance in rats (15,27). Oxygen tolerance in the rat after both sublethal hyperoxic pre-exposure and endotoxin administration is associated with an increase in pulmonary antioxidant enzyme content (15,28). The mechanism of enzyme induction following endotoxin exposure is not entirely clear, although there is evidence that SOD mRNA content increases in the lung (29). Cytokines that may be increased after endotoxin administration (30,31), such as tumor necrosis factor and interleukin-1, have been shown to increase mRNA expression for manganese SOD (32).

Oxygen tolerance that does not depend on increases

in antioxidant enzymes has been described. Administration of agents that induce cytochrome P-450 has been reported to result in both tolerance and increased oxygen sensitivity in rats (33–35). Increased quantities of phospholipid in alveolar lavage fluid have been recovered in rabbits rendered oxygen tolerant by sublethal hyperoxic exposure, providing evidence that an increase in surfactant may be important (36). Pretreatment of rats with tumor necrosis factor and interleukin-1 has been shown to produce oxygen tolerance without an increase in antioxidant enzymes (37). Although several mechanisms are undoubtedly involved in oxygen tolerance, demonstration of substantial elevations of native antioxidant enzymes provides evidence that enzyme induction is one important mediator of oxygen tolerance. Of note, neither the development of oxygen tolerance nor the induction of antioxidant enzymes in response to hyperoxia has thus far been documented in humans.

CLINICAL MANIFESTATIONS AND FUNCTIONAL ABNORMALITIES

The earliest manifestation of pulmonary oxygen toxicity in normal humans is the development of a mild chest discomfort exacerbated by inspiration and associated with cough (1,38). Symptoms of chest discomfort developing within the first 24 hr may remit initially; however, continued exposure results in progressively intense substernal burning discomfort and increased coughing. This is thought to reflect development of tracheobronchitis. With increasing durations of oxygen administration, functional abnormalities can be detected, such as progressive impairment of vital capacity, compliance, and DLCO, accompanied by an increasing alveolar–arterial oxygen tension difference (38,39). Human data on the consequences of more prolonged oxygen exposure uncomplicated by coexisting pulmonary disease are, appropriately, quite limited. Pathological data obtained from humans with irreversible brain damage and relatively normal lungs, ventilated with 100% oxygen, are the closest to sole oxygen injury. However, the data are difficult to interpret because the patients had significant trauma and were all receiving parenteral corticosteroids (40). These subjects showed a declining arterial oxygen tension, increased shunt fraction, and increased dead space with prolonged hyperoxia. In human volunteers, hyperoxia for an average of 17 hr has resulted in an increase in albumin and transferrin in alveolar lavage without quantitative changes in inflammatory cell recovery, although alveolar macrophages were found to release increased amounts of fibroblast growth factor. The increased lavageable protein is no longer present after a 2-week recovery period (18).

THERAPEUTIC IMPLICATIONS

The cornerstone of the clinical approach to oxygen toxicity is prevention. Oxygen concentrations beyond those required to ensure adequate arterial oxygen content should be avoided. In most cases, brief periods of exposure to 100% oxygen do not produce substantial injury and can be lifesaving when used as part of the treatment of acute respiratory failure and cardiopulmonary arrest. It should be noted that patients recently treated with bleomycin are particularly sensitive to oxygen, and every effort should be made to minimize unnecessary oxygen exposure to them (41,42).

With prolonged hypoxemic respiratory failure, attempts should be made to improve the efficiency of pulmonary gas exchange. These include optimizing tidal volume, use of positive end-expiratory pressure, and patient position. Efforts should be made to reduce systemic oxygen consumption by control of fever and sedation. The events that precipitated hypoxemia must be thoroughly evaluated and treated aggressively to restore more normal pulmonary gas exchange.

At present, the only effective treatment to prevent or reverse oxygen toxicity is to reduce the level of oxygen exposure whenever possible. The lack of effective clinical interventions to ameliorate pulmonary oxygen toxicity means that any effective new therapy has the potential to result in significant benefit with widespread utilization. Some promising experimental approaches to protect against hyperoxic pulmonary injury include the administration of exogenous antioxidant enzymes and free-radical scavengers which may be helpful by blocking the initiation of cellular injury. Administration of exogenous surfactant to patients with acute lung injury may improve gas exchange and allow lower inspired oxygen tensions. Surfactant therapy could both reverse some functional abnormalities resulting from hyperoxia and prevent subsequent hyperoxic injury by allowing lower inspired oxygen concentrations. Finally, the use of newer artificial membrane oxygenators, either intravascular or extracorporeal, may improve blood oxygenation and decrease ventilator pressures without excessive pulmonary oxygen exposure. Past clinical trials of extracorporeal membrane oxygenation, however, have failed to demonstrate an improved survival in acute respiratory failure (43).

ACKNOWLEDGEMENT

This work was supported, in part, by NIH grants HL-31992 and HL-42609.

REFERENCES

1. Clark JM, Lambertsen CJ. Pulmonary oxygen toxicity: a review. *Pharmacol Rev* 1971;23:37–133.

2. Kapanci Y, Weibel ER, Kaplan HP, Robinson FR. Pathogenesis and reversibility of the pulmonary lesions of oxygen toxicity in monkeys. II. Ultrastructural and morphometric studies. *Lab Invest* 1969;20:101–117.

3. Gould VE, Tosco R, Wheelis R, Gould NS, Kapanci Y. Oxygen pneumonitis in man: ultrastructural observations on the development of alveolar lesions. *Lab Invest* 1972;26:499–508.

4. Gerschman R, Gilbert DL, Nye SW, Dwyer P, Fenn WO. Oxygen poisoning and x-irradiation: a mechanism in common. *Science* 1954;119:623–626.

5. Jamieson D, Chance B, Cadenas E, Boveris A. The relationship of free radical production to hyperoxia. *Annu Rev Physiol* 1986;48:703–719.

6. Freeman BA, Topolsky MK, Crapo JD. Hyperoxia increases oxygen radical production in rat lung homogenates. *Arch Biochem Biophys* 1982;216:477–484.

7. Boveris A, Chance B. The mitochondrial generation of hydrogen peroxide. General properties and effect of hyperbaric oxygen. *Biochem J* 1973;134:707–716.

8. Turrens JF, Freeman BA, Crapo JD. Hyperoxia increases in H_2O_2 release by lung mitochondria and microsomes. *Arch Biochem Biophys* 1982;217:411–421.

9. Turrens JF, Boveris A. Generation of superoxide anion by the NADH dehydrogenase of bovine heart mitochondria. *Biochem J* 1980;191:421–427.

10. Freeman BA, Crapo JD. Biology of disease. Free radicals and tissue injury. *Lab Invest* 1982;47:412–426.

11. Weiss SJ, Peppin G, Ortiz X, Ragsdale C, Test ST. Reports: oxidative autoactivation of latent collagenase by human neutrophils. *Science* 1985;227:747–749.

12. Baird BR, Cheronis JC, Sandhaus RA, Berger EM, White CW, Repine JE. O_2 metabolites and neutrophil elastase synergistically cause edematous injury in isolated rat lungs. *Am Physiol Soc* 1986;61(6):2224–2229.

13. Speer CP, Pabst MJ, Hedegaard HB, Rest RF, Johnston RB Jr. Enhanced release of oxygen metabolites by monocyte-derived macrophages exposed to proteolytic enzymes: activity of neutrophil elastase and cathepsin G. *J Immunol* 1984;133:2151–2156.

14. Carp H, Janoff A. *In vitro* suppression of serum elastase-inhibitory capacity by reactive oxygen species generated by phagocytosing polymorphonuclear leukocytes. *J Clin Invest* 1979;63:793–797.

15. Crapo JD, Barry BE, Foscue HA, Shelburne J. Structural and biochemical changes in rat lungs occurring during exposure to lethal and adaptive doses of oxygen. *Am Rev Respir Dis* 1980;122:123–143.

16. Crapo JD. Morphologic changes in pulmonary oxygen toxicity. *Annu Rev Physiol* 1986;48:721–731.

17. Fracica PJ, Knapp MJ, Crapo JD. Patterns of progression and markers of lung injury in rodents and subhuman primates exposed to hyperoxia. *Exp Lung Res* 1988;14:869–885.

18. Davis WB, Rennard SI, Bitterman PB, Crystal RG. Pulmonary oxygen toxicity. Early reversible changes in human alveolar structures induced by hyperoxia. *N Engl J Med* 1983;309:878–883.

19. Matalon S, Cesar MA. Effects of 100% oxygen breathing on permeability of alveolar epithelium to solute. *J Appl Physiol* 1981;50:859–863.

20. Fridovich I. Superoxide radical and superoxide dismutases. In: Gilbert DL, ed. *Oxygen and living processes.* New York: Springer-Verlag, 1981;250–272.

21. Marklund SL, Holme E, Hellner L. Superoxide dismutase in extracellular fluids. *Clin Chim Acta* 1982;126:41–54.

22. Chance B, Sies H, Boveris A. Hydroperoxide metabolism in mammalian organs. *Physiol Rev* 1979;59:527–605.

23. Cohen G, Hochstein P. Glutathione peroxidase: the primary agent for the elimination of hydrogen peroxide in erythrocytes. *Biochemistry* 1963;2:1420–1428.

24. Tappel AL. Vitamin E as the biological lipid antioxidant. *Vitam Horm* 1969;20:493–510.

25. Arias IM, Jakoby WB, eds. *Glutathione: metabolism and function.* New York: Raven Press, 1976.

26. Nishikimi M. Oxidation of ascorbic acid with superoxide ion generated by the xanthine-oxidase system. *Biochem Biophys Res Commun* 1975;63:463–468.

27. Frank L, Yam J, Roberts RJ. The role of endotoxin in production of adult rats from oxygen-induced lung toxicity. *J Clin Invest* 1978;61:269–275.

28. Frank L, Summerville J, Massaro D. Protection from oxygen toxicity with endotoxin: the role of the endogenous antioxidant enzymes of the lung. *J Clin Invest* 1980;65:1104–1110.

29. Iqbal J, Clerch LB, Hass MA, Frank L, Massaro D. Endotoxin increases lung Cu,Zn superoxide dismutase mRNA: O_2 raises enzyme synthesis. *Am J Physiol* 1989;257:L61–L64.

30. Hesse DG, Tracey KJ, Fong Y, et al. Cytokine appearance in human endotoxemia and primate bacteremia. *Surg Gynecol Obstet* 1988;166:147–153.

31. Michie HR, Manogue KR, Spriggs DR, et al. Detection of circulating tumor necrosis factor after endotoxin administration. *N Engl J Med* 1988;318:1481–1486.

32. Wong GHW, Goeddel DV. Induction of manganous superoxide dismutase by tumor necrosis factor: possible protective mechanism. *Science* 1988;242:941–944.

33. Gonder JC, Proctor RA, Will JA. Genetic differences in oxygen toxicity are correlated with cytochrome P-450 inducibility. *Proc Natl Acad Sci USA* 1985;82:6315–6319.

34. Mansour H, Brun-Pascaud M, Marquetty C, Gougerot-Pocidalo MA, Hakim J, Pocidalo JJ. Protection of rat from oxygen toxicity by inducers of cytochrome P-450 system. *Am Rev Respir Dis* 1988;137:688–694.

35. Tindberg N, Ingelman-Sundberg M. Cytochrome P-450 and oxygen toxicity. Oxygen-dependent induction of ethanol-inducible cytochrome P-450 (IIE1) in rat liver and lung. *Biochemistry* 1989;28:4499–4504.

36. Baker RR, Holm BA, Panus PC, Matalon S. Development of O_2 tolerance in rabbits with no increase in antioxidant enzymes. *J Appl Physiol* 1989;66(4):1679–1684.

37. White CW, Ghezzi P, Dinarello CA, Caldwell SA, McMurray IF, Repine JE. Recombinant tumor necrosis factor/cachectin and interleukin 1 pretreatment decreases lung oxidized glutathione accumulation, lung injury, and mortality in rats exposed to hyperoxia. *J Clin Invest* 1987;79:1868–1873.

38. Caldwell PRB, Lee WL Jr, Schildkraut HS, Archibald ER. Changes in lung volume, diffusing capacity, and blood gases in men breathing oxygen. *J Appl Physiol* 1966, 21:1477–1483.

39. Sackner MA, Landa J, Hirsch J, Zapata A. Pulmonary effects of oxygen breathing. A 6-hour study in normal men. *Ann Intern Med* 1975;82:40–43.

40. Barber RE, Lee J, Hamilton WK. Oxygen toxicity in man: a prospective study in patients with irreversible brain damage. *N Engl J Med* 1970;283:1478–1481.

41. Goldiner PL, Carlon GC, Cvitkovic E, Schweizer O, Howland WS. Factors influencing postoperative morbidity and mortality in patients treated with bleomycin. *Br Med J* 1978;1:1664–1667.

42. Rinaldo J, Goldstein RH, Snider GL. Modification of oxygen toxicity after lung injury by bleomycin in hamsters. *Am Rev Respir Dis* 1982;126:1030–1033.

43. Zapol WM, Snider MT, Hill JD, et al. Extracorporeal membrane oxygenation in severe acute respiratory failure. A randomized prospective study. *JAMA* 1979;242:2193–2196.

THE LUNG: Scientific Foundations
edited by R.G. Crystal, J.B. West et al.
Raven Press, Ltd., New York © 1991.

CHAPTER 8.2.3

Mechanical Ventilation

Arthur S. Slutsky

HISTORICAL PERSPECTIVE

Although the major advances in mechanical ventilation have been made over the past 50 years, the concept of endotracheal intubation and positive-pressure ventilation was first described in 1543 in Vesalius' treatise entitled "De Humani Corporis Fabrica" (1,2). In that treatise, Vesalius stated: "But that life may . . . be restored to the animal, an opening must be attempted in the trachea, into which a tube should be put; you will then blow into this, so that the lung may rise again and the animal take in air" (2). Despite this elegant description of what now would be considered standard principles of resuscitation, the widespread utilization of these concepts was not applied for approximately 350 years. No further progress was made for approximately a century, until Robert Hooke's experiments in 1667 in which he ventilated a dog using a constant flow arrangement (3). Another century was to pass before John Fothergill's report of the successful application of mouth-to-mouth resuscitation (4). Although Fothergill was one of the founders of the British Humane Society, this approach was not adopted, possibly because of the fear of touching the dead.

From the mid-nineteenth century to the beginning of the twentieth century, a large number of negative-pressure ventilators were developed (5,6). At that time, it was believed that negative-pressure ventilation had major advantages over positive-pressure ventilation. It was not appreciated that from a physiological point of view, there was no difference in hemodynamics or in pulmonary barotrauma between these two techniques when the negative pressure was applied around the entire body. Although some of these ventilators were useful, such as the first workable iron lung

built by Woillez in 1876, many of the other devices were essentially of no use at all. The first practically useful and widely used iron lung was developed in 1928 by Drinker and Shaw (7). The iron lung consisted of a cylinder which had a number of portholes in it and which could be used to nurse the patient. Positive and negative pressures within the tank were produced by pumps which ran continuously, and the pressure changes were caused by the adjustment of a series of valves. This original ventilator was improved upon by the Kroghs and by J. H. Emerson in 1932.

These ventilators proved to be extremely useful during the polio epidemics in the mid-1950s, but since then the approach to mechanical ventilation has changed tremendously, although negative-pressure ventilators continue to be used successfully for long-term ventilatory support. Over the past 30–40 years there has been a great increase in the number of different types of ventilators and radical changes in the design of ventilators. The remainder of this chapter will review currently used ventilators, with a specific focus on new developments in mechanical ventilation. The next section will deal with ventilatory techniques, which, although different from negative-pressure ventilators, are based on the same basic physiological concept of gas exchange in the lung. The subsequent section will deal with nonconventional ventilatory techniques that have been developed in an attempt to overcome some of the problems such as barotrauma and hemodynamic compromise associated with these conventional techniques.

CONVENTIONAL VENTILATION

Modes of Ventilation

Controlled and Assist-Control Ventilation

Controlled mechanical ventilation is one of the simplest forms of artificial ventilation and was first applied

A. S. Slutsky: Mount Sinai Hospital, Toronto, Ontario M5G 1X5, Canada.

during the polio epidemics. As the name implies, with controlled mechanical ventilation the patient's alveolar ventilation is determined solely by the settings on the ventilator. The technique is effective for patients with relatively normal lungs whose disease process is very stable, or for patients who are totally paralyzed.

The major problem with controlled ventilation is that to use it effectively, the patient's spontaneous breathing efforts must be eliminated either by inducing respiratory alkalosis or by pharmacological means (sedation, paralysis) (8). This leads to two problems. First, since the patient no longer has control over his ventilation, the medical staff must determine the exact alveolar ventilation that is required by the patient. In patients who have multiple medical problems, the exact level of alveolar ventilation required is not necessarily easy to determine. The second problem is that if one has sedated or paralyzed the patient, a very important defense system is removed; also, if the patient is inadvertently disconnected from the ventilator, he may not be able to sustain any ventilation on his own.

For these reasons, the more common mode of ventilation is assist-control ventilation. With this technique, the patient can trigger a breath by creating a small negative pressure at the airway opening. Thus with this technique the patient controls his own ventilation, and if, for whatever reason, the patient does not trigger the ventilator, a fixed number of breaths are given per minute. Initially, it was felt that with this technique the patient's energy costs of breathing would be kept to a minimum. However, a number of studies have shown that the patient's spontaneous work of breathing is often greater than expected (9,10) because many ventilator circuits contain components that have a high impedance, thus necessitating a relatively large effort on the patient's part. Furthermore, the patient continues to produce inspiratory efforts even after the ventilator starts to cycle, because the gas is often not delivered quickly enough to "satisfy" the patient.

Intermittent Mandatory Ventilation

Intermittent mandatory ventilation (IMV) was developed largely because of dissatisfaction with the previously discussed methods of controlled ventilation (11a,11b). With IMV the patient is able to breathe spontaneously and is thus able to maintain a certain proportion of his required alveolar ventilation. Weaning from artificial ventilation can easily be performed using IMV (11c) by slowly decreasing the number of breaths delivered by the ventilator and letting the patient take over an increasingly greater percentage of the required alveolar ventilation as he improves. This approach has recently been tested in a prospective trial comparing IMV and T-piece weaning from mechanical ventilation (11). The major conclusion of the study was that clinically stable patients who met standard bedside weaning criteria could be weaned efficiently by protocol using either the IMV approach or the T-piece approach.

One of the proposed advantages of IMV was that the mean airway and pleural pressures would be decreased when the patient was breathing spontaneously. This should have a beneficial effect on hemodynamics. However, one of the major problems in the widespread acceptance of IMV was poor ventilator performance. Because of inadequate circuit design, the patient's spontaneous work of breathing during the spontaneous breaths was often greatly increased. Thus, patients had a tendency to fatigue.

A potential problem that surfaced with the use of IMV was the possibility that the ventilator might deliver a breath at the end of a patient's spontaneous inspiration. This might result in the delivery of a relatively large tidal volume which could potentially cause pulmonary barotrauma and hemodynamic compromise. This is unlikely to be a major difficulty, since most patients who require mechanical ventilation do not take very large breaths; furthermore, the addition of a second tidal volume should not be injurious, because "sighs" equivalent to 2–3 times the tidal volume were delivered routinely to many ventilated patients for a number of years. However, to overcome this problem, a technique called "synchronized intermittent mandatory ventilation" (SIMV) was developed (12). During SIMV, an assist mode is superimposed on the patient's spontaneous breathing pattern in order to avoid this problem. Whether this technique has any advantages over IMV is uncertain.

Mandatory Minute Ventilation

The basic concept using mandatory minute ventilation (MMV) is that the minute ventilation delivered to the patient is maintained at a set level. With the original technique, a constant flow of gas was supplied (13); the patient breathed as much as he was able to, and the remainder of that constant flow was accumulated in a bellows. When a particular set volume was reached in the ventilator, it was then delivered to the patient by the ventilator. If the patient's spontaneous ventilation increased, the gas would accumulate more slowly in the bellows; hence the breaths delivered by the ventilator would also decrease. The major advantage of this technique was purported to be improved weaning, since the weaning process was easily and precisely controlled by the patient. If the patient was doing well, he would produce more spontaneous ventilation and would thus continue to wean.

There are a number of problems with this technique,

as with all techniques. First, the minute ventilation is set relatively arbitrarily. In this regard, it is similar to controlled mechanical ventilation. Second, many patients who require mechanical ventilation have a breathing pattern which is characterized by rapid shallow breaths. Because the ventilator is set to deliver a constant minute ventilation, the actual alveolar ventilation delivered may vary considerably, depending on the patient's breathing pattern.

Pressure-Support Ventilation

Pressure-support ventilation (PSV) is a relatively new form of mechanical ventilation in which the patient's spontaneous breaths are assisted by having the pressure at the airway opening held relatively constant during inspiration (14,15). It is similar to older forms of pressure-assisted ventilatory support in that the assist is delivered during spontaneous breathing efforts, but it differs in that airway pressure is held constant during PSV. With this technique, the patient spontaneously controls respiratory timing, and the airway pressure is maintained at the predetermined level as long as there is a minimal inspiratory flow. This differs from continuous positive airway pressure (CPAP) in that PSV is primarily a mode of delivering ventilatory support, and hence the pressure is applied only during the inspiratory phase. When PSV is used at relatively high levels of airway pressure it can be used to supply the patient's full ventilatory demands, and the patient's energy costs of breathing are essentially zero.

PSV can also be used as a means of weaning patients from mechanical ventilation. By decreasing the level of pressure support, the patient gradually can increase his own spontaneous efforts. One of the major theoretical advantages of this approach is that patient–ventilator asynchrony should be decreased because the patient has control over the flow and volume of each breath. Furthermore, the workload of the ventilatory muscles during pressure support is more physiologic in the sense that the pressure–volume load on the respiratory muscles is similar to that observed during normal ventilation (14).

Positive End-Expiratory Pressure

Positive end-expiratory pressure (PEEP) is the maintenance of a pressure greater than atmospheric at the airway opening at the end of expiration during positive-pressure ventilation. Although the basic concept was proposed in the 1930s by Barach et al. (16) and Fulton and Oxon (17), for the treatment of pulmonary edema, it was not until the late 1960s and early 1970s that the technique became popular (18). In a large number of studies, PEEP has been shown to improve oxygena-

tion, especially in patients with the adult respiratory distress syndrome (ARDS) (19). Despite the intense research on PEEP over the past 20 years, it is only in the last few years that the mechanisms by which PEEP improves oxygenation have been elucidated.

A number of possible mechanisms have been proposed to explain the beneficial effect of PEEP:

1. *The stabilization of fluid-filled alveoli so that the edema fluid forms a relatively thinner layer in the alveolar wall, thus decreasing the diffusion distances* (20). The precise mechanism for this change from relatively small alveoli full of fluid to larger alveoli containing the same amount of fluid is not entirely clear (21). In addition, this does not explain the increase in interstitial fluid that has been observed by some investigators using PEEP (21).

2. *A decrease in extravascular lung liquid.* A number of studies have repudiated this hypothesis, demonstrating that PEEP increases oxygenation and reduces shunt without reducing the amount of edema (22,23).

3. *Reduced perfusion of nonventilated lung regions which are edematous.* Although this is a physiologically attractive explanation, it is unlikely to be correct based on the studies of Malo et al. (21), who showed that unilateral PEEP to an edematous lobe did not reduce its perfusion.

4. *Redistribution of pulmonary edema.* This mechanism seems like the most plausible one to explain the mechanism of action of PEEP. During the application of PEEP there is redistribution of edema away from the interstitial space near alveolar vessels to the perivascular cuff areas surrounding extra-alveolar vessels. These represent a compliant interstitial space which thus does not interfere with gas exchange (21,24).

The optimal approach to applying PEEP has been extremely controversial. This is largely because various investigators have used different endpoints to define the optimum PEEP. The general approach appears to increase PEEP in a step-like fashion with monitoring of oxygen transport or some other index of peripheral oxygen utilization until a point at which the inspired O_2 concentration can be decreased to an F_{IO_2} of 60% or 50%. Whether any further increases in PEEP are beneficial after this point is not clear. There are a number of definitions of the optimal PEEP. Suter et al. (25) designated the optimal PEEP as the level of PEEP at which the oxygen transport was at maximum (25). They found that at this level, respiratory system compliance was also at a maximum. This was an attractive observation, since theoretically it would have been possible to obtain the optimum PEEP without the need for measurements of cardiac output. It was also physiologically attractive because it was reasonable that an improvement in oxygenation would occur as alveoli were recruited, and it would be at this point that the compliance would be near the maximum. However, the correlation that was observed between oxygen delivery and compliance was obtained using mean values and was not proved in individual patients (26). In addition, Suter et al. did not increase intravascular volume as they increased PEEP. The decrease in cardiac output with PEEP usually responds to intravascular repletion. A number of other approaches to the issue of determining the appropriate level of PEEP have been suggested, including (a) using a level of PEEP at which intrapulmonary shunt is decreased to less than 15% (27) and (b) using "super-PEEP" (28).

In the publication describing this latter approach, the investigators suggested that PEEP was "a fundamental means of aborting lung injury in ARDS." For a number of years, this statement that PEEP alters the pathophysiology of lung injury in ARDS was controversial. Several clinical studies had suggested that the incidence of ARDS might be reduced by applying PEEP in patients at high risk for the syndrome. In a recent prospective, randomized study examining this issue, a number of patients at high risk for ARDS received mechanical ventilation either without PEEP or with PEEP of 8 cm H_2O applied early in the progression of the disease (29). ARDS developed in 25% of the patients given early PEEP and in 27% of the patients not given PEEP. The incidence of atelectasis, pneumonia, and barotrauma was similar in both groups, as was the mortality. Thus, it appears that the early use of prophylactic PEEP has no effect in reducing the incidence of ARDS or its complications (29).

NONCONVENTIONAL VENTILATORY TECHNIQUES

Background

As described elsewhere in this book (see Chapters 5.1.2.5, 5.3.1, and 5.3.3), the traditional concept of gas exchange in the lung is based on the principle that transport of gas takes place in two physically distinct regions: the anatomic dead space and the alveolar region. Based on this construct, for adequate gas exchange to take place, the tidal volume must exceed the dead space. This approach is the principle underlying the design of most of the ventilators which have been described in the previous section. These have been extremely useful in the treatment of respiratory failure, but because of the large tidal volumes that are required to exceed the dead space, they are associated with a number of hemodynamic and pulmonary complications. In the National Heart, Lung and Blood Institute study examining the use of extracorporeal membrane

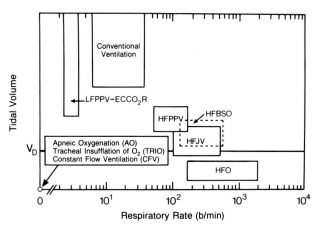

FIG. 1. Plot of tidal volume versus respiratory rate for various methods of ventilation. The ranges shown in the rectangles are rough estimates. Note that most of the x-axis has a logarithmic scale. The methods with a constant flow of gas are indicated at the origin, since there is no defined tidal volume or respiratory rate. HFPPV, high-frequency positive-pressure ventilation; HFJV, high-frequency jet ventilation; HFBSO, high-frequency body-surface oscillations; HFO, high-frequency oscillations; LPPV–$ECCO_2R$, low-frequency positive-pressure ventilation with extracorporeal CO_2 removal; V_D, dead space. (From ref. 31.)

oxygenators in the treatment of respiratory failure, over half of the deaths in the group assigned to conventional ventilation were attributed to complications of the ventilator therapy (30). For this reason, a number of investigators have been studying alternate techniques of providing adequate alveolar ventilation (31). A large number of these studies have shown that adequate gas exchange can occur under conditions in which the traditional concepts would predict no adequate alveolar ventilation.

These techniques thus represent a relatively new approach to the management of patients with respiratory failure. Because a number of these techniques use very small tidal volumes or no tidal volume (constant flow), they provide the potential for fewer complications than conventional mechanical ventilation. This section will focus on a number of nonconventional methods of ventilation. For purposes of this chapter, conventional ventilation will be defined as any technique in which the tidal volumes and frequencies are comparable to those observed during normal tidal ventilation (Fig. 1). Of course, this definition is a flexible one, since children, adults, and various animal species have a substantially different resting respiratory rate.

High-Frequency Ventilation

In the past 20 years, a number of different techniques have been developed in which the ventilatory frequencies are substantially greater than those observed during conventional ventilation (60–2000 breaths/min). This group of techniques is collectively known as "high-frequency ventilation" (HFV) (Fig. 1). Although the specific techniques and principles vary considerably, they all have in common a reduced tidal volume applied at relatively high frequency. For purposes of description, it is convenient to subdivide the HFV techniques into two categories: (i) those in which pressure changes are generated at the airway opening and (ii) those in which the pressure changes are generated at the chest wall or pleural surface.

HFV Applied at the Airway Opening

The various techniques of applying HFV at the airway opening can be grouped into those in which exhalation of gas is similar to that occurring during resting ventilation (i.e., passive exhalation) and those in which exhalation is an active process. The techniques of high-frequency positive-pressure ventilation (HFPPV) (32) and high-frequency jet ventilation (HFJV) (33) are techniques in which exhalation is passive (Fig. 2). HFPPV was originally developed by Sjöstrand and co-workers (34) as a ventilatory mode that could be used

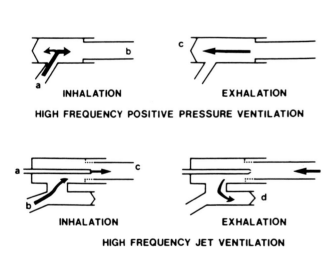

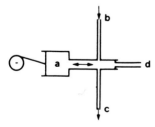

FIG. 2. Schematic diagrams indicating various high-frequency ventilatory circuits. **Top:** During HFPPV, gas is delivered from a low-compliance circuit. **Middle:** With HFJV, gas is entrained from around the catheter. **Bottom:** Bias flow is indicated as b–c. (From ref. 112.)

to study hemodynamic phenomena without the complications of large changes in pleural pressure caused by mechanical ventilation. The major feature of the ventilator was that it consisted of a relatively low compressible volume and that the tidal volume was delivered at rates of approximately 60–120 breaths/min. The tidal volumes used were small, and although they were not measured in most studies, they probably exceeded the anatomic dead space. HFPPV was first used as a physiological tool; subsequently, it was used as a clinical tool, especially for ventilation during bronchoscopy and laryngoscopy as well as in patients with respiratory failure. Among the reported advantages over conventional ventilation were the reduced need for patient sedation and reduced ventilator–patient asynchrony.

HFJV was an extension of a technique developed by Sanders in which the tidal volume was delivered to the airway via a small-bore catheter (Fig. 2). The actual ventilator can consist of any pressure or flow source in which the flow can be intermittently interrupted. The usual approach is to use a solenoid valve or a fluid-controlled valve. The tidal volume entering the patient is greater than the flow leaving the catheter; this is because of the jet effect produced as the gas leaves the narrow orifice of the catheter, thus entraining gas from around the catheter. With HFJV, respiratory frequencies usually range between 100 and 400 breaths/min, with a variable inspiratory-to-expiratory (I/E) ratio ranging from approximately 1:2 to 1:8. Tidal volumes are probably greater than the dead space (35) but are usually not measured, partly due to the difficulty in accurately measuring the entrained volume.

Unlike conventional ventilation in which the tidal volume and frequency are altered to change alveolar ventilation, during HFJV the variables that are changed include the driving pressure, frequency, and I/E ratio. Changes in these cause changes in tidal volume and airway pressures and hence affect gas exchange and hemodynamic performance. The particular tidal volume generated depends on the ventilatory–endotracheal circuit as well as on the patient's pulmonary mechanics (36). In general, increases in driving pressure produce an increase in tidal volume and hence increase alveolar ventilation (35,37). However, this increased driving pressure also causes an increase in mean airway pressure and functional residual capacity (FRC). Conversely, at a constant driving pressure, increasing the frequency or decreasing the I/E ratio decreases alveolar ventilation. This is attributable to both a decrease in the volume delivered to the jet and the entrained volume.

High-frequency oscillation (HFO) is different from the techniques described above in that both the inspiratory and expiratory phases are active; that is, on inspiration, gas is forced into the lungs, whereas on expiration, gas is actively sucked out of the lung by the ventilator (38–40). A number of different devices have been used to produce the oscillations, including piston pumps, loud speakers, and linear magnetic motors. Another major difference between HFO and the other two techniques described is that usually during HFO the ventilator does not supply fresh gas to the subject. Most systems therefore have a fresh gas flow, often termed a "bias flow," to supply oxygen and remove the CO_2 (Fig. 2). The bias flows are usually of either a relatively low impedance or high impedance to the oscillations. The low-impedance system has achieved wider clinical utility because it is simpler to use, allows spontaneous breathing by the patient, and is probably somewhat safer. The problem with this system is that the fraction of the stroke volume (generated by the ventilator) that actually enters the patient is dependent on relative impedance of the circuit and of the patient's respiratory system. With a high-impedance circuit, there is no loss of the oscillation volume to the bias flow, and thus it is easier to measure the gas entering the lungs. This explains the use of the high-impedance system for many studies investigating gas transport mechanisms during HFV. A number of studies have shown that adequate gas exchange can occur during HFO with tidal volumes considerably less than the anatomic dead space, clearly showing that the conventional concepts governing gas exchange in the lung are not entirely correct.

High-Frequency Body-Surface Oscillations

In an attempt to develop a technique in which it is possible to ventilate patients who are not intubated, a number of investigators have applied oscillations at the

pleural surface or chest wall (41–43). These techniques have been used either as a method for total ventilatory support or as a means of augmenting ventilation in patients with chronic airflow obstruction. The various techniques used have included direct compression of the chest via bladder cuffs, direct vibration using a mechanical device, and pneumatic compression in a plethysmograph. The most difficult problem with these techniques has been mechanical coupling between the ventilatory apparatus and the body surface.

Mechanisms of Gas Transport

In 1915, Henderson et al. (44) suggested that adequate gas exchange could take place with tidal volumes smaller than the dead space. They based this conclusion on the observation that dogs often used very small tidal volumes during panting. They proposed an elegant explanation for this phenomenon, suggesting that during inspiration a parabolic concentration profile of fresh gas might exist and that the tip of this parabolic cone might reach all the way into the alveolar zone, hence bringing fresh gas to the alveoli. Although this concept was an intriguing one, it does not provide the full explanation for a number of reasons. First, the development of a parabolic profile requires laminar flow. This condition is not likely to be met in the large airways. Furthermore, even if such a parabolic profile were to develop, it would be repeatedly disrupted at the multiple bifurcations as the gas traverses the conducting airways before reaching the alveolar zone.

To explain the intriguing result that adequate gas exchange is possible at small tidal volumes, a number of gas transport mechanisms have been proposed (40,45–49)(Fig. 3). In general, these gas transport

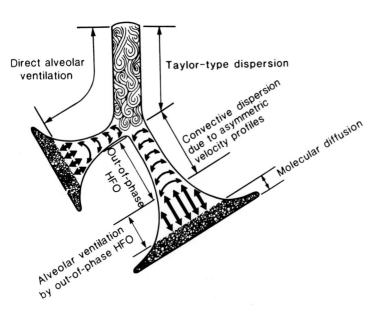

FIG. 3. Schematic representation of gas transport mechanisms during high-frequency ventilation. In reality, these various mechanisms are not mutually exclusive. Out-of-phase high-frequency oscillation (HFO) is equivalent to pendelluft.

mechanisms are dependent on two fundamental physical processes: convection and molecular diffusion.

Convective Gas Transport Mechanisms

Direct Alveolar Ventilation. During normal tidal breathing, bulk movement (convection) moves inspired gas directly to the respiratory zone, where molecular diffusion becomes the dominant gas transport mechanism. During HFV, the tidal volume is reduced to a level that is on the order of the anatomic dead space, and a smaller fraction of the inspired gas reaches the alveolar zone; thus the direct transport of gas to the alveolar region decreases in importance as a gas transport mechanism. However, because of the asymmetries in the lung and also because the velocity profiles in the airways are not uniform, even with tidal volumes on the order of the dead space, direct alveolar ventilation can occur to regions of the lung that are "relatively close" to the airway opening (46).

Convective Streaming. Haselton and Scherer (49,51) showed that because of the differences in velocity profiles on inspiration and expiration, there can be net convective flow into and out of the lung over the course of several oscillations. With this mechanism, the efficiency of gas transport is worsened by processes that tend to cause radial mixing, such as molecular diffusion and complex secondary flow patterns.

Pendelluft. Because of the differences in respiratory impedance of parallel pathways, the pulmonary gas flow entering adjacent lung regions may become out of phase. This would result in a back-and-forth motion of gas within the lung, which has been called "pendelluft." Thus, gas can flow between adjacent alveolar regions which would tend to mix the gas in the two compartments and hence decrease the nonhomogeneities in concentration profiles in the lung (52).

Augmented Dispersion. This mechanism is due to a combination of axial convection by a nonuniform velocity profile coupled to radial mixing from other convective transport mechanisms such as turbulence (46). The key factor is that the net transport of gas that occurs over a cycle is critically dependent on the lateral mixing, since without this lateral mixing there would be no net transport of gas at the end of any cycle.

Molecular Diffusion

Pure Molecular Diffusion. As during normal tidal ventilation, in the regions of the lung where the cross-sectional area becomes very large and velocities are very small, the major gas transport mechanism is molecular diffusion. The major problem during HFV is to overcome the large gas transport resistance of the conducting airways to bring the gas from the airway opening to the alveolar region. During HFV the residence time within the alveolar region is reduced, and thus the time available for equilibration of gas on a per cycle basis is also reduced. If this were to become a rate-limiting step, then the molecular diffusivity of the gas could play an important role in gas transport during HFV.

Augmented Dispersion. This mechanism is similar to that of the augmented dispersion discussed in the section on convective mechanisms above. However, in this case the radial mixing occurs not by a convective process such as turbulence, but by molecular diffusion. This is the problem that has been solved analytically by Taylor (53) for steady flow and by Watson (54) for oscillatory flow. It is interesting that under certain conditions, with Taylor dispersion, the efficacy of the gas transport can actually decrease as molecular diffusivity of the gas increases. This apparent paradox is due to the fact that if the radial movement of the gas is enhanced greatly as molecular diffusivity increases, the convective effect of the transport is relatively diminished.

In addition to the specific gas transport mechanisms, a number of theoretical models encompassing these mechanisms have been developed. Most of these models have made simplifying assumptions concerning the geometry of the lung and have assumed that plotting the cross-sectional area versus the distance from the airway opening gives a trumpet-shaped curve. In general, these models predict that gas transport would vary as the frequency times the tidal volume raised to some power, where this power ranges between 1 and 2 (39,40,45–50).

A large number of experimental studies examining gas transport mechanisms have also been performed. The main findings of these studies can be summarized as follows: First, alveolar ventilation or CO_2 transport varies as $f^a V_T^b$, where f = frequency, V_T = tidal volume, and $a = 1$, and $1.5 \leq b \leq 2.5$ (55–60). Second, the placement of the bias flow is important, since there is greater alveolar ventilation as the bias flow is positioned more distally (56,61). Third, above a certain bias flow rate, the flow rate is not very important, but below this value the flow rate is a major determinant of CO_2 transport (61). Fourth, the mechanical properties of the lungs may greatly affect gas transport (62,63). The particular properties that may be important are different than those operative during conventional ventilation. For example, because of the relatively high ventilatory frequencies, the compliance of the airways can play a role in limiting gas exchange by acting as a shunt compliance, directing a fraction of the tidal volume away from the gas-exchange regions of the lung (62,63). Fifth, in most (but not all) studies, gas transport is not greatly affected by using gases with different densities and different molecular diffusivities (64–66). Finally, the pressures measured at the airway opening may not accurately reflect pressures that exist in the alveoli (67,68). This is true for both the dynamic and static pressures. It is possible for the mean alveolar pressure to be substantially higher than the mean airway opening pressure, thus reflecting inadvertent hyperinflation of the lungs.

Potential Utility of HFV

Because of the relatively small tidal volumes used during HFV, the alveolar pressure swings should theoretically also be decreased, thus minimizing the risk of pulmonary barotrauma. In addition, it is possible to maintain higher mean lung volumes without the need for high peak alveolar pressures. These concepts underlie the rationale for a number of studies examining the effect of HFV in models of lung injury. A number of studies have shown that in various animal models of respiratory distress syndrome, HFV was associated with improved oxygenation as well as decreased pathologic evidence for lung injury (69,70,71). The mechanism responsible for these beneficial effects is likely related to an interaction between the static and dynamic properties of the lung. The optimum strategy in models with stiff lungs appears to be to provide an initial inflation to total lung capacity (TLC), thus opening up various regions of the lung, and then to apply HFV at a mean pressure which is above the closing pressure of the lung. In this way it is possible to maintain adequate oxygenation without having to use very large peak pressures. A similar concept is applied during conventional ventilation when PEEP is used to keep the lung "open." However, during conventional ventilation, because the tidal volumes are large, the peak pressures that exist during conventional ventilation become very high and may cause barotrauma.

Despite these theoretical advantages and experimental evidence in animal models showing improvement in gas exchange and pulmonary pathology, the only large, controlled, multicentered trial investigating HFV in patients with infant respiratory distress syndrome (IRDS) was not encouraging (72). The main findings were as follows: (a) There was no significant difference in the incidence of bronchopulmonary dysplasia between the two modes of ventilation; (b) HFV did not produce any significant reduction in the need for ventilatory support; and (c) there appeared to be an increased risk for intracranial hemorrhage and air leaks in the infants treated with HFV. Although these results were discouraging, the lack of efficacy may be related to the particular ventilation strategies used during the trial. In the trial, HFV was applied using only a single modality, that of high-frequency oscillations.

More importantly, the techniques for volume recruitment were relatively conservative: "Sighs" were limited to about 1 sec, and mean airway pressures in both ventilation groups were kept equal. However, as discussed above, the studies in animal models of lung injury suggest that longer periods of sighs and higher mean airway pressures are necessary to re-expand the lung and keep it open. These concepts are supported by a preliminary report which used HFO and an aggressive volume recruitment protocol in premature infants (73).

One of the disease states in which HFV has proved to be successful is in the treatment of patients with bronchopleural fistulae (74,75). The reason for the effectiveness of HFV in this disease may relate to the changes in pulmonary impedance with frequency. At relatively low frequencies, the distribution of ventilation is determined by the regional resistance of the airways and compliance of the parenchyma (76). However, at relatively high frequencies such as during HFV, the distribution of ventilation is less dependent on the regional resistance–compliance time constants but is more dependent on the regional resistance–inertance properties of the airways. Thus, it is possible to distribute the inspired tidal volume differently with HFV than with conventional mechanical ventilation. A bronchopleural fistula can be viewed as the communication to a region of increased compliance such that during conventional ventilation a large percentage of the ventilation goes to the highly compliant, non-gas-exchanging region. During HFV, with the airway properties dominating, the tidal volume may no longer be shunted to these highly compliant regions.

During HFV the respiratory rates can range from 50 to 2000/min and hence can encompass the range of heart rates. By synchronizing the delivery of the tidal volume with the electrocardiogram, HFV has also been investigated as a means of augmenting cardiac output (77,78). This approach has met with mixed success, with one study showing an increase in cardiac output of greater than 25% when synchronous HFV was compared with conventional ventilation or asynchronous HFJV (79). The mechanism by which this technique is effective may be related to the increased pleural pressures which can decrease left ventricular afterload with each tidal volume. However, because the tidal volumes are relatively small, the changes in pleural pressure are also likely to be small, and this may explain the mixed success that this approach has experienced.

HFV has been used during surgical procedures to maintain a relatively quiet surgical field (80,81) and may also be useful in decreasing intracranial pressure in patients with head trauma (82,83). In addition, HFJV is relatively easy to apply via a small catheter which can be introduced through a crycothyroid approach and thus may be a very useful technique for patients who are difficult to intubate (84).

Problems with HFV

During HFV, the flow rates used are usually substantially greater than the rates used during conventional ventilation. These large flow rates make the use of HFV inherently more dangerous, because the driving pressures are higher and any outlet obstruction can lead to a rapid increase in lung volume and intrathoracic pressures. In addition, a number of investigators have found that inadvertent gas trapping can occur in the lung even under normal operating conditions (85–88). The precise mechanisms for this are not clear but are likely related to airflow limitation occurring on exhalation. This problem is especially important in patients who have compliant respiratory systems (e.g., patients with chronic airflow obstruction) and in ventilator systems which use relatively large I/E ratios. In humans with respiratory distress syndrome and in animal models of noncompliant lungs, this problem is usually not a major one (89). The extent of gas trapping can be assessed by measuring the airway opening pressure under static conditions after airway occlusion, by estimating lung volume from measurements made at the chest wall, or by monitoring esophageal pressure.

There have been a number of reports of necrotizing tracheal bronchitis (NTB) in infants and animals ventilated with HFV (90–92). The problem of NTB is also observed during conventional ventilation, although the anatomic distribution of the lesions is different from that observed during HFV. The precise mechanisms causing NTB are unknown; however, they appear to be related to lack of humidification and may be ventilator- or frequency-dependent.

Techniques with Decreased Frequencies

Apneic Oxygenation

In the mid- to late 1940s, Draper and Whitehead (93) developed a technique called "diffusion respiration," which was able to maintain adequate oxygenation for short periods of time in apneic dogs. The application of apneic oxygenation involves ventilating the animal with 100% oxygen for approximately 30 min to de-nitrogenate the lungs. Thereafter, the source of oxygen is placed at the airway opening and the paralyzed dog remains apneic. The first minute after the apneic period begins, $P_a\mathrm{CO_2}$ increases approximately 6–8 mmHg due to the incorporation of arterial with mixed venous blood. Thereafter, $P_a\mathrm{CO_2}$ rises at a rate of 3–6 mmHg/min (8) and $P_a\mathrm{O_2}$ decreases from its initial value of greater than 500 mmHg, at roughly the same rate at

which $P_a\mathrm{CO_2}$ increases. With this technique it is possible to keep animals alive for approximately 90 min, at which point they die with a severe respiratory acidosis. The technique has also been applied in humans (95); in one study, $P\mathrm{CO_2}$ values as high as 250 mmHg and pH values of less than 6.8 were achieved with apparently no detrimental effects in the patients.

The mechanism by which this technique allows adequate oxygenation is related to the large CO_2 storage capacity of the tissues. During the apneic period, approximately 90% of the CO_2 production is stored in tissues, with the remainder entering the lungs. However, the O_2 uptake from the lungs remains essentially unchanged, thus leading to a net movement of gas from the lung to the blood. This creates a subatmospheric alveolar pressure, thus causing oxygen to flow into the lung from the airway opening by convection. No CO_2 is removed from the lungs because of this large convective flow into the lungs. Since the gas transport mechanism is not diffusion and because adequate respiration is not achieved during this technique, it is now called "apneic oxygenation."

Techniques of Constant Flow Ventilation

The concept of providing adequate alveolar ventilation with constant flows is a very old one. As mentioned earlier, in 1667 Robert Hooke, the curator of the Royal Society of London, published a classic study in which he showed that movement of the lungs was not necessary to provide adequate circulation (3). Hooke pierced the lungs and chest wall of a dog so that the constant flow of gas introduced into the trachea could leave via these puncture wounds. In a beautiful description, he then recounted how the dog was kept alive using this technique of constant flow ventilation (CFV). In the early 1900s, a number of investigators developed techniques in which constant flow was introduced into the trachea; in most situations there was a rapidly progressive increase in $P\mathrm{CO_2}$, and the animals died after approximately 30 min (96). In 1985, a technique called "tracheal insufflation of oxygen" (TRIO) was presented in which it was possible to keep animals alive for relatively long periods of time using a simple experimental setup (97). A relatively narrow lumen catheter (approximately 2 mm i.d.) was inserted until it was approximately 1 cm proximal to the tracheal carina, or deeper into the lung. By using an oxygen flow of 2 liters/min or greater, it was possible to keep apneic paralyzed dogs alive for at least 5 hr, although the steady-state $P\mathrm{CO_2}$ levels were approximately 150–200 mmHg, associated with pH values of about 6.9. The mechanisms of gas transport were thought to be cardiogenic oscillations and turbulence generated by the jet (97,98). Clearly, this technique would not be suitable for routine mechanical ventilation in hospitals, but it could be used for difficult intubations or for the treatment of mass casualties.

A technique of constant ventilation in which it was possible to maintain normal blood gases was described in 1982 (99). The equipment consisted of two catheters placed in the mainstem bronchi. A constant gas flow of 2–3 liters min^{-1} kg^{-1} was delivered through the catheters and exited from the lungs via a tracheostomy tube. With this technique, it was possible to maintain normal gas exchange for hours in dogs and cats (100,101). Its use in humans has met with mixed success: It was not possible to achieve normal levels of P_{CO_2}, but up to one-half of the normal alveolar ventilation was obtained (102).

Gas transport during CFV has been modeled conceptually by dividing the lung into two zones (103). Zone I represents the region of the lung which is affected by the jet leaving the catheters. This zone can be further divided into two regions: (i) zone Ia, in which bidirectional flows exist, and (ii) zone Ib, in which the turbulence generated by the flow leaving the catheters is the major gas transport mechanism. Zone II is the region of the lung distal to zone I in which the primary gas transport mechanisms are thought to be molecular diffusion and cardiogenic oscillations (103–106). This construct has been addressed by a number of studies which have used different carrier gases (107) or different catheter positions (104), as well as by studies in which the effect of cardiogenic oscillations has been partially to totally removed (106).

Flow through collateral channels may also be an important mechanism providing adequate gas exchange during CFV. CFV provides essentially no alveolar ventilation in pigs (108), animals which have very high resistances to collateral ventilation (109). These data might also explain why CFV is relatively ineffective in humans, since humans have values of collateral resistance which are greater than that of the dog but less than that of the pig (109).

Potential Application of Constant Flow Techniques

The application of a constant flow through a single catheter (TRIO) may be useful for the oxygenation of patients who are difficult to intubate. The technique can be applied relatively simply through a crycothyroid puncture; thus it would be possible to oxygenate patients, albeit with a relative respiratory acidosis. As such, this technique could also be applied for the mechanical ventilation of mass casualties. CFV has been used as a tool to investigate physiological phenomena affected by breathing. It has been used to study (a) the effect of phasic afferent information on control of breathing and (b) mechanisms that mediate the heart

rate response to hypoxemia (110,111). CFV also has a number of theoretical advantages which suggest that it might be an ideal ventilatory modality, since one hypothesis underlying the development of a number of ventilatory techniques is that lung injury is worsened by cyclic lung stretch. With CFV, the lung is kept completely motionless with sufficiently large pressures to maintain patency of airways and alveoli. The feasibility of the clinical test of this hypothesis awaits studies indicating the efficacy of CFV in humans.

REFERENCES

1. Vesalius AW. *De Humani Corporis Fabrica*. 1555.
2. Morch ET. History of mechanical ventilation. In: Kirby RR, Smith RA, Desautels DA, eds. *Mechanical ventilation*. New York: Churchill Livingstone, 1985, 1–58.
3. Hooke R. Account of an experiment, made by R. Hooke, of preserving animals alive by blowing through their lungs with bellows. *Philos Trans R Soc Lond* 1667;2:539–540.
4. Fothergill J. A case published in the last volume of Medical Essays of recovery of a man dead in appearance, by distending the lungs with air. In: Lettsam JC, ed. *The works of John Fotheringham, M.D.* London: C Dilly, 1784.
5. Emerson JH. *The evolution of the "iron lung."* Cambridge, MA: JH Emerson Company, 1978.
6. Woolman CHM. The development of apparatus for intermittent negative pressure respiration. *Anaesthesia* 1976;31:537–547.
7. Drinker P, Shaw LA. An apparatus for the administration of artificial respiration. *J Clin Invest* 1927;7:229–247.
8. Kirby RR. Modes of mechanical ventilation. In: Kacmarek RM, Stoller JK, eds. *Current respiratory care*. Toronto: BC Decker, 1988;128–131.
9. Marini JJ, Capps JS, Culver BH. The inspiratory work of breathing during assisted mechanical ventilation. *Chest* 1985; 87:612–618.
10. Marini JJ, Rodriguez RM, Lamb V. The inspiratory workload of patient-initiated mechanical ventilation. *Am Rev Respir Dis* 1986;134:902–909.
11a. Downs JB, Klein EF, Desautels D, et al. Intermittent mandatory ventilation: a new approach to weaning patients from mechanical ventilators. *Chest* 1973;64:331–335.
11b. Weisman IM, Rinaldo JE, Rogers RM, et al. State of the art: intermittent mandatory ventilation. *Am Rev Respir Dis* 1983; 127:641–647.
11c. Tomlinson JR, Miller KS, Lorch DG, Smith L, Reines HD, Sahn SA. A prospective comparison of IMV and T-piece weaning from mechanical ventilation. *Chest* 1989;96:348–352.
12. Hasten RW, Downs JB, Heenan TJ. A comparison of synchronized and nonsynchronized intermittent mandatory ventilation. *Respir Care* 1980;25:554–557.
13. Hewlett AM, Platt AS, Terry VG. Mandatory minute ventilation: a new concept in weaning from mechanical ventilation. *Anaesthesia* 1977;32:163–169.
14. MacIntyre NR. Respiratory function during pressure support ventilation. *Chest* 1986;89:677–683.
15. Brochard L, Harf A, Lorino H, Lemaire F. Inspiratory pressure support prevents diaphragmatic fatigue during weaning from mechanical ventilation. *Am Rev Respir Dis* 1989;139:513–521.
16. Barach AL, Martin J, Eckman M. Positive pressure respiration and its application to the treatment of acute pulmonary edema. *Ann Intern Med* 1938;12:754–795.
17. Fulton EP, Oxon DM. Left sided heart failure with pulmonary edema: its treatment with the "pulmonary plus pressure machine." *Lancet* 1936;231:981–983.
18. Ashbaugh DG, Bigelow DB, Petty TL, Levine BE. Acute respiratory distress in adults. *Lancet* 1967;2:319–323.
19. Gong H Jr. Positive-pressure ventilation in the adult respiratory distress syndrome. *Clin Chest Med* 1982;3:69–88.

20. Staub N. Pulmonary edema. *Physiol Rev* 1974;54:678–811.
21. Malo J, Ali J, Wood LDH. How does positive pressure end-expiratory pressure reduce intrapulmonary shunt in canine pulmonary edema? *J Appl Physiol* 1984;57:1002–1010.
22. Hopewell PC, Murray J. Effects of continuous positive pressure ventilation in experimental pulmonary edema. *J Appl Physiol* 1976;40:568–574.
23. Prewitt RM, McCarthy J, Wood LDH. Treatment of acute low pressure pulmonary edema in dogs: relative effects of hydrostatic and oncotic pressure, nitroprusside, and positive end-expiratory pressure. *J Clin Invest* 1981;67:409–418.
24. Pare PD, Warriner B, Baile EM, Hogg JC. Redistribution of pulmonary extravascular water with positive end expiratory pressure in canine pulmonary edema. *Am Rev Respir Dis* 1983;127:590–593.
25. Suter PM, Fairley HB, Isenberg MD. Optimum end-expiratory pressure in patients with acute pulmonary failure. *N Engl J Med* 1975;292:284–289.
26. Weisman IM, Rinaldo JE, Rogers RM. Positive end-expiratory pressure in adult respiratory failure. *N Engl J Med* 1982;307:1381–1384.
27. Gallagher TJ, Civetta JM, Kirby RR. Terminology update: optimum PEEP. *Crit Care Med* 1978;6:323–326.
28. Kirby RR, Downs JB, Civetta JM, et al. High level positive end expiratory pressure (PEEP) in acute respiratory insufficiency. *Chest* 1975;67:156–163.
29. Pepe PE, Hudson LD, Carrico CJ. Early application of positive end-expiratory pressure in patients at risk for the adult respiratory distress syndrome. *N Engl J Med* 1984;311:281–286.
30. National Heart, Lung and Blood Institute. Extracorporeal support for respiratory insufficiency. Bethesda, MD: National Heart, Lung and Blood Institute, RFP-NHLI-73-20, 1979.
31. Slutsky AS. Nonconventional methods of ventilation. *Am Rev Respir Dis* 1988;138:175–183.
32. Sjostrand U, Eriksson IA. High rates and low volumes in mechanical ventilation—not just a matter of ventilatory frequency. *Anesth Analg* 1980;59:567–575.
33. Klain M, Smith RB. High frequency percutaneous transtracheal jet ventilation. *Crit Care Med* 1977;5:280–287.
34. Borg U, Eriksson I, Sjostrand. High-frequency positive-pressure ventilation (HFPPV): a review based upon its use during bronchoscopy and for laryngoscopy and microlaryngeal surgery under general anesthesia. *Anesth Analg* 1980;59:594–603.
35. Rouby JJ, Simonneau G, Benhamou D, et al. Factors influencing pulmonary volumes and CO_2 elimination during high-frequency jet ventilation. *Anesthesiology* 1985;63:473–482.
36. Fredberg JJ, Glass GM, Boynton BR, Frantz ID III. Factors influencing mechanical performance of neonatal high-frequency ventilators. *J Appl Physiol* 1987;62:2485–2490.
37. Calkins JM, Waterson CK, Hameroff SR, Kamel J. Jet pulse characteristics for high-frequency jet ventilation in dogs. *Anesth Analg* 1982;61:293–300.
38. Bohn DJ, Miyasaka K, Marchak BE, Thompson WK, Froese AB, Bryan AC. Ventilation by high-frequency oscillation. *J Appl Physiol* 1980;48:710–716.
39. Slutsky AS, Drazen JM, Ingram RH Jr, et al. Effective pulmonary ventilation with small-volume oscillations at high frequency. *Science* 1980;208:69–71.
40. Drazen JM, Kamm RD, Slutsky AS. High frequency ventilation. *Physiol Rev* 1984;64:505–543.
41. Ward HE, Power JHT, Nicholas TE. High-frequency oscillations via the pleural surface: an alternative mode of ventilation? *J Appl Physiol* 1983;54:427–433.
42. Zidulka A, Gross D, Minami H, Vartian V, Chang HK. Ventilation by high-frequency chest wall compression in dogs with normal lungs. *Am Rev Respir Dis* 1983;127:709–713.
43. Harf A, Zidulka A, Chang HK. Nitrogen washout curves in humans during normal tidal breathing with superimposed oscillations of the chest wall. *Am Rev Respir Dis* 1985;132:350–353.
44. Henderson Y, Chillingsworth FP, Whitney JL. The respiratory dead space. *Am J Physiol* 1915;38:1–19.
45. Fredberg JJ. Augmented diffusion in the airways can support pulmonary gas exchange. *J Appl Physiol* 1980;49:232–238.
46. Kamm RD, Slutsky AS, Drazen JM. High-frequency ventilation. *Crit Rev Biomed Eng* 1984;9:347–379.
47. Chang HK. Mechanisms of gas transport during high-frequency oscillation. *J Appl Physiol* 1984;56:553–563.
48. Permutt S, Mitzner W, Weinmann G. Model of gas transport during high-frequency ventilation. *J Appl Physiol* 1985;58:1956–1970.
49. Haselton FR, Scherer PW. Bronchial bifurcations and respiratory mass transport. *Science* 1980;208:69–71.
50. Khoo MCK, Slutsky AS, Drazen JM, Solway J, Gavriely N, Kamm RD. Gas mixing during high-frequency ventilation: an improved model. *J Appl Physiol* 1984;57:493–506.
51. Haselton FR, Scherer PW. Flow visualization of steady streaming in oscillatory flow through a bifurcating tube. *J Fluid Mech* 1982;123:315–333.
52. Lehr JL, Butler JP, Westerman PA, Zatz SL, Drazen JM. Photographic measurement of pleural surface motion during lung oscillation. *J Appl Physiol* 1985;59:623–633.
53. Taylor GI. Dispersion of soluble matter in solvent flowing slowly through a tube. *Proc R Soc Lond Ser A* 1953;219:186–193.
54. Watson EJ. Diffusion in oscillatory pipe flow. *J Fluid Mech* 1983;133:233–244.
55. Slutsky AS, Kamm RD, Rossing TH, et al. Effects of frequency, tidal volume, and lung volume on CO_2 elimination in dogs by high frequency (2–30 Hz), low tidal volume ventilation. *J Clin Invest* 1981;68:1475–1484.
56. Wright K, Lyrene RK, Truong WE, Standaert TA, Murphy J, Woodrum DE. Ventilation by high frequency oscillation in rabbits with oleic acid lung disease. *J Appl Physiol* 1981;50:1056–1060.
57. Jaeger MJ, Kurzweg UH, Banner MJ. Transport of gases in high frequency ventilation. *Crit Care Med* 1984;12:708–710.
58. Solway J, Gavriely N, Kamm RD, et al. Intra-airway gas mixing during high frequency ventilation. *J Appl Physiol* 1984;56:343–354.
59. Venegas JG, Custer J, Kamm RD, Hales CA. Relationship for gas transport during high frequency ventilation in dogs. *J Appl Physiol* 1985;59:1539–1547.
60. Mitzner W, Permutt S, Weinmann G. Gas transport during high frequency ventilation: theoretical model and experimental validation. *Ann Biomed Eng* 1984;12:407–419.
61. Solway J, Gavriely N, Slutsky AS, et al. Effect of bias flow rate during HFV. *Respir Physiol* 1985;60:267–276.
62. Rossing TH, Slutsky AS, Lehr JL, et al. Tidal volume and frequency dependence of carbon dioxide elimination by high frequency ventilation. *N Engl J Med* 1981;305:1375–1379.
63. Rossing TH, Slutsky AS, Loring RH, et al. CO_2 elimination by HFV in dogs: effects of histamine infusion. *J Appl Physiol* 1982;53:1256–1262.
64. Knopp TJ, Kaethner T, Meyer M, Behden K, Scheid P. Gas mixing in the airways of dog lung during high frequency ventilation. *J Appl Physiol* 1983;55:1141–1146.
65. Kaethner T, Kohl J, Scheid P. Gas concentration profiles along airways of dog lungs during high frequency ventilation. *J Appl Physiol* 1984;56:1491–1499.
66. Robertson HT, Coffey RL, Hlastala HP. Influence of carrier gas density on gas exchange during high frequency ventilation. *Bull Eur Physiopathol Respir* 1982;18:381–387.
67. Allen JL, Fredberg JJ, Keefe DH, Frantz ID III. Alveolar pressures magnitude and asynchrony during high frequency oscillations of excised rabbit lungs. *Am Rev Respir Dis* 1985;132:343–349.
68. Fredberg JJ, Keefe DH, Glass G, Castile RG, Frantz ID III. Alveolar pressure nonhomogeneity during small-amplitude high frequency ventilation. *J Appl Physiol* 1984;57:788–800.
69. Kolton M, Cattran EB, Kent G, Volgyesi G, Froese AB, Bryan AC. Oxygenation during high frequency ventilation compared with conventional mechanical ventilation in two models of lung injury. *Anesth Analg* 1982;61:323–332.
70. Hamilton PP, Onayemi A, Smyth JA, et al. Comparison of conventional and high frequency ventilation, oxygenation, and lung pathology. *J Appl Physiol* 1983;55:131–138.

71. Froese AB, Bryan AC. High frequency ventilation. *Am Rev Respir Dis* 1987;135:1363–1374.
72. The HIFI study group. High-frequency oscillatory ventilation compared with conventional mechanical ventilation in the treatment of respiratory failure in preterm infants. *N Engl J Med* 1989;320:88–93.
73. Froese AB, Butler PO, Fletcher WA, Byford LJ. High frequency oscillatory ventilation in premature infants with respiratory failure: a preliminary report. *Anesth Analg* 1987;66:814–824.
74. Carlon G, Ray C Jr, Klain M, McCormick PM. High frequency positive pressure ventilation in management of a patient with bronchopleural fistula. *Anesthesiology* 1980;52:160–162.
75. Hoff BH, Wilson E, Smith RB, Bennett E, Philips W. Intermittent positive pressure ventilation in dogs with experimental bronchopleural fistulae. *Crit Care Med* 1983;11:598–602.
76. Mead J. The distribution of gas flow in the lungs. In: Wolstenholme GEW, Knight J, eds. *Circulatory and respiratory mass transport.* London: Churchill, 1969;204–209.
77. Matuschak GM, Pinsky MR, Klain M. Hemodynamic effects of synchronous high frequency jet ventilation during acute hypovolemia. *J Appl Physiol* 1986;61:44–53.
78. Otto CW, Quan SF, Conahan TJ, Calkins JM, Waterson CK, Hameroff SR. Hemodynamic effects of high frequency jet ventilation. *Anesth Analg* 1983;62:298–304.
79. Pinsky MR, Marquez J, Martin D, Klain M. Ventricular assist by cardiac cycle-specific increases in intrathoracic pressure. *Chest* 1987;91:709–715.
80. Heijman K, Heijman L, Jonzon A, Sedin G, Sjostrand U, Widman B. High frequency positive pressure ventilation during anaesthesia and routine surgery in man. *Acta Anaesthesiol Scand* 1972;16:176–187.
81. El-Baz N, El-Ganzouri A, Gottschalk W, Jensik R. One-lung high frequency positive pressure ventilation for slave pneumonectomy: an alternative technique. *Anesth Analg* 1981;60:683–686.
82. Todd MM, Toutant SM, Shapiro HM. The effects of high frequency positive pressure ventilation on intracranial pressure and brain surface movement in cats. *Anesthesiology* 1981;54:496–504.
83. Grasberger RC, Spatz EL, Mortara RW, Ordia JI, Yeston NS. Effect of high frequency ventilation versus conventional mechanical ventilation on ICP in head-injured dogs. *J Neurosurg* 1984;60:1214–1218.
84. Klain M, Kesler H. High frequency jet ventilation. *Surg Clin North Am* 1985;65:917–930.
85. Fusciardi J, Rouby JJ, Benhamou D, Viars D. Hemodynamic consequences of increasing mean airway pressure during high frequency jet ventilation. *Chest* 1984;86:30–34.
86. Simon B, Weinmann G, Mitzner W. Mean airway pressure and alveolar pressure during high frequency ventilation. *J Appl Physiol* 1984;57:1069–1078.
87. Saari AF, Rossing TH, Solway J, Drazen JM. Lung inflation during high frequency ventilation. *Am Rev Respir Dis* 1984;129:333–336.
88. Solway J, Rossing TH, Saari AF, Drazen JM. Expiratory flow limitation and dynamic pulmonary hyperinflation during high frequency ventilation. *J Appl Physiol* 1986;60:2071–2078.
89. Bryan AC, Slutsky AS. Lung volume during high frequency ventilation. *Am Rev Respir Dis* 1986;133:928–930.
90. Kirpalani H, Higa T, Perlman M, Friedberg J, Cutz E. Diagnosis and therapy of necrotizing tracheobronchitis in ventilated neonates. *Crit Care Med* 1985;13:792–797.
91. Boros SJ, Mammel MC, Lewallen PK, Coleman JM, Gordon MJ, Ophoven J. Necrotizing tracheobronchitis: a complication of high frequency ventilation. *J Pediatr* 1986;109:95–100.
92. Mammel MC, Ophoven JP, Lewallen PK, Gordon MJ, Sutton MC, Boros SJ. High frequency ventilation and tracheal injuries. *Pediatrics* 1986;77:608–613.
93. Draper WB, Whitehead RW. Diffusion respiration in the dog anesthetized by pentothal sodium. *Anesthesiology* 1944;5:262–273.
94. Holmdahl MH. Pulmonary uptake of oxygen, acid-base metabolism and circulation during prolonged apnea. *Acta Chir Scand [Suppl]* 1956;212:1–128.
95. Frumin MJ, Epstein RM, Cohen G. Apneic oxygenation in man. *Anesthesiology* 1959;20:789–798.
96. Meltzer SJ, Auer J. Continuous respiration without respiratory movements. *J Exp Med* 1909;11:622–625.
97. Slutsky AS, Watson J, Leith DE, Brown R. Tracheal insufflation of O_2 (TRIO) at low flow rates sustains life for several hours. *Anesthesiology* 1985;63:278–286.
98. Burwen DR, Watson J, Brown R, Josa M, Slutsky AS. Effect of cardiogenic oscillations on gas mixing during tracheal insufflation of O_2. *J Appl Physiol* 1986;60:965–91.
99. Lehnert BE, Oberdorster G, Slutsky AS. Constant flow ventilation of apneic dogs. *J Appl Physiol* 1982;53:483–489.
100. Chakrabarti MK, Whitwam JG. Pulmonary ventilation by continuous flow using a modified Carlen's tube. *Crit Care Med* 1984;12:354–356.
101. Smith RB, Babinski M, Bunegin L, Gilbert J, Swartzman S, Dirting J. Continuous flow apneic ventilation. *Acta Anaesthesiol Scand* 1984;28:631–639.
102. Breen PH, Sznajder JI, Morrison P, Hatch D, Wood LDH, Craig DB. Constant flow ventilation in anesthetized patients: efficacy and safety. *Anesth Analg* 1986;65:1161–1169.
103. Watson JW, Burwen DR, Kamm RD, Brown R, Slutsky AS. Effect of flow rate on blood gases during constant flow ventilation in dogs. *Am Rev Respir Dis* 1986;133:626–629.
104. Slutsky AS, Menon AS. Catheter position and blood gases during constant flow ventilation. *J Appl Physiol* 1987;62:513–519.
105. Ingenito E, Kamm RD, Watson JW, Slutsky AS. Model of constant flow ventilation in a dog lung. *J Appl Physiol* 1988;64:2150–2159.
106. Cybulsky I, Abel J, Menon AS, Salerno T, Lichtenstein S, Slutsky AS. Contribution of cardiogenic oscillations to gas mixing during constant flow ventilation. *J Appl Physiol* 1987;63:564–570.
107. Watson JW, Kamm RD, Burwen D, Brown R, Ingenito E, Slutsky AS. Gas exchange during constant flow ventilation with different gases. *Am Rev Respir Dis* 1987;136:420–425.
108. Webster P, Menon AS, Slutsky AS. Constant flow ventilation in pigs. *J Appl Physiol* 1986;61:2238–2242.
109. Macklem PT. Airways obstruction and collateral ventilation. *Physiol Rev* 1971;51:368–436.
110. Kato H, Menon AS, Slutsky AS. Mechanisms mediating the heart rate response to hypoxemia. *Circulation* 1988;77:407–414.
111. Menon AS, England SJ, Vallieres E, Rebuck AS, Slutsky AS. Influence of phasic afferent information on phrenic neural output during hypercapnia. *J Appl Physiol* 1988;65:563–569.
112. Saari A, Rossing TH, Drazen JM. Physiological bases for new approaches to mechanical ventilation. *Annu Rev Med* 1984;35:165–174.

THE LUNG: Scientific Foundations
edited by R.G. Crystal, J.B. West et al.
Raven Press, Ltd., New York © 1991.

CHAPTER 8.2.4

Anesthesia

Göran Hedenstierna and Leif Tokics

Anesthesia, both in the sense of general anesthesia and regional analgesia, affects respiration and circulation. Since 1847, when John Snow (1) observed that respiratory movement decreases with deepening anesthesia, data have accumulated, and still do, on the diversified effects of anesthetic agents and the way in which they interact to reduce the gas exchanging capacity of the lungs. The various effects are reviewed in this chapter.

HISTORICAL REVIEW UNTIL 1960

Within a year after William Morton's demonstration of ether anesthesia in 1846, the first deaths attributable to anesthesia were reported. Most of these early events seem to have been caused by cardiac complications, rather than respiratory depression. The pioneers of anesthesia were aware of the influence of anesthesia on ventilation, and John Snow collected his observations in a monograph published in 1847 (1). He divided the progress of anesthesia into five stages. At that time, the patients were spontaneously breathing during all kinds of operation, even after tracheal intubation had been introduced in 1880. Artificial ventilation as a means of preventing atelectasis during thoracic procedures was not employed until the 1890s and it was not until 1938 that mechanical ventilation was introduced in thoracic surgery (2). Defective arterial oxygenation after pulmonary resections was reported by Maier and Cournand in 1943 (3). After the evolution of electrode systems for measuring oxygen and carbon dioxide tensions in blood, several important contributions to the understanding of lung function during anesthesia appeared. In 1958 Campbell et al. (4) dem-

onstrated that in some individuals anesthesia is associated with an increase of the alveolo-arterial oxygen tension difference, and it was speculated that increased right-to-left shunting of blood occurs during uneventful anesthesia. In 1955 Nims et al. (5) showed that the compliance of the respiratory system decreased during anesthesia; however, a few more years were to elapse before the partitioning of this change to the lung and the thorax had been clarified and before concepts to link gas exchange impairment to mechanical alterations had been established.

GENERAL ANESTHESIA

Ventilation

Ventilation and Respiratory Muscle Function

Spontaneous ventilation is frequently reduced during anesthesia. Thus, inhalational anesthetics (6) as well as barbiturates for intravenous use (7) reduce the sensitivity to CO_2. The response is dose dependent, entailing decreasing ventilation with deepening anesthesia.

Anesthesia also reduces the response to hypoxia. As early as 1945 this was observed by Gordh (8), but it was not generally recognized until 30 years later (9). The attenuation of the hypoxic response may be attributed to an effect on the carotid body chemoreceptor (10).

The effect of an anesthetic on the respiratory muscles is nonuniform. Thus, as observed by Snow as early as 1847 (1) and analyzed in more detail more than 100 years later (11), rib-cage excursions diminish with deepening anesthesia. The normal ventilatory response to CO_2 is produced by the intercostal muscles as shown by Tusiewicz and co-workers (12), who also showed that no clear increase in rib-cage motion was

G. Hedenstierna: Department of Clinical Physiology, Uppsala University Hospital, S-751 85 Uppsala, Sweden.
L. Tokies: Department of Anesthesia, Huddinge University Hospital, S-14186 Huddinge, Sweden.

seen on CO_2 rebreathing during halothane anesthesia. Thus, the reduced ventilatory response to CO_2 during anesthesia is due to an impeded function of the intercostal muscles.

FRC and Thoracoabdominal Dimensions

Anesthesia is accompanied by a reduced functional residual capacity (FRC) or resting lung volume. This was demonstrated for the first time by Bergman (13), who used a multiple breath nitrogen wash-out technique for the assessment of gas distribution. This finding passed rather unnoticed and was not confirmed until 5 years later by Laws (14). Since then, several studies have shown a more or less consistent decrease in FRC during anesthesia by a mean of 20% during anesthesia, whether breathing is spontaneous or mechanical after muscle paralysis, and whether the recording technique is based on gas dilution recording (nitrogen wash-out, helium rebreathing) or body plethysmography (for a review see ref. 15).

With reduced FRC a shift in the position of the rib cage or the diaphragm may be anticipated. Using cineradiography, Froese and Bryan (16) demonstrated in a group of three patients a cranial shift of the diaphragm during anesthesia with no further shift after muscle paralysis. However, the recording of thoracoabdominal dimensions by means of external sensors (11) did not show any significant change in the shape of either chest or abdomen. In a more recent study, however, combining transverse exposures of the chest and abdomen by computed tomography with central blood volume measurement by dye dilution and FRC recording by multiple breath nitrogen wash-out, a rather complex pattern of changes was noted during anesthesia with muscle paralysis and mechanical ventilation (17) (Fig. 1). Thus, the cranial shift of the diaphragm was confirmed, and, in addition, it was seen that the transverse area of the chest was reduced. At the same time blood was moved from the thorax and probably pooled in the abdomen together with a small amount of blood from the extremities (18). The net effect on the external dimensions of the chest and abdomen was only 0.1–0.2 liter. All these changes could thus pass undetected by the recording with surface sensors.

Compliance of the Thorax

In 1955, Nims and co-workers (5) found that the static compliance in the total respiratory system (lungs and chest wall) was reduced from 95 to 60 ml/cmH$_2$O during anesthesia. Several studies have since then confirmed this observation (for a review see ref. 19). Nims and co-workers proposed that the reduction in compliance was due to relaxation of the inspiratory mus-

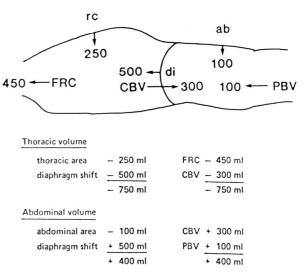

FIG. 1. Mean changes in thoracic and abdominal dimensions and in gas and blood volumes after induction of general anesthesia and mechanical ventilation. Volumes are given in milliliters. rc, rib cage; di, diaphragm; ab, abdomen; CBV, central blood volume; PBV, peripheral blood volume. (From ref. 17.)

cles and thus that there was an effect on the chest wall compliance. There are few studies on chest wall compliance in the literature and they do not clearly support Nims' conclusion (19). Westbrook and co-workers (20) suggested a right shift of the pressure–volume curve but unaltered compliance of the chest wall on induction of anesthesia (reduced "expansion pressure"), which may contribute to the reduction of the FRC.

Several studies on lung compliance have been carried out during anesthesia and the vast majority of studies indicate a decrease compared to the awake state [e.g., static compliance fell from a mean of 187 ml/cmH$_2$O awake to 149 ml/cmH$_2$O during anesthesia in the review by Don (19)]. Rehder and co-workers (15) analyzed possible sources of reduced compliance during anesthesia in their 1976 review. They considered direct anesthetic effects on the lung tissue rather unlikely but were unable at that time to evaluate possible effects of airway closure and atelectasis. These two phenomena are discussed in more detail in the following sections.

Airway Closure

In the late 1960s, Milic-Emili and associates (21) observed that airways close during a deep expiration. Don and co-workers (22) found that a certain amount of gas was trapped in the lungs during anesthesia and could be released only by deep inflations. This suggested the occurrence of airway closure during anesthesia, which was also demonstrated some years later (23), although different results have indeed been obtained (24). No good correlation between the degree of airway closure and impairment of arterial oxygenation has been seen during anesthesia (23,25). On the other hand, a decrease of FRC during anesthesia below the *awake* closing capacity (the lung volume at which airways close) was accompanied by a significantly larger shunt (mean 11%) than when FRC during anesthesia was larger than awake CC (mean 2%) (26). It may thus be concluded that there is evidence of airway closure during anesthesia but that its importance for developing gas exchange impairment is not fully established. There may be additional or more important functional disturbances that impede arterial oxygenation.

Atelectasis

In a study by Mead and Collier (27) a progressive reduction in lung compliance was seen during anesthesia in either spontaneously breathing or mechanically ventilated dogs. Compliance could be restored to initial values by hyperinflation. Bendixen and co-workers (28) made similar observations in anesthetized humans and found that the decreasing compliance was accompanied by a decreasing Pa_{O_2}. In their classical paper they put forward the "concept of atelectasis" (28). However, other research groups found an immediate decrease in lung compliance on induction of anesthesia, with no further deterioration during the anesthesia period (29). Moreover, it has not been possible to demonstrate regular occurrence of atelectasis during anesthesia by means of conventional x-ray. This has turned opinion away from atelectasis being the cause of altered lung mechanics and impaired gas exchange during anesthesia.

It was not until recently that new observations were made that may explain the altered mechanical behavior of the lung during anesthesia. Using CT with transverse exposures of the chest, Brismar and co-workers (30) demonstrated prompt development of densities in dependent regions of both lungs during anesthesia (Fig. 2, left panels). The densities appeared in more than 90% of studied, lung-healthy patients with no correlation to sex or age, and there was only a weak correlation to body configuration (31). Similar densities had previously been seen in anesthetized infants (32). The densities appear both during spontaneous breathing and after muscle paralysis and mechanical ventilation, and whether anesthesia is inhalational or intravenous (barbiturates) (33). By applying a positive end-expiratory pressure (PEEP) of 10 cmH₂O, the densities were reduced or eliminated but they reappeared within 1 min after discontinuation of PEEP (30). When the patient was turned from the supine to the lateral position, the densities in the dependent lung remained

where they had initially appeared (30). In anesthetized sheep similar densities in dependent lung regions could be demonstrated, and subsequent morphological analyses showed these regions to be atelectatic with minor interstitial edema and only moderate vascular congestion (34). If these findings are extrapolated to humans, it can be concluded that anesthesia causes atelectasis. The rapid appearance of the densities on induction of anesthesia and after discontinuation of PEEP speaks against slow resorption of gas as the cause of atelectasis, and another, as yet unclear, mechanism has to be found. Interestingly, thoracoabdominal restriction by means of a corset so that the FRC in awake volunteers was reduced as much, or more, as during anesthesia, did not produce any changes on CT scans (35). Thus, the reduced FRC during anesthesia need not per se produce atelectasis, but there must be an additional factor to produce it. This may be relaxation of the diaphragm, permitting the transmission of the higher intra-abdominal pressure into the thoracic cavity. Support for this hypothesis can be found in earlier studies on diaphragm tone and regional lung volume. Thus, an increased vertical gradient of regional volume has been observed on relaxing the diaphragm from a voluntarily tense state in awake subjects (36). Findings on regional lung volume in anesthetized subjects in the lateral position suggest an increased vertical gradient compared to the awake state (37), and the authors attribute this to relaxation of the diaphragm.

Resistance of the Lung

There are several studies on the resistance of the total respiratory system and the lungs during anesthesia, most of them showing a considerable increase during both spontaneous breathing and mechanical ventilation (for reviews see refs. 15 and 19). Clements and co-workers (38) used a flow interrupter technique that, under suitable conditions, enables the calculation of airway resistance, which was shown to be increased. However, the studies on resistance during anesthesia have been hampered by different experimental conditions during the awake and anesthetized situations. Thus, a study that enables comparison of resistance under both isovolume and isoflow conditions is still missing. The possibility remains that the increased lung resistance merely reflects the reduced FRC.

Ventilation Distribution

Multiple breath nitrogen wash-out studies in anesthetized, supine humans during spontaneous breathing and mechanical ventilation were first undertaken by Bergman (13), who found no clear change in the overall ventilation distribution index (i.e., gas mixing efficiency) compared to the awake state. Somewhat vary-

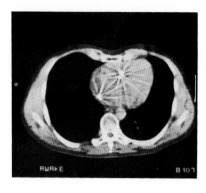
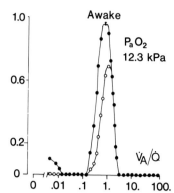

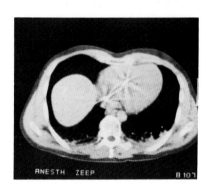
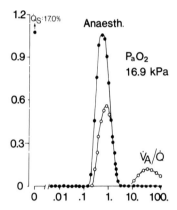

FIG. 2. Transverse CT scans of the chest and $\dot{V}_A/\dot{Q}$ distributions (○, ventilation; ●, blood flow in liters/min) in a patient in the awake state (**upper panel**) and during anesthesia with mechanical ventilation (**lower panel**). There was a small mode within low $\dot{V}_A\dot{Q}$ regions in the awake state. Note the appearance of densities in the dependent lung regions and a large shunt during anesthesia. The large white area in the right hemithorax is the diaphragm that has been moved cranially during anesthesia. (From ref. 85.)

ing results have been obtained in succeeding studies, although the majority point to an essentially maintained, or only to a small extent affected, distribution (39). More interesting data have been obtained when studying gas distribution in each lung separately in the lateral position during anesthesia by means of a double lumen endobronchial catheter. These studies indicate a larger ventilation of the upper lung (40) than has been seen in awake, spontaneously breathing subjects studied by the same technique (41). Using isotope techniques, a similar redistribution of inspired gas away from dependent to nondependent lung regions has been observed in anesthetized supine humans (37). A PEEP of 10 cmH₂O increased dependent lung ventilation in anesthetized subjects in the lateral position (42). Hulands and co-workers (43) studied ventilation distribution in supine anesthetized humans by isotope techniques but found no change in ventilation distribution compared to the awake situation, contrary to the other studies. However, they did their measurements simultaneously with an inflation of the lungs and their data should therefore be compared with those obtained during PEEP ventilation. Thus, restoration of overall FRC toward, or beyond, the awake level returns gas distribution toward the awake pattern. It is tempting to attribute this to recruitment of collapsed lung regions (dependent atelectasis) and reopening of closed airways in lower lung regions, and possibly even to

increased expansion of upper lung regions so that these became less compliant.

Circulation

Cardiac Output

All presently used inhalational anesthetic agents depress myocardial contractility *in vitro* (44). During clinical anesthesia their effects on the heart are modified by numerous factors such as depth of anesthesia, fitness of the patient, stimulation by surgical trauma, mode of ventilation, and peripheral vascular effects. The halogenated anesthetic agents all induce a decrease of systemic arterial pressure by varying effects on cardiac output and arteriolar vascular tone (44,45).

Hypoventilation increases cardiac output, whereas mechanical ventilation, especially at a low arterial carbon dioxide tension, decreases cardiac output (46). Nitrous oxide exerts a slight cardiodepressant action in humans but also causes an adrenergically mediated vasoconstriction (44). The halogenated anesthetic agents in combination with nitrous oxide have less influence on the circulation than these agents alone at the same anesthetic depth (44). In patients with congestive or ischemic heart disease, however, the use of nitrous oxide may be deleterious (47). Among intravenous anesthetic agents, thiopentone depresses the heart and causes venous dilatation, which is accompanied by a reduction of cardiac output (44). Narcotic analgesics and benzodiazepines have little effect on cardiac contractility (44,47). Ketamine is exceptional among anesthetics in use today by its activation of the sympathetic nervous system and increase of cardiac output and systemic arterial pressure (48).

Pulmonary Vascular Pressures

Modern anesthetics have little effect on pressures in the pulmonary circulation, and most investigators have reported no change at all or only minor decreases (45,49–51). Major increases may occur as a response to stress caused by surgery or intubation (52), or hypoxemia (53), or following an increase in left atrial pressure (52). Mechanical ventilation usually does not cause much change at normocapnea unless a PEEP is applied (50,51). Ketamine anesthesia, however, is sometimes accompanied by a marked increase in pulmonary artery pressure (48).

Distribution of Lung Blood Flow

Detailed information on the distribution of lung blood flow during anesthesia is only available from studies on animals, but these lack control measurements in the awake state (54,55). They all show a vertical distribution profile of blood flow during anesthesia, consistent with the concept of zone I–IV (56). In humans, measurements have been made in the awake state and during anesthesia with different modes of ventilation, applying scintillation detection of radioactive xenon, which has a rather low spatial resolution and is more or less unable to detect blood flow through nonaerated lung tissue. Two studies show no effect (57) or a small increase (43) of blood flow in dependent lung regions with mechanical ventilation and low end-expiratory airway pressure in the supine position. In the lateral position, spontaneous and mechanical ventilation did not alter the distribution of blood flow between the two lungs (42,57). PEEP causes a marked redistribution of blood flow toward dependent lung regions (42,57). Applying PEEP to the dependent lung with the subject in the lateral position creates a more even distribution of blood flow between the lungs (42). To summarize the human studies, there is only little effect of anesthesia on lung blood flow distribution at atmospheric end-expiratory pressure. However, as atelectasis regularly forms in dependent lung regions shortly after the induction of anesthesia (30), the technique so far used has probably underestimated dependent lung blood flow during anesthesia.

Hypoxic Pulmonary Vasoconstriction

Several inhalational anesthetics have been found to inhibit the hypoxic pulmonary vasoconstriction (HPV) in isolated lung preparations (58). However, no such effect has been seen with intravenous anesthetics (barbiturates) (59). Results from human studies are varying, reasonably explained by the complexity of the experiment, which causes several variables to change at the same time. The HPV response may thus be obscured by simultaneous changes in cardiac output, myocardial contractility, vascular tone, blood volume distribution, blood pH, and CO_2 tension and lung mechanics (53). In studies with no gross changes in cardiac output, the inhalational anesthetics isoflurane and halothane depress the HPV response by 50% at 2 MAC (minimum alveolar concentration) (53). There is a curved dose–response relationship, flattening off at higher alveolar concentrations of the anesthetic (Fig. 3). The HPV response acts efficiently both in the atelectatic lung (where HPV seems to be more important than mechanical kinking of vessels) and during ventilation with hypoxic gases (60).

Pulmonary Gas Exchange

Arterial Oxygenation

Arterial oxygenation is impaired in most patients during anesthesia, whether breathing is spontaneous or mechanical (29,61). It is generally held that the impairment of arterial oxygenation during anesthesia is more severe at higher ages (29). Obesity worsens the oxygenation of blood (62), and smokers show more gas exchange impairment than nonsmokers (63). The impairment in arterial oxygenation has made it a routine procedure to increase the inspired oxygen fraction during anesthesia to 0.3–0.4 in an uncomplicated anesthetic procedure, and even higher during anesthesia in obese, bronchitic, or elderly patients.

Ventilation/Perfusion Relationships

The gas exchange impairment corresponds to a venous admixture of approximately 10% (for a review see ref. 64). Using the multiple inert gas elimination technique, the ventilation/perfusion relationships ($\dot{V}_A/\dot{Q}$) have been studied in the anesthetized subject. In young, healthy volunteers only a small $\dot{V}_A/\dot{Q}$ mismatch was seen, with a widened $\dot{V}_A/\dot{Q}$ mode and the appearance of a small shunt (65). However, in a similar group, Prutow et al. (66) described a much larger shunt of mean 8% in anesthetized patients who were to undergo surgery. In a study by Bindslev and co-workers (50) of a middle-aged group of patients during anesthesia

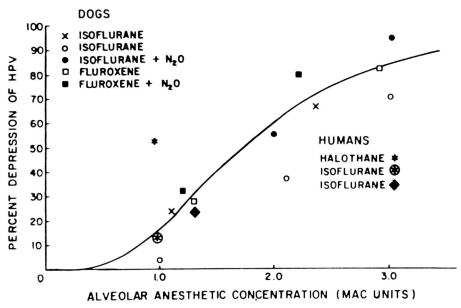

FIG. 3. Inhibition of HPV by inhalational anesthetics. Various data from humans and animals are shown. (From ref. 53.)

(spontaneous breathing), shunt was increased from 1% awake to approximately 8%, and there was a certain widening of the $\dot{V}A/\dot{Q}$ distribution. During mechanical ventilation of the same patients, regions with high $\dot{V}A/\dot{Q}$ ratios could be seen, and the ratios increased further during ventilation with PEEP. The additional high $\dot{V}A/\dot{Q}$ mode may be explained by the tiny perfusion of corner vessels in the interalveolar septa of lung tissue in upper lung regions, where alveolar pressure may exceed pulmonary vascular pressure (zone I) (67). In a group of elderly patients with a more marked deterioration of pulmonary function, anesthesia caused considerable widening of the $\dot{V}A/\dot{Q}$ distribution with large increases both in low $\dot{V}A/\dot{Q}$ regions and in shunt (63).

Recently, $\dot{V}A/\dot{Q}$ distributions have been correlated to CT scan data of the chest during anesthesia. In lung-healthy subjects, the major $\dot{V}A/\dot{Q}$ disturbance was once again the appearance of shunt and very little of low $\dot{V}A/\dot{Q}$. Atelectasis was seen in most patients (11 of 13 patients) and there was a good correlation between the magnitude of shunt and size of the atelectasis (51). In the two patients who did not develop any atelectasis during anesthesia, no shunt and no clear impairment of arterial oxygenation were seen. Both subjects were young (20–24 years) but for the whole material no age dependence of atelectasis or shunt was seen. Interestingly, a few patients with a smoking history and mild spirometric abnormalities had smaller atelectasis and less shunt but more of perfusion in low $\dot{V}A/\dot{Q}$ regions than the average patient during anesthesia (51). A PEEP of 10 cmH$_2$O reduced the atelectatic area but the effect on shunt varied: in some patients it fell and in others it increased, probably explained by a redistribution of blood flow toward the dependent, still ate-

lectatic regions (68). In summary, these studies confirm the previous observation that shunt is the major cause of gas exchange impairment in lung-healthy subjects during anesthesia, and they maintain that it is reasonably explained by perfusion of blood through the atelectatic zone in dependent lung regions. It is also interesting to note that the intravenous anesthetic agent ketamine, which does not reduce muscle tone the way other anesthetics do, did not produce atelectasis or shunt or any other gas exchange impairment, whereas both atelectasis and shunt were seen when the same patients were paralyzed with a muscle relaxant (69).

Elimination of Carbon Dioxide

In 1957 Severinghaus and Stupfel (70) showed that anesthesia results in an impaired elimination of CO$_2$. A year later Campbell and co-workers described an increase in physiological dead space during anesthesia (4). Single breath wash-out recordings showed "anatomical" dead space to be unchanged (71), indicating that the "alveolar" or parallel dead space must have been increased during anesthesia. However, the impaired CO$_2$ elimination is easily accounted for by increasing the ventilation and is seldom a problem in routine anesthesia with mechanical ventilation.

REGIONAL ANESTHESIA

Ventilation and Lung Volume

There is an uptake of local anesthetic agents in the lung; in fact, the highest concentrations in the body are found in lung tissue (72). Although toxic arterial concentrations may produce respiratory arrest in healthy volunteers, intravenous infusions of local anesthetic agents in subconvulsive doses produce no change in pulmonary gas exchange (73). Ventilatory effects of regional anesthesia depend on the type and extension of motor blockade. Epidural and subarachnoid blocks below the 5th thoracic segment and segmental epidural blockade confined to the thorax have little effect on tidal volume, respiratory rate, vital capacity, and functional residual capacity (49,74,75). With extensive blocks including all thoracic and lumbar segments, inspiratory capacity is reduced by 20% and expiratory reserve volume approaches zero (74).

Diaphragmatic function is often spared even in cases of inadvertent extension of subarachnoid or epidural sensory blocking of cervical segments (74). Opioids administered intradurally or extradurally may result in prolonged respiratory depression (76). Bilateral intercostal block of the 5th through the 11th intercostal nerves is associated with only small decreases of V_C, FRC, and maximal respiratory pressure; maximal inspiratory pressure and lung compliance are unchanged (77).

Circulation

Intravenous infusions of local anesthetic agents in healthy subjects entail only minor changes in the systemic and pulmonary circulations (73). In clinical anesthesia the circulatory reaction to uncomplicated regional anesthesia depends mainly on the extension of sympathetic blockade, which induces an increase of venous capacitance and a decrease of arteriolar vascular tone in blocked regions and reversed reactions in other regions (78). The result may be an unchanged or decreased systemic vascular resistance (49,78). Epidural anesthesia with addition of epinephrine to the local anesthetic solution causes a profound reduction of the systemic vascular resistance and an increase of cardiac output, with the net result of a reduced systemic arterial pressure (79). Adequate blood volume supplementation and the use of vasopressors restore arterial blood pressure close to the preanesthetic level in most cases (80).

Gas Exchange

Skillfully handled regional anesthesia affects pulmonary gas exchange only insignificantly. Arterial oxygenation and carbon dioxide elimination are well maintained during spinal (49,79) and epidural anesthesia (75,79) and during bilateral intercostal nerve blocks (77). This is in line with the findings of unchanged relations of closing capacity to FRC (75,77), and with the finding during epidural anesthesia of unaltered dis-

tributions of ventilation/perfusion ratios assessed with the multiple inert gas elimination technique (75).

POSTOPERATIVE LUNG FUNCTION

Lung function, both in the context of ventilation and of gas exchange, remains impaired in the postoperative period (61). The most important factors determining the degree of postoperative pulmonary dysfunction are the site of operation and the age and clinical status of the patient (61,81). Short procedures not involving the trunk cause minor and short-lasting reductions of ventilatory function and FRC with small effects on arterial oxygenation (61,81). These effects are more pronounced after lower laparotomies and are greatly magnified after upper laparotomies and thoracotomies and may not be restored even by the fifth postoperative day (81). Forced expiratory vital capacity and peak flows are often reduced to half and the FRC to below 70% of their preoperative values (81,82). The reduction of the FRC and its relation to closing volume correlated to arterial hypoxemia (81), indicating that airway, and possibly alveolar, collapse contributes to the gas exchange impairment. The reduced vital capacity and the reduction of the FRC are mainly consequent to an impaired diaphragmatic function (83). The diaphragm is displaced cranially and the tidal volume contribution of this muscle is greatly reduced (83) because of reflex inhibition (unless it has sustained direct surgical trauma) to concentration (82).

Numerous studies have tried to determine the incidence of postoperative pulmonary complications, and the estimates vary widely. Clinical (i.e., observed) complications that have required some kind of intervention are fairly rare, occurring in about 1–10% of patients scheduled for elective surgery.

The majority of studies of postoperative pulmonary dysfunction have focused on subclinical complications, for example, radiographic evidence of atelectasis with or without pleural fluid, excessive cough, and slight fever. With this broader definition of complication, the incidence of postoperative pulmonary complications increases dramatically, to 25–75% after abdominal surgery (61,84). Surgery on the extremities, however, is associated with a lower complication rate. Interestingly, the incidence of postoperative pulmonary complication has remained the same for the last 30 years (61,84).

REFERENCES

1. Snow J. *The inhalation of the vapour of ether in surgical operations.* London: John Churchill, September 1847.
2. Crafoord C. On the technique of pneumonectomy in man. *Acta Clin Scand* 1938; suppl 54:43–70.
3. Maier HC, Cournand A. Studies of the arterial oxygen saturation

in the postoperative period after pulmonary resection. *Surgery* 1943;13:199–213.

4. Campbell EJM, Nunn JF, Peckett BW. A comparison of artificial ventilation and spontaneous respiration with particular reference to ventilation–blood-flow relationships. *Br J Anaesth* 1958; 30:166–175.

5. Nims RG, Conner EH, Comroe JH. The compliance of the human thorax in anesthetized patients. *J Clin Invest* 1955;34:744–750.

6. Eger EI. Isoflurane: a review. *Anaesthesiology* 1981;55:559–576.

7. Bellville JW, Seed JC. The effect of drugs on the respiratory response to carbon dioxide. *Anesthesiology* 1960;21:727–741.

8. Gordh T. Postural circulatory and respiratory changes during ether and intravenous anesthesia. *Acta Chir Scand* 1945; 92(suppl 102):26.

9. Weisskopf RB, Severinghaus JW. Lack of effect of high altitude on hemoglobin oxygen affinity. *J Appl Physiol* 1972;33:276–277.

10. Davies RO, Edwards MW, Lahiri S. Halothane depresses the response of carotid body chemoreceptors to hypoxia and hypercapnia in the cat. *Anesthesiology* 1982;57:153–159.

11. Jones JG, Faithfull D, Jordan C. Rib cage movement during halothane anesthesia in man. *Br J Anaesth* 1979;51:399–407.

12. Tusiewicz K, Bryan AC, Froese AB. Contributions of changing rib cage–diaphragm interactions to the ventilatory depression of halothane anesthesia. *Anesthesiology* 1977;47:327–337.

13. Bergman NA. Distribution of inspired gas during anesthesia and artificial ventilation. *J Appl Physiol* 1963;18:1085–1089.

14. Laws AK. Effect of induction of anesthesia and muscle paralysis on functional residual capacity of the lungs. *Can Anaesth Soc J* 1968;15:325–331.

15. Rehder K, Sessler AD, Marsch HM. General anesthesia and the lung. In: Murray JF, ed. *Lung disease state of the art*. New York: American Lung Association, 1975–1976;367–389.

16. Froese AB, Bryan CH. Effects of anesthesia and paralysis on diaphragmatic mechanics in man. *Anesthesiology* 1974;41:242–255.

17. Hedenstierna G, Strandberg Å, Brismar B, et al. Functional residual capacity, thoraco-abdominal dimensions and central blood volume during general anesthesia with muscle paralysis and mechanical ventilation. *Anesthesiology* 1985;62:247–254.

18. Hedenstierna G, Johansson H, Linde B. Central blood pooling as an explanation for lowered FRC during anaesthesia? Thigh volume measurements by plethysmography. *Acta Anaesthesiol Scand* 1982;26:633–637.

19. Don H. The mechanical properties of the respiratory system during anesthesia. *Int Anesthesiol Clin* 1977;15:113–136.

20. Westbrook PR, Stubbs SE, Sessler AD, et al. Effects of anesthesia and muscle paralysis on respiratory mechanics in normal man. *J Appl Physiol* 1973;34:81–86.

21. Milic-Emili J, Henderson JAM, Dolovich MB, et al. Regional distribution of inspired gas in the lung. *J Appl Physiol* 1966;21:749–759.

22. Don HF, Wahba WM, Craig DB. Airway closure, gas trapping, and the functional residual capacity during anesthesia. *Anesthesiology* 1972;36:533–539.

23. Hedenstierna G, McCarthy G, Bergström M. Airway closure during mechanical ventilation. *Anesthesiology* 1976;44:114–123.

24. Juno P, Marsh M, Knopp TJ, et al. Closing capacity in awake and anesthetized-paralysed man. *J Appl Physiol* 1978;44:238–244.

25. Bergman NA, Tien YK. Contribution of the closure of pulmonary units to impaired oxygenation during anesthesia. *Anesthesiology* 1983;59:395–401.

26. Dueck R, Prutow RJ, Davies NJH, et al. The lung volume at which shunting occurs with inhalation anesthesia. *Anesthesiology* 1988;69:854–861.

27. Mead J, Collier C. Relation of volume history of lungs to respiratory mechanics in anesthetized dogs. *J Appl Physiol* 1959;14:669–678.

28. Bendixen HH, Hedley-Whyte J, Laver MB. Impaired oxygenation in surgical patients during general anesthesia with controlled ventilation: a concept of atelectasis. *N Engl J Med* 1963;269:991–996.

29. Nunn JF, Bergman NA, Coleman AJ. Factors influencing the arterial oxygen tension during anaesthesia with artificial ventilation. *Br J Anaesth* 1965;37:898–914.

30. Brismar B, Hedenstierna G, Lundqvist H, et al. Pulmonary densities during anesthesia with muscular relaxation—a proposal of atelectasis. *Anesthesiology* 1985;62:422–428.

31. Strandberg Å, Tokics L, Brismar B, et al. Constitutional factors promoting development of atelectasis during anaesthesia. *Acta Anaesthesiol Scand* 1987;31:21–24.

32. Damgaard-Pedersen K, Qvist T. Pediatric pulmonary CT-scanning. *Pediatr Radiol* 1980;9:145–148.

33. Strandberg Å, Brismar B, Hedenstierna G, et al. Atelectasis during anaesthesia and in the postoperative period. *Acta Anaesthesiol Scand* 1986;30:154–158.

34. Hedenstierna G, Tokics L, Lundh B, et al. Pulmonary densities during anaesthesia. An experimental study on lung histology and gas exchange. *Eur Respir J* 1989;2:528–535.

35. Tokics L, Hedenstierna G, Brismar B, et al. Thoraco-abdominal restriction in supine man. Computerized tomography and lung function measurements. *J Appl Physiol* 1988;64:599–604.

36. Roussos CS, Yoshinosuke F, Macklem PT, et al. Influence of diaphragmatic contraction on ventilation distribution in horizontal man. *J Appl Physiol* 1976;40:417–424.

37. Rehder K, Sessler AD, Rodarte JR. Regional intra-pulmonary gas distribution in awake and anaesthetized-paralysed man. *J Appl Physiol* 1977;42:391–402.

38. Clements JA, Sharp JT, Johnson RP, et al. Estimation of pulmonary resistance by repetitive interruption of airflow. *J Clin Invest* 1959;38:1262–1270.

39. Larsson A, Linnarsson C, Jonmarker B, et al. Measurements of lung volume by sulfur hexafluoride washout during spontaneous and controlled ventilation. Further development of a method. *Anesthesiology* 1987;67:543–550.

40. Rehder K, Hatch DJ, Sessler A, et al. The function of each lung of anesthetized and paralysed man during mechanical ventilation. *Anesthesiology* 1972;37:16–26.

41. Lillington GA, Fowler WS, Miller RD, et al. Nitrogen clearance rates of right and left lungs in different positions. *J Clin Invest* 1959;38:2026–2034.

42. Hedenstierna G, Baerendtz S, Klingstedt C, et al. Ventilation and perfusion of each lung during differential ventilation with selective PEEP. *Anesthesiology* 1984;61:369–376.

43. Hulands GH, Greene R, Iliff LD, et al. Influence of anaesthesia on the regional distribution of perfusion and ventilation in the lung. *Clin Sci* 1970;38:451–460.

44. Merin RG. Effects of anesthetics on the heart. *Surg Clin North Am* 1975;55(4):759–774.

45. Tarnow J, Eberlein HJ, Oser G, et al. Hämodynamik, Myokardkontraktilität, Ventrikelvolumina und Sauerstoffversorgung des Herzens unter verschiedenen Inhalationsanaesthetika. *Anaesthesist* 1977;26:220–230.

46. Prys-Roberts C, Kelman GR, Greenbaum R, et al. Haemodynamics and alveolar–arterial P_{O_2} differences at varying Pa_{CO_2} in anesthetized man. *J Appl Physiol* 1968;25(1):80–87.

47. Stoelting RK, Gibbs PS. Hemodynamic effects of morphine and morphine–nitrous oxide in valvular heart disease and coronary-artery disease. *Anesthesiology* 1973;38(1):45–52.

48. White PF, Way WL, Trevor AJ. Ketamine—its pharmacology and therapeutic uses. *Anesthesiology* 1982;56:119–136.

49. Johnson SR. The effect of some anaesthetic agents on the circulation in man. *Acta Chir Scand* 1951;suppl 158:59–101.

50. Bindslev L, Hedenstierna G, Santesson J, et al. Ventilation-perfusion distribution during inhalation anaesthesia. Effect of spontaneous breathing, mechanical ventilation and positive end-expiratory pressure. *Acta Anaesthesiol Scand* 1981;25:360–371.

51. Tokics L, Hedenstierna G, Strandberg Å, et al. Lung collapse and gas exchange during general anaesthesia—effects of spontaneous breathing, muscle paralysis and positive end-expiratory pressure. *Anesthesiology* 1987;66:157–167.

52. Sörensen MB, Jacobsen E. Pulmonary hemodynamics during induction of anesthesia. *Anesthesiology* 1977;46:246–251.

53. Marshall BE. Effects of anesthetics on pulmonary gas exchange. In: Stanley TH, Sperry RJ, eds. *Anesthesia and the lung*. London: Kluwer Academic Publishers, 1989;117–125.

54. Reed JH, Wood EH. Effect of body position on vertical distribution of pulmonary blood flow. *J Appl Physiol* 1970;28(3):303–311.

55. Hakim TS, Dean GW, Lisbona R. Effect of body posture on spatial distribution of pulmonary blood flow. *J Appl Physiol* 1988;64(3):1160–1170.

56. Hughes JMB, Glazier JB, Maloney JE, et al. Effect of lung volume on the distribution of pulmonary blood flow in man. *Respir Physiol* 1968;4:58–72.

57. Landmark SJ, Knopp TJ, Rehder K, et al. Regional pulmonary perfusion and V/Q in awake and anaesthetized-paralyzed man. *J Appl Physiol* 1977;43(6):993–1000.

58. Sykes MK, Loh L, Seed RF, et al. The effect of inhalational anaesthetics on hypoxic pulmonary vasoconstriction and pulmonary vascular resistance in the perfused lungs of the dog and cat. *Br J Anaesth* 1972;44:776–788.

59. Bjertnaes LJ. Hypoxia induced vasoconstriction in isolated perfused lungs exposed to injectable or inhalation anaesthetics. *Acta Anaesthesiol Scand* 1977;21:133–147.

60. Miller FL, Chen L, Malmkvist G, et al. Mechanical factors do not influence blood flow distribution in atelectasis. *Anesthesiology* 1989;70:481–488.

61. Marshall BE, Wyche MO Jr. Hypoxemia during and after anesthesia. *Anesthesiology* 1972;37:178–209.

62. Vaughan RW, Wise L. Intraoperative arterial oxygenation in obese patients. *Ann Surg* 1976;184:35–42.

63. Dueck R, Young I, Clausen J, et al. Altered distribution of pulmonary ventilation and blood flow following induction of inhalational anesthesia. *Anesthesiology* 1980;52:113–125.

64. Nunn JF. *Applied respiratory physiology,* 3rd ed. London: Butterworth, 1987;270–271.

65. Rehder K, Knopp TJ, Sessler AD, et al. Ventilation–perfusion relationships in young healthy awake and anesthetized-paralyzed man. *J Appl Physiol* 1979;47:745–753.

66. Prutow RJ, Dueck R, Davies NJH, et al. Shunt development in young adult surgical patients due to inhalational anesthesia. *Anesthesiology* 1982;57:A477.

67. Hedenstierna G, White FC, Mazzone R, et al. Redistribution of pulmonary blood flow in the dog with positive end-expiratory pressure ventilation. *J Appl Physiol* 1979;46:278–287.

68. West JB, Dollery CT, Naimark A. Distribution of blood flow in isolated lung: relations to vascular and alveolar pressures. *J Appl Physiol* 1964;19:713–724.

69. Tokics L, Strandberg Å, Brismar B, et al. Computerized tomography of the chest and gas exchange measurements during ketamine anaesthesia. *Acta Anaesthesiol Scand* 1987;32:684–692.

70. Severinghaus JW, Stupfel M. Alveolar dead space as an index of distribution of blood flow in pulmonary capillaries. *J Appl Physiol* 1957;10:335–348.

71. Nunn JF, Hill DW. Respiratory dead space and arterial to end-tidal CO_2 tension difference in anaesthetized man. *J Appl Physiol* 1960;15:383–389.

72. Jorfeldt L, Lewis DH, Löfström JB, et al. Lung uptake of lidocaine in healthy volunteers. *Acta Anaesthesiol Scand* 1979;23:567–574.

73. Jorfeldt L, Löfström B, Pernow B, et al. The effect of local anaesthetics on the central circulation and respiration in man and dog. *Acta Anaesthesiol Scand* 1968;12:153–169.

74. Freund FG, Bonica JJ, Ward RJ, et al. Ventilatory reserve and level of motor block during high spinal and epidural anesthesia. *Anesthesiology* 1967;28:834–837.

75. Lundh R, Hedenstierna G, Johansson H. Ventilation–perfusion relationships during epidural analgesia. *Acta Anaesthesiol Scand* 1983;27:410–416.

76. Editorial. Epidural opiates. *Lancet* 1980;i:962–963.

77. Jakobson S, Fridrikson H, Hedenström H, et al. Effects of intercostal nerve blocks on pulmonary mechanics in healthy man. *Acta Anaesthesiol Scand* 1980;24:482–486.

78. Shimasato S, Etsten BE. The role of the venous system in cardiocirculatory dynamics during spinal and epidural anesthesia in man. *Anesthesiology* 1969;30:619–628.

79. Ward RJ, Bonica JJ, Freund FG, et al. Epidural and subarachnoid anesthesia. *JAMA* 1965;191(4):99–102.

80. Bonica JJ. *Principle and practice of obstetric analgesia and anesthesia.* Philadelphia: FA Davis Co, 1972.

81. Alexander JI, Spencer AA, Parikh RK, et al. The role of airway closure in postoperative hypoxaemia. *Br J Anaesth* 1973;45:34–40.

82. Dureuil B, Viires N, Contineau J-P, et al. Diaphragmatic contractility after upper abdominal surgery. *J Appl Physiol* 1986;61(5):1775–1780.

83. Simonneau G, Vivien A, Sartene R, et al. Diaphragm dysfunction induced by upper abdominal surgery. Role of postoperative pain. *Am Rev Respir Dis* 1983;128:899–903.

84. Celli BR, Rodriguez KS, Snider GL. A controlled trial of intermittent positive pressure breathing, incentive spirometry, and deep breathing exercises in preventing pulmonary complications after abdominal surgery. *Am Rev Respir Dis* 1984;130:12–15.

85. Hedenstierna G, Strandberg Å, Tokics L, Lundqvist H, Brismar B. Correlation of gas exchange impairment to development of atelectasis during anaesthesia and muscle paralysis. *Acta Anaesthesiol Scand* 1986;30:183–191.

THE LUNG: Scientific Foundations
edited by R.G. Crystal, J.B. West et al.
Raven Press, Ltd., New York © 1991.

CHAPTER 8.2.5

The Lung in the Intensive Care Unit

Robert M. Smith and Roger G. Spragg

The individual disorders and stresses that affect the lungs of critically ill patients are not unique. However, the magnitude of the stresses and the cumulative impact of many disorders can make the intensive care unit (ICU) environment exceptional. Complex pathologic events interact to alter profoundly ventilation and gas exchange in the critically ill. Use of oxygen, the most commonly prescribed drug in the ICU, the goals and rationale for mechanical ventilation, various metabolic stresses and their impact on gas exchange, and the major pulmonary disorders that occur with increased frequency in the ICU environment must all be understood in order to provide rational care to the ICU patient with pulmonary disease.

USE OF SUPPLEMENTAL OXYGEN

Indications and Rationale

The primary goal of supplemental oxygen therapy in the ICU is to ensure adequate delivery of oxygen at the cellular level. Tissue hypoxia can occur because oxygen utilization is excessively high (e.g., thyrotoxicosis) or because delivered oxygen cannot be utilized (e.g., cyanide poisoning), but more commonly it is due to diminished oxygen delivery. Oxygen delivery depends on transport of blood to tissues (determined by cardiac output and distribution of blood flow) and on the oxygen content of delivered arterial blood (determined by hemoglobin concentration, hemoglobin oxygen saturation, and hemoglobin oxygen capacity). Thus, tissue hypoxia can result from processes that

R. M. Smith and R. G. Spragg: Department of Medicine, Division of Pulmonary and Critical Care Medicine, University of California–San Diego, La Jolla, California 92093.

decrease cardiac output (e.g., myocardial dysfunction or hypovolemia), decrease local perfusion, decrease Sa_{O_2} (ventilation–perfusion imbalance, shunt, or hypoventilation), or decrease blood oxygen carrying capacity (e.g., anemia or carboxyhemoglobinemia). Appropriate intervention to treat or to prevent tissue hypoxia will therefore depend on the etiology of any actual or anticipated decrease in oxygen delivery. If tissue hypoxia is occurring solely due to decreased cardiac output or to decreased hemoglobin level, then supplemental oxygen will have little benefit, and therapy should primarily be directed at correcting the underlying defect in oxygen delivery.

Patients who have arterial hypoxemia should receive supplemental oxygen when the Pa_{O_2} falls to 60 mmHg or less ($Sa_{O_2} < 90\%$). At this Pa_{O_2} the percentage of hemoglobin combined with oxygen is at the upper shoulder of the sigmoidal oxyhemoglobin dissociation curve and any further decrease in Pa_{O_2} will cause a large drop in Sa_{O_2}. In patients with chronic hypercapnia who have hypoxemia as their major ventilatory stimulus (e.g., central hypoventilation syndromes and some patients with chronic bronchitis), the administration of oxygen may cause a further reduction of alveolar ventilation. In this setting, low-flow oxygen is necessary but should be given in the least amount necessary to achieve a $Pa_{O_2} > 60$ mmHg. If worsened hypercapnia occurs despite cautious step-by-step administration of supplemental oxygen, then intubation and mechanical ventilation are needed. In contrast, the patient with hypoxemia and hypocapnia can receive oxygen without fear of suppression of the ventilatory drive. The goal of therapy is a Pa_{O_2} of 60–80 mmHg. A Pa_{O_2} above 80 mmHg does not result in significantly increased oxygen delivery and offers no benefit to most patients. Endotracheal intubation and mechanical ventilation should be considered if the Pa_{O_2} is consistently below 60 mmHg despite a Fi_{O_2} of 0.6 or greater.

Methodology

Delivery of oxygen can be by low-flow or high-flow systems. The former consist of nasal or tracheal cannulae, simple face masks, and face masks with reservoir bags. Nasal cannulae are the simplest method of supplemental oxygen delivery; flow rates of 1–4 liters/min of 100% oxygen are usually well tolerated. Although the increase in FI_{O_2} is often estimated at 0.04 for every liter of flow through the cannula, the increase actually varies with the patient's tidal volume, inspiratory flow rate, and minute ventilation, and not just with the oxygen flow rate. Simple face masks can deliver a higher FI_{O_2} (0.40–0.50) than is achievable with nasal cannulae since flow rates of 6–8 liters/min are well tolerated and are sufficient to displace most of the exhaled gases from the mask. Still higher FI_{O_2} (0.7–0.8) can only be achieved through the use of an oxygen reservoir attached to the mask with a nonrebreathing valve to prevent exhaled gases from entering the reservoir. To achieve maximal FI_{O_2}, oxygen flow rates must be high enough to prevent collapse of the reservoir during inspiration as well as to displace exhaled gas from the mask. Tightly fitting masks are available that allow a FI_{O_2} close to 1.0 and maintain low levels of continuously positive airway pressure (CPAP), but these masks are rarely tolerated for more than a few hours. Consistent delivery of a constant FI_{O_2} from 0.24 to 0.40 can be achieved with a high-flow venturi-type mask. This system is most appropriate in situations such as chronic hypercapnia when delivery of a gas mixture with a known and constant FI_{O_2} may be critical.

Monitoring

Evaluation of the efficacy of supplemental oxygen has historically relied on the measurement of arterial blood gases (ABG). The reliability and reproducibility of Pa_{O_2} measurement in arterial blood plus the added information from pH and P_{CO_2} values has made the ABG the standard against which other techniques are measured. Continuous noninvasive measurement of oxygen saturation is possible with ear or finger-oximetry. Oximetry can be useful for detecting marked unexpected arterial desaturations during a procedure or during endotracheal suctioning, but it is insensitive to small changes in Pa_{O_2} on the upper (flat) portion of the oxyhemoglobin desaturation curve. Furthermore, capillary blood flow to the skin can affect oximetry so that reliable measurement of the exact Sa_{O_2} is not possible. For these reasons, oximetry is of limited usefulness in the initial management of hemodynamically unstable hypoxemic patients.

Measurement of arterial oxygen content alone is inadequate to establish whether sufficient oxygen is being transported to the tissues of critically ill patients. The difference in oxygen content between arterial and a mixed venous sample ($Ca_{O_2} - C\bar{v}_{O_2}$) has been suggested as one way of establishing the adequacy of oxygen delivery (1,2). The necessity of using a *mixed* venous sample must be stressed, since venous measurements from the right atrium or central veins may only reflect a limited distribution of blood flow and oxygen utilization. Under the best conditions, measurement of $Ca_{O_2} - C\bar{v}_{O_2}$ provides an estimate of the overall adequacy of oxygen delivery. It does not reveal the presence or absence of impaired oxygen delivery to any one critical organ. In critically ill patients, $P\bar{v}_{O_2}$ (and thus $C\bar{v}_{O_2}$) does not correlate well with oxygen transport. In these individuals oxygen uptake by tissues depends in part on oxygen delivery (3) and therefore the relationship between $P\bar{v}_{O_2}$ and oxygen transport is complex and unpredictable at best.

USE OF MECHANICAL VENTILATION

Indications and Rationale

Intubation and mechanical ventilation are probably best viewed as supportive measures that sustain ventilation and/or respiration and prolong survival, allowing time for therapy directed at the underlying disease process to take effect. Therefore, the indications for ventilatory support will vary depending on exactly what aspect of lung function is failing. Patients can be broadly grouped into (a) those with normal lungs who have depression of ventilatory drive or failure of the thoracic pump, (b) those with airway or parenchymal disease resulting in hypercarbic ventilatory failure ($\downarrow \dot{V}_A$, $\uparrow Pa_{CO_2}$), and (c) those with parenchymal disease and predominantly hypoxemic respiratory failure ($\downarrow Pa_{O_2}$).

For patients in the first category, the goals of ventilatory support are twofold: protection of the airway and maintenance of adequate alveolar ventilation. The need for ventilatory support can be obvious in a patient who is apneic following a drug overdose. However, the need for and timing of intubation and mechanical ventilation may be less obvious in the alert patient with progressive neuromuscular disease. A resting respiratory rate ≥ 30, a maximal inspiratory effort ≤ 35 cmH_2O, or a vital capacity $\leq 35\%$ predicted are some of the guidelines that may be useful in deciding when to provide ventilatory support; a progressive decline in any of these parameters is of more significance than any single value. For some patients with intact bulbar muscle function, negative pressure ventilation may be useful to supplement or replace weakened respiratory muscles without the added risks of endotracheal intubation (4).

The approach to hypercarbic respiratory failure due to obstructive airway disease will depend on the presence, severity, and reversibility of any underlying chronic lung disease. The young asthmatic patient who develops hypercarbia during an episode of acute bronchospasm represents one end of a spectrum that ranges from sudden fully reversible disease to chronic progressive disease with little or no reversible component. In acute status asthmaticus, elevation of Pa_{CO_2} occurs because of severe airway obstruction and resulting inability to maintain adequate $\dot{V}_A$; endotracheal intubation should be performed promptly (see section on Bronchospasm). For patients with longstanding obstructive airway disease and worsening of chronic hypercapnia, the decision to intubate should be made cautiously and should, in part, be based on the proven or assumed presence of reversible precipitating factors such as infection, pneumothorax, aspiration pneumonia, pulmonary edema, thromboembolism, or depression of respiratory drive due to supplemental oxygen, metabolic abnormalities, or drugs. For all patients, once ventilatory support is instituted, attention should be directed at maximizing bronchodilator therapy, treating reversible factors, and restoring respiratory muscles to optimum function by correcting nutritional deficiency and allowing time for fatigue to resolve (5). Ventilatory support must be carefully tailored to avoid pulmonary barotrauma or other complications induced by positive-pressure ventilation.

In hypoxemic respiratory failure due to diffuse parenchymal disease, the determining factor in the decision to intubate and provide ventilatory support will be the severity of hypoxemia and its response to supplemental oxygen. If a Pa_{O_2} of 60 mmHg cannot be maintained with a $F_{I_{O_2}}$ of 0.60 or less, intubation should usually be performed. In most cases, an $F_{I_{O_2}}$ of 1.0 is used initially following intubation, and CPAP or positive end-expiratory airway pressure (PEEP) is instituted to optimize Pa_{O_2} (see section on ARDS). The $F_{I_{O_2}}$ is then reduced to levels that are less likely to result in pulmonary oxygen toxicity (typically a $F_{I_{O_2}} \leq 0.60$). Rarely, a patient with modest reductions of lung compliance (C_L) will respond well to low levels of CPAP and may not require mechanical ventilation. In the majority of patients, however, the need for high levels of minute ventilation and the greatly increased work of breathing mean that mechanical ventilatory support will be necessary to prevent respiratory muscle fatigue and subsequent failure. Pressure-support ventilation may be useful in certain cooperative patients. By reducing the work of breathing while maintaining use of the patient's own respiratory muscles, pressure-support ventilation can reduce intrathoracic pressure and minimize the impact of positive-pressure ventilation on venous return and cardiac function (6). Patients with severe abnormalities of gas exchange,

particularly those requiring higher levels of PEEP, usually require total support of ventilation. Assist-control mode ventilation is appropriate for the majority of these patients; IMV mode ventilation is of minimal benefit since the intermittent spontaneous breaths generated by the patient are unlikely to contribute to oxygenation or ventilation. Muscle paralysis should be instituted if reduction in oxygen utilization is needed or if the patient is unable to synchronize his or her own respiratory efforts with the ventilator.

Impact of Positive-Pressure Ventilation on Extrapulmonary Physiology

Changes in organ function due to positive-pressure breaths can vary with the nature and severity of the pulmonary disease and can be unpredictable. Mechanical ventilation can increase intracranial pressure (ICP) by raising central venous pressure and impeding cerebral venous return. Not surprisingly, the probability that ICP will rise during positive-pressure ventilation is greatest in patients with highly compliant lungs. Patients with head trauma, who may have baseline elevations in ICP, are particularly susceptible to the deleterious consequences of positive-pressure breaths since a modest fall in mean arterial pressure due to mechanical ventilation, coupled with a rise in ICP, can markedly decrease cerebral perfusion pressure (7).

A number of explanations have been invoked to explain the oliguria, positive fluid and sodium balance, and hyponatremia that are often observed during positive-pressure ventilation. Leithner and his associates (8) have proposed that altered renal excretion of salt and water may be due to decreased plasma levels of atrial natriuretic peptides (ANPs). ANPs are secreted by the cardiac atria in response to stretch or increased transmural pressure and act to increase natriuresis by redistribution of renal blood flow and inhibition of the renin–angiotensin system. A fall in the levels of αANPs has been noted when 15 cmH_2O PEEP is applied to the airway of patients with acute respiratory failure; concurrent falls were noted in cardiac index, creatinine clearance, urine flow, and urine sodium excretion (8). Increased intrathoracic pressure and secondary increase of central venous pressures may also cause a redistribution of renal blood flow to juxtamedullary nephrons even in the absence of change in total renal blood flow (9). The application of 15 cmH_2O PEEP to patients receiving positive-pressure ventilation does not, however, elevate antidiuretic hormone (ADH) despite significant reductions in cardiac output, sodium and potassium excretion, and renal blood flow (10). The role that reduction in cardiac index alone may play in the alteration of renal function during positive-pressure ventilation remains uncertain. However, infusion of low-dose dopamine may minimize some of the effects of positive-pressure ventilation by restoring renal blood flow and redirecting distribution of blood flow to cortical nephrons (11).

A number of theories have been offered to explain the fall in cardiac output that is commonly seen during positive-pressure ventilation. While the event may be multidetermined, the greatest evidence suggests that impairment of venous return secondary to elevated intrathoracic pressures is responsible for the decline in cardiac output (1,2).

METABOLIC STRESSES AND GAS EXCHANGE

Metabolic stresses have their dominant impact on gas exchange through alterations in oxygen utilization, CO_2 production ($\dot{V}_{CO_2}$), or both. The magnitude of the changes in these two parameters will depend to a large extent on the energy source that is being utilized. Oxidation of carbohydrates produces 4 kcal/g while producing 1 mol of CO_2 for each mole of oxygen consumed (the respiratory exchange ratio R = 1.0). Oxidation of lipids as an energy source produces 9 kcal/g with R = 0.7, and proteins yield 4 kcal/g with R = 0.8. When carbohydrate calories are given in excess of metabolic requirements, they are stored either as glycogen or as fat; lipogenesis requires oxygen and has an overall stoichiometry of 8.8 mol CO_2 produced for each mole of oxygen consumed. Therefore, in the nutritionally depleted patient, the relationship between oxygen consumption and CO_2 production will depend on whether carbohydrate calories are administered appropriately or in excess of requirements. When excess carbohydrate calories are administered, they may be diverted to lipogenesis, resulting in a marked increased in $\dot{V}_{CO_2}$ with little to no change in $\dot{V}_{O_2}$ (12). This increment in $\dot{V}_{CO_2}$ may be tolerated if minute ventilation can increase (either spontaneously or with mechanical ventilation). However, in patients unable to increment their minute ventilation, increased $\dot{V}_{CO_2}$ can precipitate acute hypercapnia and acidosis (13) or it can impair attempts to wean patients who have impaired ventilatory reserve from the ventilator (14). The administration of 50% of nonprotein calories as a fat emulsion rather than as carbohydrate may avoid an intolerable increase in $\dot{V}_{CO_2}$ (15).

PULMONARY COMPLICATIONS THAT MAY DEVELOP DURING INTENSIVE CARE

Nosocomial Infection

Nosocomial pneumonia develops in 12% of general medical ICU patients and in over 20% of mechanically ventilated patients (16,17). In the presence of ARDS or of preexisting pulmonary disease, the incidence rises to 68–70% (18,19). The onset of nosocomial pneumonia is associated with increased mortality, deterioration in pulmonary hemodynamics and function, increased length of ICU stay in survivors, and the eventual development of multiple organ failure. The pathogens responsible for nosocomial pneumonia are diverse and the infections are frequently polymicrobial. Gram-negative or gram-positive bacteria are responsible for 57% and 36% of cases, respectively. Less frequently, other organisms including *Pneumocystis pneumoniae*, viruses, invasive fungi, *Legionella* sp., and yeast may also cause nosocomial pneumonia.

Predisposing factors in an ICU environment include tracheal intubation, altered mental status, preexisting pulmonary disease, neutralization of gastric acid, and altered host defenses due to azotemia, acidosis, or leukopenia. Although direct introduction of a potential pathogen into the lung can occur with contaminated nebulizers or ventilator tubing, most nosocomial infections appear to originate from endogenous organisms. Serial cultures of the oropharynx and trachea of ICU patients show that colonization by gram-negative organisms typically occurs within 3 days of admission to the ICU (20). This colonization is not initially present in patients transferred from elsewhere in the hospital and develops because of patient factors, more common in critically ill individuals, which predispose to colonization by pathogenic organisms. These factors are incompletely understood, but colonization is strongly associated with increased adherence of gram-negative bacteria, especially *P. aeruginosa*, to the epithelial cells of the oropharynx and the trachea (20). The reasons for the increased adherence include the exposure of epithelial cell-surface attachment sites by the action of salivary proteases (21) and alterations of *in vitro* pH (22); the loss of normal interbacterial inhibition and poor nutritional status may also play a role (23). The use of antacids or H_2-receptor antagonists to raise gastric pH has also been shown to result in gastric colonization by gram-negative organisms (24); the same organisms can subsequently be found in cultures of the oropharynx or trachea (25). The use of an H_2-receptor antagonist in mechanically ventilated patients is strongly associated with the subsequent development of nosocomial pneumonias, presumably by alteration of the gastric pH and the creation of a more hospitable gastric environment for bacteria (17).

Diagnosis of nosocomial pneumonia in the ICU can be extraordinarily difficult. Elevated leukocyte counts, fever, and radiographic infiltrates may exist in the presence or absence of nosocomial pneumonia. The incidence of tracheal colonization in ICU patients makes sputum culture futile as a method of diagnosing pneumonia. Use of a bronchoscopically positioned protected specimen brush (PSB) to bypass the upper airways and directly sample organisms present in the lower airways can improve diagnostic accuracy. Quantitative cultures of PSB in animal models and in postmortem studies suggest that a growth threshold of 10^3 colony-forming units per brush correctly predicts the pathogens present in infected lung tissue (26,27). Small-volume bronchoalveolar lavage (BAL) may also assist in the diagnosis of nosocomial pneumonia. In addition to being simpler to perform, BAL does not introduce the small but significant risk of pneumothorax which follows PSB. Quantitative cultures of returned lavage fluid appear to accurately reflect the number and identity of lung pathogens in baboons with diffuse lung injury, in immunocompromised patients with new infiltrates, and in patients presenting with acute bacterial pneumonia. The utility of BAL in intubated patients undergoing mechanical ventilation remains uncertain, although at least one group has found excellent correlation between quantitative cultures of BAL and of PSB (27). The utility of PSB or BAL in the patient receiving systemic antibiotics is controversial, though some studies suggest that the specificity and sensitivity for both techniques remain high (26,27). Additional findings that have indicated the presence of nosocomial pneumonia include the presence of intracellular organisms in more than 25% of the cells recovered by BAL (28), the ELISA detection of bacterial lipid A in BAL (29), and the presence of elastin fibrils in KOH preparations of tracheal aspirate or sputum (30). Although promising, all these techniques require further examination in patients with respiratory failure.

Treatment of nosocomial infection relies on the use of antibiotics to cover the identified pathogens. If culture results are not available, antibiotics should be selected to provide broad coverage of gram-negative organisms. Unfortunately, administration of antibiotics appropriate for identified organisms does not improve the survival in patients with ARDS and nosocomial pneumonia in comparison to patients whose antibiotic therapy was judged inadequate (19). Allowing gastric pH to remain low may prevent nosocomial pneumonia by reducing gastric colonization. Sucralfate, a cytoprotective agent that binds to mucosal proteins, does not markedly alter gastric pH but is as effective as H_2 blockers and antacids in preventing stress-induced gastric bleeding. The use of sucralfate in mechanically ventilated patients is associated with reduced bacterial colonization of the stomach, pharynx, and trachea, and with reduced rates of gram-negative nosocomial pneumonia (24,31).

Barotraumatic Lung Injury

Overdistension of an alveolus during a mechanically generated breath may lead to rupture and release of gas into the interstitium where it can then spread along tissue planes. Gas traversing the pulmonary hilum can lead to pneumomediastinum or pneumopericardium; further spreading may result in subcutaneous emphysema or in pneumoperitoneum. Gas rupturing from visceral or parietal pleura will lead to pneumothorax. The incidence of barotrauma during positive-pressure ventilation is highly variable and depends on the length of ventilatory support and the nature of underlying lung disease. Preexisting emphysematous lung disease, necrotizing pneumonia, aspiration of gastric contents, bronchospasm, and ARDS are all associated with increased rates of barotrauma (32). Alveolar volume may be more important than intra-alveolar pressure per se in the development of alveolar rupture (33). If alveolar expansion is limited by fibrotic processes in the interstitium or if lung volumes are constrained by the thoracic cage, then alveolar pressures are transmitted to the interstitium and little or no pressure gradient across the alveolar–capillary membrane will exist. Although the addition of PEEP may increase peak airway pressures, it is not clear that PEEP itself is an independent risk factor for barotrauma.

Palpation for subcutaneous emphysema may provide the earliest physical finding in barotraumatic lung injury. The earliest radiographic sign of barotrauma is thought to be pulmonary interstitial emphysema, visible as perivascular halos, streaks of air radiating from the hilum, small parenchymal air cysts, or larger subpleural cysts (34). The occurrence of interstitial emphysema during mechanical ventilation is a strong predictor for the subsequent development of tension pneumothorax. In patients with acute respiratory failure, the radiographic changes of pneumothorax may be subtle because the films are usually obtained with the patient supine, and because areas of parenchymal consolidation, extensive interstitial emphysema, or extensive pleural adhesions may prevent the lung from completely collapsing. Thus, pneumothorax may manifest only as an anteromedial, subpulmonic, or posterior collection of gas, any of which may have a misleading radiographic appearance.

Pneumothorax in critically ill patients requires tube thoracostomy to allow lung expansion and restore function. The development of further barotrauma may be minimized through the use of lower tidal volumes, reduction in peak flow, the use of ventilator modes that synchronize with patients' breaths, or the induction of neuromuscular blockade in patients who are unable to synchronize with the machine breaths (see Chapter 8.2.3). Localized areas of pneumothorax can be under tension despite an ipsilateral chest tube and can cause severe cardiovascular and pulmonary compromise in patients with markedly impaired pulmonary function (35); multiple ipsilateral chest tubes may sometimes be necessary. A persistent air leak through a chest tube

TABLE 1. *Conditions that may precipitate the adult respiratory distress syndrome*

Nonpulmonary	Pulmonary
Septicemia	Aspiration: gastric contents, hydrocarbons, seawater (near-drowning)
Shock	
Nonthoracic trauma	
Blood transfusion	
Pancreatitis	Inhalation injury: NO_2, Cl_2, SO_2, NH_3, O_2, smoke
Disseminated intravascular coagulation	
Reaction to contrast injection	Diffuse pulmonary infection: bacterial, viral, other
Drug ingestion: narcotic, paraquat, aspirin	Chest irradiation
Uremia	
Acute intracranial pathology	
Fat or amniotic fluid embolism	

indicates the presence of a bronchopleural fistula. The resulting loss of alveolar ventilation can be life-threatening in patients with severely compromised pulmonary function; the volume of air leak may be minimized through the use of valves that transmit airway pressure to the chest tube or through the use of high-frequency ventilation (36).

The Adult Respiratory Distress Syndrome (ARDS)

Increased permeability of the alveolar–capillary membrane to water, solutes, and plasma proteins appears to be the underlying defect in ARDS (37). Events that may cause ARDS (see Table 1) include sepsis, aspiration, shock, and multiple transfusions—common complications in the care of ICU patients. The presentation of ARDS tends to have a number of common characteristics. These include (a) a history of a preceding noxious event, (b) a symptom-free interval lasting hours to days, and (c) the subsequent progression of severe hypoxemia, decreased lung compliance, and diffuse noncardiogenic pulmonary edema. Although the pathways that result in the development of ARDS are unknown, the incidence of ARDS increases with the presence of multiple risk factors (38). It is not known whether these different risk factors act independently or via some common pathway, but it is likely that no single agent or mechanism of injury is responsible for all the manifestations of ARDS (see Chapters 7.2.1 and 7.7.3.1).

ARDS typically progresses through successive stages of initial injury, progressive inflammation and destruction of lung architecture, and subacute fibrosis (39). The first stage, from onset to 48–72 hr is marked by rapidly worsening gas exchange, marked falls in lung compliance, pathologic changes of alveolar and interstitial edema, and platelet–leukocyte–fibrin aggregate trapping in the microcirculation. Lung function may then improve or may show further deterioration marked by difficulty in maintaining ventilatory support, increased VD/VT, and by increased pulmonary vascular resistance. Finally, from 10 to 30 days, the patient may enter a stage in which pulmonary function has stabilized (with persistent functional impairment), and organized fibrous changes have distorted or obliterated the normal alveolar architecture. If the patient survives through this latter stage there is gradual slow improvement in lung function over weeks to months. Multiple organ system failure may occur at any point in clinical course, although it is more often seen in the earlier stages. Abnormalities of left ventricular performance are present in the majority of patients with ARDS, although the etiology is poorly understood (40). Circulating myocardial depressant factors have been described in the plasma of patients with septic shock and may account for depression of left ventricular function in some patients with ARDS (41).

Steroids have not been effective as prevention or treatment for ARDS (42). The administration of PEEP to patients at risk for ARDS has been suggested as a means of preventing or modifying the development of subsequent respiratory failure, but clinical trials have not consistently supported this hypothesis (43). Advances in our understanding of the biochemical alterations that take place in the lungs of patients with ARDS (see Chapter 7.7.3.1) have led to ongoing evaluations of the use of cyclo-oxygenase inhibitors, antibodies directed against endotoxin or C5a, surfactant replacement therapy, and antiprotease and antioxidant therapy; as yet, no specific therapy for ARDS is available.

Of concern is the possibility that ARDS may be a response to barotrauma, and that use of high airway pressures to ventilate patients with ARDS may result in injury to formerly uninvolved parts of the lung (44). Thus, use of extracorporeal CO_2 removal with low-pressure/low-frequency ventilation has been suggested as a rational means of respiratory support for ARDS patients (45,46); this modality is currently undergoing clinical trial (see Chapter 8.2.6).

Pulmonary Thromboembolism

Autopsy studies have disclosed the presence of pulmonary thromboemboli in 27% of patients who die while receiving mechanical ventilation in the ICU; only one-half of these were diagnosed antemortem. Clinical and radiographic signs are neither sensitive nor specific for pulmonary emboli in ambulatory patients and are even less useful in patients with respiratory failure. Although thrombosis associated with indwelling catheters has been implicated as a source for some emboli, most thromboemboli appear to arise from the lower extremities. ICU patients can be subject to a number of influences (prolonged bed rest, left or right ventricular failure, dehydration, obesity, muscle paralysis, or recent surgical procedures) that cause lower extremity venous stasis and thereby increase the risk of deep venous thrombosis.

The diagnosis of thromboembolic disease can be extraordinarily difficult in the ICU patient. ^{125}I fibrinogen scanning may give false positive results in patients with the diffuse capillary leak occasionally seen in ARDS and is insensitive for thigh thrombus (47,48). Positive intrathoracic pressures during mechanical ventilation may impede venous return and cause a bilaterally abnormal impedance plethysmographic or doppler study of the legs. Radioisotopic lung perfusion scans have considerably less specificity in the presence of preexisting lung disease but are still valuable as a screening technique to exclude the diagnosis of thromboembolism. Some patients will have remarkably normal perfusion scans despite a very abnormal chest radiograph; any observed perfusion defects can direct selective angiographic studies, allowing the use of smaller volumes of contrast.

Treatment for pulmonary emboli in critically ill patients is guided by the presence of other organ system disease and the risk of hemorrhage with treatment. In patients with hemodynamic compromise from pulmonary emboli and with no bleeding predispositions, thrombolytic therapy may be indicated (49). However, systemic anticoagulation with heparin is the treatment of choice in most patients. When anticoagulation is contraindicated because of recent surgery, GI bleeding, or cerebral injury, consideration should be given to preventing further embolic events by interruption of vena caval blood flow. Percutaneously placed devices such as a Greenfield filter can be inserted under local anesthesia and typically remain patent while limiting the incidence of recurrent thromboembolism to approximately 2% (50).

The risk of therapy and the difficulty of diagnosing thromboembolism in an ICU patient suggest that prevention of the initial thrombosis is crucial. Oral warfarin anticoagulation, the administration of antiplatelet agents, and the use of elastic compression stockings either impose a risk of serious GI hemorrhage or are ineffective. Subcutaneous heparin successfully reduces the incidence of pulmonary emboli in patients with respiratory failure and has an acceptably low rate of GI bleeding (51). Although the efficacy of intermittent pneumatic calf compression is not known in patients with respiratory failure, its success in preventing deep venous thrombosis in other high risk groups

(52,53) suggests it may also be effective in ICU patients.

Bronchospasm

Severe airway obstruction may be a presenting complaint to the ICU or may complicate the course of respiratory failure from other causes. Tracheobronchitis from bacterial infection, irritation from endotracheal suctioning, unanticipated drug allergy, or simple anxiety may all precipitate bronchospasm (see Chapters 5.1.2.1.2 and 5.1.2.1.7). Therapy for bronchospasm in intubated ICU patients is little different from therapy for bronchospasm in other settings and includes the use of supplemental oxygen, inhaled β agonists, and parenteral aminophylline.

Patients whose bronchospasm is severe enough to precipitate respiratory failure and who require mechanical ventilation can be difficult to support. Markedly increased airway resistance leads to high peak airway pressures when conventional tidal volumes and frequencies are used. Coupled with maldistribution of ventilation and hyperventilation, the increased pressures lead to a greatly increased risk of pulmonary barotrauma. Expiratory time at usual ventilatory frequencies may be insufficient to allow alveolar pressures to return to zero prior to the next positive-pressure breath; successive ventilator breaths are stacked one on another. The level of alveolar end-expiratory pressure is not reflected in downstream airway pressures but can be detected by noting continuing airflow throughout the expiratory phase. Noninvasive methods for quantifying this phenomenon include measurement of exhaled volume during a 20-sec expiratory pause, and detection of an increase in airway pressure when expiratory gas flow is transiently blocked just prior to the time the next breath would normally be delivered (54,55). Using these techniques, unanticipated positive end-expiratory alveolar pressures are found in a large percentage of patients with acute respiratory failure and can lead to reduction in cardiac output, inaccurate measures of static lung compliance, and prolonged efforts to wean the patient from mechanical ventilation (55–57). Mechanical hypoventilation (using neuromuscular blockade, increased F_{IO_2}, small tidal volumes, and reduced respiratory frequency to minimize peak airway pressures) may reduce barotrauma in patients with status asthmaticus when bicarbonate is administered to maintain physiologic pH (58,59); Pa_{CO_2} values as high as 70–90 are surprisingly well tolerated if bicarbonate buffering is adequate.

Complications of Hemodialysis

Renal failure often occurs in critically ill patients with multiple system failure and hemodialysis may be required to preserve appropriate fluid and electrolyte balance or to minimize the end-organ effects of uremia. Unfortunately, frequent hemodialysis is often necessary because of the highly catabolic state of many critically ill patients as well as the need to remove large volumes of fluids administered with medications and nutritional support. The process of dialysis has a number of unique effects on cardiopulmonary function that can go unrecognized. These effects can be subdivided into three broad areas: (a) alteration of V/Q relationships, (b) reduction in alveolar ventilation due to CO_2 losses in the dialysate, and (c) acute alterations in cardiac function. Mild to moderate degrees of hypoxemia are found in spontaneously breathing patients undergoing hemodialysis. Neutrophil sequestration in the lung, one potential cause of this hypoxemia, has been ascribed to a sequence of events initiated by the passage of blood across a relatively bioincompatible dialysis membrane (usually cellulose derived) with subsequent complement activation. Complement activation in turn leads to neutrophil activation and agglutination, sequestration of leukocyte aggregates in the pulmonary microcirculation with peripheral neutropenia, V/Q mismatching, and increase in A-aD_{O_2}. The use of more biocompatible membranes may minimize pulmonary leukosequestration (60) but, even when present, leukosequestration frequently is inadequate to explain dialysis-associated alterations in arterial blood gases, since A-aD_{O_2} may be unchanged in the presence of a significant drop in Pa$_{O_2}$ (61,62).

Hemodialysis against an acetate-buffered dialysate results in removal of CO_2 from the dialyzed blood; the magnitude of this CO_2 removal can approach 30% of the total body CO_2 production. Due to extracorporeal CO_2 removal, a compensatory reduction occurs in $\dot{V}_A$ to maintain a constant Pa$_{CO_2}$. Analysis of expired gases during dialysis has shown that $\dot{V}_{O_2}$ does not change significantly and thus there is a marked fall in R, the respiratory gas exchange ratio. In many studies, the drop in Pa$_{O_2}$ during dialysis is attributable almost solely to this hypoventilation and drop in R. This phenomenon will not occur in the patient whose minute ventilation is controlled by a ventilator but, in other patients, the use of HCO_3^--buffered dialysate prevents the removal of CO_2 and avoids the observed hypoxemia (61,63). HCO_3^--containing dialysate may also cause an increase in the hemoglobin P_{50} (64), although the mechanism of this change is obscure since it is limited to HCO_3^--containing dialysates and is not caused by a change in pH or 2,3-diphosphoglycerate. In theory, such a change in P_{50} may promote increased

tissue oxygen delivery and may provide an additional rationale for the use of HCO_3^--buffered dialysate.

Aspiration of Gastric Contents

The aspiration of gastric contents can cause a spectrum of pulmonary injuries depending on the consistency (fluid or particulate) and content (gastric acid, mineral oil, bacterial pathogens, or enteral feedings) of the aspirated material. Gastric secretions, even with a pH up to 5.9, can cause intense pulmonary inflammation if aspirated. Infiltrates and deterioration of pulmonary function typically progress for 24–36 hr and cause early mortality in approximately 10% of cases. In survivors, infiltrates may then improve rapidly, although initial improvement may be followed by bacterial infection and secondary deterioration in one-fourth of patients (65). Aspiration of large volumes of gastric secretions can cause pan-lobar consolidation and progression to frank necrosis. The risk of aspiration is increased by loss of consciousness, presence of a nasogastric tube, gastric distension, and paralysis and remains despite a continuously inflated cuffed endotracheal or tracheostomy tube (66). Conservative measures (maintenance of a clear airway, arterial oxygenation, and normal intravascular volume; ventilatory support if necessary) are often sufficient treatment for aspiration (67). For severely compromised patients or for those who fail to improve rapidly, antibiotic therapy should be initiated: anaerobic organisms are the usual pathogens in the community; gram-negative organisms or staphylococci cause infection in the hospital setting. The use of extensive pulmonary lavage to remove aspirated fluids or of corticosteroids to reduce inflammation is ineffective and possibly harmful (67). Fiberoptic bronchoscopy should be considered if there is a possibility that particulates were aspirated and could cause airway obstruction. Prophylactic measures to limit aspiration include elevating the patient's head, frequent surveillance for large gastric residuals, and maintenance of proper nasogastric tube position.

Hemoptysis

Admission to an ICU is usual for any episode of hemoptysis severe enough to compromise pulmonary function. The absolute volume of blood is of less significance than the severity of any preexisting pulmonary disease and the impact of the hemoptysis on respiratory function. Significant hemoptysis usually originates in highly vascularized tissues such as the wall of a tuberculous or necrotizing bacterial cavity, the site of chronic bronchiectasis, a bronchial adenoma, or, rarely, from mucosa containing venous varicosities due to chronic mitral stenosis; the majority of these bleeding sites are supplied by bronchial artery collaterals. Uncommon causes are Goodpasture's syndrome, systemic bleeding diatheses including anticoagulant therapy and uremia, cystic fibrosis, and localized lung bullae. In ICU patients, potential iatrogenic causes of massive hemoptysis include tracheal-innominate artery fistula following tracheostomy, rupture of the pulmonary artery during inflation of a balloon tipped catheter, and transbronchial lung biopsy.

Initial management of hemoptysis consists of stabilization of the airway. Intubation of the main stem bronchus of the uninvolved lung may be necessary to preserve function; the use of a double lumen endotracheal tube has been suggested for this but the smaller lumen may not allow adequate suctioning of clots. Reducing the risk of further bleeding may be accomplished by moderate sedation, bed rest with the bleeding site dependent, and administration of antibiotics if an infectious etiology is present. Identification of the bleeding source is an immediate concern if early surgical intervention is considered, as well as to guide other therapeutic interventions. Use of a fiberoptic bronchoscope is safe and informative in most patients; a fiberoptic bronchoscope can also be used to place a Fogarty catheter to tamponade the bronchus supplying the bleeding site (68). Bronchial artery embolization achieves immediate, though often temporary, control of bleeding in 75–90% of patients and is the treatment of choice in patients unable to tolerate surgery (69); failure occurs when the appropriate vessels cannot be identified, when the position of vertebral arteries precludes embolization, and when all vessels supplying a bleeding source are not embolized.

Hypoventilation

A rising Pa_{CO_2} in a seriously ill patient may result from a decrease in minute ventilation due to respiratory muscle failure, or, if alveolar ventilation cannot increase, from an increase in CO_2 production (see section on Metabolic Stresses and Gas Exchange). Respiratory muscle failure can come about from drugs or disease processes that cause neuromuscular blockade, or from processes that lead to decreased respiratory muscle strength. Attenuation of neuromuscular blockade upon discontinuation of curariform agents may take significantly longer than anticipated following prolonged use in ARDS. Unintentional neuromuscular blockade, mediated through a prejunctional depression of acetylcholine release at the motor end-plate, may follow the administration of certain antibiotics including a number of aminoglycosides, some tetracycline derivatives, and colistin (70). Only rarely a cause of significant paralysis on their own, these drugs can pre-

cipitate muscular failure in patients with Guillain–Barré syndrome, Eaton–Lambert syndrome, or myasthenia gravis and can act synergistically with other neuromuscular blocking agents to enhance the magnitude and duration of neuromuscular blockade.

Nutritional deprivation diminishes respiratory muscle strength in patients without underlying lung disease (71) and has been correlated with decreased diaphragmatic mass and strength in patients with emphysema (72). Impaired ventilatory drive has also been found in semistarved patients and may be an additional factor leading to a rising CO_2 (73). Nutritional support is frequently inadequate in hospitalized patients with acute respiratory failure (74), making the deleterious effects of acute or subacute malnutrition more likely to appear during an ICU stay. Starvation is unlikely to be the sole factor responsible for respiratory failure, but it does increase the need for prolonged ventilatory support and is associated with increased mortality in patients with respiratory failure (75). Hypophosphatemia can independently decrease diaphragmatic strength and, if severe, may prolong weaning attempts or precipitate respiratory failure (76). The mechanism for this effect appears to be diminished precursors for the synthesis of high-energy phosphate compounds (77). Occult hypothyroidism may result in central hyporesponsiveness to hypoxemia and hypercarbia (see Chapters 5.4.4 and 5.4.5), phrenic nerve conduction defects, and muscular weakness. These effects frequently will cause significant hypoventilatory respiratory failure (78) and require treatment with exogenous hormone.

Vascular Gas Embolism

Air gains access to the circulation in ICU patients more frequently than is usually appreciated (79). During pacemaker insertion, 4 of 10 patients were found by echocardiography to have air bubbles in the right heart chambers, even though the procedure was performed in reverse Trendelenberg position (80). Vascular gas embolism may occur in the ICU during placement of intravascular catheters, following malfunction of a hemodialysis device, during administration of blood or fluids under pressure, or in association with traumatic lung injury or pulmonary barotrauma.

Although the lung is generally a competent filter, passage of gas bubbles across the pulmonary circulation can follow the introduction of as little as 20 ml of air as a bolus or 0.15 ml/min·kg as a continuous infusion into the venous circulation (79). Transpulmonary passage of bubbles is enhanced when pulmonary artery pressures are raised, during oxygen breathing, or with theophylline treatment. Elevation of right atrial pressures from gas bubbles occluding the pulmonary circulation or from preexisting pulmonary disease may allow passage of bubbles through a patent foramen ovale. Obstruction of the microcirculation by bubbles can lead to increased pulmonary vascular resistance and shunting of blood through unventilated lung or, in the arterial circulation, to ischemic damage to multiple organs. Venous gas embolization also causes increased alveolar capillary membrane permeability in animal models (81–84). Trapped bubbles in the pulmonary microcirculation may injure the alveolar-capillary directly or may cause activation of neutrophils, resulting indirectly in injury and capillary leakage due to released oxidants (81,82). The diagnosis of vascular gas embolism may be made clinically if a large volume of gas was witnessed to pass into the circulation but typically relies on the visualization of bubbles. This can be accomplished by M-mode ultrasonography of the heart or great vessels or rarely by observation of bubbles in retinal or, by x-ray, cerebral vessels (85,86). Skin or lingual changes due to gas embolism occur but are not sufficiently specific to allow their diagnostic use. Treatment of intravascular gas embolism relies on (a) hyperbaric reduction of bubble size and (b) administration of oxygen ($F_{I_{O_2}} = 1.0$), thereby decreasing arterial Pa_{N_2} and increasing the rate of N_2 diffusion out of bubbles. Adjunctive measures such as corticosteroids, anticoagulants, lidocaine, and prostaglandin inhibitors have been useful in animal studies but are not known to be effective in a clinical setting.

GAS EXCHANGE DURING CARDIOPULMONARY RESUSCITATION (CPR)

The initial hypothesis that generation of forward blood flow during CPR was due to direct compression of the heart between sternum and thoracic spine has been called into question. Alternately, blood flow during CPR may be attributed to a generalized increase in intrathoracic pressure, which is then transmitted to systemic arteries. Peripheral valves and the high compliance of the central veins may minimize backward flow and allow creation of the required arterial–venous pressure gradient. Recent work, however, shows that mitral valve movement and intrathoracic pressure gradients are more consistent with direct compression of the heart. Thus, standard CPR techniques are safer and more effective than those that attempt to maximize intrathoracic pressure (87).

Forward blood flow can be maintained by these techniques during CPR, but only at 25–30% of baseline values. Continued tissue uptake of oxygen, coupled with the marked reduction in systemic blood flow, accounts for the observed increase in the arterial–venous Po_2 gradient. If alveolar ventilation is maintained during CPR, delivery of CO_2 to the lung limits CO_2 excretion, and Pa_{CO_2} typically falls (88,89). Although relatively normal arterial values for pH and Pco_2 may be maintained, there are large differences between arterial and venous values for pH and Pco_2 (0.31 unit and -60 mmHg, respectively) during CPR (88). The venous values more accurately reflect the actual tissue environment. End-tidal CO_2 (Pet_{CO_2}), an indirect measure of Pa_{CO_2}, can provide a noninvasive assessment of CO_2 delivery to the lung and therefore of cardiac output during CPR (90). A fall in Pet_{CO_2} below 1.0% during CPR suggests inadequate cardiac output, and an abrupt increase in Pet_{CO_2} to prearrest levels (approximately 4.0%) may be the first sign of the resumption of spontaneous circulation. Limitation of tissue perfusion during CPR suggests that use of CO_2-producing buffers (such as bicarbonate) may result in enhanced tissue acidosis compared to the use of non-CO_2-producing buffers (such as carbonate–bicarbonate or TRIS). However, animal studies have failed to show benefit from use of selected buffers during CPR (91,92). In animal models of cardiac arrest, Pa_{CO_2} correlates closely with Pet_{CO_2} and can also serve as an indirect measure of cardiac output (91)—the applicability of this observation to cardiac arrest in patients, especially those with lung disease, is not known.

In summary, the acutely ill patient experiences a variety of stresses that may challenge or overwhelm the adaptive capacities of the lung. Currently, many of these are understood at a phenomenologic level rather than at a mechanistic level. As a result, diagnostic and therapeutic efforts remain relatively empiric and nonspecific. As the biology of the lung and of the lung's response to stress become better understood at the cellular and molecular level, clinical studies defining the lung's responses to stresses encountered in the ICU will become more sophisticated. Identification of defense mechanisms and response mechanisms of clinical importance will occur, with eventual benefit for critically ill patients.

ACKNOWLEDGMENTS

This work was supported in part by NIH SCOR HL-23584 and by an ALA research grant. RMS is the recipient of a Parker B. Francis Fellowship in Pulmonary Research.

REFERENCES

1. Wood LDH, Prewitt RM. Cardiovascular management in acute hypoxemic respiratory failure. *Am J Cardiol* 1981;47:963–971.
2. Biondi JW, Schulman DS, Matthay RA. Effects of mechanical ventilation on right and left ventricular function. *Clin Chest Med* 1988;9:55–71.
3. Danek SJ, Lynch JP, Weg JG, Dantzker DR. The dependence

of oxygen uptake on oxygen delivery in the adult respiratory distress syndrome. *Am Rev Respir Dis* 1980;122:387–395.

4. Braun SR, Sufit RL, Giavannoni R, O'Connor M, Peters H. Intermittent negative pressure ventilation in the treatment of respiratory failure in progressive neuromuscular disease. *Neurology* 1987;37:1874–1875.

5. Wilson DO, Rogers RM. The role of nutrition in weaning from mechanical ventilation. *J Intensive Care Med* 1989;4:124–133.

6. Brochard L, Pluskwa F, Lemaire F. Improved efficacy of spontaneous breathing with inspiratory pressure support. *Am Rev Respir Dis* 1987;136:411–415.

7. Shapiro HM. Intracranial hypertension: therapeutic and anesthetic considerations. *Anesthesiology* 1975;43:445–471.

8. Leithner C, Frass M, Pacher R, Hartter E, Pesl H, Woloszczuk W. Mechanical ventilation with positive end-expiratory pressure decreases release of alpha-atrial natriuretic peptide. *Crit Care Med* 1987;15:484–488.

9. Hall SV, Johnson EE, Hedley-White J. Renal hemodynamics and function with continuous positive pressure ventilation in dogs. *Anesthesiology* 1974;41:452–460.

10. Payen DM, Farge D, Beloucif S, et al. No involvement of antidiuretic hormone in acute antidiuresis during PEEP ventilation in humans. *Anesthesiology* 1987;66:17–23.

11. Hemmer M, Suter PM. Treatment of cardiac and renal effects of PEEP with dopamine in patients with acute respiratory failure. *Anesthesiology* 1979;50:399–403.

12. Askanazi J, Rosenbaum SH, Hyman AI, Silverberg PA, Milic-Emili J, Kinney JM. Respiratory changes induced by the large glucose loads of total parenteral nutrition. *JAMA* 1980;243:1444–1447.

13. Covelli HD, Black JW, Olsen MS, Beekman JF. Respiratory failure precipitated by high carbohydrate loads. *Ann Intern Med* 1981;95:579–581.

14. Dark DS, Pingleton SK, Kerby GR. Hypercapnia during weaning. A complication of nutritional support. *Chest* 1985;88:141–143.

15. Herve P, Simonneau G, Girard P, Cerrina J, Mathieu M, Duroux P. Hypercapnic acidosis induced by nutrition in mechanically ventilated patients: glucose versus fat. *Crit Care Med* 1985;13:537–542.

16. Johanson WG, Pierce AK, Sanford JP, Thomas GD. Nosocomial respiratory infections with gram negative bacilli: the significance of colonization of the respiratory tract. *Am Rev Respir Dis* 1972;77:701–706.

17. Craven DE, Kunches LM, Kilinsky V, Lichtenberg DA, Make BJ, McCabe WR. Risk factors for pneumonia and fatality in patients receiving continuous mechanical ventilation. *Am Rev Respir Dis* 1986;133:792–796.

18. Ashbaugh DG, Petty TL. Sepsis complicating the adult respiratory distress syndrome. *Surg Gynecol Obstet* 1972;135:865–869.

19. Seidenfeld JJ, Pohl DF, Bell RC, Harris GD, Johanson WG. Incidence, site, and outcome of infections in patients with the adult respiratory distress syndrome. *Am Rev Respir Dis* 1986;134:12–16.

20. Johanson WG, Higuchi JH, Chaudhuri TR, Woods DE. Bacterial adherence to epithelial cells in bacterial colonization of the respiratory tract. *Am Rev Respir Dis* 1980;121:55–61.

21. Dal Nogare AR, Toews GB, Pierce AK. Increased salivary elastase precedes gram-negative bacillary colonization in the postoperative patient. *Am Rev Respir Dis* 1987;135:671–675.

22. Palmer LB, Merrill WW, Niederman MS, Ferranti RD, Reynolds HY. Bacterial adherence to respiratory tract cells. Relationships between *in vivo* and *in vitro* pH and bacterial attachment. *Am Rev Respir Dis* 1986;133:384–388.

23. Niederman MS, Mantovani R, Schoch P, Papas J, Fein AM. Patterns and routes of tracheobronchial colonization in mechanically ventilated patients. The role of nutritional status in colonization by *Pseudomonas* species. *Chest* 1989;95:155–161.

24. Driks MR, Craven DE, Celli BR, et al. Nosocomial pneumonia in intubated patients given sucralfate as compared with antacids or histamine type 2 blockers. *N Engl J Med* 1987;317:1376–1382.

25. Du Moulin GC, Hedley-White J, Paterson DG, Lisbon A. Aspiration of gastric bacteria in antacid treated patients. *Lancet* 1982;2:242–245.

26. Johanson WG, Seidenfeld JJ, Gomez P, de los Santos R, Coalson JJ. Bacteriologic diagnosis of nosocomial pneumonia following prolonged mechanical ventilation. *Am Rev Respir Dis* 1988;137:259–264.

27. Torres A, De la Bellacasa JP, Xaubet A, et al. Diagnostic value of quantitative cultures of bronchoalveolar lavage and telescoping plugged catheters in mechanically ventilated patients with bacterial pneumonia. *Am Rev Respir Dis* 1989;140:306–310.

28. Chastre J, Fagon J-Y, Soler P, et al. Diagnosis of nosocomial bacterial pneumonia in intubated patients undergoing ventilation: comparison of the usefulness of bronchoalveolar lavage and the protected specimen brush. *Am J Med* 1988;85:499–506.

29. Campbell GD, Woods DE. Diagnosis of gram-negative bacillary pneumonia in an animal model using a competitive ELISA technique to detect the presence of lipid A. *Am Rev Respir Dis* 1986;133:861–865.

30. Salata RA, Lederman MM, Shlaes DM, et al. Diagnosis of nosocomial pneumonia in intubated, intensive care unit patients. *Am Rev Respir Dis* 1987;135:426–432.

31. Tryba M. Risk of acute stress bleeding and nosocomial pneumonia in ventilated intensive care unit patients: sucralfate vs antacids. *Am J Med* 1987;83(suppl 3B):117–124.

32. Haake R, Schlichtig R, Ulstad DR, Henschen RR. Barotrauma: pathophysiology, risk factors, and prevention. *Chest* 1987;91:608–613.

33. Macklin MT, Macklin CC. Malignant interstitial emphysema of the lungs and mediastinum as an important occult complication in many respiratory diseases and other conditions. *Medicine (Baltimore)* 1944;23:281–352.

34. Woodring JH. Pulmonary interstitial emphysema in the adult respiratory distress syndrome. *Crit Care Med* 1985;13:786–791.

35. Gobien RP, Reines HD, Schabel SI. Localized tension pneumothorax: unrecognized form of barotrauma in adult respiratory distress syndrome. *Radiology* 1982;142:15–19.

36. Pierson DJ. Persistent bronchopleural air leak during mechanical ventilation: a review. *Respir Care* 1982;27:408–416.

37. Zapol WM, Falke KJ. *Acute respiratory failure.* New York: Marcel Dekker, 1985.

38. Fowler AA, Hamman RF, Good JT, et al. Adult respiratory distress syndrome: risk with common predispositions. *Ann Intern Med* 1983;98:593–597.

39. Bachofen M, Weibel ER. Alterations of the gas exchange apparatus in adult respiratory insufficiency associated with septicemia. *Am Rev Respir Dis* 1977;116:589–615.

40. Zimmerman GA. Cardiovascular alterations in the adult respiratory distress syndrome. *Am J Med* 1982;73:25–34.

41. Parillo JE, Burch C, Shelhamer JH, Parker MM, Natanson C, Schuette W. A circulating myocardial depressant substance in humans with septic shock. *J Clin Invest* 1985;76:1539–1553.

42. Bernard GR, Luce JM, Sprung CL, et al. High-dose corticosteroids in patients with the adult respiratory distress syndrome. *N Engl J Med* 1987;317:1565–1570.

43. Pepe PE, Hudson LD, Carrico CJ. Early application of positive end-expiratory pressure in patients at risk for the adult respiratory distress syndrome. *N Engl J Med* 1984;311:281–286.

44. Kolobow T, Moretti MP, Fumagalli R, et al. Severe impairment in lung function induced by high peak airway pressure during mechanical ventilation. An experimental study. *Am Rev Respir Dis* 1987;135:312–315.

45. Borelli M, Kolobow T, Spatola R, Prato P, Tsuno K. Severe acute respiratory failure managed with continuous positive airway pressure and partial extracorporeal carbon dioxide removal by an artificial membrane lung. A controlled randomized animal study. *Am Rev Respir Dis* 1988;138:1480–1487.

46. Pesenti A, Kolobow T, Gattinoni L. Extracorporeal respiratory support in the adult. *ASAIO Trans* 1988;34:1006–1008.

47. Hull R, Hirsh J, Sackett DL. The combined use of leg scanning and impedance plethysmography in suspected venous thrombosis: an alternative to venography. *N Engl J Med* 1977;296:1497–1502.

48. Kakkar VV. The diagnosis of deep vein thrombosis using the [^{125}I]fibrinogen test. *Arch Surg* 1972;104:152–156.

49. Goldhaber SZ, Vaughan DE, Markis JE, et al. Acute pulmonary

embolism treated with tissue plasminogen activator. *Lancet* 1986;2:886–889.

50. Kanter B, Moser KM. The Greenfield venal cava filter. *Chest* 1989;93:170–175.

51. Pingleton SK, Bone RC, Pingleton WW, Ruth WE. Prevention of pulmonary emboli in a respiratory intensive care unit. Efficacy of low dose heparin. *Chest* 1981;79:647–650.

52. Butson ARC. Intermittent pneumatic calf compression for prevention of deep venous thrombosis in general abdominal surgery. *Am J Surg* 1981;142:525–527.

53. Skillman JJ, Collins REC, Coe NP, et al. Prevention of deep vein thrombosis in neurosurgical patients: a controlled, randomized trial of external compression boots. *Surgery* 1978;83:354–358.

54. Murciano D, Aubier M, Bussi S, Derenne J-P, Pariente R, Milic-Emili J. Comparison of esophageal, tracheal, and mouth occlusion pressure in patients with chronic obstructive pulmonary disease during acute respiratory failure. *Am Rev Respir Dis* 1982;126:837–841.

55. Tuxen DV, Lane S. The effects of ventilatory pattern on hyperinflation, airway pressures, and circulation in mechanical ventilation of patients with severe air-flow obstruction. *Am Rev Respir Dis* 1987;136:872–879.

56. Pepe PE, Marini JJ. Occult positive end-expiratory pressure in mechanically ventilated patients with airflow obstruction. *Am Rev Respir Dis* 1982;126:166–170.

57. Rossi A, Gottfried SB, Zocchi L, et al. Measurement of static compliance of the total respiratory system in patients with acute respiratory failure during mechanical ventilation. *Am Rev Respir Dis* 1985;131:672–677.

58. Mathru M, Rao TLK, Venus B. Ventilator-induced barotrauma in controlled mechanical ventilation versus intermittent mandatory ventilation. *Crit Care Med* 1983;11:359–361.

59. Darioli R, Perret C. Mechanical controlled hypoventilation in status asthmaticus. *Am Rev Respir Dis* 1984;129:385–387.

60. Ross EA, Tashkin D, Chenoweth D, Webber MM, Nissenson AR. Pulmonary leukosequestration without hypoxemia during hemodialysis. *Int J Artif Organs* 1987;10:367–374.

61. Dolan MJ, Whipp BJ, Davidson WD, Weitzman RE, Wasserman K. Hypopnea associated with acetate hemodialysis: carbon dioxide-flow-dependent ventilation. *N Engl J Med* 1981;305:72–75.

62. Patterson RW, Nissenson AR, Miller J, Smith RT, Narins RG, Sullivan SF. Hypoxemia and pulmonary gas exchange during hemodialysis. *J Appl Physiol* 1981;50:259–264.

63. Leunissen KML, Hoorntje SJ, Fiers HA, Dekkers WT, Mulder AW. Acetate versus bicarbonate hemodialysis in critically ill patients. *Nephron* 1986;42:146–151.

64. Ramirez G, Collice GL, James S, Johns CC, Nelson WP. Increase in P_{50} with the use of bicarbonate hemodialysis. *Int J Artif Organs* 1987;10:361–366.

65. Bynum LJ, Pierce AK. Pulmonary aspiration of gastric contents. *Am Rev Respir Dis* 1976;114:1129–1136.

66. Winterbauer RH, Durning RB, Barron E, McFadden MC. Aspirated nasogastric feeding solution detected by glucose strips. *Ann Intern Med* 1981;95:67–68.

67. Hickling KG, Howard R. A retrospective survey of treatment and mortality in aspiration pneumonia. *Intensive Care Med* 1988;14:617–622.

68. Saw EC, Gottlieb LS, Yokoyama T, Lee BC. Flexible fiberoptic bronchoscopy and endobronchial tamponade in the management of massive hemoptysis. *Chest* 1976;70:589–591.

69. Stoll JF, Bettman MA. Bronchial artery embolization to control hemoptysis: a review. *Cardiovasc Intervent Radiol* 1988; 11:263–269.

70. Pittinger C, Adamson R. Antibiotic blockade of neuromuscular function. *Annu Rev Pharmacol* 1972;120:169–184.

71. Arora NS, Rochester DF. Effect of body weight and muscularity on human diaphragm muscle mass, thickness, and area. *J Appl Physiol* 1982;52:64–70.

72. Thurlbeck WM. Diaphragm and body weight in emphysema. *Thorax* 1978;33:483–487.

73. Doekel RC, Zwillich CW, Scoggin CH, Kryger M, Weil JV. Clinical semistarvation: depression of hypoxic ventilatory response. *N Engl J Med* 1976;295:358–361.

74. Driver AG, LeBrun M. Iatrogenic malnutrition in patients receiving ventilatory support. *JAMA* 1980;244:2195–2196.

75. Bassili HR, Deitel M. Effect of nutritional support on weaning patients off mechanical ventilators. *J Parenter Ent Nutr* 1981; 5:161–163.

76. Aubier M, Murciano D, Lecocguic Y, et al. Effect of hypophosphatemia on diaphragmatic contractility in patients with acute respiratory failure. *N Engl J Med* 1985;313:420–424.

77. Knochel JP. Hypophosphatemia. *West J Med* 1981;134:15–26.

78. Laroche CM, Cairns T, Moxham J, Green M. Hypothyroidism presenting with respiratory muscle weakness. *Am Rev Respir Dis* 1988;138:472–474.

79. Murphy BP, Harford FJ, Cramer FS. Cerebral air embolism resulting from invasive medical procedures. Treatment with hyperbaric oxygen. *Ann Surg* 1985;201:242–245.

80. Gottdiener JS, Papademetriou V, Notargiacomo A, Park WY, Cutler DJ. Incidence and cardiac effects of systemic venous air embolism. Echocardiographic evidence of arterial embolization via noncardiac shunt. *Arch Intern Med* 1988;148:795–800.

81. Flick MR, Hoeffel JM, Staub NC. Superoxide dismutase with heparin prevents increased lung vascular permeability during air emboli in sheep. *J Appl Physiol* 1983;55:1284–1291.

82. Flick MR, Milligan SA, Hoeffel JM, Goldstein IM. Catalase prevents increased lung vascular permeability during air emboli in unanesthetized sheep. *J Appl Physiol* 1988;64:929–935.

83. Kobayashi H, Kobayashi T, Kukushima M. Effects of dibutyryl cAMP on pulmonary air embolism-induced lung injury in awake sheep. *J Appl Physiol* 1987;63:2201–2207.

84. Bonsignore MR, Jerome EH, Culver PL, Dodek PM, Staub NC. Effects of beta-adrenergic agents in lungs of normal and air-embolized awake sheep. *J Appl Physiol* 1988;64:2647–2652.

85. Oka Y, Moriwaki KM, Hong Y, et al. Detection of air emboli in the left heart by M-mode transesophageal echocardiography following cardiopulmonary bypass. *Anesthesiology* 1985; 63:109–113.

86. Horrow JC. Coronary air embolism during venous cannulation. *Anaesthesia* 1982;56:212–214.

87. Swenson RD, Weaver D, Niskanen RA, Martin J, Dahlberg S. Hemodynamics in humans during conventional and experimental methods of cardiopulmonary resuscitation. *Circulation* 1988; 78:630–639.

88. Nowak RM, Martin GB, Carden DL, Tomlanovich MC. Selective venous hypercarbia during human CPR: implications regarding blood flow. *Ann Emerg Med* 1987;16:527–530.

89. Gudipati CV, Weil MH, Bisera J, Deshmukh HG, Rackow EC. Expired carbon dioxide: a noninvasive monitor of cardiopulmonary resuscitation. *Circulation* 1988;77:234–239.

90. Garnett AR, Ornato JP, Gonzalez ER, Johnson EB. End-tidal carbon dioxide monitoring during cardiopulmonary resuscitation. *JAMA* 1987;257:512–515.

91. Gazmuri RJ, von Planta M, Weil MH, Rackow EC. Arterial P_{CO_2} as an indicator of systemic perfusion during cardiopulmonary resuscitation. *Crit Care Med* 1989;17:237–240.

92. von Planta M, Gudipati CV, Weil MH, Kraus LJ, Rackow EC. Effects of tromethamine and sodium bicarbonate buffers during cardiac resuscitation. *J Clin Pharmacol* 1988;28:594–599.

THE LUNG: Scientific Foundations
edited by R.G. Crystal, J.B. West et al.
Raven Press, Ltd., New York © 1991.

CHAPTER 8.2.6

Extracorporeal Membrane Lung Gas Exchange

Warren M. Zapol and Theodor Kolobow

Extracorporeal membrane oxygenation (ECMO) for the support of patients with severe acute respiratory failure (ARF) has been practiced for over 20 years (1). Perfusion with a membrane lung corrects hypoxemia and hypercapnia while relieving the patient's lungs of their primary burden of respiratory gas exchange. During perfusion the F_IO_2 and peak ventilator pressure, possible sources of pulmonary injury, can be lowered, while access to the airway permits safe tracheal suctioning and pulmonary lavage. In addition, venoarterial perfusion provides hemodynamic support. Recent clinical experience has shown that membrane lung venovenous bypass for 1–4 weeks can provide time for the injured adult lung to heal and that about half the patients recover (2). The present goals of adult extracorporeal gas exchange primarily focus on removing large amounts of CO_2 with the membrane lung while greatly reducing the respiratory rate and peak airway pressure (3). Lungs slowly inflated at high levels of positive end-expiratory pressure (PEEP) may provide better conditions for healing without producing barotrauma. In contrast, ECMO support of term newborns with reversible respiratory failure is nearly 90% successful (4). This chapter will review relevant membrane lung technology, modes of clinical perfusion and cannulation, hemodynamic adaptation to bypass, and the management of bypass. The results of treating pulmonary disorders with bypass are discussed.

ARTIFICIAL LUNG TECHNOLOGY

The artificial lung or blood oxygenator was clinically introduced in the early 1950s and opened the field of

W. M. Zapol: Department of Anesthesia, Massachusetts General Hospital, Boston, Massachusetts 02114.

T. Kolobow: Section on Pulmonary and Cardiac Assist Devices, NHLBI, National Institutes of Health, Bethesda, Maryland 20892.

modern cardiovascular surgery. The early disc oxygenators were soon replaced by bubble oxygenators because the latter were easier to use, produced acceptable blood trauma, and, most importantly, were disposable. Unfortunately, clinical use of bubble or disc oxygenators for over 12–24 hr was impossible because of progressive toxic effects; hence, prolonged extracorporeal support of respiratory failure patients was impossible.

Artificial lungs based upon the diffusion of respiratory gases across plastic membranes were first proven safe for respiratory assistance in animals for days to weeks (5). However, clinical use of the artificial lung was delayed until the early 1970s, when devices were developed that were efficient and leak-free, did not clot with heparinization, and were disposable after a single use. Currently, disposable membrane lungs are used for both short-term cardiovascular surgery and long-term extracorporeal gas exchange for respiratory failure. The membrane lung excels because of superior blood compatibility, excellent control of respiratory blood gas transport, low priming volume, low overall cost, and the future possibility of rendering blood contacting surfaces nonthrombogenic.

MEMBRANE PERMEABILITY TO GASES

Permselective Membranes

Transport of gases through synthetic membranes occurs via a process of activated diffusion and involves three steps. First, gas dissolves in the membrane at the side of higher concentration; it then diffuses through the membrane to the side of lowest concentration through a process that depends on the formation of "holes" in the polymer network due to thermal agitation of the chain segments; and finally, gas is desorbed into blood. The rate of gas transport depends upon the precise chemical composition of the polymer membrane and upon the nature of the gas. For example, the permeability of CO_2 in most synthetic membranes is nearly five times greater than that of oxygen (hence, the term *permselective membrane*). Diffusion is related to partial pressure gradient alone, not to external pressure, and rises exponentially with increasing temperature.

Total transport of gases through a polymer membrane is proportional to the total surface area and is inversely proportional to the thickness of the membrane. After it was discovered that the permeability to respiratory gases of silicone rubber membranes was several orders of magnitude greater than that of polyethylene or polytetrafluoroethylene, the modern membrane lung became a practical device.

Microporous Membranes

Gas transport across porous polymeric membranes is not selective, in contrast to that across permselective membranes. Gas transport increases with an increased pressure gradient, and it greatly decreases with increasing temperature.

Microporous polymeric membranes were first introduced into membrane lungs to overcome the limitation of a low gas diffusion rate of permselective membranes. Microporous membranes could be produced from polymers that exhibited virtually no gas transport as a solid sheet. Membrane thickness could be greatly increased, thereby augmenting the strength of the membrane. The micropores range from 0.01 to 1.0 μm and have heterogeneous sizes and shapes: They can be round or oval, slit-like or fibrillar passages. The hydrophobic nature of many microporous membranes prevents the passage of plasma and water across pores. However, there is always a critical pressure beyond which plasma and water will pass through micropores, causing a precipitous loss of gas transport. This pressure varies with time and may depend on the duration of use as well as on other uncertain factors. To avoid such a sudden decline of gas transport while taking advantage of a nonthrombogenic surface treatment, one can coat microporous membranes with an ultrathin layer of a permselective polymer, such as silicone rubber or polyalkylsulfone (6).

MEMBRANE LUNG DESIGN

It remains impossible to produce prosthetic capillary networks like the human lung, which has (a) a blood film thickness on the order of one red blood cell and (b) a length of under 1000 μm.

In plate and sheet membrane lungs, as well as in capillary-type membrane lungs, the usual width of the blood flow channel is near 200 μm, with a 20- to 40-cm blood path length. This yields a compromise between blood layer thickness, gas transport, and resistance to blood flow. As noted in the discussion of permselective membranes, diffusion of oxygen across membranes is highly dependent upon the properties of the membrane. Unfortunately, a layer of oxygenated blood adjacent to the membrane provides an additional barrier to the diffusion of oxygen and greatly reduces the efficiency of oxygen transport. Hence, great efforts are made to mix the stagnant layer of well-oxygenated blood, thereby exposing the membrane to desaturated red blood cells. This can be accomplished by making the surfaces of the membrane irregular (e.g., by incorporating a thin fabric mesh) or by imparting pulsatile motion to blood near the membrane (i.e., creating secondary flow patterns to stir up the stagnant boundary film) (7).

Unlike oxygen transport, the movement of CO_2 from red blood cells to plasma, and across the polymeric membrane, is much less impaired by the presence of a stagnant ''oxygenated blood membrane.'' As occurs with the natural lung, CO_2 removal primarily depends upon the ventilation rate of the membrane lung. Less CO_2 is removed when the membrane lung is hypoventilated.

The transport of oxygen across membrane lungs with permselective membranes is usually limited by the resistance of the imperfectly stirred layer of oxygenated blood adjacent to the permselective membrane; because of the far greater solubility of CO_2 in plasma, the transfer of CO_2 is primarily membrane-limited—that is, more CO_2 will be removed through thinner membranes. In membrane lungs with microporous membranes, the membrane poses no practical limitation to gas transport. Instead, virtually all diffusion resistance is due to the poorly stirred layer of blood adjacent to the microporous membrane.

REFERENCE BLOOD FLOW

Membrane lungs are rated by their oxygen and CO_2 transport under standard input and output conditions—that is, the *reference blood flow*.

1. *Oxygen reference blood flow.* This is the flow rate of whole blood at 37°C with a hemoglobin content of 12 g%, zero base excess, and an oxygen saturation of 65%, which has its oxygen content increased by 45 ml oxygen (STPD) per liter of blood flow by a single passage through the membrane lung.

2. *Carbon dioxide reference blood flow.* This is the flow rate of whole blood at 37°C when the CO_2 transfer rate is 45 ml CO_2 (STPD) per liter, with a mean input P_{CO_2} of 41 mmHg.

In essence, for an artificial lung the reference blood

flow for oxygen defines the maximum blood flow providing an output blood oxygen saturation above 95% (i.e., near full saturation). This reference flow does not allow distinguishing between the efficiency rates of devices needing more or less surface area to accomplish this task. The same holds true for the reference flow value of CO_2 transfer across the membrane lung.

In long-term clinical perfusion, it is worthwhile choosing a membrane lung with excess gas transport capacity to compensate for any increased metabolic demands and also to compensate for any deterioration of membrane lung performance. For enhanced performance, such as extensive CO_2 removal to reduce the need for tidal ventilation, several membrane lungs may be placed in series.

CANNULAS

Membrane lung perfusion of adults usually requires large extracorporeal blood flows of 40–90 ml/kg/min; large-bore cannulas must be used. We insert a specially fabricated thin-walled, steel-wire-reinforced, segmented polyurethane venous cannula [average adult size: 9.50-mm inside diameter (ID), 10.35-mm outside diameter (OD)] in the femoral vein (1). Proper placement of the cannula is confirmed radiologically at the time of cannulation. Locating the tip of the drainage cannula at the level of the diaphragm and the return catheter in the superior vena cava ensures minimal blood recirculation and adequate blood flow (3–6 liters/min). The tip of the drainage cannula can be placed in the right atrium for venoarterial perfusion.

For venovenous (VV) perfusion, Gattinoni et al. (8) have used (a) a double-lumen polyurethane-reinforced catheter, with an external lumen (10.5-mm OD) for inferior vena cava blood drainage, and (b) an internal catheter (6.5-mm OD) for blood return. This technique has the advantage of requiring only a single venous cannulation but with reduced blood flow (1.5 to 2 liters/min). Saphenous vein percutaneous cannulation has also been recently performed in adults (9). In newborn infants, Bartlett et al. (10) report using thin-walled vinyl chest tubes for venous drainage and arterial return (12- to 14-French drain, 8- to 10-French arterial return). Kolobow et al. (11) have reported single-catheter venovenous bypass in premature lambs, using an alternating 1.2-sec drainage period and 0.8-sec return period provided by specially programmed occluding clamps.

PUMP AND LUNG

For adult perfusion we use silicone rubber tubing: 12.7-mm ID for the venous drain line and 9.5-mm ID for other tubing. Blood drains into a 75-ml collapsible ser-

voregulated silicone reservoir bag, which limits blood suction and avoids hemolysis. From the reservoir, blood is occlusively pumped by a roller pump using an extruded polyurethane pump chamber. This chamber can be safely used for periods of up to a month without rupture. It is not safe to use polyvinylchloride tubing for prolonged pumping periods, since it may rupture. Other groups report using a centrifugal blood pump for long-term bypass.

MEMBRANE LUNG

Most clinical groups now employ the Kolobow spiral-coil membrane lung for long-term perfusions (see Fig. 1); this discussion is limited to that device. We suggest a minimum of 0.5-m^2 membrane surface be used per 10 kg of body weight for partial assistance. For total pulmonary failure, a minimum of 1 m^2/10 kg body weight is required. Gattinoni et al. (8) report using two 3.5-m^2 spiral-coil lungs in series for venovenous perfusion with near total CO_2 transport. Bartlett et al. (10) report using 0.4- and 0.8-m^2 spiral-coil lungs for newborn perfusion. In our experience, spiral-coil silicone membrane lungs can withstand 1 atmosphere of transmembrane hydrostatic pressure for prolonged periods without rupture. Because pressure drop across this lung is low (a drop of 75–150 mmHg across a 3.5-m^2 device at 3 liters/min blood flow), it is safe to use a single pump for any perfusion route. The return cannula should be short and have a large diameter (greater than 6.4-mm ID in adults). Pressures greater than 400 torr in the blood return line are unsafe.

Spiral-coil membrane lungs have been used for clinical perfusion for over 2 weeks without thrombosis or deterioration of gas exchange. If a visible thrombus appears on the clear plastic outflow surface, or outflow saturation falls below 90%, suggesting decreased performance, the membrane lung should be changed.

The extracorporeal priming volume of the adult circuit is approximately 1350 ml. We prime with fresh whole blood with heparin added (4500 units/liter). We do not use an in-line filter, since the membrane lung itself acts as a filter for large thrombi. We incorporate an electromagnetic flow probe to measure extracorporeal blood flow. For newborn perfusion, Bartlett et al. (10) employ a heat exchanger. In adults we enclose the extracorporeal apparatus in a vinyl canopy and thermoregulate the ambient air temperature, thereby obviating the need for a heat exchanger. The patient's core temperature is maintained at 34–37°C.

Large-bore Y connectors (12.7-mm ID) occluded by tetrafluoroethylene plugs are placed in the blood tubing to permit replacement of the reservoir and pump chamber or to permit substitution or addition of membrane lungs, without stopping perfusion. These access points

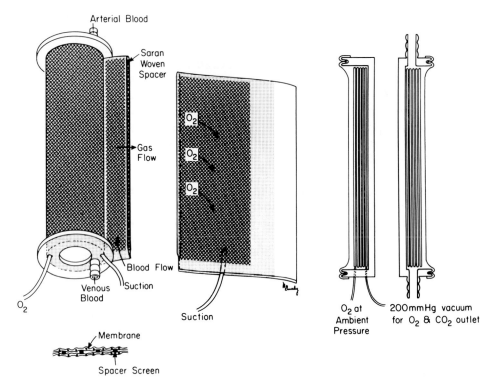

FIG. 1. Spiral coil. A 50-μm-thick, fabric-reinforced silicone rubber membrane surrounds a spacer screen and forms a closed envelope, equipped with gas inlet and gas outlet tubes. The envelope is wrapped around a central spool and is then covered with an elastic jacket. Blood flows between the layers of the membrane envelope. Gas (oxygen, or a mixture of oxygen and nitrogen) flows through the membrane lung either by suction or under slight positive pressure. Currently, the spiral-coiled membrane lung is the most widely employed artificial lung for long-term extracorporeal bypass for ARF. Under physiologic input conditions, it has a rated oxygen transport of 60–80 ml/m²·min and has comparable CO_2 transport rates.

are a necessity, especially for patients in whom there is progression to near-total pulmonary failure. Several silicone tubes (3.2-mm ID, 6.4-mm OD) are bonded to the circuit to allow heparin infusion, rapid volume transfusion, sampling, and pressure monitoring. Because blood cultures are required frequently, and venipuncture sites can bleed excessively during bypass, a self-sealing latex tube is attached to allow sterile needle puncture for bacteriological culture. All connecting tubes are continuously flushed with heparinized saline solution (10 ml/hr). The circuitry should be carefully inspected for defects, thrombosis, and other problems every 12 hr during perfusion.

CANNULATIONS

Cannulations can be performed under morphine analgesia (1 mg/kg). Extensive electrocautery is used to achieve hemostasis followed by a 30-min wait for coagulation before heparinization. The main drainage catheter is placed through the common femoral vein. The distal vein is drained to prevent venous hyperten-

sion and bleeding. If the proximal common femoral artery is cannulated, a single arteriotomy should be performed and a small catheter placed to provide arterial blood to the distal area of the leg. Femoral venipunctures should be avoided during the care of patients with acute respiratory failure; hematomas make cannulation far more difficult. No intramuscular or subcutaneous injections should be permitted. Incisions are closed in layers and then the skin is sutured. Antibacterial ointment and dry dressings are applied and changed daily. If bleeding occurs at a rate of more than 25 ml/hr from incision sites, the sites should be explored and electrocauterized. Recently, Pesenti (9) has performed percutaneous venous cannulation. Wound bleeding during bypass is then minimized.

PERFUSION ROUTES

There are now only two commonly used perfusion routes. Both require only one blood pump when used with the spiral-coil membrane lung (1).

Venovenous Perfusion

Venovenous (VV) perfusion is used in adults and children; VV or prepulmonary oxygenation allows the arterial tree to distribute oxygenated blood in a uniform pattern through the left ventricle. Venous blood can be drained from the inferior vena cava through the common femoral vein, and oxygenated blood is returned to the superior vena cava (see Fig. 2). Gattinoni et al. (8) have reported using a double-lumen catheter for venous blood drainage and arterialized return to the thoracic inferior vena cava (see section entitled "Cannulas," above, for description). Pesenti (9) has extensively used percutaneous saphenous perfusion route. In newborn infants, Bartlett et al. (10) have explored VV bypass using a double-lumen catheter placed in the internal jugular vein.

Venoarterial Perfusion (Femoral Artery Return)

Venoarterial (VA) perfusion decreases pulmonary blood flow. If mean pulmonary artery pressure decreases, the blood supply to lung regions with high pulmonary vascular resistance will be reduced and

smaller transcapillary filtration pressures can be expected. Hill et al. (12) reported that high-flow VA perfusion decreases the mean pulmonary artery pressure, but this was rarely observed in our VA or VV–VA perfusions, possibly because of extensive destruction of the lung's vasculature. Pulmonary necrosis may occur if pulmonary blood flow is markedly lowered during the adult respiratory distress syndrome (ARDS). VA perfusion is usually indicated when pulmonary artery pressures are high and right ventricular failure is present.

VA perfusion is more complex than VV perfusion and requires cannulation of the arterial system with a large-bore cannula. The common femoral artery is transected and cannulated both proximally and distally. After perfusion the artery is anastomosed end to end. False-aneurysm formation can occur after perfusion and may necessitate a vein graft. It may at times be advisable to replace the cannulated segment with a vein graft when the bypass is completed.

The major flaw of VA bypass is inappropriate distribution of arterialized blood. The highest arterial oxygen tensions occur in the region of femoral artery inflow. Oxygenated blood returned to the distal aorta is distributed to the kidneys, mesenteric bed, and lower

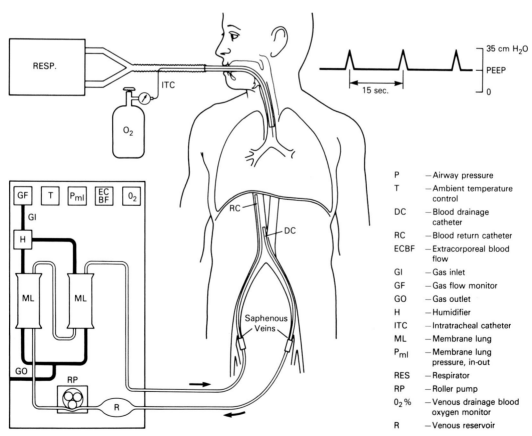

FIG. 2. Venovenous (VV) perfusion route with saphenosaphenous percutaneous cannulation. (From ref. 8.)

limbs (6). In severe acute respiratory failure, we frequently observed the combination of a large cardiac index, intrapulmonary right-to-left shunt greater than 50%, and a small arteriovenous oxygen content difference ($C_{A\bar{V}O_2}$). In these circumstances, the modest increase in venous oxygen saturation afforded by VA partial perfusion does not sufficiently increase the arterial oxygen tension of blood delivered to the heart and brain. Bartlett et al. (10) have reported using right common carotid artery return to the aorta in infant perfusion to improve cerebral oxygenation.

Placement of the return cannula tip at the aortic root permits uniform oxygenation of the systemic circulation, and the coronary arteries are perfused during diastole by extracorporeal oxygenated blood. Complete aortic root mixing of ECMO and pulmonary bloodstreams is established with this route. Thus, left ventricular blood gas tensions—and therefore natural pulmonary function—can be estimated during bypass from gas tensions of arterial blood (1).

Unlike during VV perfusion, a decrease in cardiac output during VA perfusion may alter the gas-exchange characteristics of the diseased lung. Hill et al. (12) have reported that VA perfusion occasionally decreases mean pulmonary artery pressure in severe ARF. When bypass is associated with a decrease in pulmonary blood flow, then the intrapulmonary right-to-left shunt (Q_S/Q_P) may decrease (13). This blood-flow-dependent increase in pulmonary efficiency must not be confused with improvement of pulmonary function resulting from resolution of the disease process. Markedly reduced pulmonary blood flow may promote thrombosis and necrosis of the injured lung as suggested by Ratliff et al. (14).

HEMODYNAMIC RESPONSE TO PARTIAL BYPASS

In ARF the circulatory response to bypass is complex and depends upon the site of cannulation, extracorporeal blood flow rate, distribution of oxygenated blood, and metabolic status (hypoxemia, acidosis, etc.). In addition, the following factors will modify the circulatory response to bypass: positive airway pressure; blood volume; drugs such as *d*-tubocurarine, pancuronium, and morphine; and inotropic and vasoactive agents. Disease-related changes in cardiac function, as well as injury to the pulmonary and systemic vascular beds, may also alter the circulatory response. Snider and Galletti (15) measured the normoxic circulatory response to bypass in anesthetized animals. Table 1 illustrates the hemodynamic changes with the two common bypass modes. The magnitude of change is proportional to extracorporeal blood flow. With a large-bore venous drainage cannula, over 80% of the

TABLE 1. *Hemodynamic responses to extracorporeal perfusion in normoxic normal animals by the venovenous (VV) and venoarterial (VA) routes*

	VA	VV
Heart rate	↓	→
Cardiac output	↓	→
Total systemic flow	→	→
Mean pulmonary artery pressure	↓	→
Mean systemic artery pressure	↑	→
Contractility	↓	→
Systemic vascular resistance	→	→
Pulmonary vascular resistance	→	→
Right ventricular end-diastolic volume	↓	→
Left ventricular end-diastolic volume	↓	→

pre-bypass cardiac output can be pumped from vein to artery. VA bypass partially empties, whereas arteriovenous (AV) bypass increases the filling of, the right ventricle. Ventricular filling determines cardiac output by the Frank–Starling mechanism. Heart rate, afterload, and contractile state are modified by changes in arterial baroreceptor stimulation. Decreased cardiac output at constant systemic blood flow during VA bypass in animals is accompanied by diminished end-diastolic right and left ventricular volumes, bradycardia, decreased myocardial contractility, narrowed arterial pulse pressure, increased mean arterial pressure, and decreased pulmonary arterial pressure. Increased cardiac output with AV bypass is accompanied by opposite changes.

In VA perfusion in dogs the cardiac output and extracorporeal blood flow rates increase during hypervolemia, whereas cardiac output and extracorporeal flow rate are decreased during hypovolemia (16). In contrast, VV pumping does not modify hemodynamic values of normoxic anesthetized animals. The effects relate to altered blood gas tensions.

Hypoxemia and hypercapnia are common in severe ARF. Hultgren and Grover (16) describe the major hemodynamic responses to alveolar hypoxia as tachycardia, increased cardiac output, and pulmonary hypertension with unchanged systemic arterial blood pressure. Hypoxemic changes become marked when $P_{a}O_2$ is less than 40 mmHg. During severe ARF, hypercapnia can cause systemic hypertension as a result of an elevated systemic vascular resistance. Hemodynamic changes accompanying bypass for ARF may be partly due to the amelioration of hypoxemia and hypercapnia.

PULMONARY VASCULAR RESISTANCE

Severe ARF is generally accompanied by a two- to fivefold increase in pulmonary vascular resistance (17). Bachofen and Weibel (18) used morphometric techniques and demonstrated reduced alveolar vascular volume in specimens of lung after severe clinical ARF. Greene et al. (19) demonstrated widespread occlusion of the pulmonary vascular bed in ARF. The causes of diffuse vascular obstruction are poorly understood, yet its clinical consequences are clear: pulmonary hypertension, increased right ventricular dysfunction, and an inability to lower pulmonary arterial pressures significantly despite a 50% reduction of pulmonary blood flow rate (17).

MEASUREMENT OF PULMONARY BLOOD FLOW

Accurate measurements of cardiac output during VA and VV bypass may be difficult to obtain. Right atrial injection of indicator can cause diversion of part of the bolus into the extracorporeal drainage cannula. Advancing the injection site into the right ventricle minimizes this problem. Indicator dilution techniques are usually accurate when right ventricular or pulmonary-artery injection is performed during VV bypass or VA bypass with aortic root return; they are often erroneous when performed during VA femoral perfusion, because the aorta is no longer a homogeneous compartment. Using a thermal indicator with pulmonary-artery temperature monitoring allows estimation of right ventricular end-diastolic volume and ejection fraction (20).

COAGULATION CONTROL

Although hemolysis and protein denaturation are minimal during membrane lung bypass, thrombocytopenia and hemorrhage are problems caused by both pulmonary disease and bypass. Many patients who have severe ARF develop thrombocytopenia (platelet count $<100,000/\mu l$). Diffuse intravascular coagulation (low platelet count, elevated partial thromboplastin time, and fibrin and fibrinogen degradation products) is present in 70% of ARF patients (21). All severe ARF patients studied have had a shortened platelet lifespan and increased platelet turnover (21).

Plasma coagulation factors are maintained during prolonged bypass in sheep, with minimal fibrin and fibrinogen breakdown; however, both sheep and human platelet counts decrease by 50–75% after 24 hr, and ^{51}Cr-labeled platelet lifespan is markedly shortened. Platelet aggregation in the bypass circuit and removal by the liver and spleen have been suggested as causes.

For safe clinical perfusion, the following factors appear to be helpful in maintaining adequate circulating platelet levels and in minimizing hemorrhage:

1. Highly thromboresistant materials should be used for pump chambers, tubing, connectors, and membrane lungs.

2. CO_2 or vacuum pre-priming of the circuit and lung is preferred to remove all air bubbles.

3. Extensive electrocautery of cannulation sites should be performed before heparinization to minimize surgical bleeding. A waiting period of 30 min or more is suggested before anticoagulation.

4. Initial anticoagulation in adults with 100 units heparin/kg body weight at the time of cannulation should be followed by precise control of heparin infusion to maintain the activated coagulation time (ACT) at 120–150 sec (normal: 90–110 sec) (22). The ACT measures kaolin-activated whole-blood clotting time and is a rapid method of monitoring the status of anticoagulation.

For infants, Andrews et al. (23) report maintaining the ACT at approximately 250 sec. Bartlett et al. (10) report measuring infant platelet concentration twice daily and maintaining the count above 50,000/mm^3 during infant perfusion.

RESULTS OF CLINICAL PARTIAL BYPASS FOR ARF

Since 1980 it can be estimated that 150 adult patients have undergone long-term VV bypass with membrane lungs for ARF.

About the time the NIH-sponsored, prospective, randomized VA bypass trial ended (24), Gattinoni et al. (3,8) reported animal and clinical studies with a modification of VV bypass. They employed large surface areas of membrane lungs (7 m^2 for an adult) at low blood flow rates (mean: 1.5 liters/min) with the goal of removing CO_2. This enabled them to employ extremely low ventilatory rates (4/min) with long inspiratory and expiratory periods. Pesenti et al. (2) have recently reported a review of prolonged VV bypass with this technique of 61 ARDS patients, 29 of whom are long-term survivors; on average, survivors underwent bypass for 7 days. In addition to hypoxemia refractory to an elevated $F_{I}O_2$ and 10–15 cmH$_2$O PEEP, these investigators required a total static lung compliance of less than 30 ml/cmH$_2$O in the ARDS patients they managed with VV bypass. Their belief that CO_2 removal is more beneficial than standard VV long-term bypass is based upon their desire to "rest" the diseased lungs and "assure in static conditions an optimal intrapulmonary distribution of gases and to avoid pressure-related complications of continuous positive pressure ventilation (CPPV)" (8). They note that alveolar units in ARDS lungs have various ventilatory gas flow time constants due to varying compliance and airway resistance. High lung volumes and pressures produced by CPPV produce hyperventilated and hypoventilated zones with blood flow diversion. They believe that low-frequency pulmonary ventilation with apneic diffusion and static inflation during VV bypass may allow a more even distribution of ventilatory gas with an improved V/Q distribution (2). Our group has reported angiographic (25) and pathological evidence (19) for widespread vascular occlusion in ARDS that causes regions of ischemic pulmonary necrosis. Alterations of ventilatory management alone are unlikely to alter this pathway to major lung injury, although bypass may reduce added pulmonary injury due to high-pressure mechanical ventilation.

One must admire the determination and effort of Gattinoni's group in Milan as well as that of the group in Marburg, West Germany, with 40 perfusions and 22 survivors (2). A randomized prospective study comparing VV bypass with a control group using standard mechanical ventilation is now in progress in the United States.

In a review of 715 newborns treated by ECMO in 18 neonatal care centers during 1980–1987, Toomasian et al. (4) reported an overall survival of 81%. The most common diagnoses were meconium aspiration (91% survival), respiratory distress syndrome (78% survival), congenital diaphragmatic hernia (65% survival), and sepsis (72% survival). Average pre-ECMO values were: age 59 hr, $P_{a}O_2$ 42 mmHg, $P_{a}CO_2$ 41 mmHg, pH 7.40, $F_{I}O_2$ 1.0, airway pressure 45/4 cmH$_2$O, and respiratory rate 93 breaths/min. They concluded that ECMO and lung rest were successful in the treatment of neonates unresponsive to conventional respiratory therapy. They also concluded that many etiologies of respiratory failure were potentially reversible in term and near-term neonates.

We believe that the single-catheter VV perfusion technique of Kolobow et al. (11) and the double-lumen catheters of Bartlett should be studied during infant perfusion. Such VV perfusion techniques may obviate the necessity for internal carotid ligation during newborn VA perfusion.

In the future, clinical studies of bypass will proceed in tandem with efforts to understand and reverse the acute destructive processes in the natural lung. Only in this manner will we learn to prevent death from overwhelming acute lung injury.

REFERENCES

1. Zapol WM, Snider MT, Schneider RC. Extracorporeal membrane oxygenation for acute respiratory failure. *Anesthesiology* 1977;46(4):272–285.
2. Pesenti A, Kolobow T, Gattinoni L. Extracorporeal respiratory support in the adult. *ASAIO Trans* 1988;34:1006–1008.
3. Gattinoni L, Pesenti A, Kolobow T, Damia G. A new look at
3. Gattinoni L, Pesenti A, Kolobow T, Damia G. A new look at therapy of the adult respiratory distress syndrome: motionless lungs. *Int Anesthesiol Clin* 1983;21:97–117.
4. Toomasian JM, Snedecor SM, Cornell RG, Cilley RE, Bartlett RH. National experience with extracorporeal membrane oxygenation for newborn respiratory failure. *ASAIO Trans* 1988;34:140–147.
5. Boucher R, Zapol WM, Snider MT. Week long partial pulmonary bypass with an artificial lung pumped by the right ventricle. *Trans Am Soc Artif Intern Organs* 1977;23:445–448.
6. Ketteringham JM, Zapol W, Gray DN, Stevenson KK, Massucco AA, Nelson LL, Cullen CP. Polyalkysulfone: a new polymer for membrane oxygenators. *Trans Am Soc Artif Intern Organs* 1973;19:61.
7. Bellhouse BJ, Bellhouse FH, Curl CM, et al. A high efficiency membrane oxygenator and pulsatile pumping system, and its application to animal trials. *Trans Am Soc Artif Intern Organs* 1973;19:72–79.
8. Gattinoni L, Pesenti A, Caspani ML, et al. The role of total static lung compliance in the management of severe ARDS unresponsive to conventional treatment. *Intensive Care Med* 1984;10:121–126.
9. Pesenti A. Saphenous vein percutaneous cannulation. Personal communication.
10. Bartlett RH, Andrews AR, Toomasian JM, et al. Extracorporeal membrane oxygenation for newborn respiratory failure: forty-five cases. *Surgery* 1982;92:425–433.
11. Kolobow T, Fumagalli R, Arosio P, et al. The use of the extracorporeal membrane lung in the successful resuscitation of severely hypoxic and hypercapnic fetal lambs. *Trans Am Soc Artif Intern Organs* 1982;28:365–368.
12. Hill JD, DeLaval MR, Fallat RJ, et al. Acute respiratory insufficiency: treatment with prolonged extracorporeal oxygenation. *J Thorac Cardiovas Surg* 1972;64:551.
13. Zapol WM, Qvist J, Pontoppidan H, et al. Extracorporeal perfusion for acute respiratory failure: recent experience with the spiral coil membrane lung. *J Thorac Cardiovasc Surg* 1975;69:439–449.
14. Ratliff JL, Hill JD, Fallat RJ, et al. Complications associated with membrane lung support by venoarterial perfusion. *Ann Thorac Surg* 1975;19:537–539.
15. Snider MT, Galletti PM. Left ventricular adaptation to partial heart–lung bypass and arteriovenous pumping. *Trans Am Soc Artif Intern Organs* 1968;15:311–315.
16. Hultgren HN, Grover RT. Circulatory adaptation to high altitude. *Annu Rev Med* 1968;19:119–166.
17. Zapol WM, Snider MT. Pulmonary hypertension in severe acute respiratory failure. *N Engl J Med* 1977;296:476–480.
18. Bachofen M, Weibel E. Basic pattern of tissue repair in human lungs following unspecific injury. *Chest* 1974;65:145–195.
19. Tomashefski JF, Davies P, Boggis C, Greene R, Zapol WM, Reid LM. The pulmonary vascular lesions of the adult respiratory distress syndrome. *Am J Pathol* 1983;112:112–126.
20. Hurford WE, Zapol WM. The right ventricle and critical illness: a review of anatomy, physiology, and clinical evaluation of its function. *Int Care Med* 1987;2:270–281.
21. Schneider R, Zapol WM, Carvalho A. Platelet consumption and sequestration in severe acute respiratory failure. *Am Rev Respir Dis* 1980;122:445–451.
22. Hatterslea PG. Activated coagulation time in whole blood. *JAMA* 1966;196:436.
23. Andrews AF, Klein MD. Toomasian JM, et al. Venovenous extracorporeal membrane oxygenation in neonates with respiratory failure. *J Pediatr Surg* 1983;18:339–346.
24. Zapol WM, Snider MT, Hill JD, et al. Extracorporeal membrane oxygenation in severe acute respiratory failure: a randomized prospective study. *JAMA* 1979;242:2193–2196.
25. Greene R, Zapol WM, Snider MT, et al. Early bedside detection of pulmonary vascular occlusion during acute respiratory failure. *Am Rev Respir Dis* 1981;124:593–601.

THE LUNG: *Scientific Foundations*
edited by R.G. Crystal, J.B. West et al.
Raven Press, Ltd., New York © 1991.

CHAPTER 8.2.7

The Lung Following Transplantation

Thomas M. Egan and J. D. Cooper

Following Hardy's initial attempt at human lung transplantation in 1963 (1), thoracic surgeons were frustrated for 20 years in their attempt to successfully transplant the lung. By 1980, kidney, liver, and heart transplantation were established as appropriate procedures for some types of irreversible failure of these organs. Progress with lung transplantation lagged behind these other organs, in part because of problems unique to the lung. The lung is a delicate organ that can develop significant dysfunction in response to minor insult. The interface of the outside environment to the large surface area that the lung affords is potentially dangerous in an immunocompromised host. The lung is the only solid organ that is transplanted without restoration of systemic arterial supply.

The resultant airway ischemia was identified as a reason for failed healing at the airway anastomosis in animal studies (2,3). The deleterious effect of high-dose steroids on wound healing was also a contributing factor to bronchial anastomotic disruption (4). Following the demonstration that omentopexy could provide systemic blood supply to an airway anastomosis (5) and the demonstration that cyclosporine-A did not interfere with bronchial healing (6), success in single-lung transplantation in the animal laboratory was demonstrated, even when steroids were withheld for 3 weeks (7). These techniques were applied successfully in humans in 1983 (8) in a patient with end-stage pulmonary fibrosis. Single-lung transplantation has become an option for selected individuals with end-stage fibrosis (9).

Heart–lung transplantation, pioneered by Reitz et al. (10) at Stanford University, provided another potential option for patients with end-stage lung disease. We reasoned that it should be possible to transplant a double-lung block without the heart, and thus we developed this procedure in an animal model (11). In 1986 the first successful double-lung transplant was performed at the University of Toronto (12) for end-stage chronic obstructive pulmonary disease (COPD). This has become an option for selected patients with end-stage obstructive or infective lung disease (13). Recently, single-lung transplantation for COPD has met with some success (14,15).

We have established a registry of isolated lung transplantation. Of the first 76 single-lung transplants performed between 1983 and April 1989, 60% of recipients are currently alive and well. Similar survival is the result of 49 double-lung transplants performed since 1986 (16). This chapter will review what is known about lung function following reimplantation or transplantation and will outline clinical problems peculiar to lung transplant recipients.

LUNG TRANSPLANTATION: INDICATIONS AND TECHNIQUE

Single-lung transplantation has become a therapeutic alternative for selected patients with end-stage restrictive lung disease (9). Double-lung transplant has been a therapeutic option in COPD and cystic fibrosis (i.e., patients with primarily obstructive physiology or infective end-stage lung disease) (13). Heart–lung transplantation has been utilized in patients with end-stage lung disease (17) but has had its largest application in patients with end-stage lung disease associated with right heart failure, including patients with primary pulmonary hypertension and Eisenmenger's syndrome. There is considerably more clinical experience with heart–lung transplantation than with isolated lung transplantation (18).

The technique of single-lung transplantation has

T. M. Egan: Department of Surgery, University of North Carolina at Chapel Hill School of Medicine, Chapel Hill, North Carolina 27599.

J. D. Cooper: Department of Thoracic Surgery, Washington University School of Medicine, St. Louis, Missouri 63110.

been detailed elsewhere (19). Briefly, it involves pneumonectomy through a thoracotomy with or without the aid of partial cardiopulmonary bypass. Following pneumonectomy the donor lung is reimplanted, using a cuff of donor left atrium that contains both pulmonary veins, a main pulmonary artery trunk, and a bronchial anastomosis that is protected by omentopexy. The technique for single-lung transplantation employed in humans differs little from that described by Metras (20) and Hardin and Kittle (21) almost 40 years ago. Double-lung transplant is a more complex operation, involving total cardiopulmonary bypass and bilateral pneumonectomy through a sternotomy, with positioning of a double-lung block through generous pericardial windows into each thorax. A circumferential left atrial anastomosis reconstructs the back wall of the recipient left atrium, the main pulmonary artery is anastomosed to the donor main pulmonary artery, and the airway anastomosis is performed either as a tracheal anastomosis or as two separate bronchial anastomoses (22,23). This technique evolved from methods first employed by Vanderhoeft et al. (24) and was adapted by the University of Toronto group for clinical application (11). In either case, omentopexy is used to protect the airway anastomoses.

Techniques of heart–lung transplantation were first successfully employed in humans by the Stanford group (10) and involve right atrial anastomosis, an aortic anastomosis, and a tracheal anastomosis. Omentopexy has generally not been required to protect the airway, presumably because of collateral circulation to the airway from pericardium and the coronary circulation.

All methods of lung transplantation result in denervation of the organs, interruption of the hilar lymphatics, and disruption of the arterial bronchial supply. Derangements of pulmonary physiology following transplantation can be related to one or more of these three features.

THE REIMPLANTED LUNG

An increase in extravascular water accompanies lung reimplantation in dogs (25). The data from these classic experiments are reproduced as Fig. 1. This increase in extravascular water persists for approximately 3 weeks and corresponds to the observation that lymphatics regenerate across the hilum in this time frame (26,27). Clinically, this corresponds to the observation that following double-lung transplantation, chest tubes frequently drain excessively for periods of more than 2 weeks. The effect of reimplantation on permeability is less clear. There is some evidence that permeability to radiolabeled sodium ions is altered in the reimplanted dog lung (28).

THE DENERVATED LUNG

The high mortality of early ligation of the opposite pulmonary artery following reimplantation in experimental animals confounded the role of pulmonary innervation. Vieth and Richards (29) very elegantly demonstrated that the increase in pulmonary vascular resistance that generally accompanied pulmonary reimplantation in laboratory animals was related to technical factors and could be entirely alleviated by providing a large enough outflow tract for the right ventricle. It was noted that late ligation of the pulmonary artery was better tolerated in laboratory animals. Potentially, this is related to the alterations in extravascular lung water alluded to above. Nagae et al. (30) clearly demonstrated a species difference with respect to the importance of pulmonary innervation. Whereas cats and dogs had very abnormal breathing patterns following bilateral pneumonectomy, primates breathed normally and short-term survival was possible following bilateral pulmonary reimplantation. Evidence of reenervation in dogs comes from documentation of bronchoconstriction following vagal stimulation 3–6 months post-reimplantation (31). Sympathetic reenervation can be demonstrated in dogs 45 months following pulmonary reimplantation (32).

In humans, the pattern of breathing following heart–lung transplantation or isolated lung transplantation is normal. Curiously, the pattern of breathing is unaffected in humans following bupivacaine inhalation (33), and sleep studies in survivors of heart–lung transplantation have documented normal breathing patterns (34).

Hyperresponsiveness to methacholine or histamine can be demonstrated in humans following heart–lung transplantation. Presumably, the loss of innervation may lead to an up-regulation of airway smooth muscle muscarinic receptor, a form of postdenervation hypersensitivity (35) (see Fig. 2). The clinical corollary is that inhaled bronchodilators may play a role in the jmanagement of patients following transplantation.

Mucociliary clearance is abnormal following transplantation. This can be demonstrated by tantalum bronchography in laboratory animals (36) and has been documented in humans (37). Altered mucociliary clearance may contribute to an increased susceptibility to infection in the early postoperative period. Mucociliary clearance does not appear to be related to ciliary beat frequency but may be a result of defective mucus. In dogs subjected to hilar stripping, pulmonary denervation, and bronchial division, mucus production is decreased in response to pilocapine administration (38).

Surfactant production appears not to be affected by reimplantation (39). Figure 3 supports the notion that

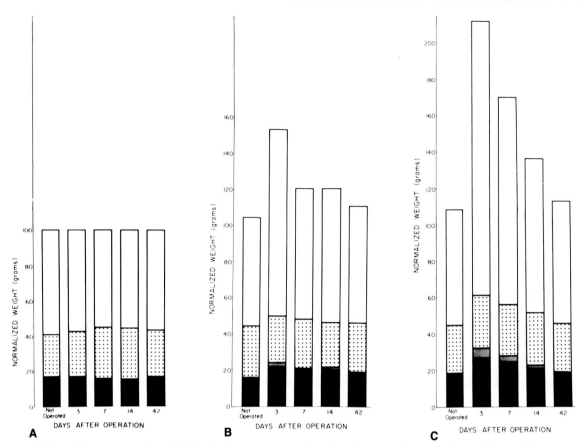

FIG. 1. Measurements of fluid in tissue compartments of canine lung subjected to left lung reimplantation. Solid black indicates dry weight, stippled area indicates circulating blood mass, cross-hatched area indicates non-circulating red cell mass, and white indicates extravascular lung water. Each bar represents the mean of five measurements. **A:** Graph showing data from the unoperated right lung of dogs subjected to a left lung reimplantation. No compartments in any group of right lungs differed significantly from the corresponding compartments in lungs of unoperated dogs. **B:** Graph showing the mean of five measurements of fluid in tissue compartments of left lower lobes from each group of dogs per 100 g predicted normal lobe weight. All compartments in reimplanted lobes studied 3–7 days after operation were significantly increased except for circulating blood mass and dry weight 7 days after operation. **C:** Graph showing similar data for the left upper middle lobes of dogs subjected to left lung reimplantation. The left upper middle lobe is the dependent lobe in the dog. All compartments in reimplanted left upper middle lobes studied 3–14 days after operation were significantly increased except for circulating blood mass. (Adapted from ref. 25.)

surfactant turnover is unaffected by reimplantation but may be adversely affected by transplantation. The resultant loss of surface tension and lung extracts can be prevented experimentally by immunosuppression, suggesting that surfactant production per se is not related to denervation.

Hypoxic pulmonary vasoconstriction following reimplantation may be species-specific, and it appears to be a recoverable phenomenon (40). In human recipients of heart–lung blocks tested 1 year postoperatively, the hypoxic vasoconstrictive reflex in the pulmonary circulation persists (41). No data are currently available on the early response to hypoxia.

To some extent the importance of pulmonary innervation has become moot following the clinical success of isolated lung and heart–lung transplantation. Nevertheless, the consequences of denervation may render the implanted lung more susceptible to infection and may promote a ventilation–perfusion imbalance until recovery of autonomic function occurs.

Recent studies have demonstrated a variable degree of cardiac denervation following double-lung transplantation (42). Evaluation of maximal heart rate after carotid sinus massage, after Valsalva maneuver, after intravenous atropine, and during the first 3 min of rest following a standardized exercise test was performed in four double-lung recipients and revealed a normal response in two patients, but the other two patients had minimal response, indicating at least some degree of cardiac denervation.

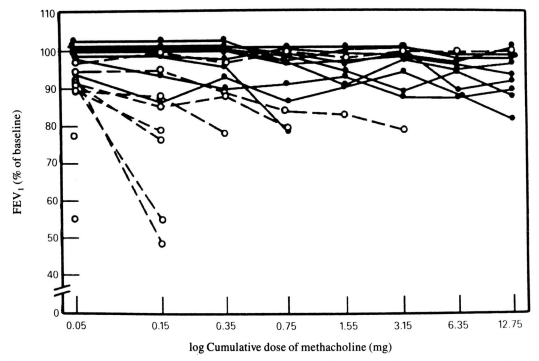

FIG. 2. Response of heart–lung transplant recipients (○) to inhaled methacholine compared with that of eight matched controls (●). Most heart–lung recipients demonstrate hypersensitivity to inhaled methacholine. (From ref. 35.)

EFFECTIVE PRESERVATION TECHNIQUES ON LUNG FUNCTION

Until recently we have utilized atelectatic cold immersion as a method of preserving lung blocks in humans. This has resulted in satisfactory lung function following transplantation that is unrelated to the degree of ischemic time (Fig. 4) up to 5 hr. We have begun to perfuse lung blocks at the time of harvesting in an effort to promote more uniform cooling. In addition, it is hoped that perfusion with the appropriate substance might prolong tolerable periods of ischemia. Currently no data are available to support this concept.

REJECTION FOLLOWING LUNG TRANSPLANTATION

The histology of pulmonary rejection has been defined extensively in canine models (43,44). The light-microscopic appearance of perivascular lymphocytic infiltration appears as early as the third or fourth postoperative day in dogs when no immunosuppression is used following lung transplantation (45). The predominance of perivascular inflammatory response corresponds to the localization of IgG and IgM deposits in subendothelial areas following canine lung transplantation (46).

Open-lung biopsy remains the "gold standard" for diagnosing rejection following transplantation, but it is impractical to employ this technique with any frequency. This has led to the evaluation of other techniques to monitor rejection. Transbronchial lung biopsy was evaluated in a canine model by Koerner et al. (47) and was found to be unreliable for documentation of rejection when compared with open-lung biopsy. Higenbottam et al. (48) have relied on this technique on heart–lung recipients. Although this is likely a specific method, its sensitivity remains unknown in the clinical setting. Because of the concern of morbidity associated with transbronchial lung biopsy, other, less invasive methods have been studied. The study of bronchoalveolar lavage (BAL) fluid in a canine model of single-lung transplant demonstrated that rejection was accompanied by an increase in the absolute number of lymphocytes recovered (49). In addition, lymphocytes recovered from the transplanted lung demonstrate a greater amount of cell-mediated lympholysis than do those recovered from the native (control) lung. This alteration in lymphocyte behavior appears to precede the radiographic changes of documented rejection (50). In a nonimmunosuppressed rat allograft model, an early increase in neutrophils (day 2) along with an increase in lymphocytes by day 4 was demonstrated in BAL fluid. The increase in BAL lymphocytes was reduced by treatment with cyclosporine-A (51). The earliest lymphocyte rise is related to an increase in T cells followed by an increase in B cells (52).

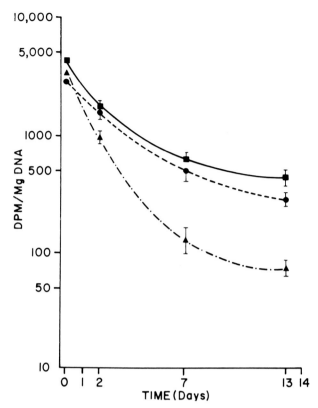

FIG. 3. Lung reimplantation had no effect on lipid radio-activity, as a reflection of surfactant turnover in dogs. Normal dogs (●) and dogs with reimplanted lungs (■) had similar surfactant turnover. Dogs with allotransplanted lungs (▲) had reduced surfactant turnover, presumably from consolidation in the rejected lung. DPM, lipid radioactivity decomposition rate per minute, an index of surfacant turnover. (From ref. 39.)

In human heart–lung recipients, observed proportions of macrophages, polymorphonuclear leukocytes, and lymphocytes are similar to those seen in animals. Unfortunately, cell profiles noted during rejection and infection frequently overlap (53). Zeevi et al. (54) doc-cumented the presence of activated T cells in BAL fluid following heart–lung transplantation, but the presence of these cells did not correlate with clinical episodes of rejection. Episodes of rejection were associated with an increase in the suppressor–cytotoxic cell population in BAL fluid, but similar increases in lymphocyte subsets were observed in the presence of cytomegalovirus (CMV) or pneumocystis infection (55).

Donor-specific assays show some promise at differentiating between infection and rejection in BAL fluid. Moeschl et al. (56) described a rosette-forming cell test and an indirect immunofluorescent test in an attempt to identify cellular and humoral immune response activity in a canine model of single-lung transplantation. Sections of the nontransplanted donor lung served as a target for indirect immunofluorescence. Organ-specific sensitization was detected as early as the fourth postoperative day. Dal Col and colleagues at the University of Pittsburgh have developed a donor-specific cytotoxicity test in a canine single-lung transplant model. Lymphocytes from the BAL are grown in culture and assessed for cytotoxicity by testing a responsiveness to lymphocytes obtained from the spleen of the donor animal (57). Another assay developed by this group involves incubation of BAL lymphocytes with irradiated lymphocytes obtained from the donor spleen. An index of proliferation of lymphocytes is obtained by measuring the incorporation of tritiated thymidine, with proliferation representing the degree of alloreactivity present in a particular culture (58). Application of these techniques following human lung transplantation may allow distinction between rejection and infection, but this remains to be established.

The search for a serum marker of rejection is complicated by the overlap of responses stimulated by rejection and infection. Soluble interleukin-2 (IL-2) receptor was shown to be elevated in human lung or

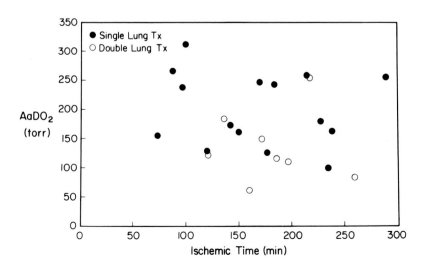

FIG. 4. Scattergram of arterial–alveolar gradient (AaDO$_2$) versus ischemic time in a human lung transplant recipient when the lung was preserved with cold atelectasis and topical cooling. There is no relationship between early AaDO$_2$ and ischemic time up to 300 min. (From ref. 16.)

heart–lung recipients during clinically suspicious episodes of rejection (59). However, in six heart transplant recipients, IL-2 receptor levels did not reflect rejection, but they increased during episodes of documented infection (60).

Rejection in dogs following single-lung transplantation is accompanied by reduced perfusion to the transplanted lung, documented by radionuclide perfusion scans (61). This implies that an increase in vascular resistance accompanies rejection. A similar reduction in perfusion is seen in humans during episodes of presumed rejection. The specificity of this response has not been established.

Clinical features of pulmonary rejection include a low-grade fever, increasing arterial–alveolar (Aa) gradient, reduced exercise capacity, and a leukocytosis. These are entirely nonspecific and can also accompany acute infection. Accordingly, every effort must be made to eliminate a diagnosis of infection, including quantitative culture methods and protected brushing (62). Ultimately, the response to a bolus of steroids is indirect evidence to secure a diagnosis of pulmonary rejection. The diagnosis of rejection remains illusory. To date, serum markers or BAL markers have not been able to distinguish between rejection and infection. Transbronchial biopsy may be useful but has not been evaluated extensively in isolated-lung transplants.

There is some reason to suspect that isolated-lung grafts may be immunologically distinct from heart–lung grafts. In support of this notion, the incidence of bronchiolitis obliterans, a common development following heart–lung transplantation (63), is markedly less in patients who have received an isolated-lung transplant. Recent work suggests an immune-mediated mechanism operative in the development of obliterative bronchiolitis, since the process may be attenuated by enhanced immunosuppression (64,65). Following heart–lung transplantation, the immune response engendered by the presence of both donor heart and lungs is different, since cardiac rejection occurs significantly less frequently than after isolated heart transplantation and is not correlated with lung rejection (66,67).

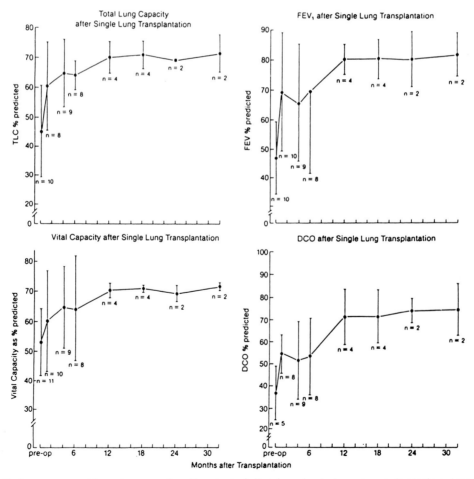

FIG. 5. Improvement in pulmonary function tests following single-lung transplantation. Improvement persists up to 30 months following transplantation. TLC, total lung capacity. (From ref. 16.)

INFECTION IN THE TRANSPLANTED LUNG

Infection is a serious hazard to the lung transplant recipient. All prospective lung donors are intubated and ventilated for a variable period of time, resulting in contamination of the airway. The denervated organ is impaired in its attempts to clear secretions, lymphatic clearance is abnormal, and the host is immunosuppressed to accommodate the new graft. These factors, along with the obligatory exposure of the air spaces to the outside environment, culminate in a high incidence of early postoperative infection. Recipients are routinely treated with antibiotics directed either at (a) pathogens identified from donor washings or (b) pathogens isolated early in the postoperative course. This aggressive approach has resulted in few cases of fulminant pneumonia following lung transplantation.

Infectious complications following lung transplantation have recently been reviewed (H. Vellend, *personal communication*). In the first 30 single- or double-lung transplants performed by the Toronto Lung Transplant Group, 32 infections occurred in 19 patients, most within 6 months of transplantation. Twenty of these 32 infections involved the chest. Seven patients who were seronegative for CMV received seropositive lungs. Two of these patients seroconverted but had no evidence of clinical infection. The only patient who developed fatal CMV pneumonia was seropositive and received a seronegative graft. CMV pneumonia has been a serious problem in heart–lung transplant recipients, leading to the recommendation that CMV status be matched between donor and recipient, just as ABO compatibility is required for a successful outcome (68). We have routinely employed pneumocystis prophylaxis with septra in all recipients and have begun to employ herpes prophylaxis with acyclovir.

CLINICAL COURSE FOLLOWING LUNG TRANSPLANTATION

Early gas exchange in the transplanted lung is variable and probably relates to both (a) the adequacy of preservation and (b) the use of cardiopulmonary bypass and its deleterious effects on the pulmonary circulation. Pulmonary compliance is less than normal in the early postoperative period, manifested by airway pressures that are mildly elevated. Mechanical ventilation is mandatory, usually for 2–3 days following single-lung transplant and frequently longer following double-lung transplant.

As a group, these patients present peculiar weaning problems. In particular, patients with obstructive lung disease develop poor inspiratory force that is often in-

adequate to allow them to ventilate their relatively noncompliant, small transplanted lungs. As a result, ventilatory weaning can be a demanding, exhausting process. Efforts must be made to allow patients to acquire both enough sleep and enough nutrition to facilitate weaning. We believe that these debilitated patients benefit from pretransplant reconditioning, which is performed routinely on prospective transplant recipients in a supervised setting where pulse rate and oximetry can be safely monitored.

Following extubation, the Aa gradient continues to improve as the radiologic evidence of congestion diminishes. Pleural drainage is required for prolonged periods, up to 2 weeks in some cases. This is likely a reflection of severed pulmonary lymphatics that require at least this amount of time for reestablishment at the hilum (69).

Improvement in pulmonary function following single-lung transplant is depicted in Fig. 5. This is paralleled by improvement in exercise capacity, assessed by 6-min walk tests in single-lung transplant recipients (Fig. 6) (70). Similar improvements in pulmonary function and exercise tolerance have been documented following double-lung transplantation (Figs. 7 and 8) (71). Following heart–lung transplantation, the Stanford group has documented a mild restrictive defect evidenced by a reduced vital capacity (72). The discrepancy between heart–lung recipients and double-lung recipients (73) is likely a reflection of the different patient populations and their chest sizes prior to transplantation. In general, double-lung recipients have had obstructive lung disease that has provided them with

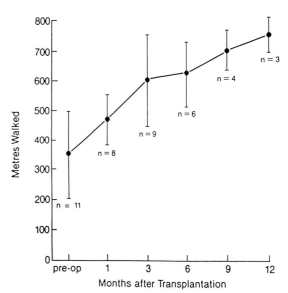

FIG. 6. Changes in exercise capacity following single-lung transplant as measured by performance in 6-min walk test. (From ref. 16.)

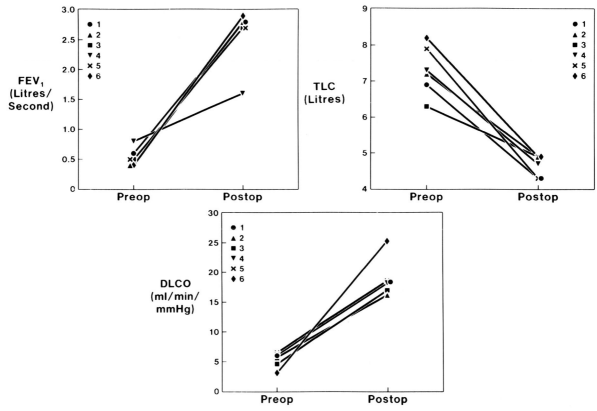

FIG. 7. Improvement in pulmonary function following double-lung transplant in the first six recipients of double-lung transplantation by the Toronto Lung Transplant Group. TLC, total lung capacity. (From ref. 16.)

an increased chest volume. In contrast, patients with pulmonary hypertension or Eisenmenger's syndrome frequently have a mild restrictive component at the time of their transplantation.

Following successful single-lung transplantation there is a progressive increase in blood flow to the transplanted lung, as documented by serial perfusion lung scans (70). In our experience, the mean perfusion to the transplanted lung is 66% at 1 week and 72% at 3 weeks, with subsequent gradual increase (9). Perfusion to the transplanted lung has been in excess of 80% in the first 24 hr in patients with elevated vascular resistance in the native lung (see Fig. 9).

AIRWAY HEALING FOLLOWING LUNG TRANSPLANTATION

High-dose methylprednisolone has a deleterious effect on wound healing, as evidenced by reduced breaking strength of skin wounds and of bronchial anastomoses in animals treated with methylprednisolone (4). Scanning electron micrographs of collagen bundles in wounds of animals treated with methylprednisolone show disorganized bundles that are markedly reduced in size (6). Neither cyclosporine nor azathioprine has any demonstrable deleterious effect on wound healing.

Interference with bronchoanastomotic healing because of steroids, coupled with the ischemia related to lack of arterial blood supply, undoubtedly contributed to early airway failures in the pre-cyclosporine era.

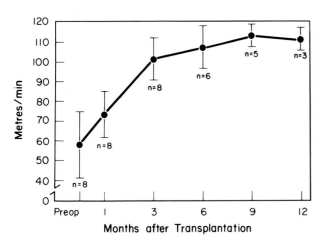

FIG. 8. Improvement in exercise following double-lung transplant as measured by performance in 6-min walk test. (From ref. 16.)

Bronchial omentopexy, coupled with cyclosporine immunosuppression and avoidance of steroids in the first 3 weeks following transplantation, has enabled lung transplantation to become a viable therapeutic option. Other methods to improve bronchial blood supply could potentially include wrapping the airway anastomosis with an intercostal muscle pedicle (74). The presence of pulmonary–bronchial collaterals has been documented in dogs (75,76), but it is unlikely that these are sufficient to allow for adequate airway healing. We have begun to evaluate a method of reimplantation of the right intercostal–bronchial artery as a pedicle following double-lung transplantation (77).

Despite these efforts, healing of the airway remains a source of morbidity following pulmonary transplantation. In a series of 17 single-lung transplants, airway necrosis caused one death. Two patients required insertion of silastic stents for anastomotic stenoses (78). One of these patients subsequently died from chronic rejection. Of 16 double-lung recipients in our experience, there have been three deaths directly related to airway necrosis or dehiscence, and two additional patients have required placement of silastic airway stents (79). Intraluminal silastic stents have been utilized as T tubes, as well as stents across stenoses in main-stem bronchi or stenoses involving the carina (80). These can be inserted endoscopically following dilatation and have been tolerated *in situ* for many months. Underlying airway healing has been documented.

THE FUTURE OF LUNG TRANSPLANTATION

Current areas of intense research include improved methods of preservation of the lung for extended periods. This research is providing insight into the mech-

anisms of lung injury following ischemia and potentially will allow improved donor and recipient matching. The search for a specific marker of rejection, either in serum or in BAL fluid, is ongoing in an effort to diagnose rejection earlier. Further characterization of bronchiolitis obliterans in heart–lung recipients may provide some insight into the mechanism of rejection following heart–lung transplantation.

The advent of isolated lung transplantation has provided hope for patients with end-stage lung disease of varying etiology. It would seem that it is now appropriate to offer single-lung transplant, double-lung transplant, or heart–lung transplant to selected patients with spectrums of end-stage lung disease. These immunosuppressed transplant patients will provide new challenges to transplant surgeons and pulmonologists. They will also provide a fascinating opportunity to learn more about pulmonary physiology and the natural history of the underlying pretransplant diseases of these patients.

REFERENCES

1. Hardy JD, Webb WR, Dalton ML, Walker GR. Lung homotransplantation in man. *JAMA* 1963;186:1065–1074.
2. Lima O, Goldberg M, Peters WJ, Ayabe H, Townsend E, Cooper JD. Bronchial omentopexy in canine lung transplantation. *J Thorac Cardiovasc Surg* 1982;83:418–421.
3. Mills NL, Boyd AD, Gheranpong C, Spencer F. The significance of bronchial circulation in lung transplantation. *J Thorac Cardiovasc Surg* 1970;60:866–878.
4. Lima O, Cooper JD, Peters WJ, Ayabe H, Townsend E, Luk SC, Goldberg M. Effects of methylprednisolone and azathioprine on bronchial healing following lung transplantation. *J Thorac Cardiovasc Surg* 1981;82:211–215.
5. Morgan E, Lima O, Goldberg M, Ferdman A, Luk SK, Cooper JD. Successful revascularization of totally ischemic bronchial autografts with omental pedicle flaps in dogs. *J Thorac Cardiovasc Surg* 1982;84:204–210.
6. Goldberg M, Lima O, Morgan E, Ayabe HA, Luk S, Ferdman A, Peters WJ, Cooper JD. A comparison between cyclosporin A and methylprednisolone plus azathioprine on bronchial healing following canine lung autotransplantation. *J Thorac Cardiovasc Surg* 1983;85:821–826.
7. Saunders NR, Egan TM, Chamberlain D, Cooper JD. Cyclosporine and bronchial healing in canine lung transplantation. *J Thorac Cardiovasc Surg* 1984;88:993–999.
8. The Toronto Lung Transplant Group. Unilateral lung transplantation for pulmonary fibrosis. *N Engl J Med* 1986;314:1140–1145.
9. The Toronto Lung Transplant Group. Experience with single lung transplantation for pulmonary fibrosis. *JAMA* 1988;259:2258–2262.
10. Reitz BA, Wallwork JL, Hunt SA, Pennock JL, Billingham ME, Oyer PE, Stinson EB, Shumway NE. Heart–lung transplantation: successful therapy for patients with pulmonary vascular disease. *N Engl J Med* 1982;306:557–564.
11. Dark JH, Patterson GA, Al-Jilaihawi AN, Hsu H, Egan T, Cooper JD. Experimental en bloc double-lung transplantation. *Ann Thorac Surg* 1986;42:394–398.
12. Patterson GA, Cooper JD, Dark JH, Jones MT, the Toronto Lung Transplant Group. Experimental and clinical double lung transplantation. *J Thorac Cardiovasc Surg* 1988;95:70–74.
13. Cooper JD, Patterson GA, Grossman R, Maurer J, the Toronto Lung Transplant Group. Double-lung transplant for advanced

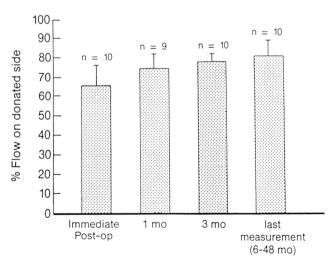

FIG. 9. Percents of perfusion to the transplanted side following single-lung transplant. At 3 months, the average perfusion to the transplanted lung approaches 80%.

chronic obstructive lung disease. *Am Rev Respir Dis* 1989;139:303–307.

14. Mal H, Andreassin B, Fabrice P, Duchatelle JP, Rondeau E, Dubois F, Baldeyrou P, Kitzis M, Sleiman C, Pariente R. Unilateral lung transplantation in end stage pulmonary emphysema. *Am Rev Respir Dis* 1989;140:797–802.

15. Trulock EP, Egan TM, Kouchoukos NT, Kaiser LR, Pasque MK, Cooper JD, the Washington University Lung Transplant Group. Single lung transplantation for severe chronic obstructive pulmonary disease: a case report. *Chest* 1989;96:738–742.

16. Egan TM, Kaiser LR, Cooper JD. Lung transplantation. *Curr Prob Surg* 1989;26:675–751.

17. Penketh A, Higenbottam T, Hakim M, Wallwork J. Heart and lung transplantation in patients with end stage lung disease. *Br Med J* 1987;295:311–314.

18. Heck CF, Shumway SJ, Kaye MP. The Registry of the International Society for Heart Transplantation: Sixth Official Report—1989. *J Heart Transplant* 1989;8:271–276.

19. Egan TM, Cooper JD. Technique of single lung transplantation. *Clin Chest Med* 1990;11:195–205.

20. Metras H. Note preliminaire sur la greffe totale du poumon chez le chien. *C R Acad Sci (Paris)* 1950;231:1176–1178.

21. Hardin CA, Kittle CF. Experiences with transplantation of the lung. *Science* 1954;119:97–98.

22. Noiclerc M, Metras D, Vaillant A, Cambouilives J, Couvely JP, Pannetier A, Garby O, Chazalette JP, Goudard A, Carcassone M. Technique chiururgicale de la transplantation bi-pulmonaire. *J Lyon Chir* 1989;3:247–251.

23. Patterson GA, Cooper JD, Goldman B, Weisel RD, Pearson FG, Waters PF, Todd TR, Scully H, Goldberg M, Ginsberg RJ. Technique of successful clinical double-lung transplantation. *Ann Thorac Surg* 1988;45:626–633.

24. Vanderhoeft P, Dubois A, Lauvau N, de Francquen P, Carpentier Y, Rocmans P, Nelson R, Kaufman S, Brickman L, Gyhra A, Ectors P. Block allotransplantation of both lungs with pulmonary trunk and left atrium in dogs. *Thorax* 1972;27:415–419.

25. Cowan GS, Staub NC, Edmunds LH. Changes in the fluid compartments and dry weights of reimplanted dog lungs. *J Appl Physiol* 1976;40:962–970.

26. Kline IK, Thomas PA. Canine lung allograft lymphatic alterations. *Ann Thorac Surg* 1976;21:532–535.

27. Eraslan S, Turner MD, Hardy JD. Lymphatic regeneration following lung reimplantation in dogs. *Surgery* 1964;56:970–973.

28. Yipintsoi T, Hagstrom JWC, Veith FJ. Pulmonary capillary permeability to sodium in unilateral transplanted canine lungs. *J Surg Res* 1979;27:353–358.

29. Veith FJ, Richards K. Lung transplantation with simultaneous contralateral pulmonary artery ligation. *Surg Gynecol Obstet* 1969;129:768–774.

30. Nagae S, Webb WR, Theodorides T, Sugg WL. Respiratory function following cardiopulmonary denervation in dog, cat, and monkey. *Surg Gynecol Obstet* 1967;125:1285–1292.

31. Edmunds LH, Graf PD, Nadel JA. Reinnervation of the reimplanted canine lung. *J Appl Physiol* 1971;31:722–727.

32. Lall A, Graf PD, Nadel JA, Edmunds LH. Adrenergic reinnervation of the reimplanted dog lung. *J Appl Physiol* 1973;35:439–442.

33. Winning AJ, Hamilton RD, Shea SA, Knott C, Guz A. The effect of airway anaesthesia on the control of breathing and the sensation of breathlessness in man. *Clin Sci* 1985;68:215–225.

34. Higenbottam T. Physiology of the transplanted lung and the results. In: Wallwork J, ed. *Heart and heart–lung transplantation.* Philadelphia: WB Saunders, 1989;533–544.

35. Glanville AR, Burke CM, Theodore J, Baldwin JC, Harvey J, Vankessel A, Robin ED. Bronchial hyper-responsiveness after human cardiopulmonary transplantation. *Clin Sci* 1987;73:299–303.

36. Edmunds LH, Stallone RJ, Graf PD, Sagel SS, Greenspan RH. Mucus transport in transplanted lungs of dogs. *Surgery* 1969;66:15–22.

37. Dolovich M, Rossman C, Chambers C, Grossman RF, Newhouse M, the Toronto Lung Transplant Group, Maurer J. Mucociliary function in patients following single lung or lung/heart transplantation [Abstract]. *Am Rev Respir Dis* 1987;135:A363.

38. Brody JS, Klempfner G, Staum MM, Vidyasagar D, Kuhl DE, Waldhausen JA. Mucociliary clearance after lung denervation and bronchial transection. *J Appl Physiol* 1972;32:160–164.

39. Drews JA, Tierney DF, Benfield JR. Effect of lung transplantation on surfactant. *Surg Forum* 1973;24:334–336.

40. Valenca LM, Lincoln JCR, Strieder DJ, Kazemi H. Pulmonary vascular response of the reimplanted dog lung to hypoxia. *J Thorac Cardiovasc Surg* 1971;61:857–862.

41. Robin ED, Theodore J, Burke CM, Oesterle SN, Fowler MB, Jamieson SW, Baldwin JC, Morris AJ, Hunt SA, Vankessel A, Stinson EB, Shumway NE. Hypoxic pulmonary vasoconstriction persists in the human transplanted lung. *Clin Sci* 1987;72:283–287.

42. Schafers JH, Frost AE, Waxman MB, Maurer JR, Grossman RF, Patterson GA, the Toronto Lung Transplant Group. Cardiac innervation following double lung transplantation [Abstract]. *Am Rev Respir Dis* 1988;137:245.

43. Veith FJ, Sinha SBP, Blumcke S, Dougherty JC, Becker NH, Siegleman SS, Hagstrom JWC. Nature and evolution of lung allograft rejection with and without immunosuppression. *J Thorac Cardiovasc Surg* 1972;63:509–520.

44. Fujimara S, Rosen V, Adomian GE, Parmley WW, Suzuki C, Matloff JM. Cellular characteristics of the rejection response to canine lung allotransplants. *J Thorac Cardiovasc Surg* 1973;65:438–448.

45. Molokhia FA, Ponn RB, Aaimacopoulos PJ, Norman JC. Microscopic and ultrastructural changes in unmodified canine lung allografts. *Arch Surg* 1971;103:490–495.

46. Moeschl P, Lubec G, Keiler A, Salem G, Gloeckler M. Donor and organ specific evaluation of antibodies eluted from canine lung allografts rejected by immunosuppressively treated and untreated recipients. *Respiration* 1979;38:12–17.

47. Koerner SK, Hagstrom JWC, Veith FJ. Transbronchial biopsy for the diagnosis of lung transplant rejection. *Am Rev Respir Dis* 1976;14:575–579.

48. Higenbottam T, Stewart S, Wallwork J. Transbronchial lung biopsy to diagnose lung rejection and infection of heart–lung transplants. *Transplant Proc* 1988;20(Suppl 1):767–769.

49. Herlan D, Kormos R, Zeevi A, Paradis I, Wei L, Nalesnik M, Hardesty R, Griffith B. Dynamics of bronchoalveolar lavage in the canine lung transplant. *Transplant Proc* 1988;20(Suppl 1):832–835.

50. Rabinovich H, Zeevi A, Herlan D, Dal Col R, Griffith BP, Hardesty RL, Kormos B, Paradis IL, Dauber JH, Duquesnoy RJ. Functional studies on lymphocytes in bronchoalveolar lavages from canine lung allografts. *Transplant Proc* 1988;20(Suppl 1):836–838.

51. Prop J, Wagenaar-Hilbers JPA, Petersen AH, Wildevuur CRH. Diagnosis of rejection in rat lung allografts by bronchoalveolar lavage. *Transplant Proc* 1987;19:3779–3780.

52. Prop J, Wagenaar-Hilbers JPA, Petersen AH, Wildevuur CRH. Characteristics of cells lavaged from rejecting lung allografts in rats. *Transplant Proc* 1988;20:217–218.

53. Gryzan S, Paradis IL, Hardesty RL, Griffith BP, Dauber H. Bronchoalveolar lavage in heart–lung transplantation. *J Heart Transplant* 1985;4:414–416.

54. Zeevi A, Fung JJ, Paradis IL, Dauber JH, Griffith BP, Hardesty RL, Duquesnoy RJ. Lymphocytes of bronchoalveolar lavages from heart–lung transplant recipients. *J Heart Transplant* 1985;4:417–421.

55. Gryzan S, Paradis I, Griffith BP, Hardesty RL, Trento A, Dauber J. T-lymphocyte subset recovery by bronchoalveolar lavage during infection and rejection of the transplanted lung [Abstract]. *J Heart Transplant* 1985;4:611.

56. Moeschl P, Lubec G, Keiler A, Salem G, Gloeckler M. *In vitro* evidence of cellular and humoral immune responses following lung allotransplantation in canine recipients with and without immunosuppressive treatment. *Eur Surg Res* 1979;11:234–242.

57. Dal Col RH, Rabinovich H, Herlan DB, Kormos RL, Zeevi A, Yousem SA, Paradis IL, Dauber JH, Griffith BP. Donor specimen cytotoxicity testing: an advance in detecting pulmonary allograft rejection. *Ann Thorac Surg* 1990;49:754–758.

58. Griffith BP, Paradis IL, Zeevi A, Rabinovitch H, Yousem SA, Duquesnoy RJ, Dauber JH, Hardesty RL. Immunologically me-

diated disease of the airways after pulmonary transplantation. *Ann Surg* 1988;208:371–378.

59. Lawrence EC, Brousseau KP, Kurman CC, Nelson DL, Young JB, Short HD, Whisenhand HH, Noon GP, Debakey ME. Soluble interleukin-2 receptor levels in serum as a marker of rejection in heart–lung transplantation [Abstract]. *Chest* 1986;89:S526.

60. Stolc V, Krause JR. Interleukin-1 receptor levels are increased in blood of heart transplant patients during infections. *Diagn Clin Immunol* 1987;5:171–174.

61. Pio Roda CL, Strandberg JD, Baker JW, Baker RR. Serial changes in pulmonary blood flow occurring during acute rejection of a lung allograft. *J Thorac Cardiovasc Surg* 1973;65:88–93.

62. Chastre J, Fagon JY, Soler P, Bornet M, Domart Y, Trouillet JL, Gibert C, Hance AJ. Diagnosis of nosocomial bacterial pneumonia in intubated patients undergoing ventilation: comparison of the usefulness of bronchoalveolar lavage and the protected specimen brush. *Am J Med* 1988;85:499–506.

63. Burke CM, Morris AJR, Dawkins KD, McGregor CGA, Yousem SA, Allen M, Theodore J, Harvey J, Billingham ME, Oyer PE, Stinson EB, Baldwin JC, Shumway NE, Jamieson SW. Late airflow obstruction in heart–lung transplantation recipients. *J Heart Transplant* 1985;4:437–440.

64. Allen MD, Burke CM, McGregor CGA, Baldwin JC, Jamieson SW, Theodore J. Steroid-responsive bronchiolitis after human heart lung transplantation. *J Thorac Cardiovasc Surg* 1986;92:449–451.

65. Tazelaar HD, Prop J, Niewenhuis P, Billingham ME, Wildevuur CRH. Obliterative bronchiolitis in the transplanted rat lung. *Transplant Proc* 1987;19:1052.

66. Baldwin JC, Oyer PE, Stinson EB, Starnes VA, Billingham ME, Shumway NE. Comparison of cardiac rejection in heart and heart–lung transplantation. *J Heart Transplant* 1987;6:352–356.

67. Higenbottam T, Hutter JA, Stewart S, Wallwork J. Transbronchial biopsy has eliminated the need for endomyocardial biopsy in heart–lung recipients. *J Heart Transpl* 1988;7:435–439.

68. Wreghitt TG, Hakim M. Donor-transmitted disease. In: Wallwork J, ed. *Heart and heart–lung transplantation.* Philadelphia: WB Saunders, 1989;341–358.

69. Bogardus GM. Evaluation in dogs of the relationship of pulmonary, bronchial and hilar adventitial circulation to the problem of lung transplantation. *Surgery* 1958;43:849–856.

70. Grossman RF, Frost A, Zamel N, Patterson GA, Cooper JD, Myron PC, Dear CL, Maurer JR, and the Toronto Lung Transplant Group. Results of single-lung transplantation for bilateral pulmonary fibrosis. *New Engl J Med* 1990;322:727–733.

71. Frost A, Dear CL, Grossman RF, Cooper JD, Maurer JR, the Toronto Lung Transplant Group. Exercise tolerance in patients undergoing double lung transplant for end stage pulmonary disease [Abstract]. *Am Rev Respir Dis* 1988;137:336.

72. Theodore J, Jamieson SW, Burke CM, Reitz BA, Stinson EB, Van Kessel A, Dawkins KD, Herran JJ, Oyer PE, Hunt SA, Shumway NE, Robin ED. Physiologic aspects of human heart-lung transplantation: pulmonary function status of the posttransplanted lung. *Chest* 1984;86:349–357.

73. Maurer JR, Myron CPR, Frost AE, Patterson GA, Grossman RF, the Toronto Lung Transplant Group. Pulmonary function following double lung transplant [Abstract]. *Am Rev Respir Dis* 1988;137:213.

74. Legal YM, Chittal SM, Wright ES. Early bronchial revascularization with an intercostal pedicle graft following canine lung autotransplantation. *Can J Surg* 1985;28:518–522.

75. Barman SA, Ardell JL, Parker JC, Perry ML, Taylor AE. Pulmonary and systemic blood flow contributions to upper airways in canine lung. *Am J Physiol* 1988 (*Heart Circ Physiol* 24);255:H1130–H1135.

76. Michelassi F, Schuette A, Landa L, Zapol WM, Grillo HC. Pulmonary and systemic contribution to canine tracheobronchial blood flow. *Ital J Surg Sci* 1987;17:105–112.

77. Schreinemakers HJ, Weder W, Miyoshi S, Harper BD, Shimokawa S, Egan TM, McKnight R, Cooper JD. Direct revascularization of bronchial arteries for lung transplantation. *Ann Thorac Surg* 1990;49:44–54.

78. Schafers HJ, Todd TR, Ginsberg RJ, Goldberg MJ, Patterson GA, Pearson FG, Cooper JD. Bronchial complications following single lung transplantation. *J Thorac Cardiovasc Surg* 1990;in press.

79. Patterson GA, Todd TR, Cooper JD, Pearson FG, Winton TL, Maurer J, the Toronto Lung Transplant Group. Airway complications following double lung transplantation. *J Thorac Cardiovasc Surg* 1990;99:14–21.

80. Cooper JD, Pearson FG, Patterson GA, Todd TRJ, Ginsberg RJ, Goldberg M, Waters P. Use of silicone stents in the management of airway problems. *Ann Thorac Surg* 1989;47:371–378.

THE LUNG: Scientific Foundations
edited by R.G. Crystal, J.B. West et al.
Raven Press, Ltd., New York © 1991.

CHAPTER 8.2.8

Acid–Base Balance in Hypothermia

Robert Blake Reeves

Classical acid–base balance theory principally focused on the human as an isothermal system at a regulated core temperature of 37°C (1). Despite the amply documented and commonplace occurrence of regional, organ, and superficial tissue temperatures far removed from core temperature (2), the acid–base state of tissues warmer or cooler than core temperature and of blood perfusing them has only recently begun to receive attention (3). With enthusiastic adoption and widespread use of deep hypothermia in cardiopulmonary bypass procedures, the need for a better understanding of the role that temperature plays in determining acid–base state became more urgent. One unexpected immediate result of such enquiry has been to challenge the cardinal tenet of all acid–base theory—that a plasma pH of 7.4 is the central regulated variable. New evidence developed from temperature studies supports the concept that preservation of protein charge state may be the regulated variable in acid–base regulation (4). The close relationship between protein charge state and functional expression of protein enzymatic and ligand binding properties makes this interpretation logically appealing.

Theory and experience as yet do not provide a proven optimal scheme for acid–base management for humans in acute hypothermia. This brief chapter chiefly addresses three areas that currently dominate discussion concerning choice of an optimal scheme. First, the required background to further discussion is the question of how temperature affects fundamental proton equilibria of all CO_2–protein solutions like plasma and intracellular fluid. Second, temperature-dependent acid–base regulatory patterns found in lower vertebrates are concisely surveyed as these re-

late to alternative models for possible human application. Finally, currently recognized consequences for patients of alternative acid–base management models are assessed.

TEMPERATURE EFFECTS ON BLOOD ACID–BASE EQUILIBRIA

Acid–Base Conditions for Blood at Constant CO_2 Content

The principles that underlie the consequences for acid–base equilibria in any aqueous biological compartment when temperature changes are best illustrated from measurements on whole blood. It is instructive to consider first the acid–base state of blood perfusing tissues operating at temperatures differing from regulated normothermic core temperature. Blood perfusing a hand in 7°C cold water, a far from uncommon event among commercial fishermen, cools intraarterially in transit. Under these conditions, blood gas content is unchanged as cooling proceeds; total carbon dioxide content in particular is constant until blood arrives at the exchange vessels of the microcirculation. Cooling at constant CO_2 content significantly alters equilibria governing both blood pH and carbon dioxide tension (P_{CO_2}) in a readily predictable fashion.

Temperature-induced changes in blood pH and P_{CO_2} shown in Fig. 1 are conveniently measured on *in vitro* blood samples. Blood that at 37°C has a pH of 7.38 when cooled to 8°C without contact with air has a pH 0.5 unit higher (i.e., pH 7.88); the rate of change of pH with temperature (dpH/dT) is not constant but decreases from -0.019 unit/°C at 7–19°C to -0.0145 at 27–37°C (4,5). The simultaneous change in CO_2 tension is a nonlinear decrease from 40 to 8 torr. From the viewpoint of classical isothermal principles of acid–base regulation, these are large changes. Such large variations of pH when carried out *at con-*

R. B. Reeves: Department of Physiology, School of Medicine, State University of New York, Buffalo, New York 14226.

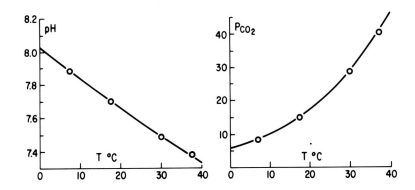

FIG. 1. Simultaneously measured pH values and CO_2 partial pressures (Pco_2, torr) of human blood at constant CO_2 content plotted separately against blood temperature. (Modified from refs. 3 and 4.)

stant temperature have conspicuous consequences for cells as illustrated by changes in red cell volume and anion distribution across red cell membranes shown in Fig. 2. An increase in plasma pH decreases r_{Cl^-}, the ratio of intracellular to extracellular $[Cl^-]$ (6). Inasmuch as ion distribution affects cell volume because of osmotic shifts in water, decreases in Donnan r_{Cl^-} for diffusible ions decreases red cell volume (and hematocrit).

Changes in pH of the same magnitude, however, when brought about solely by changing temperature (at constant CO_2 content), preserve rather than alter cell volume and r_{Cl^-} (6). For changes in temperature at constant gas content, such as occur for blood in transit from a warm normothermic core to a cooled hand, Fig. 2 shows that Donnan ratios are unaltered. Donnan distribution of diffusible anions across the red cell membrane arises as a consequence of the net negative charge on proteins, principally hemoglobin, within the red cell. The absence of a Donnan change in intracellular anion concentration when temperature is varied at constant gas content signifies that protein net charge is preserved under these conditions.

Protein Charge State Determinants

Protein net charge state does not figure prominently in the analysis of acid–base regulation at constant temperature; its importance for consequences of temperature change on acid–base systems merits brief review at this juncture. The net charge (Z) on protein molecules is the algebraic sum of cationic (n^+) and anionic groups (n^-) per molecule. Most of these amino acid side chain ionizations do not change as pH is varied in the physiological range of 6–8 because their respective pK values are far removed from this range. Two proton binding groups, however, possess pK values that fall in the physiological pH range: the imidazole moiety of histidine and the N-terminal amino group of peptide chains (7). Quantitatively, histidine imidazole groups are the major contributor to protein buffering; hence, the combined contribution from both

groups is designated collectively as histidine imidazole for convenience. The histidine imidazole proton equilibrium can be written

$$K_{Im} \times [HIm^+] = [H^+] \times [Im].$$

The fraction (α_{Im}) of total titratable histidines ($[n_{Im}] = [HIm^+] + [Im]$) lacking a proton, defined as

$$\alpha_{Im} = \frac{[Im]}{[n_{Im}]},$$

is computed as

$$\alpha_{Im} = \frac{10^{pH-pK_{Im}}}{1 + 10^{pH-pK_{Im}}}.$$

Hence, the fraction of cationically charged (HIm^+) groups is ($1 - \alpha_{Im}$). Total net charge Z per mole protein in the physiological pH range can then be written

$$Z = [n^+] - [n^-] + [n_{Im}](1 - \alpha_{Im}),$$

where $[n^+]$ now refers to cationically charged groups (mol/mol protein) other than histidine imidazole. As physiological systems contain many different proteins and Z varies from one protein to another depending on amino acid composition, evaluation of Z for each protein is not useful. However, if α_{Im} is constant as temperature changes, all proteins maintain their net charge Z constant regardless of the absolute magnitude of Z of each. Thus, α_{Im} provides a sensitive index of the changing contribution of histidine imidazole cationic groups to Z of every protein species present.

Average Values for Protein pK_{Im} and dpK_{Im}/dT

Physiological analysis requires simplifying assumptions concerning protein histidine imidazole's pK_{Im} and dpK_{Im}/dT. Charge–charge interactions between adjacent ionizing groups in proteins strongly affect the magnitude of any particular microscopic histidine pK_{Im}; in any protein a range of microscopic pK_{Im} values is encountered. For convenience in computing α_{Im}, the representative but arbitrary value for pK_{Im} of 7.0 (at 22.5°C with a ΔH°_{Im} of 7 kcal/mol) has been adopted.

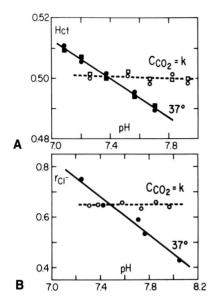

FIG. 2. The effect of pH on red cell volume **(A)** expressed as hematocrit ratio (Hct) and Donnan chloride ratio **(B)**. The ratio of chloride ion concentrations (mEq/liter water) in red cells to plasma ($r_{Cl^-} = [Cl_c^-]/[Cl_p^-]$) defines the Donnan Cl^- ratio. Plasma pH was varied in two ways: at 37°C the partial pressure of CO_2 was varied (isothermal pH variation); alternatively, the temperature was changed at constant CO_2 content ($CO_2 = k$). (Modified from refs. 3 and 5.)

The principal physiological buffering groups of proteins, histidine imidazole and α-amino groups, contrast markedly with other biological buffers, phosphate and CO_2–bicarbonate, in having a large enthalpy of ionization ($\Delta H°$) (7). Large $\Delta H°$ implies significant change in pK′ with temperature. For protein histidine imidazole, the dpK_{Im}/dT is about -0.017 unit/°C ($\Delta H°_{Im} = 7$ kcal/mol); the dpK/dT for peptide α-amino is even greater, -0.026 unit/°C ($\Delta H° = 11$ kcal/mol) (7,8). Values for $\Delta H°_{Im}$ among particular histidines within a given protein are no less variable than are pK_{Im} values (9,10); in this case, however, direct experimental demonstration that the dpH/dT measured on isolated stripped protein mixtures equals a dpK_{Im}/dT of -0.017 unit/°C is proof that an average value for $\Delta H°_{Im}$ of 7 kcal/mol obtains under physiological conditions (4).

α_{Im} and the CO_2 Equilibrium Curve

The activities of proteins always occur in the presence of carbon dioxide. Proteins and CO_2–bicarbonate constitute a binary buffer system whose acid–base responses are strongly affected by temperature change. The CO_2 combining curve of plasma or whole blood can be modeled effectively as simple binary buffer because the contribution to total buffering of phosphates

is minimal in plasma and red cells. The aim of this analysis is to predict the effect of temperature change on the pH, P_{CO_2}, and α_{Im} when CO_2 content (C_{CO_2}) is kept invariant.

In the model the protein buffer is replaced by an equivalent imidazole concentration as though proteins were simply polyhistidine dissolved in a sodium chloride solution. A pK_{Im} of 7.0 (at 22.5°C) and $\Delta H°_{Im}$ of 7 kcal/mol are assumed. This buffer system is defined by five equations (7,11).

The first is the dissociation of water:

$$K_w = [H^+] \times [OH^-].$$

Next, the dissociation of carbonic acid can be written

$$K_1 \times [q \times P_{CO_2}] = [H^+] \times [HCO_3^-],$$

where K_1 is the dissociation constant, and P_{CO_2} and q are the partial pressure (torr) and solubility (mol/liter·torr) of CO_2, respectively. The third equation is an equilibrium already cited, the proton equilibrium of histidine imidazole:

$$K_{Im} \times [HIm^+] = [H^+] \times [Im].$$

A conservation statement for the total imidazole concentration ($[c_{Im}]$) is also required:

$$[c_{Im}] = [HIm^+] + [Im].$$

Finally, the electroneutrality constraint is expressed as

$$[Na^+] + [H^+] + [HIm^+] - [Cl^-]$$
$$- [OH^-] - [HCO_3^-] = 0.$$

Since concentrations of $[H^+]$ and $[OH^-]$ are three orders of magnitude smaller than other components, this relation can be approximated as

$$[SID] = [Na^+] - [Cl^-] = [HCO_3^-] - [HIm^+] = 0,$$

where [SID] is termed the strong ion difference (11). In the calculations that follow, $[c_{Im}] = 0.130$ M/liter and $[SID] = -0.026$ Eq/liter.

At constant temperature and in an open system where CO_2 content can change, when carbon dioxide partial pressure increases bicarbonate is produced; the CO_2 titration of histidine imidazole can be written

$$Im + H_2CO_3 = HIm^+ + HCO_3^-$$

As shown in Fig. 3 (lower panel) increasing P_{CO_2} increases total CO_2 content (C_{CO_2}), bicarbonate plus some dissolved CO_2; the change, however, in dissolved CO_2 is quantitatively small compared to changes in bicarbonate concentration. In the plot of C_{CO_2} versus P_{CO_2} in Fig. 3, a line connecting any point along the CO_2 content curve with the origin describes a pH isopleth (12). Line segments connect the ends of three pH isopleths of the CO_2 equilibrium curve at

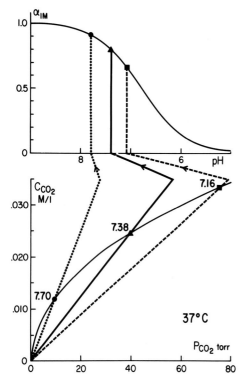

FIG. 3. Bottom: The CO_2 equilibrium of a binary buffer approximating normal human whole blood ([c_{Im}] = 0.130 M/liter and strong ion difference [SID] = −0.026 M/liter). **Top:** Fractional dissociation of imidazole groups (α_{Im}) plotted as a function of pH for same solution.

three CO_2 tensions with the corresponding pH abscissa values of the α_{Im} versus pH curve shown in the upper panel of Fig. 3. This graphic device indicates that when P_{CO_2} increases, α_{Im} decreases. At constant temperature, the effect of increasing P_{CO_2} is to create new bicarbonate ions at the expense of unprotonated histidine imidazole groups. Thus, as P_{CO_2} increases, C_{CO_2} increases and α_{Im} decreases (3).

Temperature Changes CO_2 Equilibrium Curve

The consequence of changing temperature on the CO_2 equilibrium curve of the model system is shown in Fig. 4; curves indicated are model solutions at the temperatures indicated. As temperature decreases, more CO_2 is taken up at any given P_{CO_2}; at a P_{CO_2} of 40 torr, for instance, the CO_2 content at 10°C is about twice its value at 37°C. This response occurs principally because temperature decrease has a prominent effect, increasing pK_{Im}. The temperature-driven increase in pK_{Im} causes more protons from carbonic acid to be taken up by protein histidine imidazole, forming additional bicarbonate ions. The solubility of CO_2 is also increased by a fall in temperature (7); however, the contribution to total CO_2 content from dissolved CO_2

is minor. The solid points shown in Fig. 4 plot measured CO_2 content data for normal whole blood (13); reasonable agreement is found between measured C_{CO_2} values and calculated quantities based on the simple model described.

Temperature Alters Blood Acid–Base Equilibria

Applying concepts developed in previous sections, the temperature dependence of acid–base behavior of blood at constant gas content can now be comprehended. Figure 5 presents an analysis of how the principal acid–base variables interreact when a temperature change is imposed on the model system. In the lower left panel, a line of constant CO_2 content at 0.0245 M/liter intersects three CO_2 equilibrium curves at 0, 20, and 40°C; each point of intersection is characterized by a different pair of pH and P_{CO_2} values. The pH isopleths for each intersection point are connected to the pH abscissa of the histidine imidazole dissociation curves shown in the upper left panel. The corresponding α_{Im} is indicated on the appropriate imidazole titration curve at each temperature; α_{Im} remains constant independent of temperature. Panels at the right separately plot pH and P_{CO_2} values of the intersecting points directly against temperature; values from the calculated model fall along the same experimentally measured curves for human whole blood presented in Fig. 1.

Solutions like plasma and intracellular fluid are predominantly buffered by protein. At constant gas content the change in pK_{Im} with temperature changes solution pH in the same direction and by the same

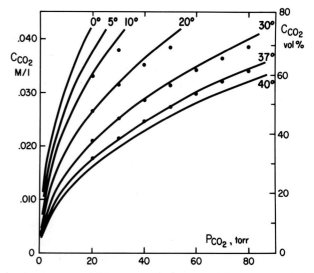

FIG. 4. The effect of temperature on the CO_2 equilibrium curve of Fig. 3. Points are C_{CO_2} measurements on normal human blood (13) at the indicated temperature and P_{CO_2} values. (Modified from ref. 3.)

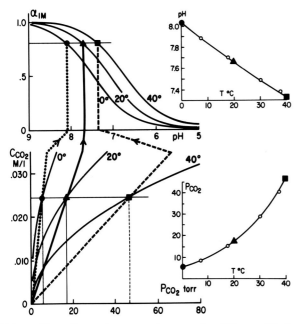

FIG. 5. The effect of temperature on the CO_2 equilibrium curve **(lower left)** and on the titration curves for imidazole groups **(upper left)**. Values for pH and P_{CO_2} from the left panels are plotted against temperature on the right. Also indicated on the pH and P_{CO_2} temperature plots are measurements on normal whole blood of Fig. 1. (Modified from ref. 3.)

amount. Consequently, since the difference (pK_{Im} − pH) in the equation

$$\alpha_{Im} = \frac{10^{pH-pK_{Im}}}{1 + 10^{pH-pK_{Im}}}$$

is maintained essentially constant, α_{Im} is also constant. Thus, protein charge state in both plasma and intra-erythrocyte compartments is preserved as temperature changes, in spite of changes in pH and P_{CO_2}. As a consequence, red cells in whole blood can change temperature under these conditions with constant ion and water composition.

Adjustments of all proton equilibria to a primary temperature-induced change in pK_{Im} not only alter pH but alter P_{CO_2} values as well. As P_{CO_2} falls with decreasing temperature, CO_2 solubility rises; their product, dissolved CO_2, does not remain quite constant. However, the contribution of dissolved CO_2 to total CO_2 content is small in magnitude.

Relative Alkalinity: An Alternative Theoretical Context

Since protein–CO_2 binary buffers are aqueous systems, the effect of temperature on the dissociation of water has been posited as critical to their acid–base

behavior (14–16). The dissociation of water can again be written

$$H_2O = H^+ + OH^-,$$

where

$$K_w = [OH^-] \times [H^+].$$

If the pH of neutrality (where $[H^+] = [OH^-]$) is designated by pN, the ratio of $[OH^-]/[H^+]$, termed the *relative alkalinity,* is given by

$$\frac{[OH^-]}{[H^+]} = 10^{2(pH-pN)}.$$

Temperature has a prominent effect on K_w, and consequently on pN, such that

$$\frac{dpN}{dT} = \frac{1}{2}(dpK_w/dT) = \frac{1}{2}(\Delta H_w^\circ/2.3RT^2),$$

and, expressed in terms of the enthalpy of ionization of water (17) (ΔH_w°),

$$\frac{1}{2}\Delta H_w^\circ = 7 \text{ kcal/mol}$$

Thus, in what may only be an astonishing coincidence,

$$\Delta H_{Im}^\circ = \frac{1}{2}\Delta H_w^\circ$$

and dpK_{Im}/dT and dpN/dT are equal; the observed pH in a CO_2–protein binary buffer system at constant CO_2 content changes with temperature so that both quantities, (pK_{Im} − pH) and (pH − pN), remain constant. Hence, when a CO_2–protein buffer changes temperature at constant α_{Im}, it is also at constant relative alkalinity (18).

Superficially, these alternative descriptions of the temperature response of CO_2–protein buffers appear equally valid; however, further analysis demonstrates that only the histidine imidazole mechanism is quantitatively compelling. Whenever, as in the physiological case, binary buffer component concentrations are in the millimolar to decimolar concentration range, water's contribution to buffering is negligible. Under these conditions, the effect of water's enthalpy of ionization in determining the system's temperature behavior is vanishingly small. It is protein's dpK_{Im}/dT that acts as the overwhelming driving force in determining the temperature behavior of CO_2–protein binary buffers. Consequently, binary buffer behavior with temperature change is better described as constant α_{Im} rather than as constant relative alkalinity (19).

IN VIVO ACID–BASE REGULATION WITH VARIABLE BODY TEMPERATURE

The effect of temperature on blood at constant gas content demonstrates that *in vivo* normal extracellular acid–base conditions for human tissues operating at temperatures removed from core temperature are not characterized by a constant plasma pH of 7.4 (4). Instead, a constant α_{Im} obtains. When whole body temperature is changed, as in the case of hypothermia induced for cardiopulmonary bypass, the question is raised anew: What are the appropriate measures for control of acid–base state? Is the acid–base behavior of tissues not at core temperature a sufficient guide for control of acid–base balance in profound whole body hypothermia? Since direct measurement of normal regulation during whole body cooling in unanesthetized mammals is precluded by thermogenesis responses, additional models have been sought. Two models predominate. One derives from the behavior of certain poikilothermic vertebrates; the second takes a true mammalian hibernator species as its model.

Alphastat Regulation

Extensive studies now available on acid–base regulation in poikilothermic vertebrates involving more than 11 fish, 8 amphibian, and 15 reptilian species have recently been reviewed (20). Sixty percent of all studies report values for blood dpH/dT falling between -0.013 and -0.020 unit/°C. The responses of these species to an increase in body temperature fall reasonably within the range of blood values that would be seen for blood *in vitro*: a decrease in pH of approximately -0.015 unit/°C, a significant increase in Pco_2, constant Cco_2 stores, and a constant α_{Im}. In these species the only temperature-independent variable is protein histidine α_{Im}; hence, their pattern of acid–base control has been designated *alphastat* regulation (21). Since measurements from these species are made on open metabolizing systems in which the animal controls ventilation and exchange of strong ions with the environment, these responses represent normal regulatory control. Noteworthy, too, is the fact that in alphastat regulation no strong ion concentration change is observed in extracellular fluid. Consequently, the principal regulatory objective is to achieve the appropriate ventilation at each body temperature that yields the Pco_2 required to keep α_{Im} constant. In the best studied alphastat species, a freshwater turtle, *Pseudemys scripta*, values for regulated blood pH and Pco_2 as body temperature changes follow closely the changes seen for turtle blood *in vitro* as a closed system at constant CO_2 (19).

pH-Stat Regulation

The second model describes the regulation of true mammalian hibernators. Data from these species can only be collected at two steady-state temperatures,

euthermic (normal core 37–39°C) awake versus hypothermia of hibernation (5–10°C). These species exhibit only minimal changes in blood pH (dpH/dT = -0.004 ± 0.002), much smaller than would be required to keep α_{Im} constant (22); hence, the approximate descriptive term *pH-stat* has been applied. To achieve a near constant blood pH, hibernators on cooling load CO_2 to increase blood and tissue Cco_2 significantly. This process may or may not include an increase in ECF strong ion difference. The Pco_2 falls only modestly in hibernation but bicarbonate concentration is strongly elevated. From the viewpoint of alphastat regulation, this pattern of acid–base control invokes a severe respiratory acidosis in order to induce and remain at the low body temperature characteristic of hibernation. The respiratory acidosis of hibernation may have a central role in the induction and maintenance of torpid states in hibernators (23). This acidosis may be critical to resetting the temperature set point and to the inhibition (via an altered α_{Im}) of metabolic pathways, including cold-induced thermogenesis. These interpretations are compatible with the finding of intracellular acidosis in most hibernator body tissues with the significant exception of heart muscle and liver, which follow alphastat regulation (24).

Acid–Base Regulation Lacking Any Identified Regulated Variable

As indicated previously, only 60% of the poikilotherm species studied achieve a dpH/dT in the range required for true alphastat behavior. Among air-breathing vertebrates the best studied exception to alphastat regulation is the Varanid lizard, *Varanus exanthematicus* (25,26). In this species, blood pH decreased only 0.005 unit/°C as body temperature increased over the range 15–38°C. Simultaneously, blood Pco_2 increased only moderately, while Cco_2 and $[HCO_3]$ decreased significantly. These responses require a regulated change in plasma strong ion concentrations together with ventilatory control as body temperature changes. This pattern more closely resembles pH-stat rather than alphastat regulation (26). In other species in which blood dpH/dT does not approach zero and yet does not reach the criterion (-0.015 unit/°C) for alphastat control, no acid–base variable can be identified as a candidate for the controlled variable (20).

No single pattern of acid–base control for vertebrates with variable body temperature emerges (20). Hibernating mammals can perhaps be exempted from consideration because they cannot exist in a steady state at temperatures intermediate between euthermic and hypothermic hibernation temperatures. However, even among the true poikilotherm vertebrates the extremes of control strategies are given by alphastat and pH-stat patterns. Hence, these are suitable alternatives to test in seeking for an optimal pattern appropriate for humans in hypothermia.

ALPHASTAT VERSUS pH-STAT: FUNCTIONAL CONSEQUENCES

The organs most likely at risk during extended periods of hypothermia are arguably the heart and brain. Numerous studies have addressed the consequences for cardiac excitability and for cerebral blood flow of acidosis and hypothermia, separately and combined (for reviews see refs. 27 and 28). Few studies have directly compared alphastat versus pH-stat acid–base management in hypothermia using a common experimental protocol. Caution must be exercised in assessing even these studies for at least two reasons. First, the temperature range over which measurements are made is necessarily a relatively limited one, typically only 10–12°C, a range over which measured changes are small. Second, the difference in key acid–base variables between normothermic and hypothermic states is also small; in the case of blood pH for a 10°C temperature differential, the alphastat pH difference is only 0.150 unit for a comparison of 7.55 with 7.40. Such relatively small differences are difficult to achieve cleanly in experimental practice. Nevertheless, in two critical areas—prevention of cardiac arrest and maintenance of cerebral blood flow—direct comparison of alphastat and pH-stat management has yielded noteworthy results.

Ventricular fibrillation has commonly been encountered during hypothermic induction particularly when accompanied by metabolic acidosis. Swain et al. (29) measured the threshold for induced ventricular fibrillation in hypothermia (25°C) versus normothermia in dogs under alphastat and pH-stat conditions. No significant change in threshold was observed under alphastat conditions whereas a 27% decrease in threshold was observed under pH-stat management. Swain et al. concluded that alphastat management improved cardiac function and electrical stability.

These results have been extended to human studies. Kroncke et al. (30) examined the incidence of ventricular fibrillation in a series of 181 patients undergoing open heart surgery during hypothermia to 24°C. pH-stat conditions were followed for the first 121 cases of which 40% fibrillated; in the remaining 60 consecutive cases alphastat conditions were employed but fibrillation occurred in only 20% of these patients. Kroncke et al. concluded that alphastat conditions significantly decreased incidence of ventricular fibrillation.

The problem of possible cerebral ischemic damage and of potential for posthypothermic neurological complications has repeatedly been discussed with regard to acid–base management strategies (28). A long-held view suggested that higher CO_2 partial pressures during hypothermia protect cerebral blood flow (CBF). Murkin et al. (31) have shed important new light on this area by direct comparison of alphastat (21 patients) versus constant Pa_{CO_2} of 40 torr (17 patients) acid–base management during hypothermia to 26°C on cerebral blood flow regulation and flow–metabolism coupling. Cerebral oxygen consumption at 26°C was the same in both groups. In the alphastat group, CBF was reduced to 60% of normothermic value and was independent of cerebral perfusion pressure over the range 20–100 mmHg but correlated with oxygen consumption. In the constant Pa_{CO_2} 40– torr group, CBF was as great as the normothermic value but flow–metabolism coupling was not maintained. Murkin et al. conclude that alphastat maintains a more physiologic relationship between cerebral oxygen uptake and CBF. Higher blood flow of the high Pa_{CO_2} group also raises questions about increasing intracranial pressure.

Alphastat control appears to have modest functional advantages over pH-stat control when judged by the small number of studies that directly compare the two management schemes. In future studies the consequences for intracellular pH of a choice between these two approaches to management of acid–base state merit examination. Linkages between extracellular and intracellular acid–base state are poorly comprehended now in any cell type at any temperature. A number of membrane processes, like the sodium–proton antiport, that control intracellular pH are now well characterized (32); however, cells may have more than one type of active proton transport protein. How activities of multiple transport proteins are coordinated to optimize cell function and particularly how regulation of the ECF acid–base state as temperature varies affects integrated function are major questions yet unanswered. Since the vast majority of enzymes are found within cells, alphastat regulation of intracellular compartments in order to optimize or control macromolecular function might be expected. In order to sustain high fluxes through metabolic integrated pathways, regulatory responsiveness, and a precise balance between stability and lability of protein structure (tertiary conformation, subunit assembly, and multiprotein complexes), some adaptation to accommodate temperature change seems likely (33). Only as knotty problems such as these begin to unravel will a fully reasoned approach emerge to acid–base management in induced surgical hypothermia in humans.

ACKNOWLEDGMENT

This work was supported by National Institutes of Health grant PO-1-HL-28542, awarded by the National Heart, Lung and Blood Institute.

REFERENCES

1. Peters JP, Van Slyke DD. *Quantitative clinical chemistry*, vol. I, *Interpretations*. Baltimore: Williams & Wilkins, 1931.
2. Bazett HC, Love L, Newton M, Eisenberg L, Day R, Forster R. Temperature changes in blood flowing in arteries and veins in man. *J Appl Physiol* 1948;1:3–19.
3. Reeves RB, Rahn H. Patterns in vertebrate acid–base regulation. In: Wood SC, Lenfant C, eds. *Evolution of respiratory processes: a comparative approach*. New York: Marcel Dekker, 1979;225–252.
4. Reeves RB. Temperature-induced changes in blood acid–base status: pH and P_{CO_2} in a binary buffer. *J Appl Physiol* 1976;40:752–761.
5. Rosenthal TB. The effect of temperature on the pH of blood and plasma *in vitro*. *J Biol Chem* 1948;173:25–30.
6. Reeves RB. Temperature-induced changes in blood acid–base status: Donnan r_{Cl} and red cell volume. *J Appl Physiol* 1976;40:762–767.
7. Edsall JT, Wyman J. *Biophysical chemistry*. New York: Academic Press, 1958.
8. Fersht A. *Enzyme structure and mechanism*. San Francisco: Freeman, 1985.
9. Matthew JB, Hanania GIH, Gurd FRN. Electrostatic effects in hemoglobin: hydrogen ion equilibria in human deoxy- and oxyhemoglobin A. *Biochemistry* 1979;18:1919–1928.
10. Matthew JB, Hanania GIH, Gurd FRN. Electrostatic effects in hemoglobin: Bohr effect and ionic strength dependence of individual groups. *Biochemistry* 1979;18:1928–1936.
11. Stewart PA. *How to understand acid–base: A quantitative acid–base primer for biology and medicine*. New York: Elsevier, 1981.
12. Henderson LJ. *Blood: a study in general physiology*. New Haven: Yale University Press, 1928.
13. Harms H, Bartels H. CO_2-Dissoziationskurven des menschlichen Blutes bei Temperaturen von 5–37°C und unterschiedlicher O_2-Sattigung. *Pflugers Arch* 1961;272:384–392.
14. Howell BJ, Baumgardner FW, Bondi K, Rahn H. Acid–base balance in poikilotherms as a function of body temperature. *Am J Physiol* 1970;218:600–606.
15. Rahn H. Gas transport from the external environment to the cell. In: deReuck AVS, Porter R, eds. *Development of the lung*, Ciba Foundation Symposium. London: Churchill, 1967;3–23.
16. Rahn H. Acid–base regulation and temperature in the evolution of vertebrates. *Proc Int Union Physiol Sci* 1971;8:91–92.
17. Weast RC, Astle MJ, eds. *Handbook of chemistry and physics*. Boca Raton: CRC Press, 1981;D-145.
18. Rahn H. Introduction. In: Rahn H, Prakash O, eds. *Acid–base regulation and body temperature*. Boston: Martinus Nijhoff, 1985;1–11.
19. Reeves RB. The interaction of body temperature and acid–base balance in ectothermic vertebrates. *Annu Rev Physiol* 1977;39:559–586.
20. Truchot J-P. *Comparative aspects of extracellular acid–base balance*. Berlin: Springer, 1987.
21. Reeves RB. An imidazole alphastat hypothesis for vertebrate acid–base regulation: tissue carbon dioxide content and body temperature in bullfrogs. *Respir Physiol* 1972;14:219–236.
22. Malan A. Respiration and acid–base state in hibernation. In: Lyman CP, Willis JS, Malan A, Wang LCH, eds. *Hibernation and torpor in mammals and birds*. New York: Academic Press, 1982;237–282.
23. Malan A. Enzyme regulation, metabolic rate and acid–base state in hibernation. In: Gilles R, ed. *Animals and environmental fitness*. Oxford: Pergamon Press, 1980;487–501.
24. Malan A, Rodeau JL, Daull F. Intracellular pH in hibernation and respiratory acidosis in the European hamster. *J Comp Physiol B* 1985;156:251–258.
25. Wood SC, Glass ML, Johansen K. Effect of temperature on respiration and acid–base balance in a monitor lizard. *J Comp Physiol* 1977;116:287–296.
26. Wood SC, Johansen K, Glass ML, Hoyt RW. Acid–base regulation during heating and cooling in the lizard, *Varanus exanthematicus*. *J Appl Physiol* 1981;50:779–783.
27. Swan H. The importance of acid–base management for cardiac and cerebral preservation during open heart operations. *Surg Gynecol Obstet* 1984;158:391–414.
28. Hickey PR, Andersen NP. Deep hypothermic circulatory arrest: a review of pathophysiology and clinical experience as a basis for anesthetic management. *J Cardiothorac Anesth* 1987;1:137–155.
29. Swain JA, White FN, Peters RM. The effect of pH on the hypothermic ventricular fibrillation threshold. *J Thorac Cardiovasc Surg* 1984;87:445–451.
30. Kroncke GM, Nichols RD, Mendenhall JT, Meyerowitz PD, Starling JR. Ectothermic philosophy of acid–base balance to prevent fibrillation during hypothermia. *Arch Surg* 1986;121:303–304.
31. Murkin JM, Farrar JK, Tweed WA, McKenzie FN, Guiradon G. Cerebral autoregulation and flow/metabolism coupling during cardiopulmonary bypass: the influence of Pa_{CO_2}. *Anesth Analg* 1987;66:825–832.
32. Seifter JL, Aronson PS. Properties and physiologic roles of the plasma membrane sodium–hydrogen exchanger. *J Clin Invest* 1986;78:859–864.
33. Somero GN. Protons, osmolytes, and fitness of internal milieu for protein function. *Am J Physiol* 1986;251:R197–R213.

Subject Index